AF538325

July 12, 1989

Presented to Gerald J. Marks, M.D., –
a contributing author, longtime colleague
and friend, –
by

Frederick B. Wagner, Jr., M.D.

THOMAS JEFFERSON UNIVERSITY

Tradition and Heritage

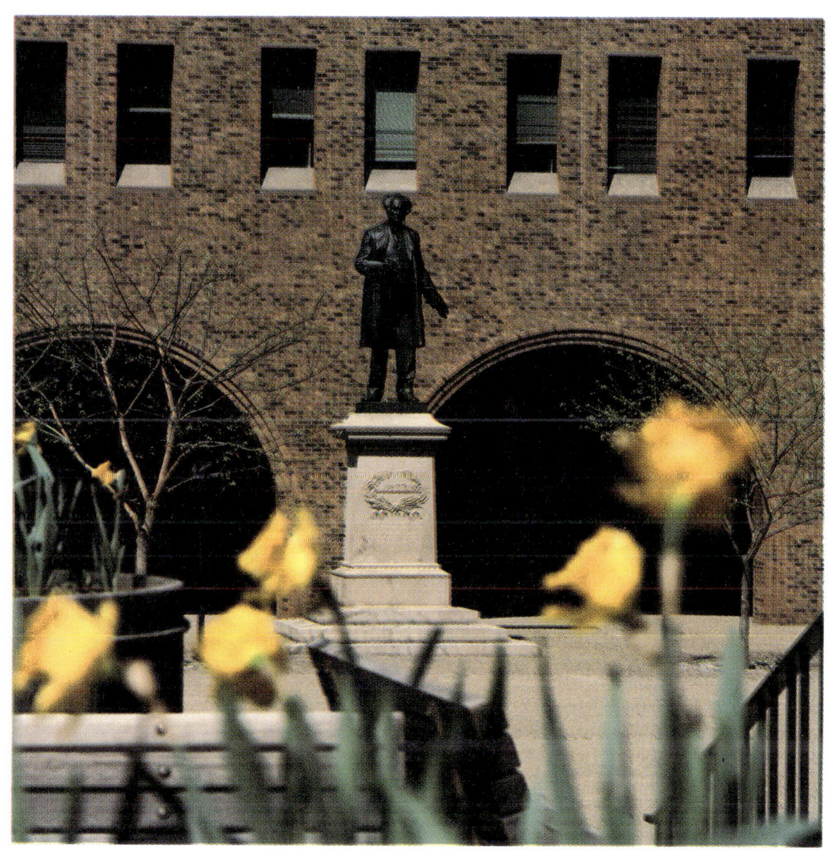

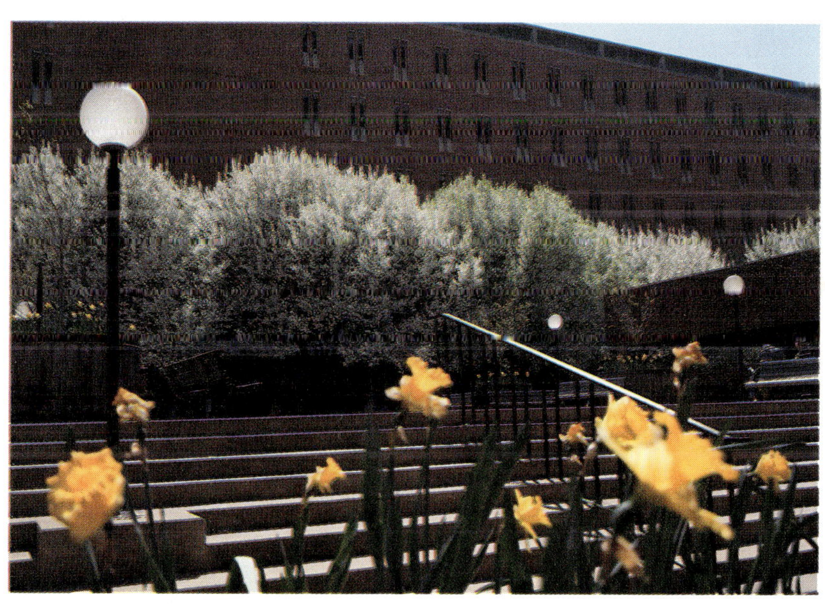

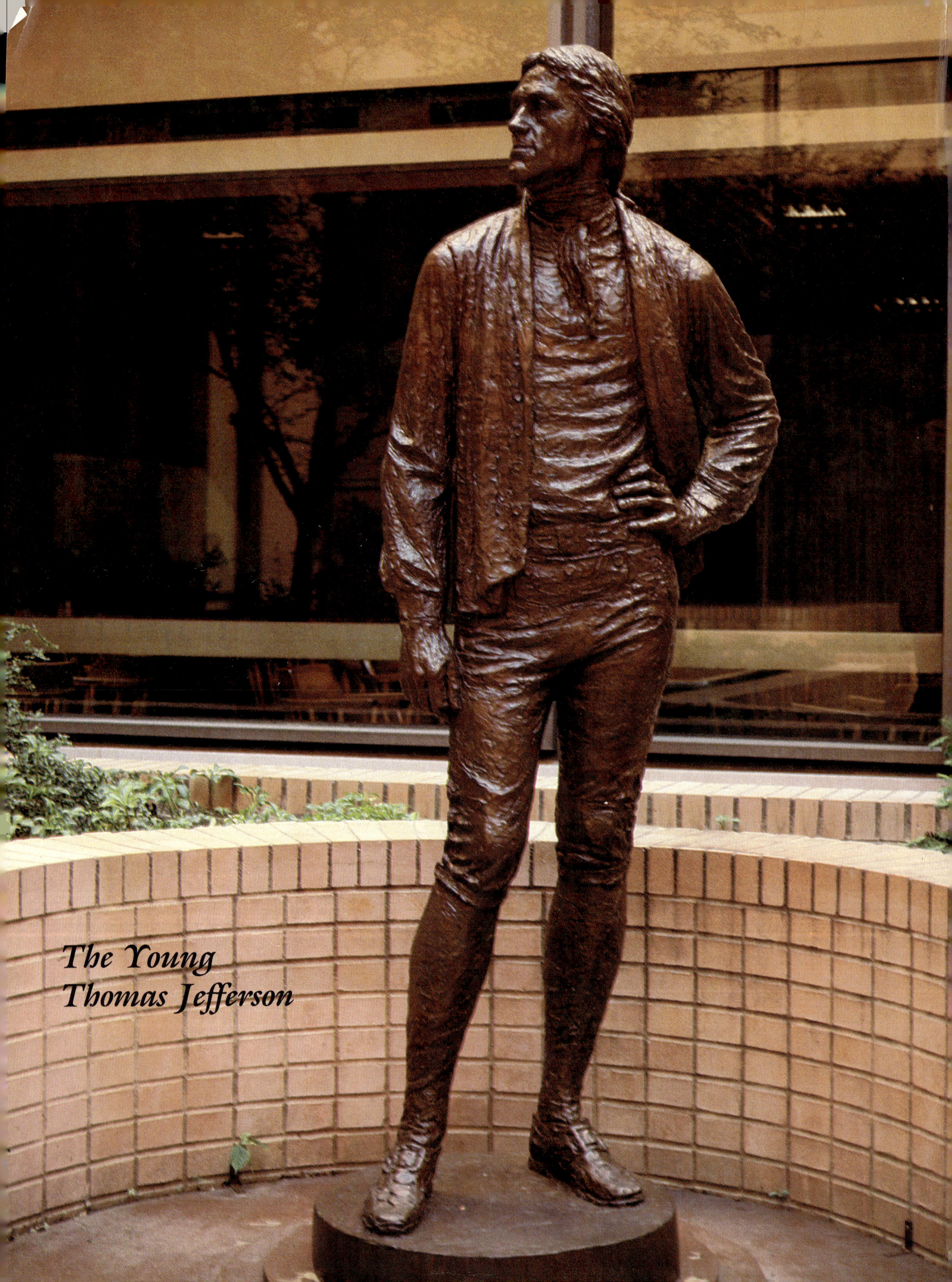
*The Young
Thomas Jefferson*

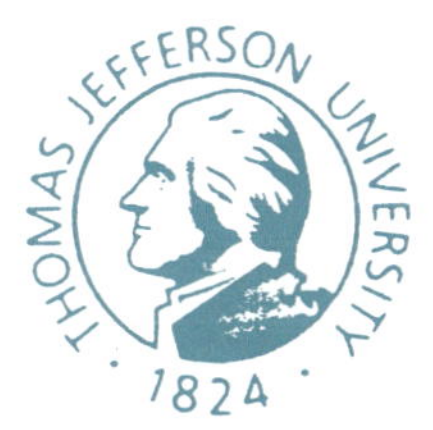

Thomas Jefferson University

TRADITION AND HERITAGE

Edited by
FREDERICK B. WAGNER, JR., M.D.
Grace Revere Osler Professor Emeritus of Surgery and University Historian
Thomas Jefferson University
Philadelphia, Pennsylvania

Foreword by LEWIS W. BLUEMLE, JR., M.D.
President, Thomas Jefferson University
Philadelphia, Pennsylvania

With editorial assistance of
J. Woodrow Savacool, M.D.,
and collaboration of 63 colleagues.

LEA & FEBIGER 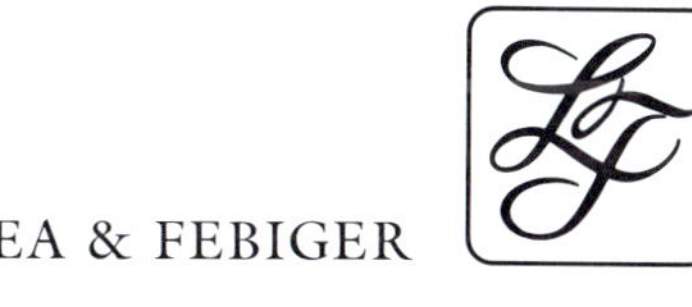 PHILADELPHIA • LONDON
1989

Lea & Febiger
600 South Washington Square
Philadelphia, PA 19106-4198
(215) 922-1330

Library of Congress Cataloging in Publication Data

Thomas Jefferson University.

Includes bibliographies and indexes.
1. Thomas Jefferson University—History.
I. Wagner, Frederick B. Jr., 1916– .
R747.T496T46 1989 610′.7′1174811 88-8338
ISBN 0-8121-1210-5

Copyright © 1989 by Thomas Jefferson University. Copyright under the International Copyright Union. All Rights Reserved. This book is protected by copyright. No part of it may be reproduced in any manner or by any means without written permission of the Publisher.

PRINTED IN THE UNITED STATES OF AMERICA
Print Number: 5 4 3 2 1

Foreword

FOR THE WELL-being of a mature university, heritage is as valuable as a creative faculty, a bright student body, or a balanced budget. Heritage goes beyond tradition. Tradition by itself may enhance a feeling of belonging but heritage reflects a core of durable values that unite the academic family not only with the past but with itself. Heritage is the flywheel in the machinery of university progress, giving us needed momentum when the engine slows down, assuring us in troubled times that problems are neither insoluble nor the exclusive province of our particular generation. It adds a patina of modesty and depth to the pride we all feel in our own accomplishments. In short, heritage is a university's spiritual endowment.

The principal vehicle for the preservation of heritage is history. To serve its purpose well the historical record must be interesting, well researched, accurate, and as comprehensive as possible. It should not gloss over the hard times that give character to the long struggle for excellence. The following account of the evolution of Thomas Jefferson University from the early 1800s to the late 1900s meets these standards. It is also a warm, affectionate story crafted by a Jeffersonian whose perceptive observations have spanned five decades as a student, house officer, teacher, staff physician, department chairman, alumni leader, trustee, and historian.

Frederick B. Wagner, Jr., M.D., University Historian and Grace Revere Osler Professor Emeritus of Surgery, was asked to write this history for several practical reasons. First, he is a relentless searcher for old records, stories, and photographs scattered among memories and dusty files of time. Second, he has a scholarly reverence for truth. Third, he is a master in the art of inducing, at times cajoling, his contributing authors to complete their assignments. But the real reason Doctor Wagner was encouraged to take on this monumental task was that we knew he would do it well, as a labor of love for his alma mater.

Three previous histories of our institution have been written. Gayley's *A History of the Jefferson Medical College of Philadelphia* (1858) and Gould's *The Jefferson Medical College of Philadelphia* (1904) covered the early years. Bauer's story (1963) entitled *Doctors Made in America*, while told with interesting flair, lacks rigor and cohesive sequence. The Wagner history goes well beyond these earlier accounts in depth, breadth, and illustrations. Indeed, it may well be regarded as the definitive literary companion piece to Thomas Eakins' portrait of Professor Samuel D. Gross, more commonly known as *The Gross Clinic,* reproduced on the cover. Thomas Eakins captured the heroic essence of early medical care and teaching at Jefferson. Frederick Wagner has recorded its maturation through two centuries. Together these two contributions document the proud heritage of Thomas Jefferson University.

In time, of course, the current work will itself become history, a reference for succeeding scholars to update as the process of medical discovery, teaching, and practice at Jefferson goes on. Hopefully these scholars will record the past, our future, with the same care and grace as are reflected here.

Doctor Gross himself captured the timeless value of historical perspective in his address entitled "Then and Now," delivered in 1868 to the Jefferson students who were beginning their course in surgery. Reflecting on the remarkable progress made since his own graduation in 1828, he said, "The advances in our knowledge in medical science within the last forty years are without parallel in any age. It would almost seem that the millenium were close at hand."

Then, following a thorough assessment of these advances, including "the most curious and interesting discovery in anatomy in modern times . . . that all animal and vegetable substances essentially consist of cells, of variable size, shape, and structures, and so minute, as to be visible only with the aid of the microscope . . . ," Gross adds, "We are too much disposed to look with contempt at the knowledge of our predecessors, as if, in reality they had worked and lived in vain, as if all true science had been reserved as a kind of special gift to the present generation."

In our own fast-moving era of molecular medicine, when even the minute cell is now considered a relatively massive unit of life, it would appear that yet another millenium is close at hand. And in another hundred years will our special gift of knowledge be eclipsed by the vision of the next millenium to follow? Probably so. But, however powerful our basic understanding of health and disease may become, its application will always depend on the institutions that create that understanding and pass it on to the next generation of students. This is the story of one such institution.

Philadelphia, Pennsylvania

LEWIS W. BLUEMLE, JR.,
M.D., L.H.D., Sc.D., F.R.C.P. (Edin.)
President, Thomas Jefferson University

Preface

JEFFERSON'S tradition and heritage, rich in ideals and achievements, span more than a century and a half. Much has been chronicled and preserved in books, articles, addresses, ceremonial occasions, archives, and art. Passage of time, accompanied by progress in science and emphasis on humanism, encouraged a new look at Jefferson's past. Creation of the post of University Historian was the idea of President Bluemle. His gentle mandate and unrestricted support led to this book.

It was the responsibility of the editor to orchestrate this endeavor. A plan was conceived to assemble a team of Thomas Jefferson University scholars not only with expertise in their fields but who themselves were a part of the history. The "honor and privilege" that the authors expressed on being asked to participate translated into a labor of four and a half years.

Jefferson is fortunate in that from its inception, careful records have been preserved without break of continuity. Minutes of the Board of Trustees and Executive Faculty, Alumni Bulletins, Student Yearbooks, College Announcements and Catalogs, and Annual Reports of the Hospital provided a wealth of detail in the archival treasure trove. Jefferson Alumni of the past who were outstanding historians include Samuel D. Gross (Class of 1828), John H. Brinton (Class of 1852), William W. Keen (Class of 1862), John Chalmers DaCosta (Class of 1885), George M. Gould (Class of 1888), and Edward L. Bauer (Class of 1914). The first librarian, Mr. Charles Frankenberger (appointed 1907), also made historical contributions in his time.

This is a long and complex history. Where to draw the line between thoroughness and excessive detail was a task of the editor, for which forgiveness in judgmental error is requested. With so many names involved, fairness in recognition is impossible. As might be expected, there are unintended omissions and perhaps unwarranted inclusions. All Jefferson Presidents and Chairmen, not merely who they were but what they did, are sketched. Activities in organization, policy, merger initiatives, finances, and proliferation of buildings are interwoven throughout. Contributions in the basic sciences and clinical area previously unnoticed are given attention. In order to avoid a strictly parochial approach, an editorial policy was adopted to place the various segments of Jefferson's history in the perspective of what was taking place in the medical world of the time.

A unique feature of this book is the profusion of illustrations. For those without time or inclination to read the entire text, the photographs alone will provide a pictorial history. Ms. Theresa Powers and her audiovisual staff performed outstanding service in reproducing old photographs and printed material. While most were obtained within Jefferson's own archives, valuable additional help is acknowledged from the College of Physicians of Philadelphia's Historical Collections, the Historical Society of Pennsylvania, the Free Library of Philadelphia, the Jenkins Law Library, the Presbyterian Historical Society, and the National Library of Medicine.

The editor interviewed historically oriented Alumni such as Baldwin L. Keyes (1917), Frederick E. Keller (1917), Reynold S. Griffith (1918), Henry H. Perlman (1918), Thaddeus L. Montgomery (1920), Benjamin F. Haskell (1923), John B. Montgomery (1926), and Joe H. Coley (1934). Board member William Potter Wear, shortly before his death in 1984, generously shared some of his memories and impressions. The editor's mentor, Thomas A. Shallow (1911), was the Class Historian and reminisced frequently about the professors of his era. The editor's interest in Jefferson History was early stimulated by this association.

The editorial assistance of J. Woodrow Savacool (Jefferson, 1938) is gratefully acknowledged. In addition to writing several of the chapters, he improved the content and quality of a number of the manuscripts along with much valuable proofreading. His aid advanced publication time by more than a year.

Mr. Samuel Davis, the Special Collections Librarian, saved much of the editor's time by his quick location of references, photocopying of source material, and aiding the search for photographs. Dr. Robert T. Lentz, Librarian Emeritus and Professor Emeritus of Bibliography and Library Science, and Ms. Judith Robins, the University Archivist, made files, documents, and photographs available which unearthed previously unrecognized items of significance. Ms. Nancy Groseclose and Joan Schott in the Alumni Office answered many queries. The word-processing secretaries, especially Mrs. Connie Buccella, tolerated the frustrations of the editor with equanimity.

Finally Mrs. Jean Lockwood Wagner (Jefferson, R.N., 1941), always a severe critic and sharp proofreader, cheerfully relinquished many leisure hours to aid in this task.

Philadelphia, Pennsylvania

FREDERICK B. WAGNER, JR., M.D.

Contributors

Abrams, Lawrence, Ed.D., Dean, College of Allied Health Sciences and Professor of Education, Department of General Studies

Abrams, William B., B.S., M.D., Adjunct Professor of Medicine

Baltzell, William H., B.A., M.D., Clinical Professor of Otolaryngology

Beadenkopf, F. Scott, B.A., M.Ed., Educational Design Specialist

Bergquist, Erick J., M.S., Ph.D., M.D., Clinical Associate Professor of Medicine and Assistant Professor of Microbiology

Bowers, Mrs. Paul A., President of Women's Board of Thomas Jefferson University Hospital (1981–1984)

Bowers, Paul A., B.S., M.D., Professor Emeritus of Obstetrics and Gynecology

Bowman, Doris E., R.N., M.S.(Ed.), Director, School of Nursing (1958–1982), Professor Emeritus of Nursing (1982)

Brent, Robert L., M.D., Ph.D., The Louis and Bess Stein Professor of Pediatrics and Chairman of the Department, Professor of Radiology (Radiation Biology), and Professor of Anatomy

Brucker, Paul C., B.S., M.D., The Alumni Professor of Family Medicine and Chairman of the Department; Clinical Professor of Medicine

Conly, Samuel S., Jr., A.B., M.D., Associate Dean Emeritus and Honorary Associate Professor of Physiology

Coon, Julius M., Ph.D., M.D., Professor Emeritus of Pharmacology

Delaney, William E., B.S., M.D., Professor of Medicine and Associate Professor of Pathology and Cell Biology

Donovan, Joseph, M.A., Coordinator of Public Relations, College of Allied Health Sciences

Erslev, Allen J., M.D., The Distinguished Professor of Medicine. Director of Cardeza Foundation and Division of Hematology (1963–1985)

Fong, Jonathan C., M.D., Jefferson, 1987

Fox, James W., IV, M.D., Assistant Professor of Surgery (Plastic)

Gartland, John J., M.D., James Edwards Professor Emeritus of Orthopaedic Surgery

Goepp, Carla E., M.D., Clinical Associate Professor of Medicine and Associate Dean of Student Affairs, Student Counseling and Career Planning

Gold, Lionel, D.D.S., Associate Professor of Otolaryngology (Oral Surgery)

Goldburgh, Warren L., M.D., Clinical Professor of Medicine

Groseclose, Nancy S., B.A., Executive Director, Jefferson Medical College Alumni Association

Hervada, Arturo R., M.D., Professor of Pediatrics

Hodges, John H., M.D., The Ludwig A. Kind Professor Emeritus of Medicine

Jackson, Laird G., M.D., Professor of Medicine, Director of Division of Genetics (Medical), Professor of Pediatrics and Professor of Obstetrics and Gynecology

Jacoby, Jay, M.B., M.D., Professor of Anesthesiology and Chairman of the Department

Jarrell, Bruce E., B.Ch.E., M.D., Associate Professor of Surgery

Koltes, John A., M.D., Clinical Professor of Psychiatry and Human Behavior

Kramer, Simon, M.D., F.F.R., Distinguished Professor of Radiation Therapy and Nuclear Medicine

Krehl, Willard A., M.S., Ph.D., M.D., Chairman of Department of Preventive Medicine,

Professor Emeritus of Medicine

Lee, James H., M.D., Professor of Obstetrics and Gynecology and Chairman of the Department

Lentz, Robert T., M.S.(L.S.), Sc.D. Librarian Emeritus and Professor Emeritus of Bibliography and Library Science

Lindquist, John N., M.D., Honorary Clinical Associate Professor of Medicine

Lowry, Louis D., M.D., Professor of Otolarygology and Chairman of the Department

Mandle, Robert J., B.S., Ph.D., Professor Emeritus of Microbiology

Mansmann, Herbert C., Jr., M.D., Professor of Pediatrics, Director of Division of Allergy and Clinical Immunology, and Associate Professor of Medicine

Marks, Gerald J., M.D., Professor of Surgery and Director of the Division of Colorectal Surgery

Miller, Bernard J., M.D., Professor of Anatomy and Clinical Associate Professor of Surgery

Murray, Austin P., M.D., Clinical Assistant Professor of Ophthalmology

Naso, Francis, M.D., Professor of Rehabilitation Medicine and Assistant Professor of Medicine

Parish, Lawrence C., M.D., Clinical Professor of Dermatology

Powers, Theresa M., B.S., Director of Audiovisual Services

Ramsay, Andrew J., Ph.D., Sc.D., The Daniel Baugh Professor Emeritus of Anatomy

Rosenfeld, Leonard M., M.A., Ph.D., Assistant Professor of Physiology

Rupp, Joseph J., M.D., Professor Emeritus of Medicine

Saukkonen, Jussi J., M.D., Professor of Microbiology, Dean of College of Graduate Studies, and Senior Associate Dean of Scientific and Faculty Affairs of Jefferson Medical College

Savacool, J. Woodrow, M.D., Honorary Clinical Associate Professor of Medicine

Schaedler, Russell W., M.D., The Plimpton-Pugh Professor of Microbiology and Chairman of the Department

Schepartz, Bernard, M.S., Ph.D., Professor Emeritus of Biochemistry

Schlezinger, Nathan S., M.D., Sc.D.(Med.), Professor Emeritus of Neurology

Simenhoff, Michael L., M.B., Ch.B., M.D., Professor of Medicine and Director of Division of Nephrology and Hypertension

Simpson, Lance L., B.A., Ph.D., Professor of Medicine and Director of Division of Environmental Medicine and Toxicology, and Professor of Pharmacology

Smith, Harry L., Ph.D., Professor of Microbiology

Smukler, Nathan M., M.D., Professor of Medicine

Steiner, Robert M., M.D., Professor of Radiology, Co-director of Division of General Diagnostic Radiology, and Associate Professor of Medicine

Varano, Nicholas R., M.D., Honorary Assistant Professor of Urology

Vernick, Jerome J., M.Sc., M.D., Clinical Professor of Surgery and Clinical Associate Professor of Radiology

Vlasses, Peter H., B.SC.(Pharm.), Pharm.D., Research Associate Professor of Medicine and Associate Professor of Pharmacology

Wagner, Frederick B., Jr., M.D., The Grace Revere Osler Professor Emeritus of Surgery and University Historian

Whiteley, William H., III, M.D., Honorary Clinical Professor of Neurosurgery

Wirts, C. Wilmer, Jr., M.D., Professor Emeritus of Medicine

Wise, Robert I., M.S., Ph.D., M.D., The Magee Professor Emeritus of Medicine

Wolfson, Philip J., M.D., Assistant Professor of Surgery and Assistant Professor of Pediatrics

Contents

PART II
The Basic Sciences

PART III
Clinical Departments and Divisions

PART III

Clinical Departments and Divisions
Continued

PART IV

University Components and Activities

George McClellan

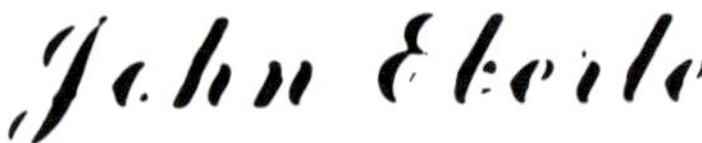

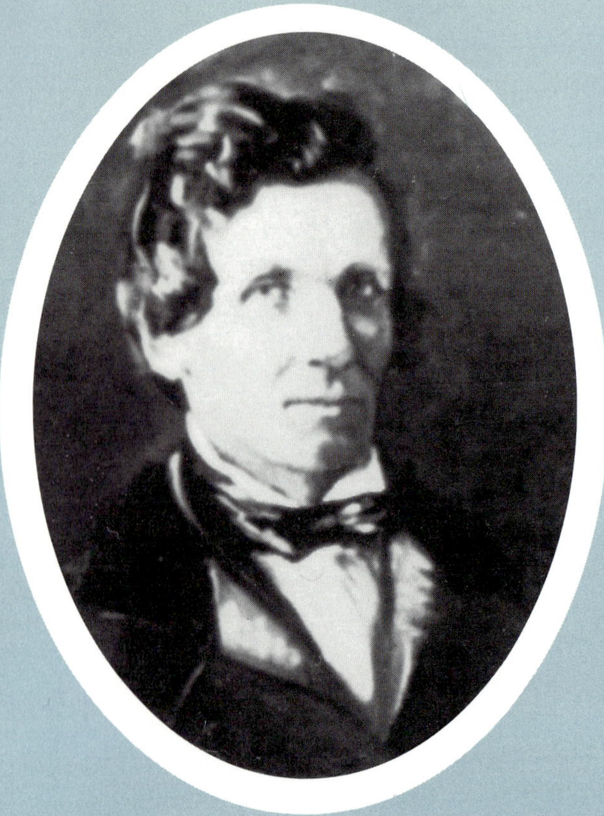

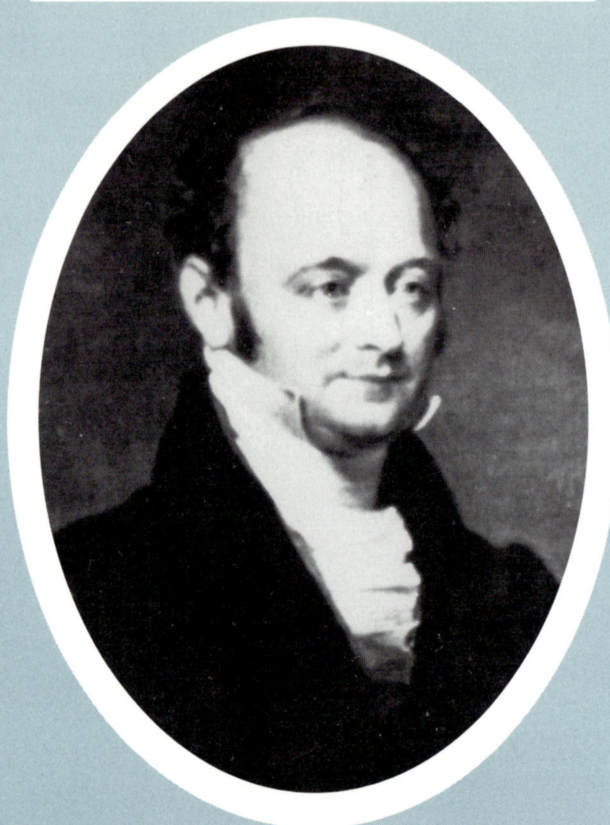

The Founders (1824)

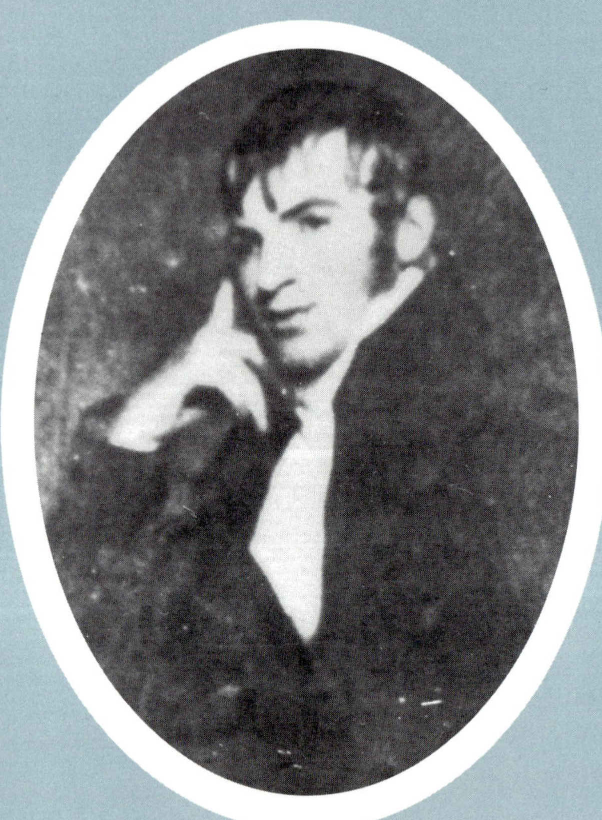

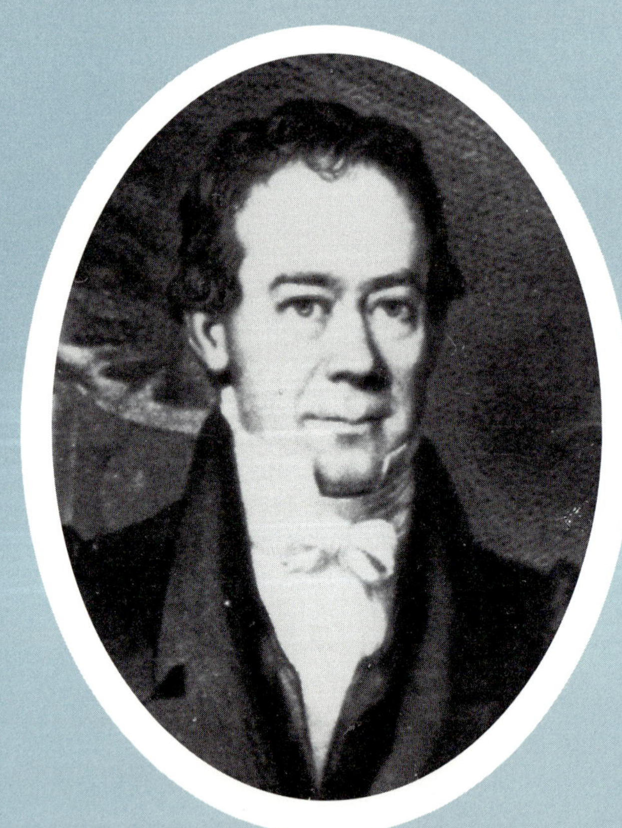

Joseph Klapp

Jacob Green

PART I

The Proprietary Years of Jefferson Medical College (1824–1895)

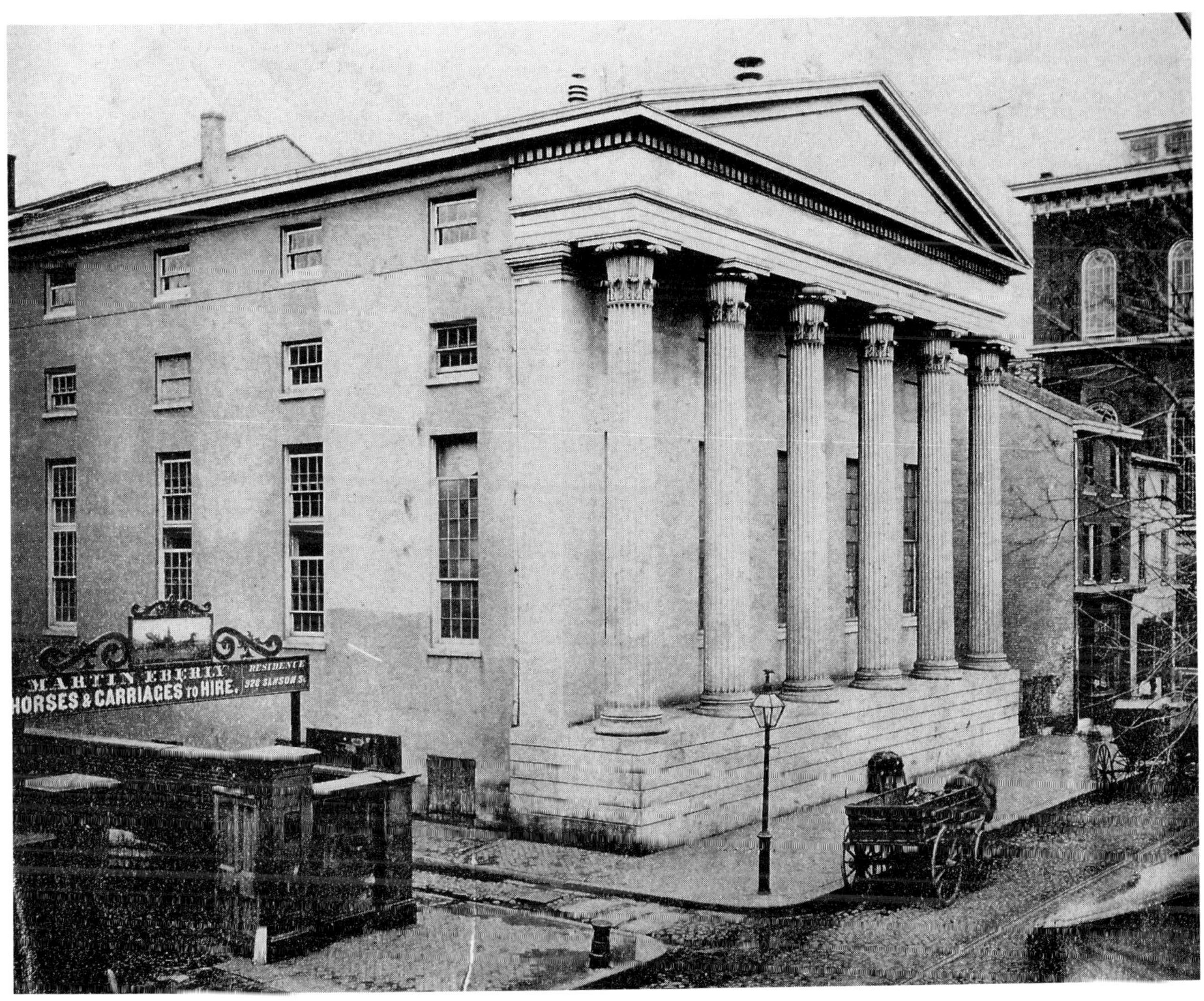

Jefferson Medical College (ca. 1850s)

CHAPTER ONE

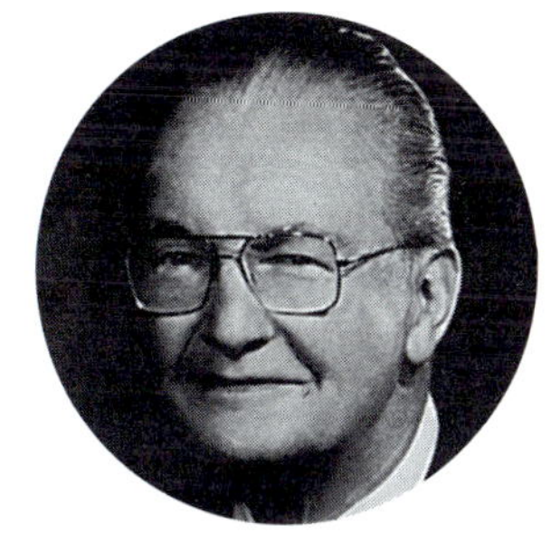

The Early Struggles

Frederick B. Wagner, Jr., M.D.

"If there is no struggle, there is no progress." —Frederick Douglass (1817–1895)

The Jefferson Connection: An Overview

How the medical institution we call Jefferson today actually got its name is a complex narrative. It involves a relationship of three cities—Canonsburg, Charlottesville, and Philadelphia. It also involves a relationship of three men—Thomas Jefferson, the namesake; George McClellan, the founder; and Robley Dunglison, the bridge (Figure 1-1).

The first root of the gigantic family tree may be traced to about 1773, when an itinerant Presbyterian minister named John McMillen (1752–1833) traveled to western Pennsylvania to preach the gospel to the Scottish settlers of that area. After founding the Chartiers Hill Presbyterian Church near Canonsburg, he founded Canonsburg Academy in a log cabin around 1780, the first chartered literary institution west of the Alleghenies.[1] The only good road into the area was a military one from Virginia, constructed in 1754 through the forest by General Braddock's pioneer battalion of 300 axemen. Because the western part of Pennsylvania was largely blocked by impassable mountains, this area was more closely linked to Virginia than to Philadelphia. The Reverend Mr. McMillen's appeal to prominent citizens of Virginia and Pennsylvania for funds and books included Benjamin Franklin, who sent £50 and some books. Shortly after Franklin's death in 1790 his portrait was sent.[2]

In 1802 the trustees chartered the institution as a college and gave it the name of Jefferson in honor of the then third President of the United States (1801–1809).[1] As a token of appreciation Jefferson made a gift of some books, and in 1803 sent a portrait of himself by an unknown artist.[2] In spite of the great statesman's reputed wealth, generosity, and interest in education, he had serious financial troubles. Because of a flamboyant life style, lavish maintenance resulted in a personal debt of $20,000 by the time Jefferson left the presidency. After the British destroyed the Library of Congress in 1814, the former President sold 13,000 volumes from his own library to the nation for $23,950. This temporary relief was erased by the hordes of relatives, guests, and strangers who unashamedly wined, dined, and boarded at his expense, even keeping their horses in his stables. His threatened bankruptcy was saved by a national subscription of $16,500 in 1826, the year of his death. A few months later Monticello itself (now a national memorial) with its furniture, pictures, and silver, was sold to cover the debts.[3] Small wonder that Jefferson was unable to send any money to the college honoring his name.

In 1824 events took place in Canonsburg, Philadelphia, and Charlottesville that marked the

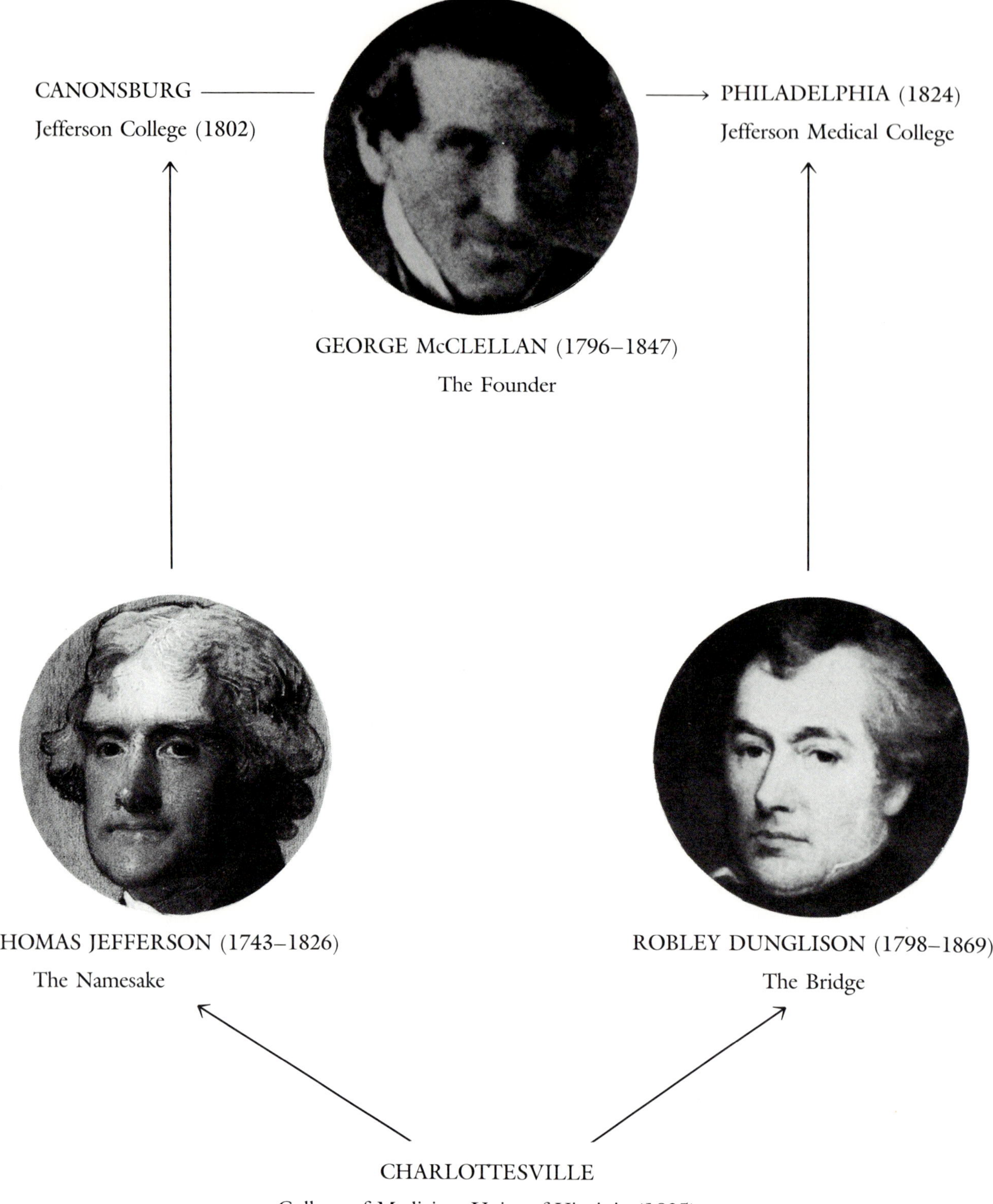

FIG. 1-1. The Jefferson–Dunglison–McClellan Connection.

birth and aided the future of Jefferson Medical College. It was the year in which Dr. George McClellan negotiated the establishment of the Medical Department of Jefferson College at Canonsburg as the Jefferson Medical College of Philadelphia.[4] His attempts to obtain a separate charter from the Pennsylvania legislature for a second medical college in Philadelphia had been unsuccessful.

In the same year at Charlottesville, Thomas Jefferson was busy with the creation of a medical school for the University of Virginia, which had first opened its doors in 1819.[5] At age 76 Jefferson had already designed much of the physical structure and curriculum of the University. Now at 81 years, in full possession of the intellectual energy and humanitarian spirit that characterized his genius, he was searching for the best possible young man "to teach medicine on historical lines with explanations of its successive theories since the time of Hippocrates for the purpose of affording such information as educated persons would want for the sake of culture." The post was deemed of such importance that the search extended to London, where Francis E. Gilmer, Esq., Jefferson's representative, enlisted Dr. Robley Dunglison.[6] Dunglison was given academic tenure, with $1,500 annual salary, free rent in one of the University pavilions, and a five-year covenant secured by a guarantee of $5,000. It was the first full-time clinical teaching position in a university medical school in this country.

Within two months of Dunglison's arrival at Charlottesville, he was summoned to become the personal physician of Thomas Jefferson. Until then Jefferson had distrusted the medical profession, preferring nature's healing. Yet in his twenties, Dunglison found himself attending the former President of the United States and serving as faculty head in the School of Medicine of the University of Virginia. He faithfully attended Jefferson's last two years and closed his eyelids at his death on July 4, 1826. Jefferson had arranged for Dunglison to receive as a gift the grandfather clock in his bedroom. The clock is now displayed in the main exhibition hall of the Historical Society of Pennsylvania, and its replica stands in the Board of Trustees' Room of the Scott Administration Building.[7]

Dunglison became a professor at the University of Maryland in 1833 and, in 1836, at Jefferson Medical College, where he remained for the rest of his life. He was just two years younger than McClellan the founder and was the bridge between Jefferson the man and Jefferson the institution.

In 1838 Jefferson Medical College obtained its independent charter from the Pennsylvania State Legislature, "with all of the rights and privileges of the University of Pennsylvania."

In 1870 Samuel D. Gross founded the Jefferson Alumni Association, which spearheaded a building fund campaign for a new detached hospital that was completed in 1877. The goal of $250,000 was oversubscribed at $350,000 in two months.

Until 1895 Jefferson Medical College, like most other medical schools, was a proprietary institution, in that the students paid the faculty professors directly for tickets to the lectures as well as for clinical instruction in the hospital. The professors in turn paid rent to the College to cover taxes and maintenance. On June 1, 1895, under Board President Joseph B. Townsend, Esq., Jefferson became a nonprofit-sharing corporation with a single board of trustees responsible for the complete integration and management of the College and Hospital. In 1949 the first President of the Corporation, Vice Admiral James L. Kauffman, U.S.N. Ret., was appointed. Through this new office the Medical College began to benefit from yearly appropriations from the Commonwealth of Pennsylvania. Also in 1949, a graduate program in various basic medical sciences was organized that led to the formation of the College of Graduate Studies in 1969.

In 1961 Jefferson Medical College first admitted women students, and in 1965 seven received their M.D. degrees. Increasing numbers and involvement of women in all aspects of the institution have most favorably enhanced its welfare and prestige.

A College of Allied Health Sciences was chartered in 1967 to provide both academic and clinical education in the health professions and occupations.

Through the untiring efforts of President Peter A. Herbut, M.D., the scope of Jefferson Medical College of Philadelphia was expanded with a new charter and the adoption of the name Thomas

Jefferson University in April, 1969.[8] Jefferson is a privately endowed, tuition- and gift-supported, nonsectarian, nonprofit corporation, which also receives certain grants and appropriations from the federal government, the Commonwealth of Pennsylvania, and the State of Delaware. The Jefferson Medical College of Philadelphia retains its original identity and is officially known as the Jefferson Medical College of Thomas Jefferson University. The three other components of the University are the College of Graduate Studies, the College of Allied Health Sciences, and the Thomas Jefferson University Hospital.

On January 18, 1972, at the second session of the Ninety-second Congress, it was "Resolved, by the Senate and House of Representatives of the United States of America in Congress assembled, That the Thomas Jefferson University, Philadelphia, Pennsylvania, be and is hereby recognized as the first university in the United States to bear the full name of the third President of the United States." Further, on November 18, 1974, at the Ninety-third Congress, second session, it was "Resolved, That the Senate congratulates Thomas Jefferson University on its one hundred and fiftieth anniversary, commends the faculty, staff, employees, and graduates of its colleges and hospital on their dedication, vision, exemplary professionalism, and extends to them every good wish for continued growth and impact on the health care needs of the Nation."

The history, tradition, and heritage of Jefferson may in some measure explain the mystique or spirit that evokes the wonderment of alumni of other institutions.

References

1. Coleman, H.T.W., *Banners in the Wilderness: Early Years of Washington and Jefferson College*. Univ. of Pittsburgh Press, 1956.
2. Corwin, J.D., "Jefferson Portraits: History and Enigma," *Jeff. Al. Bull.* Winter 1974.
3. *Encyclopedia Britannica,* 1959 ed., Vol. 12, p. 992.
4. Bluemle, L.W., Jr., "Jefferson College and Thomas Jefferson University," *Medical-Science Colloquium, Sp. Ed. of Topic: A Journal of the Liberal Arts.* Washington and Jefferson Coll. 1983.
5. Hart, A.D., "Thomas Jefferson's Influence on the Foundation of Medical Instruction at the University of Virginia," *Ann. Med. Hist.* 10:47–60, 1938.
6. Radbill, S.X., "Dr. Robley Dunglison and Jefferson," *Trans. Coll. Phys. Phila.* 27:40–44, 1959.
7. Wagner, F.B., Jr., "The Jefferson–Dunglison Clock," *Trans. Stud. Coll. Phys. Phila.* 3(2), June 1981, pp. 151–157.
8. "Report of the Committee for Master Planning, Thomas Jefferson University," December 1972.

Thomas Jefferson: Influence on Medical Theory and Practice

In the context of their times, Thomas Jefferson remains unchallenged as the most informed and versatile of all U.S. presidents. His well-known services in politics and diplomacy may be summarized as follows: member, Virginia Assembly, 1769–1775; member, Continental Congress, 1775–1776, author, Declaration of Independence (at age 33); member, Virginia Assembly, 1776–1779; Governor of Virginia, 1779–1781; minister to France, 1782–1789; Secretary of State under George Washington, 1790–1797; Vice President of the United States under John Adams, 1797–1801; President of the United States, 1801–1809; elder statesman and educator, 1809–1826.

Science was equally a lifelong pursuit of Jefferson's. Cohn[1] credits him as contributor to the fields of meteorology (United States Weather Bureau), paleontology (father of American paleontology, with study of the *Mammoth maglongx jeffersoni*), ethology, archeology, astronomy (United States Naval Observatory and Hydrographic Office), architecture (designed Monticello and University of Virginia), chemistry, agriculture, geology, exploration (Lewis and Clark Expedition and Louisiana Purchase), botany, and mechanical engineering. While U.S. Vice President he also served as President of the American Philosophical Society.

Jefferson included medical theory and practice in his preoccupation with the applications of science. Numerous articles[1–8] attest to his influence on medical education. His opinions and warnings have their relevance not solely within the profession but also with respect to increasing governmental involvement. As regards the latter, he wished to separate science from government equally as well as church from state. He believed in governmental powers to prevent injury to others and to promote scientific investigation for protection against foreign powers, but he sought to preserve scientists' privilege to arrive at independent unbiased conclusions supported by proper observation. In this sense he probably would have approved of the scientific studies sections of the present National Institutes of Health, which are administered by nongovernment experts.

Jefferson was always curious about the structure and function of the human body. His library contained the best medical books of the time, many of them presented to him by their authors, and he read the available American medical journals, which began their appearance just before the turn of the eighteenth century. He admired a number of physicians for their compassion for the sick, but in general held a poor opinion of those who practiced the internal medicine of his day. He had suffered the great personal loss of his wife in 1782 and only the eldest of his six children, Martha, reached adulthood. Jefferson articulated distrust of physicians in 1807 in an oft-quoted letter to Dr. Caspar Wistar, in which he asked for supervision of his grandson, who was to study in Philadelphia. The youth's subjects were to include botany, natural history, anatomy, and possibly surgery, but not medicine. The salient reasons were as follows:

> "We know, from what we see and feel, that the animal body is in its organs and functions subject to derangement inducing pain, and tending to its destruction. In this disordered state, we observe nature providing for the reestablishment of order, by exciting some salutary evacuation of the morbific matter or by some other operation which escapes our imperfect senses and researches. . . . Experience has taught us, also, that there are certain substances, by which, applied to the living body, internally or externally, we can at will produce these same evacuations, and thus do, in a short time, what nature would do but slowly, and do effectually, what perhaps she would not have the strength to accomplish. . . . So far, I bow to the utility of medicine. It goes to the well-defined forms of disease, and happily, to those the most frequent. But the disorders of the animal body and the symptoms indicating them are as various as the elements of which the body is composed. The combinations too of these symptoms are so infinitely diversified, that many associations of them appear too rarely to establish a definite disease, and to an unknown disease there cannot be a known remedy. Here then, the judicious, the moral, the humane physician should stop. . . . Or if the appearance of doing something be necessary to keep alive the hope and spirits of the patient, it should be of the most innocent character.
>
> But the adventurous physician goes on, and substitutes presumption for knowledge. From the scanty field of what is known, he launches into the boundless region of what is unknown. He establishes for his guide some fanciful theory . . . which lets him into all nature's secrets at short hand. On the principle which he thus assumes, he forms his table of nosology, arrays his disease into families, and extends his curative treatment, by analogy, to all the cases he has thus arbitrarily marshalled together. . . . The patient, treated on the fashionable theory, sometimes gets well in spite of the medicine. The medicine, therefore, restored him, and the young doctor receives new courage to proceed in his bold experiments on the lives of his fellow-creatures. I believe we may safely affirm, that the inexperienced and presumptuous band of medical tyros let loose upon the world, destroys more of human life in one year, than all the Robinhoods, Cartouches, and Macbeths do in a century. It is on this part of medicine that I wish to see a reform, an abandonment of hypothesis for sober facts, the first degree of value set on clinical observation, and the lowest on visionary theories. I would wish the young practitioner, especially, to have deeply impressed on his mind, the real limits of his art, and that when the state of his patient gets beyond these, his office is to be a watchful, but quiet spectator of the operations of nature, giving them fair play by a well-regulated regimen, and by all the aid they can derive from the excitement of good spirits and hope in the patient. . . . The only sure foundations of medicine are, an intimate knowledge of the human body and observation on the effects of medicinal substances on that. The anatomical and clinical schools, therefore, are those on which the young physician should be formed. If he enters with innocence that of the theory of medicine, it is scarcely possible he should come out but untainted with error. His mind must be strong indeed, if rising above juvenile credulity, it can maintain a wise infidelity against the authority of his instructors, and the bewitching delusions of their theories."

One example of medical treatment based on scientific fact was vaccination. Jefferson, as a practical man, quickly appreciated the importance of this discovery. In 1766, at age 23, he traveled to

Philadelphia where Dr. William Shippen of the newly opened medical school (subsequently University of Pennsylvania) inoculated him by direct arm to arm. In 1800 Jefferson learned about Edward Jenner's success with the much milder cowpox vaccination and its introduction into the United States by Dr. Benjamin Waterhouse, Professor of Medicine at Harvard Medical School.[9] After studying the experimental and clinical data, Jefferson was convinced of its scientific and therapeutic validity. Upon assuming the presidency in 1801, he introduced generalized vaccination into the southern states.[10] He personally diagrammed the various stages of vaccine reaction in both the whites and blacks and sent this information to a large number of influential physicians. His relatives and plantation population, numbering more than 200, were vaccinated and he kept detailed reports of each reaction. He even improved the vaccine samples by suggesting that some might have been killed in transportation by excessive heat and that larger amounts of nutrient material should be used. Indian chiefs and their wives were encouraged to be inoculated, and Captain Lewis was ordered to take cowpox vaccine on his expedition to vaccinate Indians and settlers. Cohn[1] points out that Jefferson's presidential role in the vaccination program created a precedent for President Gerald Ford's swine flu vaccine program in 1975.

An example of a medical practice not founded on scientific fact was bloodletting. Jefferson was its strong opponent, never allowing the practice to be done in his family or on the workers in his plantation. He thought that his personal friend, Dr. Benjamin Rush, had done much harm in his frequent venesections while erroneously believing he was saving lives. Medical theorists without the slightest scientific support had promulgated many ingenious arguments in its favor. The prominent current British medical journal *The Lancet* (named for bloodletting), which appeared shortly before Jefferson's death, remains a medical anachronism.

Bean[2] describes Jefferson's contributions to the training of physicians as exemplified at the University of Virginia: (1) development of a medical school in a university setting; (2) encouragement of state funding to support the medical school, in order to abolish proprietary medical schools for profit; (3) development of a forum for sharing medical knowledge; (4) encouragement of the study of physiology in order to promote conservatism against nonscientific drug therapy; and (5) promotion of honor in the maturity of physicians.

It took Robley Dunglison to disarm Jefferson of his lifelong distrust of physicians. Dunglison was the perfect model for Jefferson's teaching principles. He believed in giving nature the first chance in the cure of disease, and he was scientifically oriented. As the physician to presidents, the "Father of American Physiology," and the unique pride of Jefferson Medical College, a great deal more is to be said of Robley Dunglison.

References

1. Cohn, L.H., "Contributions of Thomas Jefferson to American Medicine," *Am. J. Surg.* 138:286–292, 1979.
2. Bean, W.B., "Mr. Jefferson's Influence on American Medical Education: Some Notes on the Medical School of the University of Virginia," *Va. Med. Mo.* 8:669–680, December 1960.
3. Rosen, G., "Political Order and Human Health in Jeffersonian Thought," *Bull. Hist. Med.* 26:32–44, 1952.
4. Hall, C.R., "Jefferson on the Medical Theory and Practice Stud. of His Day," *Bull. Hist. Med.* 31:235–245, 1957.
5. Hart, A.D. Jr., "Thomas Jefferson's Influence on the Foundation of Medical Instruction at the University of Virginia," *Ann. Med. Hist.* 10:47–60, 1938.
6. Radbill, S.X., "Thomas Jefferson and the Doctors," *Trans. Coll. Phys. Phila.* 37(2):106–114, 1969.
7. Thorup, B.A., Jr., "Thomas Jefferson and Academic Medicine," *The Pharos.* April 1977, pp. 16–23.
8. Radbill, S.X., "Dr. Robley Dunglison and Jefferson," *Trans. Coll. Phys. Phila.* 27:40–44, 1959.
9. Waterhouse, B., *A Prospect of Exterminating the Small Pox: Part II,* Cambridge Univ. Press, 1802.
10. Martin, H.A., "Jefferson as a Vaccinator" *N.C. Med. Jour.* 7:1, 1881.

Philadelphia circa 1824: Environment for a Second Medical School

Philadelphia in the 1820s was a garden spot of the United States, commercially bustling, culturally sophisticated, historically prestigious, and exciting to live in or visit. Despite the devastation by epidemics, especially yellow fever in 1793, the population nearly doubled during the first two decades of the nineteenth century, yielding the lead only slightly to New York. In 1820 the City of Brotherly Love spread its 113,000 citizens along the Delaware River; Tenth and Eleventh Streets represented the western borderland beyond which a physician's sign was rarely seen.[1] By 1825 the thriving city with 138,000 people had 69 physicians, about a dozen more than 30 years previously; 10 midwives; 78 so-called nurses; and 18 dentists,[2] although in the few years before and after 1825 there were fewer physicians in proportion to the general population than in any past or future history of the city.

In the election year 1824, John Quincy Adams defeated Jackson, Clay, and Crawford, and Lafayette was concluding his final tour of America. Benjamin Rush had signed the Declaration of Independence, but in the 1820s physicians were turning from political activities to scientific scepticism. Samuel D. Gross, 19 years old in 1824, had little interest in politics, although he later came to know or administer to six presidents of the United States.

In industry, a revolution was under way. Machinery was replacing hand labor, but the social adjustments to that change were only beginning. Entrepreneurs and mechanics had little technical training. The crying need of the time was for education, particularly in the crafts and sciences, but in 1824 there was as yet no high school in Philadelphia.

Culturally, Philadelphia was already established. The Pennsylvania Academy of the Fine Arts had been in existence since 1805 and had assembled a fine collection of paintings. The Philadelphia Museum Company was three years old. The Musical Fund Society of Philadelphia had erected a hall on Locust Street between Eighth and Ninth that could handle large-scale performances. Shakespeare's plays were being performed at the Walnut Street theater; built in 1809, it is today the oldest surviving theater in the English-speaking world. Philadelphians had formed important literary and scientific societies, such as the Library Company of Philadelphia, founded in 1731 (the first subscription library in America); the American Philosophical Society, founded in 1743; the College of Physicians of Philadelphia founded in 1787; and the Philadelphia Medical Society (1789–1846), a precursor of the Philadelphia County Medical Society. The year 1824 saw the incorporation of the Franklin Institute, the Historical Society of Pennsylvania, the Pennsylvania Horticultural Society, and the Mercantile Library. From a public health standpoint 1824 was the year of the introduction of Schuylkill River water into nearly 4,000 private homes and 185 factories. Many families were to run their first tubful of bathwater from a tap, although most likely that bath was cold. Hospital facilities included Pennsylvania Hospital (the oldest hospital in the United States, founded in 1751), Christ Church Hospital for Poor Widows, Philadelphia Almshouse (precursor of "Old Blockley," the now defunct Philadelphia General Hospital), Philadelphia Dispensary (established in 1786), Northern Dispensary, and Friends Asylum for the Insane.

The 1820s was a period of reconstruction, of resistance to old systems, and of an awakening to a new era of scientific spirit. Many of the prominent leaders were Southerners from Virginia and the Carolinas, for example, Nathaniel Chapman, William Horner, John Kearsley Mitchell, Joseph Hartshorne, Charles Caldwell, Charles Delucena Meigs, and Thomas Dent Mütter. Many students from the South were to come north and account for as much as one-half to two-thirds of medical school enrollment. A new generation of Philadelphia physicians started to locate on Chestnut, Walnut, and Spruce Streets. Most were below 55 years of age and many were scarcely 30.

Philadelphia's only medical school was at the University of Pennsylvania, the oldest in the United States, founded in 1765. It was located on the west side of Ninth Street between Market and Chestnut. Its faculty comprised Nathaniel Chapman in Theory and Practice of Medicine, with Samuel Jackson two years later as his assistant for the Institutes; William Gibson in Surgery; Philip Syng Physick (in ill health) in Anatomy with William Horner as adjunct; Thomas James and William Dewees, both in questionable health, in Midwifery; Robert Hare, inventor of the oxyhydrogen blowpipe, in Chemistry; John Coxe in Materia Medica; and

W.P.C. Barton (later at Jefferson) in Botany. At this time the University had more than twice as many medical students as any other school, 480 enrolled out of 1,970 in the entire fifteen medical colleges of the country. The only competitors were Transylvania in Lexington, Kentucky with 235; University of Maryland with 215; and College of Physicians and Surgeons of New York with 196.[3] This enlarging enrollment in a growing city encouraged provision of larger facilities.

Various threats to the monopoly held by the University of Pennsylvania began to develop. Dr. W.P.C. Barton, appointed Professor of Botany at the University in 1816, conceived plans for a second school and applied to the State Legislature in the session of 1818–1819, creating such concern that a meeting of the University students was called for an expression of views. John Kearsley Mitchell, then a student and later to become Professor of Theory and Practice of Medicine at Jefferson, as well as the father of the even more eminent Silas Weir Mitchell, was chairman, and he presented a strong resolution against a second school. Unexpectedly, another student, Benjamin Rush Rhees, subsequently to become Professor of Materia Medica and Institutes of Medicine as well as the first Dean of Jefferson Medical College, arose to argue against Mitchell. The resolution was defeated at the next meeting, but discussions continued in the Philadelphia Medical Society and in the press.

Eminent practitioners had private pupils, and many gave private and public lectures, which enhanced their prestige as well as their income. One of these, Nathaniel Chapman, collaborated in 1817 with several practitioners in other areas of medical education to give a more generalized course. He renovated the second floor of his stable and created an organization known as The Medical Institute. This systematic course of instruction attracted over 100 students and by 1837 developed into Franklin Medical College, which became extinct in 1848.[4]

In 1818 another private practitioner, Dr. Joseph Parrish, developed after several years of outstanding teaching a following of more than 30 students and engaged an assistant, Dr. George B. Wood. In the next 12 years it was necessary to add two more assistants, and in 1830 it became the Philadelphia Association for Medical Instruction with a distinguished faculty. This school gave certificates instead of degrees and passed into oblivion around 1840.

In 1820 Dr. Jason V. Lawrence began the longest lasting and most useful of these ancillary private institutions, The Philadelphia Anatomical Rooms, later to become The Philadelphia School of Anatomy.[5] It was located at the upper end of Chant Street (then College Avenue) on the north side, near St. Stephen's Episcopal Church on Tenth Street between Market and Chestnut, as well as near the University on Ninth. The lecture rooms were originally intended as a summer school to extend medical education as well as scientific investigation during the University's long vacation between April and November.

Although European education at Edinburgh, London, Paris, Leyden, Vienna, or Berlin was the common route to medical fame, Philadelphia was the acknowledged place to study in the United States. London and Paris each had only one medical college, too, but Philadelphia was ripe for a second. In this setting of 1824 a young surgeon of genius had the outrageous temerity to found Jefferson Medical College, destined to become the largest private institution of its kind in the country. That surgeon was George McClellan.

References

1. Konkle, B.A., and Henry F.P., *Standard History of the Medical Profession of Philadelphia,* 2d ed., New York: AMS Press, 1977, p. 149.
2. Wilson, Thos., *The Philadelphia Directory and Stranger's Guide.* John Bioren, Printer, 1825, pp. 158–160.
3. Sewall, T., "Opening Address at Columbian College, D.C., March 30, 1825." Quoted in Konkle and Henry (see footnote 1), p. 152.
4. Abrahams, H.J., *Extinct Medical Schools of Nineteenth-Century Philadelphia.* Univ. of Pennsylvania Press, 1966, pp. 161–175.
5. Keen, W.W., *The History of the Philadelphia School of Anatomy and Its Relation to Medical Teaching: Addresses and Other Papers.* Philadelphia: W.B. Saunders and Co., 1905, pp. 41–67.

McClellan's Private School: Founding of Jefferson Medical College

Physicians at the time of George McClellan were general practitioners who treated the ill with emetics, cathartics, and bloodletting. General anesthesia was a generation away and Listerian principles of antisepsis two generations yet to come. Brilliant men of this era could attain prominence by studying anatomy from obsolete textbooks and then, as was becoming possible, dissect cadavers and perform their own postmortem examinations. Such a man was George McClellan and the men he gathered about himself. It was a simple matter for the medical scholar of that day to switch his lectures from anatomy to surgery, to chemistry, to materia medica, or to midwifery, because established medical facts were limited and controversial theories abounded. Most of the medical literature was British or French, with few of Philadelphia's physicians contributing anything at all. Medical journals were practically nonexistent, the mainstay being the *American Medical Recorder*. The only library resources were in the College of Physicians or Pennsylvania Hospital. A medical library was a luxury of the times; the only other medical library of importance in the United States was in New York.

In those days, if one wished to study medicine in the grand manner, it was necessary to come from a relatively well-to-do family. Such was the good fortune of George McClellan, whose father, James, was a respected merchant in the wool business and also the principal of an academy of elementary education.

"The Founder" was born in Woodstock, Connecticut in 1796. His ancestry was noteworthy—he inherited the genes of battling Highlanders and American Revolutionary patriots. His great grandfather, Samuel McClellan, fought at the side of Charles Edward, the Young Pretender, who attempted the recovery of the English throne for the Stuarts but was defeated at Culloden Moor in 1746. This forced Samuel to escape for his life to America. The founder's grandfather, Samuel, Jr., fought in the French and Indian War, later moved to Woodstock, Connecticut, and became a Brigadier General under Washington. The founder's maternal grandfather had also fought in that war. The military heritage of the family was to continue in the founder's son, George Brinton McClellan, General of the Union Army of the Potomac during the early part of the Civil War.

"Little Mac," as George McClellan was called in boyhood because of his short stature, early displayed the traits that were galvanized throughout his life—tireless energy, positive character that emanated as leader rather than teamworker, excellence in mathematics and language, instant comprehension, quick movements, promptness of opinion, and enthusiasm for whatever cause he espoused. One is reminded of the young Napoleon Bonaparte from this description.

McClellan's preliminary education at his father's Woodstock Academy grounded him well in Latin, Greek, and mathematics. He entered Yale University at age 16, where he studied the natural sciences with much zeal. After graduation in 1815 he commenced the study of medicine near his home town in the office of Dr. Thomas Hubbard, subsequently Professor of Surgery in Yale Medical School. In 1817 McClellan came to Philadelphia both to be a private pupil of Dr. John Syng Dorsey, Professor of Materia Medica and Anatomy at the University of Pennsylvania, and to enroll in the University. In 1818, one year before obtaining his doctorate degree, McClellan was elected Resident Physician to the Hospital of the Philadelphia Almshouse. Few physicians of that era had as thorough a foundation for a successful career as did McClellan during his student years. His avid reading, capacious memory, copious note-taking, and long hours in the dissecting room placed him in the front rank against all competitors.

Following graduation from the University in 1819 at age 23, McClellan opened clinical practice in an office at the corner of Walnut and Swanwick Streets, just beyond Sixth. Swanwick Street (running north and south between Sixth and Seventh) no longer exists—the Public Ledger Building occupies the entire block from Sixth to Seventh. This area was directly north of Potter's Field (now Washington Square). Success was immediate, enabling McClellan the following year to marry Elizabeth Brinton, the daughter of a prominent Philadelphia lawyer. McClellan's reputation attracted a large following of private students for lectures in anatomy and surgery, requiring a move to the corner of George (now Sansom) and Swanwick Streets. The rear of this house was next to the Apollodorian Gallery of Paintings, which Rembrandt Peale had remodeled from an old stable at Walnut and Swanwick. When more space was needed, McClellan was able to rent the rear of the gallery. It was the spot where the embryo of Jefferson Medical College would develop.

With mounting increase in size and usefulness of his private school, McClellan called on Dr. John Eberle for assistance. Eberle was a former editor of the *American Medical Recorder* and a teacher of principles of medicine. Philadelphia possessed other talented practitioners and teachers that McClellan knew and could assemble to complete a medical curriculum. Around 1823, at age 27, he began thinking about founding a new school, but needed the approval of the State Legislature to grant the M.D. degree. The University of Pennsylvania had strong influence with the legislators and had successfully blocked all previous attempts as well as McClellan's to obtain a charter. McClellan resorted to an ingenious strategy.[1] None of the credit for initiative, boldness, persistence, or drama can be denied him. On June 2, 1824, he (age 28), along with Dr. John Eberle (age 38), Dr. Joseph Klapp (age 41), and Mr. Jacob Green, A.M. (age 35), the son of the Rev. Dr. Ashbel Green (former President of Princeton), sent a formal application to the Trustees of Jefferson College at Canonsburg, Pennsylvania (Figure 1-2):

> "Gentlemen:
> The undersigned, believing upon mature consideration, that the establishment of a second Medical School in the city of Philadelphia would be advantageous to the public not less than themselves, have formed themselves into a Medical Faculty, with the intention of establishing such a school; and they hereby offer to the Trustees of Jefferson College to become connected with that institution on the conditions herewith submitted, subject to such modifications as on a full and free explanation shall be found satisfactory to the parties severally concerned. The undersigned beg leave to submit a plan which they have devised for forming the faculty contemplated, and for conducting the concerns of the same, open to amendments and alterations in the manner already proposed."[2–5]

The Jefferson College at Canonsburg was controlled by Scotch Presbyterians who may have given McClellan more favorable attention as a member of the same denomination. The following affirmative action was taken:

> "The Board of Trustees of Jefferson College situated in Canonsburg, Washington County, Pennsylvania, deeming the creation of a Medical Faculty, in connection with that institution, expedient, passed at their stated meeting held in the month of June, 1824, the following resolutions, viz:
>
> That the Board of Trustees of Jefferson College hereby establish a Medical School in connection with and as a part of the Institution of which they the said Trustees are the legal Guardians and Directors.
>
> That the Medical School if established be located in the city of Philadelphia.
>
> Agreeable to the foregoing resolution, the following Gentlemen were duly appointed to the respective Professorships attached to their names, viz:
>
> Joseph Klapp, M.D., Professor of Theory and Practice
>
> John Eberle, M.D., Professor of Obstetrics
>
> Jacob Green, A.M., Professor of Chemistry
>
> George McClellan, M.D., Professor of Surgery and Anatomy"

At the same meeting articles of union were also drafted and transmitted to the Professors so appointed, in the form of an official document founded on the mutual agreement of the parties thus connected.

The "articles of union" are quoted in full, since they succinctly stated the contract that was amicably held for the next 14 years.

> "1. That it is expedient to establish in the city of Philadelphia a Medical Faculty, as a constitutent part of Jefferson College, to be styled the JEFFERSON MEDICAL COLLEGE.
>
> 2. That the Faculty of the Medical College shall consist of the following professorships: 1st, a Professor of Anatomy; 2nd, of Surgery; 3rd, of the Theory and Practice of Medicine; 4th, of Materia Medica, Botany, and the Institutes; 5th, of Chemistry, Mineralogy and Pharmacy; 6th, of Midwifery and the Diseases of Women and Children.
>
> 3. That whenever a vacancy shall occur by death, resignation, or otherwise, it shall be filled by a gentleman who shall be nominated by the remaining professors, or a majority of them, and appointed by the trustees of the College.

4. That a professor may be removed by the Board of Trustees with the consent of a majority of the other medical professors, and after a full and fair investigation of the alleged causes for the removal, but in no other way.

5. That the Medical School shall have no claims whatever on the funds of Jefferson College.

6. That the medical professors shall make arrangements among themselves for the time and place of lecturing, for examinations, and for the general benefit of the school. The time for conferring medical degrees shall be determined by the trustees, on the representation of the Medical Faculty. The same fee shall be paid to the President of the College by the graduates for degree as for a degree in the arts.

7. That this college shall use all suitable influence to send medical pupils to the Medical School connected with it in Philadelphia; and the Medical Faculty shall promote in every way the interest and prosperity of the College.

8. That the young men who have attended the course of lectures in any respectable medical institution shall be admitted to a standing in all respects equal to the one they had left.

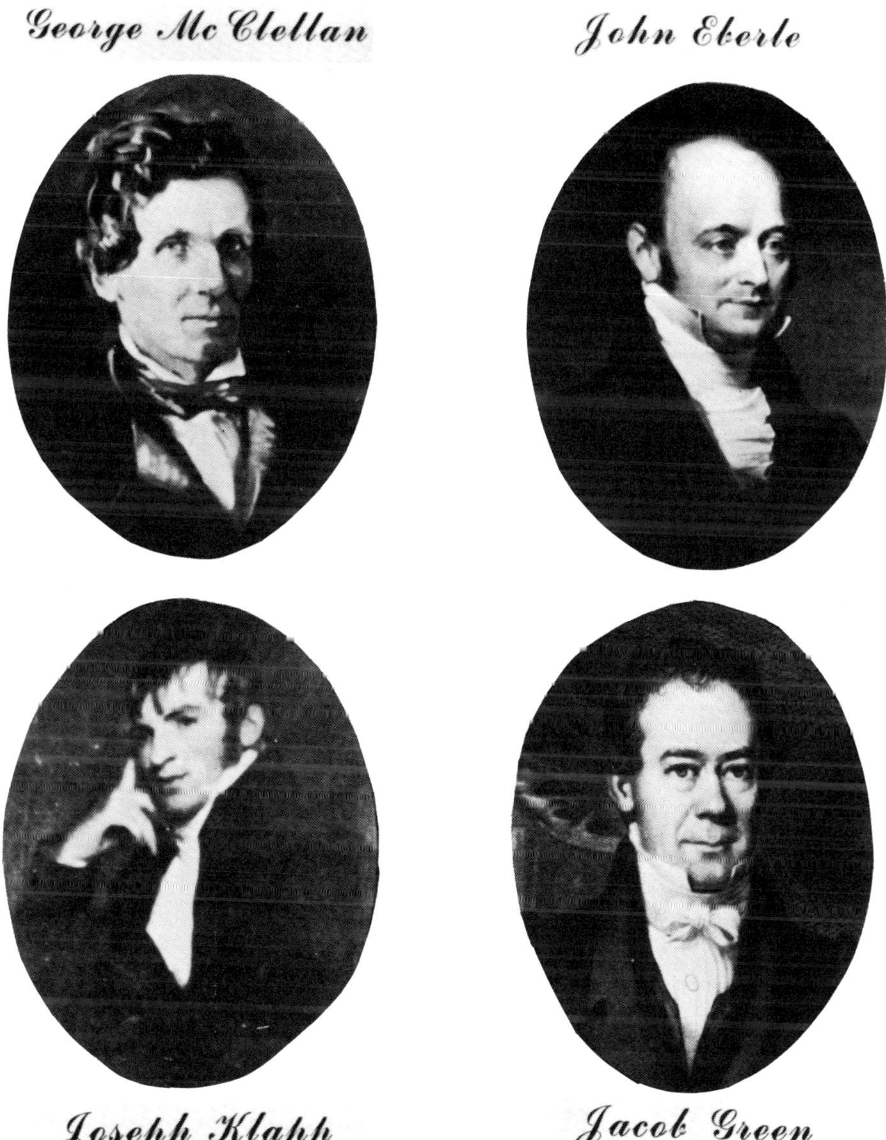

FIG. 1-2. Founders of the Medical Department of Jefferson College at Canonsburg (Jefferson Medical College).

9. That ten indigent young men of talent, who shall bring to the Medical Faculty satisfactory testimonials and certificates shall be annually admitted into the Medical School, receive its medical instructions, and be entitled its honors, without any charge.

10. That the following persons duly elected be, and they are hereby appointed to the following professorships, viz: Doctor George McClellan, Professor of Surgery; Doctor Joseph Klapp, Professor of Theory and Practice of Medicine; Doctor John Eberle, Professor of Materia Medica; Jacob Green, Esq., Professor of Chemistry, Mineralogy and Pharmacy.

11. That the President of the board be, and is hereby, appointed to forward these resolutions to the professors elect, and to hold any necessary correspondence with them on the subject until the next meeting of the board."

In October, 1824, these resolutions consummated the founding of the Jefferson Medical College of Philadelphia as the Medical Department of Jefferson College of Canonsburg.

References

1. Corner, G.W., *Two Centuries of Medicine: A History of the School of Medicine, University of Pennsylvania.* Philadelphia: J.B. Lippincott, 1965, p. 77.
2. Smith, J., *History of Jefferson College, Including an Account of the Early Log-Cabin Schools, and the Canonsburg Academy.* Pittsburgh: J.T. Shryock, 1857, pp. 113–115.
3. Gayley, J.F., *History of the Jefferson Medical College of Philadelphia.* Philadelphia: J.M. Wilson, 1858, p. 16.
4. Gould, G.M., *The Jefferson Medical College of Philadelphia.* New York: Lewis, 1904, pp. 32–34.
5. Konkle, B.A., and Henry, F.P., *Standard History of the Medical Profession of Philadelphia.* New York: AMS Press, 1977, pp. 162–164.
6. Bauer, E.L., *Doctors Made in America.* Philadelphia: J.B. Lippincott, 1963, p. 6.

The First Home: Tivoli Theater

The birthplace of Jefferson Medical College was in McClellan's office (Figure 1-3) and the rented portion of the Apollodorian gallery; the charter had been granted by a parent institution, almost a week distant by stagecoach, but not by the State Legislature; and the six professors stipulated in the "articles of union" were represented by only four. To transform a paper existence into a reality it was necessary to complete a faculty, find a suitable home, and regulate the finances. The founders were on their own in matters of management, with only moral support from the Trustees at Canonsburg.

With vestment of authority from the parent body the skeleton faculty proceeded promptly to implement its plan. Lectures continued without interruption in the former buildings, and the first lecture under the charter was given by McClellan himself on October 11, 1824. Dr. Klapp resigned because of poor health, and Drs. Benjamin Rush Rhees and Francis S. Beattie joined the group. The first regular faculty meeting, with still only five members, was held December 20, 1824. Dr. Rhees was appointed as Dean and Drs. Eberle and Beattie and Mr. Green charged as a committee to procure "the building formerly the Tivoli Theater, on Prune street (now 518 Locust Walk), near Washington Square, and owned by George Shaw."

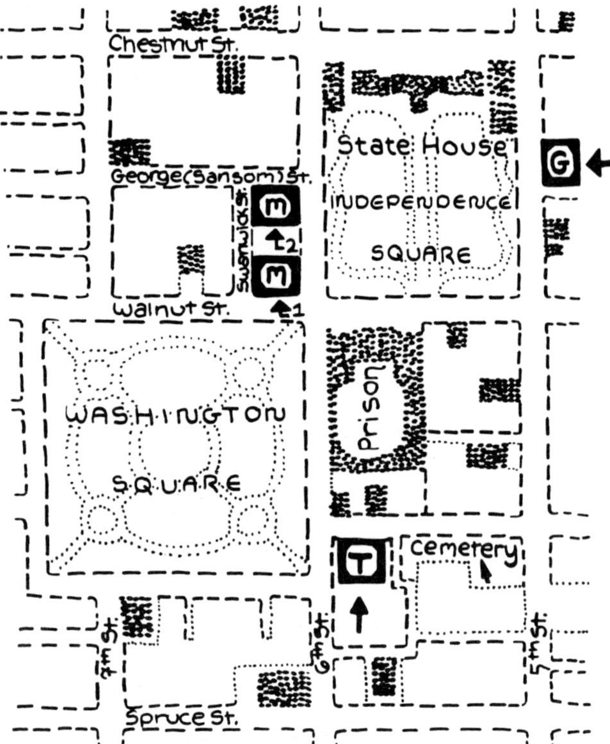

FIG. 1-3. The Jefferson Medical College Birthplace

M[1] George McClellan's first office, north of Washington Square.

M[2] McClellan's second office, corner of George (Sansom) and Swanwick Streets.

T Tivoli Theater, 518 Prune Street (Locust Walk), first home of Jefferson Medical College.

G First office (1828–1830) of Samuel D. Gross.

(See Figure 1-3.) On December 31 a lease was signed for a period of four years and three months, effective January 1, 1825, at an annual rental of $550.[1]

The building (Figure 1-4) was originally a cotton warehouse that in 1820 had been converted to a playhouse known as the Winter Tivoli (Tivoli) Theater. Many American plays premiered there with some of the favorite actors of the period. For three years the house was fairly successful, owing perhaps to the absence of competition from the old Chestnut Street Theater at Sixth and Chestnut, which had burned to the ground. On October 29, 1823, John Howard Payne's melodrama, *Clari, the Maid of Milan,* played in which the world-famous song, *Home Sweet Home,* was sung for the first time in America. In December of that year the rebuilt Chestnut Street Theater opened again, and thereafter the Tivoli Theater declined rapidly.

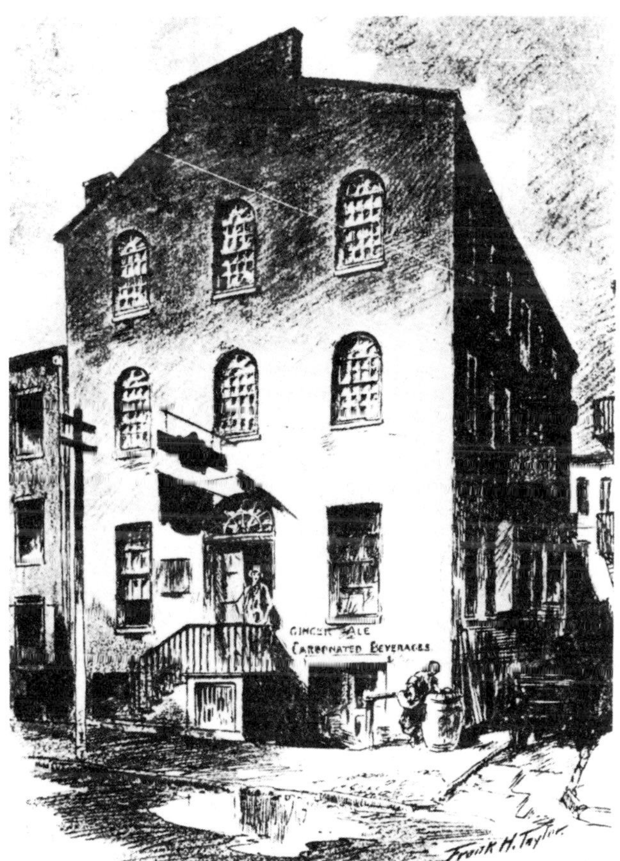

FIG. 1-4. The Prune Street Tivoli Theater (518–520 Locust Walk), first home (1825–1828) of Jefferson Medical College.

At their next meeting, in January, 1825, the faculty assigned the remodeling of the interior of the theater. Green and Beattie were responsible for the carpentry and Eberle for the masonry. Green, as treasurer, was able to collect the assessment of $20 from each faculty member except Dr. Beattie. The latter's default led to recriminations and misunderstandings.

The Hall of the Jefferson Medical College was opened on March 8, 1825, with prayer by the Reverend Ashbel Green and an address by the Dean, Dr. Benjamin Rush Rhees. The audience may have been struck by the unusual surroundings of the neighborhood. To the north and directly in front was the "infamous Walnut Street prison," built in the 1770s. Only the narrow street and a yard for the criminals and debtors separated the two buildings. Potter's Field (now Washington Square) with its 3,000 bodies of British and Continental soldiers, paupers, and Walnut Street prisoners lay to the west. The Free Quaker Cemetery, for those of the sect who had been expelled for fighting in the Revolutionary War, flanked the east. At the rear was a popular ale house, and within a block or two were St. Mary's, St. Peter's, and Holy Trinity Church.

Washington L. Atlee (Jefferson, 1829) describes the opening:[2]

> "Truly a portentious beginning! How like the poor newly fledged doctor—an abundance of penniless patients; all work and no pay; in debt, with prison staring him in the face and a convenient graveyard to bury from sight the victims of his inexperience! Here, driven as it were, into a corner, with nothing but death and the dungeon to contemplate, overshadowed and opposed by the most renowned medical school of that day, and unsupported by the medical men of the country, a few bold and enterprising adventurers threw down the gauntlet either to conquer or to die."[2]

John Chalmers DaCosta (Jefferson, 1885) aptly wrote: "There was crime and misery in front, death on either side, and consolation in the rear."[3]

The building, long after being vacated by Jefferson for its definitive home in 1828, was used by a bottling concern for carbonated beverages. It was destroyed by fire in the 1920s. The nostalgic visitor can find a bronze plaque commemorating this site placed by the Alumni Association on

October 22, 1987 (Figure 1-5). Locust Street in this area is now a brick-paved pedestrian walk overshadowed by the Penn Mutual Towers.

References

1. Gould, G.M., *The Jefferson Medical College of Philadelphia.* New York: Lewis, 1904, p. 45.
2. Atlee, W.L., *Reminiscences of the Earliest Days of Jefferson Medical College.* Philadelphia: P. Madeira, 1873, p. 6.
3. DaCosta, J.C., *Selections from the Papers and Speeches of John Chalmers DaCosta.* Philadelphia: W.B. Saunders, 1931, p. 326.

The Infirmary Department: A First in Medical Instruction

McClellan was always generous in his care of the poor. These patients were frequently presented for instruction of the students in his private school. A provision was made to continue this method by the faculty of the newly formed Medical College. On January 27, 1825, it was resolved that "in addition to their present arrangements, the committee be instructed to prepare an apartment to be used by the Dean as an office, and to be also appropriated to the reception of indigent patients, whom it is hereby determined to supply with medicine gratuitously." This action was a new idea for a professional faculty and a historical event for medical colleges in America.

The involvement of students in the care of patients, under supervision, was a deviation from the standard curriculum, which consisted of four months of lectures in each of two successive years. The lectures were the same in the second year, the concept being that a second hearing would allow better comprehension and longer remembrance. This clinical instruction, McClellan's signal contribution to medical education, was first hailed as "misleading, ineffectual, and superficial." Enhancement of didactic lectures with clinical experience not only brought Jefferson a widespread reputation for educating excellent doctors but was a model that came to be adopted by all medical colleges.

On April 20, 1825, the Faculty resolved: "That

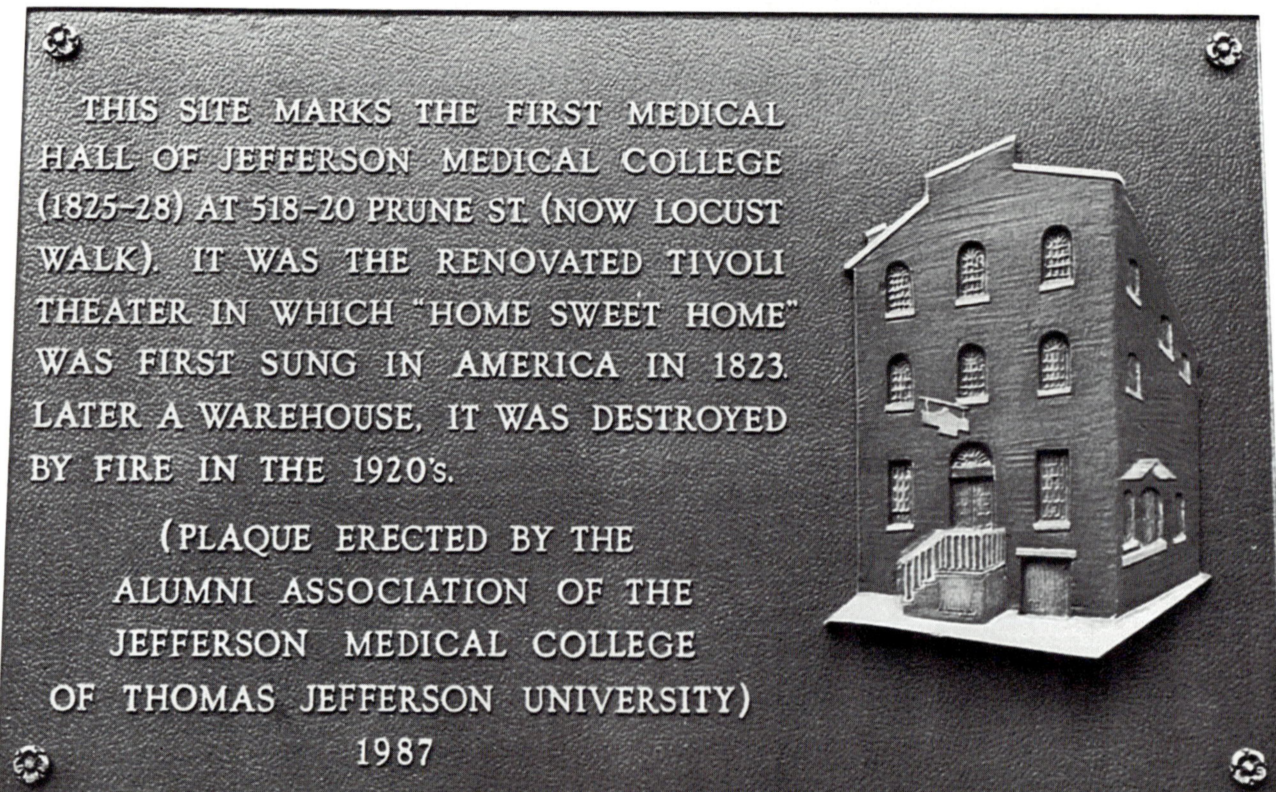

FIG. 1-5. Commemorative plaque of Tivoli Theater, first home of Jefferson Medical College (1825–1828).

circulars be published setting forth that the Infirmary of the Jefferson Medical College will be opened for the reception of patients on the 16th of May, when all medical cases will be prescribed for by Dr. Eberle and all of a surgical character attended to by Dr. McClellan between the hours of 5 and 6 P.M. every day, Sunday excepted." All other members of the faculty, except Mr. Green, who at that time lacked the M.D. degree, were to lend their services as needed. One week ahead of schedule, on May 9, the impatient and energetic Dr. McClellan performed his first operation in the Infirmary. The formal opening did occur on May 16, at which time a register was established, showing the names of those receiving prescriptions and operations. The first benefactions to the project were supplies from a Mr. George Glentworth and medicinal articles to the amount of $20 from a Mr. Jacob Bigonet. This Infirmary, the first clinic established in any college in the country, was the forerunner of the Jefferson Medical College Hospital and the ultimate Thomas Jefferson University Hospital.

The First Faculty: The Troublesome Dr. Beattie

George McClellan's sagacity in founding the "new school," as it was called, his promptness in acquiring a home for it, and his care in the choice of a faculty were notable achievements. In a strict sense, "the first Faculty," as named in the charter from Canonsburg, was theoretical in that Joseph Klapp resigned before formal classes began. Three new professors had to be added, and the curriculum had to be equitably reassigned. Conveniently, medical scholars of that era were general practitioners, knowledgeable in all the branches, and capable of switching courses or filling in the gaps. Accordingly, John Eberle changed his Chair from Midwifery to Theory and Practice, and Midwifery was taken by Francis S. Beattie to include Diseases of Women and Children. Benjamin Rush Rhees was appointed to occupy the Chair of Materia Medica, Botany and Institutes, and Nathan R. Smith the Chair of Anatomy. Four of the six men constituting this first faculty—Drs. McClellan, Eberle, Rhees, and Mr. Green—were pillars of strength who supported the College during its critical formative period and endured its subsequent harassments. A resume of the group reveals that in most respects it was outstanding, in spite of financial difficulties and personal disagreements.

George McClellan

The founder was the star teacher and main attraction to the school. His lectures were delivered extemporaneously and with an exuberance of thought that stimulated and individually communicated with every member of the class. He carried his students through his thought process and made them part of it. The material was lucid, forceful, and authentic for that time. His talent was in speaking, not at his writing desk (Figure 1-6), although he did

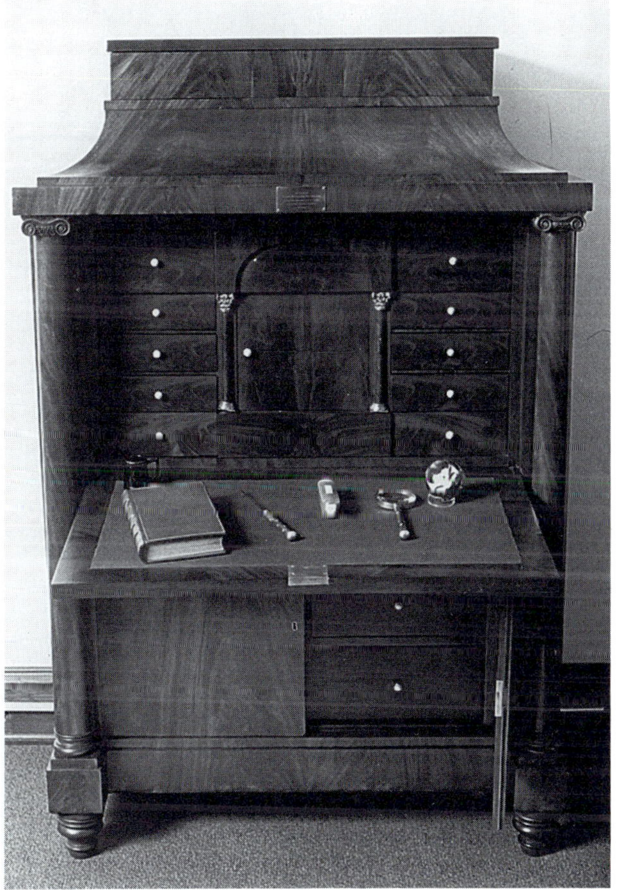

FIG. 1-6. The desk of Dr. George McClellan.

contribute a few articles to several of the existing medical periodicals (Figure 1-7). He edited an edition of John Eberle's *Theory and Practice of Physic* with notes and additions. A one-volume *Principles and Practice of Surgery* (1848) was published one year after his death; it was of practical value but greatly dwarfed by the prestigious *System of Surgery* published less than ten years later by his eminent pupil, Dr. Samuel D. Gross. A textbook of anatomy in collaboration with his brother Samuel was never completed. His greatest contribution to medical education was the involvement of students in the care of patients under suitable guidance. This came to be the greatest strength of Jefferson Medical College and was the basis of its traditional reputation for turning out excellent clinicians.

■ John Eberle

The Professor of Theory and Practice (Medicine) had studied medicine in the office of Joseph Klapp and, like McClellan, was a graduate of the University of Pennsylvania (1809). His pedagogic talents were the opposite of McClellan's—he was a gifted writer but a dull speaker. Eberle's sobriquet, "The Tripod," was due to his stance while lecturing; he stood immobile with his legs spread far apart and his right hand resting on the podium. He rarely raised his eyes from a prepared manuscript that was informative but usually monotonous. His lectures suffered from the quotation of too many authorities without giving his own decisive opinion as to which was the best for the students to follow. On the other hand, his books on *Materia Medica* and the *Practice of Medicine* went through several editions as standard texts of their day, gaining him a wide reputation at home and abroad. A German translation made of his work on *Materia Medica and Therapeutics* secured him a membership in the Medical Society of Berlin. His treatise on *The Diseases and Physical Education of Children* stamped him as a pioneer in pediatrics.

Eberle spent the happiest years of his professional life at Jefferson. Daniel Drake enticed him in the fall of 1831 to leave for Cincinnati to aid in forming another school of medicine. There Eberle encountered disappointments, vexations, and declining health. He accepted a professorship at Transylvania University in Lexington, Kentucky, in 1837. By then his weakness was such that he could not lecture for even half an hour. He died in 1838 at age 50.

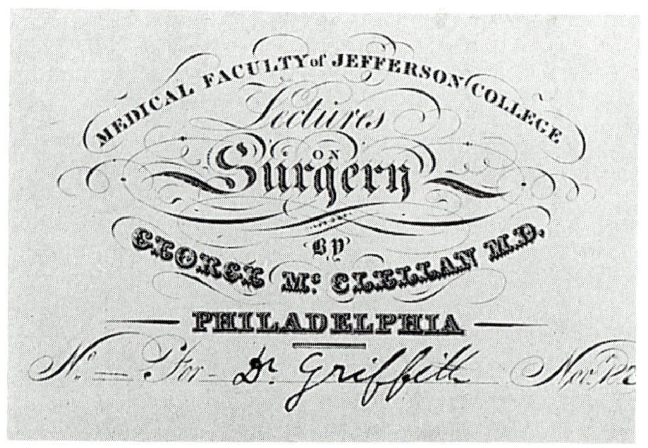

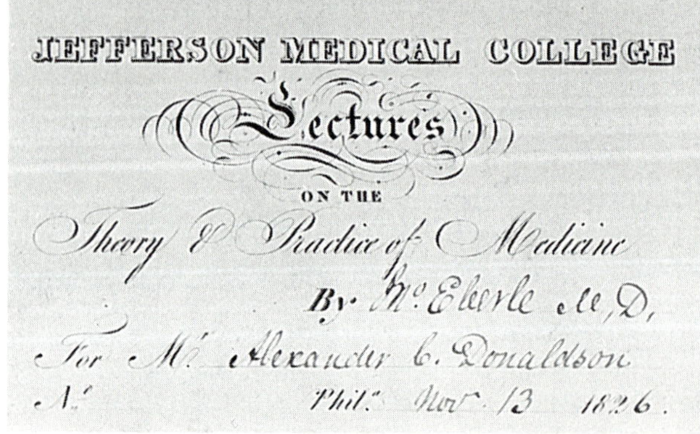

Fig. 1-7. Tickets for George McClellan's lectures on Surgery (1825–1826) and John Eberle's lectures on Theory and Practice of Medicine (1826–1827).

■ Jacob Green

The first Professor of Chemistry, although not a graduate physician at the time, held an A.M. degree from the University of Pennsylvania, was licensed to practice law in the State of New York, and had studied theology. Since 1818 he had been Professor of Chemistry, Experimental Philosophy, and Natural History at Princeton University, of which his father was the president. In 1827 he obtained an M.D. degree from Yale, and the following year traveled in Britain, France, Switzerland, and Germany. His lifetime interests remained in basic science rather than clinical practice. He published *A Text Book of Chemical Philosophy* (1829), and most of his writings were during the 13 years that followed his return from Europe until his death at age 50. Of the four founders he survived the longest at Jefferson and was endearingly called "Old Jaky." The students under his instruction attended his funeral as a group in February, 1841.

Green's lectures were carefully organized, delivered without notes, and articulated impressively (Figure 1-8). His experiments before the class were always for instruction and never for show or amusement.

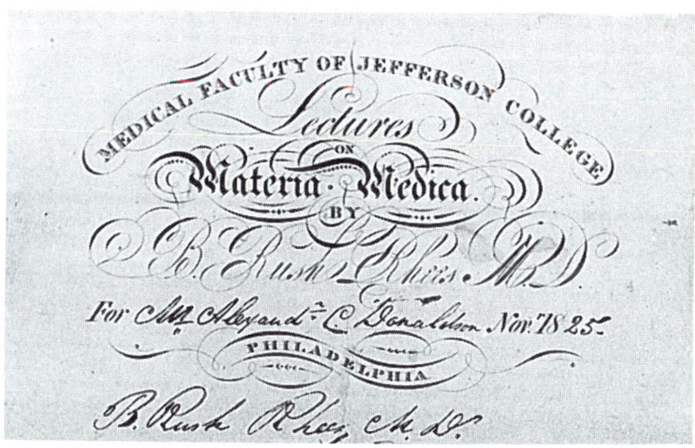

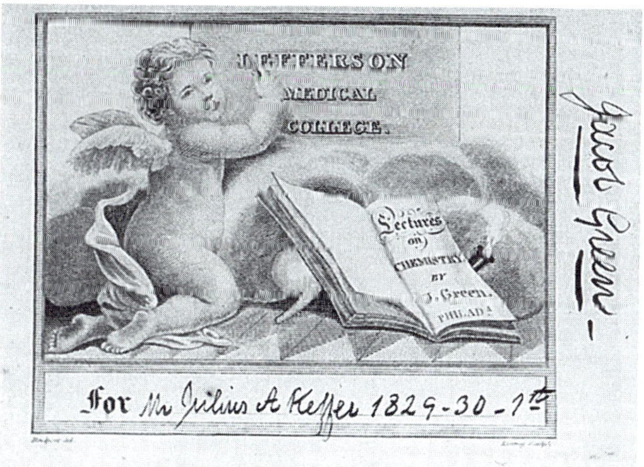

FIG. 1-8. Tickets for Benjamin Rush Rhees' lectures on Materia Medica (1825–1826) and Jacob Green's lectures on Chemistry (1829–1830).

■ Benjamin Rush Rhees

As a first-year student at the Medical School of the University of Pennsylvania in 1818, Rhees had the temerity at a class rally to argue in favor of a second medical school in Philadelphia. Little was "the dapper little fellow"[1] to know that only seven years later he would become Professor of Institutes and Dean of that rival school (Figure 1-9). Institutes is the English equivalent of *Institutiones Medicae,* the title of a book by the celebrated Dutch physician, Hermann Boerhaave, published in Leyden in 1708. It was the first work in which the study of bodily function was treated as a separate scientific discipline. The Chair of Physiology founded at Edinburgh in 1726, the first in the world, was given the name of Institutes in recognition of Boerhaave's book. Samuel D. Gross never liked the term and denounced it as follows: "This title still disfigures the annual announcement of the College. Literally interpreted, the Institutes embraces—besides Physiology—pathology and therapeutics, or the general principles of medicine."[2] Despite his objections, this title was to persist at Jefferson until the appointment of

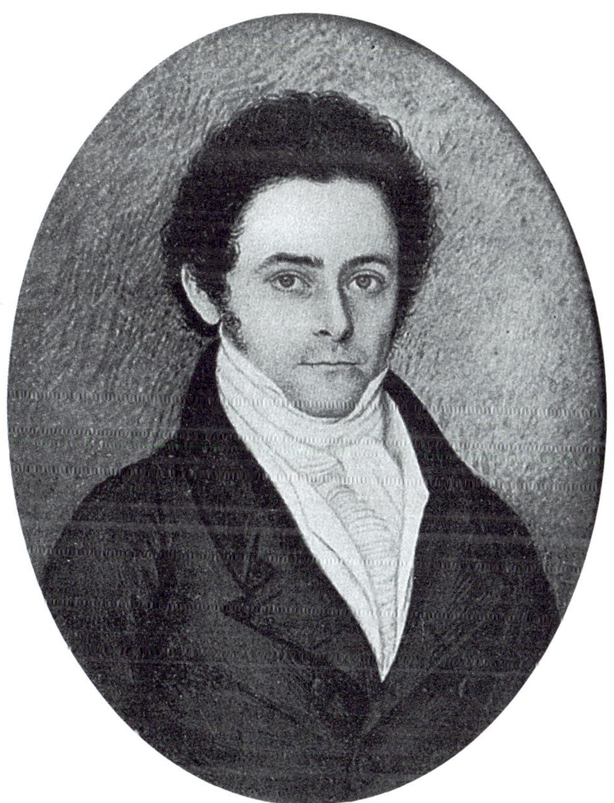

FIG. 1-9. Benjamin Rush Rhees, M.D. (1798–1831); Professor of Materia Medica and Institutes of Medicine (1825–1830); First Dean (1825–1827).

Albert B. Brubaker as Professor of Physiology in 1904.

Rhees' preceptor was Dr. James Rush,[3] son of Dr. Benjamin Rush, who outlived his eminent pupil by 38 years. After graduation from the University of Pennsylvania in 1821, Rhees took a voyage to the East Indies. There he gained experience as a physician for the various vessels in that area. On his return to Philadelphia he took care of numerous cases of smallpox and yellow fever. In his private office he prescribed for the poor, gave a course of lectures on Materia Medica and clinical instruction to a class of young men who had chosen him for preceptor, and systematically arranged a cabinet of botanical specimens. He was on the staff of the Philadelphia Hospital when McClellan appointed him to the Jefferson Faculty.

Unfortunately, Rhees died in 1831 at the age of 33 from tuberculosis, without a literary legacy to perpetuate his name. Physically he was small and frail. His voice, although somewhat weak, held the attention of his class. He always read his lectures but delivered them enthusiastically. The students respected him as a capable instructor, as well as a person erudite and cultivated in belles lettres.

■ Nathan Ryno Smith

Born in New Hampshire in 1797, Smith took his classical and medical education at Yale, receiving the M.D. degree in 1823. While attending additional lectures at the University of Pennsylvania in 1825 he met McClellan, who enlisted him to teach anatomy at the newly organizing school. Smith was only 29 years of age, but of imposing stature and possessing academic and clinical acumen (Figure 1-10). Although an excellent teacher and well accepted by the students, Smith remained only for two years. The fees from his course were barely adequate, and because he was a stranger in Philadelphia, where many of the best physicians in the country were located, he had little or no practice. In 1827 the University of Maryland offered him the advantage of the Chair of Anatomy with assurance of succession to the Chair of Surgery upon resignation of the old and infirm incumbent. He became an immense success in Baltimore during the next 50 years and was considered by Samuel D. Gross to be a great surgeon. Smith lived to be 80 years of age.

■ Francis Smith Beattie

After graduation from the University of Pennsylvania Medical School in 1821 and spending several years in naval service on the frigate *Constellation,* Beattie came to Philadelphia in November, 1824. His acquaintance with medical classmate Rhees, who had just been appointed to the new faculty, led to McClellan, who needed a Professor of Midwifery. Beattie with slim qualifications accepted the Chair. It was soon obvious that he was contentious, incompatible with his colleagues, and beset by financial difficulties. During renovation of the Tivoli Theater he suggested fixtures that were beyond the budget and was insulted when Green, the

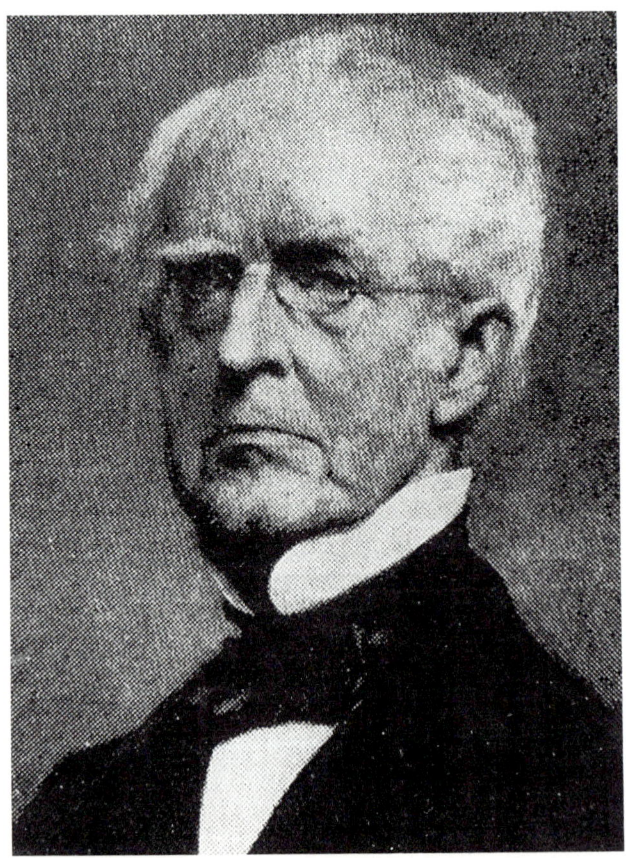

FIG. 1-10. Nathan R. Smith, M.D. (1797–1877); Professor of Anatomy (1825–1827).

treasurer, reminded him that he had not paid his own $20 assessment. In short order he alienated himself by naming Green "a dull fellow," characterizing Rhees as having "a captious and petulant temper" and Smith as "supercilious" with "offensive demeanour," calling Eberle a "tale-bearer," and faulting McClellan for "a most rude and unhandsome reception" in his home. On charges of "uncourteous deportment towards colleagues and incapacity" he received a resolution of dismissal from the President of Jefferson College at Canonsburg on October 28, 1826, after completion of one term of service.

On November 10, 1826, Beattie published a 39-page pamphlet entitled "Statement of Proceedings on the Part of the Members of the Faculty and the Trustees of the Jefferson Medical College against Francis S. Beattie, M.D., Professor of Obstetrics and the Diseases of Women and Children in that Institution" in which he claimed that dismissal was received by him without warning or trial.[4] On November 14, 1826, just four days later, Eberle published an 8-page pamphlet entitled "A Reply to Certain Calumnious Statements Uttered and Published by Francis S. Beattie, M.D." It stated: "The exposition which Dr. Beattie has published of the circumstances connected with his dismission from our Faculty, is marked throughout with misrepresentations, prevarication, and unparalleled malignity. The Trustees, the professors, and the students of our school have much reason to rejoice in having got rid of him at any price."[5]

After dismissal, Beattie continued to harass McClellan, which, on March 10, 1829, led to "Trial of a Suit brought in the District Court for the City and County of Philadelphia by George McClellan, M.D. against Francis S. Beattie, M.D. for a Libel." As a result of this trial, McClellan's professional ethics were vindicated.

It is likely that Beattie's problems were more of an emotional than an intellectual nature. Gould[6] states that "he is remembered favorably by the older alumni." On November 22, 1831, Beattie and six other physicians attended the formal organization of the Lying-in Charity,[7] a society for aiding maternity cases in their own homes. In 1833 he edited *The American Lancet,* published every two weeks. After that he faded into obscurity and died in 1841 at age 47.

Such were the men who conducted the academic session of 1825–1826. All considered, they were as competent as any similar group of teachers in the schools of this country at that period. The lecture notes of Nathan Lewis Hatfield (1804–1887) from this pioneer class are preserved in the College of Physicians of Philadelphia.[8] One can judge by reading them that he was an excellent student and that his Professors covered their subjects systematically. Hatfield became a prominent physician in the city, was on the staff of the Philadelphia Hospital, and served as President of the Board of Health in 1845 and the County Medical Society in 1865.

References

1. Gross, S.D., *Autobiography with Sketches of His Contemporaries,* Vol. I. New York: Arno Press, p. 37.
2. Gross, S.D., *Autobiography,* Vol. II, p. 410.
3. *The Jeffersonian,* 14:113, p. 17.
4. Pamphlet by Beattie, *Hist. Coll. of Coll. Phys. Phila.*
5. Pamphlet by Eberle, *Hist. Coll. of Coll. Phys. Phila.*
6. Gould, G.M., *The Jefferson Medical College of Philadelphia,* Vol. I. New York: Lewis, 1904, p. 42.
7. Konkle, B.H. and Henry, F.P., *Standard History of the Medical Profession of Philadelphia,* 2d ed., New York: AMS Press, 1977, pp. 420–421.
8. Hatfield, Nathan Lewis, "Papers: Excerpts from Notes on Lectures by Members of the First Faculty of the Jefferson Medical College." *Fugitive Leaves from Library of Coll. Phys. Phila.,* N.S., No. 72.

The Legislative Act of 1826: McClellan's Legendary Ride

Under the patronage and charter of the Jefferson College at Canonsburg, the Faculty of the Medical Department were able to open their school in Philadelphia. The venture was audacious, experimental, and lacked financial backing from the parent institution. Without guarantee of survival, success or failure rested on the medical faculty alone—it was only a foot in the door. Not unexpectedly, the right and power to grant diplomas to graduates of the Jefferson Medical College, either by its Faculty or the parent College, were challenged and disputed by the University of Pennsylvania. Legal entanglements led to confrontation when, on advice of Counsellors Edward Ingersoll and J. Coudy, a petition was introduced into the State Legislature on October 25, 1825, that would specifically enable Jefferson College at Canonsburg to grant the medical degree and to create an additional Board of Trustees in Philadelphia on behalf of its Medical Department.

The issue was debated off and on in the Legislature during the next five months, with Drs. McClellan and Eberle making occasional trips to Harrisburg on behalf of favorable passage of the bill. On January 30, 1826, William Tilghman, Chairman of the Board of Trustees of the University of Pennsylvania and Chief Justice of the Pennsylvania Supreme Court, read a protest before the Senate setting forth reasons for the opposition.

> "The medical department of Jefferson College is required by no public necessity and will be followed by very injurious consequences, not only to the University of Pennsylvania, so long and so justly cherished by the state, but to that pre-eminence in medical science and instruction which our city has hitherto enjoyed. . . . the city should not lose this pre-eminence which has been obtained by a concentration of all her force in the support of our medical school, and will inevitably be lost if it shall be distracted and divided among rival institutions. . . . At this moment, a large and essential portion of the revenue of the university is derived from the medical school, and supplied to the support of the collegiate department; and the security and continuance of this revenue depend upon the success and prosperity of that school. . . . The division of the public patronage and support between two rival institutions will necessarily weaken both; while the rivalship, judging from other similar cases, will degenerate into a sort of hostility, honorable to neither and injurious to both. . . . The competition will probably produce a facility in granting degrees, which will destroy their value, and render them no longer accredited testimonials of professional knowledge and skill. . . . In Paris there is but one chartered medical college; and but two in France, with her immense population. In Edinburgh there is but one, and in Great Britain but three in actual operation, that is, at Edinburgh, Glasgow, and Dublin; and in no instance are two established in the same place. . . . granting that there are now upwards of five hundred in this school. . . . At the college at Edinburgh, where the means of affording instruction are not superior to ours, there are this year upwards of nine hundred students; at Paris are about fifteen hundred; and, in neither place is it supposed that these numbers render the establishment of another seminary necessary or expedient."[1]

Who could refute these objections as other than logical and honorable?

McClellan learned that a vote was finally to be taken on April 7. Early on the morning of the previous day he decided to make a dash to Harrisburg for one last plea. Some have likened it in fantasy to the ride of Paul Revere. Several versions exist but the eyewitness account of a portion of the incident by Dr. Washington L. Atlee is probably the most accurate. Washington Atlee was later to be a fellow student at Jefferson with Samuel D. Gross, and his brother John had been a fellow student at the University with McClellan. Atlee's reminiscence:

> "In the spring of 1826, nearly half a century ago, four young medical students were assembled in the office of Dr. John L. Atlee, of Lancaster, for the purpose of forming a quizzing club. Quietly engaged in our deliberations, we were suddenly disturbed by a startling rap at the door. In a moment a young man, breathless and excited, bounded into our midst. He was a stranger to us, but our preceptor, soon entering, recognized him as a classmate and introduced us severally by name. His features were strongly marked, his gray, penetrating eyes deeply set, and his tongue and body were in constant motion. He seemed to be the embodiment of strong will, indomitable energy and determination, and every action of his small, wiry frame bore the impress of a restless and vigorous brain. At the door stood a sulky, with a sweating, panting horse, which he had driven without mercy over sixty miles that very day, having left Philadelphia the same morning. He *must* be in Harrisburg, thirty-six miles beyond, that night. His horse could go no further. He *must* have another. . . . My preceptor's horse and sulky were soon at the door and at his service. Hector, a noble animal, did his work well that momentous night, and before twenty-four hours had elapsed after he had left Philadelphia, this young M.D. was hammering at the door of our legislature! His mission in Harrisburg was soon accomplished, and,

> as before, he arrived at Lancaster that night. It was very dark, yet, in spite of all remonstrances, he ordered out his horse and off he flew for Philadelphia. He had driven but a few miles, when, while dashing along, he upset in the highway. Here was a predicament from which he could not extricate himself without assistance. It was night and the honest country people were in bed. After repeated halloos a farmer made his appearance with a lantern, which threw some light on the dismal scene. Quite naturally, the farmer began to inquire into all the particulars of the accident instead of at once attempting to right the difficulties. "Come, come, good friend, that won't do. Let us put our shoulder to the wheel and leave explanations until another time." Things were soon put in driving order, and the next day the charter of the Medical Department of Jefferson College was in the city of Philadelphia. . . . Need I say that this genius was young McClellan?"[2]

The bill was approved by Governor J. Andrew Shultze, becoming law on April 7, 1826. Just one week later, on April 14, the first Jefferson Medical College Commencement, which had been under postponement, was held.

The Act of April 7, 1826, was the first state legislative recognition and approval of the existence of Jefferson Medical College. It ratified all previous actions by the parent College at Canonsburg, gave permanence to all that had thus far been accomplished by the Faculty of its Medical Department, legalized the granting of the M.D. degree, and provided for the election of ten Additional Trustees at Philadelphia. It was a stunning victory for the new school.

James Fyfe Gayley (1818–1894), a graduate of the University of Pennsylvania Medical School in 1848, vindicated the existence of a second rival school in his *History of the Jefferson Medical College of Philadelphia* as follows: "The College deserves her full share of the honour of preserving to Philadelphia the proud position of being still (1858) the Mecca of the medical profession on the Western continent. This prosperity has not been at the expense of any other institution."[3] The occasional reference to Jefferson as the "Mecca" that persists among alumni to this day may be traced to Gayley's use of the expression.

References

1. Full text in *The National Gazette and Literary Register*, Philadelphia, Tuesday, February 7, 1826; also Bauer, E.L.: *Doctors Made in America*. Philadelphia: Lippincott, 1973, pp. 344–349.
2. Atlee, Washington L., *Reminiscences of the Earliest Days of Jefferson Medical College*. Philadelphia: P. Madeira, 1873, pp. 3–4.
3. Gayley, J.F., *History of the Jefferson Medical College of Philadelphia, with Biographical Sketches of the Early Professors*. Philadelphia: Joseph M. Wilson, 1858, p. 22.

The First Class (1825–1826): Enrollment of More than 100

Although the Medical Department of Jefferson College at Canonsburg was founded by Articles of Union in October, 1824, it must be realized that the lectures in McClellan's private school were not interrupted by the proceedings for the new school. On the contrary, McClellan continued to enlarge his classes and add lectures by the men who were forming his faculty while, indeed, the Tivoli Theater was being remodeled and opened on March 8, 1825. In reality that period constituted an unofficial first session for which students could receive a year's credit toward the three years of medical study required for the M.D. degree.

What is officially designated as the first session took place in the rented and renovated Medical Hall (Tivoli Theater) in the winter of 1825–1826. It was a lecture course of four months from the last Thursday in October until the end of February, by the six professors of the first faculty, and with clinical supervision in the Infirmary. As the time for the opening of the session drew near, much effort was made to attract the attention of new students arriving in the city to the merits and advantages of the rival school. McClellan, Eberle, or Rhees lectured every evening except Sunday, without charge or obligation, and undoubtedly made fine impressions. The University of Pennsylvania followed the same practice, thus affording the students a choice between the two schools.

The cost of tuition was calculated by the amount paid to each professor for a ticket to his lectures. In those times it was not necessary to have an M.D. degree to practice medicine, so some students merely took courses to certify that they had attended certain lectures at Jefferson. That was enough to qualify for a practice in many localities. Because the school was proprietary, the fees were paid directly to the professors. Popular teachers who could attract a larger following naturally did better financially.

The cost of tickets was as follows:

Anatomy	$14
Surgery	14
Materia Medica and Institutes	14
Chemistry	14
Theory and Practice of Medicine	12
Midwifery and Diseases of Women and Children	10

In June, 1826, the Board at Canonsburg separated Institutes from Materia Medica with appointment of Dr. William P.C. Barton to the latter Chair. Institutes and Medical Jurisprudence was continued by Dr. Rhees at $12 per ticket. Thus, whereas the tuition for the first session had been $78, the cost thereafter was $90.

It was stipulated in the Canonsburg agreement that each year ten free scholarships would be provided for indigent men of talent with satisfactory testimonials. Applicants for admission received a letter from the dean inquiring about financial ability and, if hardship could be established, the facts were to be submitted in writing. Students with "free tickets" would be unknown to their classmates and to the professors from whom the tickets were issued. Recipients, however, were required to pay $20 toward upkeep of the building. When the Ely Building (New Medical Hall) was opened in 1828, these letters were addressed to the Rose Chamber.[1] This was a room in the basement used by the dean and faculty for meetings and examination of candidates. It was called the Green Room or Rose Chamber because the walls were green and a rose was painted upon the center of the ceiling. The hypothesis held by Gould[2] and Bauer[3] that the Rose Room was so called because the awards were "sub rosa" should be discredited. When Jefferson became entirely independent of its parent institution in 1838, these scholarships were gradually discontinued.

At this time admission requirements were very lax, and it was necessary only to supply sufficient evidence of preliminary education that would enable one to comprehend the lecture material. Emphasis instead was placed upon the requirements for obtaining the M.D. degree. These were as follows:

1. The candidate must be 21 years of age.
2. The candidate must have attended at least two full courses of lectures, one of which must have been in the Jefferson Medical College.
3. The candidate must have studied three years (including the two full courses of lectures) under the direction of a respectable practitioner of medicine.
4. The candidate must write a thesis either in Latin, French, or English on some medical subject, selected by himself, and sent to the dean of the medical faculty before the final examination.
5. At an examination by the entire faculty as a group, the candidate must furnish satisfactory evidence of his medical knowledge and of his being qualified for the practice of his profession.

The matriculates of this pioneer class numbered 109. Fourteen states were represented as follows: Pennsylvania (63); New Jersey (10); New York (6); Delaware and Virginia (each 4); Maryland (3); Vermont, Massachusetts, Connecticut, South Carolina and Mississippi (each 2); Ohio, Tennessee, and Kentucky (each 1). There was 1 from the District of Columbia and 1 from Germany, and 4 were from Ireland. The first matriculate, Henry D. Smith of Pennsylvania, a cousin and pupil of Dr. Rhees, did not graduate. He is remembered for having cultivated a garden of rare medicinal plants.

Notice of exercises for the first commencement on April 14, 1826, at Medical Hall on Prune Street, was made public, and private invitations were sent to the clergy. The Rev. Dr. Ashbel Green opened the event with prayer, and Professor Smith gave the graduation address. Twenty of the matriculates received the M.D. degree. Their names, native areas, and theses are worth noting.

George Baldwin, Pennsylvania, "Cholera Infantum"

Peter Q. Beckman, New Jersey, "Syphilis"

John Bowen Brinton, Pennsylvania, "Cholera"

George Carll, Pennsylvania, "Anthrax"

Benjamin B. Coit, Connecticut, "Tetanus"

Thomas M. Dick, South Carolina, "Epidemics"

Joel Foster, Vermont, "Neuroses"

Ralph Glover, New Jersey, "Hernia"

Charles Graff, Pennsylvania, "Rheumatism"

John Graham, Ireland, "Epilepsy"

Charles M. Griffiths, Pennsylvania, "Cholera Infantum"

Jesse W. Griffiths, Pennsylvania, "Dysentery"

Nathan L. Hatfield, Pennsylvania, "Dysentery"

William Johnson, Pennsylvania, "Extra-Uterine Pregnancy"

M. L. Knapp, New York, "Apocynum Cannabinum"

Thomas B. Maxwell, Pennsylvania, "Lobelia Inflata"

Atkinson Pelham, Kentucky, "Mania a Potu"

Benjamin Shaw, Pennsylvania, "Medical Practice"

J. Frederick Stadiger, Pennsylvania, "Epilepsy"

James Swan, Massachusetts, "Scrofula"

There is no difficulty in explaining why only 20 graduated in the first class. These men should have been at least 21 years of age and should have had two previous years of study with a preceptor and one previous course of lectures. Thus most of the matriculates needed one or two more years of qualifications. Others might well have matriculated without intention of obtaining the M.D. degree, and still others might have failed or dropped out.

Because there were no state boards of licensure it was possible to practice as a "doctor" without the M.D. degree, merely with a certificate from a preceptor, or by showing evidence of having attended some lectures, or as an "eclectic," or, as was common, as a "quack." The truly elite of the medical profession had a preliminary college degree, the M.D. degree, took postgraduate work for a year in one or more of the famous clinics of Europe, wrote a textbook at an early age, and became a professor in a medical school. Many of Jefferson's future chairmen did this very thing.

References

1. Atlee, W.L., *Reminiscences of the Earliest Days of Jefferson Medical College*. Philadelphia: P. Madeira, 1873, pp. 10–11.
2. Gould, G.M., *History of the Jefferson Medical College of Philadelphia*. New York: Lewis, 1904, p. 75.
3. Bauer, E.L., *Doctors Made in America*. Philadelphia: Lippincott Co., 1963, pp. 16–17.

Additional Trustees: Changes and Dissensions (1826–1828)

The Act of April 7, 1826, gave the Trustees at Canonsburg the authority to elect ten "Additional Trustees, who may be residents of the city or county of Philadelphia." Any six of them could constitute a committee to superintend Jefferson Medical College, with the power to appoint and remove their fellow trustees, to hold public commencements, and to confer the M.D. degree as the General Board at Canonsburg might direct. The powers and proceedings of the "Additional Trustees" were thus subject to the censorship and approval of the parent Board, and they would have no voice in the councils of the Board at Canonsburg. The first ten chosen were a notable body from outstanding members of the religious, legal, military, and business community of Philadelphia. William Tilghman, Chief Justice of the Supreme Court of Pennsylvania, who had led the opposition in the senate on behalf of the University of Pennsylvania, had what must have been the embarrassing duty to administer the oath of office of Trustee to Edward King, LL.D., President Judge of First District Court of Common Pleas of Philadelphia. This empowered the latter to give the oath of office to Samuel Badger, James M. Broom, Joel B. Sutherland, Samuel Humphreys, Edward Ingersoll, Charles S. Cox, General William Duncan, the Rev. Dr. Ashbel Green, D.D., LL.D., and Reverend Ezra Stiles Ely, D.D. All were of the highest personal integrity with full cognizance of their responsibilities. They established the tradition of strength, sacrifice, and wisdom without which the College could not have survived and that led to its ever-increasing stature.

The Rev. Dr. Ashbel Green had already been serving on the Board at Canonsburg, had witnessed the founding of its Medical Department, and had offered prayer at the opening of the Prune Street Medical Hall in 1825.[1] His election as an "Additional Trustee" in Philadelphia made him liaison as well as the member called upon to preside over the deliberations of the newly established body. His service as President ultimately covered a period of 23 years.

Born in New Jersey in 1762, Dr. Green graduated from Princeton in 1783, entered the ministry, and served as Professor of Mathematics and Natural Philosophy at Princeton from 1785 to 1787. From 1792 to 1800 he was Chaplain to Congress in Philadelphia, which brought him into relationship with George Washington. In 1812, he was elected to the presidency of Princeton, which position he held for ten years until taking retirement at age 60. He then conducted a Presbyterian religious journal, *The Christian Advocate,* for 12 years. Green's other writings consisted of discourses, a history of Princeton College with tributes to its presidents, and a posthumously published autobiography. At death in 1848, age eighty-six, he had outlived his professional son at Jefferson, "Old Jaky," by seven years.

On August 9, 1826, the Additional Trustees convened in the College "to inquire into and report whether any changes in the then existing Professorships were necessary or expedient." At the meeting of September 28 it was recommended that the Chair of Midwifery held by Dr. Francis S. Beattie be vacated, and that Dr. John Barnes (Figure 1-11) be appointed to fill it temporarily during the ensuing session. Dr. Beattie was notified of his dismissal by the President of the Board at Canonsburg October 28 and on November 10 he published his strong objection in the pamphlet referred to earlier in this chapter. Dr. Barnes fared no better. According to Dr. Samuel D. Gross, who attended Barnes' lectures as a student in the session of 1826–1827, "he was the dullest lecturer that it was my lot ever to hear, destitute of all the attributes of a successful teacher."[2] Barnes was not reappointed the following year, and he likewise published a pamphlet of 39 pages in objection to the action of the Trustees and members of the faculty.[3] In 1826 Dr. William Paul Crillon Barton (Figure 1-12) was appointed to the Chair of Materia Medica, thus relieving Dr. Rhees of this subject and free to continue in Institutes and Medical Jurisprudence.

The appointment of Dr. William P.C. Barton strengthened the school at this crucial point in its survival.[4] He came from a distinguished family—his uncle, Benjamin Smith Barton, had been a Professor of Materia Medica at the University of Pennsylvania; his brother was John Rhea Barton, an esteemed surgeon of the Pennsylvania Hospital, in whose honor an endowed Chair of Surgery was established in 1876 at the University of Pennsylvania as its first endowed medical

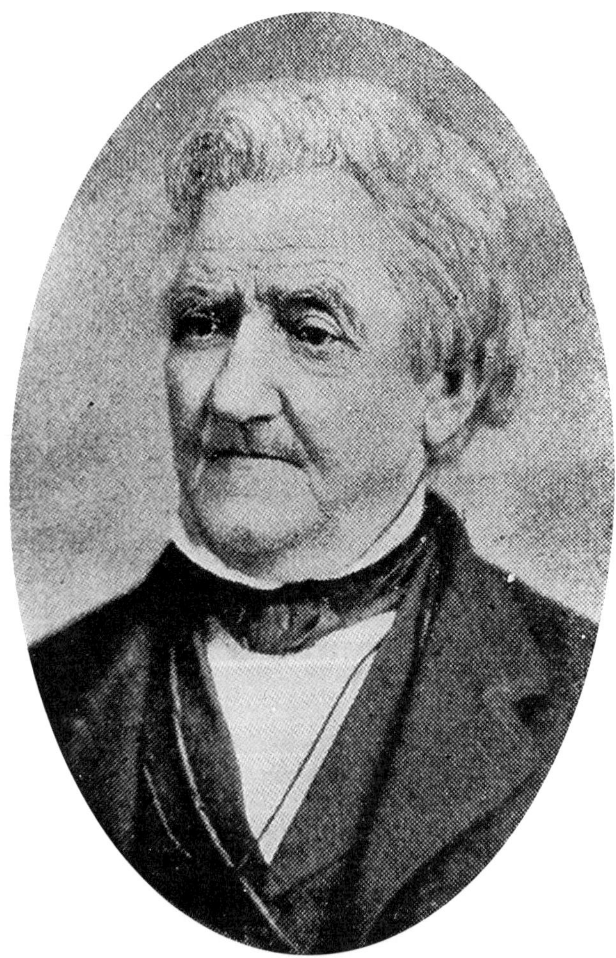

Fig. 1-11. John Barnes, M.D. (1891–?); Professor of Midwifery (1826–1827).

professorship;[5] his father who had designed the United States Seal, was a member of the bar; and his grandfather was an Episcopal clergyman. Barton graduated with distinction from Princeton in 1805 and received his M.D. degree from the University of Pennsylvania in 1808. After practice in Philadelphia for a year as one of the surgeons to the Pennsylvania Hospital, he received an appointment as Surgeon in the Navy on the recommendation of Drs. Benjamin Rush and Philip Syng Physick. He maintained a career in the Navy for the rest of his life, but had so many periods of shore duty that he was able to secure long periods of leave for academic activities. In 1815 he was chosen Professor of Botany at the University of Pennsylvania, but in a new "Faculty of Natural Sciences" rather than the Medical School. In 1818 he tried to get a charter from the State Legislature for a second Medical School but failed because of opposition from the University of Pennsylvania. In 1826 Barton was sharply rebuffed by the University Trustees when he petitioned them to reunite his College Chair of Botany with the Medical Department. At this point McClellan offered him the Chair of Materia Medica at Jefferson.

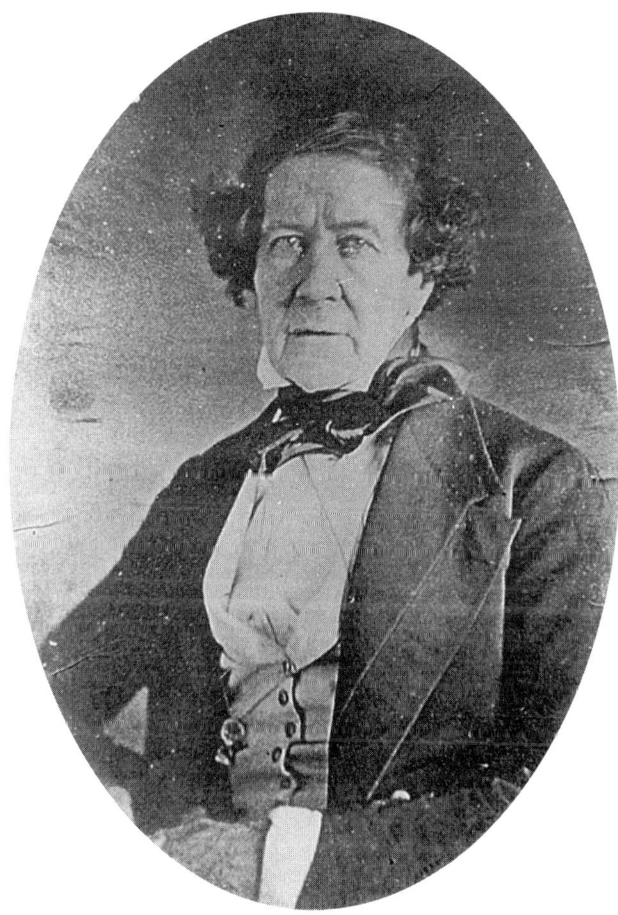

FIG. 1-12. William P.C. Barton, M.D. (1786–1856); Professor of Materia Medica (1826–1829) and Dean (1828–1829).

Dr. Barton was one of the best botanists of his time, distinguished in early life by a two-volume *Flora of North America* (1821). His lectures were interesting, authoritative, and delivered without notes. The students regarded him with awe. His style of dress was flamboyant in spite of his limited finances. He usually appeared in class wearing two vests of different colors at the same time and seldom wore the same ones on successive days. A contemptuous smile or a curl of the upper lip frequently accompanied his criticism of students or colleagues. In 1830 after having served for three years he was ordered to sea duty by the Navy. This terminated his connections with Jefferson.

Barton continued his brilliant career in the Navy. In 1842 he was appointed Chief of Medicine and Surgery of the Navy. He wrote a valuable treatise for organization and government of Marine Hospitals. In 1852 he was made President of the Board of Examiners for the Navy in Philadelphia where he remained until his death in 1856. A detachment of marines was detailed to fire over his grave in East Laurel Hill Cemetery—a simple weather-worn headstone marks the site, overlooking the Schuylkill River, not far from the more imposing stones for George McClellan and Robley Dunglison. The Barton family continued in importance to Jefferson; its bequests aided the purchase of the old Broad Street Hospital (Barton Memorial) for diseases of the chest and funded research in cancer, and the Barton Committee of the Women's Board bears its name. (Dr. James M. Barton, depicted on Eakins' *Gross Clinic,* is from a different family.)

An unfortunate phase in the history of the College had a disastrous effect on the class of 1826–1827. Numbers diminished considerably even though the graduates numbered 34, an increase of 14 over the previous year due to a carryover of students who now could satisfy the requirement of two years of lectures necessary for the M.D. degree. The decreased student enrollment can be ascribed to institutional financial problems, harassment from the University of Pennsylvania, and infighting among the faculty. The troubled feelings of the faculty have been attributed to jealousies arising from the fee system of charges for the lectures. According to the pamphlet of the disgruntled Dr. Barnes: "Language can scarcely convey an adequate idea of the appearance of the faculty meetings at this time; each meeting rather resembled a kennel of strange dogs let loose upon each other than an assemblage of professional gentlemen. Tantalizing remarks, insulting observations, and school-boy challenges constituted the prominent features."

A meeting of the Board of Trustees was held on March 22, 1827, at which time the cost of tickets for the lectures was set as follows: Anatomy, Surgery, Materia Medica, and Chemistry, each $14; Theory and Practice, Institutes, and Medical Jurisprudence, each $12; and Midwifery, $10, "so that the whole paid by each student to the seven Professors shall not exceed annually 90 dollars."

In June a code was adopted as "Rules of Government." On August 6, Professor Green was elected Chairman and Treasurer of the Faculty. The deanship held by Dr. Rhees was taken by Dr. Eberle under a former rule that this position could not be held by the same incumbent for two successive years.

Two other problems that retarded the progress of the College were its undesirable location across from the Walnut Street prison and insufficient space for the students. The first official mention of the need for a new medical hall was in February, 1827, just before the close of the second session. It was proposed that the cost should not exceed $20,000 and that funds could be "procured by subscription of joint stock." The faculty delegated Dr. McClellan and Professor Green to confer with the Trustees on this matter. Agreement was unanimous with all parties, but the funds were lacking. There was no one of wealth on the faculty. There was no endowment, and the original stipulation with the Trustees at Canonsburg expressed that there should be no claims on funds of the parent institution. The second academic session was discouraging in that attendance had decreased with associated loss of student tuition. One member of the Board of Additional Trustees of the College had the benevolence and faith to cast aside calculations of poor financial risk and assume responsibility for erecting a new building. That man was the Rev. Dr. Ezra Stiles Ely, D.D., Jefferson's first major benefactor.

References

1. Simpson, H., *The Lives of Eminent Philadelphians.* Philadelphia: Wm. Brotherhead, 1859, pp. 451–452.
2. Gross, S.D., *Autobiography.* Philadelphia: Barrie, 1887, p. 36.
3. Barnes, J., *Jefferson Medical College: A Representation of the Conduct of the Trustees and Faculty and Circumstances Connected Therewith.* Philadelphia: 1828.
4. Pleadwell, F.L., "William Paul Crillon Barton (1786–1856), Surgeon, United States Navy—A Pioneer in American Naval Medicine," *The Military Surgeon.* 46: 241–281, 1920.
5. Corner, G.W., *Two Centuries of Medicine.* Philadelphia: Lippincott Co., 1965, p. 147.

New Medical Hall (1828): The Reverend Ely's Benefaction

Ezra Stiles Ely (Figure 1-13) was born in Connecticut in 1786, the son of a Presbyterian minister. His father named him after his greatly admired preceptor, Ezra Stiles, a famous President of Yale University. This young man represented the third generation of the family to be graduated from that institution and the seventeenth member to be educated there. Ezra followed in his father's footsteps and became an ordained Presbyterian minister. After two years of service in a local church he moved to New York City as Chaplain of the New York City Hospital and Almshouse. His experience in this ministry provided material for a two-volume book entitled *Visits of Mercy,* which went through six editions until 1829 and sold thousands of copies. The volumes were compilations of case histories of beggars, thieves, prostitutes, and alcoholics and dealt with their spiritual rather than physical ills. He edited a religious paper called *The Philadelphian* and wrote a *Memoir of the Rev. Zebulon Ely,* his father. His writings on polemic theology were important in their day and included *The Contrast, Ely's Journal, Sermons on Faith, The Science of the Human Mind, Contrast Between Calvinism and Hopkinsonianism,* and *Endless Punishment*. He was coeditor of a *Collateral Bible or Key to the Holy Scriptures* (three volumes), and left in manuscript a *History of the Churches of Philadelphia*. It is speculated that these literary labors provided some of the funds for the Rev. Dr. Ely's tireless activity in the multitude of his good causes. Later events revealed that he was an obsessive entrepreneur whose extensive business empire finally collapsed and almost sent him to prison. He recorded that fascinating account in his memoirs.[1]

The Rev. Dr. Ely became pastor in 1814 of Old Pine Street Presbyterian Church, located between Fourth and Fifth Streets, only two blocks away from Jefferson's first College building, the Prune Street Medical Hall. Thus in 1826, when he became one of the "Additional Trustees," Ely came face to face with the physical problems of the school as well as its academic ones. It was he who listened with a sympathetic ear and felt the call to aid the school during its struggle for survival.

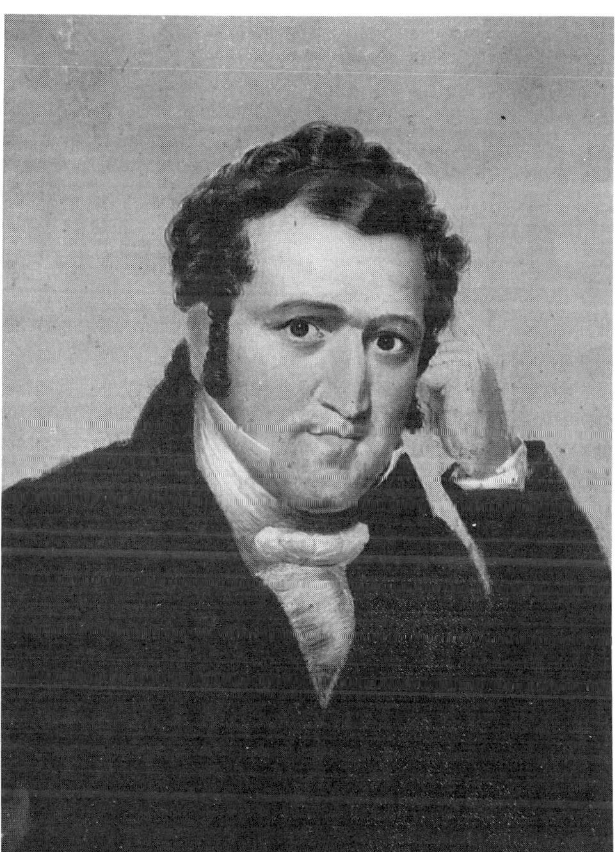

FIG. 1-13. The Reverend Ezra Stiles Ely, D.D. (1786–1861) provided the new Medical Hall (Ely Building) on Tenth Street (1828).

On March 27, 1827, Dr. Ely expressed his willingness to erect a suitable building, and one month later the Board resolved

> ". . . that the Additional Trustees of Jefferson College, in their capacity as Trustees, and not otherwise, do hereby agree with the Rev. Dr. Ely, that if he will cause to be erected a Medical Hall for the use of the Medical School, on such plan as shall be approved by this Board, the Additional Trustees will rent the same of him and such persons, if any, as he may associate with him as proprietors of said hall, for a term of time not less than five years, at a rent of one thousand dollars a year, to be paid in the month of November in each of the said five years—after said building shall be fitted for use."

On May 12, 1827, Dr. Ely reported that he had purchased a lot on Tenth Street between Juniper Alley (later Moravian) and George Street (later Sansom) at the cost of $6,500 (Figure 1-14). The dimensions were approved as well as his exhibit of plans for the building. As further endorsement, the trustees, in their capacity as a body and not as individuals, agreed to add another $200 a year rent to the $1,000 previously promised. Beyond rent, there would be expenses for the janitor's salary, heat, light, and incidentals. Because the school was proprietary, the financial responsibility rested upon the faculty. Accordingly, the professors were assessed the following sums to be paid each November: Anatomy, Surgery, Materia Medica, and Chemistry, each $250 (covering the faculty rent of $1,000); Theory and Practice, $137.50; and Midwifery, $125 (the $262.50 for expenses beyond rent). Any professor failing to pay his share would automatically be considered to have vacated his chair and be replaced. Each faculty member signed a statement binding himself to the regulations of the Board.

By August, 1828, the cornerstone had been laid by Board President the Rev. Dr. Ashbel Green; a dedication address had been delivered by Jacob Green (now M.D.), Professor of Chemistry; and the building was ready for occupancy. With periodic renovations and modifications it remained for 70 years in active use, until 1898. This site is still occupied by the old 1907 Jefferson Hospital.

There is no photograph of New Medical Hall as it appeared originally or during the 1830s, because the daguerreotype process was not announced until 1839. Fortunately, however, an architectural depiction of the exterior exists (Figure 1-15).

The building was 51 feet wide, 57 feet deep, and with a five-foot alley on the north. It was well proportioned, two and one-half floors high, with the basement rising seven feet above ground level. The first-floor facade had an arched window panel opening over the two windows and central door. The central second-floor window extended through the floor above to a niche for a statue that formed the focal point of the front. It is not known whether the statue was ever placed. There is no record of the original architect.[2] Cost of the building itself was $10,500. Yearly rent was set at $1,200. The upper lecture hall, or "pit," is depicted in Eakins' *Gross Clinic* (1875). The lower lecture hall with the *Gross Clinic* hanging on the south wall is seen in Figure 1-16.

Dr. Ely's benefaction was a provision rather than a gift, and not financed principally by his own funds. He created shares of Jefferson Medical College stock for which he was the trustee. On March 27, 1827, it was "resolved that any surplus funds which may remain in the hands of the additional trustees after discharging the rent of the Hall and other occupancy expenses, shall by the same trustees be invested in said Medical Hall as often as they deem it expedient, with the intent that they may ultimately become proprietors of the building and hold it in trust for the promotion of the objects and interests of the said school." With subsequent renovations and enlargements it was not until 1870 that the cost was repaid.

The beginning of Dr. Ely's ruinous financial entanglements may be traced to his first marriage to Mary Ann Carswell, the daughter of one of his prominent Old Pine Street Church members. Samuel Carswell, the father-in-law, was a merchant of wealth who in later life became involved in fiscal difficulties. At his death in 1822, Dr. Ely

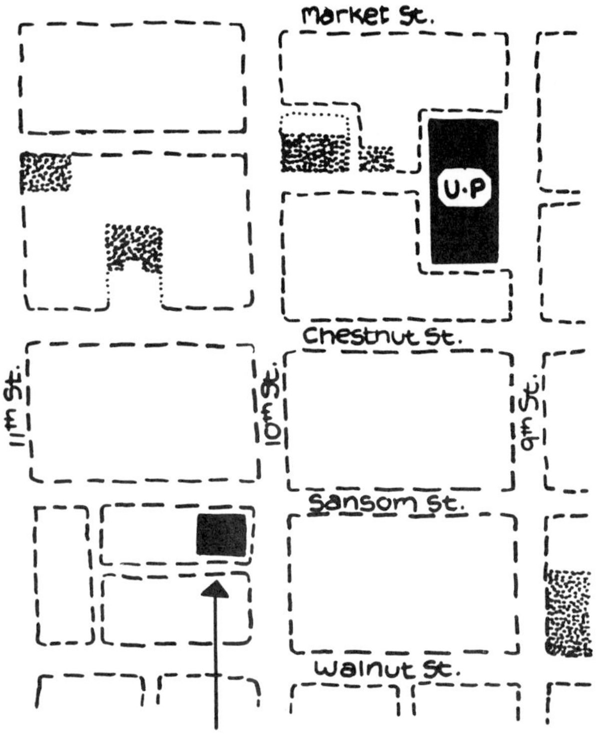

Market St.
U.P
Chestnut St.
11th St.
10th St.
9th St.
Sansom St.
Walnut St.

Fig. 1-14. Sectional map showing proximity of Jefferson Medical College (on Tenth near Sansom) to the School of Medicine of the University of Pennsylvania (on Ninth between Market and Chestnut) from 1828 to 1874.

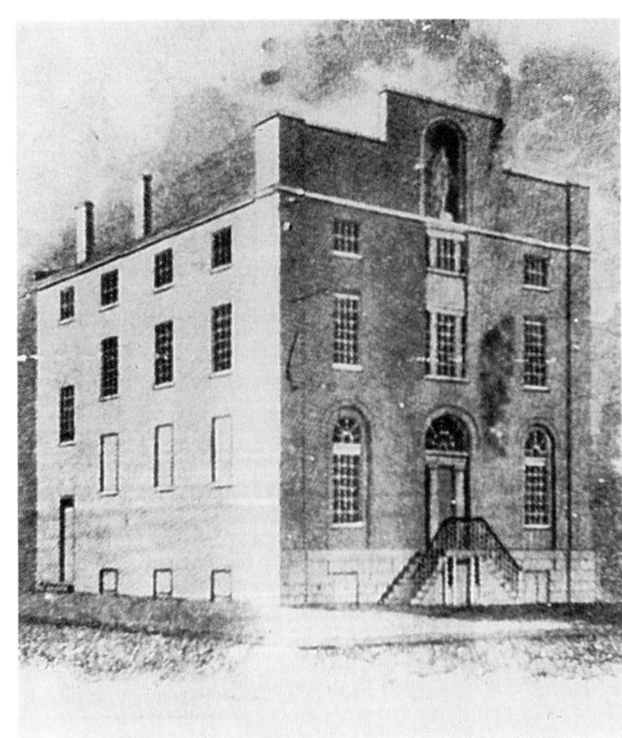

Fig. 1-15. New Medical Hall (Ely Building, 1828), located at Tenth and Moravian Streets. With enlargements and renovations it served until 1898, when replaced by the present Old Main Hospital of 1907.

became executor of the estate as well as trustee for Carswell's son who also had financial trouble and fled to the West Indies to escape his creditors. Dr. Ely also became the trustee for Mary Ann Ely Carswell, the son's daughter and his own niece through marriage. The mother-in-law, the niece, and Dr. Samuel McClellan (related to the Elys and brother of Jefferson's founder) all resided in the Ely parsonage. Matters went smoothly enough until 1835 during which he improved the Old Pine Street Church both in congregation size and physical aspects.

At this time he felt the call of a great opportunity to establish a Presbyterian college and theological seminary in Marion County, Missouri, along with two other Presbyterian ministers. Land was selling at $9 an acre and was predicted to double in value quickly. In 1836 he moved to Missouri with his wife, his mother-in-law, and his ward, Mary Ann Ely Carswell. There he plunged into what he conceived to be the most important work of his life. He became Professor of Polemic Theology, Biblical Literature, and Sacred Criticism in the Theological Department of Marion College.

Dr. Ely built a large land empire, buying thousands of acres in the Marion area with funds from his presbyters, trustee accounts, notes, mortgages, and bonds. His dreams of vast profits for benefit of his religious enterprises were shattered by Andrew Jackson's attack on the Bank of the United States, the flooding of the Mississippi River, and malaria. Land value depreciated to $6 an acre. There was a financial panic in 1837, with failures of banks and many of the richest merchants. This continued through President Van Buren's administration (1837–1841). Dr. Ely had endorsed a note of $50,000 on behalf of Marion College. A judgment bond of $100,000 was called with a lien on all his real estate. His creditors accused him of dishonesty and fraud in transferring property to family ownership. By an unforeseen change of times, those he had tried to help were clamoring for money and blaming everything on him.

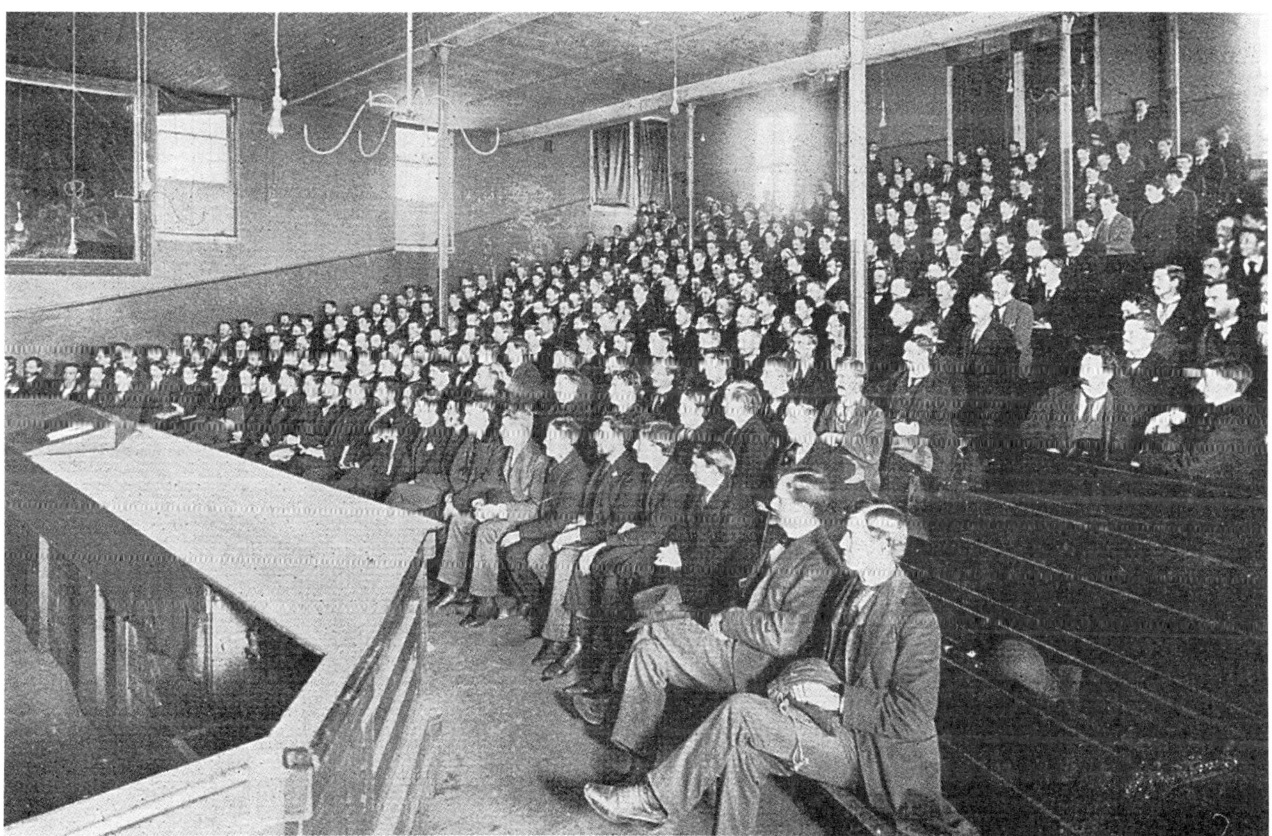

Fig. 1-16. Lower lecture hall of Ely Building (ca. 1880s) showing large class and *Gross Clinic* on south wall.

In 1843 Dr. Ely entered into a second marriage with Caroline Thompson Holmes, whose father was Dr. Thompson Holmes of Abington, Pennsylvania. In 1845, after much difficulty with creditors, Dr. Ely was cleared of dishonesty in his financial transactions by the Presbytery of Northern Missouri and returned permanently to Philadelphia for another beginning in the Presbyterian Church of the Northern Liberties (a district along the Delaware, north of Vine Street). Mr. Thomas J. Miles, who had married Dr. Ely's ward, Mary Ann Ely Carswell, now relentlessly pursued Dr. Ely into court. In her estate were listed 44 shares of Jefferson Medical College stock at $500 each, for a total $22,000. On November 1, 1846, the auditors found Dr. Ely indebted to his late ward, Mary Ann Ely Miles, to the sum of $57,409.55, for which a judgment of $49,861.51 was made against him.

The next effort of Mr. Miles was to remove Dr. Ely from the Trusteeship of the Jefferson Medical College stock, which Ely had created by the purchase of the lot and erection of the College edifice. On November 9, 1846, Judge A.V. Parsons ordered and directed "that money due this month from the Board of Trustees of Jefferson College be paid by their treasurer into court for distribution: and that the holders of the stock be permitted to take out of court their respective proportions when proper applications are made." This created needless delay and expense for the stockholders.

The copy of a protest to the Court of Common Pleas for the City and County of Philadelphia on November 16, 1846, was as follows: "The subscribers respectfully present, that they are stockholders in the stock of the Jefferson Medical College Edifice, on South Tenth Street, Philadelphia; that the Rev. Ezra Stiles Ely, D.D., Trustee of said stock has ever paid us punctually our interest on the same; and that we protest against his removal from said Trusteeship, and another in his place." In spite of other written stockholder support as well as protest from Dr. Ely's legal counsel, the judge on the bench was unyielding. He delivered a lecture complimenting Dr. Ely for his skill in theology but deplored his lack of legal knowledge in the management of money. The firm of Raybold and Sharswood was appointed to the office created and formerly held by him. The firm requested and received from Dr. Ely "all the books, papers, documents, certificates, moneys, and property remaining in your hands and under your control, belonging or in any way appertaining to the said Trusteeship."

On Saturday, March 20, 1847, the time of procuring $50,000 bail for financial insolvency expired. On that day Mr. Miles urged the sheriff to seize Dr. Ely. Dr. Ely, to comply, met Mr. Hancock, the sheriff, in the street and took him to the parsonage. There he read the warrant of arrest and was released on parole so as to be able to conduct his church services the following day. A member of the congregation who had noticed Dr. Ely with Mr. Hancock jokingly asked if he knew he was walking with the deputy sheriff. Dr. Ely replied that he had the pleasure of an acquaintance with him. The insolvent laws of that time meant going to prison if bond was not given. On Sunday, Dr. Ely, while a prisoner but yet at liberty, preached twice with his usual freedom and composure, while none of the congregation except his wife and father-in-law knew the situation. On Monday, March 22, Dr. Thompson Holmes (his father-in-law), Dr. Samuel McClellan, and a friend, Mr. John C. Farr, united to complete the bond. Dr. Ely was thus free, the sheriff bowed in departure, and Dr. Ely paid a few small necessary fees.

In this month of March 1847, Dr. Ely had 23 claims against him ranging from $60 to $49,861.51, for a total of $119,918.18. In May he agreed to settle with his creditors by turning over all estates, real, personal, and mixed, and all effects of whatever kind and wheresoever situated, especially all houses, lands, claims, and credits in the state of Missouri, and to sell and dispose of the same in any manner that was best and in conformity with law and equity.

In November 1847, Dr. Ely was considerably depressed and had lost 34 pounds as a result of his legal harassments. His memoirs relate: "I rode past the Eastern Penitentiary and reflected on the pain it would give my friends, should I, in the course of a few weeks, be confined there, at hard labour. . . . The worst I had to dread, so far as I know, must be the Eastern Penitentiary for a work-shop, a bed-chamber, a place for prayer, and a house of death." On November 15, 1847, Dr. Ely's case was argued in court before three judges. On November 27 he was discharged from all liability to be imprisoned for past debts, the opinion being unanimous that he had committed no penal offense or suffered any defamation of moral character. Fortunately, his misadventures in business had no ill effect on Jefferson Medical College.

Not long afterward the Trustees of Jefferson Medical College elected Dr. Ely President pro tempore to fill the place of the very aged and venerable Dr. Ashbel Green, who was past the power of attending to his duties and who died the following year. Dr. Ely wrote in his memoirs: "My earnest prayer is, that henceforth I may have little to do with worldly business, and may be more unreservedly devoted to the ministry of reconciliation than in any former part of my life."

A recount of Dr. Ely's colorful career would be incomplete without mention of the famous social and political furor he created in 1829 over Peggy Eaton, the wife of President Andrew Jackson's Secretary of War.[3] On March 18 of that year Dr. Ely wrote Jackson a long accusatory letter in which one of the charges was that Eaton and Peggy before their marriage had registered together as man and wife in a New York boarding house. By early 1830 Dr. Ely had been called to Washington at least three times to substantiate his claims, but in 1831 the matter led to the resignation of Jackson's whole cabinet. Ex-President John Quincy Adams in his memoirs for February 6, 1830, wrote "A busybody Presbyterian clergyman of Philadelphia is the principal mischief-maker in the affair."

Dr. Ely, who held northern antislavery views, became involved in 1831 in a controversy over establishing a school for free negroes in New Haven, Connecticut. He became further involved by his purchase of a slave named Ambrose in order to save Ambrose from being sold into the South away from his home and family. A heated controversy promptly ensued in the northern papers over whether a Presbyterian minister, for whatever reason, could morally be a slaveholder.

The members of Dr. Ely's first family never forgave him for marrying a second time. In the two marriages he had 12 children. Some must have died early, but others were notable: Samuel Carswell Ely, presumably a son, is listed as a graduate of Jefferson Medical College in the class of 1836. The Rev. Dr. Ely's son, Ben Ezra Stiles Ely, went to sea at 18, went to California with the forty-niners, and subsequently became a Presbyterian minister.[4] He wrote a narrative of his whaling voyage, *There She Blows,* edited by Curtis Dahl (Dr. Ely's great-great-grandson).[5] Ben Ezra Stiles Ely had a son, Francis Argyle Ely, M.D., who although not a Jefferson graduate was made an honorary alumnus in 1940.

The "black sheep" among Dr. Ely's children was a daughter of his second marriage, Harriet Elizabeth Ely. At age 16, two years after her father's death, she eloped with a railway clerk named Blackford. Her husband died within a short time, presumably of tuberculosis. Without visible financial support, and possessed of unusual physical beauty and cleverness, she was able to establish a residence off fashionable Rittenhouse Square in Philadelphia. Seeking an even more exciting existence, she transferred to the Boulevard Malesherbes in Paris and became a well-known courtesan to the French court under the assumed name of Madame Fanny Lear. With the fall of Paris in the Franco-Prussian war in 1871 she followed some of her Russian patrons to St. Petersburg. There she became the acknowledged mistress of the Czar's nephew, Grand-Duke Nicholas. As one of the most famous courtesans of all Europe she published her memoirs in 1875 in French. A book, *The Scandalous Mrs. Blackford,* published in 1951, revived the spicy details.

However, Dr. Ely did not live to see his little daughter's teenage elopement. Physically and financially ruined, he preached at the smaller Northern Liberties Church until 1852, when at age 66 he suffered a stroke. Living only on a meager pension and spending the next nine years partially paralyzed, the theologian, author, editor, would-be politician, philanthropist, entrepreneur, and first benefactor of Jefferson Medical College died on June 18, 1861.[8] The survival of Jefferson past its darkest hours may well have been due to the largesse of Dr. Ezra Stiles Ely. As Secretary of the Board of Trustees for many years, he recorded the minutes in a beautiful script that combined beauty with clarity.

References

1. Ely, E.S., *Memoirs of His Own Life and Times.* Manuscript and typescript in Presbyterian Historical Society.

2. Teitelman, E., "Jefferson's Architecture: Past, Present and Future," *Jeff. Al. Bull.,* Fall 1965, pp. 12–18.
3. Dahl, C., "The Clergyman, the Hussy, and Old Hickory: Ezra Stiles Ely and the Peggy Eaton Affair," *Jour. of Presbyterian Hist.* 52: 137–155, 1974.
4. Ely, B.E.S., *Autobiography:* In manuscript, Presbyterian Historical Society.
5. Ely, B.E.S., *There She Blows: A Narrative of a Whaling Voyage.* Curtis Dahl, ed., Middletown, Conn.: Wesleyan Univ. Press, 1971.
6. Blackford, H.E., *Le Roman d'une Americaine en Russie, accompagne de lettres originales.* Bruxelles, 1875.
7. Kane, H.T., and Leclerc, V., *The Scandalous Mrs. Blackford.* New York: J. Messner, Inc., 1951.
8. Throckmorton, T.B., "Ezra Stiles Ely: Benefactor of Jefferson Medical College." *Jour. Iowa State Med. Soc.* 29: 135–140, 1939.

Faculty Reconstruction (1828–1832): Struggle for Survival

Among the 27 graduates in the third class of 1828 was Samuel D. Gross, destined to become one of the most outstanding alumni in Jefferson's history. The ceremony was held on March 18 in the Prune Street Building because construction of the new Medical Hall would not be completed until the fall session. The Rev. Dr. Ashbel Green conferred the degrees, and Thomas J. O'Flaherty read in Latin his thesis entitled "De Ebrietas" (drunkenness). The main address was delivered by Dr. George McClellan. Gross related: "McClellan on this as on many other occasions was not on time. He kept the audience waiting for at least ten minutes, much to the annoyance of President Green, an old man; and when, at length, he made his appearance, he could hardly read the manuscript, so badly was it written. In fact, as I afterward learned, he had been engaged upon the composition of his address up to the very moment of leaving his house for the college."[1]

In June, 1828, all the Chairs were declared vacant and it was "resolved that all elections of persons to be professors in this institution shall be made by ballot in the Board of Additional Trustees." Secretary Ely was "to inform those gentlemen who were lately Professors and wish to be candidates [that they] must make application or [they] will not be considered as candidates." It was the apparent intent of the board to update the faculty to coincide with opening of the new Medical Hall.

At this time many predictions were afloat that the existence of Jefferson Medical College would be of short duration. An editorial comment in the *American Medical Recorder* on June 19, 1828, declared: "We are informed that the whole of the Medical Professors in Jefferson College have been *removed:* the cause of these proceedings we do not know, but if we were to give an opinion, we should say that a *few* of the *old* Professors, who no doubt understand they are to be re-elected, have been at their *old tricks*. We shall notice the proceedings in a future number, and shall conclude for the present by remarking, that we cannot conceive it possible men of *standing* if elected (pro tem it can only be) will serve in an institution where confusion, irregularity, and discord have prevailed from the moment of its birth."[2]

There were so many changes in the faculty during the critical period of 1828 to 1832 that Bauer refers to "the game of musical chairs."[3] It was a period of instability that threatened the survival of the College. Nathan R. Smith had resigned the Chair of Anatomy at the beginning of the 1827–1828 session. An attempt to secure Dr. Robert M. Patterson for the Chair was unsuccessful in consequence of his accepting a more advantageous offer from the University of Virginia. George McClellan as Professor of Surgery was then called upon to double for the vacant Chair of Anatomy. At this juncture he resourcefully solicited the aid of his brother Samuel who was appointed an Assistant Demonstrator of Anatomy.

Samuel McClellan (Figure 1-17) possessed the same intellectual capacities as his more famous brother, but his personality was entirely different. Four years younger, he was a lamb rather than a lion, shrinking from applause, avoiding political intrigue, and unassuming in character. His educational background was excellent in that he had studied anatomy in 1819 with a respectable physician from his native Woodstock, Connecticut. In 1820 he entered the office of his brother George in Philadelphia while he pursued two years of clinical lectures and practice in the Almshouse and Pennsylvania Hospital, as well as lectures at the University of Pennsylvania. He obtained his medical degree from Yale in 1823. After spending the next three years traveling through Mexico in the company of an English naturalist, he became interested in diseases of the eye. He returned to Pennsylvania and was practicing successfully in nearby Bristol when called upon by his brother. Samuel McClellan was promoted to Adjunct Professor of Anatomy in 1829 and to the Chair in 1830. In 1831 he gracefully yielded the Chair to the internationally famous anatomist Granville Sharpe Pattison and took the Chair of Institutes, Medical Jurisprudence, and Midwifery. He also served as dean from 1830 to 1834. In the teaching of all his assigned subjects Dr. Samuel McClellan earned the respect and affection of the students, colleagues, and Board of Trustees. He cooperated well in all the stopgap measures that were so important in the survival of the College.

Jefferson lost the McClellan brothers when restless George in 1839 founded another medical school in Philadelphia with the same strategy he had used for Jefferson. That rival school was created as the Medical Department of Pennsylvania College at Gettysburg.

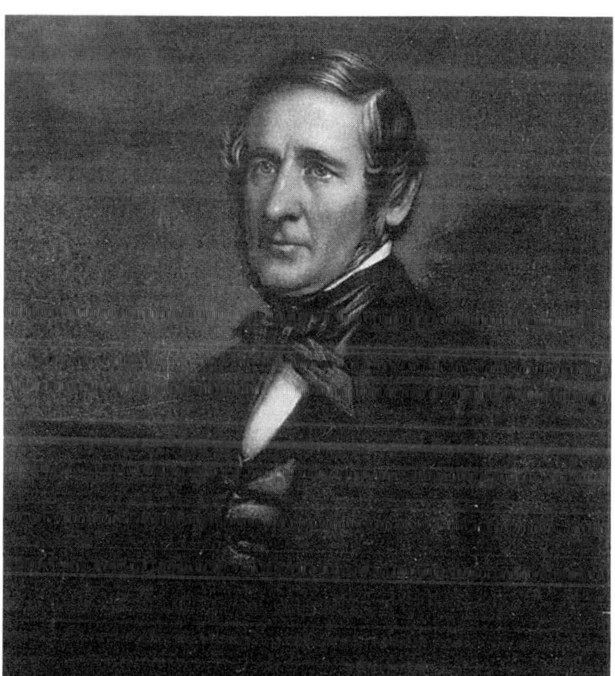

FIG. 1-17. Samuel McClellan, M.D. (1800–1854); Assistant Demonstrator of Anatomy (1828), Adjunct Professor of Anatomy (1829), Professor of Anatomy (1830), Professor of Institutes and Medical Jurisprudence (1831), Professor of Midwifery (1832–1839), and Dean (1830–1834).

The Chair of Midwifery at the occasion of opening New Medical Hall was also in difficulty; Dr. John Barnes had proven unsatisfactory in the 1827–1828 session. Another doubling of Chairs occurred in 1828 when Dr. John Eberle was appointed Professor of Theory and Practice of Physic as well as Professor of Midwifery and Diseases of Women and Children. Green, Rhees, and Barton retained their prior appointments. A squabble in the Board of Trustees on June 26, 1828, over the reelection of Dr. John Eberle versus Dr. James Rush led to the resignation of two members, Judge Coxe and Edward Ingersoll. At this juncture the Rev. Dr. Ely was appointed Secretary and Treasurer of the Board. Thus, when the new building was finished in August, 1828, the Chairs in the Faculty were not completely filled. Despite the internal strife, an optimistic announcement was made on August 6, 1828, in which "the public is informed that the new Jefferson Medical Hall in south Tenth Street is now completed and furnishes accommodations, which it is believed are surpassed by no building of the kind in our country."

The parent Board of Trustees at Canonsburg reasserted its authority on October 8, 1828, when President Samuel Ralston announced "that the Board retains power of reversing decisions of the Additional Trustees when in their opinion the interests of the institution demand."

New tuition fees for students were set at $15 each for Surgery, Anatomy, Chemistry, Materia Medicia, Theory and Practice of Physic, Institutes, and Medical Jurisprudence, and $5 for Midwifery and Diseases of Women and Children, for a total of $95.

Before November 15 each Chairman was to pay to Treasurer Ely the sum of $225, except for the Professor of Midwifery, whose assessment was $75. This amounted to a yearly budget of $1,425 for rent, repairs, and janitorial services.

On March 11, 1829, the fourth commencement but the first in the new Medical Hall was held at noon. Of the 25 graduates Washington L. Atlee (Figure 1-18) became the most prominent alumnus, "the man who did more than anyone in the world to establish ovariotomy as a legitimate practice."[4,5] The public exercises commenced with prayer by Board Member, the Rev. Mr. Gilbert R. Livingston; degrees were conferred by President

Green; and the address was delivered by Professor Benjamin Rush Rhees.

In early 1830, Dr. W.P.C. Barton, who had held the Chair of Materia Medica with distinction since 1826 and served as Dean, 1828–1829, was called to naval duty on the frigate *Brandywine*. Dr. Rhees was appointed to complete the course, and Dr. Eberle was transferred from the Chair of Practice to that of Materia Medica to take effect at the beginning of the next session (November 1, 1831). Drs. James and William Rush were appointed Professor and Adjunct Professor respectively of Theory and Practice. The two Drs. Rush declined the appointment, and Dr. Daniel Drake (Figure 1-19) of Cincinnati agreed to fill the vacant Chair.

The session of 1830–1831 opened with all Chairs filled for the first time in three years. The addition of Dr. Daniel Drake offered much promise.[6] He had already been prominent in the medical history of the West and brought students with him. His fame as a teacher was only further enhanced at Jefferson by his brilliant lectures, which he delivered spontaneously in a strong clear voice. Drake had risen from the abject poverty of log cabin residence to medical preceptorship under Dr. William Goforth, Jr., of Cincinnati, and a medical degree from the University of Pennsylvania in 1815. The rest of his life was spent in professorships in Ohio, Kentucky, and Philadelphia, as well as private practice, attempts to found medical schools in Ohio, and considerable writing. The most notable of his published works was *Diseases of the Interior Valley of North America*. Dreaming of founding his own medical school in Cincinnati, he stayed at Jefferson only one year, and then took Eberle with him.

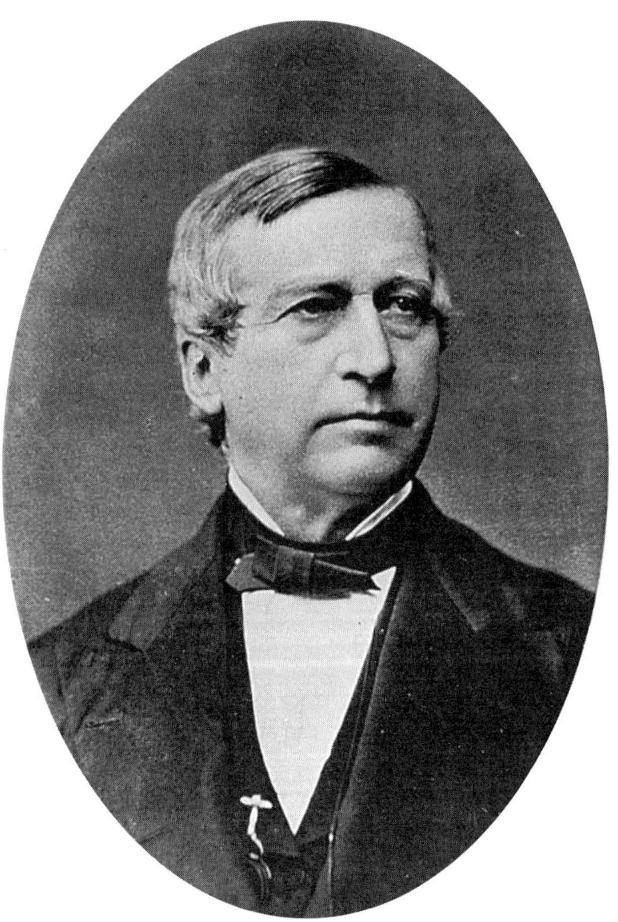

FIG. 1-18. Washington L. Atlee, M.D. (1808–1878); Jefferson Class of 1829, established ovariotomy (oophorectomy) as a legitimate procedure.

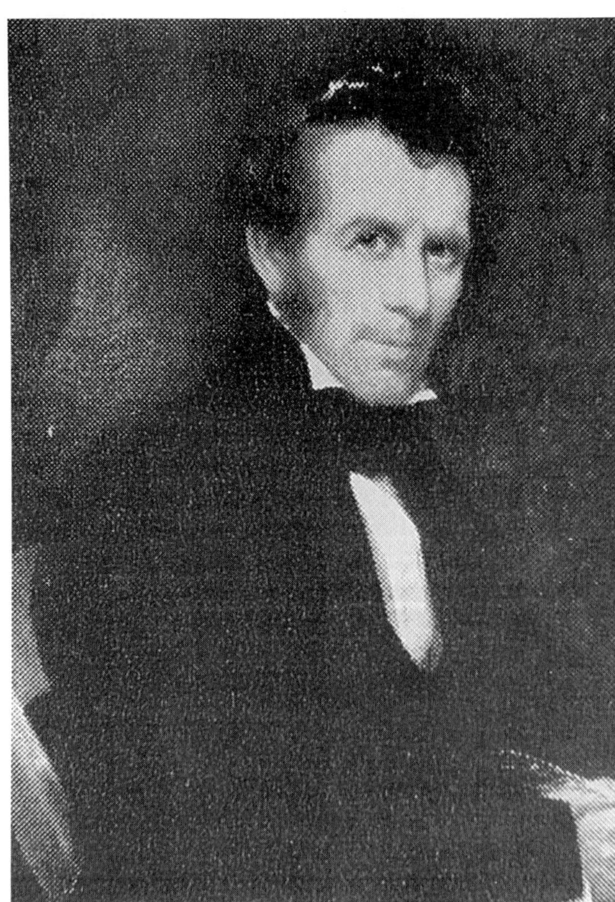

FIG. 1-19. Daniel Drake, M.D. (1785–1852); Professor of Theory and Practice of Medicine (1830–1831).

Losing these two eminent men at one time was the most serious loss of prestige the institution had thus far endured. To make matters worse, Dr. Benjamin Rush Rhees, who only recently had had a pulmonary hemorrhage from tuberculosis and whose lectures on midwifery had been transferred to Dr. Eberle, died in October, 1831.

The much-vacated Chair of Midwifery was accepted by Dr. Usher Parsons (Figure 1-20) in 1831.[7] Parsons came from Providence, Rhode Island, and had received his medical degree from Harvard in 1817. He was primarily a surgeon and anatomist rather than an obstetrician. Nevertheless his undramatic but well-prepared lectures and demonstrations were praised by the students. He taught for only one year but during this time published a paper on *The Art of Making Anatomical Preparations.* His departure was a disappointment to the students and another blow to Jefferson. The Trustees united the Chair for the time being to that of the Institutes, left vacant by the death of Rhees, and transferred Dr. Samuel McClellan from Anatomy.

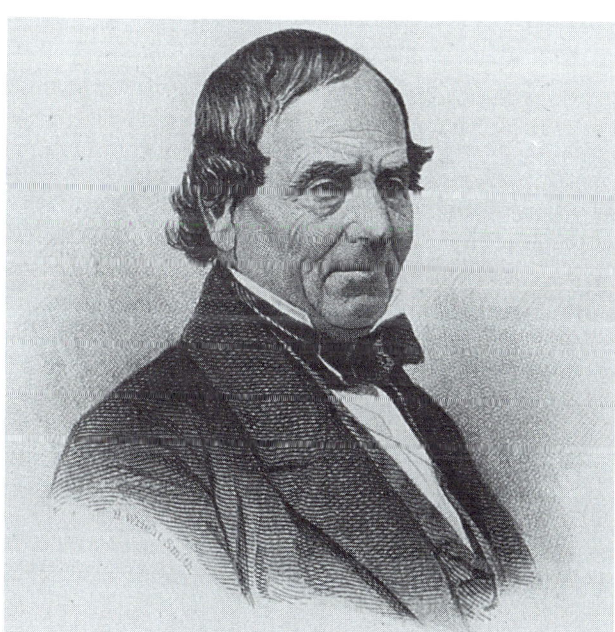

FIG. 1-20. Usher Parsons, M.D. (1788–1868); Professor of Midwifery (1831–1832).

The frequent faculty changes and reconstructions of this period resulted in diminishing enrollment with only 18 graduates in March, 1833. Those who had spread rumors that the school would fail had reason to be pleased. It was one of Jefferson's darkest hours, but the sun was soon to burst through the clouds.

References

1. Gross, S.D., *Autobiography,* Vol. I, p. 39.
2. "Editorial comment," *Am. Med. Recorder,* Vol. XIV:247–248, June 19, 1828.
3. Bauer, E.L., *Doctors Made in America.* p. 24.
4. Atlee, W.L., *Reminiscences of the Earliest Days of Jefferson Medical College.* Philadelphia: P. Madeira, 1873.
5. Kelly, H.A., and Burrage, W.L., "Washington L. Atlee," *American Medical Biographies,* Baltimore: Remington Co., 1920, p. 46.
6. Flexner, J.T., *Doctors on Horseback: Pioneers of American Medicine.* New York: Viking Press, 1937, pp. 165–234.
7. Parsons, C.W., *Memoir of Usher Parsons, M.D., (1788–1868).* Providence: Hammond, Angell and Co., 1870.

Stability Established (1832–1838): Robley Dunglison, the Peacemaker

For the six years from 1832 to 1838 the appointed professors kept their chairs. This stability was reflected in an increase in size of the classes and a growing respect by the medical profession. The graduating class of 1834 numbered 52; 1835 had 58; 1836 had 72; 1837 had 125 and 1838 graduated 108.

The Chair of Anatomy was held by Dr. Granville Sharpe Pattison (Fig. 1-21) who had been elected in 1831. He was a native of Scotland who took his preceptorship at the age of 17 under an anatomist, Dr. Allan Burns, celebrated for his lectures, anatomical rooms, and museum. Pattison then taught anatomy himself in the Andersonian Institute of Glasgow for four years before leaving for the United States in 1818 at the age of 26. He sought the Chair of Anatomy in the University of Pennsylvania recently vacated by the death of Dr. John Syng Dorsey. Dr. Nathaniel Chapman, Professor of Medicine, opposed the appointment on the basis that his letters of recommendation were "extravagant and hyperbolical" and because of a divorce case in Scotland in which Pattison, although exonerated by the court, had been accused as a correspondent. Pattison, "the vivacious and pugnacious Scot" then espoused the movement in 1818 agitated by Dr. W.P.C. Barton for the establishment of a second medical school in Philadelphia.[1]

Bitterness between Chapman and Pattison attained public exposure in 1820. At this time a University of Pennsylvania student, John Galloway Whilldin, was required to delete some passages from his graduation thesis because they reflected adversely on several members of the faculty. Pattison, as editor of the *Medical Recorder,* not only published the thesis as originally written but emphasized the objectionable passages in italics. In retaliation Dr. Chapman obtained from Glasgow a transcript of the trial brought by Professor Ure against Dr. Pattison and distributed 8,000 copies in pamphlet form. Pattison, maintaining that the divorce trial was a conspiracy against him by a colleague, challenged Chapman to a duel that apparently did not take place. He did, however, fight a duel in 1822 with General Thomas Cadwalader, a graduate in Arts from the University of Pennsylvania in 1795 and Chapman's brother-in-law, wounding him in the right arm. These difficulties in Philadelphia did not prevent his acceptance in 1820 of the Chair of Anatomy in the University of Maryland, a post he held for six years. In Baltimore, Pattison achieved professional, social, and financial success, but returned to his native country because of an illness of which it was rumored he would not recover. With restored health he took the Chair of Anatomy at the first organization of the University of London in 1827. As a result of infighting he withdrew shortly thereafter and returned to America. His assumption of the Chair of Anatomy at Jefferson at age 39 added to his established stature. He was an eloquent teacher who enlivened his subject by integrating it with physiology and surgery. Enthusiasm, sound scholarship, and sonorous delivery of his lectures enthralled his students. During his ten-year connection with Jefferson, Pattison founded the museum, enlarged the anatomical rooms, and increased the popularity of the institution. He edited *The Register and Library of Medical and Chirurgical Science,* Burn's *Surgical Anatomy of the Arteries of the Head and Neck,* Masse's *Anatomical Atlas,* Cruveilhier's *Anatomy,* and *The American Medical Recorder.* He left Jefferson in 1841 to join in the founding of the Medical Department of the University of New York. His death ten years later was caused by obstruction of the common bile duct. He was much interested in art and participated in establishing the Grand Opera House in New York. At Jefferson his stellar teaching was the precursor for a greater era to follow.

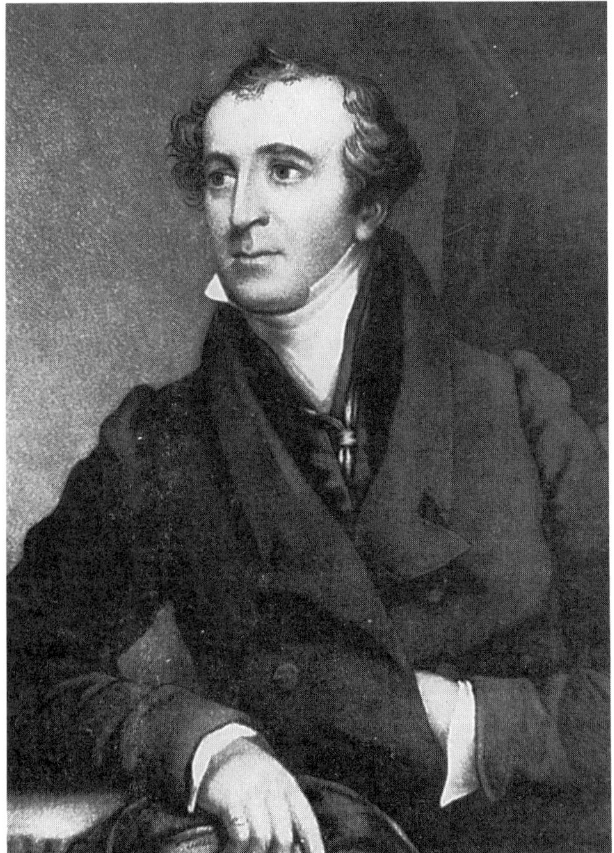

FIG. 1-21. Granville Sharpe Pattison, M.D. (1792–1851), Professor of Anatomy (1831–1841).

The Chair of Theory and Practice of Medicine vacated by Daniel Drake was filled by Dr. John Revere (Figure 1-22),[2] the son of Paul Revere, famous silversmith and Revolutionary War patriot. After graduating with honors from Harvard College in 1807, John Revere studied medicine in the office of James Jackson, M.D., of Boston. Visits to various medical centers of Europe culminated at Edinburgh University from which he received his doctorate in 1811. He returned to Boston for private practice but failing health, most likely due to tuberculosis, forced him to Virginia for rest and the sea air of the Chesapeake Bay. With improved health he moved to Baltimore, where he engaged in a small practice, studied chemistry, translated Magendie's *Physiology,* and published a few papers. Revere visited England in 1829 to solicit interest in his discovery of a process to protect the bottoms of seagoing vessels. Shortly after returning to Baltimore in 1831 he received the call to Jefferson. For a decade in the Chair of Medicine he was highly respected for his scholarship and considered one of the best lecturers of the faculty. His personal traits of faithful study, accuracy, honesty, courtesy, amiability, and command of language gained Revere high rank among teachers in the country and increasing credit to the College, for which he also served as Dean from 1839 to 1841. In his Philadelphia years he edited *The Medical Record.* In 1841, Revere accompanied Dr. Pattison to New York, having been elected to the same Chair in the newly founded University of that city. Six years later, at age 60, Revere died of typhoid fever. The Revere family name became further entrenched in Jefferson history when his grandniece, Grace Linzee Revere, married the younger Gross, Samuel W. The latter was attended by William Osler at death in 1889. The "Widow Gross" married Osler in 1892, and the couple named their son (Edward) Revere.

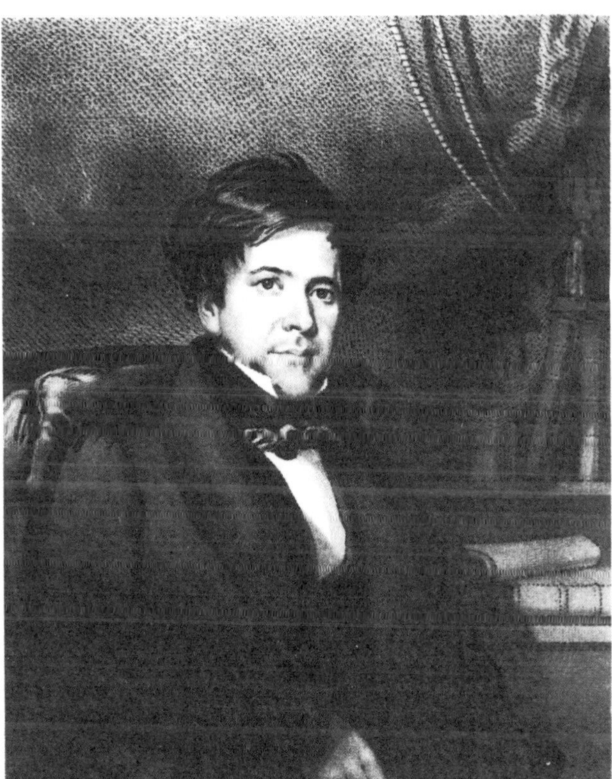

FIG. 1-22. John Revere, M.D. (1787–1847), Professor of Theory and Practice of Medicine (1831–1841) and Dean (1839–1841).

Samuel Colhoun (Figure 1-23) in 1831 took the Chair of Materia Medica, necessitated by the departure of Eberle for Cincinnati. A native of Chambersburg, Pennsylvania, he became well founded in Latin and Greek in his local Academy. He graduated from Princeton in 1804 and from the University of Pennsylvania Medical School in 1808. Despite his broad cultural background, excellent medical qualifications, handsome appearance, and courteous manners, he was not eminently successful in private practice. Dr. Colhoun contributed largely to the various periodicals of his day and was an avid reader of the medical literature. He looked on Dr. George McClellan as a medical idol and was pleased to accept the connection with Jefferson Medical College that lasted for nine years.

Unfortunately, Colhoun's lectures were dull and

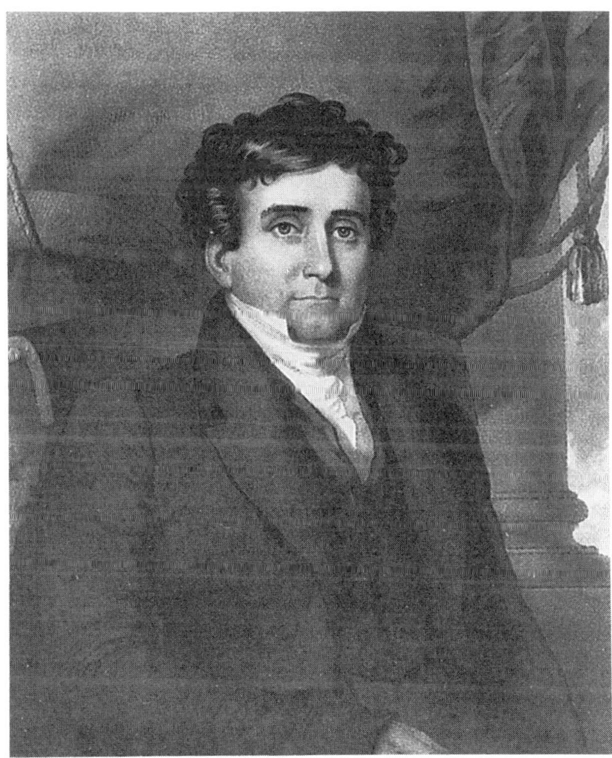

FIG. 1-23. Samuel Colhoun, M.D. (1778–1841); Professor of Materia Medica (1831–1839) and Dean (1835–1839).

delivered in a monotonous tone. Furthermore, he dwelled more on theory than on its practical application. He was characteristically unable to condense his vast store of knowledge into usable conclusions, thus leaving his students uninspired and at times confused. Nevertheless his kindly manner endeared him to the students, his unquestioned capacity as a physician commanded respect, and he served as Dean from 1835 to 1839. He published an edition of notes with Prout's *Calculus* and another with Gregory's *Practice,* notes frequently more voluminous than the original text. Colhoun was a loyal ally of the McClellan brothers in the various internal struggles of the school and accompanied them in 1839 when they left to found another medical school. He remained unmarried throughout life and, following a brief illness, died in 1841 at the age of 54.

George McClellan in Surgery and Jacob Green in Chemistry represented the founders in the climb toward stability of the school. Samuel McClellan held the Chair of Midwifery, Diseases of Women and Children, and Medical Jurisprudence. An unhealthy situation existed internally in the faculty in that the six professors divided themselves into two camps on points of issue. The McClellan brothers, with Colhoun always on their side, were usually pitched against Pattison, Revere, and Green.[3] In June, 1836, Dr. Robley Dunglison (Figure 1-24) was appointed to the Chair of Institutes of Medicine and Medical Jurisprudence, thus completing the faculty and providing an all-inclusive curriculum. This giant scholar was a connecting link between British and American medicine; he was the bridge between Thomas Jefferson, the namesake, and Jefferson, the Medical College; then he became a fulcrum that balanced the old with the new Jefferson Medical College. If McClellan was the George Washington, Dunglison was the Abraham Lincoln of Jefferson.

Before arrival at Jefferson, Dunglison had already achieved a remarkable series of innovative "firsts," as credited by Radbill.[4] At the University of Virginia, Dunglison had limited his practice to consultation only, thus making him the first full-time Professor of Medicine in the United States. His annual salary was $1,500, with supplementary tuition fees and free rent in one of the University pavilions. A five-year covenant of $5,000 guaranteed the arrangement, an early example of academic tenure. Also, when at the University of Virginia, Dunglison was the first in the country to give a formal series of lectures on Medical History in the curriculum. His treatise on *Human Physiology* (1832) was the first of its kind in America. His medical dictionary in 1833 was the first book of this type in the United States; it went through 23 editions, earning for Dunglison the sobriquet "walking dictionary." When appointed Professor of Hygiene at the University of Maryland in 1833 he became in fact the first Professor of Preventive Medicine and Public Health in the nation, and the publishing of his systematic lectures created the first formal textbook of hygiene on this side of the Atlantic.

Dunglison was warned of the jealousy and pettiness he would encounter among six faculty members of much stature and repute. Undaunted, he was convinced that as a natural peacemaker and by direct intent he could remain nonpartisan in the quarrels. In pursuing an independent course, totally devoid of political innuendo or personal

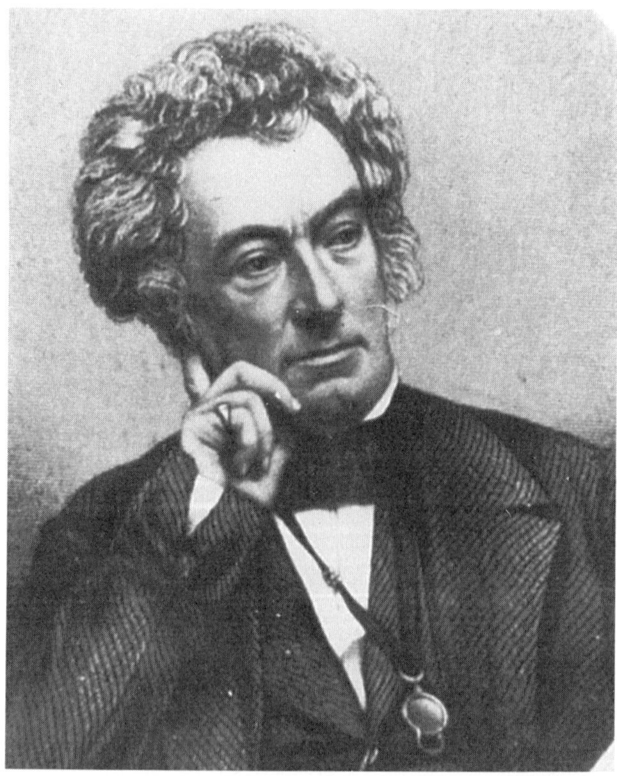

FIG. 1-24. Robley Dunglison, M.D. (1798–1869); Professor of Institutes of Medicine and Medical Jurisprudence (1836–1868) and Dean (1854–1868).

gain, neither clique could count on his support. He refused especially to take sides in the increasing tensions developing between George McClellan and the Board of Trustees.

At the time of his arrival, Dunglison was 38 years old, and he devoted the remaining 33 years of his life to Jefferson's welfare as, in Samuel D. Gross' words, "an illustrious man, a great scholar, a facile writer, a lucid erudite, and abundant author." Gross also wrote: "Of all the colleagues—nearly forty in number—with whom I have been associated, Robley Dunglison was by far the most learned." To confirm that Gross did not exaggerate Dunglison's virtues in a one-sided view, he also stated: "Dunglison was always brimful of his subject as he stood before his class, but he was monotonous, and did not sufficiently emphasize the great points of his discourse."

The classes had increased to such size that enlargement of the lecture room was necessary. Alternatives were a new, more spacious building or extension of the existing one. A mature deliberation of the Board of Trustees favored an enlargement and renovation of the current building. This apparently simple "growing pain" was to develop significant ramifications.

References

1. Landis, H.R.M., "Granville Sharpe Pattison," *The Jeffersonian,* Vol. 11, No. 88, 1910, pp. 1–6.
2. Channing, W., "John Revere." *Bos. Med. & Surg. J.* 36:292–295, 1847.
3. Senseney, A.H., "Biographical Sketch of Samuel Colhoun, M.D.," from Gayley, J.F.: *History of the Jefferson Medical College of Philadelphia with Biographical Sketches of the Early Professors.* Philadelphia: J.M. Wilson, 1858.
4. Radbill, S.X., "Autobiographical ANA of Robley Dunglison, M.D.," *Trans. Am. Phil. Soc.* (N.S.), Vol. 53, P. 8, 1964, p. 4.

The Charter of 1838: Independence of Jefferson Medical College

The contemplated modifications and additions to the existing Medical Hall involved a considerable outlay of money that could no longer be advanced by the Reverend Ely, who was in serious financial difficulties in Missouri. The faculty likewise were without funds for the purpose. It devolved upon the Board of Trustees to acquire the title to the property then vested in Ezra Stiles Ely. Unfortunately, as legally constituted, the Trustees in Philadelphia were "Additional Trustees" of Jefferson College at Canonsburg and therefore a part of the parent Board. Whatever property they acquired would belong to the parent Board, which from the very beginning had absolved itself from any financial responsibility for its Medical Department. The only solution lay in a new charter that would separate Jefferson Medical College from its parent at Canonsburg.

In the spring of 1838 an application to the State Legislature received prompt and favorable action. The fifth section of the Legislative Act of April 7, 1826, permitted the right to amend or repeal one portion of the charter. The fifth section of an act passed June 13, 1836, related to the general system of education, facilitated the transaction even more smoothly. The new Section V was as follows: "That the Medical Department of Jefferson College be and hereby is, created a separate and independent body corporate, under the name, style, and title of 'The Jefferson Medical College of Philadelphia,' with the same powers and restrictions as the University of Pennsylvania; the present additional Trustees . . . to be Trustees of the College created by this Section, with power to increase their number to fifteen."

At a last meeting of the Board of Additional Trustees on April 19, 1838, the new charter was accepted and the following resolution adopted before final adjournment:

> "That the president be directed to communicate to the mother board at Canonsburg, that in accepting the charter which separates them from the Jefferson College at Canonsburg, the additional trustees are influenced by the conviction that such a separation is for the mutual benefit and convenience of both bodies, and desired it for no other reason, and that this board will retain a grateful sense of the kind and fostering care ever exhibited towards them by the parent institution, and will in their new capacity be always ready to acknowledge their past obligations, and to exchange in every way in their power, kind offices with Jefferson College at Canonsburg."

Fortunately, although the Trustees at Canonsburg were loath to sever relationship with their flourishing Medical Department, they raised no serious objections. On the contrary, they sent the Trustees of the new College a "warm God-speed and a prayer for continued usefulness and prosperity."

It must be reiterated at this juncture that the new independent Jefferson Medical College of 1838 was not the nonprofit corporation that we know today. It was a proprietary school, like most medical schools of the time. As a business venture the professors collected fees for their lectures, paid the rent, and kept the profit. The Rev. Dr. Ely's benefaction of providing a building at rental to the professors was in itself a business venture on his part. Indeed, in 1831 two of the professors were conjointly delinquent for $403.35, and at the August 31 meeting of the Board, Dr. Ely threatened to forfeit the lease to the "Additional Trustees" and claimed "the right of renting the said College to any other agreeable to his own judgment." It must also be understood that these were hard economic times; none of the professors became affluent; and most had trouble meeting their financial obligations.

The United States in 1838 was far from the mighty nation it is today. There were 26 states and two territories of Florida and Wisconsin. Most of the land beyond the Mississippi was a vast wilderness, and much of it belonged to Mexico. Texas was a republic with Samuel Houston as President. The population of the country was around 15,000,000, of which approximately one-sixth were slaves. There was no national debt, and income tax was practically unknown. Pennsylvania had only 120 miles of railroad in operation.

The University of Pennsylvania at this time was the most famous among the 28 medical schools of the country because of its age, location, and able faculty. Its building was at Ninth between Market and Chestnut Streets, and the student enrollment numbered 400, representing over one-seventh of the total number of medical students in the land. Philip Syng Physick (1768–1837), a pupil of John Hunter and "the Father of American Surgery," had recently died as Emeritus Professor of Surgery and Anatomy. He was succeeded in 1819 by William Gibson, the first surgeon to tie the common iliac artery and who had performed two cesarean operations on the same patient with survival of the mother and both children. Nathaniel Chapman, Professor of Physic and Clinical Medicine, was one of the greatest teachers in America and was destined to become the first President of the American Medical Association. George B. Wood taught Materia Medica and with Franklin Bache edited the *U.S. Dispensatory*. William E. Horner was the Professor of Anatomy as well as the founder of St. Joseph's Hospital. Samuel Jackson, Professor of Institutes of Medicine, introduced the principles of Laennec and Louis from France to America. Hugh L. Hodge, whose forceps and pessaries were known internationally, was Professor of Midwifery. Robert Hare, inventor of the oxyhydrogen blowpipe, was the distinguished Professor of Chemistry.

In the national and local setting just described, the Board of Trustees under its new charter settled upon its first task, namely to increase its number to 15. Jesse R. Burden, Joseph B. Smith, John R. Jones, Colonel Samuel Miller, and John R. Vodges were elected. A few days later they arranged for the renovations of Medical Hall.

Thomas Ustick Walter was chosen as the architect. He was a native Philadelphian and pupil of William Strickland, who might have been the original architect. He had designed the Girard College buildings as well as the House and Senate wings and central dome of the national Capitol. His plan, which involved extensive interior and exterior remodeling, included two lecture rooms, each with seating capacity for 450 students. There were rooms for dissecting, for the museum, for the professors, and for the janitor. Improvements in natural lighting, ventilation, heat, and gas illumination were provided. No drawings of the exterior have remained, but the studies of Teitelman[1] suggest a Greek Revival style with Ionic colonnades. On June 15, 1838, the building committee reported the final estimated cost at $7,500, but the Board approved only $5,000 as the maximal expenditure.

The Rev. Ely, although in Missouri, maintained his position and interest on the Board. He made an offer, which was agreeable with the Trustees, to execute a lease on Medical Hall for 20 years, granting the privilege of paying off the principal of the yearly rent at any time before expiration of the lease. This lease was effective as of November 24, 1838, with annual rent increased to $1,770 and the property appraised at $29,500 before renovation. It represented a 6 percent return on the investment. Work commenced promptly and the building was ready for the 1838–1839 session.

By unanimous vote the Board of Trustees elected all the professors to the chairs they previously held under the old arrangement. The condition of the College seemed optimal. There was a stable faculty of respected professors, the building was ample and updated; student enrollment was increasing; and professional and public confidence was widespread. However, the session of 1838 that started so auspiciously developed problems of major proportions.

References

1. Teitelman, E., "Jefferson's Architecture: Past, Present and Future." *Jeff. Al. Bull.,* Fall 1965, p. 13.

Dissolution of the Faculty (1839): McClellan Dismissed

During the session of 1838–1839 serious dissensions arose within the faculty that cost Jefferson much of the prestige it had gained during the preceding six years. The old infighting over policy and fees had previously been kept under control by the faculty itself. For complex reasons, purely conjectural and poorly documented but certainly involving conflicts of personalities, all attempts at amicable resolution within the faculty failed. Whatever might be unknown about the inner history of this pivotal affair, it is certain that McClellan was the central figure. As the founder he had enjoyed unchallenged power and had come to regard the school as his own. A growing inclination to rebel against his authority by newer forces in the teaching corps was stubbornly repelled by the dictatorial Chairman of Surgery. His professional ability and fame, his magnetic personality, and his popularity with the students were tempered with certain characteristic faults. "Mac" was compulsive in action, easily provoked, often erratic, and obstinate. The 15 members of the Board of Trustees of the newly independent Medical School became more directly involved in its interests and more disposed to exercise authority than in the former years when they were merely "Additional Trustees." In the increasing tensions for administrative domination by the founder versus that of the Board, McClellan, in uncontrolled frustration, publically proclaimed the Board a "parcel of politicians" and "a blackguard Board of Trustees." He asserted further that the institution was "rotten and going to the dogs" and "with the rascally Board, Jefferson must go down."

On April 2, 1839, Dr. Robley Dunglison wrote a "Letter of Appeal to the Faculty" and on the same date the Dean, Dr. John Revere, presented this communication to the Board of Trustees for consideration. The far-reaching consequences of the issue justify a quotation of the salient portions:

> "I would call attention to the fact that not among the students but throughout the city, and members of the faculty were grieved to be told by some of the latter, that they had authority for stating that the Institution was "going to the Dogs," and that for certain reasons it must do so.
>
> It is far from the object as it is from the province of the undersigned to lay charges against anyone of his colleagues of desiring to injure an institution to which he is attached. . . . It is the report, that these sinister statements rest on the authority of a member or members of the Faculty, which is deplored and which is calculated to exert as baneful an influence on the Institution as if it were founded in truth.
>
> The acts of the Board have met with the most unqualified approbation of the undersigned, and it is not less gratifying to himself than it is just to that body, to attest the devotion and disinterestedness which they appear to him to have exhibited in the cause of the College. . . . The power of managing the affairs of the institution is vested in the hands of the Trustees, and all experience shows that they will not be driven from its exercise by a hostile movement on the part of the Faculty. It is scarcely to be expected, that, in directing the complicated machinery of an extensive institution, the Board of Trustees can *always* act in such a manner as to give entire satisfaction, but where this is not the result, it is with the Faculty respectfully to represent the matter to the Board and not to allow their objections to become public; still less the impression to go abroad that the acts

> of the Board are objected to by the Professors, and likely to interfere with the prosperity of the school.
>
> In like manner it is scarcely to be expected that entire harmony of sentiment can exist amongst all the members of a Faculty accidentally brought together, owing to their possessing certain intellectual requisites. Yet *harmony of action* is essential as it is practicable, and this is all that can be meant, when the importance of harmony amongst the members of an institution is spoken of. . . . The undersigned has always thought, that under an energetic Faculty actuated by ordinary prudence and judgment, there is ample space in the city of Philadelphia, for two noble Institutions, and he sees no reason whatever to modify that opinion."[1]

The Board referred the issue to a committee of three of its members "to inquire into the existing state and condition of the medical faculty of the College, and to report to this Board whether any and what measures are required to be adopted in reference thereto; and that said committee have power to call the Professors and such other persons before them as will enable them to accomplish the duties assigned to them and require the production by the Faculty of all its books, papers, and archives."

The committee composed of the Reverend C.C. Cuyler, D.D., J.B. Smith, Esq., and the Hon. John R. Jones recommended on May 2, 1839, that the faculty be dissolved, and this was accepted on June 10. All the faculty wrote letters requesting reappointment except the two McClellans, but the Board ignored their implied protest. Indeed, Samuel McClellan was reelected to the Chair of Midwifery. It took until July 10 to reconstitute the entire faculty. Colhoun was voted out and replaced by Dr. Robert M. Huston in Materia Medica. Two new candidates applied to the Board for the Chair of Surgery. One was Dr. Thomas Tickell Hewson (1773–1848), son of a celebrated London anatomist. He had conducted a private anatomical room and was currently president of the College of Physicians of Philadelphia.[2] The other was Dr. Joseph Pancoast (1805–1882), who had reopened the Philadelphia Anatomical Rooms in 1831 and was a widely respected surgeon in the city. Hewson at age 66 did get one vote. Pancoast at 34 fared better and won over George McClellan with a vote of seven to five.

Colhoun was shocked, George McClellan was mortified, and Samuel McClellan resigned. Dr. Robert Huston was transferred to Midwifery, and Dunglison took the duties of Materia Medica in addition to that of the Institutes. Pattison remained in Anatomy, Green in Chemistry, and Revere in Theory and Practice.

"Every institution," Ralph Waldo Emerson has said, "was once the act of a single man." Alas for McClellan; the institution dismissed him. It would be unfair to lose interest in the further career of the founder who had done so much for Jefferson. This irrepressible man immediately used the same strategy to found another school. By going to them in person he again obtained a Charter from the State Legislature for an institution called "The Medical Department of Pennsylvania College" at Gettysburg. McClellan, with brother Samuel, Dr. Colhoun, and three other associates, assembled a good faculty and commenced the first course of lectures with nearly 100 pupils in November, 1839. A quarrel arose in 1843 and McClellan reluctantly had to resign this final professorship. Nevertheless, his second school survived for almost two decades, and many in Philadelphia rated it the best of the three schools. Closed by attrition during the Civil War, it remains associated with Jefferson's history because the three schools were involved in a nationwide effort for the reform of medical education that got under way in 1839 and culminated in the organization of the American Medical Association in 1847.

Retired from lecturing, McClellan spent the rest of his life in practice. He treated all classes of people, but his kindness to the poor spread his name as a household word. He developed a facial neuralgia that gradually involved his lower extremities. Death struck suddenly on May 8, 1847, when he was 51. On that morning he had performed two operations. By noon he was forced home by acute abdominal pain. At midnight he went into shock and died shortly thereafter. Postmortem examination revealed a perforated sigmoid colon. McClellan was buried in East Laurel Hill Cemetery, overlooking the East River (Kelly) Drive in Philadelphia, Section L, Lot 46 (Figure 1-25). The prominent granite tombstone that also bears his wife's name shows little sign of wear.[3]

The strife in the faculty with its associated changes was reflected in the class of 1839–1840, in which the number of graduates fell to 56. This was 40 percent below the previous class and 60 percent below that of 1836. On February 1, 1841, Dr. Jacob Green, the beloved Professor of Chemistry, died suddenly. "Old Jaky" was only 51 years of age, but he represented the last of the original faculty. On returning from Dr. Green's funeral, Revere (also serving as dean at the time) and Pattison told Dunglison they were resigning to join a new Medical Department of New York University. In one swoop the Jefferson Faculty was again cut in half, but the see-saw of ups and downs was miraculously to raise Jefferson to new and previously unsurpassed heights.

References

1. Dunglison, R., *The Running Diary,* Vol. 5, Manuscript in Coll. Phys. Philadelphia.
2. Konkle, B.A., and Henry, F.P., *Standard History of the Medical Profession of Philadelphia.* New York: AMS Press, 1977, pp. 158–159.
3. Wagner, F.B. Jr, "The Making of a Medical School," *Jeff. Al. Bull.,* Winter 1980, pp. 16–18.

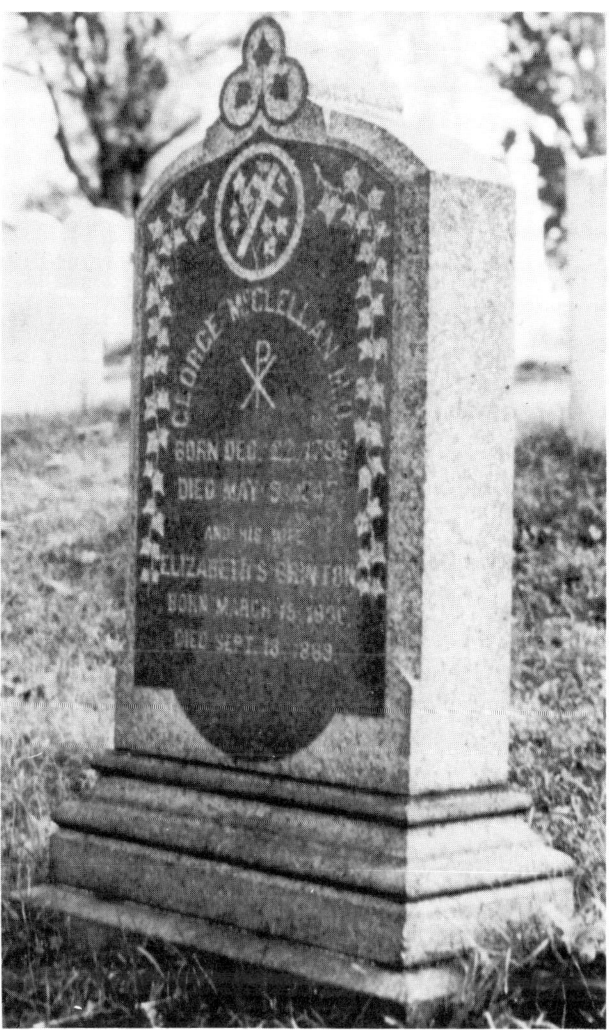

FIG. 1-25. Gravesite of George McClellan, M.D. (1796–1847) in East Laurel Hill Cemetery.

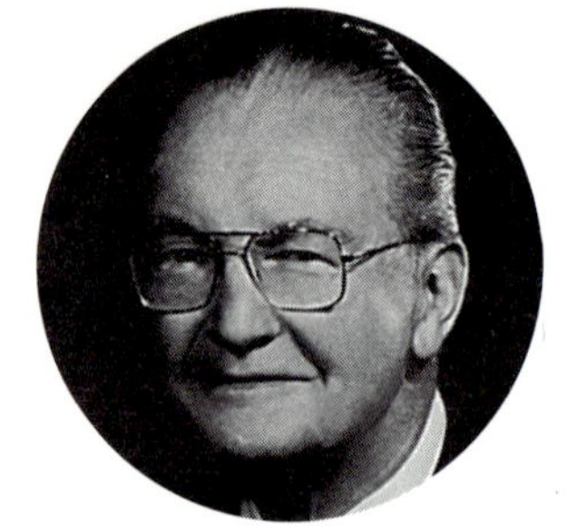

CHAPTER TWO

Growth and Consolidation

FREDERICK B. WAGNER, JR., M.D.

"Enter to grow in wisdom. Depart to serve mankind." —MODIFIED FROM CHARLES W. ELIOT (1834–1926)

The Faculty of 1841–1856: An Illustrious Harmonious Team

After an uneventful graduation on March 6, 1841, the Board of Trustees set themselves to the task of organizing a new faculty. The stated goal was to obtain "the services of gentlemen who are known throughout this country as practical teachers; and who have likewise a widespread reputation as writers on different subjects of their profession; whose very name, indeed, would be a source of confidence, and a presage of success. With this view they have banished all personal feelings, and in the appointment of Professors have endeavored to keep singly in view that which appeared to them to be the most conducive to the stability, dignity, and reputation of the school." Fifteen candidates were considered for the seven vacated Chairs. Surgery had become such an important subject that a division into one Chair of Principles and one Chair of Practice was contemplated. Dr. Jacob Randolph, son-in-law of Philip Syng Physick and a surgeon of the Pennsylvania Hospital noted for his skill in lithotomy, was elected to the latter Chair but declined because he could not reconcile a difference between principles and practice. This division would not occur until the resignation of Dr. Samuel D. Gross in 1882, but union into one Chair would resume with the appointment of Dr. John H. Gibbon, Jr., in 1956.

In April, 1841, the same Chairs were filled as follows: Robley Dunglison, M.D., Institutes of Medicine and Medical Jurisprudence; Robert M. Huston, M.D., Materia Medica and Therapeutics, and Dean; Joseph Pancoast, M.D., General, Descriptive, and Surgical Anatomy; John K. Mitchell, M.D., Practice of Medicine; Thomas D. Mütter, M.D., Principles and Practice of Surgery; Charles D. Meigs, M.D., Obstetrics and Diseases of Women and Children; and Franklin Bache, M.D., Chemistry (Figure 2-1).

The speed, thoroughness and wisdom of the Board of Trustees in organizing this truly prestigious faculty was an amazing accomplishment. It marked the entry of Jefferson into a second epoch of its history. The first epoch, from 1824 to 1841, witnessed contests for personal advantage, changes in the faculty, both voluntary and involuntary, and financial problems. The College suffered from poverty, infighting and harassment. The faculty of the second epoch brought fifteen years of unparalleled friendliness, cooperation, and progress. Jealousy was conspicuously absent. The combined outstanding achievements of each member lifted Jefferson to the forefront of medical schools of the country.

Throughout the courses of lectures, Jefferson

students had the additional opportunity to observe and participate in the care of patients in the General Dispensary attached to the College and to receive instruction in clinical medicine and surgery at the Blockley Almshouse (Philadelphia Hospital), Pennsylvania Hospital, and Wills Hospital for diseases of the eye. In the General Dispensary of the College where more than 1,000 cases were treated each year, the students were entrusted to patient care under the supervision of the professor who examined and prescribed. There likewise were opportunities in obstetrical practice. This was a strong point in Jefferson's training of excellent practical physicians for that era. Outside critics deprecated this type of pedagogy as superficial, ineffectual, and even misleading. They believed that single cases might slant the student's perception of disease in a tubular rather than wide-angle direction. Notwithstanding, the new faculty made the medical and surgical collegiate clinics a prominent feature of the weekly curriculum. Horse-drawn omnibuses carried students to the various clinics twice a week. Behavior at times was boisterous, and squabbles with students from the University of Pennsylvania occurred occasionally but never had serious consequences.

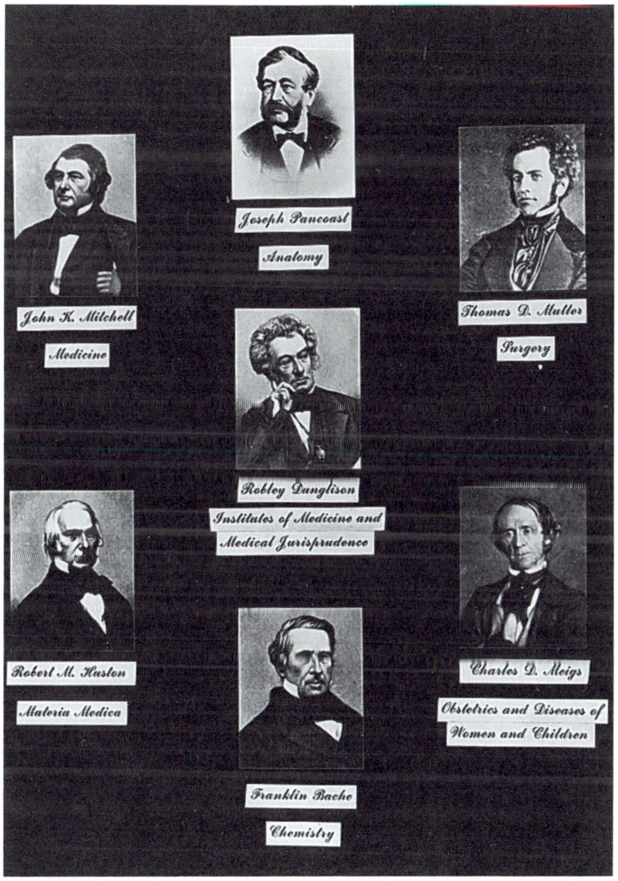

FIG. 2-1. The Faculty of 1841.

Medical instruction was significantly enhanced in this epoch by Jefferson's museum of anatomical, pathological, and obstetrical preparations. There also were drawings, plates, specimens, and reproductions for illustration in Materia Medica. Private collections from members of the faculty enriched the cabinets and displays.

John Hill Brinton, one of Jefferson's past historians, eulogized his teachers in *The Faculty of 1841*, delivered as a lecture before the Alumni Association on March 11, 1880.[1] A few highlights from this classical treatise as well as individual memoirs provide information on the achievements that made these men so notable.

Robley Dunglison (1798–1869)

No one on the list was more outstanding than Dr. Robley Dunglison, whose academic prowess benefited Jefferson for the 32 years between 1836 and 1868. He was a physician to presidents (Jefferson and Madison), a giant author and editor, a "peacemaker," a "walking dictionary," the "Father of American Physiology," and Dean for 14 years (1854–1868) who signed thousands of Jefferson diplomas. Samuel D. Gross, himself one of Jefferson's great historians, wrote the definitive memoir of Dunglison's life and also included him in the biographical sketches of his contemporaries in his *Autobiography*.[2,3] His role at Jefferson is further detailed in the section on the history of the Department of Physiology.

Dunglison was one of the most popular medical writers of his generation, sales of his books totaling more than 150,000 copies. Equally amazing were his contributions to lay journals on such topics as road making, English fashions in the seventeenth century, construction of words from sounds, English pronounciations, penitentiary descipline, universities, legends of the English lakes, Richard the Lion-hearted and Blondel, superstitions, Americanism, early German poetry, etymological history, Sanskrit language, ancient and modern gymnasia, cradle of mankind, English orthoepy (correct diction), canals of the ancients, Jeffersoniana, biographical and obituary notes, and a voluminous dictionary for the blind in raised type.

Two of Dunglison's four sons graduated from Jefferson—Richard J. in 1856 and Thomas R. in 1859. The former continued later editions of his father's medical dictionary and edited *Gray's Anatomy* in 1884. Thomas Jefferson University in 1984 honored the memory of Dunglison by restoring his grave in historic East Laurel Hill cemetery.[4]

Robert M. Huston (1794–1864)

Dr. Robert M. Huston had been previously appointed at the dissolution of the faculty of 1839 as Professor of Obstetrics, and then as Professor of Therapeutics and Materia Medica in 1841.[5] A native Virginian, Huston had served during the War of 1812 as an Assistant Surgeon in the Army. As most Jefferson chairmen since its founding, he had studied at the University of Pennsylvania (1823–1825) and then entered into practice in Philadelphia. His lectures, read from manuscript, in which he warned against the heroic use and abuse of medicines, revealed conservatism. He did less writing than the other members of his faculty, but edited the American edition of Fleetwood Churchill's *Theory and Practice of Midwifery* in 1843, and was a coeditor of the *Medical Examiner* from 1844 to 1848. In 1850 he contributed notes to Churchill's textbook on *Diseases of Females*, and in the same year Churchill dedicated his book on *Diseases of Infants and Children* to Huston, Isaac Hays, and George Shattuck.

The faculty honored Huston by choosing him as Dean, which position he held much longer than anyone prior to that time (1841–1854). He was recognized for an excellent business ability that put the financial affairs of the College on a sound basis. In 1857 Huston resigned his Chair to become Emeritus.

Joseph Pancoast (1805–1882)

Dr. Joseph Pancoast, who had proven a worthy surgical successor to George McClellan in 1839, was elected to the Chair of Anatomy in the new faculty.[6] The details of his success in these two Chairs are covered in the histories of the Departments of Surgery and Anatomy. Suffice it to say that his teaching of anatomy was medically and surgically oriented to the greatest practical advantage of his students. Pancoast's retirement in 1874 was finally accepted with the utmost reluctance by the Board of Trustees. His son, William H., succeeded him in the same Chair and was the first of three father-son chairmanships, the later two being those of Gross and Gibbon. As Emeritus Professor, Pancoast inaugurated in 1877 the opening of the new detached first Jefferson Hospital in an eloquent address. The United States mint struck a medal in his honor in 1870 at the instigation of its director, James Pollock, and it is still listed in the latest national historic series (Figure 2-2).

John Kearsley Mitchell (1793–1858)

Dr. John Kearsley Mitchell, another Virginian, was the son and grandson of a physician.[7] He in succession would also be the father and grandfather of physicians—S. Weir Mitchell and

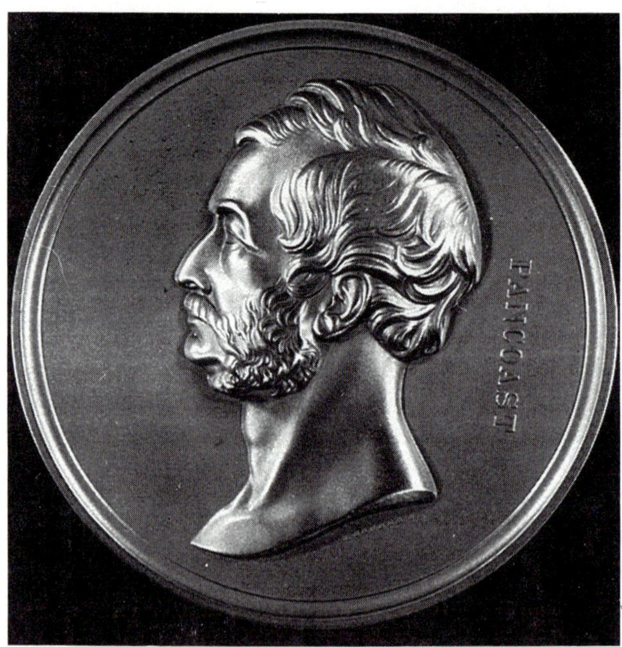

FIG. 2-2. Medal in honor of Joseph Pancoast, M.D. struck by U.S. Mint in 1870.

another John Kearsley Mitchell. As a matter of historic irony, he was a pupil of Nathaniel Chapman and while a student at the University of Pennsylvania had been a leader in the classroom opposition to the founding of a second medical school. It was he who clashed with fellow student Benjamin Rush Rhees over the matter. Mitchell made three voyages to China to improve his health, and by 1822 he was lecturing on Medical Chemistry in Chapman's summer school, the Medical Institute of Philadelphia. As a further stepping-stone in his appointment to Jefferson, Mitchell served as Professor of Chemistry in the Franklin Institute. His research in chemistry led to the discovery of solvents for rubber, tests for arsenic, and an apparatus for solidification of carbon dioxide.

In 1849 Mitchell published his views on the origins of malaria, cholera, plague, and yellow fever. As a polished litterateur he published a volume of poems and addresses such as "The Wisdom of God as Displayed in the Formation of Water," "The Practical Interrogation of Nature," and "The Means of Elevating the Character of the Working Classes." Mitchell's lectures were clear, well illustrated, enlivened by anecdotes, and projected with friendliness. He held his professorship during failing health and gave a reception at his home for the graduating class of 1858 just one month before his death.

■ Charles Delucena Meigs (1792–1869)

Charles Delucena Meigs was born into a family of culture and refinement in Bermuda, where his father was a Proctor in the English Courts of Admiralty.[8] The father in 1796 was appointed Professor of Mathematics and Natural Philosphy at Yale College and in 1801 as President of the University of Georgia. Young Charles Meigs received a classical education enhanced by a Professor of French who taught him the language well. As a boy he also spent some time in the nearby wild Indian country inhabited by Cherokees.

After graduation from the University of Georgia in 1809 Meigs took courses in the lectures of the University of Pennsylvania, 1812–1813, and 1814–1815. Although he did not receive his medical degree until 1817, Meigs started practice in Augusta, Georgia, in 1815. Two years later he moved to Philadelphia, where he began writing for the *North American Medical and Surgical Journal* and engaged actively in the debates at the Philadelphia Medical Society. Initially he seems to have had an aversion to the practice of obstetrics, but with time he devoted himself largely to this branch. By 1831 he had translated, from the French, *Velpeau's Treatise on Midwifery*, and he published in 1838 his own work *Philadelphia Practice of Midwifery*. During Meigs' twenty-two years at Jefferson he translated the treatise of Colombat de L'Isere on *Diseases and Hygiene of Females* (1845) and published his own book on *Females and Their Diseases* (1848), *Obstetrics, the Science and the Art* (1849), *Childbed Fevers* (1854), and *Acute and Chronic Diseases of the Neck of the Uterus* (1854). His book on *Certain Diseases of Young Children* (1850) established him in medical history as a pioneer in pediatrics.

Meigs' lectures stressed that beyond the purely medical aspects, a physician should be a cultured man. The charm of his words, poetic expressions, quaint humor, and philosophic reasoning never failed to instruct or impress his students. He was an enemy of anesthesia for childbirth and stressed that ether givers practiced "criminal foolhardiness." Meigs and Dr. Hodge, from the University of Pennsylvania, strongly opposed the work of Oliver Wendell Holmes (1843) and Ignaz Philipp Semmelweiss (1848) on the contagiousness of puerperal fever. This attitude was defensible in terms of the era—Pasteur's works on fermentation (1857), spontaneous generation (1862), microorganisms in the virulent diseases of anthrax and chicken cholera (1877), and vaccination (1880) were to come later. Furthermore, Joseph Lister's epochal contribution (1867) *On the Antiseptic Principle in the Practice of Surgery* would have to go through fifteen years of trial, doubt, and ultimate belief. Although the achromatic microscope was perfected in 1830, its use in medicine at this time was mainly a curiosity.

Meigs was much interested in pulmonary embolism and gave lengthy discussion to it in his lectures. In 1860, at age 68, he resigned his Professorship to become Emeritus and retire to a country home in Delaware County. He died suddenly in 1869. Portraits of Meigs hang in the halls of Jefferson and the College of Physicians of Philadelphia. His son, John Forsyth, and grandson, Arthur Vincent, followed in his footsteps, especially in pediatrics, but were not associated with Jefferson.

■ Franklin Bache (1792–1864)

Dr. Franklin Bache was the great-grandson of Benjamin Franklin. Franklin's only daughter, Sarah, married an Englishman by the name of Richard Bache.[9,10] Franklin Bache was born in Benjamin Franklin's Philadelphia home on the south side of Market Street between Third and Fourth. He obtained a B.A. degree from the University of Pennsylvania in 1810. Dr. Benjamin Rush accepted him for preceptorship in medicine, and Rush's son, Dr. James Rush, continued training young Bache after the senior Rush's death in 1813. During this period Bache also served as an Army Assistant Surgeon in the War of 1812. He received his M.D. degree from the University of Pennsylvania in 1814, engaged in private practice, and for many years was physician to the Old Walnut Street Prison and later to the Eastern Penitentiary.

From early youth Bache evinced a special proclivity for chemistry and the physical sciences. His contributions to this field and his career at Jefferson are covered in this book in the chapter on the history of the Department of Chemistry. Precision and austerity awed Bache's students, but an occasional touch of quaint humor enlivened his otherwise dull lectures. His best friend was Dr. George B. Wood of the University of Pennsylvania, with whom he coauthored the monumental *United States Dispensatory,* commonly known as the *Wood and Bache*. Bache retained his professorship until his death in 1864.

■ Thomas Dent Mütter (1811–1859)

The last star in the galaxy of famous Professors in the famous 1841 faculty was Thomas Dent Mütter.[11] He was born in Richmond, Virginia, and received his degree in medicine from the University of Pennsylvania in 1831. The following year Mütter mainly spent in Paris, at that time the medical center of the world, where he was influenced by the great surgeons, Dupuytren, Roux, Lisfranc and Velpeau. His special interest in plastic and orthopedic surgery was aroused, as well as his lifetime preference for French medical thinking. Mütter settled in Philadelphia in 1832 and immediately began teaching his newly acquired knowledge from abroad, at first in a private class for medical examinations. In 1833 he joined Dr. Paul Goddard in private instruction of a large class of medical students, and in 1835 was appointed Assistant Lecturer in Surgery at the Philadelphia Medical Institute, a summer school formed by Nathaniel Chapman in 1819. The Medical Institute was a vehicle for his academic development and a stage that focused on him as worthy of the Chair of Surgery at Jefferson. Mütter's success in that Chair is covered in the history of the Surgery Department. His eloquent lectures were illustrated with copious diagrams, models, and specimens that constituted his personal museum.

Poor health forced Mütter to resign prematurely in 1856 at the age of 45. He donated his private museum to the College of Physicians of Philadelphia along with an endowment of $30,000 for a Lectureship on Surgical Pathology.[12] His Museum and Lectureship are not only active until the present time, but have so overshadowed his career that many are surprised to learn that he ever was Professor of Surgery at Jefferson. This man, who so benefited the school as well as posterity, was the first in fifteen years of the solid faculty to die. He died in 1859, at age 48.

As with many past and later chairmen, Jefferson gained much strength from the University of Pennsylvania School of Medicine; albeit as an unwanted child, but with time the two would be regarded as sister institutions.

With appointment of the faculty of 1841 the number of students increased and would have been even greater had it not been that George McClellan's new school of 1839 had subtracted somewhat from Jefferson's attendance. The number for the session of 1840–1841 was 163; for 1841, an increase to 209; for 1842, 229; for 1843, 341; for 1844, 409; and for 1845, 469 students, the largest class in any institution of its kind in the United States. Graduates in 1843 numbered 47; in 1845 there were 116; and 170 in 1846. The College

Catalogue of Instruction for 1851 pointed with justifiable pride to the large number of students who, having taken at least one medical session at another school, came to Jefferson to study (162 of a student body of 516). In addition, approximately 100 graduates of other schools were in regular attendance at the lectures, many of them practitioners of mature age and experience. Some of these subjected themselves to fresh examinations and received a second medical diploma from Jefferson. Graduates instructed by this faculty who later became Chairmen at Jefferson were Benjamin Howard Rand (Class of 1848), Chemistry; James Aitken Meigs (1851), Institutes (Physiology); John Hill Brinton (1852), Practice of Surgery; and William Smith Forbes (1852), Anatomy.

The increasing attendance that developed within a few years of the appointment of this exceptional faculty taxed the physical capacity of the College and necessitated considerable enlargements (Figure 2-3).

References

1. Brinton, J.H., *The Faculty of 1841.* Philadelphia: Collins, 1880. (Extracted from the College and Clinical Record, March 15, 1880).
2. Gross, S.D., "Memoir of Robley Dunglison," *Trans. Coll. Phys. Phila.*, No. 4, 1869, pp. 294–313.
3. Gross, S.D., "Robley Dunglison." *Autobiography*, Vol. II, pp. 329–335.
4. Wagner, F.B. Jr., "The Dunglison Grave Revisited," *Jeff. Al. Bull.*, Fall 1984, pp. 7–10.
5. Kelly, H.A., and Burrage, W.L., "Robert Mendenhall Huston," *Dict. Am. Med. Biog.* New York: D. Appleton & Co., 1928, p. 624.
6. Kelly, H.A., and Burrage, W.L., "Joseph Pancoast" *American Medical Biographies.* Baltimore: Remington Co., 1920, pp. 879–880.
7. Gross. S.D., "John K. Mitchell," *Autobiography*, Vol. II, pp. 295–297.
8. Meigs, J.F., "Memoir of Charles D. Meigs, M.D.," *Trans. Stud. Coll. Phys. Phila.*, N.S. 4, 1872, pp. 417–448.
9. Gross, S.D., "Franklin Bache," *Autobiography*, Vol. II, pp. 306–307.
10. Wood, G.B., *Biographical Memoir of Franklin Bache.* Philadelphia: J.B. Lippincott Co., 1865.
11. Pancoast, J., "A Discourse Commemorative of the Late Professor T.D. Mütter, M.D., LL.D., Being the Introductory Lecture to the Course of Anatomy in the Jefferson Medical College of Philadelphia. Delivered Oct. 14, 1859." Philadelphia: Joseph M. Wilson, 1859.
12. Mitchell, J.S., "Mütter Museum." *Jeff. Al. Bull.*, Vol. 27, No. 3, Spring 1978.

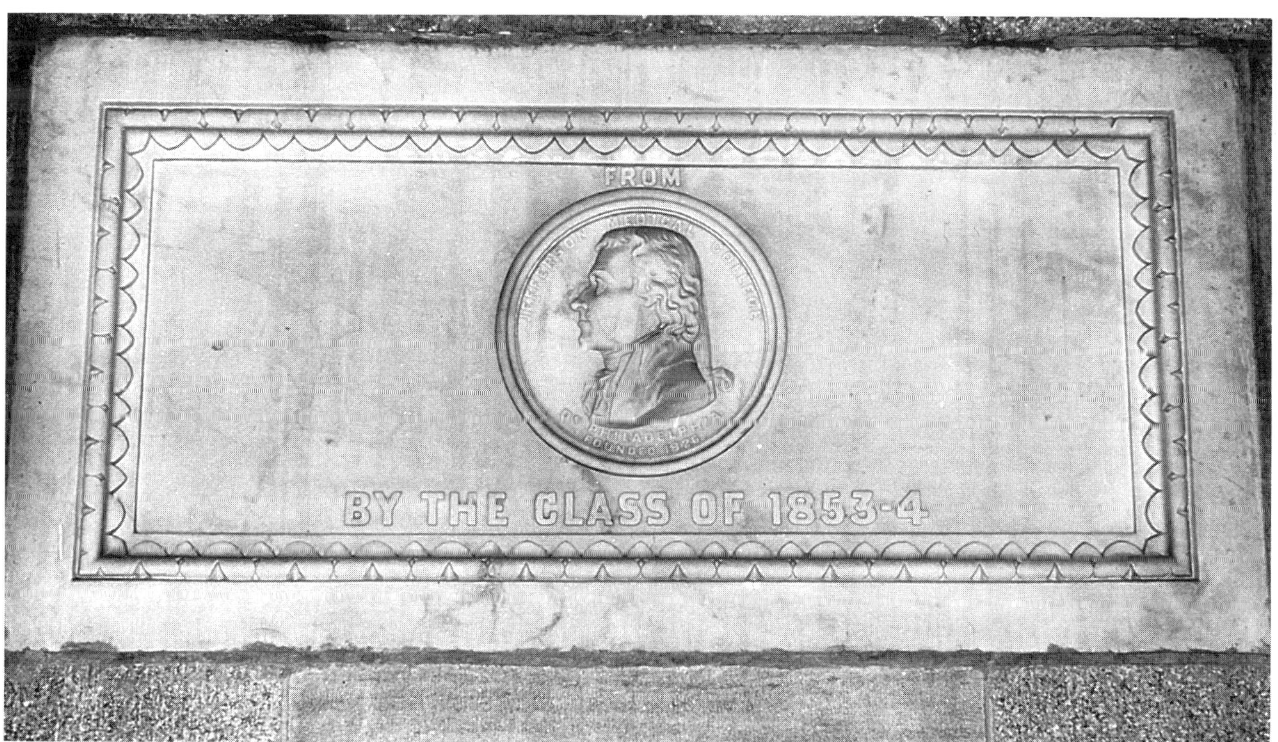

FIG. 2-3. Stone in Washington Monument, Washington, D.C., at the 280-foot landing donated by the Jefferson Class of 1853–1854. (Courtesy of U.S. Department of Interior, National Park Service.)

The Attached Miniature Hospital Ward (1843–1877): Renovation of Medical Hall (1846)

The use of collegiate clinics, which was a strong feature of the instruction at Jefferson, continued to flourish, especially with the expansion in surgery after 1841. Patients who underwent operations before students in the amphitheater of the College were sent home in a carriage, with further care by an assistant or the surgeon himself. Around 1843 the rooms over the shop of a stove-maker at the southwest corner of Tenth and Sansom Streets were rented for the stay of patients after more serious operations. A few years later the upper floors over a bottling establishment between the corner store and the College (Figure 2-4) were rented for the same purpose.[1] Remodeling was inevitable with the increased demands, and eventuated in a meager but comfortable miniature hospital capable of accommodating about fifteen patients. The store ownership may have changed hands, for DaCosta refers to the little hospital "pleasantly placed over a cigar store and oyster saloon."[2] A fireproof door connected this facility directly with the second-floor clinical amphitheater of the College where the surgery took place. This small hospital served from 1843 until 1877, when the new first detached Jefferson Medical College Hospital was opened for extended clinical purposes.

The attached hospital facilities proved sufficient for the needs of the day, although it was occasionally necessary to rent the rooms from other nearby properties. The kitchen stove of the family below furnished much of the food for the patients, and nearby restaurants could be called upon. The medical students acted as clinical clerks and watched the patients' condition under the supervision of the surgeon or his assistant. A nurse on a weekly salary was employed later. Relays of students remained on day and night duty. The faculty provided them a midnight meal of oysters with steaming coffee to ensure their wakefulness, and other hearty refreshments with cigars might be their reward.

Within eight years of the 1838 Independent Charter and the enlargement of Medical Hall by Thomas Ustick Walter, another expansion of the College was required. A change of location for the school was considered, but the decision was made to stay and remodel. The architect chosen was the 26-year-old Napoleon LeBrun, who had trained under Walter.[3] Even at this early age LeBrun was designing the interior of the Cathedral of Saints Peter and Paul at Eighteenth and Race, and his later work would include the Academy of Music in which Jefferson's graduation exercises would be held. A property to the north side of the College was acquired and cleared, allowing for a nine-foot extension of the north wall. The front was rebuilt in the form of a Roman temple with six Corinthian columns resting on a base seven feet above the street level and supporting a handsome pediment and entablature (Figure 2-4). The basement was faced with marble in which the grooves were deeply placed to make the segments more prominent. The upper facade was covered with a coating of cement painted a light stone color to match the base. An exterior connection to the remaining property fronting on Tenth Street was established by a railing and iron gateway. This passage led to the rear where the entrance and stairway to all the floors was relocated in a

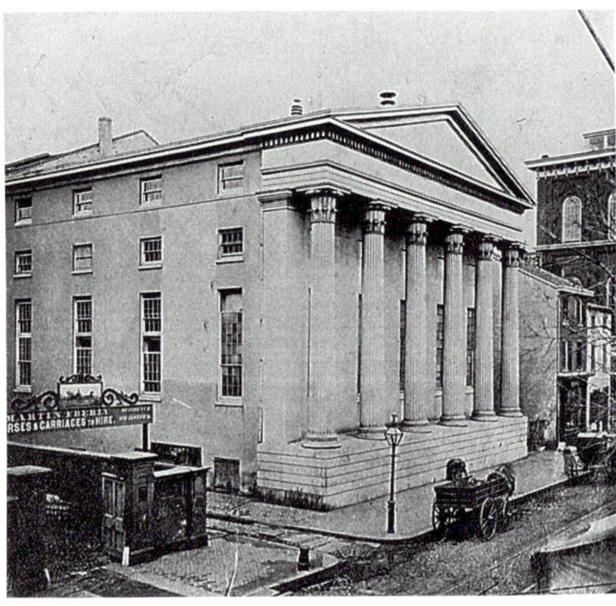

FIG. 2-4. The renovated Medical Hall with Grecian facade (1846). The upper floors of two stores became a miniature hospital ward.

backward extension of the original building. The remodeled building was considered "an ornament to the city."

On the first floor was a lecture hall in which the seating capacity was increased from 450 to 600. Special attention was paid to lighting, ventilation, and acoustics considered optimal for that time. The upper amphitheater, or "pit," was located on the second and third floors, in which the skylight provided illumination for surgery. It likewise was enlarged to accommodate 600 students. The museum at the rear of the second floor provided ample materials for osseous, neurologic, vascular, muscular, ligamentous, and other preparations for anatomical demonstrations. It also contained a large number of wet preparations relating to pathology, obstetrics, and surgery. An extensive collection of diseased bones, calculi, models in wood, plaster, and wax, together with a series of paintings and engravings of healthy and morbid organs, fractures, dislocations, and tumors completed this section. The anatomical dissecting room was over the museum on the third story and pronounced the very best for its purpose. Convenient rooms for the faculty and private chambers for the professors and students were placed in the rear of the stairways of all three floors.

It was in the upper amphitheater that on December 23, 1846, Thomas Dent Mütter was the first in Philadelphia to demonstrate the anesthetic power of sulphuric ether.[3] The operation was for the removal of a tumor from the cheek, possibly a sebaceous cyst. This epoch-making discovery which became a permanent part of operative surgery had only been demonstrated by Morton in Boston on November 19, 1846. Tragic squabbles over the legal rights led to dentist Horace Wells' suicide in 1848, dentist William T.G. Morton's death in 1868 from apoplexy while enraged at learning of attempts to deprive him of the glory of his discovery, and chemist Charles T. Jackson's insanity and death in 1880.[4] Ironically, Edward R. Squibb (Jefferson graduate in the Class of 1845) made his fortune in the manufacture of ether.

Surgery at midcentury was performed only for wounds and abscesses, amputations, removal of superficial tumors and bladder stones, ligation for aneurysm, and trephination of the skull for depressed fractures or extradural abscess. Appendicitis was called peritonitis and patients were watched to die, although some did recover. Abdominal surgery, if performed at all, might be for wounds, intestinal obstruction, strangulated hernia, or large ovarian tumors. Radical cure for hernia was more than a generation away. Chest surgery did not exist except for empyema, and drainage was so often fatal that many clinicians declined to recommend it. Catgut ligatures were not used. Almost all wounds suppurated. The mortality from compound fractures was 60 to 80 percent. Wound healing after breast amputation required three to six months and did not result in cure. Limb amputations required several months. Hemostats were not used and bleeding to death on the operating table was not unusual. Operating lights were undreamed of, and Edison's incandescent lamp would not be invented until 1879. Ether and chloroform were distrusted novelties. Bacteriology was unknown. Cerebral localization was not imagined, and it was believed that the brain, like the liver, functioned as a whole.

The physician of 1849 was without the ophthalmoscope, practical laryngoscope, endoscope, cystoscope, or X-rays. Hypodermic medication was yet to be devised. Therapeutics was empirical. Bloodletting was still employed, although not as frequently. Huge doses of purgatives were administered. Calomel was given as a general cure-all. There were only a few competent dentists, and the Pennsylvania Dental College was not to open until 1850. There was not a single woman physician, and the Woman's Medical College was not founded until 1850.

The American Medical Association was organized in 1847, with Dr. Nathaniel Chapman elected by acclamation as first President. The Committee on Constitution for the Philadelphia County Medical Society met on January 16, 1848, and Dr. Samuel Jackson, Professor of Institutes of Medicine at the University of Pennsylvania, was its first President. By 1853 it had 220 members; and fifty years later it would have 700. Prominent Jeffersonians who later in the century would become Presidents were Samuel D. Gross, James A. Meigs, Washington L. Atlee, Richard J. Levis, and William W. Keen. The profession in 1849 was opposed to women physicians and the County Medical Society recommended not to consult with them. The first woman would not be elected into membership until 1888.

Philadelphia at this time was the medical center of the country. An ambitious physician could regard a Chair in one of its Colleges as the crowning point of his career. In 1849 the University of Pennsylvania had 508 students, Jefferson Medical College had 480, Philadelphia College of Medicine, 91, Pennsylvania Medical College, 90, and the Franklin Medical College, about 40. The three last-named schools have not survived.

The city proper lay between the Delaware and the Schuylkill Rivers and between Vine and South Streets, with a population of 120,000. The various adjacent districts and townships such as the Northern Liberties, Frankford, Kensington, Southwark, Moyamensing, West Philadelphia, and Germantown swelled the total to 400,000. Philadelphia was quiet and unostentatious, but nurtured a highly cultured society. Houses of the affluent were built of brick with white marble facings. The rear yards were grass covered. Shutters were closed at sundown. Each front door contained a plate with the owner's name. Outside steps and pavements were washed daily. The pavements were of brick and the streets of cobblestones. Houses of the poor were of frame and fires were frequent. There were no street cars, but horse-drawn carriages and omnibuses served for transportation.

There were 30 states in the Union, Wisconsin having most recently been admitted. The territories of California and New Mexico had been added by the Mexican War. Famine in Ireland and political discontent in European countries were drawing tens of thousands of immigrants to America. Gold had been discovered in California and 200,000 hopeful people were heading west for quick fortunes. Locomotives were beginning to link cities, but in many sections of the country travel was by foot, emigrant wagon, stagecoach, or canal boat. Slavery and antislavery forces had begun to clash and already were threatening to split the nation.

In the currents of this local and national climate the famous faculty of 1841 remained unbroken until the 1856 resignation of Professor Thomas Dent Mütter, who was in poor health. For all his brilliant and beneficent qualities, he was but the torchbearer for the arrival of the "greatest American surgeon of his time," Dr. Samuel D. Gross.[5]

References

1. Brinton, J.H., *The Faculty of 1841.* Philadelphia: Collins, Printer, 1980, p. 5.
2. DaCosta, J.C., *The Papers and Speeches.* Philadelphia: W.B. Saunders Co., 1931, p. 353.
3. Teitelman, E., "Jefferson's Architecture," *Jeff. Al. Bull.*, Fall 1965, p. 13.
4. Garrison, F.H., *An Introduction to the History of Medicine.* 4th ed., Philadelphia: W.B. Saunders Co., 1929, p. 506.
5. Idem 4, p. 599.

Samuel D. Gross, M.D., LL.D., D.C.L.: A Third Epoch (1856–1882)

The first epoch in Jefferson's history (1824–1841) was a struggle for survival. The second (1841–1856) was an epoch of achievement due to the unbroken faculty of 1841. The third epoch (1856–1882) was one of prestige that encompassed the Professorship of Samuel D. Gross (Figure 2-5). He, as a son of Jefferson Medical College in the class of 1828, was the first alumnus to be called to a Professorship in his alma mater. Most of the previous professors had been graduates of the University of Pennsylvania. In a plenitude of superb attributes Gross brought lasting fame to Jefferson and worldwide recognition to American medicine as a whole. An unflagging intellectual energy placed him in the undisputed position of leader of academic surgery of his era and served him well as teacher, investigator, writer, anatomist, pathologist, clinician, and surgeon. Numerous accounts have eulogized his life, but the chronicle was best told by Gross himself in his two-volume *Autobiography* of more than 1,000 pages.[1–3] Lionized by the alumni of Jefferson, honored at home and abroad, immortalized in art and sculpture, and regarded as the "Emperor of

American Surgery" of his era, Gross clearly delineated a third epoch.

Gross's ancestry was German, his great-grandfather having emigrated from the Lower Palatinate in the seventeenth century. Samuel Gross was born on July 8, 1805, on a farm of 200 acres within four miles of Easton, Pennsylvania. This was Pennsylvania Dutch country, in which the Americanized German patois was the dominant language. Until adolescence Gross spoke only this unique Pennsylvania Dutch dialect, which is unintelligible even to native Germans. He first learned English after the age of 12 and

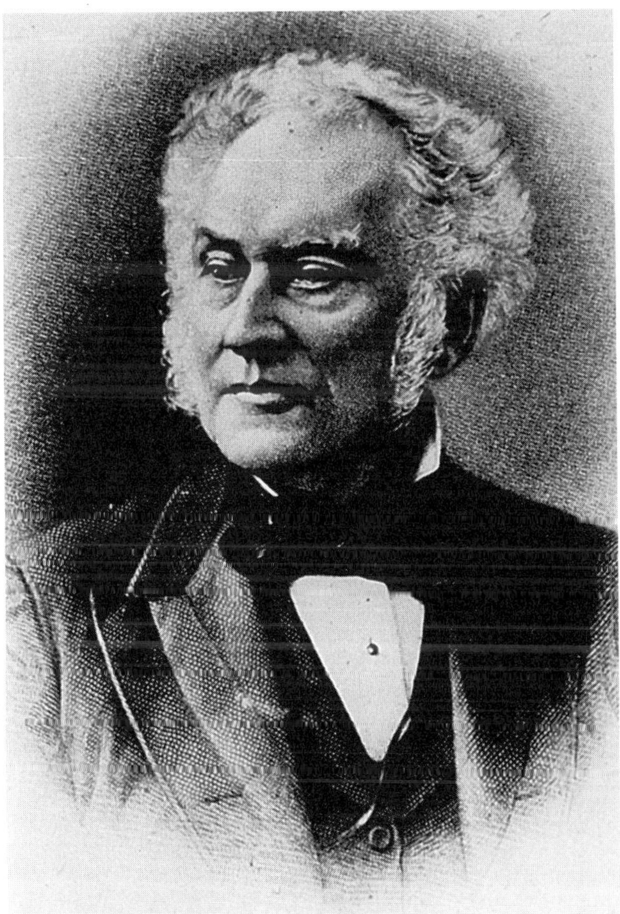

FIG. 2-5. Samuel D. Gross, M.D., LL.D., D.C.L.; Professor of Surgery (1856–1882).

subsequently studied the true German language, which left him with a slight foreign accent for the rest of his life.

Philip and Juliana Gross had six children of which Samuel David was the fifth. Of his three brothers, one, Joseph B., became a minister in the Lutheran Church. The mother was a devoted Lutheran, but the father had no strong religious orientation. Gross ascribed his strong moral character to the good training by his mother. Following a long illness, his father died in 1813 at age 56 from cerebral apoplexy when Samuel was nine. The mother lived to be 86 and died in 1853 while Gross was still at Louisville, Kentucky.

Gross enjoyed the usual pleasures of a country boy, such as hunting birds and squirrels with a blow gun, searching for beehives, and pitching quoits or pennies—he believed that tossing pennies developed coordination of eye and hand that aided his surgery of later years. His fondness for flowers throughout life was later shared by Grace Revere, who married his son Samuel W.

Although Gross acquired the nickname "Judge" in childhood, he recognized the desire to become a doctor at the age of six. From then on he considered himself to be a "born doctor." He began public school in a log cabin. There was but a single class for boys and girls of all ages. The teacher was a tyrant who used the rod freely. Gross preferred languages to mathematics and geometry. He realized his education was desultory, but improved it by avid reading of the *Bible, Aesop's Fables,* almanacs, geography, and history. To this he added extra hours for the study of English, German, and Latin. By the age of 17 he considered himself ready to study medicine.

The custom was to read medicine in the office of a preceptor physician. The books were usually scant and obsolete. Gross was quickly dissatisfied with his first two preceptors but then stayed with Dr. Joseph K. Swift of Easton, who was a graduate of the University of Pennsylvania. He studied anatomy from a skeleton with use of Fyfe's *Anatomy.* At this juncture Gross determined to prepare himself for a first-class medical career by attending the famous Academy at Lawrenceville, New Jersey. There he carefully studied Latin as well as Greek from a grammar written in Latin. He learned sufficient French to enable him to translate the texts into English, and a smattering of Italian. Considering himself to be properly prepared he resumed his preceptor studies with Dr. Swift with such zeal that his health broke down. For a remedy he rode by horseback to Niagara Falls with a brother. This six weeks was well spent, for he was restored to a vigorous state of health that lasted until he was 77.

Gross left for Philadelphia in October 1826, with letters of recommendation from Dr. Swift to Professors Dewees and Horner of the University of Pennsylvania. The brilliant achievements of Dr. George McClellan were of such repute, however, that he disregarded the wishes of his preceptor and enlisted as McClellan's private pupil. Several weeks later he matriculated in the "new school" as it was called. Gross never returned to his preceptor's office in Easton and believed he had given Dr. Swift offense, although he had paid his fee in full.

After adjusting to the revolting sight and odor of the dissecting room, Gross became intrigued by the dissections and made a special study of practical anatomy. Beyond the regular course he spent an extra month dissecting in the spring and fall. In addition to surgical anatomy he developed a deep interest in the structure of the brain and distribution of the peripheral and sympathetic nerves.

As a Jefferson student attending the renovated Prune Street Tivoli Theater, Gross seldom retired before a late hour. In his words, he became ". . . a stranger to all amusements, and medicine was the goddess of my idolatry." His Professors were George McClellan in Surgery, Nathan Smith in Anatomy, John Eberle in Medicine, William Barton in Materia Medica, Jacob Green in Chemistry, John Barnes in Obstetrics and Benjamin Rush Rhees in Institutes and Medical Jurisprudence. Gross's opinion of his teachers after two courses of lectures was as follows:

> "They were perhaps, in the main, as competent instructors as any similar number of teachers in the schools of this country at that period; for, after all, everything depends upon the student himself, his industry, his habits of attention, his culture, and his natural capacity. His knowledge must come chiefly through his own personal exertion. Lectures, however able or erudite, are only aids. They never can make a good physician or a great man out of a dunce."

Gross received his M.D. degree in 1828 in a class of 27; his graduation thesis was *The Nature and Treatment of Cataract*. The exercises were held in the spring for the last time in the Tivoli Theater Building. Little could Gross foretell that 28 years later he would return to his alma mater and become recognized as "the greatest American surgeon of his time."

Shortly after graduation Gross married Louisa Ann Weissel, a widow 21 years of age with a child that subsequently died. Deeply in love, they consummated nearly 48 years of happy family life. Of their eight children, two boys and two girls survived into adulthood, and they inherited the intellectual energy of their father. Samuel W. succeeded the elder Gross in 1882 as Professor of the Principles of Surgery and Clinical Surgery. The other son, A. Haller, matriculated at Jefferson for one year but abandoned medicine to become a prominent member of the Philadelphia Bar. Maria Rives Gross married Orville Horwitz, a Baltimore lawyer, and was a distinguished litterateur, linguist, and musician. She endowed the first Chair of Surgery at Jefferson in 1910 in honor of her father. Louisa Gross married Benjamin Horwitz, the brother of Orville, also a Baltimore lawyer. The Louisa Gross Horwitz Prize of Columbia University was endowed in her honor by her son, S. Gross Horwitz, the grandson of Samuel D. Gross. It has been awarded annually as an honorarium of $25,000 with a citation at a special presentation for outstanding basic research in the fields of biology or biochemistry. Of the 18 recipients between 1967 and 1984, eight have subsequently received Nobel prizes.

Gross decided to practice in Philadelphia after graduation and opened his office at the corner of Fifth and Library Streets, opposite Independence Square. The first year he earned only $300, which scarcely covered expenses. During this lean time he translated Bayle and Hollard's *General Anatomy* and Hatin's *Manual of Practical Obstetrics* from the French. The second year he continued translating foreign texts with Tavernier's *Operative Surgery* from French and Hildenbrand's *Treatise on Contagious Typhus* from German. His knowledge of languages gained him extra funds, initiated his academic reputation, and aroused a desire to write books on his own. He never again made translations because his conviction was that America should have its own medical texts. The financial return from his practice and literary work was so poor for the second year that his only alternative was to try for success in his native Easton.

In April, 1830, he opened an office opposite that of his old preceptor, Dr. Swift. A respectable practice developed promptly, as well as a reputation as a scientific physician. In 1832 an epidemic of Asiatic cholera broke out with extreme virulence in New York City, just 80 miles away from Easton. Gross was appointed by his town council to visit New York to possibly learn how to aid his fellow citizens. He visited the hospitals and charnel houses during a hot week in July. Fortunately, Gross did not contract the scourge, nor did it strike Easton.

Gross erected a small stone building in the garden at the rear of his Easton house for anatomic dissection and animal experimentation. Stray dogs and cats were absorbed into this laboratory and he would occasionally transfer a cadaver from Philadelphia by horse and buggy. At this time Gross was working on a book of descriptive anatomy in which he intended to change the nomenclature from Latin to English. Despite the spending of his leisure time in dissection and composition, the book was not completed. On the other hand, within three months of his arrival in Easton he readied his first original text, *Anatomy, Physiology, and Diseases of the Bones and Joints*. This octavo volume of almost 400 pages sold 2,000 copies in less than four years, but he never received a penny of remuneration. In his *Autobiography* he states: "I went little into society and took hardly any recreation. I labored day and night under the stimulus both of ambition and of poverty."

Gross struggled in Philadelphia against debt and in Easton against mediocrity. Like his role model, Dr. George McClellan, he longed to teach anatomy. In the spring of 1833 he made this desire known to his former Jefferson Professor of Medicine, Dr. John Eberle, who was now lecturing in the Medical College of Ohio at Cincinnati. Through this connection he obtained an appointment as Demonstrator of Anatomy by October of that year. He taught for two years in this capacity. By 1835 the Medical Department of Cincinnati College was organized to include a Chair of Pathological Anatomy. After unanimous appointment to that Chair by the Trustees, Gross delivered the first systematic course of lectures on morbid anatomy ever given in the United States. The teaching, dissecting, reading, and visiting of the slaughterhouses provided material for his next textbook, *Elements of Pathological Anatomy,* which was published in 1838. In two octavo volumes of over 500 pages each, with numerous woodcuts and several colored engravings, it represented the first systematic work on this subject ever produced on either side of the Atlantic. A second edition, much enlarged and extensively revised, appeared in 1845. It was a single octavo volume of 822 pages with colored engravings, 252 woodcuts and marginal references. Dr. Rudolf Virchow, the famed German pathologist, declared his admiration for the book at a dinner given for Dr. Gross in Berlin in 1868. The Imperial Royal Society of Vienna recognized its merit by making him an honorary member.

The closing of Cincinnati College in 1839 only helped to broaden Gross's career. He was offered the Chair of Anatomy at the University of Louisiana as well as the Professorship of Medicine at the University of Virginia. His ultimate goal of a Professorship of Surgery was realized by his acceptance of the Chair at the Louisville Medical Institute, later the University of Louisville. He made this move in October 1840, when he was 35 years old.

Gross's Louisville years, 1840 to 1856, were fruitful and happy except for a temporary interruption in 1850. A controversy regarding the government of the Medical School led Gross in that year to accept the Chair of Surgery at the University of New York just vacated by the retirement of the prestigious Valentine Mott (1787–1865). The latter was one of the most eminent physicians of the first half of the nineteenth century. Mott's ligations of major arteries for aneurysmal disease, performed before the discovery of anesthesia, antisepsis, and use of transfusions, subsequently earned him the title "Father of American Vascular Surgery."[14] This turned out to be a sabbatical year in that it relieved Gross of his large private practice, provided time to write most of two books, and allowed visits to surgical clinics, one of which was to Mütter's at Jefferson. After Gross served for only one academic session the management of the Louisville school was corrected. At the urgent request of his old colleagues he returned to his former post. His successor, Dr. Paul F. Eve, graciously stepped aside for him and the New York Chair was taken by Dr. Alfred C. Post.

In Louisville, Gross was beloved, trusted, and popular with patients, colleagues, and nonprofessional friends. His spacious home provided traditional southern hospitality for distinguished American and foreign guests in medicine, science, law, arts, literature, politics, and the military. His charming wife kept an ample table ready for reunions in which "the strains of music mingled with flashes of wit and humor."

By 1855, at the age of 50, Gross had planned to spend the rest of his days in Louisville. Fate decreed otherwise, for Philadelphia called that year from the University of Pennsylvania and the following year from his Jefferson alma mater.

In 1855, Dr. Rene LaRoche, a member of the Board of Trustees of the University of Pennsylvania, solicited Gross to allow his name to be placed as a candidate for the Chair of Surgery vacated by the resignation of Dr. William Gibson (1788–1868), a former bitter rival of Gross's teacher, George McClellan. Gross held America's oldest medical school in the highest esteem but could not persuade himself to pursue the offer, especially since the income would be less than he was receiving at Louisville. Instead, he wrote, at the request of Dr. Agnew D. Hays, a warm testimonial in favor of Dr. Henry H. Smith, who was elected. Agnew (1818–1892), who himself in 1871 succeeded to the Chair and in 1877 became the first John Rhea Barton Professor of Surgery, remained one of Gross's warmest friends and served as chairman of a complimentary dinner given in honor of Gross at the St. George Hotel (Bellevue) in Philadelphia in April 1879.[3] The University conferred an LL.D. degree on Gross in 1884, although he was on his deathbed. With the resignation in 1856 of Professor Thomas Dent Mütter due to poor health, the Board of Trustees of Jefferson turned unanimously to Gross as successor. He was taken by surprise but much flattered by the election, which occurred in May. His family was averse to leaving Louisville, so before accepting, Gross visited Philadelphia to ascertain the state of affairs at Jefferson. He found the College in an eminently flourishing condition and therefore accepted the Chair without further hesitation.

Gross and his family on arrival in Philadelphia in September, 1856, rented Mütter's furnished house at the southeast corner of Eleventh and Walnut Streets, now the location of the Martin Residence Building. For their first dinner Dr. Dunglison sent a bottle of champagne, a beverage heartily approved by Gross. Rent was continued annually for two years at $2,000, at the end of which time Gross purchased the property for $25,000 cash. He was obliged to spend nearly $2,000 for repairs. At his death in 1884 the house passed into other ownership, since his son, Dr. Samuel W., had previously purchased a house at 1112 Walnut Street for $39,000. Dr. Joe Henry Coley (Jefferson, 1934) witnessed the demolition of the house in the early 1930s and regretted not having saved a brick as a relic for the Jefferson archives.

In his inaugural address of the opening of the 1856–1857 session of the College, Gross concluded: "Whatever of life, and of health, and of strength remains to me, I hereby, in the presence of Almighty God and of the large assemblage dedicate to the cause of my Alma Mater, to the interests of Medical Science, and to the good of my fellow-creatures." For the next 26 years of his active Chairmanship no pledge was better kept.

As Gross was about to go before his class on the day before Christmas of the first year, the janitor handed him a telegram that read: "The University (of Louisville) was totally consumed by fire early this morning, including all your books and minerals." This represented a loss of about 2,000 books, which contained the most extensive collection on the genitourinary organs ever assembled in this country. They were not insured. Another 2,000 books had fortunately been previously brought to Philadelphia.

In coming to Jefferson as the fourth Chairman of Surgery, Gross had to compete with the charm, teaching, and surgical skill for which the idolized Mütter had acquired an enviable reputation. Gross immediately commanded a respect and popularity with the students that exceeded Mütter's zenith. A growing fame of the Gross Clinic attracted visitors from home and abroad. The class that winter was very large, such that the income for each Chair exceeded $5,000. From then on until the start of the Civil War the number of students varied between 475 and 631.

During Gross's second year at Jefferson (1857–1858) there were four medical schools in Philadelphia, with a total of 1,139 students. Jefferson had 501, the University of Pennsylvania 435, Pennsylvania College (founded by George McClellan in 1839), 140, and the Philadelphia College, 63. The total number of graduates at that period from these institutions was 407, with distribution in the same order: 209, 145, 35, and 18. The last two institutions would merge and become extinct by attrition during the Civil War.

It was customary at this time for each professor to deliver an introductory lecture at the opening session of his course, with the result that the first week was an academic waste to the students. Gross felt that only one general introductory was sufficient and that the didactic courses should commence the next day. With repeated interviews between Jefferson and the University of Pennsylvania, he was able after four years to effect this change for the two institutions. Gross declared: "It was almost as hard to move the two Faculties of the schools in this matter as it would be for a regiment of soldiers to move the rock of Gibraltar, so completely steeped were they in fogyism."

The phenomenal success of Gross as teacher, author, surgeon, investigator, historian, and founder of societies will be detailed in the history of the Department of Surgery. The "Emperor of Surgery" or "Nestor of Surgery," as he is frequently remembered, retired in 1882 and died two years later. His Professorship was divided between two successors, which elicited the comment that "it took two pegs to fill one hole."

As with the replacement of Mütter by Gross, the withdrawal or death of the other members of the faculty of 1841 did not weaken the school. The real threat was the Civil War.

References

1. Bauer, E.L., *Doctors Made in America.* Philadelphia: J.B. Lippincott Co., 1963, pp. 123–140.
2. Cohen, A.E., "The Samuel D. Gross Sesquicentennial," *Jour. Ky. Med. Assoc.,* 53:981, 1955.
3. "Complimentary Dinner Given to Professor S.D. Gross, on 10 April, 1879." Philadelphia: Lindsay and Blakiston Co., 1879.
4. DaCosta, J.C., "Samuel David Gross." *Surg. Gynec. and Obst.,* 35:115, 1922.
5. Garrison, F.H., *An Introduction to the History of Medicine.* Philadelphia: W.B. Saunders Co., 1929, p. 599.
6. Gibbon, J.H., "Samuel D. Gross," *Ann. Med. Hist.,* 8:136, 1926.
7. Hays, I.M., "Memoir of Samuel D. Gross," *Trans. Stud. Coll. Phys. Phila.,* 7:85, 1884.
8. Keen, W.W., "Samuel David Gross: The Lesson of His Life and Labors." Eulogy Pronounced at 85th Annual Commencement of the Jefferson Medical College of Philadelphia, 6 June, 1910.
9. Kotz, A.L., "Samuel David Gross," *Pennsylvania German Society,* 39:5–20, 1930.
10. Ono, J., "The Life of Samuel D. Gross, Presented at Japanese Society of Medical History, 1969." Manuscript supplied by author in Japanese and English translation to Scott Library of Thomas Jefferson University, Special Collections.
11. Rohrer, C.W.G., "Professor Samuel D. Gross: America's Foremost Surgeon." *Bull. Johns Hopkins Hosp.,* 23:83, 1912.
12. Wagner, F.B. Jr., "Revisit of Samuel D. Gross, M.D." *Surg. Gynec. and Obst.,* 152:663–674, 1981.
13. Gross, S.D., *Autobiography of Samuel D. Gross, M.D., with Sketches of His Contemporaries.* Vols. I and II. Philadelphia: W.B. Saunders Co., 1887. Reprinted by Arno Press and the *New York Times,* 1972.
14. Ruthow, I.M., "Valentine Mott (1785–1865), the Father of American Vascular Surgery; A Historical Perspective." *Surgery,* 85:441–450, 1979.

The Ante-Bellum Years: Philadelphia circa 1860

The progress and fame of Jefferson Medical College continued even as resignation and death gradually claimed the seven members of the unbroken faculty of 1841–1856. The resignation of Mütter in 1856 and replacement by Gross in surgery was followed by the retirement of Huston in 1857 and replacement by Thomas Duché Mitchell in Materia Medica and Therapeutics. (Mitchell was not related to Dr. John Kearsley Mitchell, Professor of Medicine, who died the following year.)

■ Thomas Duché Mitchell (1791–1865)

Thomas Duché Mitchell was 66 years of age when appointed to the Professorship (Figure 2-6). He came from an old Philadelphia family, received his early education in the Quaker schools, served a preceptorship with Dr. Joseph Parrish—followed by six months in a drug store and chemical laboratory of Dr. Adam Seybert—and obtained his M.D. degree from the University of Pennsylvania in 1812. Mitchell immediately started an academic career as Instructor in Vegetable and

Animal Physiology in St. John's College on Race Street. The following year he was appointed Lazaretto Physician to the pest house on the west bank of the mouth of the Schuylkill River. His reputation as a medical writer started in 1819 when he published a volume on medical chemistry.

From 1822 to 1831 Mitchell engaged in medical practice in Philadelphia and its suburbs, established the Total Abstinence Society, in which even the use of alcohol in tinctures was deprecated, and was honored by Princeton with the Master's degree in 1830. In 1831 he joined Drs. Drake and Eberle in Cincinnati, taking the Chair of Chemistry. In 1832 he published an octavo volume of 553 pages entitled *Chemical Philosophy* and, subsequently, a volume on *Hints to Students,* and became coeditor of the *Western Medical Gazette* and editor of the *Journal of Medical and Associate Sciences.* From 1837 to 1847, Mitchell filled the Chairs of Materia Medica and Chemistry in Transylvania University, Lexington, Kentucky.

Mitchell returned in 1847 to his native Philadelphia for the Chair of Theory and Practice of Medicine in the recently organized Philadelphia College of Medicine, where he remained for the next ten years. In 1850 he published an octavo volume of 750 pages on *Materia Medica* as well as an edition of *Eberle on the Diseases of Children,* to which he contributed 200 pages of notes. His manuscript of 600 pages on the *Fevers of the United States* was never published. He wrote the biography of Dr. John Eberle for Samuel D. Gross's *American Medical Biography,* and spent the last eight years of his life at Jefferson as a clear and impressive lecturer, a classical and scientific scholar, and a highly respected gentleman.

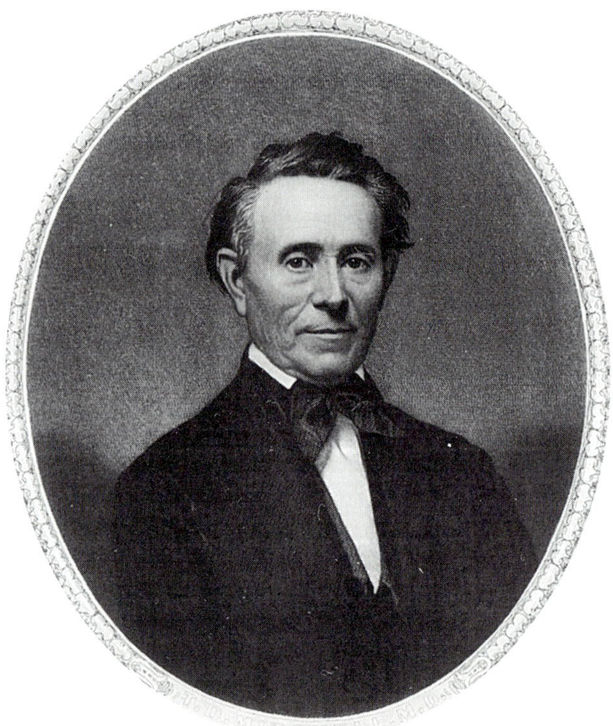

FIG. 2-6. Thomas Duché Mitchell, M.D. (1791–1865); Professor of Materia Medica and Therapeutics (1857–1865).

Samuel Henry Dickson (1798–1872)

The Chair vacated by the death of John Kearsley Mitchell in 1858 was also taken by a man well advanced in years, Samuel Henry Dickson, age 60 (Figure 2-7).[2] Dickson was born in Charleston,

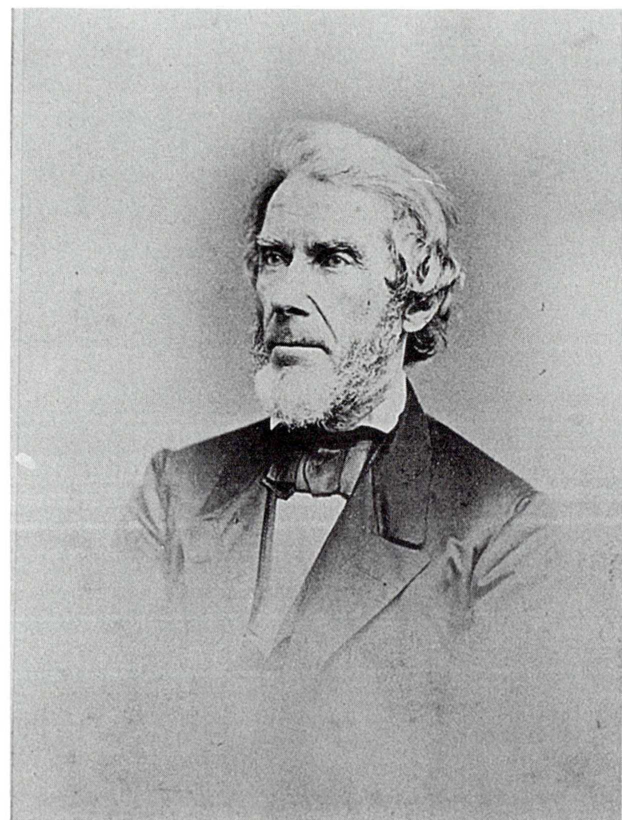

FIG. 2-7. Samuel Henry Dickson, M.D. (1798–1872); Professor of Medicine (1858–1872).

South Carolina, and was graduated from Yale College in 1814. He engaged in a preceptorship in his native city and practiced medicine without a degree during an outbreak of yellow fever there. He subsequently obtained his M.D. degree from the University of Pennsylvania in 1819 and returned to Charleston. In 1824, at the time George McClellan was founding Jefferson Medical College, Dickson joined Drs. David Ramsay and H.R. Frost in organizing the Charleston Medical College, which in 1833 was reorganized as the Medical College of South Carolina. There for 22 years he occupied the Chair of Institutes and Practice of Medicine. In 1847 Dickson replaced Dr. John Revere as Professor of Theory and Practice of Medicine at the University of the City of New York, but returned to Charleston three years later in 1850. The New York University conferred an honorary LL.D. degree on him the following year. After conducting consultation services until 1858, Dickson was called to Jefferson for the Chair of Theory and Practice of Medicine, which he filled for the next 14 years until his death at age 73.

Dr. Dickson was a man of ability and influence in medical, literary, and philanthropic circles. He was a superb orator in medicine, philosophy, and poetry. His writings, which appeared in the *Southern Quarterly Review,* Charleston, and in the *American Journal of the Medical Sciences,* were elegant in style and almost poetic. He reported upon the yellow fever in Charleston in 1817 and 1827, dengue fever in 1828, and heat stroke in 1829. His books were standards in their day and included *Manual of Pathology and Practice of Medicine, Essays on Pathology and Therapeutics,* and *Elements of Medicine.*

William Valentine Keating (1823–1894)

Charles Delucena Meigs, Professor of Obstetrics and Diseases of Women and Children, who retired in 1860, was replaced by William Valentine Keating (1823–1894). Keating, only 37 years old, was compelled to relinquish his position within the year because of poor health.[3] He was a native Philadelphian who studied under the preceptorship of Dr. Charles Delucena Meigs and graduated in medicine from the University of Pennsylvania in 1844. Keating's practice in Philadelphia gave special attention to obstetrics. He lectured in the Philadelphia Association for Medical Instruction and Agnew D. Hays Philadelphia School of Anatomy. In 1856 he edited Churchill's *Diseases of Children* and Ramsbotham's *Obstetrics.*

While abroad in Paris in 1861 in an effort to regain his health, Keating's trunk containing an original manuscript on obstetrics that represented several years of labor was stolen from a railway station and was irretrievably lost. Despite his misfortunes, the rest abroad restored his health and he returned during the Civil War with renewed vigor to serve as surgeon on the staff of the Satterlee Army Hospital in Philadelphia and also in the post of Medical Director of the Broad and Cherry Street Hospital. He was one of the founders of St. Joseph's Hospital in 1844, and at the time of his death at age 71 from a heart attack was the Medical Director of St. Joseph's and St. Agnes's Hospitals. Though Dr. Keating showed every indication of promise as the successor to Dr. Charles Meigs, he was replaced by Dr. Ellerslie Wallace in 1862.

The Philadelphia census of 1860 recorded a population of 568,000. The city was most densely settled along the Delaware River, but the citizens were dispersing west of Broad Street. The ratio of physicians to the population was increasing. The private medical schools of Philadelphia had proven so attractive that by 1860 there were 551 regular physicians for the population of over one-half million. The medical organizations consisted of the College of Physicians, the Philadelphia County Medical Society, the Pathological Society, and the Northern Medical Association. In addition to the Pennsylvania and Philadelphia Hospital (Blockley) were the Charity Hospital, St. Joseph's, the Protestant Episcopal, Children's, the Philadelphia Lying-In Charity, the Wills, the Preston Retreat, and the Howard. The two main medical schools were the University of Pennsylvania on Ninth Street and Jefferson on Tenth, whereas the remaining similar institutions were concluding their final struggle for existence. Philadelphia was the great medical center of the country, and a large student population was mainly from the South. Abraham Lincoln was elected president in 1860, and the Confederacy formed almost before the North could realize what was happening.

References

1. Kelly, H.A., and Burrage, W.L., "Thomas Duché Mitchell," *Dict. Am. Med. Biog.* New York: D. Appleton & Co., 1928, p. 857.
2. Konkle, B.A., and Henry, F.P., "Samuel Henry Dickson," *Standard History of the Medical Profession of Philadelphia.* New York: AMS Press, 1977, pp. 257–258.
3. Idem 1, p. 686.

Exodus of Southern Students: Hunter H. McGuire, M.D., LL.D.

In 1859–1860 the matriculates at Jefferson Medical College numbered 630, exceeding all records of medical schools of any country or time. The University of Pennsylvania also attained its largest enrollment in that year with an attendance of 528. This total of 1,158, plus students from the other medical schools and private students not yet enrolled, probably brought the number of Philadelphia students to about 1,300. Just two years earlier, the enrollment for Jefferson had been 501; for the University of Pennsylvania, 435; for the Pennsylvania College (McClellan's second school), 140; and the Philadelphia College, 63. Jefferson's gain in students was chiefly from the country at large, whereas gain at the University was mainly from the state of Pennsylvania. With the largest proportion of out-of-state students coming from the South, it is readily apparent that Jefferson occupied the more vulnerable position in terms of losing students in the Civil War.

Although most of the Jefferson professors had been graduates of the University of Pennsylvania, some of its most able teachers were also from the South and West, which explains the large number of students from these regions. In the record year of 630 students enrolled, the largest state contributor was still Pennsylvania, but with only 120. Then came Virginia, with 94; Alabama, with 50; Mississippi, 49; Georgia and North Carolina, 44 each; South Carolina, 36; Tennessee, 35; Kentucky, 22; and Maryland, 15. The students from Southern states, not counting states with fewer than 15, totaled 389—thus nearly 400 of the 630 were from the South.

Polarization of Northern and Southern attitudes was enhanced by press and pulpit. In this crucial atmosphere, John Brown marched into Harpers Ferry on October 17, 1859, with a body of armed men to instigate insurrection of the slaves against their masters. This rabid abolitionist was captured by federal troops, turned over to Virginia authorities, tried, and hung in Charles Town, Virginia, on December 2, 1859.

As part of a public funeral through some of the principal cities, John Brown's body was paraded through Philadelphia. Animosity flared into fights between the Southern medical students and Northern men on the streets. Some were injured and others put in jail. In this intolerable situation Drs. Hunter McGuire (Figure 2-8) and Robert Luckett called a meeting of their "quiz class" to discuss appropriate action on Tuesday, December 20, 1859, at 9 A.M. at the Assembly Building at the corner of Tenth and Chestnut Streets.[1] This

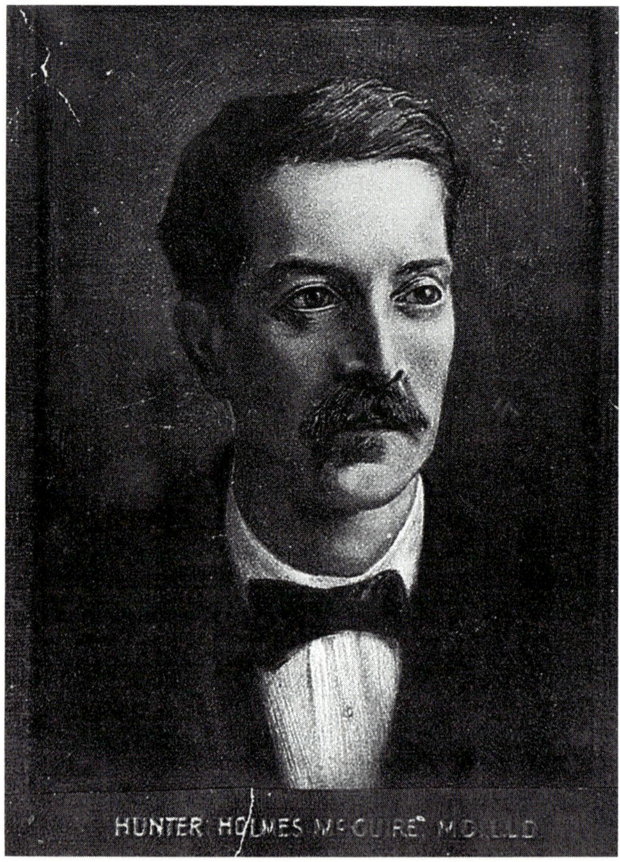

FIG. 2-8. Hunter H. McGuire, M.D., LL.D. (1835–1900); led the exodus of Southern medical students from Philadelphia to the Confederate cause.

popular "quiz class" was patronized by both Jefferson and University of Pennsylvania students, and the Assembly Building was a stone's throw from both institutions. With nearly all the Southern students present, a telegram from Governor Wise of Virginia was read, offering cordial welcome to all who would attend the College in Richmond, give credit for all previous work, and pay the expenses of transportation. Over 200 students, led in a body by Dr. McGuire, left on the evening of December 23rd. After an enthusiastic reception in Richmond, with a parade, speeches, and banquet, 140 students matriculated at the Medical College of Virginia, 56 of whom graduated in March 1860. The remaining students went to Atlanta and schools further south. The day before the great exodus Dr. Samuel D. Gross urged the importance of remaining until the end of the academic session "but, although my address was well received, the most profound silence prevailed during the delivery."

Dr. Hunter H. McGuire (1835–1900)

Dr. Hunter Holmes McGuire was a man of highest integrity and motivated only by the most genuine loyalty to his native state of Virginia.[2] His father, Dr. Hugh Holmes McGuire (1801–1873), was a graduate of the University of Pennsylvania, one of the first surgeons in the country to operate for clubfoot, President of the American Society of Surgeons, one of the founders of the Winchester Medical College, and an enlisted surgeon in the Confederate Army of Northern Virginia at the age of 60.

After preliminary education at Winchester Academy in Virginia, Hunter McGuire graduated in 1855 from the Winchester Medical College in which his father was the Professor of Surgery. To the surprise of his family and friends he decided to come to Philadelphia for wider knowledge and experience. He matriculated at Jefferson Medical College for the 1855–1856 session but accepted an invitation from Drs. Robert Luckett and Joseph Pancoast to join in the operation of a "quiz class." Because of the paucity of adequate textbooks and the limited didactic lectures of the Professors of the Medical Colleges, the students flocked to "quiz masters" to keep up with their studies and accustom themselves to examination questions. Many let their hair grow long, wore black slouch hats, and even carried bowie knives. Dr. McGuire became very popular as their advisor and leader. He even matriculated once more at Jefferson, but in the fateful session of 1859–1860; thus, despite two abortive matriculations at Jefferson he did not obtain the M.D. degree there. Dr. McGuire did matriculate in the Medical College of Virginia along with the students he brought from Philadelphia, and he received his M.D. degree for the second time at the end of the session in the spring of 1860. He then went to New Orleans where he established another "quiz class" for the students of Tulane University.

At the imminent secession of Virginia, McGuire at age 26 returned to Winchester, volunteered for army duty, and was promptly commissioned as Medical Director of the Army of the Shenandoah with General Thomas J. ("Stonewall") Jackson. He amputated Jackson's arm after the famous general was mortally wounded through a tragic mistake at Chancellorsville when the bullets of his own men felled him. Dr. McGuire was the first to advocate and practice the release of captured medical officers. He was with General Lee at Appomattox in the surrender.

In July, 1865, Dr. McGuire was elected Professor of Surgery in the Medical College of Virginia, which had been the only medical school in the Confederacy to continue operation throughout the war. In 1866 he married Mary Stuart, the daughter of a distinguished Virginia statesman. He hoped to support his wife on a salary from the Medical College of Virginia, but during the 12 years he taught in that institution he never received any.

In addition to extensive private practice in Richmond, Dr. McGuire established a Retreat for the Sick and organized St. Luke's Home for the Sick, which in 1886 developed a training school for nurses, the second one south of the Mason–Dixon line (there was one at New Orleans). Old Confederate soldiers were treated in this hospital without charge.

McGuire's literary contributions included reports of cases, clinical lectures, scientific papers, articles for standard systems and encyclopedias of medicine and surgery, presidential addresses to regional, state, and national medical societies, and reports to Confederate veteran associations with lectures on Stonewall Jackson. He was President of the American Surgical Association in 1887 and of the American Medical Association in 1893.

In 1887 the University of North Carolina conferred on McGuire an honorary LL.D. degree. According to Dr. John Chalmers DaCosta, Dr. McGuire lectured in the pit of the amphitheater of the first detached Jefferson Hospital of 1877.[3] He was awarded an LL.D. degree from Jefferson in 1888.

Friendship and affection existed between Drs. McGuire and William Osler for many years.[4] Dr. Osler visited him during his last illness, a stroke at age 65, and was one of the honorary pallbearers at the funeral. McGuire's monument is in the Capitol Square of Richmond.

References

1. Konkle, B.A., and Henry, F.P., *Standard History of the Medical Profession of Philadelphia.* 2d ed. New York: AMS Press, 1977, p. 220.
2. McGuire, S., "Hunter Holmes McGuire, M.D., LL.D.," *Ann. Med. Hist.*, N.S., 10:1–14, 136–161; 1938.
3. DaCosta, J.C., *Selections from the Papers and Speeches of John Chalmers DaCosta, M.D., LL.D.* Philadelphia: W.B., Saunders Co., 1931, p. 351.
4. Cushing, H., *The Life of Sir William Osler,* Vol. I. Oxford: Clarendon Press, 1925, pp. 277, 416, and 575.

Civil War Years (1861–1865): Jefferson Contributions

Although the triumvirate of Gross, Dunglison, and Pancoast convinced some students from the South to stay at Jefferson, more than 200 defected. The record enrollment of 630 in 1860 fell to 433 in 1861 and to 238 in 1862. This drop was also occasioned by Northern students who enlisted in the Union Army. Despite these adverse circumstances student enrollment increased to 275 in 1863, to 351 in 1864, and to 380 in 1865. Closing of the College was not threatened nor considered by the Board of Trustees or the Faculty. Robley Dunglison, one of Jefferson's greatest Deans, continued to preside throughout this period.

■ Ellerslie Wallace (1818–1885)

Only two replacements in the major faculty were required during these critical years, despite the enormous demands of the war. The first, in 1862, occurred in Obstetrics by the retirement of Charles Delucena Meigs in 1861 and the short-lived replacement by Dr. Valentine Keating, who resigned because of poor health. Ellerslie Wallace was a wise choice, for he had already taught at Jefferson for 16 years as a Demonstrator of Anatomy and would occupy the Chair of Obstetrics for 20 more, acting also as Dean during the last four of those years (Figure 2-9).[1] Wallace was a native Philadelphian, of English and Scottish ancestry, whose earlier education was at Bristol College in civil engineering and surveying. A change of interest to medicine led him to study with his brother, Joshua, who was a Demonstrator of Anatomy at Jefferson. After graduation from Jefferson in 1843 at the age of 24 he spent three years as a Resident Physician at the Pennsylvania Hospital. He then took his brother's place as Demonstrator of Anatomy at Jefferson and conducted a private practice. Wallace was only 43 when called to the Chair of Obstetrics and Diseases of Women and Children, a deserved promotion.

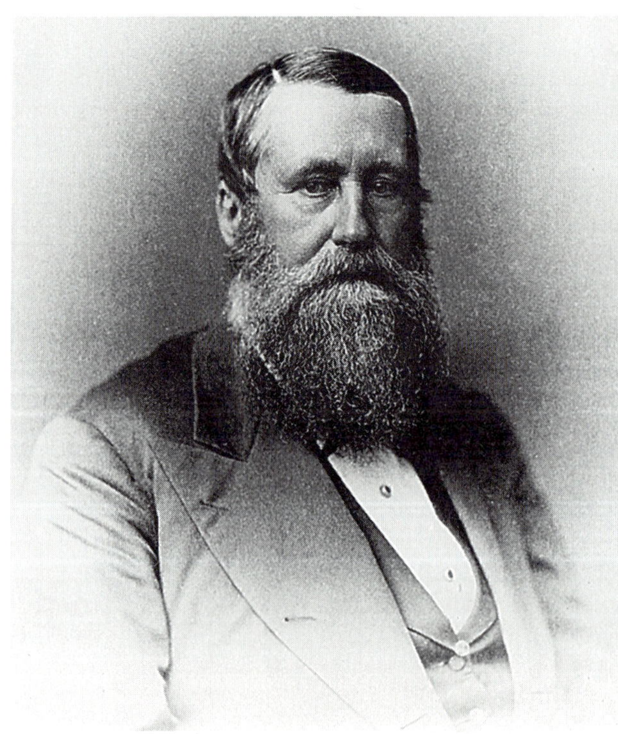

FIG. 2-9. Ellerslie Wallace, M.D. (1818–1885); Professor of Obstetrics (1862–1883) and Dean (1879–1883).

Dr. Wallace's powerful physique added to the impression of his clear lectures, which gave him recognition as one of the ablest Professors of Obstetrics in the country. He emphasized the structure of the pelvis as related to the size of the baby's head. To facilitate difficult labor he devised his own modification of forceps. He also invented a cephalotribe (head crusher) for instances when the head was too large for the birth canal, as in hydrocephalus. His writings were modest in amount and possibly retarded by his heavy load of teaching and the Deanship from 1879 to 1883.

During the war Dr. Wallace was an active member of the Union League of Philadelphia, which had been organized on November 22, 1862, as "The Union Club of Philadelphia." Membership required "unqualified loyalty to the Government of the United States, and unwavering support for the suppression of the Rebellion."[2] He served on the Board of Directors during 1865–1866.

Ellerslie Wallace, Jr., was graduated from Jefferson in 1879, the year his father became Dean. The elder Wallace resigned in 1883 and died in 1885 before he reached 66.

Philadelphia was a gigantic hospital center throughout the entire Civil War. On the Union side there were 16 hospital departments with an eventual total of 118,057 beds. Washington, D.C., was the largest department with 21,426 beds, and Philadelphia was next largest at 18,709. By December, 1864, there were 15 military hospitals in Philadelphia and its environs. With few exceptions all the best known Philadelphia physicians served for various lengths of time in these large hospitals as volunteers, regular army, or contract physicians and surgeons.

The first military hospital in Philadelphia was organized at the Christian Street commissioner's hall, May 6, 1861, at about the same time the first military hospital was opened in Washington. Additional buildings were secured to constitute the Military Hospital of Philadelphia. Previous commercial structures were renovated, such as the railroad depot at Broad and Cherry Streets, a coach factory at Fifth and Buttonwood, an old arsenal at Sixteenth and Filbert made famous by Dr. S. Weir Mitchell's novel *In War Time,* and a former silk factory at South and Twenty-fourth Streets. In May 1862, the Satterlee Hospital, the largest military hospital in the country, was begun in West Philadelphia at Forty-fourth and Spruce Streets. It was intended to care for 2,000, but by October it accommodated 2,458, and by the end of the war had a capacity of over 3,500. In December, 1862, the Mower Hospital in Chestnut Hill opened as the third largest in the country. In February, 1863, the McClellan Hospital was established about four miles from Philadelphia on the Germantown turnpike, near Nicetown. In these hospitals nearly all the most skillful physicians and surgeons of Philadelphia added greatly to the Union cause and their own fame. Unfortunately, the records of these hospitals were withheld from the public by the War Department in an order of February 23, 1879, so that a complete list is not obtainable. The work at Turner's Lane Hospital on *Gunshot Wounds and Other Injuries of Nerves* by S. Weir Mitchell (Jefferson, class of 1850), George R. Morehouse (Jefferson, 1850) and W.W. Keen (Jefferson, 1862) was published and an excellent article on this hospital was authored by Middleton.[3,4]

General George Brinton McClellan (1826–1885)

It is inescapable to mention that the son of the founder of Jefferson, General George Brinton McClellan, was summoned to Washington on July 24, 1861, by President Lincoln to command the Army of the Potomac. On November 1, 1861, at age 34, McClellan was appointed General-in-Chief of all the Armies of the Union. General Lee stated after the war that McClellan was the ablest of his opponents.[5] "No union general was so beloved as 'Little Mac' was by the untrained volunteers whom he turned into a superb instrument of war, the Army of the Potomac."[6] McClellan expected to crush the rebels in one campaign. By the middle of 1862 victory seemed in sight. After some delay he brought his army within a few miles of Richmond and the Confederate Capitol appeared doomed. Suddenly stunning reverses struck the Union Army. The Seven Days' Battle demanded a withdrawal from the peninsula between the James and York Rivers and relieved the Union threat to Richmond. General Pope was defeated at the Second Battle of Bull Run. The bloody sacrifices at Antietam on September 17, 1862, followed. It was not a decisive victory for either army.

Lincoln chose the week after Antietam to issue

the *Emancipation Proclamation.* McClellan refused to continue the Antietam battle the following day, leading eventually to rumors that Lee would take Philadelphia and locate his headquarters in the Dundas mansion at Broad and Walnut Streets. On November 7, 1862, McClellan was dismissed and replaced by General Ambrose E. Burnside. "Little Mac," as his father had also been called, became Governor of New Jersey and unsuccessfully ran against Lincoln on the Democratic ticket in 1864. He was buried in Trenton, New Jersey.

Samuel D. Gross (1805–1884)

It is remarkable that as early as May 1861, Samuel D. Gross published his *Manual of Military Surgery,* for it was only on April 12, 1861, that the first guns of the Civil War were fired against Fort Sumter. It is claimed that he completed this book in nine days, but Gross in the preface indicated that he had previously started the manuscript. It contained "hints on the emergencies of field, camp, and hospital practice." Pocket-sized (6 × 4 × 1/2 inches), lightweight, and containing 186 pages, Gross's *Manual* encompassed the care of medical and surgical casualties. It was republished in Richmond the following year—the so-called pirated edition—for the Confederate Army and became the only mutual communication in the strife between North and South. Gross visited the wounded on the field and government steamboats immediately after the battle of Shiloh at Pittsburg Landing, Tennessee, which occurred on April 12, 1862. This added nothing new to his second edition of 1862, an exact copy of the first, and eventually it was translated into German, and from German into Japanese in 1874.

Samuel W. Gross (1837–1889)

The younger Gross, Samuel W. (Jefferson, class of 1857), to whom the *Manual of Military Surgery* was dedicated, entered the United States service as a Volunteer Brigade Surgeon. In the summer of 1862 he was Medical Director of the Fifth Division of the Army of the Ohio. He next served in DeCamp General Hospital, New York Harbor, until the following summer, when he was placed in charge of hospitals in South Carolina and Florida and rose to Chief Medical Officer of the Northern District of that Department. In 1864 he was in charge of the Haddington Hospital of Philadelphia and brevetted as a Lieutenant-Colonel for his services. His sword later was donated by his widow (subsequently Lady Osler) to the College of Physicians of Philadelphia (Figure 2-10).

John Hill Brinton (1832–1907)

Dr. John Hill Brinton (Jefferson, class of 1852), the boon companion of Samuel W. Gross, had a most distinguished Civil War career. He was 29 years old and a prime candidate for military service when the war broke out. His commission as Brigade Surgeon of Volunteers was signed by Abraham Lincoln, and the original document is preserved in Jefferson's archives; all of his army orders and communications from Generals Grant, Rosecrans, McPherson, and Sheridan, as well as the office of the Surgeon General, are likewise contained in a bound volume, and his frequent letters home are also preserved in two bound volumes. These served him well for his later book, *Personal Memoirs,* completed in 1891 but not published until 1914, seven years after his death. This work with arresting literary aplomb recounts the early chaos in the organization of both the military and medical branches of the army, Brinton's insights into the personalities of his commanders, the pitiful plight of the wounded soldiers to which he was committed, the difficulties in setting up hospitals and supplies, the ineptness and inexperience of many of the medical officers, battlefield combat as viewed through the eyes of a Volunteer Surgeon, Brinton's efforts to collect specimens for the Army Medical Museum, his service on examining boards, and his collecting of statistics for the *Medical and Surgical History of the War of the Rebellion.*[8] Dr. Brinton had a cousin, Dr. Daniel Garrison Brinton (Jefferson, class of 1860), who left a diary of his own Civil War experiences that was published 100 years later.[9] General George Brinton McClellan and Dr. John Hill Brinton were first cousins but pursued independent war careers.

Duly commissioned in August, 1861, Brinton reported to the Department of the West where he came under the command of General Ulysses S.

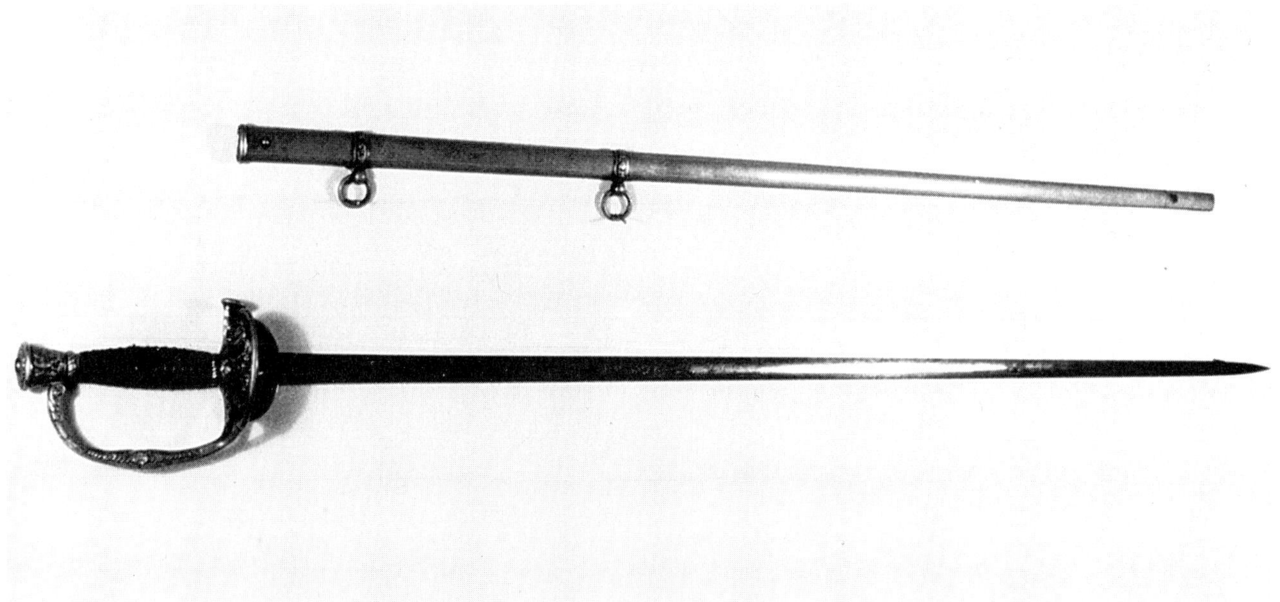

FIG. 2-10. The sword of Samuel W. Gross, M.D. during the Civil War (courtesy of College of Physicians of Philadelphia).

Grant. This marked the beginning of a mutual respect and a regard for each other's abilities that extended well beyond the war years. A letter to Dr. Brinton from Mrs. Julia Grant expresses comfort that her husband was under his medical auspices.

Brinton's first real test came under General Grant at the battle of Belmont, Missouri, during which he had the misfortune to lose all of his surgical instruments. Many of these had been brought from Paris, and others had belonged to his old preceptor at Jefferson, the late Professor Thomas Dent Mütter. In the hurry of leaving for the field at Belmont, Brinton gathered them into a single package that he entrusted to a young orderly. The latter panicked from the enemy artillery fire and was seen to rush from the open into the woods with the heavy load held on his head by two hands. The orderly was captured and the instruments fell into the hands of a Mississippi surgeon. General Grant on a flag of truce attempted to barter a captured Arabian pony for the instruments, but the exchange was never consummated.

Brinton was distressed by the inexperience and surgical ignorance of his fellow medical officers. In an effort to remedy this situation he organized the Army Medical and Surgical Society of Cairo, bringing surgeons together chiefly from Illinois, Iowa, Michigan, and Missouri for mutual improvement. The members met weekly and the society flourished long after Brinton left Cairo, Illinois.

In June, 1862, Brinton was ordered to prepare *The Surgical History of the Rebellion*. This was intended to remedy the insufficient and defective statistics on the sick and wounded that became evident in the first year of the war. In August 1862, he was assigned also to collect and arrange all specimens of morbid anatomy that had accumulated in the various hospitals or that might have been retained by any of the medical officers. In carrying out this order, Surgeon Brinton thus established the United States Army Medical Museum. His visits to headquarters of the armies in the field and different hospitals provided data and illustrations for the book and specimens for the museum. The beginning of the museum in that August of 1862 consisted of three dried and varnished specimens placed on a shelf above the ink stand of Brinton's desk. In January, 1863, a preliminary catalogue was printed with brief descriptions of 1,349 objects that had been collected within a five-month period. Of the total, 985 were surgical, 106 medical, 133 missiles, and 125 miscellaneous. By July 1, 1863, Brinton was able to submit a "Consolidated Statement of Gunshot Wounds" for publication by the Surgeon General's Office. It would be misleading and grandiose to give Brinton credit for more than the start of these monumental projects that required additional years and teams of workers, but his name is indelibly linked with them. As a result of his Civil War experiences he delivered the Mütter Lecture in 1869 at the College of Physicians of Philadelphia on *Gunshot Injuries, Their Surgery and Pathology*.

William Williams Keen (1837–1932)

William Williams Keen entered Jefferson Medical College in 1860, and after completing only ten months of his course was requested by Dr. John Hill Brinton to join the Fifth Massachusetts Regiment. Although not a graduate in medicine, and without taking any examination whatever, he was sworn into service at Washington, D.C. on July 4, 1861, as an Assistant Surgeon. He was then sent to camp at Alexandria, Virginia, and two weeks later saw action at the Union defeat in the Battle of Bull Run on July 21, when Jackson made his "stone wall" stand. It was there that he saw the woefully unorganized condition of the Medical Department, for he did not receive a single order from anyone. The enlistment in his regiment expired on August 1, 1861, and with an honorable discharge he returned to Jefferson to receive his medical degree in March, 1862. Two months later, this time after an examination, he was again commissioned as Acting Assistant Surgeon in the U.S. Army, and put in charge of the Eckington Hospital in the outskirts of Washington. Shortly thereafter he was ordered to fit up two churches as hospitals, which he accomplished in the incredible period of only five days. His unusual executive ability in organizing hospitals led to a rotation of assignments that culminated at Turner's Lane in Philadelphia, where he carried out the study on injuries of nerves in collaboration with his fellow Jeffersonians, Mitchell and Morehouse. For Keen this was only the beginning of a surgical career that would mark him as a giant of his era on a par with Harvey Cushing and William Halsted.

Jonathan Letterman (1824–1873)

As a unique coincidence, Jonathan Letterman was born in 1824 (the year Jefferson Medical College was founded) and in Canonsburg, Pennsylvania (the location of the mother institution from which Jefferson originated). Following graduation from Jefferson in 1849 he pursued a military career in the Army as Assistant Surgeon. With outbreak of the War between the States in 1861 he was assigned to duty with the Army of the Potomac. In July, 1862, he was made Medical Director of this division under the command of Major-General George McClellan. His remarkable administrative ability led to the more rapid rehabilitation of the sick and wounded, a reorganization of medical service in the field, and a more effective military hospital system. His greatest contribution was a revival of rapid evacuation of the wounded as originated by Dominique-Jean Larrey (1776–1842), Napoleon's world-renowned military surgeon. These improvements were invaluable at the Battles of Chancellorsville and Gettysburg. They formed the basis of a permanent system throughout all subsequent U.S. military engagements.

In 1866 Letterman wrote *Medical Recollections of the Army of the Potomac*. The following year he was elected coroner of San Francisco and served for two years. He died prematurely in 1872 at the age of 47. In 1911 the U.S. War Department named a government hospital of 180 beds in his honor as the Letterman General Hospital in San Francisco near the Golden Gate Bridge.

Benjamin Howard Rand (1827–1883)

Back at Jefferson, it became necessary to choose a successor to Franklin Bache, Professor of Chemistry who died in 1864 at the age of 72. It was imperative to find a teacher of unquestioned reputation, for he was to replace a member of the prestigious faculty of 1841. The selection of Benjamin Howard Rand was ideal.[10] He had taken his preceptorship under Dr. Robert M. Huston of the 1841 Jefferson Faculty and also served as Clinical Assistant to Mütter and Pancoast for two years before his graduation from Jefferson in 1848. Two years later, at the age of 23, Rand was elected

Professor of Chemistry of the Franklin Institute. He subsequently taught chemistry at Central High School and the Pennsylvaia Medical College, founded by Dr. George McClellan after he left Jefferson. Rand taught at McClellan's school from its inception in 1839 until its complete attrition in 1861.

Of the seven Jefferson Professors painted by Thomas Eakins, Rand was the first in 1874. The fathers of both Rand and Eakins were writing masters in Philadelphia and probably knew each other. Rand had taught Eakins at Central High and was in the Chair of Chemistry at Jefferson when the latter held cards of admission to the anatomy lectures for the years 1864 and 1865. The Rand portrait in Jefferson's Eakins Gallery was Eakins' first try at painting a scientist. His previous portraits had been of relatives and friends. By asking Rand to sit for this work in 1874 Eakins made himself the unofficial portraitist for the College and proceeded the following year, again without a commission, to paint the Gross Clinic.

Rand's lectures emphasized the application of chemistry to the practical aspects of clinical medicine. He was liked by the students, respected as a scholar, and served as a capable Dean (1869–1873). He authored *Chemistry for Students* (1855), and *Elements of Medical Chemistry* (1867), and edited two volumes of Metcalf's *Caloric* (1859). Rand's health became impaired in 1875 due to a pulmonary problem, which he ascribed to accidentally inhaling "arsenuated hydrogen" during a medicolegal investigation. Because of the effect on his speech he was obliged to resign in 1877 at the age of 50. He died six years later of pneumonia.

▪ Thomas Eakins (1844–1916)

The Civil War years at Jefferson carry a significant relationship in the context of "medicine in art" to the life of Thomas Eakins. When he graduated from Central High School on July 11, 1861, the class had diminished to 24 because the war had started during his senior year. He was fifth in academic rank among the students who received a degree of Bachelor of Arts, with a four-year average of 88.4.[11] As already mentioned, Eakins' Professor of Chemistry had been Dr. Benjamin Howard Rand, whose portrait he painted 15 years later. In 1862, at age 18, Eakins was a candidate for the Professorship of Drawing and Writing at Central High but was defeated by another applicant. That same year he enrolled as a student at the Pennsylvania Academy of the Fine Arts, which at that time was located on Chestnut Street between Tenth and Eleventh. This was but a stone's throw away from Jefferson Medical College. The classes emphasized drawing from casts of ancient classical figures, and there was a weekly anatomy lecture by a physician. The genius of Eakins drove him to seek a deeper knowledge of the structure of the human body than was provided by his limited drawing from life at the Academy. It is known that he held cards of admission for the years 1864 and 1865 when Professor Joseph Pancoast was at the height of his fame as an anatomist-surgeon. Pancoast not only emphasized the clinical aspects of anatomy in his lectures but aided the students in the practical anatomy of the dissecting rooms. Eakins did not participate in the Civil War. His Quaker heritage could have been a factor, but undoubtedly he was marching to the beat of a different drummer. Like most aspiring artists, and not unlike physicians of the same era, he went to Europe (Paris and Spain) for further study between 1866 and 1870. Eakins returned to Jefferson for further study of anatomy in 1873. One admission card was signed by Joseph Pancoast and a second (1874–1875) by his son, William Henry Pancoast, who succeeded to the Chair at that time. In these years Eakins painted Benjamin Howard Rand (1874) and the Gross Clinic (1875). Although Eakins never matriculated as a student for the degree of medicine, Jefferson and Eakins represented the perfect union of medicine and art.

▪ William Henry Pancoast (1835–1897)

It should be pointed out that Eakins' first courses in anatomy at Jefferson during the Civil War years were times when extra stress was placed upon the Chairs of Surgery and Anatomy to train surgeons for the Union Army. The position of Demonstrator of Anatomy was important enough to be the only teaching position listed in the

College announcement of 1863–1864 after the Board of Trustees and Professors. The vacancy created by appointment of Ellerslie Wallace to the Chair of Obstetrics and Diseases of Women and Children was filled by Joseph Pancoast's son, William Henry, who had graduated from Jefferson and just returned from study in Paris. He served in the Anatomy Department for 11 years before election to the Professorship in 1874.

William Smith Forbes (1831–1905)

An unsung hero was William Smith Forbes (Jefferson, class of 1852). He was a classmate of John Hill Brinton and Jacob Mendes DaCosta, all of whom later became Professors at Jefferson and were painted by Eakins. Forbes gave up his popular private school of anatomy just beyond the rear of St. Stephen's Episcopal Church at Tenth and College Avenue to enlist as Surgeon of the United States Volunteers in 1862. As Medical Director of the 13th Army he was in charge of the surgeons at Vicksburg. Later he served in the Summit Hospital of Philadelphia. His Civil War experiences afforded him ample opportunity to observe the lack of knowledge of practical anatomy on the part of many surgeons and the inability of many to profit from Gross's *Manual of Military Surgery*. This motivated him shortly after the war to advocate the passage of an anatomical act to provide bodies legally for dissection.

This brief narrative touches only some highlights of careers and events that affected the lives of everyone. As in all wars the demands on the medical profession led to certain improvements such as in the treatment of fractures, better experience in the use of anesthetics, and more efficient design of hospitals. Research in pathology and physiology was stimulated. On the other hand, defects in the training of medical students were tragically revealed in the field and the military hospitals. Hygiene and sanitation were primitive, with germs killing more soldiers on either side than bullets did. There were more American deaths than in any war before or since. About 620,000 men died, two-thirds from disease and one-third killed in battle or subsequently of battle injuries. It was still the pre-Listerian era.

References

1. Kelly, H.A., and Burrage, W.L., "Ellerslie Wallace," *Dict. of Am. Med. Biog.* New York: D. Appleton and Co., 1928, p. 1254.
2. Whiteman, M., *Gentlemen in Crisis*. Philadelphia: Winchell Co., 1975, p. 18.
3. Mitchell, S.W., Morehouse, G.R., and Keen, W.W., *Gunshot Wounds and Other Injuries of Nerves*. Philadelphia: J.B. Lippincott and Co., 1864.
4. Middleton, W.S., "Turner's Lane Hospital." *Bull. Hist. Med.* 60:14–42, 1966.
5. Morison, S.W., *The Oxford History of the American People*. New York: Oxford Univ. Press, 1965, p. 635.
6. Ibid., p. 635.
7. Brinton, J.H., *Personal Memoirs*. New York: Neale Pub. Co., 1914.
8. "The Medical and Surgical History of the War of the Rebellion (1861–65)." Prepared in Accordance with Acts of Congress, Under the Direction of Surgeon General Joseph K. Barnes, U.S. Army. Washington: Government Printing Office, 1870.
9. Brinton, D.G., "From Chancellorsville to Gettysburg, A Doctor's Diary." *The Pennsylvania Magazine of History and Biography*. July 1965, pp. 292–315.
10. Kelly and Burrage, "Benjamin Howard Rand." p. 1008.
11. Hendricks, G., *The Life and Work of Thomas Eakins*. New York: Grossman Pub., 1974, p. 13.

Curricular Changes: Summer Courses Started (1866)

Expansion of the curriculum by the introduction of a "Summer Course" in 1866 invites a review of the gradual changes in the preceding years.[1] Before 1832 the longest term allotted for the year's "Session" of lectures was four months (November through February). This was the standard curriculum in the medical colleges of the United States, although in the principal medical schools of Europe the term was six months. The Trustees and Professors of Jefferson were deeply aware of the necessity for a six-month term but felt that singly to attempt so great an innovation by a young institution was "scarcely prudent." Convinced, however, that the time was not far off when American medical schools would extend their courses of study, they took a first step in 1832, chiefly through the influence of Dr. Granville Sharpe Pattison, by adding an optional course of two months, during April and May, for which no extra tuition was charged. The lectures were structured to review or give greater detail to the subjects covered in the regular course.

To stimulate interest in the extra two months, an examination was held to award "to the more distinguished pupils, Medals and Certificates of Honour." The first of the three medals was given to the student whose written answers placed him at the head of the class. Certificates of Honour were given to those the excellence of whose answers entitled them to such a distinction. The examination publicized in the "College Announcement" was for an incredible eight hours. Understandably, this program was modified after two years.

In 1834 the optional two months of instruction were changed to March and October, with elimination of the examination. The March session included dissection and demonstrations in anatomy as well as twice-weekly lectures by the Professors of Surgery, Medicine, Materia Medica, and Obstetrics. The October session was similar and also included Chemistry. A fee of $10 was charged for the March session, but the October session was free. Both sessions included opportunities in the Dispensary. This was a new feature in the medical schools of the United States. In the first year, 50 out of 172 students took the extra two months, and the following year nearly 100 did.

The M.D. degree still required three years of study "under the direction of a respectable Practitioner of Medicine," including two regular "Sessions" of lectures. The optional sessions did not count toward the degree. The candidates had to be at least 21 years of age, pass an examination, and submit a satisfactory thesis.

In 1836 the March course was discontinued and not resumed until 1847. October courses, including dissection and demonstrations in anatomy, were continued without extra tuition, and lectures were increased from three to four daily. Clinical instruction and opportunities to witness operations were available at the Pennsylvania and Philadelphia (Blockley) Hospitals. The October courses were suspended in 1838 because of renovations in the College building. By 1845 there were clinical opportunities for Jefferson students in the Wills Hospital, and Saturday lectures by Dunglison in Clinical Medicine and by Pancoast in Clinical Surgery at the Philadelphia Hospital. In 1848 it was announced that the College Clinic would be kept open the whole year for the experience of the students.

In 1849 the regular required "Session" added two weeks by starting in mid-October instead of the first Monday of November. The optional dissecting room and lectures still began at the beginning of October, with the Clinic open all year. The October date for official opening was gradually shifted to the second Monday of October, and the term continued until the last of February.

In 1866, for students who were able to attend in the interval between the winter courses of lectures, the Faculty instituted a "Summer Course" conducted by the Professors in conjunction with additional staff, and made to comprise not only branches regularly taught during the winter but others. The term "Summer Course" was a misnomer, because there was a recess during the intolerably hot Philadelphia months of July and August. The course otherwise extended from the first Monday of April until the first Monday of October. It was of practical character, embracing important specialties in Medicine and Surgery, with clinical illustrations, including the following subjects: Clinical Surgery by Professors Samuel D. Gross and Joseph Pancoast, Clinical Obstetrics by Professor Ellerslie Wallace, Pathology by Professor Samuel H. Dickson, Hygiene and Meteorology by Professor Benjamin H. Rand, Materia Medica and Therapeutics by Professor John B. Biddle, Clinical Medicine by Dr. Jacob M. DaCosta, Visceral and Surgical Anatomy by Dr. William H. Pancoast, Minor and Operative Surgery by Dr. Samuel W. Gross, Physiology by Dr. J. Aitken Meigs, Ophthalmic and Aural Surgery by Dr. Richard J Levis, and Venereal Diseases by Dr. Francis F. Maury.

During the entire year, and especially in the winter, private examinations or "quiz sessions" were in operation under capable instructors who closely followed and elucidated the lectures delivered in the College. A majority of these instructors in the "Summer Course" and quiz classes subsequently became Professors at Jefferson.

References

1. "Annual Announcements of the Jefferson Medical College of Philadelphia, 1832–1866."

Post-Bellum Progress (1865–1876): End of the Civil War to the Centennial Exhibition

Jefferson took on added vigor after the War. In the immediate five years between 1865 and 1870 there was representation from 36 states, nine territories, and the countries of Germany, Sweden, India, China, Japan, Central and South America, the West Indies, and Canada. Student registration in 1866 numbered 425, with 311 from 29 states. Enrollment from the South and Southwest increased to 98 because almost all of the Southern medical schools had collapsed and were financially depleted.

■ John Barclay Biddle (1815–1879)

Dr. Thomas D. Mitchell died in 1865, the year after Rand took the Chair of Chemistry. His successor in Materia Medica was John Barclay Biddle (Figure 2-11).[1] He was the son of Clement C. Biddle and Mary Barclay, both from prominent old Philadelphia families representative of "American Aristocracy."[2] Biddle and Cadwalader names (later to appear in Professor Henry Cadwalader Chapman) were so typically Philadelphian in heritage that a saying arose: "When a Biddle gets drunk he thinks he's a Cadwalader." The prestigious Nathaniel Chapman (a successor to Rush in the Chair of Medicine at the University of Pennsylvania and later to be the first President of the American Medical Association in 1847) was his uncle through marriage to Rebecca Biddle. After an excellent education in the classics and languages at St. Mary's College in Baltimore, Biddle became a private pupil of Dr. Chapman and enrolled at the University. While there he studied with John Syng Dorsey, George Bacon Wood, Philip Syng Physick, Samuel Jackson, and William Gibson, all acknowledged leaders in their fields. After graduation in 1836 Biddle enhanced his elite education with a year of study in Paris. While establishing himself in practice in 1838, he founded *The Medical Examiner* with Dr. Meredith Clymer (1817–1902). At age 23 Biddle almost immediately became a journalist of distinction. *The Medical Examiner*, which appeared fortnightly, was subsequently issued weekly. Its success demanded additions to the editorial staff in the persons of Drs. W.W. Gerhard and Francis Gurney Smith. These youthful writers excelled in their editorials and bibliographical notices. In 1846 the journal merged with *The Medico-Chirurgical Review*.

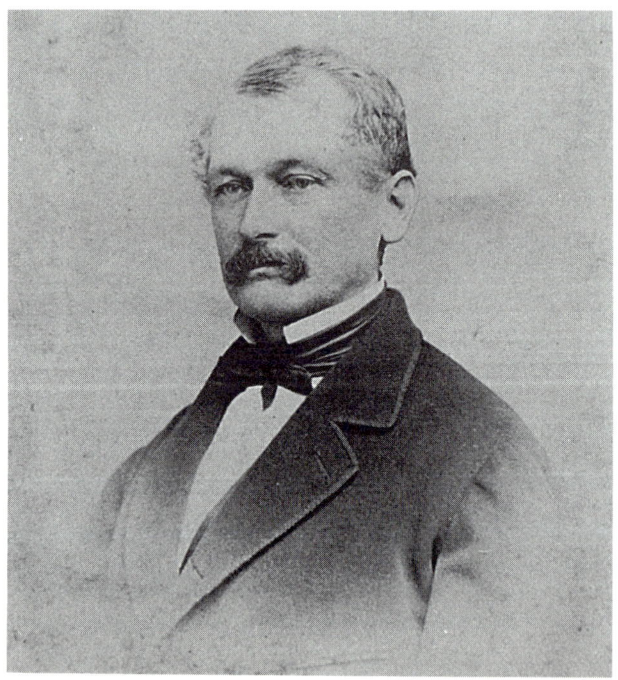

FIG. 2-11. John Barclay Biddle, M.D. (1815–1879); Professor of Materia Medica (1865–1878) and Dean (1873–1879).

In 1846 Biddle with some editorial and other colleagues founded the Franklin Medical College at Locust Street above Eleventh, where he took the Chair of Materia Medica until the College closed two years later. He also assumed the same Chair in the Pennsylvania Medical College. In 1852 he authored one of the most popular books on materia medica that had ever been published. Under the title of a *Review of the Materia Medica, for the Use of Students*, it contained about 300 pages; a second edition in 1865, when Biddle came to Jefferson, was titled *Materia Medica, for the Use of Students*. Eight additional editions followed, the last of which appeared in 1878 and had expanded to 462 pages. A later successor at Jefferson, Dr. Hobart A. Hare, would also conduct a dominant textbook of therapeutics through 21 editions. Both of these men, as most Jefferson Professors to this time, had studied at the University of Pennsylvania.

Biddle's talent as a writer was matched by his excellent lectures. His pleasing appearance added grace to his clear and authoritative teaching. He held the Chair for thirteen years (1865–1878) during the last six of which he served as Dean. Shortly after assuming the Deanship in 1873, Biddle was confronted with the first known woman applicant to Jefferson. In accord with the general sentiment of the times, he turned down her application and referred to the incident in his introductory speech to the students at the opening of the College that year:

> "Women entering medicine must be willing to subordinate love and marriage to the stern requirements of the most exciting vocation . . . . If they come into the arena they must come as equals . . . . We would spare them the conquest because we know that whatever their talent . . . the inferiority of a feebler and more delicate physical organization is insurmountable . . . . The cry for new rights is loud, but it comes from the few . . . . The clatter of all the female men in the world cannot alter the laws of nature!"[3]

In Biddle's defense it can be stated that "at the meeting of the Medical Society of the State of Pennsylvania, held in 1866, there was passed a resolution to the effect that it was considered unprofessional to consult with the professors and graduates of female medical colleges, as at that time organized."[4] Not until 1961 would Jefferson admit women applicants.

In answer to a general call from Louisville, Kentucky, to the various medical colleges of the United States, 22 representatives met at Jefferson Medical College on June 2, 1876. The object of the convention was "to consider all matters relating to reform in medical college work." This was the founding meeting of the Association of American Medical Colleges, and Dean John B. Biddle was elected the first President. He served until 1879 and was succeeded by Dr. Samuel D. Gross for the years 1879–1881. Later, Jefferson's Dean James W. Holland served as President for 1897–1898 and Dean Ross V. Patterson for 1933–1935.

Biddle was a strong supporter of the first detached Jefferson Hospital erected in 1877. Failing health forced him to retire in 1878. He died the following year at age 64. The autopsy performed by Dr. John Hill Brinton revealed a ruptured appendix with peritonitis.

Jacob Mendes DaCosta (1833–1900)

In 1866, Jacob Mendes DaCosta (Figure 2-12) became a Lecturer in Clinical Medicine. Although not related to the illustrious surgeon, John Chalmers DaCosta, who followed a generation later, his fame and benefit to the institution were just as significant. Rising through the ranks, he was the first Jefferson alumnus to occupy the Chair of Medicine. In 1872, as successor to Samuel Dickson in whose Department he had taught, he was also the first to be so appointed from the Faculty of that Department.

DaCosta was born on the island of Saint Thomas on February 7, 1833, a descendant of a Portuguese family that had immigrated to London in the 16th century. His preliminary education in Dresden led to proficiency in both ancient and

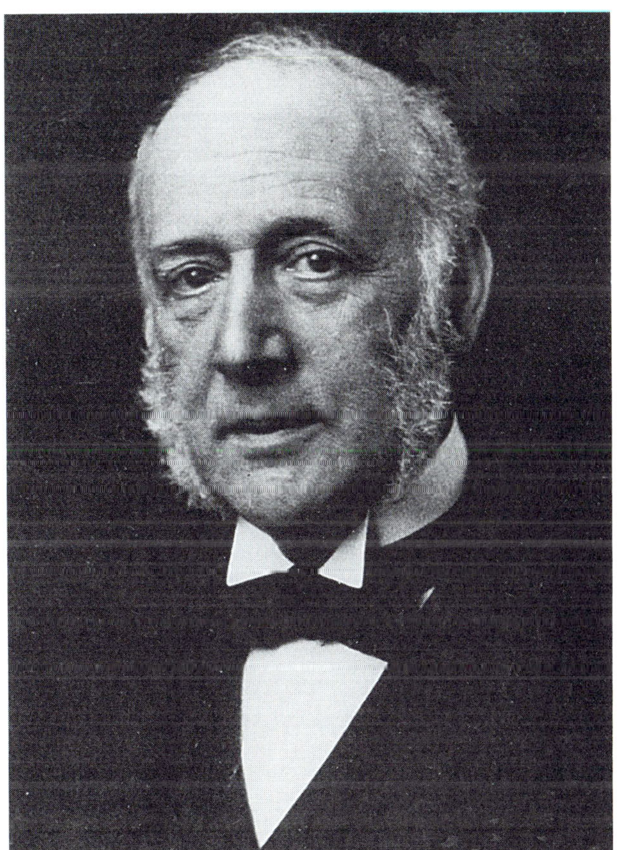

FIG. 2-12. Jacob Mendes DaCosta, M.D. (1833–1900); Professor of Medicine (1872–1891).

modern languages as well as classical literature. DaCosta immigrated to Philadelphia in 1849, where he studied at Jefferson as a pupil of Professor Mütter and with the other members of the famous faculty of 1841. His diligence was noted by Mütter, who allowed him to demonstrate the surgical specimens to his classmates twice weekly in the evenings. After graduation in 1852 DaCosta returned to Europe for study in the clinics of Paris, Prague, and Vienna. Some of this experience was in the company of his outstanding classmate, John Hill Brinton (a successor to Samuel D. Gross), whose sister he subsequently married.

On returning to Philadelphia in 1854, DaCosta began office practice, coupled with teaching of physical diagnosis both privately and in the Summer Association for Medical Instruction. In addition, he wrote papers on his clinical observations. DaCosta's textbook, *Medical Diagnosis,* first published in 1864, went through nine editions until 1900, with translations into several foreign languages. He served on the staff of Jefferson, Episocopal, Philadelphia, Children's and the Pennsylvania Hospitals. In 1857 he was active in organizing the Pathological Society of Philadelphia (President, 1864–1867). DaCosta became an Honorary Member of the Medical Society of New York and London, a fellow of the College of Physicians of Philadelphia (President, 1884–1885 and 1895–1898), original member of the Association of American Physicians (President, 1897), and a Fellow of the American Philosophical Society.

DaCosta's reputation as a physician was prestigious and his clinics were models of information, clarity, and interest. His description of "irritable heart" was a classic, marking him as a pioneer in cardiology.[5] His professional contributions were recognized by the award of the degree of LL.D. by Jefferson, the University of Pennsylvania, and Harvard. After 19 years of distinguished service as Professor, DaCosta resigned in 1891 to become Emeritus. He died quickly of a heart attack in June 1900, at his home and office at 1700 Walnut Street. Of the several memoirs for this illustrious Jeffersonian, none is surpassed by that of his faithful secretary for many years, Miss Mary Clarke.[6] DaCosta's portrait by Thomas Eakins, painted in 1893, hangs in the Pennsylvania Hospital, and the two by Robert Vonnoh in the same year are on display at Jefferson and the College of Physicians.

Wooley, in historical articles as recent as 1982 and 1985, states: "It seems fitting to recall Jacob Mendes DaCosta for many reasons—as an early American clinical investigator working in a clinical research center (Turner's Lane), as a patron for unsung clinicians and teachers in medical schools, as an example of the finest qualities of the Philadelphia medical spirit, and a noble man and physician."[7,8]

▪ Pathology and Infection

Until 1867, a smattering of pathology was taught through the medical and surgical courses of Drs. Samuel H. Dickson and Samuel D. Gross. Harvard was the only medical school in the country with a separate Chair of Pathological Anatomy (Pathology). An innovation occurred in the "Summer Course" of 1867 when William Williams Keen (Jefferson, class of 1862) lectured on pathological anatomy then and in consecutive years until 1876. The lectures were continued by Dr. Morris Longstreth, who eventually became the first incumbant of a separate Chair of Pathology (1891).

In surgery, the arrest of hemorrhage by use of the ligature was a French contribution (around 1556 by Ambroise Pare); the avoidance of pain through anesthesia was an American contribution (Crawford Long in 1842 and Thomas Morton in 1846); and the control of infection was a British one (Joseph Lister in 1867). Unfortunately, most of Lister's contemporaries failed to recognize that his paper *On the Antiseptic Principle in the Practice of Surgery* was truly innovative. Instead, they looked upon it as nothing more than the introduction of some new form of wound dressing in which the number and variety already in use were legion. Whereas Samuel D. Gross's predecessor, Professor Mütter, had been quick to adopt the use of ether, Gross himself, America's foremost surgeon, was loathe to accept Lister's new method, as is plainly evident in Eakins' depiction of the *Gross Clinic* in 1875. As late as 1882, in the last edition of his *System of Surgery,* Gross wrote:

> "When the wound is very large, as after the amputation of a limb, or the extirpation of the mammary gland, I generally cover the surface with a pledget of lint wet with olive oil or cosmoline, to prevent the contact of the air and thus diminish the chances of profuse suppuration. I have never found any appreciable benefit in such a case from the use of antiseptic dressings, although they are regarded by many surgeons as most valuable accessories. The antiseptic method, when strictly adhered to, demands rigid attention to minute details, so that it has been modified in various ways, of which the most popular appears to consist in irrigating or washing the wound with a solution of carbolic acid, boracic acid, salicyclic acid, benzoic acid, thymol, oil of eucalyptus, chloride of zinc, or pure alcohol, and afterwards enveloping the part in cotton-wool or absorbent cotton . . . . At the present day, carbolic acid is falling into deseutude. As I have pointed out in the section on septicemia and pyemia, it does not prevent the development of micrococci and bacteria in the pus of wounds, and its employment has not only frequently given rise to serious symptoms of poisoning, but it has been followed by death in a number of instances."[9]

It is gratifying to record, however, that two of Gross's pupils at Jefferson, William W. Keen (Class of 1862) and J. Ewing Mears (Class of 1865) pioneered in Listerian methods during the 1870s.

In May of 1868, forty years after graduation from Jefferson, Samuel D. Gross made his first trip to Europe. He was warmly received by many of the distinguished physicians and surgeons of the great clinics of the continent as a representative of what was best in the American medical profession. An example of the hospitality extended to him may be quoted from his *Autobiography:*

> "The evening before leaving Berlin I had the pleasure of meeting Virchow at his own table, at his elegant residence in a fashionable part of the city. The gentlemen who were invited to meet me were among others, Professor Von Langenbeck, Von Graefe, the famous oculist, Donders, the celebrated ophthalmologist of Utrecht, and Dr. Gurlt, Professor of Surgery in the University of Berlin. Our time was occupied in agreeable and instructive conversation. At ten o'clock the folding doors were thrown open, and we sat down to a bountiful repast. After the viands were pretty well disposed of, our host, availing himself of a lull in the conversation, drew forth a large volume from under the table, and rising he took me by the hand, and made me an address in German, complimenting me upon my labors as a pathological anatomist, and referring to the work, which happened to be the second edition of my *Elements of Pathological Anatomy,* as one from the study of which he had derived much useful instruction, and one which he always consulted with much pleasure. I need not say how deeply flattered I felt by this great honor, so unexpectedly and so handsomely bestowed upon me by this renowned man. I felt that I had not labored in vain, and that the compliment was more than an equivalent for all the toil and anxiety which the work had cost me."[10]

At Oxford, during August of this five-month visit, Gross was commissioned to represent the American Medical Association, of which he was the President, at the meeting of the British Medical Association. If it had been known earlier that Gross was coming to Oxford, he would have received the honorary degree of Doctor of Civil Law, which was conferred upon him in a second visit of 1872.

On the return from his first European visit in October, 1868, Gross, along with Dr. Joseph Pancoast, who had also been on an extended European tour, was further honored by a public reception in the foyer of the Academy of Music. Among several hundred men and women in attendance were colleagues, alumni, distinguished physicians from Pennsylvania and other states, as well as prominient members of the bar, pulpit, military, and business community.

Although Gross and Pancoast were at their zenith in 1868, the third member of the renowned triumvirate, Robley Dunglison, was suffering from congestive heart failure. He resigned to become Emeritus and died one year later. Samuel H. Dickson took the Deanship and James Aitken Meigs was elected to Dunglison's Chair.

■ James Aitkin Meigs (1829–1879)

James Aitken Meigs (Figure 2-13) was not related to his Professor of Obstetrics at Jefferson, Charles

Delucena Meigs, even though the latter had encouraged him to take a preceptorship with Dr. Francis Gurney Smith, who strongly influenced his interest in the natural sciences.[11] A Philadelphian of humble birth on July 31, 1829, he evidenced even in childhood a love for books, an interest in science, and a talent for poetry. As valedictorian of his class at Central High School in 1848, his address, *The Destination of Philosophy*, was couched partly in verse. Endowed with a capacious memory, inquisitiveness, and philosophical inclinations, Meigs was attracted to a career linking the study and treatment of both emotional and physical illness. While studying at Jefferson, from which he graduated in 1851, he took notes of the lectures and debates of the Philadelphia County Medical Society, gave clinical reports of cases treated at Jefferson Medical College and the Pennsylvania Hospital, and presented papers on the mortuary statistics of Philadelphia that were published in the *Medical Examiner*. Meigs' pregraduation relations with the Philadelphia County Medical Society led to his joining upon receiving his degree. He served as corresponding secretary for many years and as President in 1871.

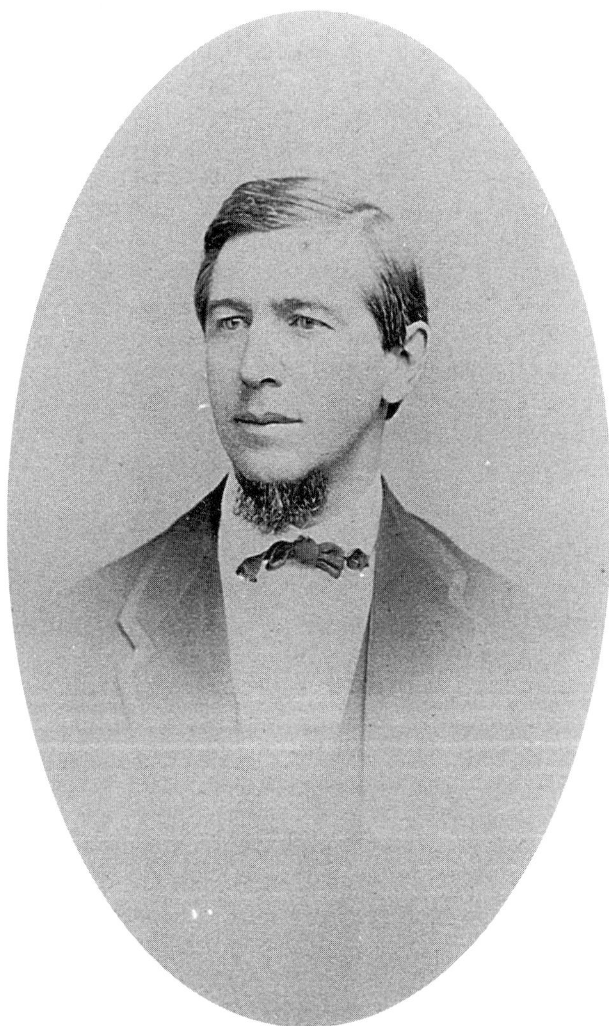

FIG. 2-13. James Aitken Meigs, M.D. (1829–1879); Professor of Institutes of Medicine (1868–1879).

Meigs' graduation thesis, *The Hygiene and Therapeutics of Temperament,* revealed his special interest in physiology. At this time he passed the examination given by the lecturers of the Philadelphia Association for Medical Instruction and was awarded a certificate. Driven both by economic and academic ambitions, he started an active practice, yet found time to study at the College of Physicians and the Academy of Natural Sciences, to the latter of which he was elected a member at the age of 22. Two years later he became a member of the Academy's Standing Committee on Ethnology, served for several years as the Librarian, and in 1857 became Chairman in Anthropology. His sustained interest in the Academy was evidenced by his delivery of a scholarly address when the cornerstone of the new building at Nineteenth Street and the Parkway was placed in 1872. Meigs sytematically catalogued the Academy's collection of human crania, which contained more than a 1,000 specimens. (This collection is not to be confused with the crania displayed in the Mütter Museum of the College of Physicians.) Meigs' publication of *Cranial Characteristics of the Races of Man,* along with other articles in this field, earned him worldwide recognition as an ethnologist.

In 1854, only three years after graduation, Meigs was appointed Professor of Climatology and Physiology in the Franklin Institute, a position he held for eight years. Two years later he assisted in the editing of William Benjamin Carpenter's *The Microscope and Its Revelations.* His own microscope, the finest then available, was a handsome binocular model accompanied by an impressive set of accessories. It was similar to the one depicted in Eakins' portrait of Benjamin Howard Rand.

In 1857, at age 28, Meigs was elected to the Chair of the Institutes of Medicine in the

Philadelphia College of Medicine. Two years later he succeeded his former preceptor, Dr. Francis G. Smith, in the Chair of Physiology in the Medical Department of the Pennsylvania College, with which the other school had been merged. In 1866 Meigs was engaged as a Lecturer in Physiology in Jefferson's "Summer Course," and in 1868 was appointed to the Chair of the Institutes of Medicine and Medical Jurisprudence, which had acquired prestige by the long and distinguished service of Professor Dunglison. Dr. Silas Weir Mitchell (Jefferson, class of 1850), the famous experimental physiologist, neurologist, and novelist, was a rival candidate for the position. Letters supporting Meigs poured in from the medical Professors of Philadelphia and scientists throughout the world. The latter included Professor William Turner of the University of Edinburgh, Dr. Paul Broca of the Academy of Medicine in Paris, and the scholars Von Duben of Stockholm and Pruner Bey of Cairo. S. Weir Mitchell had lost out to Francis G. Smith for the Chair at the University of Pennsylvania in 1863 and then at Jefferson in 1868. History has shown that Mitchell was "Philadelphia's Lost Physiologist" who wanted a faculty appointment and to start a laboratory for research at a time when the medical schools gave little priority to this type of endeavor.[12]

As an introduction to his course in physiology at Jefferson, Meigs gave a dissertation entitled *The Correlation of the Physical and Vital Forces*. He was among the first to illustrate his lectures by means of the stereopticon. His presentations were prepared thoroughly and delivered without notes. Samuel D. Gross stated that if Meigs did indeed have a fault, it was that his lectures were prepared in too great detail, and often contained more than the students could assimilate. Gross further was of the opinion that Meigs' life was on a suicidal course in that he carried on an exhausting practice mostly devoted to obstetrics while engaging in strenuous academic work. Meigs held memberships in a host of international scientific societies and collected at least 800 books on natural science and physiology.

On March 12, 1879, in the year of his death, Meigs delivered before the fifty-fourth graduating class of Jefferson at the Academy of Music a valedictory address written entirely in iambic pentameter. This classic composition of 534 lines challenged the students to cultivate the science and the art of medicine, to struggle tirelessly against disease, to show compassion toward patients, and to strive both for personal success and for elevation of the profession. The details of his death on November 9 remain obscure. He was only 50 years of age and had held the Chair for but eleven years. His case was called one of "blood poisoning" with pulmonary embolism as a terminal event. On April 20, 1880, eight recent graduates of Jefferson who had been his pupils perpetuated his memory by founding the Meigs Medical Association, which is still active beyond its centennial year.[13]

■ Alumni Association Organized (1870)

Called by distribution of circulars among the graduates, an historic meeting took place on the evening of March 12, 1870, in the lower lecture room of the College. It was well attended with the proclaimed purpose of organizing an Alumni Association. The idea and guiding spirit was that of Samuel D. Gross, who at age 65 and greatly venerated, realized the power and benefit to the college by mustering together its several thousand graduates. At that first meeting, Dr. Nathan L. Hatfield, a graduate of the first class of 1826, was elected Chairman, and the committee of five appointed to submit a plan of organization were Samuel D. Gross, 1828; Ellerslie Wallace, 1843; Benjamin H. Rand, 1848; Addinell Hewson, 1850, and J. Ewing Mears, 1865. Gross, the founder, was elected President and served from 1870 to 1874 and again from 1878 until his death in 1884. The contributions to the welfare of the school and the mystique of loyalty evidenced by what became the largest organization of its kind in the country, have remained the astonishment and curiosity of alumni of other medical schools.

Although the history of the Alumni Association is detailed in a separate chapter, it is appropriate to mention that one of its earliest actions was to initiate an art collection by commissioning Samuel Bell Waugh, a prominent Philadelphia artist, to paint the portraits of five of its favorite professors—Charles D. Meigs in 1872, Joseph

Pancoast in 1872, Samuel D. Gross in 1874, Robley Dunglison in 1876, and John B. Biddle in 1880—three of whom were deceased. These portraits grace the halls of Jefferson in excellent condition more than a century later. On the other hand, without a commission, Thomas Eakins, America's greatest portrait artist, painted Benjamin Howard Rand in 1874, *The Gross Clinic* in 1875, and John Hill Brinton (a successor to Gross) in 1876.

The Middle 1870s

The graduating class of 1870 numbered 160, and in March of that year the commencement exercises underwent a permanent change from Musical Fund Hall to the Academy of Music. In 1873 the faculty planned a series of prizes for outstanding scholarship that were first awarded at the Annual Commencement of March, 1874; before that time prizes had been awarded on a sporadic basis. The five prizes were as follows: $100, by a friend of the school, for the best graduation thesis; $50 by the Professor of Anatomy (Pancoast) for the best anatomical preparation contributed to the College museum; $50 by the Professor of Surgery (Gross) for the best report of his surgical clinic; $50 by the Professor of Practice (DaCosta) for the best report of clinical cases or original inquiry; and $50 by the Professor of Physiology (Meigs) for the best paper on original physiological investigation. The following year the prizes increased to nine. With gradual increase in recent years to more than 30 prizes, it became necessary to make the awards at special class day exercises on the day before Commencement.

In June, 1873, the famous Dr. Joseph Pancoast resigned as Chairman of the Department of Anatomy, a post he had held with great distinction since 1841, and as successor to George McClellan as Professor of Surgery in 1839. Initially nine candidates were placed in nomination. Five Jeffersonians were interested—William H. Pancoast (the retiring Professor's son), John Hill Brinton, William W. Keen, William S. Forbes, and Addinell Hewson, all of whom were well qualified anatomist-surgeons. Seventeen ballots were taken in succession without any candidate receiving a majority vote. The elder Pancoast was induced to continue, relieved of evening lectures. At another meeting in April, 1874, William H. Pancoast received a majority vote on the fifteenth ballot.

The younger Pancoast was graduated from Haverford College in 1853 and from Jefferson in 1856. As was customary at that time, he did postgraduate work for two and one-half years in London, Paris, Vienna, and Berlin. During the Civil War he was appointed Surgeon-in-Chief in charge of the Military Hospital in Philadelphia. While serving throughout the war he also aided his father's Department at Jefferson as Demonstrator of Anatomy from 1862 until his full Professorship in 1874. William Pancoast also found time to lecture on surgical anatomy in Jefferson's Summer Course. In his clinical practice he was a brilliant diagnostician and skillful operator, serving on the staff of the Charity and Philadelphia Hospitals. He published many papers on surgical subjects. In 1874, after the death at age 63 of the famous Siamese twins, Chang and Eng Bunker, he obtained permission for their autopsy under the auspices of the College of Physicians of Philadelphia. His report, in conjunction with Dr. Harrison Allen of the University of Pennsylvania, stated that no separation would have been successful except perhaps in early childhood. From 1886 until his death in 1897 at age 62 Pancoast was Professor of the combined Chairs of Anatomy and Surgery at the newly formed Medico-Chirurgical College of Philadelphia, which he helped to found.

In the early 1870s economic and psychological recovery from the Civil War was underway but far from resolved. Ulysses S. Grant was in the White House. Railroads crossed the country from coast to coast, and new cities were springing up everywhere, associated with tides of immigrants. An enlarging middle class was enjoying a better standard of living as industrial progress burgeoned. Physicians and scientists who had studied in Europe in increasing numbers added to the new achievements and rising standards. America's stature was becoming evident in a variety of fields in which the United States was emerging ahead of its European counterparts. The country was moving toward its centennial celebration, to be held in Philadelphia. Exhibitions were expected from throughout the world.

In the winter of 1874 the Philadelphia County Medical Society appointed a Centennial Medical Commission with Samuel D. Gross as Chairman to devise plans for the organization of an International Medical Congress. At the Congress, which convened for a week starting September 4, 1876, Gross was unanimously elected President. A large number of distinguished American and foreign delegates were in attendance, including Professor Miyake from the Medical College of Tokyo. Drs. William B. Atkinson (Jefferson, class of 1853), Richard J. Dunglison (Jefferson, 1856), and William W. Keen (Jefferson, 1862) were assistant secretaries. The Surgeon General, Dr. Joseph K. Barnes, was an Honorary Vice-President. At the banquet of the Congress on September 8th, Gross presided with Professor Joseph Lister of Edinburgh on his right and Governor Hartranft on the left. In the previous year Gross had published a *History of American Medical Literature from 1776 to the Present Time,* "designed to show our people how much earnest work we have done during the century now about to close of our existence as an independent power in the interests of medical science, and in upholding the national honor."[14] Gross wrote the history of American surgery from 1776 to 1876 especially for the Centennial.[15]

In addition to the seven Professional Chairs, the "Announcements" of 1875 and 1876 included the names of an enlarging faculty: Thomas H. Andrews, M.D., Demonstrator of Anatomy; J. Ewing Mears, M.D., Demonstrator of Surgery; William H. Green, M.D., Demonstrator of Chemistry, Henry Lean, M.D., Prosector to the Professor of Anatomy; Franklin West, M.D. (recorder on Eakins's *Gross Clinic*), Prosector to the Professor of Surgery and Curator of the Museum; William Thomson, M.D., Clinical Lecturer in Diseases of the Eye and Ear; Samuel W. Gross, M.D., assisting the elder Gross as Lecturer in Clinical Surgery; John H. Brinton, M.D., Lecturer on Operative Surgery; Francis F. Maury, M.D., Lecturer on Venereal and Cutaneous Diseases; Morris Longstreth, M.D., Lecturer on Pathological Anatomy; Jacob Solis-Cohen, M.D., Lecturer in Laryngoscopy and Diseases of the Throat; F.H. Getchell, M.D., Lecturer on Clinical Midwifery with Cases; J. Eneu Loughlin, M.D., Lecturer on Chemistry and Pathology of the Urine and Blood; Stanley Smith, M.D., Lecturer on Physical Diagnosis, including auscultation and percussion; and H. Osgood, M.D., Lecturer on General Symptomatology and also the Microscope.

Acceleration of teaching and clinical demands on Jefferson in the exciting atmosphere of the Centennial Celebration were echoed in the construction of the 1877 first detached hospital.

References

1. Konkle, B.A., and Henry, F.P., *Standard History of the Medical Profession of Philadelphia*, New York: AMS Press, 1977, pp. 259–260.
2. Burt, N., *The Perennial Philadelphians*. Boston: Little, Brown and Co., 1963, pp. 44–59.
3. Bauer, E.L., *Doctors Made in America*. Philadelphia: J.B. Lippincott Co., 1963, pp. 159–160.
4. *The Medical Record*. Vol. II, 1867, p. 69.
5. DaCosta, J.M., "On Irritable Heart," *Am. J. Med. Sci.* 1871, 61:17–52.
6. Clarke, M.D., "Memoir of J.M. DaCosta, M.D.," *Am. J. Med. Sci.* 1903, 125:318–329.
7. Wooley, C.F., "Jacob Mendez DaCosta: Medical Teacher, Clinician, and Clinical Investigator," *Am. J. Card.* 1982, 50:1145 1148.
8. Wooley, C.F., "From Irritable Heart to Mitral Valve Prolapse: British Army Medical Reports, 1860 to 1870," *Am. J. Card.* 1985, 55:1107–1109.
9. Gross, S.D., *System of Surgery*. 6th ed., 1882, p. 346.
10. Gross, S.D., *Autobiography*. Vol. I, p. 234.
11. Wagner, F.B. Jr., "Centennial Memoir of James Aitken Meigs, M.D," *Trans. Stud. Coll. Phys. Phila.* September 1982, Vol. 4, No. 3, pp. 171–178.
12. Fye, W.B., "S. Weir Mitchell, Philadelphia's 'Lost Physiologist,'" *Bull. Hist. Med.* 1983, 57:188–202.
13. Wagner, F.B. Jr., "Meigs Medical Association: A Jefferson Tradition." *Jeff. Med. Coll. Al. Bull.* Fall 1983, pp. 20–22.
14. Gross, S.D., *A History of American Medical Literature from 1776 to the Present Time*. Philadelphia: Collins, Printer, 1875.
15. Gross, S.D., "A Century of American Medicine: II: Surgery," *Am. J. Med. Sci.* Vol. 71, 72:431–84, 1876.

The First Jefferson Medical College Hospital (1877): Science Begins to Enhance the Art of Medicine

For fifty-three years (1824–1877) Jefferson Medical College was without a regular hospital, but, although there was no building especially devoted to hospital purposes until 1877, there was a sort of hospital from the very beginning. Even in the Tivoli Theater building on Prune Street (518–520 Locust) outpatients were cared for and operations were regularly performed before the class by

George McClellan, the first on May 9, 1825. Up to the year 1844, patients with serious operations were driven to their homes in carriages and cared for by the Professor of Surgery and his assistants. By that time the upper floors of the two stores on the southwest corner of Tenth and Sansom Streets were rented and gradually renovated into a miniature surgical hospital, and in 1852 a doorway was made to connect them with the arena of the upper lecture room of the adjacent Medical Hall (the Ely building). It was in this upper lecture room that the Professor of Anatomy taught and where Samuel D. Gross was operating in Eakins's famous masterpiece, *The Gross Clinic* (1875). The "old operating table" depicted in the painting was rescued and restored several times until permanently maintained as an archival treasure in the Samuel D. Gross Conference Room of the Department of Surgery. The two rooms over the stores, one for men and one for women, accommodated about 15 patients—they constituted the hospital until 1877 as used by Mütter, the elder Pancoast, and the elder Gross. The concept of a hospital as a place to teach medical students was new and had been preceded only by the University of Pennsylvania in 1874.

In 1877 not a building in Philadelphia was over eight stories high. Steel was not used in construction. Street cars were drawn by horses over Belgian blocks and cobblestones. Bicycles with huge front wheels were just appearing and the first automobiles were 20 years away. Streets were illuminated by flickering gas jets, tended by lamplighters who as watchmen were precursors of a police force that did not yet exist.

The telephone had been exhibited the previous year at the Centennial Celebration and was regarded only as an intriguing toy. Edison was perfecting the incandescent electric light that would appear two years later, and was inventing the phonograph. Letters and records were written with pen and ink; handwriting was a valued art in the absence of typewriters. Newspapers were without photographs, and pictures in magazines were woodcuts. Preservation of food by canning was in its infancy but on its way to becoming a large industry. Jules Verne's, book *Twenty Thousand Leagues Under the Sea,* just published, imagined submarines in the way that the twentieth-century comic strip *Buck Rogers* would regard space travel. The United States Army numbered 20,000 men, and the Navy was practically nonexistent. The Philippine Islands were little known except in connection with hemp and unusual looking cigars. Express trains ran 30 miles per hour, and the fastest passage across the Atlantic required more than seven days.

The Doctor of Medicine degree was still obtained in a three-year preceptorship with a "regular" physician, which included two years of medical college and only the simplest preliminary education. The Jefferson Professors divided the students' fees, and the College was run as a proprietary institution for private gain of the faculty, like most medical schools in the country. There was not a genuinely trained nurse in any hospital in Philadelphia. Surgery was limited mainly to the surface of the body. Serious operations consisted of ligating for aneurysm, amputation, stone in the bladder, and extirpating tumors. The abdomen was seldom entered except by a few surgeons, namely Washington L. Atlee (Jefferson, class of 1829) and J. Marion Sims (Jefferson, 1835). Gunshot wounds of the abdomen were not explored. There was tracheotomy, operating for empyema and strangulated hernia, bone diseases (*Gross Clinic*), reducing dislocations, setting and dressing of fractures, trephining for head injuries, and removal of superficial foreign bodies and tumors. Operations were performed between the hours of 11 A.M. and 3 P.M. on sunny days with natural light from a skylight. Edison's platinum wire incandescent electric lamp was not invented until 1878. Antisepsis was in its infancy, although described a decade previously. In 1877 only two surgeons in Philadelphia employed Listerian methods. They were W.W. Keen (Jefferson, 1862) and J. Ewing Mears (Jefferson, 1865) at St. Mary's Hospital. Patients were afraid of hospitals with good reason and would go only as a last resort. In 1877, medicine notably was moving toward adding science in the form of laboratories to the art. In that year Louis Pasteur discovered the bacillus of anthrax. The following year Robert Koch discovered causes of infection, and William Henry Welch introduced bacteriology in the United States. In 1879 Albert Neisser discovered the gonococcus and with Armauer Hansen described the lepra bacillus. In 1880 Pasteur discovered the streptococcus, staphylococcus, and pneumococcus, and a year later Alexander Ogston found staphylococci in abscesses. Robert Koch's discovery of the tubercle bacillus was awaiting the year 1882. Local anesthesia would not be introduced by William Stewart Halsted until 1885. Appendicitis was unrecognized until 1886 when Reginald Fitz of Boston published his epoch-making description.

The need for a separate hospital to relieve increasing encroachments on the space of the College was perceived in 1873. Trustees, Faculty, and Alumni were equally desirous and enthusiastic about getting on with the project. By 1871 the $29,000 debt on the original Ely building (Medical Hall) was liquidated and the drive for new funds could begin. A committee for public appeal was formed from five members of the Board, two from the Faculty, and two from the Alumni. In 1873 Dr. Francis Fontaine Maury (Jefferson, 1862) approached the Pennsylvania State Legislature and obtained an appropriation of $100,000 on the conditions that it be matched by a similar sum, that the money would not be available until construction was started, that only $25,000 could be used in any six months, and that the building be completed within three years. Dr. John Hill Brinton (Jefferson, 1852) undertook to raise $150,000 through the Alumni, and in this effort he surpassed even Samuel D. Gross. The Trustees and friends of the school gave generously. Consideration was given to the desirability of moving to a different location in the city, but fortunately the two stores at the corner of Tenth and Sansom (for a subsequent new laboratory) and ground (107 by 106 feet) on Sansom Street between Tenth and Eleventh (for the hospital) were available. The hospital (and grounds), at a cost of $186,000, was completed within the stipulated three years by March 1876.

At this time the population of Philadelphia was 820,000. In the following decades immigrants pouring into the city would swell the population to 1,300,000 by the end of the century. The first wave came mainly from Germany and Ireland, accompanied by many blacks from the South. Toward the end of the century the influx of Irish was matched by a sixfold increase in the Italian population. Many immigrants from Russia and Eastern Europe contributed to the "melting pot." Jefferson had not prepared too soon for the care of an expanding community.

Frank Furness (1839–1912) was the chosen architect for the new hospital. His style was Victorian Gothic, as still extant in the Pennsylvania Academy of the Fine Arts (Broad and Cherry), which he planned as part of the 1876 Centennial. Although architectural tastes turned to the Classical Revival, and although his accomplishments were subsequently ignored for more than 50 years, he is recognized today as one of Philadelphia's greatest architects.

With all the modifications, refinements, and added costs, the first detached Jefferson Medical College Hospital was formally opened on September 17, 1877 (Figure 2-14). Dr. Samuel D. Gross had been approached to give the address, but he induced Dr. Joseph Pancoast to deliver it instead. Pancoast spoke graphically about the founder of the College, Dr. George McClellan,

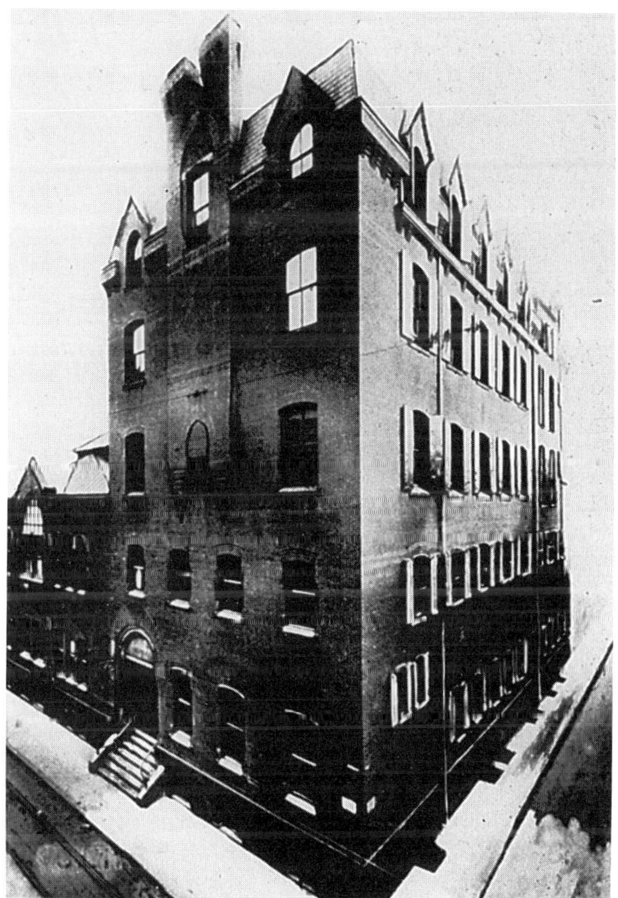

FIG. 2-14. The first detached Jefferson Medical College Hospital (1877).

and emphasized the advantages of clinical instruction that McClellan instituted at Jefferson. Pancoast at the time had already retired, and it was his last official act in the school after nearly 40 years of attachment.

The building was modern, well equipped, architecturally attractive, and the pride of the School. A two-story shed-roofed structure to the left accommodated the clinical amphitheater, and a five-story structure to the side and rear housed the hospital proper. The basement functioned for kitchens (Figure 2-15), laundry, and storerooms. The first floor of the hospital provided a public lobby, administrative offices (Figure 2-16), apothecary (Figure 2-17), and surgical-preparation rooms for the adjacent "pit." The second floor was assigned to the clinics (Figures 2-18 and 2-19), while the third and fourth floors each contained two wards (Figures 2-20, 2-21, and 2-22).

The fifth floor contained ten private rooms, a suite of three rooms with a fireplace for the Resident Physician, and a matron's room. The elevator and stairs were at the rear of the "L" where the two structures adjoined. The total bed capacity was 125.

It could only have been a coincidence that on August 30, 1877, several weeks before formal opening, Dr. Francis F. Maury, who had successfully solicited the State Legislature for funds, performed the first operation. It was an amputation of the left middle finger on Malcolm Meyer, son of the Speaker of the House. Maury was a brilliant rising star in the Samuel D. Gross Surgical Staff who tragically died of tuberculosis in 1879 at the age of 39. In addition to his prowess in the most complex surgery of his time, he was

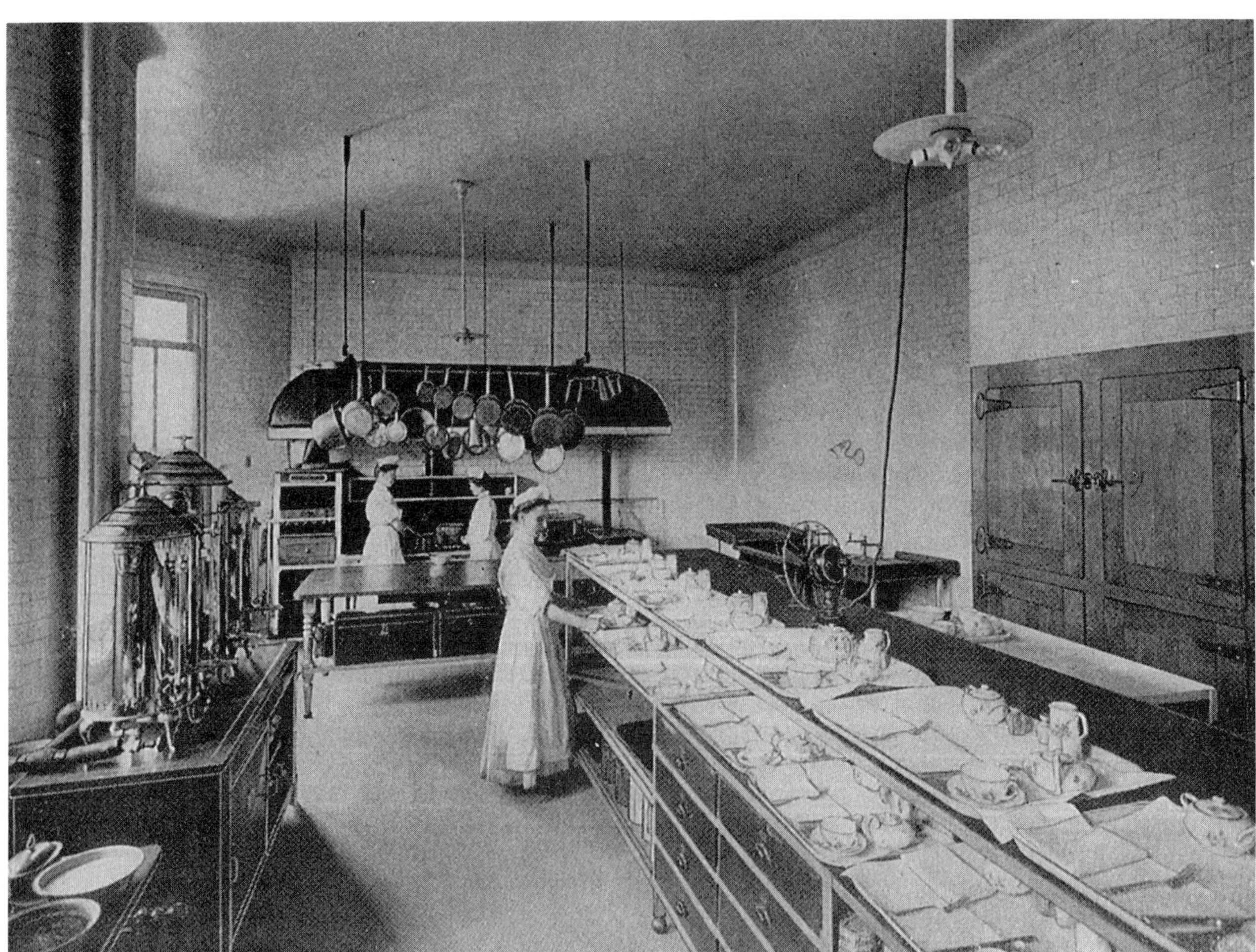

FIG. 2-15. The kitchen of the 1877 hospital.

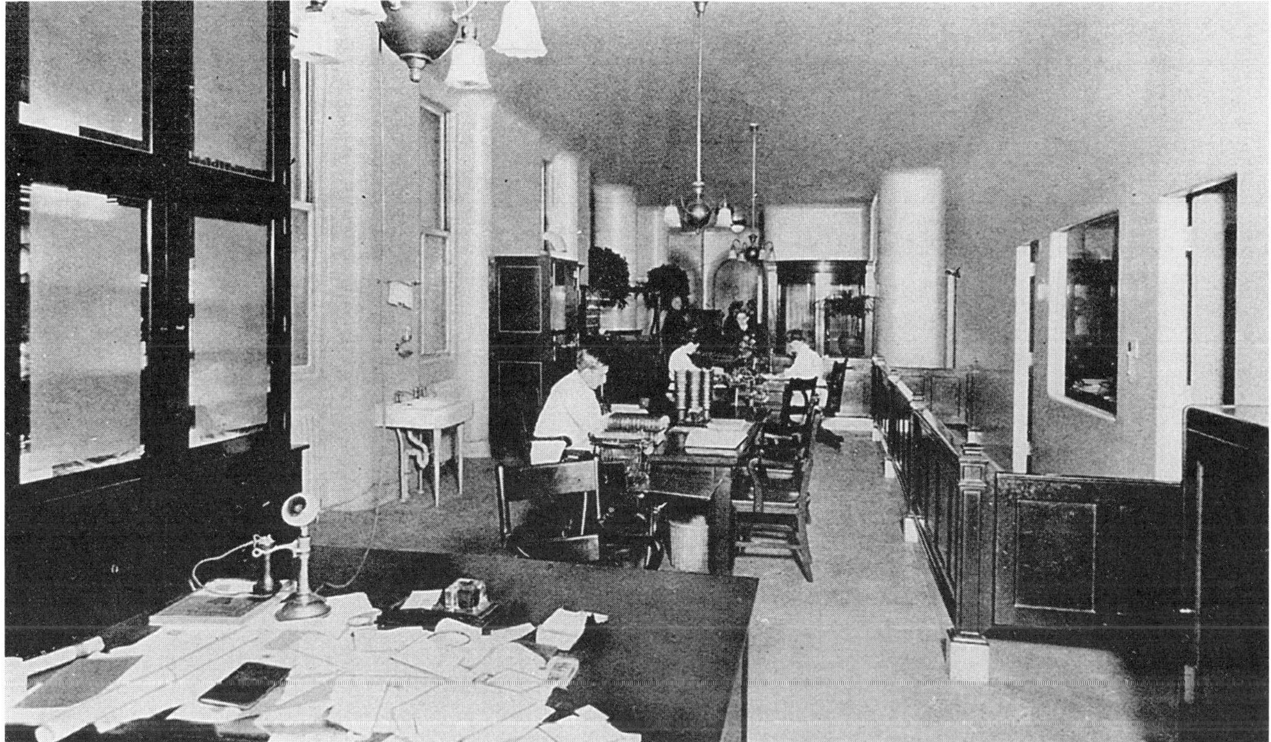

FIG. 2-16. Administrative offices of the 1877 hospital.

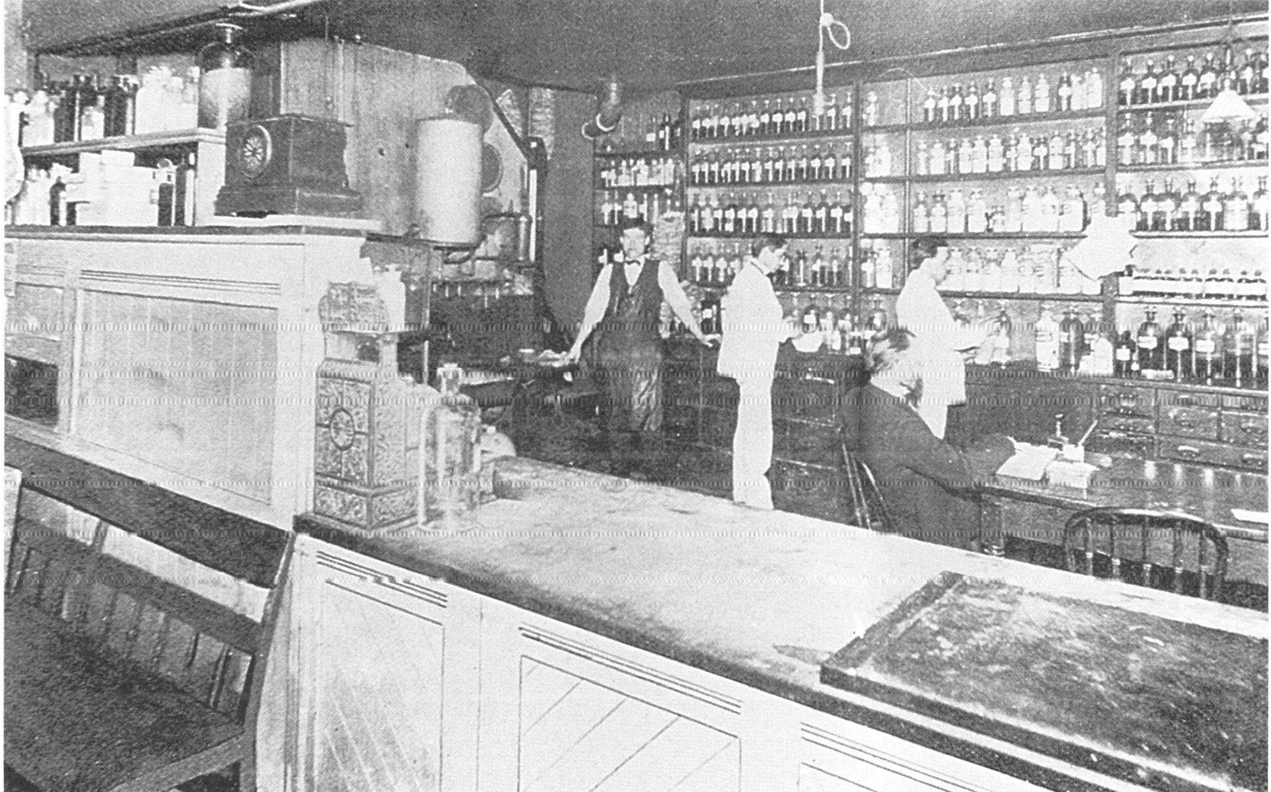

FIG. 2-17. Apothecary (1877 hospital).

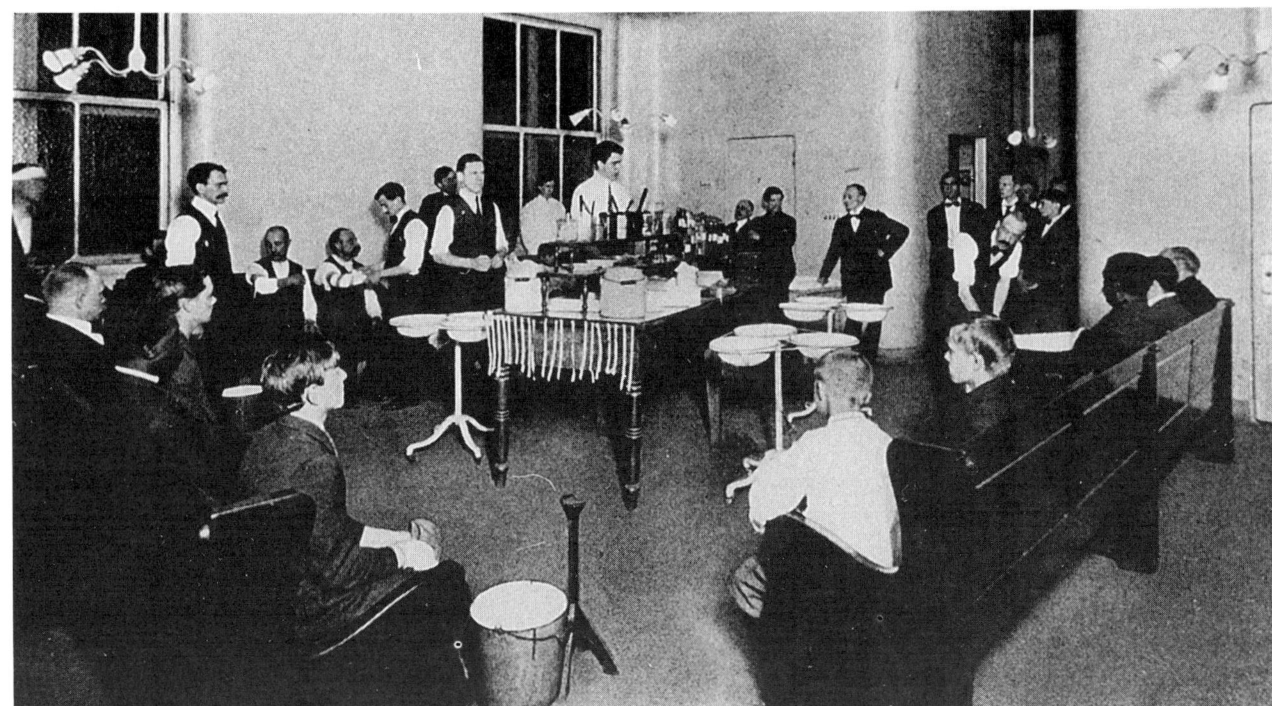

FIG. 2-18. Surgical Clinic (1877 hospital).

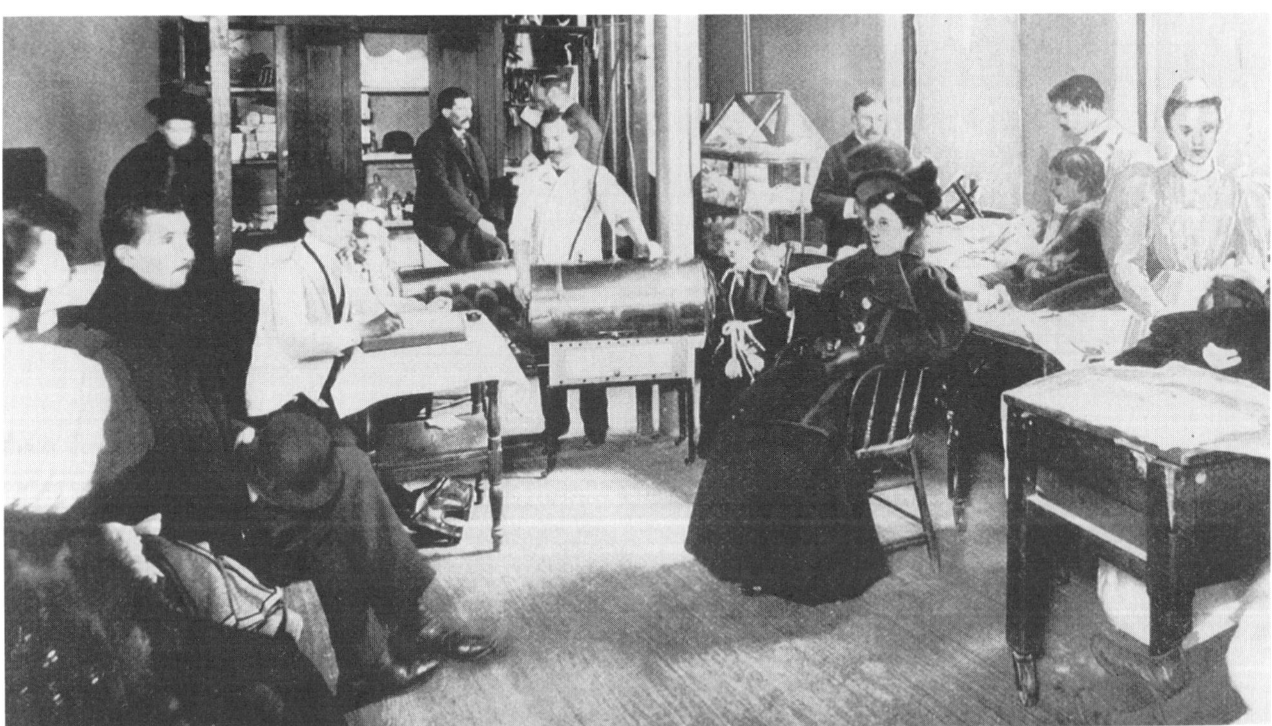

FIG. 2-19. Orthopaedic Clinic (1877 hospital).

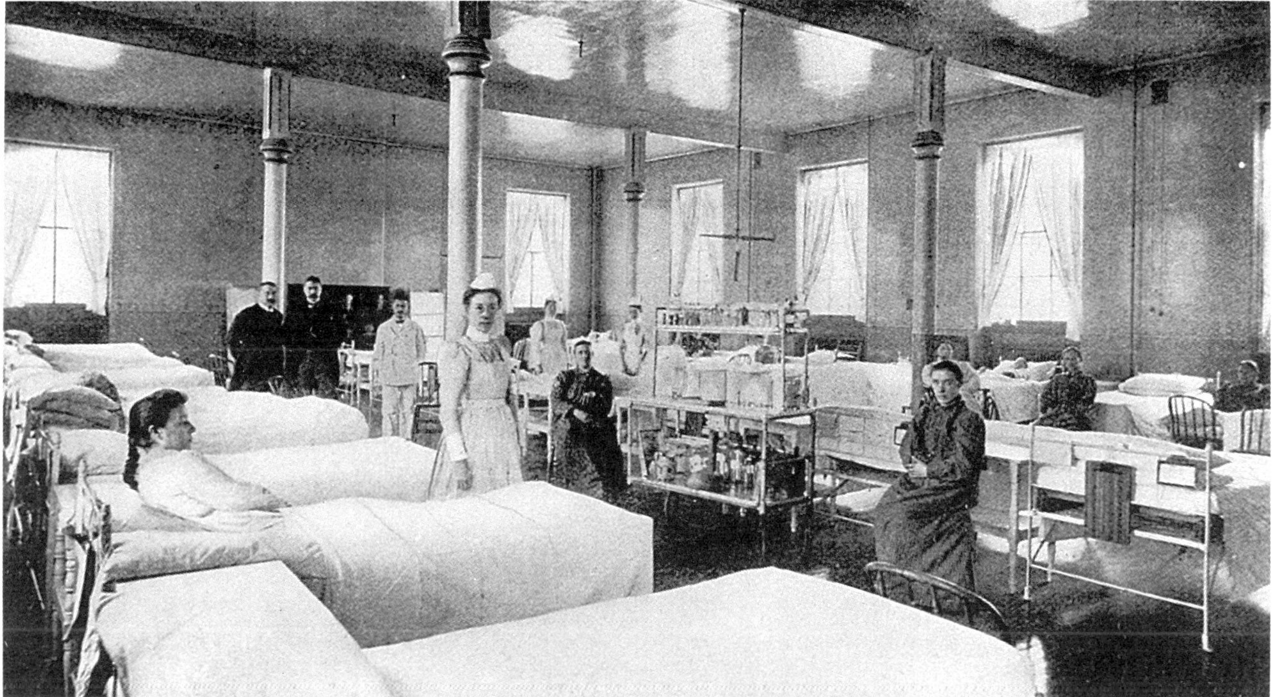

Fig. 2-20. Women's Surgical Ward (1877 hospital).

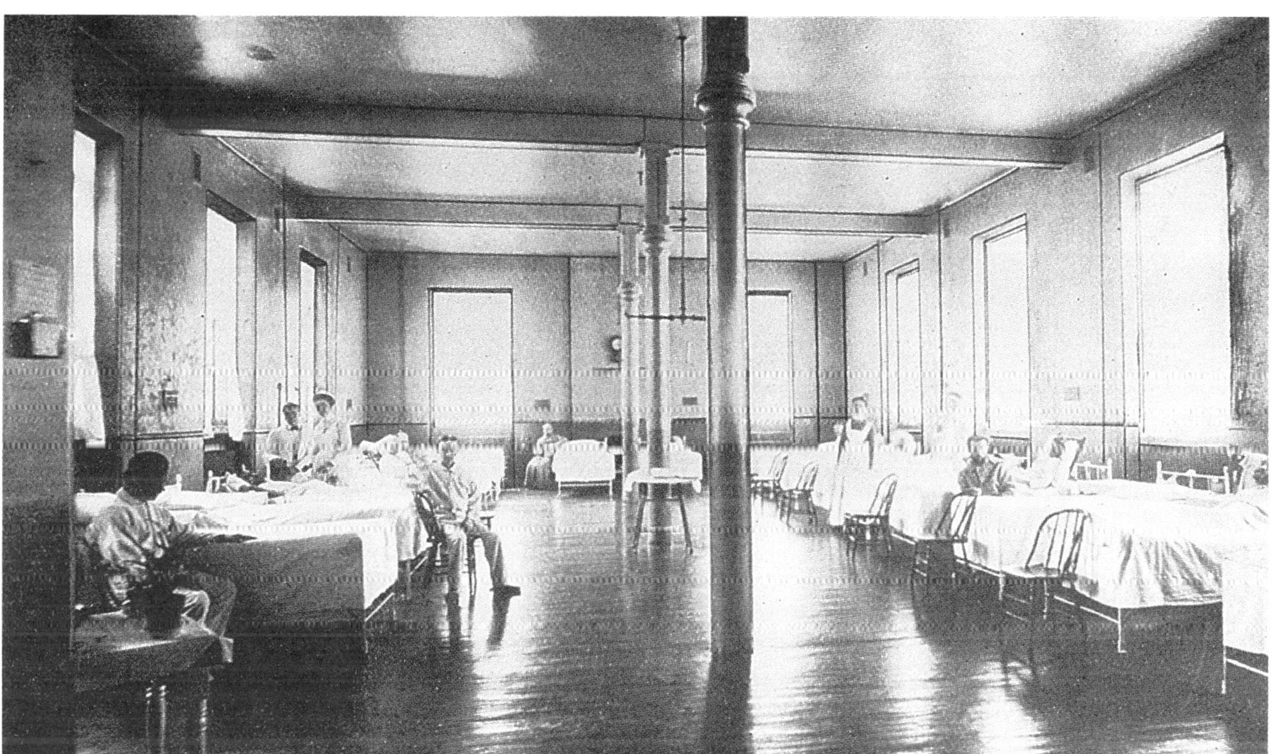

Fig. 2-21. Men's Medical Ward (1877 hospital).

also a pioneer in dermatology. His portrait is among the finest in Jefferson's art collection (Figure 2-23).

The Hospital was of immediate benefit to patients and student teaching. The first seven months witnessed the admission of 642 patients, who came not only from local areas but from distant parts of the country. The United States government established a Marine Ward in which the government paid 85 cents a day per patient. Private patients were charged $2 a day, and ward patients, when able, paid from $5 to $7 per week. Ward patients were not charged a physician's fee. Growth in the clinics was phenomenal and simultaneously showed 6,254 new outpatients for a total of 23,510 visits.

The College Professors of Medicine, Surgery, and Obstetrics each had a clinical teaching ward for student instruction, with the privilege of having assistants for whom they were responsible. Appointees to the Hospital Staff up to 1879 were: John H. Brinton, Samuel W. Gross, Francis F. Maury, and Richard J. Levis (Surgery); Jacob Solis-Cohen (Laryngology); James C. Wilson, John B. Roberts, followed in 1878 by W.W. Alzach and Oliver Rex (Medicine); Frank H. Getchell and J. Ewing Mears (Gynecology); Laurence S. Turnbull (Aural Surgery); William Thomson (Ophthalmology); and Morris Longstreth (Pathology). This select and highest calibre group of physicians was well qualified for the challenges of the new Hospital.

So rapid was medical progress and so strong the demand for more space that within thirty years this ornament to the city and the Medical College became antiquated. In 1907 another new Jefferson Medical College Hospital, the most modern possible to that time, was opened at the corner of Tenth and Sansom (now Old Main Hospital). At that time the 1877 hospital was converted for nurses' purposes, but the connected amphitheater ("pit") had a more glorious survival until the last surgical clinic was held there by Dr. John Chalmers DaCosta before the junior and senior classes on May 10, 1922.[3]

There have been three clinical amphitheaters ("pits") in Jefferson's history, each with a life span of fewer than 50 years. The first one (1828–1877), in which McClellan, Pancoast, Mütter, and Gross operated, constituted the upper lecture room of the College. The only pictorial representation of this first pit was in Eakins' masterpiece, *The Gross*

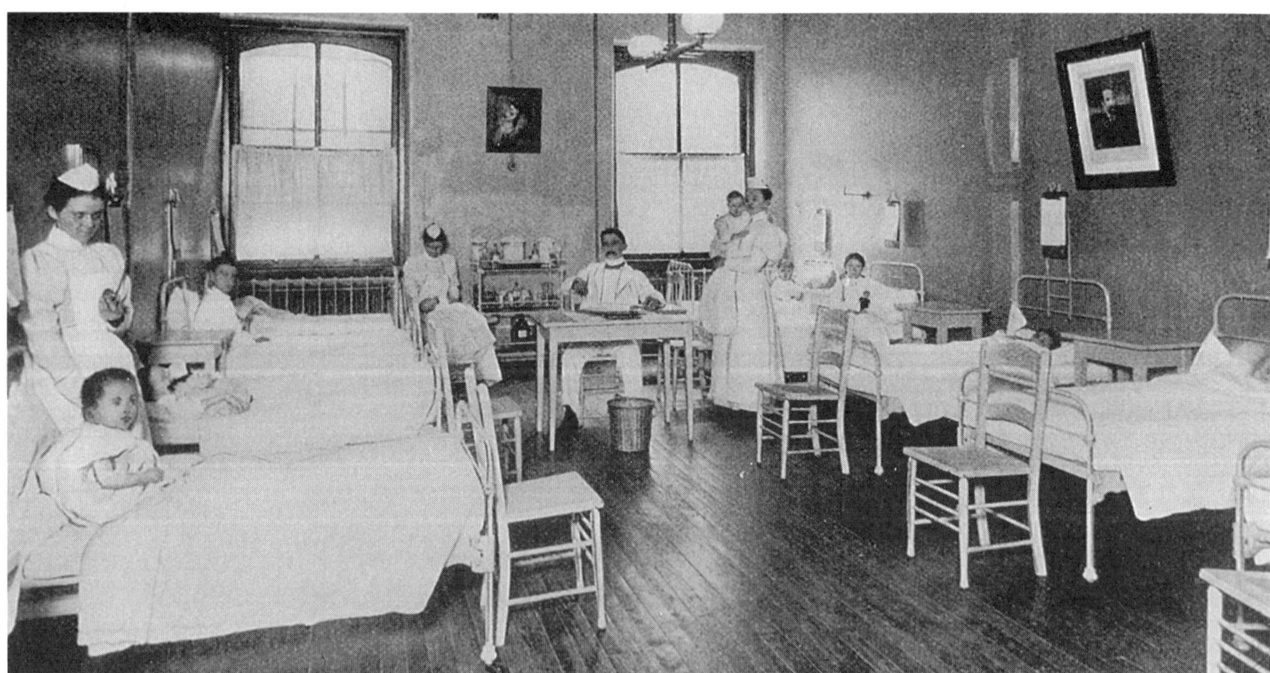

FIG. 2-22. Children's Ward (1877 hospital).

Clinic. The second pit (1877–1922) was in the left wing of the detached Hospital described in this chapter. The third (1924–1966), in the Thompson Annex, was designed to replace the previous one of the 1877 Hospital. The editor vividly recalls performing his first gastroenterostomy in that last pit before the senior class in 1945 at the end of one of Dr. Thomas Shallow's Wednesday afternoon clinics. None of the amphitheaters was limited to surgery, however, but included collegiate sessions in most branches of instruction.

The second pit, which is a main theme in this chapter, was considered to be "holy ground" by Dr. John Chalmers DaCosta because of what "man has wrought for his fellow man." The first

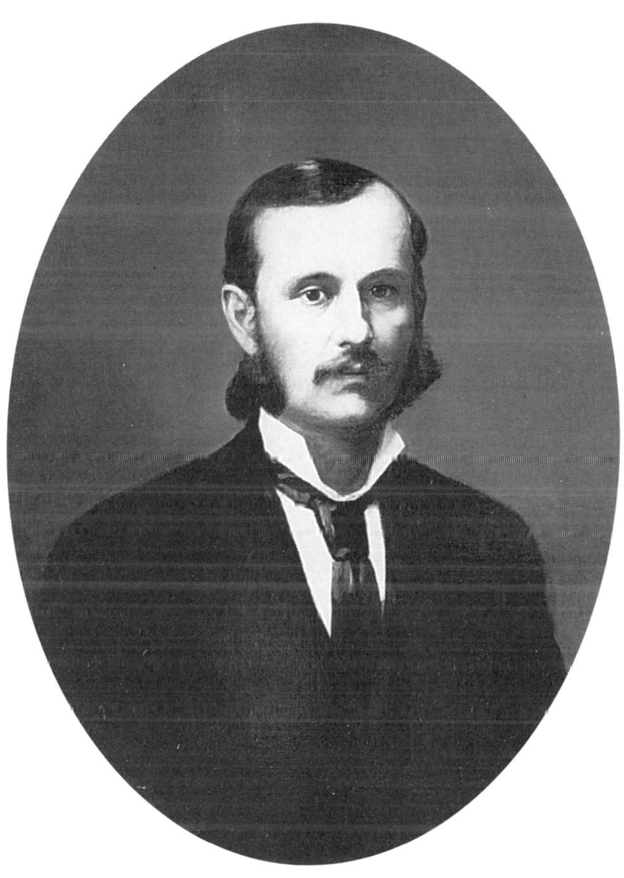

FIG. 2-23. Francis F. Maury, M.D. (1840–1879) solicited funds from the state legislature for the 1877 hospital. He was a pioneer in surgery and dermatology.

clinic of this new amphitheater was held by the elder Gross. The first surgeon to use Listerian antisepsis in this arena was the younger Gross. The first operation in Philadelphia for stone in the kidney was also performed here by the younger Gross. In addition to the two Grosses, the two Pancoasts, and John Brinton, Francis Maury, W. Joseph Hearn, James Barton, Richard Levis, W.W. Keen, and John Chalmers DaCosta, many other eminent surgeons operated here. Jacob Mendes DaCosta, Roberts Bartholow, Theophilus Parvin, Ellerslie Wallace, and John Barclay Biddle were only a few of the Jefferson notables who taught there. Guest lecturers from abroad included Esmarch of Kiel, Mikulicz of Breslau, Fauré of Paris, Lorenz of Vienna, MacEwen of Glasgow, Lawson Tait of Birmingham, Annandale and Chien of Edinburgh, and, from London, Bryant, Durham, Horsley, Ballance, and MacCormac. Jefferson's illustrious graduate, J. Marion Sims, "Father of American Gynecology," lectured here, as well as did Hunter McGuire. The latter was forgiven for having led many Philadelphia medical students to the Confederate side and was granted an LL.D. degree by Jefferson in 1888.

Good photographs of Jefferson's second pit exist (Figure 2-24), but the general features bear description. It was completely circular and seated 600 on stiff wooden benches with straight high backs. Above the northern doorway, which opened into a corridor, was a marble bust of Joseph Pancoast (now in Scott Library). By this doorway was the sink. Above the southern doorway was a marble bust of George McClellan (now in Scott Library). The floor of the arena was wood, and the sides of the center were tiled. In the middle of the pit stood the famous wooden operating table, a hand-down from the first pit and portrayed by Eakins in *The Gross Clinic*. It miraculously survived through various stages of storage, rediscovery and restoration, until its present preservation as an archival treasure in the Samuel D. Gross Conference Room of the Surgery Department.

A surgical clinic in the later years of the first College pit and early years of the second one in the new detached Hospital would have been much the same. One typical of the elder Gross could not be better described than in the words of John Chalmers DaCosta, who participated and became the first Samuel D. Gross Professor of Surgery:

"As a preliminary to the clinic a number of little tables would be brought in to hold the cases of instruments. The knives had ivory handles and were beautiful tools. Assistants set out different sizes of silk, various shapes and sizes of needles, marine sponges in basins, wax for strengthening ligatures, and perhaps a furnace for the actual cautery, such a furnace as is used by the tin roofer. Suppose the case was lithotomy. The patient was brought in under ether (Doctor Joseph Hearn administering the anesthetic), and he was pulled down to the end of the table, put into the lithotomy position and held in it by a frame and straps. On the floor, at the foot of the bed, was a wooden box of sawdust placed to catch as much of the blood as possible. Doctor Gross wore a long blue coat, a costume worn in many previous combats. Dr. James M. Barton was the chief assistant. The bladder was filled with water. A stone sound was passed into the bladder and was held by the chief assistant. Doctor Gross bent down on one knee, picked up the knife, passed it into the urethra until it struck the sound, carried it on into the bladder. As he withdrew the knife he inserted a finger, thus blocking the wound and the stone dropped right on the end of the finger. The whole operation was performed with a speed and dexterity simply marvelous, from twenty to thirty seconds being usually sufficient for the procedure. Of course, before the operation was begun, the case was lectured on and the contemplated procedure was carefully explained. Doctor Gross talked during the operation, demonstrating every step of it. Gathered around in the arena one could usually see Drs. William Keen, Oscar Allis, Richard J. Levis, John Brinton, the younger Gross, Frank Maury, Joseph Pancoast, Thomas A. Andrews, and others. Any distinguished surgeon visiting Philadelphia at that time was certain to be there. In fact, it was seldom that Doctor Gross did not have some eminent man to introduce to the class. It was the foremost surgical clinic in America."[4]

Over a period of 30 years (1877–1907) this Hospital trained 5,000 doctors in its halls; cared for 2,000,000 patients in wards and dispensaries; treated nearly 50,000 accident cases (Figure 2-25); and graduated 148 nurses. By the turn of the century the hospital was antiquated; 125 beds were insufficient for the demand; it was too small for

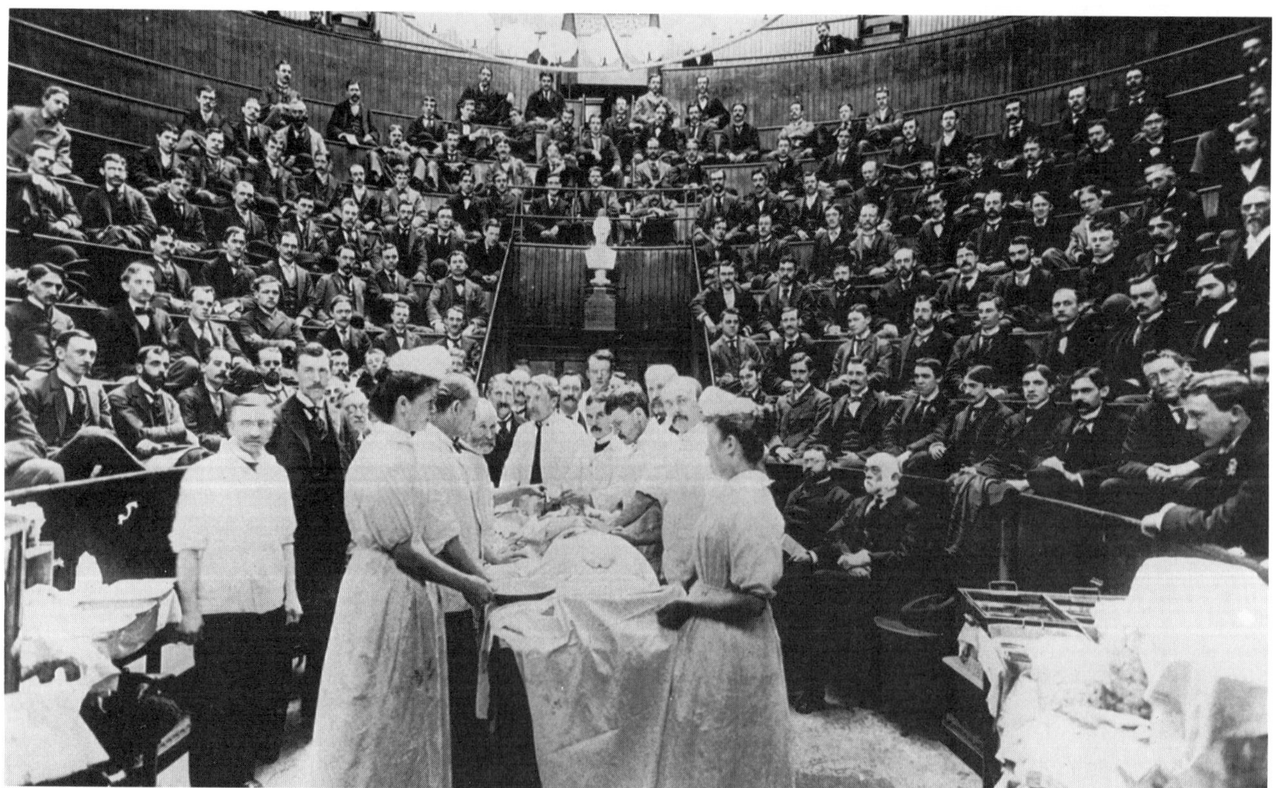

FIG. 2-24. The "pit" of the 1877 hospital.

the volume of work and not fireproof. By 1902 it was possible to demolish the old Medical School building at Tenth and Sansom and erect the new Hospital ("Old Main"). The 1877 Hospital was maintained for nurses' educational purposes and quarters, and the clinical amphitheater was continued for surgery and teaching until the Thompson Annex replaced it in 1924.

References

1. *Philadelphia Architecture: A Guide to the City. A publication of the Foundation for Architecture, Philadelphia, Pennsylvania.* Cambridge: The MIT Press, 1984.
2. Teitelman, E., "Jefferson's Architecture: Past, Present and Future." *Jeff. Al. Bull.*, Fall 1966, pp. 16–17.
3. DaCosta, J.C., *The Papers and Speeches of John Chalmers DaCosta, M.D., LL.D.* Philadelphia: W.B. Saunders Co., 1931, pp. 334–352.
4. Ibid., p. 38.

The Scientific Transition: Laboratory Courses and Specialization

The first Jefferson Medical College Hospital of 1877 was devoted not only to patient care but to the teaching of its medical students. In sharing this concept with the University of Pennsylvania, Philadelphia remained in the forefront of medical education for at least another decade before Johns Hopkins in Baltimore would spring forth with further innovations. Toward the end of the 1870s, as Lister's *Principle of Antisepsis* (1867) received wider acceptance, and as bacteriology as an entity became recognized, a transitional period was developing in which science began to enhance the art of medicine. Until this time, the laboratory instruction of Jefferson students had been limited to anatomy and study of specimens in the pathology museum.

After construction of the 1877 Hospital, the Board of Trustees accelerated its plans by purchasing the property at the southwest corner of Tenth and Sansom Streets, adjacent to the Grecian-

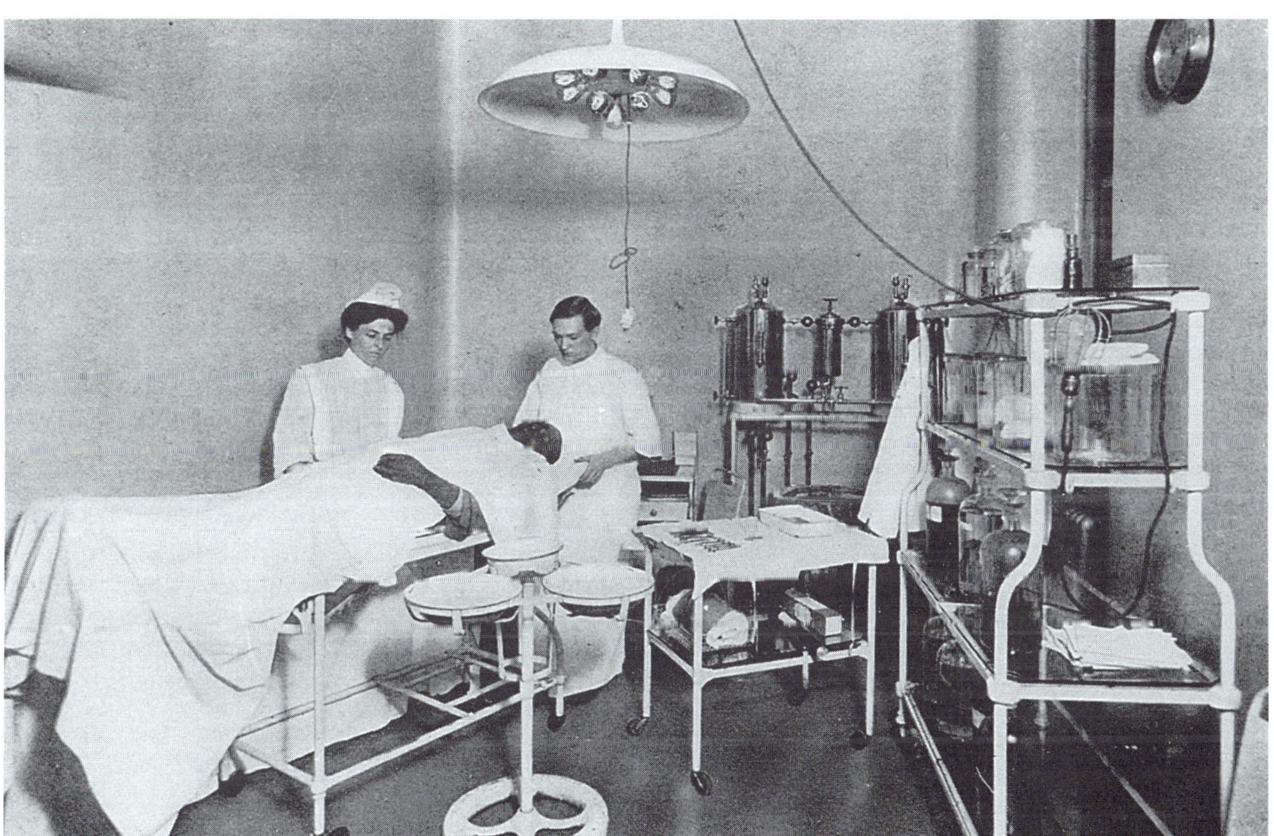

FIG. 2-25. The emergency room of the 1877 hospital.

columned College, for erection of a laboratory facility in the basic sciences. The President of the Board at that time was Dr. Emile B. Gardette, himself a graduate of Jefferson in the Class of 1838. The new building, which was completed for the 1879–1880 session, provided laboratories for operative and minor surgery, practical chemistry, microscopy, and physiology (Figure 2-26).

In 1877, Benjamin Howard Rand had to resign as Professor of Chemistry because of failing health and was succeeded by Dr. Robert Empie Rogers (Figure 2-27). The latter brought with him an experience of 25 years at the University of Pennsylvania. Rogers established the first student laboratory course at Jefferson and oriented his teaching to the newly arrived era of physiological chemistry.

John Barclay Biddle, Professor of Materia Medica and Therapeutics as well as dean (1873–1879), died in 1879. His vacant Chair was filled by Roberts Bartholow (Figure 2-28), and the Deanship was taken by Ellerslie Wallace. Bartholow came to Jefferson from the Ohio Medical College with a strong reputation as teacher and author of a well-known work *Materia Medica and Therapeutics*. While active at Jefferson until 1890 he published his *Treatise on the Practice of Medicine* and served as Dean from 1883 to 1887.[1] His handsome portrait is in Jefferson's art collection.

The College suffered the premature death of Professor James Aitken Meigs in 1879. Dr. Henry C. Chapman accordingly was promoted from Demonstrator of Physiology to the Chair. In that capacity he was successful both as teacher and investigator.[2] Professor Chapman took advantage of the new Laboratory Building to make liberal expenditures year by year for even better and newer apparatus for study and research.

In 1879, Dr. Morris Longstreth (Figure 2-29) was appointed Demonstrator of Pathological Anatomy. His instruction, which also included

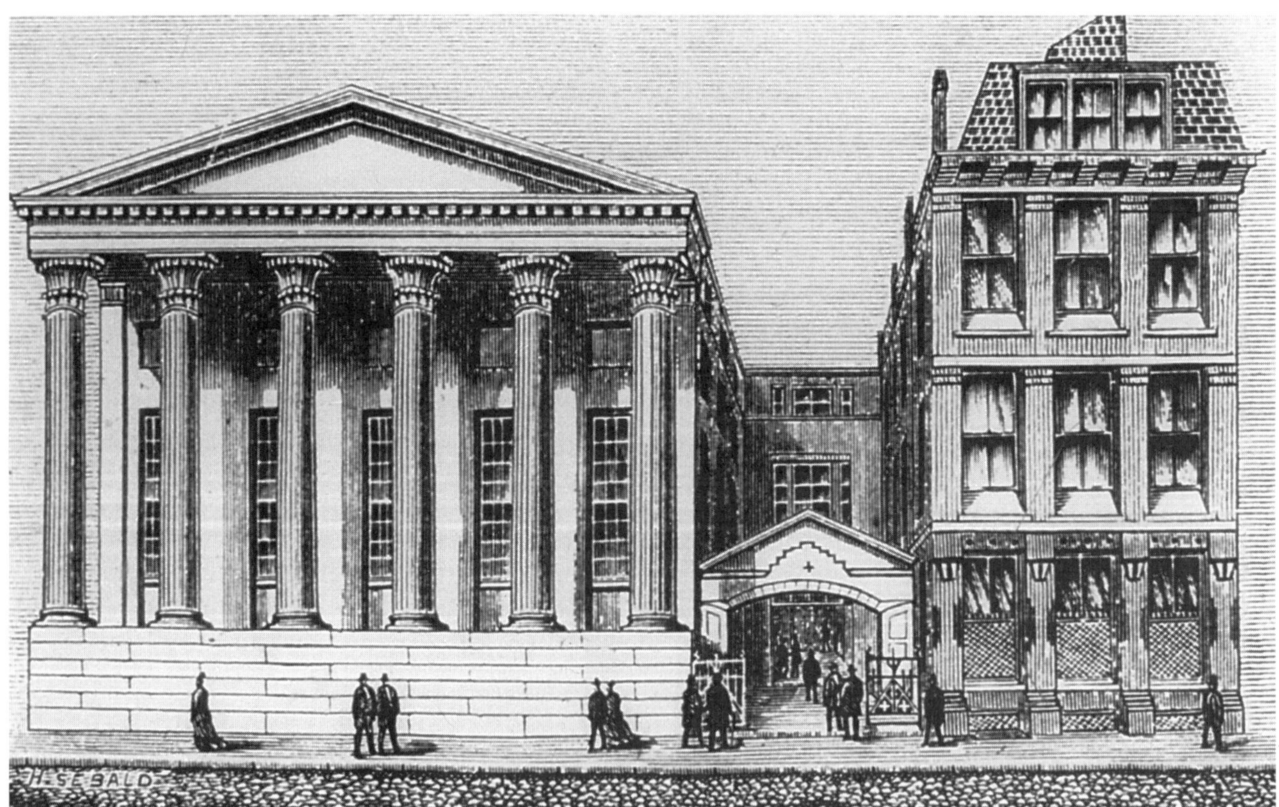

FIG. 2-26. The new Laboratory Building erected adjacent to Medical Hall at Tenth and Sansom Streets (1879). The site was previously occupied by two stores.

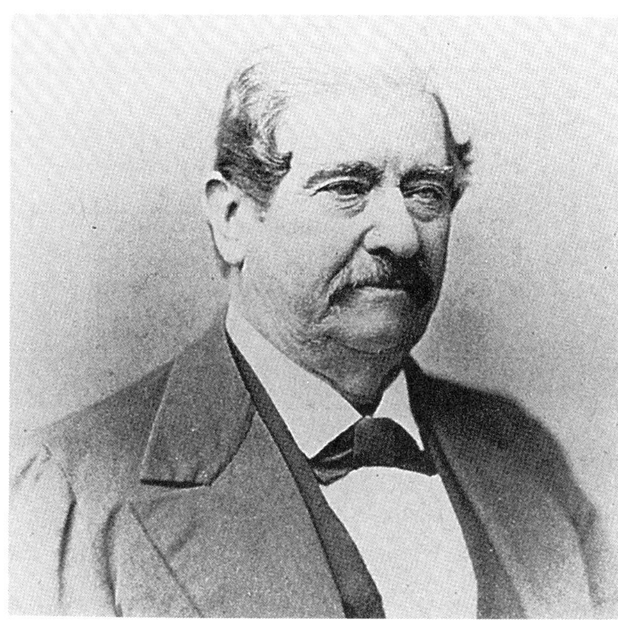

FIG. 2-27. Robert Empie Rogers, M.D. (1813–1884), Professor of Chemistry (1879–1884), established the first student laboratory course in chemistry.

histology, was aided by autopsy material from the Pennsylvania and Jefferson Hospitals. The laboratory of materia medica and pharmacy in the Medical Hall was equipped in the following year. Necessary appliances for the practical course, as well as a room for special research in the physiological action of drugs, were provided (Figure 2-30). All the new laboratories were put in charge of Demonstrators under the supervision of the Professors of each branch.

No sooner was the Laboratory Building erected than more space was needed. By 1881 the classical Grecian facade of the College was replaced by one of Victorian style to match the new Laboratory Building. This permitted a forward expansion of space that increased the seating capacity of the lecture rooms (Figure 2-31). An additional story was added to provide even more laboratory rooms.

In 1882, Dr. William S. Forbes (Figure 2-32), while Demonstrator of Anatomy at Jefferson, was prosecuted in criminal court as an alleged

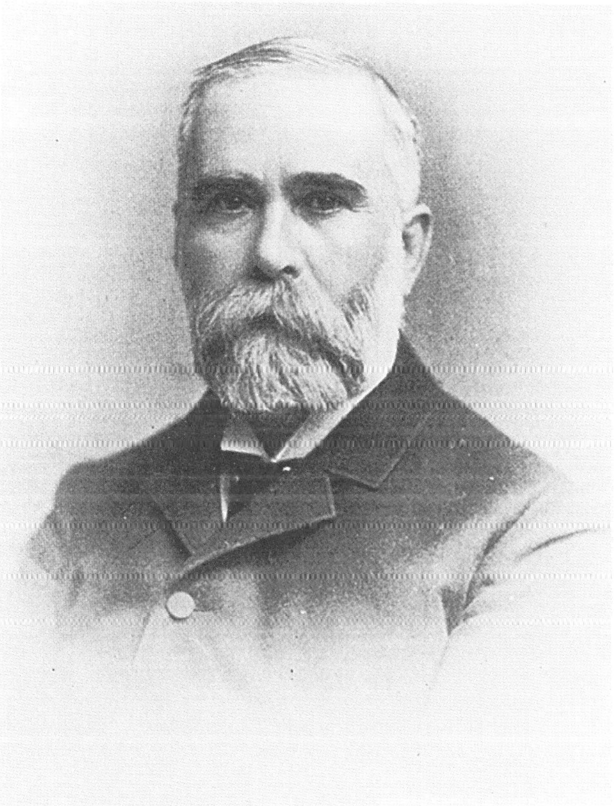

FIG. 2-28. Roberts Bartholow, M.D. (1831–1904); Professor of Materia Medica (1879–1891) and Dean (1883–1887).

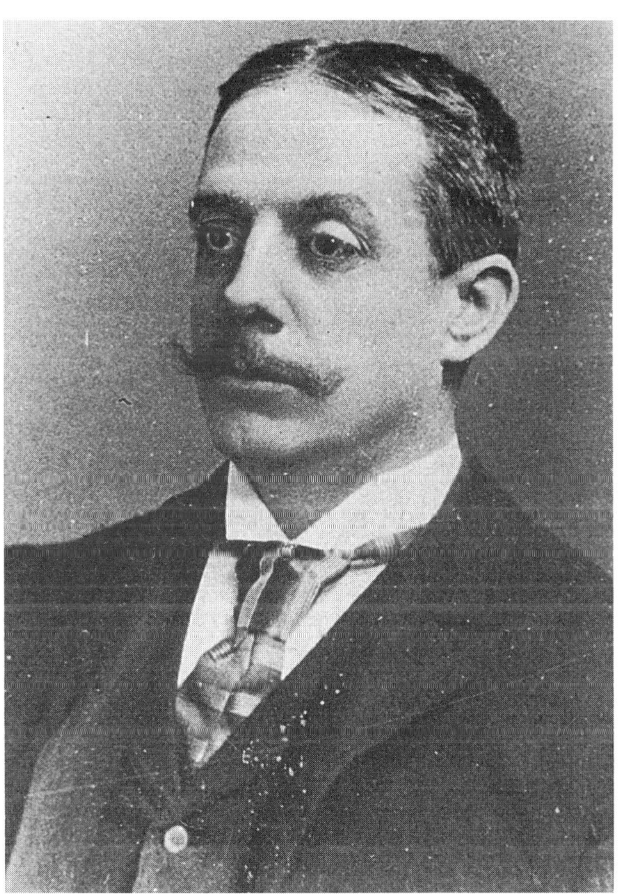

FIG. 2-29. Morris Longstreth, M.D. (1846–1914); Curator of the Jefferson Museum and the first Professor of Pathology (1891).

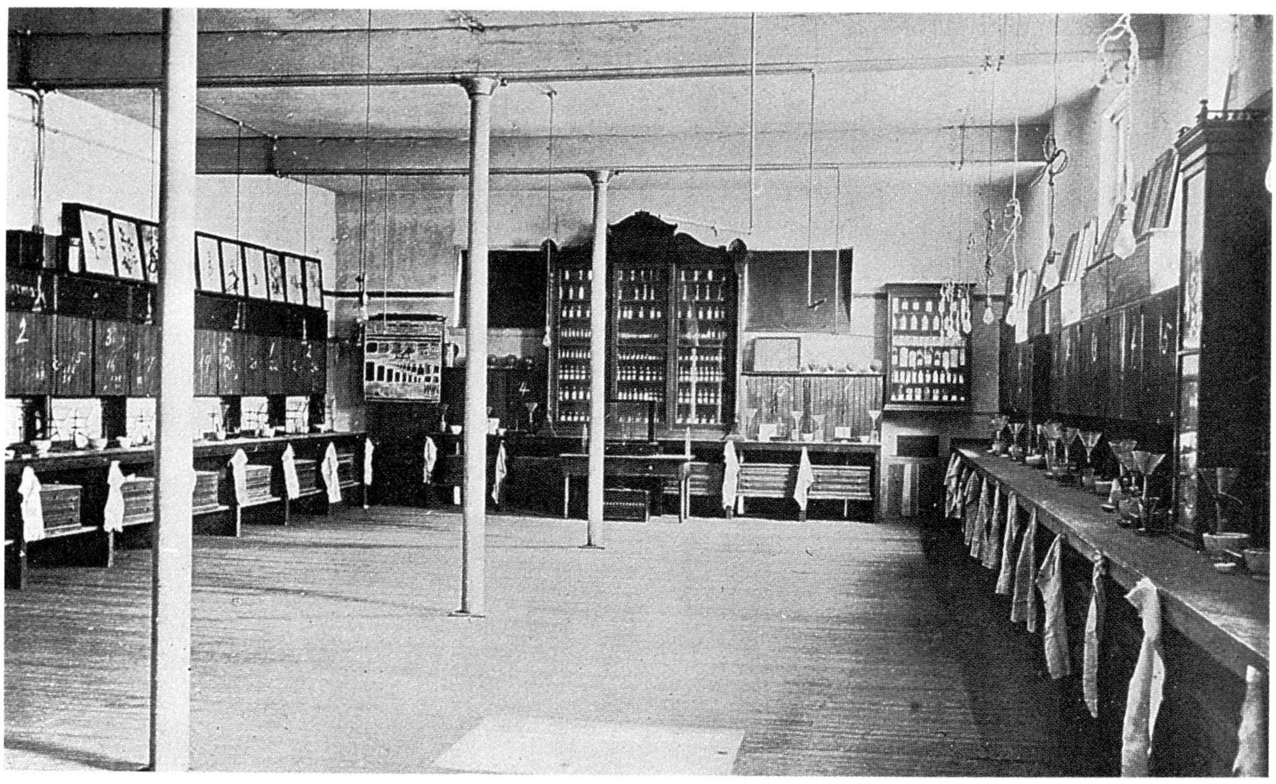

FIG. 2-30. The Laboratory of Pharmacy (ca. 1880).

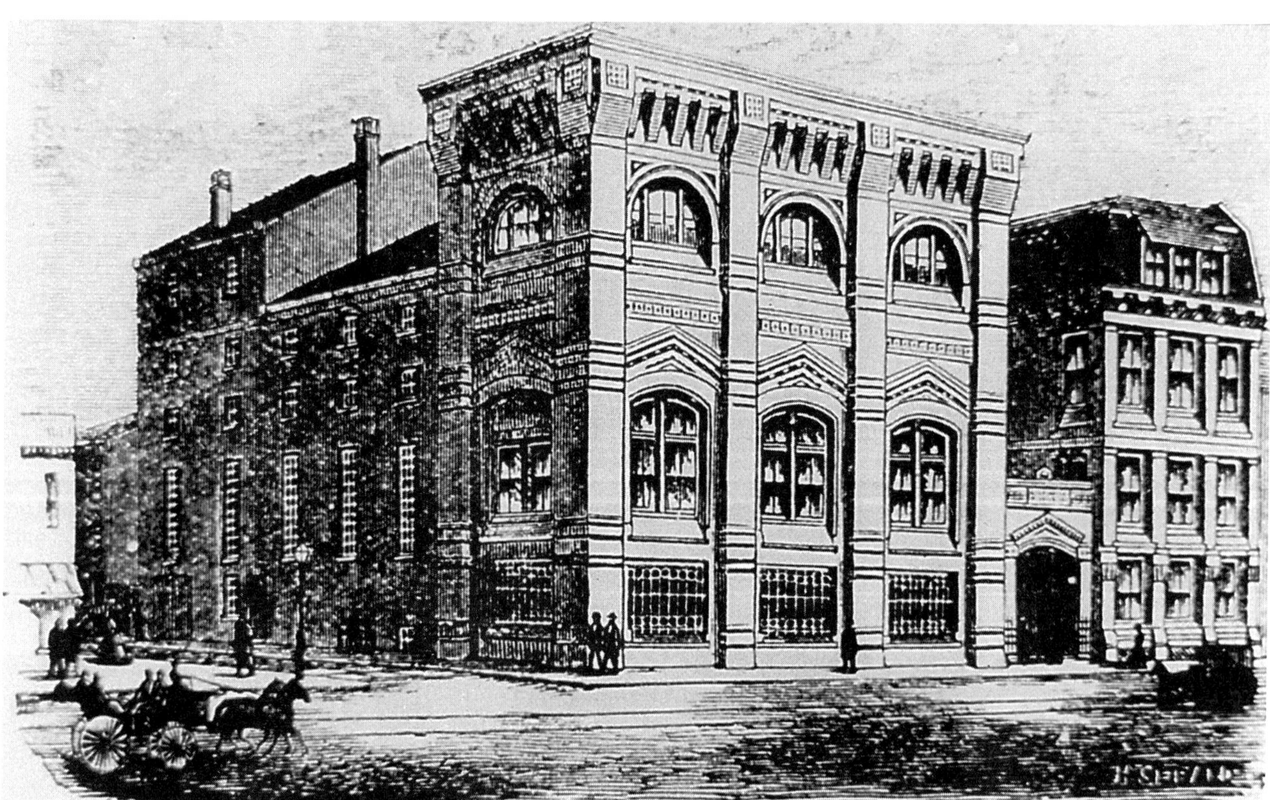

FIG. 2-31. Renovation of Medical Hall (Ely Building) in 1881, replacing the Grecian facade with a Victorian styled one.

"resurrectionist," or body snatcher, in connection with obtaining cadavers for dissection by the students. In 1866 he had previously influenced the passage of a law that permitted dissection of unclaimed bodies in Philadelphia County, but the distribution was inequitable and was not sufficient for the large classes at Jefferson. At trial he was not only vindicated but thereby caused enactment of a perfected anatomical bill that provided compulsory distribution of unclaimed bodies in fair ratio to the needs of the various medical schools.[3] The Eakins portrait of Dr. Forbes in Jefferson's collection shows his hand resting on the anatomical act that he fostered.

Also in 1882, the venerable Samuel D. Gross retired from the Chair of Surgery he had held for the past 26 years. In that capacity he had not only made Jefferson famous but promoted American medicine as a whole throughout the world. By then the subject matter in surgery had expanded to such an extent that it was necessary to divide the Surgical Chair. The younger Gross (Samuel W.) (Figure 2-33) was appointed to the Chair for Principles of Surgery and Clinical Surgery, and John Hill Brinton (Figure 2-34) filled the Chair for Practice of Surgery and Clinical Surgery. Samuel W. Gross died prematurely in 1889 and was succeeded by William Williams Keen (Figure 2-35). The latter had performed the first removal of a brain tumor with permanent cure in 1887 and in 1893 aided in the secret operation upon President Cleveland on a yacht for excision of a verrucous carcinoma in the roof of the mouth.[4]

In 1883 the declining health of Dr. Ellerslie Wallace compelled him to resign the Chair of Obstetrics in which he had served for 21 years and as Dean (1879–1883). Theophilus Parvin, M.D., LL.D., of Indianapolis, a widely known writer and previous Professor in several medical colleges, filled the vacancy (Figure 2-36). His textbook *Science and Art of Obstetrics* (1886) went into a second edition (1890). At Jefferson he promptly agitated for a separate Lying-In Building because the 1877 Hospital did not have sufficient available room. After the failure of makeshift changes, in 1889 he finally obtained a building at Second and Pine Streets where he established the first obstetrical clinic in America.[5] Thirty-four cases in which the students were given practical instruction were delivered without a maternal death. Parvin

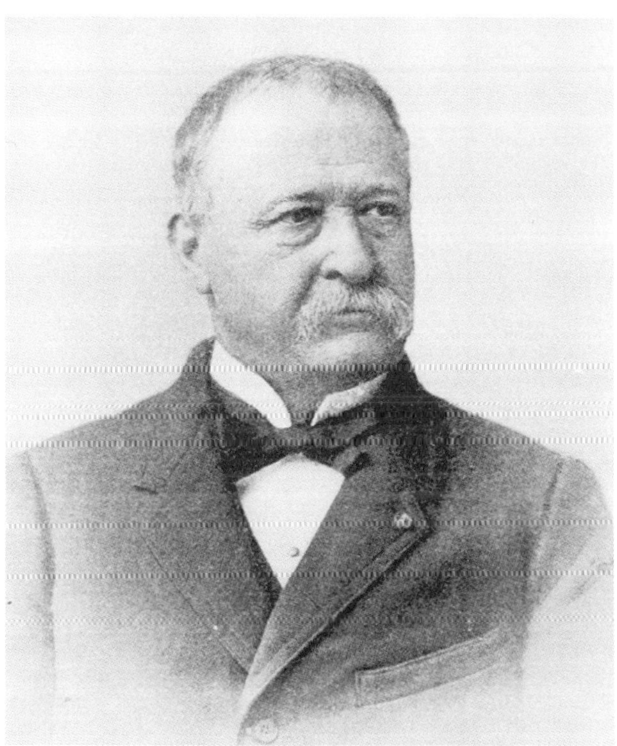

FIG. 2-32. William S. Forbes, M.D. (1831–1905), Professor of Anatomy (1886–1905), secured passage of the Anatomy Act of 1882, which legalized equitable distribution of cadavers in Pennsylvania for medical schools.

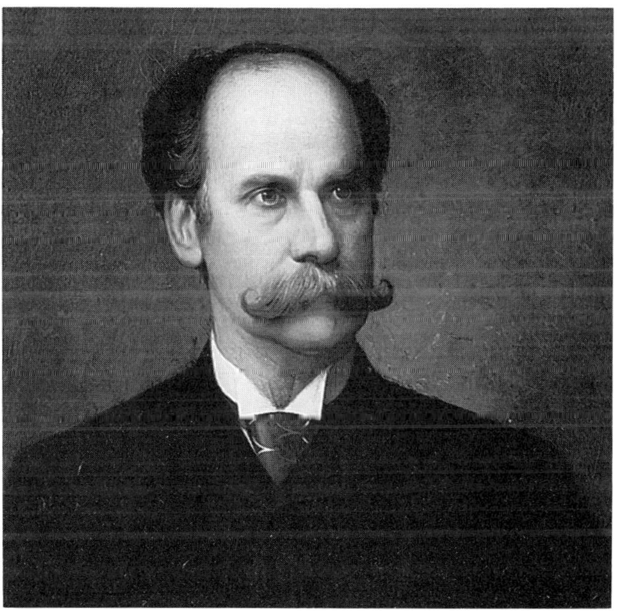

FIG. 2-33. Samuel W. Gross, M.D. (1837–1889); Professor of Principles of Surgery and Clinical Surgery (1882–1889).

reported this experience before the New York Academy of Medicine where he urged the making of clinical obstetrics a part of the curriculum of all medical schools. In 1894 the maternity facility moved to larger quarters at 224 West Washington Square, where it remained until 1924 when ample space was provided in the new Thompson Annex.

During 15 years of Professorship at Jefferson (1883–1898), Dr. Parvin was acknowledged as a national leader in his field and also was considered as one of the greatest gynecologists in his day. His death in 1898 at age 69 was a serious loss to the school and the many important organizations of which he was a member.

After the retirement of Robert E. Rogers, Professor of Chemistry, in 1884 and the succession of Dr. John W. Mallet for only one year, James W. Holland (Figure 2-37) was appointed Professor of Medical Chemistry and Toxicology in 1885. Dr. Holland, a native of Kentucky, had graduated from Jefferson in 1868 and served for 13 years as Chairman of the Practice of Medicine and Clinical Medicine at the University of Louisville. His lectures at Jefferson were remarkable for their thoroughness and practical application to clinical medicine. He served in this Chair for 27 years until 1912 and also as Dean for 29 years from 1887 to 1916. During his incumbency he improved the chemical laboratory course from an elementary status to one of relevance with physiology and clinical medicine. His literary contributions consisted of *Diet for the Sick, Common Poisons and the Urine, Inorganic Poisons, Medical Chemistry and Toxicology,* and many scientific papers. Among many important organizations, he served as Member of the Council of Medicine of the American Medical Association and as President of the Association of American Medical Colleges. Eakins painted Holland reading the "Roll Call" of students graduating from Jefferson. The original is in the Boston Museum of Art, and a copy resides in the Eakins Gallery at Jefferson. An original in oil by Adolph Borie also hangs in the Dean's office suite.

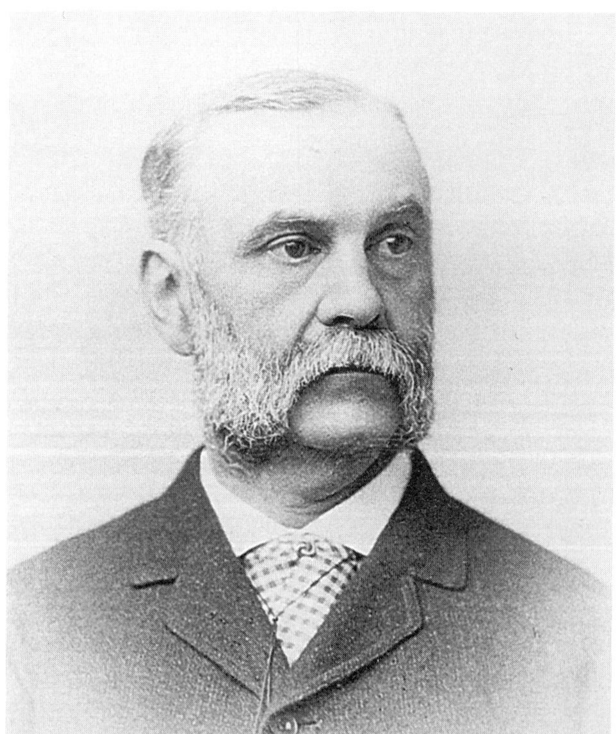

Fig. 2-34. John H. Brinton, M.D. (1832–1907); Professor of Practice of Surgery and Clinical Surgery (1882–1907).

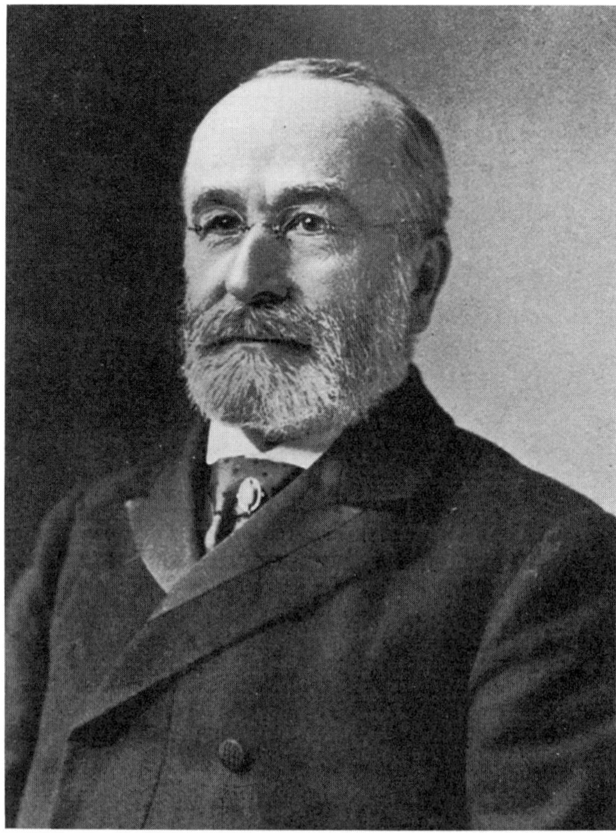

Fig. 2-35. William W. Keen, M.D. (1837–1932), Professor of Surgery (1889–1907), performed the first removal of a brain tumor with permanent cure.

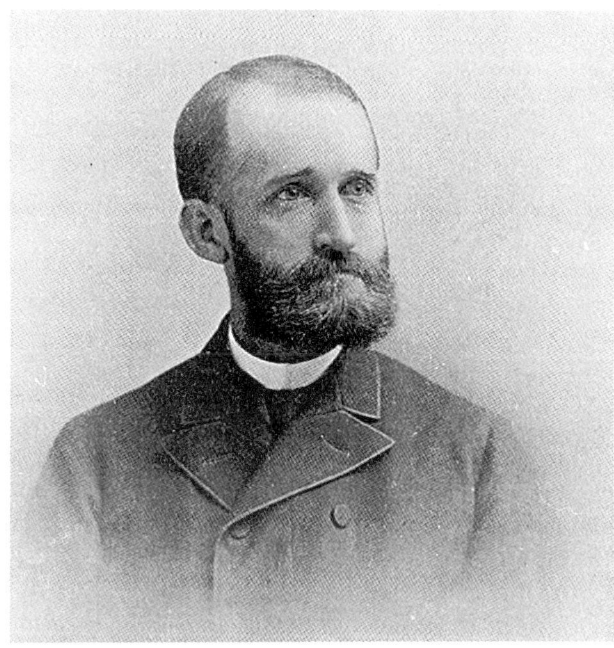

FIG. 2-37. James W. Holland, M.D. (1849–1922); Professor of Chemistry (1885–1912) and Dean (1887–1916).

In the 1888–1889 session, five clinical lectureships were established within the Hospital to provide students with latest instruction in the evolving specialties of the times. The lectureships were administered as follows: Oscar H. Allis (Orthopedic Surgery), Charles E. de Medici Sajous (Laryngology), Oliver P. Rex (Children's Diseases), A. Van Harlingen (Dermatology), and James C. Wilson (Renal Diseases). Practical instruction was also given in the use of the laryngoscope and the ophthalmoscope.

In the session of 1890–1891 an Honorary Professorship of Laryngology was created for Dr. Jacob da Silva Solis-Cohen (Figure 2-38), whose reputation in this field was nationwide. At the close of this session, Dr. Jacob Mendes DaCosta resigned his Chair of Theory and Practice of Medicine after having taught admiring classes for 24 years. He was considered one of Philadelphia's ablest clinicians, an outstanding contributor to the medical literature, and a pioneer in cardiology.

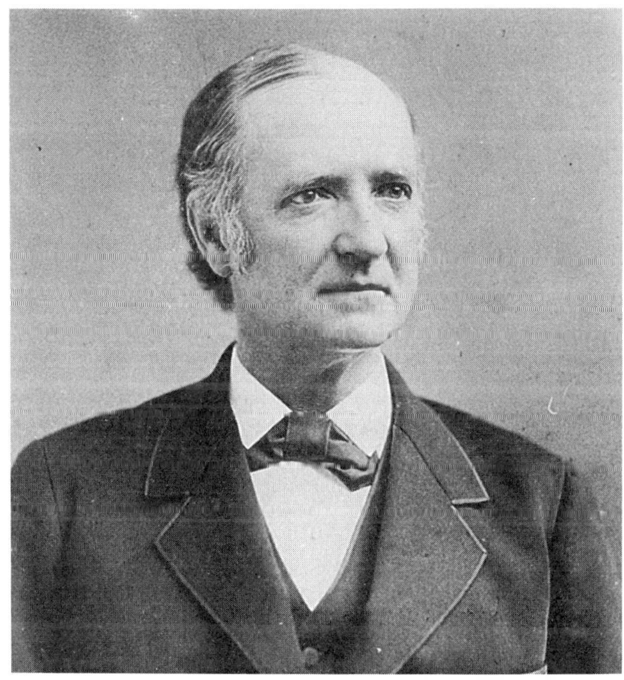

FIG. 2-36. Theophilus Parvin, M.D. (1829–1899), Professor of Obstetrics (1883–1898), established the first obstetrical clinic in America.

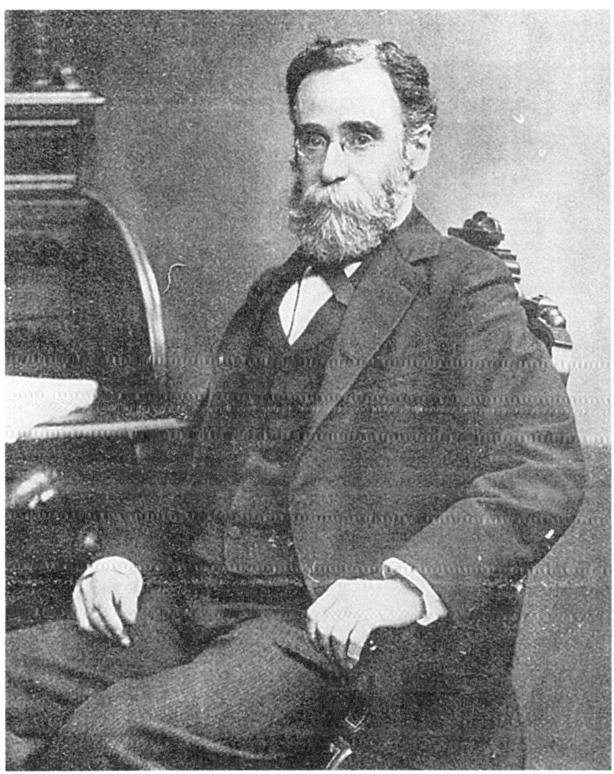

FIG. 2-38. Jacob da Silva Solis-Cohen, M.D. (1838–1927), Honorary Professor of Laryngology (1891), was a pioneer in that field.

Dr. James Cornelius Wilson (Jefferson, 1869) succeeded Dr. Jacob DaCosta in the Chair of Medicine (Figure 2-39). Two of his brothers also were Jefferson graduates, and his father, Dr. Ellwood Wilson (Jefferson, 1845), had served on the Board of Trustees. Wilson was a close friend of Dr. William Osler, and he joined Osler and Samuel W. Gross's widow for lunch on their wedding day. Wilson served for 20 years with great distinction as teacher, author, and busy clinician. His patient, Miss Anna J. Magee, endowed the Professorship of the Chair of Medicine in 1916.

Dr. Roberts Bartholow suffered a breakdown in his health in 1890, and his course in Materia Medica and Therapeutics was taught for that year by Dr. Albert P. Brubaker, who in later years succeeded Dr. Henry Chapman as Professor of Physiology. Bartholow was made an Emeritus Professor in 1891 and was succeeded by Dr. Hobart Amory Hare (Figure 2-40).

Born in Philadelphia, the son of an Episcopalian bishop, Hare graduated in medicine from the University of Pennsylvania in 1884. After receiving the additional degree of Bachelor of Science from the University in 1885 he traveled to Leipzig where he pursued physiologic research under Ludwig. This was followed by work in Berne and London. These early years were marked by his award of an unusual number of prizes. At his medical graduation he was awarded the Faculty Prize for his thesis; he was twice the recipient of the Fiske Fund Prize of the Rhode Island Medical Society (in 1885 and 1886); and he won the Cartwright Prize of the New York College of Physicians and Surgeons in 1889 (with Dr. Martin); the Warren Triennial Prize of the Massachusetts General Hospital in 1889 (with Dr. Martin); the prize offered by the Royal Academy of Belgium for the best essay on epilepsy in 1889; and the Boylston Prize of Harvard University in 1890. Hare's supreme honor was the award of the Fothergillian Gold Medal of the Medical Society of London in 1888 for his work on *Mediastinal Tumors*; he was the only American ever to attain this distinction. The medal was bequeathed to the College of Physicians of Philadelphia (Figure 2-41). Within six years of graduation Hare was elected Clinical Professor of Diseases of Children at the University of Pennsylvania.

Hare's appointment at Jefferson was to last for 40 years, until 1931, the longest of any Chairman

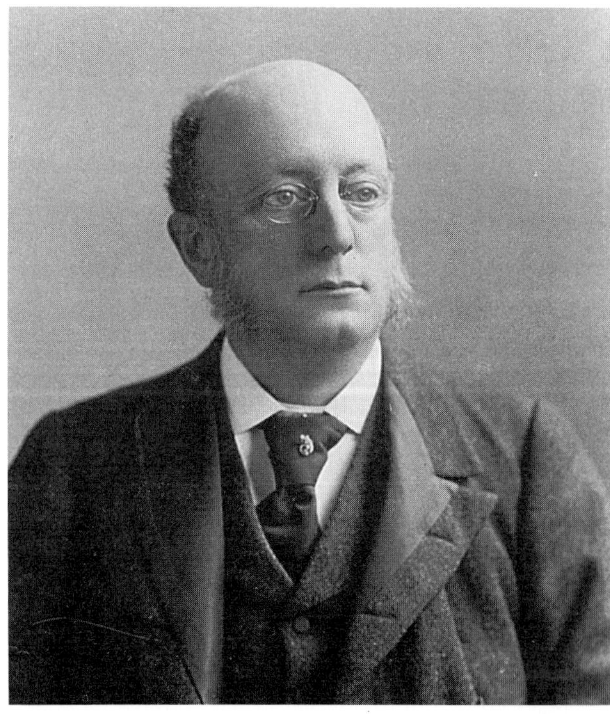

FIG. 2-39. James C. Wilson, M.D. (1847–1934); Professor of Medicine (1891–1911).

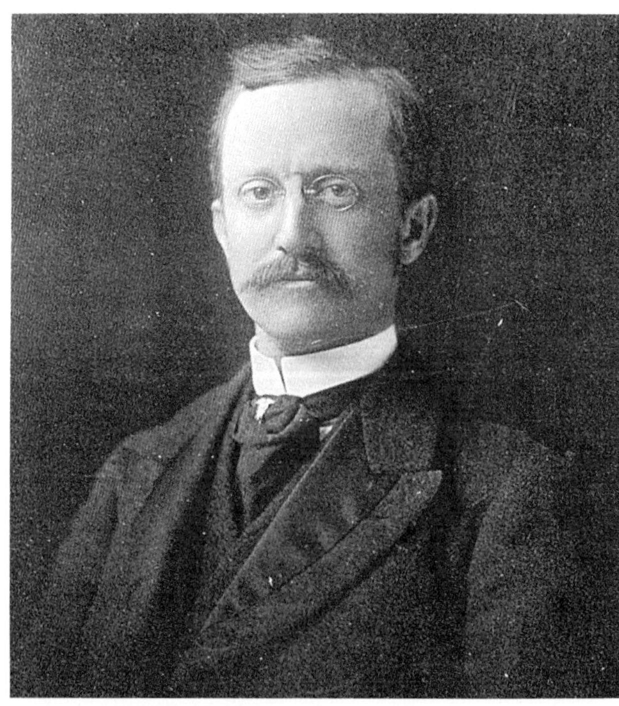

FIG. 2-40. Hobart A. Hare, M.D. (1862–1931); Professor of Materia Medica and Therapeutics (1891–1931).

in its history. His lectures were clear and emphatic, with a wealth of illustration and anecdotes. With unique skill he treated thoracic aneurysms by wiring and electrolysis, even in the clinical amphitheater (Figure 2-42). One outstanding piece of his research was done as a member of the Hyderabad Chloroform Commission in 1894, for which he and his collaborator in that work, Dr. E. Quinn Thornton, each received sterling silver platters from the Nizam (India). Hare's *Practical Therapeutics* was a best seller that went through 21 editions. His *Textbook of Practice of Medicine* went through three editions, *Symptoms and Diagnosis of Disease*, nine editions, and his *Modern Treatment* comprised two volumes. A monograph on *Medical Complications and Sequelae of Typhoid Fever and Other Exanthemata* went through two editions.

Hare supplemented his M.D. degree from the University of Pennsylvania (1884) by taking a second at Jefferson in 1893. This accounts for his membership in and later 1909 Presidency of the Alumni Association. He served as President of the College of Physicians of Philadelphia from 1925 to 1928. He was a member of the Board of City Trusts and received an LL.D. degree from the University of Pennsylvania in 1921. The Class of 1927 presented Hare's portrait to the College.

The death of Hare in 1931 at age 69 from carcinoma of the prostate was the end of the era of materia medica at Jefferson. This year marked the establishment of the Department of Pharmacology in the basic sciences, which then covered the subject material of materia medica and pharmacy during the first and second years of the four-year course. The remaining portion of therapeutics became a clinical subject in the last two years of the curriculum that was taught successively by Drs. Elmer Funk, E. Quinn Thornton, Ross V. Patterson, and finally by Martin E. Rehfuss.

Dr. Hare kept a high profile and leadership position in the Executive Faculty from the very beginning of his long tenure of service. In this respect he worked closely with Mr. William

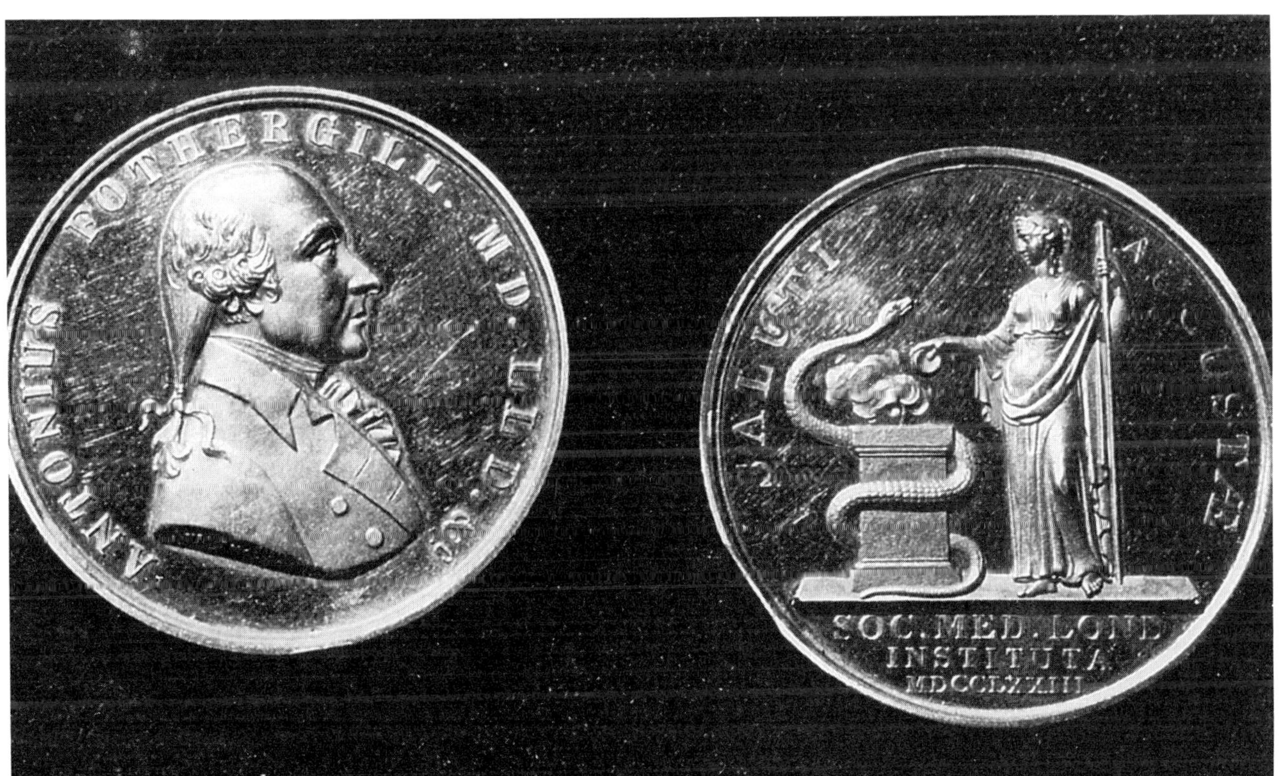

FIG. 2-41. Fothergillian Gold Medal of the Medical Society of London was awarded in 1888 to Dr. Hobart A. Hare, the only American ever to be so honored.

Potter, who became a member of the Board of Trustees in 1894. It was mainly through the efforts of Mr. Potter that Jefferson ended its just more than 70 years as a proprietary school and reorganized into a nonprofit Jefferson Medical College and Hospital under the unified control of the Board of Trustees.

References

1. Holland, J.W., "Memoir of Roberts Bartholow, M.D., Read before the College of Physicians of Philadelphia, Dec. 17, 1904." (In archives of Thomas Jefferson University).
2. Nolan, E.J., "A Biographical Notice of Henry Cadwalader Chapman, M.D., Sc.D.," *Proc. Ac. Nat. Sc. Phila.* April 1910, pp. 255–270.
3. Forbes, W.S., "History of the Anatomy Act of Pennsylvania." *Phila. Med. Pub. Co.* 1898. (In archives of Thomas Jefferson University).
4. Keen, W.W., *The Surgical Operation on President Cleveland in 1893, Together with Six Additional Papers of Reminiscences.* Philadelphia: J.B. Lippincott Co., 1928.
5. Mosher, G.C., "Theophilus Parvin," *Surg., Gynec. & Obst.,* October 1928, pp. 569–572.
6. McCrae, T., "Memoir of Hobart Amory Hare, M.D.," *Trans. Stud. Coll. Phys. Ph.*, Ser. 3, Vol. 54, 1932, pp. lxxii–lxxv.

College Reorganized: End of Proprietary Years (1895)

In the session of 1894–1895 the total number of students was 711. There were 219 in the first year, 237 in the second, 229 in the third, and 26 special students. At the annual commencement on May 15,

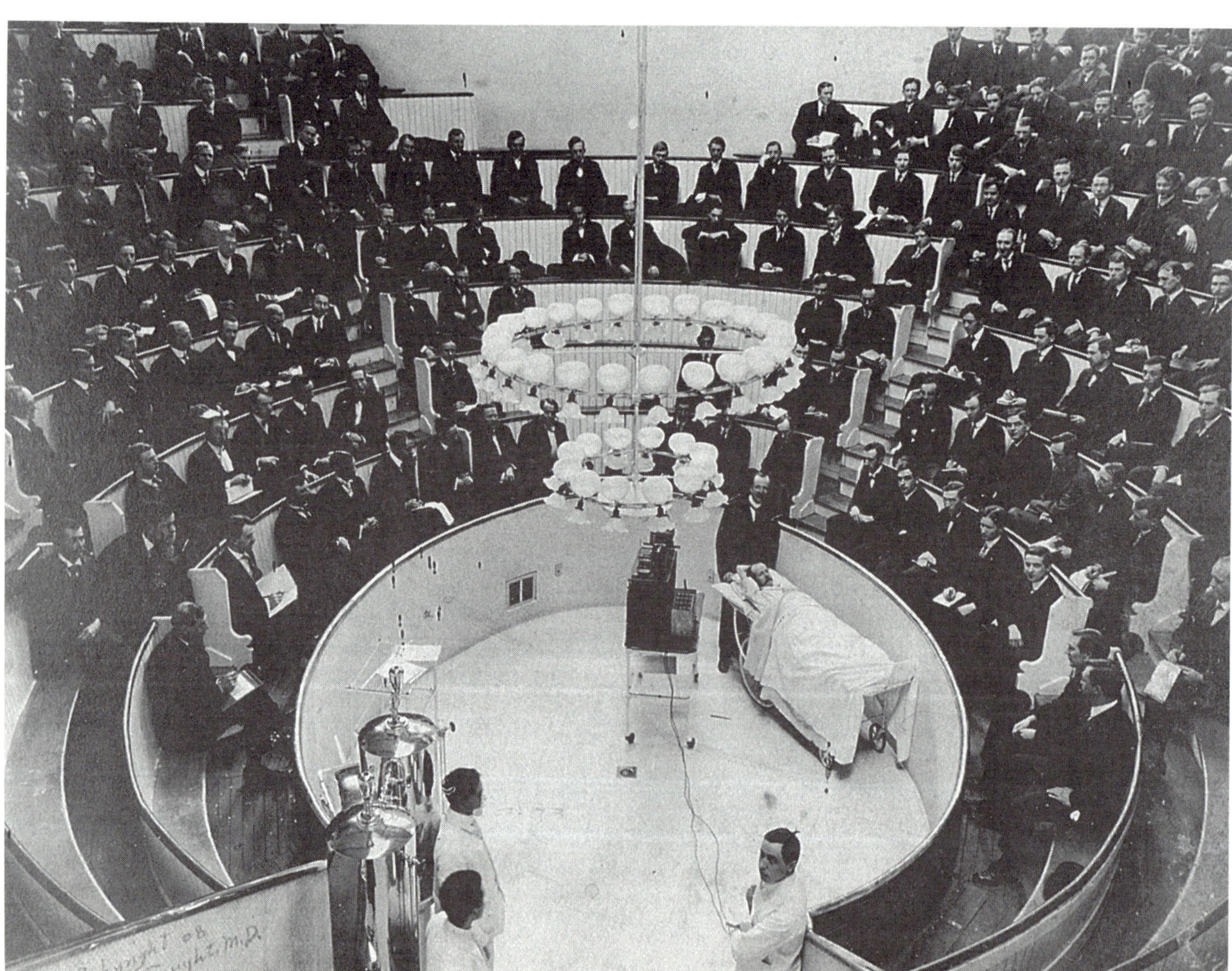

FIG. 2-42. Dr. Hobart A. Hare wiring a thoracic aneurysm in the "pit" of the 1877 hospital.

1895, the degree of Doctor of Medicine was conferred on 148 graduates. This brought the total number since inception of the College to 10,398.[1]

There was no external evidence that the great reform of 1895 was taking place and that a tradition of 70 years would belong to a bygone era. The issue was the reorganization of the College from a proprietary school, in which the profits were divided among the Professors, to a nonprofit organization of combined College and Hospital under absolute unified control of the Board of Trustees. The Professors would no longer share profits and would serve on fixed salaries. The time had come when Jefferson Medical College must be such not only in name but in fact, dedicated solely to the welfare of the community and devoid of personal benefit.

James W. Holland, Dean at the time, alluded clearly to this subject in his history of the College: "When attempting to raise endowments to carry out the expensive improvements they had projected, the Trustees and the Faculty often encountered the objection that as the receipts in excess of expenditures were divided among the Faculty, they were practically asking for money to be given to the Faculty and not to the cause of medical education or suffering humanity. In order to end this system, complete reorganization was effected by the Trustees, which was cheerfully accepted by the Faculty."[2]

Since 1893, the Trustees had been seriously considering replacement of the antiquated and undersized Ely Medical Hall of 1828 that had undergone successive renovations and expansions. As would be expected, some members of the Board did not favor the continued plans for improvement and the measures required to implement them. Others also were not quick to endorse the abolition of the established system in which the College had been operated directly by the Faculty and only indirectly by the Board. The minority of "status quo" proponents were peacefully won over by the missionary work and enlightened agitation of the progressive members of the Board.

In 1894, the members of the Board of Trustees were Edwin H. Fitler, President; George W. Fairman, Secretary; Edward H. Weil, Treasurer; and Joseph B. Townsend, Joseph Allison, Simon Gratz, Michael Arnold, Henry D. Welsh, Sutherland M. Prevost, George D. McCreary, Thomas B. Wanamaker, Edward V. Morrell, and Luther B. Bent. Later that year, Mr. Townsend became President and Mr. William Potter was elected a member. The latter championed and spearheaded the reorganization drive, and served for thirty years (1896–1926) as President of the Board with outstanding energy and advancements for Jefferson.

In the pivotal year of 1895 other members who came into the Board were Joseph de F. Junkin, Louis C. Vanuxem, Samuel Gustine Thompson, Louis H. Biddle and William H. Newbold. They aided in the special issue of reorganization of the business management and educational mission of the College. In so doing it was not necessary to create waves, to shatter previously held ideals, to remove Professors from their held positions, or to correct abuses. The Trustees rightly assumed absolute management of the property and policy of the institution. The reorganization act was adopted by the Board on February 1, 1895, to become effective on June 1 of that year.

The Faculty voiced no dissent at the action of the Board. They had been paying a rental fee of $3,993 a year for use of the College and Hospital. Although shared profits had sometimes been alluded to as the "Professorial Jackpot," none of the Professors became affluent in this system. Indeed, they increasingly had to add funds from their own resources to maintain a Department in accord with the progress of the times. This was especially true for the laboratories. Public appeals could not be ethically solicited if the Professors were to benefit personally from the donors.

To the added credit of a dedicated Faculty, the Jefferson Professors were seeking at the same time to upgrade the curriculum. In 1891, a three-year course became mandatory, although the requirement for admission was still only a high school diploma or its equivalent. It would be 1914 before the requirement would be raised to one year of college. The Faculty subsequently in the 1894–1895 session stated in the 70th "Annual Announcement" that "all persons beginning their medical studies by matriculation after June 1, 1895, must take four annual courses."

Thus, in the 1895–1896 session the College was no longer proprietary, and the curriculum was a four-year graded course. It was expected that the lengthened course of study would temporarily affect the financial status of the school. On the contrary, the popularity of the College increased at once. The aggregate attendance was 623, of which 95 were first-year students. The first-year students increased to 112 by 1897 and to 185 by 1899. By 1898 the designation of classes as freshman, sophomore, junior and senior was adopted as in other collegiate institutions.

The salary of "non-practicing Chairmen" was set at $5,000, but by 1898 was reduced to $3,700. The following year it was stipulated at $4,000 and continued at this level for several years. Mr. Daniel Baugh, a Trustee from 1896 to 1927, induced his fellow trustees to restore the $5,000 level and pledged to cover any deficit from his own private funds.

The active Professorial Faculty of 1895–1896 was composed of Drs. James C. Wilson (Medicine), John H. Brinton (Practice of Surgery), William W. Keen (Principles of Surgery), Theophilus Parvin (Obstetrics), Edward E. Montgomery (Gynecology), Hobart A. Hare (Materia Medica and Therapeutics), William Thomson (Ophthalmology), William S. Forbes (Anatomy), James W. Holland (Chemistry and Dean) and Henry C. Chapman (Physiology). The Chair of Pathology was vacant but would be filled the following year by Dr. William M.L. Coplin.

In its newly constituted authority the Board functioned with four standing committees—College Committee, Hospital Committee, Committee on the Training School for Nurses, and Committee on Finance. The subsequent history of Jefferson will be detailed through the various Departments and Divisions that progressed until and beyond the University status, which was achieved in 1969.

References

1. Gould, G.M., *The Jefferson Medical College of Philadelphia, 1826–1904*. New York: Lewis Pub. Co., 1904, p. 256.
2. Holland, J.W., *The Jefferson Medical College of Philadelphia, from 1825 to 1908. Founders' Week Memorial Volume*. Pub. by City of Philadelphia, 1909, p. 280.

PART II

Basic Sciences

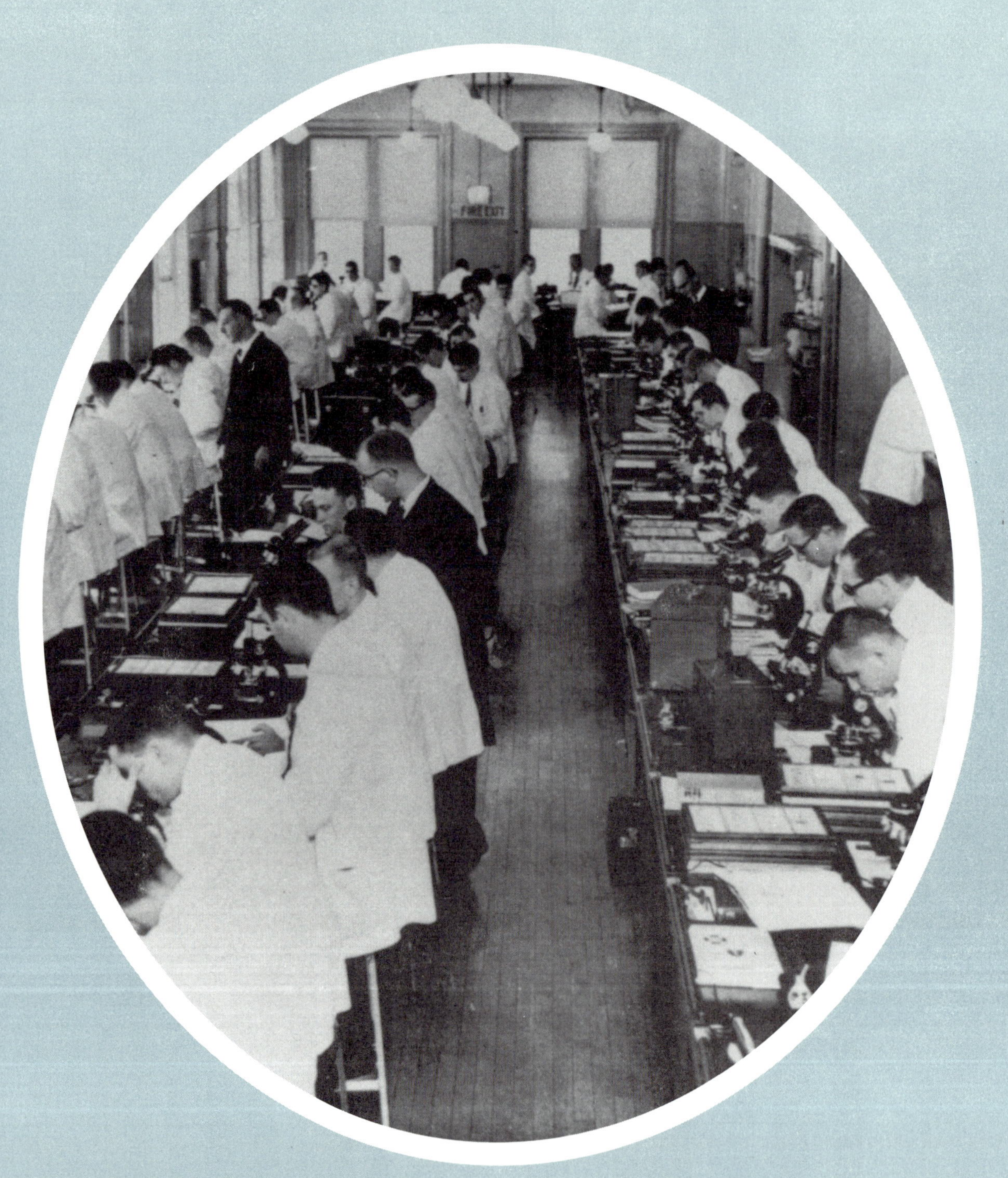

PART II

Basic Sciences

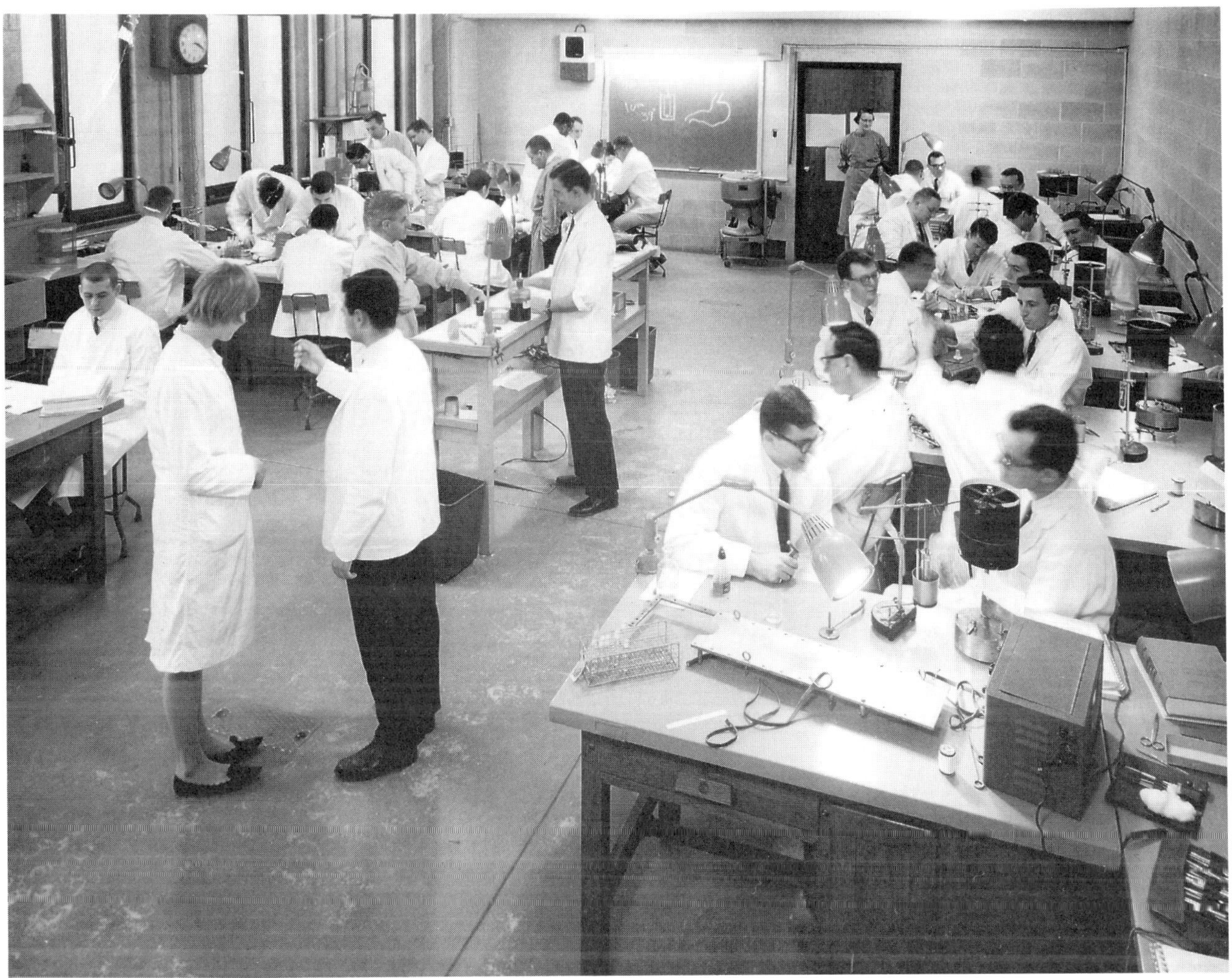

Physiology Laboratory in 1025 Walnut Street College

← *Opposite page:* Histology Laboratory in the Daniel Baugh Institute

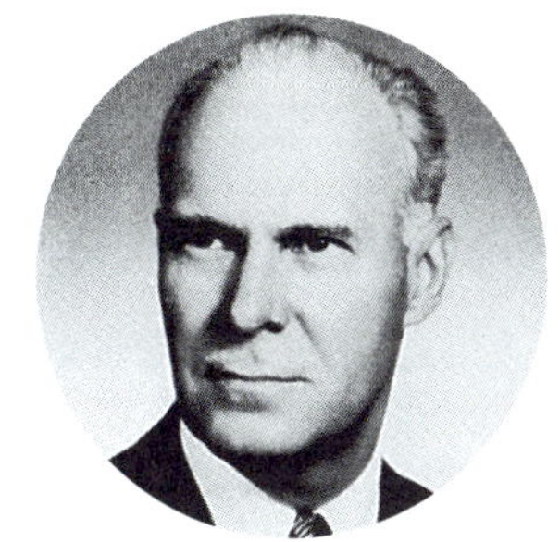

CHAPTER THREE

Department of Anatomy

ANDREW J. RAMSAY, PH.D., SC.D.

"Anatomy is to physiology as geography to history; it describes the theater of events."

—JEAN FERNEL (1497–1558)

THE SUBJECT of anatomy in American medical school curricula until late in the nineteenth century was taught primarily as gross anatomy and amounted to little more than a handmaiden to surgery. At a few universities and institutes in Europe some anatomical research was occurring and bases for the various future subdivisions of the science were being established.

Teachers of anatomy in America were really surgeon-anatomists who applied their anatomic knowledge directly to their surgical practices. With anesthetic measures not yet available, the surgeon had to operate rapidly and boldly, and detailed knowledge of the normal structure of the parts involved was essential. Histology and embryology were in their infancy, even in Europe, and were not considered to be essential components of American medical curricula.

George McClellan, M.D. (1797–1847), First Chairman (1824–1825) and Interim Chairman (1827–1830)

When George McClellan (Figure 3-1) started Philadelphia's "second" medical school, the mammalian ovum had not yet been seen; the cellular basis of living organisms was still unknown; blood capillaries and their significance had not been completely recognized; and achromatic microscope lenses would not be available for two decades (although Amici and Lister in Europe were making progress in their design). Thus, American surgeon-anatomists had to look to Europe for newly discovered advances in their science.

McClellan firmly believed in the value of dissection of the cadaver. Shortly after receiving his M.D. degree from the University of Pennsylvania (1819), he opened his private school of anatomy and insisted on individual student participation in dissection. The immediate success of this venture drew both students and physicians in increasing numbers to his laboratory.

It had become obvious that the University of Pennsylvania could not by itself provide medical education for all who desired to study in Philadelphia. George McClellan, aided by his colleagues John Eberle, Joseph Klapp, and Jacob Green provided the answer through a second medical school, a venture that others had attempted to accomplish previously but without success because of opposition from the University of Pennsylvania. Joseph Klapp was given the Chair in Anatomy in the school's first faculty but had to withdraw before the first academic session because of ill health. George McClellan, while also holding the Chair of Surgery, assumed the Anatomy Chair.

Nathan Ryno Smith, M.D. (1797–1877), Second Chairman (1825–1827)

Nathan Ryno Smith (Figure 3-2) was called to the Jefferson Chair in 1825. A medical graduate of Yale (1823), Dr. Smith was the son of the famous Nathan Smith (founder of early medical schools). He remained at Jefferson until 1827, when he was called to the Anatomy Chair at the University of Maryland where he served with great distinction for 40 years, first in anatomy, then in surgery. During Smith's short tenure at Jefferson, important advances were being made in Europe. Karl Ernst von Baer reported seeing the mammalian ovum within the ovarian follicle, a discovery that corrected DeGraaf's belief that the entire (Graafian) follicle constituted the ovum. The role of the spermatozoon and ovum in actual fertilization would not be clarified until 1875.

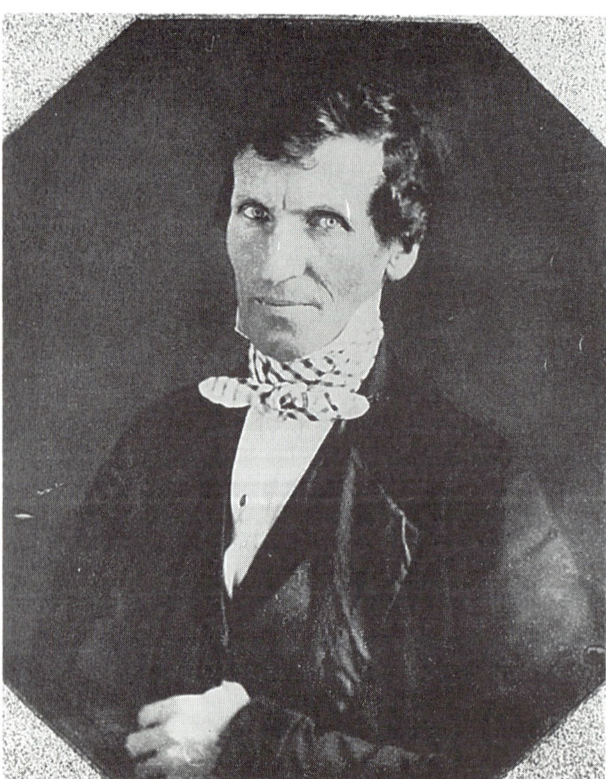

FIG. 3-1. George McClellan, M.D. (1797–1847), First Chairman (1824–1825) and Interim Chairman (1827–1830).

Samuel McClellan, M.D. (1800–1854), Third Chairman (1830–1831)

Following Smith's resignation, there being little time to seek a successor, George McClellan resumed the Anatomy Chair, assisted by his brother Samuel, first as Assistant Demonstrator (1828), then Adjunct Professor (1829). Samuel McClellan (Figure 3-3) was elected to the Anatomy Chair in 1830, succeeding his brother George. Samuel (M.D., Yale, 1823) continued in the Chair

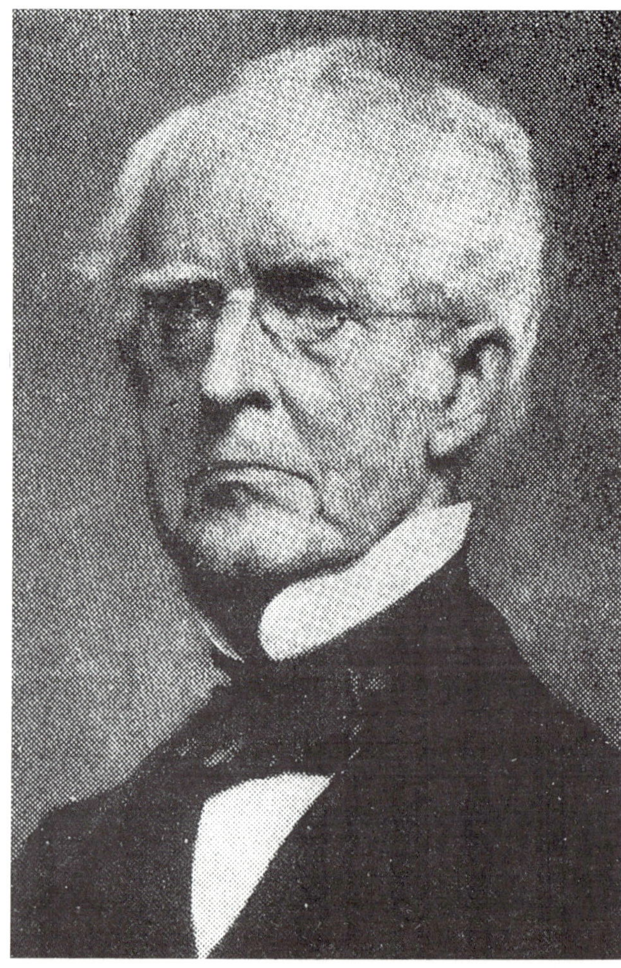

FIG. 3-2. Nathan Ryno Smith, M.D. (1797–1877), Second Chairman (1825–1827).

and served with considerable distinction until he resigned in 1831 to accept the Chair of Institutes, Midwifery and Diseases of Women and Children. He also served as Dean of the College (1830–1834).

Granville Sharpe Pattison, M.D. (1792–1857), Fourth Chairman (1831–1841)

Samuel McClellan was succeeded in 1831 by Dr. Granville Sharpe Pattison (Figure 3-4), a dynamic and gifted anatomist-surgeon who soon earned the nickname "the turbulent Scot." Dr. Pattison studied medicine in Glasgow, Scotland, came to the United States in 1818, and accepted the Chair of Anatomy at the University of Maryland. He returned to England in 1827 to take the Anatomy Chair at the newly organized University of London, a post he held until called back to America to the Anatomy Chair at Jefferson. He rapidly gained the reputation of the most effective teacher and lecturer of his day. His writings included a text, *Surgical Anatomy of the Head and Neck* and another, *Visceral Anatomy*; both became classics in their fields. In 1841 Pattison was called to New York, together with Jefferson's Professor of Medicine, Dr. John Revere (son of the patriot Paul Revere), to assist in the organization of the Medical Department of the University of New York and to accept the Chair of Anatomy.

Meanwhile, anatomic research continued in Europe, stimulated by the improvements in microscope lenses and the heightening interest in microscopic and developmental anatomy. Purkinje and others were reporting advances in embryology (e.g., the "germinal vesicles" of the ovary that had aided von Baer in his search for the ovum of mammals, cilia and their distribution in the animal kingdom, the structure and function of nerve fibers, the large "Purkinje cells" of the cerebellum, structural and functional analysis of the eye and

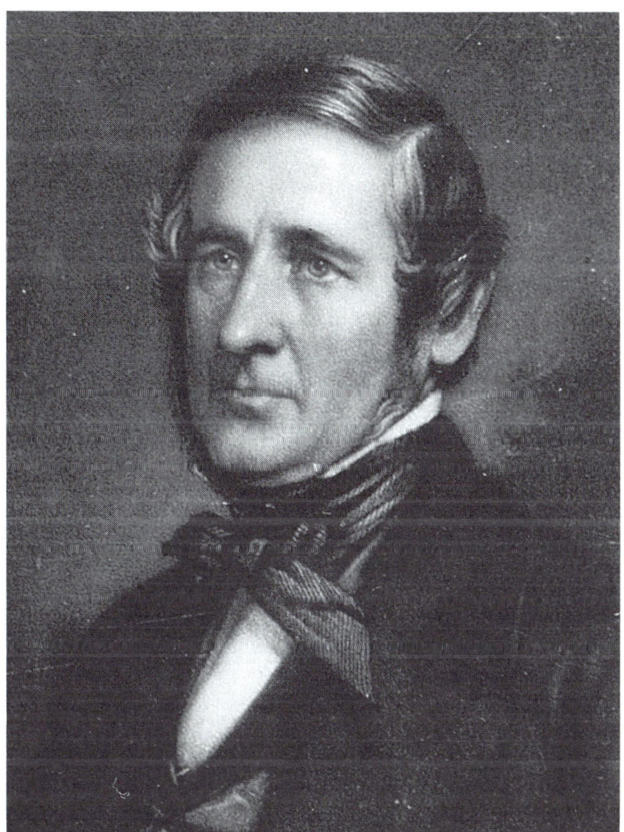

FIG. 3-3. Samuel McClellan, M.D. (1800–1854), Third Chairman (1830–1831).

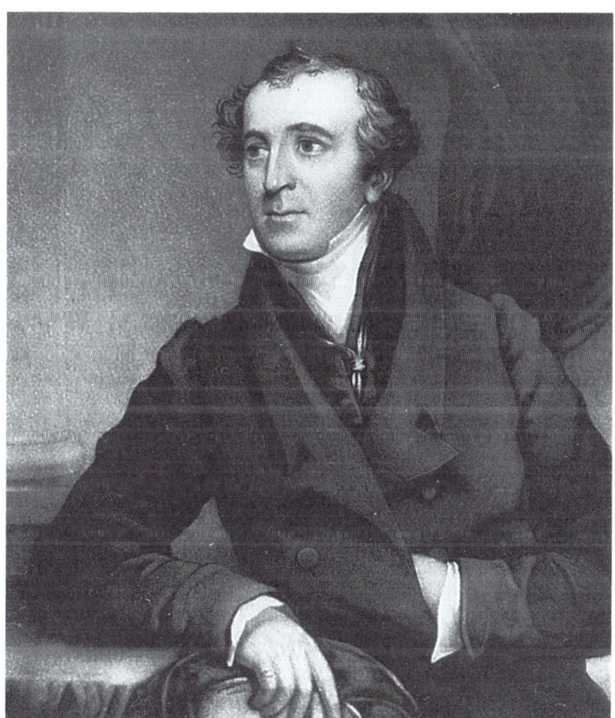

FIG. 3-4. Granville Sharpe Pattison, M.D. (1792–1857), Fourth Chairman (1831–1841).

the visual system, and the digestive process). Schleiden and Schwann were formulating their cell theory as the structural and functional units of living organisms, although they still erroneously believed in "free cell formation out of moisture." Robert Brown reported that every cell contained an "areola" which he named *nucleus*, but its significance in mitosis was still to be discovered.

George McClellan Dismissed from the Faculty (1839)

It is sad to reflect that when many fundamental advances were occurring overseas an interest in basic scientific inquiry was essentially lacking in the American medical colleges. At Jefferson there was a preoccupation of the faculty in senseless bickerings and, to a degree, to the behind-the-scenes harassment of George McClellan and the entire Jefferson Medical College enterprise by the secret Kappa Lambda Medical Society of Hippocrates.[1] The Trustees reacted firmly by vacating all the Chairs and reconstituting the faculty. In the process, George McClellan in 1839 was excluded from the faculty of the College he had brought into existence.

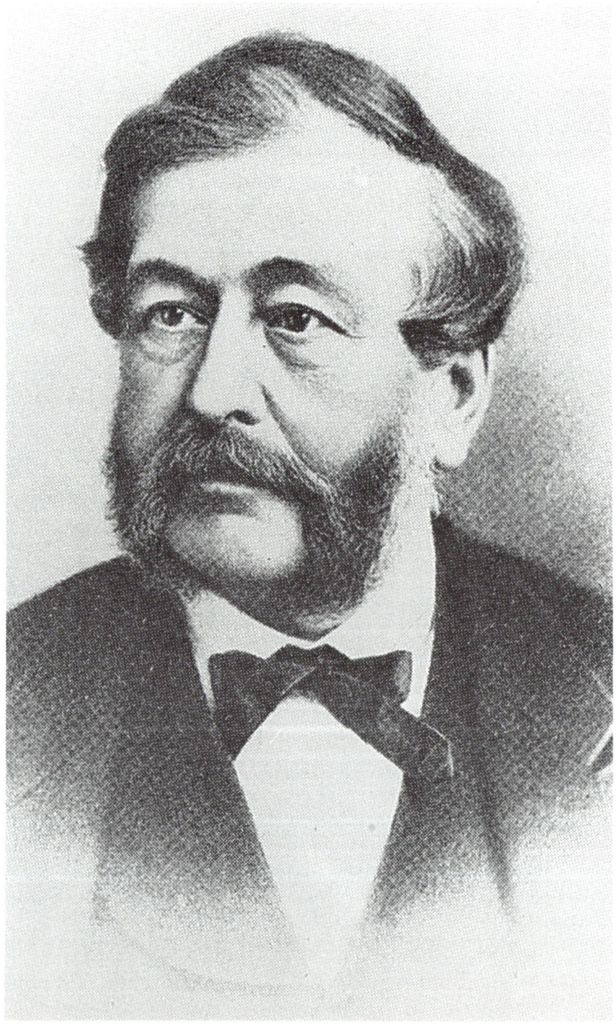

FIG. 3-5. Joseph Pancoast, M.D. (1805–1882), Fifth Chairman (1841–1874).

McClellan had little time for investigative activity, although he started a textbook of surgery and with Dr. John Eberle founded the journal, *Medical and Analytical Review,* to which he contributed articles. He published as well in other journals, but his chief professional contributions were his extraordinary teaching from patients, his stimulating effect on his students and associates, and his pioneering surgical procedures. Undaunted by the exclusion from the faculty of "his" college, McClellan forthwith started another, Philadelphia's third medical school: the Medical Department of Pennsylvania College at Gettysburg, whose instruction was held in Philadelphia. This highly respected medical school flourished until the onset of the Civil War, when occurred a resultant withdrawal of a large segment of its students to the southern states.

Joseph Pancoast, M.D. (1805–1882), Fifth Chairman (1841–1874)

At the time of George McClellan's exclusion from Jefferson's faculty, the Chair of Surgery went to Dr. Joseph Pancoast (Figure 3-5). With Pattison's move to New York in 1841, Pancoast's Chair was switched from Surgery to Anatomy. Pancoast remained in the Anatomy Chair but also continued as an active surgeon until his retirement in 1874 terminated 33 years as a member of Jefferson's famous faculty of 1841. An exceptional teacher, he had few equals in gaining respect and popularity among students and colleagues alike. His textbook, *Operative Surgery*, was eagerly received, as was his 1831 translation from the Latin of Lobstein's famous work, *Structure, Functions, and Diseases of the Human Sympathetic Nerve*. Pancoast also edited *Quain's Anatomical Plates* and, with many additions of his own, Caspar Wistar's *Anatomy*, which led its field impressively until the introduction of *Gray's Anatomy* from England. Pancoast's outstanding reputation attracted the attention of the artist Thomas Eakins, who came to Jefferson to study anatomy and is thought by some to have considered seriously but briefly a career in surgery. The Alumni Association commissioned Samuel Bell Waugh, a prominent Philadelphia artist, to paint Pancoast's portrait, which was presented to the College in 1874. In his honor, in 1870 the U.S. Mint struck a commemorative medal that is still obtainable more than a century later.

Anatomic research was continuing rapidly in Europe and England. Bowman had described the essential structure of the kidney and set forth the basic principles of renal excretion. Staining for microscopic study of biologic materials was accidentally discovered by Gerlack in 1854, after he injected a carmine solution to demonstrate the blood vessels in the mesentery and omentum and noted that the nuclei of cells also turned red. This technique was immediately followed by the use of aniline and vegetable dyes for microscopy. Gegenbauer (1861) proved that all ova of vertebrates were single cells. Wilhelm His' sliding microtome (1866) made possible the examination of very thin tissue sections, thus enhancing microscopy and cytology; Golgi and Cajal (1873) were applying "photographic" processes, using gold and silver methods to study neurohistological materials.

William Henry Pancoast, M.D. (1835–1897), Sixth Chairman (1874–1886)

William Henry Pancoast (Figure 3-6), a Jefferson graduate in 1856, succeeded his famous father in the Anatomy Chair in 1874. Like his father, William was a surgeon-anatomist and a highly competent teacher in his own right, but no doubt because he lived in the shadow of his illustrious father, he never was accorded commensurate recognition. In addition to his regular teaching, William Pancoast initiated courses in visceral and surgical anatomy in Jefferson's innovative and signally successful special Summer Course (1866) that also attracted students from other schools and became a major factor in the resultant lengthening of the entire curriculum. His portrait was commissioned for the College by the Class of 1886. Dr. William Pancoast resigned in 1886 to accept the combined Anatomy and Surgery Chair in the newly organized Medico-Chirurgical College in Philadelphia.

Advances in anatomic science were still coming mainly from Europe and England. The cell theory was finally being clarified, and cell division (mitosis) and the behavior of somatic and sex cells were being explained. In 1885 chromosomes were described, and Fleming and Van Beneden were observing the commingling of sperm and ova

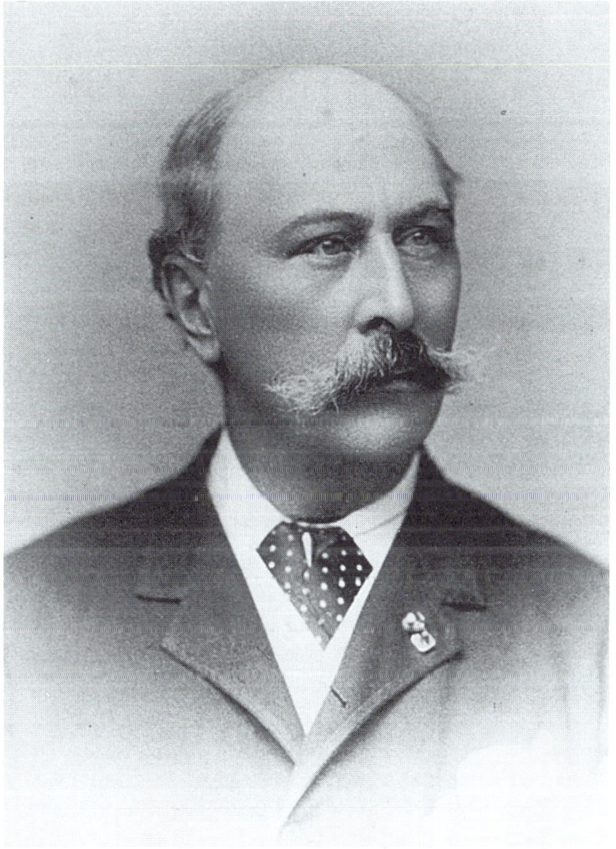

FIG. 3-6. William Henry Pancoast (1835–1897), Sixth Chairman (1874–1886).

chromosomes at fertilization, which initiated the science of cytogenetics. Attention was being directed to histo- and cytochemistry and the concept of "continuity of germ plasm," to cytophysiology, and to tissue-imbedding methods (paraffin and celloidin) for which Dr. Minot's rotatory microtome (1893) greatly aided microscopists in high-magnification studies. Experimental embryology was emerging (Wilhelm Roux in 1885, and others). Specific classification and clarification of cell types in normal, pathological, and experimentally altered tissues were also occurring.

William Smith Forbes, M.D. (1831–1905), Seventh Chairman (1886–1905)

(George) William Smith Forbes (Figure 3-7) was one of the most notable alumni of Jefferson Medical College. The last of the continuous line of famous surgeon-anatomists at Jefferson, he succeeded in initiating the transition to our present full-time scientific researcher-teacher-anatomist role.

Dr. Forbes joined the faculty as Demonstrator of Anatomy (1879) and was given the Chair in 1886 that he held until his death in 1905. Perhaps his greatest contribution was his success in achieving, through the Pennsylvania Legislature, the Anatomy Act of 1867 (amended in 1882 and 1883), which provided legally for procurement and equitable distribution of cadavers for teaching and scientific investigation in Pennsylvania's medical schools.[2] This act served as a model for other states and successfully put an end to the practice of body snatching and the activities of resurrectionists in Pennsylvania.

Born in Virginia, Forbes started his study of medicine at the University of Virginia and obtained his M.D. degree from Jefferson in 1852; the University of Pennsylvania also conferred on him an M.D. degree in 1866. It was not unusual for men of that era to obtain M.D. degrees from more than one medical school. The title of his thesis was *On the Treatment of the Wounded Men of the 13th Army Corps During the Siege of Vicksburg*. Forbes joined the staff at the Pennsylvania Hospital and soon became a Resident Physician, then served as physician-officer in the British Army during the Crimean War.

Following studies in several European countries Forbes returned to Philadelphia and opened his own School of Anatomy. He served also in the Civil War as Medical Director of the Thirteenth Army under General Grant. After the war, on his return to Philadelphia, Forbes was Senior Surgeon at Episcopal Hospital and Professor of Anatomy at the Pennsylvania College of Dental Surgery (later the Daniel Baugh Institute at Eleventh and Clinton Streets) while engaging in medical and scientific research and writing.

Dr. Forbes introduced the formal course in histology at Jefferson in 1896, for which he personally provided 40 microscopes, and he added the course in embryology in 1900. Realizing that the chairman of a basic medical science department should be full-time, he had petitioned the Trustees to be relieved of his responsibilities in

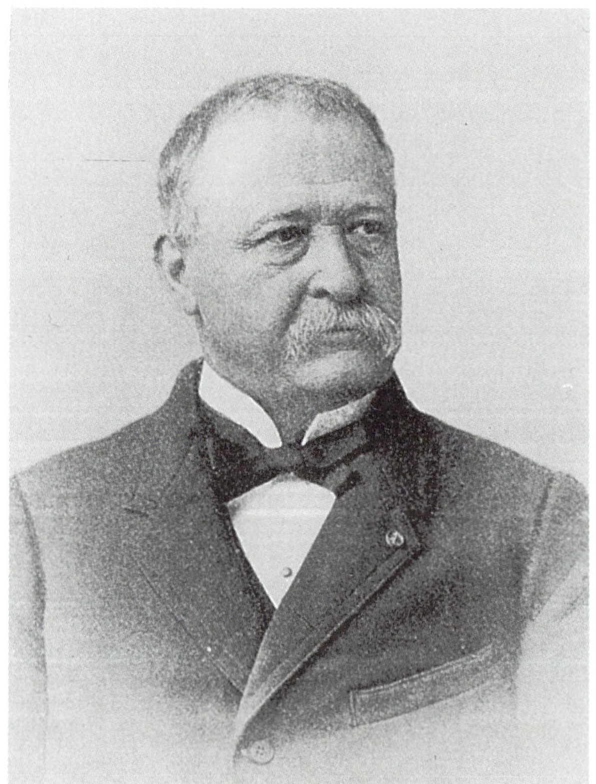

FIG. 3-7. William Smith Forbes, M.D. (1831–1905), Seventh Chairman (1886–1905).

surgery and in some surgical clinics. Death came to Forbes in 1905 while he was still actively teaching.

The portrait of Forbes painted by Thomas Eakins in 1905 hangs in the Eakins Gallery of Jefferson Alumni Hall.

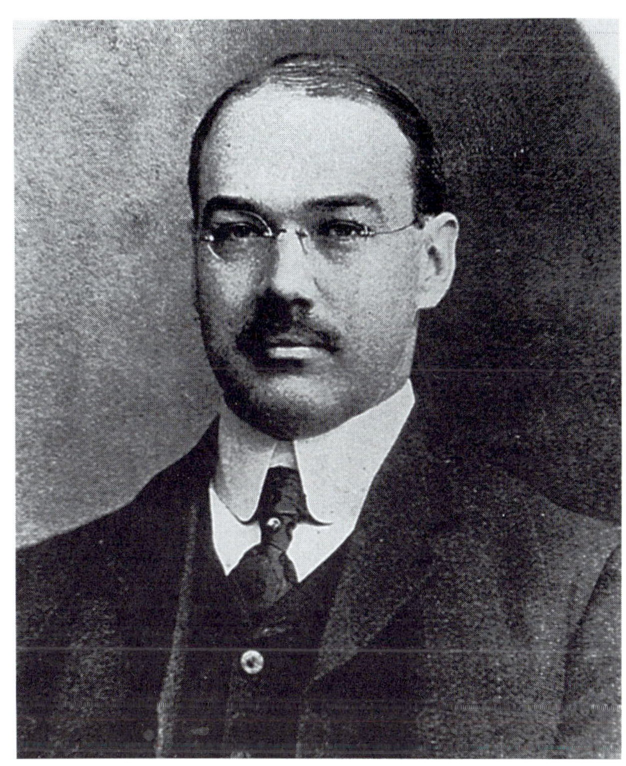

FIG. 3-8. Edward A. Spitzka, M.D. (1876–1922), Eighth Chairman (1905–1914).

Eighth Chairmanship (Divided): Edward A. Spitzka, M.D. (1876–1922), Chairman of General Anatomy (1905–1914); and George McClellan, M.D. (1849–1913), Chairman of Applied and Topographic Anatomy (1905–1913)

Following the death of Dr. Forbes and after much debate, the Chair in Anatomy was divided between Edward Anthony Spitzka (Figure 3-8), in the Chair of General Anatomy, and George McClellan (Figure 3-9), grandson of the founder, in the Chair of Applied Anatomy. Dr. Spitzka's Chair was to be responsible for the courses in gross anatomy and histology and embryology. Dr. McClellan was to teach applied and topographic anatomy and their application to medicine, surgery, and the subspecialties. The dividing of the Chair was an arbitrary action of the Board of Trustees, which seized the opportunity to appoint a young man (Spitzka, age 29), to conduct research and an older man (McClellan, age 56), to teach practical anatomy. McClellan had aspired to the Chair of General (Gross) Anatomy and never felt happy with a Co-chairman 27 years his junior.

Edward Anthony Spitzka was Jefferson's first full-time Anatomy Chairman (with no outside practice permitted) and the first Chairman to conduct basic anatomic research. Dr. Spitzka

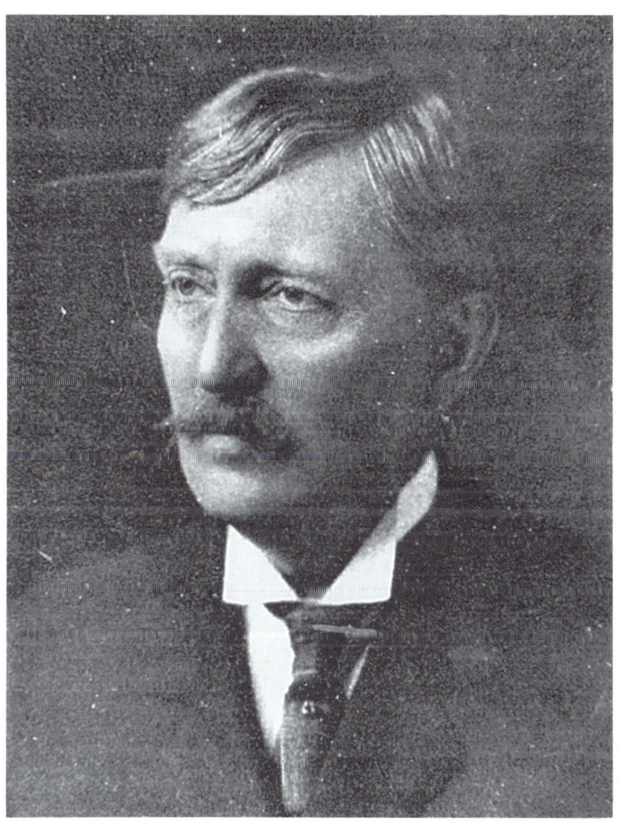

FIG. 3-9. George McClellan, M.D. (1849–1913), Chairman of Applied and Topographic Anatomy (1905–1913).

received the M.D. degree from Columbia University in 1901 and came to Jefferson four years later, succeeding Professor Forbes. Following the purchase by Daniel Baugh of the property at 11th and Clinton Streets (formerly Pennsylvania College of Dental Surgery), Spitzka helped plan its conversion into a modern facility for anatomic teaching and research (Figures 3-10 and 3-11). Mr. Baugh then presented the facility to the College.[3,4] The Trustees immediately named the building and its functional concepts The Daniel Baugh Institute of Anatomy. Soon realizing the added administrative responsibilities of the Professor of General Anatomy, they changed his title to Professor of General Anatomy, Head of the Department, and Director of the Daniel Baugh Institute of Anatomy. The Institute was opened and dedicated in September, 1911. From 1913 to 1916, when Jefferson was giving a premedical preparatory course and the biology courses were given at the Institute, the Director's title and the name of the Institute were changed to include "and Biology."

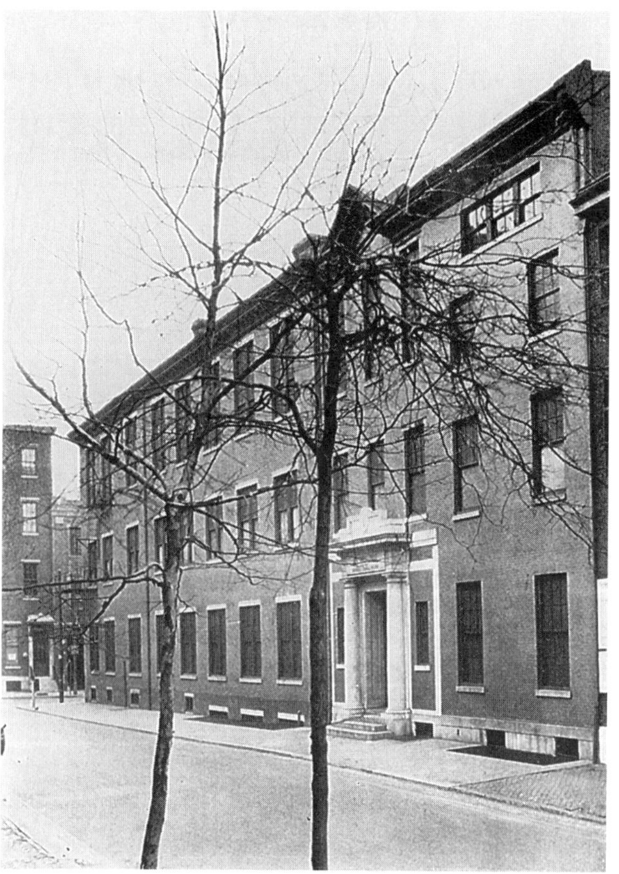

FIG. 3-10. The Daniel Baugh Institute of Anatomy.

Dr. Spitzka's research centered upon the nervous system in health and disease and included the effects of electrocution on brains of convicted criminals (one of whom was the anarchist Czolgosz, President McKinley's assassin). In addition to prolific contributions to anatomic research journals, Spitzka edited the eighteenth and nineteenth American editions of *Gray's Anatomy,* after having assisted John Chalmers DaCosta in editing the seventeenth edition.

A psychiatric disorder with paranoid behavior forced Dr. Spitzka's resignation in 1914. After regaining his health he returned to New York and opened a practice in nervous and mental diseases. Spitzka also served as a Lieutenant Colonel in World War I. Death came in 1922 at the early age of 46.

George McClellan (Jefferson, 1870), grandson of the founder, was an impressive teacher, an artist, and the author of the leading book of its kind, *Anatomy in Relation to Art* (1901). His *Regional Anatomy* (1892) in two volumes was translated into foreign languages and enjoyed widespread use. These books were beautifully illustrated with original photographs of drawings of his dissections. In 1890 McClellan held the Chair of Artistic Anatomy in the Pennsylvania Academy of the Fine Arts while concurrently conducting his own small private school of anatomy for students in medicine, dentistry, and art, which he closed upon receiving the Chair in Applied Anatomy at Jefferson. Dr. McClellan illustrated his lectures with remarkably accurate blackboard sketches of the anatomic parts under discussion. It is said that "he dissected a body as a great sculptor would carve a statue." His portrait was presented in 1914 to the College of Physicians of Philadelphia, of which he was a member. In 1982, another portrait of McClellan was donated to the Jefferson art collection by a descendant.

Unfortunately, there was very little cooperation between McClellan and Spitzka—in fact, they rarely spoke to each other. Following the death of McClellan (1913), the anatomy courses and the two Chairs were united under Spitzka.

J. Parsons Schaeffer, M.D., Ph.D., Sc.D. (1878–1970), Ninth Chairman (1914–1948)

Jacob Parsons Schaeffer, B.E., M.E., A.M., M.D., Ph.D., Sc.D. (Figure 3-12), succeeded Dr. Spitzka in 1914 as Professor of Anatomy, Head of the Department, and Director of the Daniel Baugh Institute of Anatomy. A gifted, dynamic teacher, productive investigator and author, Dr. Schaeffer served Jefferson with extraordinary distinction until his retirement 34 years later. Impeccable in appearance, dignified in manner and bearing, he personified the most desirable traits of the profession for thousands of medical students and colleagues.

Dr. Schaeffer's numerous scientific contributions and publications included all branches of anatomy as well as genetics, rhinology, and radiology (Figure 3-13). He served on federal and state commissions and successfully protected, when challenged, the use of animals in medical research and teaching in Pennsylvania. His monograph, *The Nose, Lacrymal Apparatus, and Olfactory Organ in Man* (1920) is still a classic. He was coauthor with Drs. Henry Pancoast and Eugene Pendergrass of *The Head and Neck in Roentgen Diagnosis* (1940) and editor of the tenth edition of *Morris' Human Anatomy* (1942). Schaeffer continued with later editions of these books.

After receiving the M.D. degree from the University of Pennsylvania (1907), Dr. Schaeffer entered Cornell University for advanced anatomical studies, gaining the Ph.D. degree in 1910. He then joined the Faculty of Medicine at Yale, was elevated to full Professor in 1911, and answered the call to Jefferson in 1914.

Responding to Dr. Schaeffer's leadership, Anatomy at Jefferson developed rapidly and ranked with the best in America, winning for him the respectful and affectionate title of "Mr. Anatomy—U.S.A." As President of the American Association of Anatomists during World War II,

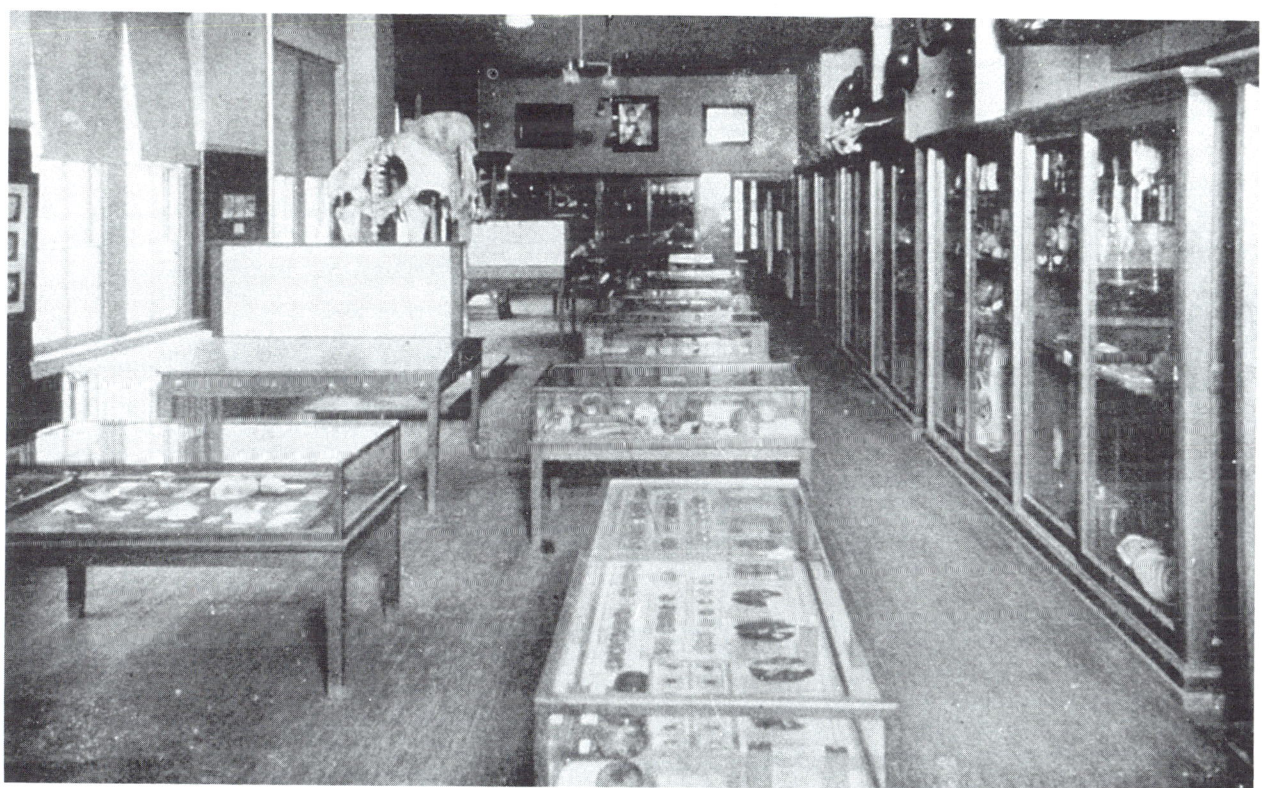

FIG. 3-11. Museum of the Daniel Baugh Institute of Anatomy.

Schaeffer also contributed guidance and direction to numerous medical and scientific organizations. For many years he administered the affairs of the Anatomical Board of Pennsylvania where he preserved the privilege of dissection of the human body for students in medical sciences in Pennsylvania. The Class of 1932 commissioned his portrait in esteem and admiration. When the Kellow Conference Area was constructed on the second floor of the main College building in 1979, one of the six rooms was named in his honor.

Following retirement in 1948, Dr. Schaeffer continued his professional activities, scientific writing, and editorships for many years, enjoying the title of Professor of Anatomy, Emeritus. His death came in 1970, at the age of 92. His wife, Mary Bobb, active on the Women's Board, lived to just a few weeks short of 100.

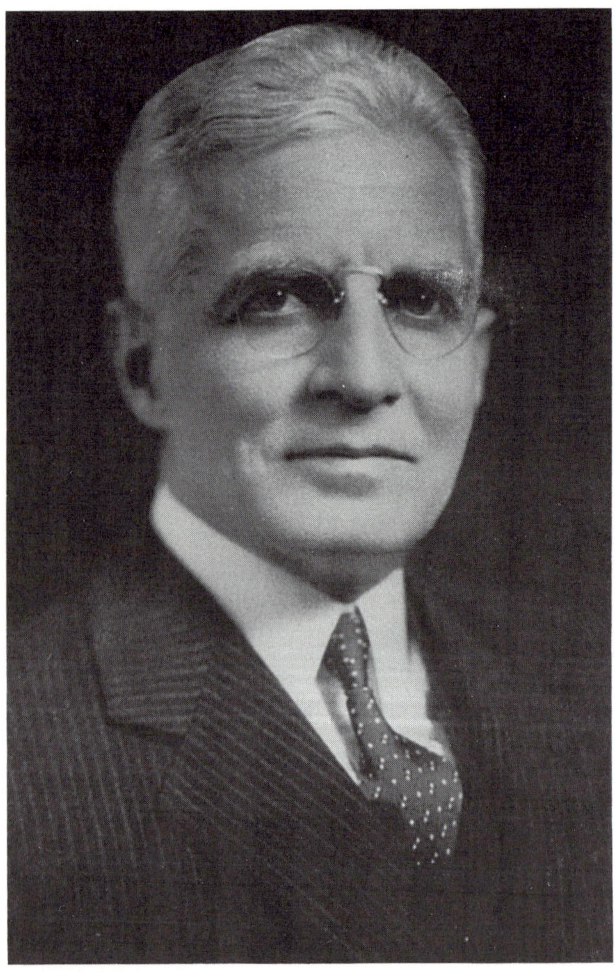

FIG. 3-12. J. Parsons Schaeffer, M.D., Ph.D., Sc.D. (1878–1970), Ninth Chairman (1914–1948).

George A. Bennett, M.D., Sc.D., LL.D. (1904–1958), Tenth Chairman (1948–1958)

George Allen Bennett, A.B., Artzt, M.D., Sc.D., LL.D. succeeded Dr. J. Parsons Schaeffer to the Chair in Anatomy and to the Directorship of the Daniel Baugh Institute of Anatomy (1948). In 1949 he was called to assist in the dean's office because of the declining health of Dean William Harvey Perkins and was appointed Dean in 1950.

Dr. Bennett's greatest contribution to Jefferson, without doubt, was his extraordinary success in teaching gross, applied, and surgical anatomy (Figure 3-14). His research program was necessarily curtailed due to the duties of the Deanship, which were complicated by administrative controversies.

Born in Mississippi in 1904, Bennett received the A.B. degree with Phi Beta Kappa honors at age 18 from Wabash College in Indiana. He pursued postgraduate study at the University of Wisconsin, the University of Athens, at Zürich, and finally at the University of Munich, where he qualified as a physician (Artzt) in 1928. Returning to his homeland, he joined the medical faculty at Baylor University and soon transferred to Harvard Medical School as a Teaching Fellow in Anatomy (1928). He then returned to Munich for continuation of his research and received the European M.D., *summa cum laude*, in 1937. Bennett also was in charge of the summer course in anatomy at Harvard and was elected Professor of Histology and Acting Head of the Biology Department at Georgetown University Medical School.

Beloved by the students, Bennett also received honors from several colleges and universities, from the U.S. government, and from professional organizations. His major scientific contributions were the experimental analysis of the action of mammalian tongue musculature (with Dr. Andrew J. Ramsay), heterochromia in relation to autonomic innervation, variational anatomy of the shoulder joint, and transplantation of muscle segments in the leg.

Death came in 1958 while Bennett was attending the February meeting of the Council on Medical Education and Licensure in Chicago. The Board of Trustees in 1959 commissioned his portrait for the dean's office suite.

Andrew J. Ramsay, Ph.D., Sc.D. (1907–), Eleventh Chairman (1958–1972)

Andrew J. Ramsay, A.B., Ph.D., Sc.D. (Figure 3-15), was called to Jefferson in 1936 by Professor J. Parsons Schaeffer as Associate in Anatomy. He was advanced to Assistant Professor (1937), Associate Professor (1942), Professor of Histology and Embryology (1948), and, following the death of Dr. George A. Bennett (1958), to Professor of Anatomy, Chairman of the Department of Anatomy, and Director of the Daniel Baugh Institute of Anatomy.

Dr. Ramsay, born in 1907 in Indiana, received the A.B. degree at DePauw University (1930) and the Ph.D. at Cornell University (1934) while teaching in the medical and graduate schools. During the tenure of Dr. George A. Bennett as Dean of the College (1950–1958), Dr. Ramsay had assumed most of the administrative duties of the Anatomy Department. His portrait was commissioned by the Class of 1966. Upon retirement (1972) he was given Emeritus status and the Honorary Degree of Doctor of Science. He was the first recipient of the title of Daniel Baugh Professor of Anatomy, awarded in 1981.

Dr. Ramsay's objectives, upon assuming the Anatomy Chair, were to strengthen the teaching programs, to foster research of a diversified nature to reflect the skills and interests of the faculty, and to maintain Jefferson's traditional excellence in anatomy.[5–7] His contributions in pedagogy included innovative curriculum adjustments and enhancement of both classroom and laboratory teaching. He initiated Jefferson's use of electronic image amplification techniques for teaching. He developed the first controlled optical lighting apparatus for color photomicrography, which resulted in the production of color transparencies for teaching and research presentations unique among all medical schools. His research contributions dealt with phylogenetic, functional, and developmental aspects of the embryonic branchial derivitives, with extramedullary myelopoiesis, and histophysiology of endocrine and digestive glands. Ramsay's pioneering work in transplanting embryonic anlagen in mammals helped to initiate the new field of experimental mammalian embryology. His research on lymph flow demonstrated, contrary to the then current opinion, that returing lymph need not all traverse a lymph node before reentering the venous system, a contribution of importance in understanding metastasis of cancer cells.

Because anatomy is probably the most "visual" of the medical courses and research, the Department developed an effective capability, including the necessary equipment, personnel, and expertise to answer its own audiovisual needs. Soon the Anatomy Department was being asked by other departments to handle their audiovisual requirements. This resulted, in 1972, in the relocation by Dean Kellow of much of the Anatomy Department's equipment, facilities, and personnel to establish Jefferson's first institutionwide Division of Audio-Visual Services, under the direction of Miss Theresa Powers, formerly of the Anatomy Department's technical staff.

Dr. Ramsay's interest in continuing medical education was expressed through the Council on Medical Television of the Institute for the Advancement of Medical Communication (now the Health Sciences Communication Association), which he served as president. His leadership in innovative pedagogic and curricular modifications occasioned his memberships on National Institutes of Health study sections to evaluate current applications for curricular experimentation.

The Anatomy Courses

The progress of the courses in anatomy may best be traced chronologically by the succession of the faculty and their activities. The courses traditionally started as gross anatomy, with later addition of histology and embryology, and still later the teaching of neuroanatomy. At this juncture, it is appropriate to review the development of these three major divisions at Jefferson.

▪ Gross Anatomy

Starting with George McClellan in 1824 and until late in the nineteenth century, anatomy was taught as gross anatomy only, with emphasis on its application to surgery. The faculty was composed of surgeon-anatomists. The last of these, Professor Forbes, asked to be relieved of his duties in the Surgery Department in order to concentrate his energies on modernizing the anatomy courses, gross and surgical, and histology and embryology. His successor, Spitzka, was Jefferson's first full-time Anatomy Chairman with no outside practice permitted.

Jefferson's traditional strength in Anatomy gained new impetus and vigor with the appointment in 1914 of Professor J. Parsons Schaeffer, both in teaching and basic anatomic research. In 1914, most of the Anatomy Faculty were part-time. By 1929, appointment of full-time teachers/researchers had begun in earnest, and soon, as in most American medical faculties, full-time appointees outnumbered part-time ones. This was highly advantageous, because part-time teachers of necessity had to depend on their medical practices for livelihood, leaving little for creative scholarship activities.

Clarence Hoffman (Jefferson, 1906) was considered by the students (from 1911–1927) to

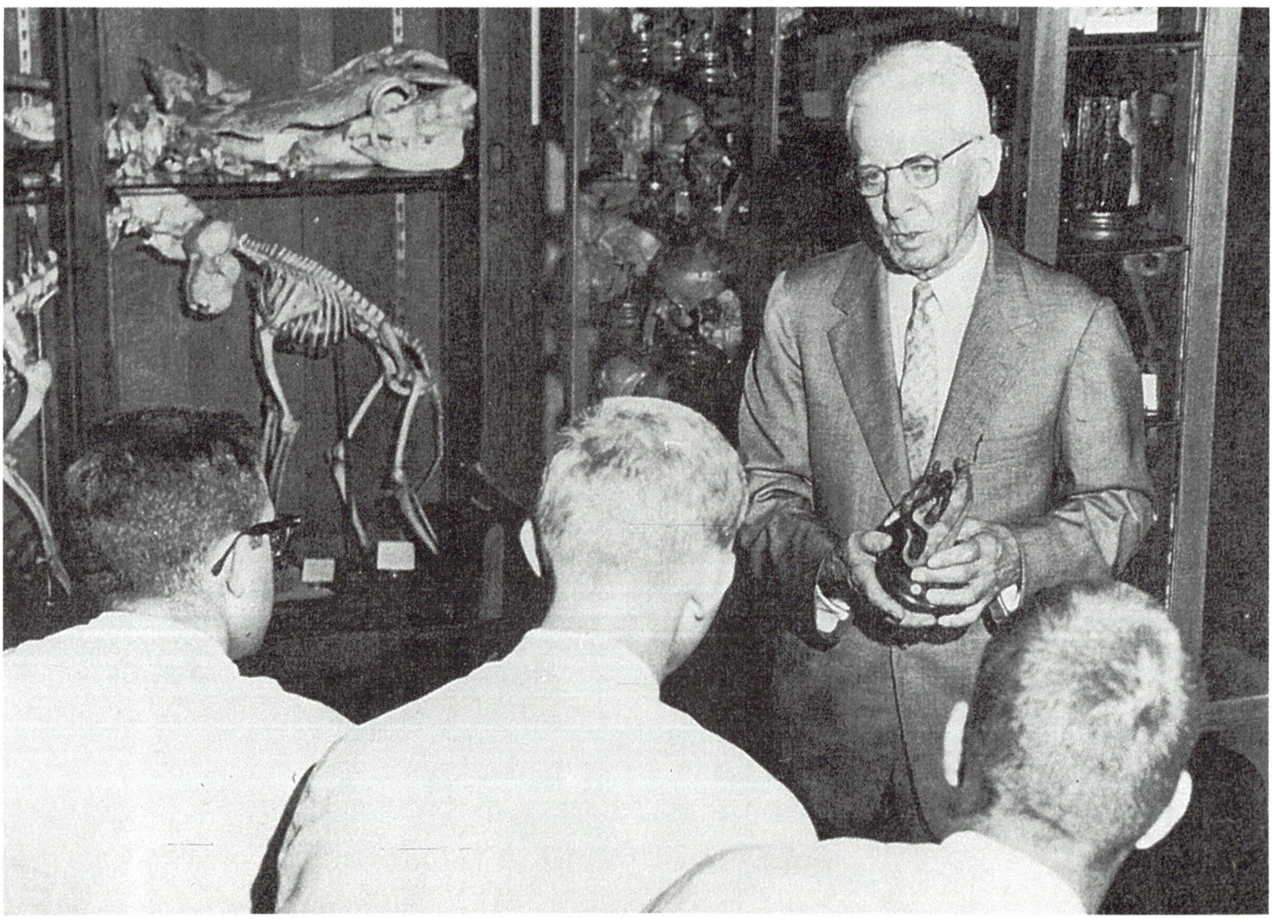

Fig. 3-13. Dr. J. Parsons Schaeffer explains the nasolacrymal apparatus and sinuses to students in the Daniel Baugh Institute.

have been an extraordinary teacher, especially in the dissecting room. His academic rank did not reflect his value to the College, unfortunately, because his main thrust was in teaching with no effort in research. Dr. Hoffman was an avid collector of unique clocks. Following his death, his widow presented to the Department one of his valuable clocks which, appropriately inscribed, is displayed in the office of the Chairman of Anatomy.

Dr. Nicholas A. Michels, M.A., Sc.D. (Figure 3-16) joined the full-time staff in 1929 after studying hematology in Belgium, France, and Italy. His original monograph on the mast cell (1924) brought him the signal honor in 1963 of being named the "Father of Mast Cell Research." On this occasion he was guest of honor at the International Congress on the Mast Cell.

Affectionately known as "The Bull," Dr. Michels influenced nearly 5,000 Jefferson students. His lecture on the embryologic rotation of the gut and the peritoneal reflections, using assorted hoses, funnels, and balloons, was a masterpiece of showmanship and pedagogy that annually filled the amphitheater beyond capacity.[8]

Dr. Michels made an impact not only in basic science but in surgery. His book, *Blood Supply and Anatomy of the Upper Abdominal Organs, with a Descriptive Atlas* (1955), became a classic. It was followed by *Celiac and Superior Mesenteric Arteries: A Correlation of Angiograms with Anatomic Dissections* (1969). Michels belonged to many learned societies and was honored in several of them. The Class of 1958 commissioned his portrait for the College, and he received the Lindback

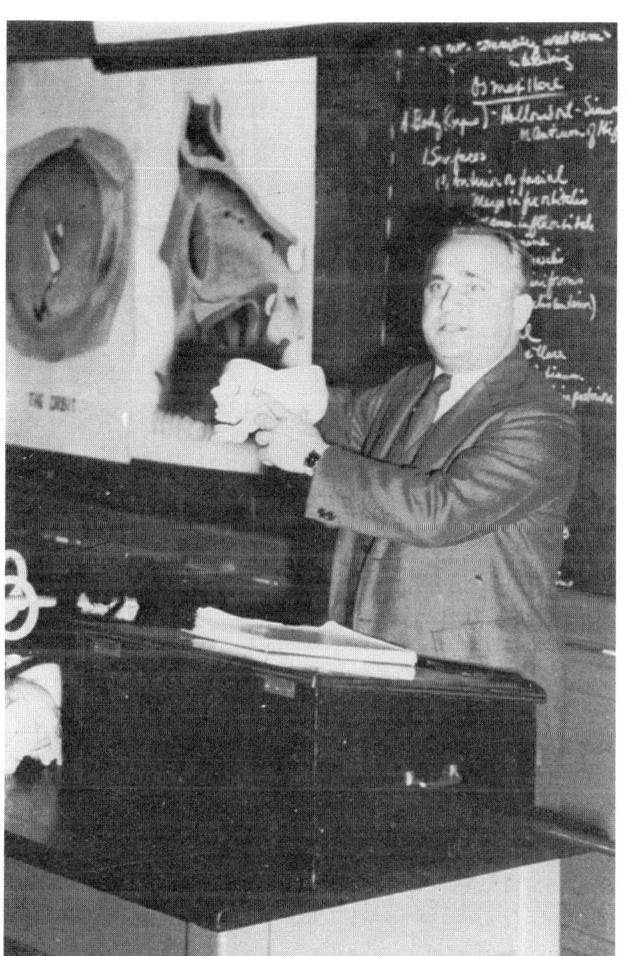

FIG. 3-14. George A. Bennett, M.D., Sc.D., LL.D. (1904–1958), Tenth Chairman (1948–1958).

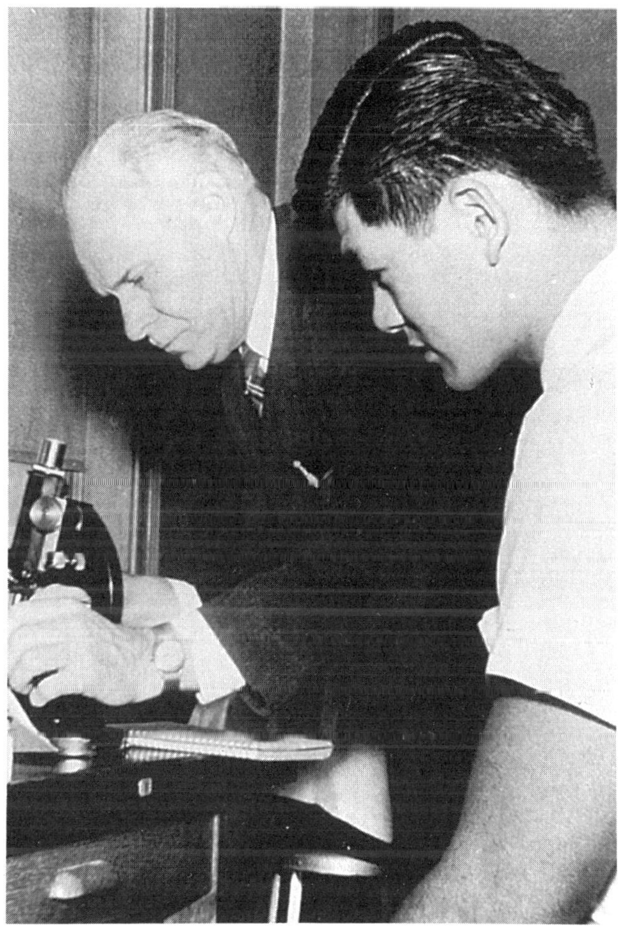

FIG. 3-15. Andrew J. Ramsay, Ph.D., Sc.D. (1907–), Eleventh Chairman (1958–1972).

Award for Distinguished Teaching in 1962. He died in 1969 as Emeritus Professor of Anatomy at the age of 78 from carcinoma of the pancreas, after 40 years of productive service as one of Jefferson's most dedicated, scholarly, and colorful faculty members.

Gross anatomy was further strengthened in 1939 by Dr. George A. Bennett, whose teaching prowess and flair for administration determined his selection to succeed Dr. Schaeffer (1948) as Professor of Anatomy, Head of the Department of Anatomy, and Director of the Daniel Baugh Institute of Anatomy. Shortly thereafter, because of ill health, Dean William Harvey Perkins called Dr. Bennett to assist him in the Dean's office, and in 1950 Dr. Bennett was elected Dean of The Jefferson Medical College, retaining, necessarily, the Chairmanship of Anatomy. (A Dean at that time, in order to attend meetings of his Faculty—that is, the Executive Faculty—was required to be a Department Chairman with a seat on the Executive Faculty.) The increasing responsibilities of the Dean's office sharply curtailed Dr. Bennett's participation in his first loves—teaching gross and surgical anatomy and conducting research.

J. Lawrence Angel, Ph.D., was appointed in 1943, bringing a refreshing physical anthropologic flavor to gross anatomy teaching. His scholarly researches in anthropology, especially in analyzing and identifying historic and prehistoric human remains, soon brought him to the forefront of American physical anthropologists. Professor Angel (Figure 3-17) was called to the Smithsonian Institution in Washington (1962) where, as Curator of Physical Anthropology, he further expanded his international reputation and enjoyed the designations of "bone doctor" and "bone detective," the latter due to his amazing analytical contributions to forensic medical matters dealing with human remains.

Also in 1943, R. Cranford Hutchinson, Ph.D., resident scientist at the Wistar Institute of Anatomy's Morris Biological Farm, joined the Department. Dr. Hutchinson continued his experimental embryologic research at Jefferson and soon, together with Dr. C. Everett Koop, currently (1988) the Surgeon General of the United States, concentrated on experimental studies on cartilage growth aimed at correcting abnormal epiphyseal cartilagenous growth problems in the developing limbs of infants and young children.

When Dr. Bennett became Dean in 1950, he called his former classmate at the University of Munich, Franz X. Hausberger, M.D., to join the Anatomy Department. Dr. Hausberger (Figure 3-18) immediately became an outstanding teacher of gross anatomy and a favorite of the students.

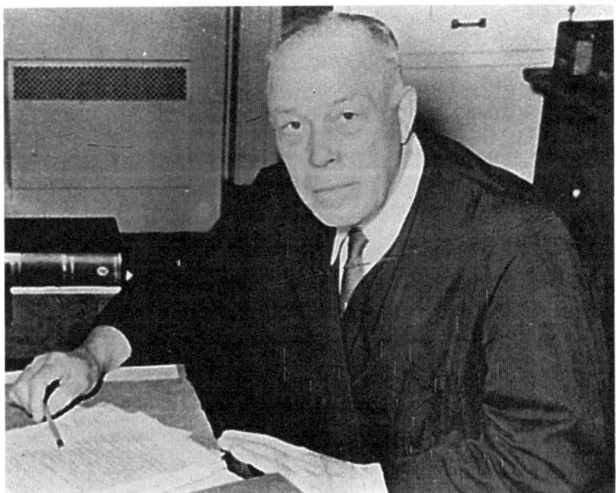

FIG. 3-16. Nicholas A. Michels, M.A., D.Sc., Professor of Anatomy and "Father of Mast Cell Research."

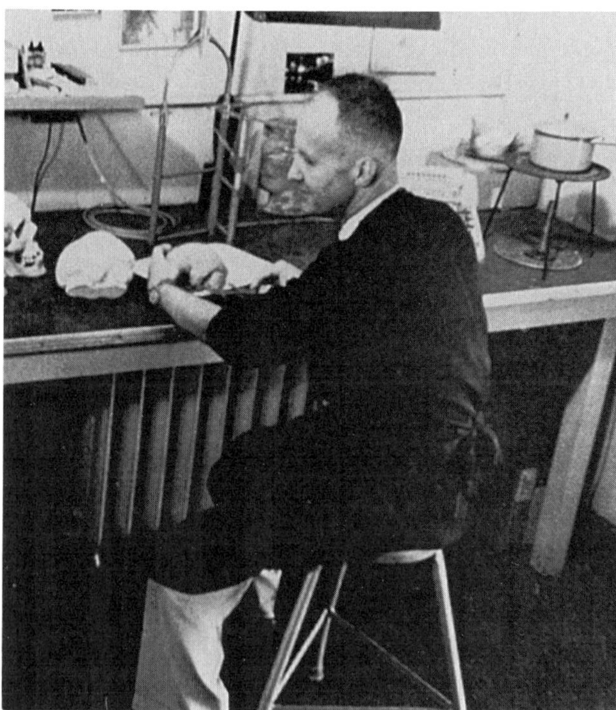

FIG. 3-17. J. Lawrence Angel, Ph.D., Professor of Anatomy (Physical Anthropology).

He received the Christian and Mary F. Lindback Award for Distinguished teaching in 1965. Hausberger's brilliant research in experimental diabetes and related fat metabolic disorders resulted in his being honored as "The Father of Adipose Tissue Research" by the *Handbook of Physiology* in 1965. The Class of 1967 commissioned his portrait for the College. Upon Professor Hausberger's retirement, he was elevated to Emeritus status.

John E. Healey (Jefferson, 1948), one of the first recipients of a Ross V. Patterson Fellowship, taught gross anatomy from 1949 to 1959 and applied the findings in anatomy of the liver of Paul C. Schroy (Jefferson, 1957, first Ph.D. graduate in Anatomy) to clinical problems.

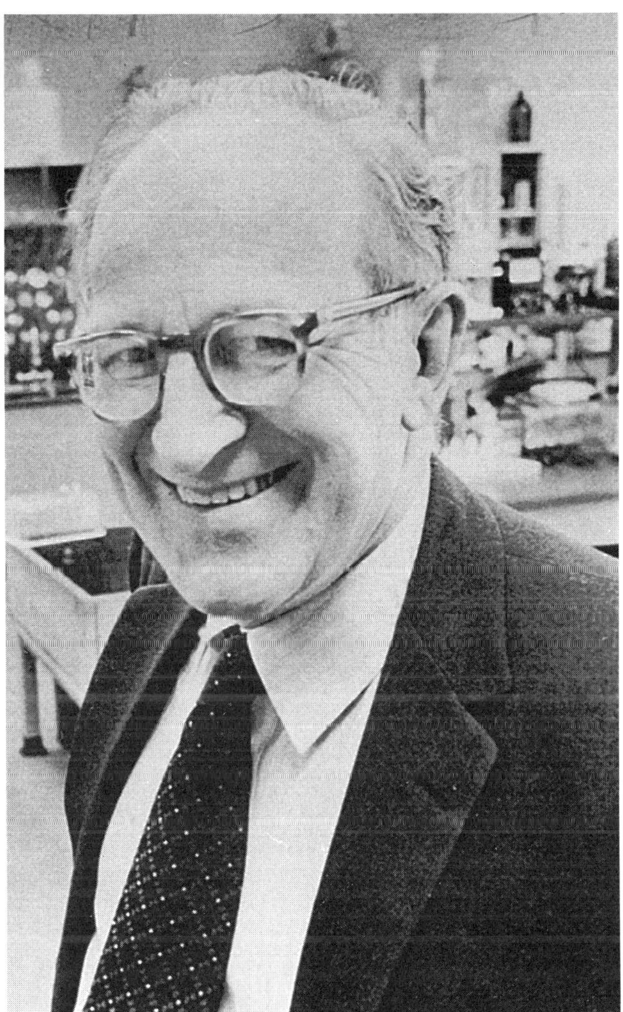

FIG. 3-18. Franz X. Hausberger, M.D., Professor of Anatomy; his portrait was presented to the College by the Class of 1967.

Robert J. Merklin, Ph.D. (Figure 3-19) was the first histochemist to join the Department (1953), adding strength to instruction in gross anatomy. Wesley W. Parke, Ph.D., arrived in 1957 to teach gross anatomy. Under the tutelege of Professor Michels, Parke made important advances in research. Later, Professor Parke moved to the University of Southern Illinois to assume Chairmanship of its Anatomy Department.

Sigfrid Zitzlsperger, D.M. (Habilitatus), the first American anatomist to apply the principles of analytical mechanics to determine stress factors in complicated joints (ankle and foot), joined the anatomy staff in 1952, later withdrawing to accept the Chairmanship in Anatomy at Chicago Medical School. Diane E. Smith, Ph.D., and Barbara F. Forbes, Ph.D., taught gross and neuroanatomy in the late 1960s and early 1970s. Dr. Smith relocated to Louisiana State University. James O. Brown, Ph.D., was appointed in 1950 to assist in gross and neuroanatomy, concentrating later on gross anatomy only, after having directed the course in neuroanatomy for several years.

The greatest impact on gross anatomy teaching following that of Professor F. X. Hausberger was contributed by John R. Shea, Jr., Ph.D., M.S. (bioengineering), beginning in 1967. Bringing a new level in lecturing, laboratory instruction, and

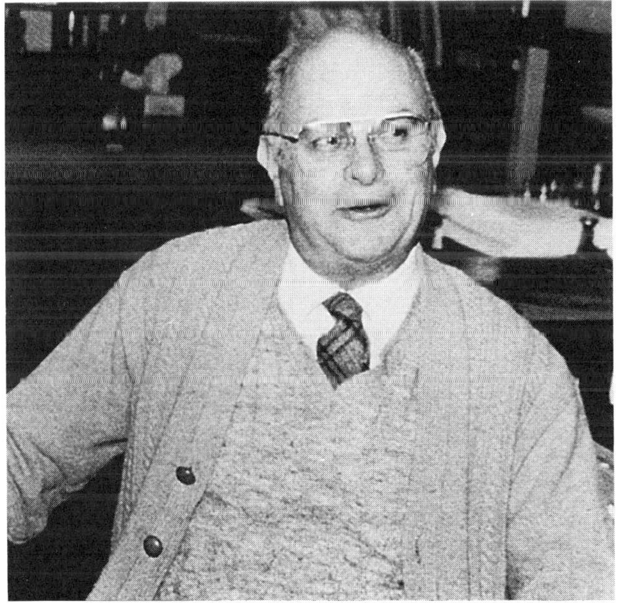

FIG. 3-19. Robert J. Merklin, Ph.D., Professor of Anatomy.

personal dedication to the needs of medical and graduate students, he immediately was honored with a variety of teaching awards, including the Mellon Faculty Award for faculty improvement in teaching, the Lindback Award for Distinguished Teaching, Outstanding Professor of the Year (1971/72), and the Outstanding Teacher Award (1980). The Class of 1983 awarded Professor Shea the honor of commissioning his portrait for presentation to the College. Dr. Shea transferred to the Department of Orthopedic Surgery in 1987.

Expansion of the Anatomy Faculty

Since its founding, the Jefferson Faculty recognized the importance of anatomy and taught it well. For over half a century anatomy was the only course that required and provided laboratory work. George McClellan and his successors insisted on student participation in dissection of the human body. By 1828 the classes in anatomy could no longer be conducted by a single teacher, and Samuel McClellan (brother of the founder) became the first Assistant Demonstrator. Thereafter, until 1875, there was one Demonstrator who received a small remuneration at the discretion of the Professor. Ellerslie Wallace (appointed Demonstrator in 1846) became Professor of Obstetrics and Diseases of Women and Children (1862–1883) and Dean of the College (1879–1883). William Henry Pancoast (appointed in 1863) rose to become Professor of Anatomy (1874). In 1875 Dr. Pancoast not only had a Demonstrator (Dr. Thomas H. Andrews) but a Prosector (Dr. Henry Leaman). In 1878 the first Demonstrator of Histology was appointed (Dr. J. Gibbons Hunt), and he was followed in 1883 by Dr. Albert Brubaker as Demonstrator of Physiology and Histology.

A growth spurt occurred in 1886, the year in which Dr. William Smith Forbes became Chairman, when four Demonstrators and four Assistant Demonstrators were appointed. Among the latter was Dr. John Chalmers DaCosta, fresh out of the Jefferson graduating Class of 1885. Another was Dr. A. J. Downes, who taught in the histology course that Dr. Forbes was establishing. By 1891 there were two Assistant Demonstrators of Histology (Drs. Howard Swayne and A. A. Eshner). Counting Professor Forbes, the Anatomy Department in 1901 encompassed ten members. Dr. Henry E. Radasch, as Demonstrator of Histology and Embryology, would become Professor of this subdivision in 1921. Dr. Charles W. Bonney, appointed Assistant Demonstrator in 1905, would become Assistant Professor of Topographical and Applied Anatomy in 1930.

In addition to the growing full-time staff, the ancillary faculty was enriched by volunteers from the Surgery Department, from the surgical specialties, and from physicians in private general practice. These men, besides their interests in anatomy, liked to teach and benefited by the enhancement of their professional skills. Before the surgical residency systems developed, the pathway to becoming a competent surgeon was to teach anatomy, work in the outpatient department, administer anesthesia, and to assist an older established surgeon. Most members of Jefferson's Surgical Department in this era taught anatomy as prosectors. Indeed, two of Jefferson's most eminent surgeons, Dr. William Williams Keen (in 1893) and John Chalmers DaCosta (in 1905 and 1908) edited American editions of *Gray's Anatomy*. The son of Robley Dunglison, Dr. Richard J. Dunglison (Jefferson, 1856) edited American editions in 1859, 1862, 1870, 1878, and 1883. Dr. Spitzka edited American editions in 1910 and 1913. Of the seven editors of the American editions of *Gray's Anatomy* (started in 1858), four were connected with Jefferson.

Part-Time and Volunteer Faculty

Many part-time and volunteer teachers complemented the staff off and on during the present century. Some of the most outstanding or well remembered were: Addinell Hewson (1903), J. Coles Brick (1903), Charles F. Nassau (1907), J. Leslie Davis (1909), George W. Miller (1910), Warren B. Davis (1912), John DeCarlo (1915), Benjamin Lipshutz (1917), Moses Behrend (1919), William J. Thudium (1920), William B. Swartley (1920), C. Calvin Fox (1921), John B. Flick (1922), Maxwell Cherner (1926), Eli R. Saleeby (1926), John T. Farrell, Jr. (1928), Thomas E. Shea (1929), George J. Willauer (1929), Herbert A. Widing (1930), Raymond B. Moore (1931), Frank J.

Ciliberti (1931), Hugh Robertson (1934), Milton Harrison (1935), James M. Surver (1935), Leon L. Berns (1935), Kelvin A. Kaspar (1936), Robert A. Matthews (1937), Sherman A. Eger (1937), John C. McNerney (1940), George J. Teplick (1941), Nicholas A. Varano (1941), Frederick B. Wagner, Jr. (1943), Russell Wigh (1946), Gerald E. Callery (1946), Armando F. Goracci (1949), Harry Subin (1949), Gerald D. Dodd (1952), Bernard J. Miller (1953), and Joseph M. Gagliardi (1954). A more complete list may be found in the Jefferson Alumni Bulletin of Fall, 1972.

Dr. Raymond B. Moore, M.D. (Figure 3-20) taught applied anatomy to the third-year students from 1930 to 1967 with the fervor of a football coach. In admiration, the Class of 1949 dedicated the *Clinic* to "Coach Moore." A great many residents were prepared successfully for board examinations by his postgraduate course at the Daniel Baugh Institute.

Dr. Bernard J. Miller (Jefferson, 1943) (Figure 3-21) carried on a combined career in clinical surgery as well as anatomy teaching and research. On the staff since 1953, and still active more than thirty years later, he investigated the role of the pancreas in carcinogenesis, the isolation of a carcinolytic factor in Sarcoma 37 mice, serum protein changes in patients showing remission from cancer, and the effect of high-energy vibration on localized tumor masses with an attempt to determine resonance frequencies of experimental tumors. He also developed electronic monitors on Dr. Gibbon's heart-lung machine.

Dr. Leon L. Berns (Jefferson, '35), Honorary Clinical Professor of Anatomy, has, since his graduation and for more than 50 years, taught gross anatomy and its clinical applications to thousands of Jefferson students. Professor Berns (Figure 3-22) has expressed his loyalty and

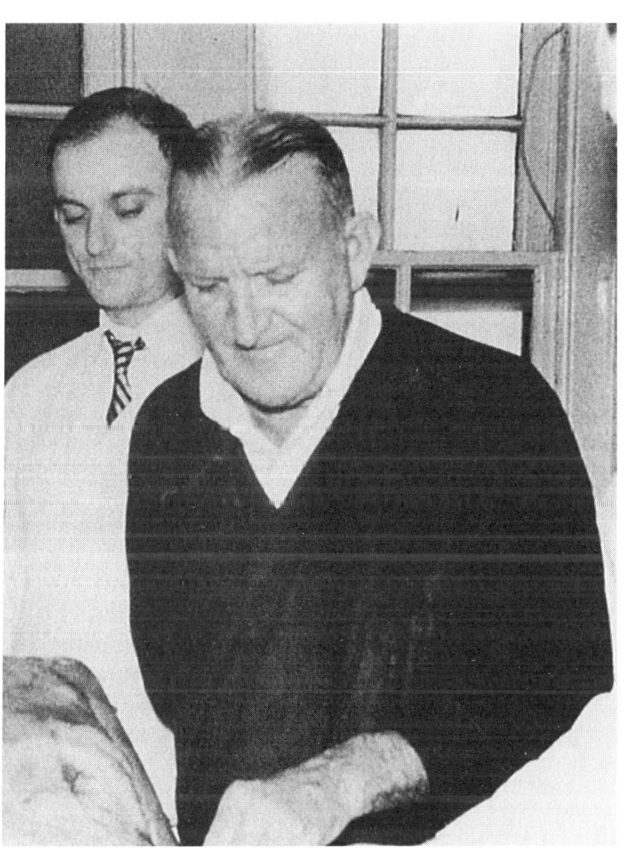

FIG. 3-20. Raymond B. Moore, M.D., a volunteer Assistant Professor of Anatomy (Applied Anatomy), affectionately called "Coach Moore."

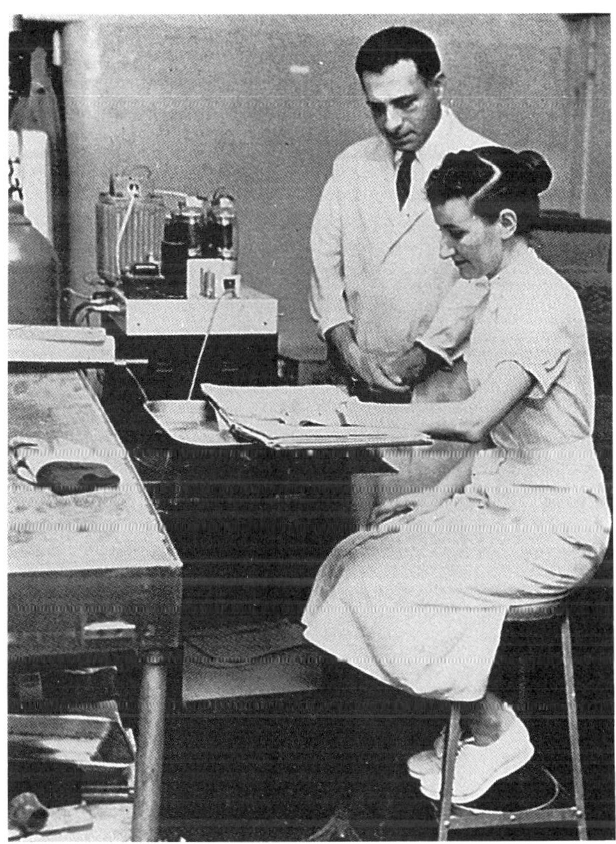

FIG. 3-21. Bernard J. Miller, M.D., volunteer and later part-time Professor of Anatomy, reviews results on studies of a carcinolytic factor in Sarcoma 37 mice with Miss Mary Pitcher, technician.

commitment to Jefferson's Anatomy Department further by always returning his honorarium stipend check to the Department Chairman for use in support of Departmental functions. His tenure has exceeded that of others in this century: J. Parsons Schaeffer (34 years); Henry E. Radasch (42 years); and Andrew J. Ramsay (36 years).

Currently in America, research into the finer aspects of gross anatomy unfortunately has come almost to a standstill.[8] Financial support for research into human gross structure, its variations and anomalies and resultant functional implications, has been virtually withdrawn. Curriculum changes in recent years, deemphasizing human structure, have reflected the controversial but widely held opinion that "following DaVinci and Vesalius there is nothing more to be discovered in human structure." As a result, some curriculum committees are openly suggesting to medical students that anatomy is of decreasing significance in their becoming qualified physicians. The folly in this misleading idea has been exposed vividly by the recent development of the many new and emerging technical diagnostic procedures (radiology, arteriography, venography, lymphangiography, and body-scanning techniques by ultrasonics, computerized tomography, and magnetic resonance). The interpretation of all these depend on thorough knowledge of normal human structure and its variations. Thus, the first division of human anatomy to be deemphasized, both in teaching and research, is experiencing a modern renaissance.

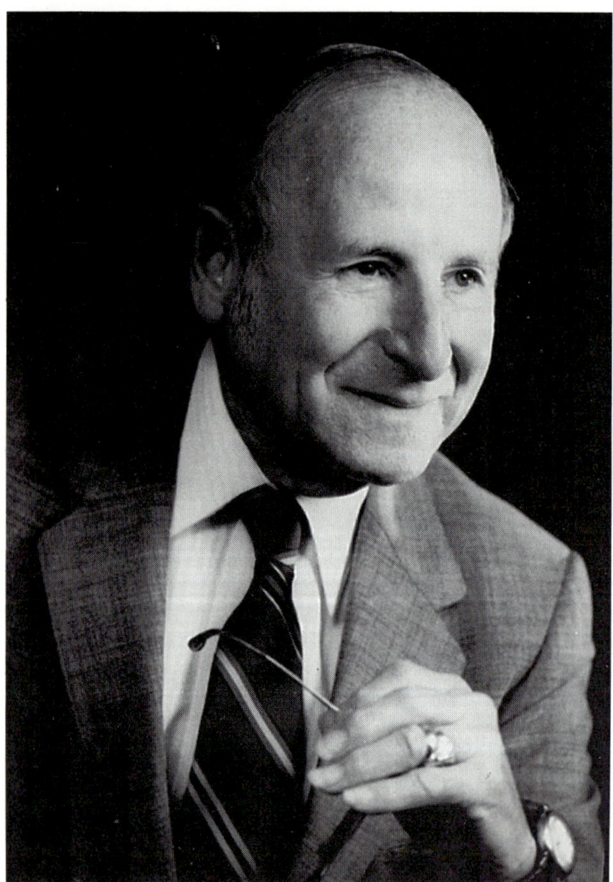

FIG. 3-22. Leon L. Berns, M.D. (1930), taught gross anatomy for more than fifty years on a volunteer basis.

Histology and Embryology

Instruction in histology at Jefferson started in 1878 as a satellite of Physiology under the Chairmanship of Dr. J. Aitken Meigs. The microscopy laboratory, conducted by Dr. J. Gibbons Hunt, Demonstrator of Histology, was "amply provided with microscopes and other appliances for thorough practical instruction." The medical course at that time consisted of two years of six months each. Because the teaching was almost entirely by lectures, the amount of instruction in histology at best had to be sparse.

In 1883, Dr. Albert P. Brubaker (Jefferson, 1874) became Demonstrator of Histology and Physiology. He taught histology for only three years, but was associated with the Department of Physiology for over fifty.

In 1886, Dr. Martin P. Rively (Jefferson, 1885) and Andrew J. Downes (Jefferson, 1885) both became Assistant Demonstrators of Histology. At this time laboratory work for "first-course students" was required. Dr. Eugene L. Vansant (Jefferson, 1884) then became Demonstrator from 1889 to 1893.

Dr. Charles S. Hearne (Jefferson, 1890) was appointed Demonstrator in 1893, and Dr. Randle C. Rosenberger (Jefferson, 1894) Assistant Demonstrator in 1894. In 1897, "Randy" Rosenberger became Demonstrator of Histology and Bacteriology and, in 1909, was elected to the Chair of Hygiene and Bacteriology.

Instruction in histology, initially under the Department of Physiology, was transferred in 1896 to Anatomy under Dr. Forbes as a separate course. In 1900, Dr. Forbes made embryology a requisite for freshmen. Dr. Herbert H. Cushing (Jefferson, 1899) was made Demonstrator of Histology and Embryology. These subjects were then taught as separate entities.

The dominant figure for 40 years in the history of histology and embryology at Jefferson was Dr. Henry Erdmann Radasch (Figure 3-23). A native of Iowa, born in 1874, he took his B.S. and M.S. degrees at the State University of Iowa and his medical degree at Jefferson. Even when a student at Jefferson (1898–1901) he was an Assistant in Histology; he was elected Demonstrator of Histology and Embryology as soon as he obtained

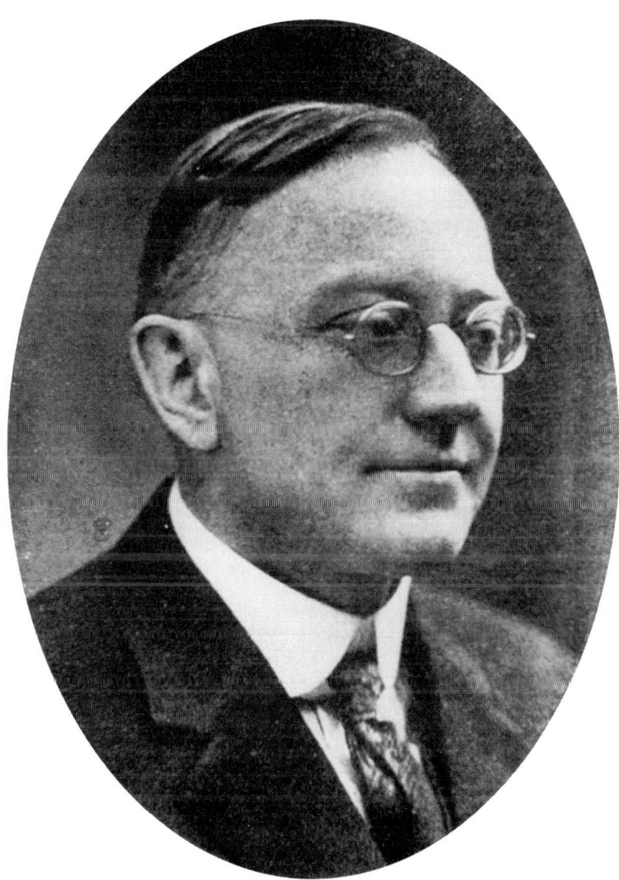

FIG. 3-23. Henry E. Radasch, M.D. (1874–1942), Professor of Histology and Embryology (1921–1942).

his M.D. degree in 1901. To further his progress, Radasch in 1903 spent several months in research in the Zoological Laboratory of the University of Leipzig. This led to his promotion to Associate the following year.

Dr. Radasch ("Rad") rose in rank to full Professor of Histology and Embryology in 1921 during the Chairmanship of Professor J. Parsons Schaeffer. In the years of Jefferson's premedical course (1913–1916) he served as Assistant Professor of Biology. He added to the literature on muscular anomalies, red blood cells, acid cells of the stomach, composition of compact bone, superfetation, and senility of bone. Between 1905 and 1924 he was the author of *Manual of Histology* (three editions) and a *Manual of Anatomy* (1917). Radasch wore a green eyeshade and lectured with machine-gun speed; all the material missed in class could be recaptured in his *Manual of Histology*, which was essential to passing the course. Professor Radasch developed the course in histology and embryology into a strong viable segment of the anatomy curriculum, aided by Dr. W. C. ("the black prince") Pritchard (1911–1930), who later moved to Temple University. Drs. Gulden Mackmull (1930–1933) and David Soloway (1932–1936) also aided in the instruction.

Dr. Radasch enjoyed an international reputation as a philatelist, specializing in balloon, rocket, and early airmail stamps and covers. The latter were carried for him to France by Colonel Charles A. Lindbergh on his historic transatlantic solo flight.

Dr. Radasch became Professor Emeritus in 1941. His death the following year was a painful shock to the some 5,000 students and graduates who held him in admiration and affection. His portrait was presented to the College by the Class of 1942.

Andrew J. Ramsay, Ph.D., joined the staff in 1936 as Associate in Anatomy to strengthen the teaching of histology and embryology (Figure 3-24). He succeeded Dr. Radasch as head of this subdivision in 1942 and became Chairman of the Department in 1958. Dr. Ramsay's lectures were greatly appreciated by the students for their clarity and ease of comprehension through the use of blackboard illustrations in different colors of chalk for the various body layers during embryological development (Figure 3-25). From 1936 to 1942 Dr. Ramsay alone conducted the laboratory sessions and gave most of the lectures. During this time he replaced the student slide sets entirely and developed a complete collection of color photomicrographs for use in lectures, the first such collection in American medical schools. In

1942, M. Noble Bates (Ph.D., Cornell) was called to assist in teaching histology and embryology. Later, Dr. Bates joined the medical faculty of Temple University. Before and during these years, there being no funds available for the support of research, a researcher had to buy with his own funds his experimental animals and their food and other necessities, take care of the animals, pay his own way to scientific meetings, buy reprints of his publications, and the like. Space in the "converted animal room" was extremely limited, so researchers kept their animals mostly in their own office-laboratories. There were as yet no "genetically identical" experimental animals available, so Dr. Ramsay developed his own strain for his mammalian embryonic transplantation experiments. The numbers of animals required for this work soon exceeded available space. With the appointment of Dr. George Bennett as Anatomy Chairman, and with the support of Dean Perkins, it became possible to add Dr. Savino A. D'Angelo to the histology-embryology faculty.

Savino A. D'Angelo, Ph.D. (Figure 3-26), was called to Jefferson in 1949 from New York University's Department of Biology to teach histology, embryology, and neuroanatomy. His research interests were in endocrine function and neurophysiology. Special interest in the thyroid gland led to his investigations on bioassay measurements, thyroid–pituitary interaction, thyroid-thyrotropic hormone balance, and radio-iodine uptake under varying conditions of cold and starvation. His neuro–endocrine integration studies employed stereotaxic apparatus for control of brain lesions and radioisotopes for histologic study of hypothalamic–hypophyseal interaction, both neural and hormonal. For one phase of this work he received, along with Dr. Ronald E. Traum (Jefferson, 1957) of the Department of Obstetrics and Gynecology, the A. Cressy Morrison Prize in 1957 from the New York Academy of Sciences. Dr. D'Angelo stimulated advanced medical students and graduate fellows to become involved in his research. He died in 1976 at the age of 66 from a dissecting aneurysm; his recently completed chapter in a book entitled *Pioneers in Endocrinology*, which depicted his exciting career, was still in press. D'Angelo's enthusiastic teaching led to his receiving the Lindback Award (1969), while his research was recognized by his receipt of the newly created Career Research Award from the National Institutes of Health, the first such honor at Jefferson and, indeed, in the northeastern United States.

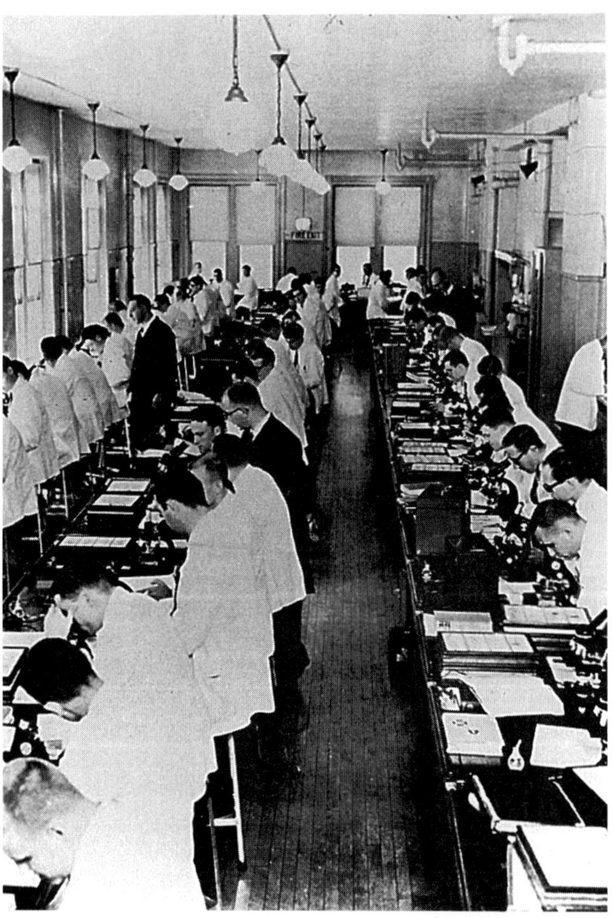

FIG. 3-24. Histology Laboratory in Daniel Baugh Institute.

Johannes P. M. Vogelaar, M.D., transferred to Jefferson in 1950 from the research facility of the United States Navy, where his research concentration was on an artificial blood plasma substitute. At Jefferson his interest was in tissue culture.

Jefferson's first electron microscope was obtained by Dr. Ramsay (1952). Charles G. Rosa, Ph.D. (Harvard), came to Jefferson in 1954 and, together with Dr. Albert W. Sedar, established ultrastructural research at Jefferson. Dr. Rosa's remarkable demonstration of the intracellular location of enzyme action (within the cristae of mitochondria), a study in which Dr. K. S. Tsou took part, was chosen by the National Institutes of Health to appear before the U.S. Congress in requesting continuing grant monies for biomedical research.

Dr. Rosa is also known for his researches on histochemical stains, endothelial transport, and thyrotroph cytophysiology, and together with Dr. J. T. Velardo he coauthored the volume on the female genital system for the German publication *Histochemie*.

Albert W. Sedar, Ph.D. joined Jefferson in 1955 from the Rockefeller Institute for Medical Research. His primary teaching interest is histology and embryology; his research centers on the cytophysiology of cell types aimed at correlating fine cell structure with functional activity. As does Dr. Rosa, Dr. Sedar uses electron microscopy plus histochemistry to accumulate data on the physiologic state of cells stimulated or inhibited pharmacologically. He collaborated with Dr. Charles G. Rosa in both teaching and research in this subdivision of the department. With Professors Sedar, Rosa, and August Epple, the course in histology and embryology pays particular attention to ultrastructural, histochemical, and histophysiological features basic to human biology and pathology. Dr. Sedar's research won funds for a second electron microscope and related facilities for the Anatomy Department and won for him the honor of a Research Development Award from the National Institutes of Health. Currently (1987), the Department has three electron microscopes.

August Epple, Ph.D., since his appointment in 1967, has stood at the forefront of research into the comparative structure and function of the pancreas and its islets throughout phylogeny of the animal kingdom. Ronald P. Jensh, Ph.D. (Jefferson, 1966), the first teratologist on the faculty, conducted research in this field and rose to the rank of full Professor and Vice-Chairman of the Department. He is one of the most successful and well known alumni of the College of Graduate Studies. Edwin M. Masters, Ph.D.

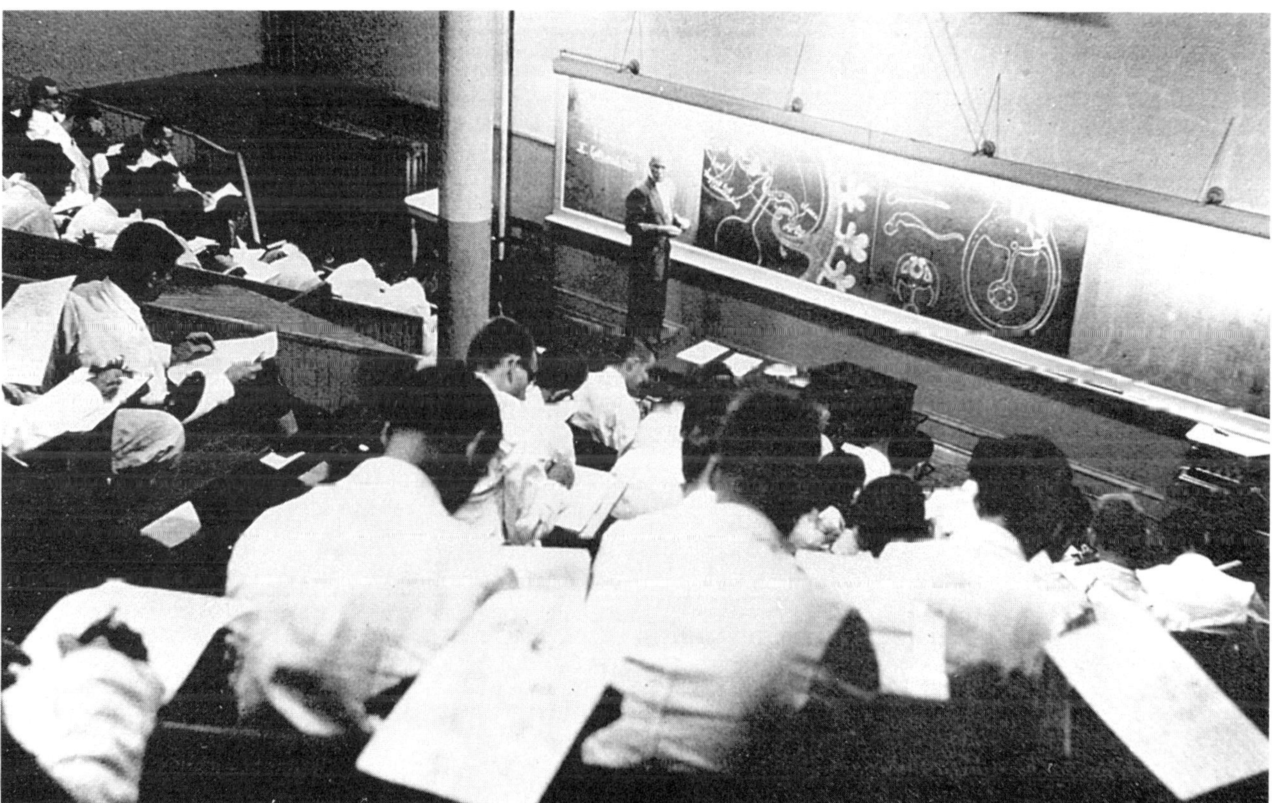

FIG. 3-25. Dr. Andrew J. Ramsay lecturing in embryology in Daniel Baugh Institute.

(Harvard), since 1964 has effectively taught histology and embryology and, later, gross anatomy. Nancy Trotter, Ph.D. (Columbia) taught histology and embryology from 1968 to 1971. Known widely for her ultrastructural studies on the liver, Trotter's career was unfortunately interrupted by illness that forced her withdrawal from scientific activity.

The Division of Neuroanatomy

Early instruction in neuroanatomy was apparently included in lectures and laboratory dissections under the division of gross anatomy. The first lectures in neuroanatomy proper were listed in 1917, given for one hour per week by Professor J. Parsons Schaeffer. The brain was dissected during the gross study of the head and neck until 1932 when laboratory sessions for one-half day per week dealing with both gross and microscopic study of the brain and spinal cord were initiated. The first faculty appointee to be identified with neuroanatomy by title was Dr. Benjamin Lipshutz in 1917, as Assistant Demonstrator of Neuroanatomy. He conducted the laboratories from 1932 until 1948, when he retired from the faculty at Associate Professorial level. A kindly, gentle, unusually competent teacher, Dr. Lipshutz for thirty years left an indelible impression on the students. In 1948, following the retirement of Professor Schaeffer, the lectures were given by Professor George A. Bennett, newly appointed Chairman. Dr. R. Frederick Becker was given charge of the course in 1949, assisted by Drs. H. Chandler Elliott and J. O. Brown (1950). The latter succeeded Dr. Becker as course director in 1952.

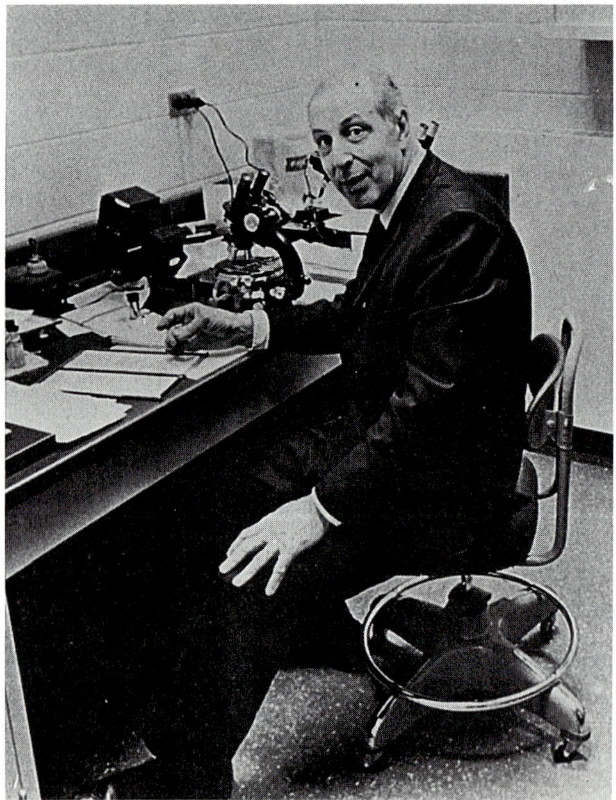

FIG. 3-26. Savino A. D'Angelo, Ph.D., Professor of Anatomy (Histology and Embryology).

To vitalize the course in neuroanatomy, and to initiate basic neuroanatomic research, Dr. Norman Moskowitz was called from Columbia University College of Physicians and Surgeons in 1962. Later, with the move into Jefferson Alumni Hall in 1969, the neuroanatomy course was revised under Dr. Moskowitz's leadership to more resemble a team effort. Dr. C. Noback, Professor of Anatomy, Columbia University, was given a visiting Professorship to help in the teaching effort. Those who provided significant contributions to the course during this period included Drs. Hausberger and Boehme.

With the revision of the curriculum to embrace the core concept, neuroanatomy became part of the interdisciplinary neuroscience course that was established in 1973. The course was given to first-year students over a period of five weeks; it was nominally extended to six weeks in 1987. In the interdisciplinary course, neuroanatomy provided about one-half of the lecture material and also the laboratory experience. The remainder of the course was divided between neurophysiology and clinical neurosciences. The course over the years has been well received by the students and remains the only interdisciplinary course of the basic sciences that has survived since its inception. Of the basic sciences' electives for seniors, instituted in 1975, those in neuroanatomy have been conducted by Dr. Moskowitz. Since 1983, a neuroscience course for students in physical therapy has been taught by Dr. Moskowitz, who also holds an appointment as Clinical Professor of

Physical Therapy in the College of Allied Health Sciences. On an ad hoc basis he has provided review programs for residents in both neurosurgery and neurology at the request of their respective departments.

The first significant award for neuroanatomical research in the Department was granted to Dr. Moskowitz in 1963 by the National Institutes of Health, under which he has made major contributions to the knowledge of the primate auditory pathways, using the monkey as his normal and experimentally altered research model. Others in the Department who have received extramural support for neuroanatomical research as principle investigators include: Dr. Diane Smith, now Professor of Anatomy, State University of Louisiana, whose grant supplied funds for relocating one of the departmental electron microscopes (after her departure); Dr. Kenna Peusner, now Associate Professor of Anatomy, George Washington University; and Drs. Eisenman and Goldowitz.

Major contributions to teaching in the interdepartmental program have been provided by Drs. Leonard M. Eisenman, Barbara Forbes, Daniel Goldowitz, Edwin M. Masters, Norman Moskowitz, Charles R. Noback, J. M. R. Shea, and more recently Gerald B. Grunwald and Kevin S. Lee.

Twentieth Century Trends

As in all fields of medical science, anatomy has developed specialties and subspecialties of its parent discipline. As more sophisticated optical, electronic, biochemical, and biophysical apparatus and technical procedures have become available, various subdivisions of basic anatomy have emerged. New titles have appeared, such as structural biology, tissue and cell biology, reproductive biology, evolutional biology, neurobiology, and so on. There evolved several dozen specialized "splinter" disciplines, some with their own professional associations and journals where, until the later years of the nineteenth century, there was but one, gross anatomy.[9] This has resulted in curriculum changes, shifting emphases, and new course content, paralleled by changes in research concentrations by the basic scientific faculty scholars, aided by significant extramural financial sources in support of research. Where once anatomy research was entirely descriptive it is now largely experimental and analytical, carried out under normal and altered functional and developmental conditions.

In 1949 the Faculty of the basic sciences Departments initiated an M.S. and Ph.D. program in their specialties and subspecialties. Some developed as interdepartmental endeavors. In 1986 Anatomy established such a Ph.D. program for Developmental Biology within the College of Graduate Studies.

Four Eras of Jefferson Anatomy

The first era of anatomy at Jefferson (1824–1905) was conducted under the Chairmanships of surgeon-anatomists from George McClellan to William Smith Forbes. The students had a laboratory for human body dissection and the professors had one or two assistants as demonstrators or prosectors. The anatomy course was a refinement of gross structure as delineated by Vesalius (1514–1564), with later, the start of instruction in histology and embryology. Research was absent to minimal.

The second era (1905–1948) witnessed the anatomist-teacher-researcher Chairmanships of Edward Anthony Spitzka and J. Parsons Schaeffer. In 1911, the Department of Anatomy moved into its newly prepared quarters, The Daniel Baugh Institute of Anatomy at Eleventh and Clinton Streets (formerly occupied by the Pennsylvania College of Dental Surgery). Dr. Spitzka expertly planned and, with Mr. Baugh, supervised the renovations and modernizations that gave Jefferson the ultimate in anatomy teaching facilities for that time. Dr. Schaeffer continued the task of renovation by transforming the Annex (a residential building adjoining the Institute on Clinton Street, which had also been purchased by Mr. Baugh) into teaching and research quarters. The first floor of the Annex was converted into a laboratory for a course in applied and topographic anatomy. Machinery and refrigeration apparatus were installed in the basement for preparing cross sections of the body. A research laboratory was equipped for operations on animals, and a photographic room was provided. Multiple dissecting rooms were converted into a single large one, and a departmental library of approximately 2,000 volumes was established. The full-time teachers and research workers increased to six.

The third era began in 1948 with the appointment of Dr. George Allen Bennett as Chairman of Anatomy and was continued by Dr. Andrew J. Ramsay. The high record for effective teaching was maintained and a thrust was accelerated in fundamental research aided by the most modern technology. The Institute was revamped for experimental work in endocrinology, neurophysiology, physical anthropology, tissue culture studies, with units for physical and chemical apparatus and equipment for applying radiographic and fluoroscopic methods. Programs were provided in 1949 for graduate students to obtain advanced degrees in the anatomical sciences. The full- and part-time staff increased to approximately 20. The move in 1968 from the old Daniel Baugh Institute building (eventually sold and converted into condominiums) to Jefferson Alumni Hall was essentially the end of the third era.

The fourth and current era in Jefferson anatomy began in 1968–1969 with new programs and with new physical facilities in Jefferson Alumni Hall, augmented in 1972 with the Chairmanship of Professor E. Marshall Johnson.

The Department's new quarters on the fifth floor of Jefferson Alumni Hall were planned to provide unusual flexibility so that they could be converted to multiple disciplinary, if desired, in the future. Instead of the traditional dissecting room with massive stationary tables and small walled-off cubicles, the laboratory contained easily removable tables, folding partitions for immediate conversion to six cubicles, and closed-circuit television with pickup from any table and individually linked to any combination of cubicles or the entire laboratory. The histology-neuroanatomy-embryology laboratory was also divisible by folding partitions. Its closed-circuit television microscopy facilities were the first in America. One room was especially insulated for use of "hot" isotopes. X-ray apparatus for cadaver study and research with closed-circuit image-intensification facilities was located in the embalming and cadaver-storage suite. Air-conditioning for the cadaver areas, the animal quarters, and the dissecting rooms was separate from the main building system so that no odors could escape.

Each faculty member's office and research laboratory accommodated at least one member, one or more graduate students and technicians, and the specific equipment required. The electron microscope suites contained three electron microscopes with facilities for microtomy, vacuum evaporating, molecular coating, and processing of the electron-exposed emulsion for recording and conversion from electron energy to visible photographic prints.

E. Marshall Johnson, Ph.D. (1930–), Twelfth Chairman (1972–)

Dr. E. Marshall Johnson (Figure 3-27) succeeded Dr. Andrew J. Ramsay as Chairman of the Department of Anatomy and Director of the Daniel Baugh Institute in the fall of 1972. He received the Ph.D. degree in anatomy from the University of California at Berkeley in 1959 and had served on the faculty of the University of Florida College of Medicine in Gainesville until 1970. He then left to assume the Chairmanship of the Department of Anatomy and accept a Professorship in the Department of Developmental and Cellular Biology at the University of California College of Medicine in Irvine.

A goal of Dr. Johnson on assuming the post at Jefferson was to use the umbrella of the Daniel Baugh Institute to develop an interdisciplinary program consistent with contemporary modes for organization of academic research-educational units. This was to be achieved by recruiting new faculty in the area of developmental biology-teratology to build a critical mass of research expertise that would be nationally and internationally competitive for extramural research support and also be a point of recognition for the College and the University. The idea was to assemble a research-teaching group that would be significantly more effective than the sum of its parts.

A second goal was to enhance the neurobiology component of the Department and to begin development of contemporary expertise in cellular biology. As new faculty were recruited to either a newly created or a newly available position, the emphasis was to recruit young people who had their primary training in medical school anatomy departments or who had significant postdoctoral experience in such circumstances. It was considered essential to maintain the excellence in anatomy, particularly in gross anatomy teaching, while recruiting individuals capable of doing the types of research at the leading edge of contemporary science.

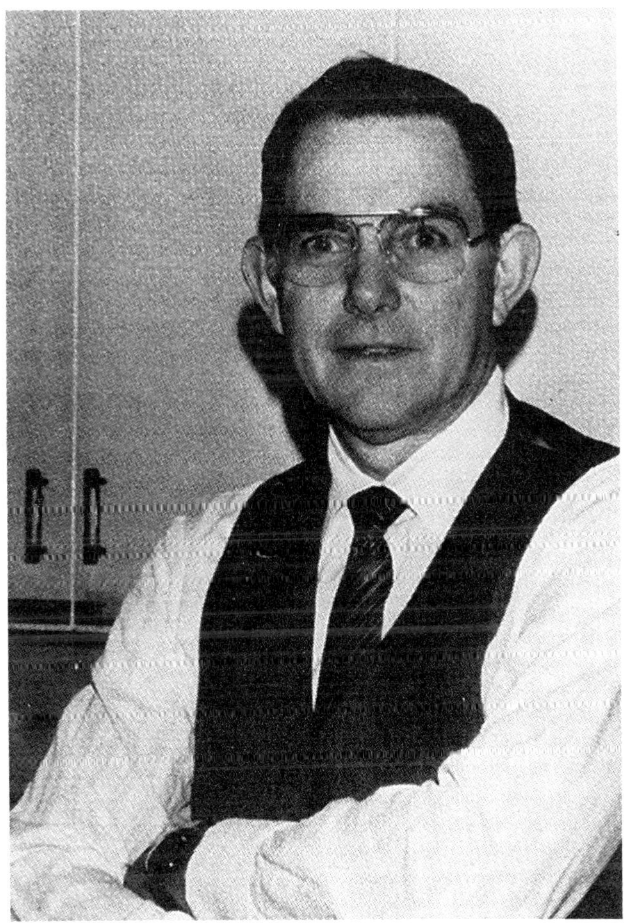

FIG. 3-27. E. Marshall Johnson, Ph.D. (1930–), Twelfth Chairman (1972–).

It was possible to begin recruiting at a very early date due to resources made available by Dean Kellow. Among these recruits were Drs. Devendra J. Kochhar and Kenneth P. Chepenik. Both were developmental biologists who were trained in anatomy departments and were competitive at the National Institutes of Health for extramural research funding. Each was then recognized as a young faculty member of considerable promise, which proved to be true as each became a full Professor in the Department with independently funded research programs in teratology. Subsequent recruits were Drs. Richard R. Schmidt and Robert M. Greene. Again, both were gross anatomists with potential for significant additional development. Dr. Greene went on to obtain a Research Career Development Award, a highly useful avenue for enhancing the growth of young faculty.

Neuroscientists were recruited who, though not uniformly expert in gross anatomy, tended to have substantial backgrounds in morphology. The first of these was Dr. Leonard M. Eisenman, and, later, Drs. Daniel Goldwitz, Gerald B. Grunwals, and Kevin S. Lee. Other faculty who either joined or returned full-time to the department were Drs. Louis M. Newman and Ronald P. Jensh. Both of these also were trained anatomists and active in their own research programs.

The philosophy of recruitment was to start at the Assistant Professor level as far as possible, thereby assuring a continuation of excellence in both teaching and research for the Department well into the twenty-first century and to avoid a situation where the entire Department would come toward retirement age simultaneously. As the research programs in the individual laboratories got up to speed, it became increasingly easy to recruit additional young people to the faculty because they sought the ferment and interaction available from a group of individuals working in the related areas of developmental biology from the viewpoint of teratogenesis or of neurosciences.

Dr. Johnson continues his own research, funded through the years at various times by pharmaceutical manufacturers and manufacturing chemical companies, the National Institutes of Health, and the March of Dimes Birth Defects Foundation. He obtained U.S. patents for research methods that began accruing royalties for the College and Department in 1985. These were methods for testing of chemicals to determine if they might cause birth defects, using an artificial embryo consisting of hydra (a small freshwater hydrozoan polyp). The purpose of the tests was to reduce the number of babies born with birth defects caused by environmental agents. Dr. Johnson estimates the existence of about 70,000 such chemicals in the environment, with 300 to 500 new ones identified each year.

A heavy concentration of young faculty developed in the Department with a high percentage of transmural funding. Through an interdisciplinary program, the anatomy faculty took the leadership and was awarded both a pre- and postdoctoral training grant in developmental biology-teratology by the Child Health and Human Development Section of the National Institutes of Health. This is the only grant of this type by the NIH and is now a degree-granting program. Having obtained approval of Jefferson's Board of Trustees, the Daniel Baugh Institute is capable of awarding the Ph.D. degree in the field of Developmental Biology-Teratology. The first predoctoral student started shortly before funding for the program began on October 1, 1986.

Dr. Johnson's activities in national and international organizations include: past advisor to the Presidential Science Advisory Board (for President Ford), member of the Environmental Protection Agency Scientific Advisory Board, Chairman of the World Health Organization Air Pollution Criteria Committee for Select Organics, member of the Department of Defense Life Sciences Advisory Committee, consultant to regulatory groups in the United States and abroad, founding President of Argus Research Laboratories, Inc. (a reproductive and developmental toxicity testing laboratory employing almost 100 workers in two states), consultant to several pharmaceutical manufacturers and chemical manufacturers here and overseas, past President of the Teratology Society, and founding President of the Specialty Section for Reprodutive and Developmental Toxicology of the Society of Toxicology.

The Department feels keenly its responsibility to maintain its enviable record in the fields of medical teaching and research, with determination to keep pace with and to participate in the inevitable advances and developments in the anatomical sciences.

References

1. Ramsay, A.J., "Kappa Lambda." *Jeff. Med. Coll. Al. Bull.*, Winter 1980, pp. 19–24.
2. Forbes, W.S., *History of the Anatomy Act of Pennsylvania.* Philadelphia Medical Publishing Company, 1898.
3. Ramsay, A.J., "The Daniel Baugh Institute of Anatomy." *Jeff. Med. Coll. Al. Bull.*, Fall 1972, pp. 4–23.
4. Ramsay, A.J., "Daniel Baugh: Benefactor." *Jeff. Med. Coll. Al. Bull.*, Fall 1981, pp. 18–21.
5. "The Department of Anatomy." *Jeff. Med. Coll. Al. Bull.*, March 1951, pp. 1–13.
6. "The Department of Anatomy, Part I." *Jeff. Med. Coll. Al. Bull.*, October 1958, pp. 14–22.
7. "The Department of Anatomy, Part II." *Jeff. Med. Coll. Al. Bull.*, December 1958, pp. 4–16.
8. Corner, G.W., *Clio Medica: Anatomy.* New York: Hafner Publishing Company, 1964.
9. Ramsay, A.J., *Directory, Anatomy Departments of the United States and Canada (Schools of Medicine, Dentistry, Osteopathic Medicine, Veterinary Medicine).* Wistar Institute Press, 1972.

CHAPTER FOUR

Department of Biochemistry

BERNARD SCHEPARTZ, PH.D.

"Let chemistry push her researches into the remotest recesses of the living economy, and let her claim, for her own, every process, every act, every transformation, over which she can establish a legitimate jurisdiction."

—ELISHA BARTLETT (1804–1855)

PREVIOUS HISTORIES of the Department of Biochemistry have been limited to a one-page summary by George R. Bancroft[1] and a somewhat lengthier essay by Abraham Cantarow,[2] both former Chairmen. Occasional mention of the affairs of the Department naturally occurred in the larger histories of the Medical College, such as those of Gayley,[3] Gould,[4] and Bauer.[5]

Most subdivisions of this history correlated with the successive tenures of chairmen. There were two reasons for this: In the early history of Jefferson, there were "Chairs" rather than Departments, and practically no staff other than the chairmen; and beginning in the 1940s the Department developed into its present form, with staff members numerous enough to render impractical any fair description of their individual contributions to the teaching and research programs. In any case, each Chairman left a sufficiently personal imprint upon the character of this Department to justify dividing the history into periods of tenure of Chairmen.

Era of Medical Chemistry (1780–1840)

Although chemistry, in its various guises, made certain contributions to medicine in ancient and medieval times, it is obvious that truly rational additions from this science to the body of medical knowledge had to await the systematization of concepts and the elimination of alchemical impedimenta, which occurred toward the end of the eighteenth century. By the turn of that century, Lavoisier and colleagues had developed an essentially modern nomenclature for chemistry, had clarified the concept of an element, had arrived at an understanding of the true nature of combustion and of animal respiration, and Proust had discovered the Law of Definite Proportions.

The quarter-century before the establishment of Jefferson Medical College saw the development of the atomic theory of Dalton, Avogadro's Law, and determination of the "combining weights" of many elements by Berzelius. In a more biological vein, one may list the discovery that urinary urea is the chief pathway of elimination of waste nitrogen (Fourcroy and Vauquelin, 1810), that nitrogen from the diet is needed for the support of the body (Magendie, 1816), the elucidation of the composition of natural fats (Chevreul, 1823), the finding of free hydrochloric acid in gastric juice (W. Prout, 1823), and the isolation of the amino acids cystine (Wollaston, 1810), leucine (J.L. Proust 1819, and Braconnot, 1820), and glycine (Braconnot, 1820).

The quarter-century coinciding with the tenure of the first Chair of Chemistry at Jefferson was a period of great activity, not only in pure chemistry, but also in its biological and medical applications. Berzelius determined accurate atomic weights for the known 50 elements (1826), Wöhler synthesized an "organic" substance, urea, from inorganic ammonium cyanate (1828), and, although little stressed in historical texts, organic analytical chemistry (begun by Lavoisier in the 1700s, carried forward by Gay-Lussac and Thenard, Berzelius, and Liebig) reached an important peak with the development of the Dumas method for nitrogen in 1833.

In the applied area, progress was made in understanding the process of digestion with the discovery of the digestive enzyme, pepsin (Schwann, 1835). The cell theory was promulgated by Schwann (1839), and fermentation was shown to be due to the action of living yeast cells (Schwann, 1837, Kützing, 1837, and Cagniard-Latour, 1838). During most of this period Justus Liebig contributed greatly to the understanding of "animal chemistry" through his papers and books, and clarified the nutritional relation of plants and animals on a global scale.

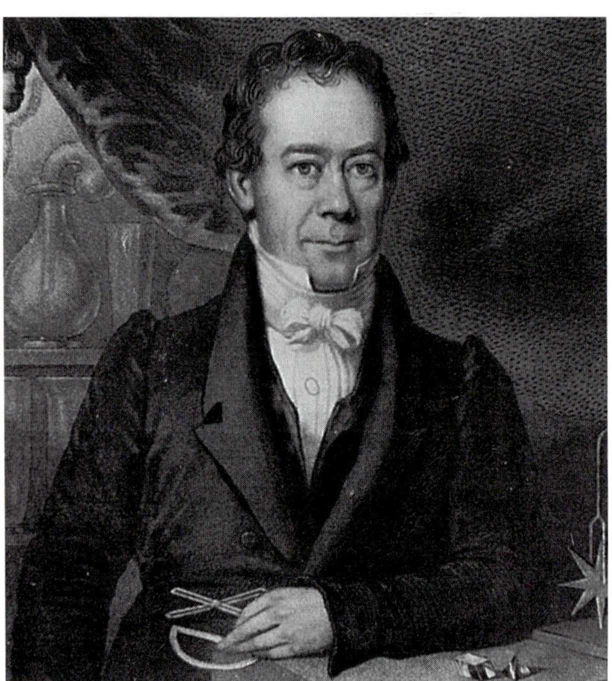

FIG. 4-1. Jacob Green, Professor of Chemistry, Mineralogy, and Pharmacy (1824–1841).

Jacob Green, M.D. Professor of Chemistry, Mineralogy, and Pharmacy (1824–1841)

Biographical information on Jacob Green ranges from the impersonal notices in the biographical dictionaries through the less systematic but warmer entries in the histories of the medical college to the very personal and poignant obituary by his father (in Gayley)[3] and the scientifically detailed biography by the noted Philadelphia historian of chemistry, Edgar Fahs Smith.[6]

Jacob Green (Figure 4-1) was born in Philadelphia on July 26, 1790, the son of Elizabeth Stockton Green and the Reverend Ashbel Green, pastor of the Second Presbyterian Church.

In terms of education and academic honors, Green, at the age of seventeen, graduated second in his class at the University of Pennsylvania and was valedictorian. Rutgers conferred another A.B. degree (honorary) upon him in 1812 and converted it to an A.M. (hon.) in 1815, in which year Green also received an A.M. (hon.) from Princeton. Finally, Yale conferred an honorary M.D. upon him in 1827.

Green had a love for all of the natural sciences. His first subject of interest was botany, but soon also encompassed electricity (in which field he and a young friend published a book, at which time Green was only 19). While preparing that book for publication, Green apprenticed himself to a local physician in order to study medicine. Exposure to a particularly gruesome surgical procedure persuaded him that medicine was not to be his life's work.

In 1809 Green left Philadelphia for Albany where he engaged in the bookselling business for seven years. The venture was not a financial success, although he made use of the time also to study law and be admitted to the New York bar. In 1816 he returned to his parents' home in Princeton, the elder Green in the meantime having been appointed President of the College of New Jersey (later Princeton University). At this time Jacob Green's interest in religion intensified, and he began a study of theology with the intention of entering the ministry. This aim, however, was subverted. While assisting the Professor of Natural Philosophy at Princeton in scientific demonstrations for classes, Green's strong inclination toward science apparently was reawakened. A reorganization of the curriculum at the College created a Professorship of Chemistry, to which Chair Jacob Green was appointed at the age of 28. The appointment proved to be temporary; another reorganization of the curriculum in 1822 resulted in the elimination of the Professorship of Chemistry. Green and his father, who had in the meantime decided to retire from the Presidency of the College, returned to live in Philadelphia.

Green joined the small group with George McClellan who founded Jefferson Medical College and accepted appointment, in 1824 at the age of 34, to the Chair of Chemistry, Mineralogy, and Pharmacy in the first faculty. His father, the Rev. Dr. Green, became President of the Board of Trustees.

In 1828 Jacob Green made a seven-month pilgrimage to the scientific centers of England, France, Switzerland, and Germany, in the course of which he met many of the leading scientists of the day, including Dalton and Faraday. He returned with chemical and physical apparatus, books, and doubtless many ideas that he was to incorporate in subsequent books and papers.

Green was well liked by his colleagues on the faculty because he remained aloof from the internal bickering that characterized the early years of the new institution. He was popular also with the students, who referred to him (as reported by Samuel D. Gross)[7] as "Old Jacky Green." (The nickname appeared also in alternative spellings: Jakey[2,5,6] and Jaky[4]).

An accurate picture of what was meant by the "Medical Chemistry" of the day can be obtained from the content of Green's course. As stated in the *Annual Announcement* of 1832, it covered physics, inorganic chemistry, and the chemistry of "organic substances" of animal and vegetable origin. Examination of his textbook,[8] which was based on Turner's *Elements of Chemistry,* revealed the following distribution of topics, expressed in terms of numbers of pages used as a percentage of the whole: Physics—15 percent, Inorganic Chemistry—58 percent, Animal and Vegetable Chemistry—23 percent, along with a small section on analytical chemistry and several useful tables of quantitative data. The distribution of topics in the textbook was exemplified by a set of lecture notes taken by Nathan L. Hatfield, a member of the first graduating Class of 1826.[9] Examination questions from the course were recorded by a student in 1832[10] and a sample set published in the *Annual Announcement* of 1836. In both instances, the emphasis was on inorganic chemistry and detection of poisons.

In general, Green's course and textbook were up to date for their time. In fact, the 1829 text referred to Wöhler's synthesis of urea from ammonium cyanate, although this had occurred only one year before publication of the book. On the other hand, Green did not use the symbols for the elements and compounds suggested by Berzelius and did not mention the discovery by Magendie that nitrogenous foods were necessary for life.

In the preface of his textbook, Green acknowledged the assistance of his friend, Charles

Davis, M.D., who was also listed as Adjunct Professor of Chemistry in the *Annual Announcements* of 1832 and 1833. There was no other evidence for a chemistry "staff" at this stage in the history of the Chair.

In addition to his lectures at Jefferson, Green also presented a series in chemistry during certain summer sessions at Jefferson College, Canonsburg, and Lafayette College, Easton.

Green made no major research discoveries, although he published scientific papers in many branches of the physical and biological sciences. His primary role was that of a disseminator of the discoveries of others. In this aspect, his roster of published books was noteworthy: *An Epitome of Electricity and Galvanism* (1809), coauthored with his friend, Erskine Hazard; *A Catalogue of the Plants Indigenous to the State of New York* (1814); *Astronomical Recreations* (1824); *Electromagnetism* (1827); *Text Book of Chemical Philosophy* (1829); *Notes of a Traveller,* 3 vols. (1830); *Consolations in Travel* (1830), by Sir Humphry Davy, edited by Green; *The Botany of the United States* (1833); *A Syllabus of a Course of Chemistry* (1835); *A Monograph* on the *Trilobites of North America* (1832, suppl. 1835); and *Chemical Diagrams* (1837). (Two biographical sources list also *Diseases of the Skin* (1841), probably an erroneous attribution—at no point in Green's career did he evidence any interest in such a topic, nor is any such book listed under his authorship in the usual bibliographic references, and furthermore, he had virtually no medical training; his M.D. from Yale was honorary. A Jonathan Green did publish a *Practical Compendium of the Diseases of the Skin* [London, 1835, 1837; Philadelphia, 1838, 1839] suggesting a possible confusion between the two "J. Greens.")

Jacob Green died February 1, 1841, at the age of 51, leaving behind a wife and two daughters. An interesting glimpse into the sometimes precarious financial state of the young Medical College is afforded by the fact that after Green's death his estate was reimbursed for the loans he had made.[5]

Era of Physiological Chemistry (1840–1880)

The tenures of the three occupants of the Chair of Chemistry following Jacob Green coincided with the period denoted "Physiological Chemistry" by historians of the subject. It was an era characterized by many advances, both conceptual and substantive.

The development of accurate methods of quantitative analysis during the preceding period had brought on a spate of feverish activity, not only in the determination of the composition of purified compounds, but also in such overly zealous endeavors as the analysis of the elemental composition of whole tissues. Such excesses provoked reactions from two directions. On the one hand, the vitalists objected to what they called "analism," on the grounds that decimation and analysis of an organism would teach nothing about the essential nature of living beings. On the other hand, researchers with a largely physiological background maintained that investigators could indeed study the phenomena of life, provided that they worked with whole organisms or, at least, intact organs.

Concurrently, the field of organic chemistry began to unfold as an independent discipline as chemists realized that their science need not restrict itself to compounds of animal or vegetable origin. This change in attitude was abetted by the rise of chemical industry, with its many areas of application of organic chemistry unrelated to biology.

The result of these events was a general abandonment of the field of biological chemistry by the organic chemists, at least for a time, leaving it in the hands of "physiological chemists," sometimes actually located within departments of physiology in the medical schools. In Germany, early in the nineteenth century, chemistry was a medical discipline, but between 1820 and 1850 "philosophical" faculties were formed in the universities, and chemistry was recognized as a "pure" science and transferred out of the medical and into the philosophical faculties.

Among the major advances in pure chemistry during this era were the discovery of the law of conservation of energy (Mayer, 1840, 1842), the mechanical equivalent of heat (Joule, 1843; Helmholtz, 1847), the periodic law (Lothar Meyer, 1868, 1870; Mendeleev, 1869, 1871), stereochemistry (van't Hoff, 1874), the law of mass action (Guldberg and Waage, 1867) and the structure of benzene (Kekule, 1865).

Discoveries and advances in physiological chemistry included the digestive enzymes (Mialhe—salivary amylase, 1845; Bernard—pancreatic enzymes, 1846 *et seq.*; and Kühne—the same, 1876), liver glycogen as the source of blood sugar (Bernard, 1848); isolation of many amino acids; the respiratory quotient (R.Q.) (Regnault and Reiset, 1849); nitrogen equilibrium (Voit, 1860s–1870s); and the beginning of the famous controversy over the necessity, or lack thereof, for living yeast cells in order that fermentation might occur (1830s–1897).

Despite these impressive accomplishments, historians were of the opinion that "Physiological Chemistry" did not have sufficient basic chemical facts and techniques at hand to stand as an independent discipline.

Franklin Bache, M.D. Professor of Chemistry (1841–1864).

Franklin Bache (Figure 4-2), a great-grandson of Benjamin Franklin, was born in Philadelphia on October 25, 1792, the son of Benjamin Franklin Bache.[12] He prepared for entrance to the University of Pennsylvania by study in the local academy of the Rev. S. B. Wylie, a well-known teacher of Latin and Greek. Bache graduated from the University with a Bachelor of Arts degree in 1810, at which time he was the class valedictorian. He then began the study of medicine as a private pupil of Dr. Benjamin Rush, after whose death he continued with Dr. James Rush, Benjamin's son. Bache then matriculated at the University of Pennsylvania, where he received his M.D. degree in 1814.

Bache served in the army during the War of 1812, but eventually resigned to take up private medical practice in 1816. He appears, however, to have had an even stronger interest in chemistry, having written articles on the subject while still a medical student. In the 1820s he lectured on chemistry to the students who were studying medicine with Dr. T.T. Hewson. Bache taught in a more formal setting beginning in 1826 when he was appointed Professor in Chemistry in the Franklin Institute, a position which he retained until 1832. He served as physician of the Walnut Street Prison beginning in 1824 and of the Eastern Penitentiary beginning in 1829, but resigned both positions in 1836. In 1830 he taught in one of the two "associations" formed for the purpose of providing private medical instruction in the city of Philadelphia. The Philadelphia College of Pharmacy appointed Bache to the Chair of Chemistry in 1831, a position he held until 1841, when he accepted the Chair in Chemistry at Jefferson.

Among professional associations, Bache was a member of the Kappa Lambda Society, the College of Physicians of Philadelphia, the American Philosophical Society (which elected him President in 1853, the first President having been his great-grandfather, Benjamin Franklin), the Academy of Natural Sciences of Philadelphia, and the National Institute at Washington, and was elected as honorary member of the Imperial Academy of Naturalists at Moscow. Among

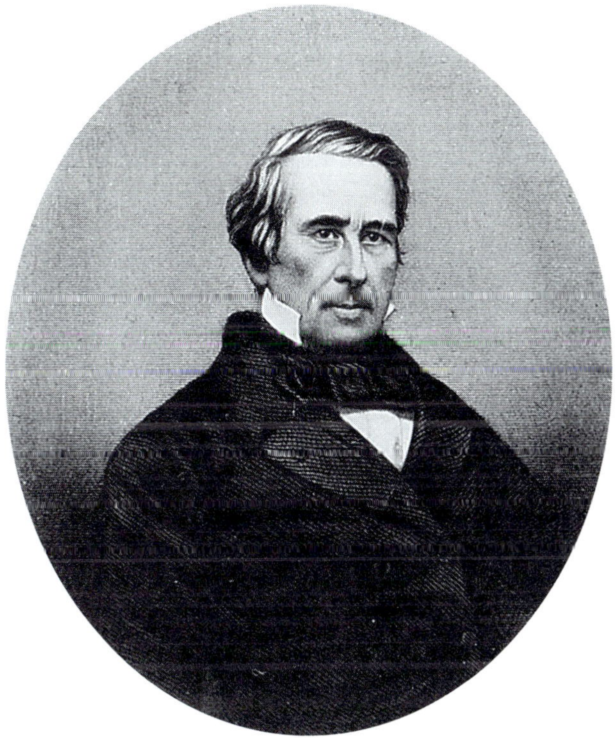

FIG. 4-2. Franklin Bache, Professor of Chemistry (1841–1864).

nonprofessional associations can be mentioned the Temperance Society.

The chemistry course taught by Bache at Jefferson, according to the *College Announcement* of 1850, included a description of "all of the important chemical preparations embraced in the United States and British Pharmacopoeias," as well as the chemistry of animal and vegetable substances. In an introductory lecture to the course, Bache went into greater detail: the course, after the usual preliminary background in basic physics, was to cover the nonmetals, laws of chemical combination, metals, and "organic substances."[13] These last were subdivided into "neuter substances (carbohydrates); oils, resins, and bitumens; alcohols and ethers; organic acids; and organic alkalis."

His friend, Dr. George Bacon Wood, from conversations with students reported that Bache's lectures were slow, deliberate, clear, and methodical.[12] His colleague, Samuel D. Gross, characterized the lectures as dull, and said that the students appeared not to know much chemistry at their final examinations.[14] On the other hand, one of his students claimed that the lectures were "not to be surpassed."[15] From an examination of the *Announcements* of 1841 through 1864, there is no indication that Bache had any assistance with his course, although a Demonstrator in Anatomy is listed frequently.

Bache is not known to have conducted any original chemical research. Wood said that Bache had "little of the imaginative or inventive faculty."[12] His chemical paper of 1811 and three in 1813 were all of a nonexperimental nature, having to do with chemical composition, the laws of chemistry, and chemical nomenclature.[16]

The major contribution of Bache to the chemistry and medicine of his time, other than through the direct impact of his teaching, was by way of his books. He published his *System of Chemistry for the Use of Students in Medicine* in 1819, edited (with Robert Hare of the University of Pennsylvania) Ure's *Dictionary of Chemistry* in 1821, prepared a supplement to Henry's *Elements of Experimental Chemistry* in 1823, anonymously edited Cutbush's *System of Pyrotechny* in 1825, served as coeditor of the *North American Medical and Surgical Journal* between 1826 and 1831, took part in revisions of the *Pharmacopoeia of the United States* in 1830, 1840, 1850, and 1860, coedited (with Wood) the *Dispensatory of the United States of America* through eleven editions from 1833 to 1864, edited Hare's *Compendium of the Course of Chemical Instruction in the Medical Department of the University of Pennsylvania* in 1836, and published four American editions of Turner's *Elements of Chemistry* between 1819 and 1841. Smith considered it likely that Bache's work on the *Dispensatory* led to his Professorship at Jefferson in 1841.[16]

Franklin Bache died on March 19, 1864, just as he was preparing to labor on yet another edition of the *Dispensatory*.

Benjamin Howard Rand, M.D. Professor of Chemistry (1864–1877); Dean (1869–1873)

Benjamin Howard Rand (Figure 4-3) was born in Philadelphia on October 1, 1827, son of a well-known educator of the same name. He graduated

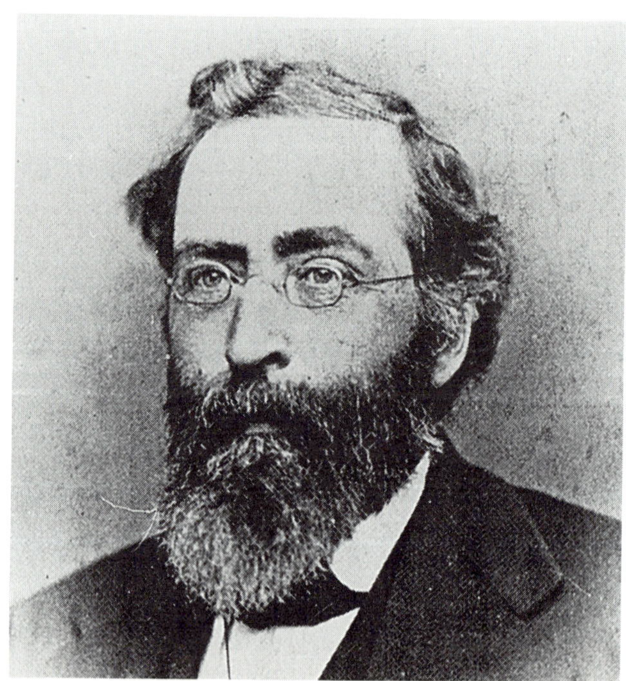

FIG. 4-3. Benjamin Howard Rand, Professor of Chemistry (1864–1877) and Dean (1869–1873).

from Central High School in 1839 at the age of twelve, worked and studied independently for four years, then began the study of medicine under Dr. Robert M. Huston.[5] During his last two years he was Clinical Assistant to Professors Thomas D. Mütter and Joseph Pancoast and graduated from Jefferson in 1848. He was named Professor of Chemistry at the Franklin Institute in 1850 and in the Philadelphia Academy of Natural Sciences (1852–1864), Fellow of the Philadelphia College of Physicians (1853), and member of the American Philosophical Society (1868). He was appointed to the Chair of Chemistry at Jefferson in 1864 and "having good business ability"[1] assumed the Deanship as well from 1869 to 1873. His portrait by Thomas Eakins in 1874, the artist's first commercial work beyond portraits of relatives and friends, is one of the highlights of the Jefferson collection.

Rand's lectures at Jefferson are said to have met with approval by the students because he emphasized the applied medical aspects of chemistry rather than the theoretical side.[5] Nevertheless, in his textbook,[17] the preface of which states that the book may be regarded as a full set of notes to the author's lectures at Jefferson, Rand did not depart from the distribution of topics found in the texts of his predecessors, Green and Bache. After the usual review of the essential bases of physics (19 percent of the text), Rand devoted 52 percent of his space to inorganic and theoretical chemistry, with only 21 percent to "organic." Furthermore, this last category was treated largely from the standpoint of descriptive chemistry and pharmaceutical applications, not from the "physiological" point of view.

In 1866 Jefferson added a summer course to the two five-month-per-year sessions that had been the standard curriculum. Rand lectured on "Applied Medical Chemistry and Toxicology."

There is no evidence that Rand had any assistance in his teaching until close to the end of his career, when William H. Green, M.D., was listed on the staff as a Demonstrator of Chemistry, and it was stated that *Practical Chemistry* was taught by the Demonstrator under the supervision of the Professor.

Rand appears not to have conducted any original research, although he contributed to medical journals, in addition to having written *An Outline of Medical Chemistry* (1855) and *Elements of Medical Chemistry* (1865), and edited the third edition of Metcalf's *Caloric: Its Agencies on the Phenomena of Nature* (1859).

Because of ill health, Rand resigned his Chair and was elected Emeritus Professor in 1877. It is sad to relate that his library of medical and other books was sold in the year following his retirement. He died in 1883.

Robert Empie Rogers, M.D. Professor of Medical Chemistry and Toxicology (1877–1884)

Robert E. Rogers (Figure 4-4) was born in Baltimore on March 29, 1813, one of four sons of Patrick Kerr Rogers. The family seems to have been exceedingly gifted in science; the father and all four sons were scientists or physicians as well as scientists.[18] Robert Rogers received his early education from his father and, after the latter's death in 1828, from his brothers, James and

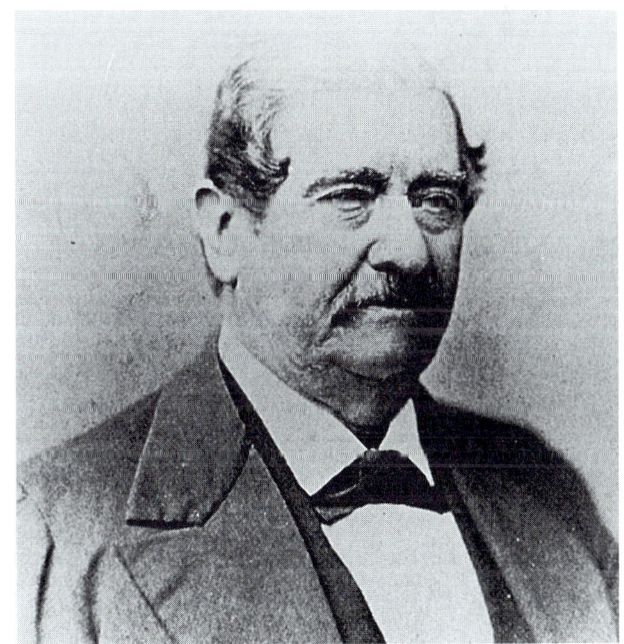

FIG. 4-4. Robert Empie Rogers, Professor of Medical Chemistry and Toxicology (1877–1884).

William. His initial professional goal was engineering, but after participating in railroad surveying in 1831 and 1832 he found the work not to his liking. He continued his own studies of botany, geology, and mineralogy, and began medical studies at the University of Pennsylvania under Robert Hare. Rogers received his medical degree in 1836 with a thesis concerning (among other topics) the diffusion of liquids and gases through animal and vegetable tissues and membranes. The thesis was of such quality that it was published as a scientific paper.

Rogers did not practice medicine after graduation. From 1836 to 1842 he was chemist of the first Geological Survey of Pennsylvania (his brother, Henry, a geologist, was head of the survey). He was then appointed Professor of General and Applied Chemistry at the University of Virginia, a position he held until 1852 when he succeeded his deceased brother, James, as Professor of Chemistry in the Medical School of the University of Pennsylvania, also becoming Dean four years later. During the Civil War, in the course of his duties as Acting Assistant Surgeon in the Army, Rogers lost his right hand while demonstrating the operation of a steam mangle in the West Philadelphia Military Hospital.[19] During his tenure at the University of Pennsylvania he advised several of the government mints concerning their metallurgical operations.

In 1874 the University of Pennsylvania was considering a number of changes, such as moving to West Philadelphia from its center city location and lengthening the medical curriculum.[5] Rogers refused to enter the ensuing controversies and, instead, accepted the Chair at Jefferson that had been left vacant by the retirement of Rand. It may be noted, in terms of views concerning age of appointees to academic positions, that Rogers entered into his duties at the age of 64, and served with distinction until the age of 71.

Rogers enjoyed both research and lecturing and performed well in both. He was "a popular teacher, loved and honored by his students, and esteemed by his colleagues of the Faculty."[4] In 1877–1878, Rogers was assisted in teaching Practical Chemistry by a Demonstrator, George M. Ward, M.D. One of Roger's major curricular achievements was the establishment of the first student laboratory course in chemistry at Jefferson. This was under the supervision of the Professor, aided by Dr. Ward, who continued in that post through 1885. In 1883–1884, a postgraduate course in Medical Chemistry was listed with the same Dr. Ward as Instructor.

Rogers was the first of Jefferson's professors of chemistry to recognize the arrival of the era of Physiological Chemistry. While still at the University of Pennsylvania, he edited an American edition of Lehmann's treatise *Physiological Chemistry*,[20] regarded as one of the most influential books of the era. In this two-volume work, inorganic chemistry occupied but three percent of the total space, descriptive organic chemistry a more usual 28 percent, but 64 percent was devoted to such topics as fluids and tissues, digestion, absorption, metabolism, oxidation, respiration, heat production, and nutrition. The attitude of the more conservative members of the profession toward such an approach can be seen in Holland's eulogy of Rogers, wherein he stated that the Lehmann treatise "contains much that is usually included in treatises on physiology."[21]

Although the weighty Lehmann text was recommended as reading material for Rogers' course (a recommendation not likely to be followed by many students, in view of the size of the work), other smaller and more usual books also were included in the list. These had the common overemphasis on inorganic chemistry and underemphasis on physiological matters. Rogers was doubtless constrained in his choices by the fact that at the time and, indeed, until the early years of the twentieth century there was no requirement of chemistry for admission to the Medical School.

By contrast to some of his predecessors, Rogers was an avid researcher. Most of his research was done prior to his arrival at Jefferson, perhaps to be expected in view of his age at the time of his appointment. While at Virginia and Pennsylvania he published in the fields of inorganic and industrial chemistry, mineralogy, and metallurgy. At Jefferson his interest was in electric generators. Smith[18] lists 20 papers without indication of coauthorship, whereas Ruschenberger lists four papers by Robert E. Rogers alone and 24 more with his brothers or other coauthors.[19] In addition

Rogers published with his brother James *A Text Book on Chemistry* (1846), based upon earlier British texts.

In June, 1883, Rogers received an Honorary LL.D. degree from Dickinson College. He resigned from his Jefferson Chair a year later due to ill health and was elected Emeritus Professor. He died on September 6, 1884, at the age of 72.[19]

Era of Biochemistry (1880–Present)

The *Era of Biochemistry,* that is, the period in which biochemistry achieved the status of an independent discipline, dates from 1880 through the present time. Signs of this achievement were the founding of the *Zeitschrift für physiologische Chemie* by Hoppe-Seyler (1877), establishment of the first Chair of Physiological Chemistry in the United States (Chittenden at Yale, 1882), founding of the two leading English language journals in the field (*Journal of Biological Chemistry* [1905]; *Biochemical Journal* [1906]), and organization of the American Society of Biological Chemists (1906 or 1907) and the Biochemical Society, London (1911).

Scientific advances that characterized this era were too many for individual citation. It can be noted, briefly, that the early years of the period saw noteworthy progress in pure chemistry along the lines of electrolytic ionization, radioactivity, osmotic pressure, valence theory, colloids, and polymers. In biological chemistry, great advances were made in the chemistry of carbohydrates, polypeptides, cell-free fermentation, nucleic acids, endocrinology, coenzymes, enzyme kinetics, biological oxidation, nutrition and vitamins, pathways of fermentation, glycolysis, oxidation of fatty acids, and inborn errors of metabolism.

At Jefferson the arrival of the era of Physiological Chemistry was recognized somewhat belatedly, and only by Professor Rogers. The era of Biochemistry, similarly, would make its appearance at Jefferson rather tardily, in the person of Philip B. Hawk. There were, nevertheless, some stirrings even before Hawk's arrival. In 1880, Drs. Richard Dunglison (Jefferson, 1856; the son of Robley) and Woodbury made the editorial comment that too much time was spent on the elementary aspects of chemistry and that the lengthy laboratory exercises in the analysis of "minerals, ores, and building stones" might better be devoted to the analysis of biological samples; in 1882, they suggested that the teaching of many of the details of chemistry in medical school could be avoided if proper attention were given to premedical education.[22]

John William Mallet, Ph.D., Professor of Medical Chemistry and Toxicology (1884–1885)

Mallet's stay at Jefferson was brief, through no fault of his or of the college. John William Mallet (Figure 4-5) was born on October 10, 1832, near Dublin, Ireland. His father was an engineer and Fellow of the Royal Society. He was educated in chemistry at the Royal College of Surgeons, in Trinity College, Dublin, and in Göttingen, where

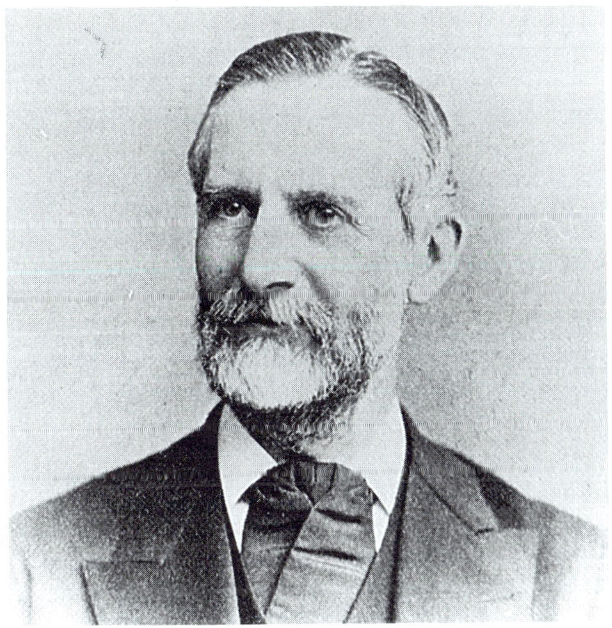

Fig. 4-5. John William Mallet, Professor of Medical Chemistry and Toxicology (1884–1885).

he obtained his Ph.D. degree under the celebrated Wöhler. Mallet came to the United States in 1853, was Assistant Professor of Analytical Chemistry at Amherst in 1854, chemist to the State Geological Survey of Alabama in 1855–1856, and Professor of Chemistry at the State University from 1855 to 1860. He worked for the Confederate Army during the Civil War and made a petroleum survey in Louisiana and Texas for a commercial group in 1865. Returning to the academic world, Mallet was Professor of Chemistry in the medical department of the University of Louisiana (1865–1867), at the University of Virginia (1867–1883), and at the University of Texas (1883–1884). His Jefferson appointment then followed but lasted only one academic year, after which he returned to the University of Virginia.

Mallet conducted much research, mostly in the field of inorganic chemistry, beginning during his college years, and totaling over 100 papers. His reputation in chemistry was attested to by his election to the presidency of the American Chemical Society in 1882.[23] His abilities in research were matched by his skills as a lecturer.

Despite his accomplishments and honors, Mallet seemed to be pursued by misfortune.[24] His move to Texas was motivated by the hope that the climate would be favorable to his son who had tuberculosis. Despite this effort, the son died. Mallet then accepted the Chair at Jefferson vacated by the retirement of Rogers. His personal and scientific possessions, stored temporarily in a Philadelphia warehouse, were destroyed by fire a few hours before the insurance was to take effect. His wife died a few months later. He returned to the University of Virginia, where he remained until retirement in 1908. Mallet died in 1912.

James William Holland, M.D., Professor of Medical Chemistry and Toxicology (1885–1912) and Dean (1887–1916)

James William Holland (Figure 4-6) was born on April 24, 1849, in Louisville, Kentucky, son of Dr. Robert Chappell Holland, a practicing physician.[25] He received his A.B. in 1865 and his A.M. in 1868, both from the University of Louisville, where he studied chemistry and toxicology under J. Lawrence Smith, noted student of Orfila and other famous European mentors.[5] In 1868 Holland graduated from Jefferson, where his M.D. degree was augmented by an honorary Sc.D. degree in 1913. Holland began the practice of medicine in partnership with his father and affiliated himself with the University of Louisville as Assistant Demonstrator of Anatomy.[4] In 1872 he became Professor of Medical Chemistry and Clinical Neurology, later successively occupying the Chairs of Materia Medica, Clinical Medicine, and the Practice of Medicine and Clinical Medicine.

Holland was called upon by Jefferson in 1885 to fill the vacancy left by the departure of Professor Mallet. Two years after becoming Professor of Medical Chemistry and Toxicology, Holland also became Dean of the Faculty, a position he held for four years beyond his retirement from the Professorship. During his tenure Holland was responsible for several significant alterations in the teaching program: In 1888, the requirement of a thesis for the M.D. degree was eliminated for

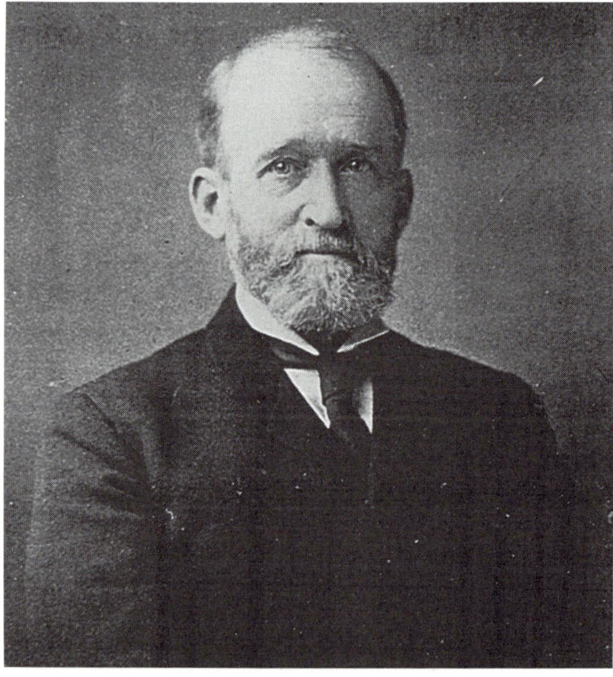

FIG. 4-6. James William Holland, Professor of Medical Chemistry and Toxicology (1885–1912) and Dean (1887–1916).

all students except those aiming at prizes. Oral examinations were replaced by written examinations, and systematic grading of courses was established.[5]

In the specific area of chemistry, the curriculum was extended to cover two years (Figure 4-7). The first year dealt with inorganic or general chemistry and toxicology. The second year covered organic chemistry and urinalysis or medical chemistry. Student laboratory courses accompanied the lectures in both years. Although the laboratory of the second year brought the student into contact with medically interesting material (e.g., bile, blood, urine, gastric contents), that of the freshman year was primarily an exercise in elementary chemistry, including acidimetry and alkalimetry, followed by toxicological tests for poisons. This part of the curriculum was not received with enthusiasm by the students, as recorded by a class historian: "We dabbled in chemistry and learned how to explode a hydrogen generator while performing the March (sic!) test for arsenic, and incidentally learned how to pay a dollar for the noise, when we got back the remnant of the breakage fee we had deposited at the beginning of the year." By 1905 the laboratory course of the second year was called Physiological Chemistry and had evolved into the following topics: chemical reactions of starches, sugars, fats, and proteins; chemistry of milk and its coagulation; salivary, gastric and intestinal digestion; and bile, blood and its coagulation. This series with modifications was the basis of the laboratory courses of several of Holland's successors.

The general outlines and order of priorities in Holland's lecture course may be surmised from examination of his textbook[26] and of the pocket "compend" of Lawrence Wolff, M.D.[27], whom Holland recruited from the "German Hospital," later to be Lankenau Hospital, to be his Demonstrator in lectures and assistant in running the student laboratory. In both, inorganic chemistry was dominant—Holland stated in his

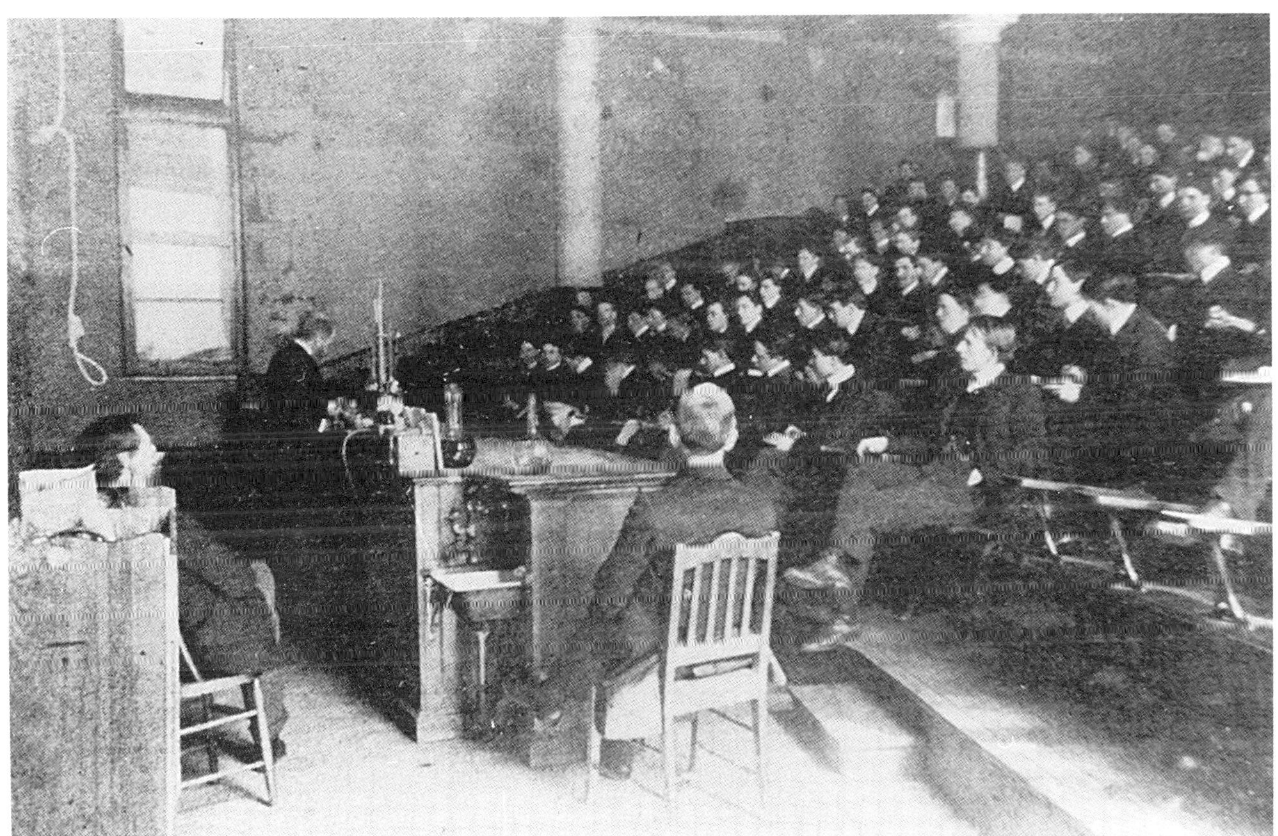

FIG. 4-7. Professor Holland's chemistry recitation in West Lecture Room, fourth floor of 1898 College (ca. 1902).

preface that the lack of proper preparation of entering medical students necessitated such coverage plus introductory physics. Holland's concept of medical chemistry, however, eschewed physiological functions and emphasized the applications of chemistry only in its toxicological, therapeutic, and diagnostic uses. Thus, although Holland's text, along with seven percent of its space devoted to physics and 48 percent to inorganic chemistry, seemed to have 42 percent designated organic and physiological chemistry, only half of this last category was truly "physiological." Digestion was covered, including laboratory experiments, in 15 pages, enzymes in four pages, and food and nutrition in three. Contemporary textbooks by others, for example, Bunge[28] (who devoted several chapters to each of these topics), more truly reflected the era of "physiological chemistry," if not yet that of "biochemistry."

As seen in the *Annual Announcements* (from 1885–1886 through 1911–1912), Holland had varying amounts of help in the teaching program. Lawrence Wolff was Demonstrator from 1885 through 1895, when he was succeeded by Albert M. Jacob, who held the position until it was taken by J.P. Bolton in 1902. In 1906, Melvin A. Saylor became Demonstrator and studied medicine while he taught, eventually obtaining his M.D. degree in 1915 and later accepting the Chair of Chemistry at Temple University Medical School.[5] During the years of his tenure Holland also employed a sizable number of Assistant Demonstrators (sometimes with M.D. degrees, sometimes with Bachelor degrees) and Assistants (usually with Bachelor degrees).

Before the arrival of Holland at Jefferson, it is probable that samples requiring chemical examinations were handled by the physicians themselves or turned over to the Professor of Chemistry. Holland established a "service" function for the chemical staff by appointing, in 1889, Henry Leffmann as "Pathological Chemist" on the Hospital staff. Leffman remained under the aegis of the Chair of Chemistry until 1910, at which time his position was absorbed by the Pathology Department of the Hospital. Leffman, who had graduated from Jefferson in 1869, had a distinguished career as a medical chemist in Philadelphia, having taught at Central High School, The Wagner Free Institute of Science, Pennsylvania College of Dental Surgery, and Woman's Medical College of Pennsylvania. In addition, he was port physician of Philadelphia, coiner of the United States Mint, chemist to the coroner of Philadelphia, and chemist to the Pennsylvania Dairy and Food Commission. He died in 1930, bequeathing in his will $30,000 to Jefferson Medical College.[29,30]

In addition to his textbook, Holland wrote *The Urine and Clinical Chemistry of the Gastric Contents, The Common Poisons, and Milk* (1908, with earlier editions under similar titles), *The Diet for the Sick* (1880), the chapter on urine in the *American Textbook of Practical Medicine,* the chapter on inorganic poisons in Peterson and Haines' *Legal Medicine and Toxicology,* and many papers.[4,25] There is no evidence that he conducted any research in the field of chemistry.

Holland retired from the Chair in 1912 and was named Emeritus but retained the Deanship until 1916. He died in 1922. His portrait, *The Dean's Roll Call,* was painted by Thomas Eakins in 1899. It depicts Holland reading the names of candidates for the M.D. degree in the Academy of Music. The original belongs to the Boston Museum of Fine Arts, and a copy hangs in Jefferson's Eakins Gallery. A second portrait by Adolph Borie, presented by the alumni at Commencement, June 6, 1910, is located in the Dean's office suite.

Philip Bovier Hawk, Ph.D., Professor of Physiological Chemistry and Toxicology (1912–1922)

Philip Bovier Hawk (Figure 4-8) was born July 18, 1874, in East Branch, New York. He obtained his B.S. degree at Wesleyan University, Connecticut, in 1898, but stayed on an additional two years as assistant to W.O. Atwater, well-known nutritional biochemist, receiving his M.S. degree in 1900. Wesleyan conferred an honorary Sc.D. upon Hawk in 1949. His second M.S. degree was received at the Yale Sheffield Scientific School in 1902, after which he transferred his studies to

Columbia University, where he served as Assistant in Physiological Chemistry to W.J. Gies, obtaining his Ph.D. degree in physiological chemistry and nutrition in 1903.[31] It is interesting that both Chittenden and Mendel at Yale considered their student, Hawk, to be an energetic worker but neither imaginative nor brilliant.[11]

Hawk's first postdoctoral position was that of Demonstrator in Physiological Chemistry in John Marshall's Department of Chemistry at the University of Pennsylvania from 1903 to 1907.[32] During this time Hawk wrote the first edition of his famous *Laboratory Manual*. From 1907 to 1912 he served as Professor of Physiological Chemistry at the University of Illinois, where he "aggressively recruited students and cranked out research."[11] Nevertheless, Hawk believed that his work did not receive sufficient recognition and in a letter of 1911 to the Chairman of the Department felt moved to state that the number of papers emanating from his laboratory, published and read before scientific meetings, exceeded that of any other laboratory in the country. In 1912 Hawk left Illinois for Jefferson, where he served as Professor of Physiological Chemistry (note the change of title) and Toxicology through 1922. After his departure from Jefferson he became headmaster of a New England preparatory school for boys in 1923, lectured on nutrition at the University of California in the summer of 1924, and founded the Food Research Laboratories in 1925, a connection that he maintained until his retirement in 1958. Hawk died September 13, 1966, at the age of 92.

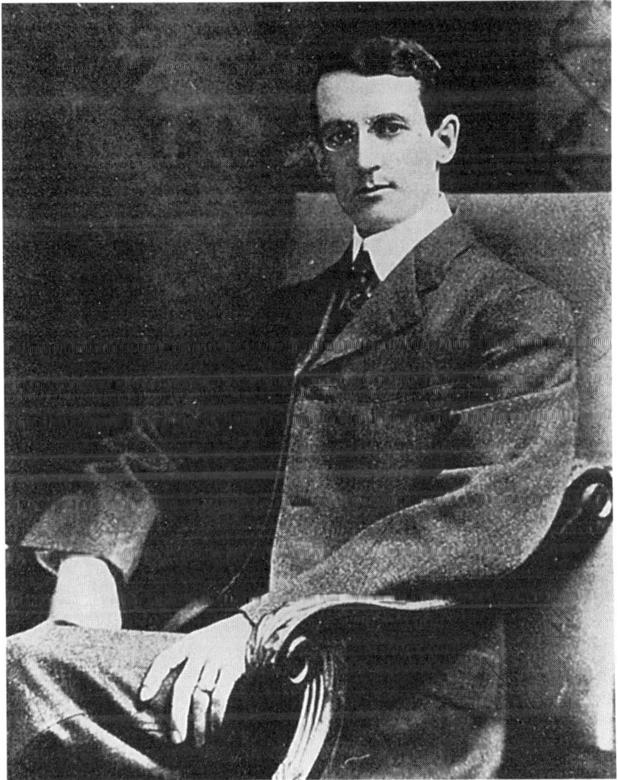

FIG. 4-8. Philip Bovier Hawk, Professor of Physiological Chemistry and Toxicology (1912–1922).

Hawk participated in the founding of the American Society of Biological Chemists and contributed his services to the American Chemical Society as abstractor and section editor for nutrition of *Chemical Abstracts* for 45 years.[23,33] He was elected to the American Philosophical Society in 1915,[31] and was one of only two Jefferson Professors of Physiological Chemistry or Biochemistry to be mentioned in Lieben's 1935 history of the subject. Mention may be made of Hawk's great interest and ability in tennis, a hobby recognized in a cartoon of Jefferson Faculty printed in the *Clinic* of 1923. He was lawn tennis champion of Delaware (1905) and Connecticut and Central New Jersey (1907–1909), veteran lawn tennis champion of the United States (1921–1923), and served on various lawn tennis committees (1908–1931). He also wrote a book on tennis, *Off the Racket* (1927).

Hawk's staff over the years included M.A. Saylor, J.A. Speed, R.M. Biddle, O. Bergeim, J.T. Leary, H.R. Fishback, C.A. Smith, M. Sillman, J.O. Halverson, and R.J. Miller, in various academic ranks. At the time of Hawk's departure, his staff consisted of Olaf Bergeim, Ph.D., as Assistant Professor, Melvin A. Saylor, M.D., as Associate, and Clarence A. Smith, Ph.D., as Associate. Bergeim and Smith had obtained their doctorates in Hawk's graduate program. Many of the staff had also been graduate students in the program. It is a curious omission that Martin Rehfuss, M.D., who participated in Hawk's researches on digestion, does not appear on the staff in any of the relevant *Announcements*, although he is listed on the Department letterhead in 1916 as Research Associate and is referred to by Hawk in a letter to the American Philosophical Society[34] as Head of the Department's research staff.

As for the Department's service function, Henry Leffmann continued as "Pathological Chemist" in the Jefferson Hospital through 1919, with Hawk also being listed as "Physiological Chemist" in the Hospital Pathology Department, beginning in 1913.

Hawk's educational activities were in three categories: medical, public, and graduate. He continued the two-year medical student curriculum begun by Holland but altered the content. By 1913, admission requirements for medical students at Jefferson included chemistry, taken to mean general or largely inorganic chemistry. To ease the transition from the former lack of this and other prerequisites, a "Medical Preparatory Course" was set up to include, along with physics, biology, German or French, a year of inorganic chemistry. Consequently, Hawk was able to omit this subject from his medical course, although organic chemistry remained part of the curriculum. In any case, the course became much more "physiological," with emphasis on the subject of nutrition.

The first-year lectures on physiological chemistry were presented by Hawk, and lectures and recitations on organic chemistry and toxicology were delegated to two of his associates. The entire staff was listed as participating in the laboratory course. In the second year, Hawk lectured on clinical chemistry and nutrition, with an associate in charge of recitations; the staff again shared the supervision of the laboratory course. It is interesting that Holland's textbook was recommended for both first- and second-year courses along with Hawk's own laboratory manual, although it could have had only limited applicability to the modernized course.

One of Hawk's major contributions to medical and biochemical education was his laboratory manual, *Practical Physiological Chemistry,* published by Blakiston (later the Blakiston Division of McGraw-Hill). The first edition of this work appeared in 1907 while Hawk was at the University of Pennsylvania. Apparently, the manual was based upon the laboratory course at Yale, where Chittenden and Mendel gave oral instructions; the shorter time available at Pennsylvania necessitated written directions.[11] The manual has had a long and illustrious history as summarized by Dr. Bernard L. Oser,[35] long-time associate of Hawk. Successive editions appeared rapidly. By the time Hawk took up his professorship at Jefferson, the fourth edition was in print; at the time of his departure, the manual had gone into its eighth edition. With the ninth edition, the authorship became "Hawk and Bergeim," with acknowledged contributions by Cole and Oser, followed by the twelfth and thirteenth under the authorship of "Hawk, Oser, and Summerson." Hawk did not actually participate in these last two. Oser took over the complete responsibility for the fourteenth edition, renamed *Hawk's Physiological Chemistry, Edited by Bernard L. Oser* 1965.

The chemistry course was well received by the students. Abraham Cantarow, M.D., then a student and destined to become one of the subsequent Chairmen of the Department, later referred to Hawk as "a dynamic, inspiring lecturer, with a remarkable gift for clarity of expression and conciseness of presentation."[2] In 1916 the students organized the Hawk Bio-Chemical Society, a group photograph of which appeared in the yearbook a year later. Despite their liking for Hawk and appreciation of his ability, various class historians have attested to the difficulty of the course, the discomfort of the "volunteers" who submitted to passage of the Rehfuss tube, and their dislike for certain of Hawk's staff, one (unnamed) individual being referred to as "the rat." In some classes the difficulty in passing the course resulted in the appellation "Bustem" Hawk.

Evidently Hawk believed that his researches on digestion and nutrition should not remain hidden from the public in scientific journals. To that end, and at the suggestion of editor Edward Bok, Hawk published a series of articles in the *Ladies' Home Journal.*[34] These were rewritten and published as a book in 1919, in the preface of which he acknowledged the financial support of his investigations by the Curtis Publishing Company, Mrs. M. H. Henderson, and Dr. L. M. Halsey.[36] This public acknowledgment was interesting, in view of certain later events. Some years after his departure from Jefferson, Hawk wrote another book for the lay public, mainly concerning obesity and diets.[37]

Hawk set up the first systematic program of graduate education at Jefferson. Shortly after his arrival he requested that a Committee on Graduate Instruction be appointed to supervise the program.

This Committee may properly be regarded as predecessor of the Board for the Regulation of Graduate Studies of many years later, which in turn evolved into the present College of Graduate Studies. It may suffice to note that, from its inception to its demise (1914–1923), Hawk's program turned out eight Masters of Science, four Doctors of Philosophy, and three Doctors of Science in Medicine.[38]

Hawk's graduate program was at once his crowning achievement at Jefferson and his undoing. The latter was chronicled in the minutes of meetings of the faculty and of the Board of Trustees toward the end of 1922.[39] It appeared that Hawk had made secret agreements with several commercial concerns for funds to support five of his graduate students, who, unaware of the sources of their support, performed analyses and other investigations of commercial products. The companies involved were given permission by Hawk to use the results of these investigations as endorsements by him and the Medical College in advertising their products.

Specifically, Dean Patterson had presented to the Board of Trustees on December 11, 1922, evidence concerning Hawk's dealings with the Postum Cereal Company of New York, although from other records additional companies involved were the Chester Kent Company of Boston and the Fleischman Yeast Company. The Board requested that the Faculty meet on this matter and present to the Board its recommendations. The Faculty met on December 15 to hear the Dean's evidence (an exchange of letters between Hawk and the Postum Company occurring during 1921) and a statement written by Hawk. Hawk was then asked to appear for the purpose of making any additional statements. He testified that he had not, at the time, considered his financial arrangements with the graduate students or the company unethical, although he admitted to having no authority to permit the company to use the name of the College in its advertisements. He pointed out, however, that similar arrangements with the Fleischman Company, evidently made previous to those under discussion, had led to no objection. Toward the end of the interview, Hawk agreed that his arrangement with the Postum Company "appeared unethical and unjustified, and should not have been made." Hawk was then excused, and after further discussion, the Faculty adopted a resolution which, among other things, recommended that Hawk's "connection with the Institution should be severed." The Dean presented this resolution to the Board of Trustees at its meeting of December 18, at which time the Board granted Dr. Hawk a hearing. The Board then concurred with the Faculty resolution, and severance of Hawk from the Faculty was carried out.

The indignation of the Faculty and Board at having been "used" was apparent in the original transcripts of the meetings. One wonders whether other factors might have exacerbated the situation. Could not the penalty have been a request to "cease and desist" plus an apology? After all, the "refined" standards of behavior must have been of relatively recent vintage, since the College apparently had permitted the publication, in the Class Book of 1899, of an advertisement for Bailey's Pure Rye Whiskey, "used by the Jefferson Medical College Hospital." Bernard Oser, who was Hawk's laboratory assistant during those trying times, mentioned other possible influences, such as Hawk's involvement in a "difficult and notorious divorce proceeding," professional jealously over the large sums of money coming to a nonclinical researcher, and an "untenable" relationship with Dean Ross V. Patterson.[35]

How persistent were the bitter feelings over this affair were evident from the minutes of a faculty meeting held March 29, 1926, in which it was resolved that papers in which the name of the Institution was used must first be submitted to the head of the Department concerned for his approval. This action was taken in response to a publication, stated as emanating from the "Laboratory of Physiologic Chemistry, Jefferson Medical College," authored by Philip B. Hawk, Martin E. Rehfuss, and Olaf Bergeim.[40] By 1953, Hawk's feelings in the matter had mellowed, at least for the public record; he wrote to the American Philosophical Society that the City of Philadelphia held a warm place in his heart, that some of his most important professional achievements were accomplished at the University of Pennsylvania and Jefferson Medical College, and that his term of service at Jefferson was particularly satisfying in this respect.[34]

Hawk left in December, 1922. Drs. Bergeim and

Smith completed the 1922–1923 teaching session. Saylor had previously left for Temple; Bergeim and Smith departed in the spring of 1922; and Earl A. Schrader, the last graduate student in the group, remained for a time as Demonstrator under Hawk's successor.

(Max) Withrow Morse, Ph.D., Professor of Physiological Chemistry and Toxicology (1923-1930)

(Max) Withrow Morse (Figure 4-9), who used the name *Max* only occasionally, was born May 7, 1880, in Dayton, Ohio, the son of a physician. He obtained his B.Sc. and A.M. degrees at Ohio State University in 1903 and 1904, respectively, followed by a Ph.D. degree at Columbia University in 1910. During this period Morse spent his summers in scientific endeavors: He was a research worker in the Lake Laboratory of Ohio State University at Lake Erie (1902–1904); a scientific assistant to the Bureau of Fisheries at Woods Hole, Massachusetts 1904–1907); an Instructor in the Marine Biological Laboratory, Woods Hole (1907–1909); and a research worker in the Harpswell Laboratory at Portland, Maine (1908–1910).

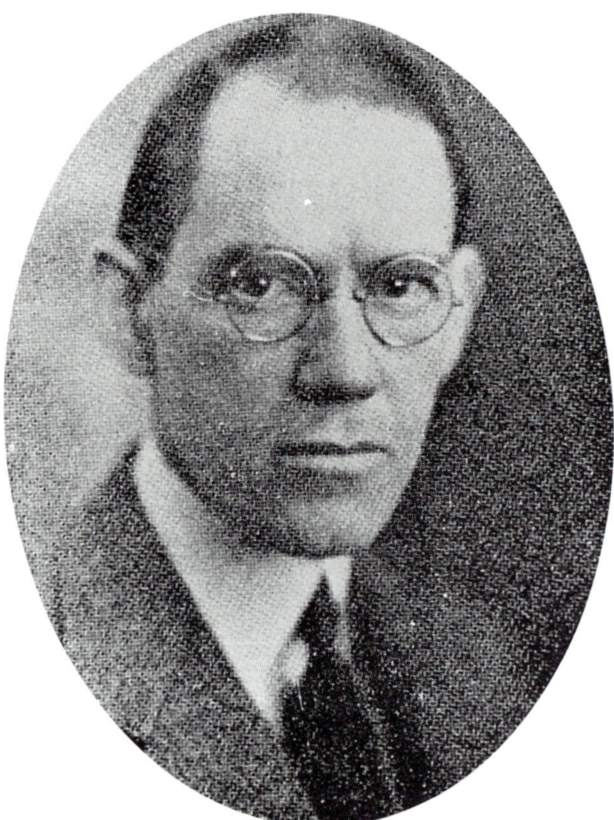

FIG. 4-9. (Max) Withrow Morse, Professor of Physiological Chemistry and Toxicology (1923–1930).

Morse's academic employment had included the following: Instructor in Physiological Chemistry at Cornell University (1906–1907); Instructor and tutor in Physiology at City College, New York (1907–1910); Morgan Professor at Trinity College, Connecticut (1910–1913); Instructor in Biochemistry, University of Wisconsin School of Medicine (1913–1916); Associate Professor of Biochemistry, University of Nebraska College of Medicine (1916–1917); Chemical Pathologist and Director of Chemical Research at the Nelson-Morris Memorial Institute for Medical Research, Michael Reese Hospital, Chicago (1917–1919); and Professor of Biochemistry in the School of Medicine, West Virginia University (1919–1923). He was appointed Professor of Physiological Chemistry and Toxicology at Jefferson in 1923. After his departure from Jefferson in 1930, Morse became investigator and consultant at Rohm and Haas Chemical Company (1930–1933), a member of the Department of Chemistry, New York State Psychiatric Institute (1932–1934), consultant for Lederle and Kalak Companies (1934), and vice-president of Vogelbach Associates. He died on February 19, 1951.

Morse's election as a first choice from a number of applicants raised high expectations at Jefferson.[41] In addition to the Chair in the College, he also became Physiological Chemist in the Hospital Pathology Department. Although Bergeim, Smith, and Schrader were listed on Morse's initial staff, Bergeim and Smith left the Department soon after Hawk. Schrader, the remaining member of the Hawk program, seems not to have endeared himself to the students, who described him as having "inherited the repulsive characteristics of his former monarch" (Hawk), taking "all of the joy out of life," and being "the source of most of our worries."

Other staff members during Morse's tenure were

Max Trumper, Samuel T. Gordy, Joseph S. DeFrates, George A. Williams, Lyle M. Nelson, Jr., Joseph M. Looney, Paul H. Roeder, John C. McNerney, David M. Farrel, Avenir Proskouriakoff, and Andrew M. Gehret. In each of the last five years of the period, one junior member of the staff was listed as "chemical resident."

Morse retained the two-year curriculum that had originated with Holland and continued with modification in content by Hawk. Two lecture series ran in parallel in the first year, one in physiological chemistry and one in toxicology. The laboratory course stressed analytical chemistry and the detection of poisons, along with practical applications of physiological chemistry. Nutrition and applied biochemistry were the topics for the second year, and the laboratory course covered clinical chemistry and nutrition.

As was frequently the case in the history of the Department, student reactions to the new regime were quite favorable at first but became more critical in later years. A "Morse Biochemical Society" was formed, interestingly including Abraham Cantarow, a later Department chairman, as a member from the faculty. Students in these early classes praised Morse's "sterling quality," "intellectual ability," and "friendliness to the students," and showed appreciation for one of Morse's innovations in teaching biochemistry, namely exhibiting patients to illustrate metabolic anomalies, although the students bemoaned the lack of a relevant textbook for the first few years (Morse's book was published in 1925). Later yearbooks, however, began to complain of the immense amount of material in the lecture course, disagreements among laboratory instructors, and the impossibility of completing the required laboratory work in the allotted time. The Class of 1932, hearing of Morse's imminent retirement, presented him with a gold watch.

Morse's textbook, *Applied Biochemistry,* which went through two editions (1925 and 1927), was more in consonance with the "era of Biochemistry" or, indeed, with the "era of Physiological Chemistry," than was Holland's. There was no attempt to provide a thorough grounding in elementary physics or inorganic chemistry. The introductory chapter covered atomic structure, ionization, pH, blood buffers, and acid-base balance. The second chapter on enzymes also included colloid chemistry, whereas organic chemistry was limited to that relevant to carbohydrates, fats, and proteins. The remainder of the text was devoted entirely to physiological chemistry, primarily digestion, nutrition, and clinical biochemistry. Although up to date in most areas, coverage ranged from poor to none on glycolysis in muscle, alcoholic fermentation, enzyme kinetics, and biological oxidations, topics that were being actively investigated and published by biochemical researchers at the time. Illustrations of chemical apparatus were borrowed with permission of the Arthur H. Thomas Company, a laboratory supply house in Philadelphia, but it was untrue, as maintained in a story circulated among students of the day, that the entire textbook was a rewritten Thomas catalog.

Morse's interests were in clinical medicine and physiological chemistry, experimental morphology and cytology, enzymes, atrophy, chemistry of the integument, reaction of tissues, proteins (especially collagen), clinical chemistry, and transfusion substitutes.[41] He published some half-dozen papers and short notes while at Jefferson.

The statements to follow, quoted verbatim or paraphrased from the minutes of meetings of the Board of Trustees or the faculty, should be regarded solely as allegations, since the records contain no actual evidence of wrongdoing, nor is there any indication that Morse, in contrast to Hawk, was given an opportunity to defend his actions before the faculty.

On December 9, 1929, the College Committee of the Board of Trustees resolved to reorganize the Department and to dismiss Professor Morse. On January 13, 1930, the committee stated that they had "considered a large number of facts bearing upon the pecuniary irregularities of Withrow Morse extending over the entire period of his connection with the Jefferson Medical College, the unsatisfactory conduct of the Department itself, the dissatisfaction of students with the Department, and other facts bearing upon the action taken." Dean Patterson was given authority to carry out the action of the Board. On January 27, 1930, the faculty approved the action of the Board and instructed the Dean to "communicate this action to Professor Morse, with discretion as to stating the reasons leading to this action," and to begin a search for a replacement for the Chair. By March 10, the College Committee of the Board decided that Morse should resign by May 31, and two days later stated that "there continue to be unpleasant matters relating to the present administration of the Department of Chemistry." On May 28, the Library, Museum, and Journal Committee informed the faculty of the receipt of a gift to the library by Professor Morse of a collection of biochemical reprints with their filing cabinets and of various journals.

Joseph Michael Looney, M.D., Acting Head of the Department (1930-1931)

Upon Morse's departure, the functions of the Department for the remainder of the academic year were directed by Joseph M. Looney, M.D., who had joined the staff as Assistant Professor in 1926. Although not recognized in the college *Announcement* as Acting Head (the Professorship was listed in 1930–1931 as "vacant"), Looney referred to himself as Acting Professor for the period, and on May 27, 1931, the faculty recommended that the board recognize Looney as having been Acting Head for the school year 1930–1931. By November, 1930, George R. Bancroft was being considered by the Board's College Committee as Morse's successor, and in March of 1931 Bancroft was appointed to take office September 1, 1931.

Looney never was considered for the Chair, possibly because of his junior professional rank. The college may, nevertheless, have overlooked a treasure in its own backyard. Although derided by the students in earlier yearbooks for some hesitancy in speech, and overdevotion to the work of Otto Folin, his mentor in clinical chemistry at Harvard, and caricatured in numerous cartoons, by the time of Morse's departure the students admitted to having "learned a great deal of Biochemistry of practical value from Dr. Looney." The students of the following year expressed sorrow at Looney's leaving.

Joseph Michael Looney (Figure 4-10) was born April 3, 1896, in Somerville, Massachusetts, and obtained his A.B. degree (1916) and M.D. (1920) at Harvard. He was Instructor in Biochemistry at Harvard (1920–1922) and Director of the Research Laboratory at the Sheppard and Enoch Pratt Hospital (1922–1926), after which time he was appointed Assistant Professor of Physiological Chemistry at Jefferson and Chemical Pathologist to the Hospital.

Looney assisted Morse with the second edition of the latter's textbook. Looney's work in research greatly exceeded that of his chief. An incomplete bibliography in the Jefferson Archives listed 17 publications in addition to the textbook. His interests were several: methods of clinical chemical analysis, some published with Otto Folin in the early 1920s; anti-pernicious anemia factors in liver, amino acid analyses of proteins in the later 1920s;

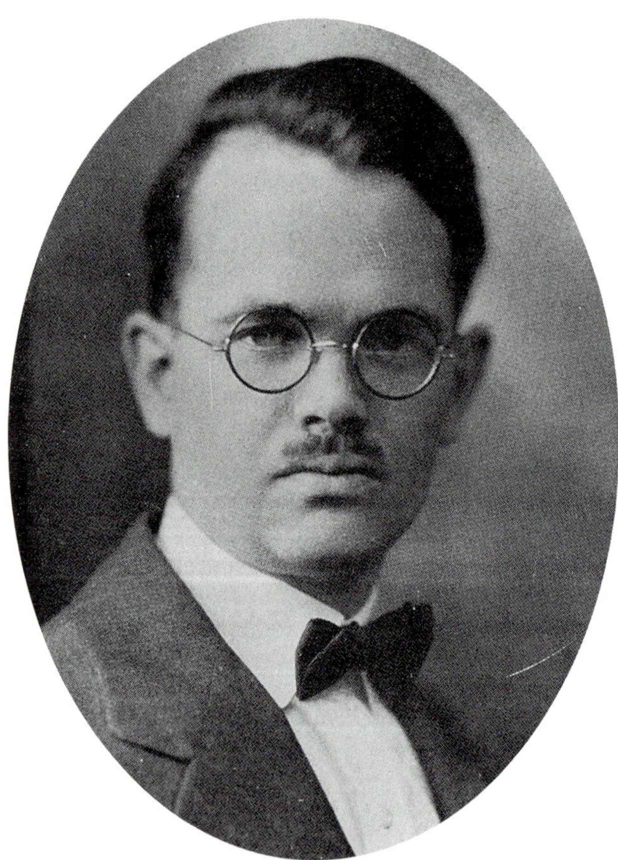

FIG. 4-10. Joseph Michael Looney, Acting Head of Chemistry Department (1930–1931).

and blood gases in schizophrenia, after leaving Jefferson in the 1930s. Looney shared with Hawk the distinction of being cited in Lieben's treatise on the history of biochemistry.

During Looney's tenure as Acting Head of the Department, the Morse Biochemical Society became simply the Biochemical Society, then disbanded.

George Russell Bancroft, Ph.D., D.Sc. Professor of Physiological Chemistry and Toxicology (1931-1945)

George Russell Bancroft (Figure 4-11) was born July 7, 1878, in Weymouth, Nova Scotia, and became naturalized in the United States in 1934. He obtained an A.B. degree from Acadia College in 1906 (where he was awarded a D.Sc. in 1934), an A.M. from Yale in 1914, and a Ph.D. from Yale in 1917. He pursued postgraduate studies at the University of Chicago in 1920 and 1924 and at Yale in 1929.

After serving as principal in the public schools of Nova Scotia (1898–1899, 1900–1903, and 1906–1907), Bancroft was Science Master at Halifax Academy, (1907–1913), Assistant Instructor in Chemistry at Yale (1914–1917), Professor of Chemistry and Physics at Transylvania College, Kentucky (1917–1918), Assistant Professor of Organic Chemistry at the University of Kentucky (1918–1920), Associate Professor of Organic Chemistry at West Virginia (1920–1923), Associate Professor of Physiological Chemistry in the School of Medicine at West Virginia (1923–1924), and Professor of Physiological Chemistry at the same institution (1924–1931). His appointment to head the department at Jefferson began in September, 1931.

Initially, Bancroft's staff consisted of Looney and Proskouriakoff from Morse's staff. These two were soon replaced by Dr. Lorenz Peter Hansen (trained mainly in organic chemistry) and Thomas Lawrence Williams (a pharmacist), both of whom were destined to remain in the Department during two successive Chairmanships. Until the last few years of Bancroft's tenure, each *Announcement* listed a different "physiological chemistry interne" in the Department roster; in most cases the same individual had an identical listing in the Hospital. Bancroft did not appoint any other staff members until 1940–1941, when Proskouriakoff made a reappearance as Fellow in Bacteriology and Chemistry, and in 1944, when Daniel Lamb Turner was named Associate in Physiological Chemistry.

In terms of the Department's service function, Bancroft was listed as Physiological Chemist in the

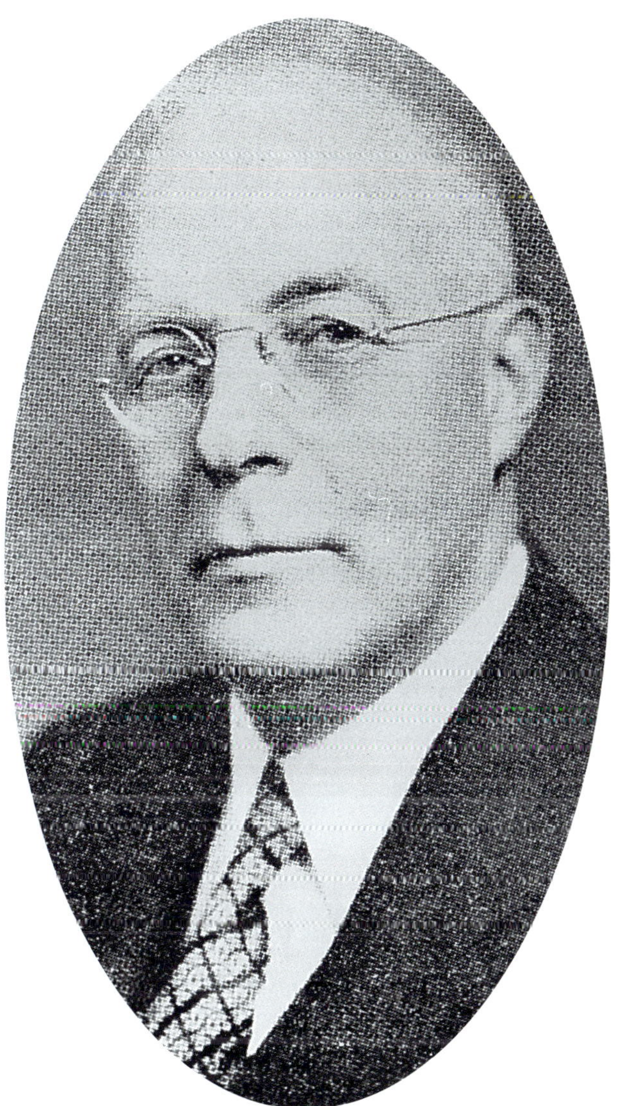

FIG. 4-11. George Russell Bancroft, Professor of Physiological Chemistry and Toxicology (1931–1945).

Hospital's Pathology Department from 1931 to 1935, along with various "internes." Abraham Cantarow appeared initially as biochemist on the Hospital staff in 1933–1934, and by 1935–1936 was listed (without Bancroft) in the Hospital Department of Clinical Laboratories with internes through 1940–1941 and then alone.

Under Bancroft the chemistry course reverted to a one-year parallel series of lectures and laboratories (Figure 4-12). Major topics of the lectures were the chemistry of carbohydrates, fats, and proteins, body fluids, digestion and metabolism, nutrition, endocrinology, and analysis of blood and urine. The laboratory experiments followed the same general scheme, with some emphasis on the use of such instruments as the microscope, colorimeter, spectroscope, and polariscope in their biochemical applications. Students made use of the laboratory manual containing review questions written by Bancroft. The recommended textbook was Mathews' *Physiological Chemistry,* one of the most widely used American texts in the early "era of Biochemistry."

Student dissatisfaction with Bancroft's course began at its inception and did not cease until his retirement. The chief sources of this discontent seem to have been the large mass of material extraneous to biochemistry that Bancroft incorporated into the course, along with dislike for Bancroft's staff. Representative complaints: "The rest of our time during the Freshman year was taken up by that one and only Dr. Bancroft and his rat terriers, Hansen and Williams. What a gang and what a course!" "We must admit that "Bandy" was at least sincere and was doing what he believed to be the right thing, whether it was or not." "Our curiosity was aroused as to why the course had been called Chemistry, since it included from the outset so many other fields, among which were Botany, Astronomy, and GREEK." These written comments were accompanied by a multitude of unflattering cartoons. It was customary for students to roll pennies down the aisle of the auditorium during his lectures, but he remained oblivious to this protest. With the retirement of Bancroft in June, 1945, an unhappy chapter in the history of chemistry at Jefferson

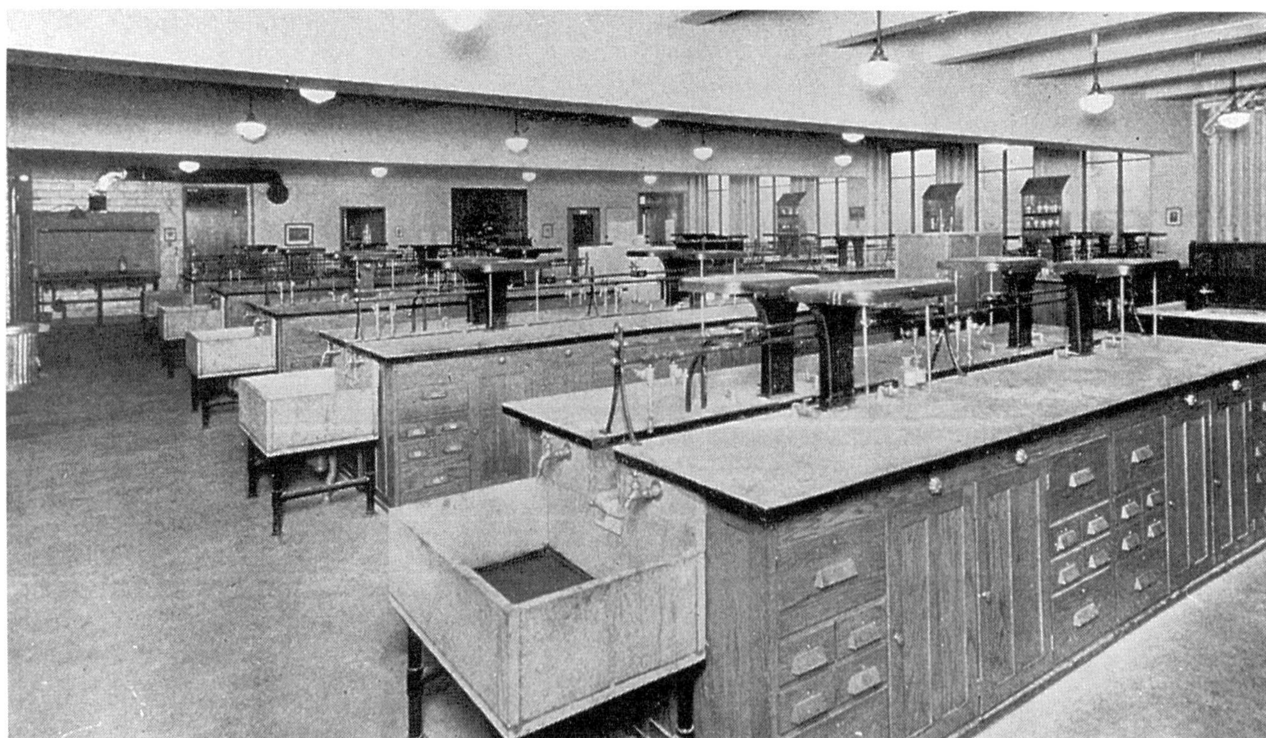

FIG. 4-12. Chemistry Laboratory on Third Floor of 1025 Walnut Street College, in 1931.

came to an end. The encyclopedic course in Physiological Chemistry, with liberal portions of etymology, botany, mineralogy, animal husbandry, and metaphysics became a memory.

There is no evidence that Bancroft carried on research during his tenure at Jefferson. Indeed, the administration of the day was cool to such endeavors. Dr. Hansen, who had a lifelong interest in the chemistry of steroids, requested permission of Dean Patterson to construct, at his own expense, a pen for chickens on an unused upper floor of the College building for the purpose of setting up the cockscomb assay for testosterone. The Dean replied: "You are here to teach, not to do research."[42] (Patterson, nevertheless, left his estate at death in 1937 to establish research fellowships at Jefferson.) Bancroft retired in 1945. At his last lecture the class presented him with a gold watch. He was not elected to Emeritus status.

Abraham Cantarow, M.D., Professor of Biochemistry and Chairman of the Department (1945–1966)

Abraham Cantarow (Figure 4-13) was born January 27, 1901, in Hartford, Connecticut, into a medically oriented family. His father, grandfather, three uncles, and an aunt were in the medical field.[43,44] After graduation from Hartford Public High School, Cantarow studied for a year at Trinity College and two years at Tufts. While there he took advanced training in violin at the Boston Conservatory of Music, at the same time becoming a top-ranking tennis player. Having decided to study medicine, Cantarow chose Jefferson—an acquaintance pointed out that the textbooks used in most medical schools of the time were written by Jefferson faculty members, and asked, "Why not get your information right from the horse's mouth?"[45] Cantarow's interest in biochemical research was stimulated by his contacts with Philip B. Hawk, Max Trumper, and Henry Leffmann and its clinical applications by Thomas McCrae and Hobart A. Hare. His roommates have reported that Cantarow finished his day's studies easily and early, then relaxed in the evening with his violin and the music of Bach. This serious music was counterbalanced by his membership in a dance orchestra. Cantarow graduated with honors in 1924.

Cantarow spent his entire professional career at Jefferson. He was, successively, Resident Chemist at Jefferson Hospital (1924–1925), Resident Physician (1925–1927), and Research Fellow in the Department of Diseases of the Chest (1927–1929), and he taught physical diagnosis in that Department (1927), was Assistant to Dr. Harold W. Jones in the Laboratory of Clinical Medicine (1930), and was Biochemist to the Hospital (1931–1945). During this time Cantarow rose in rank in the Department of Medicine from Assistant Demonstrator (1929–1931), to Instructor (1931–1934), Associate (1934–1937), Assistant Professor (1937–1939) and Associate Professor (1939–1945). He was appointed Professor of Biochemistry and Chairman of the Department in 1945.

Many honors were bestowed on Cantarow during his lifetime. Among those most closely

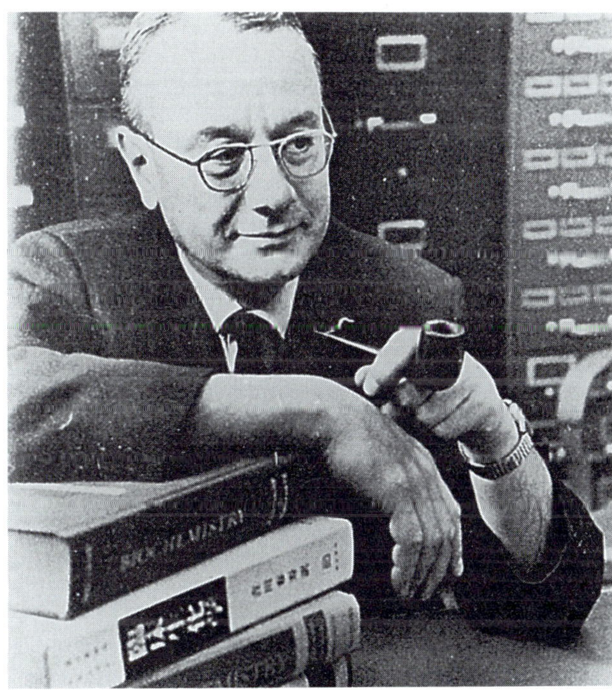

Fig. 4-13. Abraham Cantarow, Professor of Biochemistry (1945–1966).

related to Jefferson were the two issues of the *Clinic* dedicated to him (1943 and 1959), presentation of his portrait to the College by the Class of 1960, Presidency of the Alumni Association (1964–1965), recipient of the Alumni Achievement Award in 1968, an honorary Doctor of Science degree conferred by his alma mater in 1969, and appointment as alumni representative on the Board of Trustees in 1970.

Cantarow retired as Emeritus Professor of Biochemistry in 1966 and accepted a post as Research Planning Officer at the National Cancer Institute. He died in 1979.

As may be seen from its new title, the Department of Biochemistry was due to undergo extensive modernization under Cantarow's direction, although at a circumspect and evolutionary pace. One of the early changes was the elimination of the service function of the Department in the Hospital Clinical Laboratories. Although Cantarow was still listed as Biochemist or Physiological Chemist to the Hospital in both 1945–1946 and 1946–1947, this listing ceased in 1947–1948. Such a separation of biochemistry as an independent discipline, divorced from clinical chemistry, was part of a general trend in the 1940s.

Another of Cantarow's goals was the transformation of the Department from its European format of one "Geheimrat" presenting all of the lectures and performing all, if any, of the research, and one or two "dieners" handling the student laboratory. In the newer pattern the Department Head shared lectures with several staff members, who in turn might well be carrying out independent research. Cantarow inherited from Bancroft's staff Drs. Hansen and Turner and Mr. Williams. Other staff members who appeared over the years included, in chronological order, Leon L. Miller, William H. Pearlman, Romano H. DeMeio, Bernard Schepartz, Robert J. Rutman, Chiun Tong Ling, F.W. Sunderman, Sr., Leonidas Levenbook, Milton Toporek, Arthur Allen, and Sidney Weinhouse, along with several research associates or research fellows, usually graduate students. At any given time after the first few years, the Department consisted of the Chairman and some half-dozen staff members.

Although for the medical students the course differed markedly in content from that of Bancroft, the general format of lectures and laboratories remained similar for the first few years. As the Department grew to full strength, Cantarow began to share the major lectures with other staff members. During the same period, as new staff were added, each was given the opportunity to choose a program of research, either with the Chairman and his colleagues or without prejudice to embark on his own line of investigation.

The lectures were modernized with the introduction of topics such as bioenergetics, metabolic antagonism, and biochemical genetics. Essay-type examinations were eventually replaced by the multiple-choice format, although these were graded manually until the advent of the computer. An experiment in small-group teaching was instituted in which the staff member with major expertise would outline the "basics" of the topic to the entire class, after which the details would be taught simultaneously in small groups by each of the staff members. This was abandoned after much student protest because of the diverse presentations given by the various staff members.

The laboratory course, which had begun much as it had been taught under Bancroft, was also modernized. The "cookbook" experiments that involved color reactions and some physical properties of the major constituents of foods and tissues, together with extensive coverage of blood and urine analysis, were eliminated. "Problem-type" experiments were introduced, in which small groups of students were given a biochemical problem with several possible alternative approaches toward its solution, the choice of which was theirs. Many of these experiments consisted of the in vitro incubation of tissue preparations with various substrates, followed by the determination of changes in amounts of substances present by the use of paper chromatography. When possible, cooperative experiments were organized with the Department of Physiology in which "physiological" experiments upon animals were followed or accompanied by the taking of samples of fluids, tissues, or excreta for subsequent analysis in the biochemical laboratory.

Reaction of the students to the course was generally laudatory except for some unkind remarks concerning those staff members remaining from Bancroft's regime. Cantarow's lectures were uniformly praised, as was his new textbook with Bernard Schepartz, *Biochemistry,* which first appeared in 1954.

In 1949–1950 the Department announced that it would accept graduate students. In 1950–1951 special seminars in advanced biochemistry and a course in biochemical laboratory methods were offered. It was evident that, after the hiatus caused by the departure of Philip B. Hawk, the Department had returned to the twentieth century.

The Department began a course in chemistry for the diploma nurses program and participated in an interdepartmental course in cell biology for entering graduate students. Both courses were carried over into the Chairmanship succeeding Cantarow's.

In the early years of Cantarow's Chairmanship, Harrow's textbook of biochemistry was used, along with the laboratory manual of Hawk and Bergeim. At times the latter served as both text and manual. At other times the Department compiled its own manual similar to that written by Bancroft. Cantarow and Schepartz's *Biochemistry* (1954) went through four editions, the last in 1967.

Other books written by Cantarow included *Calcium Metabolism and Calcium Therapy* (1931); *Biochemistry in Internal Medicine,* with Max Trumper as senior author (1932); *Clinical Biochemistry,* with Max Trumper (1939) through five editions (1955); *Lead Poisoning,* also with Max Trumper (1944); and *Clinical Endocrinology,* with Karl E. Paschkis and Abraham E. Rakoff (1954). Textbooks for the nurses' course were written by staff member Milton Toporek.

Research in the Department eventually became more diversified. Cantarow's interests, which began with calcium metabolism, liver function, and bile pigments, finally turned toward endocrine–cancer interrelationships. This latter course of investigation was pursued with Drs. Paschkis and Rakoff and other members of the interdepartmental Division of Endocrine and Cancer Research.

A Digression; The Cold War, Faculty Dismissals, and Censure

Although the events to be described had many ramifications beyond the Biochemistry Department, their major effect was within this Department and may be included appropriately in its history. As background to this sad period in Jefferson's history, it should be noted that in the 1950s the elation following the termination of World War II gave way to a pervasive fear of communism in this country as our former ally, the U.S.S.R., began to be perceived as a political threat to the western nations. Anyone advocating so little as American–Soviet friendship was liable to be suspected of harboring more sinister thoughts, particularly during the period in which Senator Joseph McCarthy and the investigations of the House Un-American Activities Committee (HUAC) garnered much publicity.

In this atmosphere institutions of higher learning were required by the State of Pennsylvania to attest to the absence of "subversive" persons on their faculties. The Jefferson Administration never stated that it had such persons on its payroll. Nevertheless, three members were questioned before committees consisting largely of members from the Board of Trustees and Administration concerning their political beliefs and affiliations.[46] The only faculty representative was a Department Chairman. On November 30, 1953, the Executive Faculty voted unanimously that three staff members were "not deemed worthy of holding" their positions. On the same day the Board of Trustees resolved that "employment of each of them hereby is terminated, in the best interests of the institution." The Dean was empowered to make appropriate settlements. Jefferson agreed to pay each affected individual severance salary to the end of the school year, to provide each with a letter stating that dismissal was not based on a finding of subversion as defined by the Pennsylvania Loyalty Act, and each staff member in turn agreed to sign a release relinquishing all rights to future claims against Jefferson. Thus Jefferson lost two members of the Biochemistry Department and one from the Department of Physiology.

Due to the atmosphere of the time, it became habitual not to discuss "controversial" topics in the hallways for fear of being overheard. One division head of a clinical department, a professor of international repute, alleged that he had been threatened with dismissal if he continued to voice his objections to the way in which the affair was handled. The case was reviewed by the American Association of University Professors (AAUP) in 1956.[47] It was noted that two of the staff members would have qualified for tenure under the AAUP *1940* Statement of Principles on Academic Freedom and Tenure, that the dismissals were without charge or explanation, except for the statement concerning "best interests of the institution," and that faculty representation in the hearings was inadequate, as was the severance pay. As a consequence the association placed Jefferson on its "censured" list. Although certain Jeffersonians tended to take this censure lightly, others had the experience of being told at scientific meetings by well-qualified fellow scientists that they would not consider accepting a position at an institution under censure. Largely through the efforts of President Peter A. Herbut, tenure regulations at Jefferson were established that met with the approval of the AAUP, and the school was removed from the censured list in 1968.[48] Not all institutions of higher learning succumbed to the hysteria of the times; the staff members dismissed from the Department of Biochemistry found employment at other universities.

Paul Herbert Maurer, Ph.D., Professor of Biochemistry and Chairman of the Department (1966–1985)

Paul H. Maurer (Figure 4-14) was born in New York City on June 29, 1923. He earned his B.S. degree at City College, New York, in 1944 and his Ph.D. at Columbia in 1950. He worked as research biochemist at General Foods Corporation, Hoboken, New Jersey (1944–1946), Instructor at City College (1946–1951), Research Associate at the College of Physicians and Surgeons, Columbia University (1950–1951), Assistant Research Professor in the School of Medicine, University of Pittsburgh (1951–1954), and Associate Professor of Immunochemistry at the same school (1954–1960), Associate Professor of Microbiology at Seton Hall College of Medicine (1960–1962), and Professor of Microbiology at New Jersey College of Medicine (1962–1966), and was appointed Professor and Head of the Biochemistry Department at Jefferson in 1966. In 1984 Dr. Maurer announced his resignation from the Chairmanship to take effect upon the appointment of a successor.

The staff initially consisted of those remaining from Cantarow's tenure, namely DeMeio, Schepartz, Toporek, and Allen (whose portrait was presented by the Class of 1979), with the addition of George F. Kalf, Ralph Heimer, Thomas R. Koszalka, Paul Pinchuck, Arlene P. Martin, Marie L. Vorbeck, Patricia J. Walsh, Leslie G. Clark, Paul A. Liberti, Helga M. Suld, William Stylos, and Matilda Alvarez-Serra. Others associated with the Department over the years included William L. Holmes, Robert M. Metrione, Anne Steele Faust, Marianna L. Egan, Hugh James Callahan, Lorraine J. Haeffner, Yu Chen Lin, Thomas I. Diamondstone, John J. Ch'ih, Gerald Odstrchel, Robert C. Baldridge, Carmen F. Merryman, Allen R. Zeiger, George R. Hunter, Marilyn R. Fenton, Hugh McDonald, David Judd Ganfield, Robert D. Smyth, Robert E. Franzl, Fu-Li Yu, William Lawrence Long, P.V. Gopalakrishnan, Robert T. Henry, Tessa Chao, Fred D. Lublin, Stephen Joseph McGeady, Bradford Straughn Fansler, Charles S. Owen, Norman Terry Felberg, Miguel

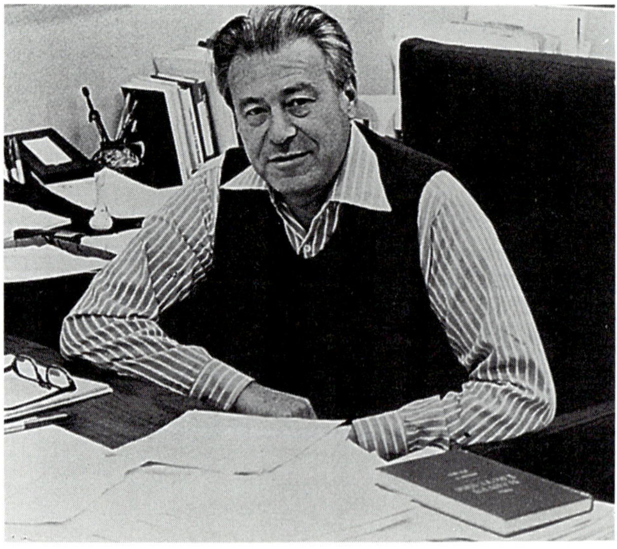

FIG. 4-14. Paul Herbert Maurer, Professor of Biochemistry (1966–1985).

Ficher, Ian Martin Zitron, Richard Douglas Baillie, Leah M. Lowenstein, Jean Kasuba Paddock, and Uma Mahesh Babu.

With the accession of Paul H. Maurer to the Chair, the Department of Biochemistry underwent a marked change in character. Because the Chairman's major interest was immunochemistry, many of the additional staff members appointed were immunochemists. On the average, the staff in subsequent years consisted of immunochemists and traditional biochemists, including "molecular biologists," in about equal proportions. This hybrid character naturally also was reflected in the various areas of teaching and research.

In the course for freshmen medical students a sequence of lectures in immunochemistry was added and remained for many years. In 1982–1983 most of this material was moved into the microbiology course of the second year. Members of clinical departments were invited to present biochemical–clinical correlation lectures. After a year or so of discussion, the medical student laboratory course in biochemistry was abolished in 1969–1970, in harmony with a national trend. In the early 1970s remedial programs were set up for students having difficulties with the course, and in the late 1970s the lecture series in nutrition was expanded. The major change in the freshman course, however, occurred in 1972–1973 when an integrated, more properly characterized as "interpolated," course in Cell and Tissue Biology was established. This combined the former course in Biochemistry with the Histology course of the Anatomy Department, in addition to contributions from several other departments or divisions of larger departments.[49]

Another innovation occurred in 1975–1976, when the senior medical students were offered a course in the clinical aspects of biochemistry and immunobiology. These fourth-year sessions, which were part of a senior-year elective program, were in the form of small-group seminars and discussions.

For many years the Department had participated in the training of diploma nurses through offering a course that included inorganic, organic, and biological chemistry. This course continued during Maurer's Chairmanship but was abolished when the diploma program for nurses was phased out in favor of a baccalaureate curriculum by 1982. The Department made a quantitatively greater commitment when, in the 1970s and extending for a decade, courses were offered to baccalaureate nurses and medical technologists in the College of Allied Health Sciences in such subjects as quantitative analysis, general biochemistry, and organic chemistry. These contributions of the Department ended in the early 1980s, when the College of Allied Health Sciences undertook to teach all of its own courses in chemistry.

The interdepartmental graduate-level course in Cell Biology, to which the Biochemistry Department had contributed a significant share, was eliminated in 1972–1973 when the Cell and Tissue Biology course of the medical curriculum became available. Courses offered within the department included a postdoctoral training program in immunochemistry; a series of seminars in biochemistry presented by graduate students, faculty, and guests; an analogous seminar series in immunochemistry; physical chemistry of proteins and enzymes; enzyme cytology; enzymology; special topics in advanced biochemistry; immunochemistry and immunology; bioorganic chemistry; advanced biochemical techniques; research in biochemical oncology; and the usual graduate credits for the students' thesis research. The hybrid nature of the Department was recognized formally in 1983–1984 when two separate programs of graduate study were listed: Biochemical Approach to Immunology and Molecular and Developmental Biochemistry. These graduate programs reflected also the divergent research interests of the two groups within the Department.

Robert C. Baldridge, Ph.D., Acting Chairman of the Department (1985–1986)

On July 1, 1985, Dr. Paul H. Maurer resigned his Chairmanship and Dr. Robert C. Baldridge was appointed Acting Chairman. Dr. Baldridge (Figure 4-15) was born January 19, 1921, in Herington, Kansas. He obtained his B.S. degree from Kansas State University in 1943, and an M.S. in 1948 and a Ph.D. in 1951 from the University of Michigan. Baldridge was Instructor in Biological Chemistry at Michigan from 1951 through 1953 and rose from Assistant Professor to Professor of Biochemistry at Temple University School of Medicine, 1953–1970, where he also became Associate Dean of the Graduate School in 1965. In 1970 he was appointed Professor of Biochemistry and Dean of the College of Graduate Studies at Jefferson, holding the latter position until 1981. Dr. Baldridge's major research interest centered on amino acid metabolism, particularly in genetic disorders such as histidinemia.

Darwin J. Prockop, M.D., Ph.D., Chairman of the Department of Biochemistry, and Director, Jefferson Institute of Molecular Medicine (1986–)

On July 22, 1985, Dr. Darwin J. Prockop (Figure 4-16) was appointed to the Chair and also named Director of the Jefferson Institute of Molecular Medicine, effective as of April, 1986. Dr. Prockop was born August 31, 1929, in Palmerton, Pennsylvania. He obtained his B.A. degree from Haverford College (1951), an M.A. from Oxford University (1953), an M.D. from the University of Pennsylvania (1956), and a Ph.D. from Washington University (1961). Prockop interned at New York Hospital–Cornell Medical Center (1956–1957), was Resident Fellow in Pharmacology at the National Heart Institute, (1957–1958), and Research Investigator in Biochemistry (1958–1961). He rose through the ranks from Associate in Biochemistry to Professor of Biochemistry and Medicine at the University of Pennsylvania (1961–1972), and was Professor of Biochemistry and Chairman of the Department at Rutgers Medical School from 1972 until his Jefferson appointment. Prockop's major

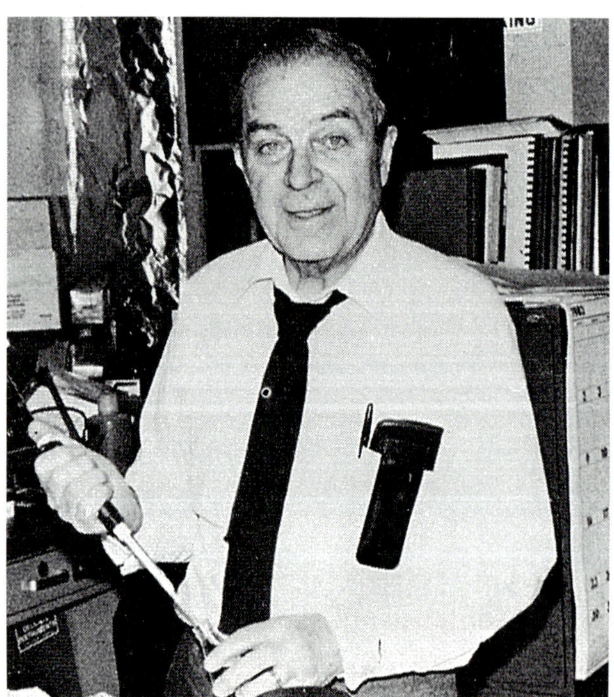

FIG. 4-15. Robert C. Baldridge, Ph.D., Acting Chairman of Chemistry Department (1985–1986).

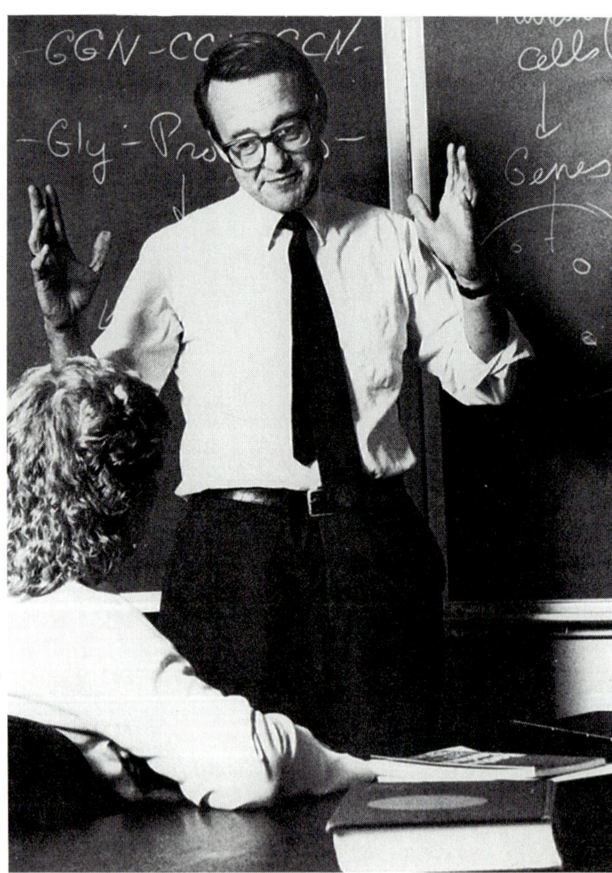

FIG. 4-16. Darwin J. Prockop, Chairman of Biochemistry Department and Director of Institute of Molecular Medicine (1986–).

research centered on the metabolism of collagen and other constitutents of connective tissue.

The Department of Biochemistry has experienced both lean and fruitful years. The last four decades, however, witnessed expansion in student and graduate programs, increase in research, and progressive enlargement of the staff. The new Institute of Molecular Medicine envisages 18 faculty appointments, extensive laboratory space and equipment, and funding for research activities. The Department is thus poised to exceed its past achievements.

References

1. Bancroft, G.R., "Department of Physiological Chemistry and Toxicology," *Clinic.* 1936, p. 81.
2. Cantarow, A., "Biochemistry at Jefferson," *Jeff. Med. Coll. Al. Bull.* Vol. 12, No. 9, October, 1962, pp. 17–27.
3. Gayley, J.F., *A History of the Jefferson Medical College of Philadelphia.* Philadelphia: Joseph M. Wilson, 1858.
4. Gould, G.M., *The Jefferson Medical College of Philadelphia: A History (1826–1904).* Vols. I and II, New York: Lewis Publishing Company, 1904.
5. Bauer, E.L., *Doctors Made in America.* Philadelphia: J.B. Lippincott Co., 1963.
6. Smith, E.F., *Jacob Green, 1790–1841, Chemist.* Philadelphia: 1923.
7. Gross, S.D., *Autobiography.* Vol. 1, Philadelphia: George Barrie, 1887, p. 36.
8. Green J., *A Text Book of Chemical Philosophy.* Philadelphia: R.H. Small, 1829.
9. Hatfield, N.L. (1804–1867), *Medical Notebooks.* In Historical Collections, Coll. Phys. Phila., Catalog No. 384, File Z10/229.
10. "Questions on Chemistry by Jacob Green, M.D., Feb. 26, 1832." Copy made by student. Jacob Green File in Archives of Thomas Jefferson University.
11. Kohler, R.E., *From Medical Chemistry to Biochemistry.* New York: Cambridge University Press, 1982.
12. Wood, G.B., *Historical and Biographical Memoirs.* Philadelphia: J.B. Lippincott Co., 1872, pp. 329–379, 381–401.
13. Bache, F., "Introductory Lecture to the Course of Chemistry, Delivered in Jefferson Medical College, October 13th, 1852." Published by the Class, Philadelphia: 1852.
14. Gross, S.D., *Autobiography.* Vol. 2, pp. 306–307.
15. Walker, J.B., "Letter to the Jefferson Alumni Association." *Jeff. Med. Coll. Al. Bull.*, Vol 1, No. 12, 1929, p. 6.
16. Smith, E.F., *Franklin Bache, 1792–1864, Chemist. Phila., 1922.* Bound in Smith's American Chemists and Chemistry, 1919–1924, as Pamphlet No. 2.
17. Rand, B.H., *Elements of Medical Chemistry.* Philadelphia: T. Ellwood Zell & Co., 1867.
18. Smith, E.F., "Biographical Memoir of Robert Empie Rogers, 1813–1884." *Jeff. Med. Coll. Addresses,* 5: 1904, pp. 291–309.
19. Ruschenberger, W.S.W., "A Sketch of the Life of Robert E. Rogers, M.D., with Biographical Notices of his Father and Brothers." Read before the American Philosophical Society, November 6, 1885.
20. Lehmann, C.G., *Physiological Chemistry.* Transl. from 2d ed. by G.E. Day, ed. by R.E. Rogers, Vol. I and II. Philadelphia: Blanchard & Lea, 1885.
21. Holland, J.W., "Introductory Lecture. A Eulogy on the Life and Character of Prof. Robt. E. Rogers, M.D., Introductory to the Course of 1885–86 at Jefferson Medical College." *The College and Clinical Record* 6: 1885, pp. 203–210.
22. Ibid. 1: 1880, p. 57; 3: 1882, p. 201.
23. Brown, C.A., and M.E. Weeks, *A History of the American Chemical Society.* Washington: American Chemical Society, 1952.
24. Eisenschiml, O., "John W. Mallet, ACS President in 1882." *Chemical and Engineering News* 29: 1951, pp. 110–111.
25. Saylor, M.A., "In Memory of Dr. James W. Holland." *Clinic,* 1923, p. 15.
26. Holland, J.W., *A Text-book of Medical Chemistry and Toxicology.* 2d ed., Philadelphia: W. B. Saunders Co., 1909.
27. Wolff, L., *Essentials of Medical Chemistry.* 4th ed., Philadelphia: W. B. Saunders Co., 1893.
28. Bunge, G., *Text-Book of Physiological and Pathological Chemistry.* 2d English ed. transl. by F.A. and E.H. Starling. Philadelphia: P. Blakiston's Son & Co., 1902.
29. *Jeff. Med. Coll. Al. Bull.*, Vol. 1, No. 15, 1931, p. 4.
30. Konkle, B.A., and F.P. Henry, *Standard History of the Medical Profession of Philadelphia,* 2d ed. Edited by L.M. Holloway, New York: AMS Press, 1977.
31. Corner, G.W., "Philip Bovier Hawk (1874–1966)," *Am. Phil. Soc. Year Book* 1966, 1967, pp. 147–148.
32. Chittenden, R.H., *The Development of Physiological Chemistry in the United States.* New York: New York Chemical Catalog Co., ACS Monograph No. 54, 1930, pp. 170–171.
33. Death notice, *Chemical and Engineering News* 44: 1966, p. 66.
34. Letter, Philip B. Hawk to the American Philosophical Society, October 26, 1953, in Am. Phil. Soc. Archives.
35. Personal communication from Bernard L. Oser, Ph.D.
36. Hawk, P.B., *What We Eat and What Happens to It.* New York: Harper & Brothers, 1919.
37. Hawk, P.B., *Streamline for Health.* New York: Harper & Brothers, 1935.
38. Letter of October 29, 1982, from Dr. A.J. Ramsay to Dr. J.J. Saukkonen, Dean, Coll. Grad. Stud., Thomas Jefferson Univ. Much of the information on this graduate program and on the events leading to Hawk's departure from Jefferson was first discovered in the University's Archives by Dr. Andrew J. Ramsay, Daniel Baugh Emeritus Professor of Anatomy, Thomas Jefferson Univ.
39. Minutes of meeting, December 15, 1922, Faculty of Jeff. Med. Coll.; Minutes of meeting, December 18, 1922, Board of Trustees, Jeff. Med. Coll.
40. Hawk, P.B., M.E. Rehfuss, and O. Bergeim, "The Response of the Normal Human Stomach to Various Standard Foods." *Am. J. Med. Sci.*, N.S. 172: 1926, pp. 359–369.
41. *Jeff. Med. Coll. Al. Bull.* 1, No. 2, 1923, p. 6.
42. Personal communication from Dr. L.P. Hansen.
43. Miller, B.J., Dedication. *Clinic,* 1943, p. 3.
44. Haskell, B.F., Talk delivered at portrait presentation, *Jeff. Med. Coll. Al. Bull.*, 11, No. 7, May 1960, pp. 26–30.
45. Personal communication from Dr. A. Cantarow.
46. Administration files of Thomas Jefferson University for 1953–1954.
47. *Bull. Am. Assoc. Univ. Prof.* 42: 1956, p. 75.
48. Ibid., 54: 1968, pp. 7 and 178–179.
49. Schepartz, B., "The Role of Biochemistry in the New Curriculum at Jefferson Medical College." *Biochem. Ed.* 2: 1974, pp. 12–14.

CHAPTER FIVE

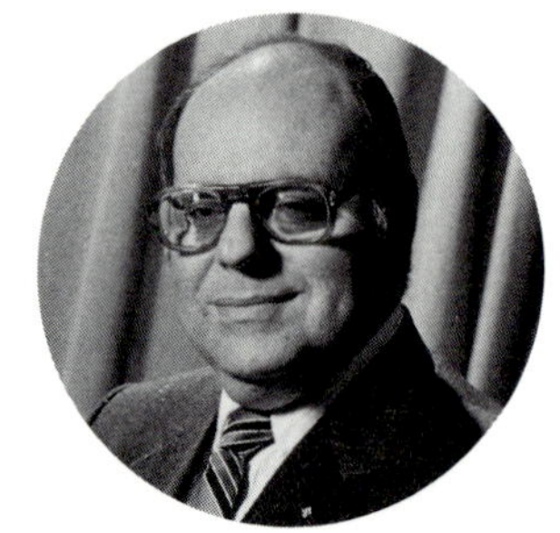

Department of Physiology

Leonard M. Rosenfeld, Ph.D.

A physician's physiology has much the same relation to his power of healing as a cleric's divinity has to his power of influencing conduct.

—Samuel Butler (1835–1902)

Although it has been said that scientific physiology emerged when primitive man first began to measure, correlate, and repeat experiences,[1] the development of medical science and its associated institutes was quite slow in Britain's thirteen North American colonies. An extensive medical treatise, with seven books devoted to physiology, was written by the noted French physician, Jean Fernel (Fernelius), as early as 1554. In 1659, Walter Charlton wrote the first English text on physiology.

The first curricular recognition of physiology was granted by the University of Edinburgh in 1726 with the appointment of Andrew Sinclair as Professor of the Institutes of Medicine. The term *Institutes of Medicine* is usually taken to mean physiology, but in practice it has actually been a composite of physiology, hygiene, physical diagnosis, experimental pathology, and even medical history and jurisprudence. The exact requirements of the Institutes were determined by the interplay between the needs of the institution and the specific interests and aptitude of the occupant of the Chair of Institutes of Medicine.

The Institutes of Medicine

In Philadelphia, a growing interest in medical affairs and progress led to the founding of Pennsylvania Hospital in 1751, its library (the first exclusively medical library in the country) in 1762, and the first school of medicine in the American colonies at the College of Philadelphia (University of Pennsylvania) in 1765. Even though the founders of the school, John Morgan and William Shippen, as graduates of the University of Edinburgh were well educated in physiology and undoubtedly shared their physiological knowledge and experiences with their students, no formal recognition of the teaching of physiology was made until Casper Wistar was appointed Professor of the Institutes of Medicine in 1789.

Once started, the medical educational infrastructure in this country developed rapidly. A medical department was established at King's College (Columbia) in 1767 and at Harvard College in 1782. As with their colleagues in Philadelphia, formalized courses in physiology were either sporadic or nonexistent for decades.

The founding of the College of Medicine of Maryland (forerunner of the University of Maryland) in 1807 established physiology as a pillar of medical education. The preamble to its charter states "that the science of medicine cannot be successfully taught under the usual organization of medical schools; that without the aids of physiology and pathology, either associated with anatomy or as a separate chair of the Institutes, the philosophy of the body in sickness or in health cannot be understood." This visionary and forceful statement of principle unfortunately was not vigorously applied in practice.

■ Physiology Formalized

Physiology was taught to the students of Jefferson Medical College at its inception, but as with other institutions of the era the subject was not presented either in depth or as a formal curricular entity. Among the tickets issued for the initial course of lectures were those bearing the inscription, "Lectures of Anatomy and Physiology by Geo. McClellan, M.D."[2] Although these lectures were undoubtedly structural in nature, with functional considerations lightly interspersed, it is nevertheless interesting to note the nineteenth-century recognition of the simultaneous consideration of structure and function (anatomy and physiology) as being the natural order. This was not a phenomenon unique at Jefferson but, rather, was the generally accepted curricular reality of the time. Later the two disciplines would go their separate ways, reuniting briefly with the reintroduction of a coordinated, integrated structure-function curricular concept nationally in the 1960s and at Jefferson in the 1970s.

Following McClellan's initial effort, whatever limited physiological instruction was presented during the organizational phase of Jefferson's existence was successfully presented by Drs. Benjamin Rush Rhees and John Revere. Revere, the youngest son of Revolutionary War patriot Paul Revere, was given the chair of Theory and Practice of Physic and as such was responsible for instruction in physiology, pathology, and therapeutics. He developed a deep interest in chemistry. In his course description, Revere identified as a prime object ". . . to point out to the student the actual state of Science; to avoid, as far as practicable, hypothetical assumptions; and to assist him in distinguishing what is known from what is conjectured."

From its inception, the Jefferson system of education combined pedagogy with practical medicine and formal lectures with exposure to actual clinical cases in both medicine and surgery. This concept was revolutionary. Belief of "the eye to be the most important organ in the acquisition of knowledge"[2] led to establishment of a prominent museum containing an extensive collection of anatomical and pathological specimens in 1834. Professors made liberal use of these specimens in illustrating their formal lectures and encouraged their students to make additional detailed observations. It was the faculty's position that they lay the foundation upon which the student subsequently, by his own diligence, observation, and study, sharpened his skills and enhanced his standing in the profession of medicine. Furthermore, as early as the academic year 1833–1834, the faculty identified the need to enhance personal interaction between professor and student. Accordingly, a series of Medical Conversaziones was established, informal gatherings of students and professors on Saturday evenings in the Hall of the Museum. The hours were 8 to 11 P.M., and light refreshments were served. The aim was to foster a unity of spirit and purpose between professor and student, stimulate enhanced diligence to study, inspire confidence, convey medical knowledge, and develop personal relationships.

Robley Dunglison, M.D., First Chairman (1836–1868)

Recognizing "the progress of Medical Science," the Board of Trustees established physiology, for the first time, as an independent course of study via the creation of a seventh Chair, a Professorship in the Institutes of Medicine and Medical Jurisprudence. Dr. Robley Dunglison[3] (Figure 5-1), distinguished physician and generally accepted

"Father of American Physiology," was elected to this chair in June, 1836. Dr. Granville Sharpe Pattison, then Professor of Anatomy at Jefferson and initiator of the negotiations that led to Dunglison's move from the University of Maryland to Jefferson, explained in a June 24, 1836, letter to Dunglison that his chair would be entitled Institutes rather than Physiology or Materia Medica so as to allow maximal latitude for his instructional program.

An Englishman by birth, Robley Dunglison studied medicine in Edinburgh and Paris, passed the examinations of the Royal College of Surgeons and the Society of Apothecaries in London, and then acquired an M.D. degree at the University of Erlangen, Bavaria, in 1823. The following year, as George McClellan set out to create a new school of medicine in Philadelphia, to the south the former president, Thomas Jefferson, was establishing a medical department in the University of Virginia, already founded in 1819. The University was to open with professors of ancient and modern languages, mathematics, natural philosophy, anatomy, and medicine. To fill this latter chair, Thomas Jefferson brought from England the young, broadly trained, and, for his youth, remarkably well-known and respected physician, Robley Dunglison.

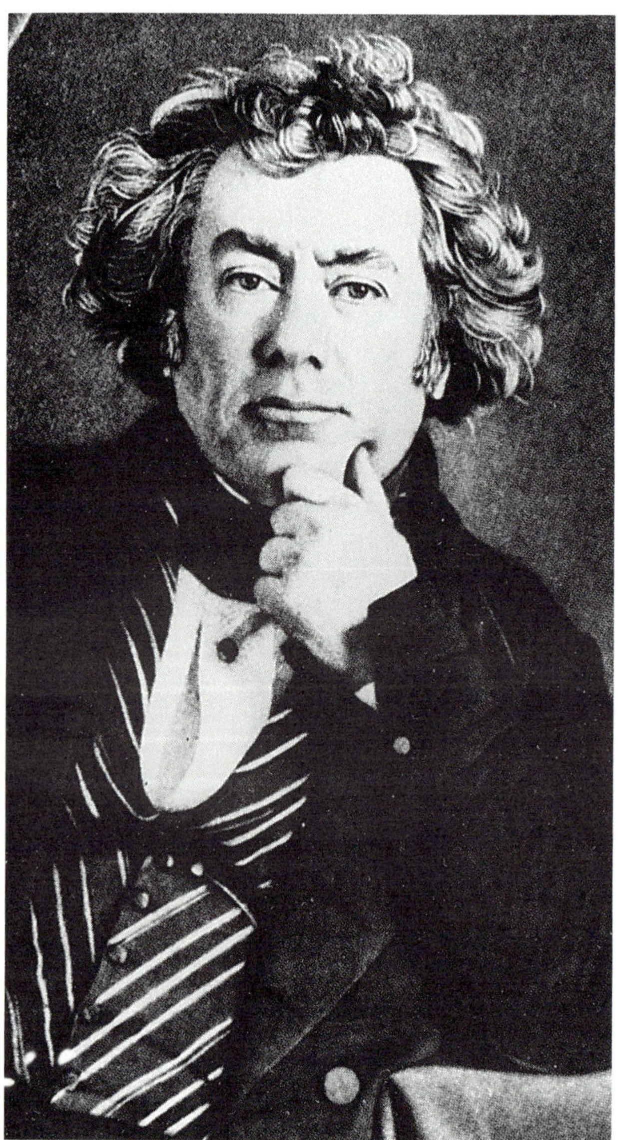

FIG. 5-1. Robley Dunglison, M.D., Professor of the Institutes of Medicine and Medical Jurisprudence (1836–1868).

■ Dunglison, Physician to Presidents

At its inception, and for the first two years of his nine-year tenure, Robley Dunglison alone was the School of Medicine of the University of Virginia. In 1827, Dunglison's responsibilities were somewhat refined as he was named Professor of Physiology, Theory, and Practice of Medicine, Obstetrics, and Medical Jurisprudence. A Professor of Chemistry and Materia Medica was simultaneously added, as was a Demonstrator of Anatomy and Surgery. A close personal and professional relationship developed between the young physician and the aging former president. Dunglison became personal physician to Thomas Jefferson, tending to his ills during the last two years of his life and actually spending the last eight days of Jefferson's life by his side. Death came to Jefferson on July 4, 1826, fifty years to the day after the signing of the Declaration of Independence. This relationship was especially unique in that, throughout his life, Jefferson was reported to have had a deep distrust of physicians.[4]

In 1833 the interaction of professional challenge, financial advancement, and desire to remove Mrs. Dunglison, who suffered from imperfect health, from the relatively primitive living conditions of Charlottesville to a different climate led to his acceptance of the professorship of Materia Medica in the University of Maryland at Baltimore. At this time, Dunglison's reputation was assured in America by the publishing in 1832 of his *Human Physiology,* a text that was to go through eight editions and become the standard in the field for many years.

In 1835 Professor Granville Sharpe Pattison set in motion forces that resulted in the Dunglisons' relocation from Baltimore to Philadelphia and the establishment of a vital role in the development of Jefferson Medical College over a period exceeding 30 years. Dunglison's establishment of a Department of Physiology was well received. Jefferson's *Catalogue of Instruction* (1839) demonstrated obvious pride when it stated, ". . . the department of physiology has been largely expanded, and it is now regarded as indispensable to make the healthy manifestations the point of departure for all enlightened pathological deductions. . . . Medical Jurisprudence, long taught in the school of continental Europe, has also taken its place as a department of instruction in our medical college."

▪ Dunglison and Beaumont

When Dunglison accepted the Institutes chair at Jefferson, he ceased practicing medicine. By devoting all his efforts to academic pursuits, he thus personified the first full-time American physiologist. Dunglison's keen mind and extensive experience continued to be highly respected in practical medical affairs, nevertheless, and resulted in 1842 in the publication of his *Practice of Medicine.* He was not an experimentalist, and he lived in an age not known for its great laboratory strengths. It is important to recognize, however, that Dunglison was involved in perhaps the most exciting and brilliant experimental contribution to the physiology of the period, the work of Dr. William Beaumont.[5]

Beaumont was the American military physician who treated woodsman Alexis St. Martin for an accidental shotgun wound. St. Martin recovered, but a permanent gastric fistula remained. Beaumont took St. Martin into his home and personally cared for him. An inquisitive mind led Beaumont into a series of innovative experiments with St. Martin that resulted in a heightened understanding of the basic physiology of the stomach. Samples of gastric juice were sent to Dunglison while he was still in Charlottesville and to Dr. Silliman at Yale. Both reported the presence of free hydrochloric acid. Dunglison and Beaumont subsequently carried on a running correspondence that Beaumont acknowledged was of great value in guiding future researchers. On at least one occasion, they met in Washington, D.C., to discuss the accumulated data and to devise additional experiments.

▪ Dunglison and Mitchell

Dunglison, the nonexperimentalist, was also a vital stimulant in the development of perhaps the greatest experimentalist, who bridged physiology and experimental medicine in the mid-nineteenth century. That man, Silas Weir Mitchell (Figure 5-2), was the son of Dr. John Kearsley Mitchell,

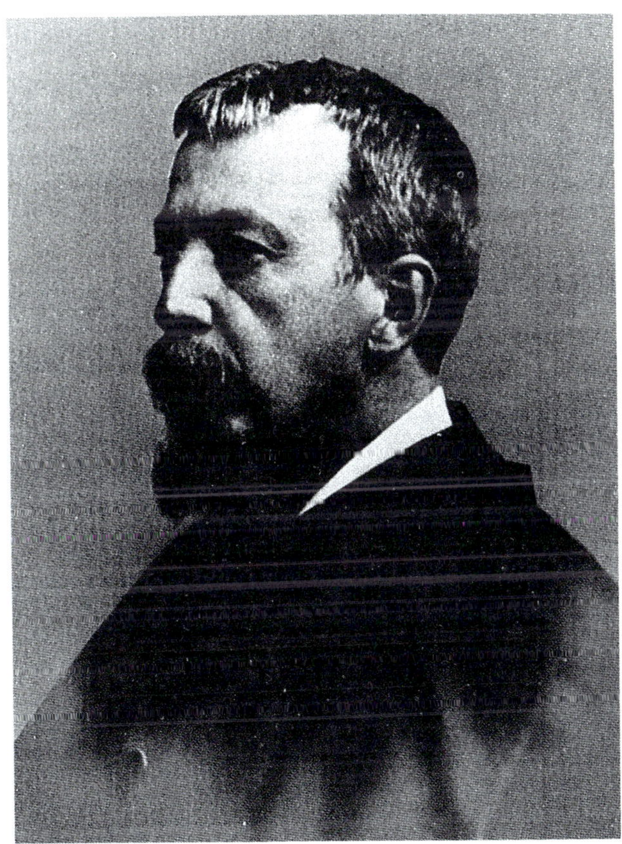

FIG. 5-2. S. Weir Mitchell, M.D., early American physiologist.

Professor of Medicine in the famous faculty of 1841. After graduating from Jefferson in 1850, Mitchell spent a year in Paris. Here he was greatly influenced by Claude Bernard, a founder of experimental medicine and originator of the *milieu interieur* concept. After investigating with Bernard the properties of rattlesnake venom, Mitchell returned to Philadelphia to continue his research. He extensively explored the physiology of the central nervous system and, via skillful union of physiology and experimental medicine, is generally credited with being the "Father of Neurology." Mitchell's experiments were revolutionary for his era. His publication in 1864 of *Gunshot Wounds and Other Injuries of Nerves,* based on his Civil War experiences and scientific observations, laid the foundation for much of the modern knowledge of neurologic symptomatology. Mitchell never held an academic appointment in physiology. A man of many talents, world-renowned clinician, premier experimental physiologist of the 1850–1875 period, man of letters and literature, he nevertheless was an unsuccessful candidate for Chairs in Physiology when those ultimately became open at the University of Pennsylvania (1863) and at Jefferson (1868). Despite this lack of a formal credential, Mitchell's influence on an emerging generation of young physicians made Philadelphia a focus of developing interest in experimental physiology.

James Aitken Meigs, M.D., Second Chairman (1868–1879)

Upon Dunglison's retirement in 1868, two of the prime candidates to succeed him were former students of his at Jefferson: Silas Weir Mitchell (Jefferson, 1850) and James Aitken Meigs (Jefferson, 1851) (Figure 5-3). Both had international reputations, Mitchell as an experimentalist and Meigs as an ethnologist. It was an era of American medicine in which there was little prestige in research. Clinical practice and teaching ability assumed much priority over the talent for investigation. Accordingly, the Trustees awarded the Chair of the Institutes of Medicine and Medical Jurisprudence to Meigs with the commencement of the 1869–1870 academic year.

Following his graduation from Jefferson, Meigs, a Philadelphian, held a series of junior teaching appointments at the Pennsylvania Medical College (founded by Dr. George McClellan) and the Philadelphia College of Medicine. He lectured at the Franklin Institute and was an active and prominent member of the Academy of Natural Sciences. Meigs had a deep interest in anthropology, and his anthropological papers were widely respected in Europe as well as in the Americas. He maintained a large private practice, which was most active in obstetrics.

In the field of medical education, Jefferson had been a leader in the concept of integrating direct clinical experience with the didactic elements. With Meigs' assumption of the Institutes Chair, his was

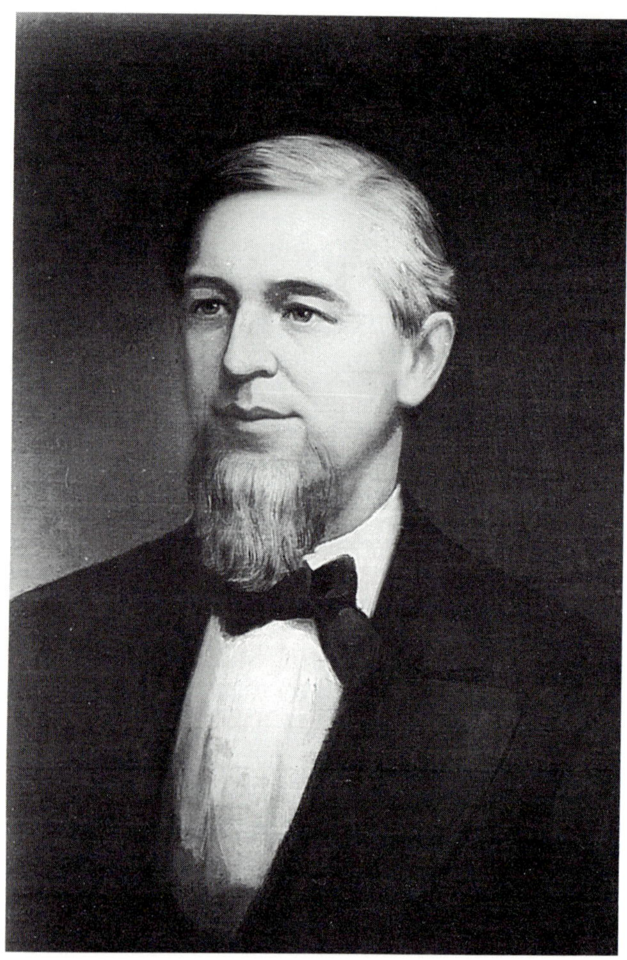

FIG. 5-3. J. Aitken Meigs, M.D., Chairman, Institutes of Medicine (1868–1879).

among the first physiology departments to use animals in demonstrations before the class. The introduction of anesthesia (ether, chloroform, nitrous oxide) further facilitated these demonstrations—such use of live animals without their suffering was quite progressive. Nevertheless, a strenuous antivivisection movement quickly developed and persisted to this day. Among those who spoke most forcefully in defense of enlightened vivisection was Silas Weir Mitchell.

Although not nearly as prolific an author as Dunglison had been, Meigs[6] nevertheless published some 30 papers, edited the American edition of Kirke's *Handbook of Physiology,* and assisted in the production of Carpenter's *The Microscope and Its Revelations*. Jefferson was among the earliest institutions to utilize seriously the microscope in medical education. A course in practical microscopy was inaugurated under the direction of Meigs as the Professor of Physiology and conducted by a Demonstrator in Histology. The laboratory was reported to be amply provided with microscopes and all other appliances requisite for thorough practical instruction.

Long a leading member of the Academy of Natural Sciences, Meigs was asked to give the address at the laying of the cornerstone of its new building in Philadelphia in 1872. He died suddenly on November 9, 1879. In April, 1880, eight recent Jefferson graduates formed in his honor the Meigs Medical Association for continuing friendship and education, which has flourished and is now one of the oldest associations of its kind in existence.[6]

Henry Cadwalader Chapman, M.D., Third Chairman (1880–1891)

With Meigs' death, the responsibilities of the department fell in midterm on his teaching assistant, Dr. H. C. Chapman. Born in Philadelphia, Henry Cadwalader Chapman (Figure 5-4), was educated at the University of Pennsylvania and its School of Medicine (M.D., 1862). Following a residency at Pennsylvania Hospital, Chapman went abroad for three years of study in London, Paris, Berlin, and Vienna. Upon his return to Philadelphia, he was named prosector (person to prepare material for demonstrations) for the Philadelphia Academy of Natural Sciences and for the Zoological Society. The latter group provided an abundance of animal material for dissection. In this work, Chapman was associated with the distinguished anatomist Dr. Joseph Leidy, of the University of Pennsylvania. The results of these studies, often performed at the Zoological Garden, appeared in the *Proceedings* of the Academy of Natural Sciences.

In 1878 Chapman was appointed Demonstrator in Physiology under Meigs and curator of the museum. He assumed complete departmental responsibility with Meigs' death. After successfully performing the duties of that department, Chapman was unanimously elected to the Chair of Institutes of Medicine and Medical Jurisprudence by the Trustees on April 12, 1880.

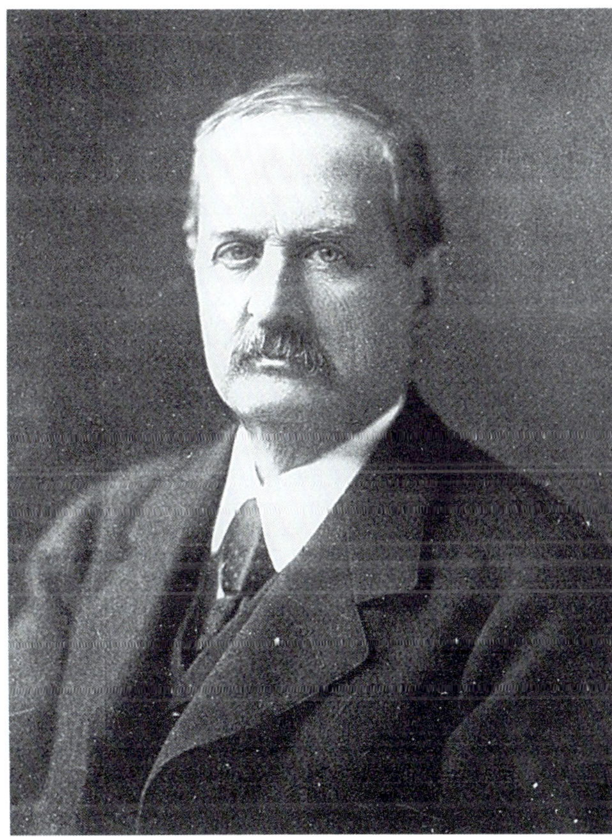

FIG. 5-4. Henry Cadwalader Chapman, M.D., Third Chairman (1880–1891).

Chapman's association with Jefferson represented historical irony. Henry Chapman was the grandson of Dr. Nathaniel Chapman. When George McClellan was struggling to establish his unprecedented second medical school in Philadelphia, it was Nathaniel Chapman who rallied his fellow faculty at the University of Pennsylvania School of Medicine to oppose Jefferson's creation. Within a year of Dunglison's arrival in Philadelphia, each of the professors of the University of Pennsylvania had paid social calls of welcome except for one: Dr. Nathaniel Chapman, despite the fact that they had previously known each other. Chapman had been entertained at Dunglison's home when he lived in Baltimore and Dunglison had visited Chapman in Philadelphia. It must be pointed out, however, that Nathaniel Chapman's opposition to Jefferson Medical College was based on purely ethical convictions. It did not tarnish his achievements as a master clinician, engaging teacher, founder of the *Philadelphia Journal of the Medical and Physical Sciences* (which became the *American Journal of the Medical Sciences*), and first President of the American Medical Association in 1847. A resolution by the Dean and Faculty of Jefferson at Nathaniel Chapman's death in 1853 attested that outward ill will no longer persisted between the two rival schools:

> "At the semi-annual meeting of the Faculty of Jefferson Medical College, held on the second day of July, 1853, the announcement of the decease of Professors Horner and Chapman having been made, it was resolved *unanimously,* that the Faculty, in common with their medical brethren, deeply deplore the loss to science of two individuals, the better part of whose valuable lives had been spent in the successful teaching of a profession of which they were distinguished ornaments, and to the advancement of which they had both so largely contributed. Resolved that a copy of this resolution be sent to the families of the deceased, and be published in the medical journals (Extracted from the minutes, R. M. Huston, M.D., Dean of the Faculty)."

The grandson's appointment to Jefferson caused no untoward reaction in either school.

As curator of the museum, Henry Chapman added significantly to its collections. When space became a problem, appropriate building modifications were made. Despite Chapman's background in prosection, he did not pursue Meigs' use of animals in teaching demonstrations with equal vigor. His postgraduate travels in Europe led to increasing utilization of the modern mechanical apparatus that was then coming into vogue for teaching purposes.

Throughout its history, Jefferson held a position of prominence in the publication of texts for medical education. Dunglison had published the standard texts in physiology and in hygiene and his *Medical Dictionary* maintained a position of supremacy for decades after his death. Meigs, in his turn, edited American editions of leading European texts. In 1887, Henry Chapman published *Human Physiology*. Subsequently, Chapman wrote the memoirs of his close friend and colleague in research, Joseph Leidy, Professor of Anatomy at the University of Pennsylvania.

S. Weir Mitchell and the American Physiological Society

The experimental elements in physiology had their foundation in Europe, primarily under the influence of Johannes Müller in Germany and Magendie and Bernard in France. With the notable exceptions of the remarkable work of Beaumont and of the enlightened S. Weir Mitchell, the experimental traditions of physiology in America would wait for the late 1870s when, almost simultaneously, three independent physiological laboratories were established: at Harvard Medical College under Bowditch, at the Graduate School of Johns Hopkins University under Newell Martin, and in physiological chemistry at Yale University under Chittenden. Within a decade of the establishment of these laboratories, a sufficient critical mass of investigators and trainees had been established, supplemented by the young medical graduates in Philadelphia, who, under the influence of S. Weir Mitchell, had sought further specialized training in physiology and medicine in Germany and France, sufficient to warrant formation of a national society of physiologists.

The American Physiological Society was formed on December 30, 1887. Although it is difficult to determine the exact origin for the concept of such a society, Howell, in the *History of the American Physiological Society*,[7] reported that the idea of forming a society of physiologists originated with Dr. S. Weir Mitchell. In November 1887, invitations to a December 30 organizational meeting were sent out over the signature of S. Weir Mitchell, H. N. Martin, and H. P. Bowditch, in that order. The organization meeting was held at the College of Physicians and Surgeons in New York with Mitchell presiding.

Of the 28 men identified in the minutes as original members of the society, three had Jefferson connections—in addition to Silas Weir Mitchell and Henry Chapman, Dr. Hobart Amory Hare was on the list. A Philadelphian by birth, Hare was educated at the University of Pennsylvania, where he received degrees in arts and in medicine (1884). Inspired by Mitchell, he pursued postgraduate experimental physiology in Leipzig and Berne and returned to Philadelphia as Lecturer in Physiology at the University of Pennsylvania. In 1890, Hare was appointed Clinical Professor of Diseases of Children at the University of Pennsylvania and in 1891 commenced a long affiliation with Jefferson as Professor of Therapeutics and Materia Medica and one of the leading medical writers in this country. Sustaining Jefferson's reputation as a leader in the publication of texts in medical education, Hare's *Practical Therapeutics* went through 22 editions.

Jefferson's importance to the founding of the American Physiological Society is further demonstrated by its hosting the first annual meeting of the Society on December 29, 1888. Mitchell was probably the most distinguished and widely known member of the Society at the time of its formation and he was elected to Council at the organization meeting but declined the offer. Had he accepted, there is little doubt that Mitchell would have been chosen president, based on his eminence and seniority of service. At the first annual meeting he was again elected to Council, accepted election, and was subsequently elected president. Mitchell served for two terms (1888–1890), when he again declined election to Council in order to serve as president of the Triennial Congress of Physicians and Surgeons. The American Physiological Society represented one of the affiliated societies of the congress, which significantly assisted the interaction between basic physiological research and experimental medicine.

At the conclusion of the inaugural meeting of the American Physiological Society, the group adjourned for the purpose of visiting Chapman's laboratory at Jefferson.[8] Seven years later, the eighth annual meeting of the Society (1895) returned to Philadelphia at the University of Pennsylvania on December 27 and at Jefferson on December 28. At this meeting, Chapman addressed the Society on "Methods of Teaching Physiology." The talk was demonstrative, illustrated by apparatus that he had previously devised. He urged the value of the comparative method and displayed a series of mammalian brains, together with other comparative anatomical preparations. Assisted by his able Demonstrator, Dr. Albert P. Brubaker, Chapman featured extensive demonstrations in digestion and absorption and in circulation, respiration, calorimetry, secretion, the nervous system, vision, voice, and hearing.

These demonstrations were effective, but Chapman and Brubaker continued to advocate that medical students perform their own laboratory experiments and thereby acquire for themselves the essential fundamentals of physiology and experimental medicine. In 1899, such a student laboratory in physiology was established at Jefferson, funded by Louis Clarke Vanuxem, Esq., a Trustee.

As reported in the February 1900 issue of the undergraduate publication, *The Jeffersonian,* the organization of the laboratory was entrusted to Professor Chapman and Dr. Brubaker, who, in conjunction with Messrs. Williams, Brown, and Earle, designed the plan, tables, and apparatus. The laboratory, 76 feet long by 22 feet wide, simultaneously accommodated two sections of 50 students each: a freshman section to investigate the fundamentals of physiological chemistry, movements of the heart, circulation of the blood, and respiration; and a section for second-year students investigating the nervous system, muscles, and special senses. From the top of each table rose substantial cases provided with sliding glass doors in which all the apparatus required by each student was kept. This obviated the necessity of carrying the apparatus from a storage room and prevented loss of time and breakage. Each case contained a kymograph, induction coil, moist chamber, electrodes, muscle levers, dissecting apparatus, physiological solutions, and drugs. For purposes of stimulating muscles and nerves, the electricity, instead of being derived from cells, came from the house current and was distributed by a controller to each station. The controller also provided each student with light, a unique feature. *The Jeffersonian,* with justifiable pride, identified this laboratory as "second to none in this country." It was a most auspicious manner in which to enter the twentieth century.

Chapman retained his chair until the conclusion of the 1908–1909 academic year, when he was made Emeritus Professor. His period of retirement was all too short, and he died on September 9, 1909, in Bar Harbor, Maine. Chosen as Chapman's successor was his long-time associate, Dr. Albert P. Brubaker. Brubaker's title was modified to that of Professor of Physiology and Medical Jurisprudence.

Albert P. Brubaker, M.D., Fourth Chairman (1904–1927)

The son of a general practitioner, Dr. Henry Brubaker of Somerset County, Pennsylvania, Albert P. Brubaker (Figure 5-5) attended Jefferson and graduated with honors in 1874. Following postgraduate training in clinical medicine at the Charity Hospital, he associated himself with Dr. Wharton Sinkler of the University of Pennsylvania at the Orthopedic Hospital. Their work involved a study of the anatomy of the nervous system and its relation to physiological and pathological processes in the body. In 1881, Henry Chapman appointed Brubaker as Demonstrator of Physiology, a position to which in 1884 Histology was added, with the further addition of Experimental Therapeutics in 1885.

When, on October 27, 1890, Jefferson's Trustees voted to vacate Dr. Roberts Bartholow's Chair of Therapeutics' Materia Medica, and Hygiene, a decision was made to postpone the election to the Chair for a year. In the interim, Brubaker was selected to give the course, the Chair of which was awarded to Dr. Hobart A. Hare in 1891.

In 1899, Brubaker was named Adjunct Professor of Physiology and Hygiene, and in 1904, Professor of Physiology and Hygiene.[9] It was the first instance of the department having two professors simultaneously. Chapman and Brubaker both gave lectures in physiology and shared duties in the weekly recitations. In addition, Brubaker gave the course in hygiene (exercise, diet, bathing and sanitation, water supply, drainage, and ventilation); Chapman gave the course in medical jurisprudence. Increased emphasis in the course of hygiene relative to the prevention of disease by measures to control microorganisms and the spread of infectious disease led to the development of later courses in bacteriology.

In addition to teaching physiology at Jefferson, Brubaker also taught at the Pennsylvania School of Dentistry and the Drexel Institute in Philadelphia.

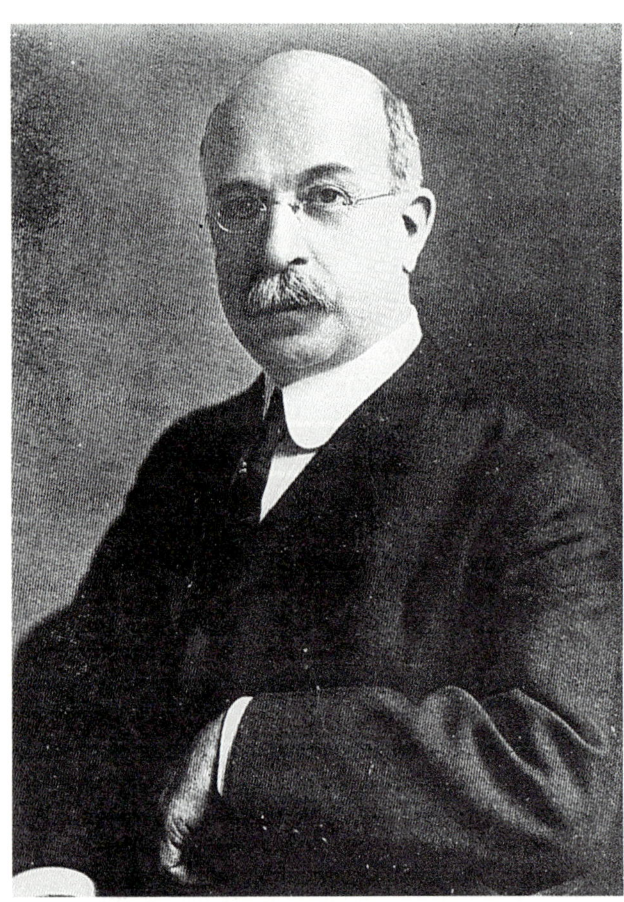

Fig. 5-5. Albert P. Brubaker, M.D., Fourth Chairman (1904–1927).

Upon Henry Chapman's relinquishment of his chair in 1909, Brubaker was elected in his stead. Brubaker was known as a kindly and fatherly person whose pedagogic style was clear, simple, and direct. Before class he would draw illustrations for the students in contrasting colors and append a synopsis to which he would strictly adhere. He was always available to his students, and in 1927 was honored by the Class of 1929 for fifty years of teaching (Figure 5-6). In keeping with the Jefferson tradition of textbook generation, Brubaker authored a *Textbook of Physiology,* which went through eight editions. In addition, to complement the emerging student laboratory in physiology, Brubaker published a *Compendium of Physiology*. A superb clarity of his lectures was evidenced in both texts. This talent for organization led to his success in numerous faculty committees and his ultimate selection as Chairman of the Faculty.

▪ The Unique Dr. Lucius Tuttle

To assist with the duties of his department, Brubaker in 1911 appointed Dr. Lucius Tuttle as Demonstrator in Physiology. Tuttle had the distinction of the longest association of any individual with the Department of Physiology, exactly fifty years (1911–1961). He was a tall, thin, moustached man, strong in mathematics, and with an introverted personality. Brubaker presented all of the lectures in physiology, while Tuttle handled the weekly recitations. Laboratory responsibilities were shared; the experiments dealt with the functions of muscles, nerves, the spinal cord, and heart, circulatory, and respiratory apparatus, as well as the pharmacological action of the more important drugs of the day.

Lucius Tuttle (Figure 5-7), a graduate of Yale,

PRESENTED TO
PROFESSOR ALBERT P. BRUBAKER M.D. LL.D.
AS AN EXPRESSION OF
ESTEEM AND AFFECTION
BY THE
CLASS OF NINETEEN-HUNDRED-TWENTY-NINE
OF THE
JEFFERSON MEDICAL COLLEGE
OF
PHILADELPHIA

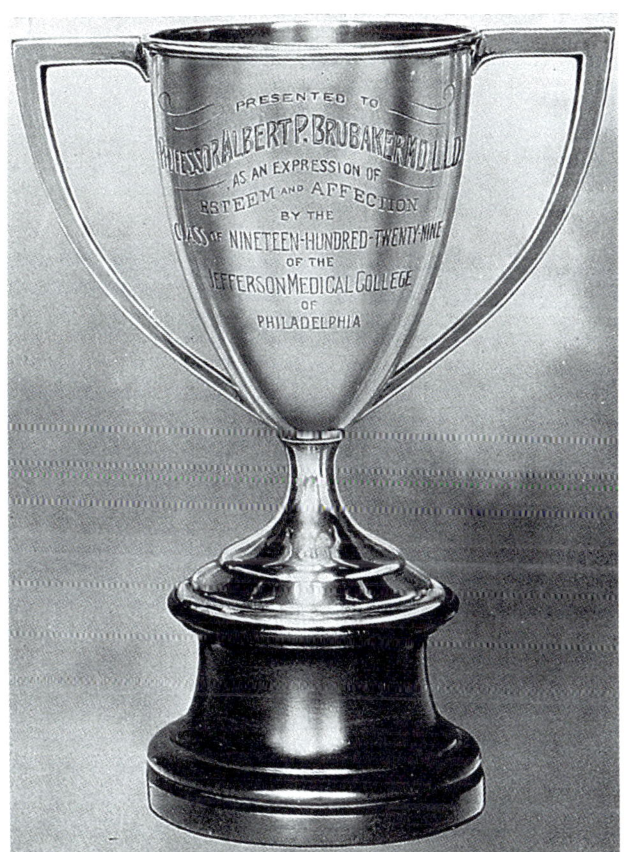

Fig. 5-6. Cup presented in 1927 honoring Professor Brubaker's fifty years of teaching.

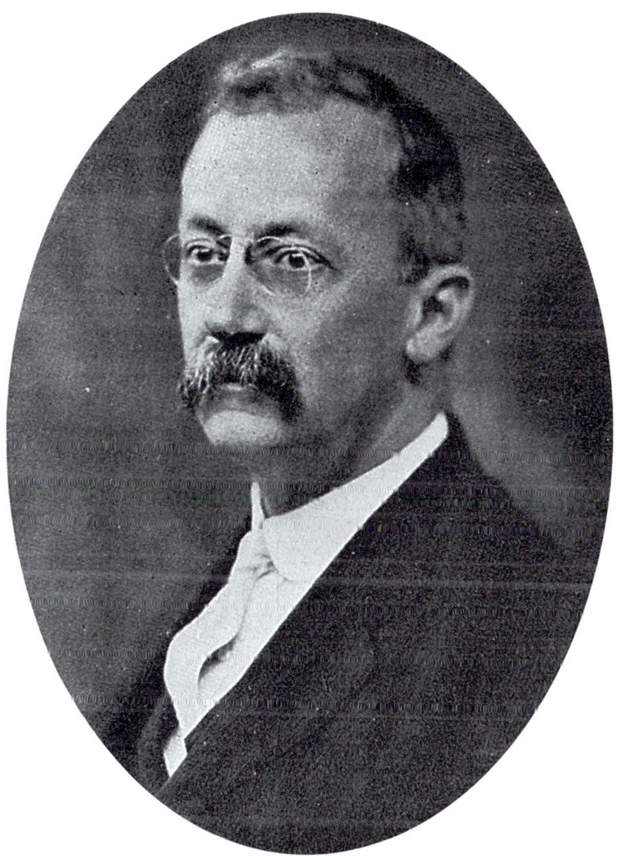

Fig. 5-7. Lucius Tuttle, M.D., Physiologist, Physicist, Mathematician.

received his M.D. degree from Johns Hopkins in 1907. His initial postgraduate position was as Assistant Demonstrator of Pathology at the University of Pennsylvania (1908–1910).[10] Having been appointed Demonstrator in Physiology at Jefferson in 1911, Tuttle's position was broadened in 1914 to Demonstrator of Physics and Physiology in recognition of his considerable mathematical aptitude. In 1915 he was named Associate in Physics and Physiology and published *Introduction to Laboratory Physics,* followed by *The Theory of Measurements* in 1916.

▪ First Graduate Education at Jefferson

In February, 1913, Jefferson's Trustees approved a resolution permitting the use of the college laboratories for holders of the bachelor's degree in arts or in science who wished to engage in special research deemed of interest and importance to medicine and surgery. This was Jefferson's first attempt at graduate education. Such persons at the end of one full year's work might be recommended by the faculty to the Trustees for the degree of Master of Science and, at the end of three years, the degree of Doctor of Philosophy. Beginning with the academic year 1914–1915, the entrance requirements for admission to Jefferson's medical course were advanced. In addition to an accredited four-year high school course, one full year of collegiate work in chemistry, physics, biology, and either German or French was necessary. In 1915, Olaf Bergeim (B.S., M.S., University of Illinois) became the first recipient of a Ph.D. from Jefferson. His dissertation, in physiological chemistry, was entitled "A Study of Calcium Metabolism in Certain Pathological Conditions." Between 1915 and 1926, a total of three Ph.D., four M.S., two D.Sc. and two B.S. degrees were awarded. After this period, graduate education did not reappear at Jefferson for over 20 years.

At the conclusion of the 1926–1927 academic year, Dr. Albert P. Brubaker retired as Professor of Physiology and Medical Jurisprudence at age 75 to become Emeritus Professor. For 30 years Brubaker was president of the Meigs Medical Association, and the Class of 1926 presented his portrait to the college. Brubaker died in 1943 at the age of 91.

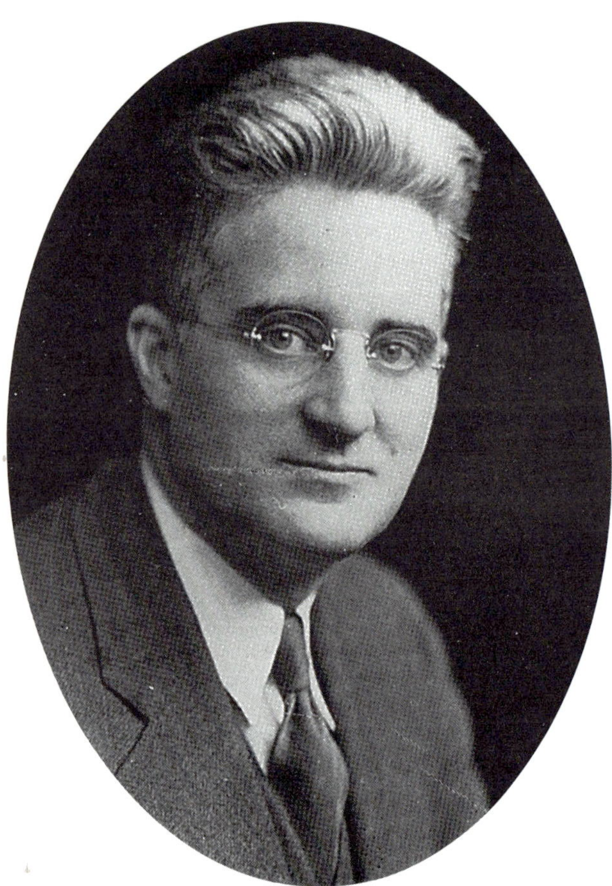

FIG. 5-8. J. Earl Thomas, M.D., Fifth Chairman (1927–1955) and Experimental Physiologist.

J. Earl Thomas, M.D., Fifth Chairman (1927–1955), Research Innovator

As Brubaker's successor, Jefferson chose Dr. J. Earl Thomas (Figure 5-8), a graduate (B.S., M.S., M.D.) of St. Louis University School of Medicine. Selecting an academic career, Thomas served as Instructor and was promoted to Assistant Professor of Physiology at St. Louis University School of Medicine (1918–1920). After an Associate Professorship in West Virginia School of Medicine (1920–1921), he returned to St. Louis University (1921–1927).

Jacob Earl Thomas[11] was a noted experimentalist, skillful experimental surgeon, and ingenious designer of research equipment. This talent for designing and making numerous pieces of laboratory equipment that came to be widely used in teaching and research has been ascribed to his boyhood experience as an apprentice in the mechanical trades. The author of more than 200 scientific papers, primarily concerning the physiology of the digestive system, Thomas materially enhanced understanding of the regulation of gastric emptying, the filling and evacuation of the gallbladder, the autoregulation of gastric secretion, the complexities of the enteroenteric reflexes, and the mechanisms of pancreatic secretion. Instrumentation and techniques that he developed to aid these advances include the Thomas drop recorder, the Thomas wrench, the Thomas intestinal cannula, the Thomas gastric pouch, and the Thomas pancreatic fistula.

In Thomas' department Tuttle assumed responsibility for approximately one-third of the lectures: the physiology of blood, muscle, and nerve, electrophysiology, and the physiology of sensation, with appropriate demonstrations to the class. In 1929, Tuttle was named Assistant Professor when Jefferson moved into the 1025 Walnut Street College. The new physiology laboratory provided facilities that fostered student experiments on larger animals and in wider variety than the earlier laboratory of 1899.

In 1931, Thomas expanded the full-time department faculty to three with the appointment of Dr. Joseph Otterbein Crider as Associate Professor. At this time Crider was already a mature academician. Born in Harrisonburg, Virginia, he received his M.D. degree in 1912 from the University of Virginia School of Medicine, Charlottesville, the institution that Robley Dunglison had first established for Thomas Jefferson. After an initial appointment as Associate Professor of Physiology and Pharmacology at the University of Virginia (1912–1913), he moved to the University of Mississippi School of Medicine where he successively served as Associate Professor of Physiology and Histology (1913–1916), Professor of Physiology and Histology and Assistant Dean (1916–1924), and Professor of Physiology and Dean (1924–1930). At Jefferson, he was concomitantly Assistant Dean. In a deep southern accent, Crider did most of the interviewing of prospective Jefferson students as admissions officer under Dean Ross V. Patterson.

Crider joined Thomas in presenting lectures and demonstrations on the physiology of the major organ systems. Recitations were conducted by Thomas, Crider, and Tuttle—the latter two shared the responsibilities of the student laboratory. As early as 1928, Thomas had introduced research as a student option: "Students may, at the discretion of the member of the staff concerned, be permitted to act as voluntary assistants in the research of the department." Such an enhancement of the program became possible not merely as a result of Thomas' interest in research but also as a reflection of the maturation of the college and of its student body. In 1929, three years of collegiate work became a prerequisite for admission to Jefferson. In 1930, these options were further enhanced by the announcement that "properly qualified candidates may, at the discretion of the Department and College administration, be granted fellowships for full or part-time research or teaching." Christopher J. Morgan, M.D. served as a Research Fellow in Physiology (1931) and assisted with both recitations and the student laboratory.

J. Earl Thomas was a man who was intellectually curious and had a deep commitment to experimental physiology. Nevertheless, he never failed to devote himself wholeheartedly to teaching. His lectures were always exceptionally well organized on small note cards and were clear, concise, and easily understood. A significant amount of material was contained within each lecture but was so well paced that the student could take excellent notes. Thomas always exhibited a sympathetic attitude toward those in scholastic difficulties and never was too busy to help a student.

▪ The Physiological Society

In 1932 Thomas assumed the presidency of perhaps the oldest local physiology society in the nation, the Physiological Society of Philadelphia. Founded October 10, 1904, as the Society of Normal and Pathological Physiology at the medical laboratories of the University of Pennsylvania, this originally "in-house" discussion group was to evolve into a strong regional and national influence in the growth and advancement of the profession. Lucius Tuttle, while still on the faculty of the University of Pennsylvania, appears in minutes of the meeting of November 23, 1908, as a guest of the society. Interestingly, the minutes of this same meeting contained an affirmation "to extend membership and usefulness outside the University of Pennsylvania." Tuttle was elected to active membership in the society on March 1, 1909. (Brubaker would appoint Tuttle to the Jefferson faculty in 1911).

The name Albert P. Brubaker first appears in the minutes of the society as a guest at the meeting of March 22, 1909. Thereafter, he was a frequent discussant of members' presentations and was elected to full membership on March 25, 1913. The January 1916 membership list of the society contained the name of Olaf Bergeim, first recipient of a Ph.D. from Jefferson (1915). On December 15, 1919, the society adopted its current name of the Physiological Society of Philadelphia.

Thomas served as president of the society, 1932–1934. He was influential in enhancing its regional status and membership. Under his auspices, the first meeting of the society at Jefferson occurred on January 16, 1933. He established the role of the Physiology Society of Philadelphia as an international forum for the most advanced physiological thought of the day. At a special meeting of the society on April 18, 1933, Sir Henry H. Dale addressed an audience of 350 on "Progress in Autopharmacology." The next year, at a similar special meeting of the society held on April 3, 1934, Dr. Corneille Heymans (Professor of Pharmacology, University of Ghent) discussed "The Role of the Carotid Sinus in the Regulation of Blood Pressure and Heart Frequency" before an overflow crowd of 400.

The society progressed, retaining its sturdy foundation at the University of Pennsylvania but incorporating the physiological strength of the entire region. Thomas had been the first Jeffersonian to lead the Physiological Society of Philadelphia, but he would not be the last. For the next 50 years, the further development of the society would be intimately intertwined with significant names of physiologists at Jefferson: Friedman, DeBias, Siegman, and Lefer.

New Relationships

The year 1940 marked the beginning of a decade of significant expansion of the Department under Thomas. The appointment of a number of truly outstanding fellows, with joint responsibilities in the Departments of Physiology and Medicine, and the expansion of the full-time faculty resulted in meaningful and continuing research that incorporated basic and clinical science. Among the earliest and most productive of these fellowships was that awarded to Dr. Karl E. Paschkis.

Viennese by birth, Karl Ernst Paschkis received his undergraduate and medical education at the University of Vienna. Following graduation (1919) he accepted positions as Assistant in Anatomy, University of Vienna Medical School (1920), and a clinical appointment at Kaiser Franz Joseph Hospital (1920–1924), and as Acting Director of its Department of Pathology (1924–1925). He held subsequent clinical appointments in the Department of Medicine at Vienna's University Hospital (1925–1931), and Allgemeine Poliklinik (1931–1938). As the political climate of Austria turned increasingly unsettled, Paschkis, at 42 years of age and with an established academic and professional reputation, emigrated from Austria to the United States.

Arriving in Philadelphia, Paschkis became a Research Associate at the Fels Institute (later a part of Temple University), where he expanded his horizons by engaging in endocrine physiological research. In 1940 he came to Jefferson as Teaching and Research Fellow in Physiology and Medicine. In the Department of Physiology, Paschkis assumed the responsibility for the lectures in endocrine physiology. His research in endocrinology developed along interdepartmental lines and resulted in Jefferson's Endocrine Clinic becoming widely recognized as an important center for research, clinical treatment, and training in endocrinology. Karl Paschkis was appointed chief of this clinic in 1942 and Associate in Physiology in 1944. As his research became more directed toward endocrinological aspects of carcinogenesis, still greater interdepartmental activity resulted, leading to eventual formation of a Division of Endocrine and Cancer Research in 1949 with Karl Paschkis as director. Principal collaborators in these interdepartmental efforts were Paschkis (physiology/medicine), Abraham Cantarow (biochemistry), and Abraham Rakoff (obstetrics/gynecology). Additional important collaboration was supplied by Romano DeMeio (biochemistry), Adolph Walkling (surgery), and Joseph Rupp (medicine). Over 100 research publications resulted from these collaborative efforts.

Clinical Physiology

At the time of Paschkis' initial appointment in 1940, two outstanding young physicians were similarly named fellows, with joint responsibilities in both the Departments of Physiology and in Medicine: Drs. C. Wilmer Wirts and J. Edward Berk. Both men shared Thomas' interest in gastroenterology and devoted their careers to its advancement in education, research, and clinical training. Aside from postgraduate training in Chicago, London, and Paris, Wirts (Jefferson, 1934) maintained his Jefferson affiliation in excess of 40 years, enhancing clinical research and training in the Gastrointestinal Division of the Department of Medicine. A pioneer in gastrointestinal endoscopy, Wirts authored approximately 150 publications and was instrumental in obtaining the first National Institutes of Health fellowship training grant in gastroenterology in Philadelphia for Jefferson. He served as president of both the American Gastroscopic Society and of the American College of Gastroenterology.

J. Edward Berk (Jefferson, 1936) took his postgraduate training at the Graduate School of Medicine of the University of Pennsylvania and at the Albert Einstein Medical Center of Philadelphia before being named a Ross V. Patterson Fellow in Physiology at Jefferson in 1940. Subsequently, Berk held academic positions at the University of Pennsylvania, Temple University (Assistant Director, Fels Research Institute), Wayne State University, and the University of California, Irvine (Head, Division of Gastroenterology, and Chairman, Department of Medicine). He authored over 250 publications. In recognition of his many talents, Berk was elected governor of the American Society for Gastrointestinal Endoscopy, chairman of the Section of Gastroenterology of the American Medical Association, president of the Bockus International Society of Gastroenterology, and president of the American College of Gastroenterology. He received the Jefferson Alumni Achievement Award in 1977.

While attending the March 1941 meetings of the Federation of American Societies for Experimental Biology in Chicago, Thomas and Crider encountered Dr. M.H.F. Friedman, then a Research Associate in Physiology at Wayne State University. Impressed with his background, and the manner in which Friedman handled potentially sensitive issues at the meetings, Thomas offered Friedman a position in his department.

A Canadian by birth (Montreal), Moe Hegby Fred Friedman was educated at McGill University (B.Sc., 1930), University of Western Ontario (M.A., 1932), and then again at McGill University (Ph.D. in Physiology, 1937). At Jefferson, Friedman's initial responsibilities included participation with Thomas, Crider, and Tuttle in recitations and with Crider and Tuttle in the physiology laboratory and demonstrations. His investigative interests, as with Thomas, focused on gastrointestinal physiology. While at Wayne State, Friedman had worked with an extract of urine that was reported to inhibit gastric secretion and to offer therapeutic possibilities for ulcer treatment. This was the work that he reported in Chicago before Thomas and Crider. At Jefferson he worked to develop a method of isolating rather pure secretin from pig intestine, a method that Wyeth Laboratories ultimately utilized as the first commercially successful method of obtaining secretin in this country. It was this preparation that Thomas and Crider utilized in their pioneering studies of pancreatic physiology.

At the outbreak of World War II (the academic session of 1941–1942), many of the staff physicians joined the Jefferson Hospital Unit. Friedman often went to the Gastrointestinal Clinic to aid the remaining short-handed staff. These contacts led to lifelong relationships that resulted in clinically relevant joint investigative projects.

Concurrent with Friedman's joining the department in 1941, Thomas named Irwin Jack

Pincus (Jefferson, 1937) as Patterson Fellow in Physiology. Pincus' postgraduate training was at the University of Pennsylvania and in Los Angeles. Following his fellowship year of 1941–1942, he accepted clinical appointments at Valley Forge General Hospital, Philadelphia General Hospital, and the Philadelphia Veterans Administration Hospital before returning to Jefferson in 1946 as Instructor in Physiology. While maintaining a clinical practice, Pincus investigated the properties of glucagon, its role in carbohydrate metabolism, and its potential relation to the etiology of diabetes mellitus.

In 1945, Thomas appointed William J. Snape (Jefferson, 1940) as Associate in Physiology. As with Pincus, Snape maintained a clinical practice while pursuing studies of gallbladder function and biliary secretion, using a newly developed type of biliary fistula (developed by Snape in cooperation with other departmental members). In addition, Snape, who went on to become Chief of Gastroenterology at Cooper Hospital (Camden, New Jersey) engaged in cooperative studies with Drs. Friedman and W. Addison Clay (Public Health Service Fellow in Physiology, 1949–1951) concerning the effect of certain antihistamines on gastric secretion, particularly the secretion induced by histamine or by gastrin.

By 1945, the effects of age and chronic illness led Lucius Tuttle to conclude that he could no longer maintain the full-time involvement in the department that he had sustained since 1911. There being no pension plan in force at the time, nor social security or other income, Tuttle was retained on the departmental roster as Assistant Professor and his salary was maintained. This special arrangement was confirmed by the Trustees on October 27, 1947, and continued until 1961 (50 years from the date when Tuttle first joined the department). On March 27, 1961, the Executive Faculty named Lucius P. Tuttle an Honorary Professor of Physiology, and on May 4, 1961, Tuttle succumbed in Jefferson Hospital.

▪ Postwar Developments

Further expansion of the Department resulted with the appointment in 1946 of Irving H. Wagman as Associate, in 1947 with Jerome M. Waldron as Instructor and Samuel Stinger Conly, Jr. as Demonstrator. A native of New York City, Dr. Wagman received his Ph.D. in Physiology in 1941 from the University of California, Berkeley. Trained as a neurophysiologist, Dr. Wagman initiated studies at the University of California and subsequently at the National Institutes of Health in vision and oculomotor mechanics. On arriving at Jefferson, Wagman joined Thomas in an investigation of degeneration and regeneration of the vagus nerves growing out of Dr. Thomas' interest in vagotomy as a potential treatment for peptic ulcer. In addition, Wagman obtained a U.S. Public Health Service grant to study the problems of aging, specifically to determine the changes that occur in the functional capacity of peripheral nerves and reflex centers from infancy to old age. In cooperation with members of the Department of Biophysics at Johns Hopkins, Wagman extended his earlier work on the function of the extraocular muscles in relation to eye movement and the measurement of light threshold of the visual sense organ.

Following graduation from the University of Pennsylvania School of Medicine (1943), Dr. Jerome Michael Waldron interned at Fitzgerald–Mercy Hospital (Darby, Pennsylvania), followed by a Fellowship in Medicine at Pennsylvania Hospital. At Jefferson, Dr. Waldron collaborated closely with Dr. Garfield Duncan of the Department of Medicine, studying the hypercoagulability of blood and the heightened danger of thrombosis following the ingestion of significant amounts of dietary lipid. Within the Department, Waldron joined Drs. Friedman and Snape in their studies on the secretion and activity of pancreatic and other digestive enzymes.

▪ Dr.Samuel S. Conly, Jr.

When Samuel Stinger Conly, Jr., and his classmates entered the first-year class at Jefferson in September, 1941, this country was about to enter World War II. As the international climate degenerated and hostilities broke out, Jefferson adjusted its curriculum to meet the emergency. Physicians were needed in large numbers and quickly. The curriculum was modified to accomodate two classes a year. Conly's class graduated in September, 1944, rather than June, 1945. At the end of their junior year most of the class entered the Army (AST, Army Student Training Program) as privates. Every morning, before class, drill was held on a field at Lombard Street between 10th and 11th Streets. After an abbreviated internship (twelve-month program shortened to nine months), they became first lieutenants. Conly interned at Bryn Mawr Hospital and then went into the Army for two years. Upon returning he informed Dr. Thomas of his interest in biology, whereupon he was offered the position of Assistant Demonstrator. Conly joined Dr. Crider in studying the secretion of bicarbonate by the pancreas in dogs with experimentally induced acidosis. For three years (1947–1950), Conly split his efforts between a developing private practice and his departmental responsibilities. This dual arrangement proved to be excessive, causing Conly to relinquish his position within the department in order to devote full time to his practice (1950–1953). In 1953 he reassumed his affiliation with the Department as Assistant Professor. Shortly thereafter, Dean George Bennett offered Conly a joint appointment in the office of the dean, and in 1956 Conly became Assistant to the Dean, reestablishing a relationship that had been held by Dr. Joseph O. Crider until 1952.

Graduate Education Formalized Again

Jefferson's postwar development was coincident with an increasing role for research. Thomas was part of the faculty nucleus of active researchers. At the time, there were concerns about how research was to be fostered as well as about the actual training of potential researchers. These concerns came to a head during Thomas' tenure as Chairman of the College Faculty. At a January 31, 1949, meeting of the faculty, chaired by Thomas, a recommendation was approved in support of Jefferson offering graduate training leading to the degrees of Master of Science and Doctor of Philosophy for qualified students in the basic medical sciences. Authority for such programs was vested in the full university charter under which Jefferson Medical College had functioned since its independent charter of 1838. This proposal was unanimously endorsed by the Board of Trustees at its meeting of February 15, 1949, providing "that the work done in these subjects shall not constitute credits for the degree of Doctor of Medicine. . . . " Thomas appointed a faculty committee, the chairs of the basic science departments, to draw up the plans for reinstitution of graduate education after a 20-year hiatus. This committee evolved into the Board of Regulation of Graduate Studies.

Throughout the decade of the 1940s Thomas had significantly enhanced the Department of Physiology by the selection of a number of truly outstanding Fellows: Paschkis, Wirts, Berk, and Pincus. In 1951 Thomas continued this tradition with the appointment of Frank Pickering Brooks as Fellow in Physiology. A 1943 graduate of the University of Pennsylvania School of Medicine, Frank Brooks took a rotating medical internship and then a two-year residency in radiology at the Hospital of the University of Pennsylvania. Following two years of active duty in the Navy (1946–1948), Dr. Brooks spent two additional years in postgraduate training as a Fellow in Gastroenterology at the Lahey Clinic, supplemented by another year of medical training at the Hospital of the University of Pennsylvania. Earl Thomas played a key role in Brooks' professional development. The year spent with Thomas (1951–1952) was pivotal in directing Brooks into a career that combined clinical medicine with investigative medicine and physiology.

At Jefferson, Brooks studied the effect of gastric juice and alcohol on pancreatic exocrine function. Returning to the University of Pennsylvania in 1952, Brooks held joint appointments in medicine and physiology, attaining the rank of professor in each in 1970. From 1962 to 1972 Brooks served as Chief of Gastroenterology at the Hospital of the University of Pennsylvania. His active research program continued the work of Thomas' laboratory: neurohumoral control of gastric secretion and the regulation of pancreatic exocrine function. The editor of several textbooks on gastrointestinal physiology and pathophysiology, he maintained an active role in national and international aspects of clinical gastroenterology and gastrointestinal physiology. Brooks served as

Chairman of the Gastrointestinal Section of the American Physiology Society, Chairman of the Gastroenterology Research Group, National Commission on Digestive Diseases, and President of the American Gastroenterological Association.

The period of the early 1950s was one of political turmoil in the United States. In reaction to the international spread of communism, a virulent movement developed, with its purpose the ferreting out of "un-American" elements from our society. Senator Joseph McCarthy became a symbol of this movement. Mere accusation, or the holding of unpopular ideas, could cost individuals their positions. It was a difficult time for civil liberties. Jefferson did not escape this turmoil, nor did the Department of Physiology.

Refusing to sign a loyalty oath in 1953, Dr. Irving H. Wagman, Associate Professor, was one of Jefferson's faculty members whose loyalty was questioned. The Medical College on reviewing Wagman's case dismissed him from the faculty. Dr. Thomas strenuously defended Wagman and was bitterly disappointed by his dismissal. After leaving Jefferson, Wagman moved to the Mount Sinai Hospital in New York City in 1954, where he pursued investigative studies on the control of eye movements. Wagman was recognized for this work by election to the Harvey Society of New York, the Association for Research in Nervous and Mental Diseases, the American Academy of Neurology, and the American Neurological Association. He was especially proud of his membership in the latter two organizations because he was one of the few basic scientists to be so recognized by these clinical societies.

Returning to California in 1961 to join the research faculty at the University of California in San Francisco, Wagman studied cutaneous sensation and sensorimotor integration. A desire to once again become involved in undergraduate teaching led Wagman in 1965 to relocate to the University of California, Davis, where until his death in 1977, he was instrumental in developing a high-caliber curriculum that included sophisticated laboratory courses and self-paced learning programs to supplement the lecture courses. In addition, he continued his research on somesthesia and somatic reflexes.

To replace Wagman, Thomas was able in 1954 to obtain the services of neurophysiologist Eugene Aserinsky as Instructor. Awarded the Ph.D. degree from the University of Chicago in 1953, Aserinsky, while still a graduate student, had been the discoverer of rapid eye movement (REM). In addition to the physiology of sleep and the role of REM therein, Aserinsky's investigative studies ranged from the activity of the spinal cord, retinal potentials in man, and the pathophysiological effects of electric shock to the nature of rhythmic biological phenomena in man.

M.H.F. Friedman, Ph.D., Sixth Chairman (1955–1974)

Not long after the Wagman incident Thomas' health deteriorated. Suffering from ulcer disease, he was advised to take a prolonged rest, whereupon he departed for a lake in Northern Ontario for a period of approximately six months. With improved health, Thomas returned to Jefferson for a final year, after which he accepted the less taxing position of Chairman of the Department of Physiology at the College of Medical Evangelists, Loma Linda, California, in 1955. Dr. M.H.F. Friedman (Figure 5-9), was designated Acting Chairman until 1957, when he formally succeeded J. Earl Thomas to the Chair. Dr. Thomas died in California on February 2, 1972, at the age of 81. His portrait, presented by the Class of 1948, hangs in Jefferson Alumni Hall.

On assuming the Chair, Friedman abolished both Saturday classes, divided student laboratories into smaller units, and added to the faculty Drs. Louis A. Kazal, as Assistant Professor, and Domenic A. DeBias as Instructor. Kazal, a 1940 graduate of Rutgers University (Ph.D., Biochemistry), was a research biochemist with the Merck, Sharp & Dohme Pharmaceutical Corporation (Director, Biological Development; Manager, Technical Information; and Technical Assistant to the Medical Director) before accepting a joint appointment in physiology and medicine (Cardeza Foundation for Hematological Research) at Jefferson in 1957. His research involved the chemistry and biophysics of blood coagulation and erythropoiesis. Kazal served Jefferson for the remainder of his professional career. In the Department of Physiology he presented lectures on the physiology of coagulation, developed laboratory exercises in coagulation, and engaged in and supervised graduate student research in coagulation and erythropoiesis. At the Cardeza Foundation, Kazal headed the Plasma Fractionation Unit from the time of his arrival, and served as Associate Director of the Cardeza Foundation from 1960 until his retirement in 1978.

Domenic DeBias received his Ph.D. degree in Physiology from Jefferson in 1956. He was the first graduate student of the Department to assume a staff position at Jefferson; his thesis research had been under the supervision of Karl Paschkis. DeBias' investigative studies involved adrenal and thyroid function stress. Later work involved hormonal factors associated with endurance to high altitude and the evaluation of sequelae to myocardial infarction with exposure to environmental pollutants (e.g., carbon monoxide).

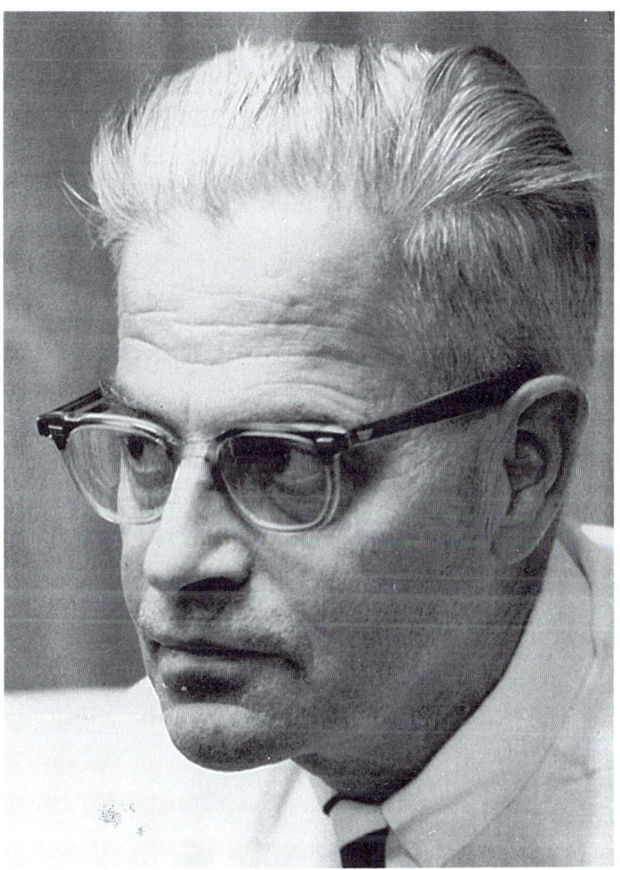

FIG. 5-9. M.H.F. Friedman, Ph.D., Sixth Chairman (1955–1974).

In the early 1970s Jefferson's curriculum embraced a concept the roots of which dated back to its earliest days: integrated teaching. After establishing a course, cell and tissue biology, that integrated biochemistry with elements of histology and genetics, anatomy and physiology were brought into an integrated course, structure and function. Dr. DeBias was selected as coordinator of this ambitious undertaking and served in this capacity until 1975, when he was named Chairman of the Department of Physiology at the Philadelphia College of Osteopathic Medicine.

The Basic Sciences Mature

Friedman responded to the increasing importance of cellular physiology and biophysics by the appointment in 1958 of Dr. June N. Barker as Instructor and in 1960 by Dr. Daniel L. Gilbert as Assistant Professor. Trained at the University of Rochester (B.S., 1952) and at Duke University (M.A., 1954, Ph.D., Physiology, 1956), Barker came to Jefferson after serving a year as Instructor in Physiology at Duke University. She was the first woman to receive a faculty appointment in physiology at Jefferson. A conservative institution, slow to change, Jefferson at the time of Barker's appointment was still three years away from admitting its first woman medical student (1961). A specialist in water and electrolyte metabolism, Barker conducted research in fetal physiology (intrauterine fluid balance, cerebral and pulmonary circulation, and metabolism). She pioneered in the development of ultramicrotechniques in fluid and tissue analysis. In 1964 Barker left Jefferson for a research career in physiology and rehabilitation medicine at the School of Medicine of New York University.

A graduate of Drew University (A.B., 1948), University of Iowa (M.S., 1950) and the University of Rochester (Ph.D. in Physiology, 1955), Daniel Gilbert held faculty appointments in physiology at the School of Medicine and Dentistry of the University of Rochester (1955–1956) and at Albany Medical College (1956–1960) before coming to Jefferson. His work in biophysics involved membrane permeability, ion distribution and equilibria, radiobiology/radiation toxicity, and the biophysics of evolution. Gilbert left Jefferson in 1963 to head the Section on Cellular Biophysics of the National Institute of Neurological Diseases and Stroke.

Friedman further strengthened the traditionally strong gastrointestinal base of the Department with the appointment in 1961 of Dr. Donald B. Doemling as Instructor. A graduate of St. Benedict's College (B.S., 1952) and the University of Illinois (M.S., 1954, and Ph.D. in Physiology, 1958), Doemling held academic appointments in physiology at the University of Illinois (1952–1957) and physiology and pharmacology at the Dental School of Northwestern University (1957–1960) before coming to Philadelphia. A dedicated teacher and skillful experimental surgeon, he took charge of and reorganized the student laboratories, in addition to his teaching responsibilities in intestinal absorption and renal physiology. His interests in intestinal absorption, inflammation, and lymph formation and flow led to the development of a surgical technique for chronic implantation of a thoracic duct cannula, allowing uninterrupted lymph collections over periods of months. Doemling returned to Chicago in 1968 to assume the Chair in Physiology and Pharmacology at the Loyola University School of Dentistry.

In recognition of the need for better understanding of smooth muscle function, Dr. Marion J. Siegman was appointed Instructor in 1967. A graduate of Tulane University (B.A., 1954) and the State University of New York (Ph.D. in Pharmacology, 1966), Dr. Siegman brought valuable laboratory experience in the study of the mechanical properties of smooth muscle. Her research interests included the energetics of contraction, excitation-contraction coupling, and cation transport and metabolism. A strong proponent of meaningful interaction among researchers, Siegman was one of the founding members of the Philadelphia Muscle Institute, an interdisciplinary areawide federally funded research center for the study of muscle, headquartered at the University of Pennsylvania. A member of the National Science Foundation Review Committee on Cell Biology and of the National Institutes of Health Physiology Study Section, in 1977 she became the first woman to be named Professor of Physiology at Jefferson.

Until 1964 Domenic DeBias had taught both the respiratory and endocrine sections of the physiology course. In that year Friedman brought in Dr. Sheldon F. Gottlieb as Assistant Professor. The era of organ system specialization was at hand. Following graduation from Brooklyn College and the University of Texas (Ph.D. in Physiology, 1959), Gottlieb joined the research laboratories of the Linde Division of Union Carbide Corporation as a research physiologist (1959–1964), investigating physiological and biochemical effects of hyperbaric gaseous environments on living systems. At Jefferson, in addition to his responsibilities in respiratory physiology, Gottlieb pursued his research interests both within the Department and through a joint appointment in the Department of Anesthesiology. In 1968 he left Jefferson to serve as Professor in the Department of Biological Sciences, Purdue University, until being named Dean of the Graduate School and Director of Research at the University of South Alabama in 1981.

Friedman continued to build up his Department through the 1960s. Departmental responsibilities were expanding, as was the degree of specialization of the staff. After bringing in Barker from Duke, Gilbert from Rochester, Doemling from Chicago, Siegman from New York, and Gottlieb from industry, Friedman added a number of Jefferson's own trainees to the faculty. Dr. Leonard M. Rosenfeld (A.B., University of Pennsylvania, 1959; Ph.D. in Physiology, Jefferson, 1964) (see Figure 5-10) was appointed Instructor in 1964. He assumed June Barker's teaching responsibilities in water and electrolyte metabolism as well as part (all, after 1974) of the gastrointestinal block. In 1975 Rosenfeld was named to replace Domenic DeBias as physiology teaching coordinator, both within the Department and within the integrated anatomy-physiology structure-and-function framework. His research included intestinal metabolism, cell population dynamics, electrolyte metabolism, and splanchnic blood flow/ischemia as well as studies on nutrition, air pollution, and myocardial infarction (diagnostic enzymology).

Dr. Eugene J. Zawoiski (Ph.D. in Physiology, Jefferson, 1963) was appointed Instructor in 1965. From 1951 to 1965, Dr. Zawoiski engaged in pathological, toxicological, physiological, pharmacological, and teratological research at Merck, Sharp & Dohme, and subsequently at the Merck Institute for Therapeutic Research. At

Jefferson, Zawoiski taught renal physiology and had extensive involvement in the teaching of physiology to student nurses in the diploma program, serving as course coordinator (1975–1980). He pursued his teratological research as well as studies on central nervous system involvement in gastrointestinal function.

In 1968, Dr. Chandra M. Banerjee was named Assistant Professor to replace Sheldon Gottlieb. Born in Calcutta, India, Banerjee received his medical education at the University of Calcutta and his physiology training at the Medical College of Virginia (Ph.D. in Physiology, 1967). After several clinical assignments in India (1955–1958) and in New York (1959–1960), Banerjee served as staff scientist in respiratory physiology at Hazelton Laboratories in Virginia (1967–1968). At Jefferson, he followed Gottlieb in holding joint appointments in physiology and anesthesiology. His research interests centered on the pulmonary effect of air pollutants, pulmonary edema, and the respiratory consequences of myocardial infarction. In 1974, Banerjee left Jefferson to take up the position of Professor of Physiology at the Southern Illinois University School of Medicine.

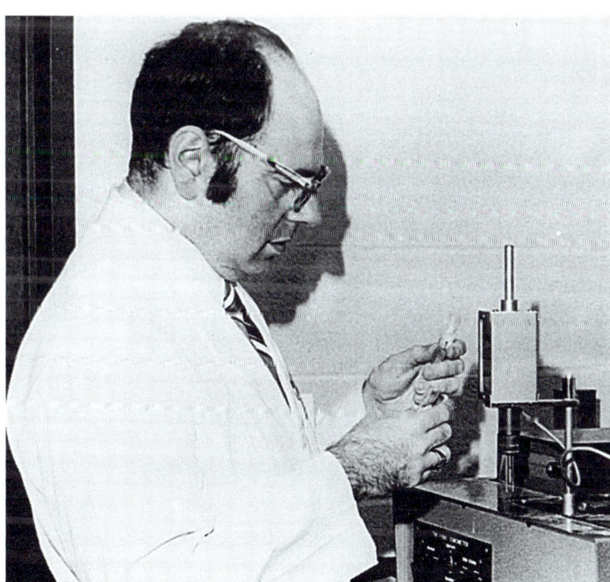

FIG. 5-10. Leonard M. Rosenfeld, Ph.D., Assistant Professor of Physiology, with main interest in the gastrointestinal system.

To fill the void created by Doemling's departure, Banerjee recommended a former colleague from Virginia to Friedman. Dr. Robert E. Thurber (University of Kansas, Ph.D. in Physiology, 1965) had served as a research associate in radiation biology at the Brookhaven National Laboratories (1956–1961) and at the Medical College of Virginia (1961–1969) before assuming an Associate Professorship at Jefferson (1969–1970). His research interests included the transfer and distribution of electrolytes, renal transport, and radiation biology. At the end of the year, Thurber was named to the Chair of Physiology at the newly established School of Medicine of East Carolina University, in Greenville, North Carolina.

Jefferson had always been one of the largest medical schools in the nation. As the class size rose from 160 to 223, concerns were raised as to how to maximize student–faculty personal contact. A system of literature clubs was inaugurated. Each faculty member was assigned 25 students. Reading assignments were established on a weekly basis. Assignment refinement led to a one-on-one interaction between staff and student, plus the obvious benefit of introducing the student to the medical and basic science literature.

Graduate education matured. Whereas from initiation of graduate training at Jefferson in 1949 until 1959 the Department of Physiology had 10 graduates (6 Ph.D., 4 M.S.), during the period of 1960–1970, 47 students received graduate degrees in physiology (24 Ph.D., 23 M.S.). As one graduate remembered the period, "Perhaps the most valuable memory I have of the time spent at Jefferson . . . [is] the spirit of collegiality among faculty and graduate students . . . . I always felt a part of the department and took away with me a real sense of pride in my accomplishments."

Dr. M.H. Friedman retired from Jefferson on June 30, 1974. He was named Emeritus Professor and then joined Domenic DeBias' Department at the Philadelphia College of Osteopathic Medicine. His portrait was presented to the College by the Class of 1974.

Allen M. Lefer, Ph.D., Seventh Chairman (1974–)

On July 1, 1974, Dr. Allan M. Lefer (Figure 5-11) became the seventh Chairman of the Department, the tenth individual to be responsible for physiology since the start of the school in 1824.

There was repeated history in this appointment. Robley Dunglison was the first occupant of the Chair (1836); he had come from the University of Virginia, the institution established by Thomas Jefferson (with an intervening Professorship at the University of Maryland, 1833–1836). Now, 138 years later, Allan Lefer, of the same University of Virginia, was following in Dunglison's footsteps as he also came to Philadelphia to occupy the Chair in Physiology.

A native New Yorker, Lefer was educated at Adelphi University (B.A., 1957), Western Reserve University (M.A., 1959), and the University of Illinois (Ph.D. in Physiology, 1962). Following an initial appointment as Instructor in Physiology at Western Reserve University (1962–1964), Lefer relocated to the University of Virginia School of Medicine at Charlottesville, rising through the academic ranks from Assistant Professor to Professor (1964–1972). He spent the year 1971–1972 as a Visiting Professor and United States Public Health Service Senior Fellow at the Hadassah Medical School, Hebrew University, Jerusalem, Israel. Allan Lefer's assumption of the Chair ended almost one-half century of special departmental emphasis on gastrointestinal function (1927–1974, through the Chairmanships of J. Earl Thomas and M.H.F. Friedman). The new departmental emphasis was to be decidedly cardiovascular. Lefer's varied cardiovascular interests, experience, and involvement included the humoral regulation of myocardial contractility, experimental myocardial infarction, and the pathogenesis of circulatory shock. His goals for the department were to "continue to promote growth and development of the quality aspects of the department" while moving aggressively to enhance capabilities and productivity in departmental research. Coincident with his appointment, Lefer recruited a previous trainee. Dr. Michael J. Rovetto, and a fellow-Virginian, Dr. James A. Spath, Jr. as Assistant Professors.

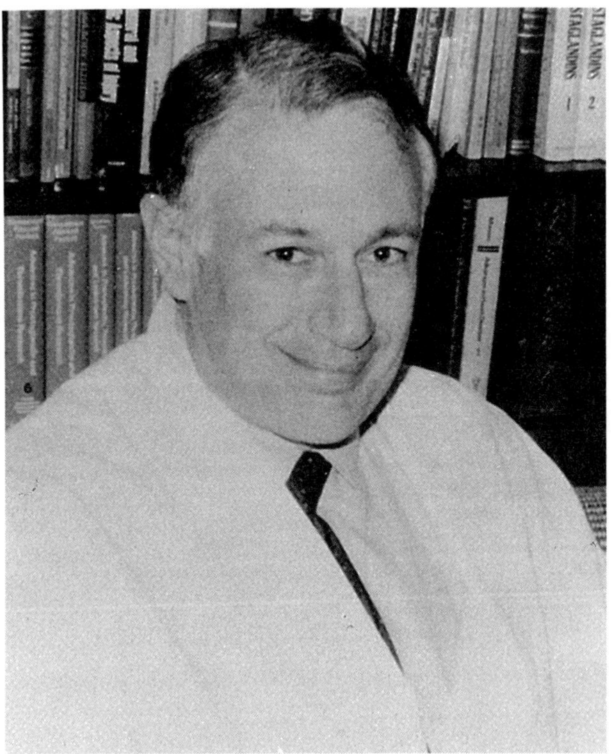

FIG. 5-11. Allen M. Lefer, Ph.D., Seventh Chairman (1974–).

Dr. Michael Rovetto received his Ph.D. in Physiology under Lefer at the University of Virginia (1970). On leaving Virginia, Rovetto served as Research Associate in Physiology at Hershey Medical Center, Pennsylvania State University (1971–1974). At Jefferson he continued his studies on myocardial metabolism and the regulation of cardiovascular function. Advanced to Associate Professorship in 1977, Rovetto resigned to accept a similar position at the University of Missouri School of Medicine (1980).

Dr. James A. Spath, Jr., trained at the University of Oklahoma Medical Center (Ph.D. in Physiology, 1966). From 1966 to 1974 he served as Assistant Professor of Physiology, Virginia Commonwealth University, Medical College of Virginia, Richmond. His research involved cardiac enzyme activity in pericardial tamponade, pharmacological limitation of ischemic heart injury, circulatory regulation in shock, and postmyocardial ischemia development of pulmonary edema.

From the start Lefer established international relationships that resulted in a continuing series of visits to the Department, for periods ranging from days up to two years, of both junior and mature scientists. The first such visitor was Dr. Minoru Okuda, an academic clinician from Japan, who served as Visiting Associate Professor and Research Associate (1974–1976), investigating glucocorticoids and the ischemic myocardium. The visit was considered extraordinarily productive, and Dr. Okuda returned to the Defense Medical College (Saitama Perfecture, Japan) better equipped to integrate basic science and clinical medicine. Other Japanese fellows that followed were Dr. Haruo Araki from Kumamoto University and Dr. Shuichi Okamatsu from Kyushu University. In addition, the research capabilities of the department were enhanced by the presence of at least one postdoctoral fellow annually. Support for such positions was made possible through enhanced extramural funding. The number of departmental research technicians similarly increased. The Department had long supported a departmental machine shop. It was this facility that had aided Thomas in the design and construction of his innovative devices. Lefer now added two additional departmental support facilities, an electronic laboratory (for design and maintenance) and a photographic laboratory for assistance in presentations and publications.

Active recruitment activities throughout 1974–1975 resulted in the appointment of Drs. Marlys H. Gee and Anatole Besarab as Assistant Professors. Marlys Gee received her graduate training at the University of Colorado School of Medicine (Ph.D. in Physiology, 1972). A three-year research fellowship (1972–1975) at the Cardiovascular Research Institute of the School of Medicine, University of California, San Francisco, preceded her 1975 arrival in Philadelphia to assume Chandra Banerjee's responsibilities in respiratory physiology. Her research interests were in the pathophysiology of pulmonary edema, pulmonary epithelial and interstitial protein transport, and postmyocardial ischemia development of lung vascular injury. This latter project involved significant collaboration with James Spath. In 1980 Dr. Gee was awarded a National Institutes of Health Career Development Research Award.

Dr. Anatole Besarab came to Philadelphia following a fellowship at Boston's Beth Israel Hospital and an Instructorship in Medicine at Harvard Medical School (1973–1975). At Jefferson, Besarab was given joint appointments in physiology and in medicine, with medicine as the primary appointment. In the department he lectured on renal physiology and acid-base balance. His research interests involved ionic modulation of parathyroid hormone action on the kidney utilizing the isolated perfused kidney.

During 1976–1977 a fourth major departmental support facility was developed, an electron microscopy suite. A departmental surgical area was converted to house a Zeiss EM-95 electron microscope, a preparation laboratory, and a photographic darkroom, along with a departmental technician to operate the facility.

Continued recruitment activity resulted in the 1976 appointment of Drs. Thomas M. Butler, John T. Flynn, and Joseph R. Sherwin as Assistant Professors. Thomas Butler received his graduate training at the University of Pennsylvania (Ph.D. in Molecular Biology, 1974) followed by a postdoctoral fellowship in the laboratory of Professor Robert E. Davis, Pennsylvania Muscle Institute at the University of Pennsylvania (1974–1976). Here Butler engaged in investigative studies of the energetics and regulation of muscle contraction. A number of these studies were collaborative among Butler, Davies, and Siegman. This cooperation continued and deepened with Butler's relocation to Jefferson. Dr. Butler received a National Institutes of Health Career Development Award in 1981.

Dr. John T. Flynn, a graduate of the Hahnemann Medical College and Hospital (Ph.D. in Physiology, 1974), came to Jefferson as Research Associate for additional postdoctoral training in cardiovascular physiology in Lefer's laboratory (1974–1976). Flynn became deeply involved in the chemistry and physiology of prostaglandins, their synthesis, and analytical methodology. He studied the development of circulatory shock and of toxemias. Several studies involved the isolated perfused liver, while others were collaborative with Lefer, Spath, or Gee.

Dr. Joseph R. Sherwin received his graduate training at the University of Pittsburgh (Ph.D. in Physiology, 1973). He remained at Pittsburgh on Research Associateship (1973–1976) until his arrival at Jefferson in 1976 to assume teaching and research in endocrine physiology. His research activities focused on the regulation of thyroid gland function, especially iodide transport and glandular blood flow. In 1980, Sherwin was named coordinator of the first-year course in medical physiology.

As Aserinsky's departure in May 1976 had left the department without a trained neurophysiologist, further recruitment resulted in the 1977 appointment of Dr. Paul S. Blum as Assistant Professor. Blum received his Ph.D. in Physiology from the University of Vermont (1973). The year 1973–1974 was spent at Duke University as a National Institute of Mental Health postdoctoral trainee in sciences related to the nervous system. Subsequently Blum served as Research Associate in Neurology at the College of Physicians and Surgeons, Columbia University (1974–1977). At Jefferson he continued his investigations pertaining to the physiological regulation of the central nervous system, with special emphasis on the function of the raphe nucleus and of the role of reticulospinal pathways in the regulation of blood pressure and the processing of sensory information.

Interdepartmental Programs

A growing research interest developed in metabolic, hemodynamic, and pathophysiological aspects of myocardial ischemias and circulatory shock. The main focus of these activities interrelated with the Departments of Pharmacology, Medicine, and Surgery. Out of this interaction was established in the fall of 1977 the Ischemia-Shock Research Center, with Allan Lefer as Director and Michael Rovetto, Marlys Gee, and Marion Siegman as the Center's Advisory Council. Monthly meetings were held to enhance scientific dialogue among the members. In addition, prominent scholars in the field were invited to give guest lectures. On April 23, 1980, the Center sponsored a minisymposium on shock. Funding for the Center was derived from donations of private industry and grants from the W. W. Smith Foundation and the Ralph and Marion Falk Foundation.

The departmental commitment to quality graduate education remained strong. The number of departmental trainees, however, dropped from its peak in the 1960s. This reflected the fact that each student received financial support and, thus, the number of incoming students was limited by the fiscal resources of the department, supplemented by institutional funds.

In 1979, the Jefferson Chapter of Sigma Xi, the scientific research society, established a separate graduate student competition as part of its annual Student Research Day. A Physiology graduate student was awarded first prize for the most outstanding poster presentation for four consecutive years (1979–1982). Edward F. Smith III, a 1981 graduate, received the first achievement award for excellence by the Alumni Association of the College of Graduate Studies. He was awarded a prestigious Alexander von Humboldt Foundation Postdoctoral Fellowship for additional study in Cologne, Germany. Further, Dr. Smith's thesis concerning pathophysiological actions of thromboxane A_2 in coronary artery disease (his thesis advisor was A.M. Lefer) was accepted into the Council of Graduate Schools' competition for their 1981 Dissertation Award. It remained in competition until the finals and was judged one of the top 12 theses of 1981.

To partially replace the loss of cardiovascular expertise experienced by Michael Rovetto's relocation to Missouri, Dr. Stuart K. Williams II was appointed Assistant Professor in 1981. Educated at the University of Delaware (Ph.D. in Cell Biology, 1979), Williams served as a postdoctoral fellow in the Department of Pathology of the Yale University School of Medicine (1979–1981). His research interests were in microcirculation and the role of micropinocytosis in capillary endothelium.

The record of 160 years of Physiology at Jefferson (1824–1984) has been impressive. It has seen the Department evolve from a basic one-man operation into a sophisticated modern system, the establishment of professional physiology, the introduction of practical application into medical education (museum, demonstrations, student laboratory, student research), meaningful clinical interaction in training and investigation, and the advancement of knowledge in varied fields of study. The challenge is to extend this record and to advance the frontiers of education and of investigation even further.

References

1. Reed, C.I., "History of Physiology." Manuscript on file at American Physiological Society, Bethesda, Md.
2. *Catalogue of Instruction*. Jefferson Medical College, 1833.

3. Radbill, S.X., *The Autobiographical Ana of Robley Dunglison, M.D.,* Trans. Physiological Soc. N. Ser., Vol. 53, Part 8, 1963, pp. 1–212.
4. Wagner, F.B., Jr., "The Jefferson-Dunglison Grandfather Clock," Trans. Stud. Coll. Phys. of Phila., Vol. 3, No. 2, June, 1981, pp. 151–157.
5. Beaumont, W., *Experiments and Observations on the Gastric Juice and the Physiology of Digestion*. Plattsburg, N.Y.: F.P. Allen, 1833.
6. Wagner, F.B. Jr., "Centennial Memoir of James Aitken Meigs, M.D.," *Trans. Stud., Coll. Phys. of Phila.,* Vol. 4, No. 3, 1982, pp. 171–178.
7. Howell, W.H., *History of the American Physiological Society: 1887–1937*. Baltimore, Md.: Am. Phil. Soc., 1938, pp. 1–89.
8. *Science,* III (56). Friday, January 24, 1896.
9. Rosenberger, R.C., "Memoir of Albert P. Brubaker," Trans. Stud., Coll. of Phys. of Phila., Vol. 1, Ser. 4, Vol. 11, 1944, pp. 136–137.
10. Rosenfeld, L.M., "Physiology at Jefferson Medical College (1842–1982)," *The Physiologist,* 27, 1984, pp. 113–127.
11. Friedman, M.H.F.: "In Memoriam—J. Earl Thomas," in *Functions: Stomach and Intestines,* edited by M.H.F. Friedman, 1975.

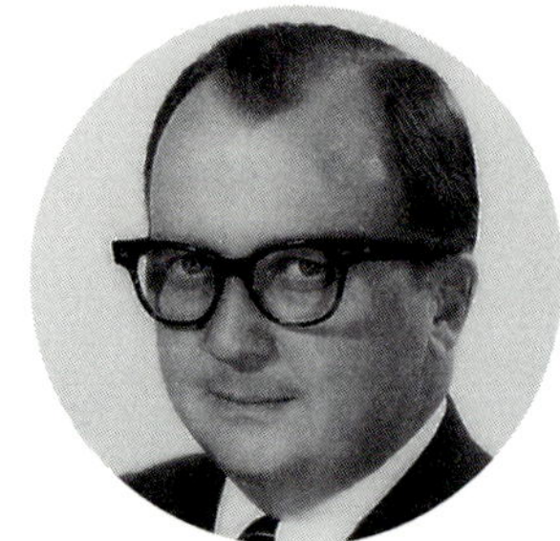

CHAPTER SIX

Department of Pathology

William E. Delaney III, M.D.

Medicine, to produce health, has to examine disease.

—Plutarch (46?–120?)

Pathology literally means "study of disease" and in its broadest sense is as old as a human's curiosity about his or her illnesses. The word *pathology* first appears in the writings of Galen (ca. 130–200).[1] Usage of the word has evolved from its broadest interpretation, which included the study of the cause, pathogenesis, abnormal function, and clinical presentation of a disease, to its narrowest application, which is limited to the gross and microscopic structural changes in disease.

Organization of the body of knowledge of disease may be said to have begun with the publication of *De sedibus et causas morborum* in 1761 by the Italian anatomist, Giovanni Batista Morgagni (1682–1771). Although the microscope had been described as early as 1646 and popularized by 1683 by Antonj van Leeuwenhoek (1632–1723), Morgagni depended solely on the changes visible to the naked eye and thus can be said to have founded modern gross pathology. The first treatise to systematize gross pathology appeared in 1793, written by the Englishman, Matthew Baillie (1761–1823), a nephew of John and William Hunter, and entitled *The Morbid Anatomy of some of the most important parts of the Human Body*. Baillie followed this with the publication of an atlas in ten parts between 1799 and 1802. *The Morbid Anatomy* went into ten English and three American editions and was widely translated into foreign languages.

The application of microscopy to pathology lagged for a century and a half because of the imperfections of early microscopes, the images of which had considerable spherical and chromatic aberration. Nevertheless, the Frenchman, Marie Francois Xavier Bichat (1771–1802), advanced the subject immensely in 1799 and 1800 with the publication of *Traite des Membranes* and may be considered the father of modern histology. The technology was vastly improved in 1824 with the invention of the achromatic microscope of Selligue, which paved the way for an understanding of the fine cellular structure of tissues. In 1831 the cellular features of plants were delineated by the German botanist, M.J. Schleiden (1804–1881). The monumental transitional step to the application of ideas of cell structure to animal tissues was taken in 1839 by the German anatomist, Theodor Schwann (1810–1882), which set the stage for real understanding of gross pathology. It is noted, however, that earlier descriptions of the universal cellular structure of plant and animal tissues were made in 1824 by Dutrochet, a French physician-biologist.

Until the new knowledge was promulgated, however, the first pathology text published in America, *Treatise on Pathological Anatomy,* written in 1829 by William Edmonds Horner (1793–1853), was based entirely on gross pathology. Horner was Professor of Anatomy at the University of Pennsylvania. The first systematic course of lectures in pathology in an American medical school was given from 1835 to 1839 by Samuel David Gross (1805–1884) at the Medical College of Ohio in Cincinnati. Gross was a graduate of Jefferson in the Class of 1828 and was a prodigious worker and reader, fluent in Greek, Latin, German, and French.[2] Largely self-taught in pathology, Gross gave credit to Baillie, Bichat, and Gabriel Andral (1797–1876) for many of the concepts in the pathology textbook that grew out of his lecture notes. His book, *Elements of Pathological Anatomy,* was published in 1839, with two further editions in 1845 and 1857.

The first edition of Gross's pathology textbook acknowledges the author's debt to Baillie and Bichat and regrets the neglect of their subject in the America of 1839.[3] Illustrations in the first edition were entirely macroscopic lesions, largely copied from other authors. By the time of the second edition six years later, one-third of the illustrations were original. They showed some understanding of microscopic pathology, albeit not of the exact role of cells (six years after Schwann's promulgation of the cell theory), as in Gross's description (page 46) of "structureless lymph" becoming organized "by arrangement of the granules, through their own vital impulse, into groups of nuclei which are converted into cells, termed cytoblasts, from which the future tissue is formed," in a description of the inflammatory process.[4]

Gross's third edition, appearing eight years after the second, exhibited considerable improvement in the comprehension of histological changes (acknowledged to have been at least partially due to the "special attention" of his young colleague, Dr. Jacob Mendes DaCosta, to microscopic features), as seen (page 64) in the microscopic description of lymph that contained cells, some of which "resemble . . . white corpuscles of the blood."[5] Gross also pointed out that "there is not, with perhaps a few exceptions, a chair of pathologic anatomy in the forty-five American medical colleges" in existence in 1857.

Indeed, teaching of the rudiments of pathologic anatomy in most nineteenth century American medical schools was left to anatomists and to surgeons. Pathology was listed in curricula of the day as "Institutes of Medicine" and was taught at Jefferson by surgeons such as Samuel D. Gross. The only American medical school prior to 1866 to have a formal course in pathologic anatomy was Harvard, but in that year the Jefferson Professor of Medicine, Samuel H. Dickson, taught pathologic anatomy in Jefferson's summer session. The course at Jefferson was then taught yearly between 1867 and 1876 by the versatile surgeon, William W. Keen.

Much of the teaching material used in the early courses in pathology consisted of specimens from anatomical museums developed largely by surgeons. One such museum was established in 1860 in the Pennsylvania Hospital, where Dr. Thomas G. Morton was the first Curator of the Museum and Pathologist to the Hospital. With the growth of his private practice and on receiving a coveted clinical appointment to the Hospital, Morton resigned as Pathologist in 1863 and was succeeded by Dr. William Pepper, who served until 1870 when Dr. Morris Longstreth became Curator and Pathologist to Pennsylvania Hospital. Longstreth eventually became the first head of the Department of Pathology at Jefferson, after starting as Keen's successor in 1876 in the delivery of pathology lectures at Jefferson.

Morris Longstreth, M.D. (1846–1914), First Chairman (1891–1895)

In the 20 years before he assumed the Chair in Pathology at Jefferson, Longstreth (Figure 6-1) had demonstrated his growing expertise at Pennsylvania Hospital, to which his Quaker background led him naturally. He came from a family that had arrived from England in 1699 and settled in what is now Hatboro, Montgomery County.[6] Born February 24, 1846, in Philadelphia, Morris Longstreth had an excellent educational background, attending Friends School and graduating from Haverford College (A.B., 1864) and also from Harvard (A.B., 1866). He received his M.D. from the University of Pennsylvania in 1869. Between 1869 and 1871 he had an 18-month appointment as Resident Physician in the Pennsylvania Hospital. Self-taught as a pathologist, although undoubtedly influenced by the pathologists at the University of Pennsylvania (Joseph G. Richardson) and the Philadelphia (General) Hospital (William Pepper), Longstreth was appointed Curator of the Museum at the Pennsylvania Hospital while still a Resident Physician. In 1872 he was appointed Physician to the Outpatient Department of Pennsylvania Hospital and began to accumulate a large private practice. In 1875 he gave a course in Pathologic Anatomy at the Hospital. In 1877 he acquired a freezing microtome. In 1879 he was promoted to Professor of Pathologic Anatomy at Jefferson after lecturing there for three years as Demonstrator of Pathology. In 1880–1881 Longstreth gave the first laboratory course in Pathologic Anatomy and Pathologic Histology at Jefferson. In 1882, after many years of study of rheumatic diseases, he published *Rheumatism, Gout and Some Allied Disorders* (New York: Wm. Woods & Co.), one of the earliest pathologic treatises in rheumatology. In 1886 he became one of the original members of the Association of American Physicians.

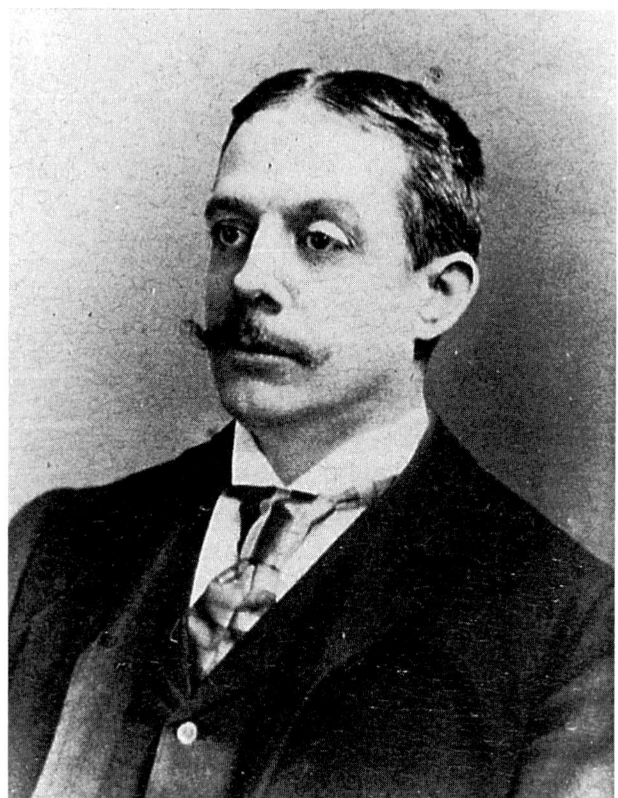

FIG. 6-1. Morris Longstreth, M.D., First Chairman (1891–1895).

Pathology became a major department at Jefferson in 1891, with Longstreth as the first Professor and Department Head. His private practice of medicine, however, continued to grow and to compete for his time with his teaching duties. From 1885 Longstreth leaned heavily on William M. L. Coplin (then only a medical student) to carry the teaching burden, shifting the duties almost completely by 1894, when Coplin became Temporary Professor. In 1895, on being asked to do so, Longstreth resigned as Professor of Pathology to continue the very large private practice he had developed.[7] The Chair was vacant from 1895 to 1896.

Longstreth continued his medical practice until late in life, interrupted by long periods of travel. He died September 18, 1914, in Barcelona, Spain, while fleeing from the opening hostilities of World War I, within a month after the death of his wife in the same city.

Longstreth's career in pathology paralleled a period in medicine that had been dominated by notable discoveries in infectious diseases. Weigert had first stained bacteria in tissues with carmine in 1871. Cohnheim had elucidated the mechanisms of inflammation and the role of leukocytes in 1873. Koch and Pasteur had inaugurated modern bacteriology in 1876–1877 with their independent investigations of anthrax. At the same time, by showing that filaria were transmitted by mosquitoes, Manson had demonstrated the role of insects as vectors of disease. Koch had discovered the tubercle bacillus in 1882. Phagocytes had been discovered in 1884 by Metchnikoff, who showed their important role in inflammation. Acute appendicitis had been established as an abdominal emergency in 1886 by Fitz, who then did the same for acute hemorrhagic pancreatitis in 1889.

As a practitioner, Longstreth became known through his advocacy of regular physical examinations to promote good health. His contributions to pathology were minimal but impressive if evaluated as those of a part-time pathologist. His generation was the last to consider pathology as a stepping-stone to clinical medicine. His major contribution may well have been the training of his successor at Jefferson, the prodigious William M.L. Coplin.

William Michael Late Coplin, M.D. (1864–1928), Second Chairman (1896–1922)

The first fulltime pathologist at Jefferson, William M. L. Coplin (Figure 6-2) was born November 1, 1864, in Clarksburg, West Virginia, of Scotch-Irish heritage. Educated in secondary schools in West Virginia, Coplin spent four years at Mount Union College in Ohio. He matriculated at Jefferson in 1883, electing to take three rather than the usual two years of medical college. He began working with pathology specimens as an undergraduate and during his senior year (1885–1886) he did much of the pathologic work on specimens from the practice of the Professor of Surgery, Samuel W. Gross. Coplin's undergraduate research thesis on *Wound Infection* won a prize in pathology.

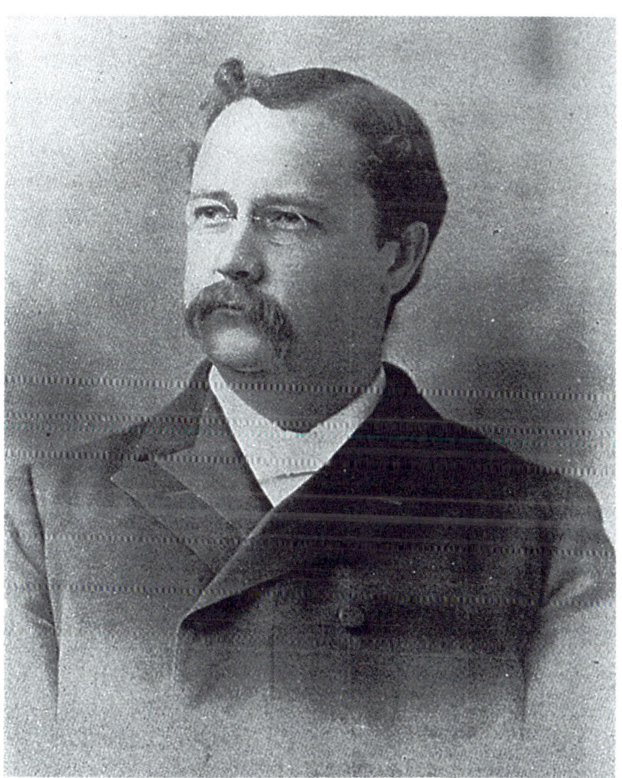

FIG. 6-2. William M.L. Coplin (1864–1928), Second Chairman (1896–1922).

On graduation in 1886, Coplin was appointed Assistant Demonstrator of Pathologic Anatomy and spent a year as Resident Physician in Jefferson Hospital. In 1887 he was appointed Assistant Pathologist to the Hospital and became a member of the surgical and gynecological staffs. In the same year he entered the private practice of pathology with a laboratory in his home, joined the staffs of many other local hospitals, and acquired expertise in infectious diseases. In 1892 he was promoted to Demonstrator of Pathology at Jefferson and made Curator of the Pathology Museum, a facility that became one of his major interests. In the same year he was appointed Pathologist to the Philadelphia (General) Hospital, a position he retained for many years. With the publication of his *Textbook of Practical Hygiene* in 1893 and *Lectures in Pathology* during the year 1894–1895, Coplin had become a well known pathologist. Although he became Temporary Professor of Pathology at Jefferson in 1894, he was not initially considered for the permanent appointment imminently to be vacated by Longstreth, so Coplin accepted the offer of the Vanderbilt University to become Professor of Pathology. He served in Nashville only during 1895–1896 when, following Longstreth's resignation, he returned to Philadelphia as Professor of Pathology and Bacteriology at Jefferson.

The career of Coplin paralleled the early growth of clinical laboratories in the United States. Until the last two decades of the nineteenth century, pathology had been a didactic subject, based in the Medical School. With the advent of microscopy and its application to clinical problems in the hospital, a need for hospital-based laboratories was generated.[8] Although the Massachusetts General Hospital had acquired a microscope in 1847, there was only one microscope in the Hospital of the University of Pennsylvania in 1887 (and that one belonged to Osler). Only three microscopic examinations are recorded during the entire year of 1866 at the Philadelphia

(General) Hospital and the number increased to only 21 by 1871. The counting of red blood cells and the quantitation of hemoglobin had become practical by 1887, when Osler was said to have had the first hemocytometer in the city of Philadelphia.[9] Johns Hopkins Hospital had a clinical laboratory, and William Osler and William Welch sought to bridge the gap between the laboratory and the patient's bedside. In 1893 George Dock organized a large clinical laboratory in the University of Michigan Hospital. In 1894 the William Pepper Laboratory of Clinical Medicine was opened in the Hospital of the University of Pennsylvania. The discoveries of bacteriology made modern clinical laboratories necessary in the hospital, as ever-increasing numbers of cultures, stained smears, and microscopic examinations became necessary for good patient care. Chemical examinations were rather primitive and low in volume. By the turn of the century, however, histological techniques were relatively advanced. By 1900 paraffin embedding was standard practice and all the basic staining methods that would be used in the following 60 years were being employed.

Coplin brought about the appointment of the first Resident Physician to train exclusively in one department at Jefferson when he named H.F. Harris as the first Resident Pathologist in 1896.[7] Coplin was everywhere in the laboratory, being found there at all hours of the day and night. He still found time to accept appointment as Bacteriologist to the Pennsylvania State Board of Health. In 1897 he published *Manual of Pathology* (a revision of *Lectures on Pathology*), which went to five editions. From 1905 to 1907, Coplin served the City of Philadelphia as Director of the Department of Public Health and Charities; he organized what became the Municipal Hospital for Contagious Diseases, and made numerous improvements at the Philadelphia General Hospital. During all this time he continued to perform his teaching and laboratory duties, but added assistants in various areas of the laboratory. In Neuropathology, appointments were given to Alfred Gordon (1906–1908), Aller G. Ellis (1908–1909), G. E. Price (1912–1913), and Michael A. Burns (Jefferson, 1907) (1913 to at least 1931). From 1908 to 1911 John W. Funke (Jefferson, 1901) was in charge of Clinical Pathology. Overlapping appointments were given in Pathologic Chemistry to Henry Leffman (1908–1919) and in Physiologic Chemistry to Philip B. Hawk (1919–1923). Gynecologic Pathology was under H.J. Hartz (1913–1919), P. Brooke Bland (1913–1921), James L. Richards (1918–1928), and James F. Carrell (1919–1921). Coplin was in charge of Bacteriology in the hospital laboratory until 1909, when Randle C. Rosenberger succeeded and remained in charge until at least 1930.

Coplin's special interest over the years was the Pathology Museum. In 1914 it was expanded with the help of an allocation of more than $100,000 from a member of the Jefferson Board of Trustees, John H. McFadden. This allowed the Museum to be moved to the top floor of Medical Hall (1898 Building) when space was vacated by the Department of Anatomy in 1914 (Figure 6-3).

Although among the lesser of Coplin's accomplishments, the invention of a grooved glass jar (the Coplin jar), which allowed slides to stand separated in a staining solution, is the only memorial to him that survives. Coplin jars continued in wide use in histology and microbiology laboratories of virtually all hospitals to this day.

With the entry of the United States into World War I, an Army hospital was organized from the Staff of Jefferson Hospital, supported by a donation of $50,000 from the Gibson family of whiskey distillers.[7] Coplin was named Commanding Officer with the rank of Colonel, U.S. Army, and served with the Hospital from 1917 to 1919, part of which time it was stationed in Nantes, France, as Base Hospital No. 38.

After the war, Coplin resumed his duties at Jefferson. He served as Head of the Pathology Department until he had a stroke in 1922, which left him disabled after 26 years as Chairman, the longest tenure of anyone. He was relieved of all duties, but in recognition of his long and distinguished service to the institution he remained on full salary for the rest of his life. He retired to his summer home in Atlantic City until he died in 1928 at age 63 of angina pectoris.

Coplin should be remembered for the diversification he brought to the Pathology Department as the general discipline of pathology developed an identity in both the Medical College and the Hospital and fostered subspecialty interests in many areas. Among those residents who received their training under Coplin were Robert M. Lukens (1910–1911), who later became a prominent bronchoesophagologist; George F. Lull (1911–1913), who became the longtime Secretary-Treasurer of the American Medical Association; and Erwin D.Funk (1913–1914), who later contributed to the development of the Reading Hospital as Pathologist and Medical Director. In addition, John B. Flick (a resident in 1916–1917) became a distinguished surgeon and Chief of Surgery in the Pennsylvania Hospital.

Aller G. Ellis, M.D. (1868–1953), Acting Chairman (1922–1923)

Aller G. Ellis (Figure 6-4), the interim successor to Coplin, was born at Cambridge Springs, Crawford County, Pennsylvania, in 1894 (B.Sc.), having been an athlete in three sports (baseball, football, and track). He graduated from Jefferson in 1900, serving as President of his class. After internship in Jefferson Hospital (1900–1902), Ellis was appointed Demonstrator of Morbid Anatomy in 1902, beginning a long association with Coplin. His rise up the career ladder began in 1903 with his appointment as Instructor in Hematology and continued in 1904 with his promotion to Associate in Pathology. In 1907 the Trustees of the Medical College honored him with the first award of the "Corinna Borden Keen Research Fellowship," founded in 1905 by W. W. Keen, Professor of Surgery. This enabled Ellis to study in Germany from 1907 to 1908. He returned to Jefferson in

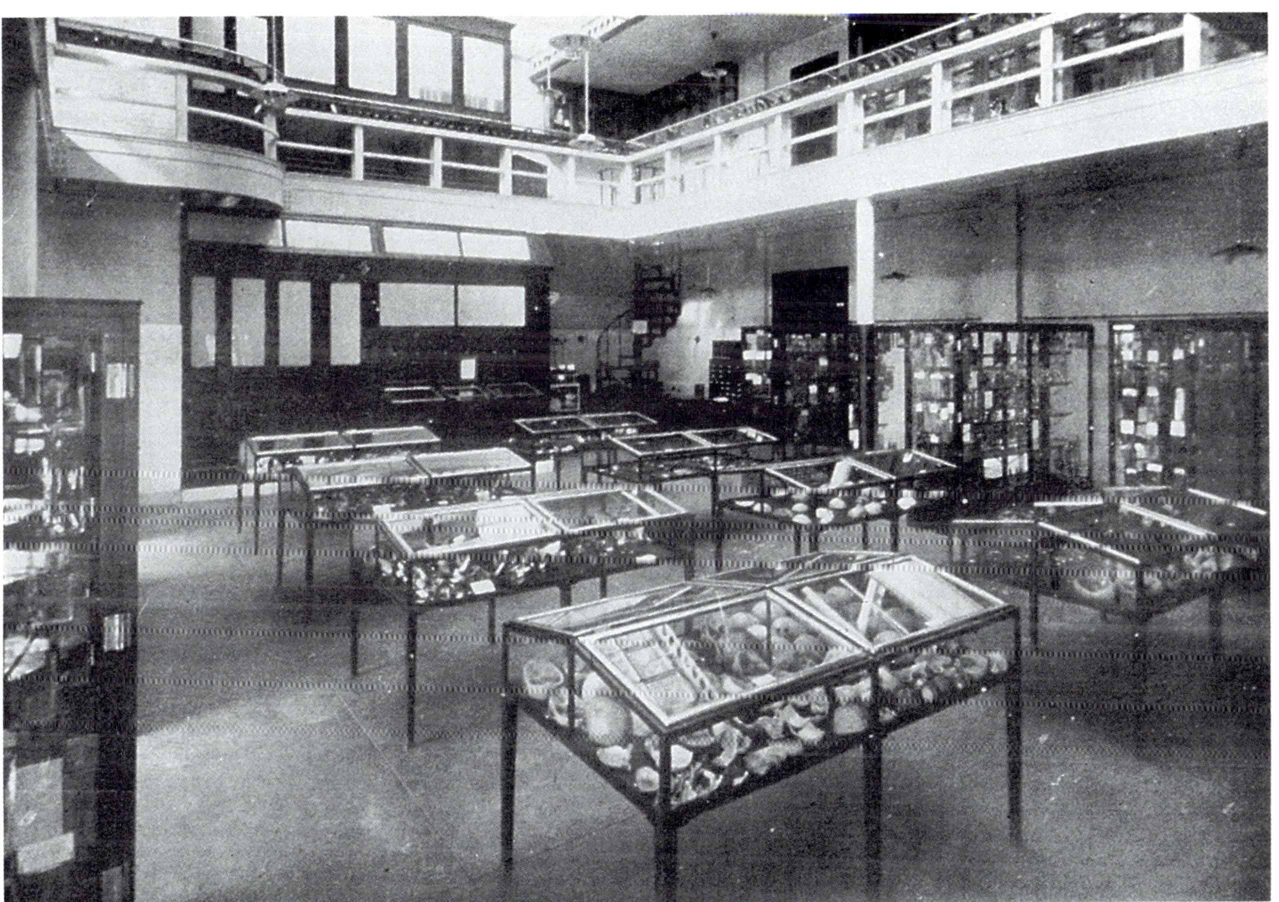

FIG. 6-3. Pathology Museum (1914), in 1898 Medical College Building.

1908 for a two year appointment in neuropathology. His status as a rising star in the Department was further confirmed in 1913 when he was sent by the Board of Trustees of Jefferson to evaluate cancer research in England and the Continent, where he visited with Ehrlich, Pick, Levaditi, and other leading researchers.

In 1917 Ellis made a trip to Lancaster to perform an historically important autopsy. The patient had been operated on 30 years previously by W. W. Keen as one of the first successful operations for a brain tumor. Keen had removed a meningioma, and the autopsy by Ellis showed that there had been no recurrence. Such a surgical achievement today would hardly be cause for comment. In those times, however, the story was a dramatic one.

From 1917 to 1919 Ellis was Director of the Ayer Clinical Laboratories at Pennsylvania Hospital. Between 1920 and 1922, under the auspices of the Rockefeller Foundation, he organized and directed the Department of Pathology of the Royal Medical College in Bangkok, Siam (Thailand). On returning to Jefferson in 1922, Ellis filled in for Coplin for one year but left in 1923 when his appointment was inexplicably not renewed. Little is known of his career beyond 1923, except that he was a member of the Colorado State Medical Society. He retained at least one tie to his alma mater, as evidenced by the memoir he wrote for the *Alumni Bulletin* in May, 1944, on the death of Randle C. Rosenberger. Ellis died on February 19, 1953, in Plainfield, New Jersey, of arteriosclerosis at the age of 84.

The contributions of Aller G. Ellis as interim Head of the Pathology Department were minimal, although he did train a pathology intern in 1922–1923, Frank Hammond Krusen, who later achieved great prominence in physical medicine and rehabilitation.

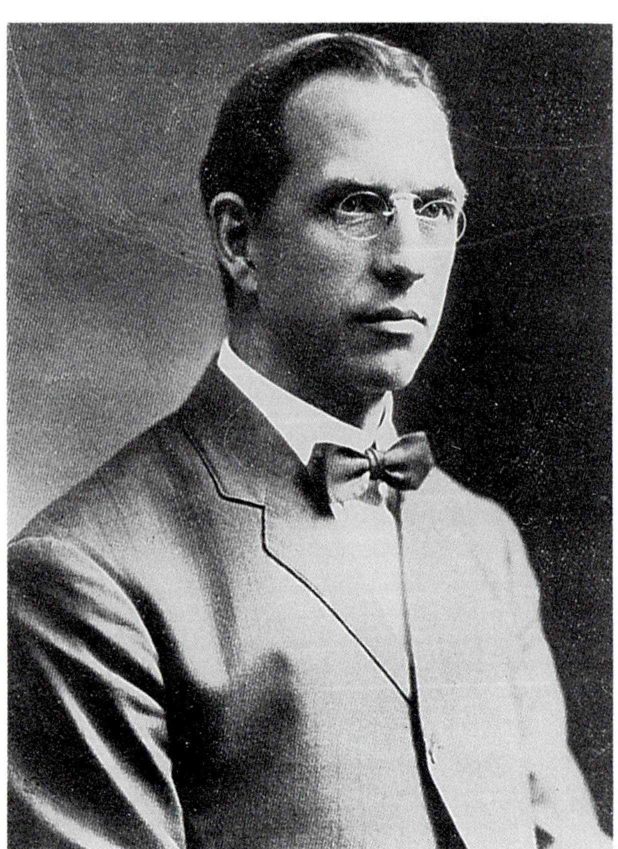

FIG. 6-4. Aller G. Ellis, M.D. (1868–1953), Acting Chairman (1922–1923).

■ Mayer Sulzberger Pathological Laboratories

The Centennial Campaign of 1924 culminated in the construction of the new hospital building on the south side of Sansom Street between Tenth and Eleventh Streets, which became known as the Samuel Gustine Thompson Annex. Toward the cost of construction of laboratories the Jewish community of Philadelphia gave $75,000 in honor of the Philadelphia jurist, Mayer Sulzberger, LL.D., a Jefferson Trustee who was related to the publishers of the *New York Times*. No plaque remains to identify with certainty the location of the Mayer Sulzberger Pathological Laboratories but it is likely that they were located on the fifteenth and sixteenth floors of the Annex, a location for laboratories until 1954.

Bowman Corning Crowell, M.D. (1879–1951), Third Chairman (1924–1926)

The first Canadian to chair the Pathology Department at Jefferson, Bowman C. Crowell (Figure 6-5) was born January 10, 1879, at

Yarmouth, Nova Scotia.[10] He was educated at McGill University, receiving a B.A. in 1900 and an M.D., C.M. in 1904. He went directly into pathology house staff training at New York City Hospital (later Bellevue) from 1904 to 1907 and then served on the staff at Bellevue until 1911. For the next eight years Crowell practiced in the Philippine Islands, culminating in his appointment as Director of the Graduate School of Medicine and Public Health of the University of the Philippines from 1916 to 1918. From 1918 to 1922 he was Chief of Pathology of the Oswaldo Cruz Institute in Rio de Janiero, Brazil. He came to Jefferson in 1923 after a year as Professor of Pathology at the Medical College of South Carolina. At Jefferson he served as Professor of Pathology and Director of Laboratories; among his residents there were Frank W. Konzelman (1923–1930), later a distinguished American pathologist; Benjamin F. Haskell (1924–1925), who became an eminent proctologist at Jefferson; John Rodman Paul (1925–1926), destined to be a prominent internist and authority on viral hepatitis; and Dr. Eli R. Saleeby (1925–1926), who served in Jefferson's Departments of Anatomy and Surgery. For many years Dr. Saleeby was the sponsor of the Kappa Beta Phi Student Society and of the Black and Blue Ball.

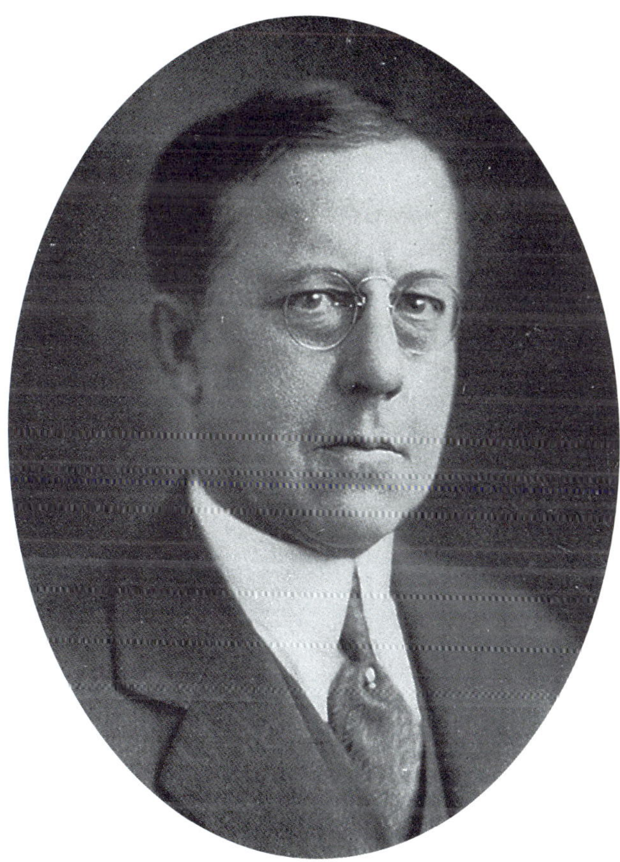

FIG. 6-5. Bowman C. Crowell (1879–1951), Third Chairman (1924–1926).

Crowell left Jefferson and pathology in 1926 when he became Associate Director of the American College of Surgeons in Chicago. He served the ACS until 1949, notably in the cancer control activities of the ACS. On his retirement he received the first gold medal of the American Cancer Society in 1949.

Baxter Lindsay Crawford, M.D. (1886–1940), Acting Chairman (1926–1927)

The second person to chair the Department in an acting capacity in the four years between 1922 and 1926, Baxter L. Crawford (Figure 6-6) was a Southerner, born February 14, 1886, at McConnelsville, South Carolina.[11] He was graduated in 1908 from Clemson College and received his M.D. from University College of Medicine, Richmond, Virginia, in 1912. Following internship in Richmond Hospital, Crawford was a Pathology Resident from 1915 to 1916 at Bellevue Hospital, New York City. He served as Major, U.S. Army, from 1916 to 1919, with assignment to various base hospitals of the American Expeditionary Forces in France and Germany. In 1919, Coplin brought Baxter to Jefferson as Assistant Professor of Pathology and Assistant Director of Clinical Laboratories. On the resignation of Crowell in 1926, Crawford was appointed Acting Chairman and served until the arrival of Dr. Virgil Holland Moon in 1927.

Crawford remained at Jefferson for the rest of his life. Because of Moon's lack of interest in the Clinical Laboratories, Crawford became Director of Clinical Laboratories during the first 13 years of Moon's tenure. Crawford's office was on the fifteenth floor of the Thompson Annex with an adjacent small laboratory, used for blood collected from private outpatients and also for Crawford's personal use. Except for Chemistry, all the rest of the laboratories were on the sixteenth floor of the Annex. Crawford's main interests were morphologic diagnosis and microbiology. His Assistant (and eventual successor as Director of Clinical Laboratories), Dr. Carl Bucher, was mainly interested in serology. They trained many Pathology Residents during this period, most notably Harold L. Stewart (Jefferson, 1926). Dr. Stewart began his Pathology Residency in 1930 and later served on the College and Hospital Pathology Staff until 1938, when he left to begin a distinguished career with the National Cancer Institute that culminated with many years of service as Chief of the Institute's Laboratory of Surgical Pathology. Stewart received Jefferson's Alumni Achievement Award in 1966. Another Pathology Resident who did well after initial training by Crawford was Hugh G. Grady (Jefferson, 1934) who later was Registrar of the Armed Forces Institute of Pathology and the founding Chairman of the Department of Pathology of Seton Hall University School of Medicine.

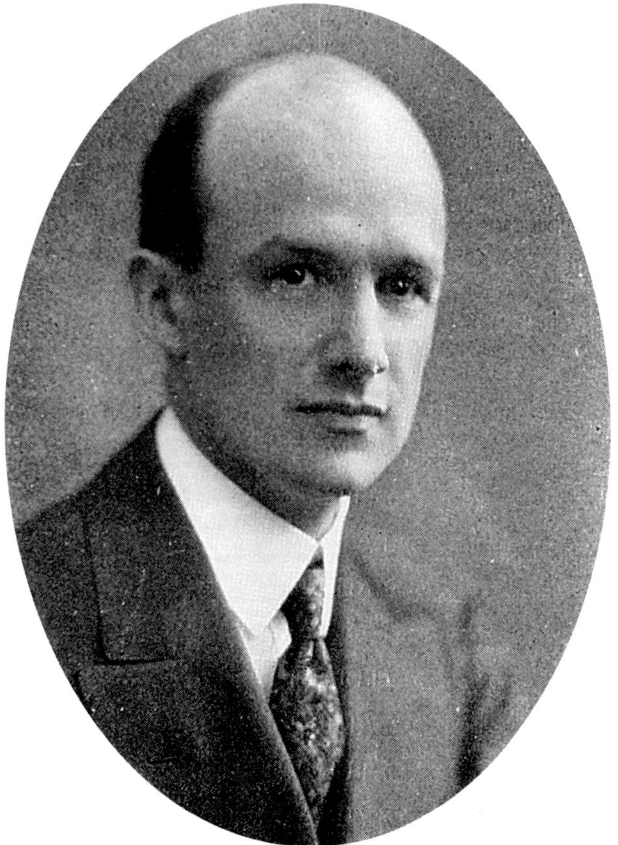

FIG. 6-6. Baxter L. Crawford (1886–1940), Acting Chairman (1926–1927).

In 1928 the Chemistry Laboratory was on the second floor of the Main Hospital opposite Men's Medical Ward. Although officially under Pathology, it was supervised by Dr. Joseph Looney of the College's Department of Biochemistry. It had one part-time technician who also performed electrocardiograms. There was also a chemistry intern (in 1928 it was David Farrel, later Professor of Obstetrics and Gynecology at Jefferson), whose duties included the collection of all blood specimens for chemistry tests. An 18-gauge needle without a syringe was used in a technique called the "drip method" of blood collection. In October of 1928 the Chemistry Laboratory ran 671 tests, mostly blood glucose and nonprotein nitrogen determinations, the latter being the kidney function test of choice in 1928. It was not until November of 1942 that blood urea nitrogen determination replaced the nonprotein nitrogen as the renal function test of choice. About 1932 Abraham Cantarow replaced Looney as Physician-in-Charge of the Chemistry Laboratory, and from that time chemistry tests expanded in numbers and complexity. Dr. Cantarow (Jefferson, 1924) had been trained in internal medicine but had interest in and understanding of chemistry and brought a clinician's sense to the Chemistry Laboratory. Eventually he became Chairman of the Department of Biochemistry at Jefferson and after retirement was in charge of Extramural Grants at the National Cancer Institute.

In May of 1932 the Chemistry Laboratory had increased its work to 830 tests; urea clearance testing for renal function had been added. Bromsulfophthalein tests of the excretory capacity of the liver were being done. All tests using colorimetric quantitation were done on the Dubosq colorimeter. A second technician (Ella Perkins, later the Laboratory's technical supervisor for many years) was added in 1928, a third in 1938, and a fourth in 1941. In October of 1938 the Chemistry Laboratory performed 1,509 tests, now including alkaline phosphatase determinations of liver function and bone activity.

Crawford's health deteriorated in the 1930s but he still found time and energy to serve as

President of the Pathology Society of Philadelphia in 1939. He died of pulmonary tuberculosis at the White Haven Sanitorium on January 3, 1940, at the age of 53.

David Reynolds Morgan, M.D. (1890–1978), Curator of the Museum (1923–1967)

One of the most revered and loved teachers at Jefferson, "Davey" Morgan (Figure 6-7) was born at Edwardsville, Pennsylvania, on October 4, 1890. Of Welsh descent, he grew up in the Wilkes-Barre area and was educated at Wyoming Seminary (1912). He graduated from Jefferson Medical College in 1916 and was elected to Alpha Omega Alpha. His Jefferson internship (May–November, 1916) was interrupted by service in the French Army, where he received a commission as a Lieutenant (Medicin-Chef of Hopital Militaire No. 10), was later promoted to Captain, and received a decoration. In September, 1917, Morgan requested discharge to transfer to the First Division, American Expeditionary Forces, but inexplicably he was denied a commission, and he enlisted as a private. His outstanding war record included a later battlefield commission as First Lieutenant in the Medical Corps, United States Army, the Distinguished Service Cross for gallantry in action, and the Croix de Guerre with Palm. A victim of wounds and mustard gas, Morgan was also awarded the Purple Heart. He was discharged in October, 1919, as a Major, the most decorated American medical officer in World War I.

Dr. Morgan returned to recuperate and in 1922 received a degree (D.P.H.) from the School of Public Health, University of Pennsylvania. An additional degree of Master of Science in Surgery was awarded by the Graduate School the following year.

Dr. Morgan's lifetime career began at Jefferson in 1923 as Demonstrator of Pathology. He became perhaps the most respected teacher in the basic sciences, always at his best in intimate section instruction. Everything he taught was done with quiet enthusiasm and good humor, with graphic demonstration of the specific lesions of diseased organs and tissues kept in formalin in large earthenware crocks (Figure 6-8). Morgan was especially skilled at relating the pathological process to clinical disease.[12]

Dr. Morgan's major interest was the Pathology Museum. In earlier decades, specimens from autopsies and later from surgery were preserved and provided the only graphic methods of instruction. The collection was organized by Longstreth in the 1880s and was nurtured by Coplin at the turn of the century as a major teaching modality, with additions during the early decades of the twentieth century (Figure 6-9). As photography and, later, color photography became generally available, the need for the demonstrations of specimens receded and by the 1950s the need for space, the difficulties of preservation, and the use of color slides for

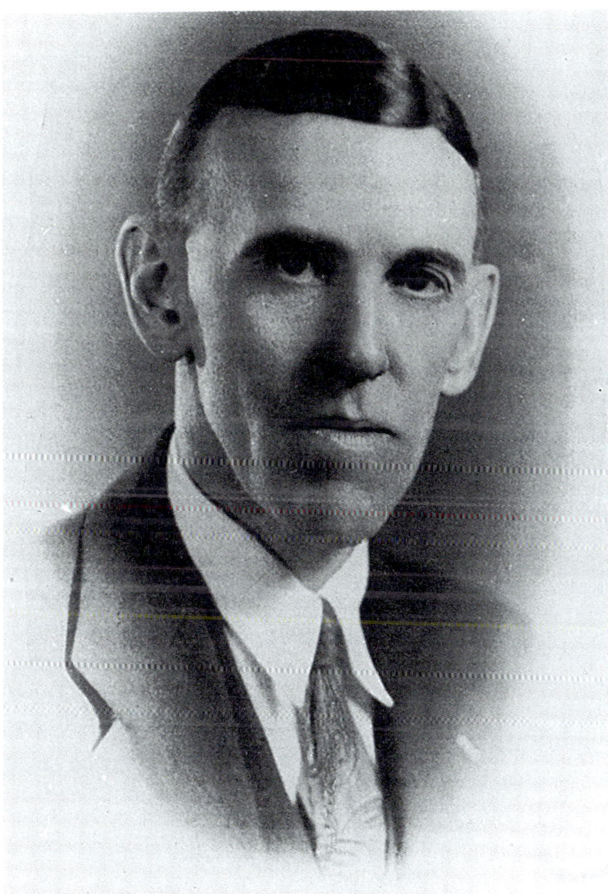

FIG. 6-7. David R. Morgan, M.D. (1890–1978), Curator of the Museum (1923–1967).

teaching both gross and microscopic pathology led to the phasing out of the Museum. When Dr. Morgan retired as Professor of Pathology in 1967, he was still the eminent teacher, but his Museum had disappeared. Dr. Morgan's career included his post as Director of Laboratories at St. Luke's and Children's Medical Center. During World War II he served as Colonel, Medical Corps, United States Army, in charge of the laboratory at Fort Belvoir, Virginia. A bachelor, he retired to a residence with a niece at Edwardsville, Pennsylvania, where he died January 18, 1978.

Carl Joseph Bucher, M.D. (1890–1951), Director of Clinical Laboratories (1940–1951)

Born in 1890 in Longansport, Indiana, Dr. Bucher (Figure 6-10) spent a year at Georgetown College, subsequently receiving his degrees at the University of Pennsylvania (B.S., 1912; M.D., 1916). Internships at St. Agnes Hospital (1916–1917) and St. Christopher's Hospital for Children (July–December, 1917), were followed by laboratory training at the U.S. Navy Medical School, Washington, D.C. (1918–1919) and by graduate study at the University of Pennsylvania, ending in 1920. Bucher then served as Medical Officer in charge of the laboratory at U.S. Naval Hospital, Newport, Rhode Island, until 1925. At that time he was appointed Assistant Pathologist at the Philadelphia General Hospital, where he continued on the staff until 1939. In 1926 he joined the staff of Jefferson Hospital as Assistant Director of the Clinical Laboratories, serving initially under Dr. Crawford and succeeding him as Director on Crawford's death in 1940. By providing stability and guidance to the Clinical Laboratories during the 25 years of their transition from low- to high-volume manual operations just prior to the emergence of automated testing, Dr. Bucher made an impressive contribution.

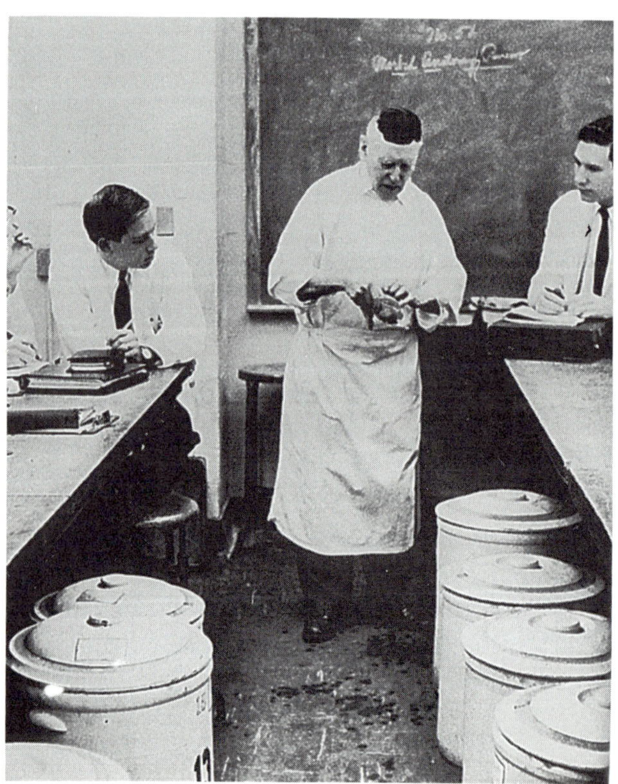

FIG. 6-8. Dr. Morgan teaching Gross Pathology.

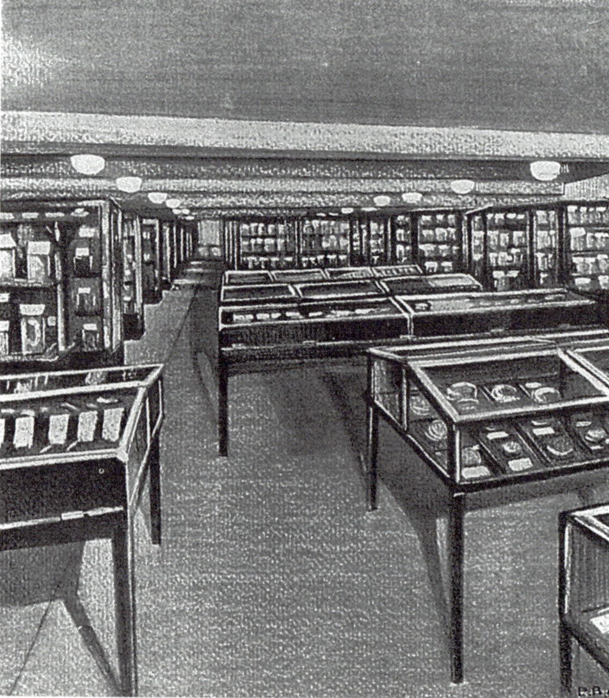

FIG. 6-9. Pathology Museum in 1025 Walnut Street Medical College (ca. 1940).

Advances in Pathology

In the 36 years between Longstreth's appointment as first Chairman in 1891 and the arrival of Moon as the fourth Chairman in 1927, enormous advances had taken place in the understanding of disease processes. The frozen-section technique, first introduced in Europe in 1818 by Pieter de Riemer,[1] was popularized in America in 1895 by the gynecologist, Thomas Cullen. Mallory and Wright's text *Pathological Technique* was published in 1897. Sternberg elucidated the histology of Hodgkins' Disease in 1899. The transmission of yellow fever by mosquitoes, first predicted in 1881 by Carlos J. Finlay (Jefferson, 1855), was established in 1900 by Walter Reed, James Carroll, Jesse Lazear, and Aristide Agramonte. Also in 1900, Karl Landsteiner laid the foundation for blood transfusion (and other transplants) by identifying the four major ABO blood groups. Eugene Opie related the islets of Langerhans to diabetes mellitus in 1901. The pathologic physiology of cardiac conduction was clarified between 1902 and 1915 by James McKenzie, Thomas Lewis, J. Erlanger, Alfred Stengel, Ludwig Aschoff, Sunao Tawara, and others. Treponema pallidum was discovered in 1905 by Fritz Richard Schaudinn and E. Hoffman. Bernard Naunyn introduced the concept of diabetic acidosis in 1906. James B. Herrick identified sickle cell anemia in 1910, the year in which tissue culture was developed by R. G. Harrison. Peyton Rous discovered the fowl sarcoma caused by a filterable agent in 1911, laying the foundation for the study of the retroviral etiology of cancer. Between 1915 and 1918 L. J. Henderson and Donald D. Van Slyke established the importance of the acid-base equilibrium in clinical medicine. Bacteriophage was described in 1917 by Felix Hubert d'Herelle. Frederick G. Banting and Charles H. Best discovered insulin in 1921. George Minot and William Murphy elucidated the deficiency nature of pernicious anemia in 1926 with their liver diet. Most of these advances were made by the application of the new sciences of microbiology and biochemistry to the clinical aspects of disease. The stage was set for the entrance of investigative pathologists typified by Virgil Holland Moon.

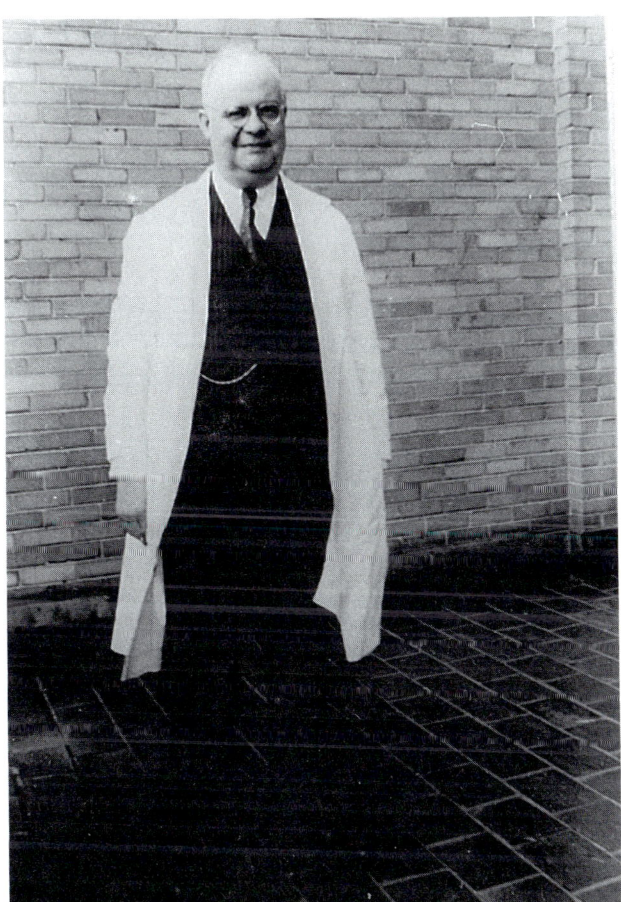

FIG. 6-10. Carl J. Bucher, M.D. (1890–1951), Director of Clinical Laboratories (1940–1951).

Virgil Holland Moon, M.D. (1879–1964), Fourth Chairman (1927–1948)

Virgil Holland Moon (Figure 6-11) was a Hoosier of Quaker stock, born in 1879 at Craig, Indiana, the son of a country doctor. An ancestor, James Moon, had come to Pennsylvania with William Penn and had settled at Morrisville, Bucks County, adjacent to Penn's estate. Virgil moved with his family to Kansas when he was two years old. He received an A.B. in 1910 and an M.Sc. in 1911, both from Kansas State Teachers College. He received his M.D. in 1913 from Rush Medical College in Chicago, having been elected to both Alpha Omega Alpha and Sigma Xi (the latter an indication of his early interest in the experimental approach to medicine). He never had an internship, but rather continued for an additional year his fellowship in infectious diseases at the McCormick Institute under the eminent Ludwig Hektoen from 1911 to 1914. This experience and Hektoen's recommendation were sufficient to enable Moon to be appointed Professor of Pathology and Bacteriology at the University of Indiana as well as Chief of Pathology at the Indianapolis City Hospital. He remained at Indiana until 1927, when he accepted the Chairmanship at Jefferson.

Dean Ross V. Patterson made it very clear to Moon what was expected of him, as seen in this excerpt from a letter to Moon on his appointment:

> "Dr. Moon, you will be expected to devote your talents and energies to the teaching of pathology. You will not be expected to do research work. In fact, I may say you will be expected NOT to do research work. A dog cannot chase two rabbits at the same time; should he try to do this, both rabbits will escape. A man cannot do good teaching and carry on successful research simultaneously."[13]

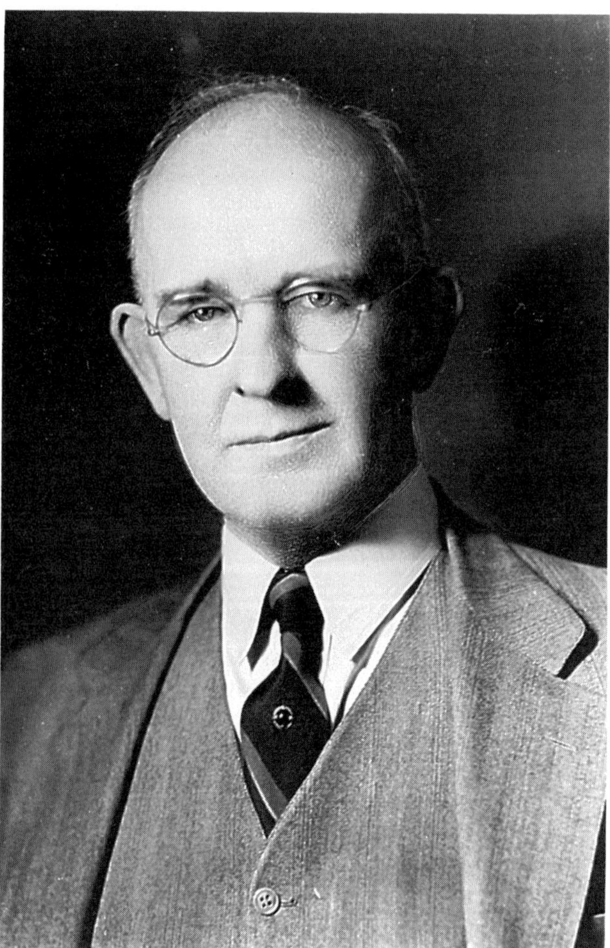

Fig. 6-11. Virgil H. Moon, M.D. (1879–1964), Fourth Chairman (1927–1948).

This does not mean that Dean Patterson was opposed to research. In point of fact, Patterson (a bachelor) left the bulk of his estate to Jefferson to establish the "Ross V. Patterson Research Fellowships."

Despite the Dean's admonition, Moon did both teaching and research, becoming an authority on shock, and writing two widely read monographs in 1938 and 1942 that profoundly influenced the way battle casualties were managed in World War II. Moon believed in 1927 that the viewpoint that research at Jefferson was dangerous to one's career was prevalent throughout the institution. Both Moon and Physiology Chairman J. Earl Thomas, who had also arrived at Jefferson in 1927, were anxious to do animal research, and they ignored the prevalent pessimistic viewpoint "partly because a few of the Trustees and of the Faculty believed as we did," according to Moon, who cited Dr. Martin E. Rehfuss as a strong supporter of research.[12] Through Rehfuss' efforts, Moon's research was initially supported by a $3,000 yearly stipend from the wife of a member of the Board of Trustees, John C. Martin. In addition, another Trustee, Percival E. Forderer, donated the building on his family's ancestral five-acre estate in the Frankford section of Philadelphia for research purposes. It evolved into animal quarters and other experimental support facilities, particularly in the immense carriage house at the rear of the estate. This animal facility proved valuable to both Moon and Thomas and was used until its sale in 1952. Moon believed that these gifts of money and property were the first expressly donated for research work at Jefferson. Despite this generous support, Moon and Thomas still had to obtain animals for research by using funds earmarked for teaching and were "ashamed that such a proud institution of higher learning should compel research workers to use clandestine methods and to bootleg their investigative work."[13]

As a result of Moon's lack of interest in the Clinical Laboratories and partly because of his failure to give any academic advancement to the Director (Dr. Bucher never rose above the rank of Assistant Professor during Moon's tenure and complained bitterly about it to all who would listen), a schism developed between the Medical School Department headed by Moon and the Clinical Laboratories (led by Bucher, who had succeeded Crawford in 1940). This made it difficult for the younger men in the Clinical Laboratories, who strove to please Bucher without offending Moon. Some of Bucher's later residents, such as Thomas Tamaki (1946–1948), did not aspire to academic advancement at Jefferson, but the new resident in 1939, Peter A. Herbut, did have academic dreams and yet managed to satisfy both masters.

During World War II the facilities and personnel of the Clinical Laboratories were severely strained. Most of the pathologists were in military service, leaving Bucher (age 51 in 1941) and Herbut (disabled by rheumatoid spondylitis) to carry the entire workload of the Hospital laboratories. The Chemistry Laboratory did an increasing number of procedures. By October 1945, test volume reached 2,879 and included such determinations as amylase, bromides, and (as a test of hepatic parenchymal cell damage) cephalin cholesterol flocculation. At this time an Evelyn photoelectric colorimeter was purchased and became the workhorse for chemical quantitation.

In 1947, Robert L. Breckenridge (Jefferson, 1944), (later Professor of Pathology at Jefferson and the 1985–1987 President of the College of American Pathologists) joined the Clinical Laboratory staff as Assistant Director. In 1946 the urinalysis laboratory was moved to the Curtis Clinic Building, freeing space for expansion of the Chemistry Laboratory, which lost its longtime mentor when Cantarow moved to the Medical College Department of Biochemistry as full-time Chairman.

Moon retired in 1948 after 21 years of service. His tenure was the second longest in the history of the Chair. He moved to Florida and was appointed Research Professor of Pathology in the Research Unit of the University of Miami Medical School. He died April 16, 1964, in his 85th year. He is remembered for his teachings on shock and for bringing respectability to basic medical research at Jefferson. He was the subject for portraiture of the Class of 1940.

Peter Andrew Herbut, M.D. (1912–1976), Fifth Chairman (1948–1966)

The second Canadian to head the Department, Peter A. Herbut (Figure 6-12) was born in Edson, Province of Alberta, Canada, on July 6, 1912. His Russian parents farmed and raised a large family. Herbut studied at the University of Alberta from 1930 to 1935 and then entered the Medical School of McGill University in Montreal, where he received his M.D., C.M. in 1937.[14] His training had included a one-year (1936–1937) internship at the Children's Memorial Hospital in Montreal, and he repeated the year of internship in 1937–1938 at Wilkes-Barre General Hospital when he decided to come to the United States for training in surgery. As further preparation for surgery, Herbut took a residency appointment in the Surgical Pathology Laboratory of the Medical

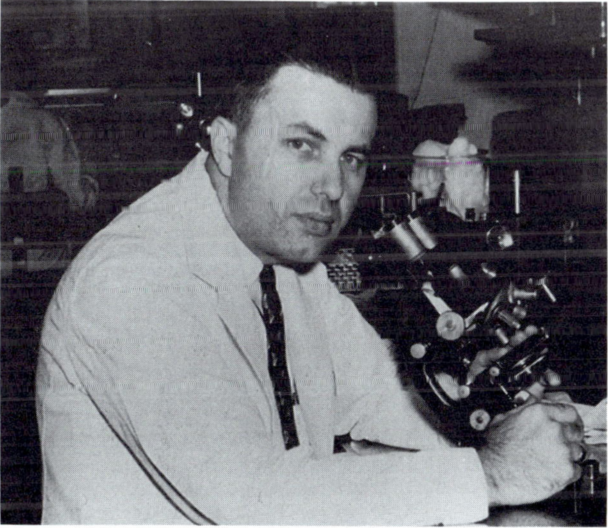

FIG. 6-12. Peter A. Herbut, M.D. (1912–1976), Fifth Chairman (1948–1966).

College of Virginia from 1938 to 1939. There he was trained by Paul Kimmelstiel, who converted Herbut to a career pathologist. Having been introduced to Virgil Moon at a convention, Herbut accepted an appointment as Assistant Demonstrator of Pathology at Jefferson, where he completed his training (1939–1940). He then joined the staff of the Clinical Laboratories as Assistant Director in 1940 and began a rise in the academic ranks of the Medical College, becoming an Assistant Professor before 1948.

Herbut had decided on first coming to Jefferson that he could be Department Chairman within ten years.[15] He made it in nine years. He resolved never to offend anyone, even the elevator operators, so there would be no impedance to his upward rise—this was no small task in a department where the Chairman and the Director of Clinical Laboratories were on poor terms. That he did not offend either one is strong testimony to Herbut's diplomatic powers. The major reasons, however, for Herbut's rise to the top by the age of 36 were his prodigious capacity for work and his great ability to concentrate. Not only did he almost single-handedly carry the anatomical pathology workload of the Clinical Laboratories during World War II, but he also found time and energy to publish 75 monographs during his first nine years at Jefferson. His colleagues looked upon him as a genius. He became a U.S. citizen in 1942. In 1948, upon Moon's retirement, Herbut was made Professor of Pathology and Chairman of the Department.

An excellent lecturer with a rapid delivery that induced writer's cramp in those students who tried (in the days before a note-taking service) to keep up, Herbut carried virtually the entire burden of 77 sophomore lectures in pathology, although he delegated the excellent lecture series on *Pathology in Internal Medicine* for juniors to William V. McDonnell and Joseph F. McCloskey, his major teaching associates in the Medical School for many years.

Always a prolific writer even when a Department Chairman, Herbut's first textbook was *Surgical Pathology,* which appeared in 1948 (and was followed by a second edition in 1954); *Urological Pathology* (two volumes), which appeared in 1952, followed by a Spanish edition in 1959; *Pathology* (a general textbook), which appeared in 1955, with a second edition in 1959; and *Obstetrical and Gynecological Pathology,* which was published in 1958.

Herbut was an excellent morphologist. His greatest fame came in the cytologic diagnosis of cancer, particularly in the lower respiratory tract, in association with Louis H. Clerf, Professor of Laryngology and Bronchoesophagology. Together they won the Ward Burdick Award (the highest honor for investigative work) of the American Society of Clinical Pathologists in 1950 for their demonstration of the efficacy of the cytologic diagnosis of bronchogenic carcinoma. Up to 80 percent accuracy was achieved by going back several times with a rigid bronchoscope to obtain more cells until the cytologic diagnosis agreed with the clinical one. Because of Herbut's reputation in the cytologic diagnosis of nongynecologic cancer and the equally excellent reputation of Abraham E. Rakoff (Professor of Obstetrical and Gynecological Endocrinology) in gynecologic cytology, Jefferson acquired an international reputation as a center for cytology training and diagnosis in the 1950s and 1960s.

With the sudden death in October, 1951, of Carl Bucher, the Directorship of the Clinical Laboratories devolved to Herbut and the schism in the Department ceased. This allowed better coordination of resources (manpower, in particular) and strengthened the Pathology Residency in a four year program of combined anatomical and clinical pathology. A steady stream of residents (usually two per year) passed through the program, most of them destined for directorships of laboratories in community hospitals.

Herbut taught his residents to think as he did, in an organized way, stressing expediency, pragmatism, and simplistics. Most of them stayed on the teaching staff after completion of their residencies.

The Clinical Laboratories expanded in both quantity and quality of work under Herbut. In 1953 a total of 343,904 tests were performed, including 8,000 surgical pathology examinations. During the year 1953–1954, in which the Foerderer Pavilion was being built, the Laboratories moved from their very crowed quarters on the fifteenth and sixteenth floors of Thompson Annex and second floor of the Main Hospital building to temporary space on the sixth floor of the Curtis Clinic. In 1954, the Clinical Laboratories moved into then-spacious quarters on the third floor of the Foerderer Pavilion, sharing the space with the Blood Bank, which was under the jurisdiction of the Cardeza Foundation. Among the Assistant Directors of Clinical Laboratories who served under Herbut were Robert L. Breckenridge (1947–1953), William C. Herrick (1948–1953), Paul N. Jernstrom (1953–1957), Henry L. Kazal (1953–1957), Richard C. Taylor (Associate Director, 1957–1970), Francis A. McKeon, Jr. (1957–1961), Paul L. Lewis (1958–1961), Simon Soumerai (1958–1961) John J. Moran (1961–1967), William E. Delaney III (1961–1968), Dennis S. O'Connor (1961–1964), and Harold L. Bauer (1964–1967). Most of these men were anatomical pathologists, but Herrick, McKeon, O'Connor, and Bauer had primary responsibilities in the Chemistry Laboratory.

In November of 1954, the Chemistry Laboratory was staffed by a supervisor, a chief technologist, seven technologists, two aides, one secretary, and numerous blood collectors (mostly medical students). The vacutainer method of blood collection had just been introduced. A flame photometer had been purchased for the ever-increasing number of electrolyte studies (replacing the Sunderman total base analyzer that had been in use since 1951). A spectrophotometer was on order. An entire room was given over to protein-bound iodine tests of thyroid function. By 1961 blood gas analysis began, using an Astrup apparatus, and a four-channel Autoanalyzer was being used for simultaneous measurement of sodium, potassium, chloride, and carbon dioxide levels in blood.

Supervision of the Microbiology Laboratory after the death of Dr. Bucher in 1951 was the responsibility on a part-time basis of Carl Clancy, Ph.D. until 1955, when it became the full-time charge of Eileen Randall, Ph.D. "Randy" brought superb professionalism and a high degree of service to Microbiology. Her departure to Evanston (Illinois) Hospital in 1969 left a great void.

No Chairman in the history of the Pathology Department had personally carried out the three major tasks of an academic department (teaching, service, and research) better than Herbut. His success in the teaching and service mission would have been predictable from his accomplishments before assuming the Chair. The remarkable expansion of the research activities for which the Department under Herbut became known could only have been anticipated after 1946, when he began his work with the Elizabeth Storck Kraemer Foundation. As discussed in detail in the chapter on Medical Oncology, the Foundation screened more than 4,000 DuPont chemicals for anti-tumor activity. Herbut and his laboratory assistant, Edward Sekula, became adept at transplanting tumors into rodents during the 18 years of work with the foundation.

The research activities of the Department in 1961 were reviewed in the March issue of the *Alumni Bulletin* that year.[16] Herbut had attracted other active, funded researchers who brought expertise in viral carcinogenesis and arteriosclerosis to the Department. The work of Drs. Robert Love and R. Gerald Suskind in the histochemistry of polyoma virus infection was supported by a $440,827 five-year grant from the U.S. Public Health Service. Their team eventually included Kay Ellem and George Studzinski. Studzinski later became Chairman of the Department of Pathology at New Jersey College of Medicine and Dentistry in Newark. Love moved to the National Cancer Institute of the National Institutes of Health, where he served as Chief of the Office of Program Planning and Analysis until his untimely death March 5, 1978. Theodore Tsaltas' area of investigation was in the field of blood lipid and lipoprotein metabolism and the development of experimental models of arteriosclerosis. It was funded by the National Institutes of Health for $200,000 over a four year period. Tsaltas also died early, having had polycystic disease of the kidneys that required prolonged dialysis treatment. Gonzalo Enrique Aponte spent the years from 1959 to 1966 not only teaching but also researching in the field of radiation carcinogenesis. He had taken a six month sabbatical leave from February to August, 1960, to study under Eugene Cronkite at the Brookhaven National Laboratory on Long Island. Aponte's research on rat mammary carcinogenesis was not funded. Herbut not only received Kraemer Foundation support through 1965, but also, as an outgrowth of those activities, received a National Institutes of Health grant renewal for three years in 1965. Unfortunately,

Herbut's later research on tumor-inhibitory principles isolated from mammalian blood and liver could not be continued beyond 1966. At that time he ceased active research and became President of Jefferson Medical College.

Herbut had occupied an increasingly responsible position in the guidance of Jefferson since election by his peers as Chairman of the Executive Faculty in 1956, a position he occupied until 1965. In this capacity he was in frequent contact with members of the Administration and in particular with Mr. William Bodine (President of the Medical College), whose confidence Herbut came to share. On September 12, 1966, after the resignation of Bodine, Herbut became the President of Jefferson Medical College. It was characteristic of this cautious man that he arranged for his salary to be paid partially as President, partly as Professor of Pathology (a title he kept although he did resign as Director of the Laboratories), and partly as Attending Pathologist in the Clinical Laboratories.

In connection with the Pathology Department, Herbut should be remembered as a man for all seasons who played all the roles expected of him with great distinction, who was a superb diagnostic morphologist and cytopathologist, a great teacher, a prolific writer, the mentor and model for the pathologists he trained, an excellent administrator, and a gifted researcher who might have achieved much more had he followed his investigative leanings to their fruition. His contributions to Jefferson began in earnest when he left pathology and laid the foundation of Thomas Jefferson University.

Gonzalo Enrique Aponte, M.D. (1929–1979), Sixth Chairman (1967–1979)

The first Pathology Chairman of Latin-American extraction, Gonzalo E. Aponte (Figure 6-13) was born July 15, 1929, at Santurce, Puerto Rico. Brilliant even at a young age, he was graduated after three years premedical study at Georgetown University, receiving his B.Sc. in 1948 at 18 years of age. Aponte received his M.D. from Jefferson in 1952, finishing first in his class. He began a rotating internship (1952–1953) in Jefferson Medical College Hospital with the intention of becoming an internist but decided to take a three month rotation in the Chemistry Laboratory (July–September, 1953) and during that time became committed to pathology as a career. He finished his four year Residency in Pathology at Jefferson in 1957. Two years of duty in the U.S. Navy as Pathologist at the Naval Hospital on Guam followed (1957–1959), and then Aponte returned to Jefferson as a full-time teacher and researcher. He was the first Jeffersonian to receive the prestigious Markle Scholarship in Medical Science, which he had from 1960 to 1965. In 1967, Dr. Aponte was named to succeed Dr. Herbut as Professor and Chairman of the Department and Director of the Clinical Laboratories.

Aponte's first love was teaching, and he was given early recognition as a gifted lecturer,

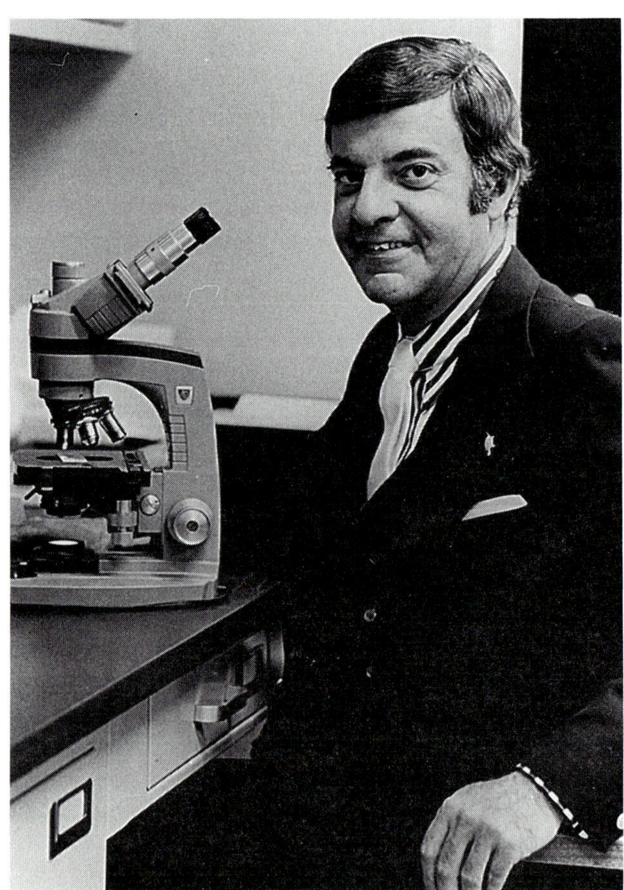

FIG. 6-13. Gonzalo E. Aponte, M.D. (1929–1979), Sixth Chairman (1967–1979).

receiving a Lindback Foundation Award for distinguished teaching in 1962, three years after joining the faculty. His extraordinary intelligence, conspicuous nervous energy, great command of the English language, stage presence, and desire to excel made him an impressive Professor in the classical sense. He put a great amount of work into the preparation of his lectures, revising them yearly and including an extraordinary amount of detail, even clinical data from the 20 medical journals he read each month. Most of his students revered him; he was consistently chosen to administer the Hippocratic Oath to each year's graduating class. The Class of 1971 commissioned his portrait to be painted when he was only 41, making him the youngest Professor ever so honored. His peers also honored him. In 1967 Aponte was named Clinical Scientist of the Year by the Association of Clinical Scientists, and in 1977 he was elected President of the Alumni Association of Jefferson Medical College.

As an extension of his interest in teaching, Aponte spent a great amount of time on the residency program in pathology. Under his leadership its size was expanded to an average of three new residents yearly in the four year program. Despite the attention he devoted to the residency program, however, his interests were primarily in the Medical College and not in the Hospital. As time went on he devoted less time to the day-to-day operations of the Clinical Laboratories, especially after the installation of new staff members, notably Heinz G. Schwartz, M.D., Ph.D. in Clinical Pathology and Arthur S. Patchefsky, M.D. in Surgical Pathology. By 1972 Schwartz was advanced from Assistant Director to Associate Director of Laboratories and in 1978 he was made Director when Aponte relinquished the Clinical Laboratory appointment.

Automation of the Clinical Laboratories proceeded rapidly through the 1960s to the 1970s. In fiscal year 1969–1970 a total of 521,834 laboratory tests were done; within six years (1970–1976) the total had risen to 919,943. The largest area of increase occurred in the Chemistry Laboratory, where test volume had gone from 261,121 to 490,000 in six years. Most of the increased workload had been accomplished with relatively small increase in manpower because of automated equipment (multiple-channel analyzers in chemistry, for example). Anatomical pathology workload had risen also, with an average of 9,673 surgical and 25,863 cytological specimens processed yearly between 1969 and 1975. During the same period the number of autopsies averaged 309 annually.

In contrast to the increasing Clinical Laboratory activity, research programs in the Medical College languished in the early years of Aponte's tenure as a result of the loss of the productive researchers (Love and Tsaltas) brought in by Herbut. At the same time, funding by the National Institutes of Health and other agencies began to be more difficult to obtain. Eventually Suskind, Ellem, and Studzinski went to other institutions, and by the mid-1970s there was no investigative activity in Jefferson's Department of Pathology.

Highlighted by the brilliance of its Chairman (but increasingly as a one-man show) the Department continued to be well regarded late in the 1970s, particularly in its teaching function. It was thus a major tragedy when Aponte died suddenly, of a cardiac arrhythmia, on June 15, 1979, at age 49, shortly after having been named the first Peter A. Herbut Professor of Pathology. It was a fitting tribute to his deserved reputation as a teacher that Gonzalo Enrique Aponte himself was honored in death by his family, hundreds of devoted friends, and students who quickly raised funds that enabled his own name to be perpetuated in an Endowed Professorship.

Warren Reichert Lang, M.D. (1918–1986), Acting Chairman (1979–1983), Seventh and First Aponte Chairman (1983–1986)

The first native Philadelphian since Longstreth to become Chairman, Dr. Warren R. Lang (Figure 6-14) was born September 18, 1918, in the Bridesburg section. Of German ancestry, Lang attended Frankford High School, from which he graduated in 1936 (third in a class of 300). He then entered Temple University, graduating in 1940 (first in a class of 460) with honors (the Owl Award). He entered Jefferson in a class that became accelerated because of World War II, enabling him to graduate in March, 1943 at the top of his class. Lang served a rotating internship at Jefferson Hospital (1943–1944) and then took a year's residency (1944–1945) in Obstetrics and Gynecology at Jefferson. From 1945 to 1947 he served as a medical officer in the U.S. Army in Korea. He returned to Jefferson in 1947, becoming associated in practice with Dr. Lewis C. Scheffey, Chairman of the Department of Obstetrics and Gynecology.

By 1963, Lang had risen to prominence in his specialty, having been appointed Professor of Obstetrics and Gynecology at Jefferson in that year after having cooperated with Drs. Scheffey and Abraham Rakoff in the early development of gynecologic cytology. Lang had served as Secretary-Treasurer of the American Society of Cytology since 1960 and had been President of the American Society of Colposcopy and Colpomicroscopy for four years. Although it surprised his acquaintances when he decided on a career change in 1968, the switch to pathology was accomplished smoothly because of Lang's many years of morphological orientation. From 1968 to 1970 he served a Pathology Residency at Jefferson under Aponte and then spent a third year (1970–1971) at Case-Western Reserve under James Reagan. Lang returned to Jefferson in 1971 as Assistant Professor of Pathology with duties in surgical pathology, cytology, and autopsies. In 1973 he became Professor of Cytotechnology in the College of Allied Health Sciences at Jefferson. In 1976 Lang was promoted to Associate Professor of Pathology, and from 1979 he served as Acting Chairman during the first four years following Aponte's death. In 1983 Lang was named the first Gonzalo Enrique Aponte Professor of Pathology and Chairman of the Department, in which post he served until June 30, 1986, when he retired from the Chairmanship and relinquished the Aponte Professorship to his successor, Emanuel Rubin. Lang continued to serve in the Department, primarily in cytopathology, until his death from pneumonia and its complications on April 19, 1987.

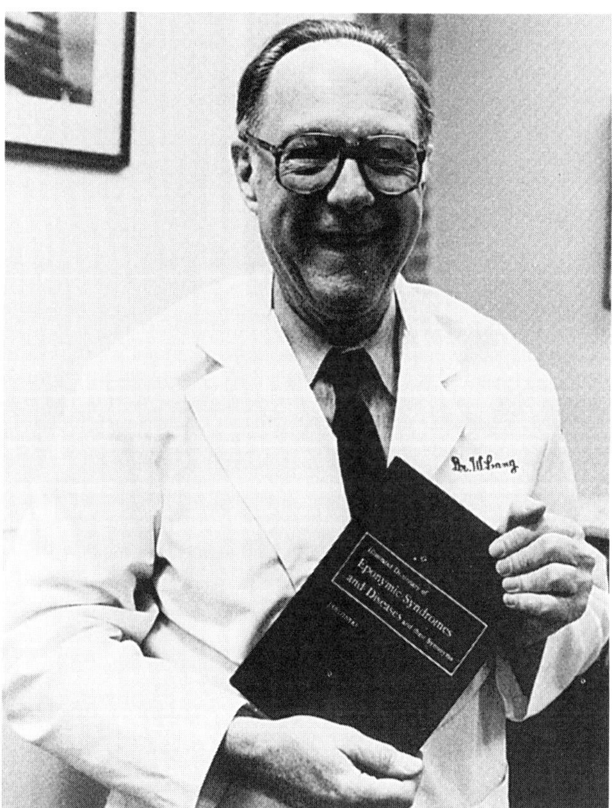

Fig. 6-14. Warren R. Lang, M.D. (1918–1986), Acting Chairman (1979–1983), Seventh and First Aponte Chairman (1983–1986).

Like his predecessor, Lang was principally renowned for his teaching ability during his years in pathology. His teaching style was unique, relying on aphorisms and wit, with lectures liberally embellished with Kodachromes. His enthusiasm for his subject was contagious, and his students reacted warmly to his teaching efforts. In 1977 he was given a Lindback Foundation Award for Distinguished Teaching. His portrait was commissioned to be painted by the Class of 1985. Lang's love for teaching carried over into his guidance of the pathology residency program. Continuing the dedication of his predecessors, he was responsible for the training of many pathologists.

A prolific writer, Lang published 147 scientific articles. His work was highly regarded, particularly in cytopathology. In 1984 he received the prestigous Papanicolaou Award of the American Society of Cytology, and he was the Society's President in 1984–1985. He was also a bibliophile, an opera lover, and a student of classical Greek literature.

Emanuel Rubin, M.D. (1928–), Eighth and Second Aponte Chairman (1986–)

Emanuel Rubin (Figure 6-15), current Chairman and second holder of the Aponte Professorship, was born in Atlantic City, New Jersey, on December 5, 1928. His status as one of the world's leading experts on alcohol-induced diseases is all the more remarkable when regarded in the light of the financing of his education. Not only was he the recipient of a scholarship from the New Jersey Association of Licensed Beverage Dealers, which was renewed yearly for each of his four years at Villanova University (B.S. in Biology with High Honors, 1950), but the beer and whiskey dealers, impressed with his extraordinary academic achievements, took the unprecedented step of paying for his entire education at Harvard Medical School (M.D., 1954). After internship in the Boston City Hospital (1954–55), Rubin served two years (1955–1957) as a Lieutenant (Medical Corps), U.S. Navy. He returned briefly (1957–1958) as a resident in Children's Hospital of Philadelphia. He then moved to New York City's Mount Sinai Hospital and Medical School, where he spent the next 18 years, receiving his clinical and research training in pathology with special emphasis on liver diseases under Dr. Hans Popper. Rubin rose to Pathologist-in-Chief of the Hospital (1971–1976) and became the Irene Heinz and John LaPorte Given Professor of Pathology and Chairman of the Department (1972–1976). He returned to Philadelphia in 1977 to become Professor and Chairman of the Department of Pathology and Laboratory Medicine and Director of Laboratories of Hahnemann Medical College and Hospital for nine years. In 1986 Rubin came to Jefferson as the Gonzalo E. Aponte Professor of Pathology, Chairman of the Department of Pathology and Cell Biology, and Attending Physician-in-Chief (Pathology) of Thomas Jefferson University Hospital. Since 1977 Rubin has also held an appointment in the University of Pennsylvania School of Medicine as Adjunct Professor of Biochemistry and Biophysics.

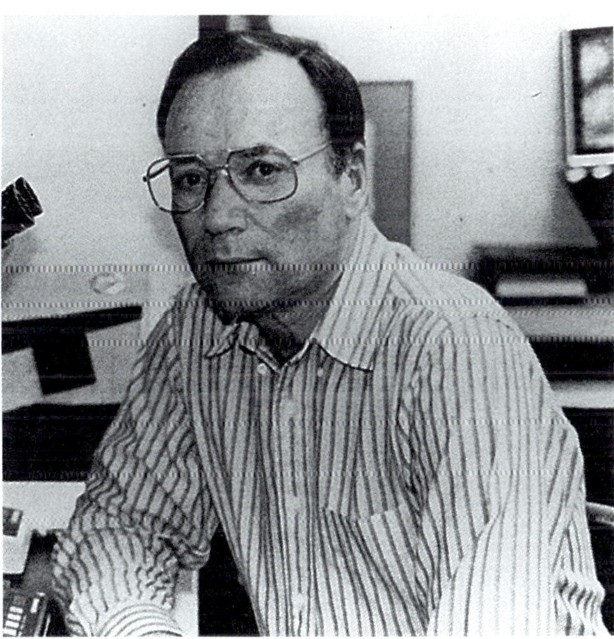

Fig. 6-15. Emanuel Rubin, M.D. (1928–), Eighth and Second Aponte Chairman (1986–).

His dual academic appointments indicate Rubin's interests. In attempting to establish a molecular basis of behavioral tolerance to alcohol and other drugs, he has become a membrane biologist, using new techniques such as nuclear magnetic resonance to learn of the biophysical principles that govern the control mechanisms for cell membranes. The change in the name of the Department reflects Rubin's belief that the boundaries between traditional pathology and biochemistry, cell physiology, and molecular pharmacology are disappearing—in the research laboratory at the moment but in routine practice in the near future. For this reason, and because skill and training in new techniques and instrumentation are needed in order to acquire new knowledge, Rubin has changed the design of the pathology residency. He has lengthened the program to five years, beginning with a core training of three years to provide competence in subspecialty areas related to clinical medicine and a final two years to complete the program with intensive training and research in one subspecialty. Rubin predicts that in ten years the changes in pathology departments of medical schools will make them unrecognizable in terms of departments of the recent past. At Jefferson, the Department is at the cutting edge in application of techniques to medicine both at the diagnostic and research levels. Though computerized teaching of pathology will be widely applied, the computer will never replace a good teacher as a role model. new biologic techniques to medicine both at the diagnostic and research levels. Though computerized teaching of pathology will be widely applied, the computer will never replace a good teacher as a role model.

In 1988, Dr. Rubin co-edited, with John L. Faber, M.D. (Professor of Pathology at Jefferson) and 40 contributors from the United States and Canada, a monumental textbook, *Pathology,* which features classical general pathology and systemic pathologic anatomy in the context of modern biology.[17]

Pathology throughout the world has assumed a distinct differentiation within the body of medicine, but at the same time it has become an integral part of disease concepts from newer aspects. Jefferson shares in this progress.

References

1. Krumbhaar, E.B., *Pathology,* Vol. 19, Clio Medica. A Series of Primers on the History of Medicine. New York: Paul B. Hoeber Medical Book Dept., Harper & Bros., 1937.
2. Wagner, F.B., Jr., "Revisit of Samuel D. Gross, M.D.," *Surg., Gynec. & Obst.* 152:1–12, 1981.
3. Gross, S.D., *Elements of Pathologic Anatomy.* Philadelphia: Blanchard & Lea, 1839.
4. Gross, S.D., *op. cit.,* 2d ed., 1845.
5. Gross, S.D., *op. cit.,* 3rd ed., 1857.
6. Tyson, J., "Memoir of Dr. Morris Longstreth," *Trans. Stud. Coll. Phys. Phila.,* 3rd Ser., Vol. 38, 1916, pp. lvii–lx.
7. Bauer, E.L., *Doctors Made in America.* Philadelphia: J. B. Lippincott Co., 1963, pp. 257–262.
8. King, L.S., "Medicine in the U.S.A.: Historical Vignettes: Clinical Laboratories Become Important, 1870–1900," *J.A.M.A.* 249: 3025–3029, 1983.
9. Morman, E.T., "Clinical Pathology in America, 1965–1915: Philadelphia as a Test Case," *Bull. Hist. Med.* 58: 198–214, 1984.
10. "Biography of Bowman Corning Crowell," 1927 CLINIC Yearbook, p. 57. (In Thomas Jefferson University Archives).
11. "Biography of Baxter Lindsay Crawford," *Jeff. Med. Coll. Al. Bull.,* Vol. 2, May, 1940, p. 49.
12. Griffith, R.S., "Biography of Dedicatee: David R. Morgan M.D.," 1935 CLINIC Yearbook, pp. 9–11. (In Thomas Jefferson University Archives).
13. Moon, V.H., "Scientific Research in Jefferson Medical College," Memoir (signed but undated) written on stationery of the University of Miami Medical Research Unit. (In Thomas Jefferson University Archives).
14. "Department of Pathology and Clinical Laboratories," *Jeff. Med. Coll. Al. Bull.,* Vol. 8, No. 7, May, 1954, pp. 3–10.
15. Herbut. P.A., "Jefferson Appointment, 1939, and Appointment, Professor of Pathology and Head of the Department, May 29, 1948," Herbut Personal Papers, Vol. 2. (In Thomas Jefferson University Archives).
16. "Expansion of Research in Department of Pathology," *Jeff. Med. Coll. Al. Bull.,* March, 1961, pp. 16–26.
17. Rubin, E., and Farber, J.L. (Editors), *Pathology,* Philadelphia: J.B. Lippincott Co., 1988.

CHAPTER SEVEN

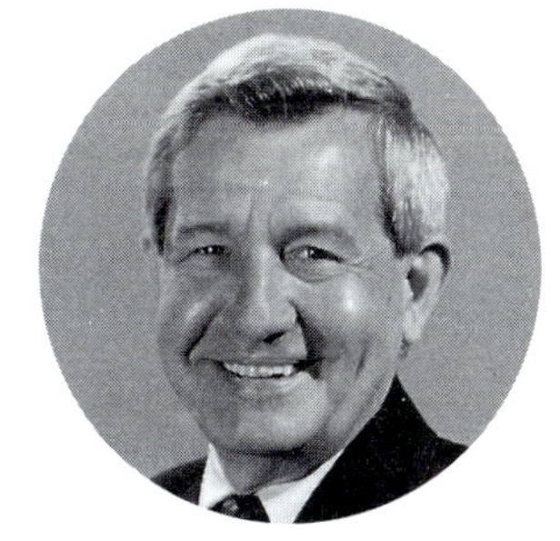

Department of Microbiology

Russell W. Schaedler, M.D.

"God grant that by my persevering labors, I may bring a little stone to the frail and ill-assured edifice of our knowledge of those deep mysteries of Life and Death where all our intellects have so lamentably failed."

—Louis Pasteur (1822–1895)

Among the "basic sciences" that provide a foundation for clinical medicine, none was more dependent upon new concepts and discoveries developed over the latter half of the nineteenth century than Bacteriology, or as later designated, Microbiology. Beginning with the low-key theories of "Contagion," the possible role of "animalcules," and continuing to firm establishment of the cause of specific diseases by microscopic agents, the subject was introduced at Jefferson by clinical lectures in several departments. Many interesting events and discussions contributed to early teaching of the subject.

Dr. John Kearsley Mitchell, Professor of Medicine, one of the early Jefferson proponents of the infectious nature of disease, presented discourses on enteric fevers, scarlet fever, consumption, measles, the pneumonias, and smallpox without being able at the time to relate these diseases to specific organisms. He wrote about the nature of malaria and "cryptogamous fevers," ascribing these diseases to minute spores and fungi.[1] In 1849 Dr. Thomas Dent Mütter, Professor of Surgery, presented a discourse on syphilis with quite accurate descriptions of chancres and the secondary stage of the disease. The following quotation from a student's notes (1849) is indicative of his views: "When gonorrhea and syphilis are produced in a patient at the same time, the respective virus (organisms) of both (diseases) have been present. One organism cannot produce the other disease." It would thus appear that Mütter was aware of John Hunter's ill-fated self-inoculation experiment in which Hunter developed syphilis from a case of gonorrhea in 1776. Jefferson professors also took part in the controversies aroused in 1843 by Oliver Wendell Holmes and in 1847 by Semmelweis, who were promoting cleanliness for prevention of puerperal sepsis and blood poisoning from contaminated wounds.

As specific discoveries confirmed the role of microorganisms in disease, the faculty gradually recognized the need to present the new development in an organized manner. Dr. W. M. L. Coplin began weekly lectures in Bacteriology in 1892 when he was Demonstrator of Pathology, and the subject continued as a part of Pathology until 1909, when the Department of Bacteriology and Hygiene was formed under Professor Randle C. Rosenberger.

Carlos Juan Finlay, M.D. (1833–1915)

In 1853, Carlos Juan Finlay (Figure 7-1), a Cuban, enrolled at age 20 in Jefferson Medical College. Only three months earlier Philadelphia had suffered its sixth yellow fever epidemic in 60 years. At that time the faculty consisted of Franklin Bache, Robley Dunglison, Robert Huston, Joseph Pancoast, John K. Mitchell, Thomas D. Mütter, and Charles D. Meigs. Pasteur was still working on crystals, Robert Koch was a young boy, and Lister was a young man working in the University

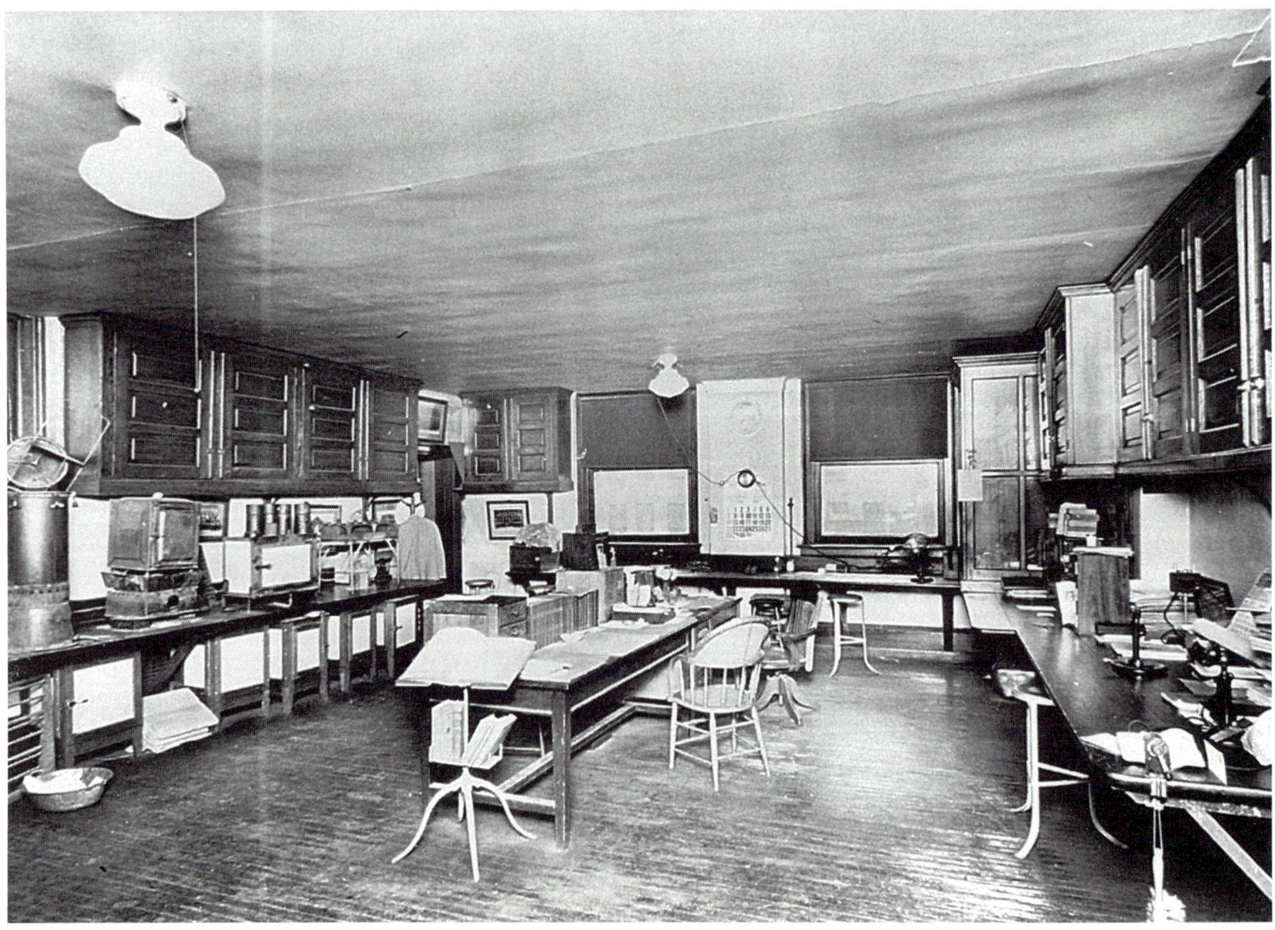

Microbiology Laboratory in the 1898 Medical College.

College Hospital in London. Surgeons prided themselves on dexterity and speed and worked in their street clothing without antisepsis.

Carlos Finlay's preceptor was John Kearsley Mitchell. The young Finlay became very close to both the senior Mitchell and his son, S. Weir Mitchell (Jefferson, 1850). They instilled in Finlay an interest in the use of the microscope and developed in him a questioning, open mind. Dr. Finlay graduated on March 10, 1855, and returned to Cuba to start a general practice. He was a well-rounded citizen, a scholar, and a physician. He wrote manuscripts on many subjects, such as leprosy, beriberi, cholera, and relapsing fever.

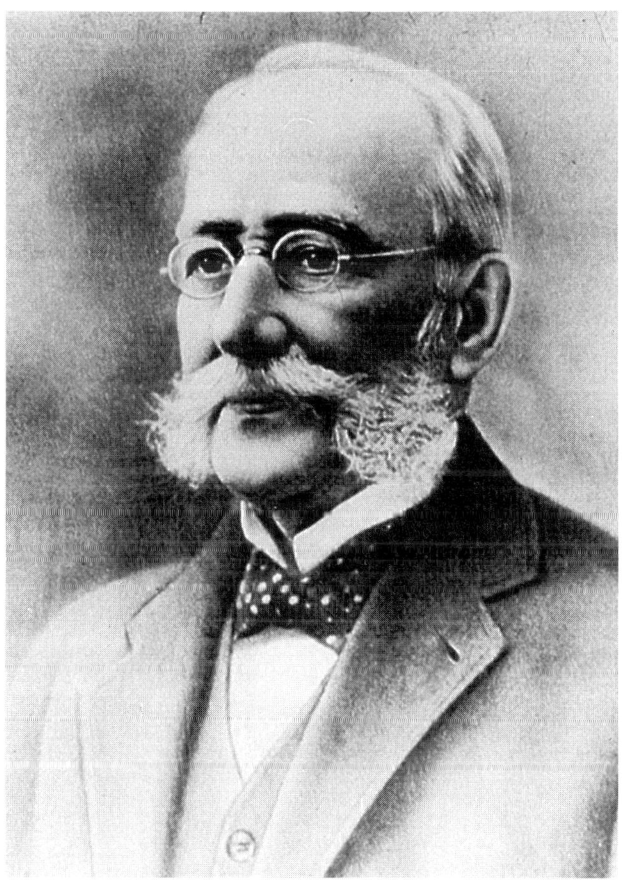

FIG. 7-1. Carlos Juan Finlay, M.D. (1833–1915). An 1855 graduate of Jefferson, Finlay incriminated the *Aedes aegypti* mosquito as the carrier of yellow fever (1881).

Between 1865 and 1881 Finlay wrote ten papers on yellow fever—his observations on the behavior and frequency of mosquitoes relative to the occurrence of yellow fever were basic. During hot weather, yellow fever occurred at low altitudes; cases diminished with higher altitudes and fewer mosquitoes. Many of his experiments were based on the hope that by mosquito inoculation he could produce a mild type of disease that would confer immunity. This line of investigation failed, but he persisted in his observations and became more convinced of the association of the disease and the mosquito.

In 1879 Dr. Finlay was appointed by the Cuban Governor General to cooperate with the United States Commission to Study Yellow Fever. At the International Sanitation Conference in Washington on February 18, 1881, Finlay proposed the three following conditions necessary for the propagation of the fever: (1) the existence of a previous case of yellow fever, (2) the presence of a subject capable of acquiring the disease, and (3) the presence of an agent necessary for its transmission. Six months later he pointed out that the mosquito, *Aedes aegypti* was the necessary agent. The Commission received all of Dr. Finlay's data and finally, in August, 1900, Lazear, working with the Commission, applied infected mosquitoes to nine American soldiers as well as to Commission members themselves. This first experiment failed, but two days later Lazear tried again and inoculated Dr. Carroll with an infected mosquito. Carroll developed yellow fever. A soldier also developed the disease after inoculation, confirming transmission of yellow fever by mosquitoes. Unfortunately, Lazear, the earliest convert of Finlay, became infected by an experimental sting of a mosquito and died of the disease. The theory proposed years before by Dr. Finlay which had been questioned and held up to ridicule for such a long period of time was proven to be correct and would have far-reaching global effects. Confirmation of his theory revealed that Dr. Finlay was a man of vision and originality, one able to accomplish basic experiments with minimal resources and without support of colleagues.

Jefferson Medical College awarded Finlay an honorary degree of Doctor of Science in 1902. His friend, Dr. S. Weir Mitchell, proposed him for membership in the College of Physicians of Philadelphia. Dr. Finlay's memory was honored at Jefferson in September, 1955, by a symposium on yellow fever in commemoration of the one hundredth anniversary of his graduation. As one remarked on this occasion, "It was a proud time for Jefferson. The institution was greatly honored by its relationship to the poor practitioner who became a prophet." In the fall of 1983 a special memorial lecture was delivered to the second-year students in honor of the 150th anniversary of Finlay's birth.

Beginning of a New Science

The groundwork for the new discipline of Bacteriology was laid mainly in Europe. Beginning in 1857, following his pioneering discoveries, Pasteur's sequential experiments finally discredited the long-held ideas of spontaneous generation. Pasteur's further work on fermentation and studies on anthrax and its prevention by immunization established him as a major pioneer. As early as 1867, Joseph Lister developed antiseptic surgery. Soon bacteriology emerged as a science for the study of specific causes of infections and for research and laboratory methods. By 1880 the organism causing typhoid fever was described by Eberth. In 1890 the Pasteur Institute was established. Rabies was transmitted to dogs, and a vaccine against rabies devised. *Vibro cholerae* was isolated and described. The tubercle bacillus was described by Koch in 1882. Diphtheria was described by Klebs and Loeffler. It was soon discovered that some diseases were caused by organisms that passed through filters that would hold back bacteria, but these organisms (viruses) could not be seen by light microscopy. By the turn of the century asepsis became a byword, and bacteria could be identified by morphological differences and fermentation reactions.

The great discoveries of the day, tuberculosis and rabies, were received in America with unbelievable skepticism. Instead of provoking experiment and investigation, the response was often controversy, hostility, and ridicule. Several individuals in the Philadelphia area, however, were exceptions. McFarland of the University of Pennsylvania became one of few American students of Pasteur, but he observed that from 1885 to 1889 there was no student teaching of bacteriology. Lawrence F. Flick, who graduated from Jefferson in 1879, readily accepted the germ theory of disease and promoted it in his valuable teachings and in his crusade against tuberculosis. He had been convinced of the infectious nature of tuberculosis by the teaching of Dr. W. H. Webb at Jefferson well before Koch's discovery of the tubercle bacillus.[2] In 1891–1892, a course in bacteriology at the University of Pennsylvania consisted of one lecture weekly for six weeks. At Jefferson, Coplin's weekly lectures were scheduled throughout the year and included hygiene.

Early Teaching At Jefferson

Having introduced the subject of bacteriology at Jefferson, Dr. Coplin included it in the evolving discipline of pathology—in 1895 the *College Catalog* listed a course entitled "Bacteriology and Clinical Microscopy." Coplin, however, left Jefferson to organize the Department of Histology, Pathology, and Bacteriology at Vanderbilt University in Nashville, Tennessee. In 1896 he returned to Jefferson to become Professor of Pathology and Bacteriology. Coplin held that title until the new Department of Bacteriology and Hygiene was established in 1909, at which time he continued a distinguished career as Professor of Pathology.

In 1897 Bacteriology was taught two days a week for six weeks by Dr. Coplin, assisted by Drs. David Biven and Randle C. Rosenberger. As new discoveries and advances came about, it was necessary to increase the teaching time in the curriculum, and a laboratory course was established. Elementary lectures were given to the first-year students to serve as an introduction to laboratory work in the third year. The latter course continued in the third year until 1917, when it was moved to the first year.

An outgrowth of the early instruction in bacteriology was the publication of the first book on Microbiology by an author from Philadelphia, Dr. Michael V. Ball (Jefferson, 1889). Entitled *Essentials of Bacteriology,* it was published by W.B. Saunders Co., Philadelphia, 1891. During the author's student years, no bacteriology was taught at Jefferson but on one occasion, Jacob M.

DaCosta introduced to the class a young physician, Julius Salinger, who had just returned from Berlin and who made a drawing of a bacillus on the blackboard. After graduation, at which he was awarded the Henry C. Lea Prize, Ball went abroad. Following a stop at the Paris Exhibition of 1889, he went on to visit clinics in London, Paris, Copenhagen, and Berlin. Because he spoke German fluently, he spent most of his time in Berlin, where he pursued a course in bacteriology at the Hygienisches Institut by Robert Koch assisted by Robert Frankel and Emil Behring. This course lasted for four weeks, ten hours daily. He returned to Philadelphia in April, 1890, and became an intern at the German (Lankenau) Hospital. Ball made the acquaintance of W. B. Saunders, a young publisher who was making a specialty of a new type of student publication, *Question Compends,* in question-and-answer form. The publisher had Ball sign a contract. Following internship, Ball took a position as a ship surgeon. With little work to do and few distractions, his manuscript for the *Essentials of Bacteriology* was completed and published in October, 1891. The question-and-answer form was not used, the text being continuous. The book became popular and went through six editions by 1908.

The teaching program continued to expand at Jefferson at the turn of the century. Gradually Dr. Coplin turned over responsibility for bacteriology to his associates. Immunology was added as new discoveries required. In addition to Dr. Rosenberger, Henry Radasch, George Nofer, and Archibald Graham became assistants while still senior medical students, and they provided instruction to underclassmen. Dr. Radasch joined the staff in Anatomy and for many years headed the teaching in Histology and Embryology. In 1903 Dr. Rosenberger was promoted to Associate in Bacteriology, and in 1904 he became an Assistant Professor. During these early years the practice of hiring student assistants led to the employment of Daniel Lewis, Henry B. Decker, Robert M. Lukens, and Erwin D. Funk, all to become well-known alumni of the College.

Randle C. Rosenberger, M.D. (1873–1944); First Chairman of Bacteriology and Hygiene (1909–1944)

Dr. Rosenberger (Figure 7-2) was born in Philadelphia, March 4, 1873. Educated at the old Central High School, he entered Jefferson in 1891 and graduated in 1894. From then until his death Rosenberger's association with Jefferson was uninterrupted. He had several early clinical appointments, but soon his attention was focused on Pathology and especially the new science of Bacteriology.

In 1897 Rosenberger became Assistant Demonstrator of Morbid Anatomy and Bacteriology and, in 1898, Assistant Pathologist to Jefferson Hospital. His career progressed at Jefferson, with advancement in 1904 to Assistant Professor of Bacteriology and ultimately to

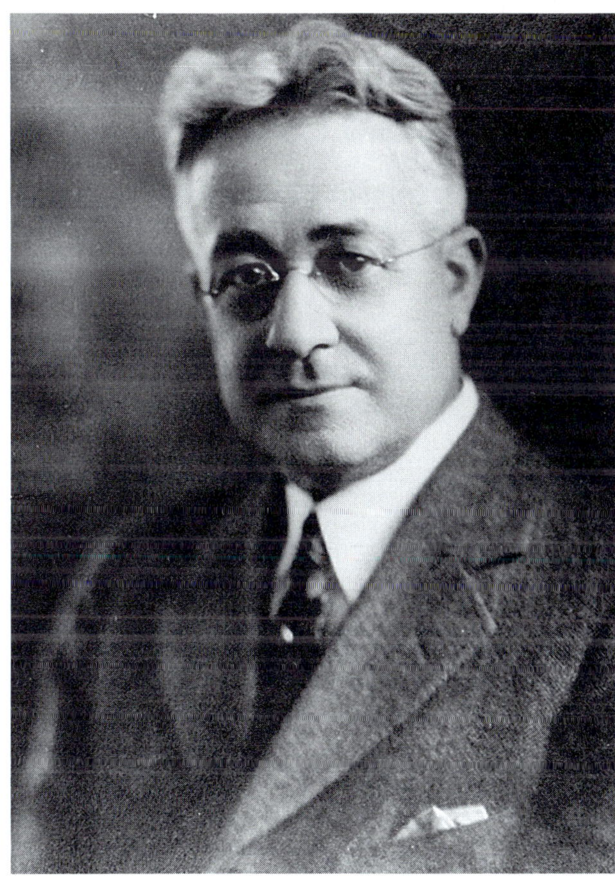

Fig. 7-2. Randle C. Rosenberger, M.D. (1873–1944); First Chairman of Bacteriology and Hygiene (1909–1944).

Professor and Head of the new Department of Bacteriology and Hygiene in 1909. Dr. Rosenberger was active in many areas in relation to developments in his field; these included the Milk Commission and the Pneumonia Commission for the City of Philadelphia. He also carried on investigation in a number of areas and published numerous papers as often as his busy teaching schedule would permit.

The early years of the Department were characterized by efforts to define the scope and limitations of the new discipline. Dr. Rosenberger himself assumed a prodigious teaching schedule in spite of other obligations that continued to demand time. He became a Lecturer and later Professor of Hygiene and Preventive Medicine at Woman's Medical College of Pennsylvania. He was also Pathologist to Philadelphia General Hospital (1903–1919) and served as Bacteriologist to the Henry Phipps Institute from 1904 to 1908.

John A. Roddy, M.D. (Jefferson, 1907), joined the Department as a Demonstrator in 1911 and was promoted to Associate in Bacteriology in 1915. He also became Demonstrator and Chief Assistant in the Department of Clinical Medicine at Jefferson Hospital as well as Professor of Hygiene and Bacteriology at the Philadelphia College of Pharmacy. His dual appointment continued until 1920. In 1917, Dr. Roddy published his book, *Medical Bacteriology,* a text for beginners and a laboratory guide for medical practitioners and pharmacists. Dr. Robert M. Lukens (Jefferson, 1911), who was an Assistant in the Department in 1911 and a former student of Dr. Rosenberger, did the illustrations. The book was published by P. Blakiston & Sons, Philadelphia.

The transfer of the laboratory course from the third to the first year in 1917 increased the need for intense student supervision, and by 1923 the course increased to 162 hours. Dr. Henry B. Decker (Jefferson, 1920), was appointed Instructor in Bacteriology in 1923 and assumed an intimate role in the laboratory course as well as sharing some of the lectures. In 1925 the Department name was changed to Preventive Medicine and Bacteriology, a title that would remain until the 1940s.

Having become established as one of the three first-year basic sciences at Jefferson, sharing those of Anatomy and Biochemistry, the Department maintained its teaching prominence in the early 1930s, its hours for laboratory increasing to 180, plus 32 hours of lecture. In addition, a third-year course was presented in preventive medicine, public health, industrial, and occupational medicine. The course covered sewage disposal, water purification, and the consideration of water and milk as vehicles for infectious diseases. Demography and vital statistics were stressed. All students presented a thesis dealing with preventive medicine in industry as a part of the third-year course.

Dr. Decker resigned in 1933 to limit himself to Dermatology, progressing to Professor and Chairman of that Department in 1950. He was succeeded by William A. Kreidler, Ph.D., who was promptly caught up in the very demanding teaching program that had become established. Dr. Kreidler was appointed Assistant Professor of Bacteriology and Immunology in 1932, and his hard work combined with his soft-spoken but authoritative manner resulted in his advancement to Associate Professor in 1936. Dr. David Meranze joined the staff in 1934 as Assistant Demonstrator, and in 1940, Dr. George Silver (Jefferson, 1938) became the first Eli Lilly Fellow. He was also appointed Assistant Demonstrator.

▪ Period of Transition (1941–1944)

The year 1941 brought major changes. Dean Henry K. Mohler died suddenly, and Dr. Rosenberger was immediately appointed Acting Dean, his long experience providing stability for the Medical School until the arrival of the new Dean, Dr. William Harvey Perkins (Jefferson, 1917) from Tulane University. Dr. Perkins, having had pioneering experience in Preventive Medicine, Public Health, and Tropical Medicine, was also appointed Professor and Chairman of a new Department of Preventive Medicine, thus removing this responsibility from Dr. Rosenberger's Department. The third-year teaching program was taken over by Dr. Perkins, but the teaching hours were increased, and the Department was renamed the Department of Bacteriology and Immunology. In 1944, a separate lecture and laboratory course in Parasitology was introduced, with the appointment of Dr. William G. Sawitz as Associate Professor. George P. Blundel, Ph.D. joined the staff as an Associate in Bacteriology and Immunology in 1942.

Wartime brought the accelerated teaching program, with its increased hours and stresses on the staff. The death of Dr. Rosenberger on February 21, 1944, marked a major change in the Department he had organized and nurtured. His professorial tenure was one of the longest in the history of Jefferson. His career had evolved with little formal training and still he was able to grow with his field, remaining abreast of developments while maintaining high standards of teaching and also conducting research. Along with his other accomplishments, Dr. Rosenberger designed several practical pieces of laboratory apparatus including a brass Petri dish holder for quick sterilization in an open flame and an exhibition test-tube stand to display the various bacterial fermentation reactions.

In spite of his dedication to Jefferson and his teaching duties, Dr. Rosenberger had a rewarding and relaxing home life. He lived for many years at Rahns, Pennsylvania, just a short distance from Collegeville, the site of Ursinus College. His funeral service was conducted by the Reverend Wharton A. Kline, Dean of Ursinus. Having been athletic in early life (baseball and tennis), Dr. Rosenberger changed to the less strenuous sports of quoits and croquet. He was fond of gardening, and for years his favorite local transportation was his horse and buggy. He was also musically talented and played a much-prized Stradivarius violin. Rosenberger's good humor and ready wit were greatly appreciated by the students. His standards were high and he did not tolerate lack of application graciously. The Class of 1928 presented his portrait to the College, and another portrait of him was painted by Dr. Robert M. Lukens (Jefferson, 1911) and later given by Mrs. Rosenberger. In his honor the Alumni Association established the Rosenberger Memorial Fellowship in March, 1944.

William A. Kreidler, Ph.D.; Acting Chairman (1944–1946)

Upon Dr. Rosenberger's death, Dr. Kreidler (Figure 7-3) was appointed Acting Chairman. He received his B.S. and M.S. from Lehigh University and proceeded to the University of Pennsylvania, where he was awarded his Ph.D. in Bacteriology and Immunology in 1926. He joined the teaching staff there, advancing to Assistant Professor before his appointment as Assistant Professor at Jefferson in 1932. As a senior member of the Department, Dr. Kreidler carried on the intensive teaching program effectively with the assistance of Dr. Grant Favorite, an Associate, and Dr. George Warren (to return in 1966 as Professor), an Instructor. Dr. Sawitz was also present as Assistant Professor to teach Parasitology.

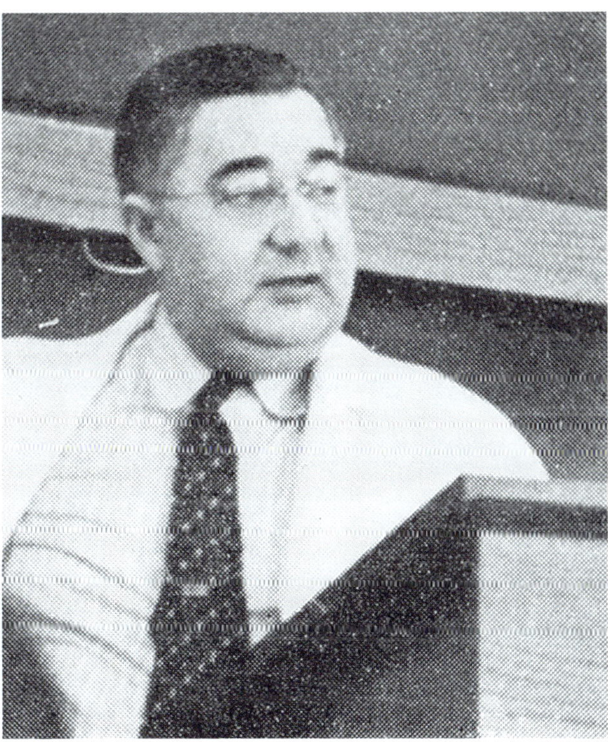

FIG. 7-3. William A. Kreidler, Ph.D.; Acting Chairman (1944–1946).

Kenneth Goodner, Ph.D.; Second Chairman (1946–1967)

Following a prolonged process of searching for a new Department Head, Kenneth Goodner, Ph.D. (Figure 7-4), was appointed Professor and Chairman of the Department of Bacteriology and Immunology in 1946, largely through the initiative of Dean Perkins. Dr. Goodner was born in 1902 in McCune, Kansas, and educated at the local schools. He received his A.B. and M.A. at the University of Kansas and proceeded to Harvard, where he studied under the eminent Hans Zinsser. Following receipt of his Ph.D. in 1929, Goodner continued as an Instructor in Bacteriology at the Harvard School of Public Health in 1930 but was then appointed to the Rockefeller Institute for Medical Research. He was one of the group of young men in Dr. Rufus Cole's program involved in the investigation of immunity to pneumococci. This ultimately led to the development of a type-specific antipneumococcal rabbit serum that was more effective and produced fewer allergic reactions in the treatment of lobar pneumonia than the previously used multivalent horse serum. Numerous publications in collaboration with his associates, Drs. Frank Horsfall, Colin MacCleod, Rene Dubos, and A. H. Harris, resulted.[3,4] The rabbit serum's period of usefulness was limited because it was soon rendered obsolete by the discovery of antimicrobial agents, beginning with the sulfa drugs in the late 1930s and soon followed by penicillin. In 1940 Dr. Goodner became a member of the staff of the Rockefeller Foundation and began his participation in the investigation of infectious diseases throughout the world, research that included further work with pneumococci and, during World War II, studies on vaccines against yellow fever. His associations with investigators from Rockefeller and government agencies formed the basis for his later studies on cholera and plague.

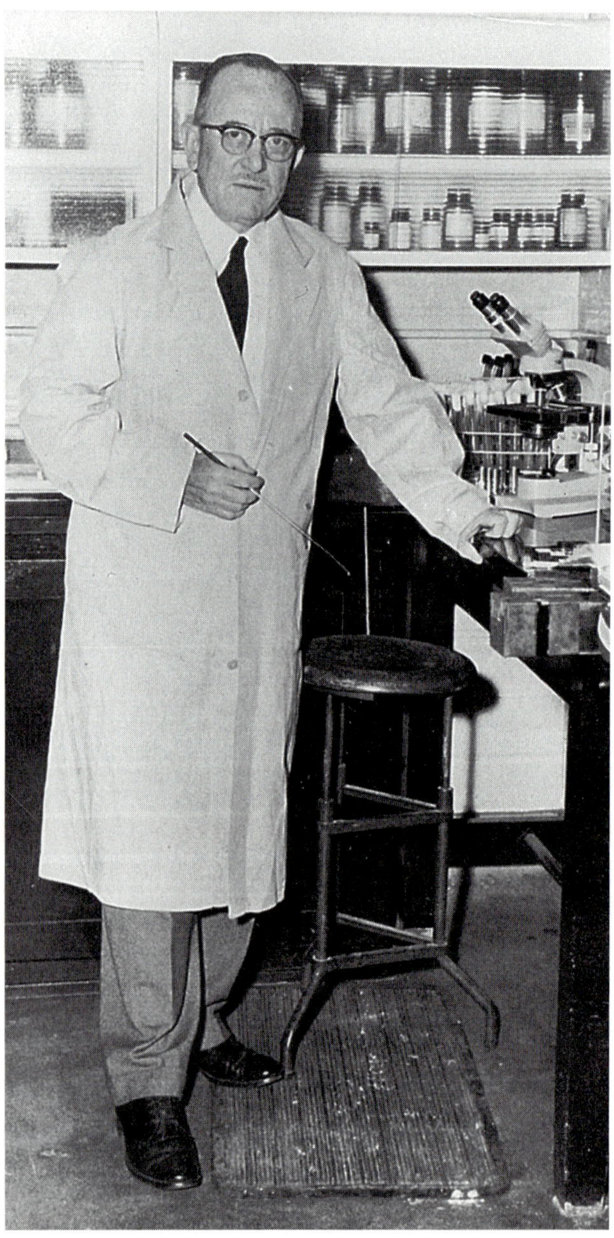

Fig. 7-4. Kenneth Goodner, Ph.D.; Second Chairman (1946–1967).

Dr. Goodner came to Jefferson as an internationally recognized scientist and a capable administrator. When Dean Perkins asked him about signing a contract, Goodner's reply was "a contract is unnecessary when two gentlemen shake hands."

The first challenge was to attract faculty, but it was also necessary to develop research programs and to revamp the courses of instruction. The latter had already begun when Dean Perkins recruited Dr. William G. Sawitz as Assistant Professor of Parasitology in 1943 and asked him to develop a new course. Dr. Sawitz came to Jefferson from Tulane University School of Medicine, having worked with Dr. Perkins there after he came to the United States from Germany in 1936 as a political refugee. Sawitz was trained in clinical medicine and tropical medicine in Rostock and Munich and was highly regarded for his skill in parasitology. He had quickly developed a course of lectures and laboratory exercises in the Bacteriology Department but his formal appointment was confirmed after the arrival of Dr. Goodner. Again at the behest of Dean Perkins, Sawitz received an appointment by Dr. Reimann in the Department of Medicine in addition to his basic status as Assistant Professor of Bacteriology and Immunology. He became a very effective laboratory instructor and investigator whose methods and skills ideally meshed with Dr. Goodner's plans for the Department. In 1949 Dr. Sawitz was promoted to Associate Professor and in 1955 to full Professor. In 1950 his book, *Medical Parasitology,* described as "the most successful condensation of the field of parasitology applicable to clinical medicine," was published by the Blakiston Company. Dr. Sawitz died in 1957.

Dr. Goodner's first new appointment was Dr. Carl F. Clancy (Ph.D., Yale University, 1942) as an Associate in 1947. Dr. Clancy was active as a bacteriologist at the Pennsylvania Hospital, so his teaching was part-time. His basic role was laboratory teaching, where he was known to students as a kind, fatherly person whose knowledge of clinical bacteriology was of practical value. Following his advancement to full-time Associate Professor in 1963, Clancy also increased teaching time and initiated a research program on the action of staphylococcal toxins. He retired in 1975.

Innovations during the early Goodner years related to teaching changes, introduction of the principles of scientific research, and the development of graduate education (Figure 7-5). The laboratory course for medical students was

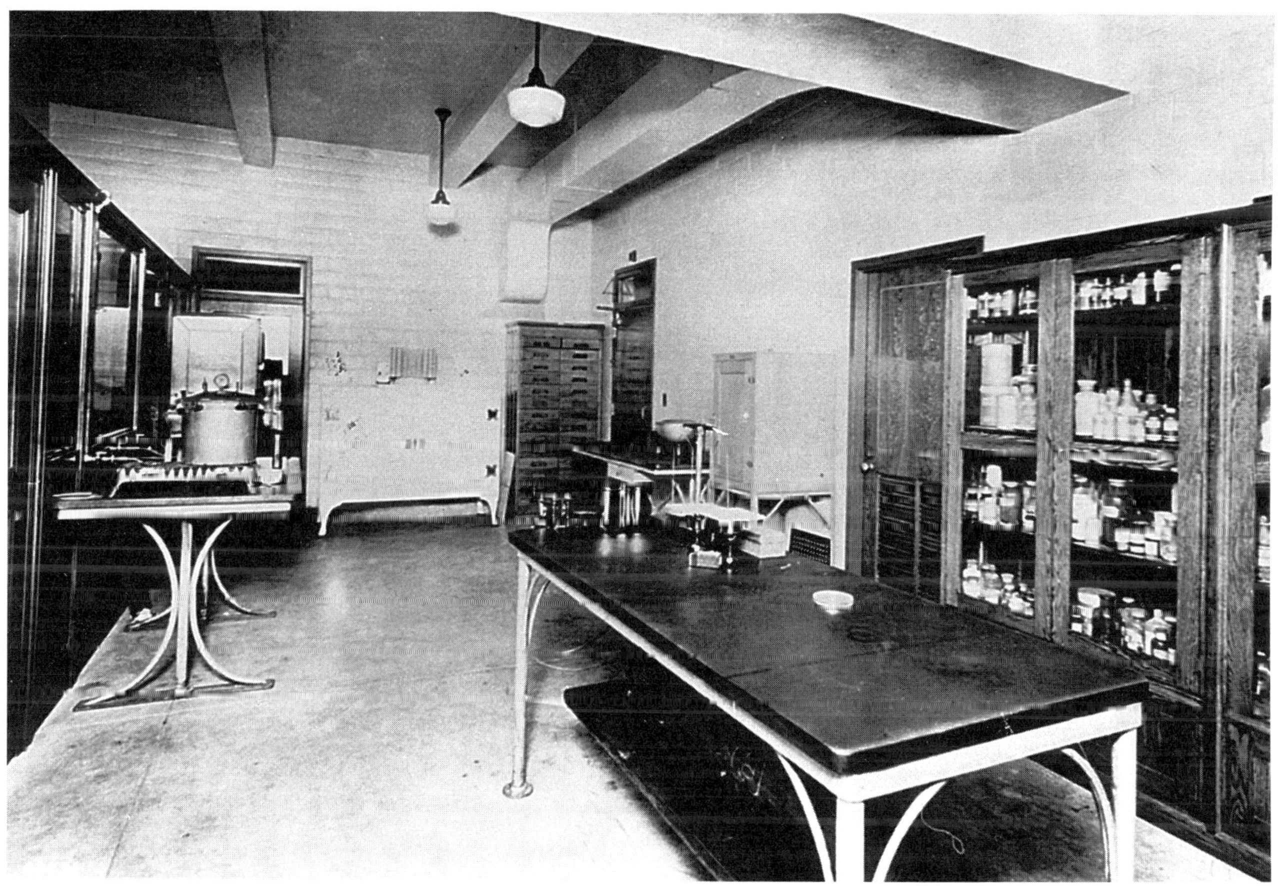

FIG. 7-5. Research microbiology laboratory in 1025 Walnut Street Medical College (ca. 1950).

changed from the first year to the second year in 1947. Dr. Goodner took his teaching obligations seriously; as a result he formed close relationships with the medical students and became their strong advocate in areas not limited to those of his discipline. Living close to the campus, he also established local relationships that enhanced his image as an academician.

▪ Research and Graduate Programs

The research program was built upon Dr. Goodner's previous activities in the international field of infectious diseases. Early involvement with studies on plague in Madagascar were followed by membership on the Cholera Committee of the National Institutes of Health. Members of this group and their associates included Drs. Joseph Smadel, Theodore Woodward, Thomas Francis, John H. Dingle, and J. Edsall. Field work was carried on in the Philippines, India, Pakistan, and Thailand. In addition, the discipline stimulated members and provided excellent material for teaching and research within the Department. In 1958 the South-East Asia Cholera Research Laboratory was established in Dacca, Pakistan (later Bangladesh), providing a regional facility for Committee activities. Dr. Goodner was a long-time consultant, continuing field trips throughout his lifetime.

The activities involving study of cholera formed an important part of the new School of Graduate Studies organized in 1949 at Jefferson through the driving efforts of Drs. Peter Herbut, Andrew Ramsay and Goodner. Along with the other basic sciences, Dr. Goodner's department was ready with programs leading toward the Ph.D. degree. The first students to enter the Ph.D. program in Bacteriology were Keith Jensen and Russell Miller, who joined the staff as Assistants in 1949 and went on to receive their degrees. The graduate program as well as the death of Dr. Kreidler in 1949 required further faculty recruitment that during the next few years proved exceptionally successful.

Dr. Goodner's first full-time faculty expansion appointee was Assistant Professor Morton Klein, Ph.D., in 1948, whose interest in virology and general bacteriology proved valuable. Klein resigned in 1950. To replace him, Dr. Goodner proposed the appointment of the first full-time woman Professor at Jefferson. Lolita Parnell, Ph.D., an experienced teacher with service in the United States Navy, was appointed Assistant Professor of Bacteriology and Immunology in 1950. Although her tenure lasted only three years, the administrative policy changes that permitted her appointment were then in place, clearing the way for the appointment of women in all departments of the Jefferson faculty.

The Department faculty was further strengthened in 1950–1951 by recruitment of three young doctoral graduates from the University of Pennsylvania. Bernard Koft (Ph.D., 1950) who was trained by Drs. A. Sevag and Stuart Mudd, was appointed Instructor in 1950 and furthered his studies on growth factors of bacteria. An effective teacher and scientist, he was promoted to Assistant Professor in 1955, but two years later became Professor and Chairman of Microbiology at Rutgers University, New Brunswick, New Jersey.

Henry Stempen, was appointed in 1950 as Instructor. His areas of investigation included the biology of *Proteus vulgaris,* fungi, and slime molds, and he introduced mycology into the departmental curriculum. Although shy and artistic, he was a well-qualified teacher and exacting in his work. Stempen advanced to Assistant Professor in 1955 and Associate Professor in 1957, but resigned in 1962 to join the Department of Biology at Rutgers University in Camden, New Jersey, where he remained until his retirement in 1988.

The third of this trio of University of Pennsylvania Ph.D. graduates, Robert J. Mandle (Figure 7-6), was appointed Instructor in 1951. He was a graduate of Lebanon Valley College (B.S., 1942), served in the Navy until 1945, then went to work as a technician for Drs. Wendell Stanley and Armand Braun in their laboratory at Rockefeller Institute's Princeton, New Jersey, Division. Mandle credits these investigators for instilling in him "the philosophy of experimentation, the philosophy of science." An exceptional biologist, his investigations included the microbiology and epidemiology of staphylococci, studies carried out with the collaboration of the Division of Infectious Diseases. He also participated in the investigation of organisms of the gut with Drs. Goodner and Freter of his department and Dr. Franz Goldstein of the Division of Gastroenterology. Dr. Mandle became expert in mycology, succeeding to responsibility for that subject upon the resignation of Dr. Stempen. Virology, bacterial physiology, and the genetics of bacterial disease were also included in his comprehensive biological skills.

Dr. Mandle progressed up the academic ladder, reaching the rank of Professor in 1965 and serving as Interim Chairman of the Department in 1967–1968. In 1979 he received the Christian R. and Mary Lindback Award for Distinguished Teaching and in 1985 the additional honor of the presentation of his portrait to Jefferson by the senior class of medical students. In 1977–1979 Mandle also was President of the Eastern Branch of the American Society for Microbiology. In 1980, he received a Fulbright–Hays Award for International Exchange of Scholars, under which he served at the Catholic University School of Medical Technology in Quito, Ecuador, for six months. After a distinguished career, Mandle retired in 1986.

Expansion continued in the 1950s. Dr. Goodner's leadership in organization was established within the Department as well as in collaborative enterprises with other Jefferson departments. Such relationships led to the appointment in 1951 of Dr. W. Paul Havens of the Department of Medicine as Associate Professor of Bacteriology and Immunology. Dr. Havens was a leader in the weekly infectious disease conferences, which became important teaching exercises in linking applied microbiology with clinical medicine. He was a pioneer in the study of viral hepatitis and served as a member of various

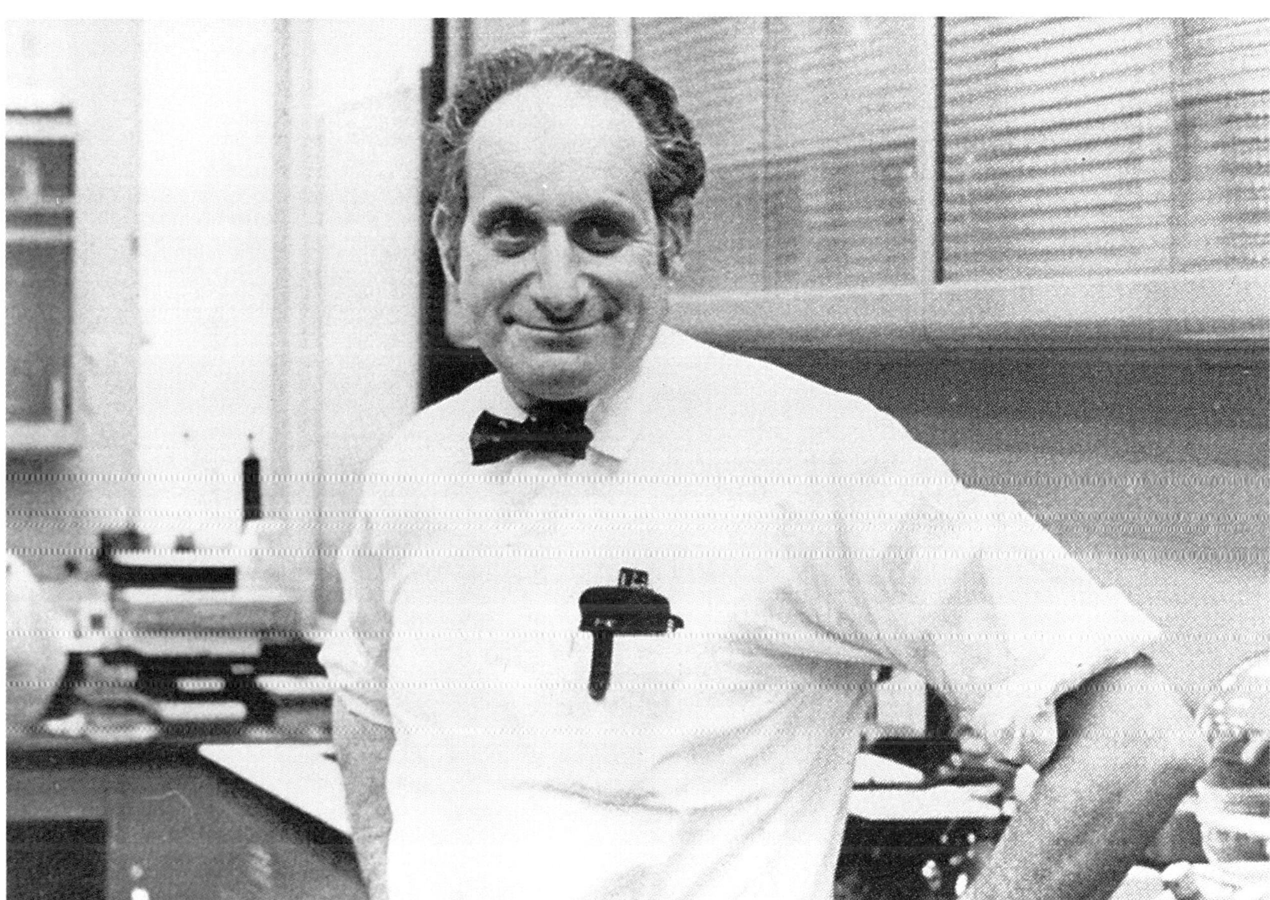

FIG. 7-6. Robert J. Mandle, Ph.D., Professor of Microbiology and Interim Chairman (1967–1968).

commissions including the Armed Forces Epidemiology Board and Consultant to the Surgeon General and to the Veterans Administration. Havens worked closely with Dr. Goodner and shared the lectures in the Microbiology course, his research laboratory being located within the Department. In 1956 he was advanced to Professor of Microbiology, and the following year to Professor of Medicine.

▪ The Middle Period of the Goodner Chairmanship

The year 1957 was eventful: Dr. Sawitz's death in March called for new approaches to the teaching of parasitology; and the first ten years of the Goodner period, even though they represented major achievements in departmental organization, outstanding instruction of medical students, and the successful development of the Graduate School program, still demanded other new emphases. The appointment of Harry L. Smith, Jr., (Figure 7-7) as Instructor in 1957 was among the first and most durable of the faculty appointments from the Graduate School. Smith (B.S., Temple University, 1952) came directly to Jefferson, where he received his M.S. in 1954 and his Ph.D. in 1957. He became intensely involved in the investigations initiated by Dr. Goodner into *Vibrio* organisms and the epidemiology of cholera. Observations on the "sticky" surface of the vibrios led him to the study of gelatin degradation by various bacterial gelatinases. Promoted to Assistant Professor in 1959 and to Associate Professor in 1964 (when he received a career development award), Dr. Smith went on to major accomplishments in international health. Field trips were carried out in the study of cholera epidemics in Thailand, the Philippines, and Pakistan. When Dr. Goodner retired, Dr. Smith took over his training and research grants. A Vibrio Reference Laboratory was established at Jefferson in 1969 with grant support from the United States/Japan Cooperative Scientific Program of the National Institutes of Health, and Smith's collection of *Vibrio* strains and serotypes was used for reference by investigators throughout the world. Grant support for this program ended in 1980, but the Laboratory has continued to function. Dr. Smith's teaching accomplishments were equally notable—he was advanced to Professor of Microbiology in 1973, for some years he was responsible for the teaching of parasitology, and he later became interested in computerized aids in teaching, especially in relation to diagnosis of infectious diseases, enabling students to manage computer-simulated cases. Dr. Smith was honored in 1988 by the senior class with the presentation of his portrait to the University.

The year 1957 was also marked by the appointment of Drs. Frank F. Katz and Rolf

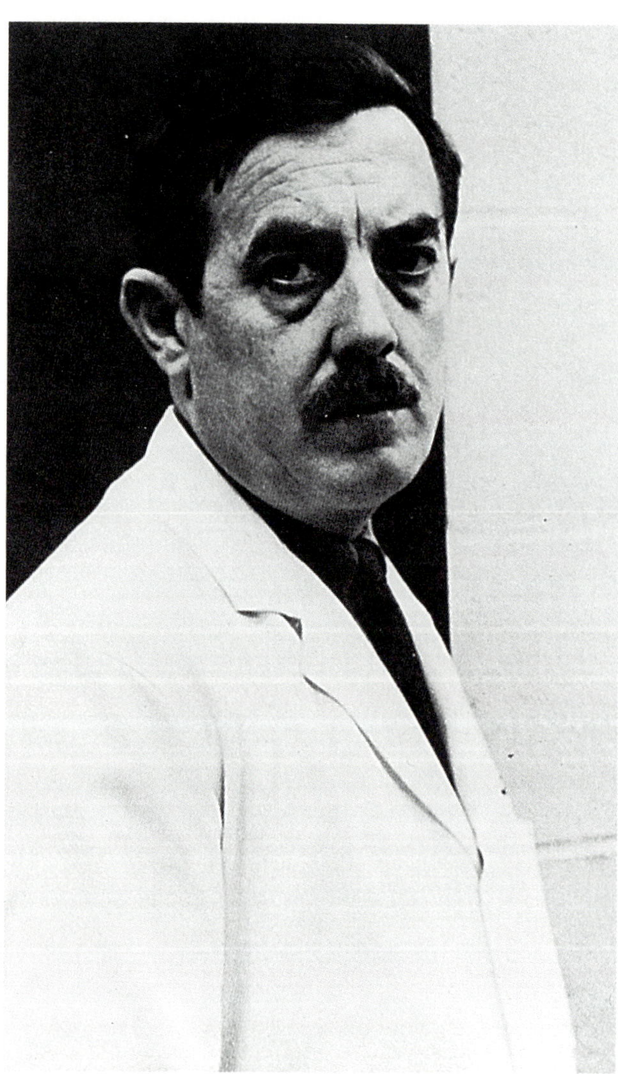

FIG. 7-7. Harry L. Smith, Jr., Ph.D., Professor of Microbiology with special interest in epidemiology of cholera.

Freter as Assistant Professors. Dr. Katz (M.S., Tulane University, 1953; Ph.D., University of Pennsylvania, 1956) had experience in teaching parasitology and took over the duties of the late Dr. Sawitz. His research centered on nematodes, especially *Stronglyloides* species, and the effects of radiation on their stages of development, studies supported by the United States Public Health Service. Katz resigned in 1962 to join the faculty at Seton Hall School of Medicine, and his teaching duties were assumed by Dr. Smith, who had also been a student of Dr. Sawitz.

Dr. Rolf Freter (Ph.D., Goethe University, Frankfurt, Germany, 1951) also came as Assistant Professor. From Loyola University, Chicago, Freter had pursued research in cholera and *Shigella,* especially characterizing the immune responses of these organisms. He was an able teacher, and his participation in the cholera programs included field work during cholera epidemics. Promoted to Associate Professor in 1960 Freter resigned in 1965 to become Professor of Microbiology at the University of Michigan.

The Department of Microbiology

Having gone through several changes of name and orientation from its inception in 1909, the designation of the Department was finally changed to Microbiology in 1959, reflecting the accretion of knowledge and the concepts of molecular biology that were then being introduced. The subject of virology was receiving increasing attention at this time, and in 1960 Dr. Paul B. Johnson (Ph.D., University of Chicago, 1957) was recruited from his former position as Chief of the Division of Virology of the United States Medical Research Unit (NAMRU-2) in Taiwan. Having published numerous papers, Dr. Johnson was co-discoverer of the "Simian Foamy Agent," and he continued his viral studies at Jefferson with a National Institutes of Health grant. Johnson left Jefferson in 1964 for a Research Professorship at the University of Louisville, Kentucky.

Of more than passing interest has been the career of Dr. Eileen Randall (B.S., Ohio State University, 1948), who entered the Graduate School program at Jefferson in 1951. She received her M.S. in 1953 while engaged as a clinical microbiologist at Jefferson Hospital, and she advanced to Director of the Clinical Microbiology Laboratory in 1955. Randall was awarded her Ph.D. in 1960. In 1963 she received a dual Medical School teaching appointment as Assistant Professor of Pathology as well as of Microbiology. Her service at Jefferson was notable for the excellence of her work in diagnostic microbiology, teaching and training of medical residents, and teaching undergraduate and graduate students, as well as for the cordial relations between her laboratory and the clinicians who required her skilled services. She continued her research as well and gained a national reputation for new laboratory techniques, including the rapid detection of bacteremia by radiometric methods. Dr. Randall was promoted to Associate Professor of Microbiology in 1969 but resigned in 1973 to become Director of Clinical Laboratories at Evanston, Illinois, Hospital and Associate Professor of Pathology at Northwestern University. In 1984 she received the Thomas Jefferson University College of Graduate Studies Alumni Achievement Award.

In 1965 Dr. Goodner appointed Dr. George Royal as Assistant Professor, the first black to hold a full-time professorial position at Jefferson. Although he was well received, he remained only one year before accepting a higher post at Howard University. The same year, Dr. George Warren returned to the faculty as Professor of Microbiology. After his brief stint at Jefferson in the 1940s he proceeded to Wyeth Laboratories as Senior Research Bacteriologist and soon as Head of the Wyeth Department of Microbiology, a position he held until his retirement. Warren's association at Jefferson was a voluntary one, and he participated in teaching and departmental affairs on this basis. Dr. Warren was an expert in the field of antimicrobial agents and was responsible for early investigations of hyaluronidase, which led to a very successful product marketed by his company. Following his retirement from Wyeth, Warren continued his teaching activities on a daily basis until being made Honorary Professor in 1987. Even then he continued his departmental connection while working on his book on antibiotics.

Dr. Goodner retired June 30, 1967, with a long

record of successes to his credit. In addition to his work in international health and infectious disease studies, his inauguration of the Ph.D. program proved a major forward step. The new Graduate School coupled with the worldwide studies of infectious diseases attracted many students from the Far East to whom Dr. Goodner was especially committed in the conviction that their training would be important in the development of their countries. Ph.D. graduates have also achieved important posts throughout the United States. The master's degree program likewise was successful in promoting the interests of the Graduate School and the useful employment of its graduates.

Dr. Goodner's sudden death on August 30, 1967 occurred only two months after his retirement. His total career contributions to microbiology, to the cause of international health, and to the teaching of a generation of medical and graduate students were summarized at a memorial service conducted at Jefferson on September 20, 1967. On that occasion he was eulogized by Dr. Theodore E. Woodward, Professor of Medicine at the University of Maryland School of Medicine and a lifetime friend and colleague. Dr. Woodward expressed appreciation for Dr. Goodner's accomplishments in the global campaign against infectious diseases, saying: "His ideas sparked enthusiasm in others; his mind and efforts were selflessly shared in the training and development of young scientists who now make their mark. Never one to shun work, he pressed his tired but willing body over the globe, to Africa for study of yellow fever, to Madagascar and problems of plague, and during the last decade to the Asian subcontinent and the Pacific Far East for cholera."

Dr. Robert Mandle in a more intimate memoir prepared for the Executive Faculty also described Dr. Goodner in these words:

> "He quickly became 'Ken' to his peers and 'K.G.' to his students. His was a truly noble spirit; he was a rare teacher, investigator, and student advisor and confidant. He was a sentimentalist by tradition, yet one on whom sentimentality was wasted. One did not have a neutral feeling about him. He was at times a charmer, an irritant, a prodding conscience or an outspoken critic. Jefferson, its halls and occupants, was his life for 21 years. He was proud of his heritage and his contemporaries as they sought together to build upon the glories of the past."

Russell W. Schaedler, M.D.; Third Chairman of Microbiology (1968–), First Plimpton-Pugh Professor (1985–)

Russell W. Schaedler, M.D. (Figure 7-8) (Jefferson, 1953, Alpha Omega Alpha) was appointed the new Chairman January 1, 1968. He was born in Hatfield, Pennsylvania, on December 17, 1927, and received his B.S. at Ursinus College in 1949. Completing his Jefferson internship in 1954, he received an appointment to the Rockefeller Institute for Medical Research and to its associated Hospital. He advanced through residency to Associate Physician to the Hospital of Rockefeller Institute in 1961 and to Physician to that Hospital in 1962. Schaedler was intimately associated with the great microbiologist, Dr. Rene J. Dubos. His early investigations centered upon the effects of bed rest in tuberculosis and upon the etiology of sarcoidosis but later focused on nutrition, infection, and host–parasite

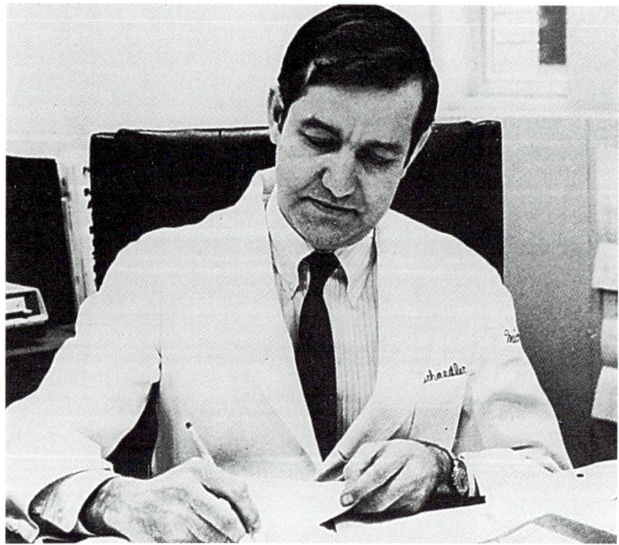

FIG. 7-8. Russell W. Schaedler, M.D.; Third Chairman of Microbiology (1968–), First Plimpton-Pugh Professor (1985–).

relationships. He became well known in the field of gastrointestinal microecology. His bibliography relative to his studies during this period provides evidence of the wide range of Schaedler's work. He developed a medium that bears his name and has been widely used for two decades for the isolation and identification of anaerobes. His work delineating the microbial flora of the mouse led to the "Schaedler Cocktail,"[5] a group of indigenous organisms of the mouse used to associate germ-free animals; these animals with a defined flora are then used to establish breeding colonies of pathogen-free animals in barrier rooms. The technique is now being used by almost all commercial breeders in the United States. Dr. Schaedler's clinical background together with his research accomplishments provided exceptional credentials for his appointment.

The Department upon Schaedler's arrival had a solid base, but personnel losses in recent years had placed a burden on the teaching staff remaining. Faculty recruitment required teaching skills as well as research plans and funding. The Department was well equipped with its own media-preparation rooms, areas for sterilizing media and equipment, and areas for decontamination of glassware and spent media. There were well-kept animal quarters, an electron microscopy suite, darkrooms for photography, a walk-in incubator room, cold rooms, and freezers. All of these facilities were enhanced by the move in May, 1969, of the Department to the newly erected Jefferson Alumni Hall, one of the best designed basic science buildings in the country.

A unique faculty appointment was made in 1969 when Dr. Jussi J. Saukkonen (Figure 7-9) joined as Associate Professor of Microbiology, advancing in 1972 to full Professor. Dr. Saukkonen, born in Helsinki, Finland (B.S., Helsinki University, 1951), had a research fellowship at the University of Heidelberg (1954–1956) and was awarded his M.D. from Helsinki University in 1955. After a postdoctoral fellowship at Columbia University College of Physicians and Surgeons (1955–1959), Saukkonen returned to Finland to become Head of the Biochemistry Laboratory of the Central Public Health Laboratory and, from 1966 to 1969, Director of Biochemistry. During a sabbatical leave served at Rockefeller University in 1966–1967, he made the acquaintance of Dr. Schaedler and in 1969 became the first academic appointee of the new Chairman at Jefferson.

Dr. Saukkonen's qualifications were ideal. In addition to training as a physician, he was a biochemist and microbiologist especially skilled in microbial genetics. His research centered on molecular biology and DNA replication. These multiple assets were to prove valuable in developing a clinically oriented curriculum in microbiology. In addition to teaching medical students, Dr. Saukkonen became a force in the Graduate School program where his students profited by his teaching and research skills, receiving excellent postdoctoral positions and making major scientific contributions. He was also active in academic government, a member of

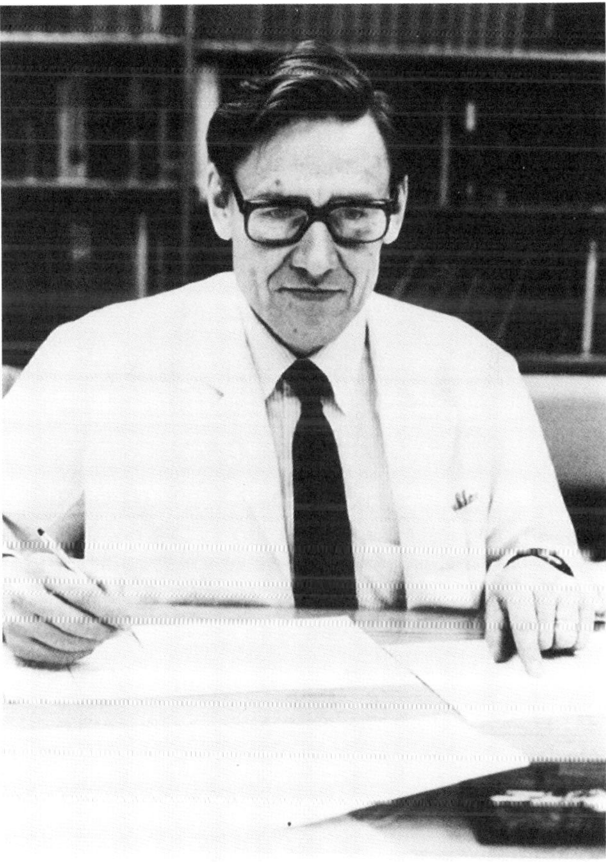

FIG. 7-9. Jussi J. Saukkonen, M.D., Professor of Microbiology, Dean of the College of Graduate Studies, and Senior Associate Dean of Scientific and Faculty Affairs of the Medical College.

various committees, and editor or associate editor of several journals. In 1976–1977, Saukkonen took a leave of absence to serve as Director of the Central Public Health Laboratories, the Finnish equivalent of the United States National Institutes of Health.

Dr. Saukkonen's involvement extended beyond the Department. In 1981, he was made Dean of the College of Graduate Studies of Thomas Jefferson University and in 1983 he was appointed Dean of Scientific Faculty Affairs in the Medical College.

The Department proceeded to seek funding for its many projects, often relative to those initiated by or programmed by new faculty members. Dr. Schaedler, in cooperation with Dr. Abraham Benenson, epidemiologist in the Department of Preventive Medicine, Dr. Dhodanand Kowlessar of the Division of Gastroenterology, and Drs. Smith and Mandle, received a large grant from the United States Navy for the study of diarrheal diseases.[6] This project was an outgrowth of studies by Drs. Mandle and Goldstein using clinical material and following through from Dr. Schaedler's investigations on the gastrointestinal flora of animals. These funds provided new equipment for research and supported graduate students in the Department.

The Clinical Masters Program was a further cooperative project of the Department and the School of Graduate Studies. Dr. Eileen Randall, in her role as Chief of the Microbiological Laboratories, with the support of Dr. Mandle brought to the attention of the Chairman the need for advanced training of medical technologists, a need also recognized by the American Academy of Microbiologists, by which agency the criteria for designation as "Specialist in Medical Laboratory Microbiology" were developed. The program was designed to emphasize laboratory management skills but included emphasis on molecular virology, immunology, biochemistry of microorganisms, and advanced diagnostic microbiology. A minimum of three years of work in a clinical microbiology laboratory (later reduced to two years) was a prerequisite. The students rotated through a number of laboratories with full-time exposure to different managerial techniques and the means of solving problems of personnel, budget, and tactics in laboratory supervision. After careful planning, the program was launched in 1972 with 15 students enrolled that year. It proved successful from the start, and its continuation was assured when Drs. Schaedler and Mandle obtained training grant support. Over 100 graduates completed the program and filled many supervisory positions in hospitals in Philadelphia and the Eastern Seaboard. Other graduates went on to the Ph.D. program, and some to the M.D. Ultimately professional opportunities for these graduates became limited and the course was discontinued except for part-time students.

In 1969, Dr. Junius Clark (Ph.D., University of Texas, 1967) joined the Department to develop the study and teaching of cellular immunology. Trained in electron microscopy as well, he became an excellent teacher for medical students and also organized a graduate course in immunology. Funded by a Merck Faculty Development Award in 1970, Clark served well in introducing modern immunology to the Department.

Another area urgently in need of development was that of virology. Although Assistant Professor Ihor Zajac had been recruited for this subject by Dr. Goodner in 1965, it needed vigorous promotion. This was provided by the appointment in 1971 of Dr. E. Frederick Wheelock (M.D., Columbia University, 1955; Ph.D., Rockefeller University, 1961) as Professor of Microbiology. His research at Rockefeller had centered on cellular responses to multiplication of the cytovirus using Newcastle Disease Virus. Having been appointed Assistant Professor of Preventive Medicine at Western Reserve School of Medicine in 1961, Wheelock received a career development award, and his research programs were well funded. He continued these studies at Jefferson with major contributions in the fields of interferons, viral interference, and Friend leukemia virus. Not regarded as a dynamic teacher but able to entice good graduate students for his research, the teaching in virology was bolstered by the appointment of Dr. Stephen Toy (Ph.D., University of Florida, 1966) who came to Jefferson with Dr. Wheelock from Western Reserve. His viral studies included the same areas as those of Dr. Wheelock, but he was also skilled in the field of molecular biology and carried the major portion of the teaching of virology to medical students. His brief tenure ended, however, in 1974, at which time his duties were taken over by Dr. Preston Marx (Ph.D., Louisiana State University, 1969), who was appointed Assistant Professor. Dr. Marx was well trained in molecular virology and the biochemistry of viral infections, and he was an able teacher. Drs. Wheelock and Marx resigned in 1981.

Another area of microbiology that required promotion was that of microbial pathogenesis. To accomplish this goal, Dr. Schaedler in 1975 appointed Dr. Charles Panos (Ph.D., University of Pittsburgh, 1952) as full Professor. Dr. Panos had broad experience in research and teaching at the University of Illinois and at the Einstein Medical Center in Philadelphia, where he became expert in the investigation of mycoplasma and L-forms. A biochemist and bacterial physiologist, Panos had a research career development award and continuing National Institutes of Health grant support through the years. He attracted individuals from all over the United States, Europe, and the Far East to work with him. Panos also participated in teaching medical students and graduate students as well as serving on the student Admission Committee and other committees of the University. His recent work has focused on the role of lipoteichoic acid of streptococci in the pathogenesis of disease.

During this period, Dr. Donald Lee Jungkind (M.S., University of Houston, 1968; Ph.D., University of Texas, Galveston Branch, 1972) succeeded Dr. Eileen Randall as Director of the Clinical Microbiology Laboratory as well as holding joint appointments in Pathology and Microbiology, first as Assistant Professor and, since 1987, as Associate Professor. Jungkind's activities in Microbiology have included participation in training and supervising the research projects for clinical masters and students, collaboration with various members of the Department in their research, and participation in the teaching programs. His own research has pursued rapid methods for the identification and susceptibility testing of bacteria, the laboratory diagnosis of sexually-transmitted diseases, and more recently, blood culture techniques by non-radiometric methods.

The departure of Dr. Junius Clark in 1977 prompted the appointment of Dr. Catherine E. Calkins (Ph.D., Purdue University, 1972) as Assistant Professor to maintain the Departmental program in immunology. Dr. Calkins received postdoctoral training at Yale University with Dr. Byron Waksman and was then a Research Associate at Sloan-Kettering Institute in cellular immunobiology. She proceeded with her research on cellular regulation of the immune response, for which she received extramural support. Calkins proved to be an excellent teacher, was promoted to Associate Professor in 1982, and was named Assistant to the Chairman in 1985. She has attracted excellent graduate students who have achieved firm footholds in the world of science.

To complement Dr. Calkins' program in immunology, Dr. Thomas T. MacDonald (Ph.D., University of Glasgow, 1976) was appointed Assistant Professor in 1978. His research focused on the immunology of the gastrointestinal tract especially relative to mucosal cell surfaces and cellular interactions of Peyer's patches. Aggressive and self-assured, MacDonald worked well with other Department members and stimulated the students with his enthusiasm as a lecturer. He made significant contributions with his studies in the priming and regulation of antibody-producing cells. He resigned in 1984, ultimately returning to Great Britain to pursue his investigations.

Further Staff Development

During the early 1980s, the explosion of biological knowledge of the previous two decades required further expansion of the Department Staff for the extensive teaching and research programs. The course in Medical Microbiology served in excess of 200 medical students annually, including laboratory experience. Each laboratory group of 16 to 20 students had a faculty member or graduate student assigned. Much staff effort was also devoted to the Graduate Teaching Program and the multiple research projects. An important appointment in 1980 was helpful in promoting the area of immunology and renewing investigative parasitology: Dr. Joye E. Jones (Ph.D., University of Florida, 1977), joined the staff as Assistant Professor. Jones had entered the Peace Corps upon her graduation from Florida State University in 1969 and was assigned to Malawi, where in addition to teaching biology, hygiene, and agriculture, she assisted in various surveys of parasitic infestations in the villages. In the Ph.D. program she studied altered immune response to trichinella and followed up as a postdoctoral fellow at the Immunology Branch of the National Cancer Institute, thus developing skills in the immunology of parasitic diseases. At Jefferson she was well received by students and colleagues while beginning her studies on altered responses during trypanosome infestation. She received a new investigator award, which was regularly renewed and funded. Her interest in general microbiology plus her special teaching skills were recognized by receipt of the Christian R. and Mary Lindback Award. Although promoted to Associate Professor in 1986, Dr. Jones resigned the same year to accept a position as grants administrator at the National Institutes of Health.

Another staff person of note during this period was Dr. Thomas J. Wade, a Ph.D. graduate of Jefferson, who returned as Assistant Professor with the special task of acting as coordinator for medical microbiology for Allied Health Science programs. He also worked with Dr. Mandle using a gas chromatograph to characterize nonfermenting gram-negative bacteria. Wade resigned in 1985.

With the departure of Drs. Wheelock, Marx, MacDonald, and Jones, the Department was reorganized in the early 1980s along three separate but interrelated groups: immunology, molecular genetics, and virology, with pathogenesis of infectious disease at the molecular level. A new biological-containment laboratory was constructed through funds provided by the Mary Smith Charity. This suite housed the latest equipment for researching hazardous biologicals, especially genetic recombinants. Dr. Robert Grafstrom (Ph.D., Hershey Medical Center of Pennsylvania State University, 1975) was appointed Assistant Professor in 1985 to head the DNA laboratory and develop the area of molecular genetics. His research respecting the mechanism in DNA repair was funded by the National Science Foundation, and he quickly achieved recognition as an able Department member with stimulating ideas.

Dr. Grafstrom, Dr. Richard Peluso (Ph.D., Rockefeller University), and Dr. Timothy Black (Ph.D., Roswell Memorial Institute of University of Buffalo School of Medicine, 1979) constituted a trio referred to as the "microbiology mob," all having been appointed about the same time. All became funded investigators, enthusiastic and hard-working. Dr. Peluso, a virologist, was early engaged with replication of the RNA genome of the vesicular stomatitis virus, and Dr. Black was studying Marek's Disease Virus genes and their gene products, as well as the molecular details of the killing of cells by the Herpes virus and how some cell types resist.

Dr. Robert Korngold (Ph.D., University of Pennsylvania, 1979), was appointed Associate Professor in 1987 as a youthful authority on graft versus host-disease problems, with experience at the Wistar Institute. Dr. David Abraham (Ph.D., University of Pennsylvania, 1983) was recruited in 1983 as an immunoparasitologist.

The teaching staff of the Department reached its full complement in the late 1980s. There were eight Professors, including two Adjunct Professors; seven Associate Professors (two Adjunct), six Assistant Professors, and three Instructors. Sophisticated research was being carried on at all levels in the field of microbiology. In addition to extramural funding for Departmental projects, an Endowed Professorship in Microbiology was established by Dr. V. Watson Pugh (Jefferson, 1953) and Mrs. Frances Plimpton-Pugh in 1985 as a family memorial. Dr. Schaedler, the Chairman, was the first incumbent of this Chair.

Microbiology has surmounted many milestones in the advancement of medicine for the prevention and cure of disease. Jefferson's past contributions have been noteworthy, but there are plans for greatly expanded research in various aspects of molecular medicine—these include erecting a Research Building with the most modern facilities at the northeast corner of Tenth and Locust Streets, an endeavor integrated in a multidisciplinary approach involving other Departments.

References

1. Mitchell, J.K., "Cryptogamous Origin of Malarious and Epidemic Fevers." Philadelphia: Lea and Blanchard, 1849.

(Included in Mitchell, S. W.: Five Essays by John Kearsley Mitchell. Philadelphia: Lippincott, 1859.)
2. Webb, W.H., "Is Phthisis Pulmonalis Contagious and Does it Belong to the Zymotic Group?" *Am. Jour. Med. Sc.* 76:426–434, 1878. (Also published as a monograph with the same title: Philadelphia: Wm. F. Fell Co., 1878. [In Historical Collections, College of Physicians of Philadelphia.])
3. Goodner, K., and Horsfall, F.L. Jr., "Type-Specific Antipneumococcus Rabbit Serum." *Science* 84:579–581, 1936.
4. Goodner, K., MacCleod, C.M., and Harris, A.H., Jr., "Antipneumococcus Rabbit Serum as Therapeutic Agent in Lobar Pneumonia." *J.A.M.A.* 108:1483–1490, 1937.
5. Schaedler, R.W., Dubos, R., Costello, R., "The Development of the Gastrointestinal Flora in the Gastrointestinal Tract of Mice." *J. Exp. Med.* 122; 59–66, 1964.
6. Schaedler, R.W., and Goldstein, F., "Bacterial Populations of the Gut in Health and Disease: Basic Microbiologic Aspects." In *Gastroenterology,* Bockus Ed., Philadelphia: W. B. Saunders Co., 1976, pp. 145–152.

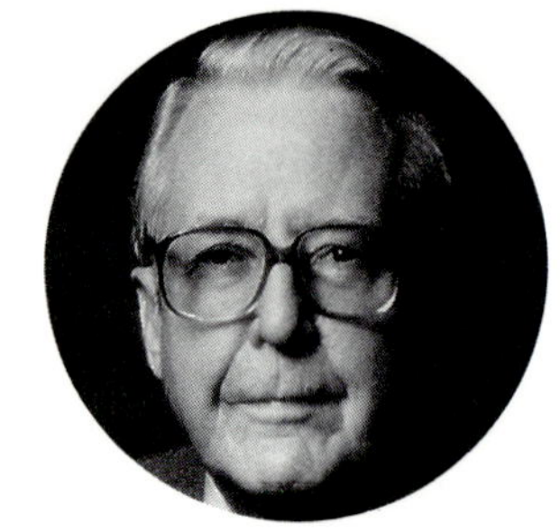

CHAPTER EIGHT

Department of Pharmacology

Julius M. Coon, Ph.D., M.D.

"Poisons and medicine are oftentimes the same substance given with different intents."

—Peter Mere Latham (1789–1875)

The minutes of the faculty meeting of September 29, 1930, stated: "Upon recommendation of the Curriculum and Roster Committee, the Faculty adopted a resolution that the Board of Trustees be advised that, in the opinion of the Faculty, it would add materially to the standing of the Jefferson Medical College and to the scope of its teaching if a course in Pharmacology be established, the course to be entirely separate from the Department of Therapeutics as now constituted." As a result of this resolution the Department of Pharmacology was founded in 1932.

Although the Department of Pharmacology was by far the latest of the basic medical science departments to be established at Jefferson, this was not inconsistent with the early status of pharmacology as a separate academic discipline in the medical schools of the United States at that time. The first Chair of Pharmacology in this country was established at the University of Michigan and was filled by John J. Abel, M.D., in 1891. His official title, however, was Professor of Materia Medica and Therapeutics in the Department of Medicine and Surgery. During his two-year tenure of that position Dr. Abel formulated a type of teaching and research program in pharmacology that finally evolved through later years as the basic design of the academic discipline of pharmacology in the medical schools of America. Abel has long been called the "Father of American Pharmacology."

It is of interest to note that the first Professorship of Pharmacology in an English medical school was filled by Arthur Cushny in 1905, 12 years after he had succeeded Abel at the University of Michigan in 1893.

After leaving Michigan, Dr. Abel became another first Professor of Pharmacology, this time in the Department of Pharmacology at the Johns Hopkins Medical School. In the next two decades there was an increasing show of interest in pharmacology as a separate subject in medical school curricula but it was not until the 1920s that it was generally accorded departmental status in American medical schools. Thus, the Jefferson Department of Pharmacology received recognition relatively early on a footing equal to that of the other five basic science departments.

Charles M. Gruber, Ph.D., M.D. (1887–1974); First Chairman of Pharmacology (1932–1953)

In the beginning the Department of Pharmacology operated on a small but productive scale. In the words of its first Professor and Head, Dr. Charles M. Gruber, in the *1936 Clinic*:

> "The teaching staff of the department has consisted from the beginning of two members: Charles M. Gruber, Ph.D., M.D., Professor, and John T. Brundage, Ph.D., M.D., Assistant Professor.
>
> The course in Pharmacology is a valuable addition to the curriculum, giving the student essential information on the action of drugs on the living cells and organs as well as some pharmacy, materia medica, toxicology, prescription writing, [etc.]
>
> The staff of the department has not limited its activities to the teaching of the course only, but has carried on active research and encouraged students to do research under its guidance. During the past three and a half years through grants of moneys from sources outside the college, original investigations in the field of pharmacology have been made possible. By co-operation with members of other departments in the institution and with the assistance of former and present medical students, the results of 16 original investigations have been published and at present six more manuscripts of original work are ready for the press."[1]

Thus Dr. Gruber planted the seeds for what grew into an extensive pharmacology program. The Departmental interest in research revealed in his 1936 statement later developed into the graduate training program leading to the Ph.D. degree in the basic medical sciences. Dr. Gruber played a leading role in the formation, in 1949, of the Board for the Regulation of Graduate Studies, which eventually evolved, in 1969, into the College of Graduate Studies of Thomas Jefferson University. A memoir of Dr. Gruber was published by the College of Physicians of Philadelphia.[2]

Charles M. Gruber (Figure 8-1) was born on March 11, 1887, in Hope, Kansas, the youngest of nine children of German immigrant parents who were homesteading a Kansas farm. He first acquired an interest in biology and medicine during his high school days, when the family physician encouraged him to come to his office to browse through *Gray's Anatomy*.

Gruber started his scientific career as a physiologist. After graduating with A.B. and M.S. degrees from the University of Kansas in 1911 and 1912, he earned the Ph.D. degree in physiology at Harvard in 1914. He subsequently held faculty positions in the Department of Pharmacology at Albany Medical College and at the University of Colorado School of Medicine. He took leave from the latter position to complete a medical education at Washington University in St. Louis, where he received the M.D. degree in 1921. After serving an internship at Barnes Hospital, Dr. Gruber remained at Washington University as Associate Professor of Pharmacology, while also serving as physician to outpatients at the University Dispensary. It was from this position that Dr. Gruber came to Jefferson in 1932.

Dr. Gruber was as tireless and enthusiastic in research as he was in teaching. When he came to Jefferson he had already authored or coauthored 82 scientific papers in the fields of physiology and pharmacology. During his 21 years at Jefferson this

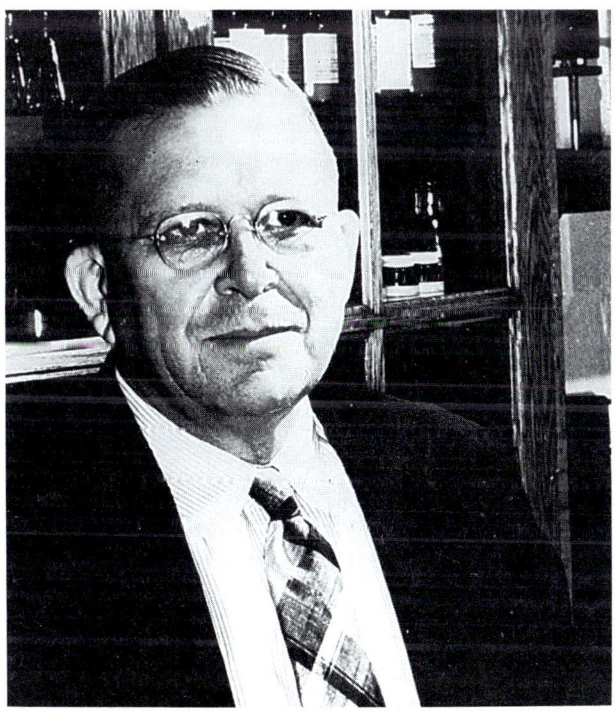

FIG. 8-1. Charles M. Gruber, Ph.D., M.D.; First Chairman (1932–1953).

number more than doubled, to 177. He was also author of the *Handbook of Treatment* and *Medical Formulary* and from 1948 to 1953 was associate editor of the *Cyclopedia of Medicine, Surgery and Specialties.* His contributions in research dealt largely with muscular and cardiovascular physiology and with the pharmacology of morphine, papaverine, quinidine, posterior pituitary hormones, the benzyl esters, meperidine, diphenylhydantoin, and the barbituric acid and thiobarbiturate derivatives.

During his long and productive professional career, Dr. Gruber played an exceedingly active role in many scientific and medical societies at the local, state, and national levels. Most notably, in 1953, he was elected President of the American Society for Pharmacology and Experimental Therapeutics, in which he had previously served as Vice-President and Treasurer. He was a member of the American Physiological Society and a charter member of the American College of Cardiology and of the Central Society for Clinical Research. Gruber served a term as Chairman of the Section of Pharmacology and Experimental Therapeutics of the American Medical Association, and for nine years as alternate delegate to its House of Delegates. Among the numerous honorary fraternities and societies of which he was a member were Alpha Omega Alpha and Phi Beta Pi. He was National Supreme Archon of the latter from 1941 to 1943 and was named Man of the Year of that fraternity in 1958.

When Dr. Gruber retired in 1953 he did not truly go into retirement. He immediately took the Chairmanship of the Department of Pharmacology at the College of Medical Evangelists in Loma Linda, where he had been invited to establish and build a new department. Four years later, in 1957, after having accomplished that mission very successfully, he resigned and became Visiting Professor of Biology at the University of Redlands in nearby Redlands, California, where he and Mrs. Gruber had established their home upon leaving the Philadelphia area. Dr. Gruber continued teaching in this capacity until 1963, when he finally retired at the age of 76, having taught continuously for 52 years, 46 of them in medical schools. By his own count he took part in the medical education of 4,976 physicians.

Typical of his indomitable spirit, after retiring from his last teaching position in 1963 Dr. Gruber remained active in numerous community affairs in Redlands. He served as a Deacon in the First Congregational Church and as a member of the Board of Directors of the Patton State Hospital. He was a leader in the Redlands Horticultural and Improvement Society. As a flower gardener he gained local fame for his eight-foot-tall delphiniums. The Redlands Day Nursery was one of his chief interests during these years. Charles M. Gruber, educator, scientist, physician, and Professor Emeritus of Pharmacology died on November 19, 1974, in Loma Linda, California. He was 87 years old.

In his long life of dedication and action Dr. Gruber played a major role in the development of the science of pharmacology, during that period in its history when it was coming into its own as an independent academic discipline and when the medical schools of this country were beginning to establish separate departments for teaching and research in this relatively new field of basic and applied science. In 1951 Dr. Gruber wrote a detailed account of the 19-year history of the Department, including the development of the physical facilities, the expansion of personnel, the medical student teaching program, the research activities, and the 1949 beginning of the graduate training program.[3]

The Departments of Physiology and Pharmacology shared the fourth floor of the College building (1025 Walnut Street) for six years (1932–1938). With the expansion of both Departments, Pharmacology then moved to the seventh floor, which, as designed by Dr. Gruber, doubled the space available for the activities of the Department. Thirteen years later, at the time of his 1951 report on the history of the Department, Dr. Gruber again expressed concern about the inadequacy of the space occupied by its present staff. From four staff members only a few years before, the space was now occupied by 16 full-time faculty, graduate students, and technical assistants.

Under Dr. Gruber's regime the pharmacology course for medical students, presented in the spring semester of their sophomore year, included 105 hours of lectures, 126 hours of laboratory work and 18 hours of recitations and examinations. The lectures covered basic pharmacology, therapeutics, and toxicology, with significant emphasis on pharmacy, prescription writing, and the memorization of dosages. In the laboratory, the students, in groups of five, tested the effects of various drugs and poisons on animals (dogs, cats, rabbits, guinea pigs, mice, turtles, frogs) and sometimes on themselves. Only half the class could occupy the laboratory at one time, so that the teaching staff was occupied for a total of 252 hours in this segment of their duties with the medical students. Thus, during the semester when classes in pharmacology were in session, practically all of the available time of all the members of the staff was devoted to teaching the medical students. The remainder of the school year and the summer months were given over to original investigations.

The graduate training program soon became a substantial component of the activities of the Department. In the short time since the inception of this program in 1949 to the time of Dr. Gruber's retirement in 1953, three Ph.D., and two M.S. degrees in pharmacology had been granted. Three other graduate students had completed most of their requirements for the Ph.D. degree, which they received in 1954. In all, the new Chairman of the Department, on his arrival in September, 1953, inherited nine candidates for the Ph.D. degree and one for the M.S. degree. It speaks well for the high standards of the original selection of these students that they all completed their degree requirements by 1956.

Julius M. Coon, Ph.D., M.D.; Second Chairman (1953–1976)

Dr. Gruber's successor to the Chairmanship of the Department was Julius M. Coon, M.D., Ph.D., from the University of Chicago, where he had been Associate Professor of Pharmacology and Director of the United States Air Force Radiation Laboratory of the University of Chicago. Some years later, when reflecting upon his arrival at Jefferson Dr. Coon stated that he "was fortunate in inheriting at Jefferson a good nucleus of staff, several outstanding graduate students, and a good physical plant. Accordingly there was little need for major reorganization, reorienting, or rebuilding in any of the principal facets of the activities and responsibilities of the Department, in teaching the medical students, in graduate education, and in research. During the last nine years, however, these activities have evolved to keep pace with modern trends."[4]

When Dr. Coon assumed the Pharmacology Chairmanship no major changes were immediately instituted in any aspect of the activities of the Department. Through subsequent years alterations in the medical and graduate student teaching programs and in research took place more by evolution than by revolution and were essentially quantitative rather than qualitative in nature. As a result of this process, the pharmacology course for the second-year medical students in 1987 included 82 lectures, four conference hours, and no laboratory work, compared with the 1957 schedule of 105 lectures, 18 conference hours, and 126 hours in the laboratory. These alterations took place gradually over that 30-year period as a result of generally changing emphases in the science of pharmacology in medical education in the United States. For medical students who developed special interests, elective courses in pharmacology and toxicology, and seminars and laboratory research for academic credit, were made available to the medical students in their junior and senior years.

Julius M. Coon (Figure 8-2) was born on October 29, 1910, in Liberty, Missouri, where his

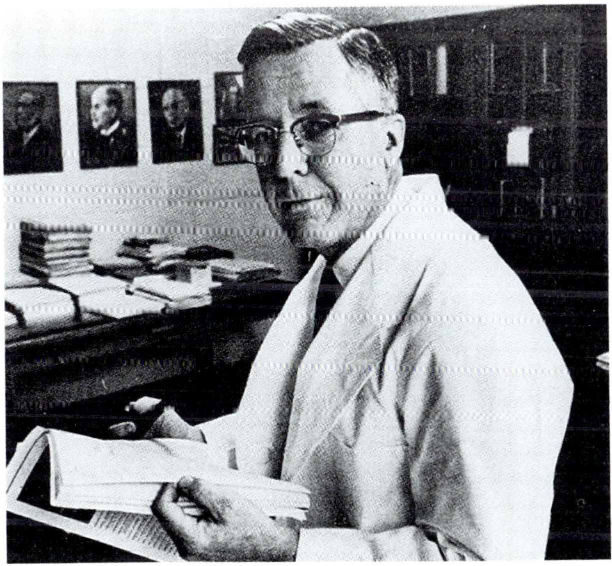

FIG. 8-2. Julius M. Coon, Ph.D., M.D.; Second Chairman (1953–1976).

father taught Latin and Greek at William Jewell College. In 1923 the family moved to Bloomington, Indiana, where in high school Coon majored in Latin. He thought this fun, like playing word games, as was also the case with both German and French later at Indiana University. He took his A.B. degree in chemistry, however, which, with courses in biology and physiology, put him on the track for graduate studies in biochemistry at the University of Chicago in 1934.

At the end of his first year at Chicago Coon took a course in pharmacology in which he recognized an exciting convergence of his prior studies in chemistry, biology, physiology, and biochemistry. Pharmacology was then the focus of his subsequent studies for the Ph.D. degree, which he obtained in 1938. The Chairman of the Department of Pharmacology at the University of Chicago and Dr. Coon's mentor was Professor Eugene Maximillian Karl Geiling, who had previously been associated for many years at Johns Hopkins University with John J. Abel, the "Father of American Pharmacology."

Dr. Coon stayed as a faculty member of the Pharmacology Department at the University of Chicago from 1938 to 1953, except for a one-year stint in 1946 as a pharmacologist with the Food and Drug Administration in Washington, D.C. His studies for the M.D. degree, which he finally received in 1945, had been interrupted by World War II, during which time he spent four years in research on the toxicology of chemical warfare agents at the University of Chicago Toxicity Laboratory, under the auspices of the Office of Scientific Research and Development of the United States Government. After World War II this laboratory continued research on the toxicology of various insecticides chemically related to some of the compounds that had been proposed as chemical warfare agents. From 1948 to 1953 Dr. Coon was Director of this laboratory, which in 1951 was renamed the U.S. Air Force Radiation Laboratory. The general nature of the research after this change remained largely toxicological.

When Dr. Coon came to Jefferson in 1953 his research activities in the preceding 12 years had been exclusively in toxicology. Though he continued his own interests and research efforts in this area, no major increase in the emphasis of toxicology in the research and teaching programs of the Department immediately resulted. Through the succeeding years, however, toxicologic issues became a substantial part of the research and graduate training activities of the Department. It is pertinent to note that the first Ph.D. degree in Pharmacology was awarded in 1952 to a student whose thesis research concerned the toxicology of acrylonitrile and who has subsequently pursued a career in toxicology. Two other students who started graduate studies before Dr. Gruber's retirement completed their thesis research on toxicological problems after Dr. Coon's arrival. During Dr. Coon's tenure as Chairman approximately half of the faculty and graduate student research activities of the Department involved toxicological issues. These activities were well supported by research and training grants from the National Institutes of Health and other government agencies. Throughout the period from 1952 to 1978, 27 of 59 Ph.D. theses involved research regarding the toxicology of chemicals that were of interest and importance not as drugs but as risks to health in the environment. Important examples of these were the organochlorine and organophosphate insecticides, benzene, toluene, benzpyrene, carbon tetrachloride, and some of the heavy metals. Numerous studies involved toxicologic interactions between these substances and, in some cases, with drugs. Many graduate students went on to respected careers in education or industry and held a variety of important offices.

The first printed notice of the new Board for the Regulation of Graduate Studies in 1949 listed pharmacology and toxicology together as major fields of study in the Department of Pharmacology. In fact, toxicology was a subject with a distant past at Jefferson. In 1866, Benjamin Howard Rand, Professor of Chemistry, lectured on "Applied Medical Chemistry and Toxicology." At the end of Rand's tenure in 1877, the name of the Department became Medical Chemistry and Toxicology. In 1912 the name was changed to the Department of Physiological Chemistry and Toxicology, which persisted until 1945 when it became the Department of Biochemistry under Dr. Abraham Cantarow.

Toxicology in the academic and research programs at Jefferson kept pace with the development of the subject internationally during the last half of the nineteenth and the early twentieth centuries. The outstanding personality in toxicology was Dr. James William Holland, Professor of Medical Chemistry and Toxicology from 1885 to 1912. Holland had previously been a student, at the University of Louisville, of J. Lawrence Smith, who had been trained in toxicology by Mateo J. B. Orfila in Europe. Orfila (1787–1853) is credited with establishing a body of knowledge that has subsequently developed into the modern science of toxicology. Before his time there existed what is commonly called the "art of poisoning." Early in the period of Dr. Gruber's Chairmanship of the Department of Pharmacology (1932–1953), it became recognized that the disciplines of pharmacology and toxicology had very pertinent overlapping basic scientific relationships, and that toxicology should be considered as a part of the pharmacology teaching curriculum. The Department of Physiological Chemistry and Toxicology had been teaching primarily the analytical chemistry of poisons, not their biological effects on living organisms. The word "toxicology," however, remained in the name of the Department from 1877 to 1945. It is of interest that Abraham Cantarow, Associate Professor in the Department at that time, published the book *Lead Poisoning* in 1944 with his associate, Max Trumper, as coauthor.

During his professional career from the early 1940s, Dr. Coon's scientific interests and activities were primarily in toxicology, with further specialization in food toxicology. His early studies of the toxicology of chemical warfare agents, some of which later were used as pesticides that became important food contaminants, led to interests in food additives, to chemical changes in foods due to processing, and to the natural chemical constituents of foods. He thus became involved with advisory panels and study committees of the National Academy of Sciences' National Research Council, National Institutes of Health, Food and Drug Administration, United States Department of Agriculture, and the Environmental Protection Agency. He served on several advisory panels for the World Health Organization and the Food and Agriculture Organization, studying the safety of food additives and pesticide residues.

Dr. Coon continued to pursue his activities in toxicology following his official retirement in 1976. Examples of these later activities included memberships on the Expert Panel on Food Safety and Nutrition of the Institute of Food Technologists, the Board of Scientific Advisors of the American Council on Science and Health, the Expert Panel on Cosmetic Ingredient Review of the Cosmetic, Toiletry, and Fragrance Association, and several task forces of the Council on Agricultural Science and Technology. In recognition of his services and contributions in toxicology Dr. Coon received from the Society of Toxicology the Merit Award in 1978 and the Education Award in 1983. He also received in 1983 the Ambassador of Toxicology Award from the Mid-Atlantic Chapter of the Society of Toxicology "in appreciation of his outstanding contribution to the international recognition of the science of toxicology."

The evolution of the primary programs of the Department of Pharmacology during Dr. Coon's chairmanship from 1953 to 1976 is reviewed in two issues of the *Alumni Bulletin* published in 1962 and 1976.[4,5] These describe the increase in the number of faculty and graduate students, the addition of courses made available to both medical and graduate students, and the general nature of the research programs. Another issue of the *Alumni Bulletin* in 1963 briefly reviews only the research activities of the Department.[6]

It should be emphasized that substantial research programs other than in toxicology were pursued. Research in progress at the time of Dr. Coon's retirement can be described as follows:

In psychopharmacology and neuropharmacology, research was directed toward the relationship between both normal and abnormal brain and nerve chemistry on the one hand, and the action and metabolism of drugs on the other hand, with the hope of revealing information leading to improvements in the drug treatment of diseases affecting the brain and nervous system. The chemical composition of the cerebrospinal fluid and its relation to various neurological and mental disorders were studied as a basis for developing drugs for the treatment of these disorders. Other research involved the micro-injection of psychoactive drugs into specific sites of the brain and the recording of the electrical activity from those and related brain centers. This "chemical dissection" to create "biochemical lesions" in the brain was designed to further the understanding of the biochemical basis of neuropsychiatric disorders and provide a basis for more effective drug therapy.

An extensive investigation was carried out on the function and importance of taurine in the central nervous system, the eye, and the heart of different species of animals. Important functions of this natural chemical component of the body were found in relation to such varied disorders as epilepsy, retinitis pigmentosa, and myocardial hypertrophy.

Other research involved studies of the roles of arachidonic acid and the prostaglandins in relation to platelet aggregation and the use of aspirin and modification of the diet to reduce platelet aggregation. Also, the role of acetaldehyde in heavy alcohol consumption and heavy cigarette smoking received concentrated attention.

During his tenure, Dr. Coon recruited a number of faculty members who served the Department and Jefferson well. Those who served for many years on a full-time basis were Drs. A. J. Triolo, R. Snyder, M. S. Silver, J. J. Kocsis, T. A. Hare, R. M. Manthei, and W. H. Vogel.

Carmine Paul Bianchi, Ph.D; Third Chairman (1976–1986)

The new Chairman of the Department, effective July 1, 1976, was Carmine Paul Bianchi, Ph.D. (Figure 8-3) from the University of Pennsylvania School of Medicine, where he had been Professor of Pharmacology since 1969 and a member of the faculty of that Department since 1961.

Dr. Bianchi was born on April 9, 1927, in Newark, New Jersey. After receiving his diploma at Columbia High School in 1945, he spent two years in the Army Medical Corps as Technical Sgt. Fourth Grade. He then attended Columbia University, where he majored in chemistry and obtained the B.A. degree in 1950. Like Dr. Gruber, the first Chairman of the Pharmacology Department at Jefferson, Bianchi earned his Ph.D. in physiology. He pursued his graduate studies at Rutgers University, supplementing his physiology major with a biochemistry minor for the M.S. degree in 1953 and with a physical chemistry minor for the Ph.D. degree in 1956. Dr. Bianchi then spent several years at the National Institutes of Health—two years as a Public Health Fellow and one as a Visiting Scientist. Following that he was Assistant Member of the Institute for Muscle Disease in New York for one year. In 1961 Dr. Bianchi became classified professionally as a pharmacologist by becoming an Associate in the Department of Pharmacology at the University of Pennsylvania School of Medicine. There he advanced to Professorship in 1969 and remained until he came to Jefferson. The evolution of Dr. Bianchi's career from physiology to pharmacology was the logical result of his investigations of the effect of various drugs on the metabolism and distribution of some of the important elements of the body, notably calcium. His major field of interest became classified and remained in electrolyte pharmacology.

Throughout his career Dr. Bianchi has been very active in the affairs of outside professional organizations. He is a member of the American Society for Pharmacology and Experimental Therapeutics, the American Physiological Society, the American Chemical Society, and the International Society of Toxicology, to name

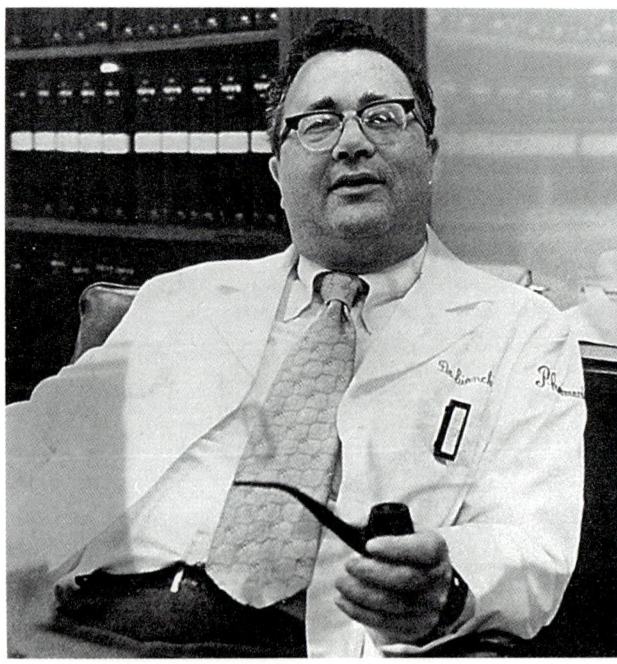

FIG. 8-3. Carmine P. Bianchi, Ph.D.; Third Chairman (1976–1986).

only a few. He served as President of both the Philadelphia Physiological Society and the John Morgan Society in the same year (1973–1974), and of the Philadelphia Chapter of the Society for Neuroscience (1979–1980). He gave much time and valuable services as Field Editor for the *Journal of Pharmacology and Experimental Therapeutics* (1970–1979) and as a member of the Pharmacology Section of the National Board of Medical Examiners (1981–1985).

After Dr. Bianchi became Chairman no immediate changes in the general structure and activities of the Department took place. He enlarged the Department and filled vacancies occasioned by the retirement of some faculty members. The didactic schedules and subject matter offered to the medical and graduate students underwent only minor annual changes. Research activities were augmented by the addition of Dr. Bianchi's specialty in electrolyte pharmacology and the appointments of new staff members for investigations in that and related fields. Through the following decade there was a marked change in the faculty structure of the Department. The 1975 Jefferson catalogue, for example, listed 15 faculty appointments in Pharmacology, of which eight were on a primary full-time basis with offices and laboratories in the Department. In 1985 there were 36 faculty appointments of which eight were on a primary full-time basis. The large increase in the total number of faculty resulted from adjunct appointments from outside organizations and from secondary appointments of faculty members of the Clinical Departments at Jefferson. This expansion reflected a broadening of interests and interactions on both the scientific and clinical fronts in clinical pharmacology and clinical toxicology.

A notable addition to the faculty of the Department in 1978 was Dr. Hyman Menduke (Figure 8-4) as Professor of Pharmacology (Biostatistics). After receiving his Ph.D. in Economic Statistics at the University of Pennsylvania, Menduke came to Jefferson in 1953 as Assistant Professor of Biostatistics with no official Departmental affiliation until 1963, when he was appointed Professor of Preventive Medicine (Biostatistics). When Dr. Menduke first came to Jefferson he gave a ten-hour course in biostatistics to the second-year medical students in time provided during their pharmacology course. Through the years his offerings expanded to a 12-hour course for freshman medical students and introductory and advanced courses for graduate students. An early and valuable contribution was a series of individual conferences with graduate students on the statistical planning of their research problems and the later analysis of their data. Dr. Menduke also became Adjunct Professor of Statistical Evaluation of Clinical Data at the Philadelphia College of Pharmacy and Science and past President of the Philadelphia Chapter of the American Statistical Association.

Graduate training leading to the Ph.D. degree in pharmacology has been a major and continuous program of the Department since its official inception in 1949. The Department takes pride in its achievements in this respect. It is interesting to note that of the 304 Ph.D. degrees awarded at Jefferson commencements through 1987, there were 91 Ph.D.s in Pharmacology. All of the senior faculty of the Department made substantial contributions in sponsoring the research efforts of candidates for the Ph.D. degree.

The interests and activities of the Department in research in toxicology have been emphasized.

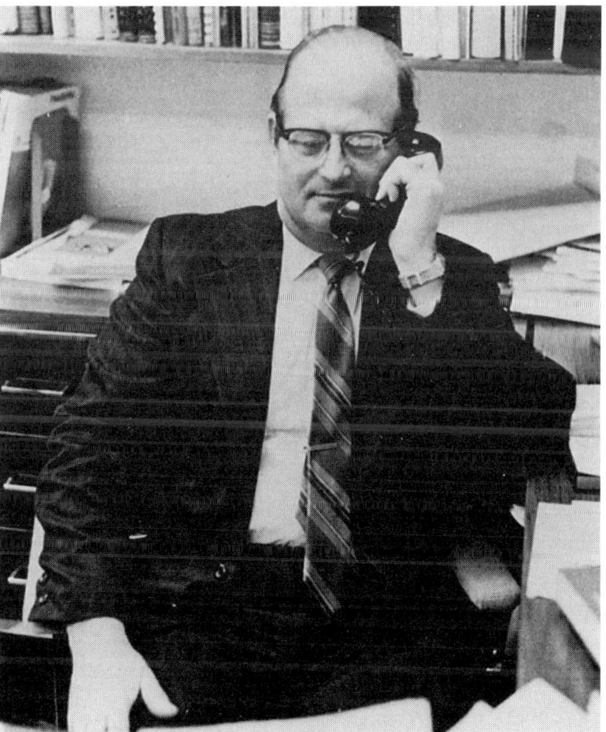

FIG. 8-4. Hyman Menduke, Ph.D.; Professor of Pharmacology (Biostatistics).

Toxicology continued as an important part of the research program after Dr. Bianchi became Chairman in 1976, although under his direction the major emphasis in research became redirected toward the general areas of cell pharmacology and neuropharmacology.

In accord with its continuing research and teaching activities in toxicology, the Department starting in 1977 organized a series of annual workshops on Industrial Toxicology sponsored by the College of Graduate Studies. These were four-day symposia on important toxicologic problems in industry and the general environment, presented by toxicologically involved Jefferson faculty and by invited experts from other universities, industry, and government.

In 1979 the Department was awarded a training grant in Industrial and Environmental Toxicology by the National Institute of Environmental Health Sciences. The purpose of this award was to provide postdoctoral training in toxicology for individuals who had previously received their Ph.D. degrees in other sciences. Ten M.S. degrees were subsequently awarded in this program through the years from 1981 to 1986.

On December 14, 1978, a full day's workshop with outside invited experts was held to discuss the formation of a Toxicology Center and the establishment of a Chair in Toxicology-Pathology to broaden the base of research and training in toxicology at Jefferson. It was envisioned that the Center would be an administrative Division within the Department of Pharmacology, with research participation from other basic science departments and the Department of Medicine. Although funds accumulated in support of a Toxicology Center, disagreements developed relating to the administrative base of the Center. The death of Dr. Gonzalo Aponte, Chairman of the Department of Pathology, and the resignation of the Professor of Pharmacology who had originally conceived the idea of the Toxicology Center further delayed the development of an organized interdisciplinary program in Toxicology. Eventually an agreement was reached between the central administration and Dr. Willis C. Maddrey, Chairman of the Department of Medicine, and approved by the Executive Council on September 6, 1983, which later resulted in the establishment of the Division of Environmental Medicine and Toxicology administered by the Department of Medicine. This became a very active and well-funded interdisciplinary research program headed by Lance L. Simpson, Ph.D., Professor of Medicine and Professor of Pharmacology. This Division occupied laboratory space in the Department of Medicine and about 20 percent of the space originally designated for the Department of Pharmacology.

Wolfgang H. Vogel, Ph.D.; Acting Chairman (1986–)

In 1986, Dr. Bianchi resigned his Chairmanship and remained as Professor to pursue his research interests more actively. Dr. Wolfgang H. Vogel (Figure 8-5), Professor of Pharmacology, then became Acting Chairman of the Department. Dr.

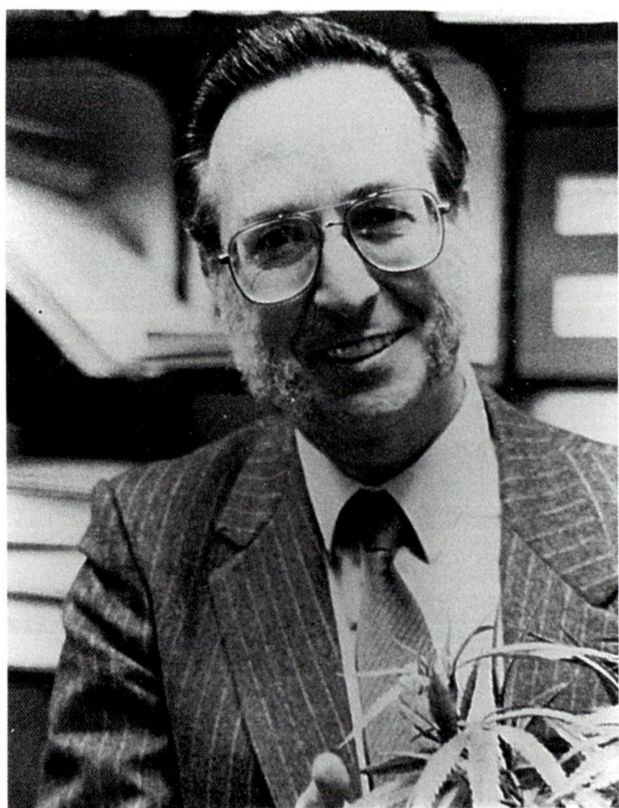

FIG. 8-5. Wolfgang H. Vogel, Ph.D.; Acting Chairman (1986–).

Upon his leaving the chairmanship, Dr. Bianchi expressed the hope that the Department would develop its primary research strength in cell and molecular pharmacology and in neuropharmacology as promising areas for future progress.

Vogel, born in 1930 and educated through the doctorate level in organic chemistry in Germany, came to the United States in 1958. He spent several years with the Department of Pharmacology at the University of Illinois College of Medicine, came to Jefferson as an Associate Professor of Pharmacology in 1967, and was appointed Professor in 1974. Dr. Vogel's primary research and teaching interests have been in the areas of psycho- and neuropharmacology. His outstanding scholarship and effective teaching were recognized by the Class of 1982, which presented his portrait to the University.

References

1. Gruber, C.M., " Department of Pharmacology." *Clinic Yearbook,* 1936, p. 83.
2. Coon, J. M., "Memoir of Charles Michael Gruber." *Trans. Stud. Coll. Phys. Ph.* 45:46–47, 1977.
3. Gruber, C.M., "The Department of Pharmacology," *Jeff. Med. Coll. Al. Bull.* October, 1951.
4. Coon, J.M., "The Department of Pharmacology." *Jeff. Med. Coll. Al. Bull.* December, 1962.
5. Coon, J.M., "Teaching and Research in the Department of Pharmacology." *Jeff. Med. Coll. Al. Bull.* Summer, 1976, pp. 4–9.
6. "Research in the Department of Pharmacology." *Jeff. Med. Coll. Al. Bull.* October, 1963, pp. 31–33.

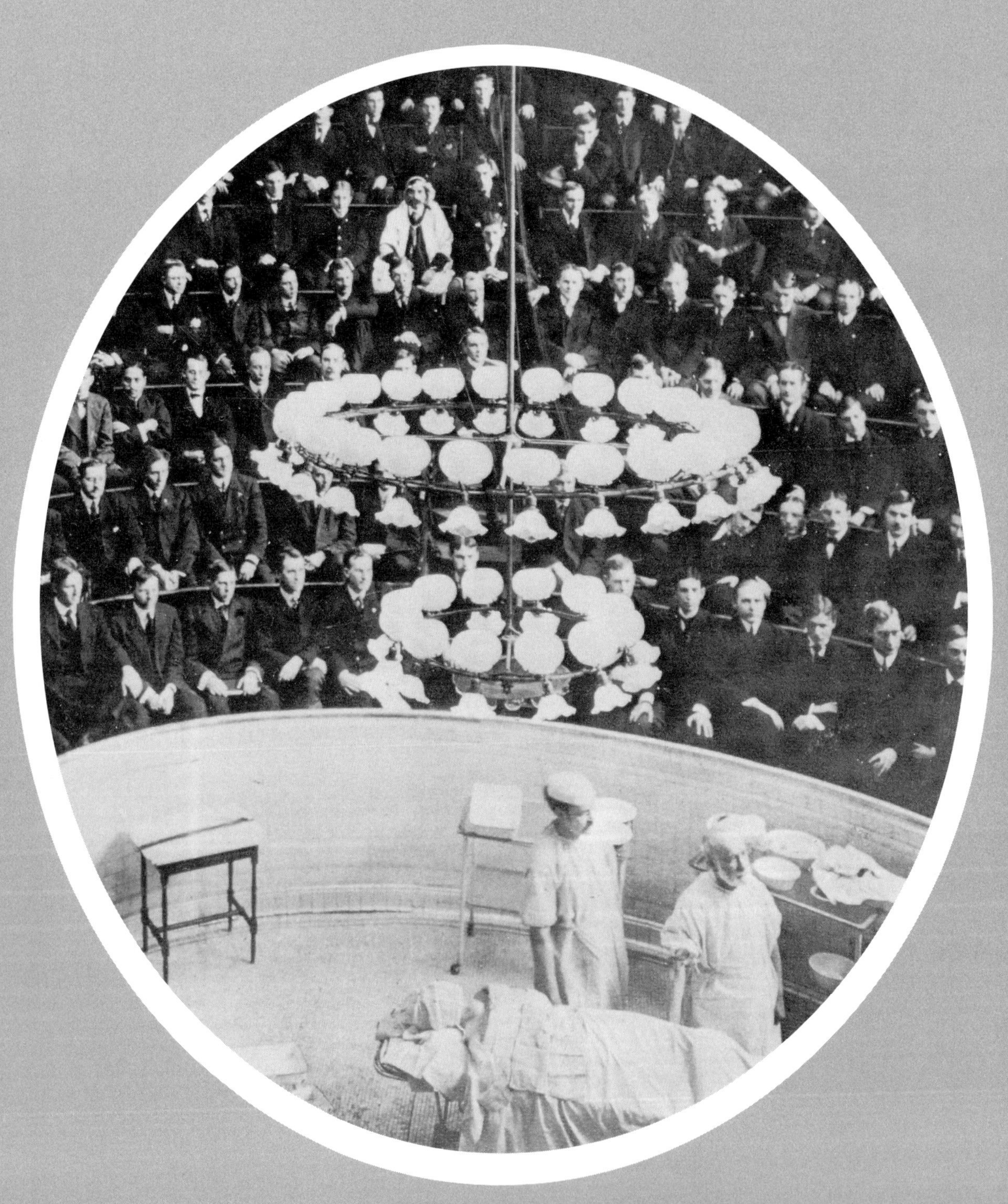

PART III

Clinical Departments and Divisions

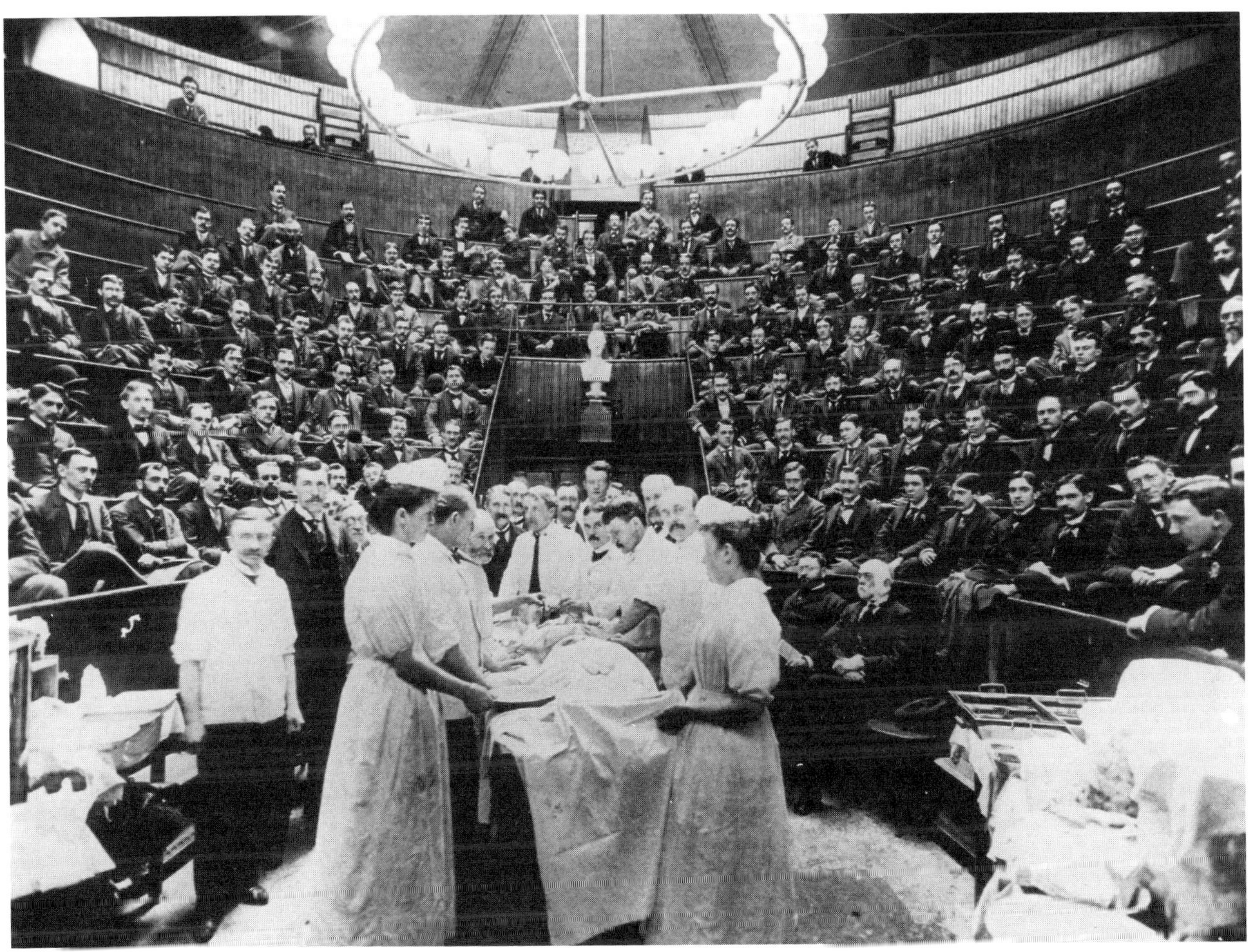

Clinical Amphitheater ("Pit") of 1877 Hospital

← *Opposite page:*
Clinic of Dr. W.W. Keen in "Pit" of 1877 Hospital (ca. 1900)

CHAPTER NINE

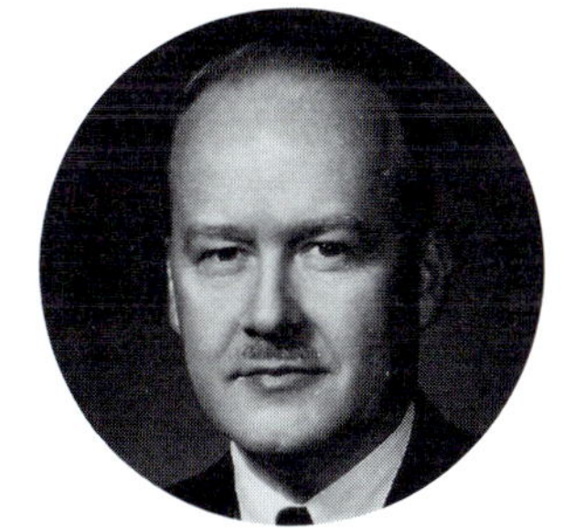

Department of Medicine

JOHN H. HODGES, M.D.

"Wherever the art of medicine is loved, there also is love of humanity."

—HIPPOCRATES (460–370 B.C.)

THE PASSAGE of over 150 years makes possible the comparison of the status of the teaching of Medicine at Jefferson. In 1985 the Department Chairman, Willis C. Maddrey, had 475 Faculty Members in 13 Divisions, 88 Residents, two Chief Residents, and 30 Fellows. The Department occupied five floors in the College Building and was assigned 219 teaching beds in Thomas Jefferson University Hospital, with additional medical teaching arrangements in ten affiliated Hospitals. Research grants totaled over $8 million. By contrast to this extensive and diversified teaching, patient service, and research group, one individual was responsible for the teaching at Jefferson's founding in 1824.

This contrast in the Medical Department's size, manpower, research, and financial capabilities was the norm in United States medical schools in the eighteenth and early nineteenth centuries. It was also true of the other partitions of medical teaching such as Surgery, Obstetrics, Chemistry, and Anatomy. The new schools of this era started a change in medical education. Before the advent of the medical school, the Preceptor had the authority to decide when a pupil was ready to practice on his own. The role of the medical school in taking over this decision was gradually accepted over a period from about 1760 to 1875. The total number of graduates of the four surviving medical schools from the eighteenth century was approximately 100 (University of Pennsylvania, Columbia, Harvard, and Dartmouth)[1] in contrast to the roughly 16,000 a year being graduated in the latter portion of the twentieth century.

In 1765 the Medical Department of the College of Philadelphia (later the University of Pennsylvania) had six members, with Dr. John Morgan as the Professor of Medicine.[2] The Medical Department of King's College, New York, (Columbia) also had six professors at the time of its establishment in 1768, each of whom had the total responsibility for the teaching of a complete subject: Physic, Midwifery, Chemistry, Surgery, Physiology, or Anatomy. As late as 1849 the total medical faculty of the University of Pennsylvania consisted of seven members, and the Medical Department of the University of the State of Missouri had nine members.[3] Thus, it was not unusual that the list of the faculty for Jefferson Medical College that was presented for a charter in 1824 contained but four names, one of whom was Dr. Joseph Klapp as the Professor of Theory and Practice.

Joseph Klapp, M.D. (1783–1843); First Chairman (1824)

Dr. Klapp (Figure 9-1), an 1805 graduate of the University of Pennsylvania, had a large practice and was one of the physicians to the Philadelphia Almshouse Infirmary. He published medical papers such as those that appeared in the *American Medical Recorder* of 1818 and which included *Sudden Death, Singultus,* and *On Tremulant Diseases* (vertigo, mania, and epilepsy).[4] He had been one of the teachers with McClellan prior to the formal establishment of the Medical College. A few months later Klapp was transferred to the Chair of Anatomy. Illness caused his resignation after only six months of association with Jefferson Medical College. His effect on the medical portion of the curriculum was nominal, at most. This busy clinician had three sons who were active physicians in Philadelphia and continued the local prominence of the family name in medicine.[5] Klapp was succeeded by Dr. John Eberle.

John Eberle, M.D. (1787–1838); Second Chairman (1824–1830)

Dr. Eberle (Figure 9-2) was listed originally as the Professor of Obstetrics, then as Professor of Materia Medica, and finally, following the transfer of Klapp to Anatomy, as Professor of Theory and Practice of Medicine (September, 1824). Subsequent to Eberle's graduation from the University of Pennsylvania (1809), he practiced medicine in Lancaster County. He returned to Philadelphia to continue practice but was destined to reach fame through his teaching and writings. He was, for a time, one of the editors of the *American Medical Recorder,* and in 1827 he published his Jefferson Medical College *Notes of Lectures on the Theory and Practice of Medicine,*[6] a book of 87 topics from anasarca to yellow fever, which was interspersed with ruled pages for notes by the students. The purchase of this treatise by the students, along with their usual lecture fees, aided his income. A prodigious reader of medical journals, Eberle wrote *A Treatise on the Practice of*

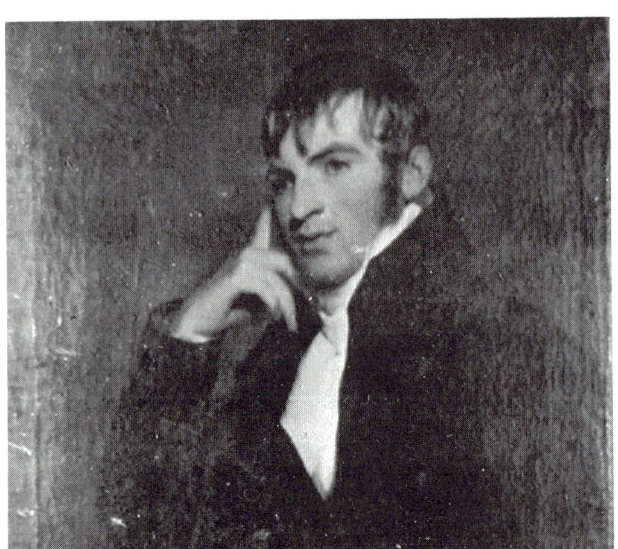

Fig. 9-1. Joseph Klapp, M.D. (1783–1843); First Chairman (1824).

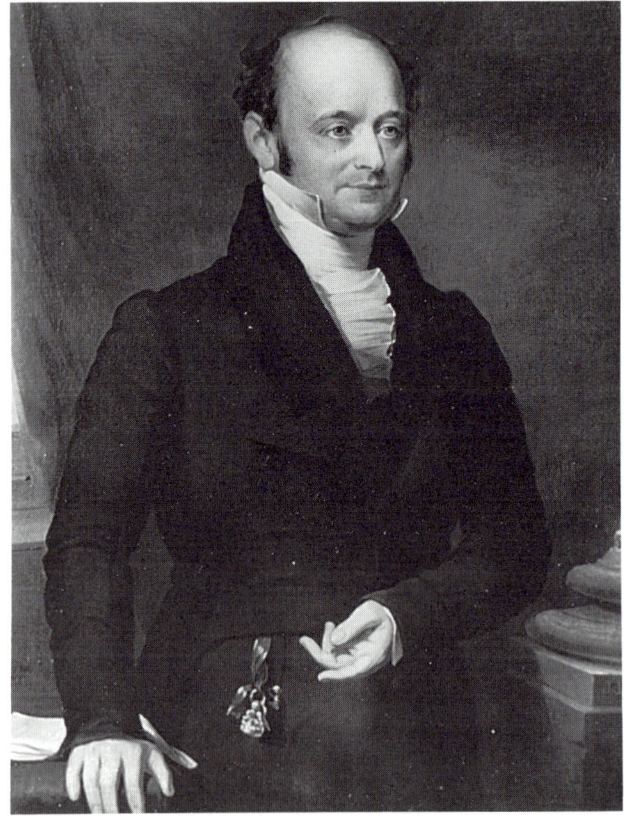

Fig. 9-2. John Eberle, M.D. (1787–1838); Second Chairman (1824–1830).

Medicine (1831),[7] a two-volume work of over 1000 pages, which was to go through six editions. The *Notes* and *Treatise* were both preceded by a two-volume work entitled *Treatise of the Materia Medica and Therapeutics* (1825).[8]

Eberle chaired the original meeting of the faculty (December 20, 1824)[9] and served as Jefferson's second Dean from 1827 to 1828 (the first was Dr. Benjamin Rush Rhees, Professor of Materia Medica). He was a regular attendant at the Infirmary in the Tivoli Theater site of the College. The constant disturbance of a chronic abdominal disorder coupled with a tendency to emotional swings probably contributed to his transfer to Materia Medica in 1830. He was succeeded in the same year by Dr. Daniel Drake.

Daniel Drake, M.D. (1785–1852); Third Chairman (1830–1831)

Daniel Drake (Figure 9-3) received the first certificate to practice medicine that was issued west of the Alleghenies (1805) and was the first to travel east and bring back a medical diploma (University of Pennsylvania, 1815). His varied career included owning a pharmacy and general store in Cincinnati, holding positions as Professor in several medical schools in Kentucky and Ohio, and aiding in the founding of the Medical College of Ohio and Cincinnati College (later the University of Cincinnati), the Cincinnati Infirmary, and the Ohio School for the Blind. An eloquent extemporaneous speaker, Drake became the favorite of the students at a time when they could attend lectures free of charge at Jefferson or the University of Pennsylvania for a fortnight before deciding at which institution they would like to matriculate.[9] His outspoken manner with colleagues was to cause repeated changes of academic position, and after one year he resigned and returned to the West where he pursued a productive life in medicine and civic activities.[10,11,12]

John Revere, M.D. (1787–1847); Fourth Chairman (1831–1841)

Dr. John Revere (Figure 9-4), a Bostonian and son of the Revolutionary patriot Paul Revere, was appointed in 1831 to succeed Drake in the Chair of Theory and Practice of Physic. An 1807 honor graduate of Harvard, he served a preceptorship in Boston and received his M.D. degree from Edinburgh, Scotland, in 1811. At the time of his appointment at Jefferson he was practicing in Baltimore, Maryland. He had translated Magendie's *Physiology* and published some papers. Revere became an editor of the *Medical Record* and served as Dean (1839–1841) during his last two years at Jefferson. His personal graciousness endeared him to his peers, and his ability as a lecturer earned him the admiration of the students. In 1832 the course of the Chairman for the class of 96 students included physiology, pathology, fever, exanthemas, functional disorders, blood-letting, and therapy for the diseases discussed. An attempt was made to differentiate what was known in

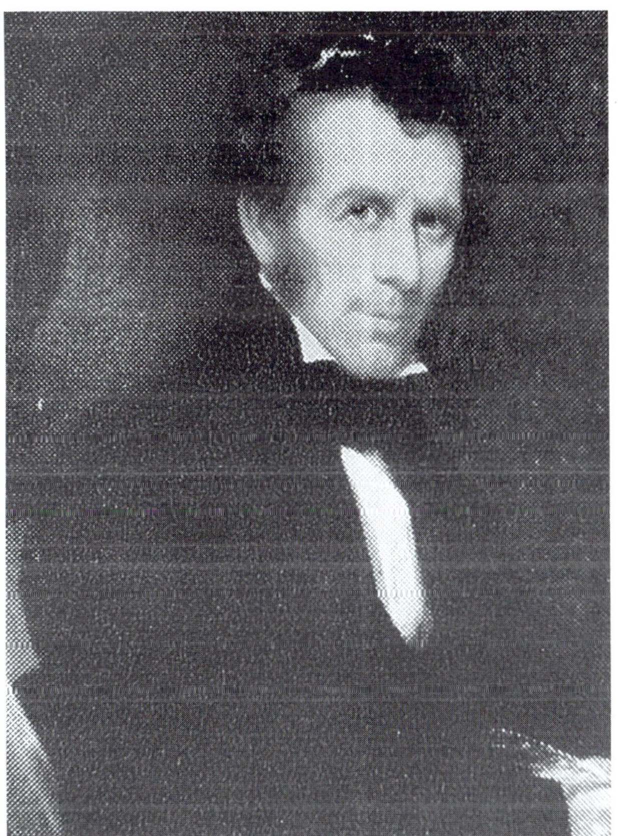

FIG. 9-3. Daniel Drake, M.D. (1785–1852); Third Chairman (1830–1831).

contrast to what was conjectured.[14] Revere resigned in 1841 to take a similar position in the founding of the Medical Department of New York University. His successor, Dr. John Kearsley Mitchell, was destined to strengthen and solidify the standards of medicine as set forth by Revere.

John K. Mitchell, M.D. (1793–1858); Fifth Chairman (1841–1858)

Dr. Mitchell (Figure 9-5) was a man of diverse talents who wrote poetry, expressed his views on social matters *(Means of Elevating the Character of the Working Classes),* combined philosophy and science *(Wisdom of God as Displayed in the Formation of Water),* and displayed his chemical talents by writing *A Study of Tests of Arseine* and by devising an apparatus for the solidification of gaseous carbonic acid. He received international acclaim with his paper *Osmosis of Fluids and Gases.* His medical work included his views on *The Cryptogamous Origin of Malarious and Epidemic Fevers.* Mitchell invented a spine appliance for cases of vertebral disease and suggested a curative treatment by extension of the trunk and support of the head. His timely teaching included hypotheses about the yet-to-be-discovered antibodies and toxins.

Mitchell was born in 1793 in Shepherdstown, Virginia (later West Virginia), the son and grandson of physicians. Of Scottish origin, he received his academic degree from the University of Edinburgh and later the M.D. degree from the University of Pennsylvania. Poor health led him to travel to China on three occasions as a ship's physician. He subsequently started what was to be a large and continuous practice in Philadelphia. In 1822 he began lecturing on Medical Chemistry at the Philadelphia Medical Institute and subsequently became a Professor of Chemistry at the Franklin Institute.

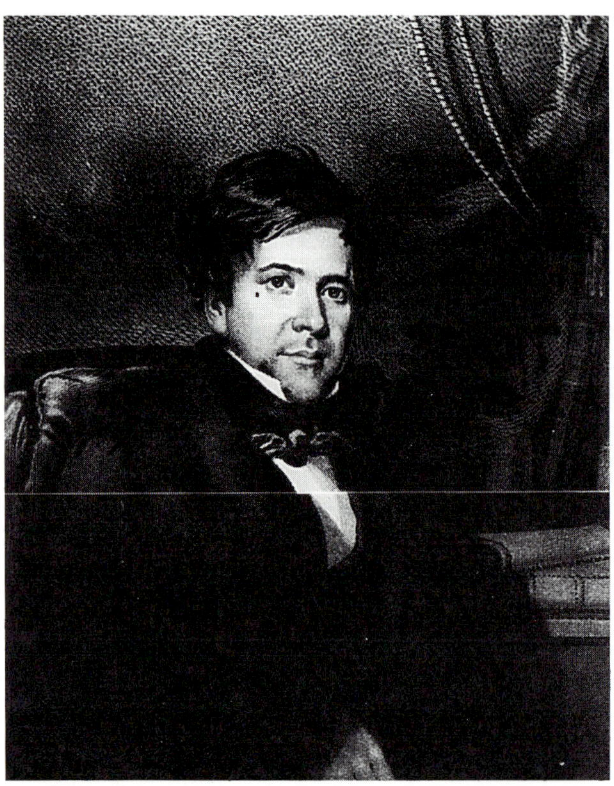

FIG. 9-4. John Revere, M.D. (1787–1847); Fourth Chairman (1831–1841).

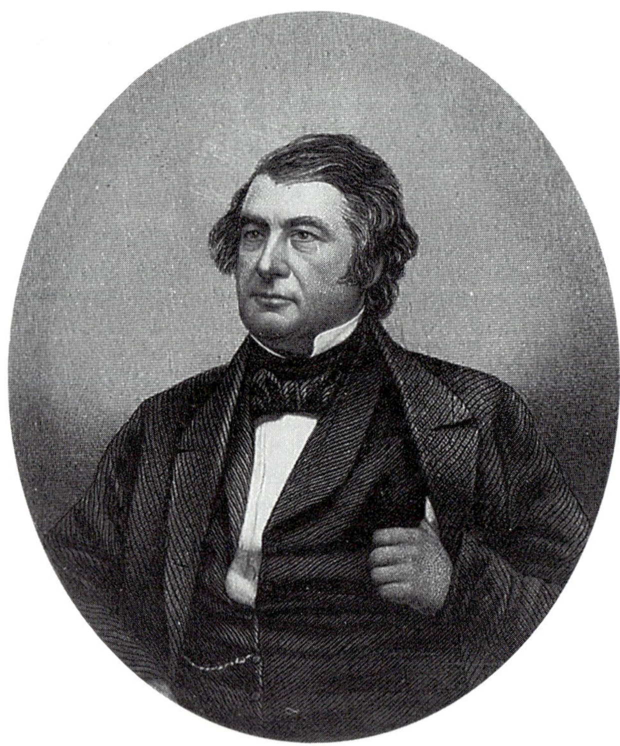

FIG. 9-5. John K. Mitchell, M.D. (1793–1858); Fifth Chairman (1841–1858).

This was a time when the clinics became "the right arm of the College."[13] The General Dispensary of Jefferson Medical College was attended regularly by the students, and the patients were entrusted to them under the direction of the Professor.[14] Students also had access to the lectures at the Pennsylvania Hospital, and the class was transported by horse-drawn "omnibuses" (on top as well as inside the vehicles) twice a week to the Philadelphia Almshouse by way of the Old Market Street Bridge, which was the chief means of getting across the Schuylkill. They had access to the facilities of the Philadelphia Dispensary and the Wills Eye Hospital following the latter's opening in 1834.

The tall, portly, charming Mitchell lectured in a polished and witty manner. As the students' friend, he cared for their illnesses, gave them advice, and assisted them financially. Although he was ill he hosted the graduating class at his home for their commencement reception a month before his death in 1858.

Robley Dunglison (1798–1869); Professor of Institutes of Medicine and Medical Jurisprudence (1836–1868)

The teaching of Medicine had been additionally strengthened by the appointment of Dr. Robley Dunglison to a position created for him, the Chair of the Institutes of Medicine and Medical Jurisprudence, which he occupied from 1836 until one year before his death in 1869. Although the "Institutes" comprised what was later more specifically delineated as "Physiology," his course included adjunct material in the field of theory and practice of medicine. This learned man, who had a keen ability to judge character, also served as Dean of the Medical School from 1854 to 1868, when he resigned the office and became Emeritus Professor.

Dunglison was born in 1798 in the Lake Region of England; he started a medical apprenticeship there at the age of 17, studied in various European medical centers, passed the examination at the Royal College of Surgeons, and obtained his medical degree in Erlangen, Germany, in 1824. Responding to an invitation from United States ex-President Thomas Jefferson, Rector of the University of Virginia, Dunglison accepted a comprehensive Chair in that institution. He stayed at Virginia for nine years, during which time he became famous as a lecturer, author, and man of letters. He was physician and friend to Presidents Jefferson and Madison. His appointment at Jefferson Medical College was preceded by three years as Professor at the Medical School of the University of Maryland. By this time the number of students at Jefferson had increased to 364 and the course had been extended to five months by including October.[15]

Dunglison, a man of broad knowledge, had an extensive personal library and wrote many professional and nonprofessional articles on such topics as road making, penitentiary discipline, early German poetry, the sanskrit language, and English fashions in the seventeenth century. He devised some of the gastric juice experiments on Alexis St. Martin that were reported by Beaumont and gained international fame from his treatises on *Practice of Medicine, Therapeutics and Materia Medica, New Remedies, Medical Dictionary,* and an edition of *Forbes Cyclopedia.* He received numerous honors and was a member of over 100 scientific societies. Dunglison was a fluent speaker whose extemporaneous lectures received the undivided attention of his class.[9] He gave clinical lectures on development, physiology, therapeutics, and jurisprudence at the Philadelphia Hospital, Blockley.[16]

Robert M. Huston, M.D. (1795–1864); Professor of Materia Medica and Therapeutics (1841–1859)

Some lectures were added to the general curriculum in April and May of 1836. Coinciding with Mitchell's appointment in 1841 was that of Robert M. Huston, M.D. as Professor of Materia Medica and General Therapeutics. The renaissance taking place in the faculty at this time thus included these additional medical subjects. By 1850 student enrollment reached 516, with 211 graduates. The following year a total of 1,074 cases were treated in the Medical Department.

Samuel H. Dickson, M.D. (1798–1872); Sixth Chairman (1858–1872)

The appointment in 1858 of Dr. Samuel H. Dickson (Figure 9-6), another Southerner, to succeed Dr. Mitchell as Professor of Theory and Practice of Medicine was a sad foreboding of the upcoming War Between the States. Dickson had been a founder of the Medical College of South Carolina and for 22 years had held the Chair of the Institutes and Practice of Medicine. This school had been for many years the only medical school of any repute in the South, east of the Alleghenies, which probably contributed to the fact that at the time of his appointment the class at Jefferson had a majority of Southern students.

Samuel Dickson was born in Charleston, South Carolina, in 1798, graduated from Yale, and following a preceptorship in Charleston earned the M.D. degree at the University of Pennsylvania in 1819. He returned to Charleston to practice medicine and to serve as Professor at the University of South Carolina. He then spent three years at the Medical College of New York, succeeding Dr. Revere. After eight more years of practice in Charleston, Dr. Dickson received the call from Jefferson. This eloquent orator was noted for his knowledge of the art as well as the science of Medicine. His outstanding work was *Elements of Medicine: A Compendium View of Pathology and Therapeutics* (1859).[17]

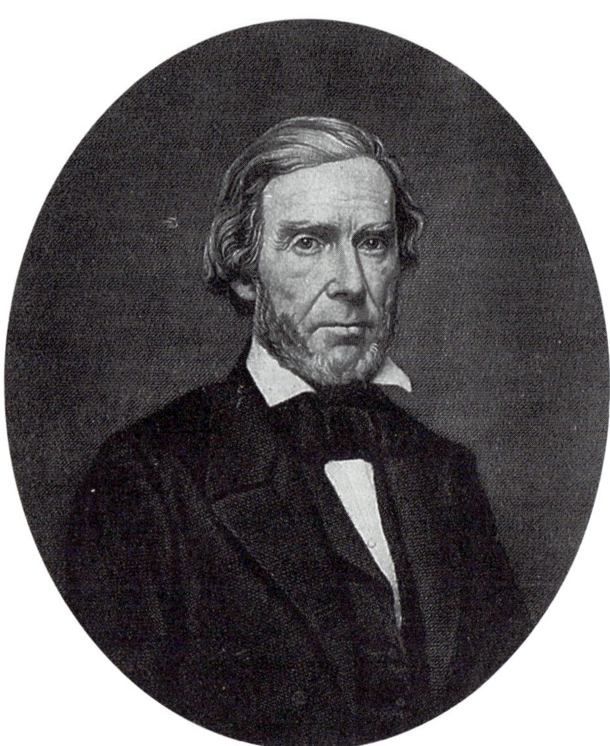

FIG. 9-6. Samuel H. Dickson; M.D. (1798–1872); Sixth Chairman (1858–1872).

The so-called "Summer Courses" were firmly established by 1866. There were specialized lectures by W. H. Pancoast in Anatomy, by S. W. Gross in Surgery, by J. Aitken Meigs in Physiology, by R. J. Levis in Eye and Ear, by F. F. Maury in Venereal Diseases, by J. M. DaCosta in Clinical Medicine, by J. H. Brinton in Surgery, and by W. W. Keen in Pathological Anatomy. This made a total of eight Lecturers in addition to the Chairmen. Each Lecturer was chosen with reference to his capacity to teach the subject assigned to him. This would seem, in essence, to herald the start of specialty teaching, but even as late as 1899 there were adverse criticisms of this form of teaching.[18] Throughout the years it would not be unusual for a Lecturer to succeed to the position of Chairman.

Jacob M. DaCosta, M.D., LL.D. (1833–1900); Seventh Chairman (1872–1891)

One of the first examples of the succession of a Lecturer to the position of Chairman was Dr. Jacob Mendes DaCosta (Figure 9-7) who succeeded to the Chair of Medicine in 1872. An 1852 recipient of the M.D. degree from Jefferson, he studied the various divisions of Medicine under the greats of Europe during the two years following his graduation. Returning to Philadelphia, he entered practice and became a Lecturer on the Jefferson Faculty in 1866. A man of broad medical knowledge, DaCosta published various papers and a treatise, *Medical Diagnosis* (1864), which went through nine editions and was translated into several foreign languages. His classic description of "irritable heart" in 1871 marked him as a pioneer in Cardiology.[19] DaCosta was noted for the excellence of his clinics. An original member of the Association of American Physicians, he was also a Fellow of the American Philosophical Society, received Honorary LL.D. degrees from Jefferson, the University of Pennsylvania, and Harvard, and became Emeritus in 1891. He and Dr. John Chalmers DaCosta, Jefferson's first Samuel D. Gross Professor of Surgery, were not related.

The expansion of facilities was keeping pace with the expansion of the faculty. A new hospital building was opened in 1877, and its Medical Division included Drs. Jacob da Silva Solis-Cohen, James C. Wilson, John B. Roberts, and Oliver P. Rex. A laboratory building at Tenth and Sansom, adjacent to the Medical Hall, was opened in 1879. This allowed for studies and demonstrations in practical chemistry, microscopy, and physiology. There was a gradual increase in the displayed objects of the Medical Museum. By 1895 the full faculty listed eight Chairmen, eight Honorary and Clinical Professors, one Adjunct Professor, seven Lecturers, nine Demonstrators, and 30 Instructors and Assistant Demonstrators.[20]

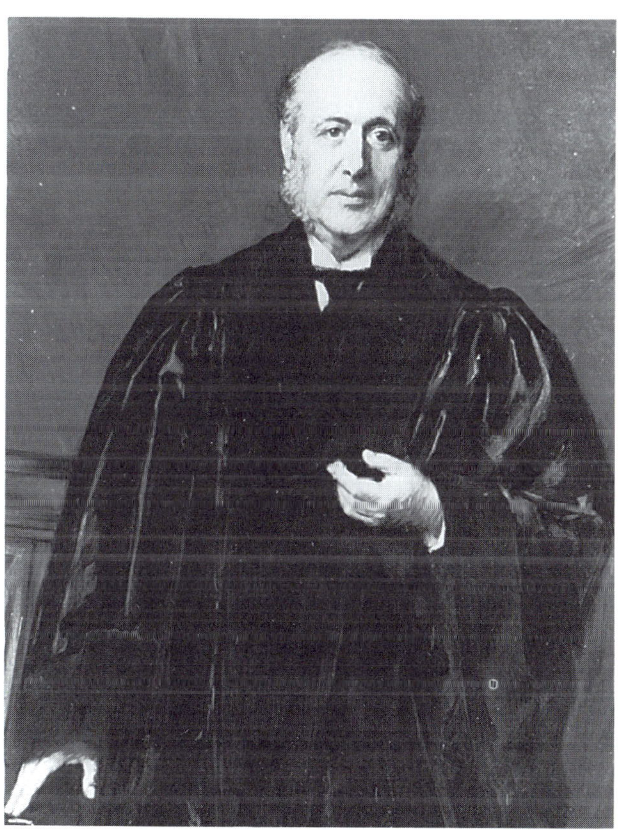

FIG. 9-7. Jacob M. DaCosta, M.D. (1833–1900); Seventh Chairman (1872–1891).

The Summer Course extended through the months of April, May, June, and September. It was voluntary, without additional tuition cost, and welcomed by most students as a desirable adjunct to the Regular Course which began in October and ran to April. The curriculum had grown to a voluntary three years by 1884, which became compulsory in 1891. At this time, Dr. James C. Wilson, previously Instructor in Physical Diagnosis and Diseases of the Chest, was appointed Chairman. Before 1885 a thesis and an oral examination were required for a diploma. At this time these were discontinued and replaced by a written examination in each branch. In 1895 the curriculum was increased to four years, and in the same year the institution changed from a proprietary school to one in which the Board of Trustees assumed the sole responsibility for financial management, including salaries of the professors.

James C. Wilson, M.D. (1847–1938); Eighth Chairman (1891–1911)

Although "Medicine" had always been a distinct part of the curriculum, it began its expansion into a Department with the appointment of Lecturers and subsequently Clinical Professors, Instructors, Demonstrators, and Assistant Demonstrators during the Chairmanships of Dickson and DaCosta. Dunglison in the Chair of Institutes of Medicine and as Dean abetted this thrust. The Department expansion continued under the Chairmanship of Dr. James Cornelius Wilson (Figure 9-8), appointed in 1891. By 1904 there were actually 19 "branches" of instruction at Jefferson. Henry C. Chapman, M.D. was Professor of the Institutes of Medicine and Medical Jurisprudence, a "branch" that later became physiology under Dr. Albert P. Brubaker but contributed some of its teaching to Medicine. Therapeutics was destined eventually to fuse into the Department of Medicine. James C. Wilson,

M.D., was the Professor of the Practice of Medicine and Clinical Medicine. Under his Chairmanship served the following members of the Department: Solomon Solis-Cohen, M.D., Professor of Clinical Medicine; Ward Brinton, M.D., Demonstrator of Physical Diagnosis; John C. DaCosta, Jr., M.D. (Figure 9-9), Demonstrator of Clinical Medicine; Frederick John Kalteyer, M.D., Demonstrator of Clinical Medicine; Aller G. Ellis, M.D., Instructor in Hematology; Henry G. Godfrey, M.D., Assistant Demonstrator of Clinical Medicine; Archibald H. Graham, M.D., Assistant Demonstrator of Clinical Medicine; and Authur Dare, M.D., Assistant Demonstrator of Physical Diagnosis.

The administration of such a department required a leader in medical sciences and one who could be captain of a "departmental ship" while he carried on a large medical practice. Dr. James C. Wilson provided this capability. Born in 1847, he was the son of Dr. Ellwood Wilson (Jefferson, 1845) who was a teacher, an assistant to Charles D. Meigs, and a member of the Jefferson Board of Trustees. Young Wilson graduated from Princeton *cum laude* and received his M.D. from Jefferson in 1869. He served as Resident Physician to the Wills Eye and Pennsylvania Hospitals before going abroad for a year to study in Dresden and Vienna. On his return he was made Chief of the Jefferson Hospital Medical Clinic and served as Physician to many of the other Philadelphia hospitals. His teaching at Jefferson included the course in Physical Diagnosis and lectures on renal and pulmonary disease. He served as Chief Clinical Assistant to Professor Jacob Mendes DaCosta, whom he succeeded in 1891. A true clinician, Wilson believed in the vigilant search for the cause of illness, attention to the comfort of the patient, the use of a minimum of drugs, and permission for nature to take its course. He contributed to medical journals and was the editor of *An American Textbook of Applied Therapies.*

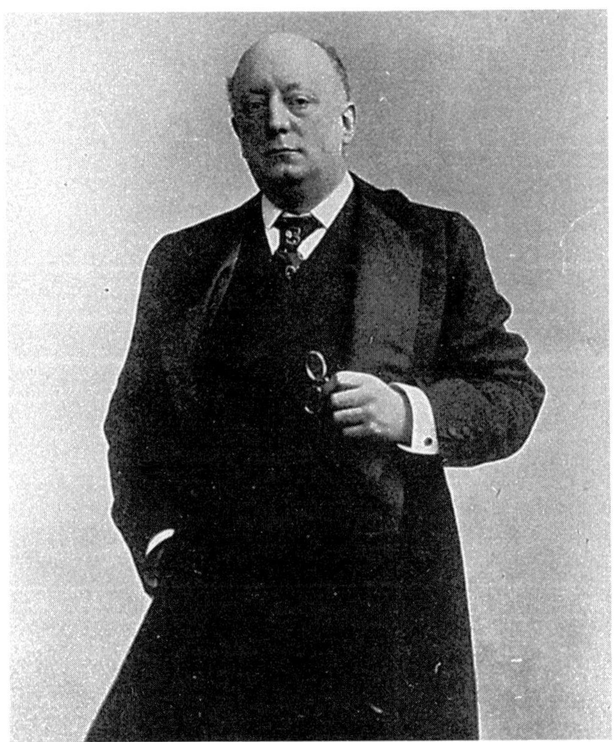

Fig. 9-8. James Cornelius Wilson, M.D. (1847–1938); Eighth Chairman (1891–1911).

It was in 1904 that the student body was delineated into two segments: the first, the Undergraduates, were candidates for the M.D. degree, and the second were special students or those graduates of medical colleges, approved by the faculty, who desired to receive instruction in one or more branches. The latter were granted a Certificate by the respective Professors whose Lectures or Clinics they attended after passing an examination in the subject. This was the origin of Specialty Certification, at the time subject to local approval, but which would be replaced over the years by the establishment of Medical Specialty Boards.

The members of the Jefferson Hospital Staff in the Department of Medicine included: James C. Wilson, M.D., Professor of Medicine and Clinical Medicine; Hobart A. Hare, M.D., Professor of Materia Medica and Therapeutics; Solomon Solis-Cohen, M.D., Professor of Clinical Medicine; John C. DaCosta, Jr., M.D., Assistant Physician; and Frederick John Kalteyer, M.D., Assistant Physician.

The Outpatient Staff included John C. DaCosta, Jr., M.D., and Frederick John Kalteyer, M.D., as Chief Clinical Assistants, and the following assistants: A. H. Graham, M.D., A. Dare, M.D., W. Brinton, M.D., H. G. Godfrey, M.D., and D. R. McCarroll, M.D.

Wilson had declared that he would resign the Chairmanship in 1911 but was not taken seriously.

When he actually resigned there had been no plans for his successor; therefore, the Board of Trustees appointed an interim committee to direct the Department until Wilson's successor could be found. This committee was made up of Drs. E. J. G. Beardsley (Jefferson, 1902), Frederick J. Kalteyer (Jefferson, 1888), Elmer H. Funk (Jefferson, 1908) and Ross V. Patterson (Jefferson, 1904).

Wilson asked his friend Dr. William Osler, at Oxford University, to recommend a suitable successor for the Chair. Osler recommended his nephew by marriage and member of his former staff at Hopkins, Dr. Thomas McCrae. Wilson had known Osler on closest terms during the latter's Philadelphia years (1884–1889) and those in Baltimore (1889–1905). Figure 9-10 shows Wilson with Osler, who was a guest of the J. C. Wilson student medical society at Jefferson in 1896. The society was founded in 1892 by admiring senior students who wished to augment their knowledge by hearing faculty or visiting professors that Wilson regularly obtained for the monthly meetings. Although Wilson retired in 1911, he faithfully attended all the meetings of the society for the next ten years.

Wilson's early retirement at age 64 was probably occasioned by an insidious decline in his health due to tuberculosis, gout, and increasing hearing loss. During the late 1890s he had spent nine months in southern France in an attempt to improve his vigor. Despite the threat of chronic illness he continued to practice for many years following his academic retirement and continued as Physician-in-Chief at the German (Lankenau) Hospital. Poetry, Shakespeare, and chess were his intellectual stimulants during this time. Wilson died on October 28, 1938, at the age of 91. He left a legacy, nationally as well as locally, of learned scholarship, able teaching and fine medical practice.

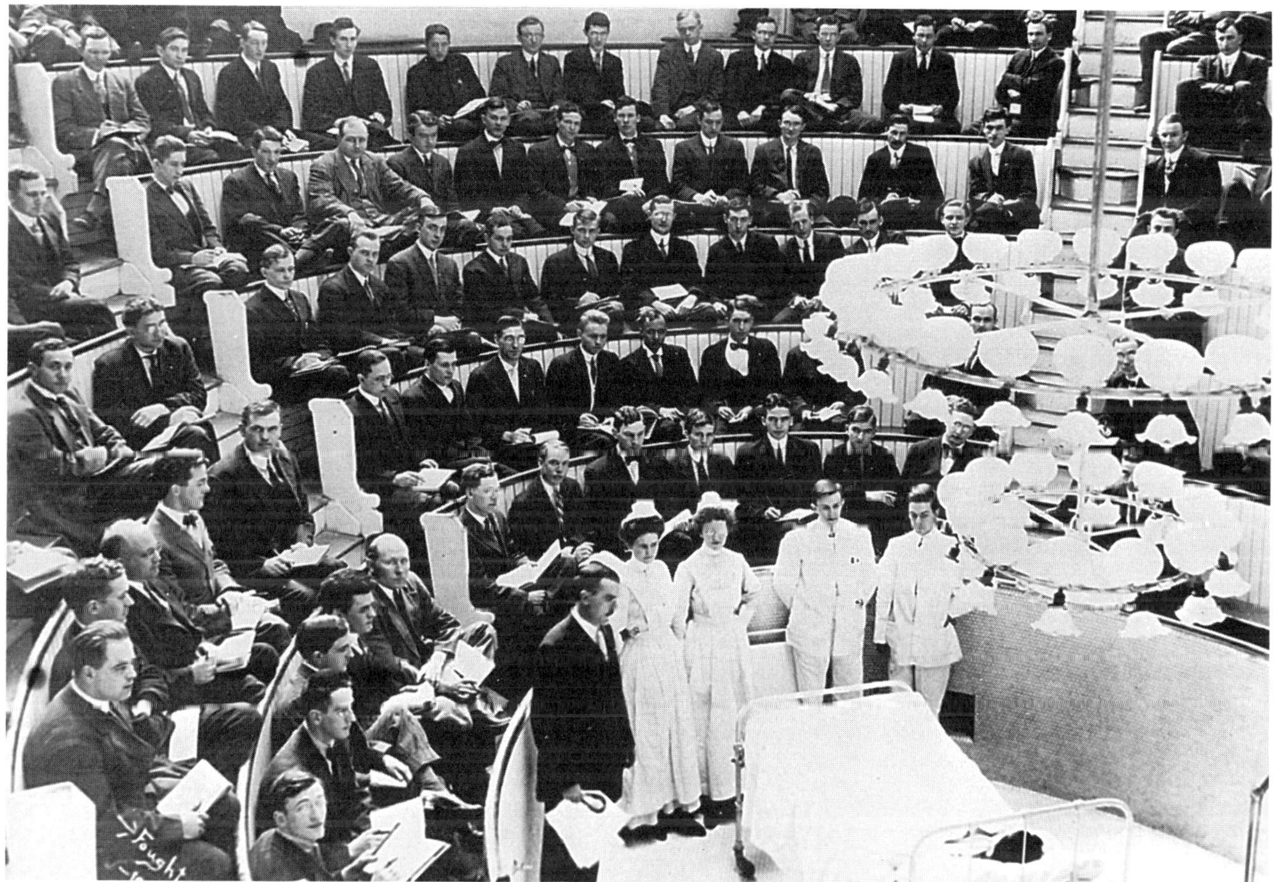

FIG. 9-9. Teaching of Clinical Diagnosis; John C. DaCosta, Jr., M.D. (1910)

▪ Magee Professorship of Medicine and Magee Memorial Hospital for Convalescents

Wilson believed that the progress of medicine had neglected "the patient who got over his sickness, but could not get well," and he delivered a paper on this subject at the College of Physicians of Philadelphia in 1924.[21] These long-held interests undoubtedly influenced a loyal and wealthy patient of Dr. Wilson, Miss Anna J. Magee, to endow in her will of 1916 the Magee Professorship of Medicine as well as the Magee Memorial Hospital for Convalescents. The Professorship was designated to be attached to the Chair of Medicine of which Dr. Thomas McCrae became the first incumbent in 1917. All future Chairmen of Medicine would carry the title of Magee Professor.

The endowment for the Magee Hospital at 6 Franklin Plaza stipulated the constitution of a Board of Trustees of 11 members to which Dr. Wilson would belong and become the first Physician to the Hospital. The exact terms stated: "In case of death, resignation or incapacity to act, the person who shall at the time be Professor of the Practice of Medicine and Clinical Medicine, in the Jefferson Medical College, shall become his successor as Physician and as a member of the Board of Trustees."

The Jefferson art collection includes the portrait of Miss Anna J. Magee.

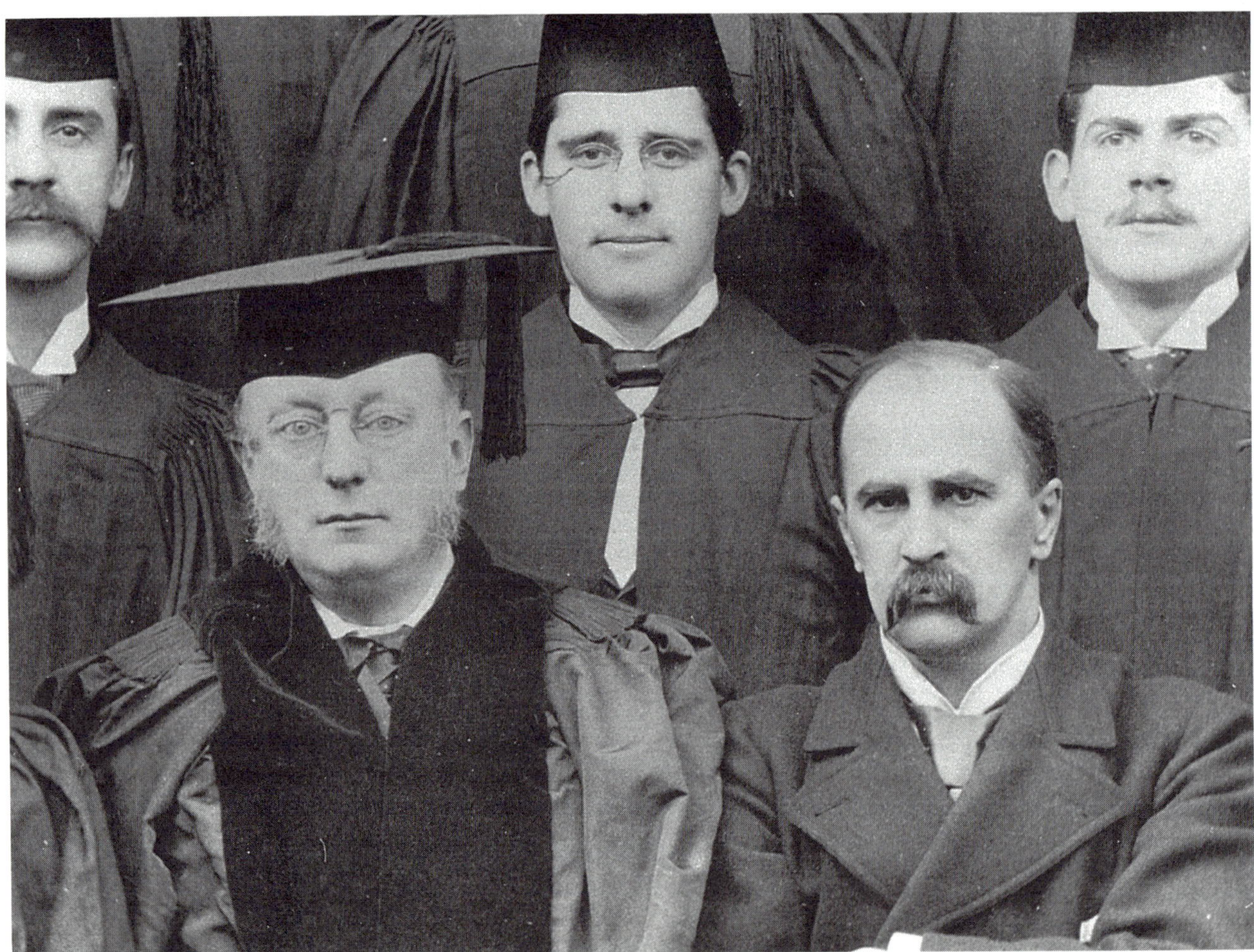

FIG. 9-10. William Osler, M.D. (first Professor of Medicine at Johns Hopkins School of Medicine) as guest of the J. C. Wilson student medical society in 1896.

■ The James Cornelius Wilson Professorship of Medicine

Wilson's beneficient influence on Jefferson continued beyond his death with the establishment of the James C. Wilson Professorship of Medicine in 1973. This evolved through the efforts of Drs. Creighton H. Turner[22] and Robert I. Wise.

Dr. Turner (Jefferson, 1909), a protegé of Dr. Wilson and prominent in teaching of physical diagnosis at Jefferson as Associate Professor of Medicine, was the family physician for Wilson's daughters, Beatrice and Helen. He conveyed to Dr. Wise, the Magee Professor of Medicine, his awareness of the love of Wilson's daughters for their father and the expression of their father's interest in the welfare of Jefferson before his death. Dr. Turner introduced the daughters to Dr. Wise, who continued their medical care and further cultivated their interest in Jefferson.[22] Beatrice Wilson bequeathed $1.5 million in her will for establishment of the James C. Wilson Professorship of Medicine to be filled by the Director of the Division of Cardiology in the Department of Medicine for research, teaching, and patient care.[23] The first appointee was Dr. Albert N. Brest in the fall of 1973.

Thomas McCrae, M.D. (1870–1935); Ninth Chairman (1912–1935) and First Magee Professor (1917–1935)

In 1912 Dr. McCrae (Figure 9-11) was appointed Professor of Theory and Practice of Medicine, a title that in 1917 would change to Magee Professor of Medicine and Clinical Medicine. He was born in 1870 of Scottish parents, Colonel David McCrae and Janet Eckford McCrae, in Guelph, Ontario, Canada. Most of his classical and medical education was obtained at the University of Toronto, where he received the Bachelor of Medicine in 1895, after which he went to Johns Hopkins as an Intern. This education was supplemented by studies in Göttingen, Germany. He started as Resident Medical Officer on the service of Dr. William Osler in 1901. (His brother John, the pathologist and physician, and the poet famous for "In Flanders Fields," who died in France in 1918, also had some of his training with Osler.) Dr. McCrae received the M.D. degree from the University of Toronto in 1903, and in 1906 was appointed Associate Professor of Medicine at Hopkins with the addition of Therapeutics in his teaching curriculum. His first scientific articles were written in this early period at Hopkins: a monograph in conjunction with Dr. Osler on *Cancer of the Stomach*[24] and later a report of five cases of lymphatic leukemia.[25] Osler had published the *Principles and Practice of Medicine* in 1892 and later enlisted McCrae's help and relied on him for further editorial assistance as well as contributing articles. This continued, after Osler's death in 1919, to the twelfth and final edition in 1935. When Osler was called upon to edit another medical book, *Modern Medicine,* a seven-volume work, he indicated that McCrae would "do all the

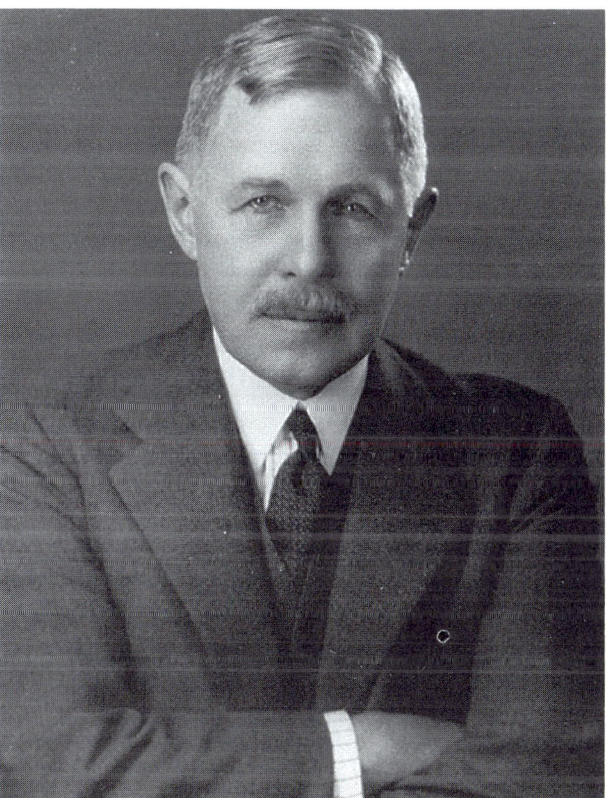

FIG. 9-11. Thomas McCrae, M.D. (1870–1935); Ninth Chairman, Department of Medicine (1912–1935), First Magee Professor (1917–1935).

dirty work."[26] McCrae contributed many articles to *Modern Medicine* and did most of the compilation of all three editions. In 1908 he married Amy Gwyn, a niece of Dr. Willian Osler.

Dr. McCrae was a dignified and polite individual who behaved in a kindly manner to his peers.[27] He disliked administrative duties and meetings, preferring to spend his time teaching. A somewhat methodical lecturer, he was at his best with small groups of students in the clinics and wards of the Jefferson and the Pennsylvania Hospitals. He stressed the importance of a complete history and physical examination with emphasis on the symptoms and signs that would lead to a diagnosis—X-rays and laboratory studies were adjuncts that would only confirm a diagnosis already made. He stressed the cases that a student would more commonly see, such as rheumatism, heart disease, syphilis, and pneumonia (Figure 9-12). The drugs McCrae usually prescribed were barbiturates, cascara, mercury, aspirin, and digitalis. He showed a personal interest in patients and had an active consulting practice, both locally and in Canada, but limited the number of patients so that his practice did not "run" him. In earlier times, he had played football for four years at Toronto; later he enjoyed vacations in Canada and the British Isles, especially visits to the Oslers at Oxford and to his beloved Scotland. Sometimes described as shy or timid, McCrae enjoyed many friends. The few persons with whom he was intimate enjoyed his wit and humor.[28]

McCrae's interest in the history of medicine led to many articles in the *Johns Hopkins Bulletin* from 1900 to 1906. He later wrote *The Early History of*

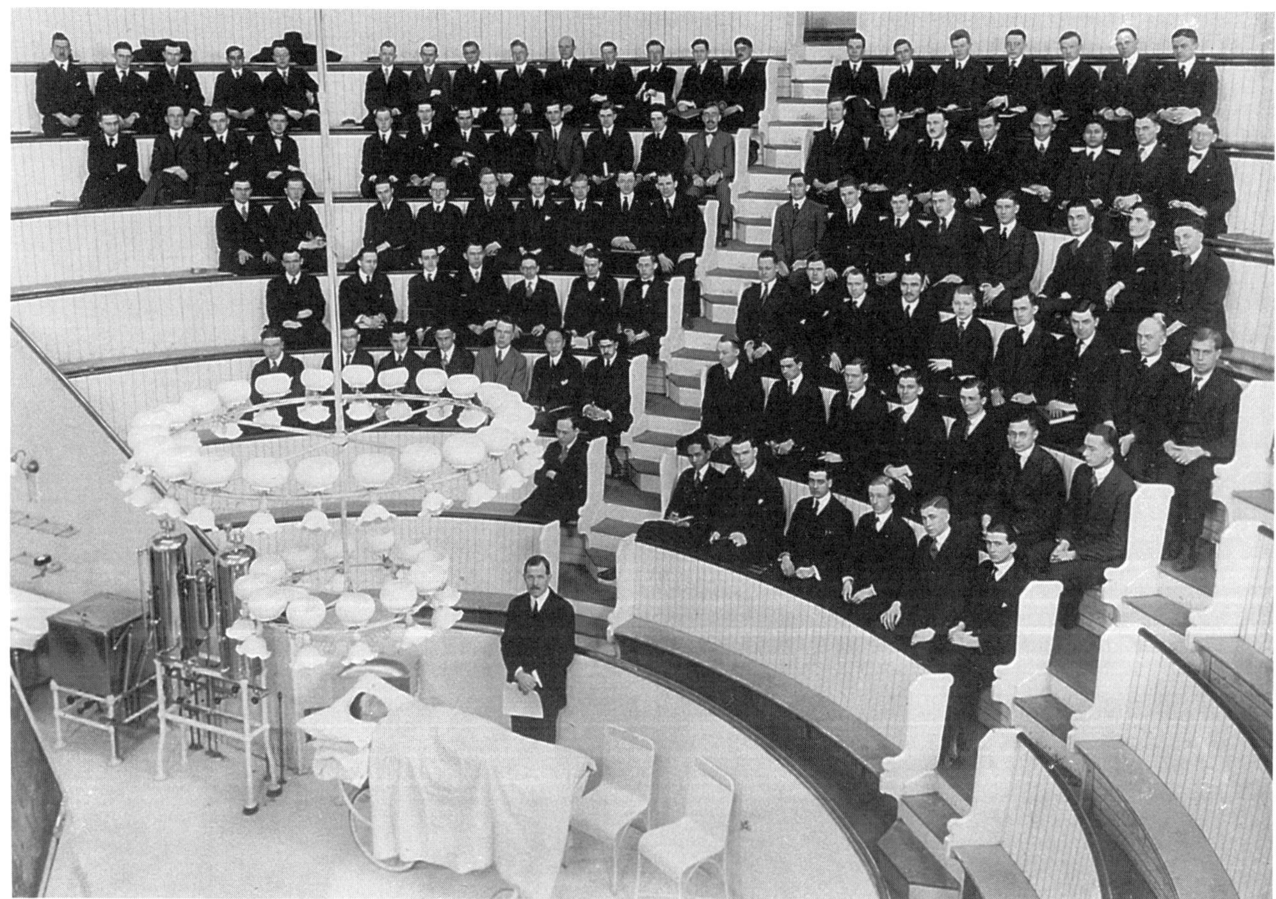

FIG. 9-12. Clinic of Professor Thomas McCrae (1918).

the Association of American Physicians following his Presidency of that organization in 1930.[29]

The interim committee of Kalteyer, Beardsley, Patterson, and Funk, together with Emeritus Professor Wilson, Professor Hobart A. Hare, Professor John C. DaCosta, Jr., Professor Solomon Solis-Cohen (Figure 9-13), and eight others made up the entire faculty of the Department of Medicine when McCrae assumed the Chairmanship. This did not take into account those with Jefferson Hospital appointments as Resident Physicians and those assigned to the Outpatient Medical Clinics.[30] His ensuing Chairmanship of 24 years was to set a record of longevity for any Department of Medicine Chairman and was accompanied by the growth of faculty to 37 members in 1935, in a pattern that saw the continued evolution of the specialities in Medicine.

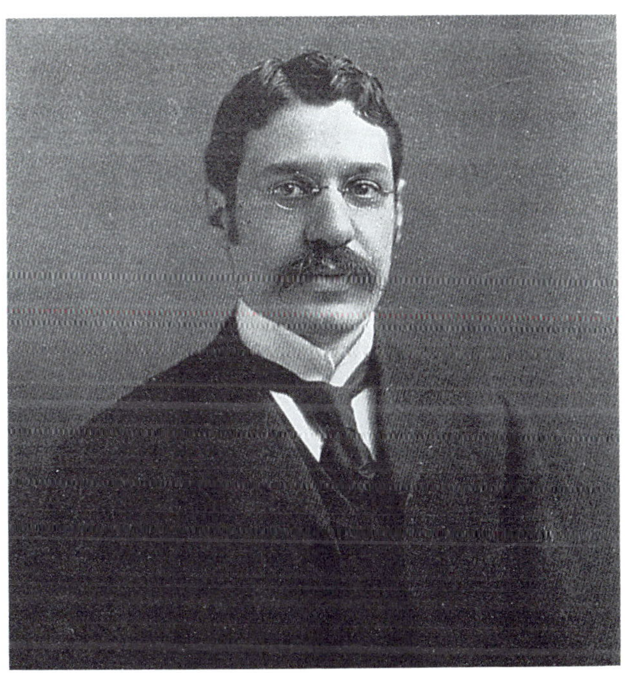

FIG. 9-13. Solomon Solis-Cohen, M.D. (1857–1948); Professor of Clinical Medicine (1904–1927).

Hobart Amory Hare, M.D. (1862–1931); Professor of Therapeutics (1891–1931)

Professor Hobart A. Hare (Figure 9-14), a graduate of the University of Pennsylvania in 1884, resigned his Chairmanship of Diseases of Children at the University of Pennsylvania to accept a Professorship of Therapeutics and Materia Medica at Jefferson in 1891.[31] This distinguished teacher and clinician, called "decisive and dogmatic" by McCrae, might be described as the Dean of the clinical teaching of the nucleus of physicians who taught Medicine at Jefferson Hospital. His textbook, *System of Practical Therapeutics*,[32] was destined to go through 21 editions, some in foreign languages that included Chinese. In 1913 Hare held the title of Professor of Therapeutics, Materia Medica and Diagnosis; in 1916 he was named the first Sutherland M. Prevost Professor of Therapeutics, Materia Medica and

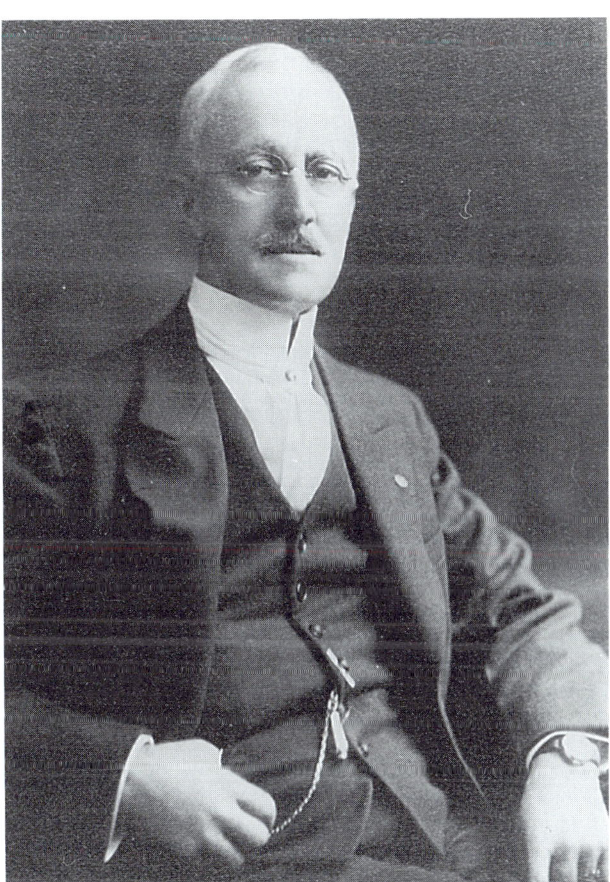

FIG. 9-14. Hobart A. Hare, M.D. (1862–1931); Professor of Therapeutics (1891–1931).

Diagnosis. Thus, even from the times of Revere and Dunglison, Therapeutics had strong ties with, or was vested in, the Department of Medicine. This Professorship was established in 1916 by the Board of Trustees from the contribution to endowment funds made by Mrs. Sutherland M. Prevost in memory of her husband who had been a Trustee of Jefferson Medical College from 1891 to 1905. The staff members who worked with Dr. Hare included Drs. Ross V. Patterson, E. Quinn Thornton, L. F. Appleman (Figure 9-15), and Reynold Griffith (Figure 9-16). Dr. Hare held this Professorship until his death from carcinoma of the prostate in 1931. He was succeeded by Dr. Elmer H. Funk, who died after one year. Then Dr. E. Quinn Thornton (Figure 9-17) held the Professorship for a year until he was succeeded by Dr. Ross V. Patterson in 1934. Professors Kalteyer and Beardsley, active clinicians at Jefferson, continued to teach into the latter portion of the 1930s, applying particular emphasis to the signs and symptoms of disease.

Dr. Elmer H. Funk (Jefferson, 1908), the bright and energetic clinician, served for a short time as Medical Director of the Hospital before Dr. McCrae asked him to be the Director (1913) of the Tuberculosis Department located in the newly purchased buildings at Third and Pine Streets, a Department that was destined to become the Division of Chest Diseases. Dr. Funk was promoted to Assistant Professor of Medicine and Therapeutics in 1926 and was succeeded by Dr. Burgess Lee Gordon (1927) as Medical Director. This relieved Dr. Funk, whom Dr. McCrae increasingly had called upon to perform various duties such as assisting with the editing of the third edition of Osler's *Modern Medicine*.[33] Dr. Gordon (Jefferson, 1919), who had extensive postgraduate training in Internal Medicine in Boston, was an interesting teacher and a strong administrator. He developed numerous inventions, among which were a pneumothorax machine, which displayed pressure readings, and the Gordon stethoscope.

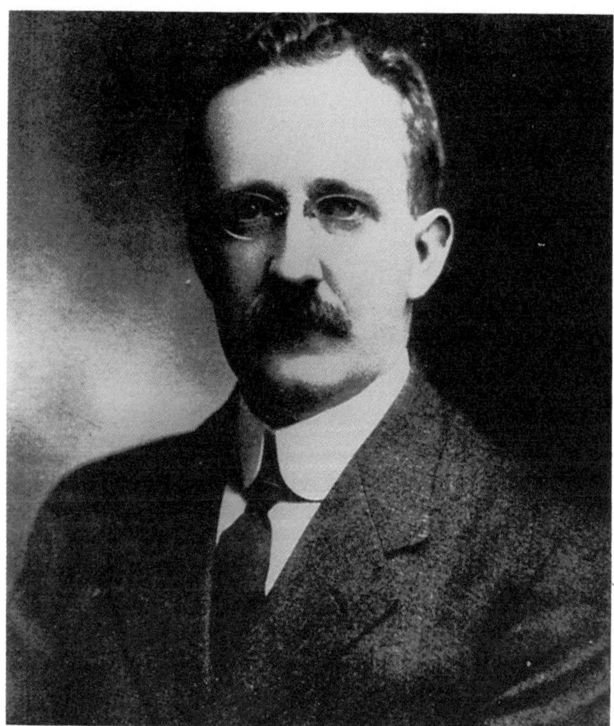

Fig. 9-15. Leighton F. Appleman, M.D., taught Pharmacy, Materia Medica, and Therapeutics (1904–1932).

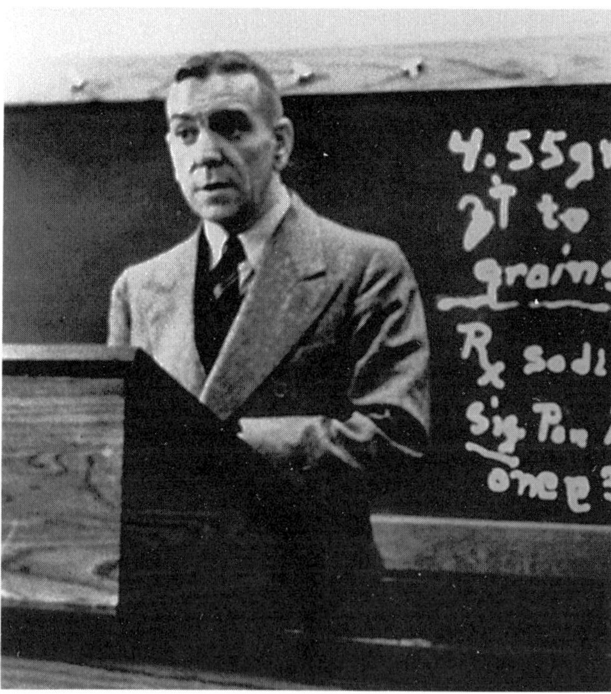

Fig. 9-16. Reynold S. Griffith, M.D., lecturing in Therapeutics (1938).

death in 1938 and succeeded Dr. E.Q. Thornton as Sutherland M. Prevost Professor of Therapeutics in 1934. This strong administrator and extemporaneous lecturer in Therapeutics left the bulk of his estate to Jefferson Medical College, one of the benefits of which was the establishment of the Ross V. Patterson Fellowships.

Ross V. Patterson, M.D. (1877–1938); Electrocardiography

Dr. Ross V. Patterson (Jefferson, 1904), who was a member of the departmental governing committee bridging the interval between the Chairmanships of Wilson and McCrae, strongly recommended the acquisition of an electrocardiogram machine. McCrae liked this idea, and when Patterson obtained the machine McCrae had him appointed to head the Subdepartment of Electrocardiography of the Medical Department of the Hospital (1918). Dr. Patterson served as Dean of Jefferson Medical College from 1916 until his

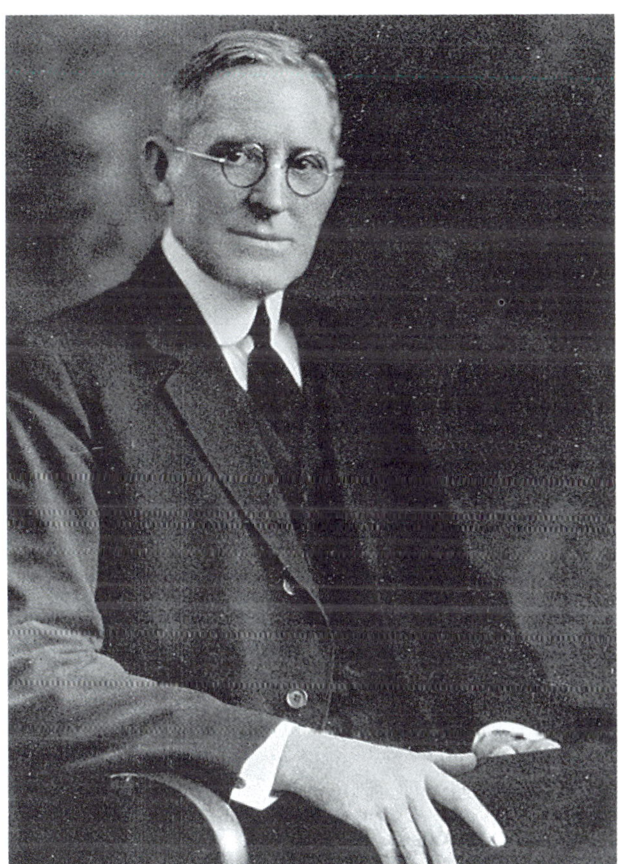

FIG. 9-17. E. Quinn Thornton, M.D. (1866–1945); Professor of Materia Medica and Therapeutics (1932).

Gastroenterology

Gastroenterology flourished in McCrae's time particularly due to the efforts of Dr. B. B. Vincent Lyon and Dr. Martin E. Rehfuss. Dr. Lyon (Johns Hopkins, 1907) studied in Europe, joined the Jefferson Faculty in 1912, and established the first Gastrointestinal Clinic at Jefferson. He was a worldwide authority on gallbladder function and disease. Dr. Rehfuss (University of Pennsylvania, 1910) spent two postgraduate years in Europe, where he developed the Rehfuss gastric tube. He joined the faculty at Jefferson in 1914 and continued his research on gastric digestion. Drs. John T. Eads (Jefferson, 1926) and Guy M. Nelson (Jefferson, 1928), two of his protégés, were fine clinical gastroenterologists. Dr. Rehfuss was appointed the Sutherland M. Prevost Lecturer in Therapeutics in 1941. His work was characterized by "old world" graciousness and charisma.

Clinical Laboratory Teaching

In 1913 the Board of Trustees established the Jacob M. DaCosta Laboratory of Clinical Medicine. It was outfitted on the second floor of the Laboratory Building with stone tables, lockers, and microscopes, by funds supplied partially by the Alumni of Jefferson Medical College. Originally, Dr. McCrae and senior students performed studies of blood, gastric contents, and urine from the patients assigned to them in the hospital. By 1921 it included instruction to the junior students, and the laboratory facilities were available to members of the faculty. Separate instruction in Hematology became a part of the curriculum in the late nineteenth century. Dr. Arthur Dare (Jefferson, 1890) invented the Dare hemoglobinometer, and Dr. John C. DaCosta, Jr. (Jefferson, 1893) published an extensive textbook, *Clinical Hematology*,[34] in 1901, with a second edition in 1905. Dr. DaCosta rose to the rank of Professor before he left Jefferson in 1915. Hematology, which had been taught through lectures by Dr. Allan E. Ellis in the Department of Bacteriology (1907) and later by Dr. Erwin D. Funk, who had dual appointments in Pathology and in Medicine, became established with the Laboratory of Clinical Medicine. By 1922 the teaching of Clinical Laboratory was under the direction of Drs. Harold W. Jones (Jefferson, 1917) and Christian W. Nissler.

Doctor Jones was a brilliant physician who had an excellent manner with patients. The more than 60 scientific articles he had published covered general medicine and laboratory studies, particularly hematology. He was one of the pioneers of blood transfusion, first direct and later by the indirect method. Jones continued to direct the Laboratory of Clinical Medicine until 1938. The following year a hematology foundation was funded by the will of Mrs. Charlotte Drake Martinez Cardeza, a patient of Dr. Jones. Mrs. Cardeza's son established the Cardeza Professorship of Clinical Medicine and Hematology, and Dr. Jones was named the first recipient of the Chair in 1941.

In 1929 the Laboratory of Clinical Medicine moved to new quarters in the New College building (1025 Walnut Street) to share the third floor with the Department of Biochemistry. Later on it moved to the sixth floor to share space with Microbiology. With the opening of Jefferson Alumni Hall, Clinical Medicine forfeited all claim to an independent teaching space and shared areas of the Basic Sciences. Dr. Leandro M. Tocantins joined Professors Cantarow and Jones in teaching in the Laboratory of Clinical Medicine. Dr. Jones stopped this teaching assignment in 1938, and several years later Dr. Karl Paschkis joined Drs. Cantarow and Tocantins.

Tradition of Clinical Instruction

The outline of studies in the Department of Medicine was characterized by courses in history taking, physical diagnosis, and symptomatology, starting in the Sophomore year with continuing emphasis on these basic disciplines throughout the next two years. The Sophomores also began having supervised teaching contact with patients. Clinical Clerkships, at first limited to the Senior year, along with lectures, became the principal method of teaching Medicine in the Junior and Senior years. This was carried out by the Jefferson group under the title "Practice of Medicine and Clinical Medicine," headed by Dr. McCrae, and the Philadelphia Hospital group titled "Clinical Medicine," under the direction of Dr. Solomon Solis-Cohen, Professor of Clinical Medicine. The latter group included Drs. Samuel A. Lowenberg, David W. Kramer, Harold L. Goldburgh, and R. Max Goepp, among others.

Dr. Solomon Solis-Cohen (Jefferson, 1883) was an excellent diagnostician, physician, and therapist, highly skilled in the use of a variety of medications. He was President of the Philadelphia County Medical Society and was prominent as a member of the Board of Education of Philadelphia.[31] Following the retirement of Dr. Solis-Cohen in 1927, the listing of the group "Clinical Medicine" was discontinued.

Academic Achievements

Dr. McCrae studied the effects of foreign bodies in the bronchi in conjunction with bronchoscopist Dr. Chevalier Jackson and later with Dr. Louis Clerf. These studies were the topic of the Lumleian Lecture, which McCrae presented before the Royal College of Physicians (of which he was a member) in London in 1924.[35] This was followed in 1927 by an article, including Doctors Funk and Jackson, on primary carcinoma of the bronchus, which detailed the findings, warned of its increasing frequency, and stressed the value of bronchoscopic diagnosis.[36]

The close bonds between Osler and McCrae continued even after Osler went to Oxford in 1905. Osler's confidence in McCrae's tenacity of purpose was evident in a July 15, 1904, letter to C. F. Martin: ". . . I have been beguiled into editing a 7(!!!) volume System of Medicine (McCrae to do the dirty work) . . ."[26] and thus began a relationship cemented by their mutual work on Osler's textbooks, which continued even after Osler's death in 1919. The last work directly inspired by Osler was a review of 80 cases of syphilis of the liver with tumor.[37] Dr. McCrae's admiration for the teaching methods of Osler,[38] the evidence of his care for the patient as an individual, and the insistence upon a careful history and physical examination, are well documented in his preface to the twelfth edition of the *Principles and Practice of Medicine* by Osler and McCrae (1935):

> "In these days it is often said that the number of thoroughly trained clinicians is growing less and that internal medicine is being split up more and more into separate compartments with walls of various thickness between them. This tends to emphasize the study of one system without sufficient attention to the patient as an individual made up of many systems. Certainly we should keep before ourselves and our students the need of emphasis on the study of the patient as a whole and as a human being, and all the manifestations of disease as shown in him. Too often the idea is held that a clinician can be made overnight, especially with the aid of instruments and laboratory procedures. In saying this the value of the aid from these is not made light of but time and effort and hard work must go to the acquiring of a knowledge of disease and the patient in whom it exists. We can not be Oslers but we can do our best to follow his steps. The physician and student should always make it a rule to learn everything possible about a patient by the use of his own senses and brains. For example, to have a roentgenologist make the diagnosis of fluid in a pleural cavity should cause a clinician to be thoroughly ashamed of himself. As far as possible a textbook of medicine should emphasize the clinical side of disease problems."

McCrae also acknowledged the assistance of his associates with this book including Drs. Rehfuss, Mohler, Jones, Gordon, Kramer, Duncan and Cantarow. This same year he wrote the preface for the book *Diabetes Mellitus and Obesity*[39] by his Associate in Medicine Dr. Garfield G. Duncan, who emphasized the teaching of metabolic diseases in the wards of the Pennsylvania Hospital. Dr. McCrae experienced increasing limitation in ambulation during the early 1930s. For two years before his death his mobility was limited to use of a wheelchair, but he continued his activities at Jefferson until the spring of 1935. His death on June 30, 1935, followed complications of a laminectomy at the Hospital of the University of Pennsylvania. The actual cause of his illness remained unclear even though his brother-in-law, Dr. Norman Gwyn, made efforts to summarize the medical findings.[40]

McCrae, this great physician, teacher, and author, was known for his dignity, wisdom, humor, and humility, and was always dedicated to his profession. His ability to impart to his students his own dedication to a knowledge of medicine and care for the patient created in them respect and admiration which lasted a lifetime.

Hobart A. Reimann, M.D., Sc.D. (1897–1986); Tenth Chairman (1936–1951)

The death of Dr. Thomas McCrae, the Magee Professor of Medicine and Chairman of the Department, in the summer of 1935, was a tragic loss to the faculty—the feeling among students, faculty, and administration was that no one could replace McCrae. His personal clinical approach to the patient and his graciousness as a physician and teacher had left its mark for the great number of alumni whom he had instructed. Thus, the appointment of his successor was awaited with anxiety. Within a year the administration brought Dr. Hobart Ansteth Reimann (Figure 9-18), Professor of Medicine and Chief of the Hospital Medical Service, University of Minnesota, to be the Magee Professor and Chairman of the Department of Medicine. This tall, slender, 38-year-old, oval-headed, acquiline-nosed individual with a wisp of a moustache strode through the halls in a military bearing with long and purposeful steps. His manner of speaking was rapid, articulate, and precise, with a sense of humor always ready in the background.

McCrae had used the gradually evolving laboratory facilities to aid in the confirmation of his carefully and patiently constructed clinical diagnosis. Reimann was to rely heavily on laboratory findings and to lay the groundwork for new fields of laboratory endeavors to confirm the precisely made diagnosis. He was to speed the evolution of the science of medicine by talks and publications at Jefferson and throughout the medical world. By this combination of the clinical and the investigative Reimann was destined to recognize and describe new entities of disease.

Hobart Reimann was born in Buffalo, New York, October 31, 1897, the son of Ottilla Ansteth and George Reimann.[41] His father was a pharmacist, and German was the language spoken in the home. Before age ten Reimann had traveled with his family to Florida, California, the western National Parks, and Cuba, a prophetic indicator of his future worldwide travels principally in his role as a Professor and Educator in the field of Medicine. He ranked fourth in a class of 160 and was President of his class in the local high school. He completed a year of pharmacy studies at the University of Buffalo, then matriculated for a year in premedical studies at Townsend Hall, obtaining his M.D. training at the University of Buffalo Medical School (1917–1921). While in medical school he occupied his summers with laboratory work, such as preparing slides for medical school teaching or aiding in the establishment of a research laboratory. At that time, as throughout later life, Reimann managed to have vacations for himself and for his family, frequently including medical writing in the vacation time. Scientific articles were to number over 300 during his lifetime. His first published paper, written while he was in medical school, reported on the study of the relative efficacy of benzidine and guaiac as a test for fecal blood. This study was accomplished by using his own blood with himself as a test subject. Medical school was followed by a year of internship and a year as Chief House Physician at the Buffalo General Hospital. During the latter year he completed a restructuring of the hospital's Clinical Laboratory. Dr. Rufus Cole invited him to be an Assistant Physician at the Rockefeller Institute, which was then under the direction of Dr. Simon Flexner. While there Reimann worked on the transformation of the pneumococcus from a rough strain to smooth and back again. The work was performed under the direction of Dr. Oswald T. Avery, who laid the groundwork for the elucidation of DNA and RNA. After three years at the Institute, Reimann accepted a previously postponed offer to study for a year at the Anton Ghon Institute in Prague. While there he worked with the tubercle bacillus and with Rocky Mountain spotted fever. He then spent two years as Associate Professor of Medicine at the Peking Union Medical College under the auspices of the Rockefeller Foundation. Ample laboratory facilities permitted him to continue to work on the pneumococcus and to study typhus, and he added Chinese to his linguistic capabilities. He joined the Medical Department of the University of Minnesota in 1930 and rose to the rank of Professor of Medicine and Chief of the Medical Department of the University Hospital.

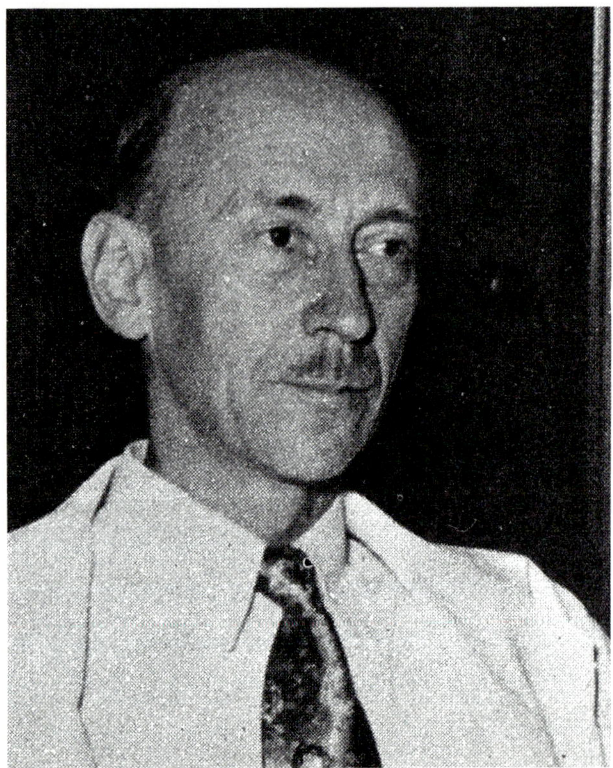

FIG. 9-18. Hobart A. Reimann, M.D., Sc.D. (1897–1986); Tenth Chairman (1936–1951).

■ Changes in Teaching Philosophy

At Minnesota Reimann started work as author and editor of a three-volume book entitled *Treatment in General Medicine*,[42] which eventually went through three editions. A longer survival is not surprising because, to Reimann, treatment was "cut and dried" and was unimportant if it was not curative. The interest in microorganisms continued and included the study of *M. tetragenous,* its infectious and variant forms,[43] and typing of the pneumococcus. Additional studies included blood proteins and amyloid disease leading to the description of primary amyloidosis.[44]

Reimann demanded exactness from his students in their pursuit of the patient's history, physical findings, and laboratory studies. The latter led to the establishment of a students' laboratory in Jefferson Hospital, and in each of the affiliated teaching hospitals, where the clinical clerk performed the basic laboratory studies on each of his assigned patients, thus carrying forward a precedent established by McCrae. In a medical environment where empirical treatment and measures of dubious value were still common, Reimann insisted upon an etiological diagnosis whenever possible. Ward rounds required that the Intern or Resident present every detail of the case history, even down to the differential leukocyte count, while the Professor held the patient's chart. A logical diagnosis and consideration for therapy was expected in the summary. His familiarity with the pneumococcus fostered the routine typing of the organism in cases of pneumonia at Jefferson, and if specific anti-serum was available, its administration was advised. The treatment had variable therapeutic efficacy and sometimes undesirable side-effects. The advent of sulfonamides in 1936 and the beginning availability of penicillin in 1941 eliminated the use of serum treatment. His interest in pneumonia continued[45] and it led him to the observation of an illness with an acute infection of the respiratory tract, or atypical pneumonia, which he felt was caused by a virus.[46] Thus the first description of virus pneumonia was published in 1938 in the *Journal of the American Medical Association* and republished in the Centennial series of the same Journal in 1985 as one of 51 *Landmark Articles in Medicine*.[47]

■ Medical Residency

The era of the late 1930s was a time of the beginning of formal residencies throughout the country. Dr. W. Paul Havens, Jr., was the first medical resident at Jefferson. A graduate of Harvard Medical College, he was destined to become an expert in the field of hepatitis. He studied and reported on the occurrence of the organism of Rocky Mountain spotted fever in ticks in the local areas and collaborated with Dr. Reimann on some of his articles published in the literature at that time and received an honorary degree from Jefferson in 1985. The second resident, Dr. Allison H. Price (Jefferson, 1938), became Dr. Reimann's direct assistant. He carried out the day-by-day management of the Department and made possible the details that entered into the accomplishment of many of Dr. Reimann's research projects.

The original Medical Department office, a room for the Chairman and a small adjoining room for the secretary, was located off the Sansom Street side of the main corridor of the first floor of the Old Hospital Building at Tenth and Sansom Streets. Dean Patterson's promise of laboratory space equal to that which he had at Minnesota finally occurred when the office was moved to the northwest corner of the eighth floor of the College Building (1025 Walnut Street). This location also provided offices and laboratories for Dr. Price and the third resident, Dr. John H. Hodges (Jefferson, 1939). (See Figure 9-19.) During the first two years of his medical residency (1942–1946), Dr. Hodges proctored in the course in Clinical Laboratory Medicine, now taught in the Sophomore year, which at that time was ably directed by Drs. Leandro Tocantins, Abraham Cantarow, and Karl Paschkis. In 1944, Dr. Hodges was given the Directorship of the course by Dr. Reimann and continued in that role for the ensuing 28 years while he performed and collaborated in research work. After 1946 he carried on an active clinical practice.

An attack of acute gastroenteritis suffered by Dr. Reimann and his family coincided with the observation on Men's Medical Ward by Dr. Hodges of eight cases of severe and acute nausea, vomiting, and diarrhea with negative studies for a bacterial or parasitic involvement. Subsequent clinical and laboratory research by Drs. Reimann, Price, and Hodges led to the establishment of viral dysentery as an entity.[48,49]

Visiting physicians were in regular attendance at Reimann's weekly "pit" sessions with the Junior and Senior students in the amphitheater of the Thompson Annex. He was always in full command at these sessions, with the students on the alert in case called upon by name from the ever-present roll book. A wide variety of cases was presented, from snake-bite and favism to infectious diseases, the latter being his particular interest, as evidenced by the fact that Reimann wrote 40 consecutive Annual Reviews of Infectious Diseases (1935–1975) published principally in the *Archives of Internal Medicine* and the *British Postgraduate Medical Journal*.[50] Research in microorganisms, perpetuated by his work at the Rockefeller Institute, in Prague, in Peking, at the University of Minnesota, and particularly with viruses at Jefferson, was coupled successfully with the study of their clinical disease counterparts. The United Nations Rehabilitation and Relief Administration called upon him in 1945 to join a cholera team in Chungking, China, and he spent a two-month leave of absence working with cholera patients in and around Chungking. His subsequent report called to the attention of the medical world the prime importance of prompt fluid replacement in lowering the mortality rate.[51]

It was Reimann's nature to take positive stands on issues in medicine, and sometimes he pursued them with considerable vigor. He spoke out publicly against the overworked theory of "focal infection" and its role in systemic disease,[52] decried the excessive practice of the removal of teeth and tonsils as a panacea for the prevention and treatment of some illnesses, and expressed concern over the unnecessary or excessive use of antibiotics, both for prophylaxis and in therapy. This stimulated the establishment of hospital committees to monitor the use and choice of antimicrobials by physicians, with the improvement in the indications for and selection of specific drugs and also, eventually, in financial saving.

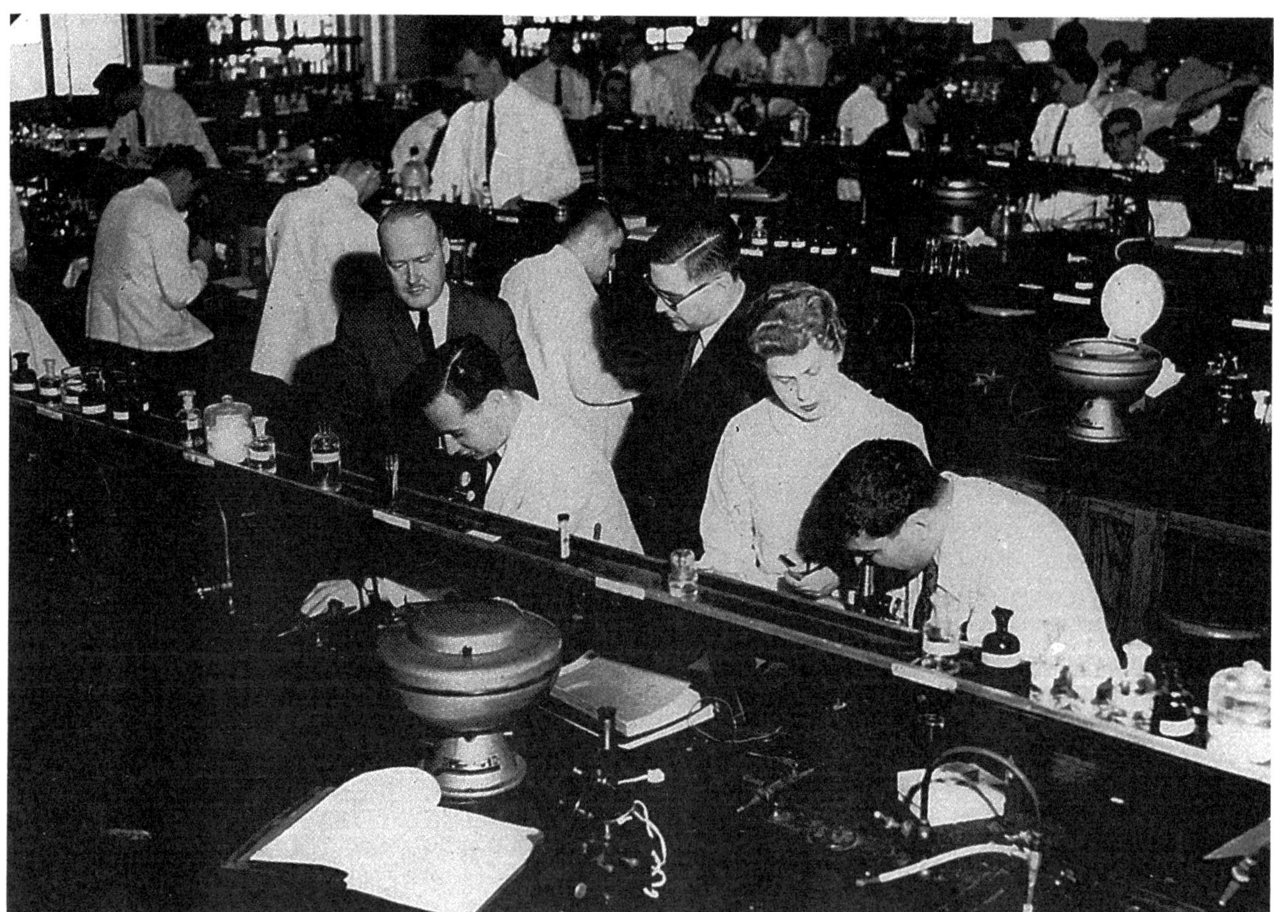

FIG. 9-19. John H. Hodges, M.D., Director of Clinical Laboratory Medicine, later the Ludwig A. Kind Professor of Medicine, with Arthur J. Weiss, M.D., and Jane E. Kirk, M.T.

Reimann's Further Career

Reimann's frustrations in the administration of his Department caused him to resign in late 1951. This started his nine-year worldwide odyssey that ended in his return to activity in Philadelphia with an appointment as Professor of Medicine at Hahnemann Medical College (University) in 1960. The initial and perhaps the most enjoyable assignment for Dr. Reimann in this era was the four years he spent in Lebanon as Visiting Professor of Medicine at the American University of Beirut. The beautiful campus and the exotic city of Beirut were at that time (1952–1956) a pleasure to experience. Subsequent assignments included the University of Indonesia, Djakarta, and the University of Shiraz, Iran. At Hahnemann he added the duties of Associate Medical Director and continued to publish and to travel. He served as Field Director (A.M.A.), Project in Medical Education, Saigon, Vietnam, and as Guest Consultant, CARE-MEDICO, Avicenna Hospital, Kabul, Afghanistan. He also served as Guest Consultant, CARE-MEDICO in Honduras, and Visiting Lecturer at military hospitals in Colombia.

The following statement occurs in the first paragraph of Reimann's paper, *The Problem of Long-Continued, Low-Grade Fever,*[53] published in 1936: "The problem of diagnosis in patients with long-continued low-grade fever occurs far more commonly than one would be led to believe by the few studies that have been reported dealing exclusively with the subject." This study at the University of Minnesota concerning 16 women without significant organic disease who had an apparent temperature range above the medically accepted normal variation, started a pursuit throughout the ensuing years of conditions with fever occurring periodically, fever accompanying periodic agranulocytosis, conditions of periodic swelling of a joint, and other with a temporal rhythmicity. Numerous reported papers resulted and culminated in the publishing (1963) of the book *Periodic Diseases.*[54] He was the author and editor of *Acute Respiratory Tract Diseases* and the editor of *Acute Respiratory Tract Infections. Infections and Parasitic Enteric Diseases* appeared in 1976. He was a contributor to *Oxford Medicine, Encyclopedia Britannica, Encyclopedia of Medicine,* Musser's and Cecil's *Textbook of Medicine,* Conn's *Current Therapy,* and *Current Diagnosis,* and others.

Reimann's first wife, Dorothy Sampson Eaton, studied as an artist and probably stimulated him to try his talents as a painter. Dorothy died in 1958. His second wife, Cecelia DeMise, who became his constant supporter and critic, fostered his artistic work in water color and pastel. There were one-person shows, and his work, particularly in pastels, received local and national acclaim in exhibits, on the cover of the *Journal of the American Medical Association,*[55] in permanent display in private homes, and in the halls of Hahnemann and Thomas Jefferson Universities.

Dr. Reimann contributed to the education of numerous students and physicians. His research in the field of medicine uncovered many "firsts" and contributed widely to the clinical practice of medicine. He, in turn, was honored as a member of Alpha Omega Alpha, Sigma Xi, the American Board of Internal Medicine (1934), and by membership in numerous prestigious local, national, and international medical societies. Awards received included the Charles V. Chapin Medal of the Rhode Island Medical Society; Citation for Distinguished Service in Medical Education, University of Buffalo; Order of Cedars, Lebanon; Shaffrey Award, Medical Alumni of St. Joseph's College (University); and Hahnemann Corporation Medals for Distinguished Service, and he was made an honorary member of the J. Aitken Meigs Medical Association (to which he presented a copy, in pastel, of Petit's painting of Dr. Meigs) Jefferson's students honored him when the Senior Class (1951) chose him as the subject of a portrait to be presented to the College; this portrait by Cameron Burnside is displayed outside the room dedicated to Dr. Reimann in the Kellow Conference Center. The Board of Trustees of Thomas Jefferson University conferred upon Reimann the Honorary Degree of Doctor of Science (1977), and perhaps one of the most appreciated of Jefferson's honors was the conferring of the title Visiting Professor of Medicine (1979). His affection for Jefferson had remained with him throughout the years, and on reception of the Professorship he stated that "it was like returning home." Reimann retired from Hahnemann in 1980 but retained his connection with Jefferson until his death from pneumonia on January 21, 1986.

■ Departmental Growth and Changes

The establishment of the Cardeza Professorship in 1941 gave strength and enduring growth to hematology in respect to teaching and research. The acquisition of a Fellow in Hematology, Dr. Welland A. Hause (Jefferson, 1938), and the appointments of Drs. Leandro M. Tocantins (1936), Franklin R. Miller (1944), and Lowell A. Erf (1945) to the staff strengthened this growing specialty under the direction of Dr. Harold Jones.

Additional changes in 1941 included the advancement of the teaching of Clinical Laboratory Medicine in the Sophomore year where it was under the direction of Professors Cantarow and Tocantins and Drs. Paschkis, Wirts, and Bucher. Doctor Tocantins had come to Jefferson in 1932 as a J. Ewing Mears Research Fellow and was becoming established as an important hematologist who in 1938 would publish a comprehensive document on platelets.[56] Dr. Karl Paschkis was an internist with a strong interest in endocrinology who had emigrated from Austria in 1938 and in 1940 was the J. Ewing Mears Teaching and Research Fellow in Physiology and Medicine. He was destined to become the Director of the Division of Endocrine and Cancer Research in the Department of Experimental Medicine, an interdepartmental complex confirmed by the Board of Trustees in 1949. This Department also had Dr. Abraham Cantarow, the Chairman of Biochemistry, and Dr. Abraham Rakoff, Department of Obstetrics and Gynecology, as prominent members. The Department was responsible for research contributions in the areas of the relationship of endocrines to carcinogenesis and in the realm of basic steroid chemistry. This Department was discontinued in 1958. Dr. Paschkis was the Director of the Division of Endocrinology in the Department of Medicine from 1942 until his death on January 27, 1961. Dr. Joseph J. Rupp succeeded him as Director of the Division and served until he assumed a position in the Dean's office in 1969.

Dr. Carl Bucher (University of Pennsylvania, 1916), a member of the Department of Pathology of the Hospital, stressed laboratory studies, such as the Wassermann and Kahn tests, and was destined to become Hospital Chief of Pathology. Dr. Charles Wirts was working in Gastroenterology under Lyon and Rehfuss. He, like Lyon and Rehfuss, had some of his postgraduate education in Europe and was the last of the twentieth-century gastroenterologists at Jefferson to exhibit this "old world" flair. Dr. Hodges was placed in charge of teaching in the Laboratory of Clinical Medicine in 1944, and he continued in that role until 1972. This course formed the union between basic science and clinical medicine. The students performed tests on blood, urine, and various other body fluids. They were instructed in pulmonary function, electrocardiography, venous pressure, forensic medicine, renal and hepatic function, endocrinology, and all laboratory procedures used in diagnosis. The knowledge of these tests was combined with the various symptoms and physical findings in disease states to lead to clinical diagnoses. Physical diagnosis was under the direction of Dr. Creighton H. Turner until 1942, when he was succeeded by Dr. Robert Charr. Clinical Clerkships were conducted on the wards in Jefferson Main (Old) Hospital, where Dr. Reimann and his staff held forth, and at the following affiliated hospitals: Methodist, Cooper, Philadelphia General, Lankenau, Germantown, Pennsylvania, Barton Memorial, and the White Haven Sanitorium. The Outpatient Clinics at Jefferson were manned by various members of the staff, principally volunteers. The General Medical Clinic came under the Directorship of Dr. John N. Lindquist (Jefferson, 1943).

Dean Patterson died in 1938, and Dr. Henry K. Mohler of the Medical Staff succeeded him as Dean and as Sutherland M. Prevost Professor of Therapeutics. Following the death of Dr. Mohler in 1940, Dr. William Harvey Perkins succeeded to the Deanship and Dr. Martin E. Rehfuss became the Sutherland M. Prevost Professor of Therapeutics. Dr. Rehfuss had been presenting clinics to the Senior students and now he also gave many of the lectures in Therapeutics. In 1949 the Board of Trustees discontinued the Professorship of Therapeutics, and Dr. Rehfuss continued the course as a lectureship in the Department of Medicine.

Tropical Medicine and World War II

The specialized teaching of Tropical Medicine started in 1913 with lectures by Dr. E. R. Stitt (U.S.N.). Dr. Stitt was succeeded after 1922 by Dr. Glen F. Clark (U.S.N.). In 1942, Dr. William Sawitz was brought from New Orleans by Dr. Perkins and started a course in Parasitology and Tropical Medicine. It was at about this time that the Mary Markle Foundation financed the teaching of tropical medicine for two representatives from each of the medical schools in the country. This was in response to the recognized needs of the Armed Services in their experiences in the tropical warfare in the Pacific, particularly the Guadalcanal campaign. The course consisted of five weeks of lecture and laboratory work at the Bethesda Naval Medical Center or at Walter Reed Army Hospital, followed by five weeks of field instruction in Central America. Doctor Hodges represented Jefferson (1943) and on completion of the course was appointed Assistant to Dr. Sawitz and aided in teaching this course for five years.

When Dr. Reimann succeeded Dr. McCrae, the Medical Staff consisted of 32 members. At the time of Dr. Reimann's resignation, late in 1951, there were 89 staff members, ten residents, and three fellows.

The Interim Committee

A committee for the administration of the Department of Medicine (Figure 9-20) was established by the Board of Trustees in 1951 following the resignation of the Chairman Dr. Hobart A. Reimann.[57] This group, like the one appointed in 1911 at the retirement of Dr. James C. Wilson, consisted of four members of the Medical Staff: Drs. Rehfuss, Jones, Duncan, and Tocantins. Dr. Martin E. Rehfuss, who with Dr. Philip B. Hawk had performed extensive studies on gastric digestion and published various books on Gastroenterology, as well as a textbook of practical therapeutics,[58] was named Chairman. Dr. Harold W. Jones was a noted hematologist and Director of the Charlotte Drake Cardeza Foundation and Laboratories. Dr. Garfield G. Duncan, a Canadian, was educated at McGill University and joined the staff of the Pennsylvania Hospital under the tutelage of Dr. McCrae. He rose to the Directorship of the Medical Service of the Pennsylvania Hospital. As a colonel in the Army in World War II, he received commendations for his work in malaria and infectious hepatitis. His publications dealt with metabolism and principally diabetes mellitus. A fine gentleman, Duncan was admired by the students as a wise and capable physician. Dr. Leandro M. Tocantins (Jefferson, 1926), was Secretary of the Committee. His particular interest was in coagulation and bleeding diseases. An outstanding hematologist, Tocantins was Head of the Department of Hematology at Pennsylvania Hospital and Assistant Director of the Division of Hematology at Jefferson.

The Committee successfully directed the functions of the Department until the appointment of the new Chairman, Dr. John E. Deitrick, in 1952.

John E. Deitrick, M.D. (1905–); Eleventh Chairman (1952–1957)

The arrival of John English Deitrick (Figure 9-21) at Jefferson was a timely one for the academic processes of the Department and the College, which needed to devise new procedures and to strengthen older channels of operation. Deitrick had just published the *Preliminary Observation of a Survey of Medical Education* and was in the process of writing the results of a *Survey of the Medical Schools in the United States at Mid-Century.*[59]

John Deitrick was born April 13, 1905, in Watsontown, Pennsylvania, the son of Edgar Dentler and Capitola (Heine) Deitrick.[60] He graduated from Wyoming Seminary, attended Princeton University, where he received his B.S. degree in 1929 (Phi Beta Kappa), and earned the M.D. degree (Alpha Omega Alpha) from Johns

Hopkins University in 1933. Following an Internship at Hopkins and four years of Residency at The New York Hospital (1934–1938) he became a member of the Staff of the Hospital and the Faculty of Cornell University, rising to the rank of Associate Professor of Clinical Medicine and Director of the Cornell Division at Bellevue Hospital. Dr. Deitrick developed a private practice, but his primary interest was directed toward medical education. In 1948, the American Medical Association and the Association of American Medical Colleges selected him to direct a national study of medical education. He moved to Chicago, set up a staff, and for the next four years was occupied in accomplishing this task.

Dr. Deitrick had a profound knowledge of the workings and interrelationships of Medical School faculties, the administration, and the hospital staff. He appointed a committee of the medical staff, chaired by Dr. Hodges, to investigate the feasibility of establishing a Hospital Intensive Care Unit. He and the committee met with the Hospital Director, Dr. Hayward Hamrick, and approval was obtained for the first Intensive Care Unit at Jefferson. Another committee, chaired by Dr. Hodges, worked out a plan to have intern and resident care of the patients of the private medical service. This was approved by the Staff on January 12, 1956. Dr. Deitrick worked persistently with Dean George A. Bennett and Dr. Hamrick to improve the status of the Medical Residents and to establish their financial support.

A Period of Rebuilding

It is possible that the resignation of Dr. Hobart A. Reimann in 1951 was an omen of future problems among the faculty, problems that reached a climax in 1955 with the resignation of Dr. Lewis C. Scheffey as Chairman of the

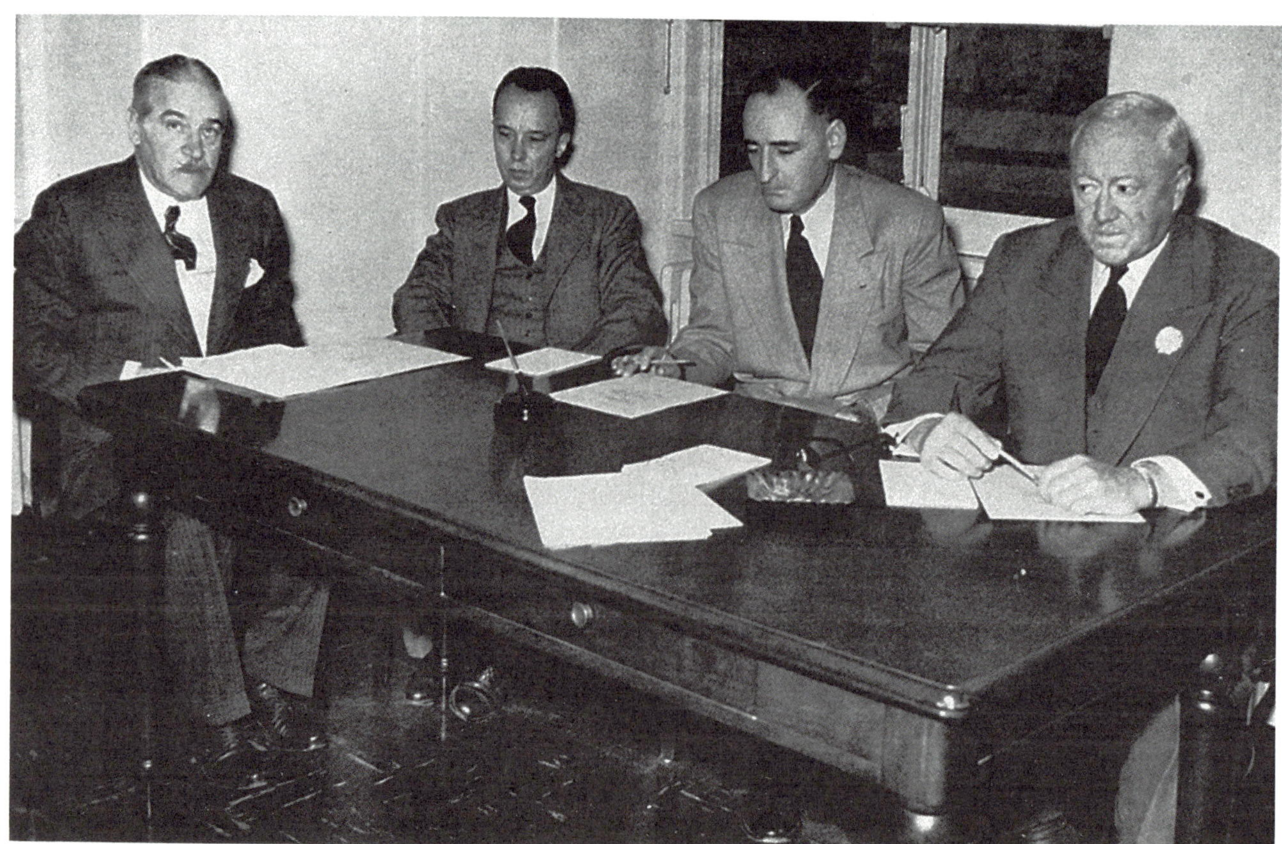

FIG. 9-20. Interim Committee (1951): Drs. Martin E. Rehfuss, Leandro M. Tocantins, Garfield G. Duncan, and Harold W. Jones.

Department of Obstetrics and Gynecology, the retirement of Dr. Louis H. Clerf as Chairman of Laryngology and Bronchoesophagology, the request of Dr. Charles F. McKhann to be relieved of his position as Chairman of the Department of Pediatrics and assigned as Professor of Pediatric Research, and the resignation of Dr. Paul C. Swenson as Chairman of the Department of Radiology. The announcement of these changes at the Annual Alumni Association Meeting (June 16, 1955) was met with boos from the audience even though there was an accompanying announcement of the formation of a new Department of Anesthesiology. This prompted Dr. Deitrick and two other members of the faculty,

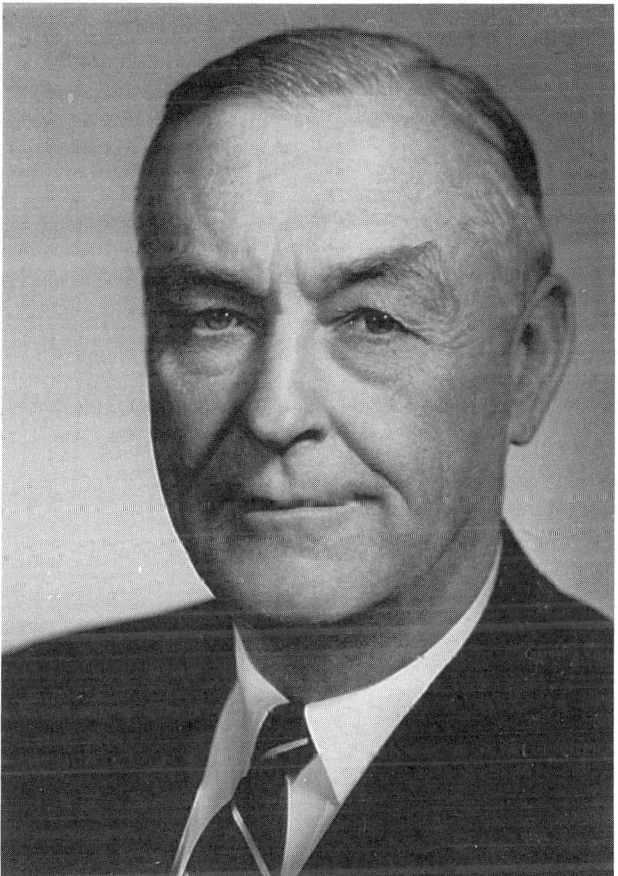

FIG. 9-21. John E. Deitrick, M.D. (1905–); Eleventh Chairman (1952–1957).

Dr. Abraham Cantarow and Dr. John H. Gibbon, Jr., to make a written appeal to Mr. Percival E. Foerderer, Chairman of the Board of Trustees (June 27, 1955).[61] They stated that situations caused by certain policies and practices were at fault: Candidates for Professorships and Heads of Departments had been selected by the administration without a voice by the faculty, the Jefferson Medical College Internship had become less attractive, the Staff of the Hospital had no influence on the Internship and the choice of interns, and the recent resignations had lessened the prestige of the institution. The loss of the Radiology staff created inconveniences in patient care. This disturbed the morale of the students, the faculty, and the alumni.

In the appeal, Deitrick, Cantarow, and Gibbon suggested that a committee of the Executive Faculty, with the Dean, choose and recommend a candidate to the faculty for approval and that this selection be recommended to the Board of Trustees for final approval. The interns should be selected by the Medical Staff of the Hospital, with the Dean and Medical Director represented ex officio, and their selection presented to the Board of Trustees for approval. The head of every major department should be provided with an operating budget that would be approved by the administration six months before the beginning of the fiscal year. A meeting might be held, possibly three times a year, between representatives of the Board of Trustees and the faculty. The passage of time has seen these principles become a reality.

One of the precedent-setting changes undertaken by Dr. Deitrick was the establishment of the Mohler Physicians Offices in 1955. This was a setting for outpatient practice for members of the faculty. The fees for participation were minimal, on an hourly basis, and directed to the younger members of the faculty to give them a site for private practice in the immediate vicinity of the College. The Board of Trustees underwrote the original costs of renovating the first floor of the Henry K. Mohler Building (formerly the Blakiston Building) at 1020 Walnut Street and outfitted it with a laboratory and fluoroscope. A secretary and nurse aided in the formal care of the patients. Dr. Hodges served as Director of the unit from its inception and continued in this role for its 20 years of existence. The unit moved to 1216 Walnut Street (St. James Annex Building) in 1966 prior to the demolition of the Mohler Building. An average of 25 physicians were members of the unit at a time and most of them moved to the Edison Building at Ninth and Sansom Streets in 1975 following the formation of practice-type offices in this building and the sale of the St. James Annex. In turn, many of the staff physicians moved to the Thomas Jefferson University Hospital when offices were made available on alternate floors of this structure at Eleventh and Chestnut Streets in 1978. These offices were supplemented in 1986 with the completion of a new outpatient building at Eleventh and Walnut Streets adjacent to the Forrest Theater.

Faculty changes were occurring. Pennsylvania Hospital became unavailable for teaching because of its academic relationship with the Medical School of the University of Pennsylvania. Dr. Garfield Duncan, however, was encouraged to continue to teach the Junior students at Jefferson. Dr. Harold Jones retired as Director of the Cardeza Foundation (1956) but retained the Professorship of Medicine until he became Emeritus in 1958. Dr. Leandro M. Tocantins succeeded Dr. Jones as Director of Cardeza. The Cardeza Foundation, with its Transfusion Unit and other facilities, moved into a specially renovated building at 1015 Sansom Street in 1956. Dr. Martin E. Rehfuss became Emeritus Professor of Clinical Medicine and Director of the Division of Therapeutics in the Department of Medicine. Dr. F. William Sunderman (Figure 9-22) who came to Jefferson during the Chairmanship of Dr. Reimann, was Director of the Division of

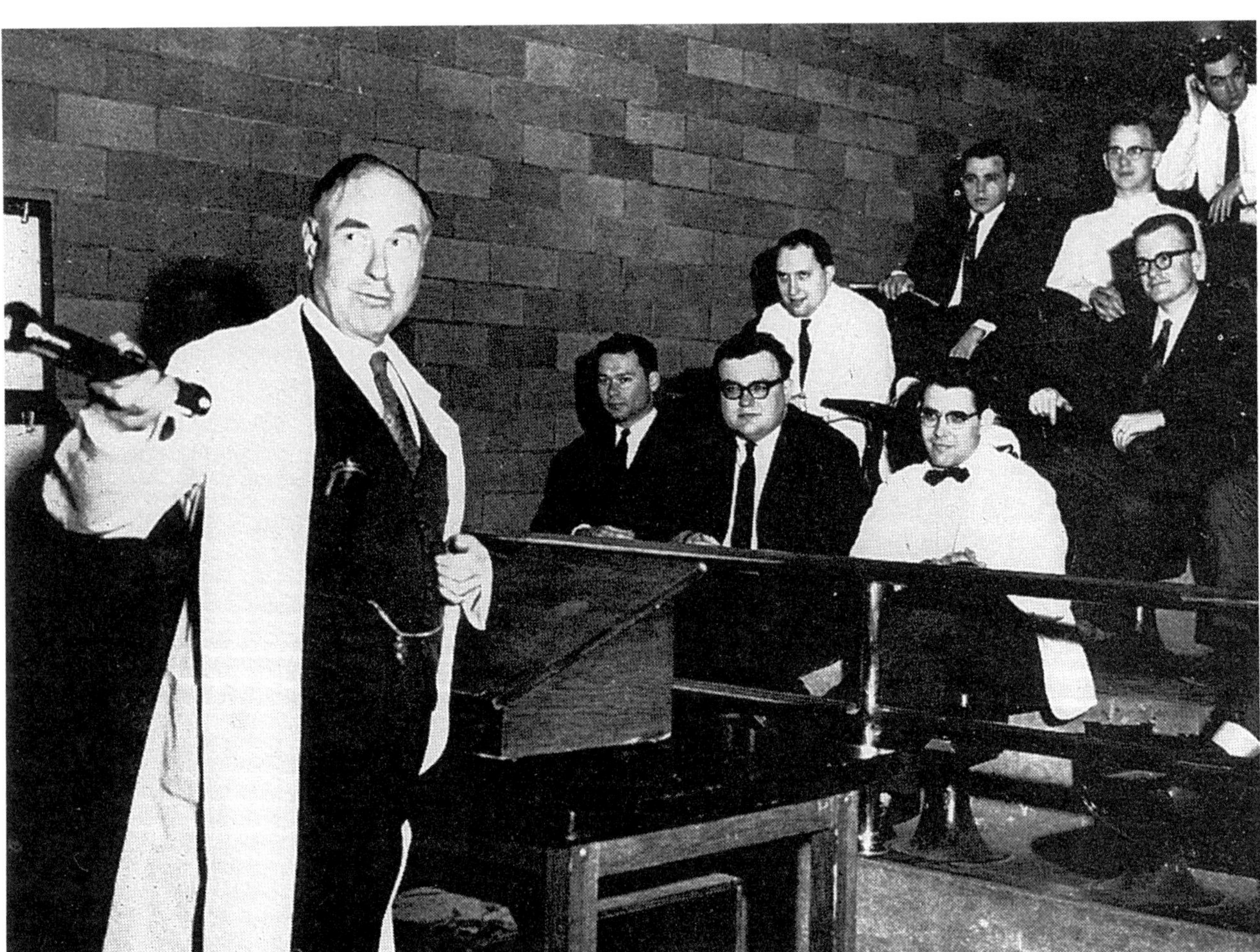

FIG. 9-22. F. William Sunderman, M.D., Director of Metabolic Research.

Metabolic Research. His chief realm of productivity was the monitoring of the nationwide standardization of laboratory tests.

Dr. Deitrick was a tall, quiet, modest physician who brought to Jefferson a much-needed realignment of its academic and administrative processes. In his words, "The period 1952–1957 was one of confusion, conflict, change, and progress at Jefferson. There was confusion between the Medical School and the Hospital Administrators. There was also conflict between the Faculty and the Administrators. The Hospital was operated primarily for the private practice of medicine with the new pavilion for private patients and the old wards for student teaching. There was very little research."[61]

Dr. Deitrick's academic abilities were recognized locally as well as nationally. He served on Committees for the Philadelphia County and State Medical Society, for the College of Physicians of Philadelphia, and for the Heart Association. In Philadelphia he became a member of the Laennec Society, the J. Aitken Meigs Society, and Sigma Xi. He was later President of the Association of American Medical Colleges and the New York Academy of Medicine, and he served on the Board of Directors of various New York Medical Associations, the Associated Medical Schools of New York and New Jersey, and the American Cancer Society. He was a member of the Advisory Committee on Medicine of the W. K. Kellogg Foundation.

Deitrick's dozens of publications covered cardiovascular research, the effects of immobilization, and perhaps the most significant, the treatises pertaining to medical education.[59,62] The experiences at Jefferson may have served as practical training for this affable and intelligent master of medical education to move on to his next academic challenge. Dr. Deitrick resigned on July 31, 1957, to accept the position of Dean and Professor of Medicine of Cornell University Medical College. During his 12 years as Dean at Cornell, two buildings were constructed, one for research and the other for a library. He was instrumental in organizing cooperative efforts for all the medical schools in New York State, obtained financial support from Governor Rockefeller for the private New York Medical Schools and established a primate colony for all the medical schools in the State. He remained Dean until 1969 and became Emeritus Professor of Medicine at Cornell in 1970.[61]

William A. Sodeman, M.D., Sc.D., L.H.D. (1906–); Twelfth Chairman (1957–1958)

It could hardly have been predicted that when Dr. William Harvey Perkins came from Tulane to Jefferson in 1941 to be Dean, his successor, Dr. William Anthony Sodeman (Figure 9-23), an associate and successor at Tulane, later would come to Jefferson as Magee Professor of Medicine (1957) and then also as the Dean (1958).[60] This forthright man, who had the ability to make a rapid summation of a situation and evolve a practical solution, was a broadly educated internist and an accomplished administrator. He was born in Charleroi, Pennsylvania, on June 13, 1906. The family moved to Toledo, Ohio, when he was six, and he received his secondary school education there.[63] Sodeman obtained the B.S. degree (Phi Beta Kappa and Phi Kappa Phi) in 1928 and the M.D. degree (Alpha Omega Alpha and *cum laude*) in 1931, both at the University of Michigan. Following an internship at St. Vincent's Hospital in Toledo he went to Tulane for a four-year residency and fellowship in Internal Medicine with Dr. John Herr Musser (1932–1936). Additional formal education was obtained as a Commonwealth Fund Fellow in Cardiology at the University of Michigan (1938–1939). Dr. Sodeman's academic career of over 20 years at Tulane started in 1932 with his appointment as Instructor in Medicine. He was appointed as Professor and Head of the Department of Preventive Medicine in 1941. In 1946 the Department of Preventive Medicine merged with the Department of Tropical Medicine and he became the Professor of Tropical Medicine and Chairman of the Department of Tropical Medicine and Public Health (William Henderson Professor), a position he held until 1953, uninterrupted except for a partial year (1951) as Visiting Professor in Medical Sciences at the Calcutta (India) School of

Tropical Medicine. He had served for four years (1953–1957) as Professor and Chairman of the Department of Internal Medicine at the University of Missouri School of Medicine when he received the call to be Chairman of the Department of Medicine at Jefferson. His colleagues at Tulane had described him as ". . . a teacher, research worker, writer, speaker, councilor, but above all a clinician who is a doctor's doctor; a person who was fair and logical in everything he did."[64] His broad talents in the field of Medicine were emphasized by his certification in the American Boards of Internal Medicine, Cardiovascular Diseases, and Preventive Medicine.

It did not take long for Dr. Sodeman to come to the conclusion that it was important for the welfare of Jefferson's Department of Medicine that it strengthen the subspecialties and that all these units remain within the Department. He was referring to Hematology with its desire for autonomy and Cardiology which did not have a Director who was certified and which was financially under the authority of the Hospital Director. Efforts to effect these changes were deferred by the untimely death of Dean Bennett in 1958. Several factors favored Sodeman's ideas for improvement of the Department. Dr. Robert I. Wise of the Division of Infectious Diseases, whom he had known in New Orleans, concurred with his thoughts. Dr. Sodeman was instrumental in encouraging the appointment of Dr. Wise as his successor in the Chairmanship of the Department of Medicine.[63] In his new role as Dean he could work with Dr. Wise in the implementation of their mutual aspirations for the Department of Medicine.

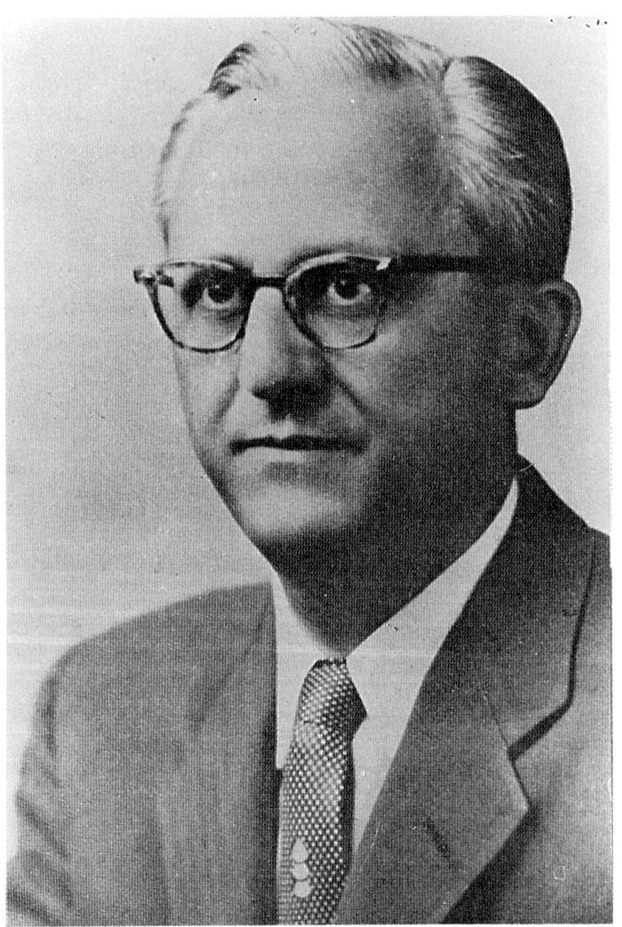

FIG. 9-23. William A. Sodeman, M.D., Sc.D., L.H.D. (1906–); Twelfth Chairman (1957–1958), Dean (1958–1967).

Dr. Ross V. Patterson had been placed in charge of a Subdepartment of Electrocardiography in the Medical Department of Jefferson Hospital in 1918. This became the Ross V. Patterson Heart Station after the death of Dr. Patterson in 1938. Its awkward administrative status was temporarily resolved through an agreement between Dean Sodeman and Hospital Director, Dr. Ellsworth Browneller, that the heart station become the responsibility of the Department of Medicine with administrative and financial power still that of the Hospital (1960).[22,60] It remained for Dr. Wise to make a final definition of the Division of Cardiology in 1964.[22] Dr. Wise was destined also to establish the Division of Hematology containing the Cardeza Foundation within the Department of Medicine.

Doctor Sodeman won respect from the Medical Staff that continued when he undertook the new role as Dean. Perhaps his change from clinician to mainly an academician was the loss to the Department of Medicine of "an unsurpassed diagnostician," in the words of John H. Killough, Ph.D., M.D., who was an early Director of the evolving Division of Cardiology and who became an Associate Dean and Director of Continuing Medical Education under Dr. Sodeman. Among Dr. Sodeman's accomplishments as Dean were the vestiture in the Admission Committee of final choice of applicants; the institution of Faculty Retreats; the introduction of National Board Examinations into the curriculum; the admission of women students; the reestablishment of a viable Department of Radiology under a new Chairman, and the removal of Jefferson from the American Association of University Professors' blacklist.[63] He and Dr. Samuel Conly, Associate Dean, were responsible for the implementation of the College and Medical School total five-year plan in combination with Penn State University. He corroborated the plans for new buildings such as the Stein Radiology Research Center and Jefferson Alumni Hall—the latter the basic science and communal building at 1020 Locust Street. Through the combined cooperation of Mr. James Large, Chairman of the Board of Trustees, and Mr. William Bodine, President of the College, he made possible the Alumni Advisory Committee, which evolved into the establishment of Alumni Trustee members of the Board of Trustees starting in 1965.

Sodeman's activities in the American Medical Association Council on Medical Education, the Chairmanship of the Liaison Committee on Medical Education, and membership on the National Board of Medical Examiners brought national acclaim to Jefferson. In 1962 he received the Clarence E. Shaffrey Medal of St. Joseph's College for Distinguished Service to Medical Science.

When Dr. Sodeman prepared for his 1967 retirement from Jefferson he conveyed to President Peter A. Herbut the idea of Jefferson becoming a Medical University.[63] His resignation as Dean and as Vice-President for Medical Affairs, a title given by the Board of Trustees in 1962, decreased the stresses on his life and allowed his taking the position of Scientific Director of the Life Insurance Medical Research Fund. This Fund was sponsored by 120 life insurance companies in the United States and Canada. His purpose was to aid in directing the funds to medical schools for the improvement of education and research.

Dr. Sodeman started a new career in 1970 as Executive Director, Commission on Foreign Medical Graduates, formed to upgrade educational standards and levels of practice of doctors trained in medical schools in other countries but who seek to practice or take additional training in the United States. He continued in this position for three years and then became Clinical Professor of Medicine of the Medical College of Ohio at Toledo, a position he continued to occupy in 1986.

Doctor Sodeman rarely limited himself to a single category of activities. Throughout his career he became consultant to medical schools, to the United States Public Health Service, and to other groups. He lectured frequently and was a Visiting Professor here and abroad. He published over 200 articles in the medical literature, primarily on cardiac and tropical medical subjects, and continued to serve on editorial boards of medical journals. His textbook, *Pathologic Physiology: Mechenisms of Disease*, has gone through seven editions (1950 to 1985). As a member of numerous scientific societies, Sodeman has served as Presidents of the American Society of Tropical Medicine, the Heart Association of Southeastern Pennsylvania, the American College of Cardiology, and the American College of Physicians. Awards have included the Sesquicentennial and the Distinguished Alumni award of the University of Michigan and the Strittmater Award of the Philadelphia County Medical Society. He was made a Distinguished Fellow of the American College of Cardiology and Emeritus President of the American College of Physicians. In 1968 his portrait was presented to the College by colleagues and friends.

Dr. Sodeman's wife, the late Agnes Wagner Sodeman, a strong and independent person, acted as his constant companion and critic. She served in the Women's groups related to the organizations in which her husband was active, and founded the Faculty Wives Club at Jefferson in 1961.

Dr. Sodeman's distinction as an individual and his many triumphs in the medical field continue to be a source of honor and pride for Jefferson.

Robert I. Wise, M.D., Ph.D., Sc.D. (1915–); Thirteenth Chairman (1959–1975)

The phrase "a demand for excellence" perhaps best describes the 16-year term of Robert Irby Wise, M.D., Ph.D. (Figure 9-24), as Magee Professor of Medicine and Chairman of the Department. A quote from the preface of his history of that period further defines his meaning of excellence: "As we approach the end of the twentieth century, the college is again in an ascendancy of achievement of excellence. The physical plant is magnificent. The faculty is creative and stimulating in educational programs. An environment exists for inquiry, which is essential for productive clinical investigation and a high quality of patient care. All are necessary if excellence in medical education is to be maintained."[23]

Dr. Wise had been a member of the Division of Infectious Diseases, directed by Dr. Paul Havens in 1955, when Dr. John E. Dietrick was Magee Professor. He was born May 19, 1915, in Barstow, Texas. He received the B.A. degree from the University of Texas in 1937 and the M.S. in 1938 from the University of Illinois, where he performed research and taught in the Departments of Animal Husbandry and Bacteriology while working there for the M.S. and the Ph.D. (1942). He spent one year as Director of the regional Public Health Laboratories of the Texas State Department of Health in Wichita Falls and Houston. The following four years he was Associate Professor of Bacteriology at the University of Texas Medical Branch, Galveston, and four years later (1950) he received the M.D. degree from the same institution.

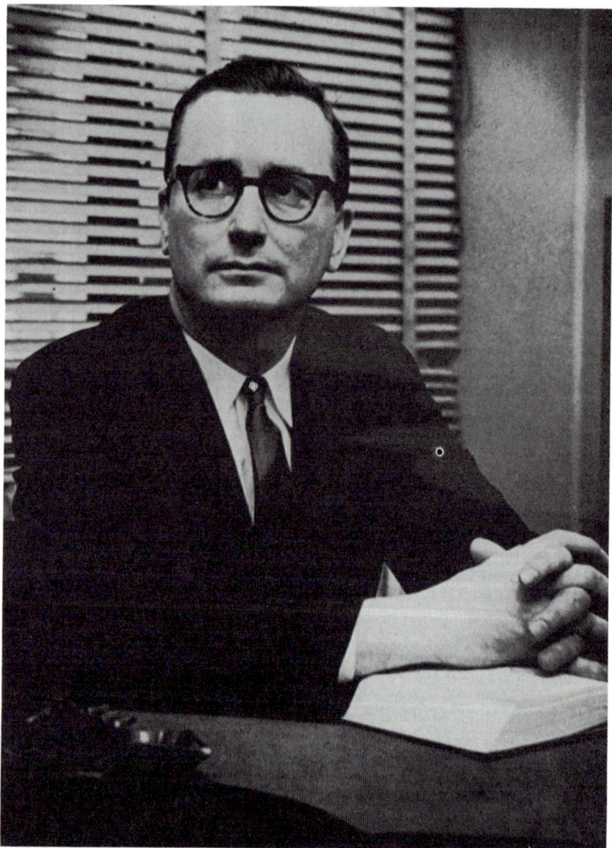

FIG. 9-24. Robert I. Wise, M.D., Ph.D., Sc.D. (1915–); Thirteenth Chairman (1959–1975).

It was during the following year's internship at the U.S. Public Health Service Hospital in New Orleans that he met Dr. William A. Sodeman, whom he was to succeed as Magee Professor. After a two-year residency in Medicine and fellowship in Infectious Diseases at the University of Minnesota Hospital, Wise was appointed Assistant Professor of Medicine and a year later acquired the additional title of Assistant Professor of Bacteriology and Director of the Bacteriological Laboratories, University of Minnesota Hospitals. He was certified by the American Board of Internal Medicine in 1957.

Thus, with this solid base in bacteriologic study, teaching, research, and administration, and with a recently acquired expertise in clinical medicine, Wise was presented with a new challenge when he was appointed the Magee Professor and Chairman of the Department in 1959 to succeed Dr. Sodeman, who had served as Acting Chairman since his appointment as Dean in 1958. Dr. Wise recognized, at the beginning, certain problems and determined to confront them. He delved into the history of the Department and assembled information about each Head of the Department from the time of Jefferson's inception in 1824. This was published in 1975.[60] He perceived that Jefferson was a model for private practice but that it should be more aggressive in the pursuit of research. The salaries for geographical full-time (partially salaried plus private practice) physicians were low and without fringe benefits or pension and lacked uniformity. General funds for the Department were low. Jefferson students were no longer assigned to the Pennsylvania Hospital and there were fewer than the ideal number of applications for the Jefferson Hospital Internship.

Clinical and Affiliated Hospital Teaching

The faculty in 1959 had 162 members. There were 15 medical Interns and ten Fellows. The

Sophomore courses were: Clinical Laboratory Medicine, under the direction of Dr. John H. Hodges with the assistance of Dr. John B. Atkinson and Miss Jane Kirk; Physical Diagnosis was conducted by Dr. Daniel W. Lewis, succeeded in 1965 by Dr. William Fraimow when Dr. Lewis transferred to St. Agnes Hospital. Much of the clinical teaching was performed on the medical wards on the second floor of the Main Hospital, but since the time of Dr. Dietrick there had been a gradual assignment of Residents and Senior students to the private side. By 1964 Junior students also were assigned to the private patients. The wards were eliminated in 1971, and an area on the sixth floor of the Main Hospital was arranged for the care of indigent patients under the supervision of a resident and staff member whose assignments were rotated systematically.

The Junior students were assigned to the General Medical Clinic, where they received practical training in history taking, physical examination, and the care of the patient under the direction of Dr. John N. Lindquist and members of the staff.

The following Clinics were active at this time:

General Medicine	Dr. John N. Lindquist
Asthma	Dr. Howard C. Leopold
Cardiac	Dr. Daniel Lewis
Arthritis No. 1	Drs. Irvin F. Hermann and Richard Smith
Arthritis No. 2	Dr. Abraham Cohen
Hypertension	Dr. Edmund L. Housel
Peripheral Vascular Diseases	Dr. David W. Kramer

The physicians assigned to these clinics were principally on a volunteer basis. Senior students were assigned to clinics other than General Medicine.

The clinical clerkships were at Jefferson Hospital and the following affiliated hospitals:

Philadelphia General	
Goldburgh Service	Dr. Harold L. Goldburgh
Kramer Service	Dr. David W. Kramer
Israel Service (1959)	Dr. Harold L. Israel
Methodist	Dr. Harold F. Robertson
Lankenau	Dr. Malcolm Miller
Germantown	Dr. Ralph W. Mays
Cooper	Dr. Edwin Murray
Atlantic City	Dr. J. Gleason

Over the ensuing years, terms of affiliation were in existence temporarily at the Veterans Administration Hosptial (Philadelphia), the Hunterdon Medical Center, the Landis State Hospital, the U.S. Naval Hospital (Philadelphia), and on a continuing basis with the Mercy Catholic Medical Center, Einstein Southern, Bryn Mawr (1972), the Wilmington Medical Center (1971), and Our Lady of Lourdes (1972). Teaching at the Philadelphia General Hospital was discontinued in 1971.

The organization of the Department consisted of the following:

Endocrinology and Cancer Research	Dr. Karl E. Paschkis
Gastroenterology	Dr. C. Wilmer Wirts
Hematology (Cardeza Foundation)	Dr. Leandro M. Tocantins
Infectious Diseases	Dr. W. Paul Havens, Jr.
Metabolic Research	Dr. F. William Sunderman
Pulmonary Diseases	Dr. Martin J. Sokoloff
Laboratory of Clinical Medicine	Dr. John H. Hodges

Dr. Robert L. Evans (Jefferson, 1950), Instructor in Clinical Medicine, was the administrative assistant to the Head of the Department and developed the teaching organization. He had been Chief Medical Resident with Dr. John E. Deitrick, then succeeded to the present position and continued until late in 1959 when he resigned to become Director of Medical Education at York Hospital in Pennsylvania.

In 1963 the rotating internship was changed to a straight intern program, the intern year thus constituting the first year of medical residency.

These programs were aided by the Martin Rehfuss Fellowships. The Chief Medical Resident was a key individual in the clinical teaching programs, and Dr. Wise had discussed with Dr. Rehfuss the importance of this position. Dr. Rehfuss' will in 1964 left a bequest of $250,000 that was to be used to supplement the salary of the Chief Medical Resident, thereby enhancing the importance and value of this position.

The library-conference room that was established during the renovation of the Chairman's office on the eighth floor of the College Building was dedicated to Dr. Martin E. Rehfuss and to Dr. John H. Gibbon, Jr. The latter had used the room as a construction laboratory for the final stages of the perfection of the heart-lung machine, which was first used on a human in 1953. It was the prototype for all heart-lung machines used throughout the world in open heart surgery.

Dr. Francis J. Sweeney (Jefferson, 1951) succeeded Dr. Evans in coordinating the senior student program for three years until his appointment to direct the medical services at the Philadelphia General Hospital. He returned in 1968 as Hospital Director and later became Vice-President for Medical Affairs. Dr. Elliott Goodman was the coordinator for the Junior year. With the change from rotating internship to Medical Residencies in 1963, the popularity of the program began to increase, and the numbers grew from 12 to 81 over the next 12 years. In 1971 residency rotations were started with Methodist, Southern Einstein, and Our Lady of Lourdes Hospitals. A Committee on Postgraduate Education coordinated this effort. A Committee on Private Medical Services gradually evolved a system with private medical patients admitted to specific areas of Jefferson Hospital. Medical rounds on this service were conducted originally by Dr. Wise, accompanied by residents and students and later by other staff physicians. By 1966 there were 230 patient beds assigned to the Medical Service. Dr. Joseph Medoff (Jefferson, 1939) developed a list of criteria for physician preference in the admission of patients and a list of illnesses that could legitimately be termed emergencies. This improved problems of priorities for hospital admissions.

Dr. William F. Kellow, who was the Dean of Hahnemann Medical College, was appointed Dean to succeed Dr. Sodeman in 1967. Both he and his assistant, Dr. Joseph Gonnella, were appointed to the staff of the Medical Department. One of the first important actions of Dr. Kellow was the establishment of a Practice Plan for full-time staff members. The first plan was devised, with his direction, by a committee in the Department of Medicine (1968). This became the guide for the rest of the College and subsequently a benefits package evolved for full-time staff members. Another Departmental Committee was Appointments and Promotions.

An administrative problem that needed to be settled was the status of the Cardeza Foundation and Division of Hematology, which Mr. J. Howard Pew, Chairman of the Cardeza Committee, and Dr. Leandro M. Tocantins, the Cardeza Professor, wished to be maintained as a Department separate from Medicine. Dr. Wise confronted them on this issue and it was resolved by their agreement to have Cardeza and Hematology be a Division of the Department of Medicine. There continued to be a Board of Trustees'–appointed Committee, which had a primary function for direction of the care of the finances of the legacy. Dr. Tocantins died in March of 1963 and was succeeded by Dr. Allan J. Erslev, a native of Denmark who received his medical education there; he came to the United States in 1946 and worked at the Sloan-Kettering Institute, Yale University, and the Thorndike Memorial Laboratories before coming to Jefferson. A fine teacher and researcher, Erslev was one of the discoverers of erythropoietin and was coauthor of the textbook *Hematology*.[65] The Cardeza Foundation moved to new quarters on the seventh, eighth, and ninth floors of the Curtis Building in 1974. Hematologic research, clinical care, and teaching had risen to a high level of excellence coincident with additions to the staff that included Dr. Scott Murphy in platelets, Dr. Sandor Shapiro in coagulation, Dr. Farid Haurani in red cell kinetics, Dr. Jose Martinez on fibrinogen, and others. Dr. Erslev retired as Director of Cardeza in 1985 and became Emeritus and Distinguished Professor. Sandor Shapiro was appointed to succeed him as Director of Cardeza.

The Pulmonary Division was experiencing a gradual reduction in emphasis on tuberculosis and a concomitant increase in the incidence of obstructive and interstitial lung diseases. Drs. Hurley Motley and Richard Cathcart, experts in pulmonary physiology, dealt with these trends. Dr. Peter Theodos served as clinical coordinator for the Anthracite Health & Welfare Fund's research project in the lung diseases of coal miners.

The appointment of Dr. Harold Israel (1959), an expert in sarcoidosis, additionally with the clinical acumen and teaching abilities of such stalwarts as Drs. Jacob J. Kirshner and J. Woodrow Savacool, contributed toward a broad-based Division of Pulmonary Diseases. Dr. Sokoloff retired as Director in 1963, to be succeeded by Dr. Richard Cathcart, who served until 1974. The latter was replaced by Dr. William Atkinson, a graduate of the Ohio State University (1964) who came to Jefferson as a Resident and Fellow in Pulmonary Disease and had studied alpha-1-antitrypsin. He introduced fiberoptic bronchoscopy and supervised the transformation of a portion of the hospital pulmonary unit into a modern pulmonary laboratory and a pulmonary intensive care unit.

Progress in Research

Dr. Karl E. Paschkis, the Director of the Division of Endocrinology and the Director of the Division of Endocrine and Cancer Research in the Department of Experimental Medicine, together with Dr. Abraham Cantarow, had been responsible for the formation of the Endocrine Clinic. The members of this Division (14 members in 1950–1951) had been active in research into the endocrinological aspects of experimental carcinogenesis. John J. Schneider, M.D., Ph.D. and Marvin L. Lewbart, M.D., Ph.D. maintained a laboratory on the eighth floor of the College Building and were nationally famous for their pioneer work in the study of steroid compounds. Dr. Ralph Carabasi (Jefferson, 1946), an oncologist, was particularly interested in breast cancer. Dr. Abraham Rakoff, prominent obstetrician and gynecologist, who contributed to research in the field, was a member of the Division. The Department of Experimental Medicine was discontinued in 1958. When Dr. Paschkis died in 1961 he was succeeded by Dr. Joseph Rupp (Jefferson, 1942) as Director of the Division of Endocrinology until he entered the Dean's Office in 1969 as Assistant Director of Continuing Medical Education.

Dr. F. William Sunderman had maintained an office and laboratory on the eighth floor of the College since the Chairmanship of Dr. Reimann. When Dr. Sunderman retired in 1966 as Director of the Division of Metabolic Research, a new Division of Endocrinology and Metabolic Diseases was established. Dr. David W. Kramer (Jefferson, 1912), an early writer on diabetes (1922) and a national authority on peripheral vascular diseases through his interest in diabetes, directed the Peripheral Vascular Disease Clinic. Kramer died in 1969, and his clinic became a part of the Division of Endocrinology and Metabolic Diseases. He had discussed with Dr. Wise his intent to support the Division of Endocrinology, and in 1973 the bequest in his will endowed the Bertha and David Kramer Professorship of Medicine to support the Director of the Division of Endocrinology and Metabolic Diseases. When Dr. Rupp retired as Director of the Division of Endocrinology in 1969, he was succeeded by Dr. Richard Field, who had been Chief of the Diabetes Unit at the Massachusetts General Hospital and was renowned in the field of diabetic retinopathy. Dr. Field resigned after a year and there was no full Director of the Division until the appointment of Dr. Glennon in 1977. Dr. Joseph A. Glennon became the first Kramer Professor of Medicine and Chief of the Division of Endocrinology and Metabolic Diseases. A graduate of the University of New York and certified in Internal Medicine, Endocrinology and Metabolism, Glennon had extensive clinical experience and was interested particularly in diabetes and obesity.

Dr. Charles Wirts, who with Dr. Franz Goldstein had developed a Fellowship program in Gastroenterology, resigned as Director of the Division of Gastroenterology in 1966. He was succeeded by Dr. O. Dhodanand Kowlessar, a native of India, who had studied at Oxford, trained in biochemistry, and obtained his M.D. degree from the University of Iowa. He held the position of Director of the Division until 1985, when he became Associate Chairman for Educational Programs. Kowlessar had replaced Dr. Laurence Wesson as head of the Clinical Research Center, a position he occupied until the closure of the Center in 1971 because of lack of funding. Dr. Franz Goldstein became Head of Gastroenterology at Lankenau Hospital in 1970, and in the same year Dr. Gordon Benson became a member of the Division to direct research in diseases of the liver with particular emphasis on the effects of alcohol. Dr. Susan J. Gordon (Jefferson, 1966) joined the Division and developed an expertise in gastroscopy.

When Dr. Wise came to Jefferson in 1955, he became a member of the Division of Infectious Diseases under the direction of Dr. W. Paul Havens, Jr. Dr. Havens, a Harvard graduate (1936), had interned at Lankenau Hospital and was the first Medical Resident in the program started by Dr. Reimann. He spent a year at the Rockefeller Institute, became noted for his work on viral hepatitis while in the armed services, and studied under Dr. John Paul in Preventive Medicine at Yale. He returned to Jefferson in 1946 as a member of the Departments of Medicine and Microbiology. Dr. Wise continued his work on the *Staphylococcus* while Dr. Francis J. Sweeney, Jr. carried on the bulk of the effort. Soon after Dr. Wise became Chairman, a hospital epidemic of *Salmonella derby,* which occurred in 1963, involved the resources of Dr. Eileen L. Randall of Microbiology and Dr. Sweeney, Dr. Wise, and Dr. Eugene Sanders of the Center for Disease Control. The results proved the efficacy of the infection control system devised by Dr. Wise in 1955, to which he had added a nurse surveillance officer the following year, had reported it to the American Medical Association in 1957, and saw it become a requirement of the Joint Commission on Accreditation of Hospitals in 1958. Subsequent members of the Division included Dr. Craig K. Wallace, who became Director of the Fogarty Institute of International Health, and Dr. Michael A. Manko, who became Chief of Medicine at Lankenau Hospital. Dr. Havens retired in 1972. Dr. Joseph S. Gonnella became Acting Director in 1975 and Dean of the Medical College in 1983.

The process of bringing the Heart Station under the control of the Department of Medicine had been started by Dr. Sodeman. Former directors succeeding Dr. Ross V. Patterson had included Drs. Hayward Hamrick (also Medical Director of the Hospital), Bruce Nye (later Associate Dean), and Charles W. Semisch III (Jefferson, 1933). Dr. Wise in 1960 combined the services of cardiac catheterization, pulmonary function, and electrocardiography, with Dr. John H. Killough as Director. Dr. Richard Cathcart and Dr. Daniel W. Lewis (Jefferson, 1944) served under him. Four years later Dr. Killough became Director of Continuing Medical Education as a member of the Dean's Office. Dr. Cathcart was appointed Director of the Pulmonary Division, and Dr. Lewis resigned to become Director of Cardiology at St. Agnes Hospital. Dr. William Eliades (Jefferson, 1958) carried on until a definitive Division of Cardiology was established in 1969, with Dr. Albert N. Brest, who transferred from Hahnemann Medical College, as Director. Soon an Intensive Cardiac Care Unit was developed. In 1973, Dr. Brest became the first James C. Wilson Professor of Medicine.

In 1959 Dr. William H. Schmidt retired as Associate Professor of Physical Medicine in the Department of Medicine after 42 years of service. He was succeeded that year by Dr. John W. Goldschmidt, who directed the construction of a new and modern area for the Division and headed the first independent Department of Physical Medicine and Rehabilitation. In 1967 he became Dean of the newly established College of Allied Health Sciences.

The Division of Rheumatology was established in 1959 with Dr. Nathan Smukler (Jefferson, 1947) as Director. Dr. John R. Patterson (Jefferson, 1954) became a member, and in 1967 Dr. John Abruzzo joined the group and later became its Director.

■ Subspecialty Developments

A Division of Medical Oncology was established in 1961, with Dr. Arthur Weiss as Director. Dr. Weiss had a strong interest in cancer, the study of anticancer drugs, and had participated in the development of the technique of lymphangiography with Dr. Laird Jackson. With Dr. Weiss' interests gradually being directed toward his large private practice in oncology, he gave up the Directorship to Dr. Chester Southam in 1971. Cancer patients utilized 56 percent of the medical hospital beds in 1975. Dr. Michael Mastrangelo, a former Medical Resident, became

Director in 1984. Acting Directors included Drs. William P. Delaney and J. Frederick Laucius. In 1958 Dr. Weiss established the Jefferson branch of the Clinical Drug Evaluation Program of the Cancer Chemotherapy National Service Center and the following year became cochairman of the Central Oncology group. Dr. Farid Haurani became Jefferson's representative of the Cancer and Acute Leukemia Group B.

Hemodialysis was started at Jefferson by Dr. James E. Clark (Jefferson, 1952) in 1959 after he had studied with Dr. Lewis W. Bluemle at the University of Pennsylvania. Dr. Lawrence G. Wesson, Jr., from New York University School of Medicine, was appointed Director of the Division of Nephrology in 1961. Dr. Clark continued in charge of dialysis until his resignation in 1968 to become Chairman of the Department of Medicine at Crozer-Chester Hospital and Professor of Medicine at Hahnemann. Dr. Wesson resigned as Director in 1974 and was succeeded by Dr. Michael Simenhoff. Dr. Wesson established and was Acting Director of the Clinical Research Center in 1964. This was a ten-bed laboratory unit backed with funds from the National Institutes of Health. Dr. Kowlessar became the Director in 1966, but the Center was closed in 1971 because of a lack of funds.

The Allergy Clinic had existed for many years, having been founded by Dr. James Alexander Clark (Jefferson, 1916) as an outpatient clinic, and was staffed by very loyal volunteers. Dr. Howard C. Leopold replaced Dr. Harry L. Rogers as Director in 1959. Dr. Frank J. Gilday, Jr. (Jefferson, 1944) was appointed Acting Director in 1974 after the death of Dr. Leopold.

The Division of Genetics was established in 1969. The motivating force for this Division was a graduate of the University of Cincinnati, Dr. Laird Jackson. Jackson completed a residency at Jefferson and started work in Oncology with Dr. Arthur Weiss. He developed a competence in chromosome study and in genetics in general, assisted in this work by Marie Barr. The Division worked with the Departments of Obstetrics, Gynecology, Pathology, and Pediatrics. In 1972 Dr. Susan Z. Cowchock (Jefferson, 1968) developed the first maternal serum-alpha-fetoprotein method in the United States to detect fetal neural tube abnormalities. Dr. Jackson was basically a member of the Department of Medicine but held secondary appointments in the other departments. He was coauthor of a textbook, *Clinical Genetics,*[66] developed programs in prenatal counseling and Tay-Sachs detection, and drew international attention with the development in 1983 of first-trimester fetal diagnosis by chorionic villus sampling.

Funds from Smith, Kline and French (Smith, Kline and Beckman) were used in 1969 to establish a Division of Pharmcology for the testing of drugs, but the Division was discontinued in 1973, to be reestablished in 1977 under the direction of Dr. Roger K. Ferguson. Dr. Francis J. Sweeney, Jr., had returned to become Medical Director of the Hospital in 1967, and through his efforts, combined with those of Dean Tice of the College of Pharmacy and Dr. Wise, a system of satellite pharmacies, manned by pharmacists and student pharmacists, was started in the Hospital. The system continues as an integral Hospital service. As a member of the Editorial Board of the *Medical Letter,* Dr. Wise had become particularly interested in Pharmacy.

Following the 1971 teaching session the Directorship of the course in Laboratory of Clinical Medicine was changed from Dr. John H. Hodges to Drs. Robert C. Mackowiak and Carla Goepp, of the Dean's office, who would coordinate with the Department of Medicine the newly evolved Sophomore course designated the "Introduction to Clinical Medicine." It was becoming apparent that specialization in Internal Medicine was causing a decrease in the education of Internists in the realm of General Medicine. Two things happened to counterbalance this change: the establishment of a Division of General Medicine (1974) with Dr. Hodges as Director and the establishment of a Department of Family Medicine. During the same period (1972) the General Medical Outpatient Clinic was being discontinued. About 40 physicians became members of the Division of General Medicine including Dr. Paul C. Brucker, Chairman of the Department of Family Medicine, and a member of his Department, Dr. Edward H. McGehee. An agreement between the Departments of Medicine and Family Medicine provided that Family Medicine hospital patients would be cared for in the Medical Department and that General Medicine outpatients would be cared for in the Family Practice Department.

During the Chairmanship of Dr. Wise, the Ludwig A. Kind Professorship of Medicine was established through an initial gift of over one-half million dollars by Mrs. Ludwig A. (Hester) Kind, in memory of her late husband. Ludwig Kind, an industrialist, had been an owner of the Kind Gelatin Company, President of the Kind Knox Gelatin Company, and President of the Board of Directors of the First Bank of Camden. He and Mrs. Kind, who lives in Cherry Hill, New Jersey, had been patients of Dr. John Hodges. The Board of Trustees confirmed the Professorship in 1964, and Dr. Hodges was made the first Ludwig A. Kind Professor.

Through the generosity of Mr. Percival Foerderer, Chairman of the Board of Trustees and former patient of Dr. Rehfuss, a Lectureship in honor of Dr. Rehfuss was established after the death of Dr. Rehfuss in 1968. A lecture is presented each year under auspices of the Percival E. and Ethel Brown Foerderer Foundation.

Accomplishments of Dr. Wise

Dr. Wise's continued striving for excellence led him to develop a system of reports from members of the Staff concerning individual students and also from students about specific instructors. This kept a steady flow of information to the office of the Chairman. This highly academic teacher was a member of Alpha Omega Alpha and the author of over 45 medical papers including articles on public health, botulism, staphylococci, brucellosis, and antibiotics. He was a member of the Association of American Physicians and was active on various committees of the American College of Physicians (of which he was a Fellow) and the College of Physicians of Philadelphia. He served on the Board of Trustees of Magee Memorial Hospital and Drexel University, the Board of Directors of the West Philadelphia Corporation, as representative of the American College of Physicians to the American Medical Association and Chairman of Internal Medicine of the American Medical Association.

Wise received the Ashbell-Smith Distinguished Alumni Award of the University of Texas at Galveston and the Julius W. Sturmer Memorial Lecture Award of the Philadelphia College of Pharmacy and Science. He was a Consultant to many organizations and a frequent Visiting Professor. His colleagues and friends presented his portrait to Jefferson in 1975, and Thomas Jefferson University awarded him the Honorary Degree of Doctor of Science in 1980.

Dr. Wise became Emeritus Professor of Medicine in 1975, and he and his wife, Catherine Dosterschill Wise, settled in Maine, where he became Chief of Staff, Veterans Administration Medical and Regional Office Center, Togus, Maine, until retirement in 1984. They then moved to Williamsburg, Virginia, and kept a summer home in Maine.

This tireless worker never ceased in his efforts to improve the Department of Medicine and Jefferson in general. The strengthening of existing divisions and establishment of new divisions, the establishment of Professorships, and the maintenance of a high level of quality of academic and clinical standards are prominent in the numerous accomplishments of his Chairmanship.

Interim Arrangements Again

It was the third time in the twentieth century that a group of four faculty members had been called upon to administer the Department of Medicine in an interval between the retirement of one and the appointment of a new Departmental Chairman. The notice of plans for the early retirement of Dr. Robert I. Wise had been announced at a regular monthly meeting of the Department on February 21, 1974, by Dr. John H. Hodges representing Dean William F. Kellow.[67] A previous similar statement of resignation of Dr. Hobart A. Reimann (1951) had come unheralded and unexpected. The departure of Dr. Wise in the fall of 1975 was followed, rather than preceded, by the appointment of a search committee for his successor, even though his intent was well known and had been preceded by the exhibition of pictures of his new home in Maine. Dr. James Wilson's statement of intent to retire had also gone unheeded (1911).

Dean Kellow appointed four Administrative Coordinators to manage the affairs of the Department until the appointment of the new Chairman. These were Professors Allan J. Erslev, John H. Hodges, Albert N. Brest, and O. Dhodanand Kowlessar. It was decided that each Coordinator rotate through the office of the Chairman for a period of three months to administer the day-by-day duties and that they meet as a group as the need for decisions arose. Dr. Erslev occupied the office from October through December of 1975, followed for three months by Dr. Hodges, who was succeeded by Dr. Brest. The latter continued through the summer months because of the imminent arrival of the new Chairman.

Frank Davis Gray, Jr., M.D. (1916–); Fourteenth Chairman (1976–1981)

Frank Davis Gray, Jr., M.D. (Figure 9-25), Director of the Division of Medicine at the Lankenau Hospital and Professor of Medicine at Jefferson, came across the City to the Jefferson campus as the new Magee Professor on September 13, 1976, following the July 2 recommendation of the Search Committee. Faculty and students had been impressed by the calm, soft-spoken, and orderly teaching methods of this Head of the Medical Division of one of Jefferson's teaching affiliates. Dr. Gray had described his impression of the role of Community Hospitals in medical student teaching.[68] He saw a student in his hospital clerkship as a deliverer of health care in a team of Attending Physician, Residents, and Interns, constituting a core group, with consultants as ancillary contributors to the learning process. It was Dr. Gray's impression that the practice of medicine should be the aim of the clerkship.

Dr. Gray's academic conclusions had evolved during his eight years at Lankenau and his prior experiences at Yale University, where he rose from Instructor (1949) to Associate Professor of Medicine (1957). This was complemented by his attendance at the Yale-New Haven Medical Center, where he served as Director of the Cardiopulmonary Laboratory, Director of the Cardiac Clinic, and Director of the Chest Clinic. During this period of time, before he came to Lankenau in 1968, Gray was consultant to the Laurel Heights, Veterans Administration and Woodruff Hospitals (Connecticut).

Born in Marshall, Minnesota, August 24, 1916, the son of Frank D. Gray and Nettie Wilhelmina Urbach, Dr. Gray remained in his home town for his secondary schooling. He received the B.S. degree (1938) from Northwestern University, Evanston, Illinois, and entered Columbia University, College of Physicians and Surgeons, New York. After two years he attempted to combine research with his medical program and studied tissue culture of leukocytes for a year in

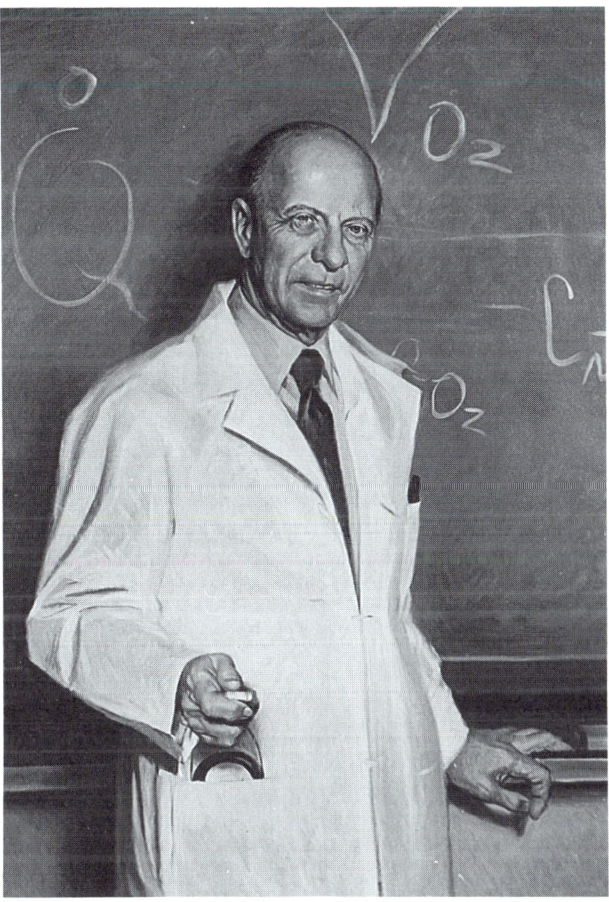

FIG. 9-25. Portrait of Frank D. Gray, Jr., M.D. (1916–); Fourteenth Chairman (1976–1981).

Columbia's Department of Microbiology. This was not an outstanding success in the realm of research but had a happy result in that he married his teacher, Frieda Gersh, who also became an internist after receiving the M.D. degree from New York University Medical College in 1944. He continued his medical studies at Columbia and received the M.D. degree in 1943. A year as Intern and Assistant Resident at the Bellevue Hospital in New York was followed by two years of active duty in the Army Medical Corps. He landed in Normandy in September of 1944 as an Infantry Battalion Surgeon. Gray progressed across Europe, and when the war ended he was stationed in southern Bavaria. He was made Regimental Surgeon and rose in rank from Lieutenant to Major at the time of retirement from active duty in 1946. It is not surprising that the military service recognized the fine training qualities of Dr. Gray and sent him to service schools at Carlisle Barracks and Fort Sam Houston. By the time of his retirement from reserve service in 1971 he had advanced to the rank of Colonel.

The year 1946–1947 was spent as Assistant in Surgery at the Johns Hopkins University, followed by a year as Assistant Resident at the Grace-New Haven Community Hospital and a year as Research Fellow in Medicine at Yale University.

Dr. Gray became a member of numerous medical societies including the American College of Chest Physicians, serving on various committees and as Vice-Chairman of the Board of Regents (1979–1981). He was President of the Connecticut Chapters of the American Thoracic Society and the American Heart Association. A Fellow of the American College of Physicians, he became Medical Advisor and Editor of their Self-Assessment Program (1983). He was a member of the American Society for Clinical Investigation, the American Federation for Clinical Research, the Association of American Medical Colleges, the Association of Military Surgeons of the United States, the Association of Professors of Medicine, and the Association of Past Professors of Medicine. A member of Alpha Omega Alpha and Sigma Xi, Gray was certified by the American Board of Internal Medicine in 1952 and recertified in 1974. He attended Special Management Schools given by the Armed Forces and was certified (1978) by the Harvard School of Public Health for the Harvard University Executive Program in Health Policy and Management for Chiefs of Clinical Services. He served on numerous administrative committees throughout his career both before, during, and after his appointment at Jefferson.[69] Fulfilling the prerogative of the Magee Professorship, Gray served on the Board of Trustees of the Magee Rehabilitation (Memorial) Hospital.

Dr. Gray's book, *Pulmonary Embolism,*[70] published in 1966, contained a concise discussion of the definition, varieties, and causes of pulmonary emboli with the resulting physical and laboratory changes. This was followed by clear presentations of the diagnosis, management, and prognosis. The book is complete with 15 concise and frankly presented illustrative case reports and nearly 700 references. Dr. Gray also contributed eight chapters and monographs plus over 54 articles in the scientific literature. Of these latter articles, the first five discussed congenital heart disease and were written while he was at Johns Hopkins. The remainder dealt with clinical and physiologic studies of cardiac and pulmonary diseases, the teaching of clinical medicine, and the educational role of the community hospital.

Dr. Gray's Chairmanship was characterized by a maintenance of the status quo in some areas and notable changes in others. The Department continued to administer the American Board of Internal Medicine Examinations, and Subspecialty Examinations were added.

▪ Associate Chairman

An innovation in the administration of the Department was the appointment of an Associate Chairman (1978). This position was incorporated in the duties of Dr. John H. Martin when he was brought from Temple University, where he had been Professor of Medicine, to be Director of the Division of General Medicine and Professor of Medicine. Dr. Martin had specific responsibilities for House Staff matters and was expected to be familiar with all of the functions of the Department so that he could take over in the Chairman's absence. The appointment carried with it supervision of the medical residency program. It was Dr. Gray's intent that the Division of General

Medicine be made up of faculty members who were interested in a practice that cut across all medical specialties and emphasized primary care. The Department of Medicine made available office space and support facilities. Dr. Martin as Division Director also assumed responsibility for the Wills Eye Hospital consultation service. The Division of General Medicine was renamed the Division of Internal Medicine under Department Chairman Dr. Willis C. Maddrey in 1983, with Dr. Martin continuing as its Director.

■ New Affiliations

The constant need for adequate numbers of patients to meet teaching needs, such as in physical diagnosis, prompted Dr. Gray to arrange with Coatesville Veterans Hospital and the Sacred Heart Hospital in Norristown to give adequate coverage to such educational disciplines. The course in Physical Diagnosis for Sophomore students was changed from minimal teaching contact spread over a large part of the year to a concentration particularly in the "miniclerkship" as directed by Dr. O.D. Kowlessar and Dr. Carla Goepp.

The affiliated hospitals continued to supplement the educational requisites for the Junior and Senior students. Visits and meetings by Dr. Gray and other members of his faculty with responsible physicians in each institution were conducted on a regular basis. The affiliation with Wills Hospital was strengthened by the establishment of a routine and an emergency consultation service, whereby a member of the Division of General Medicine would see the patient on call or by the end of the same day. The Wills Eye Hospital staff physician could call any physician who had privileges, but most availed themselves of this assured service. The Wilmington Veterans Administration Hospital became a "Dean's Hospital" in 1978. This meant that Jefferson's Dean and a joint Jefferson Medical College and Veterans Administration Committee had control over academic and professional affairs, especially the appointment of teaching faculty. The first full-time Chief of Medicine appointed under this plan was Dr. Brajesh N. Agarwal. This program made a major bid for additional resident staff, as did other affiliates, and at the same time there was increased need for resident coverage in the New Hospital at Jefferson. It was not until July of 1981 that Dr. Agarwal and Dr. Gray were able to establish a residency program at the Wilmington V. A. Hospital, and this was effected by rotation of Jefferson's residents through the Wilmington Hospital.

The number of Department of Medicine Residents, not counting Subspecialty Fellows, expanded from 56 to 82 during Dr. Gray's tenure as Chairman. The increase in residents and the increased commitment to the affiliates resulted in the decision (1980) to appoint two Chief Residents instead of one, beginning with the year 1982–1983. The other major change in the residency program was the establishment of set times for teaching rounds and conferences. This was a system that had been used previously but which seemed to fade out of usage. In 1979 a plan of geographic location of a teaching team with resident assignment that was proposed by a committee under the chairmanship of Dr. Michael Simenhoff was approved. In this plan a house staff unit had a "home floor" of approximately 32 beds with a chief, an associate chief, and several attending physicians. All patients of the members of this team were assigned to this area as far as was possible. This greatly enhanced the *esprit de corps* among the physicians, nurses, and students and contributed to patient care and the efficiency of the unit.

■ Lectureships

The Rehfuss Lecture, sponsored in 1963 by the late Mr. and Mrs. Percival Foerderer, continued as an annual event in the Department of Medicine. Prominent speakers were recruited and members of the Foerderer family were always in attendance. The Housel Lecture was also delivered annually, starting in 1981, to honor Dr. Edmund L. Housel (Jefferson, 1935). Dr. Housel had been the founder and long-time Director of the Jefferson Hypertension Clinic. A lecturer prominent in the field of cardiology was chosen accordingly, with special reference to hypertension.

Between 1977 and 1981, Dr. Mark Altschule, Emeritus Professor of Medicine at Harvard Medical School, served as annual Visiting Lecturer on varying subjects. His presentations were followed by hospital rounds with the residents. These lectures had previously been given at Lankenau during Dr. Gray's tenure there. The Department was awarded an Alpha Omega Alpha Visiting Professorship, the 1978 incumbent having been Dr. W. A. Tisdale from the University of Vermont. This visit extended for one week and included rounds, conferences, and lectures.

Progress in Departmental Divisions

Changes occurred in some of the Divisions during Dr. Gray's Chairmanship. The Division of Nephrology developed sophisticated units for inpatient and ambulatory dialysis, but the renal transplant program was still trying to reach its potential.

In 1978, the Division of Cardiology was stimulated by the opening of the Dr. Samuel Bellett Laboratory of Cardiac Catheterization in the New Hospital. New skills and equipment for physiologic studies signaled a major advance in diagnostic procedures. Dr. Sheldon Goldberg succeeded to direction of the Catheterization Laboratory in 1980. The Heart Station and Non-Invasive Laboratory were under the direction of Dr. Edward K. Chung, and the Division was directed by Dr. Albert N. Brest, since 1973 the Wilson Professor of Medicine. During Dr. Gray's Chairmanship, all of the research, clinical, and educational programs of the Division made significant progress.[71]

The Division of Infectious Diseases had been temporarily under the directorship of Dr. Joseph Gonnella because Dean Kellow had requested that the choice of a permanent director await the appointment of a new Chairman of Medicine. In 1977, Dr. Sheila A. Murphey was appointed Director of the Division. Dr. Murphey was trained in internal medicine and infectious diseases and came to Jefferson from the University of Pennsylvania. Her post at Jefferson included responsibilities as Epidemiologist to Thomas Jefferson University Hospital. In 1978 she recruited Dr. Erick J. Bergquist (Jefferson, 1973; Ph.D., University of Maryland) who quickly made his influence felt in clinical teaching and in the Antibiotic Review Program of the Hospital. Both Drs. Murphey and Bergquist had secondary appointments in the Department of Microbiology.

The Division of Rheumatology had made significant strides under the Directorship of Dr. Nathan M. Smukler. Whereas it had originally been two outpatient clinics, Smukler built a strong Division with good educational abilities, a fine consultative service, and facilities for laboratory research. Among the additions that occurred during Dr. Gray's tenure were the establishment of a Lupus Study Center in October of 1979 and the opening of new research laboratories on the sixth floor of the Curtis Building in June of 1981, under the direction of Dr. John L. Abruzzo, who had succeeded Dr. Smukler as Director the preceding year.

The treatment of malignant diseases assumed increasing importance during Dr. Gray's tenure, having reached 50 percent of admissions in the Department of Medicine. The aging population and the skills of department members were largely responsible. Dr. Gray perceived a need within and outside the Department for development of a center that would reach a level of excellence in patient care, teaching, and research, combining all of the oncologic activities of the Institution. Dr. William E. Delaney, III (Jefferson, 1953) was appointed Interim Director of the Division of Oncology in July, 1980. Dr. Delaney had previously been a member of the Surgical Pathology Staff of Jefferson Hospital, had transferred to St. Vincent's Hospital in New York City, and had then decided to become a clinician. He served an Internal Medicine Residency at the Lankenau Hospital and a two-year Fellowship in Medical Oncology at Johns Hopkins before returning to Jefferson with appointments in both Internal Medicine and Pathology. Dr. Delaney transferred to Lankenau Hospital after serving as Interim Director for just one year. Dr. Gray took over as Acting Director until he became Interim Dean, and then Dr. J. Frederick Laucius, one of Jefferson's outstanding clinical oncologists, was appointed Acting Director and served until Chairman Willis C. Maddrey appointed Dr. Michael J. Mastrangelo Director of the Division in 1983. Dr. Mastrangelo, a former Resident in Medicine at Jefferson, had been a member of the

Fox Chase Cancer Center in Suburban Philadelphia and had attained considerable acclaim for his work in immunology and malignant melanoma.

The Division of Endocrinology and Metabolic Diseases had lacked a strong guiding hand since the resignation of Dr. Joseph Rupp as Director in 1969 except for the year in which Dr. Richard Field served as Director (1970). Dr. Rupp had been Acting Director but his duties in the Dean's Office, particularly in the realm of Continuing Education, decreased the time that he could devote to the Division. Dr. Rupp had become an accomplished and popular lecturer on Continuing Education programs, traveling to many areas, especially in the State of Pennsylvania, talking mostly on endocrinological subjects. Taking matters into their own hands, the members of the Division who were interested in diabetes mellitus joined interested faculty from other departments and services to form the Interdisciplinary Diabetes Study Group, the first meeting of which was held December 1, 1976. In September of the following year Dr. Joseph A. Glennon was appointed Director of the Division and the first Kramer Professor of Medicine. This Professorship was endowed by the will of Dr. David W. Kramer (Jefferson, 1912), who had died in 1969. Dr. Glennon, a graduate of New York University, was certified in Internal Medicine, Endocrinology and Metabolism, and had particular interests in diabetes and obesity.

Intensive Care

The first Intensive Care Unit at Jefferson was established in the Thompson Annex in response to the request of Dr. John E. Deitrick while he was the Magee Professor (1952–1957). The use of the facility rather promptly came under such great demand that separate Medical and Surgical units were constructed. Dr. Gray had the final responsibility for the transfer of three of the Medical Department's Intensive Care Units to the New Hospital in 1978: the Pulmonary Intensive Care Unit, which had been established on the second floor of the Main (Old) Hospital in 1976; the General Medical Intensive Care Unit (the "first" as identified above); and the Cardiac Intensive Care Unit, which had been located in the Annex Building.

New Subdivisions

The establishment of a Clinical Pharmacology Unit at Jefferson had been considered for some time but hope for a concrete solution began with negotiations in 1976 between Jefferson and the pharmaceutical company Merck, Sharpe and Dohme. Dr. Roger K. Ferguson of the University of Eastern Michigan was appointed Director of the Clinical Pharmacology Unit and Professor of Medicine. The unit was in operation by 1977.

It was during Dr. Gray's Chairmanship that two hematologic units with close connections to the Cardeza Division of Hematology were established. The first was the completion of a contract between the Commonwealth of Pennsylvania and the Division of Hematology to establish a Sickle Cell Center at Jefferson with a satellite center at the Pennsylvania Hospital. Dr. Edward Burka was named Director. Second, the Division of Hematology/Cardeza Foundation received a federal grant in 1977 to establish a Hemophilia Center for research and service in hemophilia. Dr. Sandor S. Shapiro was the first Director of this unit. The Hemophilia Unit remained very active, with hundreds of patients registered, and in 1987 it continued to occupy its original site on the second floor of the Main (Old) Hospital. A short time after the establishment of the Sickle Cell Unit, Dr. Burka transferred to the Pennsylvania Hospital and Jefferson became the site of the satellite Clinic.

Departmental Faculty and Teaching

Dr. Gray, in his quiet and efficient manner, did many things to ensure the smooth functioning of the Medical Department and to enhance the correlation of its actions with other departments of the University. Representative activities included meetings with the Volunteer Faculty Organization, indicating his appreciation for their work in the Department, and the establishment of the Young Investigators Award (1978), a program allowing young investigators who had not hitherto had grants of their own to develop projects qualifying for federal grants. This proved more helpful as a research stimulus, especially for newly organized Divisions, than the Dean's overage research program, which was for approved but unfunded federal research grants. Dr. Gray was on hand to aid in the transfer to the New Hospital during its first year of occupancy (1978). In 1979 he established a Departmental word/text processing unit under the direction of Miss Frances Hylan, a unit that provided word processing, editorial work, storage/retrieval facilities, manuscript development, and related services for members of the Department and to other Jefferson Medical College faculty at cost.

The faculty of the Department of Medicine in 1981 totaled 445, of which 195 were based at Jefferson. The remainder were largely accounted for by the teaching programs in the affiliated hospitals (Bryn Mawr Hospital, Coatesville V.A. Hospital, Daroff Division of Albert Einstein Medical Center, Lankenau Hospital, Mercy Catholic Medical Center, Methodist Hospital, Our Lady of Lourdes Hospital, Sacred Heart Hospital, Norristown, Wilmington Medical Center, and Wilmington V.A. Hospital). Among the honors received by members of the faculty of the Department of Medicine were the presentations of portraits to Jefferson. Five were presented during Dr. Gray's Chairmanship: Charles W. Wirts, Jr., William F. Kellow, Robert C. Mackowiak, Nathan M. Smukler, and John H. Hodges.

Following a protracted illness, Dean William F. Kellow retired November 16, 1981 (he died on December 3), and Dr. Gray agreed to become Interim Dean, another instance of a member of the Department of Medicine succeeding to the Dean's Office. Dr. Gray continued as Interim Dean until the appointment of Dean Leah M. Lowenstein, D.Phil., M.D. Gray retired on June 31, 1982, and was honored by the presentation of his portrait (Figure 9-25) on that day. Dr. Gray's calm and exacting nature combined with a strong memory for facts enabled him to make a signal contribution to Jefferson's progress.

Dr. John H. Martin, the Vice-Chairman of the Department of Medicine, assumed the full duties of the Department on the day Dr. Gray occupied the Dean's Office. Dr. Martin continued in this role until the appointment of Dr. Willis C. Maddrey as Chairman and Magee Professor of the Department of Medicine became effective May 1, 1982.[67]

Willis Crocker Maddrey, M.D. (1939–); Fifteenth Chairman (1982–)

The first successful liver transplant performed at Jefferson on May 31, 1984, was an outcome of two short years of effort by the new Magee Professor of Medicine, Dr. Willis Crocker Maddrey (Figure 9-26). Thus was fulfilled one of the goals he had set forth after his May 1, 1982, arrival from the Johns Hopkins Medical School, where he had been Professor of Medicine and Associate Physician-in-Chief of the Department of Medicine. The transplant, an interdepartmental accomplishment, made possible by the temporary approval of the State Health Department, was followed by the establishment at Jefferson later that year of a permanent liver transplant center. The event signaled a milestone in the career of this brilliant, energetic, and perceptive planner. Maddrey was born March 29, 1939, in Roanoke Rapids, North Carolina, the son of Dr. Milner Crocker Maddrey (Jefferson, 1931) and Sara Jane Willis. The young Maddrey gave early evidence of his abilities when he graduated *summa cum laude* from Wake Forest University in 1960. His election to Alpha Omega Alpha followed at the Johns Hopkins School of Medicine, where he received the M.D. degree (1964). The paper on *Familial Cirrhosis*, published in 1964, concerned work he performed while in medical school and was an indication of his future pursuits.[72]

Dr. Maddrey's postgraduate training on the Hopkins Osler Service, which included one year of internship and three years of residency, was appropriately commended in his last year by appointment to the Chief Residency (1969–1970). Military service interrupted the residency (1966–1968) by duty in Calcutta, India, in the U.S.

Public Health Service under the auspices of the Office of International Research of the National Institutes of Health. A year as a Fellow in Liver Disease at Yale University under Dr. Gerald Klatskin was followed by his appointment as Assistant Professor of Medicine at Johns Hopkins. There he rose to Associate Director, Associate Physician-in-Chief, and Professor of Medicine. Honors at Johns Hopkins included the Henry Strong Denison Award in the Medical Sciences (1963–1964) and presentation by the Senior Class

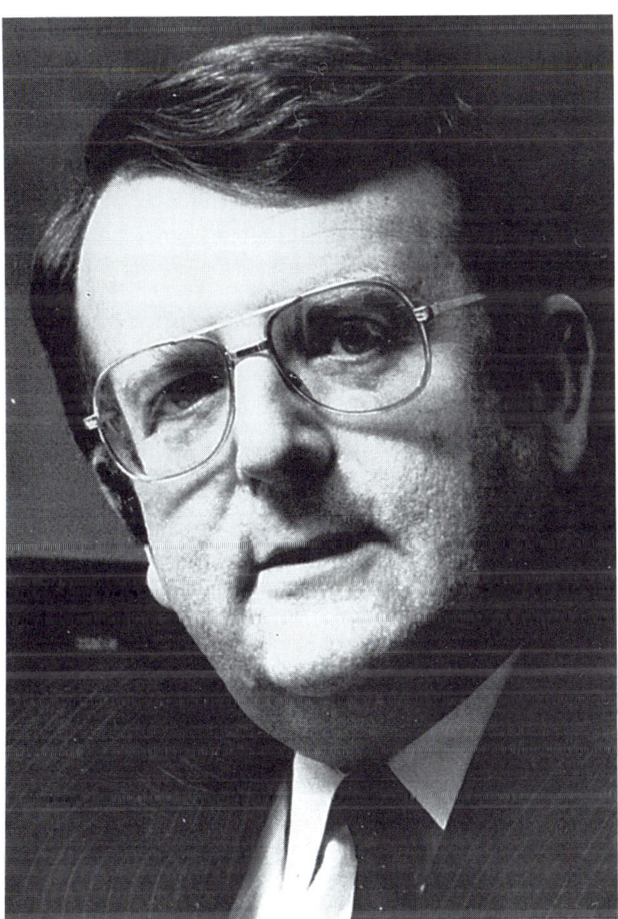

FIG. 9-26. Willis C. Maddrey, M.D. (1939–); Fifteenth Chairman (1982–).

of the George Stuart Outstanding Teacher Award (1970). An internationally recognized authority on liver disease, he coauthored a book, *Liver* (1984),[73] and contributed over 20 book chapters on hepatic topics. His early article in 1964 was followed by over 80 articles dealing principally with studies on liver-related problems. Maddrey's editorial abilities were recognized by his appointment as Associate Editor of *Medicine*, Consultant to the *American Journal of Medicine*, and membership on the editorial boards of *Viewpoints in Digestive Diseases*, *Hepatology*, and *Gastroenterology*, and the international advisory board of *Alimentary Pharmacology and Therapeutics*, as well as membership on the board of the American College of Physicians. He was also made a Regent in the latter organization.

A Diplomate of the American Board of Internal Medicine, Dr. Maddrey was a member of its Subspecialty Board and President of the Council of Subspecialty Societies. He was active in the National Institute on Alcohol Abuse and Alcoholism, and he served on the Board of Directors of the American Liver Foundation and of the Magee Hospital of Philadelphia.

Impact on Student Instruction

Schooled in the disciplines of administration and teaching, as well as patient care, Maddrey soon directed his attention to the role of the Department in its medical student instruction. It had been the custom to direct the Freshman class in first aid, emergency medicine, history taking, and physical diagnosis. By 1983 the formal teaching of freshmen by the Department was discontinued. Dr. Carla Goepp continued to direct the Sophomore course "Introduction to Clinical Medicine," which had been started in 1972. This consisted of lectures from most of the Departments of the Medical College with the aim of bringing the knowledge of the basic sciences into practical clinical application. These lectures were supplemented by case studies with slide demonstrations of laboratory findings. Physical diagnosis and history taking were taught throughout the year, with concentration toward the end of the year in a four-week miniclerkship at Jefferson or at one of 14 outlying hospitals. The Junior students had 12-week clerkships in which half of the time was spent at Jefferson and the other half at Lankenau, Our Lady of Lourdes,

Fitzgerald-Mercy, Misericordia, Medical Center of Delaware (Christiana), or Wilmington V. A. Hospital. Dr. Melissa A. McDiarmid was appointed coordinator for Junior medical affairs in 1982 and was succeeded by Dr. Joseph Majdan several years later. The Senior students served subinternships, a step above the Junior year in the hospital patient-care system. About half of the Seniors spent this time at Jefferson and the remainder at affiliated hospitals. The other activity for the Seniors was a choice of electives in the various subspecialties. In the summer of 1984, Dr. Maddrey appointed Dr. O. Dhodanand Kowlessar as Associate Chairman of the Department of Medicine for Educational Programs. Dr. Kowlessar's duties included coordination of the Departmental programs for medical students in the Sophomore, Junior, and Senior years, and active participation in the teaching program of the students both at Jefferson and the affiliated hospitals. Dr. Kowlessar was also in charge of the program for counseling the medical students regarding their curricula within Jefferson and for subsequent postdoctoral training.

The governance of the Department was further strengthened by assigning additional importance to the Executive and Advisory Committee, which met monthly and reviewed the activities of the Department for all matters relating to the medical staff. The Chairman of the Committee, Dr. Joseph Medoff (Jefferson, 1939)(Division of Gastroenterology), had played a similar role for nearly 30 years. The committee had been instrumental, more recently, in the development of the new programs regarding the Medical-Respiratory Intensive Care Unit (MRICU) and the renovations in the Hospital permitting increased facilities for the Medical Staff. The unbiased nature of Dr. Medoff's opinions made them of special value to Chairmen and Deans.

Dr. Medoff was made sponsor of the Hobart A. Hare Medical Society in 1961. Through his continuing efforts the society underwent a rejuvenation and was established as an Honor Society for the Department of Medicine. Dr. Medoff and his wife and children established the Philip and Bella Medoff Memorial Prize for a Senior member of the Hare Society in honor of Dr. Medoff's parents. The members of the Society presented Dr. Medoff's portrait to Jefferson in 1976 as a tribute to his accomplishments on its behalf. In addition, Dr. Medoff and his wife Elinor had established the Alexander and Lottie Katzman Award in Gastroenterology in honor of Mrs. Medoff's parents.

Plans and Progress

Dr. Maddrey's goals for the Department included strengthening the clinical research base while expanding the educational and patient care programs.[74] He initiated a five-year plan in pursuit of these goals through recruitment of talented new faculty. He recognized Jefferson's historical strength as a center for teaching and patient care and indicated that the development of clinical research would promote excellence in clinical care. Research support for the Department, during the first four years of Dr. Maddrey's Chairmanship, grew from approximately \$2½ million to \$8 million. Although this was good growth, it was not the desirable amount Dr. Maddrey wished to have to establish the Department as a major force in biomedical research. The Department budget increased about fourfold to nearly \$20 million a year. The full-time faculty, 50 percent of whom he had recruited, was by 1986 generating nearly \$9 million yearly for the Practice Plan.

Teaching Leadership

Teaching flowed from Dr. Maddrey as a natural talent. Medical grand rounds was a weekly exercise that had been an educational device of the Department in some form for many decades. The presentation of an actual clinical case, with discussion related to the particular medical problem, survived up to the demise of the clinical amphitheatre in the mid-1960s. Since then a case presentation, usually in the absence of the actual patient, had been the rule. Dr. Maddrey changed this to two case presentations, reminiscent of the procedure at Hammersmith Hospital in London, England, each case followed by succinct discussions by experts in the field and then audience participation in a question and answer session. Dr. Maddrey's broad knowledge, quick grasp of a situation, and wit in his role as moderator, stimulated discussion and added wisdom to these excellent teaching sessions. He cherished his contacts with the students on teaching rounds in the hospital and attempted to know each one personally. He received the Christian R. and Mary F. Lindback Award for Distinguished Teaching in the Clinical Sciences in 1986.

The Jefferson medical residency continued to grow in popularity. There were over 1,200 applicants in the 1987–1988 class for 39 positions to maintain a total of 90 house officers. This contrasted with approximately 300 applications for 31 positions in the 1981–1982 session. The residents had clinical and teaching experience at Jefferson and at one or more of these affiliated hospitals: Our Lady of Lourdes, Methodist, and Wilmington V.A. This program was under Dr. O.D. Kowlessar as part of the total Jefferson residency program under the direction of the Dean and his staff. The Departmental Selection Committee was headed by Dr. Erick Bergquist, who was later succeeded by Dr. Howard Weitz. Nine of the 13 Divisions of the Department had fellows, the highest number of fellows having reached 11 in the Division of Cardiology for the year 1985–1986.

The Divisions of the Department of Medicine

The continued maturity of the subspecialties in medicine saw their development in the Department of Medicine grow to 13 distinct Divisions by the year 1986, when a Division was defined by the Executive Council as "an academic unit structured as a major distinct but subordinate administrative unit of a department within the medical college. It shall have a high level of educational, service and research responsibilities, an appropriate administrative structure, and a function commensurate with the mission of the department." Specific criteria for the formation, cessation, membership, function, and administration of a Division were specifically delineated. Each division had a Director who was appointed by the Chairman. Each member of the Department had a primary appointment in a Division and occasionally in more than one.

As the detailed history of the specific Divisions will show in subsequent chapters, they evolved from clinics or less well-structured units under the aegis of the Department and were organized as Divisions at varying times in recent decades. A brief resume of the status of each Division as of 1987, especially relative to personnel recruited and research development, follows.

Hematology

The Division of Hematology (1941) continued to progress under Dr. Sandor Shapiro, who succeeded Dr. Allan J. Erslev as Director on June 30, 1985. Dr. Erslev was designated Distinguished Professor, one of the highest honors of the University. He had pioneered in the development of knowledge of humoral regulation of red cell production and supported the theory of the major role of the kidney in the production of the factor erythropoietin.[75,76] In 1987 his editorial was published in the *New England Journal of Medicine* in response to an accompanying article reporting successful clinical trials of recombinant human erythropoietin in the correction of the anemia of end-stage renal disease.[77,78,79] The erythropoietin work continued at Jefferson with a National Institutes of Health grant to Dr. Jaime Caro. The Division's other activities included Dr. Shapiro's studies of hemostasis and hemophilia, Dr. Scott Murphy's studies on preservation of platelets, Dr. Jose Martinez on fibrinogen, and Dr. Stephen Hauptman on lymphocyte transfusion in patients with acquired immune deficiency syndrome (AIDS). Dr. Farid Haurani retired in December of 1987

Pulmonary Medicine

The Division of Pulmonary Medicine (1946) was stimulated in 1985 by the arrival of Dr. James E. Fish and Dr. Stephen Peters as Director and Associate respectively. In 1986, Dr. Jonathan Gottlieb was recruited from Yale to head the newly developed Medicine-Respiratory Intensive Care Unit (MRICU). Drs. Fish and Gottlieb were developing a Critical Care Medicine Program while members of the Division continued research on airway resistance and inflammation. Dr. Harold L. Israel, international expert on sarcoidosis, joined the fulltime staff in 1985.

Gastroenterology and Hepatology

The Division of Gastroenterology and Hepatology (1946) was headed by Dr. Steven R. Peiken as Acting Director. Peiken spent the latter part of 1986 in England on sabbatical leave studying with Dr. Graham Dockray and further developing his research into the effects of cholecystokinin analogues on satiety. Dr. Maddrey served as Director during his absence. Early in 1987, Dr. Eckhart G. Hahn, one of the foremost world authorities on collagen metabolism and the mechanisms of cell injury, was recruited from the University of West Berlin as Director of the Division. On June 16, 1987, Dr. Hahn was formally installed as the first Rorer Professor in Medicine. The relationship of Jefferson and the Rorer Group dated back to the 1940s when members of the Department of Medicine conducted clinical trials of Rorer's prominent antacid in Jefferson Hospital. The approximate $1 million that established the Professorship in 1983 was the culmination of discussions between Rorer and the University during the Decade Fund Drive. The source of the endowment was the combination of the charitable trust contributions of Herbert C. Rorer and Gerald F. Rorer, the sons of William H. Rorer, the founder of the Company, and the corporate contribution of Rorer Group Inc. Plans for the Division included a new endoscopy and clinical area for advanced technical procedures, including the use of lasers.

Infectious Diseases

The Division of Infectious Diseases (1957) played an important role in the control of infections in the Hospital while its Director, Dr. Sheila A. Murphey, continued research on *Staphylococcus aureus*. Dr. Hans H. Liu joined the staff from Rockefeller University on March 1, 1986. His Daland Fellowship provided for the study of the mechanism of induction of bacterial drug resistance and analysis of infections in human liver transplantation. Dr. Erick Bergquist resigned his position in mid-1987.

Rheumatology

The Division of Rheumatology (1959) with Dr. John Abruzzo, Director, cooperated in the development of a comprehensive bone center with responsibility shared by Drs. Abruzzo, Joseph A. Glennon, Director of Endocrinology, and Eric L. Hume of the Department of Orthopedics. Dr. J. Bruce Smith was expanding his research into immune functions with special emphasis on the autologous mixed lymphocyte reaction and its mediation by cellular factors. Dr. Maureen H. Bocchieri continued her work studying the oncogenic aspects of T-lymphocytes.

Nephrology

The Division of Nephrology (1961) under Dr. Michael Simenhoff continued responsibilities in the field of renal transplantation, while Dr. James F. Burke, Associate Director, was responsible for dialysis. He cooperated with Dr. Bruce E. Jarrell in the renal transplant procedure with 80 transplants in 1986 compared to 70 in 1985. During the 1985–1986 period, Dr. Burke conducted approximately 1,000 acute dialysis procedures, and Dr. George C. Francos conducted the 14 chronic dialysis units for 100 patients, 20 of whom were employing home dialysis.

Oncology

The Division of Oncology (1961) continued to be highly visible and increasingly active. Dr. Michael J. Mastrangelo, who was appointed Director in 1984, relieving Acting Director Dr. J. Frederick Laucius, proceeded to develop laboratory research programs that would address central issues in the biology and treatment of cancer. The new laboratory program was headed by Dr. David Berg. Dr. Mastrangelo's primary interest was in immuno-adaptive therapy of patients with cancer with particular emphasis on melanoma. Drs. H. S. Brodovsky, L. J. Rose, C. M. Southam, and A. J. Weiss continued to be active in the Division. Financial resources of the Division, virtually nonexistent in 1982, amounted to about $1 million in 1986. The Division was well poised for skilled and sensitive approaches to this important research and clinical area of medicine.

Endocrinology and Metabolic Diseases

The Division of Endocrinology and Metabolic Diseases (1961) (which had replaced the Division of Endocrine and Cancer Research of 1949) under Dr. Joseph A. Glennon, recruited Dr. Steven B. Nagelberg, formerly of the National Institutes of Health. Dr. Nagelberg continued the study of the beta subunits of gonadotropins until he left Jefferson in January of 1987. Dr. Boas Gonen continued his work in the field of lipoprotein research and its application to clinical medicine. Dr. Joseph A. Glennon resigned in 1987 after completing ten years as Director of the Division.

Cardiology

The Division of Cardiology (1964) by 1986 had progressed to nine full-time members under Dr. Albert N. Brest, the first James C. Wilson Professor of Medicine (Cardiology). Dr. Sheldon Goldberg, who had pioneered coronary angioplasty at Jefferson, was in charge of the new cardiac catheterization laboratory that had opened in 1985. A new cardiovascular research laboratory was developed in 1986 directed toward methods of reducing the size and severity of myocardial infarcts in experimental situations. To further develop the programs in electrophysiology, Dr. Gregory Kidwell was recruited to work with Dr. Arnold J. Greenspon. The strength of this Division was maintained and enhanced by a part-time staff of 20 outstanding clinical cardiologists at Jefferson and others at affiliated hospitals.

General Internal Medicine

The Division of General Internal Medicine (1968), having been changed in name to the Division of Internal Medicine in 1983, was under the acting directorship of Dr. Geno J. Merli following the resignation of Dr. John H. Martin on March 1, 1986. Dr. Merli was appointed Director on February 23, 1987. The Division was pursuing clinical research especially in the prevention and treatment of thrombosis in postoperative states and in spinal cord–injured patients. In 1987, extensive renovation of the clinical offices was underway in the New Hospital to be used by the Chairman and the Divisions of Internal Medicine, Nephrology, Pulmonary Diseases, and Endocrinology.

Genetics

The Division of Genetics (1968) under Dr. Laird G. Jackson was responsible for the first use in this country of chorionic villus sampling for the detection of congenital defects early in gestation (1985). Dr. Jackson and members of the Division of Oncology were cooperating in research on the genetics of colon cancer. Dr. Susan Z. Cowchock, Associate Professor of Medicine, and Dr. J. Bruce Smith of the Division of Rheumatology were investigating the possibilities of an immunologic basis for recurrent abortion.

Occupational and Environmental Medicine and Toxicology

The Division of Occupational and Environmental Medicine and Toxicology (1983) was formally established in July, 1983. The new Division was an outgrowth of an earlier section of Pharmacology plus previous functions of the Department of Community Health and Preventive Medicine. Dr. Maddrey headed the new Division until October, 1984, when Dr. Lance L. Simpson became Director with the dual title of Professor of Medicine and Pharmacology.[80] Dr. Simpson was awarded a contract from the Department of Defense to continue his work on bacterial toxins, having previously received the Jacob Javits Award for outstanding research in neurobiology. Dr. Maddrey had objectives for the Division that included a student educational program, research, continuing education, and a resource for persons exposed to environmental hazards. It was also planned that the Division would participate in clinical activities of the Health Maintenance Program under Dr. Joseph F. Rodgers following the retirement of Dr. Willard A. Krehl.

Clinical Pharmacology

In 1986, Dr. Thorir D. Bjornsson, from Duke University, became Director of the Division of Clinical Pharmacology, pursuing his investigation of anticoagulants and the endothelial cell culture evaluation of mechanisms of atherogenesis.

On November 19, 1987, Dr. Maddrey appointed Dr. Lawrence Samuel Friedman as Vice-Chairman of the Department, describing him as a gifted teacher and superb clinician. A native of Newark, New Jersey, Dr. Friedman attended Princeton University, followed by studies at Johns Hopkins University where he received the B.A. in 1975, the M.D. in 1978, and his Internship and Residency training at the Johns Hopkins Hospital (1978–1981) where, like Drs. McCrae and Maddrey, he served on the Osler Service. Subsequent to a year as a Research Fellow in Medicine at Harvard he had a three-year Fellowship in Gastroenterology under Dr. Kurt J. Isselbacher at the Massachusetts General Hospital. A member of Phi Beta Kappa and Alpha Omega Alpha, Friedman received teaching awards at Hopkins and later at Jefferson following his appointment to the staff in 1984. He has been a prolific writer, with major interest in inflammatory bowel disease and liver problems, and has been prominent in national societies.

The Department of Medicine has experienced many significant changes over the years. From a single Professor in 1824, Medicine has become the largest Department, with faculty numbering in the hundreds and Divisions of subspecialties numbering 13. Included in the entire faculty, a very large number of physicians have volunteered their services to the Department. The quality and significance of their contributions have been inestimable.

The changes in Departmental functions reflect the complexity of medical progress, the evolution of hospitals, the conquest of diseases, especially infections, and major developments in medical education. Patient care at Jefferson Hospital has assumed tertiary status but the needs of students continue to command priority at all levels. Each Chairman through the years has perceived his time-related mission differently, but each has accomplished major goals during his tenure. Molecular medicine is already well established at Jefferson and in this new era the Department is substantially involved.

References

1. Williams, S.W., "Medical Improvement and Discoveries of the Last Half-Century: United States of America," *The Franklin Med. Assoc. of the State of Mass.*, 1852.
2. Henry, F.P., *Standard History of the Medical Profession of Philadelphia*. Chicago: Goodspeed Brothers, 1897.
3. Soule, S.D., *Medicine in St. Louis Medical Schools in the Nineteenth Century*. 1850.
4. *The American Medical Recorder*. Vol. 1. Philadelphia: James Webster, 1818.
5. Klapp, J.: *Trans. of the Med. Soc. of the State of Penn.*, Vol. 17, Philadelphia: 1885.
6. Eberle, J., "Notes on the Theory and Practice of Medicine delivered in the Jefferson Medical College at Philadelphia." Philadelphia: J.G. Auner, 1827.
7. Eberle, J., *A Treatise on the Practice of Medicine*. 2d ed., Philadelphia: John Grigg, 1831.
8. Eberle, J., *A Treatise on the Materia Medica and Therapeutics*. 2d ed. Baltimore: S. and W. Meeteer; and Philadelphia: James Webster, 1825.
9. Gould, G.M.: *The Jefferson Medical College of Philadelphia*. New York: Lewis, 1904.
10. Farmer, H.E., "The Golden Calf," *Bryn Mawr Hosp. Bull.*, Vol. 3, No. 2, Winter, 1981.
11. Major, R.H., "Daniel Drake," *A History of Medicine*. Vol. 2. Springfield, Mass.: Charles C. Thomas Co., 1954.
12. "Special Communications: Daniel Drake." *JAMA*, 254:2111–2118, 1985.
13. Brinton, J.H., *The Faculty of 1841*. Philadelphia: Collins, Printer, 1880.
14. *Annual Announcement of Lectures (Jefferson Medical College)*, 1832.
15. *Idem* 13, 1836.
16. *Idem* 13, 1843.
17. Dickson, S.H., *Elements of Medicine: A Compendium View of Pathology and Therapeutics; or the History and Treatment of Diseases*. Philadelphia: Blanchard and Lea, 1859.
18. Conver, P.S., "Opening Address, Jefferson Medical College," October 2, 1899.
19. DaCosta, J.M., "On Irritable Heart." *Am. J. Med. Sc.* 61:17–52, 1871.
20. "The Jefferson Medical College of Philadelphia and its Hospital," *Annual Announcement*. No. 71 (1895–1896).
21. Wilson, J.C., "The Care of the Convalescent," *Trans. Stud. Coll. Phys. Phila.*, 3d Ser. XLVI: 155–171, 1924.
22. Personal communication.
23. Wise, R.I., *Centrifugal and Centripetal Forces: A History of the Department of Medicine, The Jefferson Medical College of Thomas Jefferson University (1959–1975)*. 1986, p. 197. (In Jefferson Archives).
24. Osler, W., and McCrae, T., *Cancer of the Stomach: A Clinical Study*. Philadelphia: P. Blakiston's Son & Co., 1900, p. 157.
25. McCrae, T., "Acute Lymphatic Leukemia," *Br. Med. J.* February 25, 1905.
26. Cushing, H., *The Life of Sir William Osler*. Oxford Univ. Press, 1925.
27. Ezell, S.D., M.D. (Jefferson, 1932), "Thomas McCrae—Personal Recollections, 1985." (In Jefferson Archives).
28. Wallach, A.: "Editorial." *Ann. Med. Hist.*, New Ser. 8, 1936, pp. 371–375.
29. McCrae, T., *Trans. Assoc. Am. Phys.* 50:15–23, 1935.
30. *Jefferson Medical College Circular of Information*. 1912–1913.
31. Bauer, E.L., *Doctors Made in America*. Philadelphia: J.B. Lippincott Co., 1963.
32. Hare, H.A., *A Text-book of Practical Therapeutics*. Philadelphia: Lea Brothers & Co., 1890.
33. Osler, Sir W., McCrae, T. (Ed.), and Funk, E.H. (Asst. Ed.), *Modern Medicine*. 3d Ed., Philadelphia: Lea & Febiger, 1925.
34. DaCosta, J.C., Jr., *Clinical Hematology*. Philadelphia: P. Blakiston's Son, 1901, p. 474.

35. McCrae, T., and Jackson, C., "The Clinical Features of Foreign Bodies in the Bronchi." *Lancet*. No. 1, 1924, p. 735 (April 3), p. 787 (April 8), p. 838 (April 10).
36. McCrae, T., Funk, E.H., and Jackson, C., "Primary Carcinoma of the Bronchus," *JAMA* 89:1–20, 1927.
37. McCrae, T., *Tumors in Syphilis of the Liver—Contribution to Medicine and Biological Research*. (Dedicated to Sir William Osler), 1919, Vol. 2, p. 985–990.
38. McCrae, T., "The Influence of William Osler on Medicine in America," *Can. Med. Assoc. J.* July 1920, pp. 78–81.
39. Duncan, G.G., *Diabetis Mellitus and Obesity*. Philadelphia: Lea & Febiger, 1935, p. 215.
40. Gwyn, N., "Thomas McCrae, M.D. Memorial" *Can. Med. Assoc. J.*, 33:224, 1935.
41. Reimann, H.A., *Autobiography* (unpublished).
42. Reimann, H.A., *Treatment in General Medicine*. Philadelphia: F.A. Davis Co., 1936.
43. Reimann, H.A., "*Micrococcus Tetragenous* Infection." *J. Clin. Invest.* 14:311–319, 1935.
44. Reimann, H.A., Kouchy, A.F., and Ecklund, C.M.: "Primary Amyloidosis Limited to Tissue of Mesodermal Origin," *Am. J. Pathol.* 11:977–989, 1935.
45. Reimann, H.A., *The Pneumonias*. Philadelphia and London: Saunders and Co., 1938; Springfield: Charles C Thomas, 1954; St. Louis, Warren H. Green, Inc., 1971.
46. Reimann, H.A., "An Acute Infection of the Respiratory Tract with Atypical Pneumonia: A Disease Entity Probably Caused by a Filterable Virus," *JAMA* 111:2377–2384, December 24, 1938.
47. "Landmark Articles in Medicine." Ed. by Harriet S. Meyer and George D. Lundberg. *Am. Med. Assoc.*, 1985.
48. Reimann, H.A., Price, A.H., and Hodges, J.H., "The Cause of Epidemic Diarrhea, Nausea and Vomiting (Viral Dysentery?)," *Proc. Soc. Exper. Biol. & Med.* 59:8–9, 1945.
49. Reimann, H.A., Price, A.H., and Hodges, J.H., "Epidemic Diarrhea, Nausea and Vomiting of Unknown Cause," *JAMA* 127:1–6, 1945.
50. Reimann, H.A., "A Review of Infectious Diseases," *Arch. Intern. Med.* (1935–1962): *Postgrad. Med. J.* (1963–1975).
51. Reimann, H.A., Chang, G.C.T., Chu, L.W., Liss, P.Y., and Ou, Y.: "Asiatic cholera—Clinical Study and Experimental Therapy with Streptomycin," *Am. J. Trop. Med.* 26:631–647, 1945.
52. Reimann, H.A.: "Focal Infection and Systemic Disease: Critical Appraisal." *Address at the American Med. Assoc. Convention,"* St. Louis, May 16, 1939.
53. Reimann, H.A., "The Problems of Long-Continued Low-Grade Fever," *JAMA* 107:1089–1093, 1936.
54. Reimann, H.A., *Periodic Diseases*. Philadelphia: F.A. Davis Co., 1963, pp. 1–189.
55. *The Pretzel Vendor*. Cover, *JAMA*, Vol. 221, No. 1, July 3, 1972.
56. Tocantins, L.M., "The Mammalian Blood Platelet in Health and Disease," *Medicine* 17:175, 1938.
57. *Jeff. Med. Coll. Al. Bull.*, December, 1951, pp. 5–9.
58. Rehfuss, M.E., Albrecht, K.K. and Price, A.H., *A Course in Practical Therapeutics*. Baltimore: The Williams and Wilkins Co., 1948.
59. Deitrich, J.E. (Director), and Berson, R.C. (Assoc. Director), *Medical Schools in the United States at Mid-Century*. XXII, 380 pp., New York: McGraw-Hill, 1953.
60. Wise, R.I., "The Magee Professor—History and Heritage," *Jeff. Med. Coll. Al. Bull.*, Spring 1975, pp. 4–17.
61. Personal communications.
62. Deitrick, J.E., "Teaching of Clinical Specialities," *J. Med. Ed.* Vol. 30, No. 5, May, 1955; "The Primary Responsibilities of the Medical Schools," *Bull. N.Y. Acad. Med.* 53:473–479, 1977; "Survey of Medical Education (Preliminary Observation)," *JAMA* 124:1122–1124, 1950.
63. Personal communications.
64. William Anthony Sodeman, M.D., *Bull., Tulane Med. Fac.* 12:81, 1953.
65. Williams, W.J., Beutler, E., Erslev, A.J., and Rundles, R.W., *Hematology*. 2d Ed. New York: McGraw-Hill Book Co. 1977.
66. Jackson, L., and Schimke, R.N., *Clinical Genetics*. New York: John Wesley and Sons, 1979.
67. "Records of the Office of the Dean, Jefferson Medical College," Philadelphia.
68. Gray, F.D., Jr., "Student Programs in a Community Hospital," *AHME Journal*, 5:35–38, 1972.
69. Gray, F.D., Jr., Personal communication.
70. Gray, F.D., Jr., *Pulmonary Embolism*. Philadelphia: Lea and Febiger, 1966.
71. Gray, F.D., Jr., and Martin, J.H., *Department of Medicine Annual Report: Jefferson Medical College of Thomas Jefferson University*. July 1, 1981, to June 30, 1982.
72. Maddrey, W.C., and Iber, F.L., "Familial Cirrhosis: A Clinical and Pathological Study." *Ann. Int. Med.* 61:667–679, 1964.
73. Williams, R., and Maddrey, W.C., *Liver*. London: Butterworth, 1984.
74. Maddrey, W.C.: *Jeff. Med. Coll. Al. Bull.* Winter 1984, pp. 8–12.
75. Erslev, A., "Humoral Regulation of Red Cell Production," *Blood* 8:349–357, 1953.
76. Jacobson, L.O., et al., "Role of the kidney in erythropoiesis," *Nature* 179:633–634, 1953.
77. Erslev, Allan, "Erythropoietin Coming of Age," *N.E. Jour. Med.* 316:101–103, 1987.
78. Eschbach, J.W., et al., "Correction of the Anemia of End Stage Renal Disease with Recombinant Human Erythropoietin," *N.E. Jour. Med.* 316, 73–78, 1987
79. Winearls, C.G., et al., "Effect of Human Erythropoietin Derived from Recombinant DNA on the Anemia of Patients Maintained by Chronic Dialysis," *Lancet* 2:1175–1178, 1986.
80. *Jeff. Med. Coll. Al. Bull.* Fall 1984, p. 13.

CHAPTER TEN

Division of Hematology

Allan J. Erslev, M.D.

"The blood is the life."

—Deuteronomy 12:23

In the early part of this century medicine began to change from an art to a science, from observation and palliation to testing and treatment. This change was associated with an increasing demand for doctors to be informed and experienced in the management of all illnesses, and it became more and more difficult to live up to the Oslerian tradition of being a complete general physician. The field was too great; many physicians began to restrict their study to certain diseases and became recognized not for their breadth of knowledge but rather for their narrow competence in the malfunction of a single organ. At Jefferson, John Chalmers DaCosta, Jr., a cousin of John Chalmers DaCosta, the Gross Professor of Surgery, was the first American physician to write a textbook on hematology (Figure 10-1). This textbook, entitled *Clinical Hematology,* was first published in 1901 and predated Wintrobe's famous textbook of the same name by 41 years. A second edition appeared in 1905 and was used in the teaching of medical students during their rotation in the newly created Laboratory of Clinical Medicine. This laboratory, first installed in the Jefferson Medical College Annex building on Tenth Street, was then considered one of the first and most advanced developments in the use of a laboratory for medical teaching. It was directed in turn by Doctors Erwin D. Funk, Henry Mohler, and Harold Jones, but it was under Dr. Jones' leadership that it first became hematologically oriented.

Early Hematology at Jefferson

Dr. Harold W. Jones (1891–1959), after graduation from Jefferson in 1917, served as a Lieutenant in the Army Medical Corp at Fort Oglethorpe. From 1919 to 1921 he was Chief Resident physician at Jefferson (Figure 10-2). He practiced for a while as a general internist, but after being put in charge of the Laboratory of Clinical Medicine his interest turned to disorders of the blood. One of the main functions of the course in Laboratory Medicine then as now was to teach medical students how to examine and observe blood, but he realized that there was very little clinical or pathophysiologic follow-up. He suggested to Dr. Thomas McCrae, the Magee Professor of the Principles and Practice of Medicine, that Jefferson should establish what we now would designate as the Division of Hematology. Specifically, he suggested the development of three facilities: one for the accurate study of patients with blood disorders by specially trained technical and professional personnel; one consisting of laboratories for the long-term study of fundamental aspects of blood diseases; and one for a facility to provide transfusions of carefully matched blood.

The present Division of Hematology was an outgrowth of these early ideas, but until 1939 no organizational facility could be established because of lack of funds. Nevertheless, Dr. Jones proceeded with independent and unfunded studies of blood diseases and blood transfusions. He published widely and wrote a number of textbook articles dealing with the problems of anemia, hemorrhagic disorders, and the direct and indirect transfusion of blood.[1] Jones was one of the founders of the Jefferson Society for Clinical Investigation at his alma mater. Nationally, he was known as an outstanding physician and hematologist, was elected to fellowship in the American College of Physicians, and was made a member of the Association of American Physicians and the Interurban Club.

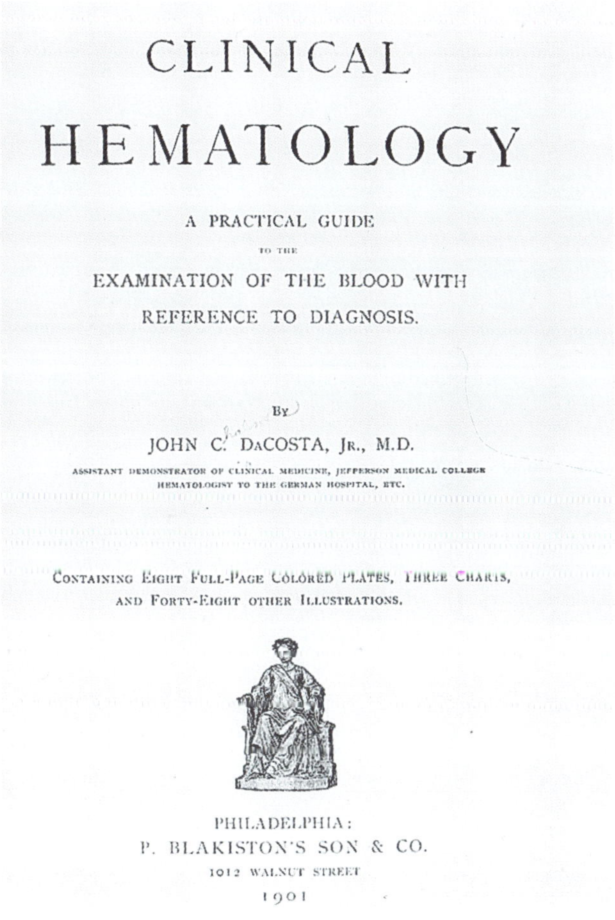

CLINICAL

HEMATOLOGY

A PRACTICAL GUIDE

TO THE

EXAMINATION OF THE BLOOD WITH

REFERENCE TO DIAGNOSIS.

BY

JOHN C. DACOSTA, JR., M.D.

ASSISTANT DEMONSTRATOR OF CLINICAL MEDICINE, JEFFERSON MEDICAL COLLEGE

HEMATOLOGIST TO THE GERMAN HOSPITAL, ETC.

CONTAINING EIGHT FULL-PAGE COLORED PLATES, THREE CHARTS,

AND FORTY-EIGHT OTHER ILLUSTRATIONS.

PHILADELPHIA:

P. BLAKISTON'S SON & CO.

1012 WALNUT STREET

1901

FIG. 10-1. First American textbook of hematology (1901), by John Chalmers DaCosta, Jr., M.D.

■ Leandro M. Tocantins (1901–1963)

In his work and hematologic interests Jones was supported by Dr. Leandro M. Tocantins (1901–1963), a young Brazilian-born physician who graduated from Jefferson Medical College in the Class of 1926 after a classic premedical education abroad and at Cornell University (Figure 10-3). He interned at Chestnut Hill Hospital and then practiced general medicine for three years in Cleveland, Ohio. Tocantins returned to Jefferson and became a J. Ewing Mears Research Teaching Fellow until 1936, after which he received a faculty appointment. Dr. Tocantins early became involved in the study of hemostasis and blood coagulation, but his interests were, like those of Dr. Jones, directed at all aspects of hematology. He published widely on such diverse subjects as anti-platelet serum, urine anti-thromboplastin, bone marrow infusions, lipid anticoagulants, and abnormal hemoglobins. As a special student of bleeding disorders, his name became linked to the effect of inhibitors of blood coagulation and especially the hypothesis that hemophilia is caused

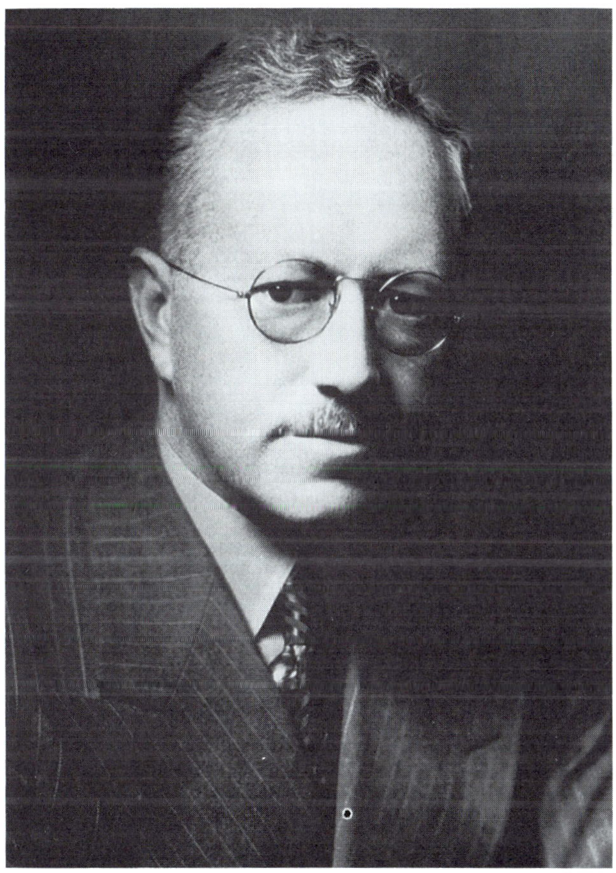

FIG. 10-2. Harold W. Jones, M.D. (1891–1959).

by such inhibitors. His work on blood platelets resulted in the classic monograph *Mammalian Blood Platelets in Health and Disease,* published in 1938, which exerted a major influence on subsequent studies of this blood component.[2] Tocantins also spearheaded the field of autoimmunity by infusing an anti-platelet serum and producing thrombocytopenia. This study led to attempts to treat both idiopathic thrombocytopenic purpura and acquired hemolytic anemia with macrophage blocking agents such as radioactive gold.

These were years in which investigators provided for their own livelihood through busy medical practice and squeezed research into spare hours and free weekends. The new Magee Professor of Medicine, Dr. Hobart A. Reimann, was keenly aware of that and hoped for a day when investigators could be released from the burden of full-time practice and devote a major part of their time to scientific investigation within their special fields. Dr. Reimann was also a strong supporter of Dr. Jones' effort to develop a Division of Hematology, but funds were needed to fulfill these dreams. It was not until 1939, when Mr. and Mrs. Thomas D. Cardeza became interested in the project, that substantial backing was obtained for the development of a research-oriented Division of Hematology.

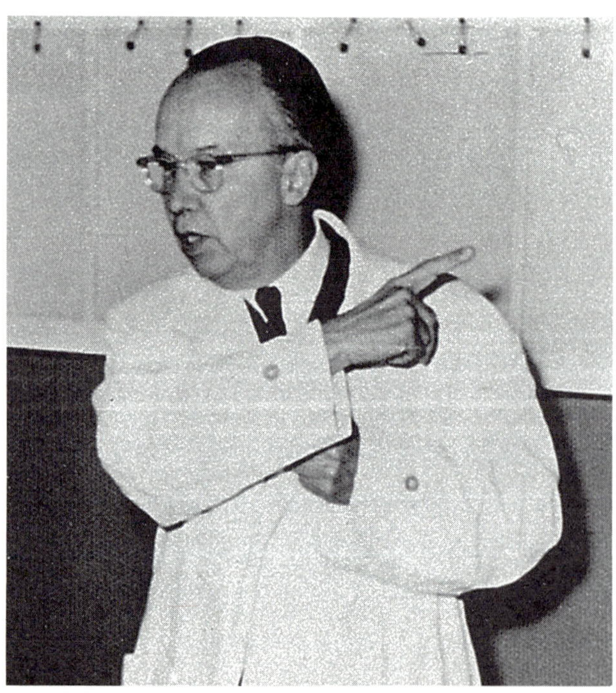

FIG. 10-3. Leandro M. Tocantins, M.D. (1901–1963).

The Cardeza Foundation

Mr. Thomas Drake Martinez Cardeza (1875–1952) was the last scion of the Drake family, which came to the United States from Leeds, England in 1828 (Figure 10-4). His ancestors Thomas Drake (1807–1890) and his brother moved to Philadelphia from Ohio in 1837 and established a small woolen mill in Manayunk. They began to manufacture jeans under the trade name of "Kentucky Jeans." Their business prospered with the establishment of

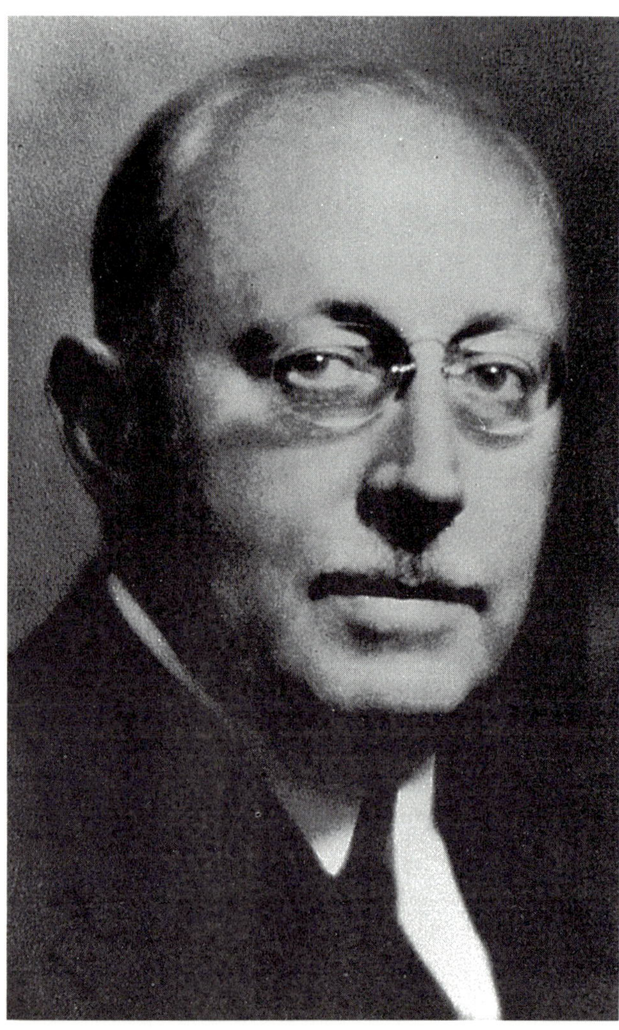

FIG. 10-4. Thomas Drake Martinez Cardeza (1875–1952).

additional mills near the present South Street Bridge and at Twenty-first and Pine Streets. With the heavy demand for woolens by the Union Army, further expansion took place, and at the end of the Civil War Thomas Drake retired a wealthy man. He was highly respected in the business community and was able to augment his fortune with successful investments in real estate. He held a number of trusteeships and was an organizer and director of the old Fidelity Trust Company, a position he held until his death in 1890. With his wife Matilda and seven children, Mr. Drake lived the style of the very rich. In his large estate in Germantown he had a small zoo, with free-roaming elks and bison, and kennels for Great Dane dogs. Sadly, six of his seven children died at a young age, many from scarlet fever, leaving Charlotte Drake (1854–1939) as the sole heiress to his fortune.

In 1874, Charlotte married James Warburton Martinez Cardeza, the grandson of Count Juan Martinez Cardeza, a nobleman from La Coruna, Spain. However, after her only son Thomas was born, she divorced and from then on devoted her life to her son and to the sports and pleasures of the leisure class (Figure 10-5). She and Thomas circumnavigated the globe on her steam ocean-going yacht, *The Eleanor,* with its crew of 39 and guest rooms for 16 (Figure 10-6). As an ardent and accomplished hunter she pursued big game in India and Africa. She and Thomas maintained a hunting lodge at Moose Head Lake in Maine, a shooting establishment in Montana, and a hunting Schloss in Austria. She was also a patron of the opera and of the Academy of Music, and was a witty and beautiful lady of high society in Philadelphia. In 1912, she and Thomas were on the *Titanic* together but both survived (Figure 10-7). All kinds of rumors were circulated afterwards about how Thomas had gotten into a lifeboat, rumors that undoubtedly made his survival difficult to enjoy.

From all accounts, it appears that Charlotte ran the family with a firm hand. When Thomas married Mary Racine (1880–1943), another determined woman (Figure 10-8), he was caught between two strong-willed ladies separated by background and religion. Mary was born in France and was a Roman Catholic. They were married in secret, and the conversion of Thomas to Catholicism was difficult for Charlotte to accept. However, both families lived in estates not far apart in Germantown and together they maintained the zoo and kennel established by Thomas Drake.

After World War I, Mary developed a chronic incapacitating illness, the nature of which is unknown, but it led her into a close personal and professional relationship with Dr. Harold Jones at Jefferson. He became a close friend of the family and treated Mrs. Cardeza both at home and in Jefferson hospital with a variety of medications, including direct infusions of small amounts of whole blood obtained from a donor at the bedside. He talked to them about his dream of establishing a transfusion and hematology research center at Jefferson. When Charlotte Drake Cardeza died in 1939, Thomas and Mary decided to support the development of such a center in her memory.

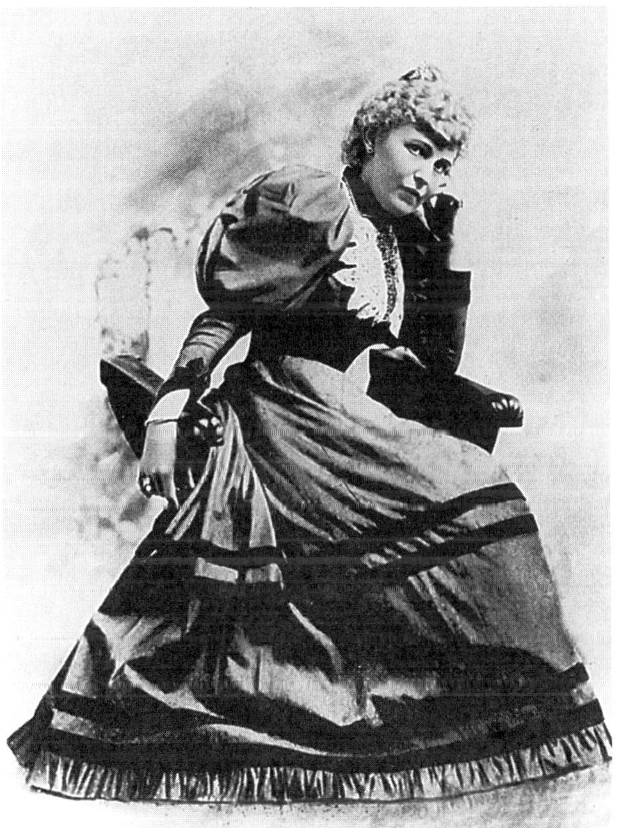

FIG. 10-5. Mrs. Charlotte Drake Cardeza (1854–1939).

On December 14, 1939, at a memorable dinner at the University Club, attended by Mr. Cardeza and many department heads, Dr. Jones toasted the establishment of a Hematology Division in the Department of Medicine (Figure 10-9), to be named The Charlotte Drake Cardeza Foundation for the Study of Diseases of the Blood and Allied Conditions. After two years of legal and academic discussions between Mr. J. Harry Wagner, legal counsel for the Cardezas, and Mr. Robert P. Hooper, President of the Board of Trustees of Jefferson, the Charlotte Drake Cardeza Foundation was formally incorporated on October 17, 1941, to be directed by Dr. Harold Jones, as the first Thomas Drake Martinez Cardeza Professor of Clinical Medicine and Hematology in the Department of Medicine (Figure 10-10). Jones was allotted a teaching service in the Department of Medicine, plus adult and pediatric hematology beds in the Hospital. Staff members for the Division of Hematology and a number of research and teaching Charlotte Drake Cardeza Fellows were recruited. The Division was to conduct and operate a Transfusion-Plasma Unit and a Biologic Photographic Unit, activities to be supported by an annual grant from the Cardezas of $50,000 for not less than ten years, $7,500 of which could be used for the salary of the Director of the Division of Hematology.

Although the Charlotte Drake Cardeza

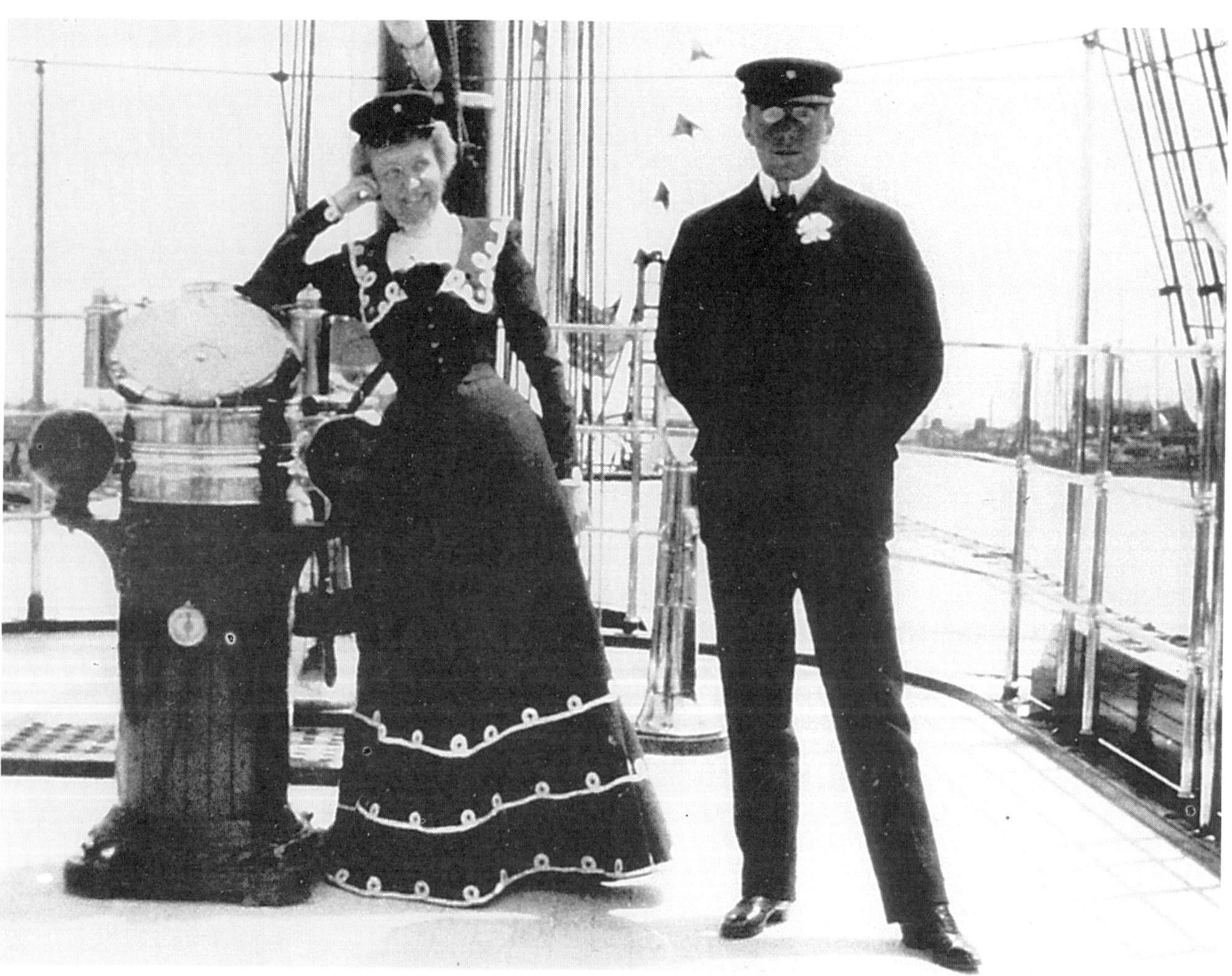

FIG. 10-6. Charlotte and Thomas Drake Cardeza on board *The Eleanor*.

Foundation served as the Division of Hematology of the Department of Medicine, the Director reported to a Cardeza Foundation Advisory Committee of the faculty appointed by the Board of Trustees, rather than to the Chairman of the Department of Medicine. The Committee in turn reported to the Board of Trustees. Subsequent changes in the line of command provided for two channels, one academic, via the Chairman of the Department of Medicine, and one fiscal, via a Cardeza Foundation Faculty Advisory Committee to a Joint Advisory Committee comprised of appropriate individuals representing the Board of Trustees, administration, faculty, and the Cardeza Trust.

Mr. Cardeza was the first Chairman of the Joint Advisory Committee, and until 1947 he had almost daily administrative contacts with Dr. Jones. At that point, he requested that Jefferson Medical College take over supervision of activities of the Foundation and changed the annual allotment of $50,000 to a corresponding amount derived from a Trust deposited at the Fidelity Bank. Mr. Horace Liversidge became Chairman, and Mr. Percival Foerderer and Mr. J. Harry Wagner were two of the more active committee members. With the additional support of a legacy of about $100,000 from the Kress brothers, considerable research was carried out in laboratories spread throughout the College.

In two small laboratories in the College Building and one in Room 247 in the Thompson Annex, Dr. Franklin A. Miller (Figure 10-11), who had been recruited as Assistant Director, and Dr. Leandro Tocantins, Co-Assistant Director, had for that period a great opportunity to pursue their research interest almost full-time. Dr. Miller's interest was in the pathogenesis of malignant lymphomas and leukemias. He succeeded in isolating from the urine of patients with these illnesses several substances that when injected into guinea pigs would alter cellular proliferation.

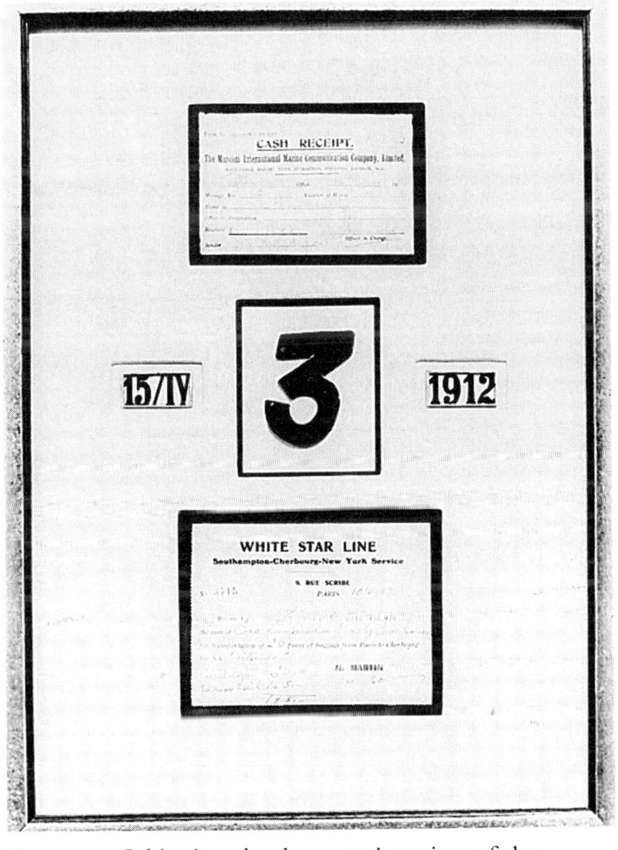

FIG. 10-7. Cabin door hardware and receipts of the Cardeza passage on the *Titanic*.

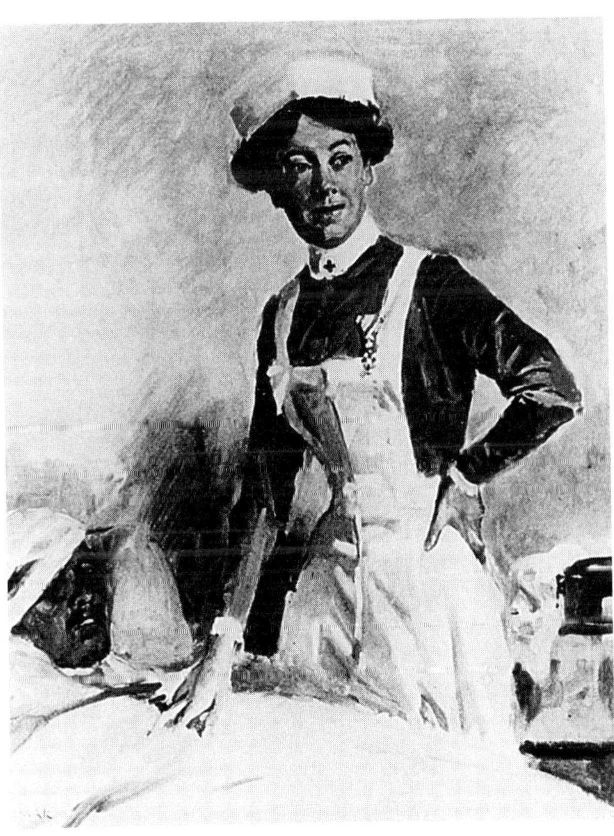

FIG. 10-8. Mary Racine (1880–1943).

Dr. Daniel Turner (Figure 10-12), an organic chemist, characterized these substances, and in many papers they hypothesized regarding their possible pathogenetic relationship to malignancy. Dr. Tocantins continued his work on platelets and the coagulation inhibitor found in some patients with hemophilia, and with Dr. Robert Carroll (Jefferson, 1952) and Dr. Ruth Holburn (Figure 10-13) he established a Hemophilia Clinic. Dr. Jones was primarily involved in patient management centered around a clinic in the Curtis Building designated the Blood, Spleen, and Bone Marrow Clinic. With Dr. Lowell A. Erf, Jones also established a Blood Bank in a small building on Eleventh Street and became deeply involved in the processing and administration of plasma.

In 1952, Mr. Cardeza died and left his estate for the support of The Charlotte Drake Cardeza Foundation. After some years of intense legal wrangling, his mansion in Germantown was bequeathed to the Archdiocese of Philadelphia, and his fortune, about $3 million, was used to establish a trust for the Foundation with Mr. Wagner and the Fidelity Bank as co-trustees. This input of funds permitted the recruitment of more staff members. When Dr. Tocantins became the new vigorous Director in 1954, he spearheaded further expansion. Dr. Tocantins and Dr. Farid I. Haurani (Figure 10-14) began studies on bone marrow transplantation. After both exciting and painful experiences they learned that although autotransplantation was possible, still unknown immunologic barriers prevented successful heterotransplantation.[3] With the help of Dr. Louis A. Kazal (Figure 10-15), Dr. Daniel Turner, and Dr. Melvin J. Silver (Figure 10-16), Dr. Tocantins continued his quest for the identification of the elusive inhibitor that he believed characterized hemophilia.[4] That quest was actually not finished until Dr. Sandor S. Shapiro (Figure 10-17), after the death of Dr. Tocantins, identified the inhibitor as a Factor VIII antibody that develops in about ten to 15 percent of treated patients with hemophilia.[5]

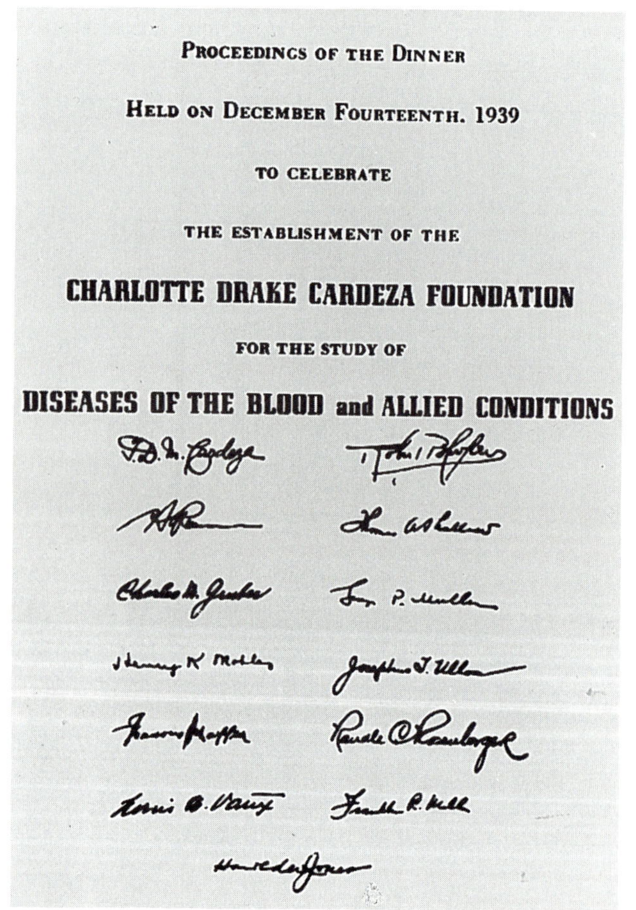

PROCEEDINGS OF THE DINNER

HELD ON DECEMBER FOURTEENTH. 1939

TO CELEBRATE

THE ESTABLISHMENT OF THE

CHARLOTTE DRAKE CARDEZA FOUNDATION

FOR THE STUDY OF

DISEASES OF THE BLOOD and ALLIED CONDITIONS

FIG. 10-9. Dinner proceedings at the establishment of Charlotte Drake Cardeza Foundation.

In 1959 Dr. Allan J. Erslev was recruited from the Thorndike Memorial Laboratory at Harvard as Associate Director. He pursued his work on erythropoietin, a renal hormone he had discovered earlier. This hormone controls the rate of red cell production and plays a major role in recovery from blood loss and in adaptation to high altitudes.[6]

The Sansom Street Center

The trust income was, according to Mr. Wagner, restricted to support personnel and provide supplies and equipment and could not be used for renovation. Fortunately, a new chairman of the Joint Advisory Committee, Mr. J. Howard Pew, President of Sun Oil Company, saw the need for providing a separate building for the Foundation, and through his generosity a three-storied property on 1015 Sansom Street was purchased and completely renovated (Figure 10-18). In 1960, the

Foundation moved in and for the first time became a coherent unit, permitting easy academic and personal interaction among its members. The move was followed by an expansion in personnel and activities, an expansion greatly enhanced by the new availability of federal research funds. In a few years, federal grant support actually matched and exceeded trust income. The new Cardeza quarters housed the Blood Donor Center, a photographic unit, and laboratories and offices for a professional staff that had increased to include 15 M.D.'s and Ph.D.'s, five to ten American and foreign clinical and Research Fellows, and a nonprofessional staff of about 60 technicians, secretaries, and maintenance personnel.

Academically, the Foundation was primarily the Division of Hematology in the Department of Medicine, but it also served as the Division of Hematology in the Departments of Pediatrics, Physiology, and Pharmacology. It was responsible for the teaching of hematology to students and house staff, and clinically its members provided consultations and care for hematologic patients in the Jefferson Medical College Hospital.

In 1963, after Dr. Tocantins' sudden death, Dr. Allan J. Erslev (Figure 10-19), a native of Denmark (born in 1919), became Director. He continued the recruitment of new investigators and expansion of federal funding. Dr. Sandor Shapiro (Figure 10-17), the first senior recruit, was trained at Harvard and Massachusetts Institute of Technology; after arrival at Cardeza he established

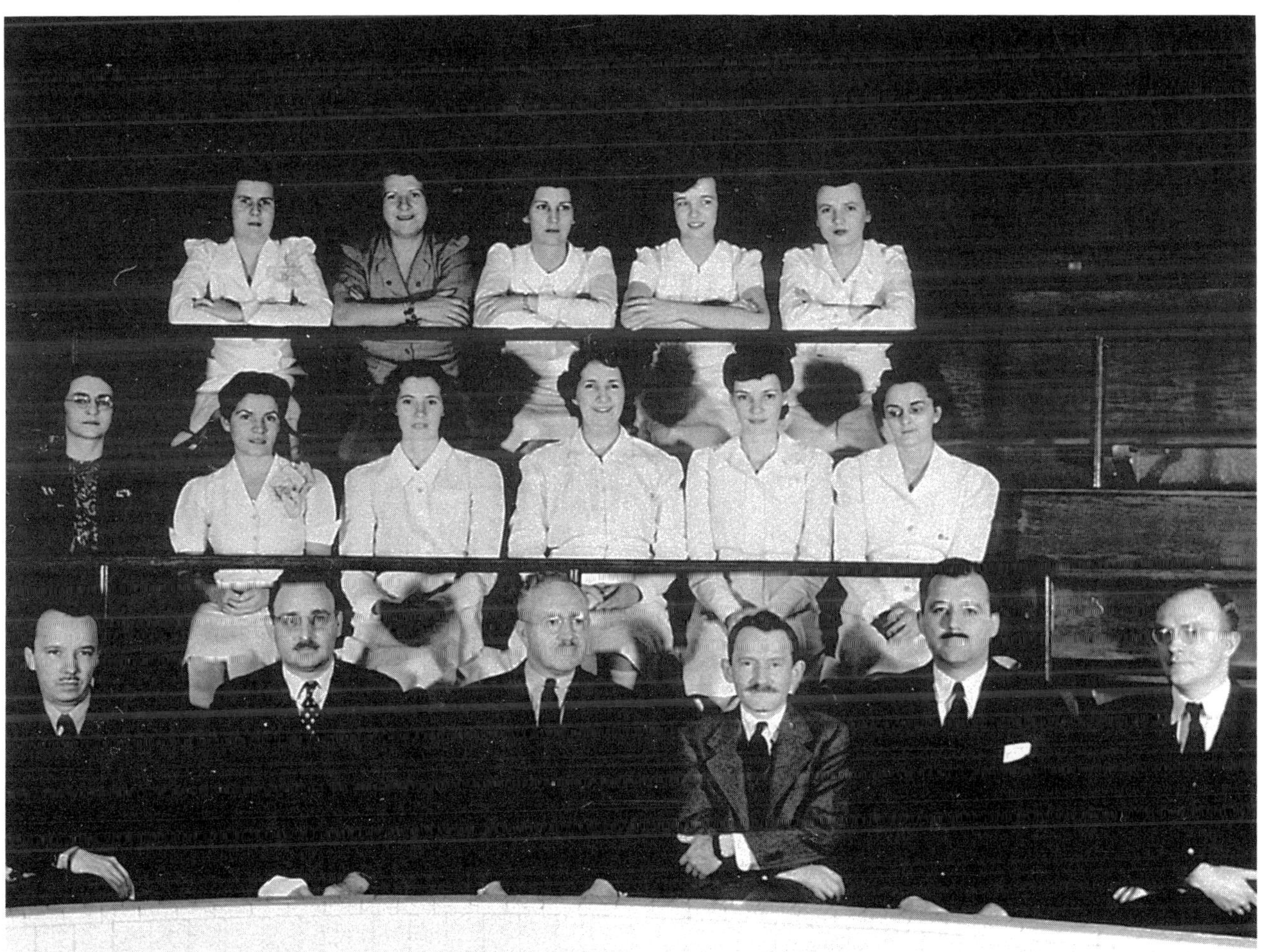

FIG. 10-10. Harold W. Jones, M.D. and his Cardeza Staff.

a Thrombosis and Hemorrhagic Disease Section and a state-supported Hemophilia Center.

With Drs. Melvin Silver, Louis Kazal, Jose Martinez (Figure 10-20), and J. Bryan Smith (Figure 10-16), Shapiro spearheaded research in coagulation-factor kinetics, the immunologic basis for some coagulation disorders, and the biochemical processes involved in platelet aggregation and release action.[7–11] Dr. Edward Burka, Dr. Elias Schwartz, Director of the Division of Pediatric Hematology, and Miss Jean Atwater (Figure 10-21), Head of Cardeza Laboratories, studied normal and abnormal hemoglobins and identified the defects responsible for several hemoglobinopathies and thalassemias.[12,13] Their laboratories served as a

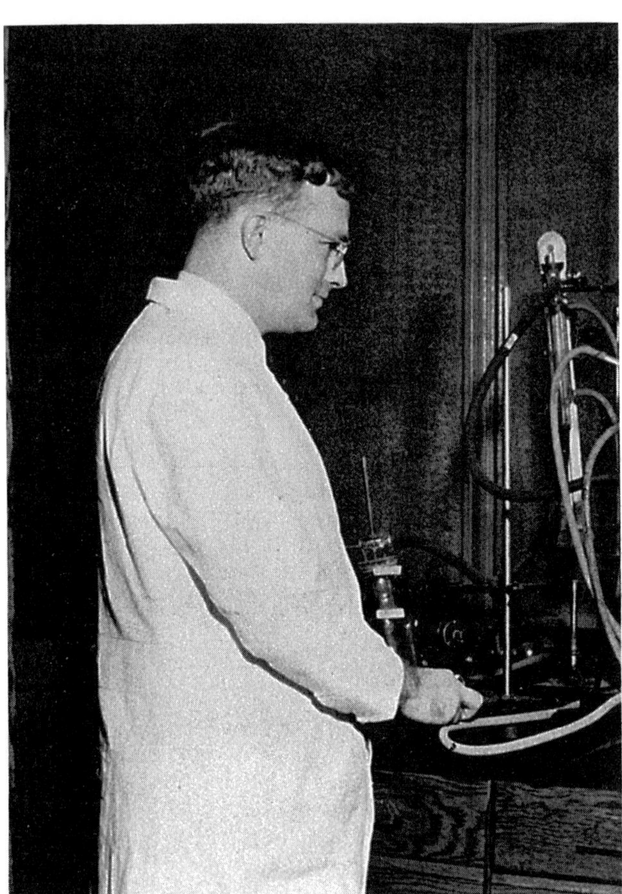

FIG. 10-12. Daniel Turner, Ph.D.

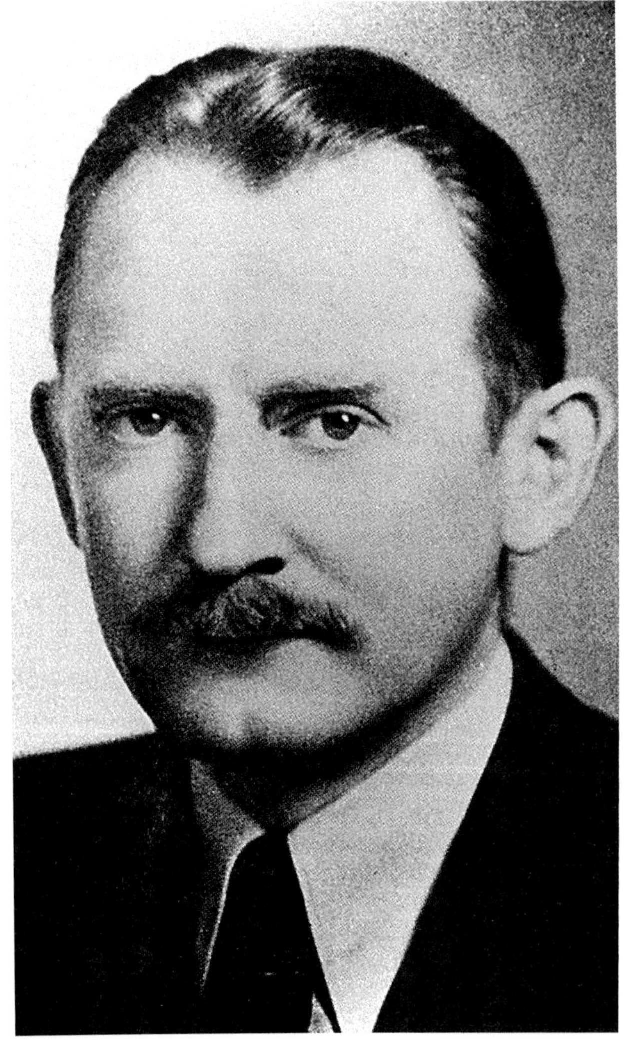

FIG. 10-11. Franklin R. Miller, M.D.

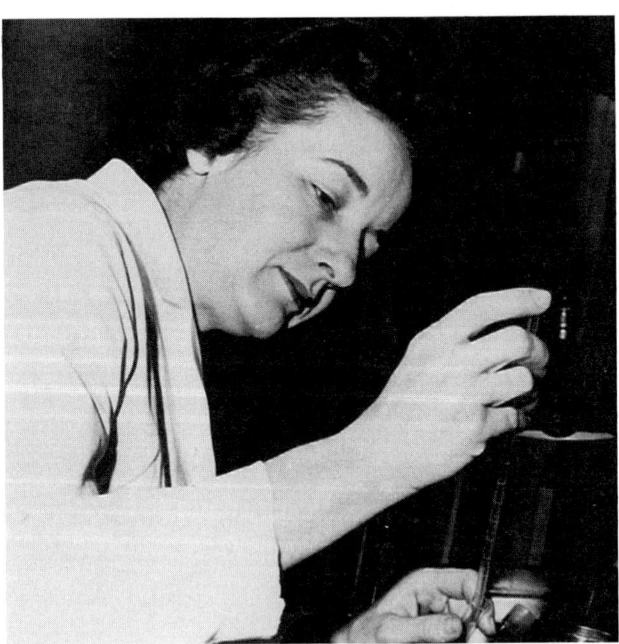

FIG. 10-13. Ruth Holburn, Ph.D.

nationally recognized referral center for abnormal hemoglobins. Dr. Burka also established a state-supported Sickle Cell Center and became Blood Bank Director. These positions were later taken by Dr. Samir K. Ballas, with the assistance of Dr. Stephen P. Hauptman for tissue typing and Dr. Scott Murphy (Figure 10-22) for blood fractionation. Dr. Ballas' interest was directed mainly at the red cell membrane with its external antigenic sites and internal structural skeleton,[14] while Dr. Hauptman studied the same membrane structures on lymphocytes.[15] Dr. Murphy's primary interest was platelets, and he established storage conditions for platelets that effectively increased their shelf life from hours to the present seven days.[16] Dr. Susan Travis, who followed Dr. Schwartz as Director of Pediatric Hematology

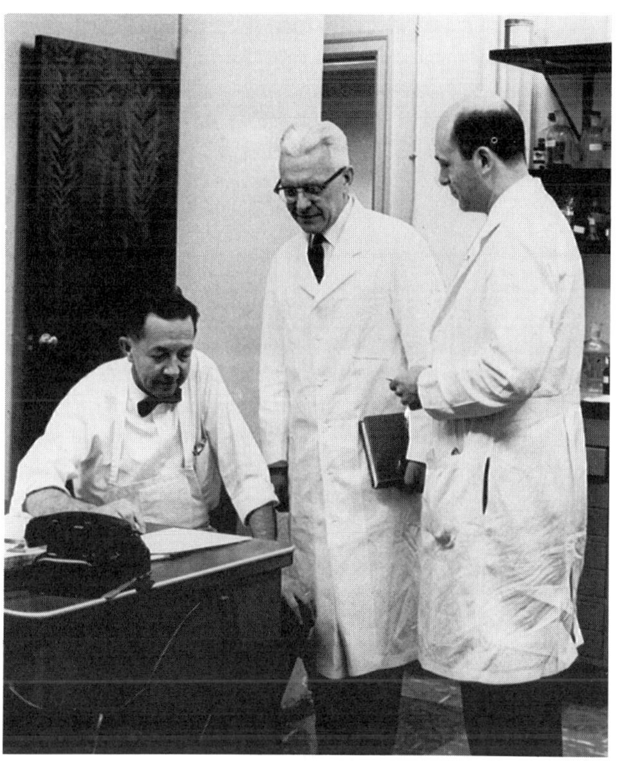

FIG. 10-15. Mr. Orin Miller (technician to Louis Kazal for 30 years), Louis A. Kazal, Ph.D., and Sandor Shapiro, M.D.

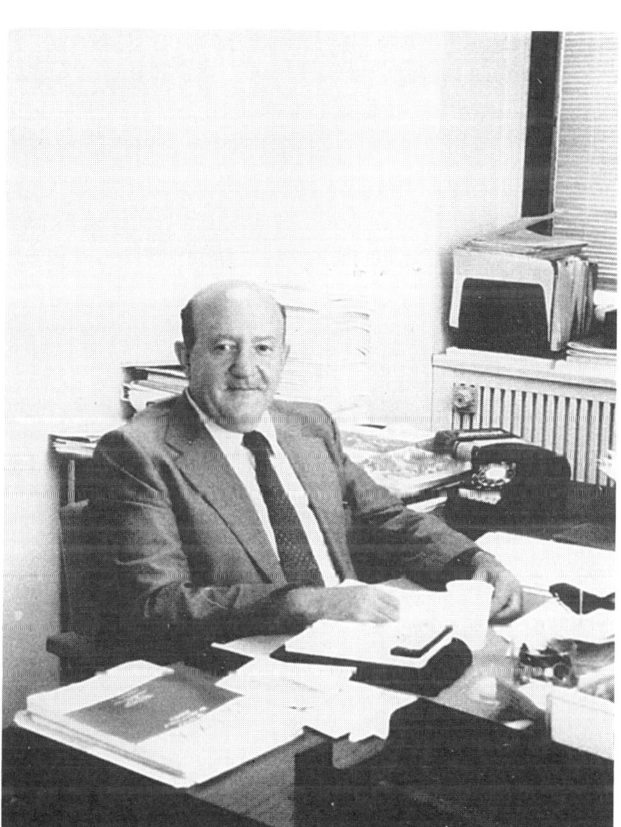

FIG. 10-14. Farid I. Haurani, M.D.

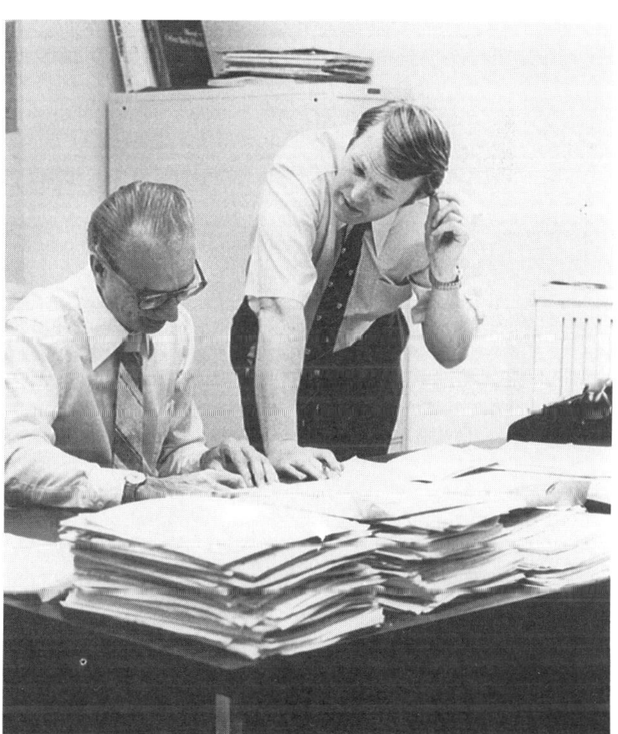

FIG. 10-16. Melvin J. Silver, D.Sc., and J. Bryan Smith, Ph.D.

was primarily involved in unraveling red cell enzyme function.[17] Dr. Haurani's interest centered on iron and B_{12} metabolism. He directed the Jefferson branch of the National Cooperative Acute Leukemia Group B (ALGB). Dr. Erslev continued his research in erythropoietin with Dr. Thomas Gabuzda, Dr. Ruth Silver, and Dr. Lewis Kazal. Later, Dr. Jaime Caro joined his team and provided further information about the renal biogenesis and bone marrow action of this hormone.[18] They also established a research and referral center for erythropoietin bioassays and for the diagnosis of polycythemia vera, secondary polycythemia, and the anemia of chronic renal disease.

Concomitantly with these research activities, all clinical members of the Cardeza Foundation were members of the Cardeza Associates of Clinical Hematology and shared in consultations at the Thomas Jefferson University Hospital. With the competent support of some outstanding nurses, (Marian Ramp and Kay Houser are excellent examples), they provided in- and outpatient management of patients with hematologic

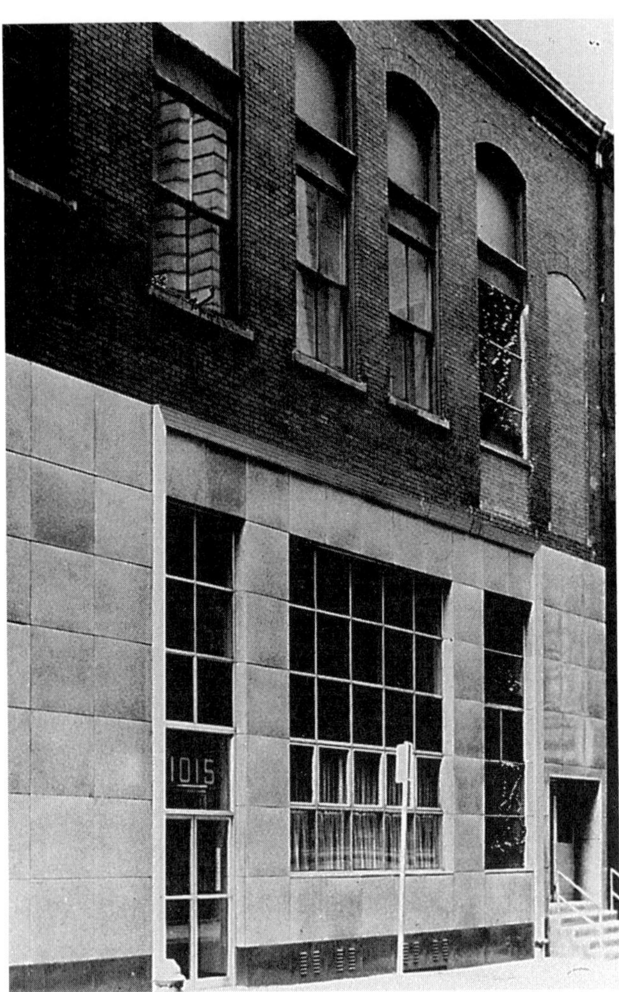

FIG. 10-18. The Cardeza Foundation at 1015 Sansom Street.

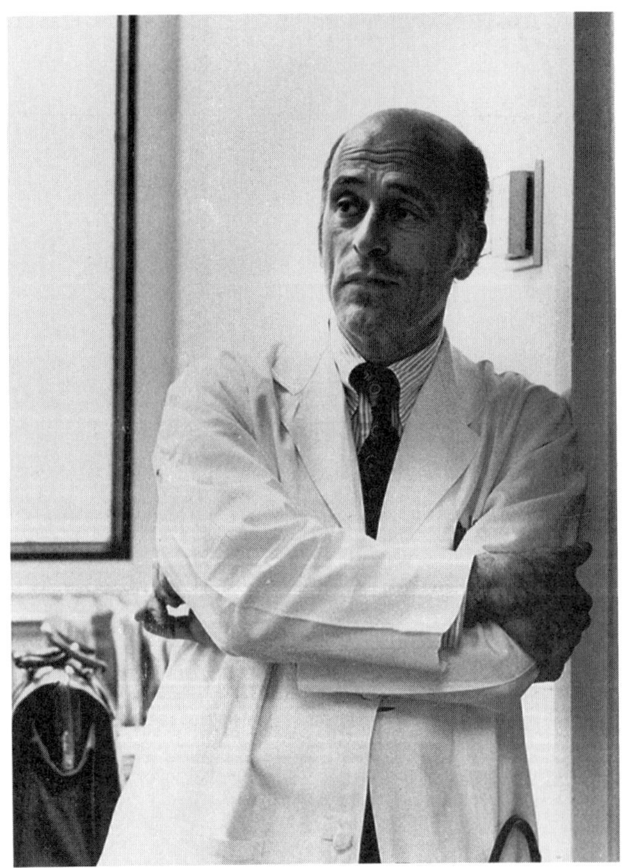

FIG. 10-17. Sandor S. Shapiro, M.D.

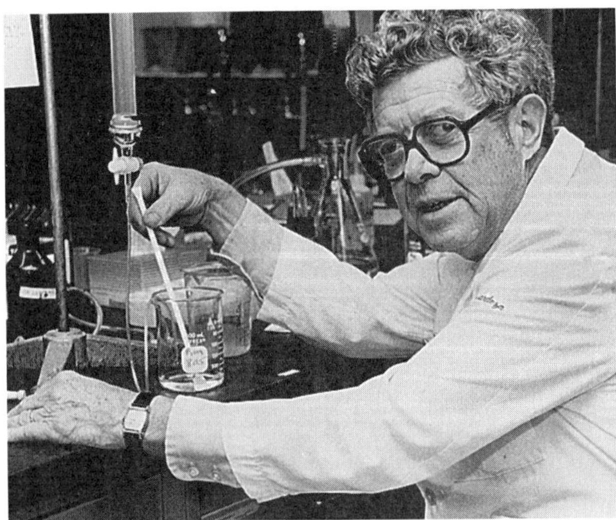

FIG. 10-19. Allan J. Erslev, M.D. (1919–).

disorders. Assisted by the more clinically oriented faculty members, Drs. John Hodges and Edward McGehee, they also taught hematology to Jefferson students and house staff and provided clinical and research instruction to Fellows supported by two National Institutes of Health Training Grants.

Numerous reviews and textbook articles resulted. Dr. Erslev became coeditor of a major textbook, *Hematology*,[19] and, with Dr. Gabuzda, coauthor of a small paperback *Pathophysiology of Blood*.[20] Both books have gone through three editions.

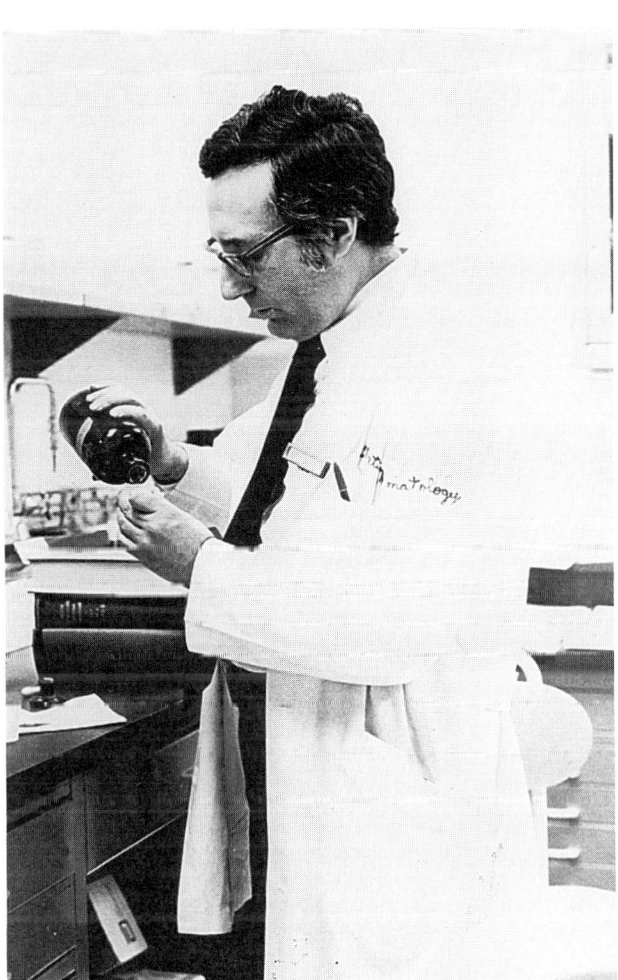

FIG. 10-20. Jose Martinez, M.D.

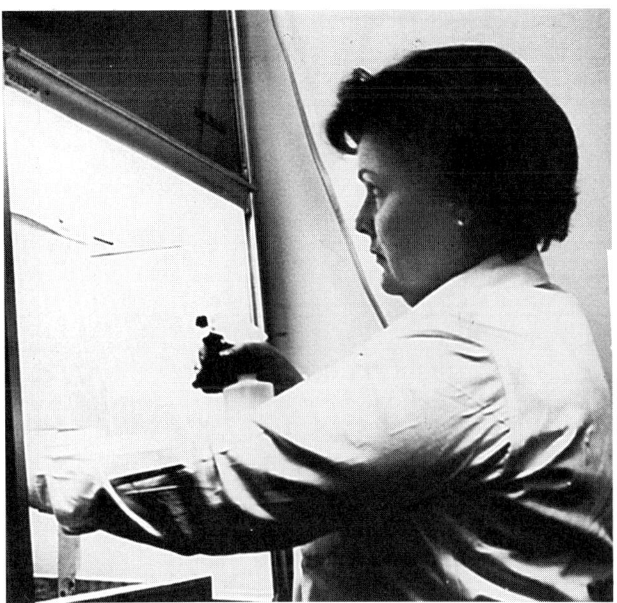

FIG. 10-21. Jean Atwater.

In 1975, the Cardeza building had to make room for the new Thomas Jefferson University Hospital. The foundation moved into 1,600 square feet of a completely renovated laboratory and office space on the seventh, eighth, and ninth floors of the

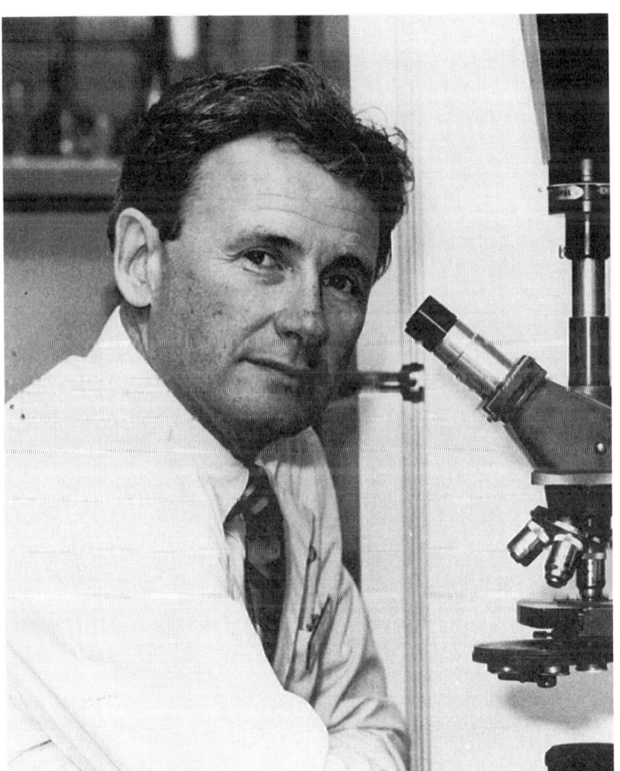

FIG. 10-22. Scott Murphy, M.D.

Curtis Building (Figure 10-23). The Cardeza Blood Donor Center and Tissue Typing Center as well as the Sickle Center moved into the first floor and the Cardeza Hemophilia Unit into the second floor of the old hospital, and the outpatient facilities were located eventually on the fourth floor of the New Hospital. The move into new laboratories symbolized the move in research from the days of traditional morphologic and pathophysiologic studies to the current phase of molecular biology. Studies became characterized by monoclonal antibodies, restriction enzyme analysis, radioimmune assays, membrane receptor analysis, cell sorting, and gene cloning. Young investigators such as Drs. Perumal Thiagarajan, Carol Ingerman-Wojenski, Patricia Catalano, Iftekhar Alam, and Jaime Caro adopted these new techniques and turned research efforts at Cardeza in that direction. Although the funding never seemed to match expenditures, the annual Cardeza budget was maintained in precarious balance by the competent juggling of the administrative assistants, Bella Sigal and Helen Gilliam. In 1984–1985, the budget reached about $3.5 million, with $2.3 million provided from federal grants and contracts.

In 1985 Dr. Erslev stepped down as Director of the Division but remained at Jefferson to continue his research on red cell diseases. He was immediately named Distinguished Professor of Medicine, the first in the Department of Medicine to be so honored. Previous awards included a Guggenheim Fellowship, presentation of his portrait by the Class of 1972, and the first

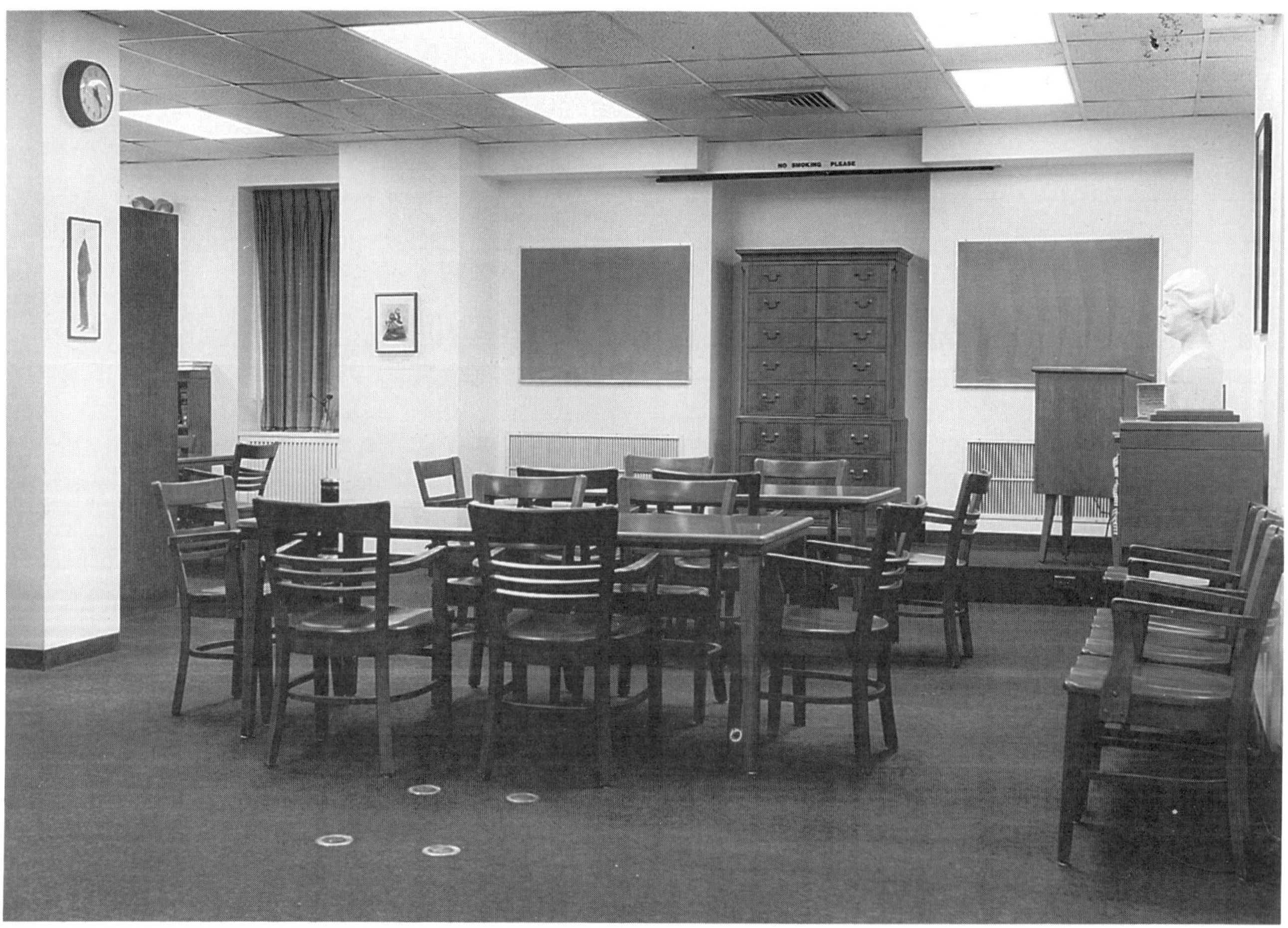

FIG. 10-23. Hematology conference room and Leandro M. Tocantins Library on the ninth floor of the Curtis Building (1975).

William B. Castle Lectureship at Boston University. He remained prominent in many of the important clinical and research societies related to his field both here and abroad.

The Division may look back with pride to its contributions to the understanding and treatment of diseases of the blood and look forward under the new leadership of Dr. Sandor Shapiro to the challenge of a future in hematologic molecular biology.

References

1. Jones, H.W,. and Tocantins, L.M., "Diseases of the Blood," *Obstetric Medicine*. F.L. Adair and E.J. Stieglits, eds. Philadelphia: Lea & Febiger, 1934, p. 623.
2. Tocantins, L.M., "The Mammalian Blood Platelet in Health and Disease," *Medicine* 17:155, 1938.
3. Haurani, F.I., Repplinger, E., and Tocantins, L.M., "Attempts at Transplantation of Human Bone Marrow in Patients with Acute Leukemia and Other Marrow-Depletion Disorders," *Am. J. Med.* 28:794–806, 1960.
4. Turner, D.L., Silver, M.J., Holburn, R.R., and Tocantins, L.M., "Phospholipid Antithromboplastin Not Related to Sphingosine," *Soc. Exp. Biol. & Med.* 96:641–643, 1957.
5. Shapiro, S.S., "The Immunologic Character of Acquired Inhibitors of Antihemophilic Globulin (Factor VIII) and the Kinetics of Their Interaction with Factor VIII," *J. Clin. Invest,* 46:147–156, 1967.
6. Erslev, A.J., "Humoral Regulation of Red Blood Cell Production," *Blood* 8:349–357, 1953.
7. Shapiro, S.S., and Martinez, J., "Human Prothrombin Metabolism in Normal Man and in Hypercoagulable Subjects," *J. Clin. Invest.* 48:1292–1298, 1969.
8. Smith, J.B., and Silver, M.J., "Prostaglandin Synthesis by Platelets and its Biologic Significance," *Platelets in Biology and Pathology*. J. Gordon, ed. New York: Elsevier, 1976, pp. 331–352.
9. Silver, M.J., "Platelet Aggregation and Plug Formation: A Model Test System," *Am. J. Physiol.* 218:384–388, 1970.
10. Kazal, L.A., Amsel, S., Miller, O.P., and Tocantins, L.M., "The Preparation and Some Properties of Fibrinogen Precipitated from Human Plasma by Glycine." *Proc. Soc. Exp. Biol. & Med.* 113:989–984, 1963.
11. Martinez, J., Palascak, J.E., and Kwansniak, D., "Abnormal Sialic Acid Content of the Dysfibrinogenemia Associated with Liver Disease," *J. Clin. Invest.* 61:535–538, 1978.
12. Schwartz, E., "The Silent Carrier of Beta Thalassemia," *New Eng. J. Med.* 281:1327–1333, 1969.
13. Atwater, J., and Schwartz, E., "Separations of Hemoglobin," *Hematology*. W.J. Williams, E. Beutler, A.J. Erslev, and R.W. Rundles, eds. New York: McGraw-Hill Book Company, 1972, pp. 1364–1369.
14. Ballas, S.K., Mohandas, N., Marton, L.J. and Shohet, S.B., "Stabilization of Erythrocyte Membranes by Polyamines," *Proc. Natl. Acad. Sci.* USA 80:1942–1946, 1983.
15. Hauptman, S.P., and Kansu, E., "T-cell Origin of Human Macromolecular Insoluble Globulin (MICG)," *Nature* 276:393–394, 1978.
16. Murphy, S., "The Preparation and Storage of Platelets for Transfusion," *Review of Hematology,* 1980.
17. Travis, S.F., Martinez, M., Garvin, J.H., Jr., Atwater, J., and Gillmer, P., "Study of a Kindred with Partial Deficiency of Red Cell 2,3 Disphosphoglycerate Mutase (2,3DPGM) and Compensated Hemolysis," *Blood* 51:1107–1116, 1978.
18. Caro, J., and Erslev, A.J., "Biologic and Immunologic Erythropoietin in Extracts from Hypoxic Whole Rat Kidneys and in Their Glomerular and Tubular Fractions," *J. Lab. Clin. Med.* 103:922–931, 1984.
19. Williams, W.J., Beutler, J., Erslev, A.J. and Rundles, R.W., *Hematology*. New York: McGraw-Hill Book Company, 1972, pp. 1–1479.
20. Erslev, A.J., and Gabuzda, T.G., *Pathophysiology of Blood*. Philadelphia: W.B. Saunders Co., 1975, pp. 1–187.

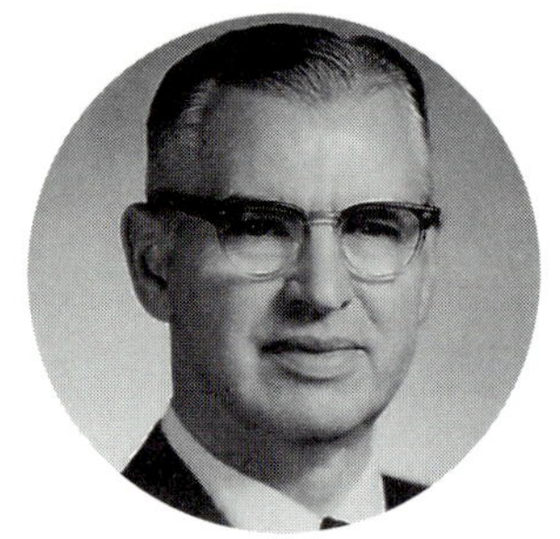

CHAPTER ELEVEN

Division of Pulmonary and Critical Care Medicine

J. Woodrow Savacool, M.D.

"Behold, I will cause breath to enter into you, and ye shall live." —Ezekiel 37:5

The decade of 1910–1920 was an eventful one. Smoldering world events culminated in World War I, with its consequent changes in governments, social upheavals, and revolutions. A new era was developing in medicine as well. Medical education was challenged by progressive educators and by the Flexner report of 1910,[1] which indicated the need for medical schools to develop meaningful teaching in response to the opening of the scientific and ultimate technological era of medical practice. Jefferson Medical College was well poised for such response; its clinical faculty was widely respected, hospital facilities were improving, and its students came from all parts of the United States as well as many foreign countries. The Department of Medicine had a new and stimulating head, Dr. Thomas McCrae, who arrived from Johns Hopkins in 1912 and brought with him the ferment of new medical educational views and practices, especially the clinical applications of laboratory procedures that were just being introduced.

Impetus for the organization of a Department for Diseases of the Chest stemmed from the perceived need for improved facilities for teaching physical and clinical diagnosis, thereby diminishing reliance on lectures. At the same time the continuing challenge presented by tuberculosis as a major cause of illness and death was recognized, as interest in its management and prevention increased both nationally and locally. The *Yearly Report of Jefferson Hospital for 1911* includes the comment that a Dispensary for Tuberculosis was organized "several years ago" but that "a facility for the care of seriously ill patients and for teaching should be acquired."[2] Then, fortuitously, the Henry Phipps Institute for the Study, Treatment, and Prevention of Tuberculosis, founded in 1903 by Dr. Lawrence F. Flick (Figure 11-1) (Jefferson, 1879),[3] moved to its new building at Seventh and Lombard Streets, and its previous buildings at 236–238 Pine Street became available. This grouping of events led to action by the Board of Trustees.

The first reference to the new department was dated February 20, 1913, when the Board, through its Hospital Committee, received a request from Professors Coplin and McCrae to "consider the advisability of obtaining the present building of the Phipps Institute for the purpose of securing a Tuberculosis Department for the Hospital thereby adding to the teaching of that branch of medicine."[4] At the same meeting it followed that the Committee had already acted, since "Mr. Potter reported that a meeting of the Hospital Committee and a Committee of the Free Hospital for Poor Consumptives has been held for the purpose of considering the acquisition by the Jefferson Medical College of the property at 3rd and Pine Sts. formerly occupied by the Phipps Institute, and the sharing of the cost of maintenance by the two institutions."

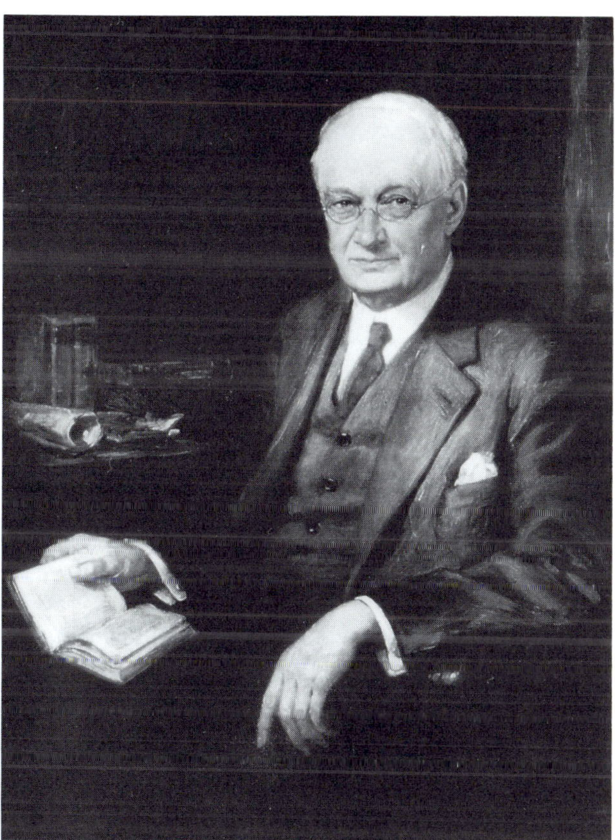

FIG. II-1. Dr. Lawrence F. Flick (Jefferson, 1879); pioneer Philadelphia crusader against tuberculosis; founder of White Haven Sanatorium (1901) and Henry Phipps Institute (1903); organizer (1892) of first State (Pennsylvania) Society for Prevention of Tuberculosis.

The Tuberculosis Control and Treatment Program

An explanatory note is appropriate. The Free Hospital for Poor Consumptives was organized as a fundraising Society in 1895 by the same Dr. Flick,[5] its purpose having been to collect and administer funds for the hospital care of patients with tuberculosis. For the first few years these funds were offered to general hospitals that would accept such patients, but prejudice against tuberculosis patients was such that only a few hospitals would do so. In 1901 the Free Hospital for Poor Consumptives opened the White Haven Sanatorium at White Haven, Pa. The Institution was ultimately officially named "The Free Hospital for Poor Consumptives and the White Haven Sanatorium." In 1903 Dr. Flick was responsible for enlisting Mr. Henry Phipps in his aggressive concerns and projects for tuberculosis treatment and control. This led to the opening of the Phipps Institute in the two buildings at 236–238 Pine Street.[6]

Between 1901 and 1913 some of the same physicians who visited White Haven were on the staff of the Phipps Institute, and patients were often transferred from one to the other facility as the need for local and/or remote treatment was perceived. Dr. Flick continued to be a driving force in the campaign against tuberculosis both with respect to hospital treatment and in the public health effort. The offer by the Free Hospital for Poor Consumptives to "share" the cost of maintenance was an apparent extension of its established policy of providing for tuberculous patients in available hospitals.

■ The Department for Diseases of the Chest

The Hospital Committee, having recommended favorable action on the proposal, was authorized to proceed with the acquisition of the property at "a cost not exceeding $20,000 and to operate the same as a branch of the Jefferson Hospital providing that a satisfactory agreement shall be entered into with the Free Hospital for Poor Consumptives to bear one-half the cost of operation not exceeding $10,000 per annum."

The buildings were duly purchased, and the minutes of the next 3 months reflect the actions preparatory to the opening of the buildings for

Jefferson's use. In view of the multiple changes in the area of Philadelphia where the hospital was located, a note about its history is of interest. In 1761 John Stamper purchased 300 acres of land from Thomas and Richard Penn, which tract included the block between Second and Third Streets. Mr. Stamper erected a mansion at 224 Pine Street and later built for his son a "castellated mansion" on the corner of Third and Pine Streets, which later became the home of Dr. Philip Syng Physick, whose interests included tuberculosis. The building at 238 Pine Street was erected by Rev. Robert Blackwell for his daughter Maria Harrison Blackwell, a granddaughter of John Stamper, on the occasion of her marriage to George Willing on November 26, 1800. The 236 property was willed to Robert Burton by the Rev. Blackwell at the latter's death in 1831 and was used as a private dwelling but also as a dispensary of the Mount Sinai Hospital for a time. The 238 Pine Street property was used as a lodge meeting hall for some years before its acquisition by the Phipps Institute[7] in 1903.

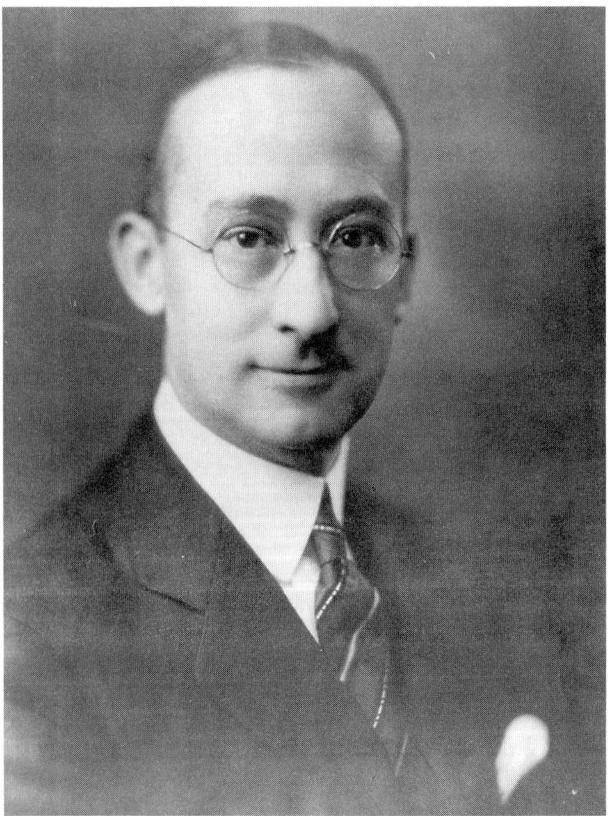

FIG. 11-2. Dr. Elmer H. Funk (Jefferson, 1908), first Medical Director and Physician-in-Charge, Department for Diseases of the Chest (1913–1926).

Dr. Elmer H. Funk (Figure 11-2) (Jefferson, 1908) had been Acting Medical Director of the Jefferson Hospital in addition to his clinical duties in the Department of Medicine. Only four years out of medical school when Dr. McCrae arrived at Jefferson in 1912, a close bond quickly developed between these two able physicians, and on April 28, 1913 Dr. Funk presented his resignation as Acting Medical Director in order to accept Dr. McCrae's offer to take medical charge of the Tuberculosis Department under his direction. The arrangement was approved by the Trustees in May, and the next month Dr. Funk was instructed to "open the Department for Diseases of the Chest as soon as it is advisable and send notice to the White Haven Association." Funds authorized for renovation of the buildings ultimately amounted to almost $20,000. A complete report by Dr. Funk and the Hospital Committee to the Board in October 1913 indicated that renovations were almost complete, staffing plans were in place, and the Hospital would soon be ready to open. Legal arrangements were not yet in order between the Hospital and the White Haven Sanatorium Association, and the exact date of that agreement is not recorded; however, the Board at its March 1914 meeting authorized execution of the contract between White Haven Sanatorium and Jefferson, "understanding between the hospital and W.H.S. having been arrived at."[8]

The Chest Department (Figure 11-3) was organized as a part of the general hospital, administratively under the hospital medical director, but Dr. Funk was also instructed to "render a monthly report to the Hospital Committee of the Board of Trustees. . . . " Dr. Funk medically served under Professor McCrae. From the beginning, plans for teaching of medical students and nursing students assumed a prominent place. Plans for nursing supervision and for social service personnel were also included, the public and social aspects of tuberculosis control having been given much greater attention than formerly.

It should be noted that although "Diseases of the Chest" still related principally to tuberculosis, the selection of the title for the new department represented a forward-looking attitude. Tuberculosis had long been the leading cause of death. With the discovery of the tubercle bacillus in 1882 and the beginning of efforts to prevent and control the disease, much activity was generated at the turn of the century. Isolation of active cases became a major factor in prevention of transmission. In addition to the organization of sanitoria like White Haven and the Trudeau Sanitarium at Saranac Lake, state and local governments were gradually becoming involved in the public health process. Some states were establishing their own institutions; other governments were contributing to the care of tuberculous patients in private sanatoria and dispensaries. City and state clinics were being established as a part of the process, mainly to apply newly conceived measures for managing tuberculous patients in view of the lack of availability of hospital beds for all needing care. These measures included the teaching of home isolation, currently perceived dietary measures, and adaptation of the "rest and fresh air treatment" to patients at home. These emerging principles of care lent themselves well to the adventure of the opening of the new Department.

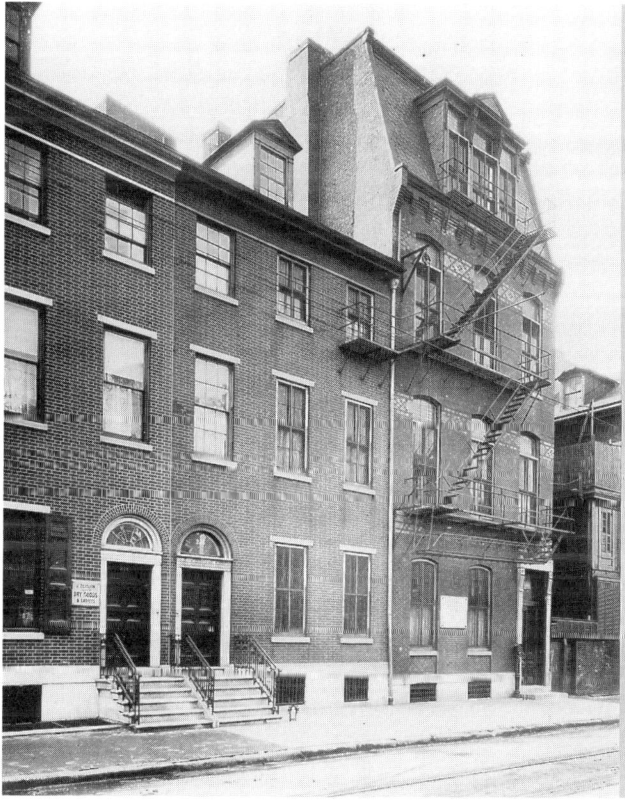

FIG. II-3. Department for Diseases of the Chest (1914–1946) at 236–238 Pine Street (main entrance at 238). (Building at left [234] is a commercial one.)

The medical students reacted with enthusiasm to the opening of the Chest Department. The student publication, *The Jeffersonian*, carried several articles during the year 1913 about the new facility.[9] In October 1913 it recorded: "The new department as stated on the marble tablet contributed by Mr. Baugh, will be known as the Jefferson Medical College Hospital, Department for Diseases of the Chest." Its direction under Dr. McCrae and Dr. Funk was noted, as well as a plan to relate to White Haven Sanatorium for patient transfer as needed. They also noted that "sociologic features" of tuberculosis would be studied and social service workers would supervise student visits to patients' homes. The college catalogue also carried through the themes of social service and home visiting for a number of years, but how much home visiting by medical students actually took place cannot be estimated.

The first few months of the operation of "Pine Street" are somewhat obscure. Some delay occurred between the time of Dr. Funk's optimistic report that the opening might occur in October 1913 and the actual date of admission of the first patients. The receipt of the first funds ($690) from White Haven Sanatorium for the month of March 1914 was acknowledged by the May meeting of the Board, so obviously patients were being treated early in 1914. Dr. Flick, although acknowledged as an important mover in the development of the department, appears not to have had a role in its operation and at no time did he hold an academic Jefferson appointment. The medical program was administered by Dr. Funk, whose energetic leadership soon led to recognition by the medical students of the excellence of his teaching. Drs. Baldwin Keyes and Reynold S. Griffith, having been medical students during the World War I period, both testified to the esteem in which Dr. Funk was held and to the popularity of his teaching program.[10] Visits of the medical students to Pine Street became important in the teaching in the Department of Medicine and some students obtained part-time appointments to perform laboratory work.

Policies with respect to patient care are not clearly recorded. The Trustees approved closing of the Department for the summer months for inpatients beginning in 1916, and this arrangement continued for some years. Continued care was available in the dispensary, which remained open for outpatients, but the ward patients were either discharged home or to another facility for the summer months. As time went on relationships with county, state, and private sanatoria in Pennsylvania and New Jersey were developed, which ultimately led to transfer both ways of patients who required more or less aggressive treatment. Important in the early policies was the Social Service Department, from the beginning a vital factor in assisting in the economics and family programs of patients with a devastating disease accompanied by inability to work and the imminent threat of death and/or invalidism. Nursing care and the teaching of nursing students also became a high priority function of the new Department.

It is of interest in connection with the career of Dr. Funk to note that although he had just graduated from Jefferson Medical College in 1908, as early as June 1911 he was appointed to a committee to administer the Department of Medicine following the resignation of its Chairman, Dr. James C. Wilson. The other members of the committee were Drs. E. J. G. Beardsley, Frederick Kalteyer, and Ross V. Patterson. This committee served until the arrival of Dr. Thomas McCrae in September, 1912. Dr. Funk also was Acting Secretary of the Board of Trustees and Acting Medical Director of the hospital as early as 1913. These appointments gave evidence of unusual abilities that became even more apparent as his career evolved.

Early in the course of operation of the Department, new plans had to be made. In December 1914, the Board of Trustees was notified by letter from Dr. Flick that the White Haven Sanatorium Association, having reached the limit of its borrowing power, would find it necessary to cancel its arrangement for support of beds in the Department for Diseases of the Chest as of March 3, 1915. Thus after one year the total care of patients rested with Jefferson. Such an event must have been anticipated, since the Board of Trustees applied for State aid in October 1914 for the years 1915 and 1916, amounts requested being $200,000 for the general hospital and $22,473.96 for the Chest Department. The latter figure represented the total estimated deficit for the new facility for two years.

There is little recorded concerning the character of the patient population of the Chest Department in its early years. The building housed the outpatient department on the first floor along with offices for reception, nursing, and social services (Figure 11-4). There were three floors for inpatient care, each one having about 12 beds (Figure 11-5). The upper floors of the 236 building accommodated the nurses. It is presumed that patients were referred from the Jefferson outpatient clinics and from public facilities and clinics. Since there were not nearly enough beds for tuberculosis patients in the city or state, it is not difficult to imagine the dissemination of information concerning the new facility and its rapid filling. Without a doubt the concerns and contacts of Dr. Flick, who continued as President of White Haven Sanatorium, played a large role in this process.

Early Clinical Research

The treatment of patients with pulmonary tuberculosis underwent little change during the early years of the Department. Diagnosis was gradually achieving more accuracy with increasing availability of culture and animal inoculation techniques for mycobacteria supplementing stained smears. Roentgen diagnosis was not well developed before the 1920s, and clinicians were often resistant to the suggestion that it was more accurate than their physical diagnosis. In spite of many medications, both systemic and topical, prescriptions of rest, exercise, climate, solar therapy, dietary measures, and psychological efforts, there was still nothing specific known to be effective in limiting death and disability. Collapse therapy, beginning with artificial pneumothorax, was gaining acceptance during the early decades of the century, but before 1920 little impact was discernible in limiting the duration of hospital treatment. The evidence suggests that patients were treated by standard methods until the 1920s when more aggressive treatment efforts were made. Dr. Funk, however, appears to have been very active in clinical investigation, having reported on numerous aspects of chest diseases in a rapidly developing series of papers in medical literature and speeches before medical groups.[11] His personal experience with tuberculosis, requiring a period of residence at White Haven Sanatorium during 1915–1916, appeared barely to interrupt his career activities. He continued as a visiting physician to White Haven until death. Increasing interest in and employment of artificial pneumothorax and other procedures at Pine Street is evident from his publication in 1929 of a paper discussing selection of patients for collapse therapy.[12]

Shortly after the opening of the Chest Department, a number of physicians joined the staff either as teaching volunteers limited to the facility or as part of a more inclusive Jefferson appointment. The earliest names to appear in the College catalogue included Drs. Halpern, N. Blumberg, M. W. Newcomb, T. S. Burwell, Maude A. Bowyer, and F. M. Dyson.[13] In 1920 Drs. S. Singer, A. R. Vaughn, A. Trasoff, and Wm. Haines were added to the list of Assistants in Medicine. Dr. R. M. Lukens was a Clinical Assistant in Medicine in 1915, but in 1917 he was listed as Chief Clinical Assistant in Laryngology, with Dr. H. S. Wider as a Clinical Assistant.[14] Lukens continued his association with the Department for many years and pioneered with bronchoscopic techniques both for tuberculosis and suppurative lung disease. In 1924 Dr. Martin J. Sokoloff joined the staff. He was destined to become Director in later years.

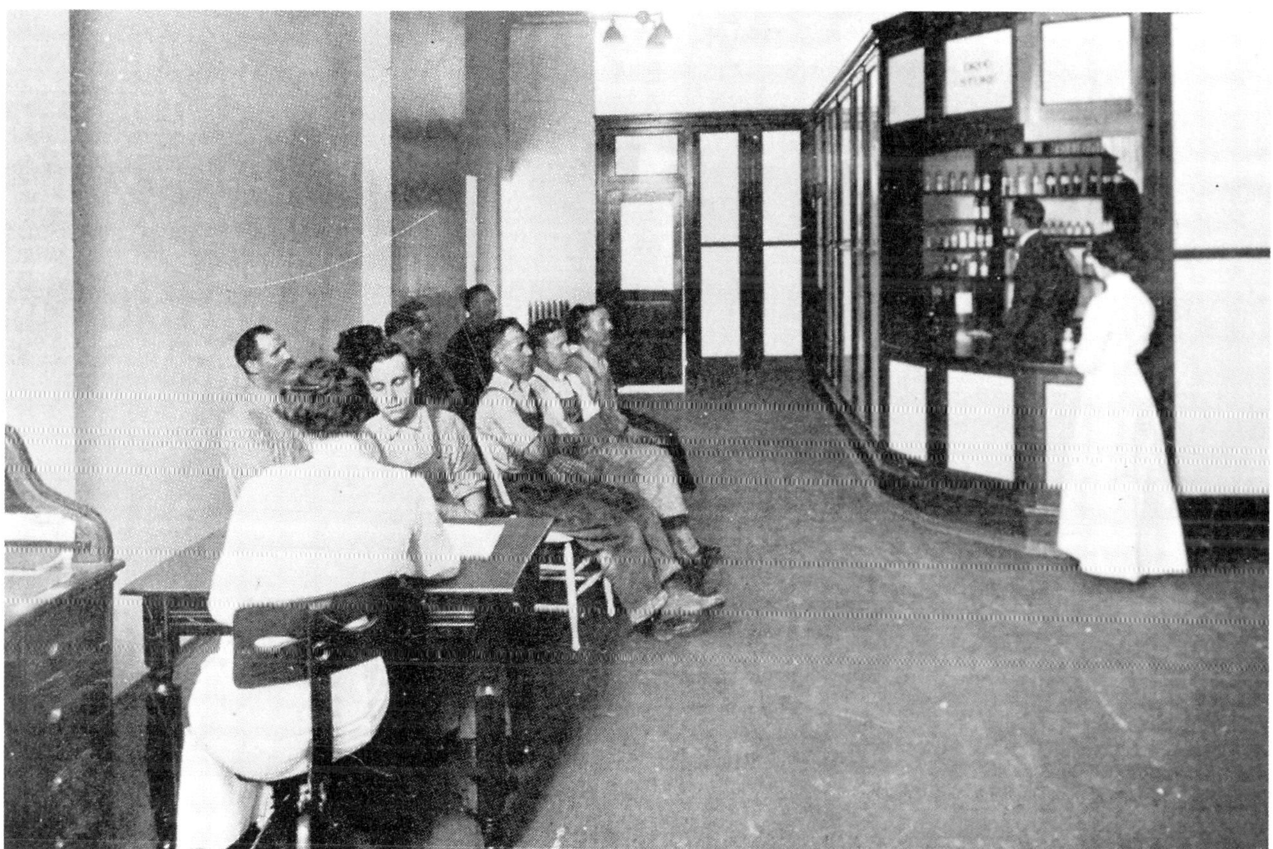

FIG. II-4. The "Pine Street" clinic and pharmacy (ca. 1915).

The Department experienced a significant benefit from the establishment of a Women's Board committee for Diseases of the Chest in 1922. Mrs. J. Dobson Altemus, President of the Board from 1921 to 1942, was increasingly interested in and supportive of the Chest Department.[15] During the 1930s especially, the committee members were very active, supplying items and activities for the comfort of inpatients and looking after recreational and decorative needs.

Miss Hedy Kern[16] provided one of the few remaining links between the present and the early years of the Chest Department. Having been employed there as a secretary for the Social Service Department between 1924 and 1927, she recalled a patient population of mainly young people, many of Polish, Irish, and Italian background, who were very susceptible to tuberculosis. Social Service personnel, led by Mrs. Millicent H. Maull, who could only be described as a great lady, warm, able, and dedicated, arranged hospital and sanatorium admissions for clinic patients, tried to implement medical and nursing orders for outpatients, planned financing for those unable to work, and related to other facilities for family care. Since far advanced disease was generally a requirement for admission, the inpatients were quite ill, and the mortality rate was high. Dr. John B. Montgomery (Jefferson, 1926)[17] remembered this well during his student years and also remarked about the skill of Dr. Sokoloff in teaching physical diagnosis. In spite of the risks inherent in close contact with tuberculous patients, the medical students and nursing students appreciated the assignment to "Pine Street."

In addition to the busy clinic for ambulatory patients operated by volunteer staff physicians, the Department also accommodated a City Chest Clinic during the middle 1920s, and in company with the Phipps Institute, a special Negro Clinic, with black physicians and nurses, in an effort to reach patients who might not otherwise obtain

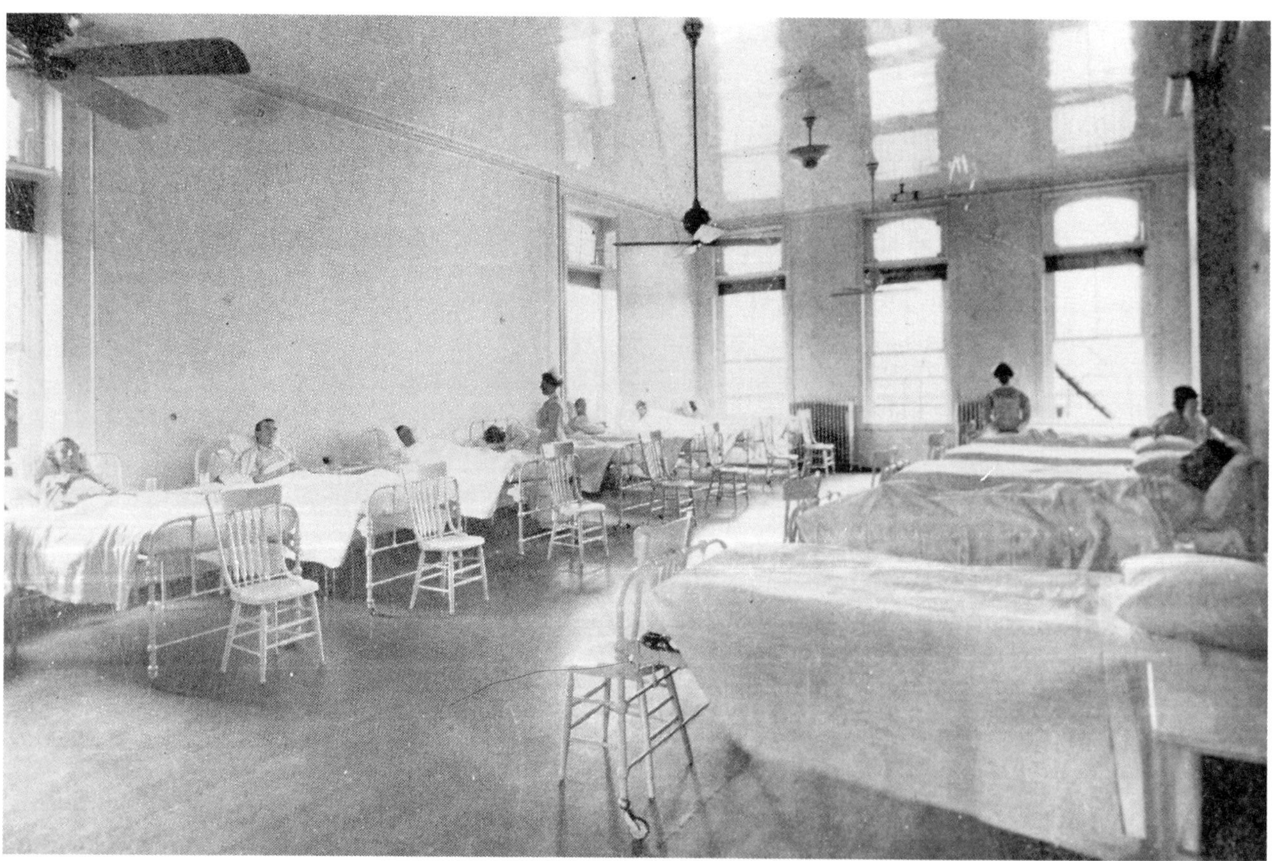

FIG. 11-5. The "Pine Street" fourth-floor men's ward (ca. 1920).

care and among whom the prevalence of tuberculosis was quite high. Among the physicians was Dr. Paul J. Taylor (Jefferson, 1906), one of the first two black graduates of Jefferson Medical College. (The other was a classmate, Henry M. Minton, who like Dr. Taylor was involved with treatment of tuberculosis.) Gradually this special clinic merged into the regular outpatient program and the City Clinic was transferred to a district facility.

Dr. Funk's activities were by no means limited to the Chest Department. His academic progress included studies in gastric function, coronary artery disease, diaphragmatic hernia, bronchogenic carcinoma, diabetes, and syphilis. These studies were often from the standpoint of treatment, since he was becoming more committed to the field of clinical therapeutics as a discipline slightly tangential to the central one of clinical diagnosis and medicine. In 1925 Funk was promoted to Assistant Professor of Medicine and Therapeutics. In 1926, Dr. McCrae decided to relieve him as Medical Director of the Chest Department to permit him to pursue his other activities more intensively. At the same time, Dr. Burgess Lee Gordon, a Jefferson graduate of 1919, who had pursued graduate training in Boston after internship, was appointed Assistant Director. Dr. Funk went on to succeed Dr. Hobart A. Hare as Sutherland M. Provost Professor of Therapeutics on September 22, 1931. His untimely death May 13, 1932, terminated a brilliant career in medical teaching, administration, clinical investigation, and patient care. His success in developing and guiding the Chest Department was an outstanding accomplishment. Elmer H. Funk, Jr., (Jefferson, 1947) strikingly inherited the physical and intellectual characteristics of his emminent father, and served as President of the Alumni Association in 1968.

New Directions

Dr. Burgess Gordon (Figure 11-6) (Jefferson, 1919), had served as Assistant Resident and later Resident in Medicine at Peter Bent Brigham Hospital in Boston from 1921 to 1926 under Dr. Henry A. Christian, Hersey Professor of Medicine at Harvard Medical School and Physician-in-Chief at the Brigham. His service there included a Teaching Fellowship in Medicine at Harvard from 1923 to 1926, which led to a major interest in clinical investigation. He was a man of many interests and talents, all of which were brought to bear promptly in his new appointment as Associate Director of the Chest Department in 1926. In addition to his Boston experience he quickly developed skills in administration and in pulmonary diseases through association with Dr. Elmer Funk, whom he succeeded as Medical Director and Physician-in-Charge in 1927. Very soon a number of physicians were added to the staff. Drs. Maurice Jacobs, C. W. Nissler, Charles S. Aitken, H. B. Slotkin, and Samuel Jaffe all became active in teaching and clinical duties. Dr. Aitken and Dr. Gordon became visiting physicians at White Haven Sanatorium in 1932, Dr. Sokoloff

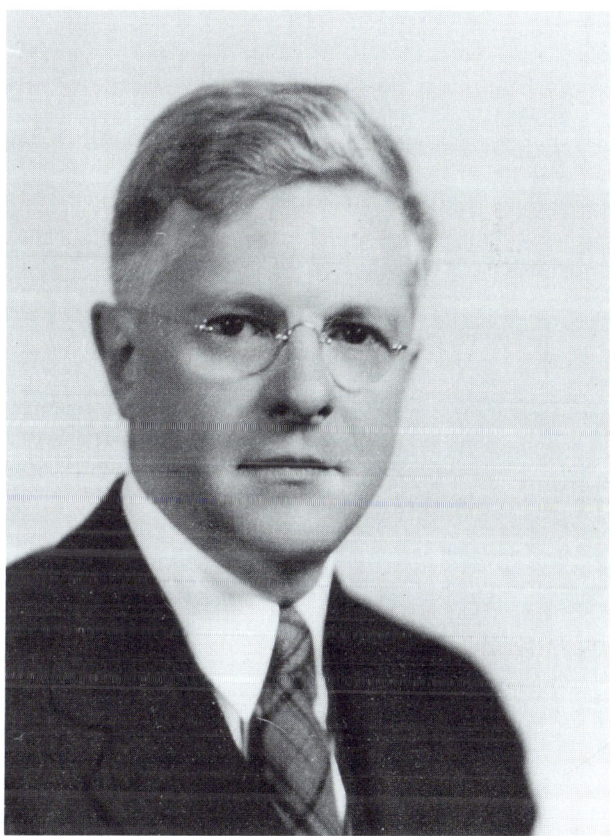

FIG. 11-6. Dr. Burgess L. Gordon (Jefferson, 1919), Medical Director and Physician-in-Charge (1927–1951).

having done so in 1924.[18] This solidified a relationship that proved beneficial to both institutions.

Change and expansion were necessary. In 1928 an annex was built in the rear of 238 Pine Street to accommodate new laboratories, an X-ray department, social service and medical examination rooms, a group of four quiet rooms for very ill patients, and a roof garden for patient recreation (Figure 11-7). Later many other changes and improvements were made to patient areas. During the 1930s the roof was redecorated and became a center for patient activities important for patient comfort and morale. Many of these were made with funds from private donors, who responded readily to Dr. Gordon's gentle urging.

During Dr. Gordon's early years at Pine Street, he was very active in clinical investigation and medical writing.[19] He continued his studies of the cardiopulmonary physiology of long-distance runners begun in Boston, studied metabolic processes related to tuberculosis and obesity, investigated the parathyroid secretion in relation to calcium metabolism with Dr. Abraham Cantarow, and followed through with studies of calcium and gold treatment for tuberculosis. He also studied Vitamin A and D deficiency and its treatment.

During these years there was evidence that the programs for tuberculosis control were showing some effect; patients were not as seriously ill at the time of first diagnosis and admission. As a consequence, more treatment measures could be brought to bear, especially collapse therapy. Dr.

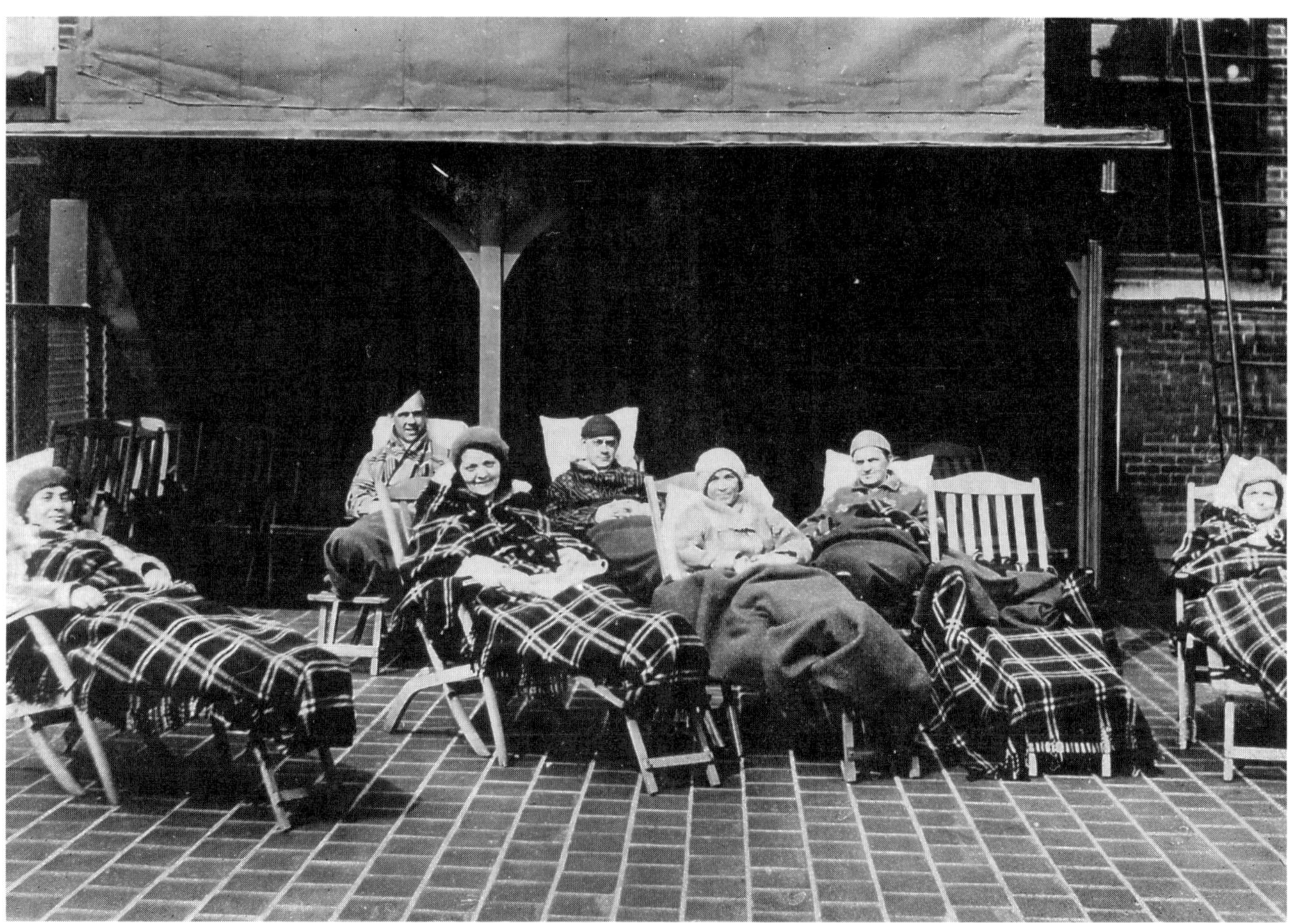

FIG. 11-7. "Taking the cure"; outdoor treatment on the roof at Pine Street (ca. 1930).

Gordon developed a new apparatus for use in administration of pneumothorax treatments that incorporated a graphic pressure record and permitted direct observation of manometric reading during the inflow of air, thus contributing to the safety of the procedure (Figure 11-8).[20] His inventive talents also led to the design of a device for decompression of pressure pneumothorax and for thoracentesis, an abdominal support for elevation of the diaphragm in people with tuberculosis and emphysema,[21] and the design of a new chest piece for the stethoscope, which became known as the Gordon Stethoscope. In 1932, he published an article entitled "Pulmonary Asbestosis,"[22] which in recent years has been regarded as a landmark observation in relation to the major hazards to the lungs that are now known to result from asbestos exposure. Along with research, he was quickly promoted from Associate in Medicine to Assistant Professor in 1930 and to Associate Professor in 1932. Gordon's writing also included revision of Hughes' *Practice of Medicine* in 1935, and he contributed to McCrae's revision (twelfth) of Osler's *Principles and Practice of Medicine* the same year. Later he joined Christian in editing *Oxford Medicine*.

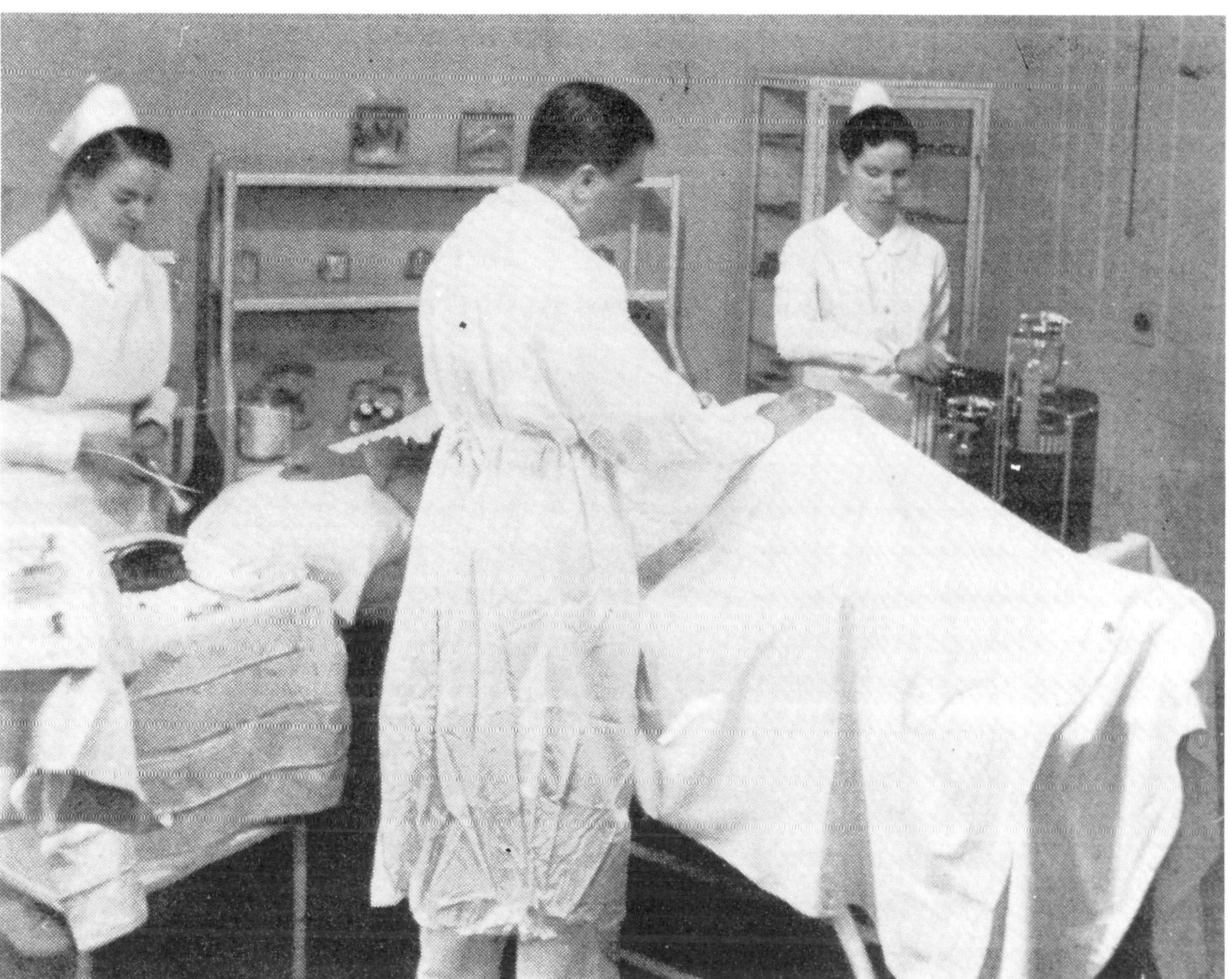

FIG. 11-8. Artificial pneumothorax treatment at White Haven Sanatorium (ca. 1936) employing the Gordon device (see text). Collapse therapy was ultimately rendered obsolete by antituberculous drugs.

The Department prospered in spite of the Great Depression of the 1930s. Although the patient census decreased in 1931, there was a great deal of activity in patient treatment, teaching, and research. A proposal to develop an animal house at Pine Street in 1931 was not adopted because facilities were becoming available in the new College building. The teaching at Pine Street for third- and fourth-year medical students continued its popularity, and the increased activities during the 1930s also made the Department attractive to student nurses. Hiring of staff nurses was never a problem.

Two important teaching modalities developed in addition to usual group teaching. Dr. Gordon conducted a clinic in the Thompson Clinical Amphitheatre once weekly where patients were shown and discussed by him and by Dr. John T. Farrell from the Department of Radiology, giving emphasis to the increasingly important role of x-ray diagnosis in lung diseases. Repartee between these two popular teachers added to the attractiveness of the hour for the medical students. The other event was the later institution of semimonthly clinical conferences held in the classroom in the basement of the Pine Street Hospital. In a sense this continued a tradition begun in the early days of the Phipps Institute in the same building. At that time all fatal cases were discussed at a weekly staff meeting but now the conferences were extended to include staff personnel, house staff, radiologists, surgeons, bronchoscopists, and at times other disciplines. Later, guests from other hospitals and sanatoria attended these conferences, which became important teaching and exchange media well before the now widely used clinical conference became popular. Dr. Peter A. Theodos (Jefferson, 1935), who joined the staff in 1938, had also been exposed to the conference system during his residency and had much to do with its effectiveness. As time went on, especially during World War II, this conference was changed to include the medical students, who found it effective and stimulating.

Research and Surgical Developments

Funds contributed for research purposes from 1929 forward played an important role in the activities of the Department. These included grants from Mrs. E. T. Bedford of New York, C. Mahlon Kline, Lessing J. Rosenwald, and Mrs. Mabel Mann Davis of Philadelphia, and one in memory of Anne Woodhill White of Newark, New Jersey. A chemist, Dr. Proskuriakoff, was added to the staff, and laboratory facilities were improved. A nutrition clinic, an allergy clinic, and at various times a bronchoscopic clinic were supported as outpatient activities flourished. A pneumothorax clinic was added so that patients discharged from the wards could receive their air "refills" as outpatients. During these years, it was still not possible to treat chest diseases totally in the Pine Street facility, and much transportation of patients to the main hospital was necessary as tuberculosis treatment became more involved. Surgical procedures were done at the main hospital, but difficulty in isolation was a problem. The need for surgical facilities at Pine Street was soon obvious, but in the depression of the 1930s funds were short. Finally in 1938, Mr. Joseph V. Horn provided a grant for a surgical unit with $5,000 that he later supplemented at the time of its completion. This made it possible to carry out pneumolysis, extrapleural pneumothorax, phrenic nerve exeresis, and thoracoplasty in the same building in which the patients were housed. X-ray facilities were also updated, and Dr. Robert Lukens continued his close relationship for bronchoscopic diagnosis and treatment, in which he had pioneered 15 years earlier. Surgeons previously appointed as consultants became much more active and participated in teaching and the clinical conferences as well. These included Drs. George J. Willauer (Jefferson, 1923) and Howard H. Bradshaw (Jefferson, 1927) who were later joined by Drs. Richard J. Chodoff (Jefferson, 1933) and Frederick W. Deardorff (Jefferson, 1932). The availability of surgical facilities also resulted in referrals of patients from regional tuberculosis institutions.

Among medical men who became important in the new endeavor were Dr. Robert Kyun-Hyun Charr (Figure 11-9) (Jefferson, 1931) in 1933 (whose appointment was interrupted by a bout with tuberculosis), Dr. Edward H. Kotin (Jefferson,

1930) in 1934, Dr. Paul Klempner (Jefferson, 1932) in 1935, Dr. J. J. Kirshner (Jefferson, 1933) in 1937, and Dr. Peter A. Theodos (Jefferson, 1935) in 1938.

Dr. Hobart A. Reimann succeeded as Attending Physician in 1936 following the death of Dr. McCrae in 1935.[24] Expanding activities required increased efforts on the part of the nursing, social service, and other personnel whose dedication was exemplary. At the same time many factors contributed to the building of patient morale. Attitudes toward tuberculosis gradually changed when the patients perceived that aggressive treatment programs resulted in higher percentage of recoveries and shortening of hospital stay. More attention was also paid to their comforts in the hospital. Wards were redecorated with pleasing colors, and pictures were hung. In 1934 the Department became a subscriber to the circulating picture library of the Philadelphia Art Alliance. The following year, Mr. Abbott of the Art Alliance gave lessons in painting and modeling. The patients responded with enthusiasm to these and other applications of arts and crafts appropriate to patients' limited potential for physical activity. Similar effort ultimately led to the acquisition of a group of landscape oil paintings by Mr. W. Emerson Baum, which were displayed in the Chest Department until 1961 and now adorn the walls of the Pulmonary Division of the Department of Medicine.

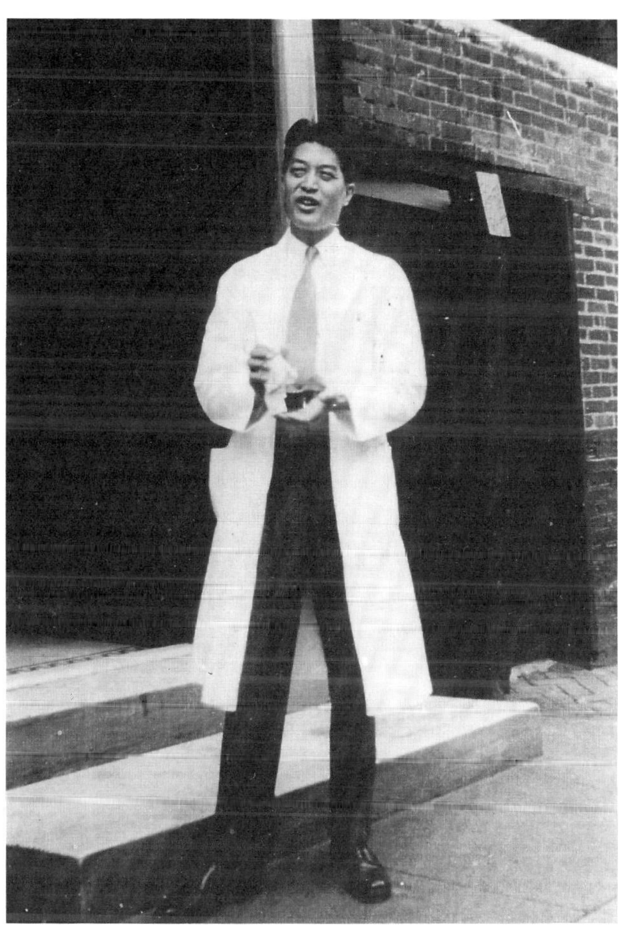

FIG. 11-9. Dr. Robert K. Charr (Jefferson, 1931) at "Pine Street" entrance (ca. 1941). Dr. Charr became highly respected as a clinician and teacher.

During these years the patients were encouraged to organize activities of their own. One result was a publication known as *The Bug*, and another in 1939 entitled *Quest* went through several editions. Also in 1939, a "Graduates' Club" was organized to dramatize the potential for recovery. Awards were given to a number of recently recovered patients to encourage current ones. All of these efforts plus the enthusiasm of the nursing staff and ancillary personnel made for an unusual "esprit de corps," readily perceptible to visitors, house staff, and students. The addition of younger staff members also contributed to a spirit of vigor and optimism.

In 1938, Dr. Charr returned from White Haven Sanatorium, where he had been a physician in residence after his recovery, and his staff appointment was reactivated as Associate in Medicine, part-time fellowship funds having been provided by Mrs. Davis and Mr. Horn. Dr. J. Woodrow Savacool (Jefferson, 1938) was awarded a similar fellowship for teaching and research in 1939 under the same auspices, and a number of projects were undertaken. These led to publications relative to the pathology of the pulmonary vascular system in tuberculosis and anthracosilicosis, the clinical aspects of pleural effusions in tuberculosis, the causes and pathology of pulmonary hemorrhage, and application of the newly discovered plasma prothrombin determination to patients with tuberculosis.[25]

In 1940 a staff dinner was held to celebrate the accomplishments of the previous decade and develop enthusiasm for continuing progress. Dr. Gordon addressed the group[26] and emphasized the role of the new surgical unit in improving the outlook for the patients. Not only did he show the excellence of results of the surgical procedures but indicated the overall improvement in the results of treatment generally. It is apparent in retrospect that the improved outlook resulted more specifically from the fact that patients on admission were less seriously ill than formerly and the potential for recovery was, therefore, greater. The dinner was attended by Trustees and major faculty, and the report was received with enthusiasm. The Department seemed poised for a period of stability, growth, and service.

Contributing greatly to the atmosphere of the Division was the excellence of the nursing care. The staff nurses were dedicated and skilled, and the student nurses rotating through the wards readily captured the spirit. When wartime strictures became the rule, it was common for both staff and student nurses to put in extra time to keep the work under control. Miss Thelma Showers, previously an outpatient department supervisor in Pediatrics, succeeded Miss Mary Cushen as Nursing Supervisor in 1940. She set the tone for the nursing service and made thereby a major contribution to the care of the patients and to the recruitment of excellent staff nurses, who came through the program as students (Figures 11-10 and 11-11). Among these were Miss Joanna Laise, Miss Jean Fluck, Miss Jean Lebkicker, Miss Anne Haines, and Miss Jean Fishel. Miss Mary Albright did yeoman service as night supervisor.

Mrs. Millicent Maull continued as the principal Social Service person, aided for some years by Louise H. Goodman and Anna B. Lutz. Frances McBlain joined in 1929, but during the 1930s Mrs. Maull carried on alone except for a secretary.[27]

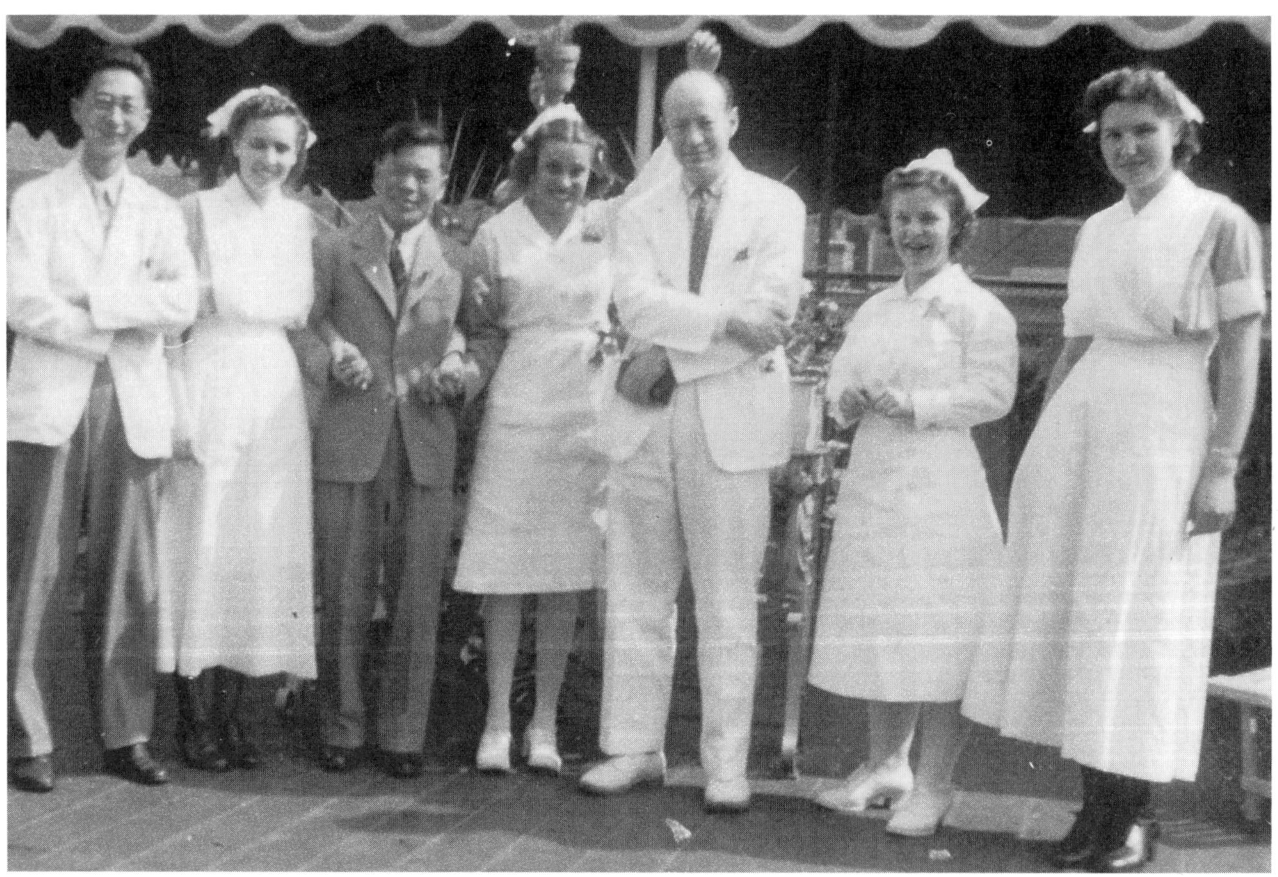

FIG. 11-10. Informal "Pine Street" staff group (ca. 1940). From left: student Thomas S. Min (Jefferson, 1942); student nurse; medical student laboratory assistant Chang Ha Kim (Jefferson, 1941); Nursing Supervisor, Miss Thelma Showers; Dr. Randolph V. Seligman (Jefferson, 1940); Staff Nurse, Mrs. Cake; student nurse.

Mrs. Margaret Flisher Arthur, a person of great talent and experience, replaced Mrs. Maull at her retirement and continued the effective, compassionate care that had become a feature of the operation of the Department.

Wartime

World War II brought about major changes in personnel and required adaptations of all sorts on the part of physicians and nurses. Drs. Gordon, Theodos, Kirshner, and Chodoff were members of the Jefferson 38th Hospital Unit that was activated in 1941, Dr. Gordon having transferred from the Harvard Unit to which he had been attached since his Boston experience. Dr. Martin Sokoloff became Acting Medical Director and Physician-in-Charge in 1942. Major teaching duties were assumed also by Drs. Charr, Nissler, Savacool, Vaughn, Cadden, and Jaffe. Dr. George J. Willauer (Figure 11-12) (Jefferson, 1923) was virtually the only surgeon to carry on the increasing workload, and at times he had to operate without assistance except from the nurses, even student nurses. During the war years research was virtually at a standstill all the while surgical procedures were increasingly utilized. These in turn were made safer by advances in anesthesia and the gradual availability of antimicrobial agents,

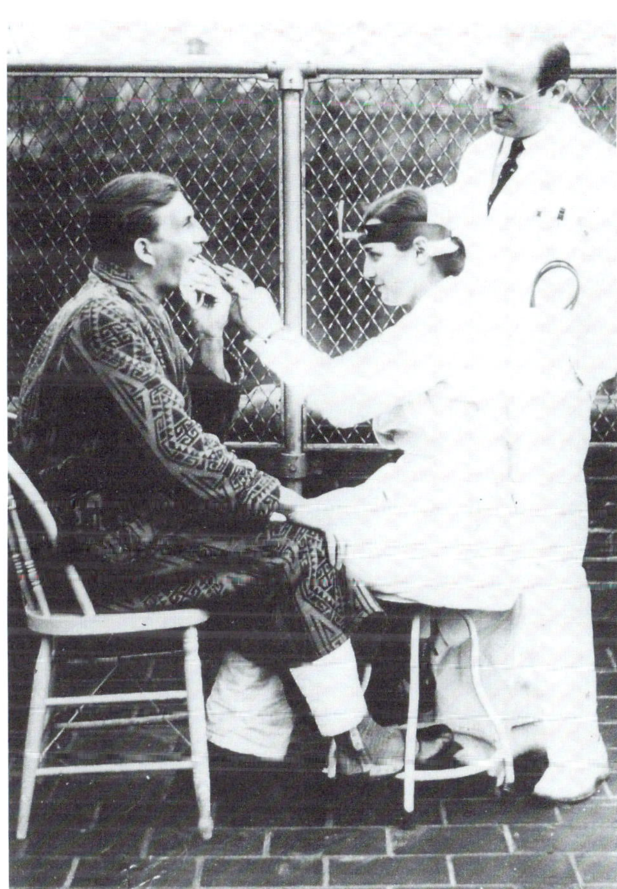

FIG. 11-11. Laryngoscopy was an important part of tuberculosis diagnosis and treatment. A staff nurse participates in the process with the laryngologist.

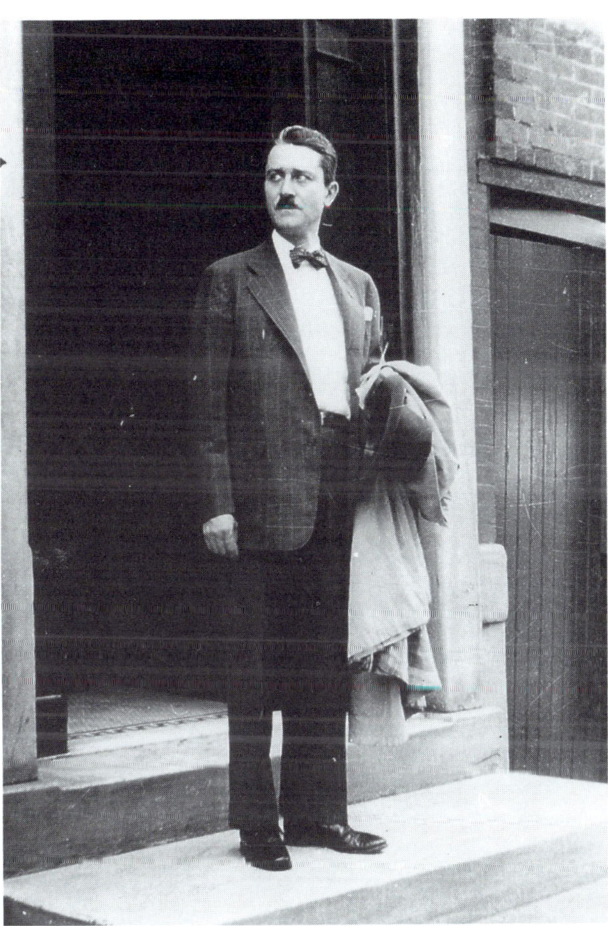

FIG. 11-12. Dr. George J. Willauer (Jefferson, 1923) at "Pine Street" (1941), pioneer thoracic surgeon, later described by a colleague from another medical school as having done the best and perhaps the most surgery for pulmonary tuberculosis in Philadelphia.

at first for control of nontuberculous infections and later for tuberculosis. Until the end of the war, however, no effective antituberculous agents played a role in treatment. The order of the day was to find early cases, begin rest treatment and, if not rapidly effective or if cavitation was present, to begin collapse with pneumothorax. When treatment was successful, patients could be discharged after a relatively few weeks to continue pneumothorax refills as outpatients. Thus patient turnover increased.

Dr. Martin J. Sokoloff (Figure 11-13) (Jefferson, 1920), having garnered experience in public health as Director of the Division of Tuberculosis Control for the City of Philadelphia just before the war, continued in that role while assuming the Acting Directorship of "Pine Street." With the momentum that had been developed in the prewar years, he proved especially effective in managing the affairs of the Department. He gave many teaching hours, continued the student–staff conferences, and with the help of the teaching staff maintained the morale of the facility.

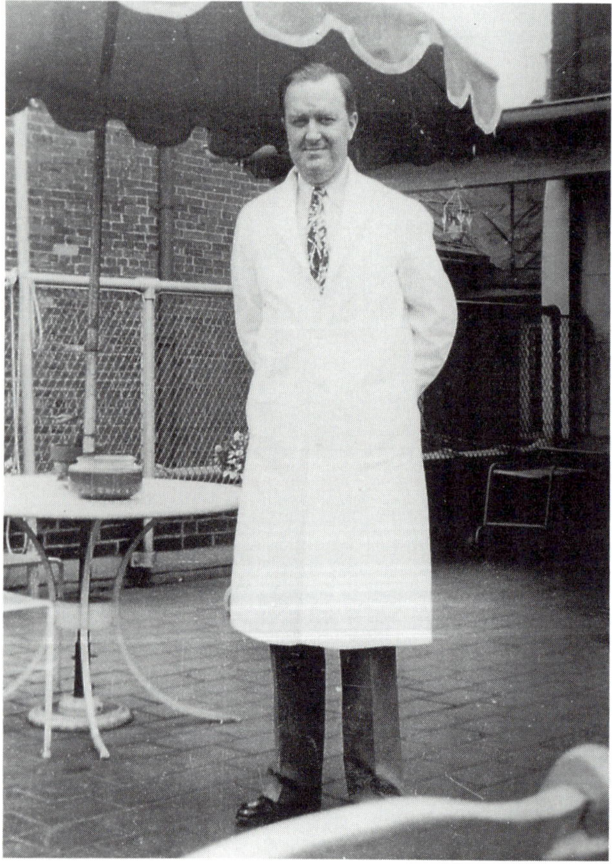

FIG. 11-13. Dr. Martin J. Sokoloff (Jefferson, 1920), staff member from 1924, Acting Medical Director (1942–1945), and Medical Director (1952–1962).

Dr. Gaetano Brindisi (Jefferson, 1940) joined the clinical staff in 1943, and Dr. James S. D. Eisenhower (Jefferson, 1943) in 1945. It is a tribute to the abilities of the local people that tuberculosis control continued to improve even during wartime. Methods devised for similar control among military personnel also proved useful in civilian life.

Return of Drs. Gordon, Theodos, and Kirshner from military service in 1945–1946 led to much new activity. Planning for progress could be resumed and long-awaited consideration for expansion of services assumed importance. Dr. Gordon was soon informed by the Trustees that a bequest from the Pendleton–Barton Family had produced funds that could be applied to create a larger facility. Negotiations were ultimately concluded for the purchase of a building at Broad and Fitzwater Streets, formerly the site of the Broad Street Hospital. The building was purchased at Sheriff's Sale for $124,000, settlement date June 10, 1946. Renovations were then undertaken to adapt the building to its new uses. The news was greeted with enthusiasm by the staff and administration with anticipation of improved facilities for patient care, nursing care, medical teaching, and research. A very orderly transition was made in January, 1947 to the new facility, which was designated the Barton Memorial Division of Jefferson Medical College Hospital (Figure 11-14).

The Barton Division for Diseases of the Chest

The Barton bequest resulted from the will of Emily Barton Pendleton, who died February 24, 1940. It left her residuary estate to Jefferson to be divided between the Edward Gray Pendleton Memorial Fund for work in cancer and the Emily C. Barton Memorial Fund for work in tuberculosis. Mrs. Pendleton's great-uncle was Dr. Wm. P. C. Barton (1786–1856), who was Dean of Jefferson from 1828 to 1830. Mrs. Pendleton's mother, Emily Chase Barton, had died of tuberculosis, and her husband, Edward Gray Pendleton, had predeceased her in 1920. The original bequest was valued at $310,000 in 1940, but careful use of the funds and investments resulted in appreciation to $1,864,128.54 in December, 1983.[28] The first funds were distributed February 28, 1941; the major distribution occurred in August 1941 and the final one in October 1944. The Barton funds thus have resulted in major contributions to medical progress, research, and patient care over virtually one-half century while still providing for the future. A court decision of October 21, 1983, has interpreted the intent of the testator in such a way that the funds could be used "to further research regarding diagnosis and treatment of respiratory and pulmonary problems. Such problems may include but are not limited to problems resulting from cancer affecting these areas and systems."[29]

The White Haven Sanatorium

A related occurrence dovetailed very well with postwar developments for the Chest Department, namely the acquisition of the White Haven Sanatorium, negotiation for which had been under way for some time. The Sanatorium was

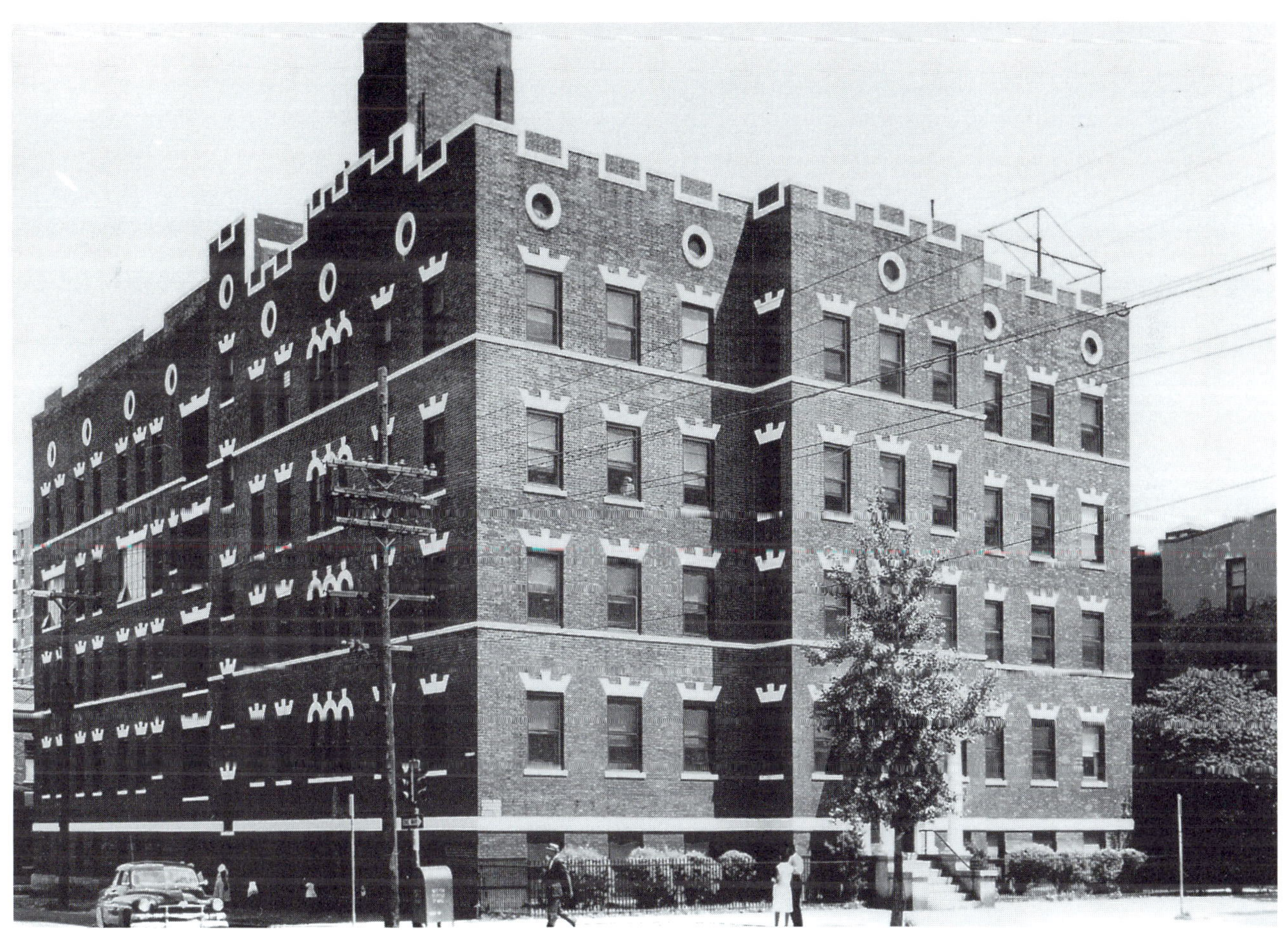

FIG. 11-14. The Barton Memorial Division of Jefferson Medical College Hospital. Located at Broad and Fitzwater Streets, the building housed the Department for Diseases of the Chest from 1946 until 1961.

founded in 1901 and had served its constituency with skill and effectiveness. During the prewar period, however, it became apparent that changes would be necessary to permit it to fulfill its mission. In company with similar institutions both private and public, especially those remote from population centers, the need for more aggressive treatment of tuberculosis became apparent. White Haven, therefore, added facilities for surgical treatment and upgraded its ancillary services in the late 1930s, a process that proved useful only for interim purposes. Thus as the war was ending and planning could be resumed, several proposals were considered for change and improvement. Ultimately the Trustees decided that the free-standing status of the Sanatorium was no longer in the best interest of modern treatment. Since association with a teaching institution was desirable, a merger with Jefferson would place White Haven in the strongest position for the pursuit of its long-term goals. Appropriate legal steps were taken, and on March 18, 1946, the Sanatorium became the White Haven Division of Jefferson Medical College Hospital (Figure 11-15). Dr. Gordon was made Director of White Haven and Barton Divisions, and the staffs were expanded to man both. Jefferson was now in a position to treat and study all aspects of pulmonary diseases, with acute and surgical treatment available at Barton and prolonged care at White Haven.

Many adaptations were needed. Housekeeping, maintenance, and nursing services required expansion for the new Barton, which provided 91 beds for care of patients with all types of lung diseases. Surgical facilities were much improved over those at Pine Street. Laboratory and x-ray facilities were likewise expanded. Dr. Sokoloff,

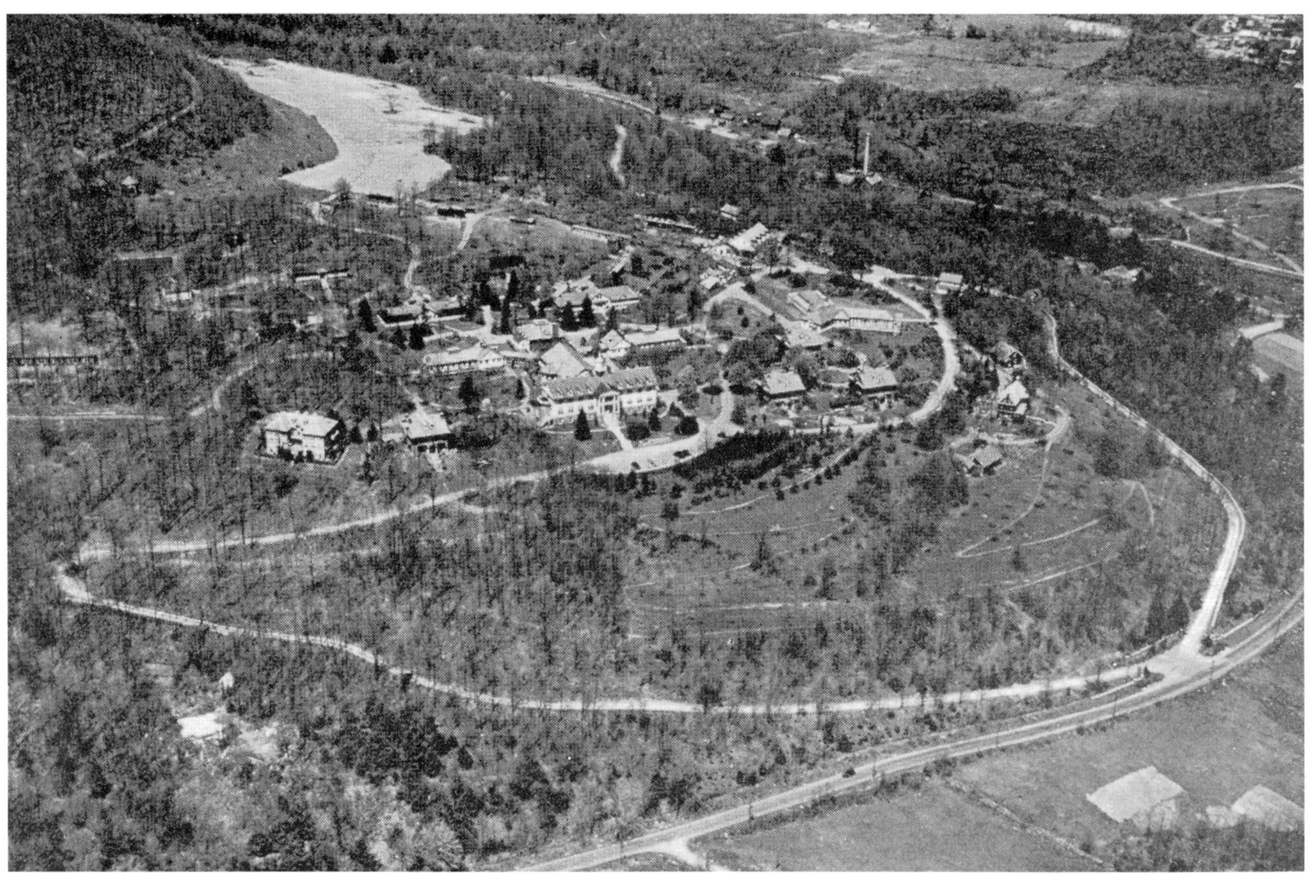

FIG. 11-15. The White Haven Sanatorium Division of Jefferson Medical College Hospital from 1946. It was sold to the State of Pennsylvania in 1956 for the White Haven State School and Hospital.

having kept the Division functioning well during the War, continued as Assistant Medical Director. Dr. Willauer was designated as Visiting Surgeon, Dr. Bradshaw having become Professor and Chairman of the Department of Surgery at the new Bowman-Gray School of Medicine. Dr. Francis F. Allbritten became Assistant Surgeon. Miss Thelma Showers organized the nursing services with increased reponsibilities for those staff nurses who had served so effectively at Pine Street. Mrs. Margaret Flisher Arthur provided experience and sensitive skill in an expanded Social Service Department. Teaching was more satisfactory, the small section program for medical students being more intimate and diverse. In addition, small student sections rotated through White Haven, usually with one of the Barton staff members accompanying them for part of a weekend. An effort to expand the staff at White Haven with visiting physicians from the region was only partly successful. Ultimately, responsibility for the care of the patients devolved upon the resident staff and the visiting staff from Barton.

The Laboratory for Pulmonary Physiology

An important development that could be realized with the availability of larger quarters at Barton was the establishment of a laboratory for pulmonary physiology. Interest in this activity had progressed during the war, especially in aviation medicine, and there was a need for basic and applied research. Studies of lung function and cardiopulmonary circulation held great promise for improvement in patient care and selection of patients for surgical and special procedures. The association with White Haven opened the possibility of improving the care of the large numbers of anthracite miners treated there for many years. Large numbers of miners were afflicted with anthracosiliosis, tuberculosis, emphysema, and combinations of processes known in the coal regions as "miner's asthma." These people were generally seriously ill, and the mortality rate was high. Symptoms of cough and dyspnea were distressing, and in the past little could be done. Tuberculosis often complicated the scarring resulting from the inhalation of silica-laden mine dust, and collapse therapy could not be used. Early in 1947, Dr. Gordon suggested to a local miner's union counsel that a major research program into the lung problems of anthracite miners could be undertaken. A visit to Mr. John L. Lewis, President of the United Mine Worker's Union, was arranged, and he proved enthusiastic about the idea. The Anthracite Health and Welfare Fund was immediately developed to initiate the program. The laboratory was established on the ground floor of the Barton Division. To direct it, Dr. Hurley L. Motley (Harvard, 1936) was recruited. Dr. Motley, previously Associate Professor of Physiology at the University of Missouri School of Medicine, had experience during World War II as an aviation physiologist and Flight Surgeon. At Wright Field, Dayton, Ohio, he pioneered in research on pressure breathing. Most recently Motley had served as a Research Fellow at Bellevue Hospital, New York, under Drs. Dickinson Richards and Andre Cournand. His qualifications were thus unusually appropriate. He arrived at Barton in September 1947 and quickly assembled the equipment needed to begin the studies. Dr. Leonard Lang (Jefferson, 1939), who was appointed to the teaching staff in 1946, became associated with Dr. Motley, and Dr. Peter A. Theodos (Jefferson, 1935) joined the group as Clinical Associate under Dr. Gordon.

The new organization proved effective, especially in the area of teaching and patient care. Medical students had opportunities not previously available, notably the ability to observe the diagnosis and management of chest diseases in a comprehensive manner, including x-ray and bronchoscopic diagnosis, which were readily at hand. Students could also appreciate the increasing role of surgery in treatment of tuberculosis and the burgeoning cases of lung carcinoma. Surgical residents rotating through the Barton Division found the experience rewarding. At this time, in 1947, adequate supplies of streptomycin, the first antimicrobial agent to prove practical in tuberculosis treatment, became available. The impact of this new modality, however, was not a major one until adjunctive agents were developed, notably para-aminosalicylic acid (PAS) in 1949 and the more definitive isonicotinic acid hydrazide (isoniazid) in 1952. Intrathoracic surgical procedures could be carried out with greater safety, increasing the frequency of lobectomy and pneumonectomy for both tuberculosis and cancer. The duration of hospital stay decreased and convalescence could be followed at White Haven. The physiology laboratory made an immediate difference in patient care and attracted patients and personnel from the main hospital for studies and observation. During the 1950s, fellows in pulmonary physiology became affiliated with the Department for training. At one time there was a proposal to convert the Barton Division into a major center for cardiac studies and surgery, but ultimately the decision was made not to take this course.

The availability of comprehensive facilities attracted patients from the Veterans Administration, since postwar needs were not met by existing veterans hospitals. This program under contract with the federal government provided material for teaching, physiological studies, and medical and surgical treatment at a reasonable daily rate and for about 6 years was a very useful arrangement. Ultimately the Veterans Administration had its own facilities, and soon the impact of anti-tuberculous medication diminished drastically the need for beds for war veterans. Also, Barton contracted with the City of Philadelphia to care for patients originating in the city chest clinics for whom state sanatorium beds were not available. This program began in 1950 and continued in numbers diminishing after 1954 until 1960. For these patients all services were included in the per diem rate.

▪ Miners' Diseases

Perhaps the most widely publicized events in the history of the Department surrounded the early studies in the cardiorespiratory laboratory. The mine workers' program, being the most visible, quickly attracted attention with the new "machines" for their study and with efforts at treatment generated by the findings. Thus the obstructive aspects of the impaired lung function were treated by the newly developed valves for positive pressure breathing applied by Drs. Motley, Gordon, Lang, and Theodos to the miners studied at Barton (Figure 11-16).[30,31] Mine workers on a regular basis were admitted to Barton and evaluated for 10–14 days (Figure 11-17). Those judged to be adaptable to mechanical treatment began it at Barton and, if necessary, continued it at White Haven. Several depots were available in the mining regions for those able to be discharged. The miners responded to these efforts with enthusiasm and cooperation, since for the first time something was being done for "miners' asthma." Publicity about the program was generated in the local newspapers[32] and national news magazines.[33] A number of scientific publications quickly followed in the medical literature.[34] It was a period of real productivity and accomplishment.

Although the pathology of anthracite miners' diseases had previously been relatively well developed, the Barton studies enlarged upon the

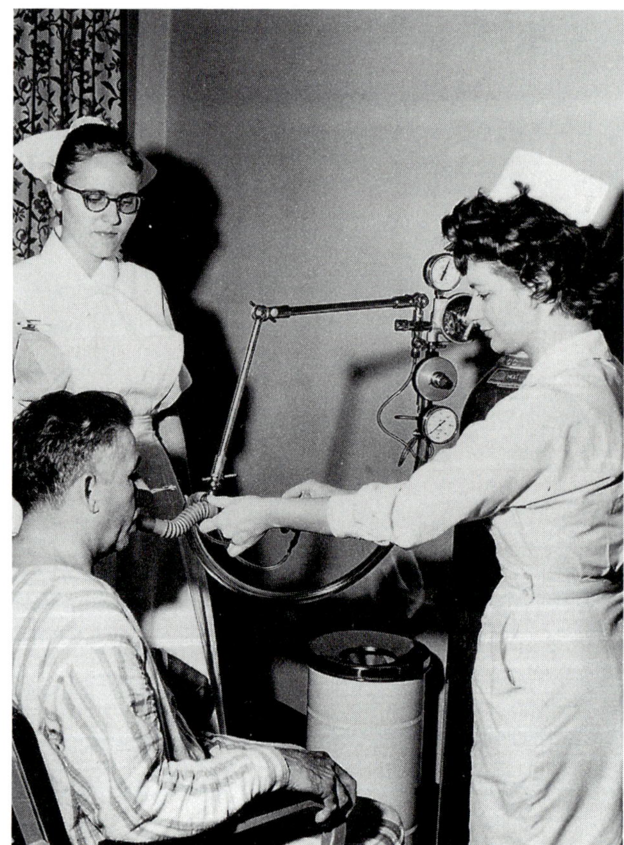

FIG. 11-16. An anthracite miner with anthracosilicosis receiving treatment with intermittent positive pressure breathing. Miss Emma Gallo (right), Barton Supervising Nurse, teaches the technique.

relationships among the lesions of silicosis, anthracosis, tuberculosis, and emphysema. Cavitating silicotic masses were described exclusive of the effects of tuberculosis by Dr. Theodos (Figure 11-18), who became nationally known for these observations that led to other concerns in environmental and industrial medicine. The studies made a significant contribution to preventive measures in all industries with dust inhalation problems. In 1949 arrangements were made for admission of bituminous miners to White Haven and Barton to permit comparison of their disease problems with those of anthracite miners. About 200 soft coal miners ultimately participated in these studies.

Progress was not achieved in total peace and quiet. Some of the plans for the expanded Department were not realized, and there were also interpersonal and institutional problems. The full staffing of the White Haven Division proved difficult. Physicians no longer were willing to limit their activities and training to remote sanatoriums, and the regional internists appointed to the staff were willing to attend occasional meetings but not to admit patients and participate in day-to-day treatment. Thus, the medical staff in residence was limited mainly to physicians themselves convalescing from tuberculosis. Dr. Edward A. Favis, one of the last Chief Resident Physicians, was one of a long list of such physicians who achieved success in internal medicine following recovery. As antituberculous treatment became available, the need for collapse therapy and surgery gradually diminished, a process that simplified the

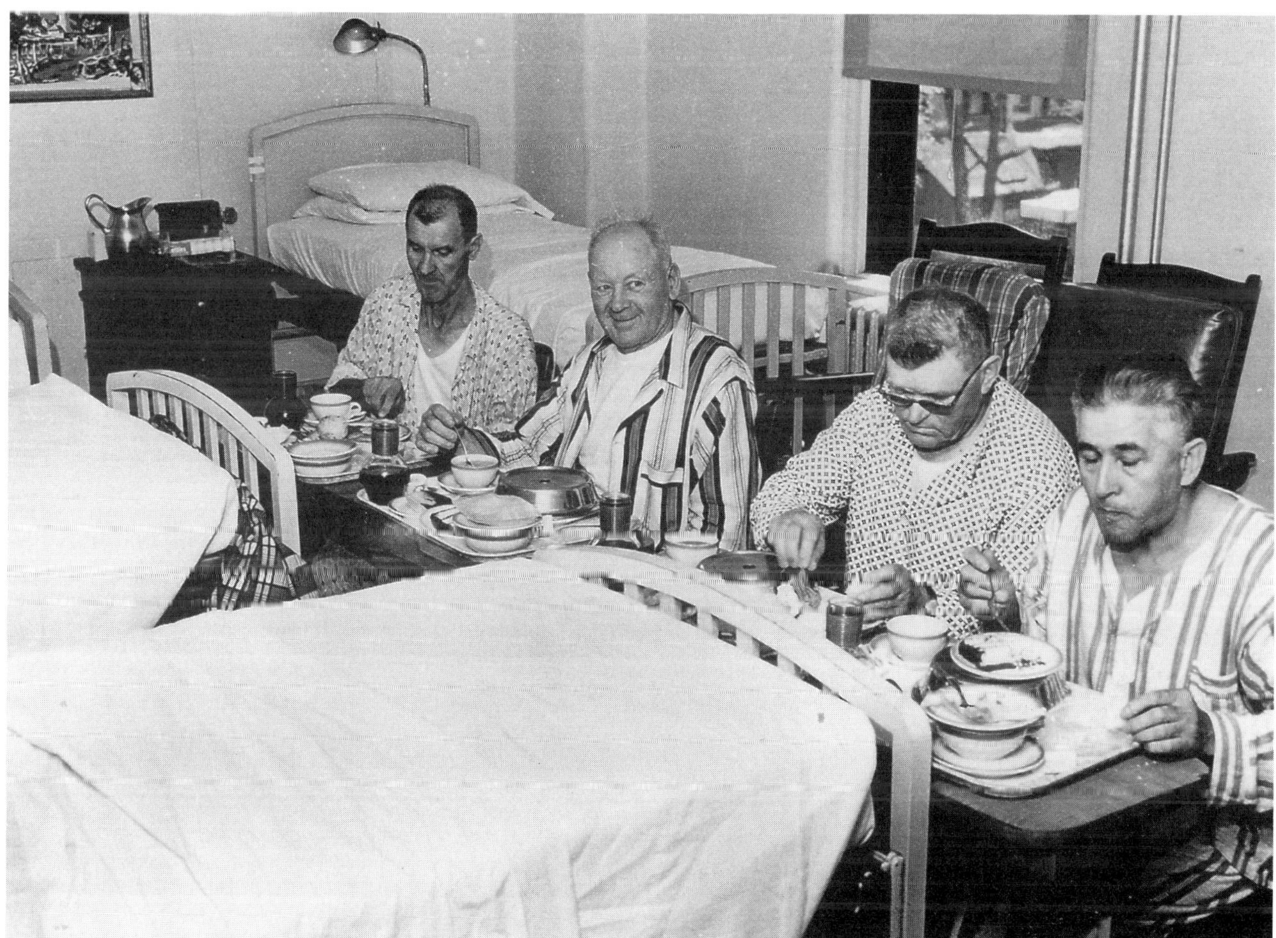

FIG. 11-17. Coal miners at Barton during study and treatment for anthracosilicosis under United Mine Workers Research Project.

care of tuberculous patients. Postwar economic expansion of industry did not include anthracite coal; alternate fuels were exploited that appeared less difficult and hazardous to bring to market. The fate of the White Haven Division, therefore, was to have stable occupancy until the middle 1950s, when fewer beds were needed, and the maintenance of a full staff could no longer be justified.

A controversy developed in the late 1940s, when the departmental acquisitions had been fulfilled, between Dr. Reimann, as Attending Physician, and Dr. Gordon. Some members of the staff found that the new relationships were not producing the intended results, and dissatisfactions came to Dr. Reimann's attention. Specifically, the use of the White Haven facility for student and resident teaching left much to be desired, especially due to its remoteness and lack of experienced staff teachers. Numerous meetings, letters, and exchanges occurred, sometimes with heat and accusatory implications. At one time, Dr. Gordon's resignation was suggested as a solution. Although some similar criticism was applied to the Barton Division, especially for training of medical residents, the effectiveness of the cardiorespiratory laboratory program and the traditional good will among members of the staff surmounted the difficulties. The Department entered the 1950s on a positive note. The surgical program was going well and a number of surgical and medical residents rotating through Barton made significant contributions in relating progress to their colleagues at the main hospital. Patients from the main hospital were increasingly brought to Barton for pulmonary function studies prior to surgery.

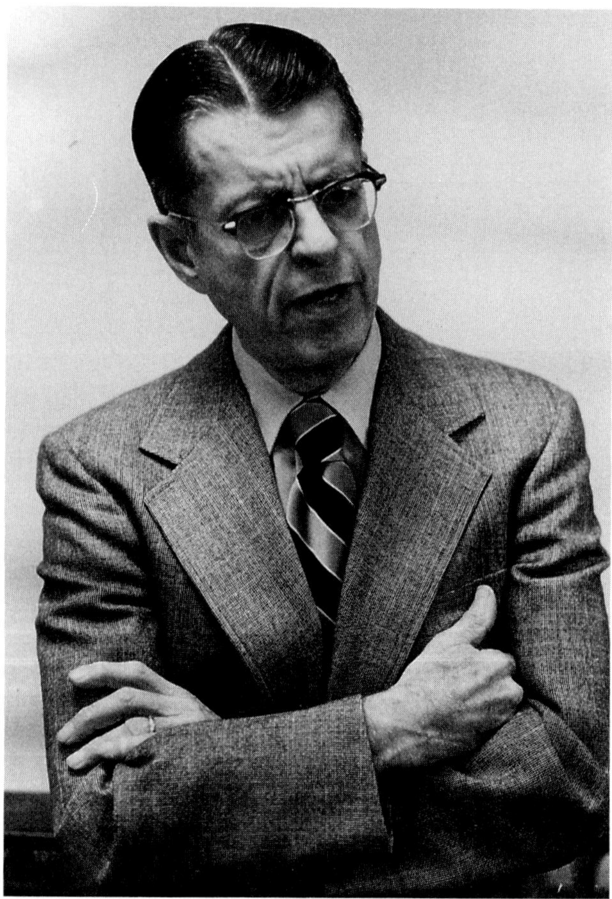

FIG. 11-18. Dr. Peter A. Theodos (Jefferson, 1935), whose studies of silicosis contributed to efforts at environmental and industrial controls of inhaled particles.

Associated with the pulmonary physiology program from the start in 1947, Dr. Leonard Lang had participated with devotion and skill in the studies and publications that followed. Upon his resignation to establish a practice in pulmonary diseases in Wilmington, Delaware, his successor, Dr. Joseph Tomashefski, a Fellow from 1949–1951, went on to a distinguished career in pulmonary medicine.

During the early 1950s many changes took place. Dr. Gordon had been advised by Dr. Christian, his mentor at Harvard, not to remain at one place too long.[35] Several opportunities for change had opened for Gordon, but in early 1951 serious negotiations for his services had begun with Womans' Medical College and Hospital. These led to his appointment as of September 1, 1951, as President of Womans' Medical College and Wm. Mullen Professor of Medicine.

Dr. Martin J. Sokoloff, who had done excellent service as Acting Director of the Chest Department during the war, was appointed as Acting Director immediately upon Dr. Gordon's resignation. He served until his appointment as Medical Director and Physician-in-Charge was affirmed as of January 1, 1953. At the same time changes were taking place in the Department of Medicine. Dr. Reimann resigned in October, 1951, and was succeeded by Dr. John E. Deitrick, whose commitment to medical teaching fitted well with the ongoing activities of the Barton Division.

While there were continuing tensions in the Department of Medicine, the early 1950s proved to be relatively stable at Barton. Research into miners' disease and several of the newly described interstitial lung diseases, and the problem of increasing incidence of obstructive lung diseases, received appropriate attention.

Changes Relating to Effective Tuberculosis Treatment

During the middle 1950s a major change in emphasis occurred with respect to lung diseases. Isoniazid, which became available in 1952, more than fulfilled its promise. After a few years it became clear that with the use of effective antituberculosis therapy, long periods of rest treatment were no longer necessary. Surgical and collapse therapy were also gradually replaced by medical measures for the routine treatment of tuberculosis. About 1954 the chronic bed shortage for city and state agencies disappeared, and soon sanatoriums could be abandoned. By the end of the decade, major emphasis could again be directed toward prevention, with total control of this previously devastating disease. The diminishing demand for chronic beds led the Trustees to seek alternative uses for the White Haven Division, and on January 26, 1956, an agreement to sell the sanatorium to the Commonwealth of Pennsylvania was concluded. The Barton program for research in the diseases of miners, however, was continued, the mine agencies and local physicians in the mining regions serving as referral sources.

At the same time the Division was more clearly defined administratively as a division of the Department of Medicine, overriding the earlier arrangement specified by the Board of Trustees requiring the Medical Director to report directly to the Trustees as well as to the Attending Physician, at that time Dr. McCrae. The designation "Department for Diseases of the Chest" gave way to that of the "Barton Memorial Division" of the Department of Medicine.

Other changes occurring during the 1950s included major increases in carcinoma of the lung and obstructive lung diseases. Both of these events are now known to have related in great measure to the increase in cigarette smoking, some of which could be ascribed to the stresses of World War II. In any event, the studies and treatment inclined more toward changes in pulmonary function as factors in acceptability for lung resection and in conservation of breathing capacity. Gradually the research aspects of pulmonary function were incorporated into established clinical procedures.

In 1953 Dr. Motley resigned to accept an appointment as Professor of Medicine and Physiology at the University of Southern California Medical School. In reviewing the experiences of the Barton staff during the 5-year period of his direction of the laboratory, many accomplishments were recorded. Fellows were trained; research was productive. Teaching of medical students was enhanced through Dr. Motley's efforts, and the miners' program achieved many of its goals. The group was in great demand for medical meetings, and much effort was devoted to making the new pulmonary physiology understandable to the physician in practice. As expected, Dr. Motley went on to major accomplishments in pulmonary medicine with national recognition, but much of the groundwork was done at Jefferson.

Dr. Motley was succeeded by Dr. Richard T. Cathcart (Figure 11-19) (A.B., Yale, M.D., Columbia), who was trained in cardiology and pulmonary physiology at Bellevue and Presbyterian Hospitals in New York. He had for 3 years been director of the Cardiorespiratory Laboratory at St. Luke's Hospital, New York, and his new duties enabled him to build upon his experience there. In addition to continuing the research program, Dr. Cathcart quickly established himself as a teacher who could reduce complicated physiological problems to an understandable level for medical students and house staff. He was appointed Assistant Professor of Medicine.

During this period, Dr. Sokoloff continued as Director of Tuberculosis Control for the City of Philadelphia and was able to coordinate his public health duties with those pertaining to Jefferson. Among the Barton staff members associated with him as consultants to the Philadelphia Department of Health were Drs. Theodos, Kirshner, Savacool, and Cohen, all of whom continued their activities throughout the 1960s. The morale of the nursing and ancillary staff remained high under his leadership. Mrs. Thelma Showers Morris resigned in 1948 and was succeeded as Director of Nursing by Miss Helen Whitney, later to be followed by Miss Grace Ronco and still later by Miss Emma Gallo. The surgical program was under the joint direction of Drs. Thomas A. Shallow, John H. Gibbon, Jr., and Frank F. Allbritten until Allbritten's resignation in 1954 to become Chairman and Professor of Surgery at the Medical School of the University of Kansas. He was succeeded at Barton by several young and able surgeons who had rotated through Barton during their training: Drs. John Y. Templeton III (Jefferson, 1941), George J. Haupt (Jefferson, 1948), Thomas F. Nealon, Jr. (Jefferson, S1944), and John J. McKeown, Jr. (Jefferson, 1947), all of whom went on to major appointments in thoracic surgery and in teaching of general surgery. Dr. Charles Fineberg, later Professor of Surgery at Jefferson, rotated through the program and contributed to its strength, also serving with Dr. George Willauer at Eagleville Sanatorium. In medicine, Dr. Robert Charr shared his activities with teaching duties at the main hospital. He was responsible for the course in physical diagnosis, where his teaching abilities came to full flower. Charr was also an Attending Physician at the Pennsylvania Hospital in the tradition of Dr. McCrae; his death in 1956 was a serious loss to Jefferson. During these years the medical teaching and clinical program was strengthened by the participation of Dr. Jacob J. Kirshner (Jefferson, 1933), whose experience and skills were highly regarded. In bronchoscopy after the war Dr. Robert M. Lukens (Jefferson, 1912), was joined by Dr. John J. O'Keefe (Jefferson, 1937), and later by Dr. William H. Baltzell (Jefferson, 1946). The high quality of work in this Department was thus maintained.

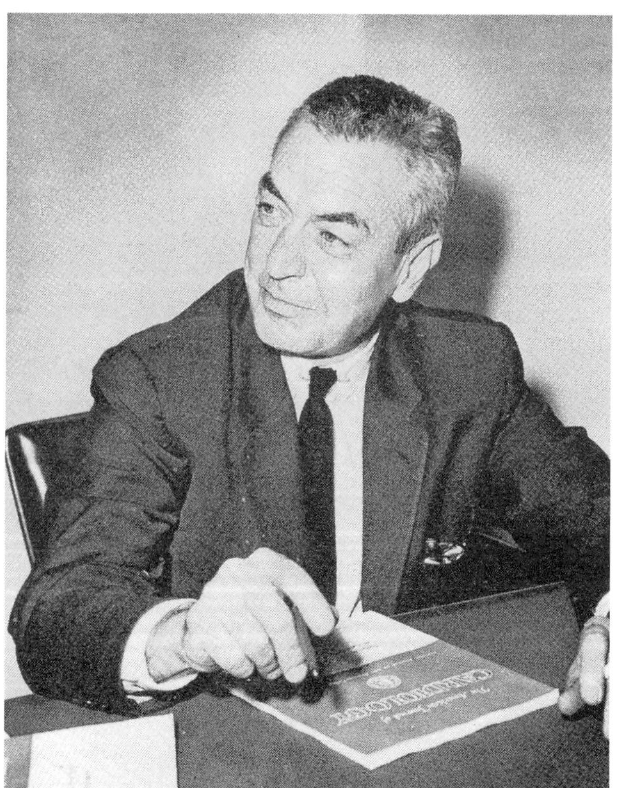

FIG. 11-19. Dr. Richard T. Cathcart, Medical Director of Barton Division (1963–1974).

In addition to his work with the miners' program, Dr. Theodos was mainly responsible for the outpatient clinic, which underwent considerable change from the experience at Old Pine Street. The reduction in incidence of tuberculosis and the availability of other agencies for its care resulted in diminishing need for outpatient services, especially since many referrals of nontuberculous lung disease patients were likely to be made to the hospital for direct admission. The Social Service program underwent a change in emphasis for similar reasons, but Mrs. Margaret Arthur continued to function with compassion and effectiveness.

Gradually in the late 1950s the diminishing census especially for tuberculosis resulted in consideration of plans for change. Dr. Deitrick had resigned as Magee Professor and thus as Attending Physician on July 31, 1957, to become Dean of the Medical College of Cornell University. He was promptly succeeded by Dr. William A. Sodeman, who in turn served only until April 2, 1958, when he was appointed Dean of Jefferson Medical College and Vice-President for Medical Affairs. His succession by Dr. Robert Irby Wise assured continuation of policies and procedures that were in the process of development and that promised progress for the Pulmonary Division.

Barton Moves to Main Hospital

In April 1959, Jefferson's President, James L. Kauffman, appointed a committee to study "the possibility of integrating the facilities now at Barton with Jefferson's main hospitals." This committee was given only one month to make its recommendations, but in spite of this stricture a report was submitted that soon gave rise to action. Some considerations were legal in character because the use of funds from the Barton bequests as well as residual endowment funds of the White Haven Sanatorium were involved. The latter proved readily adaptable to the plans that evolved, and the ultimate legal opinion regarding the Barton funds has been quoted.[29] The conclusion of negotiations and planning resulted in a move of the Barton Division to the second floor of the main hospital building (Old Main 1907).

Renovations of the second floor proceeded apace. The unit consisted of two rooms of four beds each for tuberculous patients, plus several beds planned for surgical tuberculosis, but the latter were soon converted to other uses. There were 19 semiprivate beds for nontuberculous patients, which included those needed for the miners' program. There was a centrally located nurses' station and utility area with a comfortable lounge for visitors, all of which proved effective and attractive. The tuberculosis beds were employed for the few patients still requiring admission for advanced disease as well as for transfer of patients in the general hospital requiring isolation. The pulmonary laboratory was located on the second floor of the Thompson Building adjacent to the clinical area with administrative offices and treatment rooms on the main corridor. A classroom and small conference room completed the arrangement. On June 5, 1961, the move to the new locale was accomplished with minimal disruption of patient care, especially since little change in personnel was involved.

Just before the move, a complete report (1960) of accomplishments of the mine workers' program was developed by the staff of the Barton Memorial Division to Mr. Thomas Kennedy, President of the United Mine Workers Union.[36] This report summarized and described the purposes, procedures, and accomplishments of the program that had then spanned 13 years, and it projected its continuation in the new setting with enhanced facilities. In 13 years, a total of 2,092 miners had been studied, most of them going on to continued treatment in four regional hospital centers. The report stressed the training of physicians who went on to establish laboratories at other hospitals and medical schools as well as publication of physiological and clinical findings in medical literature. During the five years from 1955 to 1960 alone, Drs. Cathcart and Theodos presented 37 speeches and papers before medical groups including the American College of Physicians, American Trudeau Society, American College of Chest Physicians, and the American Surgical Association. Scientific exhibits were shown at ten different conventions including the American Medical Association convention in Atlantic City in 1959 (where it won Honorable Mention). The entire concept of the pathophysiology of anthracosilicosis was developed and defined in detail during this period, with Jefferson acknowledged as a major center of its study and teaching.

In 1959 Dr. Harold L. Israel (Jefferson, 1934) (Figure 11-20) joined the Jefferson staff as Clinical Professor of Medicine in charge of the teaching program at Philadelphia General Hospital. The sarcoidosis clinic pioneered by him was relocated to the Curtis Clinic, and he ultimately became associated with the Barton Division. As the Philadelphia General program was phased out, he became more active in teaching and research, especially relative to training residents and fellows. His studies in sarcoidosis and Wegener's granulomatosis were basic and were internationally recognized during the next two decades. Numerous publications and presentations at national and international meetings enhanced his prestige and were important to Jefferson. His portrait was presented to the College in 1984. During this period the medical staff was also enlarged to include Dr. I. Sacks Cohen (Jefferson, 1939) and Dr. Anthony L. Forte (Jefferson, 1954).

For most members of the medical, nursing, and technical staffs the new location of the Barton Division proved a culmination of many hopes and plans. Although the facility was now much smaller, the aspects of isolation formerly perceived by personnel and reflected by main hospital people were eliminated, and the integration process was gracefully accomplished under Dr. Sokoloff's leadership. Nevertheless, the operation of the Barton unit with some administrative independence contributed to its strength. The nurses' program was carried on with more efficiency, the tuberculosis section constituted one of the very few areas in the city where private patients could be treated on a short-term basis, and the teaching facilities were improved. Admission of increasing numbers of patients with emphysema and carcinoma provided excellent materials for teaching and research. The teaching conference program was continued, and more of Jefferson's staff of attending physicians and house staff were regularly in attendance. The rotation of medical residents through the Barton program was more rewarding in view of the diversity and intensity of experience in managing lung problems.

In 1962, Dr. Sokoloff's sixty-fifth birthday signaled his retirement. In 1963 he was succeeded by Dr. Cathcart as Director of the Barton Memorial Divison of Diseases of the Chest. Dr. Sokoloff continued his association with Jefferson in patient care and teaching, having been promoted to the rank of Clinical Professor of Medicine. He was thus able to round out his career in clinical medicine, teaching, and administration, with significant influence on the careers of many Jefferson graduates and contributions to the control of tuberculosis at a critical period.

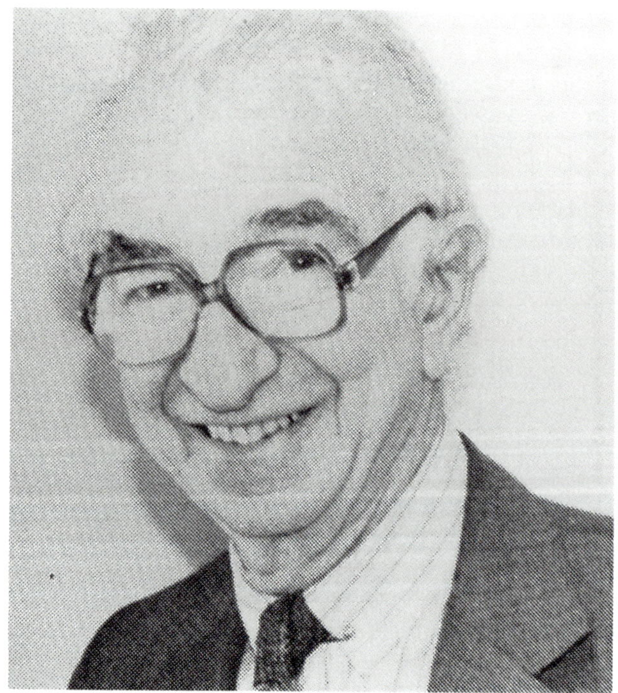

FIG. 11-20. Dr. Harold L. Israel (Jefferson, 1934), Professor of Medicine. Investigator and international authority on sarcoidosis and Wegener's granulomatosis.

Dr. William Fraimow, having served his residency in internal medicine at Veterans Hospital, Philadelphia, came to Barton as a Fellow in cardiopulmonary diseases in 1957 and then joined the medical staff as Assistant in Medicine in 1959. He continued his association with Dr. Cathcart, and both were appointed consultants to the Henry R. Landis State Hospital, at Girard and Corinthian Avenues in Philadelphia, where they served until the hospital was closed in 1973. This was the last surviving tuberculosis hospital in the area, where Dr. John Y. Templeton, III and Dr. John J. McKeown, Jr., from the Department of Surgery also served under circumstances in which diminishing demand for surgery was associated with a need for superior skills.

New Programs

The Barton group continued its studies into diffuse lung diseases. Dr. Theodos and others collected a group of patients for whom the recently introduced procedure of open lung biopsy made a crucial diagnostic difference in planning treatment and prognosis.[37,38] Dr. Cathcart, among other activities, became a member of the Governor's Committee on Pneumoconiosis and a member of the Committees on Pneumoconiosis and Tuberculosis for the Pennsylvania Department of Health. As the federal government became more involved in the lung diseases of coal miners, the extensive experience of the Barton group led to Dr. Cathcart's appointment to the Coal Mine Advisory Council of the Department of Health, Education and Welfare and as a medical advisor on Title IV, Federal Coal Mine Health and Safety Act of 1969 for the same Department.[39] Dr. Theodos also was a member of the Governor's

Committee to the Miners' Respiratory Disease and Rehabilitation Program and a medical advisor to the Bureau of Hearings and Appeals, Social Security Administration, Department of Health and Human Services. He also served the American College of Chest Physicians in various capacities, including Chairman of the Council on European Affairs, Vice-Chairman of the Board of Regents, and Chairman of the Committee on Occupational Diseases of the Chest. Later (1982) he was President of the Philadelphia County Medical Society. In 1965 Drs. Cathcart and Theodos played leading roles in Governor Scranton's Conference on Pneumoconiosis.

The teaching program proved eminently satisfactory. In addition to the third-year clinical clerkships, second-year students found the patient population well suited to their first exposure to physical diagnosis. The nursing student program continued its popularity among those rotated through the Barton Division, again providing experience not available elsewhere in a comprehensive manner. The maintenance of a few beds for tuberculosis into the 1970s proved to be a useful process that bridged the gap between the treatment of tuberculosis as the major concern in chest diseases and the relegation of tuberculosis to a minor problem infrequently requiring isolation and inpatient treatment. The release of the new drug Rifampin in 1966 further extended the effectiveness of antituberculous therapy and in time permitted reduction in the total duration of the multiple medication program. For most patients, tuberculosis could now be treated with a few generally well-tolerated pills and capsules once daily instead of parenteral and oral medication with numerous and occasionally serious ill effects. Use of isoniazid as a prophylactic medication for persons at high risk became commonplace, requiring only that circumspect judgment govern its use and that cooperation of patients be maintained.

During this period, the role of mycobacteria other than *Mycobacterium tuberculosis* was subjected to much study because the occurrence of atypical mycobacteriosis did not show a significant decrease in prevalence as did tuberculosis. The fact that these diseases proved not to be communicable from human to human was the probable reason, but it was necessary to determine in each instance whether the mycobacteria isolated were causative, contributory, or merely saprophytic. A review of the problem was presented to the Association of Clinical Scientists in 1973.[40]

It is interesting to note that during the decades of 1960 and 1980 excisional surgery for bronchiectasis declined to virtually none because control of the causes of bronchiectasis caused its incidence to diminish a great deal. Prevention of pertussis, antibiotic treatment of pneumonia, and the vaccine for measles were largely responsible for this change. At the same time emphysema and the obstructive lung diseases emerged as major concerns, resulting in the need for a change in the management of patients and in planning for the future. More patients with physiological impairment came to require intensive respiratory care, and these were transferred to the general intensive care unit when ventilatory or postoperative care was needed. With the increased use of ventilator-assisted breathing and the increased skills needed in the mechanics of treatment, it became evident that a respiratory intensive care unit should be part of the chest program. It was not possible to implement this change until funds were available.

In 1976 Dr. Robert I. Wise was succeeded as Magee Professor of Medicine by Dr. Frank A. Gray, whose background in pulmonary medicine promised to strengthen the Division. Many problems, however, prevented the uninterrupted progress that appeared certain at the time. Dr. Michael Casey joined the Division in 1978, but after one year he resigned to become Chief of the Division of Pulmonary Medicine at Pennsylvania Hospital.

In 1974 Dr. Cathcart resigned to accept a less demanding position with the Veterans Hospital, Coatesville, Pennsylvania. He was succeeded by Dr. G. William Atkinson (Figure 11-21), who had joined the Division following military service and his residency and fellowship at Jefferson. His qualifications were excellent: Chief Resident in Medicine at Jefferson (1969–1970), Pulmonary Academic Award of National Institutes of Health (1972–1977), and major research completed or in progress in fungal diseases of the lungs, especially aspergillosis; in interstitial pulmonary diseases; and in the mechanics of ventilation. He had served as director of the Pulmonary Laboratory since 1970.

Numerous publications[41] resulted from these activities, and during the next few years exhibits and presentations at national and regional conventions followed. The division regained a surge of enthusiasm, and once more medical student teaching was stimulated. The Pulmonary Fellowship under Dr. Atkinson's direction became a popular and sought-after appointment. His rank was Assistant Professor of Medicine at the time of his appointment; he was promoted to Associate Professor in 1980 and to Clinical Professor in 1982.

■ Respiratory Intensive Care Unit

Continuing progress required the development of a respiratory intensive care unit as an immediate goal. Planning included the final abandonment of beds specifically for tuberculosis and the placement of the new unit where they had been located. The miners' program terminated in 1974, so the activities of the pulmonary laboratory changed to those of a hospital service laboratory for lung consultations and continuing research. A new laboratory-office arrangement was developed on the tenth floor of the Curtis Building, and a spacious conference room adjoined. In 1977 the new intensive care unit was opened and promptly became a focus for the care of patients.

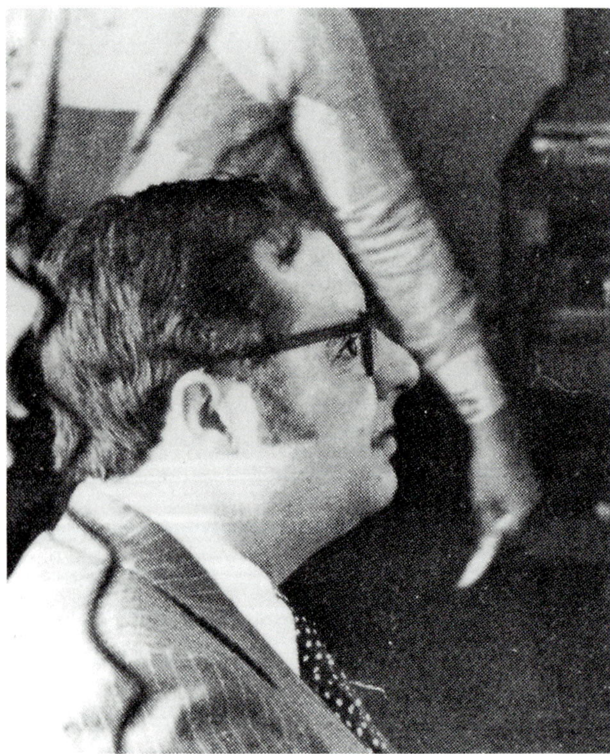

FIG. 11-21. Dr. G. William Atkinson, Medical Director of Barton Division (1974–1983).

The New Hospital and Comprehensive Pulmonary Medicine

In June, 1978, the New Hospital Building was opened. There was no longer a separate area for the Barton Memorial Division. The fifth floor was designated for pulmonary and cardiac patients. The respiratory intensive care center was in close proximity to the nursing areas of the fifth floor, and the laboratory-offices were nearby. The physical arrangements for excellent patient care were now well organized.

The practice of pulmonary medicine continued its evolution. Fellows in training, in addition to learning the intricacies of pulmonary physiology and its application to the treatment of acute respiratory failure and chronic lung diseases, were trained in bronchoscopy especially as it related to the recently developed flexible fiberoptic bronchoscope. Skills in the latter technique permitted its prompt application to diagnosis and treatment in the intensive care unit. Dr. Atkinson, having been part of the development of this program, was ideally suited for its teaching. Fellows trained in the Respiratory Division became heads of pulmonary sections in other hospital and medical school Departments of Medicine. Before long, procedures previously limited to tertiary-care hospitals became available in community hospitals. Research and progress depended upon availability of funds, and for a time the program was very productive, with numerous publications and much activity. Subjects included sarcoidosis,[42] respiratory distress syndrome,[43] and pulmonary angiitis and granulomatosis,[44] among others. These were developed under the aegis of Drs. Israel, Atkinson, and associates. In time, however, the limitation of funding and the need to devote more time to teaching and patient care caused a strain on the Pulmonary Division Staff. This was partly responsible for Dr. Atkinson's resignation in 1982 to become Chief of the Pulmonary Section at Presbyterian–University of Pennsylvania Medical Center and Clinical Professor of Medicine at the Medical School of University of Pennsylvania. Dr. Willis C. Maddrey, who succeeded Dr. Frank Gray as Magee Professor of Medicine in 1982, was faced with the urgent need to rehabilitate the Pulmonary Division. Dr. James Wilson was recruited from Tulane University in 1983, but his sudden death in the same year continued the instability. Dr. Denise Moylan and Dr. Edward S. Schulman (Jefferson, 1975) shared responsibilities as codirectors in the interval until the arrival of Dr. James E. Fish (Figure 11-22) to head the Division July 1, 1985. Dr. Krishna Mohan, also recently trained in the pulmonary fellowship program, shared clinical responsibilities during this period. Dr. Fish recruited new associates, including Drs. Stephen Peters, Herbert Patrick, and Jonathan Gottlieb. Expanding responsibilities occasioned a change of name from the Divison of Pulmonary Diseases to the Division of Pulmonary and Critical Care Medicine.

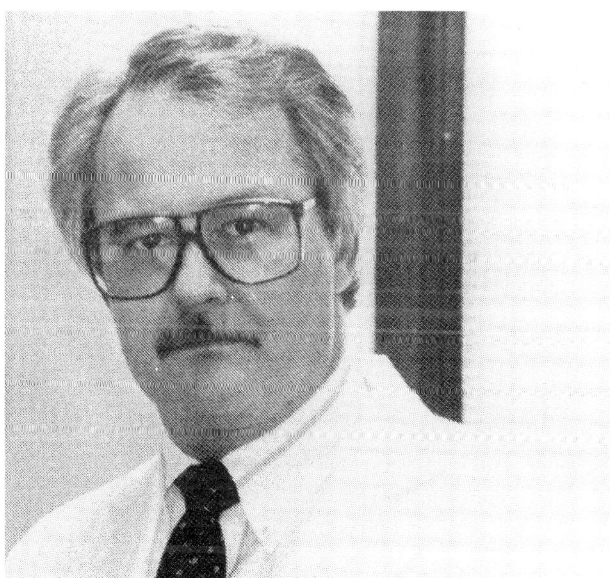

FIG. 11-22. Dr. James E. Fish, Director, Division of Pulmonary and Critical Care Medicine (1985–).

The history of the treatment of diseases of the chest at Jefferson for the past 75 years is a story of people responding effectively to the needs of individuals and society. For the first part of that period, the response related to an age-old challenge, that of the control and treatment of tuberculosis and the conservation of the lives of the usually young people so severely and frequently threatened. The perception of a need to initiate a program for that purpose early in the twentieth century set in motion plans that in retrospect were forward-looking and appropriate. Generations of Jefferson graduates benefited greatly from their experiences in the Chest Department and thereby enhanced the reputation of Jefferson as a training ground for physicians with superior clinical skills. Many professional people of great ability and high motivation, often themselves victims of tuberculosis, played a major role in these efforts, their successes at times limited and in other instances apparently enhanced by their illnesses. The total effect of the brilliant achievements in tuberculosis treatment unfortunately did not translate into the elimination of lung diseases. As the century progressed, the incidence of man-made problems, especially diseases caused by inhalation of foreign substances, was sufficiently serious to develop a new group of diseases that as yet are not controlled. Principal among these man-made problems is tobacco smoking, which now results in high morbidity from obstructive diseases and cancer; the latter is still increasing among women and overtaking cancer of the breast as the leading fatal malignant disease. The changed emphasis in management of these problems is obvious, and the role of a Division for chest diseases requires reassessment, calling for leadership in addressing these issues as well as those posed by the entire field of environmental medicine. Sophisticated technological measures for prolonging the lives of people with preventable diseases have little meaning unless coordinated with basic measures to prevent those illnesses. Jefferson has the experience and the potential to build solidly in approaching these problems for the future.

References

1. Flexner, Abraham, *Medical Education in the United States and Canada*. New York: Bulletin No. 4, Carnegie Foundation for the Advancement of Teaching, 1910.

2. *Yearly Report,* Jefferson Hospital, June 1, 1911, p. 23.
3. Savacool, J.W., "Philadelphia's Dr. Flick—Medical Crusader," *Philadelphia Medicine* 78, p. 148, 1982.
4. *Minutes.* Board of Trustees of Jefferson Hospital, March 1914.
5. Flick, Cecilia R., *Dr. Lawrence F. Flick: As I knew Him.* Dorrance & Co., 1956.
6. Craig, Frank A., *Early Days of Phipps.*
7. VanBuskirk, G.P., *The 1944 Clinic Year Book.* P. 226.
8. Idem 4.
9. *The Jeffersonian.* Vol. XIV, No. 113, April 1913, p. 18.
10. Personal interviews, 1984.
11. Funk, E.H., Collected papers.
12. Funk, E.H., "The Selection of Cases of Chronic Pulmonary Tuberculosis for Collapse Therapy," *Penn. Med. J.* 32, 1929, p. 859.
13. *College Catalogue, 1915–1916.*
14. *Hospital Annual Reports,* 1915, 1917.
15. *Hospital Annual Reports,* 1922.
16. Kern, Hedy, Personal interview, January 1985.
17. Montgomery, John B., Personal interview, January 1985.
18. Craig, Frank A., *The Story of the White Haven Sanatorium.* Privately published, 1956.
19. Gordon, B., Collected papers.
20. Gordon, B., "A Recording Type of Artificial Pneumothorax Apparatus," *Jour. Lab. and Clin. Med.* XVII, 1, 1931, p. 75.
21. Gordon, B., "The Mechanism and Use of Abdominal Supports and the Treatment of Pulmonary Diseases," *Amer. Jour. Med. Sc.* 187, 5, 1934, p. 692.
22. Gordon, B., "Pulmonary Asbestosis," *Penn. Med. J.* 35, 1932, p. 637.
23. *Jefferson Hospital Annual Reports, 1929–1931.*
24. *Jefferson Hospital Annual Reports, 1933–1936.*
25. Charr, Robert, and Savacool, J.W., Collected papers.
26. Gordon, B., "Report Given at a Dinner for the Faculty Sponsors and Staff of the Chest Department, The Wellington Hotel," Philadelphia: January 13, 1940. Unpublished.
27. *Jefferson Hospital Reports, 1926–1940.*
28. Jefferson Development Office. Courtesy of Mr. Frank McGovern and Miss Shirley Gray.
29. Bradley, Michael, Financial Records.
30. Gordon, B.L., Motley, H.L., Theodos, P.A., and Lang, L.P., "Studies of Disability in Anthracosilicosis," *Trans. Assoc. of Am. Phys.* 62, 1949, p. 270.
31. Gordon, B.L., Motley, H.L., Theodos, P.A., and Lang, L.P., "Anthracosilicosis and its Symptomatic Treatment," *W. V. Med. J.* 45, 1949, p. 125.
32. *Philadelphia Evening Bulletin.* 1948.
33. *Time.* 1948.
34. Gordon, B.L., Motley, H.L., Theodos, P.A., and Lang, L.P., Collected papers.
35. Gordon, B.L., Personal communication, May 15, 1984.
36. *Report by the Barton Memorial Division of the Jefferson Medical College Hospital to Mr. Thomas Kennedy, President of the United Mine Workers.* 1960.
37. Kirshner, J.J., Breckenridge, R.L., Allbritten, F.F., and Theodos, P.A., "Diffuse Interstitial Fibrosing Pneumonitis," *Journal A.M.A.* 154, 1954, p. 336.
38. Theodos, P.A., Allbritten, F.F. Breckenridge, R.A., "Lung Biopsy in Diffuse Pulmonary Disease," *Diseases of the Chest.* 27, 1955, p. 637.
39. Cathcart, R.T., *Curriculum Vitae.*
40. Savacool, J.W., "Status of Mycobacterial Infections of the Lungs," *Ann. Clin. Lab. Sci.* 3, 1973, p. 91.
41. Atkinson, G.W., Collected papers.
42. Steplewski, Z., Yaverbaum, S., Atkinson, G.W., Israel, H.L., Atkinson, B., and Mitchell, K.F., "Monoclonal Antibody-Defined Antigens in Sarcoidosis," *Sarcoidosis and other Granulomatous Disorders.* Paris: Pergamon Press, 1983, pp. 142–149.
43. Memon, N.A., Branca, P.A., Atkinson, G.W., Kagen, J.J., and Dave, R.J., "High I/E Ratio Ventilation with Low PEEP in Respiratory Distress Syndrome," *Respiratory Therapy.* 9, 1979, p. 6.
44. Saldana, M., Patchefsky, A.S., Israel, H.L., and Atkinson, G.W., "Pulmonary Angiitis and Granulomatosis." *Human Pathology.* 8, 1977, p. 391.

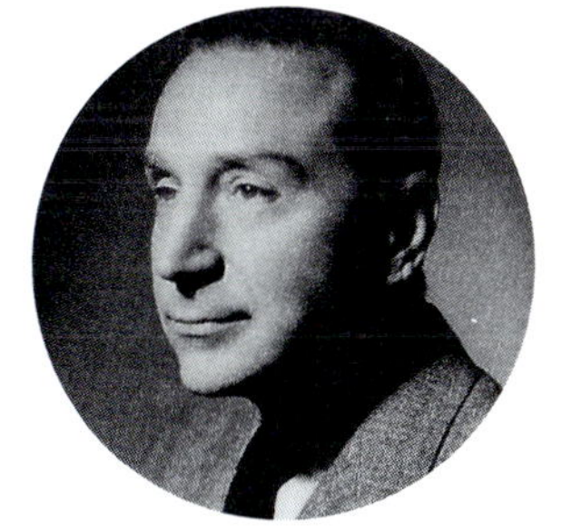

CHAPTER TWELVE

Division of Gastroenterology and Hepatology

Charles W. Wirts, Jr., M.D.

"Unquiet meals make ill digestions."

—Shakespeare (1564–1616) *The Comedy of Errors.*

Robley Dunglison (Figure 12-1) was one of the first physicians in this country to take a scientific interest in the gastrointestinal system. Dunglison was brought from England to America by Thomas Jefferson in 1825. After teaching at the University of Virginia and then at the University of Maryland, he was appointed Professor of the Institutes of Medicine at the Jefferson Medical College in 1836. Here Dr. Samuel D. Gross, Professor of Surgery, considered him the most erudite member of the faculty. He gained international recognition after the publication of his book, *Human Physiology*. As a result of this publication and the esteem in which Dunglison was held generally in the medical profession, Dr. William Beaumont sought his help in carrying out an analysis of the gastric juice obtained from his patient, Alexis St. Martin, who had a chronic gastric fistula as the result of an accidental gunshot wound. The excitement engendered by the finding of free hydrochloric acid led to further plans for collaborative experiments on digestion by Dunglison and Beaumont using St. Martin. The results were published by Beaumont in his book, *Experiments and Observations on the Gastric Juice and the Physiology of Digestion,* and in later editions of Dunglison's *Human Physiology*.[1] After a very productive career, Dunglison retired from Jefferson in 1868, having served for over 30 years, 14 of them as Dean.

Early Gastroenterology at Jefferson

It was not until the final decades of the nineteenth century that gastroenterology first emerged as a specialty, and the American Gastroenterology Association was founded in 1899. Dr. William Ward Van Valzah (Figure 12-2), an early specialist in this field, was graduated from Princeton University in 1873 and from Jefferson Medical College in 1876. For three years following his graduation, Dr. Van Valzah was connected with the German Hospital and the Blockley Hospital of Philadelphia as intern and served as a physician on the staff of Jefferson Medical College Hospital from 1879 to 1883. In 1884, after several years of traveling in Europe and America, he located in New York and began giving his attention exclusively to the treatment of diseases of the digestive tract. From 1892 until 1902 Van Valzah served as Professor of Diseases of the Digestive Organs in the New York Polyclinic College. He wrote many papers on his speciality and collaborated with Nisbet in *Diseases of the Stomach*,[2] published in 1889.

During the era just before World War I, the first activity in research and teaching in the field of gastroenterology developed at Jefferson, notably as the result of the efforts of two men, Drs. B.B. Vincent Lyon and Martin E. Rehfuss. Dr. Lyon (Figure 12-3) was a graduate of the Lawrenceville Preparatory School (1889), Williams College (A.B., 1903, Sc. D., 1931), and received his medical degree at the Johns Hopkins Medical School (1907). He served his internship at the old German (Lankenau) Hospital and later formed a Gastrointestinal Clinic there in 1910. In 1912 Lyon joined the Jefferson Medical College, where he founded the first outpatient Gastrointestinal Clinic, initially in the hospital building at Tenth and Sansom Streets. During 1914 he undertook postgraduate study in England, France, and Germany, and ultimately became well known for his pioneer work on the function of the biliary tract. He described the color sequence and characteristics of the different bile fractions after stimulation through an indwelling duodenal tube.

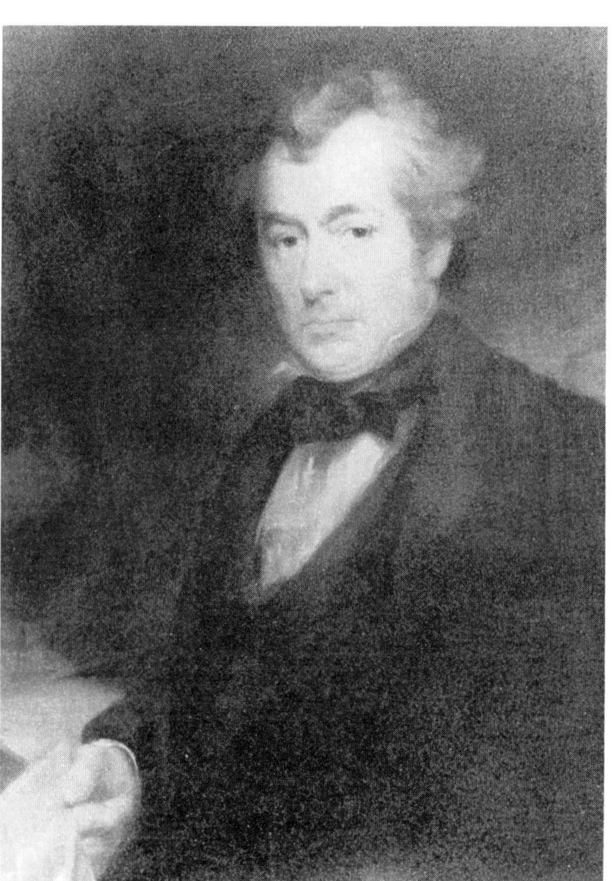

Fig. 12-1. Robley Dunglison, M.D., Professor of the Institutes of Medicine (1836–1868).

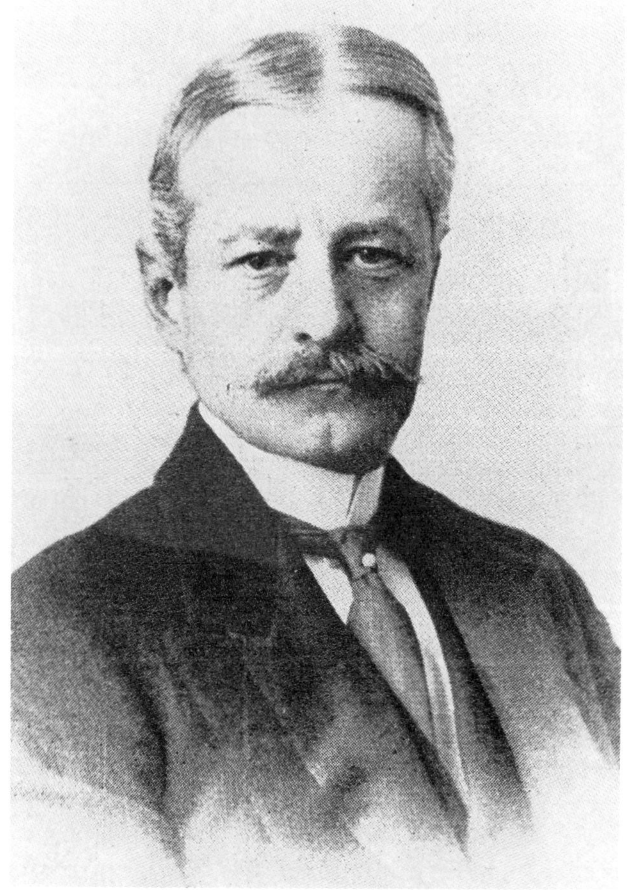

Fig. 12-2. William Ward Van Valzah, M.D. (Jefferson, 1876). Pioneer in Gastroenterology.

This method proved to be a tremendous advance in the field of gastroenterology, which previously had largely depended upon surgical exploration. His *Atlas on Biliary Drainage Microscopy*[3] emphasized the cytologic differences encountered in various forms of biliary disease. Other contributions dealt with the bacteriology of the bile and the phenomena associated with catarrhal cholangitis, jaundice, and duodenal parasitosis. Lyon also became interested in nonsurgical duodenal drainage as a therapeutic procedure not only in the biliary tract but in liver disease. His volume on *Nonsurgical Drainage of the Biliary Tract*[4] is a classic. In addition, he published 51 articles in various medical journals and textbooks, including the chapter on diseases of the digestive system in John C. DaCosta Jr.'s, *Handbook of Medical Treatment*,[5] in Tice's *Practice of Medicine*, in Osler's *Modern Medicine*, and in Sajous' *Cyclopaedia of Medicine*.

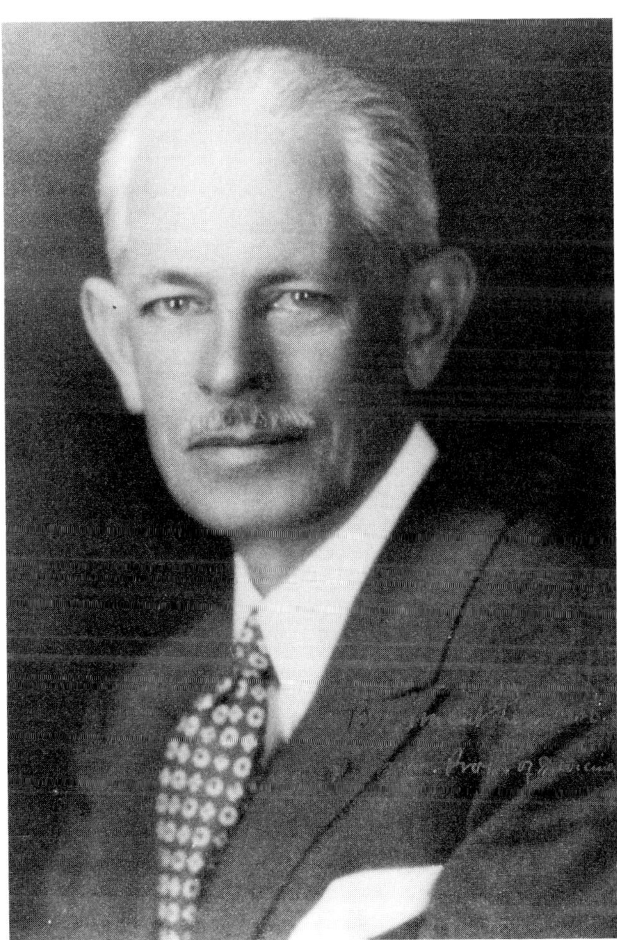

FIG. 12-3. B.B. Vincent Lyon, M.D., founder of first outpatient Gastrointestinal Clinic (1912).

Dr. Lyon was a brilliant speaker and an indefatigable worker. He was the recipient of many honors, among which were election as President of the American Gastroenterological Association in 1934 and reception of the Julius Friedenwald Medal in 1950. Lyon was steadily advanced in rank from Demonstrator in Medicine, becoming Clinical Professor of Medicine on his retirement in 1946. He died suddenly in Washington, D.C., on May 20, 1954, at the age of 73.

In 1931 the Clinic was moved to the new Curtis Building at Tenth and Walnut Streets, and the staff included Doctors Henry Bartle, Samuel Immerman, Ray Halpern, Robert Steiner, David Anderson, Paul Stroup, John DeCarlo, Clifford Arnold, and William Swalm. Dr. Charles W. Wirts joined the staff in 1939 and was appointed Chief Clinical Assistant in 1942. Dr. Joseph Medoff (Figure 12-4) (Jefferson, 1939) was a member of the Clinic staff from 1946 to 1960 and was advanced steadily until he became Emeritus Professor of Clinical Medicine in 1978. He was extremely active as Faculty Advisor to the Hare Society of Internal Medicine from 1960 to 1976, and in recognition of this his portrait was presented to the University in 1976.

Dr. Martin E. Rehfuss (Figure 12-5) attended the Central High School of Philadelphia and the University of Pennsylvania. He received his M.D. degree from its School in Medicine in 1909 and served his internship there in 1910. He was a resident physician at the American Hospital in Paris in 1911–1912 and from 1912–1913 studied in Berlin, Munich, and Vienna. It was during this time that he developed the Rehfuss tube, a modified gastric tube with which he devised the procedure known as fractional gastric analysis. In 1914 Rehfuss became associated with the Jefferson Medical College and Hospital. Over the next decade he carried out original studies on the digestion of food in the normal and abnormal stomach in association with Dr. Phillip B. Hawk. Subsequent investigations of diseases of the biliary tract were published in textbooks: *Diagnosis and Treatment of Diseases of the Stomach*,[6] *Medical Treatment of Gallbladder Disease*,[7] with Guy M.

Nelson, and *Practical Therapeutics*.[8] In addition, he contributed more than 200 articles to the medical literature.

Dr. Rehfuss was appointed an Instructor in Medicine in 1914, rose to Clinical Professor of Medicine in 1933, and was named Sutherland Prevost Lecturer in Therapeutics in 1941. He was a physically handsome man, with a John Barrymore profile, and his impeccable attire always included a white vest with a sparking gold chain. His hobby as an artist served him well in the lecture room, where his sketches of various portions of the gastrointestinal tract were vividly realistic. His private practice encompassed many socially prominent patients from suburban Philadelphia, but he was generous and kind to those in less fortunate financial circumstances. He became Professor Emeritus in 1952. A Rehfuss Lectureship was established by the Foerderer Foundation in 1963, and his bust on a pedestal is always on the stage during the presentation. Mrs. Foerderer insisted on a short organ recital before each lecture, a custom that spread into other lectureships and portrait presentations. Dr. Rehfuss died at home in 1964 after a long illness.

Dr. John T. Eads (Figure 12-6) (Jefferson, 1926) and Dr. Guy M. Nelson (Figure 12-7) (Jefferson, 1928) both served in the capacity of assistants to Dr. Rehfuss and collaborated in contributing to the literature in the field of gastrointestinal diseases.

Among other notable Jeffersonians who made major contributions to gastroenterology were Dr. Henry L. Bockus (Figure 12-8) (Jefferson, 1917, D.Sc., 1958) and Dr. J. Edward Berk (Figure 12-9)

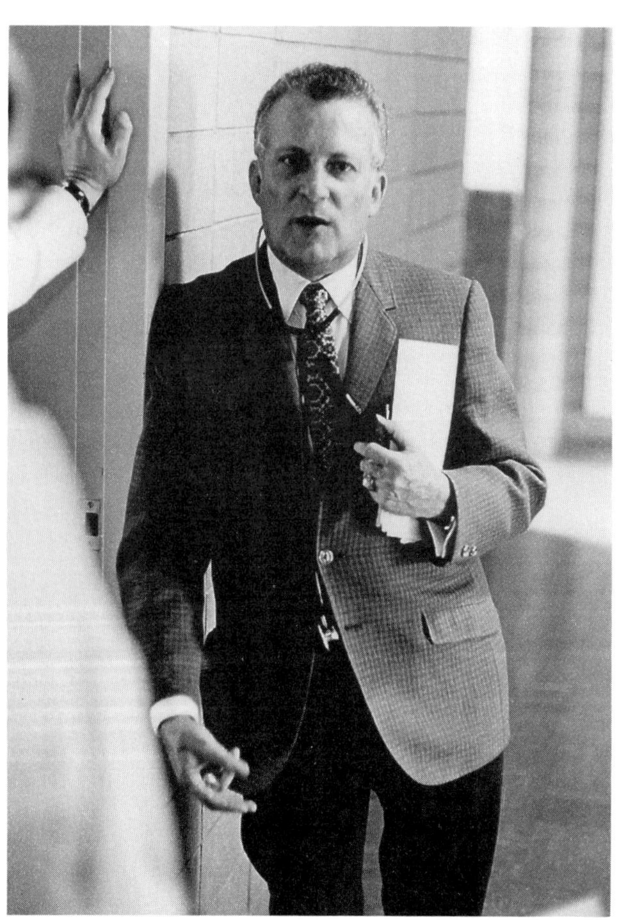

FIG. 12-4. Joseph Medoff, M.D. (Jefferson, 1939).

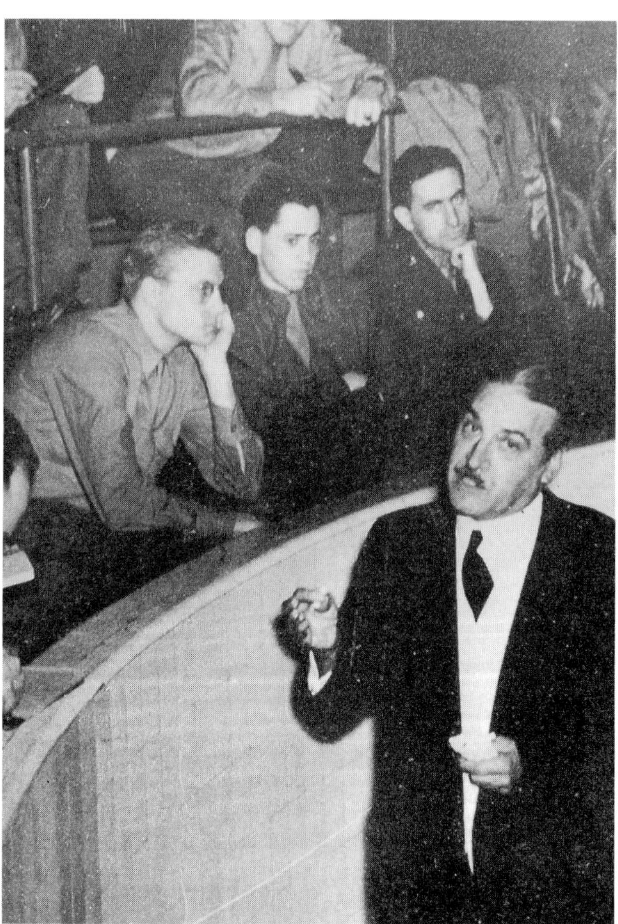

FIG. 12-5. Martin E. Rehfuss, M.D., Professor of Clinical Medicine (1914–1956).

(Jefferson, 1936). Dr. Bockus showed interest in this field when it was first being separated as a subdivision of internal medicine. He ultimately became "one of the giants of American and World medicine and gastroenterology."[9] He was internationally recognized for his teaching and medical publications, especially for his textbook *Gastroenterology,* in three volumes, published in 1943 and rewritten in 1963.[10] Dr. Berk, who took much of his training under Dr. Bockus, served as Chairman of the Department of Medicine and Head of the Division of Gastroenterology at the University of California, Irvine, and as Editor-in-Chief of the fourth edition of Bockus' *Gastroenterology.*[11]

The Gastroenterology Division

Following the retirement of Dr. Lyon in 1946, Dr. Charles W. Wirts, Jr. became Head of the Gastrointestinal Clinic and developed the first Division of Gastroenterology in the Department of Medicine. Dr. Wirts attended the Mercersburg Academy (1926), Lafayette College (B.S., 1930) and Jefferson Medical College (M.D., 1934). He took a rotating internship at St. John's General Hospital and a residency in pathology at St. Francis Hospital, both in Pittsburgh, and a residency in medicine at the American Hospital in Paris. At this time he also worked in the endoscopic clinics of the Hôpital Necker and the Hôpital Vaugiraud in Paris. Upon returning to Jefferson Wirts was appointed the first Ross V. Patterson Fellow in Gastroenterology (1940–1942) and became a Diplomate of the American Board of Internal Medicine and the subspecialty Board of Gastroenterology. After taking a course with Dr. Rudolf Schindler in Chicago and working with Professor François Moutier in Paris, Dr. Wirts

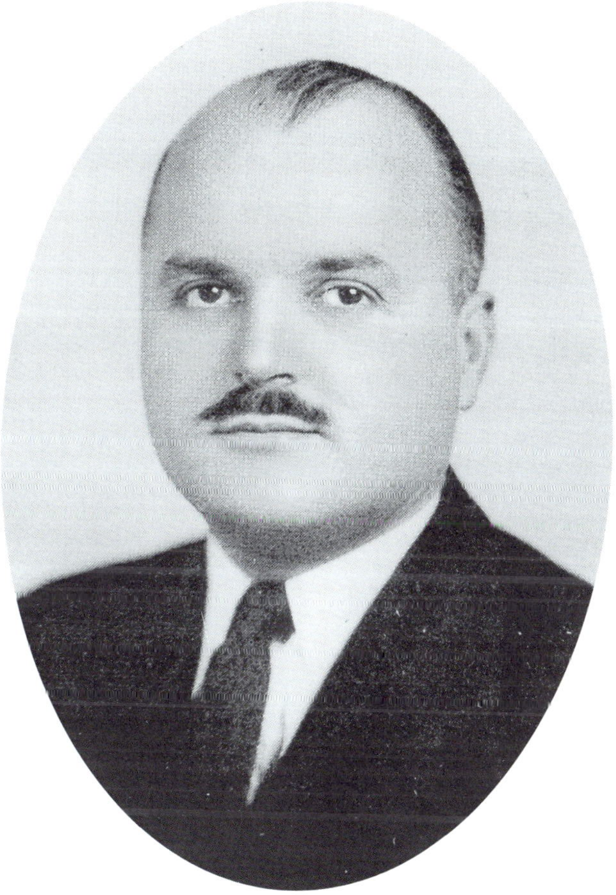

Fig. 12-6. John T. Eads, M.D. (Jefferson, 1926).

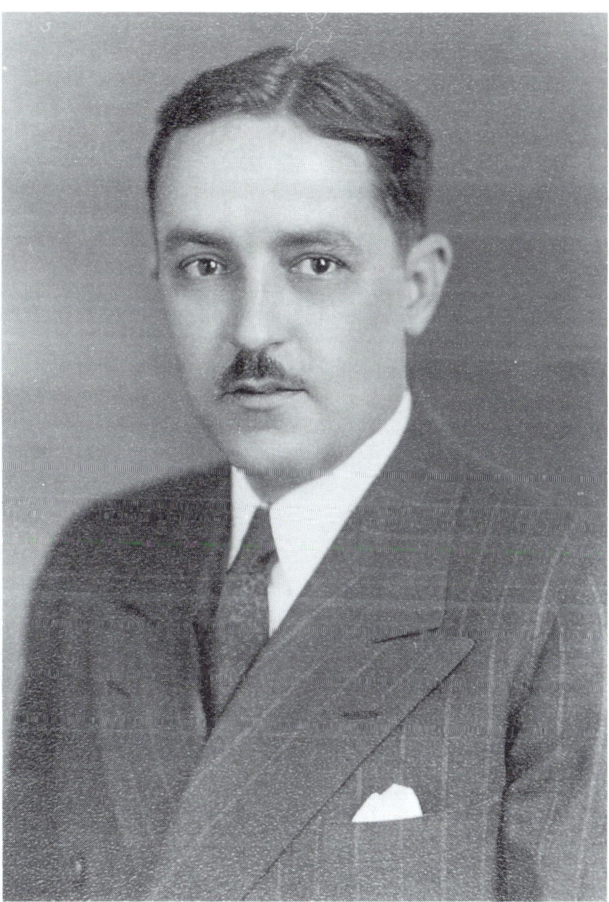

Fig. 12-7. Guy M. Nelson, M.D. (Jefferson, 1928).

introduced the use of the Schindler flexible gastroscope (not to be confused with the later fiberoptic flexible gastroscope) at Jefferson. He also collaborated with Dr. William J. Snape (Jefferson, 1940) and Dr. Abraham Cantarow (Jefferson, 1924), Professor of Biochemistry and Chairman of the Department, in carrying out a number of liver function studies in dogs in whom they had constructed a "Thomas chronic-bile-fistula." This work was carried out under the auspices of Dr. J. Earl Thomas, Professor of Physiology and Chairman of the Department (1927–1955), without whose generous help and guidance it could not have been accomplished. Dr. Thomas was a noted experimentalist and designer of research equipment primarily concerning the physiology of the digestive system. He was internationally recognized for his investigation of the regulation of gastric emptying, the filling and evacuation of the gall-bladder, the autoregulation of gastric and pancreatic secretion, and the entero–enteric reflexes.[12]

Dr. Wirts became an attending physician at the Pennsylvania Hospital and a consultant in gastroenterology at the Philadelphia General Hospital, the Veterans Administration Hospital of Philadelphia, the Walson General Hospital (U.S.Army, Fort Dix, New Jersey), and the Chester County Hospital (West Chester, Pennsylvania). He belonged to a number of medical societies, including the American Gastroenterological Association (Figure 12-10), the American College of Gastroenterology (President, 1957; Chairman of the Board, 1958), the American Gastroscopic Society (President, 1959), the American College of Physicians, and the Alpha Omega Alpha and Sigma Xi Honor Medical

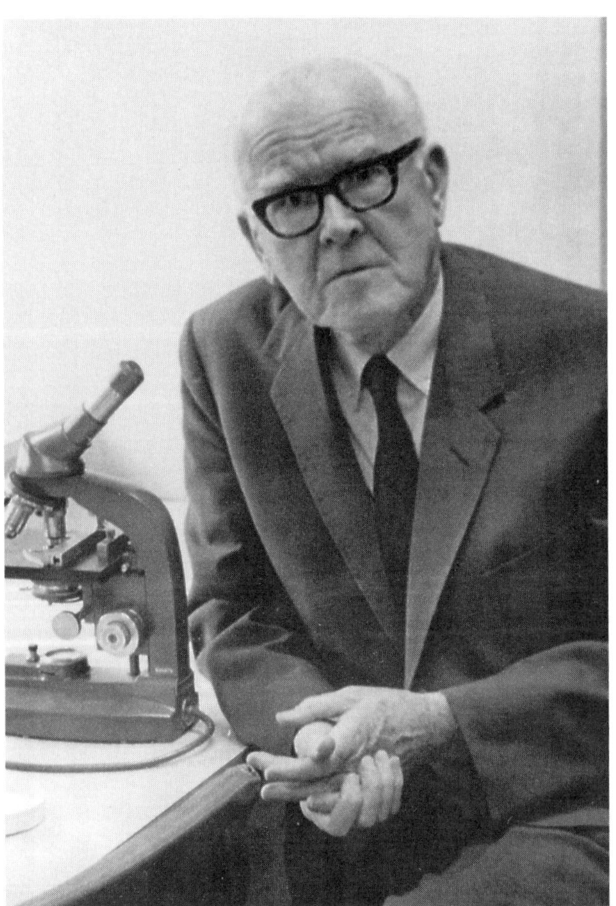

FIG. 12-8. Henry L. Bockus, M.D. (Jefferson, 1917).

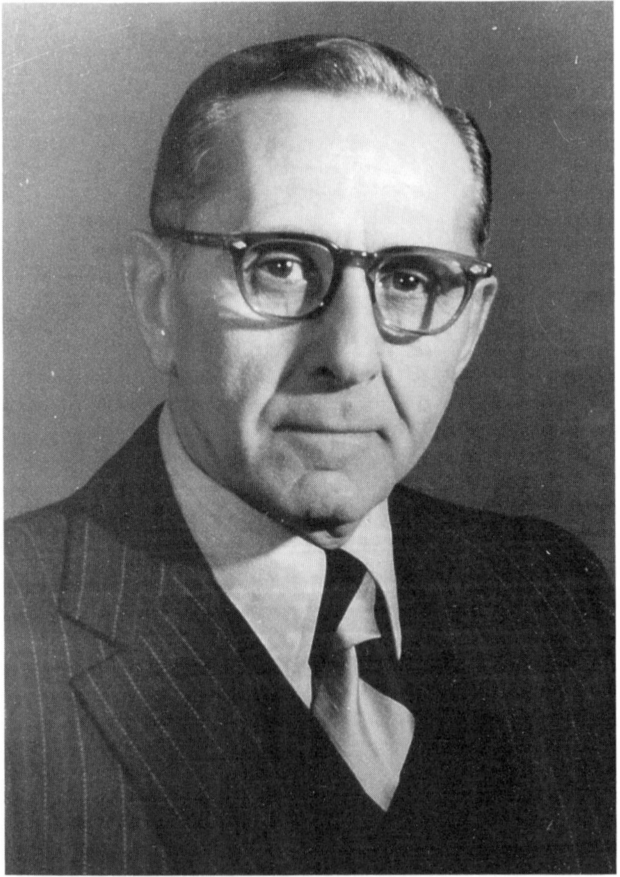

FIG. 12-9. J. Edward Berk, M.D. (Jefferson, 1936).

Societies. He was advanced in rank from Instructor to Emeritus Professor of Medicine in 1981. He retired from the Directorship of the Division of Gastroenterology in 1966 and from active practice in 1985.

Dr. Franz Goldstein (Figure 12-11) who received his premedical education at the University of Würzburg, Germany, was graduated from Jefferson Medical College in 1953. After completing his training in internal medicine and gastroenterology at the Graduate Hospital of the University of Pennsylvania under the chairmanship of Dr. Henry L. Bockus, he was appointed the first full-time member of the Division of Gastroenterology headed by Dr. Charles W. Wirts. A period of productive collaboration evolved, and the results of their numerous research projects were published in national medical journals, among them a series of studies dealing with the "blind-loop" syndrome, carried out in cooperation with Dr. Russell W. Schaedler (Jefferson, 1953), Professor of Microbiology and Chairman of the Department, and Dr. Robert Mandle, Professor of Microbiology. Dr. John Y. Templeton (Jefferson, 1941) Professor of Surgery, and Dr. Charles Fineberg, Professor of Surgery, also assisted in this project by performing the jejunal-interposition operations to correct the blind-loop that occured in some patients following a gastrojejunostomy.

Dr. Wirts and Dr. Goldstein succeeded in obtaining the first National Institutes of Health gastrointestinal research and training grant at Jefferson. This permitted the establishment of offices, research laboratories, and stipends for the trainees. Most of the Fellows trained in the

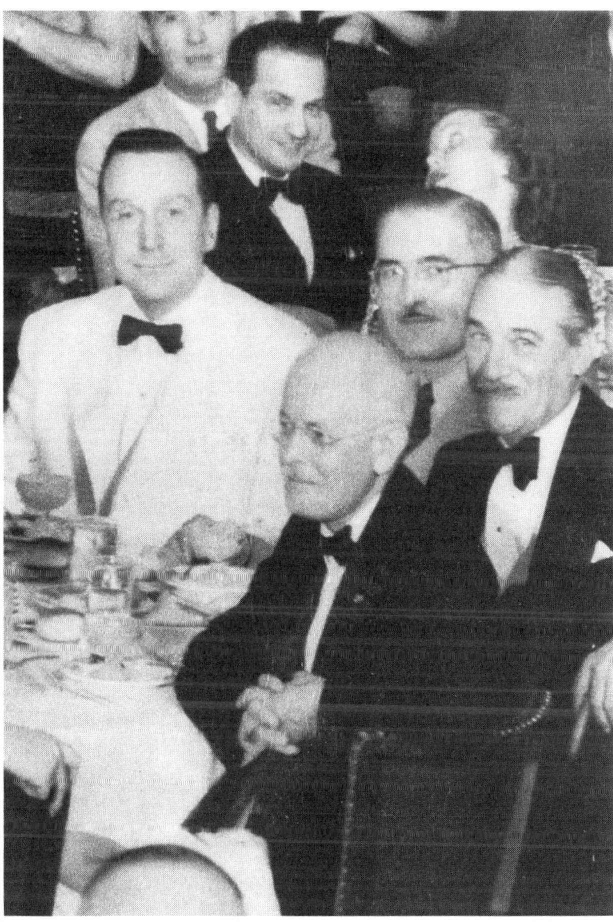

FIG. 12-10. Fiftieth Annual Banquet of the American Gastroenterological Association, The Claridge, Atlantic City, N.J. on June 3, 1949. Left to right: Dr. Wirts, Dr. Lyon, and Dr. Rehfuss. Others unidentified.

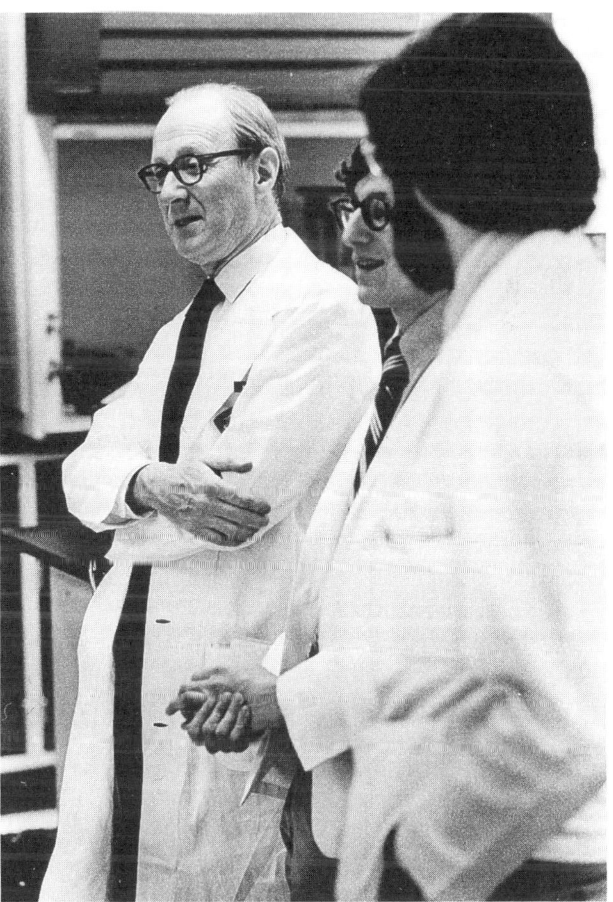

FIG. 12-11. Franz Goldstein, M.D. (Jefferson, 1953).

Division have retained a primary interest in gastroenterology. Those who practiced at hospitals affiliated with Jefferson include Dr. Francis X. Keeley, Chairman of the Department of Medicine and Chief of the Division of Gastroenterology at Our Lady of Loudes Hospital in Camden, N.J.; Dr. David Ginsberg, Chief of the Division of Gastroenterology at the Methodist Hospital; and Dr. Divo O. Messouri, in charge of Gastroenterology at the Chestnut Hill Hospital. Dr. Gerald Salen (Jefferson, 1961), a Fellow in 1965–1966, was appointed Professor of Medicine at the College of Medicine and Dentistry–New Jersey Medical School, Chief of Gastroenterology at the East Orange Veterans Hospital, and Director of Gastroenterology at the Cabrini Health Center in New York. He became a member of the American Society for Clinical Investigation, published extensively on bile salt metabolism and many of its ramifications, and was recognized as one of the outstanding experts in that area of research.

Dr. Goldstein progressed in rank from Instructor to Professor of Medicine (1970), at which time he transferred his activities to Lankenau Hospital where he became Chief of the newly created Department of Gastroenterology and a newly established gastroenterology training program. He has continued his research activities, particularly in the area of inflammatory bowel disease and its treatment. Goldstein is a member of many medical and gastrointestinal societies, including the American Gastroenterological Association, the American College of Gastroenterology (President, 1981–1982), the American Society for Gastrointestinal Endoscopy, and the Bockus International Society for Gastroenterology (President, 1986).

Dr. O. Dhodanand Kowlessar (Figure 12-12) received his Doctor of Medicine with honors from the University of Rochester School of Medicine, Rochester, New York, in 1955. He was elected to Alpha Omega Alpha during his Junior year and was the recipient of the Borden Undergraduate Award for Outstanding Research. He served his internship and residency in Internal Medicine at the New York Hospital–Cornell Medical Center, New York City. Here he became a Fellow in Gastroenterology under the directorships of Dr. Thomas Almay and Dr. Marvin Sleisenger, and in 1960 was made Assistant Professor of Medicine. In 1963 Kowlessar was appointed Associate Professor of Medicine and the Director of the Division of Gastroenterology at the New Jersey College of Medicine in Jersey City. From 1966 to 1984 he served as Professor of Medicine and the first full-time Director of the Division of Gastroenterology and the Director of the Clinical Research Center at Jefferson Medical College.

During his tenure he trained 20 Fellows, who subsequently practiced gastroenterology in many states and Canada. Dr. Susan Gordon (Jefferson, 1966) (Figure 12-13) was prominent among these and became active in the Gastroenterology Division of Jefferson. Her grandfather, Dr. Benjamin Lee Gordon (Jefferson, 1896), was a prolific writer of articles on ophthalmology and medical history. Another Fellow, Dr. Steven R. Peikin (Figure 12-14) (Jefferson, 1974), subsequently served as Acting Director of the Division following Dr. Kowlessar. Dr. James

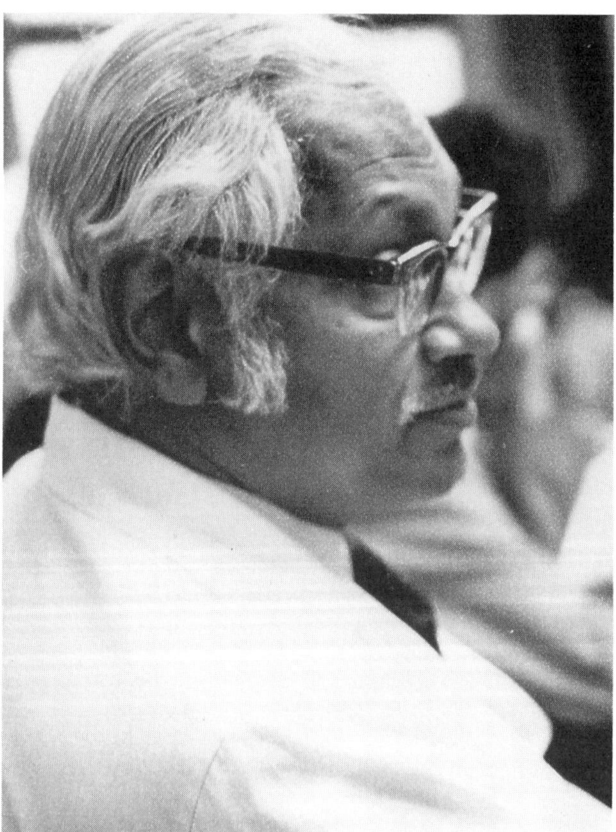

FIG. 12-12. O. Dhodanand Kowlessar, M.D., Director of Division of Gastroenterology (1966–1984).

Thornton became a member of the Department of Gastroenterology at Lankenau Hospital; Dr. William R. Long affiliated with the University of Pennsylvania School of Medicine; and Dr. William Snape, Jr., became Professor of Medicine and Director of the Division of Gastroenterology at the University of California in Los Angeles.

During the early period of Dr. Kowlessar's directorship he was aided by Dr. Charles W. Wirts, Dr. Franz Goldstein, and Dr. Philip Bralow, who assisted in the training of the Fellows. Significant contributions were made by Dr. Joseph Medoff (Jefferson, 1939) and Dr. Francis X. Keeley. Keeley spent many hours instructing the Fellows both at Thomas Jefferson University Hospital and Philadelphia General Hospital in endoscopic techniques. In 1970 Dr. Gordon Benson, who had trained as a Fellow in Hepatology with Dr. Gerald Klatskin at Yale University School of Medicine, joined the Division as Head of the Section of Liver Disease. In 1978 he was appointed Professor of Medicine and Director of the Division of Gastroenterology at Rutgers Medical School, New Brunswick, New Jersey.

Dr. Kowlessar was the cofounder with Dr. Frank Brooks, of the University of Pennsylvania School of Medicine, of the Philadelphia G.I. Training Group. He served as Secretary-Treasurer and President of this organization and later as Presidents of the Philadelphia G.I. Research Forum and the Sigma Xi Chapter of the Jefferson Medical College. He was a member of the National Institutes of Health Training Grant Committee, the Advisory Committee on Enzymes for the Food and Drug Administration, and the Scientific Review Committee for the Veterans

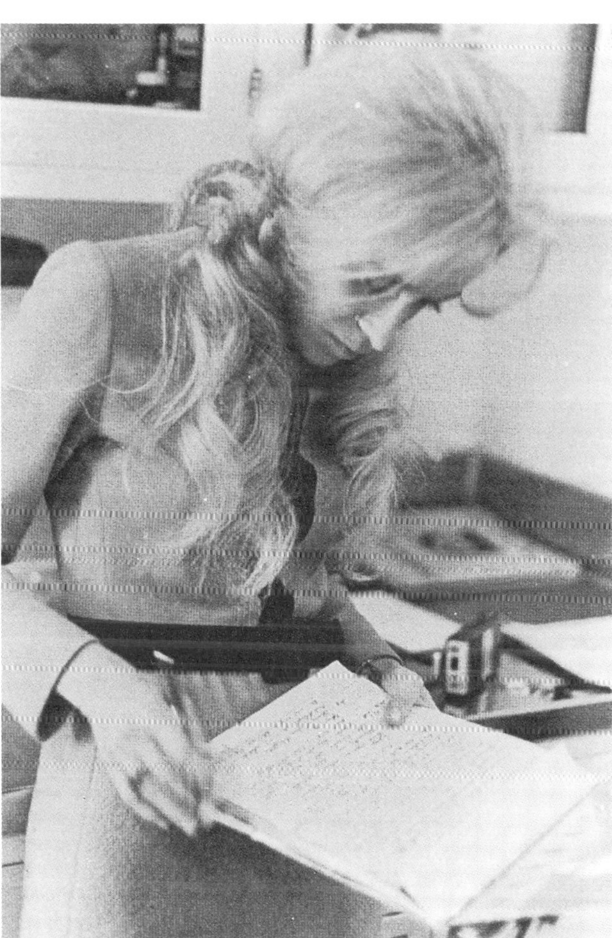

FIG. 12-13. Susan J. Gordon, M.D. (Jefferson, 1966).

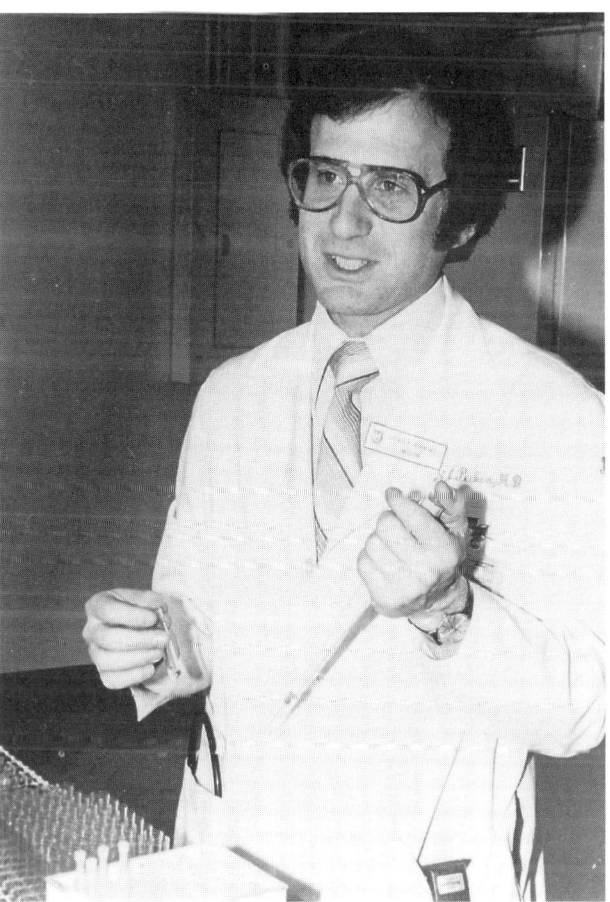

FIG. 12-14. Steven R. Peiken, M.D. (Jefferson, 1974).

Administration. He was the author and coauthor of over 80 publications including chapters in Cecil–McDermott's *Textbook of Medicine,* Sleisenger–Fordtran's *Pathophysiology of Gastrointestinal Diseases,* and Zakin and Boyer's *Hepatology.* Dr. Kowlessar was a member of the Editorial Boards of *Digestive Diseases, Science,* and the *American Journal of Gastroenterology,* and Editor of *Gastroenterology Abstracts and Citations.*

Dr. Kowlessar's research interests included the isolation and characterization of enzymatically derived gliadin peptides and their effects on patients with celiac disease. He made significant contributions in the area of pancreatic and hepatic enzymes and studied amino acids and peptides in the serum of patients with hepatic encephalopathy with Dr. Willis C. Maddrey. In October 1984 Dr. Kowlessar retired as head of the Division of Gastroenterology-Hepatology and was appointed Associate Chairman of Educational Programs.

Dr. Willis C. Maddrey (Figure 12-15), the Magee Professor of Medicine and Chairman of the Department, came to Jefferson in May 1982, from Johns Hopkins University School of Medicine, where he was Professor of Medicine and Associate Director of the Department. His father, Dr. Milner Crocker Maddrey, was a Jefferson graduate in the Class of 1931. The new Chairman had a major research interest in liver diseases in which he authored approximately 100 articles and book chapters dealing with this topic. Dr. Maddrey was President of the American Association for the Study of Liver Diseases and Chairman of the Council of Subspecialty Societies of the American College of Physicians, of which he was a member of the Board of Regents. In addition to his numerous other activities, Dr. Maddrey maintained an active interest in the Division of Gastroenterology-Hepatology. In 1984 he made two new appointments; Dr. Steven R. Peikin (see Figure 12-14) as Acting Head of the Division and Dr. Lawrence Friedman as Assistant Professor of Medicine.

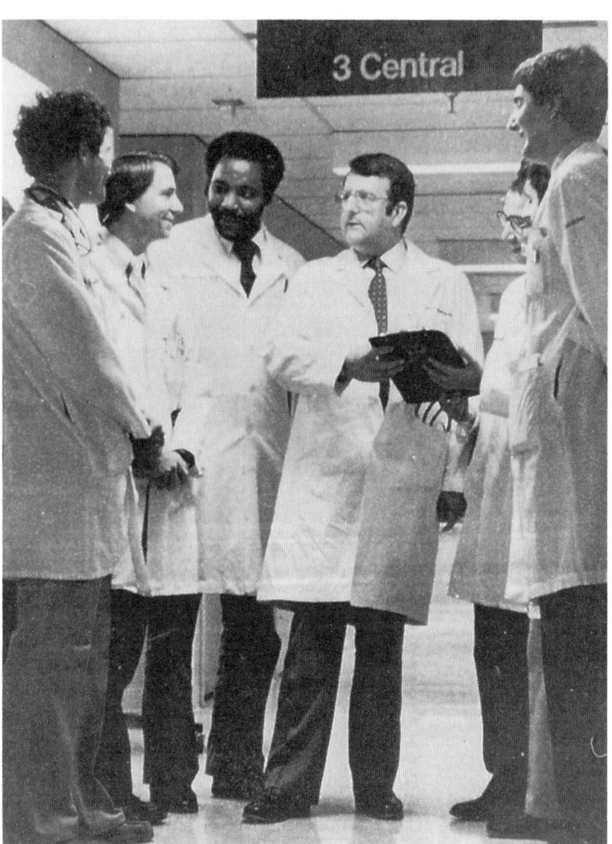

FIG. 12-15. Willis C. Maddrey, M.D., Magee Professor of Medicine and Chairman of the Department (1982).

After pursuing a Research Fellowship in Medicine at Harvard Medical School, Dr. Peikin returned to Jefferson and organized a team to investigate the broad field of obesity. In July 1982 he was promoted to Associate Professor of Medicine. Dr. Friedman, who had had extensive training at both Johns Hopkins and Harvard in addition to working in the field of hepatic disorders, began a clinic for the study of inflammatory bowel diseases.

A program in liver transplantation under the joint leadership of Drs. Willis Maddrey, the Magee Professor of Medicine and Chairman of the Department, Francis E. Rosato, the Samuel D. Gross Professor of Surgery and Chairman of the Department, and Bruce Jarrell, Associate Professor of Surgery, was initiated in 1984. On Thursday, May 31, of the same year, an emergency liver transplant operation, the first in the Delaware Valley, was successfully performed on a 30-year old man. It marked the beginning of an expanding program.

The pioneer contributions and ongoing research in gastroenterology and hepatology at Jefferson may well be a source of pride. The Division is poised with an excellence of faculty members and the latest technological aids to meet the challenge of new and changing spectrums of diseases in this field.

References

1. Dunglison, R., *Human Physiology.* 2d ed., Philadelphia: Carey, Lea and Blanchard, 1836, p. 473.
2. Van Valzah, W.W., and Nisbet, J.D., *Diseases of the Stomach.* Philadelphia: W.B. Saunders, 1898.
3. Lyon, B.B.V., *Atlas on Biliary Drainage Microscopy.* Published privately.
4. Lyon, B.B.V., *Nonsurgical Drainage of the Biliary Tract.* Philadelphia: Lea and Febiger, 1923.
5. DaCosta, J.C., Jr., "Diseases of the Digestive System," *Handbook of Medical Treatment,* Philadelphia: F.A. Davis Co., 1919, Vol. II, pp. 643–923.
6. Rehfuss, M.E., *Diagnosis and Treatment of Diseases of the Stomach.* Philadelphia: W.B. Saunders Company, 1927.
7. Rehfuss, M.E., and Nelson, G.M., *Medical Treatment of Gallbladder Disease.* Philadelphia: W.B. Saunders Company, 1935.
8. Rehfuss, M.E., *Practical Therapeutics.* 3d ed. Baltimore: Williams and Wilkins, 1956.
9. Goldstein, F., "Obituary on Henry L. Bockus," *Jeff. Med. Coll. Al. Bull.,* 31:4, Summer 1982.
10. Bockus, H.L., *Gastroenterology.* 3 Vols. Philadelphia: W.B. Saunders Company, 1943; rewritten, 1963.
11. Berk, J.E., Ed. *Bockus: Gastroenterology.* 4th ed. Philadelphia: W.B. Saunders Company, 1983.
12. Rosenfield, L.M., "Physiology at Jefferson Medical College (1842–1982)," *The Physiologist,* 27:3, 113–127. June, 1984.

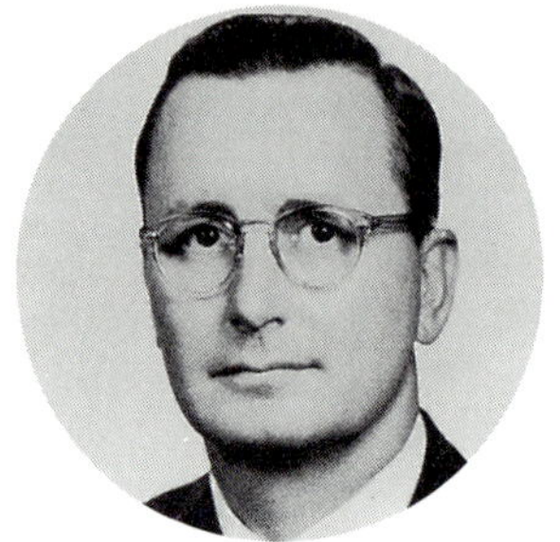

CHAPTER THIRTEEN

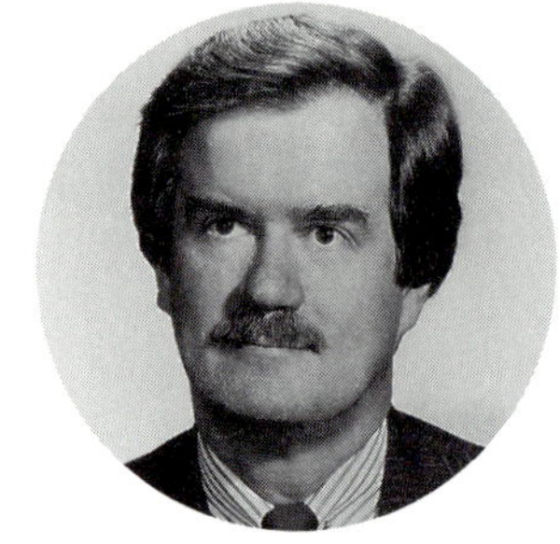

Division of Infectious Diseases

Robert I. Wise, Ph.D., M.D., D.Sc., and
Erick J. Bergquist, M.D., Ph.D.

"What timid man does not avoid contact with the sick, fearing lest he contract a disease so near?" —Ovid (43 B.C.–17 A.D.?) *Pontic Epistles* III, *ii,* 13

From earliest recorded history the causes of illness were ascribed to the whims of the gods. Spiritual leaders tried to intercede for appeasement of their anger or to seek their favor by preventive measures to maintain health.[1] The *Holy Bible,* especially in the Books of Leviticus and Deuteronomy, make frequent reference to medical subjects such as sanitation and dietary practice.

Speculation that certain febrile diseases could be transmitted from person to person started many centuries ago. Varro and Columella in the first century B.C. thought that illness was caused by living objects, "animalia minuta," which were taken into the body by food or air. During the reign of Justinian in the sixth century A.D., bubonic plague was thought to be contagious, and in the fourteenth century enforcement of quarantine in Marseilles and Venice was a practical application of this belief in contagion. Opinion that disease could pass by contact of humans with sick persons was strengthened by the epidemic spread of syphilis in Europe in the late fifteenth and early sixteenth centuries.

In his book published in 1546, Fracastorius described the transmission of disease by direct contact, by fomities, and through the air. Leeuwenhoek, who owned more than 200 microscopes with more than 400 lenses, was the first to see protozoa under the microscope (1675) and to describe bacterial chains and clumps as well as individual spirilla and bacilli among microorganisms from the teeth (1683). In 1836 Agostino Bassi showed that silkworm disease was due to the presence of microorganisms, thus ascribing a microorganism to a specific disease. In 1843 Dr. Oliver Wendell Holmes claimed that puerperal fever was frequently spread from patient to patient by physicians and nurses, but biologic evidence for his conclusions was not yet available.

Early Interest in Infection at Jefferson

In the theses that the Jefferson medical students were required to write until 1885 as a condition for graduation, the subjects most commonly chosen were those dealing with contagious illness. Dr. Samuel D. Gross in 1829, in the first year after his graduation from Jefferson, translated, from the German, Hildenbrand's *Contagious Typhus,* a disease confused with typhoid fever (the bacillus of which was not isolated until 1880 by Eberth). Gross' career encompassed the era before bacteriology became identified as a medical discipline around 1880. Lister's *Principle of Antisepsis* (1867) was opposed and required 20 years for acceptance.

At Jefferson, Dr. John K. Mitchell, Professor of Medicine, published in 1849 a small volume of six lectures to the medical students entitled *The Cryptogamous Origin of Malarious and Endemical Fevers.* Among the students was Carlos Finlay (Class of 1855) (Figure 13-1) who in 1881 advanced the theory that yellow fever was transmitted from one individual to another by the bite of a mosquito. Mitchell ascribed the causation of febrile illness to "agents possessed of organic vitality and the power of reproduction which had the power of penetrating into and germinating upon the interior tissues of the human body."

Improved understanding and prevention of hospital-acquired infections was initiated by Ignaz Phillipp Semmelweiss, the Hungarian physician who in 1846 noted the high mortality rate in puerperal cases in the Allgemeines Krankenhaus in Vienna. The following year he associated the death of his former instructor, Professor Kolletschka, with the cut from a scalpel used in a postmortem dissection. Semmelweiss demanded the washing of hands in a chlorinated lime solution as a simple expedient to the conduct of labor. It reduced the mortality rate from 9.92 percent to 1.27 percent.[2] The work of Holmes and Semmelweiss was opposed by the Professor of Obstetrics at Jefferson, Dr. Charles D. Meigs, who attributed this particular malady "to accident or to Providence."

The last half of the nineteenth century witnessed great advances in the understanding of the epidemiology of contagious diseases, associated with methods of prevention by antiseptics and aseptic methods. Despite this progress, a lack of treatment for suppurative disease persisted for 90 years following the observations of Semmelweiss. In the preantibiotic era, lack of therapy for staphylococcal infections resulted in high mortality for those with septicemia (82 percent) or prolonged disability for those who recovered. Although the mortality rates in childhood and youth were lower, the complication of chronic osteomyelitis of the long bones often ensued. Eakins employed this dreaded condition as the theme for his *Gross Clinic.*

Sulfonamides became available in 1937 and suppressed in vitro the growth of staphylococci. They appeared to be of some value in minor staphylococcal infections of the urinary tract, but often failed to eradicate or even control staphylococci. Well-timed surgical drainage of suppurative lesions, especially for osteomyelitis, remained of major importance in recovery.

Infectious diseases were the special interest of Dr. Hobart A. Reimann, Magee Professor of

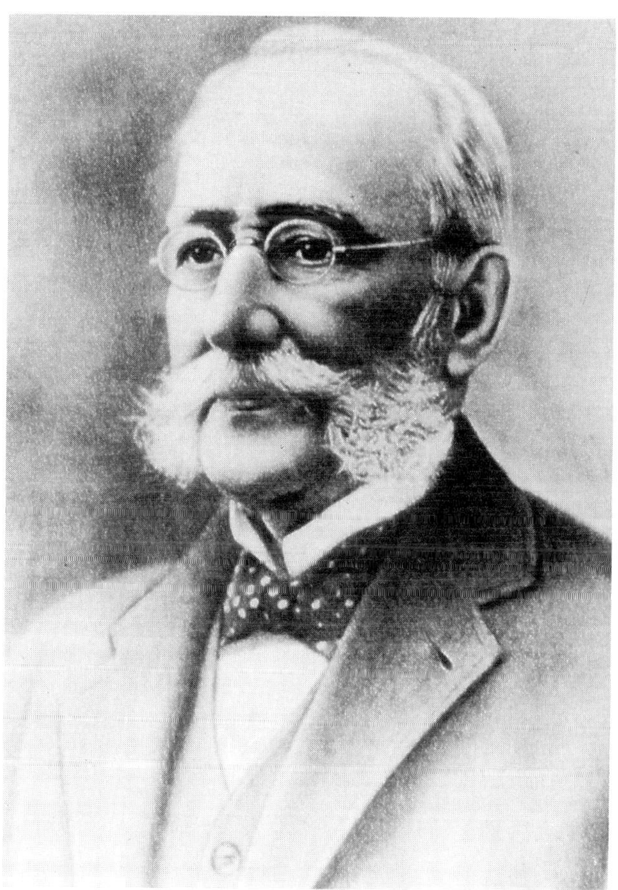

Fig. 13-1. Carlos J. Finlay, M.D. (1833–1915), Jefferson Class of 1855, who in 1881 ascribed yellow fever to the bite of a mosquito.

Medicine and Head of the Department from 1936 to 1951. He achieved worldwide fame for his many contributions to new knowledge of infections and for the 40 years of his *Annual Reviews of Infectious Diseases* (1935–1975). Dr. Reimann described viral pneumonia in a landmark 1938 article, wrote three books on pneumonia, and contributed to the confirmation of a viral etiology for some nonbacterial diseases.

Establishment of the Division of Infectious Diseases at Jefferson

The first formal resident in internal medicine at Jefferson was Dr. W. Paul Havens, Jr. (Figure 13-2), who received his M.D. degree from Harvard Medical School in 1936 and served his internship at the Lankenau Hospital. From 1938 to 1941 he trained under Dr. Reimann, whose influence led him to concentrate his future career on infectious diseases.

Following his residency at Jefferson, Dr. Havens became a National Research Council Fellow at the Rockefeller Institute (1941–1942). For the next four years, during his service in the U.S. Army Medical Corps, he investigated the problems encountered by the military with infectious hepatitis. He returned to Jefferson in 1946 as Associate in Medicine and Clinical Microbiology as well as Chief of the Section of Infectious Diseases at the Pennsylvania Hospital. His clinical investigations into the etiology and pathophysiology of infectious hepatitis and his contributions to serologic techniques, particularly complement fixation in the study of neurotropic viral diseases, were internationally respected.

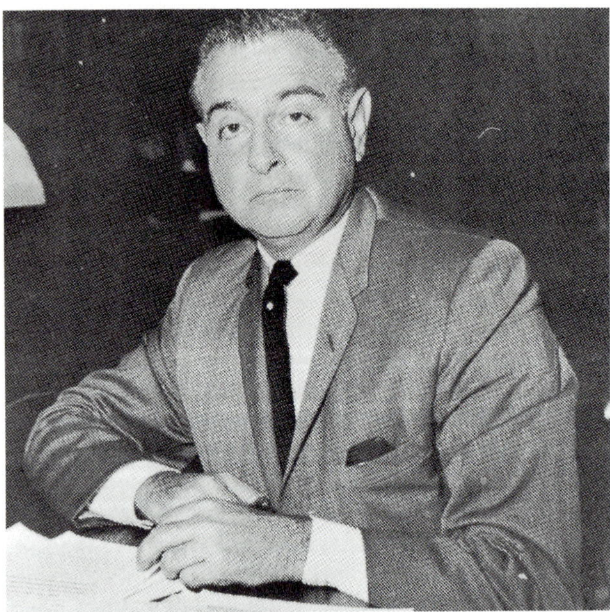

FIG. 13-2. W. Paul Havens, Jr., M.D., Jefferson's first resident in Internal Medicine (1938) and first Director of the Division of Infectious Diseases (1957).

Dr. Havens continued his equal interest in the basic science as well as the clinical aspects of infectious diseases by holding simultaneous faculty appointments in the Departments of Microbiology and Medicine. He was promoted to Associate Professor (1954) and developed the Fellowship Program in Infectious Diseases at Jefferson in 1955. Upon his promotion to Professor in 1957, Havens also was appointed the first Director of the Division of Infectious Diseases.

At retirement on January 1, 1972, Dr. Havens left an impressive list of accomplishments. His lifelong interest in hepatitis extended back to World War II in Egypt and Germany, when he was consultant to the Chief Surgeon, European Command. He was a member of the Neurotropic Virus Disease Commission of the Army Epidemiology Board on Virus and Rickettsial Diseases, the Commission on Viral Infections, the Commission on Liver Diseases of the Armed Forces Epidemiological Board, and a member of the World Health Organization Expert Panel on Viral Hepatitis. He also was editor of *The History of Internal Medicine in World War II* published by the Office of the Surgeon General, Department of the Army. In addition to the Army Commendation ribbon for research in viral hepatitis in 1946, Havens received the Outstanding Civilian Service Award from the Surgeon General of the Army in 1970.

In 1955 Dr. Havens and Dr. John E. Deitrick, Magee Professor of Medicine and Head of the Department, invited Dr. Robert I. Wise to come to Jefferson from the University of Minnesota to assist in the development of a program of education and research in infectious diseases and the utilization of antibiotics. As Assistant Professor with laboratory space on the eighth floor of the College building, Dr. Wise's research related to the epidemiology of hospital-acquired staphylococcal infections, utilizing bacteriophage typing as a tool, and to the clinical use of antibiotics.

Dr. Wise brought to Jefferson a wide previous experience in the study of infectious disease. His research in microbiology had started in 1937 at the University of Illinois, where he spent a year evaluating chemical and microbiological tests for mastitis in cows (leading to the M.S. degree in 1938). Another year was spent as Assistant in Animal Genetics of the Agriculture Experimental Station to study changes in virulence of a certain strain of *Salmonella pullorum,* and three additional years study in the survival of anaerobic pathogens in home-canned vegetables and meats while working toward a Ph.D. degree (awarded 1942). As Director of the Public Health Laboratories of Wichita Falls and Houston, Texas (1942–1943), Wise performed or supervised the tests for contagious diseases as well as quality control tests for milk and water. For four years as Assistant Professor of Microbiology at the University of Texas Medical Branch at Galveston, his research dealt with *Granuloma inguinale,* in which he demonstrated the cause to be a bacterium. He also studied the problem of sewage pollution of oysters in Galveston Bay. During four years of study for the M.D. degree (1950) at the University of Texas, he collaborated with Dr. Edgar Poth, Professor of Surgery, in developing methods for the reduction of bowel flora. This research led to the use of neomycin in the preparation of the bowel for surgery, which later was used by others in the management of hepatic encephalopathy. Dr. Wise's residency in medicine with a Fellowship in Infectious Diseases was spent at the University of Minnesota with Dr. Wesley Spink. He then served as Assistant Professor of Medicine and Director of the Microbiology Laboratory of the University Hospitals, with special attention to staphylococcal diseases.

With Dr. Havens, Dr. Wise initiated at his arrival in 1955 a weekly infectious diseases conference associated with weekly infectious diseases rounds. These were attended by the Fellows in infectious diseases, by Eileen Randall M.A. (the Hospital microbiologist, who later received a Ph.D. in Microbiology and became a national leader in its technology), by Dr. Gonzalo E. Aponte (later Chairman of Pathology) and by interested medical residents and students.

Dr. Francis J. Sweeney, Jr., (Figure 13-3) joined Dr. Wise in his research in infectious diseases in 1956. Born in Philadelphia in 1925, he obtained his B.A. degree at the University of Virginia (Charlottesville) in 1947 and his M.D. at Jefferson in 1951. He interned at Jefferson (1951–1952), took his residency in internal medicine there (1952–1953, 1955–1957, and spent 1957–1958 as Chief Medical Resident at Jefferson. He spent the years 1944–1945 enlisted in the Navy and 1953–1955 commissioned in the Navy. In 1958 Sweeney was

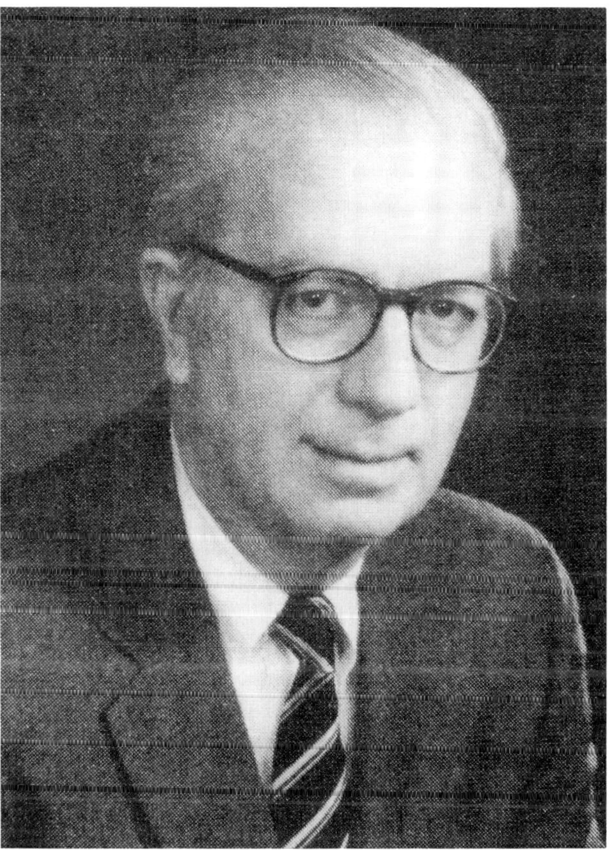

FIG. 13-3. Francis J. Sweeney, Jr., M.D. (Jefferson, 1951), Researcher and Clinician in Infectious Diseases (1956–1967), Medical Director of Jefferson Hospital (1967–1972), Vice-President for Health Services and Hospital Director (1972–1984).

appointed Instructor in Medicine and continued as a member in the Division of Infectious Diseases until his assumption of the position of Jefferson Hospital Director (1967) with promotion to Vice-President for Health Sciences and Hospital Director in 1972.

Dr. Sweeney, during the late 1950s, performed epidemiological studies of staphylococcal infections with Dr. Wise at the Norristown State Hospital in collaboration with Dr. Robert Mandle of the Department of Microbiology. Dr. Eileen Randall collaborated in similar studies at Jefferson. In 1959 Dr. Sweeney went to Thailand with the Jefferson Medical Cŏllege/U.S. Public Health Service Cholera Study Team. Between 1957 and 1967 he wrote numerous papers and three chapters in books or reviews on infectious diseases.

Dr. Sweeney was a member of the Professional Advisory Committee of the Department of Public Health of Philadelphia, 1962–1964, and Co-Director of the Victory over Polio Campaign (Philadelphia, 1962–1964). As a consultant in infectious diseases he served at Eagleville Sanatorium (1962–1966), Philadelphia General Hospital (1969–1971) and Chestnut Hill Hospital (1967–1983). Among a host of professional societies, two related to infectious diseases were the Pennsylvania Public Health Association and fellowship in the Infectious Diseases Society of America.

Dr. Sweeney's entry into hospital administration and many board memberships forced him to withdraw from his outstanding career in infectious diseases. He left Jefferson to become Vice-President for the Health Sciences Center of Temple University (1984–1986) and in June 1986 became Vice-President for Professional Affairs and Medical Director of Mercy Catholic Medical Center.

Among Dr. Sweeney's many awards and honors were: the Lindback Foundation Award for Distinguished Teaching (1963), presentation of his portrait to Thomas Jefferson University (1978), Jefferson Annual Alumni Achievement Award (1983), Jefferson's Winged Ox Award (1984), Special Presidential Citation (American College of Physicians, 1985), The Laureate Award Medal (American College of Physicians, 1985), and Mastership, American College of Physicians (1986). He also served as Chairman of the Board of Regents of the American College of Physicians (1983–1985).

A Jefferson "first" occurred in 1955 when a system for daily surveillance of all infections in the hospital was developed by Dr. Wise. A hospital staff committee including representatives from Nursing Service and all clinical services was organized to study epidemiologic data and make recommendations for prevention and control. In 1956 a nurse, Mary Ann Anderson (Waddell), R.N., who was trained in epidemiology by Dr. Wise, was appointed to conduct surveillance of hospital acquired infections. This was the beginning of the international discipline of Nurse Epidemiologists or Infection Control Practitioners. The program involved daily collection of data from all hospital head nurses and from the Chief of Microbiology, Dr. Eileen Randall, with committee review.

At a 1957 Joint Symposium on Hospital-Acquired Infections in Cleveland, Ohio, Dr. Wise was invited to discuss the Jefferson program. This led to a recommendation to the Board of Trustees of the American Medical Association "that every hospital establish a responsible officer or committee charged with the investigation and control of infections within the hospital and with the institution of procedures and practices designed to prevent such infections."[3] This plan was initiated by the Joint Commission on Accreditation of Hospitals in 1958. Visitors from medical centers from the United States and other countries as well as epidemiologists from the Center for Disease Control (CDC), came to Jefferson to learn about the program. This led to the development of a training program at CDC where Terri Camilli (Usitano), R.N., Nurse Epidemiologist at Jefferson, served as consultant and instructor at the first workshop in nurse epidemiology of nosocomial infections.

During the 18 months of March 1963 through September 1964, an epidemic of *Salmonella derby* infection occurred in the Jefferson Medical College Hospital. A total of 155 employees and over 450 patients became infected with this diarrheal disease. Dr. Sweeney and Dr. Eileen Randall developed a program for collection of rectal swabs from every patient being admitted to the hospital and every physician on the staff. Only one physician of approximately 600 tested was found to be a carrier of *Salmonella* and it was not of the epidemic strain. It was learned that the microorganisms had entered the hospital in chicken eggs. The findings were reported by Drs. Sweeney and Randall at a Conference on Salmonella at the Center for Disease Control and in the *Journal of the American Medical Association*.

When Dr. Wise was appointed Chairman of the Department of Medicine in 1959, it was necessary for him to delegate many of his research activities to Dr. Sweeney, while Dr. Havens continued his Directorship of the Division. There were grants from the National Institutes of Allergy and Infectious Diseases of the U.S. Public Health Service and the Squibb Company. Gow T. Lam, Ph.D., and Charlotte Witmer joined the laboratory staff in 1959 as Research Associates to study abscess-forming factors produced by *Staphylococcus aureus*. Funds for the training of Fellows in Infectious Diseases came from pharmaceutical grants for the investigation of antibiotics. Dr. Craig Wallace was provided a stipend by a grant from the Charles Pfizer Company in 1958–1959. Stipends were provided by Warner-Chilcott for Dr. Joseph F. Rodgers (Jefferson, 1957), and by the Hoffman LaRoche Company for Drs. Thomas G. Bell (Jefferson, 1956) and James R. Regan (Jefferson, 1956). In those early years there was some criticism of receiving funds from the pharmaceutical industry for fear of possible conflict of interest in the reporting of results.

The activities of the Division in evaluation of antibiotics led Dr. Wise to serve on the Editorial Advisory Board of the *Medical Letter on Drugs and Therapeutics,* which required critical review of every publication in the field every two weeks. He was assisted by members of the Department of Medicine and by members of other Departments for 17 years, until his retirement in 1975. The *Medical Letter* became the major force in calling attention to false advertising, in stimulating new legislation, and in bringing to physicians and pharmacists critical unbiased information on drugs in terms of effectiveness, adverse reactions, and possible alternative medications.

Following legislative changes in Congress, a Drug Efficacy Study was organized to accomplish the Herculean task of reviewing an estimated 4,000 drugs and about 7,000 formulations by members of 30 panels developed by the Drug Research Board of the National Academy of Sciences of the National Research Council. Jefferson cooperated in this endeavor for two years in a review of antibiotics by six members of the staff. Other activities of Dr. Wise, related to Jefferson's clinical investigation of antibiotics, included service as a member of the Committee on Advertising of the American College of Physicians and being invited to testify on drug combinations of antibiotics at the hearings before the Subcommittee on Monopoly of the Select Committee on Small Business of the U.S. Senate, which was investigating competitive problems in the drug industry in 1969.[4]

Dr. Joseph F. Rodgers (Figure 13-4) completed a Residency in internal medicine and a Fellowship in Infectious Diseases, and was Chief Medical Resident in 1961–1962. In 1962 he was appointed Instructor in Medicine and became a full-time

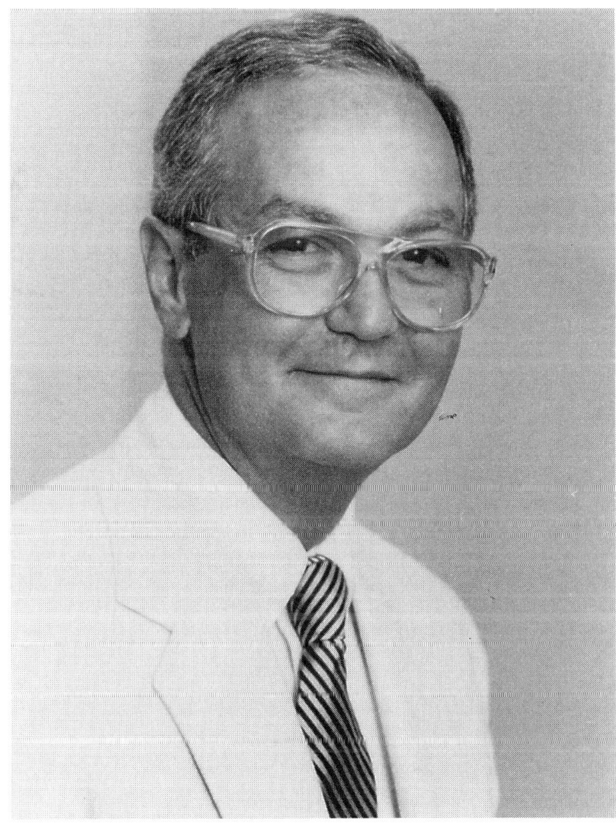

FIG. 13-4. Joseph F. Rodgers, M.D. (Jefferson, 1957), Fellow in Infectious Diseases, Researcher and Clinician in the Division, and Associate Dean, Affiliations and Residency Programs (1984).

member of the Division of Infectious Diseases. He became the Director of the new Division of Home Care, which was established in 1964, and maintained his activities in teaching in the Division of Infectious Diseases. In 1966 he resigned his full-time appointment as Director of the Division of Home Care to become a part-time member of the faculty as Associate in Medicine and continued his active participation in the educational and clinical programs of the Division. In 1984 Rodgers became Associate Dean of the Affiliations and Residency Programs. He currently holds the academic rank of Clinical Associate Professor of Medicine.

Michael Manko, M.D., became a Fellow in Infectious Diseases in 1963–1964, bringing interest and previous research experience during a military assignment with the association of Mycoplasma with primary atypical pneumonia. After completing his Fellowship, Dr. Manko was appointed Instructor in Medicine and developed a program of infectious diseases at the Lankenau Hospital. He continued actively his lectures and attendance at the weekly infectious disease conferences at Jefferson as well as his teaching at Lankenau.

In 1965 the effectiveness of gentamicin and the cephalosporins was examined as therapy for infections caused by gram negative bacteria. Attempts were made to isolate and purify enzymes of *Staphylococcus* and study their role in abscess formation. Dr. Havens was working to adapt the hepatitis viruses to tissue culture.

The Division of Infectious Diseases operated on a very low budget and was dependent on grants from the National Institutes of Health and pharmaceutical companies for studies of therapeutic agents. The programs of medical education were dependent upon the interest and cooperation of the members, who received their financial support from sources other than a Division budget. A boost occurred during the years 1967–1970 with appointments of Drs. Joseph S. Gonnella, Christopher M. Martin, Dominick N. Pasquale, and Earl B. Byrne. Drs. Gary Lattimer and Richard McCloskey were appointed in 1972. Most of these members eventually developed programs in infectious diseases in Jefferson's affiliated hospitals or elsewhere.

Dr. Paul Havens retired as Professor of Medicine, Professor of Microbiology, and Director of the Division of Infectious Diseases in 1972. Budgetary plans were initiated to recruit a full-time Director of the Division, and Dr. Wise became Acting Director. Unfortunately, the reduction of budgeted funds required Dean Kellow to rule that unfilled positions at Jefferson were frozen in 1973. This was also a year in which Dr. Wise asked to be retired, but Dean Kellow requested that the position of Director of the Division be left vacant to allow the next Head of the Department the opportunity to select the next Director. The heritage left by Dr. Reimann in infectious diseases had been maintained and expanded at Jefferson and its affiliated hospitals. At the retirement of Dr. Wise in October, 1975, Dr. Joseph Gonnella became Acting Director of the Division, but the budgeted position for new leadership in infectious diseases was left to the selection by the next Magee Professor (Dr. Frank D. Gray, Jr.). Dr. Sheila A. Murphey (Figure 13-5) was appointed in November, 1977.

When she was appointed Assistant Professor of Medicine and Director of the Division of Infectious Diseases, Dr. Sheila A. Murphey was Assistant Professor of Medicine at the University of Pennsylvania. Dr. Murphey received her M.D. degree from the Woman's Medical College (now The Medical College of Pennsylvania) and completed a residency in Internal Medicine at Mt. Sinai Hospital, New York, and an Infectious Diseases Fellowship at the Hospital of the University of Pennsylvania under Dr. Richard Root. After completing her fellowship she was an attending physician at the Philadelphia General Hospital until it was closed in 1977. She is board certified in Internal Medicine and Infectious Diseases and has been recertified in Internal Medicine. Her research interests were related to pulmonary macrophages and hospital epidemiology. In addition to her duties as Division Director she is the Hospital Epidemiologist of Thomas Jefferson University Hospital. She has received the Medical Resident teaching award on three occasions.

Dr. Murphey recruited Dr. Erick J. Bergquist (Figure 13-6) to the division in July, 1978. Dr. Bergquist (Jefferson, 1973) received some of his infectious diseases training as a student and Medical Resident at Jefferson from Doctors Paul

Havens, Joseph Rodgers, Joseph Gonnella, Robert I. Wise, and Eileen Randall. He completed an Infectious Diseases Fellowship under Dr. Richard Hornick at the University of Maryland Hospital. Prior to receiving his M.D. degree, he had also received the Ph.D. in parasitology under Dr. Gilbert F. Otto at the College Park campus of the University of Maryland. Bergquist's research at Jefferson has also been related to pulmonary host defenses and antibiotic studies. He is a coauthor with Dr. John R. Dalton, Department of Urology, of a book on urinary tract infection (in press). Dr. Bergquist has received the Medical Resident teaching award and the Alpha Omega Alpha student teaching award. Both Drs. Murphey and Bergquist have secondary appointments in the Department of Microbiology, where Dr. Bergquist has regularly been asked to lecture to classes in the Clinical Masters of Microbiology program. Dr. Bergquist chairs the Antibiotic Utilization Subcommittee of the Pharmacy and Therapeutics Committee and for four years was the Chairman of the Intern Selection Committee of the Department of Medicine.

Dr. Murphey recruited Dr. Hans H. Liu to the Division in July 1985 after he had completed a postdoctoral fellowship under Dr. Alexander Tomaz at the Rockefeller University. Dr. Liu received the M.D. degree from Harvard Medical School, completed a residency in Internal Medicine at The New York Hospital-Cornell Medical Center, and an Infectious Diseases Fellowship at the Yale-New Haven Hospital. He is board certified in Internal Medicine and Infectious Diseases. His current research activities include study of mechanisms of antibiotic action and resistance.

In 1980 the Fellowship program of the Division of Infectious Diseases was reactivated and Richard Wills, M.D., trained for one year from 1980–1981. Paul Alessi, D.O., trained from 1982–1984, Joyce Rubin, M.D., from 1984–1986, and J. Robert Williams, M.D., began his training in 1986.

The Infection Control Program has been significantly expanded in order to fulfill its multiple duties, which include routine surveillance for nosocomial infections, outbreak investigation, management of exposures of patients and of personnel to contagious diseases, teaching infection control theory and practice at all levels throughout the hospital, and infection control policy review in all departments of the hospital. Three Infection Control Practitioners, Ms. Beth

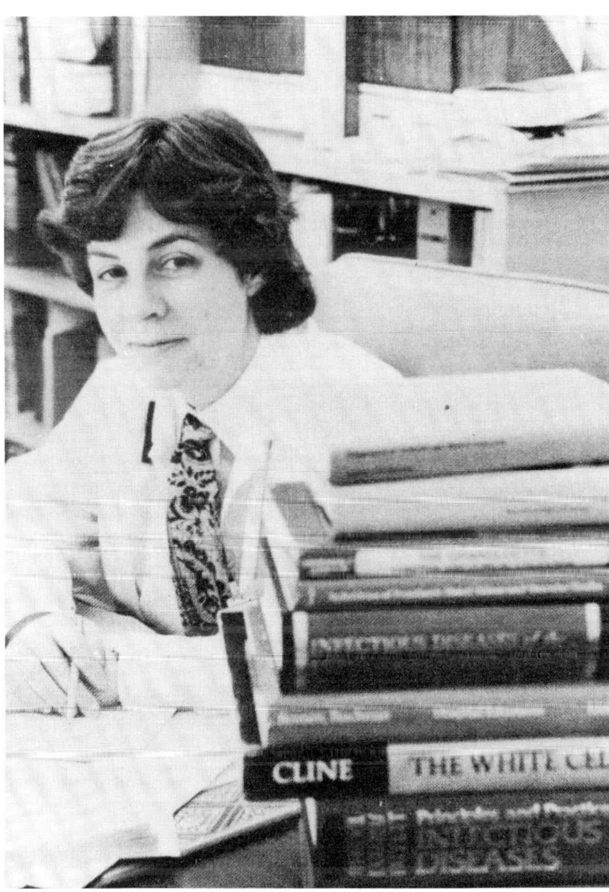

FIG. 13-5. Sheila A. Murphey, M.D., Director of Division of Infectious Diseases (1977–).

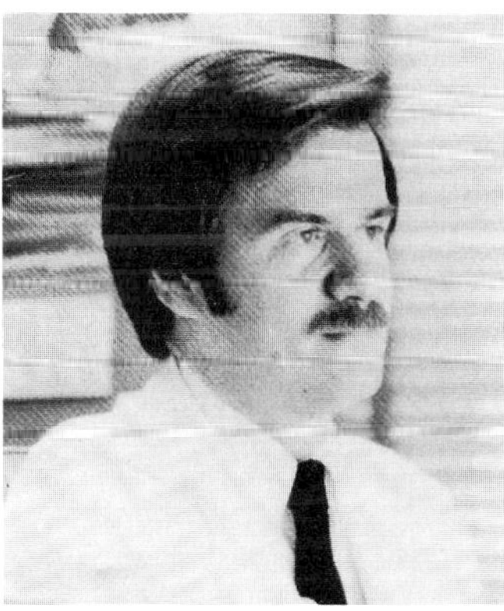

FIG. 13-6. Erick J. Bergquist, M.D. (Jefferson, 1973), Clinician, Teacher and Researcher in the Division of Infectious Diseases.

Ossman, Ms. Joan Forrer, and Mrs. Leigh Gitman now assist the Hospital Epidemiologist.

The third edition of the *Jefferson Infection Control Manual* is now in preparation. Uniform employee health policies emphasizing disease prevention have been developed in cooperation with Dr. Robert Gilbert of the Student and Employee Health Service. Computerization of the Clinical Laboratories has provided easy access to long-term as well as immediate microbiologic data and permitted long-term studies in several areas. Yearly "Infection Control Week" programs and other educational campaigns have publicized to the Hospital such topics as hand washing and needle safety.

Nosocomial infections, their natural history and their prevention, continue to provide a fertile research area for the Division. Dr. Murphey and Dr. Donald Jungkind, Director of the Clinical Microbiology Laboratory, are currently involved in a study of the epidemiology of *Mycobarterium avium-intracellulare* at Jefferson. Dr. Murphey and Dr. Alessi reviewed infectious diarrhea in Jefferson employees, finding *Campylobacter jejuni* to be the most common pathogen isolated. Dr. Murphey and Dr. Rubin studied the epidemiology of *Acinetobacter* isolates at Jefferson. Each of these studies has been reported at national scientific meetings. Currently, Drs. Liu, Williams, and Murphey are studying the epidemiology and significance of *Staphylococcus epidermidis* bacteremia and Drs. Murphey, Liu, and Jungkind are investigating the frequency and resistance mechanisms of borderline oxacillin-resistant *Staphylococcus aureus*.

Determination of causes along with the control of infectious disease has been a major factor in the prolongation of the human life span. A waging battle continues in the elimination of old diseases and the encounter with new ones. Never in the history of mankind have the resources to win this battle been more propitious. Jefferson will continue its role and contributions in this field.

References

1. Zinsser, H., and Bayne-Jones, S., *The History and Scope of Bacteriology* (Chapter 7), Textbook of Bacteriology; 7th ed. New York: D. Appleton-Century Co., 1934.
2. Semmelweiss, T.P., "The Etiology, the Concept and the Prophylaxis of Childbed Fever," Ed. and trans. by F.P. Murphy. *Med. Classics* 5:340. January–April, 1941.
3. "Dr. N. Nosoquo, Secretary, Conference on Cross Infections in Hospitals," *Memorandum to the Board of Trustees, Amer. Med. Assoc.*, November 26, 1957.
4. Wise, R.I., *Centrifugal and Centripetal Forces: A History of the Department of Medicine, The Jefferson Medical College of Thomas Jefferson University, 1959–1975*. Philadelphia: Archives of 1987, T. J. Univ.

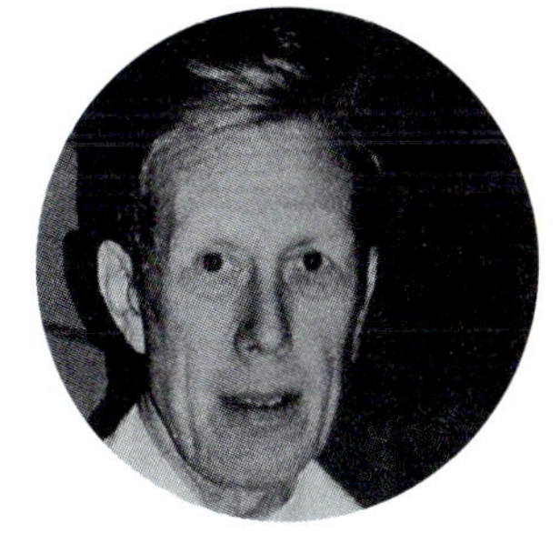

CHAPTER FOURTEEN

Division of Rheumatology

NATHAN M. SMUKLER, M.D.

"The rheumatism is a common name for many aches and pains, which have yet got no peculiar appellation, though owing to very different causes."

—WILLIAM HEBERDEN (1710–1801)

As the various subspecialties of internal medicine evolved, rheumatology developed comparatively late. In the immediate decades preceding and following World War II, Departments of Medicine of United States medical colleges generally adopted divisional or sectional formats. During this organizational period such established subspecialites as cardiology, gastroenterology, and hematology took priority, and at many institutions rheumatology was either present on a very small scale or nonexistent. In the 1950s and 60s, however, there occurred a surge of interest in rheumatology, and this subspecialty became an organized entity at many institutions. Among the factors that contributed to this rapid development of rheumatology were the discovery of the antiinflammatory properties of glucocorticoids by Hench and co-workers at the Mayo Clinic, the explosion of new knowledge in the field of immunology, the National Institutes of Health research and training grants, and the trend to subspecialization by internists during the post–World War II era.

At Jefferson the divisional organization of the Department of Medicine occurred during the tenure of Dr. Robert I. Wise as Chairman (1959–1975). In the forming of Divisions, rheumatology was among the last. Nevertheless, an arthritis clinic was established at Jefferson Hospital in 1931 and preceded the establishment of the Division by 28 years. Even before these events, a number of Jeffersonians made contributions to this specialty.

Early Rheumatology at Jefferson

In 1880, Roberts Bartholow, Professor of Materia Medica, wrote an elegant detailed description of the rheumatic diseases that constituted a chapter of his textbook *Practice of Medicine*.[1] Dr. Bartholow was born in 1831, received his M.D. degree from the University of Maryland, and was a member of the active faculty at Jefferson from 1879 to 1891. He died in 1904. Teaching and clinic activities at Jefferson did not deter him from writing; his bibliography included numerous articles and the sole authorship of a textbook of therapeutics, as well as the one of medicine.

Bartholow's chapter devoted to rheumatism was divided into discussions of acute and chronic joint disease. The portion on acute rheumatism was entirely concerned with rheumatic fever, a disease known also at the time as articular rheumatism and polyarthritis rheumatica. In his clinical description of the arthritis of rheumatic fever he detailed its migratory course, the tendency to involve large rather than small joints, and its limited duration of four to six weeks. Also cited was the propensity of those complicated with carditis to develop chronic heart disease later in life. Erythema marginatum and chorea were not mentioned. Although the temporal relationship of rhematic fever and scarlet fever was discussed, there is no indication of appreciation that acute pharyngitis frequently preceded this disease. Bartholow's lucid discussion of the differential diagnosis of rheumatic fever is entirely valid after the lapse of a century. It included pyaemia (septic arthritis), rheumatoid arthritis, acute gout, urethral rheumatism (gonococcal urethritis and Reiter's syndrome), and hysterical joint disease. A variety of treatment modalities were described, but only salicylate is still in use. Salicylate was described as being very effective, but its use caused gastrointestinal complications, tinnitus, and depression of the heart. Possibly the cardiotoxic properties attributed to salicylate reflected the carditis of rheumatic fever. However, the concept that "aspirin is bad for the heart" persisted, and many patients some 70 and 80 years later refused aspirin for this reason.

In his discussion of chronic joint disease, Bartholow presented three categories: chronic rheumatism, gout, and arthritis deformans. Chronic rheumatism was identified as a joint disorder developing in patients beyond middle age, marked by stiffness, particularly in the morning, intermittent swelling, and rarely joint inflammation. His "chronic rheumatism" appeared to be that portion of the spectrum of arthritis that is presently classified as osteoarthritis. It is of interest, however, that he failed to touch upon a key point of osteoarthritis, the predilection of the disease to involve the distal joints of the fingers, the hips, the knees, and the low spine.

Gout was classified as a chronic disease, although the acute episodes of arthritis that may precede or be superimposed upon the chronic involvement were described in detail. Bartholow listed obesity and lead nephropathy (saturnine gout) as factors that predispose to gout and also discussed the association of gout and atherosclerosis. Colchicine and salicylate were advocated for the treatment of acute gouty arthritis. After the passage of a century colchicine is still utilized for treatment and prophylaxis of this phase of gout. Also, today it is appreciated that weight reduction may lower the serum uric acid. Thus there is a rational basis for Bartholow's empiric recommendation of a sparse diet featuring fruits and vegetables and regular exercise in the treatment of this disease.

The final group of patients presented in Bartholow's chronic rheumatism section were those with destructive inflammation of multiple joints. They were discussed under the heading of arthritis deformans, which he favored over "rheumatoid arthritis," the term coined by the English physician Garrod to describe similar patients. Bartholow's arthritis deformans patients included those with limb joint involvement and also those with rigidity of the spine. These patients by present-day criteria would be categorized as having rheumatoid arthritis and ankylosing spondylitis, respectively.

In 1882, Morris Longstreth (1846–1914), Professor of Pathological Anatomy at Jefferson, authored a monograph concerned with rheumatic diseases. Dr. Longstreth was born and raised in the Philadelphia area and received an A.B. degree from both Haverford and Harvard Colleges and an M.D. degree from the University of Pennsylvania. He became a Resident at the Pennsylvania Hospital, where he developed an interest in both pathology and the rheumatic diseases.[2] After his residency he continued at the Pennsylvania Hospital as Attending Physician and Curator of the Pathological Museum. He was appointed Professor of Pathological Anatomy at Jefferson in 1879 and retained this position until 1895, when he resigned to enter private practice in Philadelphia. The William Wood publishing firm in New York City encouraged Dr. Longstreth to make known his knowledge of the rheumatic diseases and he responded with a monograph of 279 pages.[3]

The first few chapters of Longstreth's text, entitled *Gout, Rheumatism and Some Allied*

Disorders, were concerned with the spectrum of rheumatic diseases, including etiology and pathology. The middle and largest portion of the volume was devoted to the clinical, laboratory, and pathological aspects of rheumatic fever, which at the time of publication was the most prevalent of the acute rheumatic diseases. The emphasis on rheumatic fever is of interest in that present-day medical students are unlikely to encounter this disease except in relation to residual valvular heart disease.

Longstreth's chapter devoted to rheumatic fever gave an excellent description of acute arthritis associated with this disease. He and his contemporaries had a good understanding of rheumatic heart disease. They appreciated that there was involvement of the pericardium, myocardium, and endocardium. Although auscultation permitted clinical detection of endocarditis, the myocardial and pericardial disease was generally demonstrated at postmortem examination. Finally, it was clearly described that some patients with acute endocarditis went on to recovery, whereas others developed severe progressive and ultimately fatal heart disease. Longstreth noted that acute rheumatic fever was more common among the poor than in those from the higher economic classes, an observation that was made again in this country some 50 years later.

A chapter of Longstreth's book was devoted to central nervous system complications of rheumatic fever. He described neuropathological findings in the meninges and brain and also neural symptoms that were considered to reflect systemic aspects of the disease such as fever. For example, he quoted Dr. Jacob Mendes DaCosta of the Jefferson faculty, who reported that a patient may develop cerebral rheumatism during or shortly after an attack of rheumatic fever.[4] Cerebral rheumatism was described as a restlessness passing into stupor, coma, or delirium and terminating in death. In some of these patients there were focal neurological findings as seizures, palsies, or hemiplegia. This material is difficult to reconcile with present-day concepts of the central nervous system involvement in rhematic fever, which is limited to the basal ganglia, expressed as chorea. In fairness to Longstreth it is to be noted he indicated that the meninges and cerebral disease described in these rheumatic fever patients may have been due to a complicating disease such as meningitis rather than the rheumatic fever. In hindsight the "cerebral rheumatism" may have represented systemic lupus erythematosus that was not delineated from rheumatic fever, or even a phase of rheumatic fever no longer encountered. With respect to treatment, salicylate in various forms was recommended as being effective in management of the arthritis but not the carditis of rheumatic fever. A quote from Longstreth concerning salicylic acid is of interest in view of the fact that many present-day physicians favor salicylates over the other nonsteroidal antiinflammatory drugs, as they are effective and less expensive. "The acid (salicylic acid) has been known since 1844 when it was prepared from oil of wintergreen. Its scarcity and great cost prevented its use and its quality remained to a great degree unknown." He goes on to state that in the ensuing years manufacturing techniques improved, and the drug became less expensive.

Longstreth's last chapters were devoted to chronic articular rheumatism (osteoarthritis), gout, and gonorrheal arthritis. Of particular interest is the description of the natural course of gonococcal arthritis in the prepenicillin era. The attack of arthritis might last for weeks or months, and in some instances there was progression to chronic effusion, fibrous involvement, and fibrous ankylosis. In contrast to present-day rheumatology textbooks, which give top priority to rheumatoid arthritis, Dr. Longstreth was cursory in his approach to this disease and considered it primarily in subsections devoted to the differential diagnosis of arthritis. Factors to be considered in the rise in importance of rheumatoid arthritis over the course of a century include the virtual disappearance of rheumatic fever in the United States and Western European countries, the development of laboratory and radiographic techniques that facilitate the delineation of rheumatoid arthritis from other rheumatic diseases, and possibly an increased prevalence of rheumatoid arthritis in recent decades.

In 1886 representatives from Philadelphia hospitals presented their treatment programs for the rheumatic diseases.[5] Drs. J. M. DaCosta and Bartholow represented Jefferson, and Dr. Longstreth the Pennsylvania Hospital, although he also held a Professorship at Jefferson. The renowned Dr. William Osler of the University of Pennsylvania Hospital and Dr. James Tyson of the Philadelphia Hospital (Philadelphia General Hospital) also contributed. The main focus on the discussion was directed to rheumatic fever. It was generally agreed that salicylates were useful in controlling the articular but not the cardiac manifestations. For joint pain, opium or one of its derivatives was advocated both systemically and by local application.

In 1914 Dr. Solomon Solis-Cohen (Figure 14-1) (Jefferson, 1883), Professor of Clinical Medicine, authored a paper[6] that represented the first report in the English literature of the rheumatic entity now termed palindromic arthritis. It is an episodic disorder marked by attacks of pain and swelling of joints or tissues adjacent to joints, lasting for a day or a few days, with variable intervals between attacks. After months or years the attacks may cease. At times, however, they may be a harbinger of rheumatoid arthritis. Dr. Solis-Cohen's report reviewed a series of patients, many of whom manifested an episodic disorder consistent with palindromic arthritis. He attributed the articular and periarticular involvement to an autonomic imbalance, which he termed vasomotor or autonomic ataxia; however, at present this condition is considered to reflect a disorder of the immune system. He also published many additional reports dealing with clinical features or treatment of rheumatic disease.[7–9]

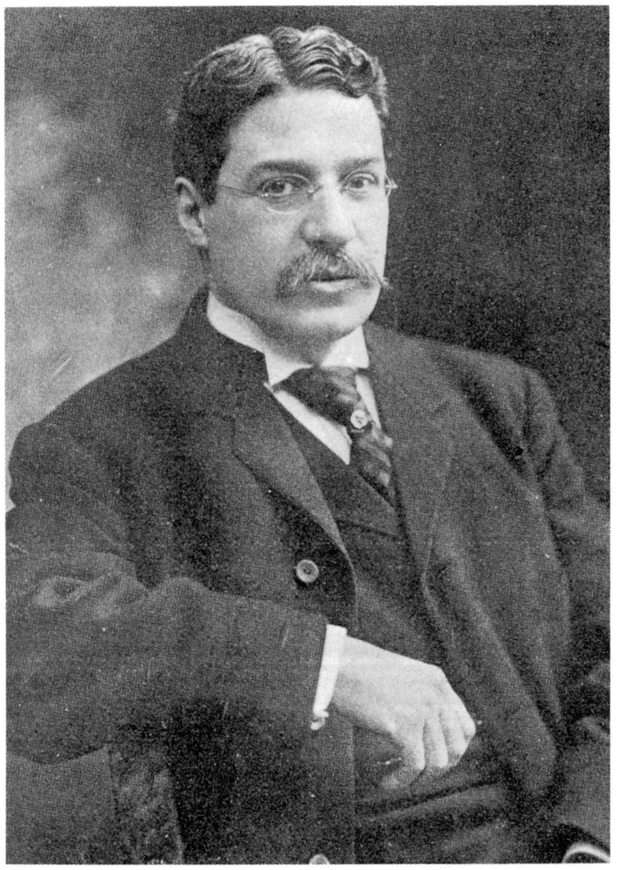

Fig. 14-1. Solomon Solis-Cohen, M.D., Professor of Clinical Medicine (1904–1927) and Jefferson pioneer in treatment of "rheumatic disorders."

Dr. Abraham Cohen (Figure 14-2) was one of the pioneer rheumatologists in the United States. Cohen (Jefferson, 1925) was a member of the staff of Jefferson Hospital with special interest in its arthritis clinic from 1931 until his death in 1969. In addition, he was active at the Philadelphia General Hospital and headed an arthritis clinic at that hospital for many years. Dr. Cohen's hospital appointments and bibliography demonstrate his

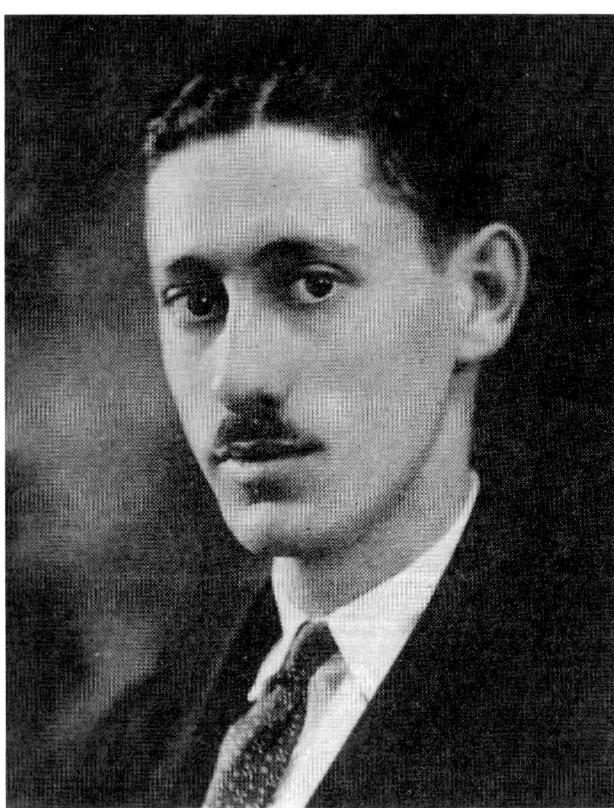

Fig. 14-2. Abraham Cohen, M.D., innovative organizer of Jefferson's first arthritis clinic (1931).

capacity as tireless worker, astute observer, and innovative therapist. In 1941 he published the first definitive description of gouty arthritis in black Americans.[10] Before that time there was only one case report of gout in a black American, which had appeared in a Scandinavian journal. Cohen also authored 20 additional papers on a variety of rheumatological topics. In the *New England Journal of Medicine,* he detailed his experience with gold therapy for rheumatoid arthritis.[11,12] He also reported a trial of an estrogenic substance for the treatment of rheumatoid arthritis. Several papers described his use of physostigmine and neostigmine for patients with musculoskeletal-articular pain and muscle spasms, as well as histamine for those with impaired peripheral circulation.[13–15] In the context of today's use of such immunosuppressive agents as azathioprine and methotrexate to manage connective tissue diseases, Dr. Cohen's effort with a trial of nitrogen mustard for patients with rheumatoid arthritis was prophetic.[16]

From 1946 until 1956 Dr. Richard T. Smith (Figure 14-3) (Jefferson, 1941) served as Chief of the Rheumatology outpatient clinic. He was a staunch advocate of gold therapy prior to the time that this agent was unequivocally established as an effective therapeutic modality for rheumatoid arthritis. Subsequent to his activity at Jefferson Hospital, Dr. Smith was the Attending Rheumatologist at Pennsylvania Hospital and also was active at the Merck Pharmaceutical Company. He died suddenly at age 58.

Dr. Irvin F. Hermann (Jefferson, 1937) assisted Dr. Smith at the arthritis clinic. Dr. Hermann's training included a fellowship with the eminent rheumatologist, Dr. Walter Bauer, at the Massachusetts General Hospital. Following his fellowship, Dr. Hermann returned to Philadelphia and was active in rheumatology at Jefferson, at Mt. Sinai Hospital of Philadelphia (the Southern Division of the Albert Einstein Medical Center), and at Pennsylvania Hospital. He later served as Medical Director of the United States Postal Service. In addition, Drs. Roy G. Hays, Edward Mazur (Jefferson, 1941), Howard Lorenz, John Blizzard (Jefferson, 1954), and Leon Weiner participated in the Jefferson Arthritis Clinic.

The Division of Rheumatology

A Division of Rheumatology within the Department of Medicine was formed in July 1959, with Nathan M. Smukler (Jefferson, 1947) as Division Head. Dr. Smukler (Figure 14-4), who had trained at the Mt. Sinai Hospital of Philadelphia (now the Southern Division of the Albert Einstein Medical Center) and in rheumatology at the Hospital of the University of Pennsylvania under Dr. Joseph Hollander, was a member of the Department of Medicine at the University of Pennsylvania School of Medicine before his appointment at Jefferson.

At the outset the only member of the Division of Rheumatology beside Dr. Smukler was Howard Lorenz, M.D., a volunteer faculty member who attended the arthritis clinic. It was thus necessary for Dr. Smukler to concentrate on teaching and patient care activities and to put aside temporarily his research interests. The teaching program included bedside teaching rounds at Jefferson Hospital, presentations of outpatients to students assigned to the arthritis clinic, and participation at medical grand rounds and formal lectures.

A particular interest of Dr. Smukler was the suspected role of psychological disorders in

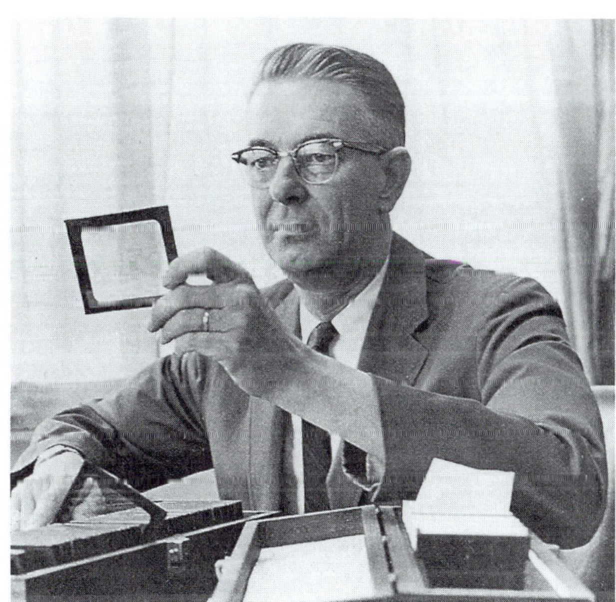

Fig. 14-3. Richard T. Smith, M.D., early advocate of gold therapy for rheumatoid arthritis.

provoking, sustaining, or aggravating rheumatoid arthritis and other systemic inflammatory rheumatic diseases. It was envisioned that a group of psychologists, psychiatrists, and rheumatologists could be organized to investigate this psychosomatic concept, and a request for support was submitted to the National Institutes of Health. Although this application was never funded, Dr. Smukler continued his observations of psychological factors upon the course of rheumatoid arthritis and other chronic rheumatic diseases. Other areas of study included the neuroanatomy and neurophysiology of pain, nonorganic musculoskeletal-articular pain, systemic vasculitis, and spinal arthritis.

Dr. John Abruzzo became the second full-time member of the Division in February, 1967. Before coming to Jefferson, Dr. Abruzzo (Figure 14-5), a graduate of Georgetown University School of Medicine, had been a resident in internal medicine at the Jersey City Medical Center, a Fellow in Rheumatology at the Columbia-Presbyterian Medical Center in New York City, and faculty member with the rank of Assistant Professor of Medicine at the New Jersey College of Medicine. During his fellowship at the Columbia-Presbyterian Rheumatic Disease Unit under Dr. Charles Christian, Dr. Abruzzo collaborated in a study that showed that chronic injection of *E. coli* into dogs induced rheumatoid factor.[17] This pioneer work is among the factors that stimulated intensive research directed to uncovering an infectious etiology for rheumatoid arthritis. After coming to Jefferson, Dr. Abruzzo engaged in teaching, reorganized and directed the outpatient center, and carried out clinical testing of nonsteroidal antiinflammatory drugs in patients

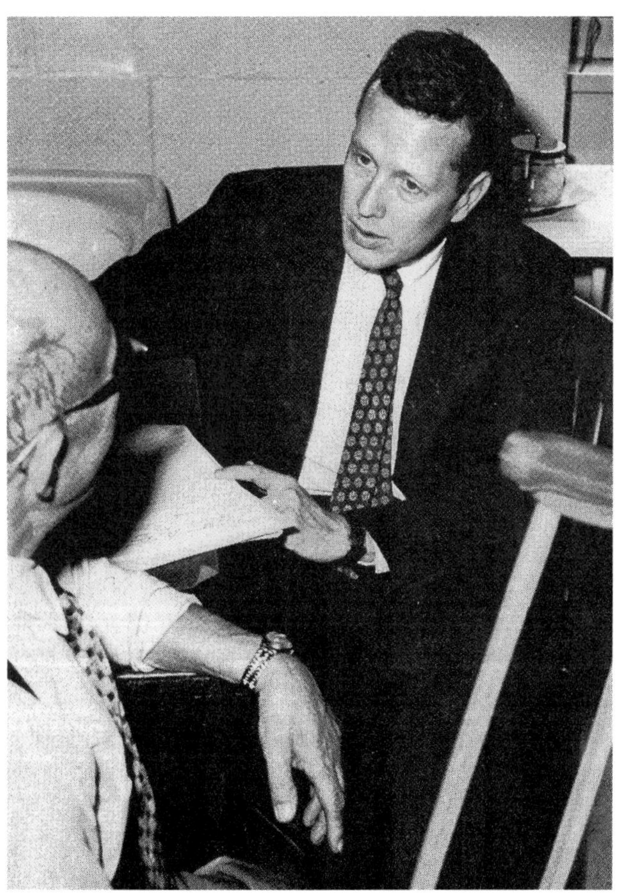

FIG. 14-4. Nathan M. Smukler, M.D., Chief of the Jefferson Rheumatology Division (1958–1980).

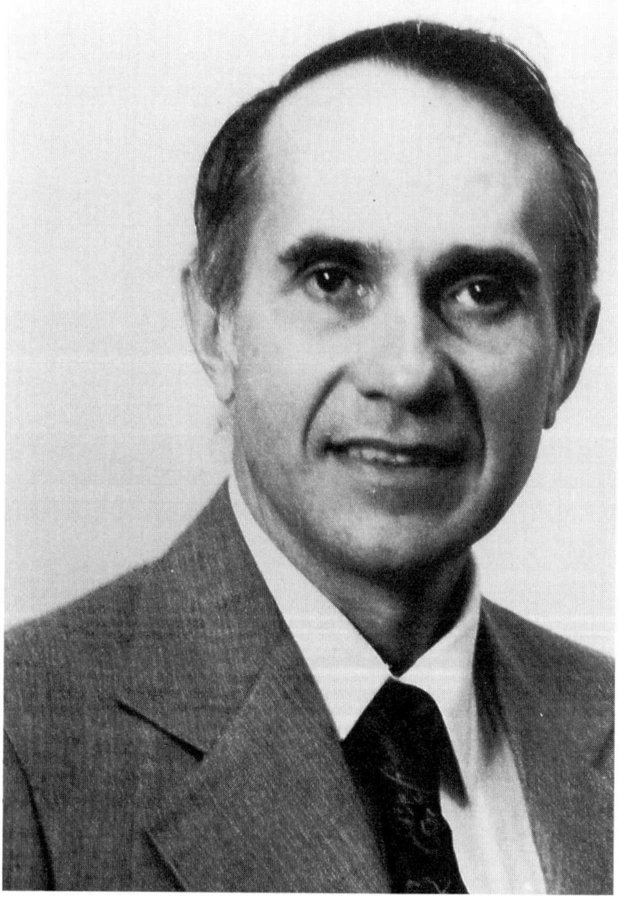

FIG. 14-5. John L. Abruzzo, M.D., Director, Division of Rheumatology (1980–).

with rheumatoid arthritis and osteoarthritis. He also collaborated with Dr. Ralph Heimer, a member of the Department of Biochemistry, in the study of alterations of serum proteins in patients with various rheumatic diseases. In 1978 Abruzzo was named Associate Editor of the *Annals of Internal Medicine*. Dr. Abruzzo was promoted to Associate Professor of Medicine in 1969 and to full Professor in 1974. He succeeded Dr. Smukler as Head of the Division in 1980.

Dr. Ralph DeHoratius (Figure 14-6) (Jefferson, 1968) became the third full-time member of the Division in 1974. He had interned at Jefferson and subsequently served a residency in internal medicine and a fellowship in rheumatology at the University of New Mexico School of Medicine under Dr. Ralph Williams. Following completion of his training, Dr. DeHoratius joined the faculty of the University of New Mexico School of Medicine with the rank of Assistant Professor. At the time, he also received a career development award from the Veterans Administration, which enabled him to pursue research concerning pathogenetic immune mechanisms in connective tissue diseases. A particular interest of Dr. DeHoratius was detection of antibodies to lymphocytes that are concerned with immune regulatory mechanisms. He demonstrated their presence in patients with systemic lupus erythematosus, in their families and household pets, and in laboratory workers exposed to their blood. After returning to Jefferson as Assistant Professor of Medicine, DeHoratius received a young investigator award from the National Institutes of Health to continue his studies of defects in immune regulation in systemic lupus erythematosus patients and their contacts. He also developed an outpatient facility for evaluation and treatment of systemic lupus erythematosus patients. As a result of his productivity he rose to the rank of full Professor in 1982. In that year DeHoratius left Jefferson to accept a position as Director of an Immunology and Rheumatology Division in the Department of Medicine at Hahnemann Medical College.

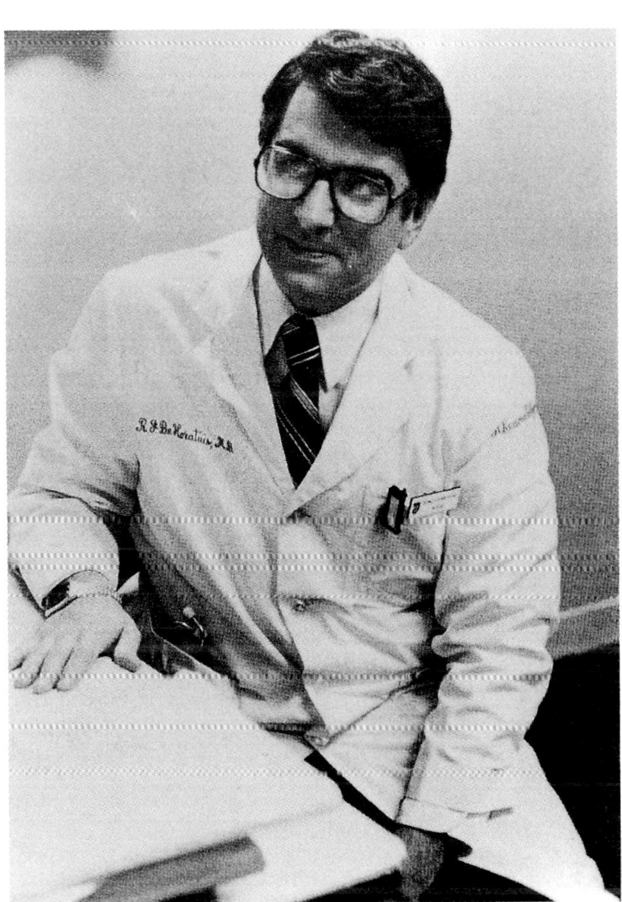

FIG. 14-6. Ralph DeHoratius, M.D., explorer of immunologic interrelationships in rheumatology.

During the 1950s and succeeding decades, intensive investigation indicated that immunological mechanisms contributed to the pathogenesis and perhaps the etiology of rheumatoid arthritis and other connective tissue diseases. Consequently, immunologically oriented research flourished at numerous rheumatology units throughout the United States. In an effort to facilitate this type of investigation at Jefferson, Dr. Frank Gray, the Magee Professor of Medicine (1976–1981), along with Drs. Abruzzo and DeHoratius, recruited Dr. J. Bruce Smith to join the Division in 1981. Dr. Smith, a graduate of the Bowman Gray School of Medicine, had trained in internal medicine at Pennsylvania Hospital and the University of Pennsylvania Hospital. He then became a Fellow in Immunology under Nobel Laureate Dr. Baruch Blumberg at the Institute for Cancer Research in Philadelphia and at University College, London, England, under Dr. N. A. Mitchison.

Following his training in immunology, Dr. Smith was appointed a Research Physician at the Institute for Cancer Research in Philadelphia (1974–

1981). During this period he received grants from the American Cancer Society and the National Institutes of Health for his studies of immune cell interactions in laboratory animals, in normal persons, and in patients with cancer. After joining the Jefferson faculty, Dr. Smith expanded his studies of immune cell interactions to patients with rheumatic diseases. His laboratory provided research opportunities for Ph.D. investigators and Fellows in Rheumatology. Dr. Smith also participated in all the clinical activities of the Division.

To enhance further the expertise of the Division in immunology, Dr. Willis Maddrey, who had succeeded Dr. Frank Gray as Magee Professor of Medicine in 1982, and Dr. Abruzzo recruited Dr. Henry Scovern. Dr. Scovern, a graduate of the George Washington University School of Medicine, had just completed a combined fellowship in allergy, immunology, and rheumatology at Yale before joining the Jefferson faculty in 1982. His research concerned the cellular actions and interactions associated with delayed hypersensitivity. In addition, he has actively engaged in teaching and patient care at the Jefferson Arthritis Center and Hospital.

Volunteer physicians have also made important contributions to the Division. Dr. John R. Patterson (Jefferson, 1959) joined the Division as a part-time member in 1961. After completion of a residency in internal medicine at Jefferson, during which he devoted nine months to training in rheumatology, Dr. Patterson limited his practice to the subspeciality of rheumatology. In addition to teaching at the arthritis clinic, he attended the sarcoid clinic directed by Dr. Harold Israel. The sarcoid clinic provided Dr. Patterson with a unique opportunity to evaluate and classify rheumatic disease among a large group of patients with sarcoidosis.

Dr. Ronald Restifo, a graduate of the Indiana University School of Medicine, who had been a fellow and staff physician in the section of rheumatology at the University of Pennsylvania Hospital, joined the Division in 1967. While at Jefferson he attended the arthritis clinic, maintained an office at the Mohler building, and was also active at Jefferson Hospital. A capable clinician and teacher, Dr. Restifo was popular with students, house staff, and colleagues. The call of the West proved irresistible, however, and Restifo left Jefferson in 1972 to enter private practice in San Jose, California.

A Fellowship Program was established in the Division in 1968. The first trainees were Drs. Walter Schwarzchild and Vincent Giuliano, both going on to the practice of rheumatology. Subsequent early Fellows varied in their pursuits with respect to practice and research. As the Division gained strength, research became more intense and innovative. Dr. Anthony Cuccinotta investigated bone density in patients with rheumatic disease. Dr. Muhammed Sadeghian, a graduate of the University of Teheran, worked with Dr. Abruzzo in the evaluation of piroxicam, a nonsteroidal antiinflammatory drug. Sadeghian has continued investigations in Iran, including the possible value of colchicine in the management of calcinosis universalis.

In 1982 the Fellowship Program was expanded so that a trainee was accepted every year rather than every two years. This format permitted the first-year Fellow to concentrate on clinical activities and the second year Fellow to devote his or her efforts to a research project. Dr. Lawrence Brent (Jefferson, 1978) became the first Fellow under the two-year program. His studies on T-lymphocytes in normal mice stimulated him to pursue further training in the field of immunology at the University of Alabama. Dr. Bruce Bender (Jefferson, 1977) studied monoclonal antibodies with specificity for HLA-DR antigens. Dr. John Fort studied the occurrence of anticardiolipin antibodies in various connective tissue diseases during his Fellowship, then joined the Jefferson full-time faculty to continue research, teaching, and patient care activities. The Division accepted its first woman Fellow in 1985, Dr. Celia Fernandez, from the Rutgers University School of Medicine.

Jefferson's history of rheumatology is replete with contributions in literature, teaching and patient care. During the 1980s, successors to its pioneer rheumatologists required an environment supportive of research for full-time investigators with relatively light teaching and patient care responsibilities. To this end Dean Joseph Gonnella and Professors Willis Maddrey, Darwin Prockop, and Jouni Uitto recruited a group of new faculty members: Drs. Sergio Jimenez, John Varga, and Reza Bashey. This trio provided research skills for the rheumatology program as well as for other departments engaged in the comprehensive study of collagen and diseases marked by collagen defects and progressive fibrosis. These newcomers are ranked along with Cornile LeRoy and his co-workers at the Medical University of South Carolina as the two groups most productive in the investigation of scleroderma in the United States. Dr. Jimenez and his colleagues joined other newcomers to Jefferson, Drs. Prockop (Biochemistry), Emanuel Rubin (Pathology), Maddrey (Medicine), and Uitto (Dermatology) for a multilateral approach to the diseases of connective tissue, particularly the collagen component. Specific diseases studied include osteoarthritis, osteogenesis imperfecta, and those associated with progressive fibrosis such as scleroderma and hepatic cirrhosis.

Dr. Sergio Jimenez, a native of Peru, received his early training there (M.D., University of San Marcos, 1964, *magna cum laude*). Following internship in Lima, he came to the United States for training in internal medicine on the University of Pennsylvania service at Philadelphia General Hospital and later at the Mayo Clinic, returning to Philadelphia General Hospital as a Research Fellow under Dr. Darwin Prockop at the Clinical Research Center. Numerous publications followed relative to the molecular structure, biochemistry, synthesis, and genetic regulation of collagen. Jimenez was appointed to a Rheumatology Fellowship under Dr. Allen Myers at the University of Pennsylvania School of Medicine and joined the teaching staff as Associate in Medicine in 1973. He advanced to full Professor in the Departments of Medicine and Orthopedic Surgery. In 1987 he was appointed Professor of Medicine and Director of Rheumatology Research at Jefferson, thus rejoining his early mentor, Dr. Prockop, who had come to Jefferson in 1986 as Chairman of Biochemistry and Director of the Jefferson Institute of Molecular Medicine.

Dr. Jimenez has published more than 100 papers and has received numerous awards including the Gerald Rodnan Award for excellence in scleroderma research.

Dr. John Varga (New York University School of Medicine, 1980) was trained in internal medicine at Rhode Island Hospital. This was followed by a Fellowship in rheumatology under Dr. Alan Cohen at Boston University and a postdoctoral fellowship at the University of Pennsylvania, where he joined Dr. Jimenez in the study of collagen. Dr. Varga has studied specifically amyloidosis and scleroderma. His publications include chapters in three textbooks.

Dr. Reza Bashey was educated at the University of Bombay (1952). He remained there for his M.S. in biochemistry and then went on to Rutgers for his Ph.D. His collagen research began at the University of Southern California and at the University of Miami, after which he had appointments at Albert Einstein College of Medicine in New York and at Hahnemann University, Philadelphia. In 1975 Bashey was appointed a senior investigator at the Philadelphia General Hospital Clinical Research Center, where he joined Dr. Jimenez and held Associate status in the Department of Medicine at the University of Pennsylvania. He continued at Pennsylvania, with appointments in both the Schools of Medicine and Dentistry, until he joined the Jefferson Faculty as Research Associate Professor of Medicine in 1987.

These recent research capabilities promise improvements in our knowledge of the etiology of rheumatic diseases, with the possibility of better methods of treatment while at the same time aiding in a more comprehensive understanding of disease in its global relationships.

References

1. Bartholow, R., "Acute Rheumatism, Chronic Rheumatism, Gout and Podagra, Arthritis Deformans," In Bartholow, R., *A Treatise on Practice of Medicine*. New York: D. Appleton, 1880, pp. 809–828.
2. Tyson, J., "Memoir of Dr. Morris Longstreth," *Trans. Stud. Coll. Phys. of Phila.* Ser. 3, 1916, 58, pp. 58–60.
3. Longsreth, M., *Rheumatism, Gout, and some Allied Disorders*. New York: William Wood and Co. 1882, pp. 1–279.
4. DaCosta, J.M., "Cerebral Rheumatism," *Am. Jour. Med.* Sc. 1875, 69, pp. 17–45.
5. *Medical News*. 1886, 49, pp. 627–629.
6. Solis-Cohen, S., "On Some Angioneural Arthroses (Periarthroses, Paraarthroses) Commonly Mistaken for Gout or Rheumatism," *Am. Jour. Med. Sc.* 1914, 147, pp. 228–243.
7. Solis-Cohen, S., "Obstinate Sciatica Cured by Deep Injection of Osmic Acid," *J. Nerv. & Ment. Disease*. 1889, 16, pp. 177–179.

8. Solis-Cohen, S., "Therapeutics of the Gouty Diathesis," *Medical News.* 1889, 54, pp. 553–556.
9. Solis-Cohen, S., "The Prophylaxis and General Management of Acute Rheumatic Fever," *Jour. Amer. Med. Assn.* 1907, 49, pp. 2049–2053.
10. Cohen, A., "Gout and the Negro," *Southern Medicine—Surgery.* 1941, 103, pp. 654–655.
11. Cohen, A., and Dubbs, A.W., "The Treatment of Rheumatoid Arthritis with Gold," *New Eng. J. Med.* 1943, 229, pp. 773–778.
12. Cohen, A., Goldman, J., and Dubbs, A.W., "The Treatment of Rheumatoid Arthritis with 417 Courses of Gold." *New Eng. J. Med.* 1945, 233, pp. 199–203.
13. Cohen, A., Goldman, J., and McBride, T. J., "Preliminary Report of 20 Patients Treated with Delta-5 Pregnenolone and Remissions in Rheumatoid Arthritis Following Gold Therapy," *Journal-Lancet.* 1950, pp. 264–265.
14. Trommer, P. R., and Cohen, A., "Use of Neostigmine in the Treatment of Muscle Spasm in Rheumatoid Arthritis and Related Conditions: Preliminary Report," *Jour. Amer. Med. Assn.* 1944, 124, pp. 1237–1239.
15. Cohen, A., Trommer, P., and Goldman, J., "Physostigmine for Muscle Spasm in Rheumatoid Arthritis." *Jour. Amer. Med. Assn.* 1946, 130, pp. 265–270.
16. Cohen, A., Rose, I., and Cooper, E., "Nitrogen Mustard in the Treatment of Rheumatoid Arthritis," *Jour. Amer. Med. Assn.* 1953, 152, pp. 402–403.
17. Abruzzo, J. L., and Christian, C. L., "The Induction of a Rheumatoid Factor-Like Substance in Rabbits." *Jour. of Exper. Med.* 1961, 114, p. 791.

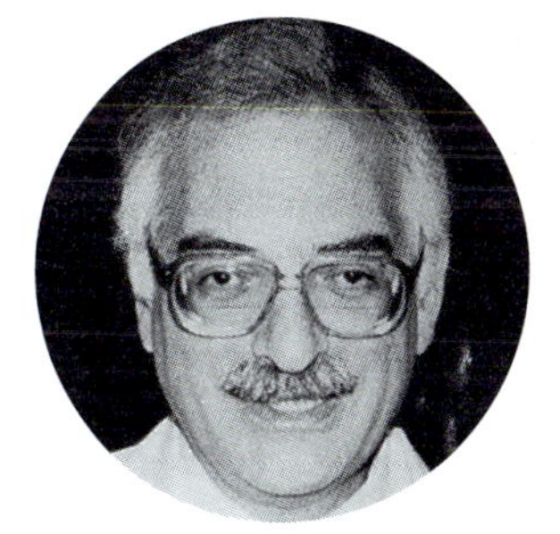

CHAPTER FIFTEEN

Division of Nephrology

Michael L. Simenhoff, M.D.

"It is no exaggeration to say that the composition of the blood is determined not by what the mouth takes in but by what the kidneys keep." —Homer W. Smith (1895–1962)

Early Nephrology at Jefferson

Nephrology has been relatively a latecomer to the disciplines of medicine as a whole. The major impetus came from the development of an artificial kidney by William Kolff, M.D., in Holland during World War II. This advance in turn derived from a series of technological steps, the first of which was the use by Abel, Rountree, and Turner in 1913 of hemodialysis to remove urea in dogs. The organization of Nephrology into a separate Division of the Department of Medicine began at Jefferson only in 1962 when Laurence G. Wesson, Jr., was appointed Professor of Medicine and Head of the Division of Nephrology. Before this, in the late 1950s and early 1960s, Dr. James E. Clark (Jefferson, 1952) had acquired an artificial kidney for hemodialysis in order to study adrenal problems, but this machine was soon commandeered to treat ill patients with acute renal failure. He held together the loose discipline of renology alone with the services of a small supplementary laboratory adjacent to the room that housed the artificial "kidney unit." Although peritoneal dialysis had been performed a few times in the 1950s, it was not an established procedure for use in acute renal failure.

Dr. Clark (Figure 15-1), together with Dr. John Y. Templeton III, (Jefferson, 1941), explored the use of isolated intestinal loops as an alternative functioning membrane to rid the body of uremic toxins, fluid, and electrolytes. A generous grant was obtained from the John A. Hartford Foundation for this study, and Dr. Miles H. Sigler, Associate Professor of Medicine, became involved in the kinetics of sodium and glucose transport across the intestinal membrane. Dr. Herbert E. Cohn (Jefferson, 1955), Associate Professor of Surgery, perfected the surgical techniques for creating the isolated small intestinal loops in man and continued the study. It soon became clear, however, that the intestinal mucosa was much too discriminating a barrier for dialysis. Uremic toxins other than urea and sodium could not be removed adequately, and uremic patients with loops came to need hemodialysis as much as patients without loops. In order to keep loop patients well enough to permit studies, a chronic dialysis unit had to be created within the Hartford Foundation research program. Just as one research program had led to the establishment of the earlier acute dialysis unit, so another research program now led to the creation of a chronic dialysis unit.

Dr. Wesson (Figure 15-2) had been recruited from the New York University Graduate School of Medicine. He had spent 15 years in close collaboration with Dr. Homer Smith, one of the pioneers of Physiological Nephrology, and himself had been instrumental in developing the concept of osmolar and free water clearance by the kidney. There was much enthusiasm in the arrival of Dr. Wesson to develop a superior nephrology program, particularly with the presence of the Clinical Research Center as well as available space and funds. Dr. Joseph Letteri was appointed Research Fellow in Medicine in January of 1962 to further this project.

Dr. Clark continued as the major renal clinician and gradually dissociated himself from his previous private partnership practice because of the time commitments to the nephrology program. He was supported by the dialyzer and research funds to obtain a technician. No one at Jefferson had special training or extensive experience related to renal problems beyond that of a general internist except Dr. F.W. Sunderman, Sr., who headed a small unit recognized as a chemical section but not a Division of Medicine. He was often asked to consult on electrolyte, water, and acid-base problems. There was no teaching program, resident rotation, or student elective featuring the kidney as a discipline until Dr. Michael Simenhoff joined the Division in 1964. Simenhoff was recruited from Dr. John Merrill's program at the Peter Bent Brigham Hospital. As Assistant

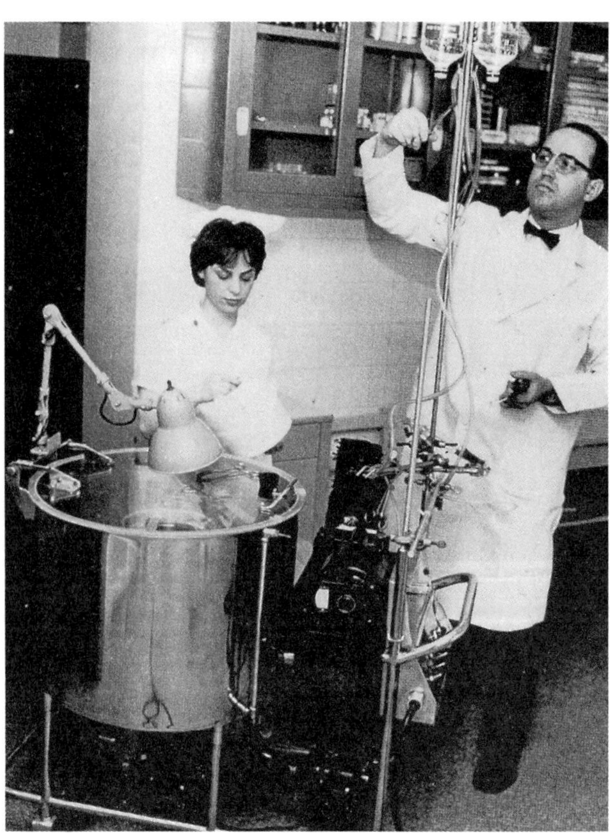

FIG. 15-1. James E. Clark, M.D., a pioneer at Jefferson in clinical nephrology and hemodialysis in the late 1950s.

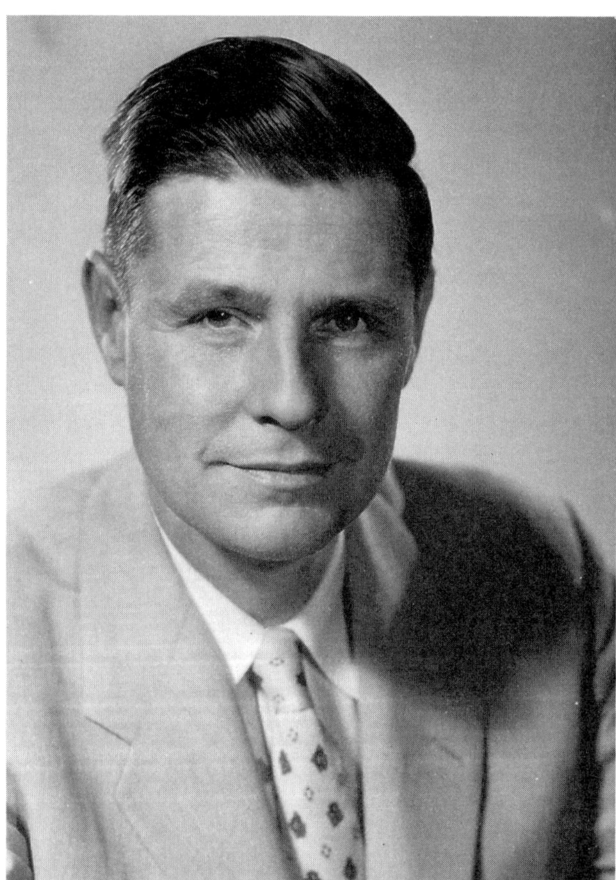

FIG. 15-2. Laurence G. Wesson, Jr., M.D., Professor of Medicine and First Head of the Nephrology Division (1962).

Director of the Clinical Research Center, he developed investigative studies in the diurnal rhythm of kidney function with Dr. Wesson. The Division was initially Renal Diseases in Fluid and Electrolyte Metabolism, next changed to Renal Disease, and finally to Nephrology in 1966.

It is germane to put nephrology in perspective in Philadelphia in 1962 when the Division of Nephrology at Jefferson was initiated. Clinical nephrology was still part of General Internal Medicine. Kidney-related research at the University of Pennsylvania was mainly out of Dr. Russell Elkinton's chemical section, where Dr. Miles Sigler took a research fellowship. Dr. Lewis W. Bluemle, Jr., destined to become the President of Thomas Jefferson University in 1977, was an outstanding pioneer in nephrology at the University of Pennsylvania from 1946 to 1968, during which time he authored or coauthored 46 articles in this field. Hahnemann Medical College had a renology section headed by Dr. Albert N. Brest, who subsequently came to Jefferson as Director of Cardiology. Neither Woman's Medical College (later Medical College of Pennsylvania) nor Temple Medical School had anything going in the line of nephrology. This paucity of nephrology services in the early 1960s soon changed, and nephrology as a subspecialty developed rapidly in many of the community as well as university hospitals.

At this time, there was an institutional move to obtain a general clinical research center for Jefferson. A committee of Drs. Wise, Sodeman, Gibbon, and Cantarow directed this effort but could find no candidate for Director. Because of Dr. Wesson's reputation he was urged to accept the position in addition to his responsibilities as Director of the Division of Nephrology.

Around 1964, Dr. Herbert Cohn became interested in renal transplantation, and a few were performed, but there was no major institutional commitment in this area. Later, in 1972, Dr. Harry Goldsmith, Chairman of the Department of Surgery, recruited Dr. James Colberg as Chief of the surgical arm of the transplantation program.

Refinement of Dialysis Technology

With the departure of Dr. Clark in 1968 to become the Chief of Medicine at Crozer Chester Hospital, Dr. Norman Lasker came to Jefferson in 1969 as Director of the Dialysis Unit. Dr. Lasker continued the development and expansion of the Unit and introduced new dialysis technologies and services, particularly in the area of peritoneal dialysis. Together with Dr. Bruce E. Jarrell (Jefferson, 1973), a peritoneal dialysis cycler was developed. Patients could thus be dialyzed while they were sleeping at night with an automated system. In 1971 the Clinical Research Center was discontinued, and many of the clinical investigative programs carried out in the Center had to be abandoned. In 1971, Dr. James F. Burke, Jr. (Jefferson, 1966) (Figure 15-3) was appointed to the faculty to assist Dr. Lasker in the dialysis program. In 1973 the Tsaltas dialysis unit with six beds was established, which was responsible for approximately 2,000 dialyses per year. Dr. Theodore Tsaltas, who was Professor of Pathology at Jefferson, had been a patient on chronic dialysis and the Center was named in his honor.

The Early Renal Transplantation Program

At this time, Dr. James E. Colberg was appointed to head the surgical arm of the transplant program. Dr. Steven Bulova was also appointed to run the tissue typing laboratory and perform the mixed lymphocyte cultures, procedures that were then important in selecting donors for renal transplantation. In those years approximately ten transplants were performed per year.

Prior to Dr. Lasker's coming, in the late 1960s an electron microscopy unit was set up with Dr. Serge W. Duckett in neuropathology. Soon after, Dr. Ruth P. Gottlieb, a pediatric nephrologist in the Department of Pediatrics and active in the nephrology programs, established a fluorescent microscopy laboratory so that these techniques could be used to detect antibody deposition in renal tissues. Thus at this time renal biopsy services incorporated light, electron, and fluorescent microscopical analysis, and wide-range diagnostic services became available.

In 1973 to 1974, while Dr. Michael Simenhoff was on sabbatical leave in London studying amine metabolism in uremia at the laboratories of Dr. Malcome Milne at Westminister Hospital Medical School in the University of London, Dr. Laurence Wesson decided to resign his position as Director. On his return, Dr. Simenhoff as made Acting Director, and Director in July 1975. At this time Dr. Anatole Besarab joined the Division with a secondary appointment in the Department of Physiology. Dr. Besarab had been trained under Dr. Franklin Epstein, an internationally known nephrologist at Harvard Medical School, where Dr. Besarab had learned the technique of perfusing isolated rat kidney under various physiological and pathophysiological conditions. Dr. Besarab's expertise, together with Dr. Wesson's background in this area, led to National Institutes of Health funding. Dr. Besarab studied the interrelationship of calcium, parathyroid hormone, and cyclic AMP, and also made contributions in the better understanding of transplantation nephropathy. This, combined with Dr. Simenhoff's funding for the production of carcinogenic nitrosamines in patients with chronic renal failure, also now funded by NIH, and Dr. Wesson's continued Career Award from the National Institutes of Health, gave the Division a solid base of support for basic research in the Division. Dr. Wesson continued his research studies on the preservation methods of the isolated kidney.

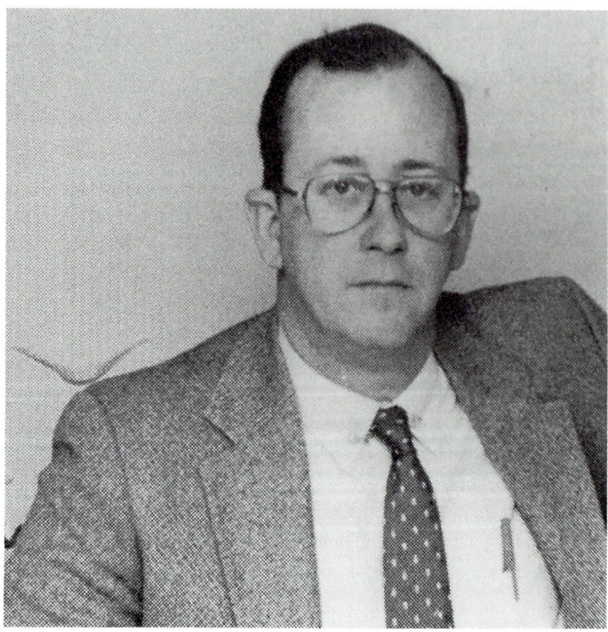

FIG. 15-3. James F. Burke, Jr., M.D., Professor of Medicine; nephrologist for renal transplantation program.

Growth of Renal Transplantation

The transplantation program accelerated with the recruitment of Dr. Bruce E. Jarrell in 1980. Dr. Jarrell's background in engineering had already facilitated contributions to the development of the cycling peritoneal dialysis machine previously mentioned, and his ability and enthusiasm gave new life to what had been a stagnant transplantation program. With Dr. James Burke as the nephrology arm of the program and Dr. Jarrell on the surgical side, the transplantation program grew vigorously, with physician referrals statewide and from nonaffiliated hospitals. With participation of Dr. Besarab many clinical studies were performed in the transplantation field, and at the basic level Dr. Jarrell was funded for studies on the role of the endothelial cell in transplantation rejection. The number of transplants per year rose to 80.

As the clinical services continued to grow in the 1980s it became essential to recruit additional personnel. Dr. Norman Lasker had left Jefferson in 1979 to take up an appointment as head of the Division of Nephrology at the New Jersey College of Medicine in Newark. Dr. Burke became head of the Dialysis Unit, but with the growing transplantation program, it became clear that the Division needed a full-time dialysis director apart from the transplantation group.

Dr. Nancy B. Jermanovich was recruited in July of 1982 to bolster the clinical services but mainly to develop a program in experimental glomerulonephritis, an area that had not been previously developed. With the emphasis on dialysis and with more than 60 percent of patients on chronic dialysis (having glomerulonephritis as the etiology of the renal disease), it was felt that this was an important area for the Division to develop. Dr. Jermanovich came from New York State University at Syracuse and had been trained by Dr. William Couser at Boston University during her fellowship. Arrangments had been made with the Department of Biochemistry to interdigitate her interests in immunology with those of the Department of Biochemistry.

Soon after this, Dr. George C. Francos (Jefferson, 1978), who had come through the Jefferson ranks, including a Fellowship, was appointed to the Division and to be the Director of the chronic dialysis program. The dialysis program was still growing, and the facilities at the Health Science Building on Ninth and Sansom Streets containing 12 stations for three daily shifts had already become cramped. Both hemodialysis and peritoneal dialysis modalities were offered, with emphasis on in-Center hemodialysis and continuous ambulatory peritoneal dialysis (CAPD).

The history of the nephrology programs at the affiliated hospitals was one of gradual independence, so that each of them acquired free-standing independent nephrology units. Earlier, intermittent involvement at Jefferson by Dr. Miles Sigler (Lankenau Hospital), Dr. John T. Magee (Jefferson, 1957; Bryn Mawr Hospital), Dr. Robert B. Flinn (Wilmington Medical Center), and Dr. John P. Capelli (Jefferson, 1962; Our Lady of Lourdes Hospital) had resulted in independent units of high caliber. This was beneficial in the teaching of Jefferson medical students and house officers when they rotated through these affiliated hospitals. The affiliated nephrology programs became important sources for transplantation referral.

Progress in the prevention and treatment of renal diseases has not only saved lives but provided a normal life span for many of its unfortunate victims.

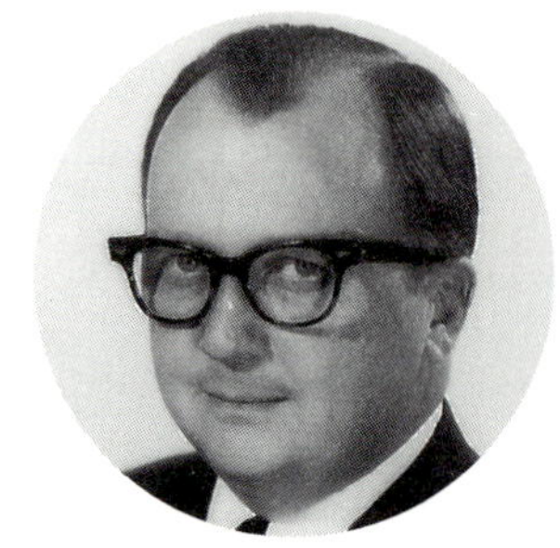

CHAPTER SIXTEEN

Division of Medical Oncology

WILLIAM E. DELANEY, M.D.

"While there are several chronic diseases more destructive to life than cancer, none is more feared."

—CHARLES H. MAYO (1865–1939)

ALTHOUGH medical oncology was first officially recognized as a medical subspecialty by the American Board of Internal Medicine in 1972, a formal Division of Medical Oncology in the Department of Medicine at Jefferson had been established since 1961. The first Director (1961–1970) was Arthur Weiss, M.D. (Figure 16-1), and the second (1970–1980) was Chester Southam, M.D. (Figure 16-2). Acting Directors were William E. Delaney, M.D. (Jefferson, 1953; 1980–1981) and J. Frederick Laucius, M.D. (Jefferson, 1967; 1981–1984). The third Director is Michael J. Mastrangelo, M.D., appointed in 1984.

The major activities of the Division since its inception have been patient care, teaching, research, and the training of medical oncology Fellows. Among the latter, the first Fellows were Laird Jackson, M.D., who was the first National Institutes of Health Postdoctoral Fellow (1961–1962), and Harvey Brodovsky, M.D. (1961–1963). Several additional Fellows have served in the Division since that time, most notably Carla Goepp, M.D. (Figure 16-3), (1965–1967), who became Associate Dean of Student Affairs and Director of the Office of Student Counseling and Career Planning, and Michael J. Mastrangelo, M.D. (1968–1970). Significant accomplishments in cancer care, research, and teaching at Jefferson occurred in the years before the establishment of the Division.

The Tumor Clinic and Elizabeth Storck Kraemer Foundation

The Tumor Clinic was informally begun in 1928 and has continued since that date as the major institutional follow-up mechanism for cancer patients. Formal establishment began in the fall of 1929 when, through the auspices of William H. Kraemer, M.D. (Figure 16-4, Jefferson, 1906),

Associate Professor of Surgery, a grant received from Mr. Pierre S. DuPont, consisting initially of $35,000 plus $10,000 annually for five years, was augmented by an initial grant of $15,000 for one year from Mr. Lammot DuPont. Through an additional 30 years (1934–1964), Pierre DuPont provided the sole support of Jefferson's Tumor Clinic through annual grants from the Longwood foundation to the Elizabeth Storck Kraemer Foundation.[1]

All of the Department Chairmen have served as Attending Physicians or Surgeons in the Tumor Clinic. Outstanding contributors to the activity of the Tumor Clinic over the years have been Drs. James M. Surver (Assistant Professor of Surgery), Harry J. Knowles (Assistant Professor of Surgery), and Gerald J. Marks (Professor of Surgery), who directed the day-to-day activities of the staff.

The Tumor Registry began as an offshoot of the Tumor Clinic in June, 1959. From that time through December 1983, as many as 28,593 patients have been accessioned, and 19,139 patients are known to have died. By June 1984, as many as 9,973 patients were under active follow-up, a rate of 92.3 percent. This Registry is the resource for all professionals interested in follow-up data over the years for Jefferson's oncology activities. Its overall direction is through the Cancer Committee of the Hospital.

The other major activity of the Elizabeth Storck Kraemer Foundation was to provide an investigative arm for the development of new cancer treatment drugs that had been isolated or synthesized by chemists of the DuPont Company.

Dr. Kraemer died in March, 1962, and on December 31, 1964, the Foundation was dissolved. For nearly 35 years it had actively supported not only the Tumor Clinic and weekly Tumor Clinic conferences but also chemical research at the DuPont experimental station in Wilmington,

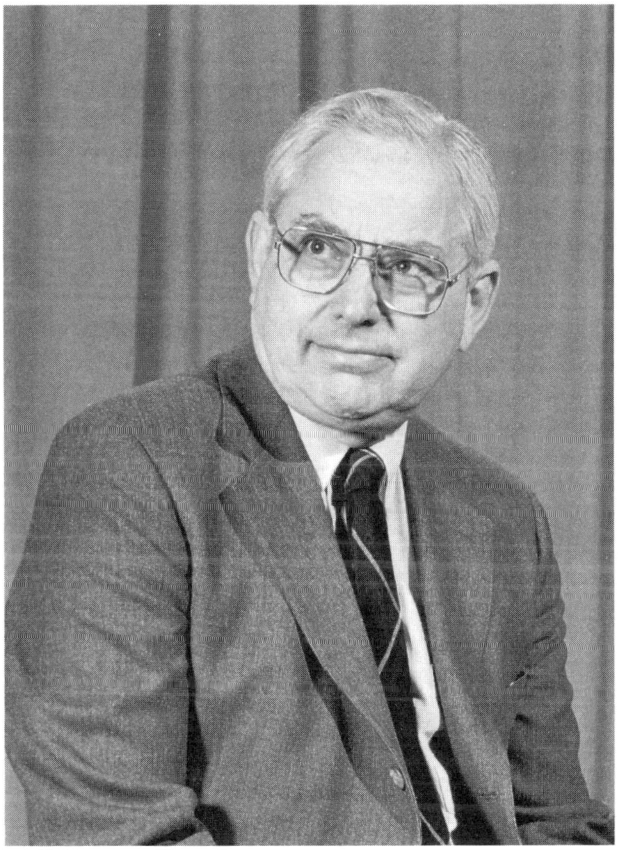

FIG. 16-1. Arthur Weiss, M.D.; First Director, Division of Oncology (1961–1970).

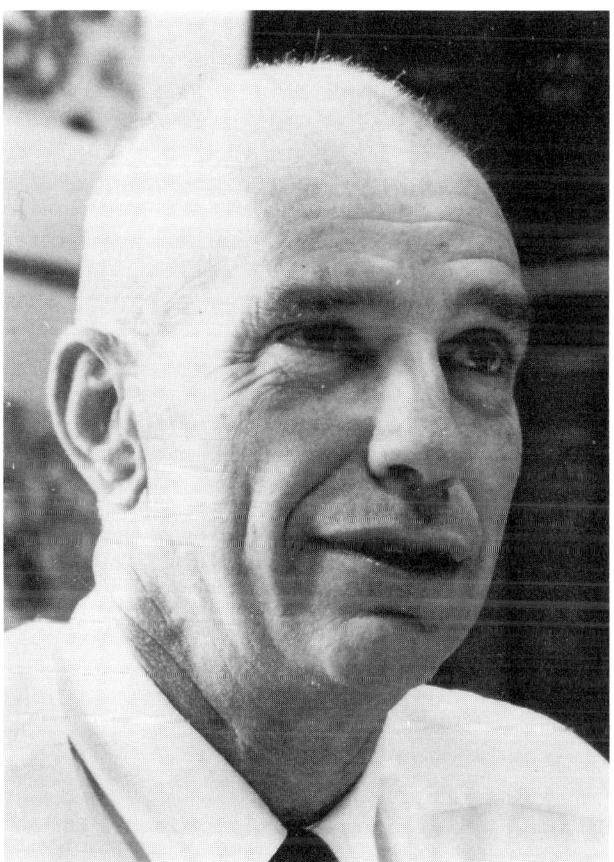

FIG. 16-2. Chester Southam, M.D.; Director, Division of Oncology (1970–1980).

Delaware, and biological research conducted by the Department of Pathology under the supervision of Dr. Peter A. Herbut. Dr. Herbut was Director of the Biological Division of the Foundation, incorporated from September, 1946, to December 31, 1964, on a stipend of $200 a month payable by the Tumor Clinic. Dr Kraemer was Director of Research from 1929 until his death. The funding after 1964 came through the Hospital budget.

The first publication from the Foundation appeared in 1931 and was a preliminary report on colloidal lead phosphate with manganese as an anticarcinogenic agent.[2] In subsequent years the Foundation was responsible for 22 publications in experimental cancer by Dr. Herbut, 14 of which were coauthored with Dr. Kraemer. In a 1955 article,[3] Herbut and Kraemer stated that the Walker Rat Mammary Carcinoma 256 had been carried in their laboratory since 1936. Dr. Kraemer's cancer research was recognized formally by his Jefferson alma mater in the award of an Honorary Degree of Doctor of Science at graduation on June 16, 1961.

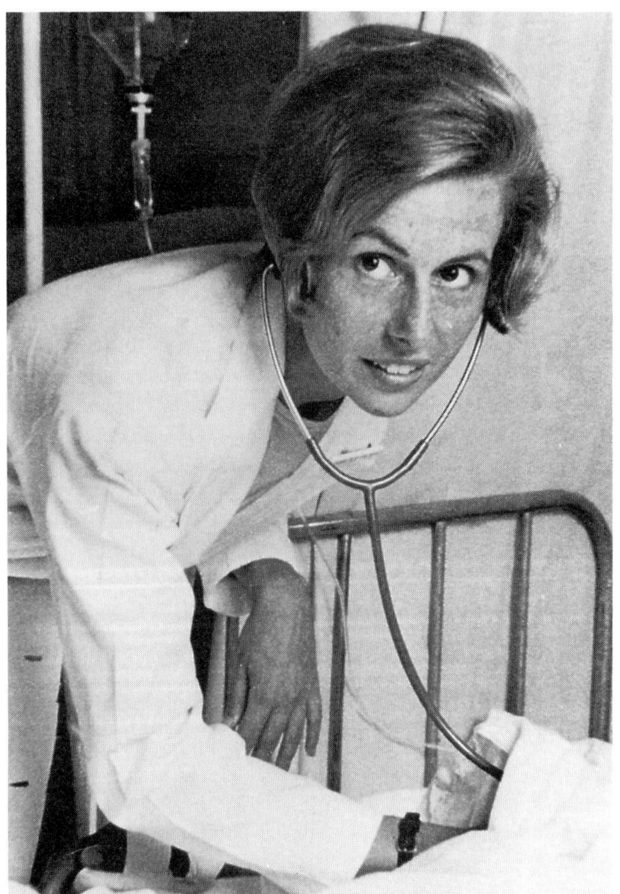

FIG. 16-3. Carla Goepp, M.D.

William H. Kraemer (born 1879) came to the United States as a boy from Germany. The family settled in West Virginia where he learned frugality and a proper set of values. He was trained as a pharmacist, and his application to Jefferson was accepted on the basis of his pharmacy credits. He worked at pharmacies during medical school and graduated in 1906. While working as a physician with the DuPont Company, he began to experiment on cancer in his garage using rats he caught there.

In 1926 Dr. Kraemer attracted the attention of Pierre S. DuPont, who requested his treatment for a leg ulcer that DuPont attributed to a kick by John J. Raskob intended to keep him awake during a General Motors Corporation board meeting. Dr. Kraemer had x-rays taken of Du Pont's teeth out of desperation because he had

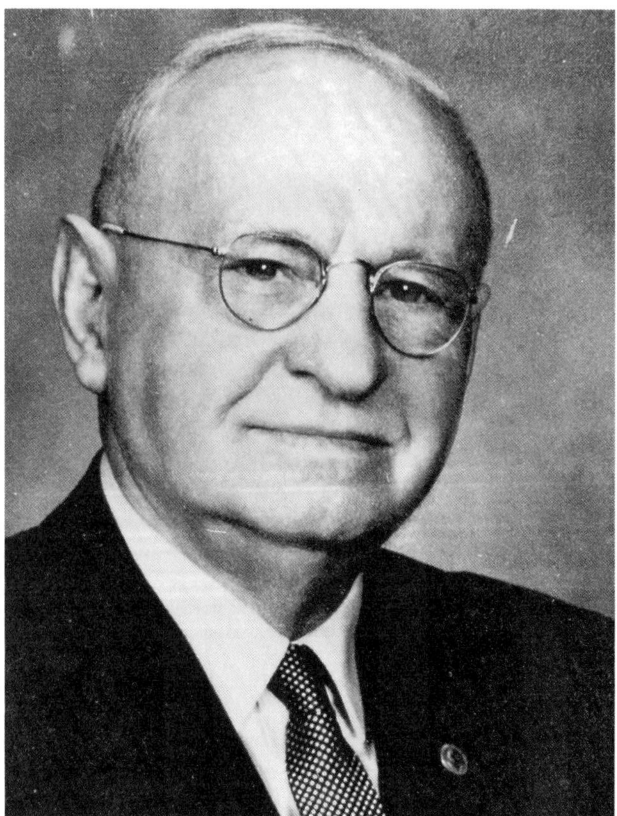

FIG. 16-4. William H. Kraemer, M.D.

found nothing systemically to account for the poor healing. The film revealed two abscessed wisdom teeth on each side, which Kraemer believed to have contributed to DuPont's somnolence. He immediately brought his patient to Jefferson, and taking a hospital room next to DuPont for himself, began to take care of all his health needs, including extraction of the teeth. Although the mandible was fractured in the extraction of the teeth, rendering DuPont speechless for a time, DuPont was grateful because his somnolence completely disappeared. While recuperating, DuPont communicated with Dr. Kraemer by written notes. In one of them he asked: "What is this I hear about your experimenting with cancer in the garage?" Dr. Kraemer told him about it and suggested that DuPont Company's vast chemical expertise be used to develop cancer chemotherapy.

In addition to personal physician, Dr. Kraemer became a friend and confidant. He played golf with DuPont, went on trips with him, and with Mrs. Kraemer moved to the DuPont area. Mr DuPont put him on a lifetime retainer of $6,000 per year and gave Mrs. Kraemer $5,000 per year for life. He also set up the Elizabeth Storck Kraemer Memorial Foundation in honor of Dr. Kraemer's second wife, who died of cancer.

In the early years, the biological aspect was carried out in New York's Memorial Hospital for Cancer, through Dr. James Ewing and later at New York University by Dr. Robert Chambers. In the mid-1940s, following Dr. Chamber's death, biological studies were centered at Jefferson. The chemical division of the Elizabeth Storck Kraemer Memorial Foundation was headquartered in the experimental station in Wilmington, Delaware. Toward the end, the annual budget of the Foundation should be funded for ten years after his death or until Dr. Kraemer died, whichever was longer. Pierre DuPont died in 1954. William H. Kraemer died March 20, 1962, and the Foundation was dissolved December 31, 1964. The Directors in 1964 are listed in Volume 2 of the *Herbut Papers* in the Scott Library's Special Collections. The Foundation was headquartered in room 2095, DuPont Building, Wilmington, Delaware. By December 3, 1959, the Foundation had completed its thirty-first year of activity, and during that time 4,000 chemicals had been screened for antitumor activity and 1,000 cancer patients had received chemotherapy. After the 1964 termination of the research support, the Trustees of the Foundation granted $24,650 to Jefferson Medical College for research at Dr. Herbut's discretion. As an outgrowth of the research activities that had been supported by the Kraemer Foundation, a National Institutes of Health grant award to Dr. Herbut was renewed for three years in 1965.

The Interdepartmental Endocrine and Cancer Research Group

The relationship between Drs. Abraham Cantarow (Biochemistry), Karl E. Paschkis (Medicine) (Figure 16-5), and Abraham E. Rakoff (Obstetrics and Gynecology) led to their formation of an informal endocrine and cancer research group in 1940. In 1945, at the close of World War II, they began to contribute significantly to the literature, and by 1959 they had realized more than 300 publications. The Board of Trustees in 1948 formally organized the Endocrine and Cancer Research Group with Dr. Paschkis as the first and only Director. He was the unique catalyst who was involved in all activities of the group. It received partial funding by the American Cancer Society on the recommendation of the Committee on Growth of the National Research Council and by the National Cancer Institute.

In the field of steroid hormone metabolism they originated the concept of the biliary excretion and enterohepatic circulation of estrogens and androgens.[4] They first showed that androgens accelerated the development of malignant hepatomas when the carcinogen 2-acetyl-amino-fluorine (AAF) was fed to rats and that thiouracil given with this chemical protected the liver exposed to testosterone; in addition, they first demonstrated the enhancement of the carcinogenic action of progesterone on the breasts of rats treated with AAF.[5] Their work on pyrimidine metabolism as related to normal growth of malignant tumors led to the synthesis by Charles

Heidelberg, Ph.D., at the University of Wisconsin, of 5-fluorouracil, a drug widely used in many cancer chemotherapy programs.[6] Their research further indicated that in the presence of regenerating liver, not only tumor growth but also a large variety of nonmalignant growth processes were stimulated; similar effects could be obtained by injection of certain liver fractions.[7] Another basic investigation was the transmission of tumor by subcellular units. Thus, injection of isolated tumor chromatin induced tumor growth in recipient animals. The effect was noted to be specific in that chromatin from malignant lymphoma cells induced malignant lymphoma after subcutaneous injection and chromatin from hepatoma cells induced hepatomas after intrahepatic injection.[8–10]

Dr. Paschkis faced his own terminal illness from bronchogenic carcinoma with composed heroism. With his death of January 27, 1961, at age 65, the Endocrine and Cancer Research Group ceased to function as a unit and was dissolved.

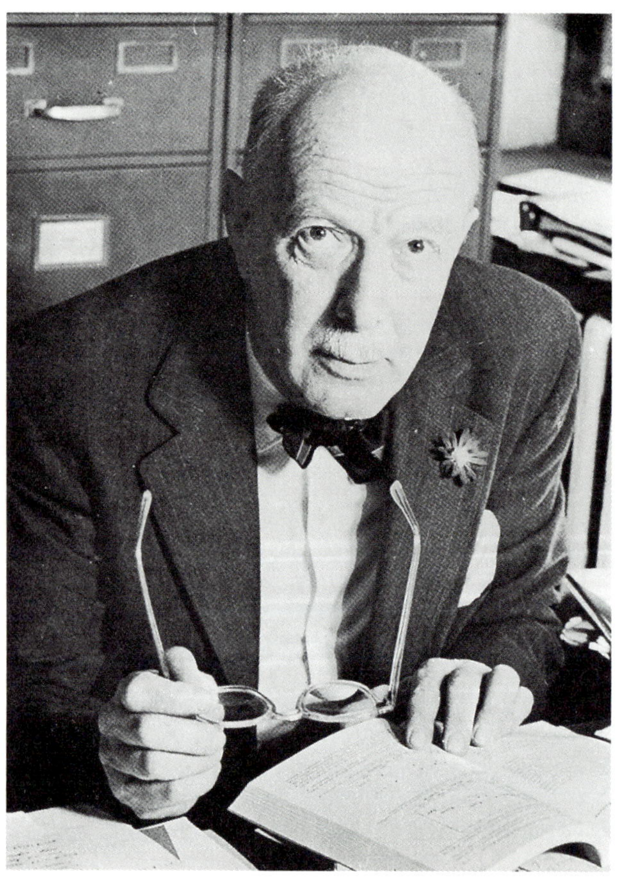

FIG. 16-5. Karl Paschkis, M.D.

Cooperative Cancer Therapy Groups

Among the earliest investigators cooperating with other institutions in the evaluation of new drugs for the management of cancer, Arthur Weiss, M.D., Assistant Professor of Medicine, was the leader at Jefferson since 1958, when he established the Jefferson branch of the Clinical Drug Evaluation Program of the Cancer Chemotherapy National Service Center, a subsidiary of the National Cancer Institute. In 1960, Dr. Weiss also led Jefferson into the Central Oncology Group as a cochairman of that body. In addition, in 1960, Farid Haurani, M.D., became the representative at Jefferson of the Cancer and Acute Leukemia Group B in an association that lasted through 1981. Eastern Cooperative Oncology Group participation has been continuous since 1968 at Jefferson under the direction of Harvey Brodovsky, M.D. He has been a coauthor of 17 papers published on ECOG trials and was a grant recipient of ECOG funding for many years until 1981.

A significant contribution to the use of adriamycin in chemotherapy occurred when the Cooperative Group, with Arthur Weiss, M.D., as the senior author and R. William Manthei, Ph.D., Professor of Pharmacology, as coauthor, reported the decrease in cardiac toxicity of low-dose infusions at frequent intervals as compared to the significant cardiac toxicity of high-dose bolus therapy with this drug.[11] This modified the approach to the use of this excellent chemotherapeutic agent and has extended its useful application in all fields of cancer chemotherapy.

Applied Research and Clinical Oncology

Shortly after exfoliative cytology was developed in the early 1940s by Dr. George Papanicolaou, its application to the detection and eradication of gynecologic tumors was led by such men at Jefferson as Lewis C. Scheffey (Jefferson, 1920), Professor of Gynecology, and Abraham E. Rakoff (Jefferson, 1937), Professor of Gynecologic and Obstetrical Endocrinology.

The bronchoscopic diagnosis in lung cancer by cytology studies of aspirated secretions won for Louis H. Clerf (Jefferson, 1912), Chairman of the Department of Otolaryngology, and Peter A. Herbut, Chairman of the Department of Pathology, the Gold Medal of the American Medical Association in 1951.

Early research into naturally occurring stimulators and inhibitors of granulocytic and lymphocytic proliferation in human leukemia was the special interest of Franklin Miller, M.D., Assistant Professor of Medicine, who was one of the early associate members of the Cardeza Foundation for Hematologic Research.

In the management of human breast cancer in the 1950s, when endocrine manipulation of the tumor was the major therapeutic modality, Ralph A. Carabasi (Jefferson, 1946) was a pioneer. Early immunologic studies in cancer were conducted by Irwin L. Stoloff (Jefferson, 1951), in addition to those performed by Chester Southam, M.D.

Lymphangiography was originally described as a unilateral procedure for the analysis of lymph flow in 1955. In 1960, Dr. Phillip Hodes, Professor and Chairman of Radiology, and Dr. Simon Kramer, Head of Radiation Therapy, realized that this technique might be adaptable to the evaluation of lymph node involvement by cancer. They encouraged Sidney Wallace, M.D., Assistant Professor of Radiology, and Laird Jackson, M.D., who was then a medical resident, to develop the procedure. Drs. Wallace and Jackson performed the first bilateral simultaneous injection of intralymphatic contrast materials in humans in 1960. This was a tedious procedure in the beginning, requiring prolonged hand-delivered injections by two people, until Dr. Jackson invented a motor-driven pump that became universally used for lymphangiography. By 1985 the information gained by lymphangiography was largely replaced by noninvasive methods.

Laird G. Jackson, M.D., Professor of Pediatrics, Director of the Division of Genetics, Professor of Medicine and Professor of Obstetrics and Gynecology, performed all of his early work in chromosomes and on the genetics of cancer while assigned to the Division of Medical Oncology of the Department of Medicine. This began in 1961 when he was a medical oncology Fellow and investigated chromosomes in leukemia. He expanded this work after he took the Bar Harbor course in medical genetics given by Victor McCusick, M.D., in 1962.

With the return of Michael J. Mastrangelo, M.D. (Figure 16-6) to Jefferson in 1984 to renew an association he had begun as a medical intern in 1964, Jefferson entered a new era of research and therapy of malignant melanomas. Dr. Mastrangelo's interest has been in the immunologic aspects of cancers in general and of malignant melanoma in particular since he took postdoctoral training in the laboratory of Richmond T. Prehn, M.D., in the Institute for Cancer Research of Philadelphia (1971–1972). Mastrangelo was an early member of the Malignant Melanoma Clinical Cooperative Group (1973–1977) and a member of the Committee on Tumor Immunotherapy of the Division of Cancer Biology and Diagnosis of the National Cancer

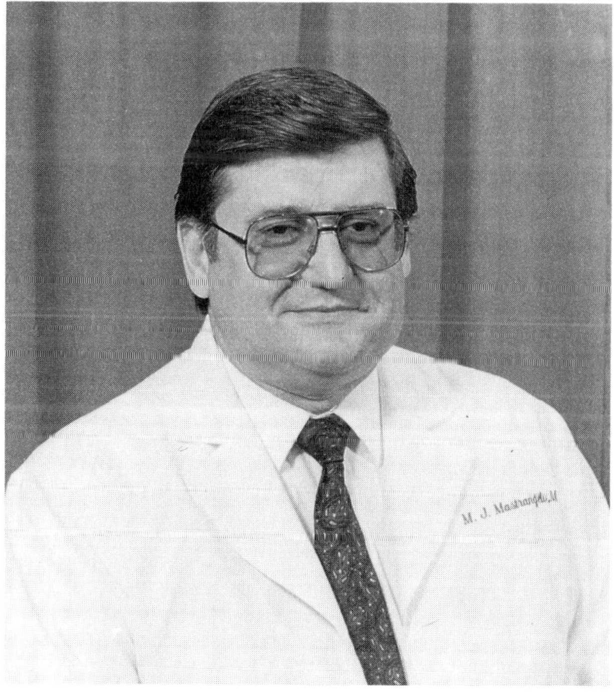

FIG. 16-6. Michael J. Mastrangelo, M.D.; Director, Division of Oncology (1984–).

Institute (1975–1979). Since 1980 he has been a member of the Experimental Therapeutic Study Section of the National Institutes of Health, serving from 1982 to 1984 as its Chairman. He continues an active program in immunologic aspects of cancer and of malignant melanoma in particular.

Medical science is still at the frontier in understanding the complex mechanisms that lead to cancer, its better palliation, and the ultimate goal of total prevention and cure. The progress thus far engendered by interdepartmental cooperation has been significant, but more intense focus on the possible role of viruses not yet isolated, genetic investigation, and study of neoplasms at the molecular level will increase Jefferson's stature in this field.

References

1. "The Jefferson Hospital Tumor Clinic," *Jeff. Med. Coll. Al. Bull.* Vol. IV, May 1947, pp. 1–4.
2. Kraemer, W.H., "A Preliminary Report on Colloidal Lead Phosphate with Manganese," *Am. J. Cancer.* 1931, 15:pp. 2357–2358.
3. Herbut, P.A., and Kraemer, W.H., "The Effect of N,N'-(4-methyl-m-phenylene)-bis-(aziridine-carboxamide) (ESK 230) on Walker Mammary Carcinoma 256," *Cancer Research.* 1955, 15:614–616.
4. Cantarow, A., Rakoff, A.E., Paschkis, K.E., Hansen, L.P., and Walkling, A.A., "Excretion of Estrogen in Bile," *Endocrinology.* 1942, 31:515–519.
5. Cantarow, A., Paschkis, K.E., Stasney, J., and Rothenberg, M.S., "The Influence of Sex Hormones upon the Hepatic Lesions Produced by "2-Acetaminofluorene." *Cancer Research.* 1946, 6:610–616.
6. Rutman, R.J., Cantarow, A., and Paschkis, K.E., "Studies in 2-Acetylaminofluorene Carcinogenesis," *Science.* 1951, 114:264–265.
7. Paschkis, K.E., Cantarow, A., Stasney, J., and Hobbs, J.H., "Tumor Growth in Partially Hepatectomized Rats," *Cancer Research.* 1955, 15:579–582.
8. Stasney, J., Cantarow, A., and Paschkis, K.E,: "Production of Neoplasms by Injection of Mammalian Neoplasms," *Cancer Research.* 1950, 10:775–782.
9. Stasney, J., Cantarow, A., and Paschkis, K.E., "Production of Neoplasms by Injection of Fractions of Mammalian Neoplasms," *Ann. N.Y. Ac. Sc.* 1952, 54:1177–1183.
10. Paschkis, K.E., Cantarow, A., and Stasney, J., "Induction of Neoplasms by Injection of Tumor Chromatin," *J. Nat. Cancer Inst.* 1955, 15:1525–1532.
11. Weiss, A.J., and Manthei, R.W., "Experience with the Use of Adriamycin in Combination with Other Anticancer Agents Using a Weekly Schedule, with Particular Reference to Lack of Cardiac Toxicity," *Cancer.* 1977, 40:2046–2052.

CHAPTER SEVENTEEN

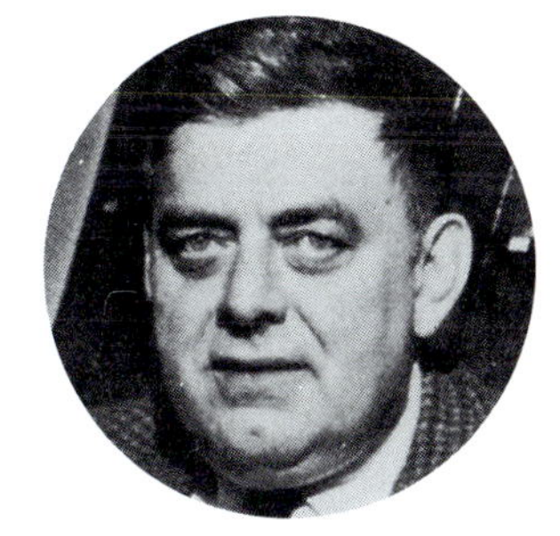

Division of Endocrine and Metabolic Diseases

JOSEPH J. RUPP, M.D.

"We may, of course, strike a balance between what a living organism takes in as nourishment and what it gives out in excretions. . . . That could be like trying to tell what happens inside a house by watching what goes in by the door and what comes out by the chimney."

—CLAUDE BERNARD (1813–1878)

THE College was 24 years old when, in 1848, A. A. Berthold,[1] of Göttingen, reported that transplantation of the testis restored secondary sex characteristics in castrated roosters. This observation established endocrine physiology as a science. During this same period Claude Bernard was studying the hepatic metabolism of sugars and in 1855 first used the phrase "internal secretions."[2] Bernard's experimental observations laid the foundations of the science of metabolism. Bernard's successor, Charles Edouard Brown-Sequard (1817–1894), continued the physiological approach and made significant observations concerning the nervous system. Best known as a neurologist, Brown-Sequard is also remembered because of the report of his marked increase in vigor and potency in 1889[3] following the self-injection of an emulsion of bull testes, one of the early observations of therapeutic trials and the beginning of a long era of the use of cell extracts in an attempt at rejuvenation.

A Famous Last de Medici at Jefferson

Modern endocrinology had its birth in Europe, especially in France, where the "Father of American Endocrinology" trained under Brown-Sequard. Charles Eucharist de Medici Sajous (Figure 17-1) was born at sea and received his early education in France. He was a descendant of the Florentine de Medicis and the royal house of France. His father died when he was two years old, and his mother remarried; Charles adopted the name of his stepfather, Sajous. During his teens the family lived in Mexico and California. He matricualted at the Medical School of the University of California, transferred to Jefferson, and received the medical degree in 1878. His initial interest was in laryngology; he was appointed Clinical Lecturer at Jefferson (1883–1891) and in 1898 published *Lectures on the Diseases of the Nose and Throat: Delivered During the Spring Session of Jefferson Medical College,* a work dedicated to Samuel D. Gross, M.D.

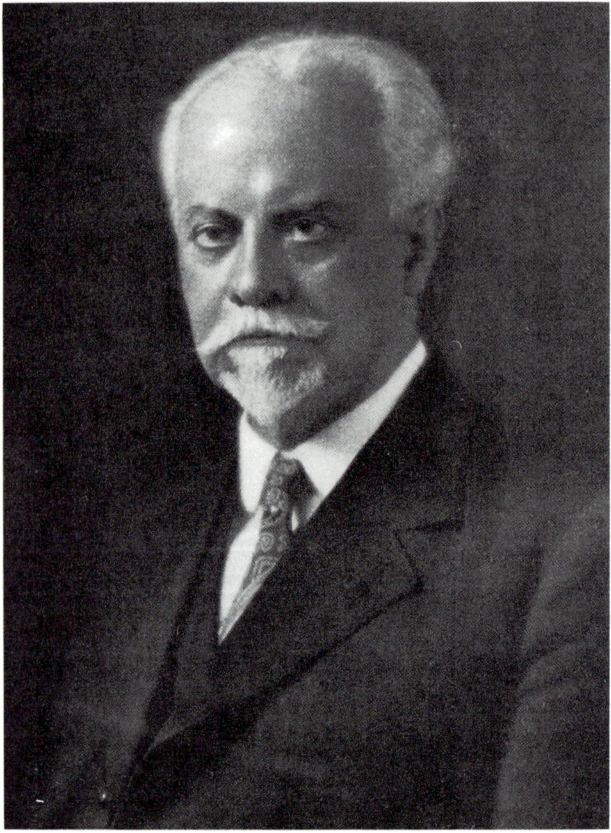

FIG. 17-1. Charles Eucharist de Medici Sajous, M.D., early investigator of internal secretions.

In 1892 Sajous abandoned his practice and teaching positions for the study of internal secretions with Brown-Sequard in France. Following his return to Philadelphia in 1897, Sajous became Professor of Laryngology and Dean of the Faculty of the Medico-Chirurgical College. From 1910 to 1922 he was Professor of Applied Therapeutics at Temple University Medical College and, from 1921 until his death in 1929, Professor of Applied Therapeutics at the Graduate School of the University of Pennsylvania. When his physician son, Louis Theodore, also an endocrinologist, died three months before the father, it was the termination of the 900-year-old name of the Medici of Florentine history.

Dr. Sajous published the first American textbook of endocrinology in 1903, *The Internal Secretions and the Principles of Medicine* (in two volumes of 1,873 pages). He held office and membership in many medical and other activities, including the American Medical Editors' Association (President, 1903), American Association for the Study of Internal Secretions (President, 1917), and American Therapeutic Society (President, 1919). He also authored the *Annual of the Universal Medical Sciences* (1888–1896), and the *Sajous Analytic Cyclopaedia of Practical Medicine* (60 volumes).

Dr. Sajous had a running battle with the physiologists and those who used the physiologic approach to the study of internal secretions. He believed that animal experimentation led to therapeutic incompetence. His major contributions were broad concepts and appreciation of the importance of internal secretions in health and disease. His specific observations were of lesser importance.

Spanning the decades at the turn of the century, Dr. Francis X. Dercum (Figure 17-2) (Clinical Professor of Nervous and Mental Diseases at

Jefferson from 1883 to 1900 and Chairman of the Department from 1900 to 1925) had dual interests in neuropsychiatry and endocrinology. He was the author of the *Biology of Internal Secretion* (1924) and wrote many articles in the field of endocrinology. In 1892 he described adiposa dolorosa (Dercum's disease), which is probably not of endocrine or metabolic origin. Dr. Milton K. Meyers (neuropsychiatrist at Jefferson, 1939–1954) published in 1915 the first American edition and English translation from the German of Wilhelm Falta's textbook, *The Ductless Glandular Diseases* (673 pages). Samuel A. Loewenberg (Figure 17-3), Clinical Professor of Medicine at Jefferson, published *Clinical Endocrinology*—the first edition in 1937 and the second in 1941.

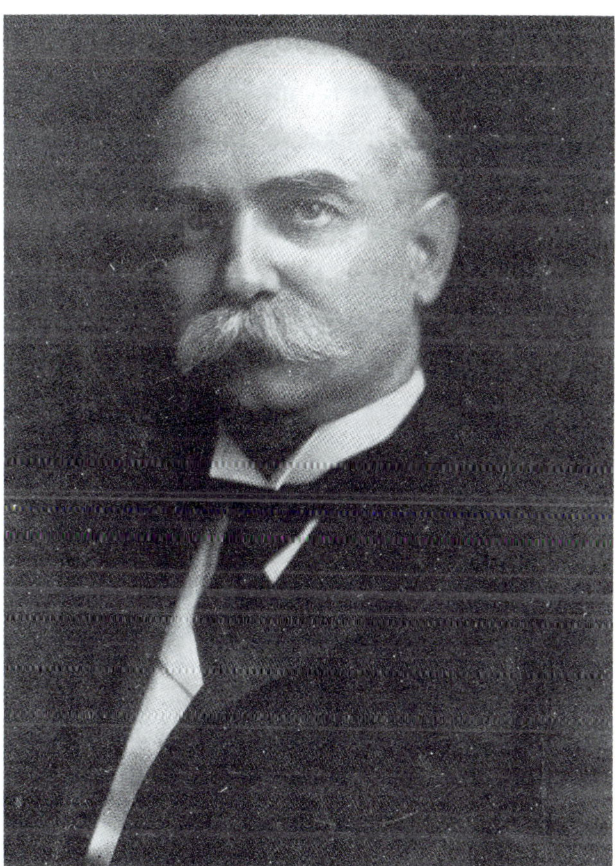

FIG. 17-2. Francis X. Dercum, M.D., studied the biology of internal secretions.

The relationship of the endocrine glands to disease states was noted by the clinicians of the nineteenth century: the adrenal by Addison (insufficiency), and the thyroid by Graves (thyrotoxicosis) and Basedow (myxedema). An understanding of the mechanisms responsible for these diseases awaited developments in biochemistry through which the hormones could be identified, purified, measured in body fluids, and satisfactory products made for pharmacologic and therapeutic experimentation. This era began in the twentieth century and matured from 1950.

David W. Kramer, M.D.

Following the report in 1889 by von Mering and Minkowski that diabetes mellitus followed pancreatectomy, a search for the hypoglycemic hormone of the pancreas began. In a talk before Jefferson's Alpha Omega Alpha Society around 1952, Dr. Charles H. Best (codiscoverer of

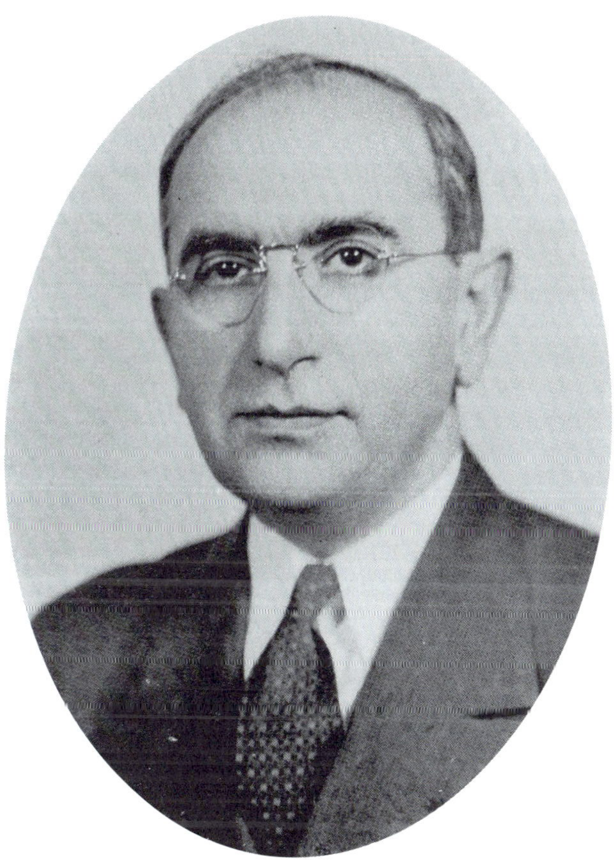

FIG. 17-3. Samuel A. Loewenberg, M.D., author of *Clinical Endocrinology*.

insulin with Dr. Frederick G. Banting in 1922) acknowledged that Dr. David W. Kramer (Figure 17-4) (Jefferson, 1912) had demonstrated the effectiveness of a pancreatic extract in humans. The marked toxicity of the product precluded its use, and the study was terminated. In 1922, just before the announcement of the discovery of insulin, Kramer[5] published a paper on *Clinical Observations on the Pathogenesis of Diabetes Mellitus.* His interest and work was thus of preliminary aid to Banting and Best in their isolation of a clinically useful product (insulin). Kramer maintained a lifelong interest in the treatment of diabetes, which, because of its vascular effects, motivated his study of peripheral vascular diseases. In this field he became a national authority, with publication of *Manual of Peripheral Vascular Disorders* in 1940 and *Peripheral Vascular Diseases* in 1948. The Bertha and David Kramer Professorship of Medicine was created in 1974 and first held by Dr. Joseph Glennon as Director of the Division of Endocrine and Metabolic Diseases in 1977.

Garfield G. Duncan, M.D., and Insulin

Shortly after the availability of insulin, a young Canadian physician, Dr. Garfield G. Duncan (Figure 17-5), joined the faculty in 1927, bringing with him skills in the treatment of diabetes mellitus acquired during the early years of the availability of insulin for human use. During his 30 years on the faculty Dr. Duncan made many important observations, not only about diabetes mellitus but also other endocrine and metabolic disorders. His many publications were important in establishing the nature, and especially the

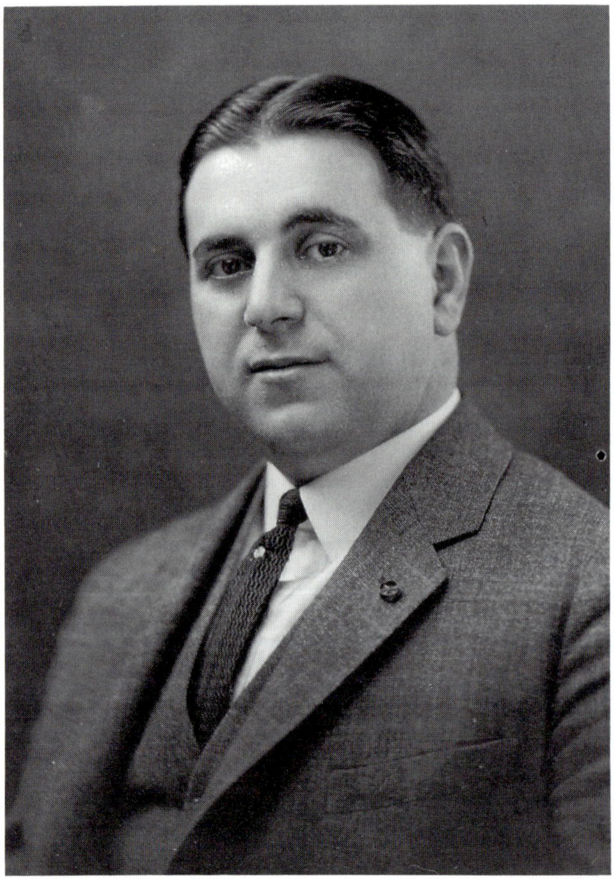

FIG. 17-4. David W. Kramer, M.D., pioneer investigator of diabetes mellitus and insulin therapy.

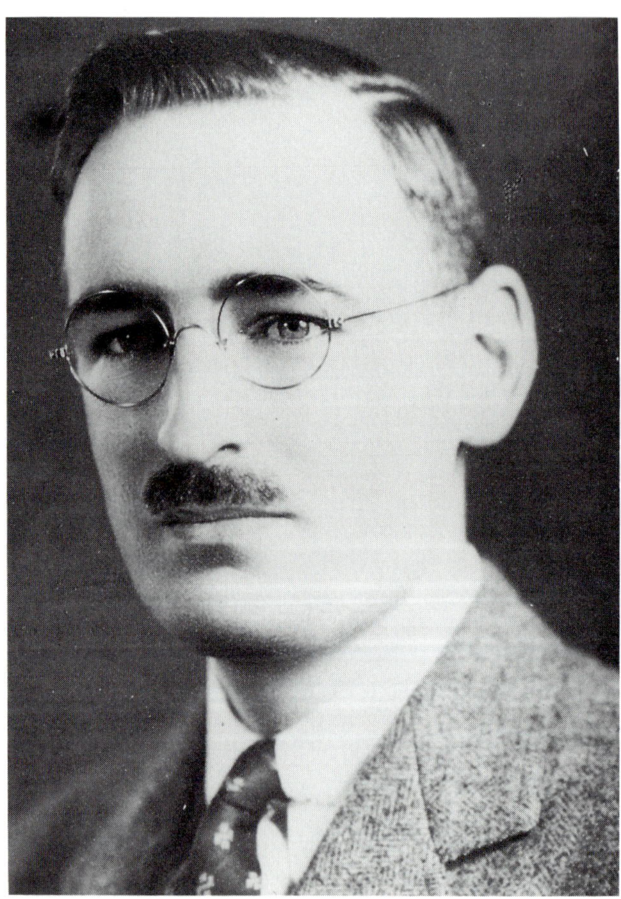

FIG. 17-5. Garfield G. Duncan, M.D., author of *Diseases of Metabolism.*

treatment, of the "whole" patient. Duncan's textbook, *Diseases of Metabolism* (1942 and 1947), was the standard text used by students and practitioners. He was more than a diabetologist. As a well-rounded clinician, his lectures, conferences, and rounds at Pennsylvania Hospital, where he was Chief of Medicine, were informative, well-prepared, and delivered with a nasal twang. Students were frightened by him; he gave the impression that he lacked a sense of humor. They knew he would not tolerate incompetence or improper bedside manner. Nevertheless, students appreciated him and learned from watching and being supervised by a dedicated teacher and clinician. Duncan elected to join the faculty of the University of Pennsylvania when it affiliated with Pennsylvania Hospital in 1957. He died in 1983 at the age of 81. Dr. Theodore G. Duncan (Jefferson, 1955) succeeded his father as Chief of Diabetes at Pennsylvania Hospital and was one of a few select physicians picked to evaluate the clinical usefulness of human insulin.

Abraham Cantarow, M.D.

After graduation from Jefferson in 1924, Abraham Cantarow (Figure 17-6) joined its faculty in clinical chemistry. It was said that he selected Jefferson as his medical school because most of the textbooks were written by Jefferson faculty (Hawk and Bergeim's *Chemistry*, Brubaker's *Physiology*, DaCosta's *Surgery*, McCrae's editions of *Osler's Principles and Practice of Medicine*, and Schaeffer's *Morris' Anatomy*). For the rest of his academic career he devoted his life to his alma mater as a teacher, researcher, and active member of the Alumni Association, of which he was President in 1964. His interest in clinical chemistry directed him to the field of endocrinology and metabolism in particular. Dr. Cantarow was a complete clinician and an excellent bedside teacher who used pathophysiology as the basis for explaining disease mechanisms. His early appreciation of metabolic alterations in carcinogenesis steered him into cancer research. Despite the duties imposed when he accepted the Chairmanship of the Department of Biochemistry, he continued his research career while delivering an excellent course in basic science. Following his Emeritus retirement in 1966, Cantarow joined the staff of the National Cancer Institute, National Institutes of Health.

Early Advances

The fourth decade of the twentieth century saw the blossoming of endocrinology. By 1940 techniques were developed that permitted investigation of the function and malfunction of the endocrine system. Bioassay for estrogens, androgens, and gonadotropins, chemical assays for 17-ketosteroids and pregnandiol, and staining methods for studying vaginal cytology were available for use in a clinical setting. About this time two men, Drs. Abraham E. Rakoff (Figure 17-7), and Karl E. Paschkis (Figure 17-8), joined the faculty and with Dr. Cantarow were to play a major role in the field of endocrinology, not only at Jefferson but nationwide.

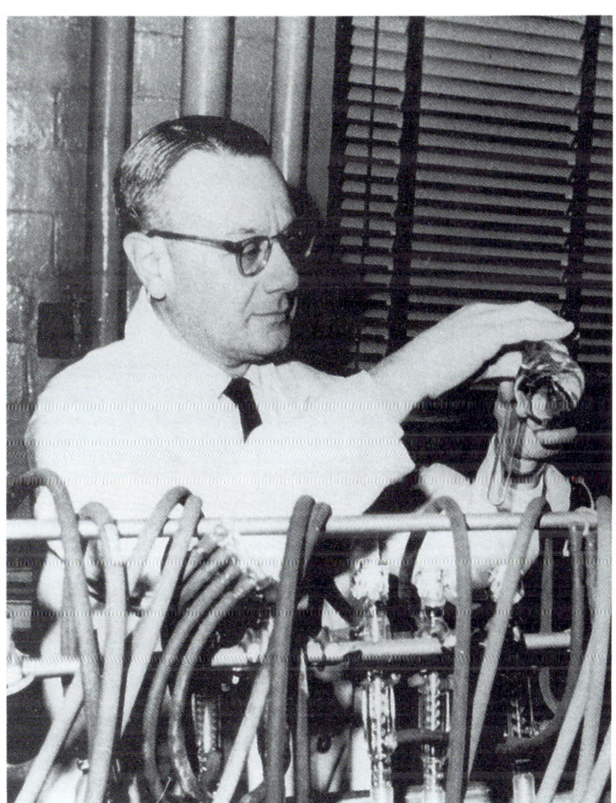

FIG. 17-6. Abraham Cantarow, M.D.; Professor of Biochemistry, researcher in metabolism and endocrinology.

■ The Paschkis Stimulus

Drs. Karl and Margaret Paschkis, the latter a pediatrician, were born and educated in Vienna. They were very vocal activists in opposition to the takeover of Austria by Nazi Germany—they escaped with nothing. Following a short period in England, the Paschkises came to the United States and settled in Philadelphia. After a year at the Fels Institute, Temple University, Dr. Karl Paschkis joined the Department of Physiology and, a little later, the Department of Medicine. He was active in each Department for the rest of his life. Dr. Paschkis was a trained internist with an interest in endocrinology and thereby a fortuitous interactor for Dr. Abraham Rakoff (Jefferson, 1937) who, following internship at Frankford Hospital, joined the Department of Obstetrics. While an undergraduate at the University of Pennsylvania, Dr. Rakoff did research in cytology and staining techniques. He had a major interest in this area for the rest of his career, refining and developing new techniques for use in gynecologic endocrinology. Like Cantarow, Rakoff was devoted to Jefferson and served as President of the Alumni Association in 1969—they both received the Alumni Achievement Award.

In 1940, Cantarow, Paschkis, and Rakoff joined to form an endocrine outpatient facility, an endocrine laboratory, and an informal research group. By 1945 they became a recognized interdepartmental group that, by action of the Board of Trustees in 1948, was formalized as the Division of Endocrine and Cancer Research. Representatives of the Departments of Surgery, Anatomy, Pathology, Physiology, Urology, Psychiatry, and Ophthalmology were members of the Division and were consulted in the planning

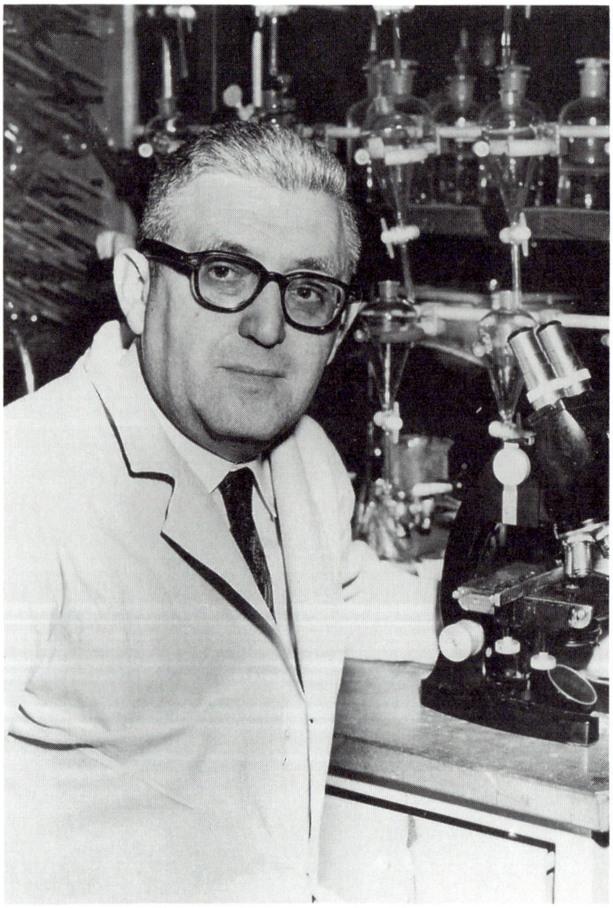

FIG. 17-7. Abraham E. Rakoff, M.D., gynecologic endocrinologist.

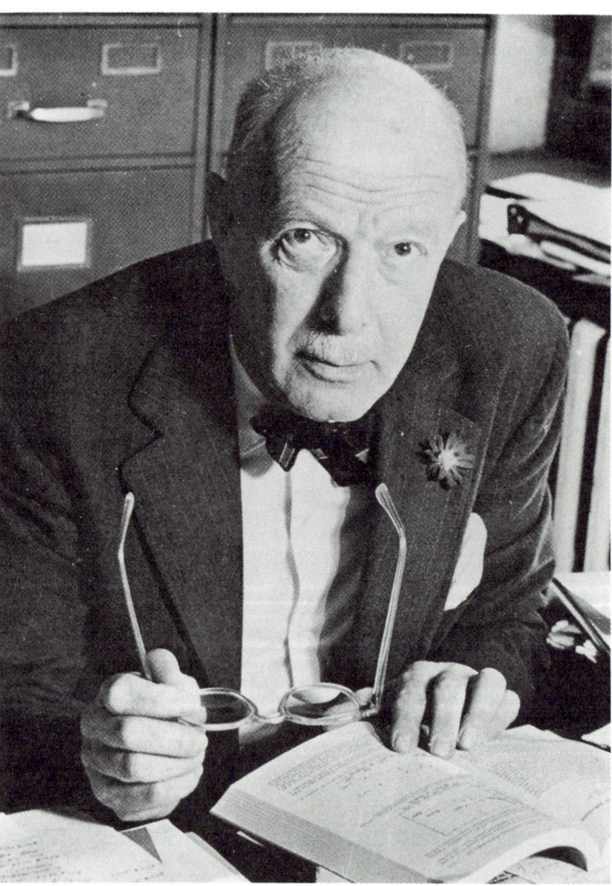

FIG. 17-8. Karl Paschkis, M.D., clinical and research endocrinologist.

and implementation of basic and clinical research. They cooperated also in the monthly research conferences. In 1948 John J. Schneider, M.D., Ph.D., and in 1951, Joseph J. Rupp (Jefferson, 1942; Figure 17-9), after a four-year period of residency and fellowship training at Jefferson, were given appointments in the Department of Medicine and joined the Division on a full-time basis.

Dr. Schneider, a graduate of the University of Chicago School of Medicine, completed his postgraduate education in the field of steroid chemistry at the Graduate School of the Mayo Clinic. At Jefferson he continued his study of steroid metabolism for the next 30 years. He had only three research associates, and no more than one at a time. Patricia Horstmann, B.A., and Constance Decourcy, Ph.D., each stayed for a few years. Dr. Marvin L. Lewbart (Jefferson, 1957), after internship at Lankenau Hospital, completed his graduate work at the Graduate School of the Mayo Clinic and returned to Jefferson as Dr. Schneider's associate, an association that lasted until the latter's retirement in 1975. This was a most productive combination. The two not only collaborated but each carried out individual projects. It was a unique laboratory in which admission was limited and often by invitation only. There were neither technicians nor housekeeping personnel. Dr. Schneider cleaned the glassware, scrubbed the floors, and painted the laboratory. His day began about 5 A.M. and continued until 9 or 10 P.M., with an interruption for breakfast with Drs. Robert Mandle and Harry Smith, for coffee with Rupp, and for lunch and dinner in the hospital cafeteria. The only distraction in the laboratory was classical music. Dr. Schneider was an avid reader of history, especially military and political, an interest that continued into his retirement.

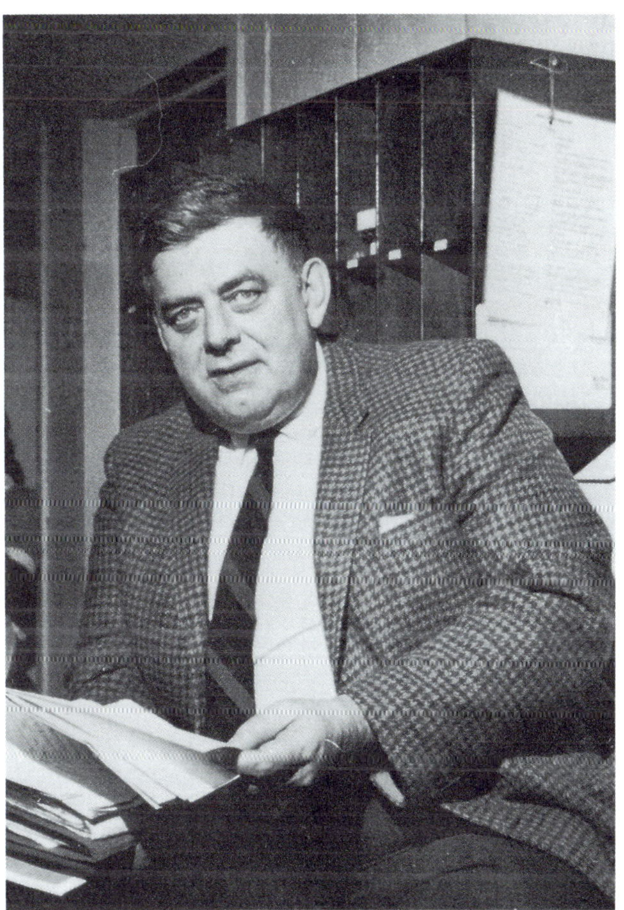

FIG. 17-9. Joseph J. Rupp, M.D., Director of the Division of Endocrine and Cancer Research, 1961.

Advanced Basic Research

Dr. Schneider enjoyed a worldwide reputation in the field of steroid chemistry. His expertise in evaluating the effects of various tissue enzymes on the steroid nucleus led to the development of methods for the isolation and identification of steroid metabolites including some not previously described. He was consulted by some for help in identification of a new compound and by others who needed a new compound to continue their endeavors. The individual and joint research of Schneider and Lewbart resulted in publication of more than 50 papers.

The activities of the members of the Division of Endocrine and Cancer Research encompassed both the fields of general and reproductive endocrinology and carcinogenesis. Dr. Paschkis was interested in all aspects of endocrinology, but to a lesser extent in reproductive endocrinology. Most of his papers were concerned with clinical and basic science aspects of the pituitary, thyroid, and adrenal glands. Dr. Rakoff, on the other hand, while well-versed in all areas, was mainly concerned with gynecologic endocrinology. He was joined by Dr. Alvin F. Goldfarb who made contributions not only in patient care and teaching but also in clinical research. Dr. Rakoff and his associates developed procedures for increasing the sensitivity of the pregnancy test, for the bioassay of pituitary and chorionic gonadotropins, and for assessment of the pituitary–ovarian–adrenal function in infertility and hirsutism. Dr. Rakoff's clinical reputation was worldwide and his patients came from afar, especially infertile couples and hirsute women. Dr. Rupp, who became Chief of the Diabetes Section, studied various aspects of thyroid function in both humans and lower animals. His was the first report of "T-3 Toxicosis."

The joint studies of Paschkis and Cantarow in the field of cancer research resulted in several important observations on the influence of tumor growth on the endocrine system, of the effects of hormones on tumor growth, and the intermediary metabolism of tumors. There were two pathologists associated with them, initially Dr. Joseph Stasney and later Dr. James W. Goddard. The studies of humoral factors in carcinogenesis and pyrimidine metabolism in malignant and normal growth indicated that malignant tissue utilized signficantly greater amounts of uracil than did normal tissue. This observation was important to the development of the antimetabolite, 5-flurouracil. More than 250 papers were published by members of the Division.

Endocrine and metabolic research at Jefferson was not limited to the active members of the Division. Dr. Savino A. D'Angelo (Department of Anatomy) made significant contributions to an understanding of hypothalamic–pituitary thyroidal function in pregnancy and other conditions. Dr. Franz X. Hausberger (Department of Anatomy) studied fat metabolism in normal and diabetic states. Drs. Irwin Jack Pincus (Jefferson, 1937; Department of Physiology) and W. Paul Havens, Jr., (Department of Medicine) reported on the influence of impaired liver function on hormonal function. Dr. Domenic A. DeBias (Department of Physiology) was actively engaged in endocrine research during his time at Jefferson. Dr. William H. Pearlman (Department of Biochemistry) made major contributions in the field of sex steroid metabolism.

Education and Patient Care

Clinical and basic research were important, but not the dominant role of most members of the Division in the overall functions of the medical school. Drs. Paschkis and Rakoff, by example and fiat, insisted that patient care and the education of undergraduate and graduate students have first priority. These clinical activities were important because they permitted a hands-on approach to inpatient and outpatient care. Each clinic session was followed by a conference where the unusual problems were discussed. Students and residents were given the opportunity to present and discuss problems of their individual interest.

Members of the Division participated in undergraduate, graduate, and continuing medical education. Dr. Paschkis gave the lectures in physiology. Dr. Rakoff was responsible for gynecologic endocrinology, and Dr. Rupp participated in teaching of the second year. Before the introduction of the new curriculum in the mid-1960s, undergraduate education in endocrinology was reinforced over the four-year period. The facilities of the Division were available to students; they came with their interests and volunteered to be summer research associates. Students enjoyed their exposure to endocrinology, and the faculty mutually delighted in the students, whom they considered to be the school's most important asset. Members of the Division were honored by the students. Three (Cantarow, Rakoff, and Rupp) had class portraits painted. Those three, as well as Dr. Paschkis, had yearbooks dedicated to them, and some were selected for the Lindback Award for outstanding teaching.

Graduate education of residents and fellows began shortly after the Division was established in 1940 and expanded after World War II. The Division was awarded a National Institutes of Health training grant. In addition to Americans, trainees came from Canada, Mexico, South American, Europe, and the Near and Far East. Most remained for one year and some for two or more. The Residents and Clinical Fellows were responsible for patient care. They also prepared clinical and teaching conferences under the supervision of the faculty, including Sidney M. Wolfe (Jefferson, 1947), Jack Zagerman, Rachmel Cherner (Jefferson, 1955), and Sheldon Gilgore

(Jefferson, 1956). Dr. Gilgore, who studied carbohydrate metabolism, reported the definitive study on the hypoglycemic effects of aspirin. He subsequently became President of Pfizer Pharmaceuticals, an Alumni member of Jefferson's Board of Trustees, and Chairman of the Board at Clark University.

Among the other trainees were Dr. Angelo DiGeorge, who became Chief of Endocrinology at St. Christopher's Hospital for Children; Dr. William A. Abelove (Jefferson, 1951), who accepted a position in the diabetic section at the University of Miami; and Dr. Agustin M. DeAndino (Jefferson, 1944), who returned to Puerto Rico where he practiced endocrinology until his untimely death. Dr. Doris Bartuska returned to the Medical College of Pennsylvania in the fields of both endocrinology and medical education. Dr. Ruth Ann Fitzpatrick became Chief of Endocrinology at the Crozer-Chester Hospital. Dr. John Aloi accepted a position at Stony Brook Medical School (SUNY) and became Professor of Medicine and Chief of Endocrinology. Dr. Joseph T. Curti (Jefferson, 1963), following his training, entered the pharmaceutical industry and became Vice-President of Roerig Company. Dr. Francis H. Sterling (Jefferson, 1960) returned to the Veterans Hospital and the University of Pennsylvania. He received many awards as an outstanding teacher. Other Jefferson graduates who were Fellows in endocrinology included Drs. Stephen L. DeFelice (1961) and Murray B. Grosky (1961). Later members of the Division were Drs. Joseph S. Fisher (Jefferson, 1970) and Edward B. Ruby (Jefferson, 1971).

Further Graduate Teaching

Dr. Ralph A. Carabasi, Jr. (Jefferson, 1946) completed his training in endocrinology and oncology at Tulane and was appointed in the Department of Medicine in 1950. He aided in the student and resident training programs and was especially active in the Diabetic Clinic.

Dr. Stanley N. Cohen, a graduate of the Medical College of Virginia (1952), served as Chief Pathologist and Head of the Clinical Laboratories at Fort Gordon, Georgia (1954–1956). He took a medical residency at the Veterans Administration Hospital in Richmond, Virginia (1956–1958) and became a National Institutes of Health Fellow in endocrine and metabolic diseases at the University of Pennsylvania (1958–1959). After joining the Jefferson faculty in the Department of Medicine in 1959, Cohen's special interest and training in diabetes mellitus led to his holding all the major positions in the local affiliate of the American Diabetes Association (President, 1978–1980; Chairman of the Board, 1980–1981; and President of the Professional Section, 1981–1983). He was a cofounder at Jefferson of the Sexual Function Center, as the outgrowth of a National Institutes of Health grant for the research into the problem of impotence in diabetes mellitus (1977–1980). This multidisciplinary center for the diagnosis and treatment of impotence in males became one of the largest of its type in the world. In 1985 he cofounded, with Dr. Steven R. Peikin, the Jefferson Nutrition Program.

Graduate training was not limited to those who could spend a year or more in the program. Residents at Jefferson and also the affiliated hospitals, especially the Naval Hospital, often elected to experience three to six months at Jefferson. The program was not limited to those concerned only with clinical training. Three candidates for the Ph.D. degree in physiology fulfilled part of the course requirements in the Division. Dr. Domenic DiBias, after receiving his degree, joined the faculty in the Physiology Department. He later accepted an appointment at the Philadelphia College of Osteopathic Medicine as Professor and Head of the Departments of Physiology and Pharmacology and became Assistant Dean. Dr. Frederick D. DeMartinis joined the staff of the Medical College of Pennsylvania and became Professor of Physiology. The late Arthur Segal, D.V.M., was Professor of Physiology at the School of Veterinary Medicine of the University of Pennsylvania.

In addition to conferences held on campus, Dr. Paschkis had "beer-and-pretzel" meetings at his home, attended by faculty, trainees, and students. Here the discussions began with endocrinology but usually more time was spent discussing history, politics, and music. A highlight for members of the Division was carol singing at the Paschkis home on the third Sunday of Advent.

Dr. Rakoff had an active training program in gynecologic endocrinology. Dr. Alvin F. Goldfarb, one of his Fellows, joined him in carrying out the research, education, and clinical activities of residents and trainees in the Department of Obstetrics and Gynecology. He accepted an appointment at Pennsylvania Hospital and became active in their endocrine division.

In 1961 Drs. Rupp, Rakoff, and Goldfarb initiated programs in continuing medical education when they presented a 13-week night course in endocrinology for the practicing physician. This course was given for several years and was replaced by a day course. Members of the Division participated in continuing medical education courses presented by other Departments and Divisions at Jefferson and its affiliated hospitals. These included three yearly Seven Springs Symposia at the Latrobe Hospital area and yearly ongoing Eastern Shore Medical Symposia with the University of Delaware.

Division Organization

Following the death of Dr. Paschkis in 1961, Dr. Rupp was appointed Director of the Division, a position he held until he was made Assistant Director of Continuing Medical Education in 1969. He was replaced by Dr. Richard A. Field, internationally known in the special area of diabetic retinopathy. The latter was responsible for bringing Dr. Nicholas Zervas to Jefferson for the transsphenoidal method of pituitary ablation for the treatment of diabetic retinopathy. Dr. Field returned to Boston in 1971. After a hiatus, Dr. Sheldon R. Schlaff became the interim Director from 1974 to 1977.

In 1977 Dr. Joseph A. Glennon (Figure 17-10) was appointed the first Kramer Professor of Medicine and Chief of the Division of Endocrinology and Metabolic Diseases. He received his M.D. degree from the State University of New York (Downstate, 1957); interned at St. Vincent's Hospital in New York (1958); and took his residency in internal medicine at St. Vincent's Hospital (1959) and Hartford Hospital (1961–1963), interrupted by United States Navy duty (1959–1961). He taught in the Department of Medicine at the University of Wisconsin (1965–1971), Tufts University (1971–1973), and as Professor at Texas Tech University School of Medicine, Lubbock, Texas (1973–1977). He became certified by the American Board of Internal Medicine in 1964, was recertified in 1974, and board certified in Endocrinology and Metabolism in 1972.

Before coming to Philadelphia, Dr. Glennon had much clinical experience as attending physician and consultant in civilian and Veteran's Administration Hospitals in Wisconsin, Massachusetts, and Texas. He was active in the pertinent professional societies of his specialty and served in the curriculum planning of several medical schools.

Dr. Glennon's main research interest has been in the fields of diabetes mellitus and obesity. His

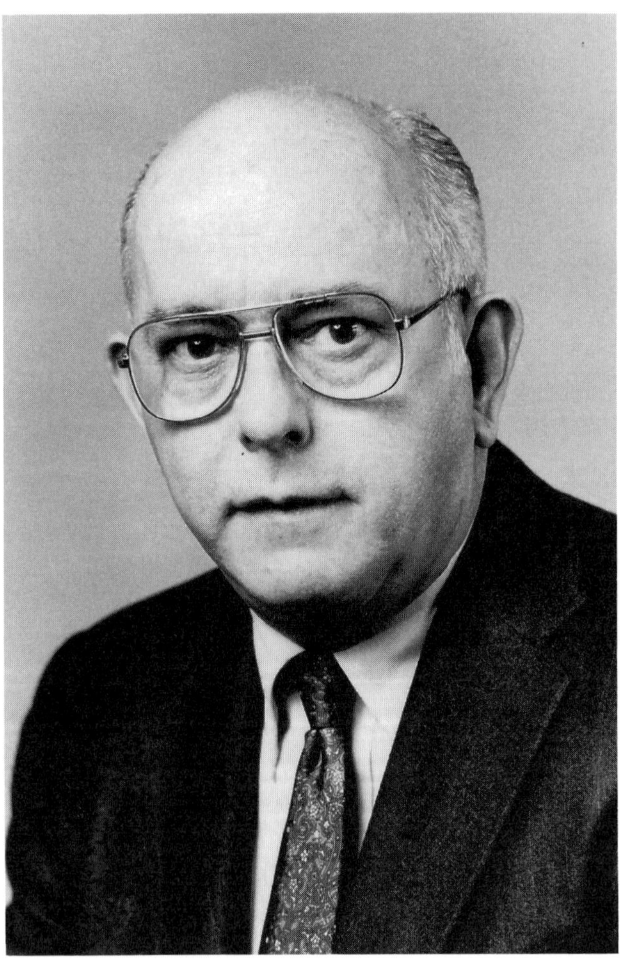

FIG. 17-10. Joseph A. Glennon, M.D.; Director of the Division of Endocrine and Metabolic Diseases (1977–). First Kramer Professor of Medicine.

studies involved also the nervous system, the liver, enzyme systems, the lungs (especially sarcoidosis), and the inevitable path of endocrine changes in carcinoma. In conjunction with Drs. Boas Gonen and Steven Nagelberg at Jefferson, research continued in the area of hyperlipoproteinemia and gonadotrophins.

While the Division remains a distinct entity within the Department of Medicine, its history is strongly one of interdepartmental cooperation in all the basic sciences as well as the clinical arena of physical and mental health. There are approximately 5,000,000 diabetics in the United States and possibly an equal number not yet diagnosed. Even the meticulous control of the blood sugar level with insulin does not prevent the vascular, neurological, renal, and ophthalmologic complications in many patients. The full understanding of obesity and its control remains open for further investigation. Continued interaction by new faculty and the added dimension of an Institute of Molecular Medicine provide the path for Jefferson's future distinction in the field of Endocrinology and Metabolism.

References

1. Loewenberg, S.A., *Clinical Endocrinology,* 2d Ed., Philadelphia: F. A. Davis Co., 1941, p. 1.
2. Idem, p. 2.
3. Robinson V., "Charles Eucharist de Medici Sajous," *Med. Life,* Vol. 32, January 1925, p. 7.
4. Anders, J. M., "Memoir of Charles Eucharist de Medici Sajous, M.D., ScD., LL.D.," *Trans. Stud. Coll. Phys. Phila.* 3d Ser., 1930, 52:65–70.
5. Kramer, D. W., "Clinical Observations on the Pathogenesis of Diabetes Mellitus," *N.Y. Med. J. and Med. Rec.* 1922, 115:472–75.

CHAPTER EIGHTEEN

Division of Cardiology

WARREN P. GOLDBURGH, M.D.

"Of all the ailments which may blow out life's little candle, heart disease is the chief."

—WILLIAM BOYD (1885–1979)

BEFORE THE establishment of a formal Division of Cardiology at Jefferson in 1964, a rich tradition of the diagnosis and treatment of heart disease existed. Dr. John Eberle, one of Jefferson's founders, while Professor of Theory and Practice of Medicine (1825–1831) wrote a *Treatise on the Practice of Medicine* (1830), which devoted 25 pages to diseases of the heart, including a section on sympathetic affections not attributable to organic lesions.[1] Robley Dunglison, Professor of the Institutes of Medicine from 1836 to 1868 and Dean during the last 14 of these years, wrote a text on *Practice of Medicine* (1842), in which he devoted 41 pages to diseases of the circulatory system. Roberts Bartholow, Professor of Materia Medica, encompassed diseases of the heart within 59 pages of his *Practice of Medicine* (1880). His successor, Dr. Hobart A. Hare, extended coverage on diseases of the heart to 70 pages in his *Practice of Medicine* (1905).

The Electrocardiographic Department

The most notable of Jefferson's Professors during the nineteenth century with respect to pioneering in heart disease was Dr. Jacob Mendes DaCosta (Jefferson, 1852) who was Chairman of Internal Medicine from 1872 to 1891. His preliminary report in 1862 and 1864 concerning "irritable heart" was the result of studies performed at the U.S. Army Hospital for Injuries and Diseases of the Nervous System at Turner's Lane Hospital in Philadelphia during the Civil War.[2] His textbook *Medical Diagnosis with Special Reference to Practical Medicine* (1864) devoted five pages to functional disorders of the heart. His classic work on "irritable heart," however, was published in 1871 and led to the naming of that condition "DaCosta's syndrome."[3] During World War I this was called "neurocirculatory asthenia" and in World War II "anxiety neurosis." The syndrome was regarded as largely of functional cause, but in retrospect some cases were more involved and included the later-to-be-identified process of mitral valve prolapse.[4]

The invention of the electrocardiograph by Einthoven in 1902 ushered in the scientific era of cardiology. It took until the 1920s for it to come into widespread clinical use. Copies of old correspondence obtained by Dr. Robert I. Wise, Magee Professor of Medicine (1959–1975), provided information on the initiation of electrocardiography at Jefferson. In 1917, Dean Ross V. Patterson accepted a proposal from the Charles F. Hindle Company of New York City to install an electrocardiograph outfit for $1,675.25 with "extra instruction—additional charge per day of $16.00." Patterson raised funds for the equipment and used it successfully in a room of the 1907 Hospital provided by the Medical Director, Dr. Henry K. Mohler. In 1918 Dr. Thomas McCrae, Chairman of Medicine (1913–1935), proposed to the Hospital Committee "the question of establishing a separate department in the Hospital to be termed 'The Electrocardiographic Department'. . . The electrocardiograph represents a great advance in the study of cardiac disease and is a very important addition to our means of diagnosis . . . If you think favorably of this suggestion, the logical man to be put in charge is Dr. Ross V. Patterson [Figure 18-1] . . . It would, of course, be a department within the General Department of Medicine." With the support of Drs. Solomon Solis-Cohen and Hobart A. Hare, the Hospital Committee on May 21, 1918, acted upon Dr. McCrae's recommendation to create a Subdepartment of Electrocardiography, placing Dr. Ross V. Patterson, Assistant Physician to the Jefferson Hospital, in charge.

Dr. Patterson, who had graduated from Jefferson (1904), took further training at the Philadelphia General Hospital until 1906, and then became a member of the Jefferson faculty for the remainder of his life. He was President of the Alumni Association (1923–1925) and served as President of the Pennsylvania Medical Society (1930–1931) as well as President of the Association of American Medical Colleges (1933–1935). He was Sub-Dean at Jefferson (1906–1916) and Dean from 1916 until his death in 1938. Dr. Patterson, who never married, left almost his entire estate to Jefferson for Fellowships in Research. A curiosity among the personal effects in his bequest was the skull of the famous English Shakespearian actor, George Frederick Cooke (1756–1812), which he had received from the widow of Dr. George McClellan, the grandson of Jefferson's founder.

The Ross V. Patterson Heart Station

In 1939, a foundation in memory of Dr. Ross V. Patterson was established. Its purpose was "for the study and treatment of diseases of the heart and circulation; to study the history and treatment of diseases of circulation; to collect literature pertaining to these subjects; to undertake experimental work—animal, chemical, physical, etc., which may throw light upon the cause and cure of diseases of the heart and circulation; and to investigate such problems as may arise during

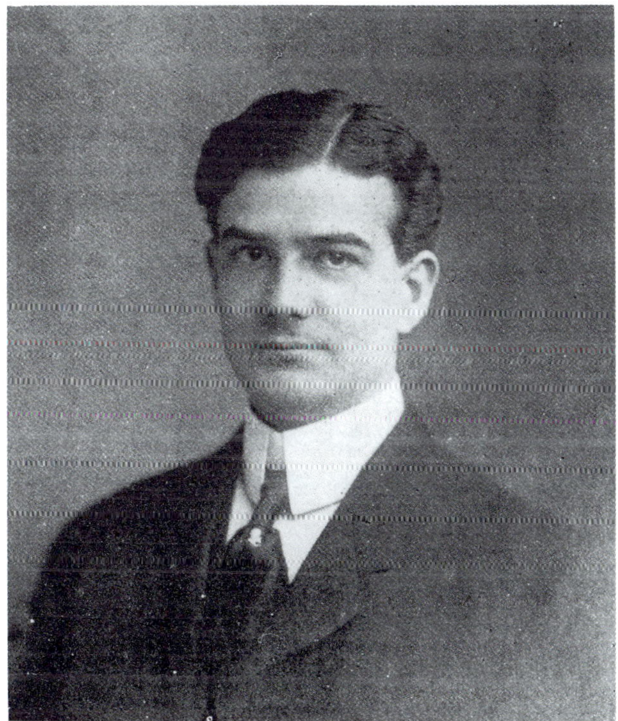

FIG. 18-1. Ross V. Patterson, M.D., First in Electrocardiography at Jefferson (1918).

the course of the aforementioned work." The Department of Electrocardiography was named the Ross V. Patterson Heart Station and headed by Dr. Henry K. Mohler (Jefferson, 1912), who, like his predecessor, was a cardiologist and the Dean. By this time, the volume of studies had increased to the point that Dr. Charles W. Semisch, III (Figure 18-2; Jefferson, 1933) was added to the staff as an Associate Cardiologist.

In 1942, the Cardiac Clinic was founded as an outpatient activity in the Curtis building. The Acting Chief Clinical Assistant was Dr. Louis B. Laplace, with Drs. Robert B. Nye (Jefferson, 1927), Hayward R. Hamrick (Jefferson, 1935), Charles W. Semisch, III, and James D. Nelson as Clinical Assistants. In the same year, following the death of Dr. Mohler, Dr. Nye became Physician-in-Charge of the Ross V. Patterson Heart Station, with Dr. Semisch continuing as Associate Cardiologist. In 1951, Dr. Louis Merves (Jefferson, 1937) joined as Assistant Cardiologist. Drs. Semisch and Merves were volunteer physicians with offices outside the hospital.

On May 6, 1953, the first open heart surgery in the world for closure of an interatrial septal defect was performed at Jefferson Hospital by Dr. John H. Gibbon, Jr., under total cardiopulmonary bypass with use of the heart-lung machine. This aspect of Jefferson history is covered in the chapter on cardiothoracic surgery, but deserves mention at this juncture as the beginning of a new era in the treatment of congenital and acquired cardiac disease. Cardiac catheterizations to study cases for cardiopulmonary bypass were at that time performed in the Department of Radiology by the Department of Surgery.

In 1956 the Heart Station was refurbished and expanded on the second floor of the Thompson Annex. Orthodiography and phonocardiography were being performed in addition to conventional electrocardiography. The administrative arrangement was loose in that it was under hospital control without the direct supervision of the Medical Department.

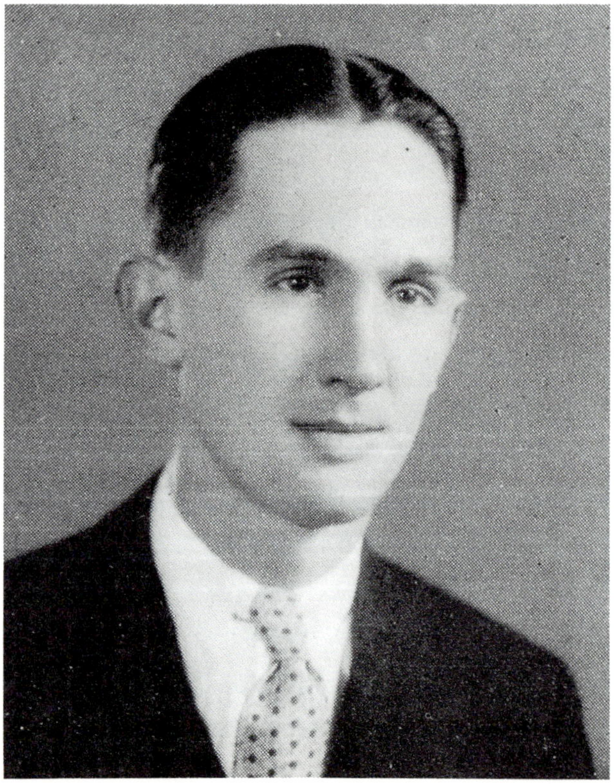

FIG. 18-2. Charles W. Semisch III, M.D.

The Division of Cardiology

Dr. Robert I. Wise, upon his appointment as Chairman of Medicine in 1959, desired clarification of the responsibilities of the Heart Station. By action of Dean William A. Sodeman and the newly appointed Hospital Director, Dr. Ellsworth R. Browneller, the appointments of professional personnel and the standards of quality for education, medical practice, and research in the Patterson Heart Station came under the aegis of the Medical Department. The administration of the physical plant, finance, and equipment remained with the Hospital Director. The Magee Professor was authorized to integrate the programs.

Cardiac catheterization, pulmonary function, and electrocardiography were unified into a single program in 1960, which allowed a single team to cooperate with the Departments of Radiology, Surgery, and Pediatrics. This enhanced the teaching of students, residents and fellows. Dr. John H. Killough (Figure 18-3), Associate Professor of Medicine, was appointed Director of Cardiopulmonary Diseases, with Dr. Richard

Cathcart of the Barton Division for Diseases of the Chest. Dr. Daniel W. Lewis (Figure 18-4) (Jefferson, J1944), Assistant Professor of Clinical Medicine, was assigned to the Heart Station and Pulmonary Function Laboratories.

In 1964 a formally recognized Division of Cardiology presented its first annual report. The cardiac clinics and conferences that had been held during the Chairmanship of Dr. John Deitrick (1952–1957) were extended by 1964 into a weekly graphic records conference, a clinical medical, pediatric, and surgical cardiology conference, daily instruction of students and residents in interpretation of electrocardiograms, and instruction in cardiac catheterization, vectorcardiography, phonocardiography, and apexcardiography. Introduction to electrocardiography for students was offered in an elective series of ten lectures. Over 1,000 electrocardiograms were being performed monthly. A cardiac catheterization laboratory had been established in the Hospital, and in 1961 Dr. Warren P. Goldburgh (Jefferson, 1952) was added to its staff. From 1967 to 1969, catheterizations were under the direction of Dr. William Eliades (Jefferson, 1958). Facilities for gas, dye, pressure, and radiologic studies were developed with a staff of three technicians and a nurse. An automatic cine-film developer was installed, and a laboratory for exercise functional studies. An animal laboratory was established with the Department of Anesthesiology. A graduate student in biomedical engineering joined the Division, and a candidate for a Master of Science was continuing his second year. In 1967, a journal club in cardiology was started. Insertion of electrical catheters for temporary cardiac pacing was initiated that same year.

In 1969, new leadership was provided to the Division with the appointment of Dr. Albert N. Brest (Figure 18-5) from Hahnemann Medical College as Director of the Division. Dr. Brest brought Drs. Hratch Kasparian and Leslie Wiener to aid as Directors of the Cardiac Catheterization Laboratory and Medical Cardiac Care Unit, respectively. They developed a modern cardiac care unit for medical and postoperative cardiac care supported by the most modern techniques for cardiac monitoring and laboratory studies. Electrocardiography with computerization and two new cardiac catheterization laboratories were constructed. Drs. Charles Semisch and William Eliades were Co-Directors of the Division for 1968–

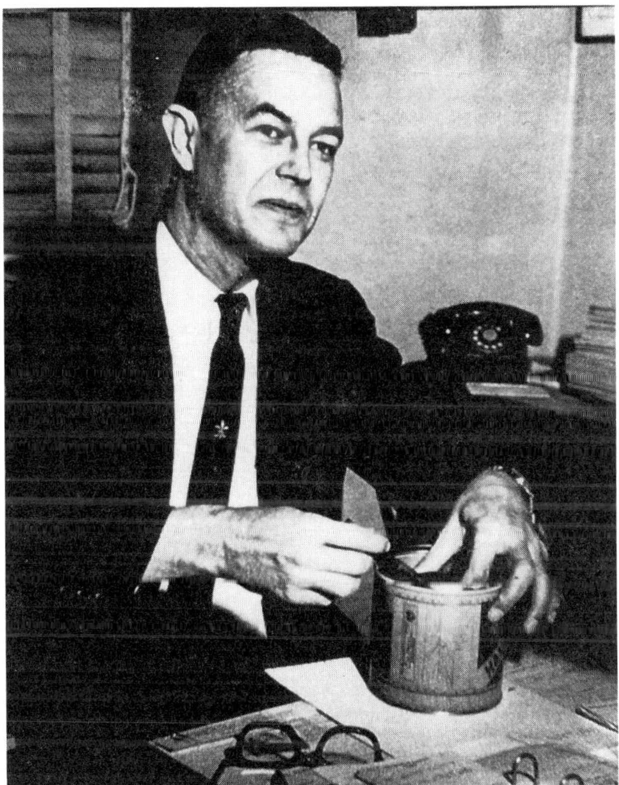

FIG. 18-3. John H. Killough, M.D., Ph.D.; Director of Cardiopulmonary Diseases (1959).

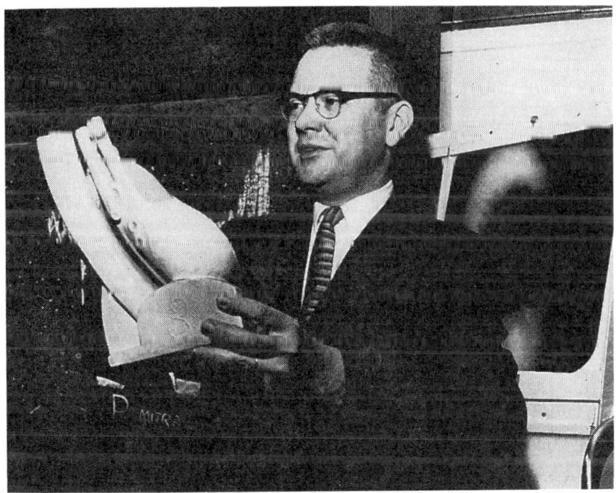

FIG. 18-4. Daniel W. Lewis, M.D.; Director of Cardiology Clinic (1954–1965).

1969 until replaced by the new team. The latest facilities became functional in 1971.

Dr. Jorge Rios of George Washington University was appointed Director of Electrocardiography in 1971 but returned after one year to Washington, eventually becoming Chairman of the Department of Medicine there. He was replaced by Dr. George Rafter until the appointment in 1973 of Dr. Edward K. Chung of West Virginia University School of Medicine. Dr. Chung, Professor of Medicine (Figure 18-6), brought to Jefferson a national reputation as a cardiologist and author of numerous scientific publications, manuals, and textbooks of electrocardiography.

In the early 1970's a formal Coronary Care Unit on the fourth floor of the Thompson Annex replaced the previous Intensive Care Unit and came under the direction of Dr. Leslie Wiener. Specialized nursing and technical staff were recruited with specific guidelines and protocols. Full-time cardiologists were assigned to the Unit with responsibility at all times for the care of the patients. Those with myocardial infarctions could be constantly monitored for disturbances of cardiac rhythm and given resuscitation within minutes in case of cardiac arrest. Studies were undertaken on the acutely ill patients with myocardial infarction by means of coronary arteriography and myocardial metabolic studies. Surgical intervention was studied as a method of treatment. The Coronary Care Unit and Cardiac Catheterization Laboratory were moved to the fifth floor of the new Thomas Jefferson University Hospital when it opened in 1978. Dr. William Frankl was Director of the Unit from 1979 until 1984.

In 1973 the Heart Station was performing more than 20,000 electrocardiograms yearly, 250

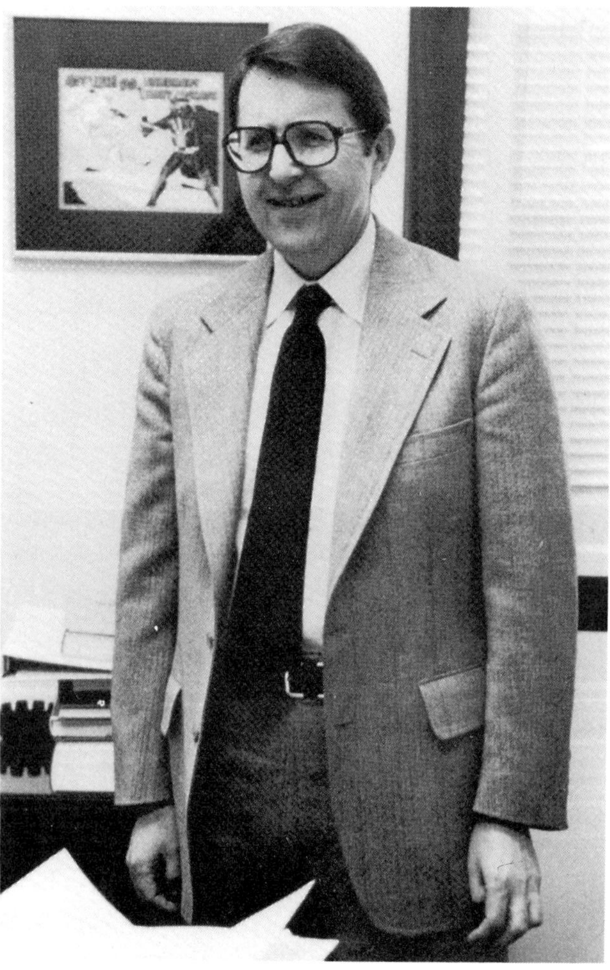

FIG. 18-5. Albert N. Brest, M.D.; Director, Division of Cardiology (1969–), and James C. Wilson Professor of Medicine (1973–).

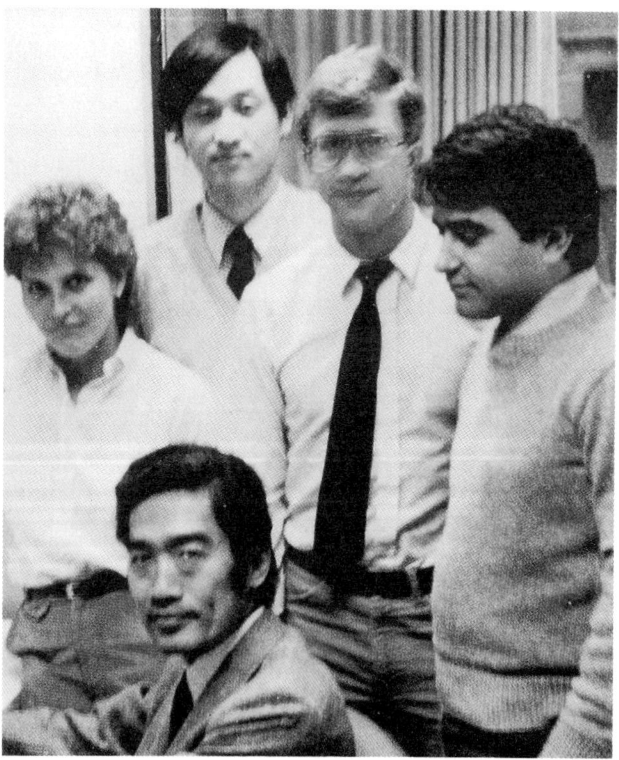

FIG. 18-6. Edward K. Chung, M.D.; Director of Electrocardiography (1973–).

phonocardiograms, 250 echocardiograms, 250 cardiac rhythm telemetry tapes, 200 vectocardiograms, and 100 cardiac work studies. Approximately 500 cardiac catheterizations were performed annually. Cardiac clinics were held twice weekly, and consultation services were in high demand. The Intensive Cardiac Care Unit, in addition to its patient care, provided education and research activities.

In 1973 a Professorship in Cardiology was established through a bequest of $1.5 million from Miss Beatrice Wilson of Haverford, Pennsylvania, in memory of her father, Dr. James Cornelius Wilson, Professor and Head of the Department of Medicine at Jefferson (1891–1911). Dr. Albert N. Brest was appointed the first James C. Wilson Professor of Medicine in the fall of 1973.

Between 1959 and 1979, twenty-seven Fellows were trained in cardiology. For the year 1975–1976 the Division attracted approximately 50 applicants for fellowships.

In 1980, Dr. Sheldon Goldberg was appointed to the Directorship of the Cardiac Catheterization Laboratory. Under his leadership the study and treatment of patients with myocardial infarction was intensified. Fibrinolysin therapy and angioplasty were employed in acute cases, and angioplasty was also introduced for treatment of chronic coronary artery disease.

The Cardiac Outpatient Clinic increased in size to become one of the largest in the Philadelphia area, and received many out of town referrals. Following the pioneer years from 1942 onward, Dr. Daniel Lewis served as Director of the Clinic from 1954 until 1965. Dr. Warren Goldburgh (Figure 18-7) headed the Clinic from 1965 until its closing in 1975. In that year the old clinic system at Jefferson was discontinued, and all patients were assigned to an attending physician. Dr. Goldburgh served Jefferson in many ways since completing his training in 1961. An able clinician and enthusiastic teacher, he received the Lindback Award for distinguished teaching. He also served as President of the Medical Staff and of the Volunteer Faculty Association. In 1987 his portrait was presented to the University by colleagues and friends.

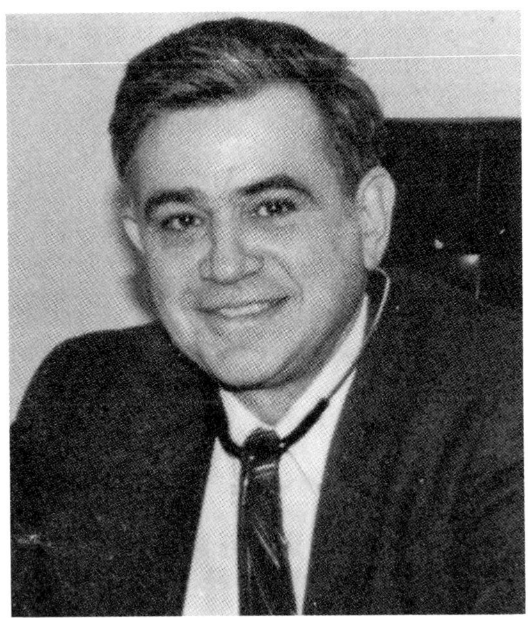

FIG. 18-7. Warren P. Goldburgh, M.D.; Director of Cardiology Clinic (1965–1975).

The Division of Cardiology by 1986 had grown to a staff of 25 members, including nine full-time cardiologists. The diagnostic capabilities encompassed ultrasonography and radionuclide studies, exercise testing, and electrocardiographic and electrophysiologic testing. Intervention cardiology was being conducted on a large scale. In July 1986, for the first time, a cardiac support team from Jefferson traveled nearly 100 miles to another hospital to place an aortic balloon in a patient with myocardial infarction complicated by failure and arrhythmia. After arrival at Jefferson, the patient underwent emergency coronary catheterization and coronary bypass with complete recovery.

Latest challenges lie in more effective prevention of heart disease along with improvements in rehabilitation following recovery from myocardial infarction or cardiac surgery.

References

1. Eberle, J.: *Treatise on the Practice of Medicine*. Vol. II, Philadelphia: John Grigg, pp. 245–247.
2. Wooley, C.F., "Jacob Mendez DaCosta: Medical Teacher, Clinician, and Clinical Investigator," *Am. J. Cardiol.* 1982, 50:1145–1148.
3. DaCosta, J.M., "On Irritable Heart," *Am. J. Med. Sci.* 1871, 61:17–52.
4. Wooley, C.F., "Where are the diseases of yesteryear?" *Circulation*. 1976, 53:749–751.
5. Wise, R.I., *Centrifugal and Centripetal Forces: A History of the Department of Medicine, The Jefferson Medical College of Thomas Jefferson University, 1959–1975*. (In T.J.U. archives)

CHAPTER NINETEEN

Division of Internal (General) Medicine

JOHN H. HODGES, M.D.

"The art has three factors, the disease, the patient, the physician. The physician is the servant of the art." —HIPPOCRATES (460–370 B.C.)

BEFORE THE establishment of the Division of General Medicine in 1968,[1] evolutionary changes in the Department of Medicine resulted in progressive subspecialization. To understand the mechanisms behind this process, it is well to recount briefly the trends of change over the past two centuries.

Art and Science

It is often not recalled that medical diagnosis was poorly organized before the development of percussion and auscultation during the first three decades of the nineteenth century. Even then, acceptance by physicians was limited so that only in the most progressive medical centers would stethoscopy and physical diagnosis have been employed as a routine. Early nineteenth century textbooks usually referred only obliquely to physical diagnosis as a part of the management of the patient or disease. Later in the century, physical diagnosis as an academic pursuit became increasingly important. When teaching was largely preceptorial, decades were often required for even such major changes to reach day-to-day practice. At Jefferson, a disciplined diagnostic process has always been esteemed. The great clinicians from Eberle (1825) to McCrae (1935) and beyond stressed the basic skills of history taking, symptomatology, and physical examination in the evaluation of disease processes and the direction of treatment.[2] Almost from the beginning, classroom, clinic, and hospital facilities were in close proximity.

▪ Laboratory Medicine for Jefferson Students

As scientific progress burgeoned toward the end of the nineteenth century, simple laboratory procedures were added to students' course content. Soon ways were sought to provide laboratory facilities for students' direct use. Dr. McCrae, upon his arrival at Jefferson in 1913, enthusiastically supported dedication of the new Laboratory of Clinical Medicine to Jacob Mendes DaCosta, M.D., who had been Chairman of Medicine from 1872 to 1891.[3] The Laboratory was located on the second floor of the Laboratory Building on Tenth Street, and its equipment was provided in part by funds from the Alumni Association.

From this time forward, the teaching of clinical laboratory methods became the responsibility of the Department of Medicine, supplementing the earlier programs conducted by pathologists and bacteriologists. From 1913 the clinical laboratory was stated to be available for use of the students relative to patients anywhere in the hospital. The instruction was provided by several of the younger members of the Department, but in 1921 Dr. Harold W. Jones (Jefferson, 1917) was appointed Director of the Clinical Laboratory. The unit combined laboratory studies of blood, urine, and other body fluids with established methods of clinical diagnosis for which Jefferson was well known. The course was then taught to Senior medical students who performed tests on hospital patients assigned to them, but later Junior students were included. From the 1940s onward, the course was taught to Sophomores only, constituting a "bridge" between the basic sciences and the clinical courses. By that time, laboratory facilities were available in the hospital for the use of students for their patients.

The Trend Toward Specialization

The teaching at Jefferson has always been directed toward imparting a broad knowledge of the art and science of medicine. As specialization advanced early in the twentieth century, along with increasing emphasis on the applied sciences, many clinicians became defensive about laboratory techniques to the exclusion of clinical skills. Dr. McCrae's Oslerian philosophy of teaching reflected this concern, but it must be recalled that upon his arrival at Jefferson he encouraged the use of chemistry and microscopy for basic blood and urine studies by the students. His insistence upon thoroughness in all aspects of general medicine may paradoxically have advanced the growth of specialties. His successors in the Department of Medicine saw the gradual establishment of 13 Divisions, each of which represented a mature specialty. Specialization was thus a relentless process.

A major change in the provision of medical care was developing. Gradually physicians who limited their practices to nonsurgical diagnosis and treatment became known as "diagnosticians," "consultants," or later, "internists" as a phase of specialization. In the 1930s the specialty boards, notably the American Board of Internal Medicine, were developed to provide standards of advanced achievement. As subspecialization progressed, especially in the 1960s, it was realized that hospital-trained board candidates were well versed in secondary and tertiary care, but there was a deficiency in the experience of taking full responsiblity for patient care in office or outpatient settings. Consequently, Departments of Medicine began to assign their members continuing primary care to divisions of "General Medicine" or "Internal Medicine." Among these faculty members were several who attempted to meet the learning deficiency by inviting residents to see patients with them in their private offices, especially in the Mohler Building. The procedure proved cumbersome and time-consuming.

▪ Formation of the Division

In 1968 Dr. Wise, recognizing the need for emphasis on the care of the entire patient, decided to form the Division of General Medicine.[1] Because the Laboratory of Clinical Medicine was already in place as a teaching section under Dr. John H. Hodges (Figure 19-1), this became the cornerstone of the new Division. Dr. Hodges, who had been appointed the first Ludwig A. Kind Professor of Medicine in 1964, was named the Director of the Division of General Medicine. He was also an Associate in the Division of Hematology, but most of the early members did not have a prior Division affiliation. With the new arrangement each member of the Department faculty was assigned to a Division. The new

Division included the General Medical Clinic under the direction of Dr. John N. Lindquist, the Emergency Ward under Dr. Joseph Keiserman, and the Laboratory of Clinical Medicine under Dr. Hodges. The membership of the Division was listed in the Department Annual Report of 1969–1970 as follows: Dr. John H. Hodges, Director; Dr. Joseph Keiserman, Miss Jane Kirk, M.T., Drs. William Allison, William V. Betsch, Adolph Borkowski, Leonard S. Davitch (Jefferson, 1943), Philip J. Dorman, Elmer H. Funk, Jr., (Jefferson, 1947; also in Clinical Pharmacology), Elliott Rosenberg, Norman G. Sloan, William Stepansky (Jefferson, 1952), William R. Thompson, and Herbert A. Yantes (Jefferson, 1950).

▪ The Clinical Laboratory Under Dr. Jones

Teaching of medicine in the 1920s was stimulated by the presence of young and able clinicians. The appointment of Dr. Harold W. Jones as Director provided a new thrust in the use of methods ancillary to clinical diagnosis and treatment. Jones proceeded in the early 1920s to organize the laboratory teaching as a vital aspect of student teaching. In company with subsequent Directors of Clinical Laboratory Medicine, he was actively involved in clinical practice. In addition, his ability to recognize and develop research opportunities along with laboratory teaching led him into the field of hematology, already pioneered at Jefferson by Dr. Arthur Dare (Jefferson, 1890) and Dr. J. C. DaCosta, Jr.,+ (Jefferson, 1893; see Hematology). With his aggressive studies in the transfusion of blood, Jones rapidly progressed to national recognition. He ultimately was responsible for the formation of the Cardeza Foundation and was advanced to Professor of Medicine.

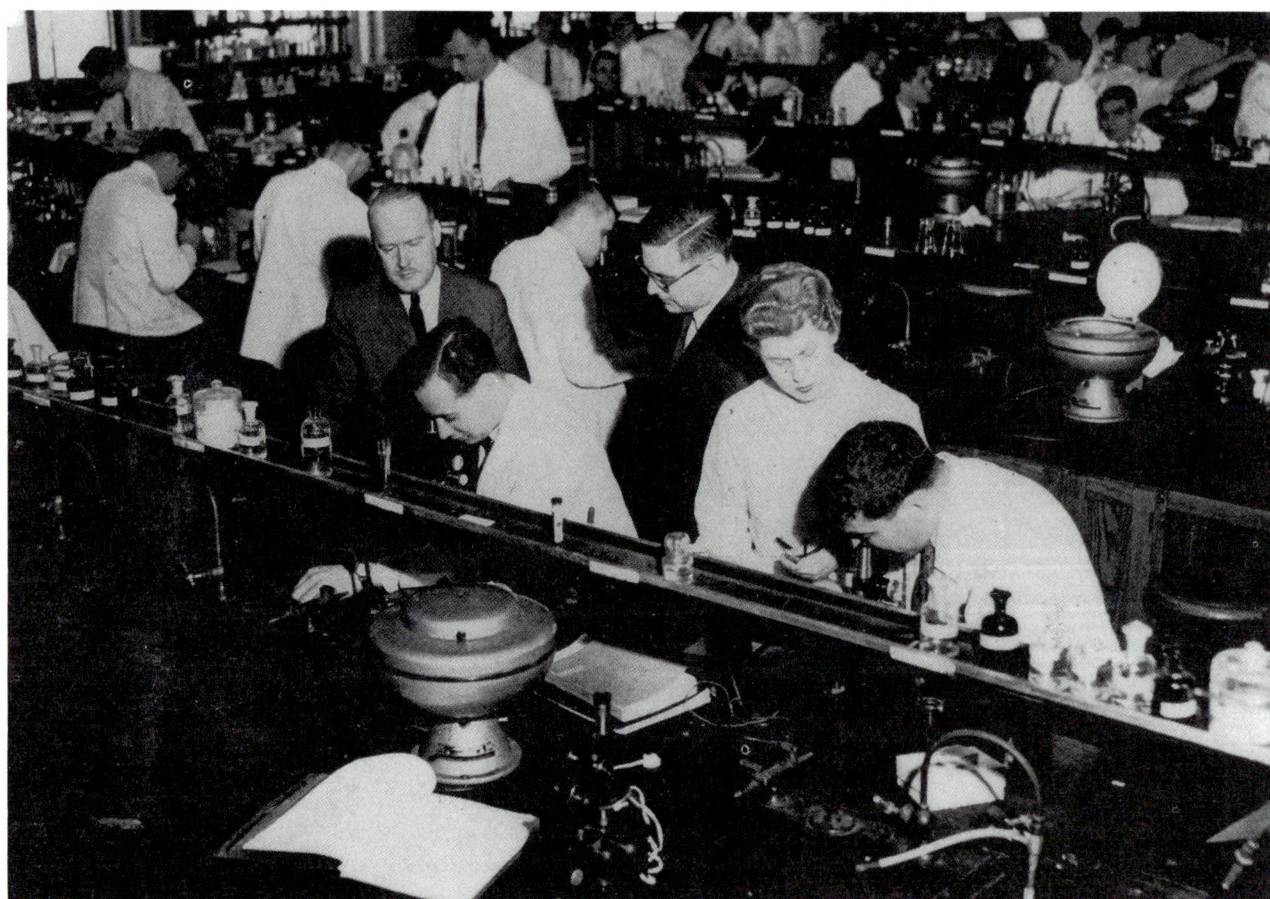

Fig. 19-1. John H. Hodges, M.D. (in suit at left); Director of Division of Internal (General) Medicine (1968–1978).

In the laboratory, Dr. Jones was assisted early by Dr. Christian W. Nissler (Jefferson, 1919). Later, Dr. Leandro M. Tocantins (Jefferson, 1928), who ultimately succeeded him as Director of Hematology, joined him in the Laboratory of Clinical Medicine and in 1937 assumed the Director's duties when Dr. Jones relinquished active responsibility for the Laboratory. In 1941, Dr. Tocantins was joined by Dr. Karl Paschkis, an endocrinologist who became Director of the Division of Endocrine and Cancer Research in the Department of Experimental Medicine, and by Dr. Abraham Cantarow, who became Chairman of the Department of Biochemistry (1945).

Dr. Charles Wirts of the Division of Gastroenterology spent several years as Proctor in the Laboratory. In 1942 Dr. John H. Hodges (Jefferson, 1939), a medical resident (1942–1946), began a two-year proctorship. In 1944 Dr. Reimann, Chairman of the Department of Medicine, appointed him Director of the course—Dr. Hodges had returned to Jefferson after a two-year rotating internship at the Philadelphia General Hospital and a year of general practice in Martinsburg, West Virginia.

Dr. John H. Hodges

Dr. Jones had written a small book, published in 1928, titled *The Application of Laboratory Methods to Clinical Medicine*. This evolved into an important guide for Clinical Laboratory Medicine with frequent revisions. By 1966 Dr. Hodges had seen it through 11 revisions, the last of which, entitled *Manual for Laboratory Medicine,* had over 300 pages and 23 contributors. The book covered the basic tests and function studies pertinent to Internal Medicine and served as a guide for the course. Specimens derived from normal individuals and hospitalized patients were studied under constant supervision in the course. The history, physical findings, and laboratory results were correlated with logical diagnostic conclusions. Laboratory discussions, demonstrations, and lectures interspersed with oral, practical, and written quizzes helped to place various diagnostic features into proper perspective. Members of various specialties were recruited for lectures and discussions to broaden and maintain the high level of educational experience.

Early in the teaching of the course, Dr. Hodges had medical technology assistance of high caliber from the very conscientious Miss Francilla Sherry. Then later, Miss Jane E. Kirk, M.T., Instructor in Medicine, made outstanding contributions for many years by directing the maintenance of the laboratory and preparing specimens. An accomplished hematologic technician, she had seen service in the Cardeza Laboratory and the hematologic division of Lankenau Hospital. In addition to expertise in blood and bone marrow techniques and morphology, Kirk became accomplished in the other procedures and was an invaluable laboratory teacher. Among those who spent some years as full-time assistants were Dr. John B. Atkinson (Jefferson, 1948), a hematologist who was a pioneer in bone marrow transfusion in the therapy of leukemia in twins, and Dr. Arthur J. Weiss, a hematologist who became Director of the Division of Oncology. Occasional assistants in the laboratory included Drs. Herbert Bowman (Jefferson, 1947), later Hematologist to the Harrisburg Hospital, Sandor Shapiro, and Allan Erslev, both of whom succeeded to the directorship of the Cardeza Foundation. Among the resident physicians who trained in this course were Dr. Michael Manko, who became Chairman of the Department of Medicine and Chief of the Division of Infectious Diseases at Lankenau Hospital, and Dr. Edward C. Bradley (Jefferson, 1955), who became a specialist in cardiovascular diseases and a Jesuit priest.

Changes in Laboratory Location and Emphasis

The location of the Laboratory changed several times early in its development, but in 1928 the new College Building at 1025 Walnut Street provided a special Laboratory of Clinical Medicine on the third floor. When the Biochemistry Department expanded, the Laboratory was moved to the sixth floor, where it shared with the Department of Microbiology the large student laboratory on the northwest side. The Director maintained an office on the eighth floor. In 1969, the Laboratory was moved to Jefferson Alumni Hall upon the completion of that building. No special provision, however, had been made for teaching space, which was shared with courses in the basic sciences and required the use of three rooms at the same time. The laboratory course was losing its identity, and for the teaching year of 1972 it came under the combined direction of the Dean's Office and the Department of Medicine. Dr. Hodges' 30-year association with the course came to an end.

The General Medical Clinic

The clinical practice aspects of the Division of General Medicine had a long and respected tradition in the Medical Clinic. Although the names of department heads are generally listed as Clinic Chiefs, others, perhaps less well known but contributing signally to the teaching, deserve mention. Drs. Frederick J. Kalteyer (Jefferson, 1899), Ward Brinton (Jefferson, 1894), E. J. G. Beardsley, H. R. M. Landis (Jefferson, 1897), C. H. Turner (Jefferson, 1909), Harold L. Goldburgh (Jefferson, 1915), Mitchell Bernstein, (Jefferson, 1914), Jacob M. Cahan (Jefferson, 1915), Reynold S. Griffith (Jefferson, 1918), and Thomas Aceto served prior to the Lindquist era. Thus the Medical Clinic played a teaching role for many years. In retrospect, the loose organization of the Clinic appears to reflect built-in ineffectiveness, but it must be remembered that all approaches to the patient were much more direct than was the case later on. Students were assigned to patients who were the responsiblity of the Clinical Assistants, and the teaching was intimate and personal. During the nineteenth century, the evidence suggests that outpatient care was directed largely toward indigent patients, many of whom required hospitalization. Separation into Medical and Surgical Clinics was followed by gradual splitting off of specialty clinics from each but especially from the Medical Clinic, leaving a group who were cared for as long-term medical patients or relative to hospital admission. Following World War II, and accompanying major changes in patient care, the General Medical Clinic assumed a new role as a primary care clinic and a source of referrals to medical Specialty Clinics and to other Departments.

The Lindquist Era

Dr. John Norman Lindquist (Jefferson, 1943) (Figure 19-2), the Director of the General Medical Clinic and the Geriatrics Clinic from 1951 to 1975 was a Pennsylvania native who was reared in Jamestown, New York. Before matriculating at Jefferson, Lindquist received a B.S. degree from Washington and Jefferson College at Washington, Pennsylvania (1939). This college had resulted from the amalgamation of Washington College and Jefferson College, the latter at Canonsburg, Pennsylvania, from which Jefferson Medical College had received its original charter. Washington and Jefferson was later to recognize Dr. Lindquist's accomplishments by bestowing

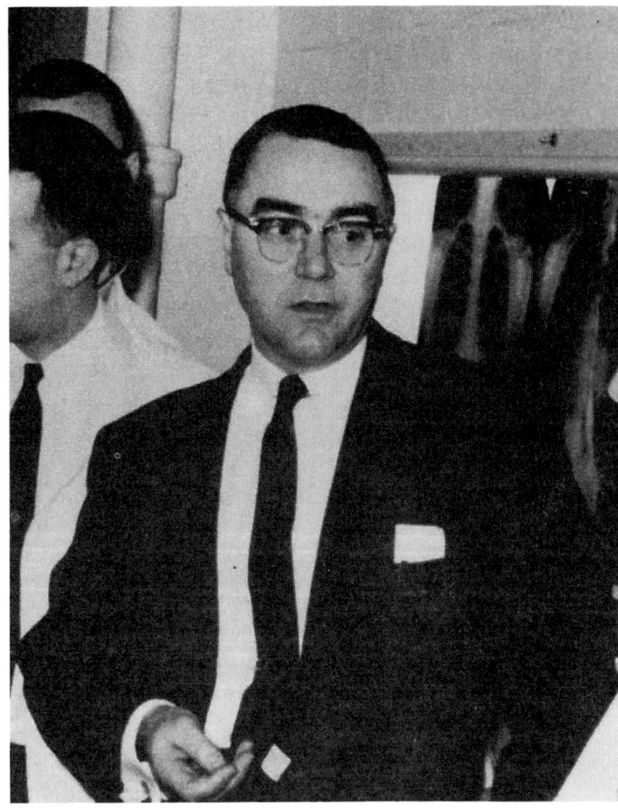

FIG. 19-2. John N. Lindquist, M.D.; Chief of the Medical Clinic (1951–1975)

upon him its Alumni Achievement Award (1967). Following a wartime internship of ten months at Jefferson Hospital, he went to Europe as a member of the United States Army Medical Service (1944–1947) and attained the rank of Major. Returning to Jefferson he served a medical residency until 1951, when he was appointed to the outpatient clinic and started a private practice. He was an Attending Physician to Jefferson Hospital as well as a Consultant in Medicine and Geriatrics to local hospitals, and he presented talks, usually on subjects relating to geriatrics and nursing home problems, to organizations locally and in neighboring states. The author of scientific articles, Lindquist was also a delegate to numerous committees and councils on aging, including Philadelphia County, the State of Pennsylvania, and the White House Conferences. Honors included dedication of the 1956 Jefferson Yearbook, the Christian R. and Mary S. Lindback Award for Distinguished Teaching (1964), and the dedication of the John N. Lindquist, M.D., Hall in the Philadelphia Center for Older People where he was a Trustee and had been Chairman of the Board. Dr. Lindquist served as President of the Alumni Association for the period 1978–1979.

Under Dr. Lindquist, the General Medical Clinic was a primary teaching area for Junior and later Senior students. Dr. Lindquist stressed history taking, physical diagnosis, the ordering of tests and consultations, proper decorum and the ideal attitude toward patients. He supplied the students with a brochure on the conduct of the Clinic. He was in constant attendance to aid the students and had a staff of 38 physicians with seven or eight in attendance each day. These Chiefs were listed as follows for the period of the late 1960s: Drs. Joseph Keiserman, Robert Gilbert, Joseph Gonnella, Edward Kotin (Jefferson, 1930), J. J. Kirshner (Jefferson, 1933), and Peter Amadio (Jefferson, 1973). The personnel of the Clinic included the head nurse, nutritionist, licensed practical nurse, nurse's aide, secretary to Dr. Lindquist, two clinic secretaries, two volunteers, and an executive secretary.

The General Medical Clinic was the first and most important facility in the student's education in the care of the ambulatory patient. It was frequently, for the patient, the beginning of the treatment process, which might include referral to specialized areas or to the hospital. Dr. Lindquist supervised all activities with a practical wisdom and an insistence on the highest of ideals.

During the post-World War II period, the personnel of the clinic came to include the Medical Residents in addition to the volunteer staff. Medical records also were organized to provide continuity of care for the patients in spite of changing personnel. For two decades, the Clinic adapted to rapidly changing conditions in a very effective manner. The establishment of Medicare and third-party programs, however, gradually caused a decline in patient numbers even though the clinic was charging minimal fees only to those who could afford to pay. The Clinic closed in 1975.

▪ The Emergency Service

The Emergency Department was for a time peripherally related to the Department of Medicine although under the administration of the Hospital. This relationship profited by the appointment in 1966 of Dr. Joseph Keiserman (Figure 19-3) as Director of the Emergency Service after long experience in the General Medical Clinic. For nine years his practical wisdom guided the care of patients with a great variety of acute and chronic problems. Instruction of students and residents was a major part of his service that he enjoyed with philosophical contentment. Dr. Keiserman, a graduate of the Medical School of the University of Pennsylvania, became associated with Jefferson in 1936 when he was appointed to the Medical Clinic by Dr. Jacob Cahan, Service Chief at the time. For several years he attended the clinic five days weekly, seeing patients and teaching students. Upon return from military service following World War II, he resumed his clinic teaching but also was appointed to Medical Ward Service, alternating at first with Dr. Louis Laplace. The combination of military experience, inpatient service, and clinic duties fitted him uniquely for his new position.

In 1968 the Emergency Service moved from the first floor of the Curtis Building to the ground level of the Thompson Annex Building, a site formerly occupied by the Clinical Amphitheater. The new location with improved accessibility and advanced design proved helpful in promoting the type of sensitive care that characterized Dr. Keiserman's medical practices. His background of interest in the arts, history, and philosophy with a light touch provided special features even in this unlikely setting. The Emergency Room was a popular teaching medium at a time when many people were using its facilities because of the diminishing availability of physician services in local neighborhoods. Jefferson students were well served in their contacts with Dr. Keiserman and his staff.

The Division and Family Medicine

Coincident with the formation of the Division of General Medicine, there was increasing public concern that doctors no longer made house calls. With the increasing numbers of specialists the availability of Primary Care or Personal Physicians was rapidly diminishing. Partially in response to this need on the national level, the American Board of Family Practice was established in 1969. This specified a three-year residency with additional training in Medicine, Pediatrics, Obstetrics-Gynecology, and Ophthalmology, with the aim of preparing the physicians for total family care. Private and government funds were becoming available for training programs in Family Practice or Family Medicine throughout the country. Dean William F. Kellow was very interested in this new specialized class of physicians, an enthusiasm that was not shared by the Chairman of Medicine, Dr. Robert I. Wise. With the persistence of Dr. Kellow and the cooperation of Dr. Willard A. Krehl, a Division of Family Medicine was established in 1971 in the Department of Community Health and Preventive Medicine, with Dr. Paul C. Brucker as Professor and Director. Dr. Brucker was a graduate of the School of Medicine of the University of Pennsylvania and organizer of a highly successful group of Family Physicians. In 1973, the new Division was reconstructed as a full Department of Family Medicine with Dr. Brucker as Professor and Chairman.

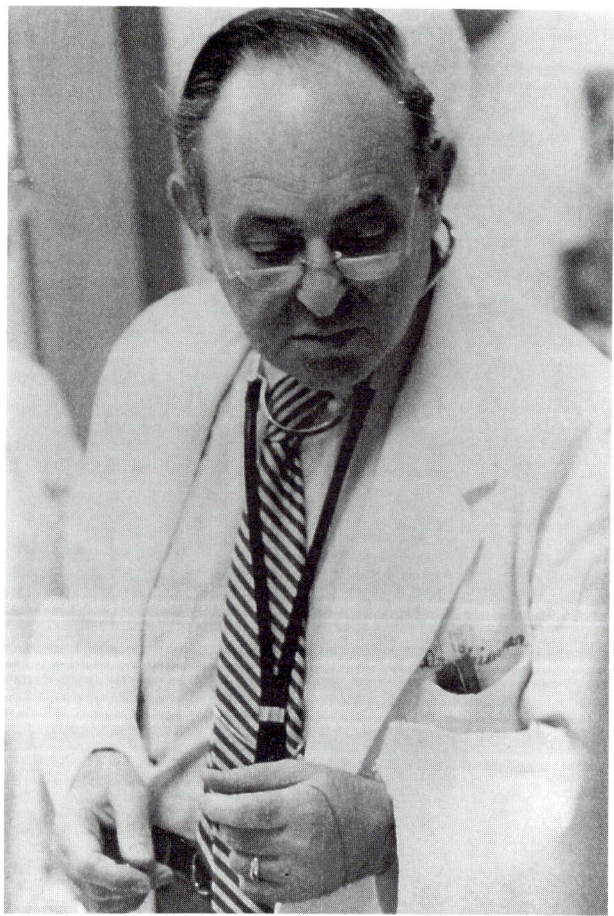

Fig. 19-3. Joseph Keiserman, M.D.; teacher, humanitarian, clinician; First Emergency Room Director (1966).

In 1973 plans were initiated to coordinate the services of the Departments of Medicine and Family Practice. It was agreed that inpatient services would be the responsibility of the Department of Medicine but utilized by both Departments. The ambulatory service would be the responsibility of Family Practice but utilized by both Family Practice and the Division of General Medicine. Reciprocal appointments to the two services were planned but not definitively realized.

Further Division Changes

The year 1972 was a time of further changes in the Division of General Medicine in the Department of Medicine.[5] There was a gradual decrease in emphasis on the Laboratory of Clinical Medicine course; outpatient clinics were gradually closing as the number of patients declined in response to the rising acquisition of medical insurance. The General Medical Clinic closed in 1975. The third element of the Division, the Emergency Ward, actually came under the Department of Surgery. Thus the Division was more a titular than a practical concept.

Residencies and Fellowships were planned for General Medicine. The changing nature of the components of this Division, however, and the announcement by Dr. Wise of plans for early retirement discouraged efforts in this direction. Outpatient offices were established so that Residents who cared for unassigned hospital patients could continue to care for them as outpatients. This was an effort to increase their experience in ambulatory care. Another effort in this direction was the assignment of 46 members of the Department of Medicine to the Division of General Medicine early in 1976. Forty of these physicians had primary appointments in other Divisions.

Dr. Hodges Retires

Dr. Hodges, who had changed from geographical full-time (partial salary plus private practice) to full-time status and membership in the practice plan in 1972, accepted leave and retirement from practice on disability, August 1, 1977, and on July 1, 1979, became the Ludwig A. Kind Emeritus Professor of Medicine. In 1981 his portrait was presented to the University by colleagues and friends. He served as Alumni Trustee for two terms on the Board of Trustees of Thomas Jefferson University (1978–1984). In 1984 the Board elected him as an Emeritus member and he continued to serve actively.

Dr. John H. Martin, Division Director

A new Director of the Division of General Medicine, Dr. John H. Martin (Figure 19-4), was appointed by Dr. Gray in 1978 along with his responsibilities as Associate Chairman of the Department of Medicine.[6] Dr. Martin (M.D., Temple University School of Medicine, 1958), had received the M.S. degree from the University of Minnesota after serving three years at the Mayo Clinic. Following two years in the Medical Corps of the Army Air Force, he returned to the Mayo Clinic as a consultant for a year and then spent a year studying rheumatology at Temple University. A recipient of the Philip S. Hench Scholarship Award, a member of Alpha Omega Alpha, and certified by the American Board of Internal Medicine and the subspecialty Rheumatology, he was well qualified when he came to Jefferson. Under Dr. Martin the Division assumed responsibility for the entire Medical Residency program, while the Department of Medicine provided office space and support personnel.[6]

New Division Responsibilities

One of the new services offered by this Division was consultation coverage for the Wills Eye Hospital. This service provided routine and emergency coverage for the internal medicine problems of the patients. It did not preclude a physician on the Wills staff from using any other Jefferson physician as a consultant, but it

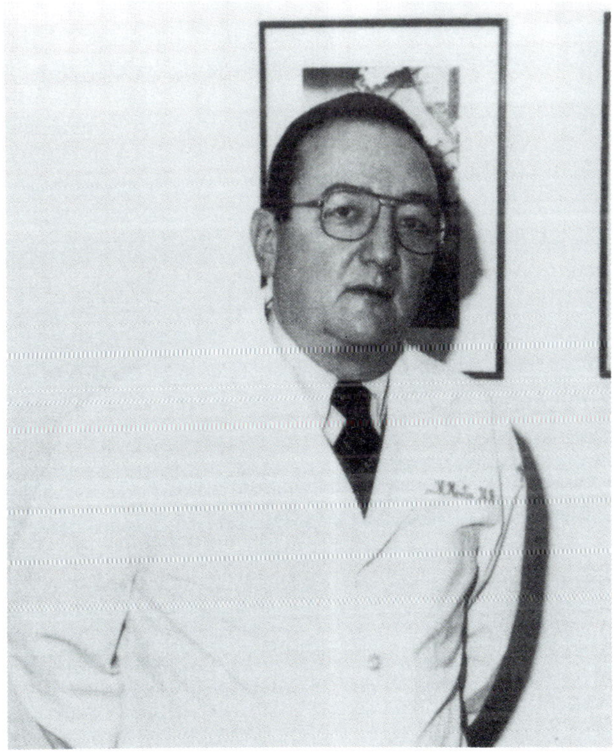

FIG. 19-4. John H. Martin, M.D.; Director, Division of Internal (General) Medicine (1978–1986).

guaranteed that, if called, a member of the Division would respond immediately to requests for emergency consultation and provide same-day response for routine consultations. Later, similar service was extended to other Jefferson programs. At the time of his appointment, Dr. Martin was the sole full-time member of the Division. In 1979 he recruited Dr. Alan G. Adler and Dr. Guy E. McElwain, Jr., as Instructors in the developing Division. Members of the Divison were also responsible for unassigned medical patients admitted to Jefferson Hospital and for monitoring the Residents' Ambulatory Patient follow-up program. Dr. Martin emphasized preoperative medical consultations, and recruited Dr. Geno J. Merli (Jefferson, 1975) to strengthen these activities.[7]

Dean William F. Kellow died December 3, 1981, having retired just a few weeks earlier. Dr. Gray was named Interim Dean. In turn, Dr. Martin assumed the duties of Interim Chairman of the Department of Medicine on November 16, 1981. He continued the dual responsibilities of the Department and of the Division of General Medicine until the appointment of Dr. Willis C. Maddrey in 1982. The Division prospered in this interval. Dr. Martin introduced innovations in house staff function with reference to order writing, weekend charting, and chart dictation. A workshop was presented at the Annual Meeting of the American College of Physicians in Philadelphia in 1982 involving all members of the Division. From this presentation there evolved a manual, a yearly course, and a publication that included instruction in Preoperative Medical Consultation. The group also evolved a course for Residents designed to instruct them in methods of teaching and in designing research projects. A teaching course was devised to be given under the auspices of the American College of Physicians and the American Organization of Program Directors.

Change of Division Name

Dr. Maddrey changed the name of the Division from General Medicine to Internal Medicine in 1983. It may be noted that the Society for Research and Education in Primary Care Internal Medicine (SREPCIM)[8] was founded in 1978 with a grant to the American College of Physicians from the Robert Wood Johnson Foundation. In January of 1986 there appeared the inaugural issue of the *Journal of General Internal Medicine,* a bimonthly journal for general and primary care internists.[9] The American College of Physicians maintained a strong interest in this group and did not wish to see it separate into a specialty fragmented from internal medicine. The new name for the Division was in accord with this ideal.

The Division continued to advance in the areas of medical consultation, ambulatory care (from offices located on the fourth floor of the New Hospital), postgraduate education, and research. Dr. Martin resigned his position in March of 1986. Dr. Geno J. Merli (Figure 19-5) was appointed Acting Director, and early in 1987, he was confirmed as Director.

Dr. Merli (Jefferson, 1975) had completed residencies at Jefferson in both Rehabilitation Medicine and in Internal Medicine. He became Clinical Assistant Professor in each Department in 1981 after having been certified by the American

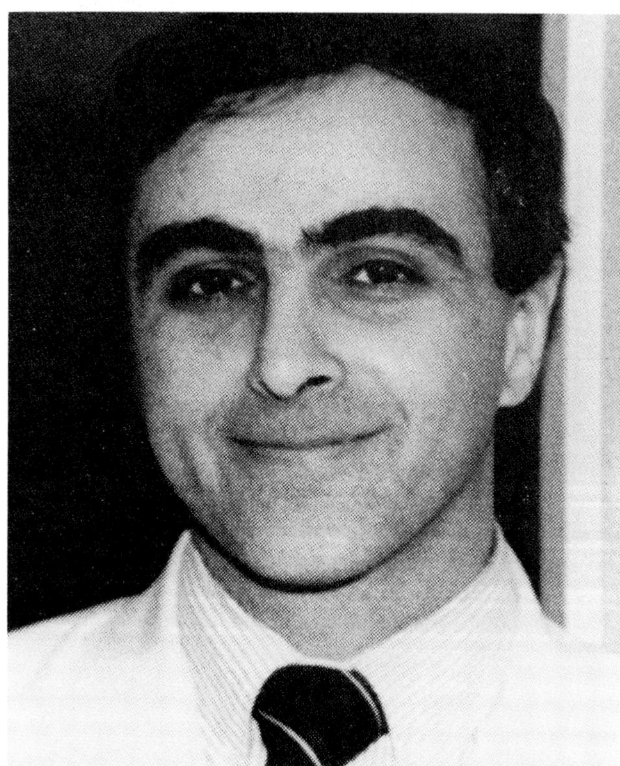

FIG. 19-5. Geno J. Merli, M.D.; Director, Division of Internal (General) Medicine (1987–).

Board of Internal Medicine in 1980. He was involved in the study of drugs, the prevention and treatment of venous thrombosis, and teaching modalities. He also developed workshops on spinal cord injury and consultation evaluation.

It is apparent that Department–Division relationships have been undergoing exploratory and innovative change as part of the pattern of academic progress. This applies particularly to Internal (General) Medicine, Family Medicine, and Preventive Medicine. Because these disciplines vary a good deal among various teaching institutions, the experience at Jefferson is not unusual. Changes in emphasis will surely continue dependent upon perception of need and propriety.

References

1. Wise, R.I., Annual Report, Department of Medicine, Jefferson Medical College of Thomas Jefferson University. July 1, 1968 to June 30, 1969.
2. Idem, 1969–1970.
3. "The Jacob M. DaCosta Memorial Laboratory of Clinical Medicine," *The Jefferson Medical College and its Hospital—Circular of Information, 1913–1914.*
4. DaCosta, J.C., Jr., *Clinical Hematology.* Philadelphia: P. Blakiston's Son & Co., 1901.
5. Wise, R.I., *A History of the Department of Medicine, the Jefferson Medical College of Thomas Jefferson University, 1959–1975.* Camden, Maine, 1986. (In T.J.U. archives)
6. Gray, F.D., Jr., Personal communication.
7. Adler, A.G., Merli, G.J., McElwain, G.E., and Martin, J.H., *Medical Evaluation of the Surgical Patient.* Philadelphia: W.B. Saunders, 1985.
8. Hook, E.W., "ACP and SREPCIM: A Vital Kinship for Internal Medicine," *Am. Coll. of Phys. Obs.* November 1985, p. 3.
9. Spanier, R., "A Home in the Literature," *Am. Coll. of Phys. Obs.* November 1985, p. 4.

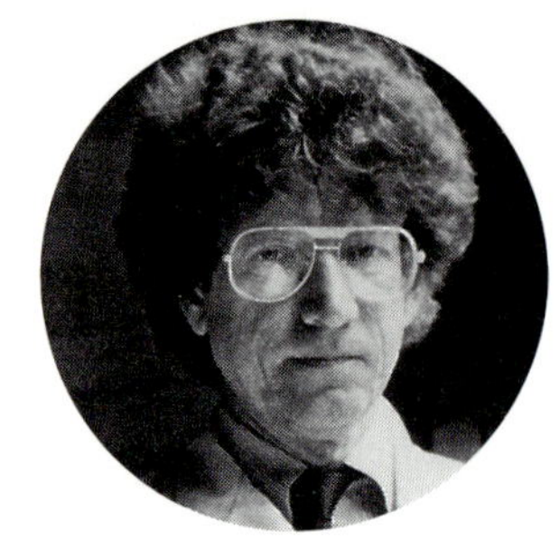

CHAPTER TWENTY

Division of Medical Genetics

Laird G. Jackson, M.D.

"Rare is the tree whose every bud develops into perfect fruit, and if there be such a family tree I find no adequate evidence of it."

—Victor C. Vaughan (1851–1929)

Genetics in the 1960s

The Division of Genetics was established within the Department of Medicine in 1969. Impetus in this field developed in 1960 with the discovery by Drs. Peter Nowell and David Hungerford[1] in Philadelphia of chromosomal changes in chronic myelocytic leukemic cells. Dr. Laird Jackson, a resident in internal medicine, who had been working with Dr. Arthur J. Weiss in 1959 and 1960 on clinical investigation of cancer chemotherapeutic agents, became interested in the cytogenetics of neoplasia. In 1961 his success with the application of cytogenetic techniques attracted requests from pediatric and obstetrical clinicians to detect cytogenetic abnormalities in their patients. The finding of such defects, with the necessity of explaining them to patients, led to the beginning of genetic counseling.

In 1962 a National Institutes of Health research grant for the study of chromosomal nucleic acid processing, and in 1964 a March of Dimes grant for the study of chromosomal histone proteins aided the research of Dr. Jackson. Subsequent fellowship support from the Leukemia Society, expanding into a five-year Leukemia Society Scholarship in 1965, extended his tissue culture and chromosomal research.

At the creation of the Genetic Division by Dr. Robert I. Wise, Chairman of Medicine, Dr. Jackson was appointed Director. Research Fellows from the Oncology Division were provided

Robert L. Brent, Chairman of Pediatrics, provided new space for clinical activity and introduced two additional members, Drs. Gary G. Carpenter (Jefferson, 1960) and Leonard E. Reisman.

training in methods used in cytogenetics and tissue culture. One of these Fellows was Dr. Carla E. Goepp.

In the late 1960s Dr. Leon A. Peris (Jefferson, 1955) of the Obstetrics Department and Dr. Irving J. Olshin of the Pediatrics Department began to combine their interest along with Dr. Jackson across departmental lines. Weekly or biweekly meetings of the three were held to share case experiences, hold informal conferences, and profit from the chromosome laboratory. In 1967, Dr. Roy B. Holly, Chairman of Obstetrics and Gynecology, supported a grant request from the March of Dimes that established a formal Genetic Counseling Clinic, which united the efforts of the Medical and Obstetric Departments. Dr.

Genetics in the 1970s

In 1971 Dr. Peris began genetic prenatal diagnosis with Dr. Jackson and Marie Barr (Figure 20-1). Dr. Peris performed the amniocentesis, and Ms. Barr and Dr. Jackson handled the genetic counseling and the cytogenetic laboratory processing of the tissue cultures and chromosome studies of the amniotic fluid cells. With the training of Dr. Ronald J. Wapner in perinatology and genetics in the mid-1970s, the collaboration with Obstetrics became complete.

Although the Directorship of the Division of Genetics was within the Department of Medicine, Dr. Jackson held Professorships in Medicine, Pediatrics, and Obstetrics and Gynecology. Dr. Susan Z. Cowchock (Jefferson, 1968) and

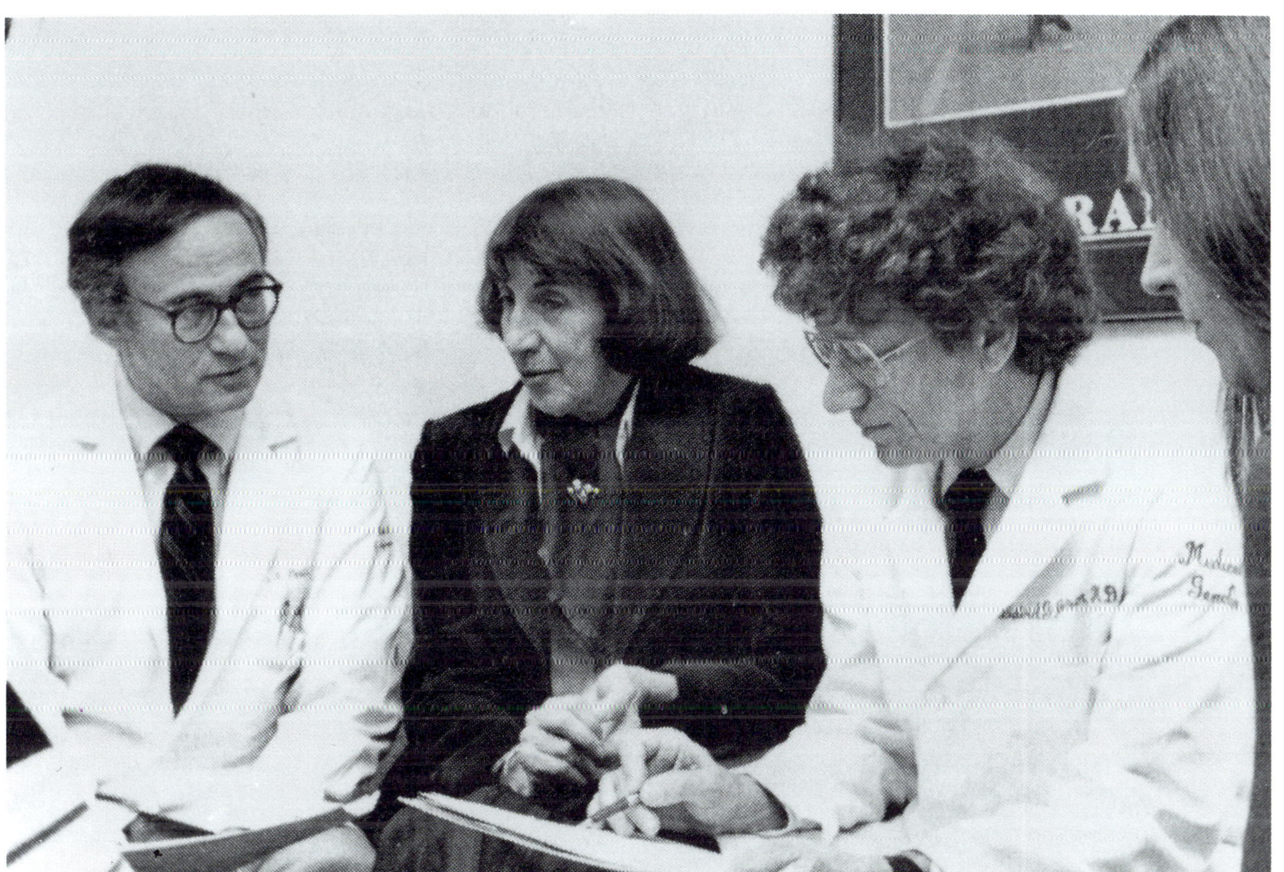

FIG. 20-1. Dr. Leon A. Peris, Ms. Marie Barr, and Dr. Laird G. Jackson conduct genetic counseling.

Eugene E. Grebner augmented the Division. The teaching of genetics was done in several departments both in the preclinical and clinical years for covering the related material in several disciplines: Dr. Arthur Allen included genetics as part of the Cell and Tissue Biology block administered by the Biochemistry Department; Pediatric Genetics and Neurology were taught by Drs. Leonard J. Graziani, Jeanette C. Mason, and Gary G. Carpenter; and Maternal Fetal Medicine was taught in the Department of Obstetrics and Gynecology by Drs. Ronald J. Wapner, Benjamin Chayen, and George Davis.

Clinical service in genetics continued to grow rapidly as applied to diagnosis and counseling. This activity involved six M.D. geneticists or Fellows and four non-M.D. genetic counselors with technical personnel varying in number between six and 14. Several new genetic tools were established within the Division. In 1972 Dr. Susan Cowchock developed the first maternal serum alpha-fetoprotein method in the United States to detect fetal neural tube defects. This program provided a service for the entire Delaware Valley region as well as many areas beyond. In 1972 the Division established one of the country's first Tay-Sachs disease prevention programs. In 1974 Dr. Eugene Grebner headed this effort, became a national leader on the scientific advisory committee, and instituted biochemical genetic research now leading toward contemporary molecular genetic research. This research program was further expanded in 1986 when Dr. David A. Wenger, an internationally known researcher in lysosomal disorders, joined the staff. Dr. Wenger brought a group of three additional laboratory research workers and established a tie with the new Institute of Molecular Medicine with cross-appointments to the Institute and the Department of Biochemistry.

In the mid-1970s Dr. Ronald Wapner established a leading prenatal diagnostic program. Collaborative work with the Division of Ultrasound led to additional innovative procedures. Fetal diagnostic work, always a major activity of the Division, was extended when Dr. Ronald J. Wapner added the fetal medicine program in the late 1970s. In collaboration with Drs. Barry B. Goldberg and Alfred B. Kurtz of the Ultrasound service, early diagnosis of fetal anatomic abnormalities was developed. The most rapidly successful accomplishment occurred when Drs. Wapner and Jackson began work on first-trimester fetal diagnosis by chorionic villus sampling in 1983.[3] This led to an international leadership position in the field of first-trimester diagnosis.

Other innovative diagnostic achievements by the entire genetics team may be anticipated in this rapidly expanding field.

References

1. Nowell, P.C., and Hungerford, D.A., "A Minute Chromosome in Human Chronic Granulocytic Leukemia," *Science* 132. September 1960, p. 1497.
2. Jackson, L., "Prenatal Genetic Diagnosis by Chorionic Villus Sampling (CVS)," *Seminars in Perinatology*. Vol. 9, No. 3, April 1985, pp. 209–217.

CHAPTER TWENTY-ONE

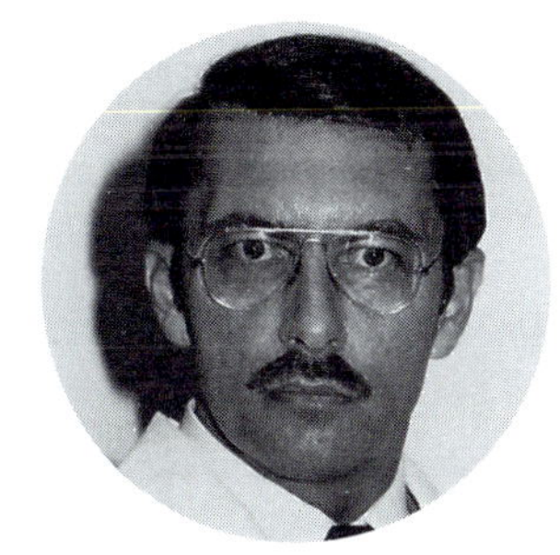

Division of Environmental Medicine and Toxicology

Lance L. Simpson, Ph.D.

"It is evident that efforts to preserve health will be most intelligently and effectually applied when they are based upon an accurate and full knowledge of the agencies which cause disease."

—William H. Welch (1850–1934)

Research, Diagnosis, and Treatment

In the fall of 1984, the Department of Medicine embarked on a new venture, the Division of Environmental Medicine and Toxicology. The Division was planned to comprise three separate but interacting components, as follows: (1) a basic science research component with scientists whose goal would be to determine the mechanism of action of toxins; (2) a clinical services component with physicians board certified in Occupational Medicine and in Medical Toxicology; and (3) a clinical toxicology unit with physicians and scientists who work collaboratively to improve and refine methods for the diagnosis and treatment of poisoned patients.

There are several reasons why the creation of this Division should be seen as a bold venture. Neither Occupational Medicine nor Medical Toxicology has typically been granted more than "backroom" status in Departments of Medicine. Also, relatively few schools of medicine have had full-fledged programs in toxicology at all, the subject usually having been treated as an appendage to the Department of Pharmacology. Flourishing groups in the basic science specialty of toxicology have generally been limited to schools of public health or pharmacy. The initiative of the Department of Medicine in developing a Division of Environmental Medicine and Toxicology equal in status to the other 12 Departmental Divisions represented a break with tradition. It was also a wise anticipation of future needs and opportunities.

Strides toward the reduction of morbidity and mortality have been made in many areas of medicine. Antibiotics and vaccines against infectious diseases, antiarrhythmic and vasoactive drugs against heart disease, anti-inflammatory drugs, and dialysis may be cited as accomplishments. Such advances have caused a refocusing of attention. With the elimination or control of some illnesses, the remaining problems, often of obscure cause, command greater attention. There is clear evidence that many forms of illness are toxin-mediated, with some of the toxins being of natural origin and some man-made. The majority of such toxin-mediated diseases have not been brought under control. It was in the hope of contributing new initiatives in this area that Jefferson embarked on this course.

The past decade has been dominated by what has been called "descriptive and regulatory toxicology." Descriptive toxicology involves the administration of potentially toxic substances to subjects and thereafter attempting to identify and quantify adverse effects. Regulatory toxicology involves the effort to translate laboratory data into risk assessment and then using this to establish guidelines for human exposure to toxic agents.

There are serious drawbacks to the overemphasis of descriptive and regulatory toxicology. Not the least of these is the fact that they involve serious decision making, such as setting limits for human exposure, without knowing the underlying mechanism of toxin action. The Division of Environmental Medicine and Toxicology has been built in a way that is calculated to avoid these difficulties. All of the newly appointed staff members are devoted to research aimed at clarifying the mechanisms by which toxins act, thus providing a more substantive basis for such measures as risk assessment. In addition, it provides the scientific basis for advances in diagnosis and treatment.

The first full-time appointment to the Division was that of Lance L. Simpson, Ph.D., (University of California, Berkeley), who is currently Professor of Medicine and Pharmacology and Chief of Environmental Medicine and Toxicology. Dr. Simpson took his undergraduate degree at Vanderbilt University in Nashville, Tennessee, and did his doctoral work at the University of California in Berkeley. He next did a postdoctoral Fellowship at the College of Physicians and Surgeons of Columbia University. His graduate work was done in the Laboratory of Chemical Biodynamics, under the supervision of Professor Melvin Calvin, a Nobel Laureate. His postgraduate work was done under the joint supervision of Dr. Maurice Rapport, Professor of Psychiatry and Biochemistry, and Dr. S. C. Wang, Professor of Pharmacology, both at the College of Physicians and Surgeons. After completing his studies in 1971, Dr. Simpson joined the staff at the Columbia-Presbyterian Medical Center. He remained there until moving to Jefferson's Medical Department in the fall of 1984.

Dr. Simpson has been working on toxins since his undergraduate days at Vanderbilt University. Most of his effort has been directed toward the study of protein toxins that act on the nervous system. These substances include poisons of microbial origin, such as botulinum toxin and tetanus toxin, as well as poisons of snake venom origin, such as alpha and beta bungarotoxin. This work has several motives, including determining the mechanism of toxin action, determining the structure of toxin molecules and then correlating structure with function, developing drugs for the treatment of poisoned patients, and constructing synthetic vaccines that can be used to immunize patients. More recently, another aspect of toxin-related research has been added. There are certain toxins, or pieces of toxins, that appear to have value as potential therapeutic agents. For example, tissue-targeted toxins that can locate and kill neoplastic cells may have clinical utility in the treatment of cancer. This area of research has now been added to the overall scope of activities.

Although work on protein toxins has been the main theme of Dr. Simpson's research, there was one stretch of time when another aspect of toxicology was undertaken. From the late 1970s until the early 1980s Dr. Simpson was involved in a collaborative research project with the New York City Police Department. The purpose of the work was to assess the effects of illicit drug use on criminal behavior, and thus the project was one in behavioral toxicology. The method used by the investigators was to observe crime while it was occurring. These observations were then compared with data on drug use by the offenders. The crimes of interest were larceny, assault, robbery, and gun-related incidents; the drugs of interest were opioids and central nervous system stimulants. A wealth of data was collected and the findings are to be published in a book that will appear in 1988.

During Dr. Simpson's relatively short tenure as Chief of the Division, he has added four members to the staff. Three of these were principally oriented toward research, and one mainly clinical. The first addition to the research staff was Kevin Chinn, Ph.D., Assistant Professor of Medicine. Dr. Chinn did his graduate work in the Department of Physiology at the University of Hawaii, where he worked under the guidance of Dr. Howard Gillary. While there he took an interest in the use of highly sophisticated electrophysiological techniques as a means for studying the effects of drugs on the nervous system.

In 1981 Dr. Chinn moved on to a postdoctoral Fellowship in the laboratory of Dr. John Lisman at Brandeis University, and two years later he joined the laboratory of Dr. Toshio Narahashi at Northwestern University. During the both of these fellowships Dr. Chinn was able to enhance his electrophysiological skills. In the fall of 1986, he moved to his present position at Jefferson.

Dr. Chinn is one of the few toxicologists in the nation who is capable of using the patch clamp technique for the study of excitable tissues. This technique in microelectrophysiology allows him to study the actions of toxins on individual ion channels in nerves and heart. He is employing the method to analyze the effects of agents such as insecticides on sodium channel behavior. Chinn is responsible for the finding that one insecticide in particular, Deltamethrin, is capable of blocking the transition of sodium channels between the open and closed states. These and other of Dr. Chinn's findings help to explain the cellular and molecular basis for the toxicity of certain poisons.

In addition to this major thrust of his work, Dr. Chinn has developed methods that permit the injection of real or suspected toxins into individual cells that are grown in tissue culture. This is an especially powerful technique, and it promises to help resolve the mechanism of action of many toxic agents. It is potentially a method for examining the effects of therapeutic agents as well.

The next member to join the Division was Dr. Charles Mactutus, Ph.D., Assistant Professor of Medicine, an investigator trained both in toxicology and in the experimental analysis of behavior. Dr. Mactutus did his graduate work with Dr. David Riccion in the Department of Psychology at Kent State University, where he did research in the area of learning and memory. In 1979 he accepted a postdoctoral Fellowship at the Johns Hopkins University, where he was able to apply his background in experimental psychology to the study of central nervous system toxicology. While at Johns Hopkins, he performed a series of experiments to examine the influence of prenatal carbon monoxide exposure on learning and memory of the offspring. This work, which was designed to provide a model of cigarette smoking during pregnancy, demonstrated persistent alterations in memory. The research was widely cited, both in the scientific press and in the lay press.

Dr. Mactutus moved from Johns Hopkins to accept a position at the National Institute for Environmental Health Sciences. He was instrumental in forming and leading a group of investigators who studied the effects of toxins on central nervous system development. The group examined a number of environmental substances, including tetraethyl and triethyl lead. In early 1987 Mactutus joined Jefferson's faculty. He is establishing a new program in central nervous system toxicology that emphasizes a multidisciplinary focus; using a lifespan approach, he will perform psychological and toxicological studies aimed at assessing the impact of prenatal or early neonatal exposure to toxins on subsequent neurological and psychological development.

The most recent recruit to the Division is Dr. Masaru Tanaka, Ph.D., who is a Research Associate. Dr. Tanaka did his entire training at the University of Tokyo, and later for many years was a member of the Faculty at the University of Hawaii. Dr. Tanaka is an expert in the field of protein chemistry. He has developed exquisite methods for the isolation, purification, and characterization of proteins from both procaryotic and eucaryotic sources. His past work has focused on substances isolated from bacteria as well as substances derived from the mammalian cardiovascular system. Dr. Tanaka has joined the Division to work with Dr. Simpson and will oversee research on the isolation and characterization of protein toxins.

■ Clinical Services

In the spring of 1987 the Division formally initiated its clinical activities by inaugurating an Occupational and Environmental Medicine Clinic. The physician who currently holds principal responsibility in the Clinic is Dr. Jack Snyder. Dr. Snyder (M.D., Northwestern) is an unusually well-trained individual. His medical degree was followed by a law degree at Georgetown University. He completed his Master's Degree in Forensic Science at George Washington University and his Master's in Public Health at Johns Hopkins University. Finally, Dr. Snyder took a Ph.D. degree in the Department of Pharmacology and Toxicology at the Medical College of Virginia. He is licensed to practice both law and medicine.

Dr. Snyder has done postgraduate work in occupational medicine, internal medicine, and pathology. He is board certified by the American Board of Pathology in Anatomic and Clinical Pathology and by the American Board of Medical Toxicology.

Dr. Snyder's main interest in the area of clinical medicine is the acutely and seriously poisoned patient. This interest finds its expression in three different settings: (1) he is responsible for seeing patients who come to the Occupational and Environmental Medicine Clinic; (2) he has a close association with the Emergency Room; poisoned patients who are treated initially in the Emergency Room and who are subsequently candidates for inpatient care are admitted to Dr. Snyder's service; and (3) he is a member of the Advisory Board of the Delaware Valley Regional Poison Control Center. In collaboration with other medical and related professionals, Snyder oversees the activities of the poison information service for Philadelphia and the surrounding areas.

In addition to clinical responsibilities, Dr. Snyder is building a research program. Following up on his Ph.D. thesis work, he is establishing a laboratory that focuses on liver pathology. He is interested in the adverse effects of alcohol on the function of liver membranes, and especially those untoward effects that might be mediated by enzymes such as phospholipase. Beyond this, he is attempting to learn whether there are adverse interactions between alcohol and environmental toxins. Snyder is pursuing the hypothesis that some aspects of what has traditionally been called alcohol-induced liver pathology is in reality the outcome of an interaction between alcohol and environmental substances.

■ A Future Clinical Research Unit

The Clinic will not function separately from teaching and research. It will provide both medical students and house staff with practical opportunities in the diagnosis and treatment of occupational and environmental health problems. The possibility that man-made substances can cause disease has given rise to two rather robust areas of research. Basic scientists have contributed a great deal to our understanding of mechanisms of toxin action. Clinical scientists and investigators trained in public health have provided a wealth of epidemiological data. Both of these have added to our growing knowledge of the link between man-made substances and human illness. However, each has its acknowledged shortcomings. Basic science focuses on the study of animals or tissues obtained from animals, and therefore the data have to be extrapolated to humans. This is sometimes appropriate, sometimes not. Epidemiology, too, has its weakness. The use of statistical techniques and large populations does help to identify broad trends and associations, but it cannot establish whether the illness of a particular individual is due to the specific hazards that surround that individual.

A consensus among investigators in occupational and environmental medicine is that there must be more physicians involved in research. The nature of the research needed is that in which the physician-scientist studies individual patients or specimens obtained from patients. There is a tendency to view patients as though they belong to one or the other of two discrete states, healthy or ill, but this clearly is an oversimplification. When one is dealing with patients exposed to hazardous substances, there is a gradation. There may well be a time when the patient is healthy and a later time when he is ill, but between these two extremes is a period of mounting vulnerability and susceptibility.

It would be a magnificent accomplishment in occupational and environmental medicine if physician-scientists, who are regularly seeing patients from the workplace, could develop chemical markers or related techniques for detecting those individuals who are in transition from a healthy to an ill state. In essence, this would be a meshing of environment medicine with preventive medicine. Not only would this safeguard the welfare of the individual worker, but it would spare what would otherwise have been lost productivity, and it would forestall the entire compensation issue and possible litigation.

The development of markers for incipient disease is a great challenge. Nevertheless, it is a legitimate undertaking for a physician-scientist, and therefore it is a part of the scope of activities of the Division of Environmental Medicine and Toxicology.

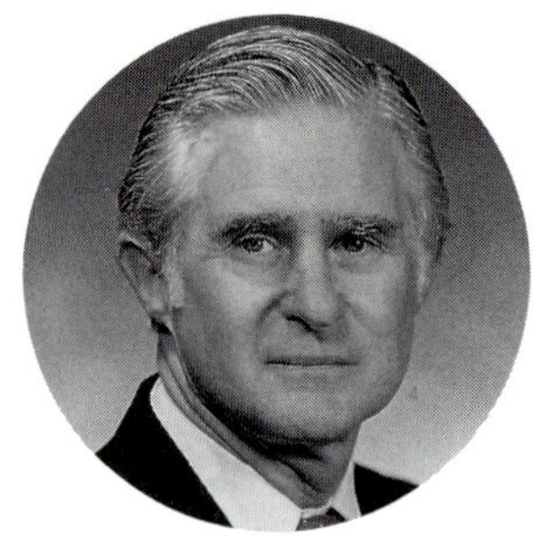

CHAPTER TWENTY-TWO

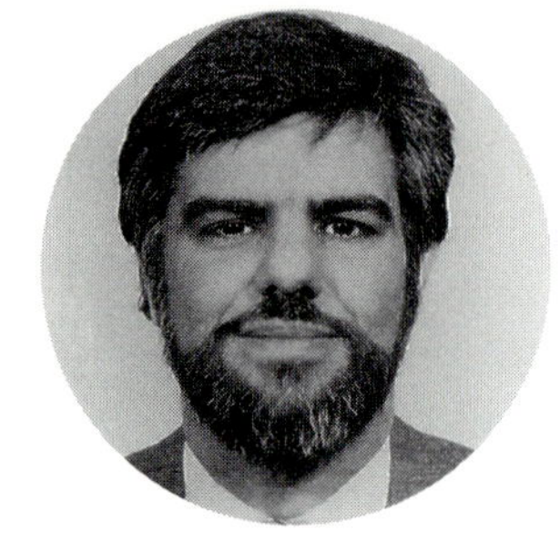

Division of Clinical Pharmacology

William B. Abrams, M.D. and Peter H. Vlasses, Pharm. D.

"The Lord hath created medicines out of the earth; and he that is wise will not abhor them."

—Ecclesiasticus 38:4

Clinical pharmacology is the study of drugs in man. Its two principal components are drug disposition (the effect of the body on the drug) and pharmacodynamics (the effect of the drug on the body). These broad categories have been expanded and combined over the years so that investigations reported under this label have ranged from receptor studies to controlled clinical trials.

The discipline of clinical pharmacology emerged in this country in the 1950s, led by studies of cardiovascular drugs by Harry Gold at Cornell and of human drug metabolism at the Goldwater Memorial Hospital in New York City, and by cardiovascular pharmacology programs at the National Institutes of Health. Academic clinical pharmacology units appeared at Johns Hopkins, Emory, Kansas, Yale, Vanderbilt, and many other universities. The study of drugs in man is, of course, of prime interest to the pharmaceutical industry. Industry-sponsored clinical pharmacology programs thus came on the scene at the same time, modeled after the Lilly unit in Indianapolis, which had been in operation since 1927. Other successful early units were sponsored by Hoffmann-La Roche, Upjohn, and Parke-Davis.

Clinical Pharmacology at Jefferson

Clinical pharmacology, as a special field, was introduced to Jefferson in 1966. In that year, the Smith, Kline & French Foundation provided funds to develop a joint Division of Clinical

Pharmacology in the Departments of Medicine and Pharmacology. Dr. John Capelli (Jefferson, 1962) was appointed Director in 1968.

Dr. Capelli pursued his fellowship training at the Michael Reese Hospital and Jefferson. Following his year as Chief Medical Resident, he was appointed Director of the Division of Clinical Pharmacology and a member of the Division of Nephrology. Dr. Lawrence Wesson was made a member of the Division of Clinical Pharmacology at that time.

Unfortunately, 1968 and 1969 were difficult years in the development of the medical practice plan for members of the full-time Faculty of the Clinical Departments at Jefferson. Dr. Capelli decided to resign his full-time position as Director of the Division of Clinical Pharmacology and enter private medical practice. Dr. Wesson was then appointed Director. Other members of the Division at that time were Drs. Peter Amadio of Wallace Laboratories, Elmer Funk, Jr., and Thomas N. Gates of Merck Sharp & Dohme, and Charles K. Gorby of Lankenau Hospital. This original Division of Clinical Pharmacology continued through June 30, 1973, when it was discontinued because of lack of financial support.

The Present Clinical Pharmacology Division

The present Clinical Pharmacology Program began in 1975 when senior officers of the Merck Sharp & Dohme Research Laboratories (MSDRL) approached their counterparts as Thomas Jefferson University with a proposal for a collaborative clinical pharmacology venture. The proposed arrangement had a number of unique characteristics. Unlike units funded by other pharmaceutical companies elsewhere, the administration and staffing of the Jefferson Unit would be entirely under the control of the University even though the major portion of the financial support would come from MSDRL. An advisory committee with representatives from both institutions initially oversaw the function and direction of the Unit. Although the major Unit effort would be committed to MSDRL studies, other projects from a variety of funding sources could be undertaken. The Unit would be a Division of the Department of Medicine and be located on the fifth floor of the 1907 Main Hospital Building. A letter of understanding that included these provisions was signed by officers from both institutions in December of 1976. Jefferson officials prominent in these early negotiations were Dr. Francis J. Sweeney, Jr., Vice-President, Medical Affairs; Dr. William Kellow, Dean of Jefferson Medical College; Mr. Byron Irwin, Associate Administrator, Thomas Jefferson University Hospital; Dr. Frank D. Gray, Chairman and Professor of Medicine; and Dr. C. Paul Bianchi, Chairman and Professor of Pharmacology. MSDRL was represented by Dr. William B. Abrams (Jefferson, 1947), Executive Director of Clinical Research; Dr. Richard O. Davies, Director, Clinical Pharmacology; Dr. Hubert C. Peltier, Vice-President for Medical Affairs; and Mr. Donald S. Brooks of MSDRL Legal. A letter of understanding was signed by Mr. George M. Norwood, Jr., interim President of Thomas Jefferson University, for Jefferson, and by Dr. P. Roy Vagelos, President of MSDRL, for Merck.

Research

A search committee was formed by the University, and in May 1977 Dr. Roger Ferguson was recruited to be the first Director. He received his medical degree at the University of Utah, then served his residency and was an M.S. in Pharmacology at the University of Iowa. Dr. Ferguson was active in antihypertensive drug research at Michigan State University. He had recently spent a sabbatical leave with Dr. Hans Brunner in Lausanne, Switzerland, where Dr. Ferguson undertook the first human investigation of a new class of agents, the angiotensin converting enzyme inhibitors (ACE inhibitors). Dr. Ferguson recruited the initial staff, and the first clinical study was undertaken in the fall of 1977. Peter H. Vlasses, Pharm.D., was appointed in 1978 as Assistant Director. Dr. Vlasses received his Doctor of Pharmacy degree from the Philadelphia College of Pharmacy and Science (PCPS); his special interest was in cardiovascular drug research.

Administratively, liaison with the Unit was the responsibility of Dr. William B. Abrams, Executive

Director of Clinical Research at Merck. Collaboration was initially implemented by Drs. David Cooper and John Schrogie through Dr. Davies. In 1980, Dr. Abrams assumed the liaison function directly. Dr. Abrams graduated from Jefferson in 1947, interned in Atlantic City, and received postgraduate training at the Children's Hospital of Philadelphia, Philadelphia General Hospital, and St. Louis University. He is a past President of the American Society for Clinical Pharmacology and Therapeutics. Dr. Abrams joined Merck in 1975, having previously been employed by Ayerst Laboratories and Hoffmann-La Roche, Inc. In order to facilitate the arrangements between the institutions, Thomas Jefferson University offered adjunct faculty positions to the Merck liaison officers. Thus, Dr. Abrams has been Adjunct Professor of Medicine since 1977. He received strong support relative to this liaison from Marvin E. Jaffe, M.D., Vice-President of Clinical Research, who was also a Jefferson Medical College graduate and a member of the adjunct faculty in neurology.

The initial direction involved active pursuit of ACE inhibitors and expansion of the Division's human research capabilities. Over the next several years, key personnel additions included Brian N. Swanson, Ph.D., Heschi H. Rotmensch, M.D., and, in a collaborative arrangement with PCPS, Mario L. Rocci, Jr., Ph.D. Dr. Swanson had expertise in assay development, especially high-performance liquid chromatography. Dr. Rotmensch brought expertise in pharmacodynamics, whereas Dr. Rocci was skilled in pharmacokinetic laboratory and data analysis. In this same period, the Unit underwent physical expansion, funded by MSDRL, to accomodate new laboratory and computer data processing facilities. With the assembling of this critical mass, the Division became very productive in its clinical research efforts.

The evaluation of ACE inhibitors in hypertension at Jefferson included dose-response, mechanism of action, comparative efficacy, and drug interaction studies with captopril, enalapril, and lisinopril. The ACE inhibitors subsequently have received extensive use in hypertension and congestive heart failure. The important Jefferson contributions to this field are summarized in a text edited by Drs. Ferguson and Vlasses, published in 1987.

Over its ten-year existence, 131 studies of new compounds were conducted by the Division of Clinical Pharmacology. Important contributors over this time also included Louis J. Reilly, Jr., M.D., and Michael D. Cressman, D.O. A wide range of therapeutic categories was represented, including diuretics, nonsteroidal anti-inflammatory drugs, antibiotics, ophthalmologic agents, and psychotherapeutic drugs. In general, this was an unprecedented period of research productivity in this field.

Many studies at Jefferson characterized the pharmacokinetics of the different investigational compounds in man. The special emphasis on pharmacodynamic assessments in these trials led to the development or application of many clinical and laboratory drug evaluation techniques. Important contributions in healthy volunteer experiments included the unraveling of the differential clinical pharmacology of the enantiomers of indacrinone, a uricosuric diuretic, and the assessment of systemic beta-blockade after dermal and ophthalmic application of timolol and other compounds. Parviz Mojaverian, Ph.D., undertook studies with the Heidelberg capsule, a pH-sensitive, radiotelemetric device. These studies led to important contributions to the understanding of the physiology of the interdigestive migrating myoelectric complex and pharmaceutical considerations dealing with gastric indigestible dosage forms (for example, enteric coated and sustained-release tablets). The nature and mechanism of many drug–drug interactions have also been evaluated. Close collaboration between Jefferson and Merck clinical and basic scientists evolved over this time. Extremely efficient processing of studies has resulted, facilitated by industrywide innovations in research data telecommunications. To date, well over 125 research and scholarly publications bearing the Jefferson affiliation have resulted from these evaluations. Recent research efforts have emphasized drugs affecting the prostaglandins and leukotrienes and their involvement in inflammation, pain, and local vascular regulation.

▪ Education, and Service

In addition to research efforts, the Division of Clinical Pharmacology has participated actively in Jefferson Medical College's education and service programs. Since 1977 the Division has offered a well-received fourth-year medical student elective course in clinical pharmacology employing a case-simulation format. Twelve postdoctoral (M.D., Ph.D., or Pharm.D.) Fellows as well as graduate and undergraduate medical and pharmacy students received training in the Division. Many faculty held cross-appointments in pharmacology, and a close working relationship evolved with many physician collaborators and the Hospital's Department of Pharmacy, directed by Joe E. Smith, Pharm.D. Unit faculty have served as teacher for the medical students, provided consultation for hospitalized and ambulatory patients on drug-related problems, served on pertinent comittees (for example, Pharmacy and Therapeutics, the Institutional Review Board) and have contributed to a variety of community services and professional organizations, both locally and nationally. In this regard, Dr. Vlasses was a founding member of the American College of Clinical Pharmacy in 1979, subsequently served as national President in 1983, and was honored as a Fellow in 1985.

Dr. Ferguson left Jefferson in 1985 to assume the Chair in Medicine at the University of Nevada at Reno. Discussions between Jefferson and MSDRL officers at that time led to a reaffirmation of the commitment of each party. The desire of both institutions was to maintain the activities in clinical research and to add investigations of a basic and mechanistic nature to this collaborative research effort. A revised letter of understanding, with funding commitment for a five-year renewal period, was executed in 1986. Key figures in the discussions leading to the continuation agreement in addition to Dr. Abrams were Willis C. Maddrey, M.D., Chairman of the Department of Medicine; Lewis W. Bluemle, M.D., President of Thomas Jefferson University; Marvin Jaffe, M.D., Vice-President of Clinical Research; and Edward Scolnick, M.D., President of MSDRL.

At this time, the role of the MSDRL Liaison was assumed by Dr. Keith H. Jones, Executive Director for Clinical Pharmacology. Dr. Jones received his medical degree at the University of Wales in 1966 and a Diploma in Pharmaceutical Medicine from the Royal College of Physicians in London in 1976. Prior to coming to MSDRL in 1979, he was employed by Beecham Pharmaceuticals, Surrey, England for ten years. Dr. Jones was appointed Adjunct Professor of Medicine at Jefferson in 1986.

A national search by Dr. Maddrey led to the recruitment of Thorir D. Bjornsson, M.D. as Director of the Division of Clinical Pharmacology in 1986. Dr. Bjornsson received his medical degree at the University of Iceland. He trained in clinical pharmacology at Stanford University and held previous faculty positions in clinical pharmacology at Duke University. He serves on the pharmacology study section of the National Institutes of Health.

As an expression of the commitment to clinical pharmacology and the desire to expand the scope of Divisional research, Dr. Maddrey provided funds for construction of a new Divisional facility encompassing 11,000 square feet of laboratory, clinical, and office space in the new Medical Office Building. The new Divisional facilities opened in April, 1987.

Dr. Bjornsson established three Sections within the Division: the Laboratory for Thrombosis and Atherosclerosis Research, which he heads; the Clinical Research Unit, headed by Dr. Vlasses; and the Laboratory for Investigative Medicine, headed by Dr. Rocci. Each Section has specific interests and functions as well as collaborative activities. Merck-funded projects as well as research programs funded through other sources (federal, foundation, and other pharmaceutical companies) are now commonly undertaken by the Divisional faculty. Divisional faculty are committed to developing a stronger program in drug development through clinical and basic research and training of future clinical pharmacologists. Dr. Bjornsson received a prestigious Pharmaceutical Manufacturers' Association Development Grant for Clinical Pharmacology in 1987 for expansion of the Division mission.

Thus, the decade spanning 1977–1987 has seen the evolution of a nationally recognized program in clinical pharmacology at Jefferson that would not have been possible without the strong collaborative venture with MSDRL. As the second decade begins, enthusiasm runs high for continued growth and recognition in an even broader realm of research as advances in biotechnology provide novel agents for the treatment of human disease.

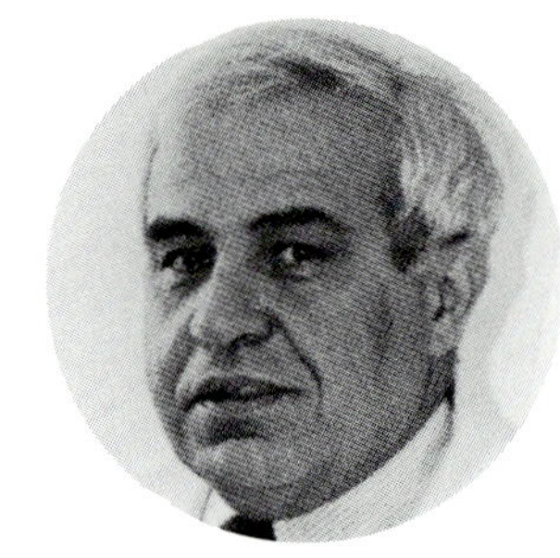

CHAPTER TWENTY-THREE

Department of Family Medicine

PAUL C. BRUCKER, M.D.

"Almost every one who goes to bed counts upon a full night's rest: Like a picket at the outposts, the doctor must be ever on call."

—KARL F. H. MARX (1796–1877)

The Specialization of Health Care

The famous Flexner report of 1910 resulted in the closing of many substandard medical schools and placed a long-needed emphasis on the scientific foundation for the practice of medicine. This shifted clinical instruction from a preceptorial, outpatient setting into the teaching hospitals. The report heralded the emphasis that was to be placed on full-time clinical faculty. As a result, most of the efforts in clinical teaching were directed to the study of life-threatening disease that necessitated hospitalization. Medical education and research dealt primarily with selected, serious problems from an unselected population. As more specific, organ-related knowledge developed, the various specialties evolved.

In the 1950s there was a tremendous infusion of federal monies into the medical schools for biomedical research and research training. Understandably, these efforts were primarily directed to the dread diseases that required hospitalization. The teaching hospitals, not the outpatient setting, were the clinical laboratories. Efforts were more directed toward the prolongation of life rather than the prevention of disease. Great strides in the technology of medicine were the result. Open-heart surgery was initiated and followed closely by dialysis and transplantation, just to mention a few of the exciting, almost miraculous accomplishments.

As a result of all of this activity and the seemingly endless supply of resources for research, the generalists in medicine began to disappear. There was a steady rise in the absolute number and proportion of specialists. The best students followed able medical school role models and were attracted to specialty careers, whereas those who were less talented became the generalists. Even the general internist, who generically viewed himself as the "doctor's doctor" or the diagnostician, began to disappear. Bright medical school graduates were attracted to specialties where the "action" and generous rewards existed. Specialty training programs forced more fragmentation of medicine, both from an organizational and practice standpoint.

By contrast, in Great Britain there were three primary care physicians for every specialist, whereas in the United States there were four specialists for every general practitioner. As a result, many United States citizens were concerned that they could not find a well-trained, available personal physician. Patients felt that the continuity and comprehensiveness of their care left much to be desired, and that medicine in general had become very fragmented and detached. Prevention, health care, and attention to the psychological needs and the effect of illness on the social unit were being ignored.

In 1964, all of this societal concern was formalized in the reports of two government-appointed commissions, the Willard and Millis Commissions. Both of these well-constructed reports proved to be a tremendous stimulus in making the medical community and the government formally aware that the disappearance of the generalist in medicine was having great negative implications. Furthermore, the allopathic physicians, most of whom were specialists and very dependent upon referrals from primary care physicians, were alarmed that such individuals were disappearing. Reluctantly, allopathic, specialty physicians in urban areas had to be more and more dependent upon the primary care osteopaths, who were rapidly becoming the only referring primary care physicians in the community.

Nationally, the general practitioners were concerned lest they disappear from the scene of American medicine. They too felt that their presence was greatly needed, but in order to improve their stature and do away with the second-class label of the "local medical doctor" (LMD), they had to upgrade their image by improving the qualifications of those entering practice. Consequently, over a five-year period they were finally able to convince organized medicine that there should be a three-year specialty training program in family practice. The American Board of Family Practice was established in 1969. This was achieved after the American Board of Internal Medicine in 1964 refused to accept family practice as a legitimate discipline or specialty subdivision. Dr. Nicholas J. Pisacano, the first Executive Secretary of the American Board of Family Practice, was largely responsible for leading organized medicine through endless negotiations to recognize that the specialty of family practice would be good for academic medicine and for health care delivery in the United States. Jefferson's Dean, Dr. William F. Kellow, and Dr. Pisacano knew each other well, for they worked together on national committees. They respected each other, and Dean Kellow frequently consulted Dr. Pisacano about the new specialty and the possibility of establishing a new family medicine program at Jefferson.

Following these national discussions, Dean Kellow and the senior faculty decided to explore the possibilities of developing a program in family practice to help meet these manpower needs. In 1967 he invited Dr. Franklin C. Kelton from Ambler and Dr. David Kistler from Wilkes-Barre, two leaders and representatives of the Pennsylvania Academy of Family Physicians, to meet with him. They discussed how the training of the primary care physician might best be accomplished. Both of these family physicians spent a great deal of time and effort at Jefferson in attempting to explain how and why family practice should be a distinct program in the Medical College.

The Beginning of Family Medicine at Jefferson

In 1971 as a result of all the societal, political, and professional influences, the faculty under the leadership of Dean Kellow agreed to establish a Division of Family Medicine in the Department of Community and Preventive Medicine. Dr. Willard Krehl, the Professor and Chairman of that Department, was most enthusiastic, supportive, and helpful. With the assistance of Dr. Franklin Kelton and Dr. David Kistler, he established elective preceptorships in family practice. The Pennsylvania Academy of Family Physicians helped to recruit 25 family physicians as preceptors. In the program's first year, 40 Jefferson students elected to take the six-week family practice elective. They were keenly interested, and the physician-preceptors were enthusiastic. Family practice had officially come to Jefferson. Shortly thereafter, in 1972 the Medical College and the University Hospital agreed to form a new Department of Family Medicine. This culminated a seven-year dialogue among all concerned, and a search committee was formed.

Dr. Joseph Gonnella, then Assistant Dean in Charge of Academic Affairs, was responsible for recommending Dr. Paul C. Brucker to the search committee for the Chairmanship. Dr. Brucker and Dr. Gonnella had worked together in helping to devise a system for the evaluation of medical care at the Chestnut Hill Hospital in Philadelphia. Over a four-year period they had established a strong professional relationship.

When Dr. Brucker was initially asked to be a candidate for such a position, he was not interested, for he was very content in his private group family practice in Ambler, Pennsylvania, a suburb of Philadelphia. There, in a 100-year-old practice, he and three other family physicians enjoyed a successful group family practice. One of his partners, Dr. Franklin C. Kelton, was the individual who had been so instrumental in helping Jefferson decide upon the formation of the new Department.

Dr. Gonnella convinced Dr. Brucker to at least meet with the search committee. Ironically, Dr. Brucker's first scheduled appearance before the search committee was well known to the entire committee, but not to Dr. Brucker. Dean Kellow discovered this oversight and called Dr. Brucker the evening before his scheduled appearance to apologize for not officially notifying him of the meeting. After a good chuckle with Dean Kellow, Dr. Brucker rearranged his schedule and appeared the next day. He was impressed by the composition of the committee and the depth of their understanding as to what a new Department would entail. This was a tribute to the preparatory work that the Medical College had done prior to deciding to form such a Department. After an enjoyable three-hour meeting with the committee, Dr. Brucker returned to Ambler, only to be called that same evening and be informed by Dean Kellow that the committee was extremely interested in him as a candidate. He wanted Dr. Brucker to meet with the various Chairmen in the College. Several stood out. Dr. Thomas Duane, the Chairman of the Curriculum Committee and Professor and Chairman of the Department of Ophthalmology, was most helpful in explaining the intent of the anticipated, revised curriculum, a curriculum that would provide a mandatory clerkship in family medicine. Dr. Robert Brent, Professor and Chairman of the Department of Pediatrics, lent additional encouragement. Dr. Robert Wise, the Magee Professor and Chairman of the Department of Medicine, cautiously supported the concept of the new Department, but did have reservations about the quality of training that the Department would be able to deliver.

Dean Kellow, Associate Dean Gonnella, and Dr. Kelton, plus the receptive atmosphere at Jefferson, all helped to convince Dr. Brucker that accepting the new position would be a true opportunity. On January 1, 1973, he was appointed the new Professor and Chairman of the Department, both in the Medical College and the University Hospital (Figure 23-1).

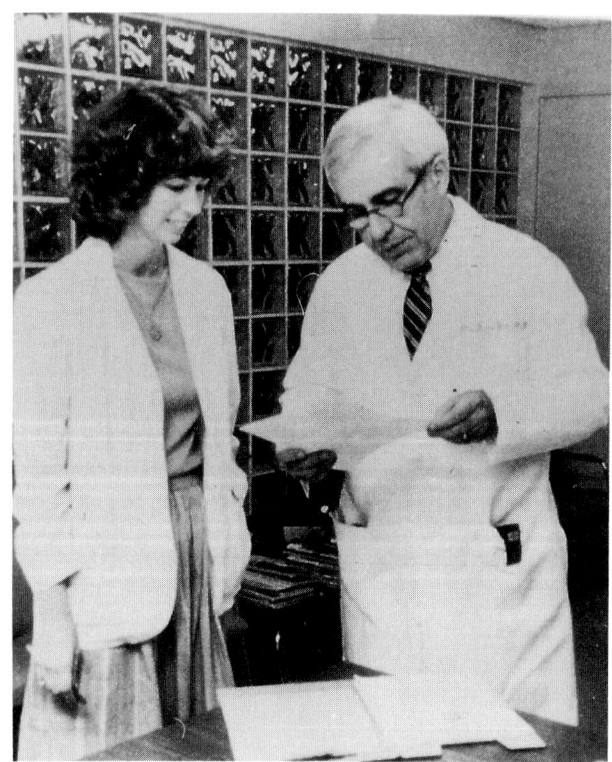

FIG. 23-1. Paul C. Brucker, M.D.; First Chairman, Department of Family Medicine, (1974–).

Almost simultaneously with Dr. Brucker's acceptance of the position, Richard Bennett, President of the Haas Community Fund, called Dean Kellow to see why a new Chairman had not been appointed and why the monies that the Foundation had donated to help form the new Department had not yet been used. When Dean Kellow informed him that Dr. Brucker had accepted the invitation to chair the Department, he was somewhat astounded, for Dr. Brucker had been his friend and personal physician for 13 years. Fortunately, this relationship continued even after Dr. Brucker moved from Ambler to Jefferson; Mr. Bennett was the first Family Practice patient at Jefferson.

▪ The Beginning of the Department

When Dr. Brucker first arrived on campus in March, 1973, newly renovated space in the old Scott Library, located on the first floor of the 1025 Walnut Street Medical College, was just about completed. This new, attractive facility consisted of five offices for faculty members, one office for the Chairman, and adequate space for clerical help. The only furniture present, however, was an old army desk and chair, for the furniture that was ordered had not arrived on time.

Dean Kellow met with Dr. Brucker on the first day and charged him with establishing undergraduate, graduate, and postgraduate educational programs, a patient service program, and eventually a research program. He extended his hand of assistance to guide Dr. Brucker through the complexities of accomplishing this. He and the other members of the Dean's Office, including Dr. Gonnella and Mr. Thomas Murray, the Business Administrator for the College, were always available for assistance.

The Undergraduate Family Medicine Curriculum

The Department constructed a curriculum for the first mandatory Family Medicine Junior Clerkship, which was initiated in the fall of 1974. This curriculum paid attention to developing an ambulatory experience that would provide ready access for patients, allow for continuity and comprehensiveness of care, and pay attention to the psychosocial needs of the family. Simultaneously, a curriculum was designed for the senior-year elective track in Family Medicine.

Initially, a big problem was where to place 223 Junior students so that the ambulatory clerkship would fulfill the curricular goals. In order to accomplish this, the Department looked to existing Jefferson affiliated institutions. An approved family practice residency existed at the Wilmington Medical Center where Dr. Dene Walters was the Program Director. It soon followed that the Wilmington Medical Center became a site for a family medicine clerkship. Likewise, because Chestnut Hill Hospital was affiliated with Jefferson, plans were made to develop a family medicine affiliation there. After some discussion, Dr. Harry Kaplan became the first director of the program at Chestnut Hill.

With the assistance of Dean Kellow and Associate Dean John Killough, an affiliation discussion was started with the Richard K. Mellon Foundation and representatives of the Latrobe Area Hospital in Latrobe, Pennsylvania. The Latrobe Area Hospital wanted to establish a medical school affiliation in order to improve the quality of care, to attract even better medical staff, and to serve as a training site for sorely needed family physicians in their community. With the help of Drs. Robert Mazero, Joseph Govi, and Robert Gordon, the affiliation materialized in 1973, and shortly thereafter an affiliate family practice residency program was established. With generous funding from the Mellon foundation, the hospital built a clinical facility in which the students could see outpatients, and also established residential housing for the undergraduate students and residents.

Sufficient clerkship spots were located for all of the students, curriculum time was granted by the Curriculum Committee and approved by the professorial faculty, and the Department was off on its undergraduate educational mission.

The Latrobe affiliation, along with a societal concern for better distribution of family physicians, led to the establishment of the Physician Shortage Area Program (PSAP) in 1974. The Medical College agreed to preferentially accept up to 12 qualified students into the Freshman class who came from urban or rural underserved physician areas in Pennsylvania, who in turn would pursue the family medicine curriculum, family medicine residency training, and upon finishing that training return to an underserved area. In 1978 the program was expanded to include 24 students. This unique program was most successful. Since 1978, many students have entered family practice in underserved areas of Pennsylvania.

■ The Residency Program

Initially, an attempt to establish an approved family practice residency at the Thomas Jefferson University Hospital failed. The residency application was not approved when reviewed in September, 1973. The same day that Chairman Brucker received notice of this disapproval he arranged an immediate consultative appointment in Kansas City, Missouri, with Dr. Robert Graham, the educational representative of the American Academy of Family Physicians. He and Dr. Graham stayed up until the early hours of the next morning rewriting the application, which was then retyped and resubmitted the next day. Finally, provisional approval was gained in December 1973, and the Department made plans to initiate the first family practice residency at Jefferson in July, 1974.

After approval was gained, Dr. Brucker tried to obtain funding for the family practice residency positions, which represented a total of 18 spots for the three-year program. This was a frustrating struggle, since each Department and residency program also wished to expand and did not wish to give up any positions. The new Chairman met with many committees, administrative persons, and Chairman of Departments. All of this was to no avail, and no funds were allocated.

Dr. Peter Herbut, President of the University, asked Dr. Brucker to give a progress report about the new Department to the Board of Trustees. When it became apparent that sharing the information about a lack of funding for the residency positions would prove embarrassing to the President, Dr. Brucker met with him three days before the scheduled meeting and asked that he be excused from giving the report to the Board. With a single phone call Dr. Herbut found the funds necessary for the residency, and Dr. Brucker was able to give a glowing progress report to the Board some three days later.

Unfortunately, the late residency approval and late source of funding did not allow the Jefferson family practice program to recruit vigorously across the nation. Consequently, in the inaugural class of residents only four out of six positions were filled through the traditional National Intern and Resident Matching Program. Two additional residents were enlisted outside of the Match. The full complement of six entered the residency in July, 1974. These pioneers in a completely new, three-year residency program and the medical schools that they graduated from were: David Cheli, M.D. (Medical College of Pennsylvania); Sandra Harmon, M.D. (Temple University); Franklin Kelton, Jr., M.D. (Jefferson, 1974); Allan Kogan, M.D. (Baylor School of Medicine); James Plumb, M.D. (Jefferson, 1974); and Margaret Stockwell, M.D. (University of Nebraska).

■ Facilities

When the Department was started, it had neither clinical space nor patient population, two requisites for both the undergraduate and graduate programs. Monies were available from the Haas Community Fund and the Department of Health, Education and Welfare for the development of the overall program. The government's funds had to be used by July 1, 1973. In early June, 1973, Dr. Brucker requested that these funds be approved for the building of the first family practice center on the fifth floor of the Jefferson-owned Edison building at Ninth and Sansom Streets. Quickly, with the assistance of the University architect he helped to design a new 8,000 square-foot family practice center that had 28 examining rooms, a small laboratory, and conference rooms. The plans were hand-delivered to Washington, D.C., for approval. This was obtained some three days before the grant expired. Although hurriedly designed, this particular clinical facility worked out very well. It was extremely practical and functional. The Department occupied this facility until 1978, when it moved to the fourth floor of the new University Hospital.

■ Faculty Recruitment

Once curriculum time, a residency program, and a clinical facility were established, Dr. Brucker had to search for qualified faculty. He turned his attention to recruiting able, senior faculty. In addition to assuring that appropriate faculty be chosen to carry out the programs, he was aware that the entire University and its alumni would be viewing his choices with close scrutiny. Faculty selection was considered to be one of the key elements in ensuring the credibility and stability of the Department.

The first person to be contacted was a friend and professional colleague of Dr. Brucker, Dr. Edward H. McGehee (Figure 23-2). Dr. McGehee was trained as an internist, with additional training in pathology and hematology. A Jefferson graduate (Class of 1945), he practiced general internal medicine in the Chestnut Hill section of Philadelphia, where he was a respected, loved "family physician." He worked long and hard, made house calls on his bicycle, had grateful students in his office almost continuously, and had chaired the Department of Medicine at the Chestnut Hill Hospital. He had also held the positions of Physician and Hematologist to the Pennsylvania Hospital and the Benjamin Franklin Clinic. It took many meetings to convince him to join the faculty. Again, Dr. Joseph Gonnella was most helpful in encouraging Dr. McGehee to join as a Professor of Family Medicine in 1974.

The next full-time faculty person to be recruited was Dr. William Mebane, a professional colleague of both Drs. Brucker and McGehee. He too required a great deal of encouragement to leave a very successful and satisfying private group pediatric practice in Chestnut Hill. In 1974 he joined the faculty until 1976, when he moved to the affiliate family medicine program at Chestnut Hill Hospital. There, he served as an Associate Director of the program until 1985, when he became the Director.

Recruiting two of Chestnut Hill's most respected physicians to Jefferson had a marked impact on the Chestnut Hill community. Dr. Brucker received many troubled calls about his recruiting two of the more valued professionals from a single community into the Jefferson program. Fortunately, most of the Chestnut Hill residents understood the importance of good role models and the training of future physicians. Many requested that they be allowed to follow their personal physicians to Jefferson. This loyalty helped to form the initial panel of patients that was so necessary for the training of students and residents.

Outpatients

In order to conduct the ambulatory care program, a large number of patients were required. Although a fair number of the full-time faculty's private patient population followed them to Jefferson, a much larger number of patients was needed.

It was fortuitous that in 1974 the Hospital decided to disband the traditional clinic system and have the clinic patients seen in a more

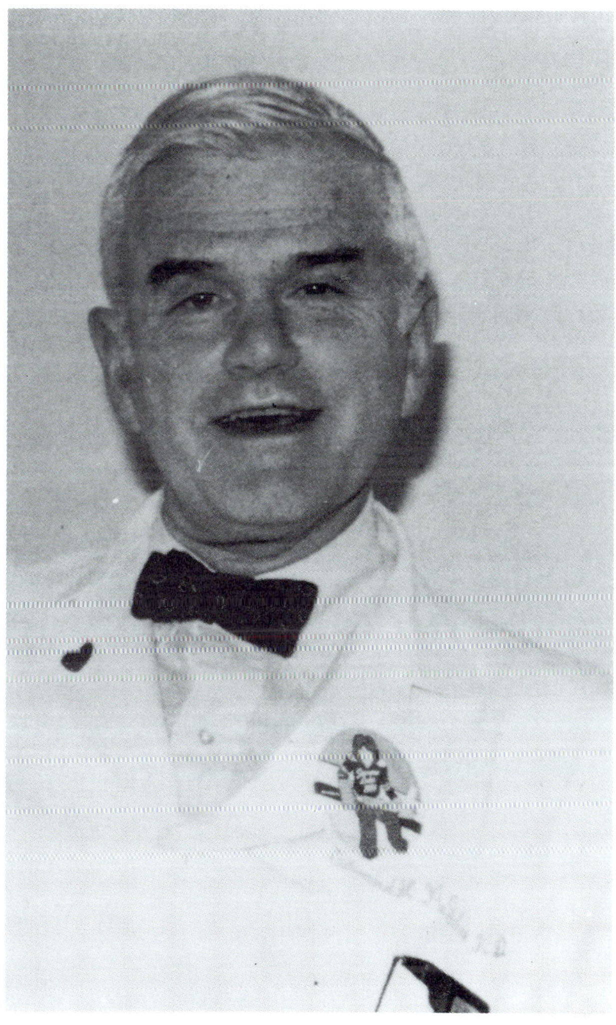

FIG. 23-2. Edward H. McGehee, M.D. (Jefferson, 1945); Ellen M. and Dale W. Garber Professor of Family Medicine.

traditional "private system." The Hospital felt fortunate that a Department existed that was so interested and so in need of adult ambulatory patients. Dean Kellow and Dr. Francis Sweeney, Vice President for Health Affairs, thought that it would be most appropriate for family medicine to assume the care of such patients. The Department of Medicine, long responsible for the Medical Clinic patients, debated about relinquishing this responsibility. Because of minimal interest in maintaining the Medical Clinic, they agreed to allow the Department of Family Medicine to care for these patients. Consequently, in 1974 the Medical Clinic was closed and the patient population referred to family medicine. Initially, the clinic population was skeptical that many of their medical needs could be cared for in a single facility. They were accustomed to many referrals to specialty clinics as well as the long waits because there was no appointment system. Family medicine developed an appointment system, provided coverage 24 hours a day, seven days a week, and attempted to assign a single doctor to each patient so that there might be continuity of care. The dramatic change was difficult for the patients to accept. When the Family Practice Center opened, 80 percent of the patients failed to keep their appointments. The faculty, the residents, and the students were disheartened. As the patients became more familiar with the system and trusted the family medicine staff, appointment compliance gradually improved. Approximately two years later, 60 percent of the patients kept their appointments.

Approximately 60 percent of the family practice patient population qualified for medical assistance. This meant that the Institution had to subsidize the family practice clinical operation. This subsidy was appreciated, but annually was the subject of considerable discussion at budget time. It was always difficult to justify how much effort was required for patient care, and how much more was required for student and resident education. It was apparent from the start that primary care training was expensive, and that the rewards for service, particularly for the indigent, were very low.

■ Inpatients

From the very beginning of the program there were Department concerns about how the inpatients generated from the outpatient population should be managed. Dr. Robert Wise, Chairman of the Department of Medicine, was concerned that family physicians may not possess the necessary knowledge and skills to care for adult patients. Other members of the Department of Medicine envisioned family practice in the United States as being similar to that in the United Kingdom, where the inpatients were always referred to the more traditional specialists. This particular issue was the most difficult one encountered in the establishment of the Department's programs. The members of the Department of Family Medicine in both the College and the Hospital felt that they were capable of handling general medicine inpatients. At no time did family medicine request obstetrical or surgical privileges. The inpatient issue resulted in many meetings. Dean Kellow and Vice President Sweeney convened the leaders in each Department in order to arrive at a satisfactory solution. Finally, thanks to Warren Lambright, M.D., who worked for Dr. Sweeney in the hospital's administrative offices, an acceptable solution was found and agreed upon. The Department of Medicine and the Department of Family Medicine agreed that all inpatients would be admitted to the Hospital on the Internal Medicine service. All qualified faculty in the Department of Family Medicine would receive secondary faculty appointments in the Department of Internal Medicine. Dr. Brucker, the Chairman of Family Medicine, would be responsible for the quality of their care, but should this not meet the usual standards, Dr. Wise, the Chairman of Internal Medicine, would have the right to intervene. (Incidentally, this never happened.) On the other hand, Dr. Brucker was held responsible for all outpatient care, and a similar arrangement for outpatient care was established between him and the Department of Medicine. This compromise allowed both Departments to pass an almost insurmountable hurdle. After ten years, in 1984 this particular inpatient care arrangement was dismantled because Dr. Willis Maddrey, the new Chairman of the Department of Medicine believed that the Department of Family Medicine had clearly demonstrated that they were able to take care of inpatients, and he suggested that family medicine have its own inpatient service.

By 1975 the Department had undergraduate and graduate programs, an outpatient facility with an adequate patient population, a faculty, and the privilege to admit and care for general adult medical patients. The first two years for the new Department were very busy. The Board of Trustees, the College, and the Hospital united in a commitment to the Department that was vital and solid.

Maturation Of The Department: Undergraduate Programs

The Department grew quickly. By 1976, six full-time faculty were recruited. In addition to the three already mentioned, they included Dr. Peter Amadio (Jefferson, 1958), Dr. Su Hain, Dr. Howard Rabinowitz, and Dr. Elmer Taylor (Jefferson, 1952). Three were trained in internal medicine, two in family medicine, and one in pediatrics (Figure 23-3). Such specialty representation lent itself well to the overall education programs. This particular faculty mix was one that attracted favorable attention nationally.

In addition to this complement of full-time faculty, the Department was always able to gain assistance from all of the other faculty in the College. Not one faculty person in the College refused to cooperate and contribute to the family medicine program. In fact, many volunteered. The result of this unparalleled cooperation was a very healthy integration of the Family Medicine Program into the University setting.

As the faculty number increased, the amount of undergraduate teaching responsibility also increased. The family medicine faculty became involved in clinical correlation courses in the first two years and eventually became responsible for a 16-week segment of the Sophomore Medicine and Society Course. Family medicine supervised the teaching of epidemiology, medicolegal and ethical issues, and health-care delivery issues, including the new emphasis being placed on the economic aspects of medicine. In addition to the mandatory Junior clerkship, a large number of students chose the Senior-year track in family medicine. In this track they were required to take an additional 12-week experience in an ambulatory setting. In order to accommodate all of the students who desired family medicine clinical experiences, the Department had to increase the number of student openings. With the help of federal funding, a rural preceptorship program was started. Students were assigned to carefully selected faculty physician preceptors in rural offices located from Vermont to North Carolina. Since 1976 this program has been supervised by Dr. Howard Rabinowitz, an Associate Professor of Family Medicine. The majority of students who take the rural preceptorship in their Senior year claim that it is one of the highlights of their medical school training. They see unselected problems in a defined community, live and participate in the community, and have one-on-one teaching. In order to ensure the quality of the teaching, the preceptors are visited on a regular basis in their offices. Each preceptor is invited back to the medical school for an annual preceptorship workshop, concerned with upgrading their medical knowledge and to discuss how the preceptorship can be improved.

Three other affiliate programs were added, bringing the total to six. The Underwood Memorial Hospital program was started in 1980, Bryn Mawr Hospital under supervision of Dr. Stratton Woodruff in 1975, and Franklin Hospital in 1978.

Residency Program

The pioneer group of Residents performed well. They proved to be excellent ambassadors for the Department. The Residency, from its beginning, enjoyed an excellent reputation both within and outside the Institution. Many applicants appreciated the advantages of training for family medicine in the medical school setting. Fortunately, the initial hurdle of recruiting Residents was overcome, and after the first year there was a large number of qualified applicants from all over the country, representing many different medical schools. All of the graduates of the Residency program have passed the American

Board of Family Practice certifying examination. They practice all over the United States and in two foreign countries.

In 1978 the Residency program received full accreditation. Nationally there was concern that family physicians trained in the northeastern part of the United States did not acquire sufficient skills to practice obstetrics and surgery. Dr. Brucker had many discussions with the Residency Review Committee about this particular issue. Finally, a compromise was reached. All of the residents received the minimal amount of training as specified in the Essentials for Family Practice, but for those who wished or were required to practice obstetrics, a six-month Obstetrical Fellowship was made available after the completion of the three-year Family Practice program.

As a result of the family medicine program, plus some national trends, the number of Jefferson graduates going into family medicine residencies increased from three per year in 1973 to 35 in 1976.

As of 1986 approximately 16 percent of the Jefferson graduating classes go into family medicine residencies. This is considerably above the national average.

Postgraduate Programs

In order to qualify for the mandatory recertification examination in family practice, all diplomats are required to take at least 150 hours of approved continuing medical education courses every three years. This particular requirement made it easy for the Department to conduct

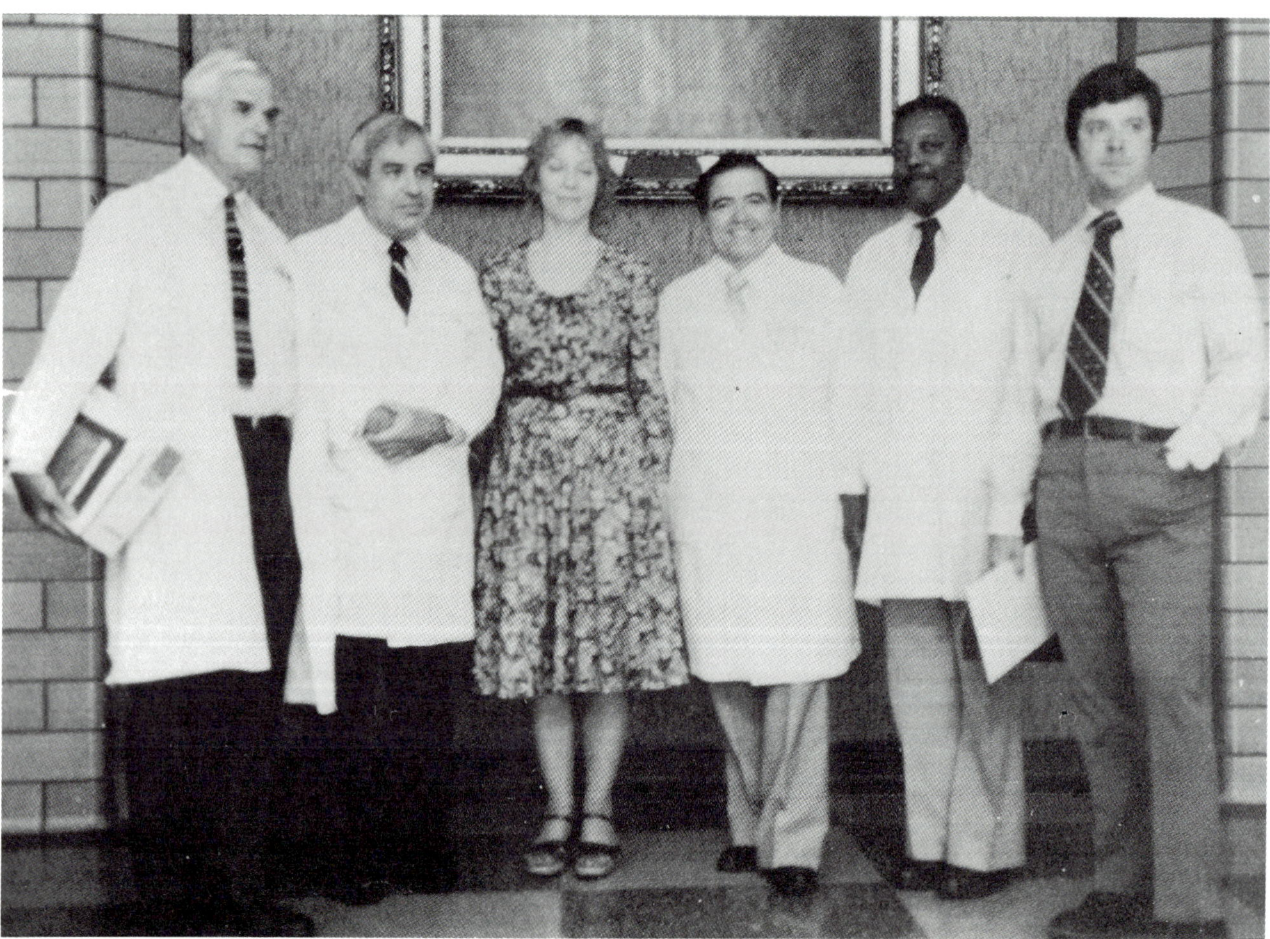

FIG. 23-3. Conference group, Department of Family Medicine, 1976; left to right, Drs. Edward H. McGehee, Paul C. Brucker, Su Carroll Hain, Peter Amadio, Jr., Elmer H. Taylor, Jr., and James D. Plumb.

successful annual continuing medical education courses. Some of these were in conjunction with the annual alumni trips, whereas others were conducted independently, both at Jefferson and in other places.

Research Programs

After establishing successful teaching and patient care programs, the Department paid more attention to developing a research program. Although the faculty in the Department conducted some clinical trials, there was no concerted research effort until 1982. It was at that time that a Research Division was formed. Dr. Donald J. Balaban, M.D., MPH, was invited to join the Department as a Research Associate Professor of Family Medicine and to head the Department's Research Division. Dr. Balaban was no stranger to Jefferson, for he had taken some of his internal medicine training there. He then took additional training in epidemiology at the University of California, where he received his MPH. Before coming to Jefferson, Dr. Balaban carried out his research at the Leonard Davis Institute of the University of Pennsylvania. There he was intimately involved in health care delivery research, particularly as it applied to studying functional outcomes in chronic conditions. Dr. Balaban brought with him an enthusiasm and expertise to carry out similar research in the Department. He was supported by the outpatient clinical practice that the Department had established, and he was anxious to train fellows and junior faculty in research methodology in order to improve their research skills. The timing for the establishment of this Division was right. The Research Division's presence lent an important academic stimulus to the Department. Appropriate research questions began to be asked, and methodologies were developed in an attempt to answer them.

Economic Influences

In 1982 with the advent of the Prospective Payment System for hospitalization, numerous significant impacts began to take place on the delivery of health care. It became readily apparent that society was going to impose limits on the cost of health care delivery. For the first time there were debates about the rationing of care and the effectiveness and efficiencies involved with certain types of care. The private corporate sector began to exert a significant effect on the organizational structure for delivering care. Medicine began to assume much more of a private enterprise or business posture. Different types of capitation systems sprung up for the well and employed. The government subsidies for the care of the poor and the elderly started to become limited. It became very apparent that hospitalization, the most expensive part of health care delivery, would be curtailed and that probably many small hospitals might be forced to close. This prospective payment system was a particular threat for teaching hospitals located in poor urban areas where so much of the care delivered was subsidized. With the medical schools turning out a surplus of physicians, "competition" and "doctor glut" came to be frequent conversation topics. For the first time in 60 years, the outpatient setting and ambulatory care took on a very new significance. Likewise, for the first time in the 1900s residents and students began to become concerned with finding a position after finishing their residency training.

Jefferson became very aware of all of these trends and in its long-range planning attempted to make sure that it would remain fiscally sound, but still heed its mission of education, research, and patient service. The Department of Family Medicine, in cooperation with the Hospital administration, began to participate in various capitation systems that were designed not only for the relatively well and employed, but also for the poor and elderly. In 1986, they established one primary care satellite in the Fairmount section of Philadelphia, and another in the South Philadelphia area. In 1988, a third satellite was started in Chinatown. Such satellites were an attempt to ensure an adequate patient population for training both in the inpatient and outpatient setting. The training of the students and the residents in a capitation model requires a great deal of skill, for intelligent use of resources and logical decision analysis are required in order to remain financially sound. It appears that this particular type of training will be even more important as the capitation models continue to grow and residency graduates become dependent upon them for employment. The Department continues to do research in this important area, so that there can be some factual basis for the decisions that will be required.

■ Benefactors

In the first 13-year period (1973–1986) of the Department's existence there have been many generous contributions. In 1973 the Alumni Association of Jefferson Medical College voted to contribute $50,000 annually to help sponsor the Alumni Professor of Family Medicine. Dr. Brucker was named the first Alumni Professor of Family Medicine, and that honor along with an honorary lifetime membership in the Alumni Association were distinctions that he prized.

One outstanding contributor was Dr. Dale W. Garber (Jefferson, 1924). He was a respected general practitioner in Delaware County, Pennsylvania. Dr. Brucker had the good fortune to first meet him in 1976 on an Alumni-sponsored continuing medical education trip to the lowlands in Europe. He became very interested in the Department of Family Medicine. After several years of finding out more about the Department and how it functioned, Dr. Garber established a Professorship in Family Medicine. This endowed chair was awarded to Dr. Edward H. McGehee in 1984 when he became the first Ellen M. and Dale S. Garber Professor of Family Medicine. The esteem in which Dr. McGehee was held among the student body was manifested when the Class of 1976 presented his portrait to the College.

In 1982, Mrs. Nell T. Haac, who had been in Jefferson Hospital repeatedly over the past 50 years, left a generous sum to the Department that adequately ensured funding for the initial year of the Research Division.

As the Department's programs rapidly expanded they became very short of administrative space. The headquarters on the first floor of the College building were no longer adequate, but there was no funding to allow a move to larger quarters, In 1982, the Glen Meade Foundation provided a generous grant for renovations to be made on the fourth floor of the Curtis Building. The Department moved to these new headquarters in 1983.

In an increasingly restrictive financial climate, the Research Division had difficulties in funding stipends for Fellows and various research projects. Mr. Gustave Amsterdam, a member of Jefferson's Board of Trustees and a member of the Etelka J. Greenfield Foundation Board, became aware of this and interceded with the Foundation to contribute a generous gift to the Research Division. In order to recognize this and the importance of the gift, in 1984 the Research Division was called the Etelka J. Greenfield Research Center of the Department of Family Medicine.

All of these gifts, plus the dedicated efforts of many individuals in an Institution that has been most supportive of this new Department, have allowed a great deal to be accomplished in a relatively short time. A solid foundation has been established to further Jefferson's and Family Medicine's mission.

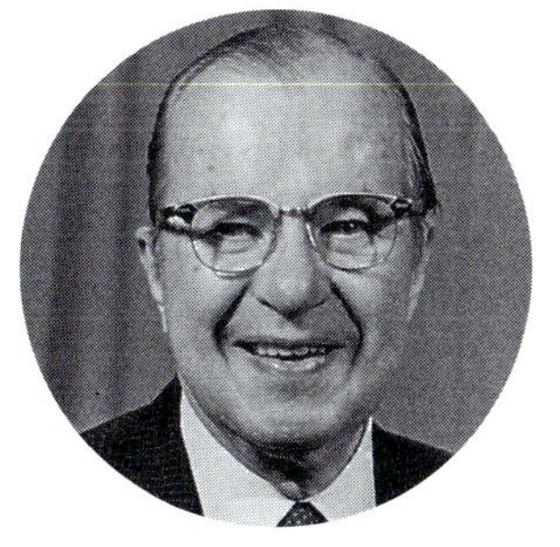

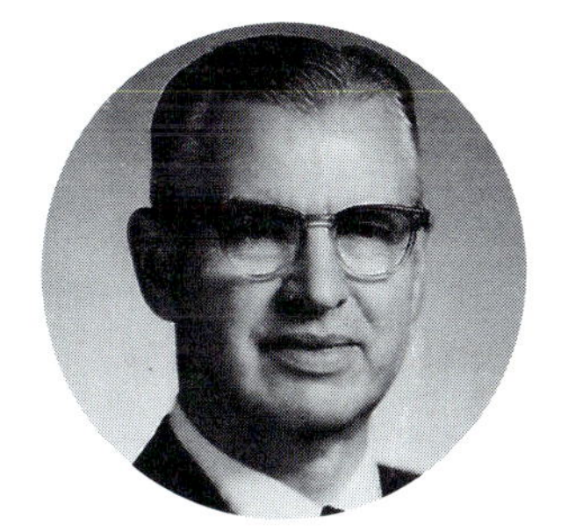

CHAPTER TWENTY-FOUR

Department of Preventive Medicine

WILLARD A. KREHL, M.D., PH.D., AND
J. WOODROW SAVACOOL, M.D.

"It is the nature of man that the case for cure is always more compelling than the case for prevention. But, it is in the nature of biology that the most effective measure against disease is PREVENTION."

—JOHN F. KENNEDY (1917–1963)

PERHAPS one reason for the difficulty of establishing Preventive Medicine in formal medical education was the nature of instruction in the nineteenth century. Teaching was principally by lecture, and the professors were largely those in medical practice. Although there were ancient precedents for the concepts of prevention, little attention was paid to them in the courses, primarily because of the general lack of understanding as to the cause of disease and because of physicians' preoccupation by necessity with sick people. To be sure, there were early organized efforts by the Marine Hospital Service, founded in 1798, and later assigned certain preventive duties such as surveillance of immigrants; it eventually evolved into the U. S. Public Health Service through an Act of Congress in 1902. Also, the American Public Health Association was organized about 1870. More specifically, smallpox prevention was established by vaccination a century before the identification of the viral cause of this disease, and scurvy could be prevented by provision of citrus sources of the factor later to be identified as vitamin C.

The tremendous impetus provided by the discovery of agents of infectious diseases at the end of the nineteenth century and the subsequent availability of vaccines and epidemiologic measures for prevention were major factors in disease control, in the evolution of Preventive Medicine as a discipline, and in the involvement of government. For a time this involvement was perceived by medical school professors as an intrusion into their prerogatives rather than as an extension of their teaching. Whereas individual professors included preventive measures in their lecture formats, there was no organized approach until the early years of the twentieth century. Graduate schools of public health ultimately filled the void, and undergraduate medical education benefited from the ferment. Lessons learned in wartime also broadened the base of the involvement of prevention.

During the early years of the twentieth century, a famous Jeffersonian, Dr. Victor Heiser (Jefferson, 1897), became one of the major pioneers in preventive medicine, public health administration, and international health (Figure 24-1). Although not on the Jefferson faculty, his innovative, imaginative skills and organizational talents provided important challenges for preventive medicine and public health that had an impact on medical education. As Associate Director, Internal Health Division for the Rockefeller Foundation (1927–1933), Heiser was able to establish policies for worldwide health programs from experiences of many years. His teachings and activities in international control of cholera, leprosy, plague, and smallpox became widely recognized among officials in high places all over the world. Dr. Heiser was awarded the Honorary Degree of Doctor of Science at Jefferson in 1911 and the Alumni Achievement Award in 1968. He was the author of many medical publications and popular magazine articles. His autobiographical book *An American Doctor's Odyssey* (1936) was a popular best-seller.[1]

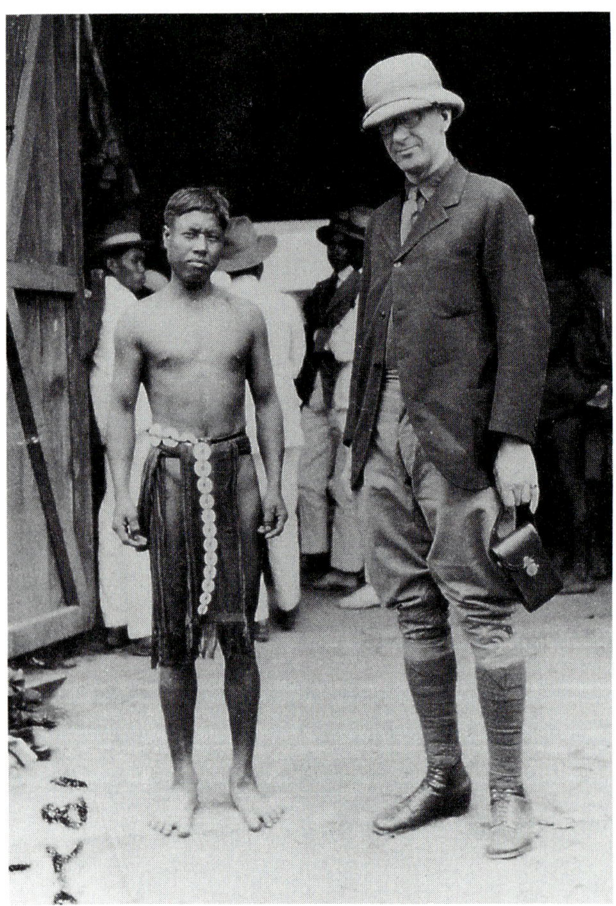

FIG. 24-1. Victor G. Heiser, M.D., a pioneer in the international approach to disease prevention in the Philippines.

Randle C. Rosenberger; M.D., First Chairman (1909–1941)

Individual lecturers at Jefferson gradually included the teaching of preventive measures, especially with respect to infectious diseases and surgical infections. Although perhaps not the first to employ organized principles, Dr. Randle C. Rosenberger (Jefferson, 1894), having already served in pathology at the Philadelphia General Hospital and in bacteriology at the Henry Phipps Institute (1904), was appointed Assistant Professor of Bacteriology and Curator of the Museum in 1906. He was advanced to Associate Professor in 1908 and the following year was appointed Professor of Bacteriology and Hygiene. Rosenberger's teaching soon included organized lectures on matters pertaining to public health, infectious disease prevention, industrial medicine, and early aspects of epidemiology. The second-year course in 1913 was described as one in Hygiene and "Preventative" Medicine and in 1918 a third-year course included public health (Figure 24-2). Dr. Rosenberger was an able lecturer with a phenomenal memory. He made it a point to recall the names of all his students, even after the passage of many years. His courses broadened the viewpoints of students regarding preventive medicine early in their training. He required a paper from each third-year student on the subject of prevention of industrial hazards, developed from a summer project.

In 1916 a first year laboratory course was begun and in 1923 was expanded to 162 hours as bacteriology dominated the program. Dr. Henry B. Decker (Jefferson, 1920) joined Dr. Rosenberger and participated in the additional 47 hours of first-year lectures. Dr. Decker instituted lectures on immunology that dealt with the expanded theories of body responses often observed in the development of vaccines against infectious disease. There was also a third-year course of 66 hours dealing with public health and sanitation as well as protection against agents and circumstances of disease. This prodigious teaching program was carried on by only two people, Drs. Rosenberger and Decker. In 1925 the Department name was changed to Preventive Medicine and

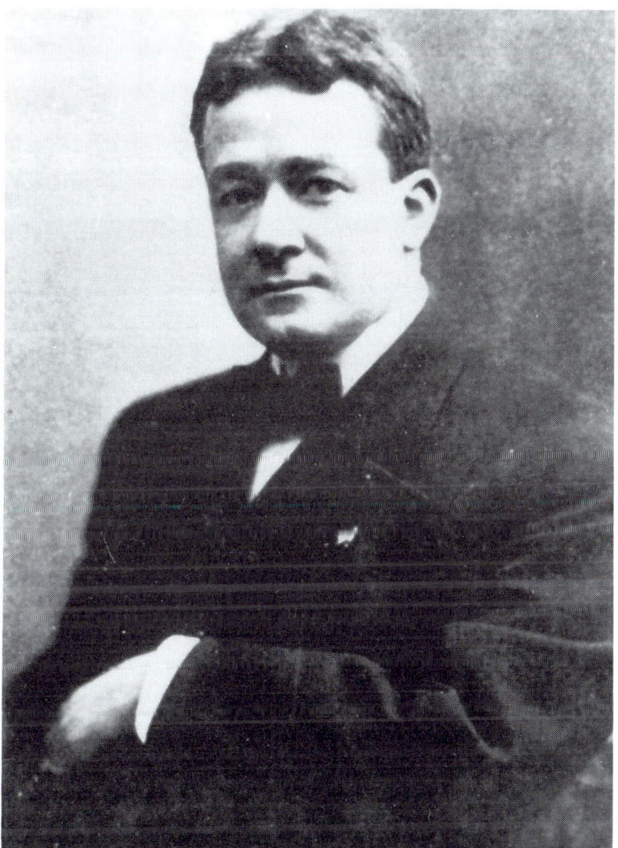

FIG. 24-2. Randle C. Rosenberger, M.D.; First Professor of Hygiene and Preventive Medicine.

Bacteriology, and Dr. Rosenberger was designated as its Professor and Head. This arrangement was continued until 1939. In 1931–1932 the first-year course was increased to 167 hours. In 1933 Dr. William A. Kreidler replaced Dr. Decker as Assistant Professor of Bacteriology, while Dr. Rosenberger continued to carry the principal lecture responsibility. Dr. Donald Meranze was added as Assistant Demonstrator of Bacteriology in 1935. In 1940 the meager staff was supplemented by the appointment of two Fellows.

Among other early preventive programs, Dr. Edward L. Bauer (Jefferson, 1914), before his appointment as Professor of Diseases of Children (1926), had responsibility for a broad range of public health problems in the Department of Health of Philadelphia.[2] He organized immunization programs for schools and orphanages, especially for diphtheria, and was for years physician to Girard College, where he was able to pursue and enlarge his experiences in preventive medicine. Following his professorial appointment Bauer organized special clinics and classes in his Department that carried forward some of the principles he developed—well-baby clinics proved among the most effective of these.

William H. Perkins, M.D.; Second Chairman (1941–1959)

Other teaching departments gradually developed principles of prevention that applied to their various specialties and that proved important in the years before their inclusion in the specific discipline. These supplemented the teachings of Dr. Rosenberger and his staff until 1941, when Dr. William Harvey Perkins (Jefferson, 1917) was appointed as Dean and Professor of Preventive Medicine (Figure 24-3); this appointment was received with enthusiasm. Serving as Acting Dean from the time of the death of Dean Mohler (1939) until Dr. Perkins' arrival, Dr. Rosenberger was at the same time designated as Professor of Preventive Medicine and Hygiene. With Dr. Perkins' arrival, Dr. Rosenberger's title changed to Professor of Bacteriology and Immunology.

Dr. Perkins was a well established educator with many innovative ideas that he had already implemented in a varied career. Following a brief period of service in the United States Army (1918–1919), Perkins served with the American

Presbyterian Mission in Thailand from 1919 to 1923. Under primitive medical conditions he encountered many serious health problems, which he quickly concluded could not be solved by traditional individual medical treatment and required public effort and health education. He returned briefly to Philadelphia, where in 1923 he served as Instructor in Medicine at Jefferson and as Assistant Pathologist at the Philadelphia General Hospital. He also worked at the Philadelphia Zoological Garden, where he studied Darwinian concepts in animals and developed interests that he enlarged upon as an intellectual hobby throughout his life. Perkins soon accepted a fellowship with the Rockefeller Foundation in Medical Education in conjunction with which he became Professor of Medicine at Chululongkorn University in Bangkok, Thailand (1926–1930). His previous experience there proved helpful. Nevertheless, the observations made earlier regarding the enormity of health problems in a primitive society, coupled with the impossible task of teaching modern medicine in such a setting, caused him to seek more comprehensive approaches. He, therefore, left Thailand in 1930, bearing with him the gratitude of his associates and the Order of the White Elephant conferred by the King.[3]

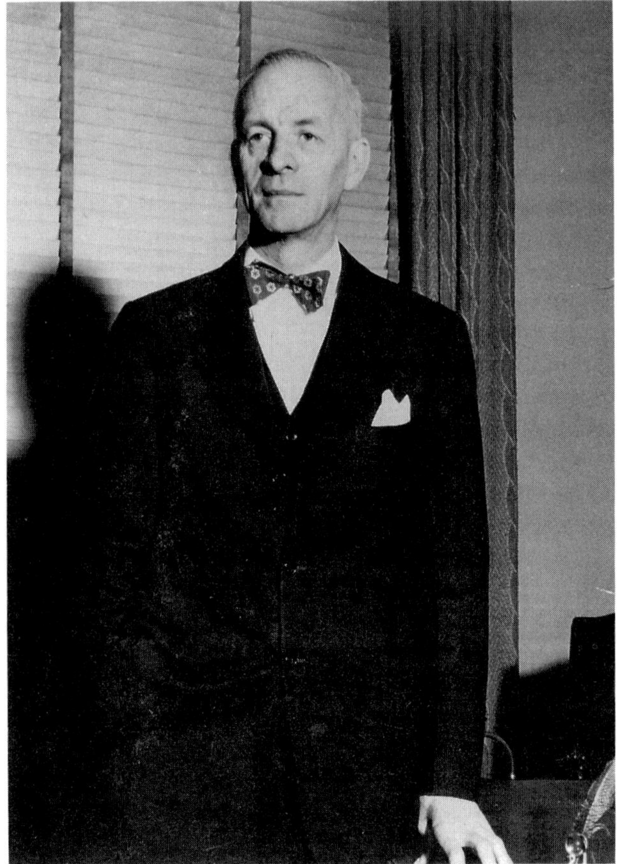

FIG. 24-3. William Harvey Perkins, M.D., Sc.D., LL.D., Litt. D.; Dean and Professor of Preventive Medicine.

Opportunities were now developing in the field of preventive medicine. Dr. Perkins was appointed Instructor in Medicine at Tulane University School of Medicine in 1930, but the following year his real challenge and purpose were realized with his appointment as Professor and Chairman of the new full-time Department of Preventive Medicine at Tulane with support from the Commonwealth Fund. There were many and varied experiences, including tropical medicine, the emerging discipline of public health administration, the efforts to define the scope of Preventive Medicine, and methods of gaining acceptance of developing principles, especially by organized medicine. In addition to these innovations he was able to implement his ideas relative to individual health by establishing a demonstration Health Maintenance Clinic where students and faculty could join in learning. In 1938 he published a major work entitled *Cause and Prevention of Disease*,[4] one of the first textbooks of preventive medicine. At Tulane Dr. Perkins made the acquaintance of Drs. William A. Sodeman, later Dean at Jefferson, and of E. Harold Hinman, later Professor and Chairman of the Department of Preventive Medicine.

Dr. Perkins was highly qualified for the task of establishing a new Department of Preventive Medicine at Jefferson as well as for the more comprehensive challenge as Dean. One of the principles emphasized by Dr. Perkins was that of "disease as a process." Whereas infections have a fairly straightforward cause–effect–cure–prevention sequence that permits their control once disease agents have been identified, most other diseases have more subtle causes and associations that generally are much more difficult to elucidate. These bear upon heredity and environment, plus chemical, physical, degenerative, neoplastic, and psychobiological factors that may be perceived variously by different individuals. Early detection of primary factors and avoidance of contributing ones may be keys to prevention of disability and death. The "disease-as-a-process" concept was a keystone of Dr. Perkins' definitive teachings. As a counterpart, he also formulated a definition of "health" that has never been improved upon: "Health is a state of relative equilibrium of body form and function which results from its successful dynamic adjustment to forces tending to disturb it."[4] This was an extension of the principle of "homeostasis" that had shortly before been promulgated by Walter B. Cannon[5] and later philosophically extended by Dickinson Richards.[6,7]

The early experience at Jefferson was constricted by the stresses of war. Dr. Perkins as Dean responded to the urgency of the time and was forced to postpone the implementation of his ideas for the development of his Department. His teaching was limited to the third-year lectures, often shared with guest lecturers (64 hours). Immediately after the war (1945), however, he recruited Dr. Heinrich Brieger, who proved a major asset to Jefferson (Figure 24-4).

Dr. Brieger had had broad experience in medicine, toxicology, medical social administration, and occupational medicine in Germany, a country he left in 1941 for political reasons. He was appointed as Associate Professor of Preventive Medicine at Jefferson. In short order, with Dr. Perkins' support, his program became established as the only one in industrial medicine in any Philadelphia school of medicine. Research grants were obtained, a laboratory established, and consultations with many regional industries were developed. Dr. Brieger spoke quietly but always with conviction and authority. Important for the progress of his Department was his ability to generate funds through industry for the support of his research and teaching activities.

In 1946 Dr. W. Paul Havens was added to the teaching staff as Associate Professor, to contribute his skills to the third-year lecture program, which continued at a modest 32 hours.

The Genesis of the Health Maintenance Program

Perhaps the most pressing of projects delayed by the war was the organization of a health maintenance program for further study of the causes of disease and problems of prevention. Exactly how the movement was initiated is not clear, but Dr. Perkins participated in discussions that led to a proposal to Jefferson by the Board of Trustees of the Babies' Hospital to develop an expanded district health center that would serve a population of about 150,000 in southeast Philadelphia. The Babies' Hospital was developed in 1911 (its definitive building was constructed at Seventh and Delancey Streets in 1923) by Philadelphia pediatricians to serve mainly as an

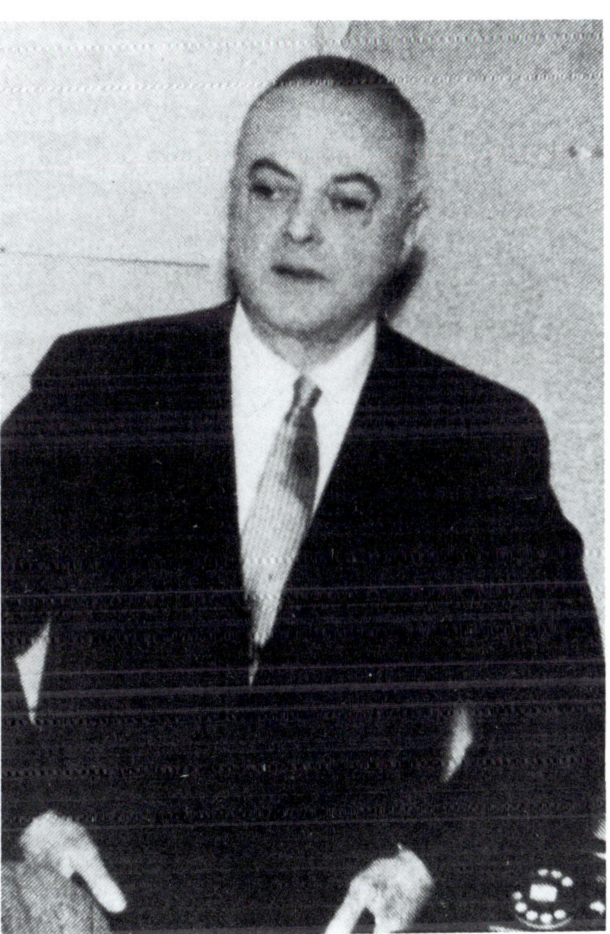

Fig. 24-4. Heinrich Brieger, M.D.; Professor of Preventive Medicine (Occupational Medicine).

outpatient center for child health, well-baby clinics, pediatric care, and public health nursing. It additionally included about 15 beds for inpatient treatment. Among the founders were Dr. Charles Andrew Fife (1871–1935) and Dr. Samuel McClintock Hamill (1864–1948), both one-time Presidents of the American Society of Pediatrics. The proposal stated ". . . that the Board of Trustees of the Babies' Hospital and the Philadelphia Child Health Society, two agencies with a long record of significant services, now pool their interests and funds to provide the basic resources for the Health Center Association, that the Babies' Hospital building be made available for the Center and that the Jefferson Medical School become a factor in this important enterprise by developing a Health Maintenance Program as a new and essential feature of this unit which might become an important part of the City Health Department center program and be a matter of civic pride."[8] Discussions progressed, at one time including the Jefferson Department of Pediatrics, but ultimately the involvement of Jefferson focused mainly on health maintenance for adults and on public health administration and teaching. The Center was named Fife–Hamill Memorial Health Center (Figure 24-5) to honor the two Babies' Hospital leaders. The Jefferson administration enthusiastically supported Dr. Perkins in approving the project, and details were worked out during 1947 and 1948.

Dr. Perkins was now enabled to implement his plan for development of a Health Maintenance Clinic along the lines he had pioneered in New Orleans a decade earlier to study the effectiveness of and to put into practice the ideas for individual and group health in which he believed so firmly. One of his most important contributions to medical education was the involvement of students in patient care under careful supervision for the specific purpose of disease prevention and health promotion and maintenance.

After building renovations, the Clinic opened in 1948. To head it Dr. Perkins appointed Dr. Gulden Mackmull (Jefferson, 1925) as Assistant Professor of Preventive Medicine and Director of the Division of Clinical Preventive Medicine. Mackmull was assisted by Dr. Joseph J. Cava. In addition to the research built into the program, Dr. Perkins planned the Clinic as a demonstration that could ultimately expand into a comprehensive public health program and be incorporated into each of the Health Centers of the Philadelphia Department of Health, which were in the stage of development at the time. Patients were largely recruited by word-of-mouth publicity, especially through the Public Health Nursing program already established at Fife–Hamill. Procedures for annual examinations were developed, supervised by Drs. Mackmull and Cava but performed by fourth-year Jefferson medical students, all of whom rotated through the clinic. The scope of the examinations and ancillary procedures was studied and modified with experience. Data collection assessed the effectiveness of the program and constituted an important aspect. The Clinic developed an enthusiastic and cooperative group of patients who returned faithfully for annual examinations. All patients were reviewed by the physicians and were given summaries of their health status including risk factors to be guarded against and preventive measures to be applied.

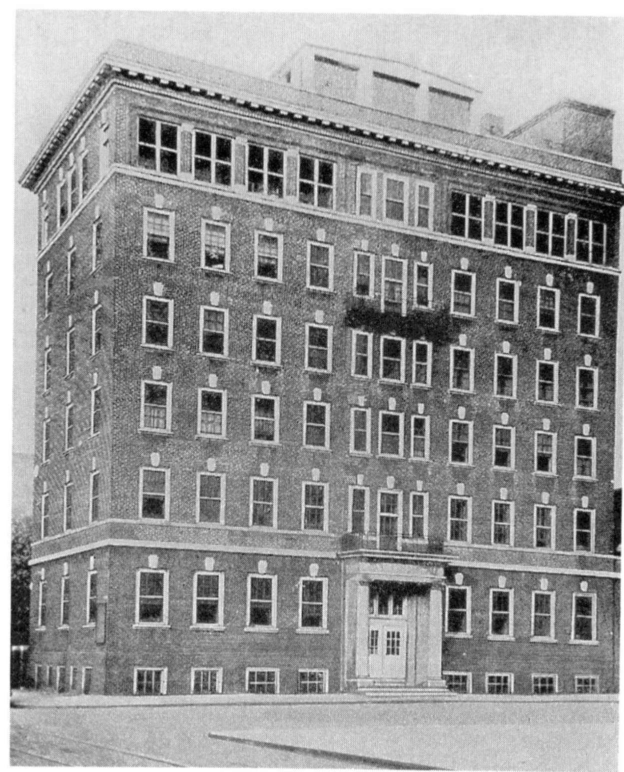

FIG. 24-5. Fife–Hamill Memorial Health Center, Seventh and Delancey Streets (formerly Babies' Hospital of Philadelphia).

Treatment of abnormalities detected was carried out by physicians of the patients' choice. After 5 years, the results of the Health Maintenance Clinic experiences were evaluated and published.[9]

Further Expansion of the Department

This was a time during which health risk and health promotion programs were being actively pursued by insurance companies, a few health-related foundations, and medical schools. The Health Maintenance Clinic at Jefferson was in the forefront of these studies, based as it was on solid principles developed by Dr. Perkins and ongoing experience. The change in emphasis from treatment of disease to active promotion of health was difficult for physicians as well as patients, especially when results of examinations often required changes in life-styles and habits rather than a temporary prescribed treatment regimen. The enthusiasm generated in the Clinic was difficult to translate into a community adventure, and results were not sufficiently spectacular to persuade government of the need for funds. Thus, the plan to include Health Maintenance Clinics in the City Health Centers ultimately failed. (However, 10 years later, the City of Philadelphia Department of Health did establish a "generalized health clinic" in each of its 10 district health centers.) Dr. Perkins noted in a 1956 letter that failure to incorporate such a plan into the design of the new Health Center at Broad and Lombard Streets would require that the tentative agreement between Jefferson and the City for a cooperative program be anulled.

Plans for the Fife–Hamill program included the recruitment of Bernard M. Blum, M.D., M.P.H. (Figure 24-6) as Professor of Public Health in the Department of Preventive Medicine and Director of the Fife–Hamill Memorial Health Center. This was the first appointment of a Professor of Public Health in a Philadelphia Medical School, and almost at once it was followed by similar appointments by others. Dr. Blum was enthusiastic about the possibilities and had plans for health center development that required only funding for realization. His teaching duties included lectures to fourth-year students, field trips for the study of environmental health and sanitation, and nutritional education.[10]

The postwar Department consisted of four Divisions under Dr. Perkins: (1) Public Health, Fife–Hamill—Dr. Blum; (2) Occupational Medicine and Hygiene—Dr. Brieger; (3) Communicable Disease Control—Dr. Havens; (4) Clinical Preventive Medicine—Dr. Mackmull. Third-year students were scheduled for 33 hours, and fourth-year students for 37 hours. It was a well-designed program but unfortunately could not be continued during the 1950s for various reasons. The infectious disease program was largely taken over by the Department of Medicine, and lack of funding limited the public health activities. The industrial program, however, prospered and enjoyed increasing prestige. Dr. Brieger was promoted to Professor of Preventive Medicine in 1952.

In 1955 Drs. Mackmull and Cava resigned and were replaced by Drs. J. Woodrow Savacool (Jefferson, 1938) and W. Bernard Kinlaw

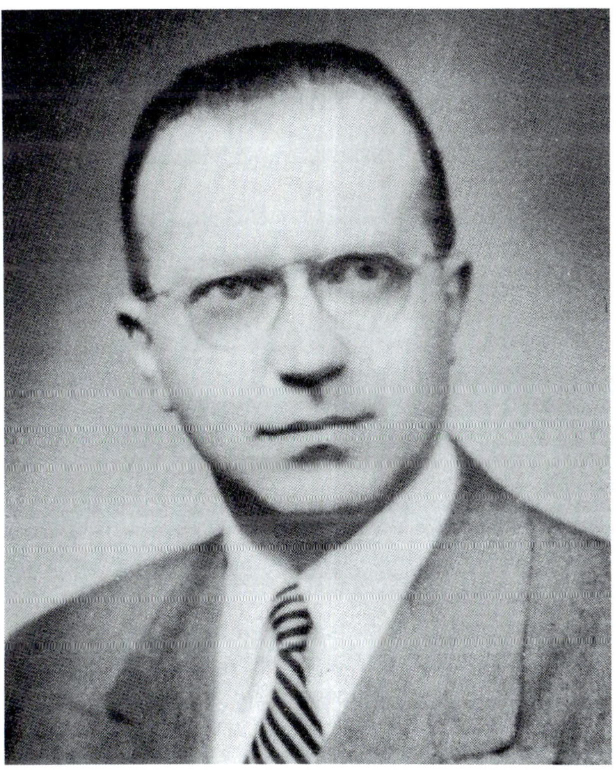

FIG. 24-6. Bernard M. Blum, M.D., M.P.H.; First Professor of Public Health, Director of the Fife–Hamill Memorial Health Center.

(Jefferson, 1949). Inevitably revisions in procedures and emphasis followed. Dr. Perkins's personal role in teaching diminished in view of his deteriorating health (he was forced to resign as Dean for health reasons in 1950), and the teaching was directed toward clinical epidemiology and methods of prevention in clinical situations. Inclusion of representatives of other Departments, especially cardiology, psychiatry, gynecology, and ophthalmology, was well received by the students. Public health nursing with personnel headquartered at Fife–Hamill permitted home visiting by medical students for further environmental evaluation. The entire program was effective and stimulating, but changes were inevitable with medical progress. In 1959 Fife–Hamill closed, and its major functions were transferred to the new City District Health Center, the first director of which was Dr. Thomas W. Georges, Jr. (Jefferson, 1955). Jefferson was no longer involved in the public health administration and nursing programs. The Health Maintenance Clinic was transferred to the Curtis Clinic building where, apart from the loss of public health experience, the program was in some respects enhanced by closer contact with other clinical departments. Efforts continued to teach the basic principles of health definition, promotion, and maintenance along the line so ably developed by Dr. Perkins. The enthusiasm and cooperation of the patients was, if anything, improved.

Dr. Perkins' resignation as Professor and Chairman of the Department also occurred in 1959 as a result of progressive disability. This ended the academic career of one of the ablest scholars ever associated with Jefferson. In spite of physical distress he resumed his studies in zoology at the Philadelphia Academy of Natural Sciences and his last academic presentation at Jefferson occurred soon after with a 75-minute scholarly lecture on Charles Darwin given completely without notes. A final publication entitled *Evolution and Progress Under Natural Law*[11] appeared in 1963. Dr. Perkins died in 1967 at the age of 73. His portrait was presented to the College in 1951 by his Class of 1917. A room in the Kellow conference area on the second floor of the College Building was named in his honor in 1979.[12]

During the mid-1930s, preventive medicine lectures included material on demography and vital statistics in the third year. This constituted the only formal mention of biostatistical material at Jefferson until the appointment of Dr. Hyman Menduke as Assistant Professor of Biostatistics in 1953, although preclinical departments made reference to the subject as it applied to their disciplines. Dr. Menduke first organized courses for graduate students but soon was given a few hours of teaching of medical students in the Department of Pharmacology. This continued for a few years as he became involved in the research programs of both clinical and preclinical departments. In 1961 he was appointed Associate Professor of Preventive Medicine (Biostatistics) and in 1963 advanced to Professor. In 1965 he was made Coordinator of Research for the Medical Center while continuing his basic teaching of biostatistics in the Department of Preventive Medicine. His association with Jefferson has been an important one, his appointment having reverted, with dismantling of the Department of Preventive Medicine, to Professor of Pharmacology (Biostatistics).

E. Harold Hinman, M.D.; Third Chairman (1962–1969)

With Dr. Perkins' resignation, the Health Maintenance Clinic and Occupational Medicine programs continued without interruption during the interval before the arrival on February 1, 1962, of the new Chairman and Professor of Preventive Medicine, E. Harold Hinman, Ph.D., M.D., M.P.H. (Figure 24-7). Dr. Hinman was a former Dean of the University of Puerto Rico School of Medicine and School of Tropical Medicine and was an authority in the whole field of tropical medicine and public health. He had served as a consultant to the Secretary of War in World War II while successively heading the Health and Sanitation Divisions in El Salvador and Mexico on assignment by the Institute of Inter-American Affairs. His extensive and distinguished background in the field of public health added a new dimension to the philosophies that had been established by Dr. Perkins.

Dr. Hinman promptly developed programs new to the Department while encouraging and promoting those already in place, especially the Health Maintenance Clinic and Dr. Brieger's Occupational Health Division. Training grants were obtained, research projects were initiated in cooperation with federal, state, and local government agencies, and these promptly led to a large number of publications. During his tenure, Dr. Hinman also conducted several consultative missions in Indonesia and East Africa for the Federal Government. He authored a book *World Eradication of Infectious Diseases* (1966).

Dr. Brieger was to continue to progress in his work in occupational medicine. He had attracted various colleagues, had been well supported under joint grants from various industries, and continued to make occupational medicine flourish in the Department. Brieger was made an honorary member of the faculty in 1966 when he reached the age of 71. During his tenure, Dr. Brieger introduced advanced educational programs, and three graduate students, Drs. Frederick Reiders, Charles W. LaBelle, and Charles Garby, received their Ph.D. degrees in Toxicology under the joint direction of the Departments of Pharmacology and Preventive Medicine.

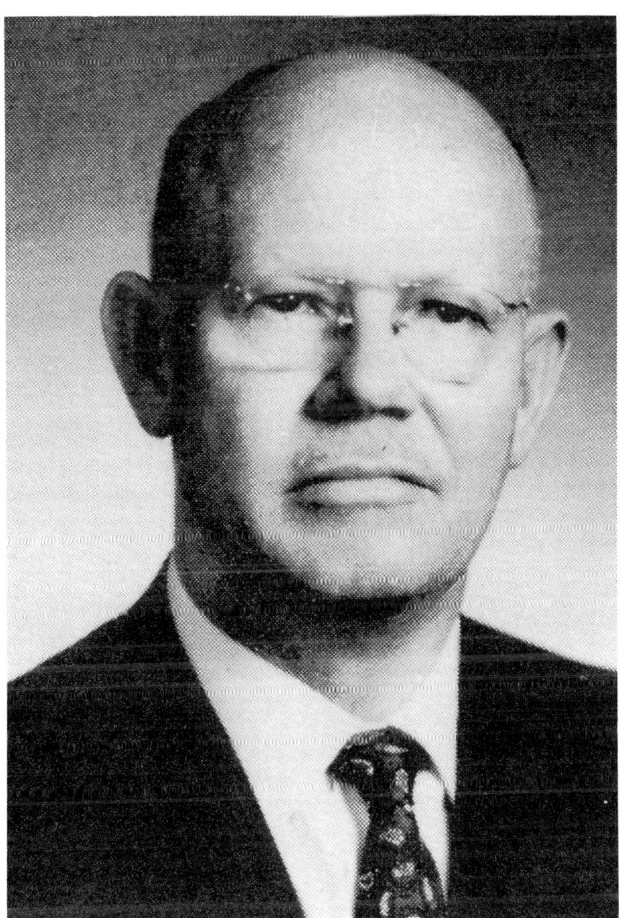

FIG. 24-7. E. Harold Hinman, Ph.D., M.D.; Professor and Chairman of the Department of Preventive Medicine.

Following Dr. Brieger's retirement late in 1966, occupational medicine remained inactive briefly until the appointment of Dr. Norman Williams in the summer of 1967. The Department's emphasis at this time changed from a major concern with industrial toxicology to the organization of services primarily involving the evaluation of health hazards, particularly of industrial plants too small to justify the employment of an industrial physician. Dr. Williams was successful in obtaining support from the U.S. Public Health Service for "Health Surveillance of Workers in Hazardous Occupations." This approach to occupational medicine was established at Jefferson in advance of the current emphasis on occupational safety and health as established in the Federal Government. Dr. Williams also served as a consultant in Occupational Medicine in the City of Philadelphia Department of Health. He organized a winter and spring postgraduate course in occupational medicine dealing with practical matters and serving the occupational medicine physicians in the area as well as graduate students. This was directly sponsored by Jefferson as the Industrial Medical Association of Philadelphia.

The Section of Biostatistics was substantially strengthened. Dr. Hyman Menduke advanced to Professor of Preventive Medicine (Biostatistics) a year after Dr. Hinman's arrival, allowing more comprehensive use of his skills in teaching and research. Although in 1965 his duties were broadened to coordinate research activities for the entire Medical Center, Menduke continued as a very active member of the Department of Preventive Medicine. The enhancement of the program permitted the introduction of several courses in the general area of biostatistics. For those students who wanted to pursue the use of statistics in their special studies, this was a welcomed addition. Dr. Menduke and his colleagues were very productive scholars, as attested to by their numerous publications. Teaching of graduate students increased. Dr. Patricia A. Kay joined the staff in 1966.

Health Maintenance

Having reconstituted the Health Maintenance Clinic in the Curtis Clinic Building in 1959 when Fife–Hamill closed, Drs. Savacool and Kinlaw continued the operation until their resignations in 1965. At that time Dr. Irwin L. Stoloff (Jefferson, 1951) assumed its direction and initiated some changes in operation while maintaining its philosophical principles. Also, Dr. William Pfischner, a public health physician in the City of Philadelphia, was appointed an Associate in Preventive Medicine in 1962 and very effectively cooperated in the teaching program in the Health Maintenance Clinic and also through small-group conferences of senior medical students at the City Health Center.

C. Earl Albrecht, M.D.

A major acquisition for the Department was the appointment in 1963 of Dr. C. Earl Albrecht (Jefferson, 1932) as Professor of Preventive Medicine (Figure 24-8) with main responsibility for development of community health programs and for coordinating research projects. Dr. Albrecht was the first Commissioner of Health for the State of Alaska after a pioneering medical career there. Later he was an Assistant Commissioner of Health for the State of Pennsylvania and was appointed a Visiting Professor of Public Health in 1961 at Jefferson. His full-time status made possible numerous projects that Dr. Hinman was able to promote. Albrecht also served in the Health Maintenance Clinic.

Increasingly, the Department and its programs became almost totally dependent upon Federal funding, and disaster was always just around the corner when the financial support was threatened. Dr. Hinman was expert in developing funding from a variety of governmental sources, one of which was to undertake a comprehensive survey to obtain a broad range of data and information on the extent of problems and needs in the neurological and sensory fields, with the development of a plan to overcome deficiencies and improve services both to patients and physicians. Eastern Pennsylvania, southern New Jersey, and Delaware were included. This was to be a cooperative undertaking of the Departments of Preventive Medicine, Neurology, Ophthalmology, and Otolaryngology. To make this expansive program work, Dr. Albrecht was appointed Director of the project in 1963. A two-volume report, *Neurological and Sensory Disease Project,* completed in 1964, served as a major policy guide for the development of regional and national neuroscience programs.

Another important study, the Lehigh Valley Pennsylvania Nursing Home Survey, was initiated in 1966, again with Dr. Albrecht in charge, and a study of stroke clinics in Delaware and Montgomery Counties in Pennsylvania in 1967 was conducted in association with the staff of the Departments of Preventive Medicine, Physical Medicine, Neurology, and Internal Medicine.

A preceptor-guided apprenticeship program initiated in 1964 through support from Public Health Service was placed under the supervision

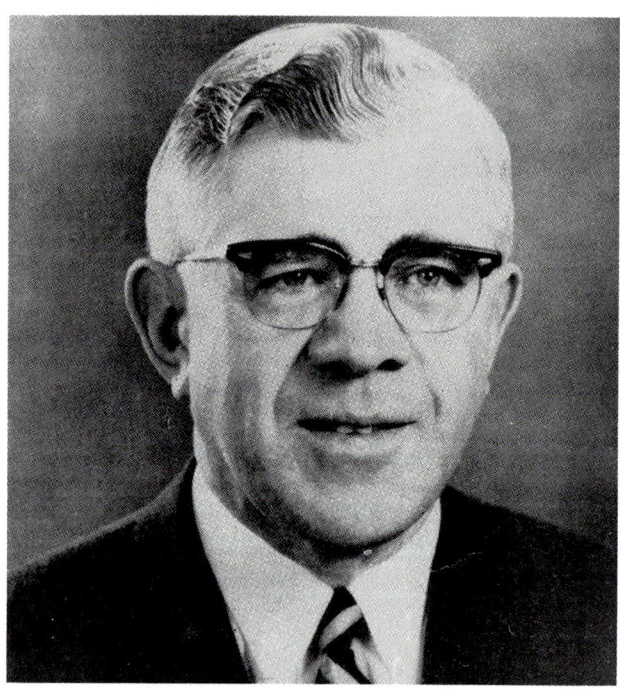

FIG. 24-8. C. Earl Albrecht, M.D.; Professor of Preventive Medicine and pioneer in Arctic Medicine and Public Health.

of Dr. Albrecht. This program continued through the Hinman and Krehl eras. Each year it supported up to 14 medical students for the minimum period of 60 days and placed them in assignments during summer vacation for a three-block project with the Department of Preventive Medicine or off-campus in public health programs.

A study of the Curtis Clinic in the years 1965 to 1968 was conducted, again with governmental research grant monies. This proved valuable in the ongoing evaluation of the contribution of the Curtis Clinic. Also developed was a cost-effective record-keeping system for alcoholism clinics in 1967–1968 under contract with the Pennsylvania Department of Health. Two individuals particularly involved with this program and given faculty appointments were Drs. Jerome Jacobs, Instructor of Preventive Medicine (1962) and Mary W. Herman, Assistant Professor of Preventive Medicine (social sciences) in 1967. The full-time services of Dr. Herman were to have a new influence and emphasis on the Department's teaching and research program. She introduced an elective, "Health, Medicine and Society," which was ultimately to lead in later years to the Medicine and Society Program. Dr. Herman was an effective proponent for the societal aspects of medical care delivery.

The instructional program in biostatistics was enhanced by the appointment to the Preventive Medicine staff of Dr. Paul B. Kanofsky. Dr. Kanofsky assumed responsibility for teaching biostatistics to the preventive medicine residents and provided consultation service.

▪ The Development of Graduate Training in Preventive Medicine

In 1965 a "Graduate Training in Public Health" grant, was made to the Department of Preventive Medicine with Dr. Hinman as Project Director and Dr. Albrecht as Supporting Director. With the introduction of health-hazard programming in the Health Maintenance Clinic, it became necessary to increase the number of preceptors. This program was to blossom and have final development in a subsequent era. It was a new approach at the graduate level for the Department and again demonstrated the close association between the clinical and basic sciences.

▪ Epidemiology and its Development in Preventive Medicine

In November 1966 the Department of Preventive Medicine appointed Dr. Abram S. Benenson as Professor of Preventive Medicine (Epidemiology). His contributions were numerous, not only in the teaching program, but in the research and hospital problems associated with the epidemiology, particularly, of infectious diseases. Unfortunately, Dr. Benenson departed after a short tenure to become Chairman of the Department of Community Medicine at the University of Kentucky School of Medicine.

Several important research projects were funded from governmental sources to conduct such epidemiology studies as *Improved Methods in Vaccination and Serology in Smallpox, Guide to the Laboratory Diagnosis of Smallpox for Smallpox Eradication Programs*, and *The Pathogenesis of Acute Diarrheal Disease*. Dr. Stoloff was a collaborator in these studies that were based on human clinical material and supported by laboratory and experimental animal efforts.

Dr. Earl B. Byrne, M.D., MPH, was brought into the Department of Preventive Medicine as Associate Professor of Epidemiology. He conducted productive research in this area with a primary emphasis on infectious diseases and their prevention. A number of residents and students participated in several of these projects, which received Federal research support.

▪ Residency in General Preventive Medicine

The experience gained in the graduate training program in public health served as the base for the approval of a three-year residency program in General Preventive Medicine awarded to the Department. The area of special competence approved was epidemiology, although clinical preventive medicine was also considered favorably. The award was made in July of 1968, and the first resident to initiate his training under this grant was Dr. David W. Faust, who began on June 1, 1969, just one month before the retirement of Dr. Hinman. This program was designed to train physicians destined for academic appointment in preventive medicine, community medicine, or those interested in associating themselves with administrative responsibility for clinical programs with national, state, or metropolitan health departments. This was a unique program in that it offered variable opportunities for training both in the basic sciences related to preventive medicine such as epidemiology, biostatistics, occupational medicine and nutrition, and in clinical responsibilities in the Health Maintenance Clinic. Related opportunities in the City Health Department on an assigned basis were included. Dr. Lawrence J. Mellon, Jr. (Jefferson, 1959) and Stanley S. Brownstein, D.O., served part-time in the residency program. Dr. Leah Z. Ziskin, M.D., participated on a part-time basis while working with the New Jersey State Health Department. Dr. Earl Wentzel joined this group to complete the allotment for training in General Preventive Medicine. All five completed their programs, prepared acceptable theses, stood for examination for their Masters in Science Degrees at Jefferson in the Basic Science Program, and became board certified in General Preventive Medicine and/or Occupational Medicine. This consumed a period of three or four years, in view of the fact that most were functioning part-time while working in their regular positions in the health care field.

Instructional Programs in Preventive Medicine

In the second year of the program, lectures were designed to acquaint medical students with the basic statistical methods as an aid in understanding scientific literature and determining the statistical significance of clinical and laboratory data as well as vital statistics in disease reporting. These were the responsibility of Dr. Menduke. In the third year a series of didactic lectures was delivered covering the broad categories on prevention of disease, principles of epidemiology and communicable disease controls, environmental health and occupational health problems, accident prevention, organization of health services at all levels from local to international, voluntary health agencies, and patterns of medical care. These teaching responsibilities utilized a full staff complement of the Department.

The quality that ran through the years of development of the Department was the specific application of the principles of environmental medicine and public health through student participation in the Health Maintenance Clinic. All of the facets of preventive medicine were funneled into these clinic responsibilities, and the great merit of this program was the opportunity for students to have a hands-on relationship with patients.

Having made innovative and important contributions to the concepts and teaching of Preventive Medicine, Dr. Hinman retired in 1969.[12] Before the arrival of his successor (Dr. Krehl), Dr. Albrecht became the Acting Chairman; with detailed knowledge and organizational skills, he carried on admirably during a difficult interlude. Harold Hinman, Emeritus Professor of Preventive Medicine, died on December 25, 1971, at the age of 67, following heart surgery necessitated by a myocardial infarction sustained in June 1971. His epitaph stated: “A man dies but his spirit has not fled nor quit the scene of his endeavors. The work of his hand, his heart and his mind lives on.”

Willard A. Krehl, Ph.D., M.D.; Fourth Chairman (1970–1979)

It has been said that the facts of history may be painful since they reveal so acutely mistakes that have been made and things that could have been done more successfully. The final phase of the Department of Preventive Medicine began with the appointment of Willard A. Krehl, M.D., Ph.D. (Figure 24-9) as Professor and Chairman on February 1, 1970, and concluded with the dissolution of the Department on June 30, 1979. It coincided with the retirement of Dr. Krehl to become Emeritus Professor of Medicine. Dr. Krehl had been with the University of Iowa as a Professor of Internal Medicine and also coordinator of the Iowa Regional Medical Program for Heart Disease, Cancer and Stroke. He had previously served in Iowa for five years as

Research Professor of Medicine and Director of the Clinical Research Center. Before those appointments Dr. Krehl taught at Marquette University School of Medicine as Associate Professor of Medicine in charge of the Hypertension and Renal Service and served as Director of Clinical Biochemistry at Milwaukee County General Hospital. He graduated from Cornell College, Mt. Vernon, Iowa, and did postgraduate work at the University of Wisconsin, where he received the M.S. and Ph.D. degrees in Biochemistry. He joined the faculty in Nutrition and Biochemistry at Yale University School of Medicine and at that institution took a leave of absence to obtain his M.D. degree in 1957. Dr. Krehl brought a new transitional phase to the Department of Preventive Medicine with an emphasis on nutrition and metabolism. His experience in the Regional Medical Program in Iowa and with the American Heart Association representing community programs was an advantage to his appointment.

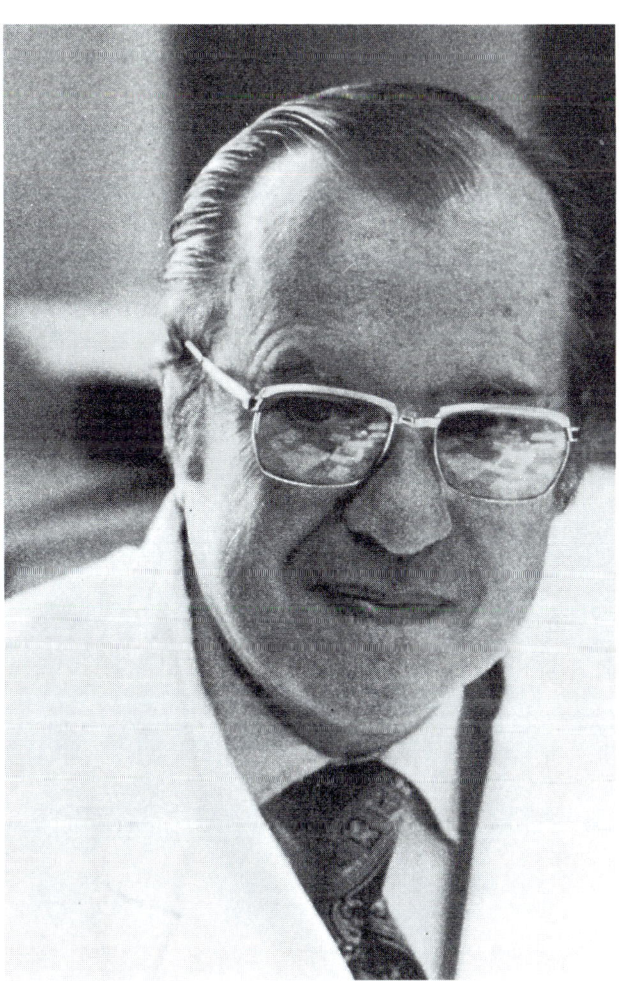

FIG. 24-9. Willard A. Krehl, Ph.D., M.D.; Chairman and Professor of Community Health and Preventive Medicine.

The Preventive Point of View

The overall objective planned for the program in preventive medicine was to ensure that students would understand the existence of a continuity between traditional crisis-oriented medical practice and emerging practices in preventive medicine. Students should come to understand the role of health hazard appraisal and health maintenance as a diagnostic process, with the results of the appraisal corresponding to the management prescribed in traditional medical practice. The role of the physician is that of helping individuals to maintain their health and of ensuring a high level of adaptive functioning.

The concept of treating health patients is rather foreign to traditional concepts of medical practice. Attention, however, to the problems of people reveals a natural history of illness that allows one to treat potential disability in selected individuals well before it produces overt signs or symptoms. Preventive medicine in the eyes of the new Chairman related to all physician behavior concerned with potential disability and associated risk reduction. When the point of intervention occurs before the appearance of signs and symptoms of disease, the practice of preventive medicine is involved.

The Development of Community Health in Preventive Medicine

In the closing phase of Dr. Hinman's Chairmanship extensive discussions were held to project the Department more actively into community affairs. Shortly after Dr. Krehl assumed the Chairmanship it was proposed and approved by the Board of Trustees that the name be changed to Community Health and Preventive Medicine.

Annual reports of the Department of Community Health and Preventive Medicine revealed that the goals and ambitions of the previous Chairmen, Perkins and Hinman, continued to be pursued. The teaching programs focused on biostatistic principles and methodology, environmental hazards to health and their control through occupational medicine practice, and the social, cultural, and behavioral factors of medicine. These principles were emphasized to the medical students through lecture programs, small-class or group-training sessions, by apprenticeship experience in the field, and most importantly through the practical clinical experience achieved in the Health Maintenance Clinic.

▪ Staff and Its Support of the Department

Dr. Albrecht, Professor of Preventive Medicine, continued to provide able support for the incoming Chairman. Dr. Norman Williams was in charge of occupational medicine. Irwin L. Stoloff, Associate Professor, continued his research activities, his teaching program, and particularly the management of the Health Maintenance Clinic. Dr. Hyman Menduke continued as Professor of Preventive Medicine (Biostatistics). Mary W. Herman, Ph.D., Assistant Professor, focused her activities predominantly in the area of social sciences.

▪ Volunteer Faculty

From the very genesis of the Department, through the many difficult years of its transitions, it was aided by a large number of individuals functioning actively in the various programs as nonpaid volunteers. Dr. Jan Lieben, M.D., was Visiting Professor of Preventive Medicine and Occupational Medicine. Louis D. Polk, M.D., Head of the Philadelphia Health Department, was Visiting Professor of Preventive Medicine, as were Albert L. Chapman, M.D., Charles M. Ledum, M.D., J. Thomas Millington, M.D., and Ralph D. Dwork, M.D. Alfred R. Stumpe, M.D., was a Visiting Associate Professor of Preventive Medicine and Aerospace Medicine. William C.E. Pfischner, Jr., M.D., was Assistant Professor of Preventive Medicine and a very active participant in the Health Maintenance Clinic. J. Wayne McFarland, M.D., Assistant Professor of Preventive Medicine, was especially interested in problems regarding cigarette smoking and other habituating problems. Edwin D. Harrington, Jr., M.D., served as Assistant Professor of Preventive Medicine, as did Patricia A.J. Kay, M.D., in the special area of biostatistics. Instructors in the Preventive Medicine Program were Drs. Jerome H. Jacobs, Kenneth J. Brosole, and James S. Urda. Heinrich Brieger continued as an Honorary Professor in the area of occupational medicine.

Although the staff of the Department was small in numbers, it measured up to its responsibilities in the basic areas of biostatistics, epidemiology, the principles and practice of preventive medicine, occupational medicine, and in the Health Maintenance Clinic.

▪ Family Practice Established

On assuming the Chairmanship of the Department, Dr. Krehl had been questioned by the Chairman of the Board of Trustees regarding the feasibility of developing a Family Practice Program at Jefferson, possibly as a Division of the Department. This appeared appropriate because discussions with Family Medicine leaders, particularly board-certified Jefferson graduates, had already taken place. Further efforts to develop such a Division proved successful through the cooperation of the Curriculum Committee, the Dean's Office, and the Jefferson administration. Franklin C. Kelton, M.D., Clinical Instructor in Community Health and Preventive Medicine, provided guidance for the practitioners of family medicine. In the first year of this program, 12 family practitioners, board certified, were additionally appointed as Clinical Instructors in the Division. Most important, 31 freshman students participated in the elective preceptorship programs sponsored by the Family Medicine Group. They met on Wednesday afternoons with mutual satisfaction of both the teachers (family physicians) and the students. Because each group evaluated the other, there was an opportunity for interchange of information regarding the course in this new adventure.

Dr. Kelton was appointed Acting Director of the Division of Family Practice. The number of Clinical Instructors under him was expanded to 29. Each member was a participant in the educational program for freshman medical students as an elective on Wednesday afternoons. The Family Practice Program received support through a generous grant from the Haas Community Fund.

Program Developments

A program in community health care needs was initiated with the cooperation of 12 students in each quarter of the school year, using elective time to bring primary health care delivery to the Gray's Ferry Multipurpose Health Care Facility. This again broadened the community approach in preventive medicine and supported the outreach concept. The Department also significantly increased its development of the South Philadelphia Health Action Program, emphasizing its concerns about community medicine and health care delivery in deprived areas.

At this time a collaborative educational program at Drexel University in the area of occupational and experimental medicine was developed, largely with the active assistance of Dr. Norman Williams. A combined program in the nutrition sciences with the Nutrition Division of Home Economics at Drexel University was also established.

Retirement of Dr. C. Earl Albrecht

Dr. Albrecht retired as of June 30, 1971. He had served the Department with vigor and was of special assistance during his last year and one-half in Dr. Krehl's new Chairmanship. Continued progress was evident in the residency program, with official approval by the College of Graduate Studies for the M.S. degree program. Dr. Albrecht with undiminished energy went on to new adventures in transpolar medicine.

Family Medicine Changes from a Division to a Department

The goal of the Department of Community Health and Preventive Medicine to sponsor a program in Family Medicine reached fruition during 1971 with the appointment of Dr. Paul C. Brucker as Professor and Director of the Division of Family Medicine. The development of the Division saw the participation of 34 part-time practitioners within the Philadelphia area and an approved elective program for freshmen, which provided a strong base for subsequent development under the leadership of Dr. Brucker. In March 1973 Dr. Brucker became Chairman of an independent Department of Family Medicine.

The Impact of Funding on Departmental Changes

A strong shock wave was felt throughout the Department and, indeed, throughout the Medical School with the termination of training grants at the Federal level. Increasingly, the schools and the departments within the medical schools had depended upon Federal support, grants and other governmental assistance to maintain their programs.

The impact of Federal funding restrictions required that the Chairman assume responsibilities representing Jefferson with the Regional Medical Program. The first responsibility was the development of a community hypertension control program in Eastern Pennsylvania. This was a major undertaking and resulted in excellent rapport with the Regional Medical Program, the American Heart Association, and the physicians involved with the latter Association.

A grant-in-aid from the Heinz Foundation permitted the development of a program of clinical and community nutrition in the Department. This was also geared to a statewide education program with Penn State University. The coordinated and linked program benefited both institutions and their students. In practical terms, from the Departmental point of view this relationship generated much-needed staff support for an M.D.-Ph.D. clinician to take on the Directorship of the Division of Clinical and Community Nutrition with appropriate support in the dietetic area.

The most encouraging development in the Department was the program of clinical and community nutrition. Robert Karp, M.D., (a pediatrician with special training in nutrition) was its Director along with Mrs. Gwendolyn Mead, a registered dietician, and Mrs. Jeanette Fairworth, R.N., who had special expertise and experience in the area of public health education. These individuals came into the Department in February of 1974 and worked effectively to develop an appropriate program for the medical students.

Teaching in Medicine and Society

A course called "Medicine and Society" became mandated for freshman and sophomore students. The Department cooperated with this, and Drs. Byrne, Herman, Krehl, and Williams participated. This was a strenuous task, since it meant a restructuring of the old teaching program and reorientation of the Department. Teaching in the Health Maintenance Clinic continued and provided an opportunity for students to evaluate at least two new patients each week for a period of 3 weeks under the direct supervision of a member of the faculty.

A significant reduction in teaching personnel occurred through the transfer of Dr. Earl Byrne from a part-time status to a volunteer clinical responsibility and the illness of Dr. Norman Williams which ended fatally on April 24, 1975. The Chairman incurred increased responsibilities when asked to participate half-time as a staff participant of the Greater Delaware Valley Regional Medical Program with a major responsibility for the community high-blood-pressure control activities. The course in Medicine and Society continued to be a heavy drain on Departmental teaching resources.

The Development of a Departmental Medical Practice Program in Health Maintenance

The success of the Health Maintenance Program was evidenced by a patient load of approximately 3,500 per year. Agreements were made with the administration to cover the costs of this program entirely through resources generated from fees from the individuals who attended. This was eminently successful and permitted the establishment of the Health Maintenance Program in the Health Sciences Center (Edison Building), all costs being borne out of medical practice earnings, and the development of a medical practice plan account. This was a new first for a Department of Preventive Medicine. It demonstrated that preventive medicine could be profitable.

Continued progress in the Health Maintenance Program was evidenced by the expansion of patient flow and by increasing arrangements with industrial groups to provide executive health evaluations. This was a benefit to Jefferson because many of the individuals found to have significant health problems were referred to the medical staff. Again, preventive medicine was fighting its way to profitability at Jefferson. The expansion of the Health Maintenance Program provided opportunities for students in the senior-track program to participate in the occupational health activities associated with some of the medical departments of the industries of the area.

The addition of Dr. Robert Sharrar to the staff in the area of infectious disease epidemiology enhanced that area significantly. A nutrition counseling program was added to the Health Maintenance Program. An alcohol management clinic operated by Dr. William F. Hushion (Jefferson, 1960), Medical Director for the Philadelphia Electric Company, was also added.

Research Activities

Research continued to occupy the interest of the staff. A major project was developed regarding the nutritional status of school children relative to their growth and mental performance. The results indicated that an important segment of the population was inadequately nourished, as manifested through poor school performance, impaired growth and development, and most significantly, serious behavior maladaptations.

The year 1975–1976 saw improvement in the status of the occupational medicine program when Dr. Jan Lieben served as Director of Community Health and Preventive Medicine on a half-time basis. Also, Dr. Ernest M. Kuhinka, Ph.D., as a Visiting Professor of Community Health and Preventive Medicine, undertook research to determine the cost of managing myocardial infarction in 10 community hospitals in the greater Delaware Valley. The area of community health was improved with the addition of Robert Levine, M.S., as an Instructor in Community Health and Preventive Medicine with an emphasis on the role of the social worker in the health care delivery system. Mr. Levine developed an effective apprenticeship program whereby medical students could work with the social workers directly and learn more specifically of their problems and the process of finding solutions, again enhancing the medical students' experience through direct patient contacts.

▪ A Year of Extensive Evaluation (1977–1978)

The Department underwent a series of in-depth reviews, first by the traditional departmental review committee, then by a special committee appointed by the Dean culminating in a special committee headed by Dr. Paul C. Brucker. The latter committee evolved an extensive report along with a series of recommendations for the future. Many areas of tension had been brought into focus in view of the forthcoming retirement of Dr. Krehl as Chairman as of June 30, 1979. Recommendations tended to favor the dissolution of Department.

All of this was somewhat tempered by the Brucker Committee's report, which suggested that the Department not be dissolved but have its focus shifted. The Jefferson Executive Council reviewed and approved the Brucker Committee's recommendation, along with some additional modifications; these were to continue to provide quality teaching programs for the students and to increase the focus on epidemiology, with a renewed emphasis on occupational medicine and environmental health.

The Final Year (1978–1979)—Dissolution of the Department of Community Health and Preventive Medicine

With the retirement of the Chairman, Dr. Krehl, on June 30, 1979, a recommendation was made and accepted by the Board of Trustees to dissolve the Department. Plans were undertaken by the Dean to accommodate the necessary changes. The Department's last year was an anxiety-provoking one.

▪ The Chairman's Reflections on Dissolution of the Department

A final conversation occurred between Dean William F. Kellow and Dr. Krehl regarding the past, present, and future of the Department of Community Health and Preventive Medicine. The Dean expressed his appreciation for the support given to him and the administration in all of the events leading to the dissolution of the Department. This had been expressed previously in a letter from him reporting on the final Departmental Annual Report for the year 1978–1979. In the course of the discussion, Dean Kellow reflected, "You know, Dr. Krehl, I don't think I ever really did understand preventive medicine." Dr. Krehl rather hastily replied, "This is one place where I agree with you completely, Dean Kellow." They both had a bit of a chuckle out of this, because neither statement was made with rancor, anger or criticism—it was just an observation of the realities of two individuals with different philosophies regarding the concept of preventive medicine and all that it should mean in medical education and the people's health.

Dean Kellow and Dr. Krehl went on to discuss in great detail the Health Maintenance Program, its obvious financial success, and its move from the Health Sciences Center to the new Jefferson Hospital. The Dean gave his full agreement and support for it to continue under the full direction and complete financial responsibility of Dr. Krehl. As such, it continued to function until June 30, 1985, when its full management and operational responsibilities were assumed by the Department of Medicine, approved by Dr. Willis Maddrey, Chairman of the Department of Medicine, and under the direct supervision of Dr. John Martin (Figure 24-10). This transfer was particularly gratifying since it gave recognition from a distinguished clinician and Chairman that preventive medicine was important and probably the medicine of the future. The old Health Maintenance Clinic, started by Dr. Perkins, continued to flourish under the direction and management of the Department of Medicine. Direct management came under Dr. Joseph F. Rodgers (Jefferson, 1957) as Medical Director.

Epilogue

Total health care costs in the United States in 1986 amounted to an estimated $445–460 billion. It is important to note that the cost of health care is increasing at the rate of over twice the annual cost of living. A point has been reached where government, corporations, and individuals want to stop this escalating burden. Unfortunately, government programs such as Medicare and Medicaid, most insurance programs, and other agencies responsible for paying health care costs refuse to accept preventive medicine and the quality and potential savings it can provide. As individuals there is a major personal responsibility for each to focus on better diet, more exercise, and avoidance of abusive drugs, including cigarette smoking and alcohol. Society itself is the major cause of excessive health care costs.

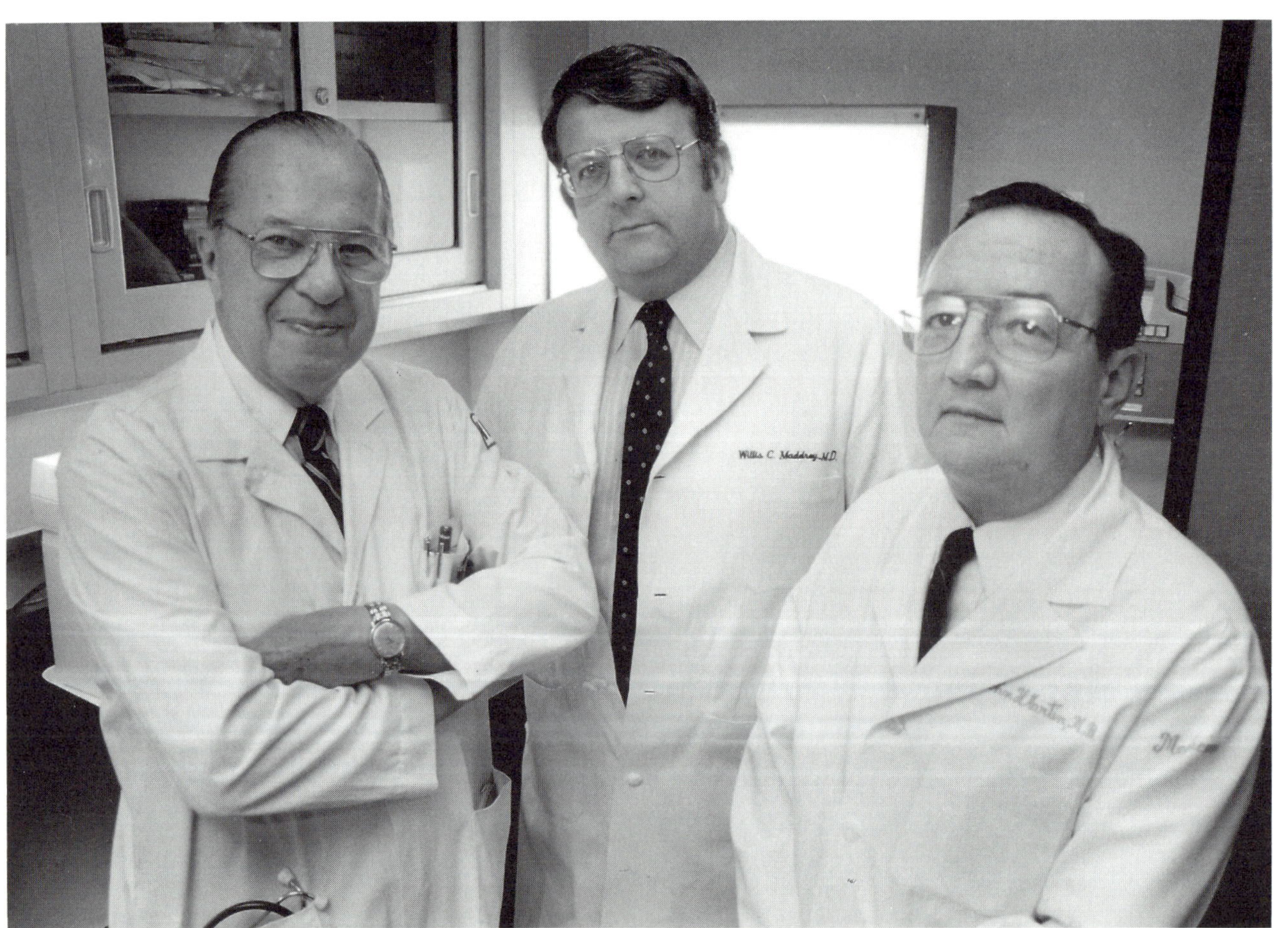

FIG. 24-10. Willard A. Krehl, M.D., Willis C. Maddrey, M.D., and John R. Martin, M.D., on the occasion of transfer of the Health Maintenance Program to the Department of Medicine.

References

1. Heiser, Victor, *An American Doctor's Odyssey*. New York: W.W. Norton & Co. Inc., 1936.
2. Bauer, Edward L., "Preventive Medicine at Jefferson," unpublished manuscript, Jefferson Archives, 1964.
3. Hinman, E. Harold, "William Harvey Perkins, M.D., Sc.D., LL.D., Litt.D., Celebrates 70th Birthday." Jefferson Archives, 1967.
4. Perkins, Wm. Harvey, *Cause and Prevention of Disease*. Philadelphia: Lea & Febiger, 1938.
5. Cannon, Walter B, *The Wisdom of the Body*. Philadelphia: W.B. Norton, 1932.
6. Richards, Dickinson W., "Homeostasis: Its Dislocations and Perturbations," *Persp. in Biol. and Med.*, 1960, pp. 238–251.
7. Richards, Dickinson W., "Homeostasis vs. Hyperexis: Or Saint George and the Dragon." *Scientific Monthly*. 1953, 77: 289–294.
8. Babies' Hospital of Philadelphia Archives. *Historical Collections, College of Physicians of Philadelphia.*
9. Mackmull, Gulden, Menduke, H., and Cava, Joseph, "The Health Maintenance Clinic Program of the Fife–Hamill Memorial Health Center," *Public Health Reports* 1955, 70: 598–604.
10. "Statement of Organization of the Fife–Hamill Memorial Health Center for Southeast Philadelphia," Jefferson Archives.
11. Perkins, Wm. Harvey, *Evolution and Progress Under Natural Law*. Privately published, 1963.
12. Hinman, E. Harold, "Department of Preventive Medicine, Jefferson Medical College 1941–1969," unpublished statement, Jefferson Archives.

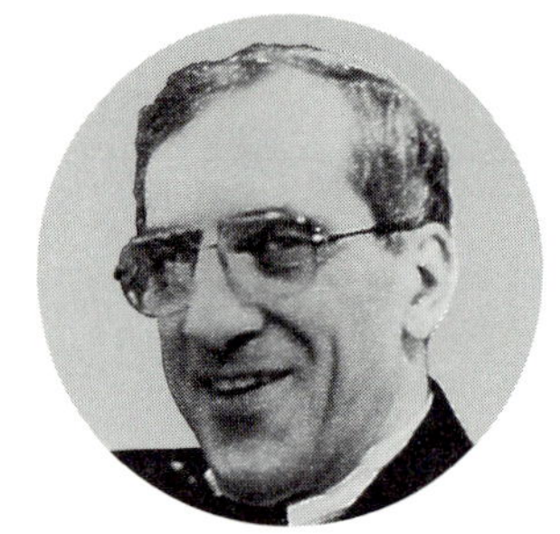

CHAPTER TWENTY-FIVE

Department of Rehabilitation Medicine

FRANCIS NASO, M.D.

"Use strengthens, disuse debilitates."

—HIPPOCRATES (460–370 B.C.)

Physical Therapy Begins as Electrotherapy

The Department of Rehabilitation Medicine had its roots in "Franklinism," the use of electricity in the treatment of disease. In 1752 Benjamin Franklin[1] in Philadelphia employed electricity with success for hysteria in a 24-year-old woman. This modality thereafter became an adjunct in the treatment of both functional and organic disorders of the central and peripheral nervous systems.

In 1881 Dr. Roberts Bartholow,[2] Professor of Materia Medica and General Therapeutics at Jefferson, published an exhaustive treatise on *Medical Electricity*[3] that included electrophysics, electrophysiology, electrodiagnosis, electrotherapeutics, and electricity in surgery. Dr. Hobart A. Hare,[4] who succeeded Dr. Bartholow from 1891 to 1931, was well known for his skill in treating syphilitic thoracic aneurysms by inserting gold wires through a needle coated with porcelain, followed by electrolysis. This was usually performed in the clinical amphitheater before the students.

The first lectures in electrotherapy were given by Max H. Bochroch[5] (Jefferson, 1880) who was listed as Instructor in Electrotherapeutics in the Jefferson Catalogue of 1895–1896 and 1900–1901. He was subsequently a Demonstrator of Neurology (Mind and Nervous System) in 1901–1902 and 1905–1906. Dr. Bochroch was also one of the eight Jefferson founders of the James Aitken Meigs Medical Association,[6] a social and scientific group that still flourishes. A lifelong interest in mental and nervous diseases led to his Professorship at Temple University around 1925.

In 1909 electrotherapy and massage were carried out in the Neurological Dispensary of what was then the new hospital (1907) at Tenth and Sansom Streets. Drs. William L. Clark and Cyril P. O'Boyle served as Chief and Assistant Electrotherapists respectively, while therapeutic massage was conducted by J.B. Briechner and Miss Liddie Keffer. The appointment of Dr. William H. Schmidt as Assistant Electrotherapist in 1920 accelerated the development of this hospital service. A "Clark Electrotherapeutic Society" of 27 students held meetings in 1923 and 1924, with Dr. Clark as Honorary President, and then disbanded.

In 1925 Dr. William H. Schmidt (Figure 25-1) became the Lecturer in Electrotherapeutics, the name of which was changed to Physical Therapy in 1930. Dr. Schmidt was promoted to Assistant Professor in 1936. He lectured rapidly without notes and never failed to fascinate the group gathered in the clinic or operating room. He was energetic, extrovertive, and dramatic as he demonstrated various modalities of treatment, including electrostatic sparks and fulgerations of skin cancers. He was popular with the students, some of whom felt that he carried an aura of Merlin the Magician (Figure 25-2).

At this time, major changes were occurring in the field of physical medicine and rehabilitation outside the Jefferson complex. A 1921 graduate of Jefferson, Dr. Frank H. Krusen formed the first Department of Physical Medicine at Temple University Hospital in 1929. In 1943 the Baruch Foundation, under the influence of Dr. Krusen as Executive Director, met for the first time to explore means of developing the field further. By this action, Dr. Krusen was credited as the "Father of the Field of Physical Medicine."[7]

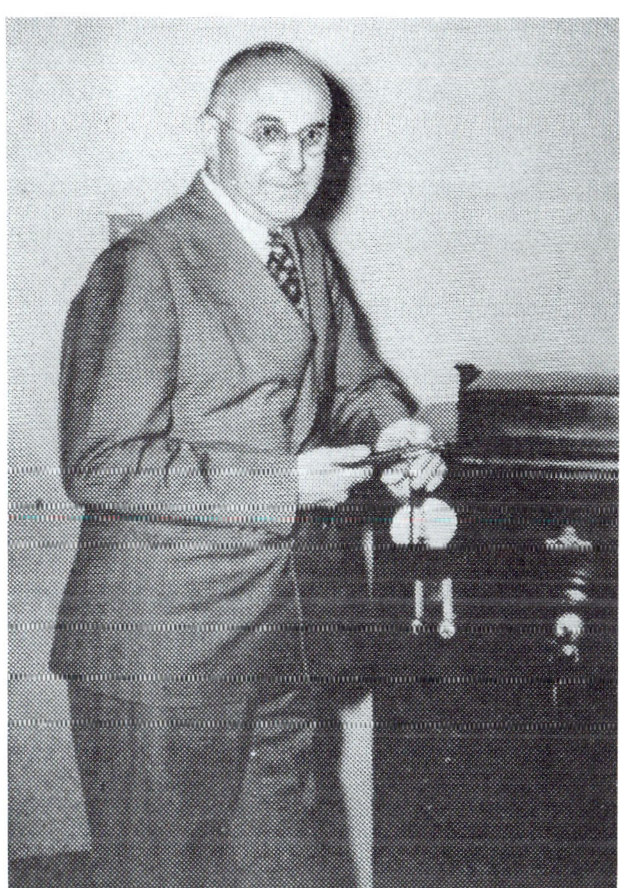

Fig. 25-1. William H. Schmidt, M.D., early proponent of electrotherapy and physical therapy.

From the experience of World War II, important changes occurred through improved management of military casualties with major trauma and spinal cord injury. Reduced mortality rates created an increased demand for rehabilitation medicine teaching because no one was quite sure what to do with those patients affected by major paralysis. The field began to stress rehabilitation and its two major principles: adjustment to disability and attainment of independence. This aspect of treatment would peak 30 years later with the development of regional spinal cord centers.

The Division of Physical Medicine and Rehabilitation

At the retirement of Dr. Schmidt in 1959, Dr. John W. Goldschmidt (Jefferson, 1954) became Director of the newly designated Division of Physical Medicine and Rehabilitation. Dr. Goldschmidt (Figure 25-3), after his internship at Fitzgerald Mercy Hospital, completed two years of medical residency. In 1957 he enrolled in the rehabilitation residency at the Hospital of the University of Pennsylvania and completed his training in 1959. He then returned to Jefferson to initiate the next step in the development of Rehabilitation Medicine at his alma mater. An advisory committee for physical medicine and rehabilitation was created, composed of the Chairmen of the major Departments, including Dean William A. Sodeman; Bernard J. Alpers, Professor of Neurology; John H. Gibbon, Jr., Professor of Surgery; Anthony F. DePalma, Professor of Orthopaedic Surgery; Robert A. Matthews, Professor of Psychiatry; and Robert I. Wise, Professor of Medicine. A Division of Rehabilitation Medicine in the Department of Medicine was established with Dr. Goldschmidt as Director. Physical therapy, which until then had been in the Department of Neurology, became a part of the new section. During this tenure, services were expanded to include physical and occupational therapies and speech pathology

(Figure 25-4). In 1963 a new Rehabilitation Unit was dedicated on the third floor of the Thompson Building, with a 32-bed inpatient unit and a new electromyography (EMG) laboratory. When Dr. Goldschmidt left the Division in 1967 to accept the Deanship of the College of Allied Health Sciences, Dr. Thomas A. Kelley, Jr., became Acting Director of the Section of Physical Medicine and Rehabilitation of the Department of Medicine.

The Department of Rehabilitation Medicine

In 1969 Rehabilitation Medicine became a separate Department with Dr. John F. Ditunno, Jr. as its first Professor and Chairman (Figure 25-5). Dr. Ditunno was a Philadelphian whose training had its roots in multiple centers throughout the country. After receiving his degree in medicine in 1958 at Hahnemann, he remained at that institution for his internship. He left the City to practice general medicine in Hot Springs, North Carolina. Although he was destined for a comprehensive approach to medical care even before these years in the South, he became more convinced that his future was neither in the technical field of surgery nor the esoteric hands-off approach of the medical subspecialties. He enjoyed the close relationship with patients and appreciated the importance of the concept that once life-and-death issues of diseases were resolved, the quality of life of the patient needed attention.

In 1962 Ditunno returned to Hahnemann for

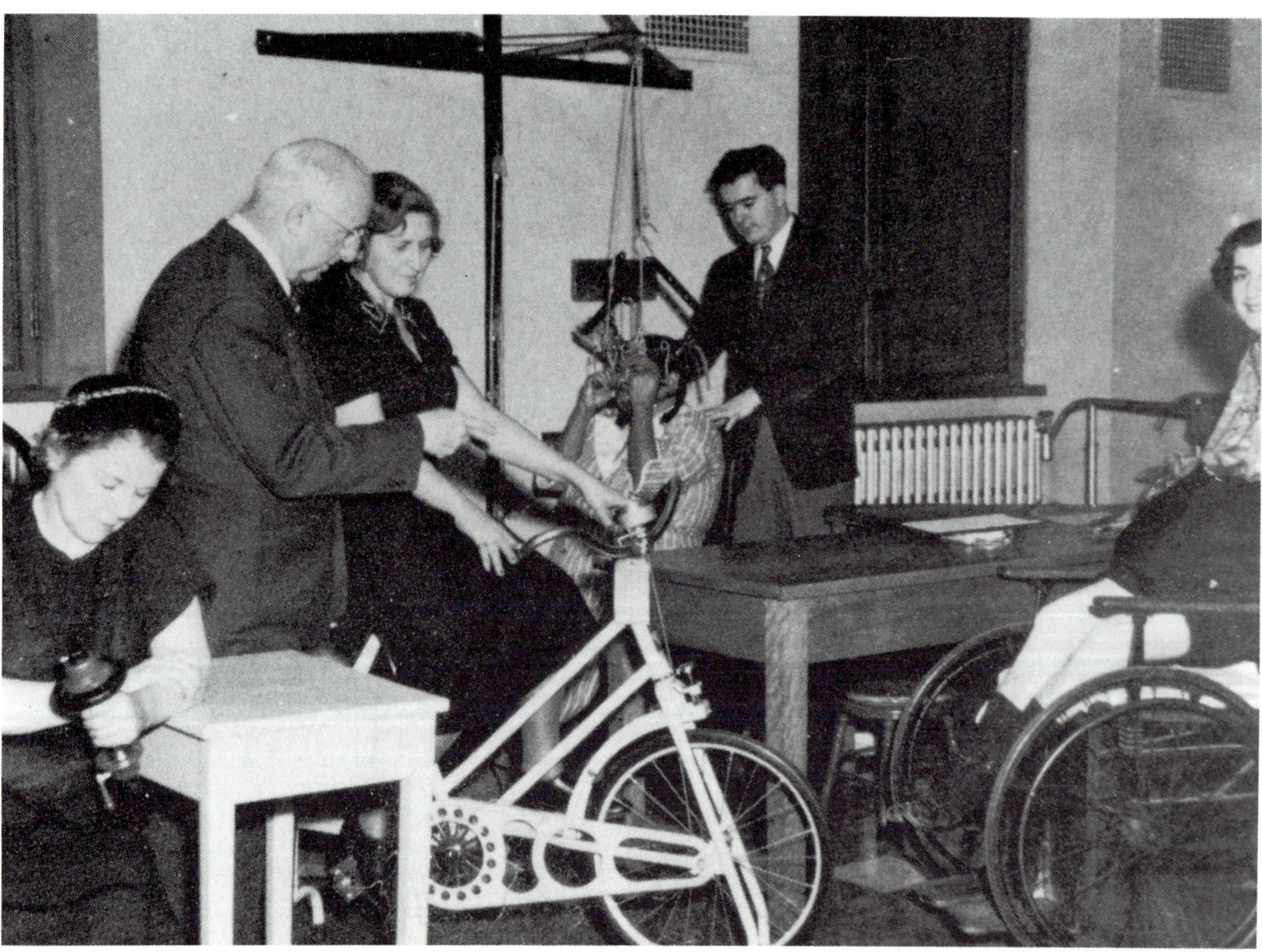

FIG. 25-2. Dr. Schmidt supervising physical therapy session (ca. 1930s).

a residency in internal medicine. The phrase "comprehensive medicine" was in vogue at this time, meaning total care of the patient—addressing psychological-social as well as physical needs. Dr. Ditunno began to familiarize himself with this aspect of medicine and read about Dr. Howard Rusk and his accomplishments. Upon deciding to enter the field of Rehabilitation Medicine, he spent six months at Jacobi Hospital at the Albert Einstein Medical School in New York under Dr. Arthur Abrams, an inspirational role model. It was here that he met Dr. Gerald J. Herbison (Figure 25-6) with whom a relationship developed that was to be of critical importance to the future program at Jefferson. Ditunno continued his residency at the University of Pennsylvania in Philadelphia and received his certification in 1965. On return to Hahnemann he began to develop the section of Physical Medicine and Rehabilitation. Unfortunately, events at that hospital prevented his expectations from reaching fulfillment and he left to become an Associate Professor of Rehabilitation Medicine at Temple University. Dr. Herbison joined the Temple staff in 1969 as Associate Director and with this the seeds were sown for the new Department at Jefferson.

As major changes continued in the field, the former Dean at Hahnemann, Dr. William F. Kellow, was now at Jefferson, and he remembered Dr. Ditunno well from his Hahnemann years. Dean Kellow was convinced that Jefferson needed a Rehabilitation Department, and he contacted Dr. Ditunno. This constituted a challenge particularly because Ditunno would be one of the youngest Chairmen in the field. Dr. Ditunno accepted Dr. Kellow's offer and set out to choose the members of the Department. He first selected

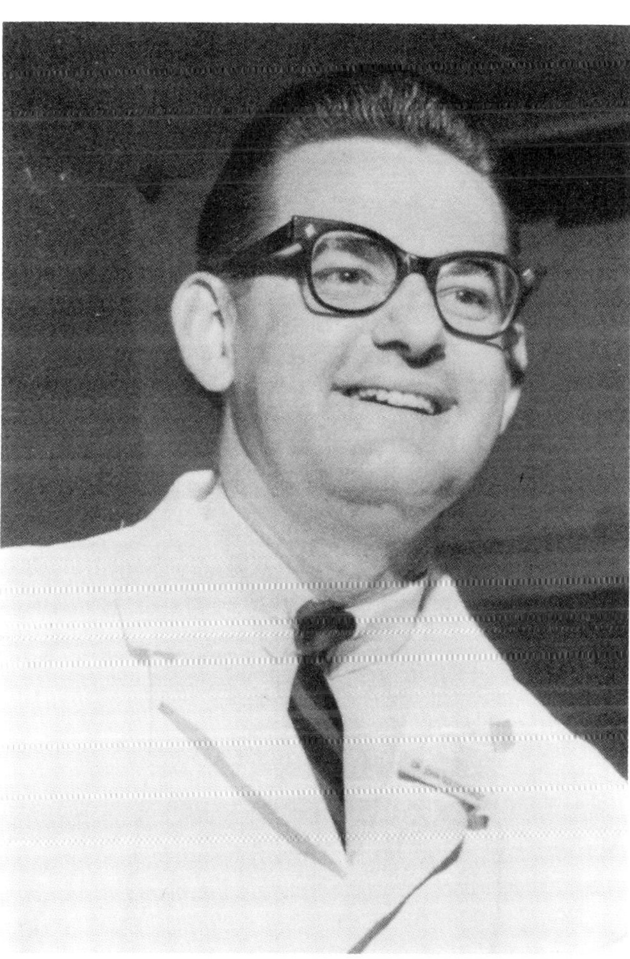

FIG. 25-3. John W. Goldschmidt, M.D.; First Director, Division of Rehabilitation in Department of Medicine, later Dean (1967), College of Allied Health Sciences.

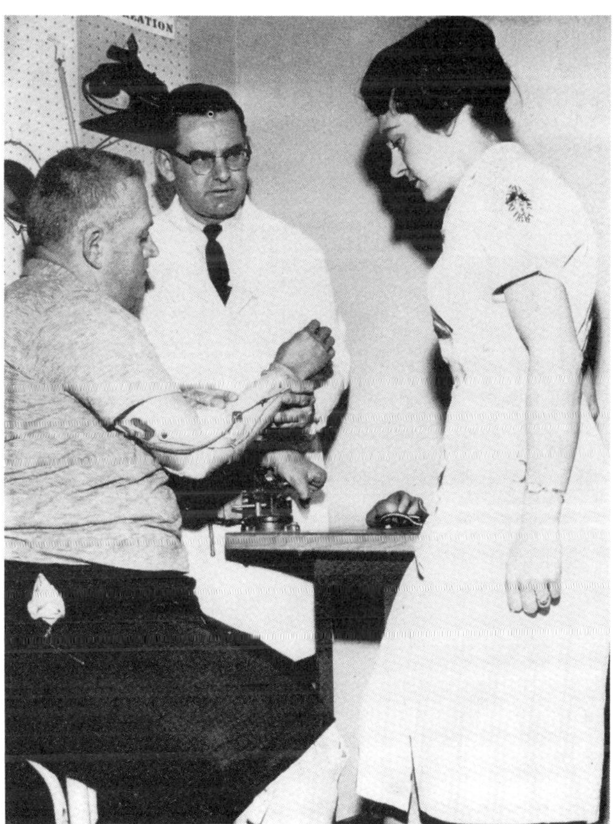

FIG. 25-4. Dr. Goldschmidt planning a treatment program.

Edward E. Gordon, M.D. as Professor and Director of Research, an extremely productive physiatrist, whose contributions to the literature and qualities as a teacher were unsurpassed. The field needed physicians of this type, and Jefferson was fortunate to have Dr. Gordon. His second choice was Dr. Herbison, the promising young man from Temple who was to become one of the leading physicians in rehabilitation medicine. As was often the case in the early development of the field, Dr. Herbison's major motivating factor that directed him into rehabilitation medicine was his own physical impairment. He had had poliomyelitis as a child and, given the proper circumstances, would relate his experiences during the almost brutal treatment that characterized the management of the disease years before. Dr. Ditunno appreciated the intensity of his commitment and knew that he would be the person to get the new program on its way.

A key position in the Department was filled by William E. Staas, M.D. (Jefferson, 1962). After spending two years with the Armed Services, Dr. Staas (Figure 25-7) trained in Rehabilitation Residency at the Hospital of the University of Pennsylvania. His rotations included a considerable time at Jefferson, because this was part of the rotation schedule for the University Residents. He joined the staff of the Section of Rehabilitation Medicine with its Acting Director, Dr. Kelly. Staas proved to be a valued addition to the new Department because he was known to the Jefferson staff and was highly respected as a clinician. The Department seemed established, only to undergo almost immediate change when Dr. Gordon left because of problems that required his return to the Midwest. Dr. Herbison was selected to continue the research program, something that he had not intended. Over the five to six years that followed, Dr. Gordon acted as consultant as the Research Program continued with the acquisition of a Research Laboratory in the Curtis Building. Although he was present in a consultation capacity only, Dr. Gordon served as a mentor for Dr. Herbison through the early phases of medical exploration in the new Department. The success of that guidance was clearly evident later.

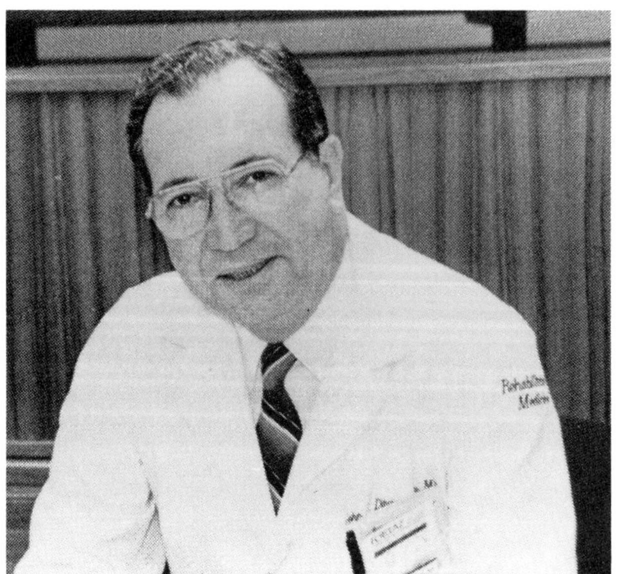

FIG. 25-5. John F. Ditunno, Jr., M.D.; First Chairman, Department of Rehabilitation Medicine (1969–).

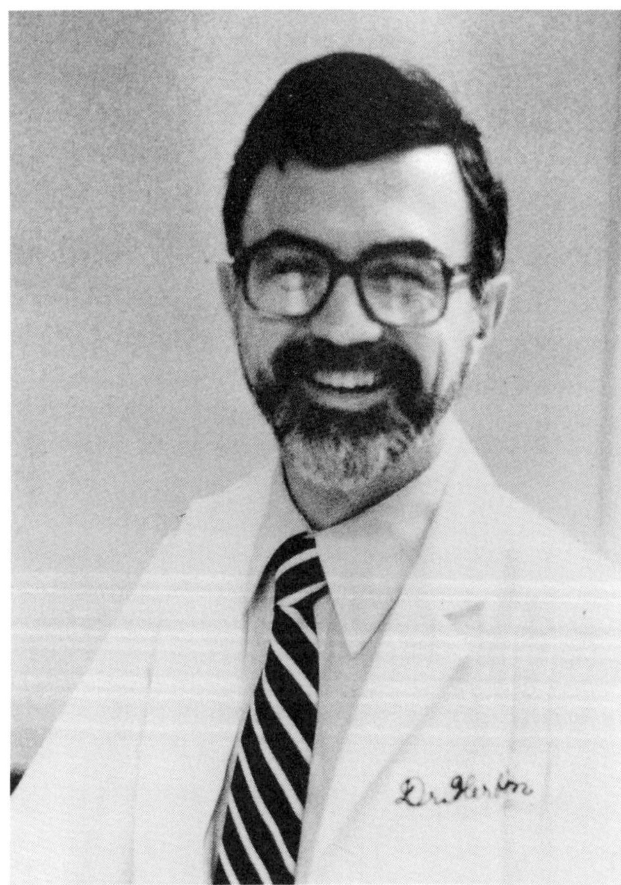

FIG. 25-6. Gerald J. Herbison, M.D., Professor of Rehabilitation and Research.

A training program was initiated with Dr. Leon Venier as the first Resident. Affiliations were established with Lankenau Hospital and with Einstein Medical Center, Daroff Division.

Expansion of the Department continued with the addition of full-time physicians and affiliations with other hospitals. In 1972 a pediatric rehabilitation affiliation was developed with Children's Heart Hospital, renamed the Children's Rehabilitation Hospital in 1986. Dr. Ditunno was also called upon to assist in the formation of a rehabilitation facility at Crozer-Chester Medical Center, and in 1974 Dr. Robert Condon became its full-time Director. This institution served as a valued rotation for the Residency program, offering experience in the care of burns and acute and chronic pain. In 1985 when it opened its ten-bed rehabilitation unit, it added a second full-time physiatrist, Dr. Peggy Abrams, a former Chief Resident in Rehabilitation at Jefferson.

An affiliation of primary importance was consummated on October 10, 1975, between Jefferson and Magee Memorial Rehabilitation Center (currently Magee Rehabilitation Hospital) at 6 Franklin Plaza in Philadelphia. This institution was founded through the 1916 bequest of Miss Anna J. Magee (Figure 25-8), whose generosity also endowed the Magee Chair of Medicine. In 1977 Dr. Staas, who served as Director of Resident and Medical Education as

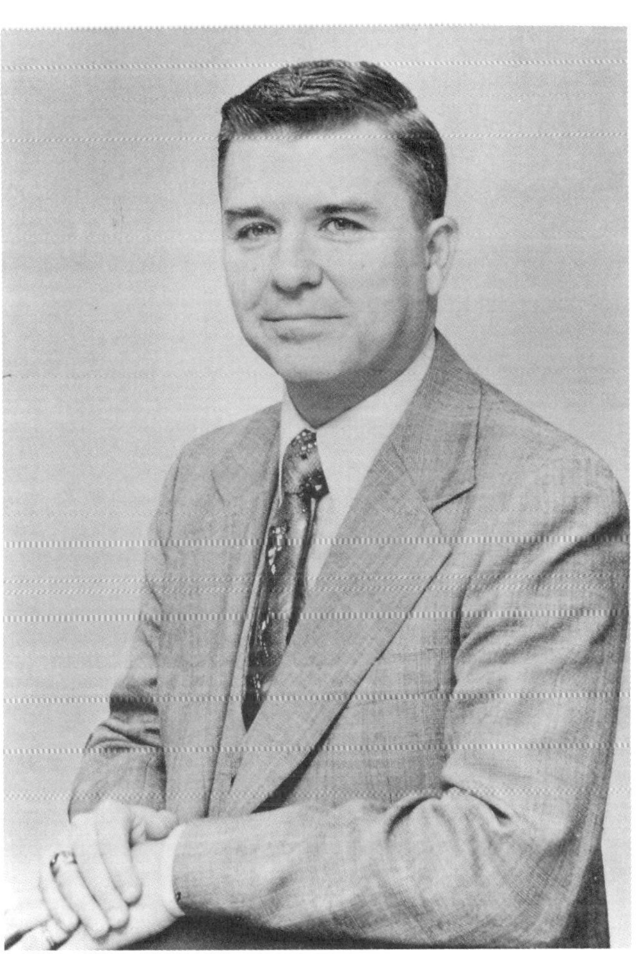

FIG. 25-7. William E. Staas, M.D., Medical Director and President of Magee Rehabilitation Hospital (1967).

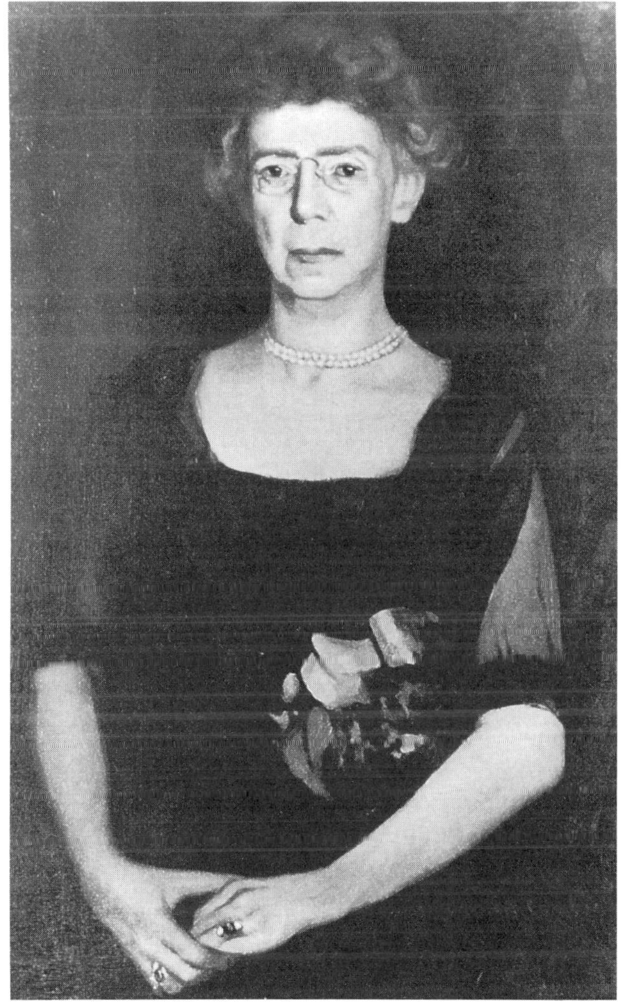

FIG. 25-8. Portrait of Miss Anna J. Magee, donor of Magee Rehabilitation Hospital.

well as Director of the Rehabilitation Unit, became the Medical Director and President of Magee. Under his tutelage the facility became an important part of the training program for residents, which expanded from the original three positions in the 1970s to 18 positions in 1987. Furthermore, Magee would serve as an essential part of the Thomas Jefferson University Hospital Program in medical student teaching and research, and its cooperative program in pain management, brain injury, and spinal cord injury. Dr. Staas' unique abilities as a superb clinician, administrator, and teacher were clearly responsible, to a major degree, for the continued growth of Magee and the refinement of its relationship with Jefferson.

Under the guidance of Drs. Nathan Smukler (Jefferson, 1947) and John Abruzzo, of the Rheumatology Division of the Department of Medicine, and Dr. Ditunno, the Arthritis Center was developed, coordinating the treatment concepts of the fields of rheumatology as well as rehabilitation medicine. Representing the Department of Rehabilitation Medicine, Dr. Stanley Jacobs (Jefferson, 1972), after his internship, became a Resident in the new Department of Rehabilitation Medicine and upon completion of his Residency remained on the staff. His preciseness and concern about detail made him one of the finest teachers in the Department. Additional programs were added such as the cardiac rehabilitation program in 1973, which, under the directorship of Dr. Frank Naso, encompassed all phases of management.

Spinal Cord Injury

A significant development was the awarding of a multiyear demonstration grant to Jefferson in 1978 for the study and treatment of spinal cord injury. This effort was to produce major changes throughout the University. Dr. Ditunno, utilizing his unique ability to relate to his surgical peers, planned a multidisciplinary approach to the treatment of spinal cord injury. With Drs. Jewell Osterholm, the Chairman of Neurosurgery, and Jerome Cotler, the Clinical Director of Orthopaedics, the team was complete. With this arrangement, the physiatrist was no longer "at the end of the line," providing treatment only when the patient was "medically stable." At the time of admission to the Spinal Cord Injury Center, each patient would be seen not only by the neurosurgeon and orthopedist, but also by the physiatrist. Evaluation would begin by each of the disciplines and follow-up would continue. The physiatrist directed the early rehabilitation program to prevent or retard those sequelae and complications so characteristic of this phase of illness. Very early in this care, these patients would be transferred to the Rehabilitation Center where the primary physician would be the physiatrist. The program continued its development through the efforts of a large staff that included Drs. Ditunno, Staas, and Posuniak.

The Regional Spinal Cord Injury Center of Delaware Valley became one of the most important in the country and has made a substantial contribution to medical practice. With over 120 new admissions each year, each of the major Departments has benefited. In addition to the areas of orthopaedics and neurosurgery, its impact was felt in medicine, urology, plastic surgery, and physiatrics. Opportunities in research became important in the further development of the Center with projects in the causes and treatment of thrombophlebitis in spinal cord injury patients. The project was carried out in cooperation with the Department of Medicine through Dr. Geno J. Merli (Jefferson, 1975) a physiatrist as well as an internist.

Departmental Expansion

In 1981 after 11 years of continued rehabilitation service expansion, Lankenau Hospital, one of the regional major medical centers and a long-time affiliate of Jefferson Hospital, recognized the importance of full-time physiatric coverage and announced the appointment of Dr. Jay Siegfried, a former Chief Resident at Jefferson, as Director of the Department. It became a major residency rotation and since 1983 has offered continued experience with electromyography as well as a consultation service. An affiliation with Bryn

Mawr Rehabilitation Hospital was formulated in 1983 and became a rotation for the Residents in 1985. Also in 1986, the former Children's Heart Hospital changed its name and orientation to become the "Children's Rehabilitation Hospital." At this time, Ditunno attracted Dr. Nadine Trainer, educated both in Pediatrics and Rehabilitation, to the staff. She was a major addition to the staff of both Jefferson and the Children's Rehabilitation Hospital. In 1984 the Department had been asked to participate in the training of medical students at the junior and senior levels. Although electives had been offered before, this was to be an obligatory rotation. The two-week rotation made Jefferson one of the few institutions that exposed all medical students to the field of Physical Medicine and Rehabilitation.

In 1987 the Department consisted of seven full-time physicians with nine additional physicians at Magee. Full services were offered in all disciplines, with 17 physical therapists, 11 occupational therapists, three speech pathologists, two psychologists, and three social workers. Treatment programs included spinal cord injury, stroke, amputations, cancer, cardiac disease, arthritis, compensable injury fitness, and cooperative programs in sexual dysfunction, sports medicine, and pain management.

The Department and its members were recognized as constituting one of the major rehabilitation facilities and training centers in the country. Its members have received recognition throughout the world. In 1983 Dr. Herbison, Director of Research and one of the most inspired physicians in the field, became editor of the *Archives of Physical Medicine and Rehabilitation*,[7] the

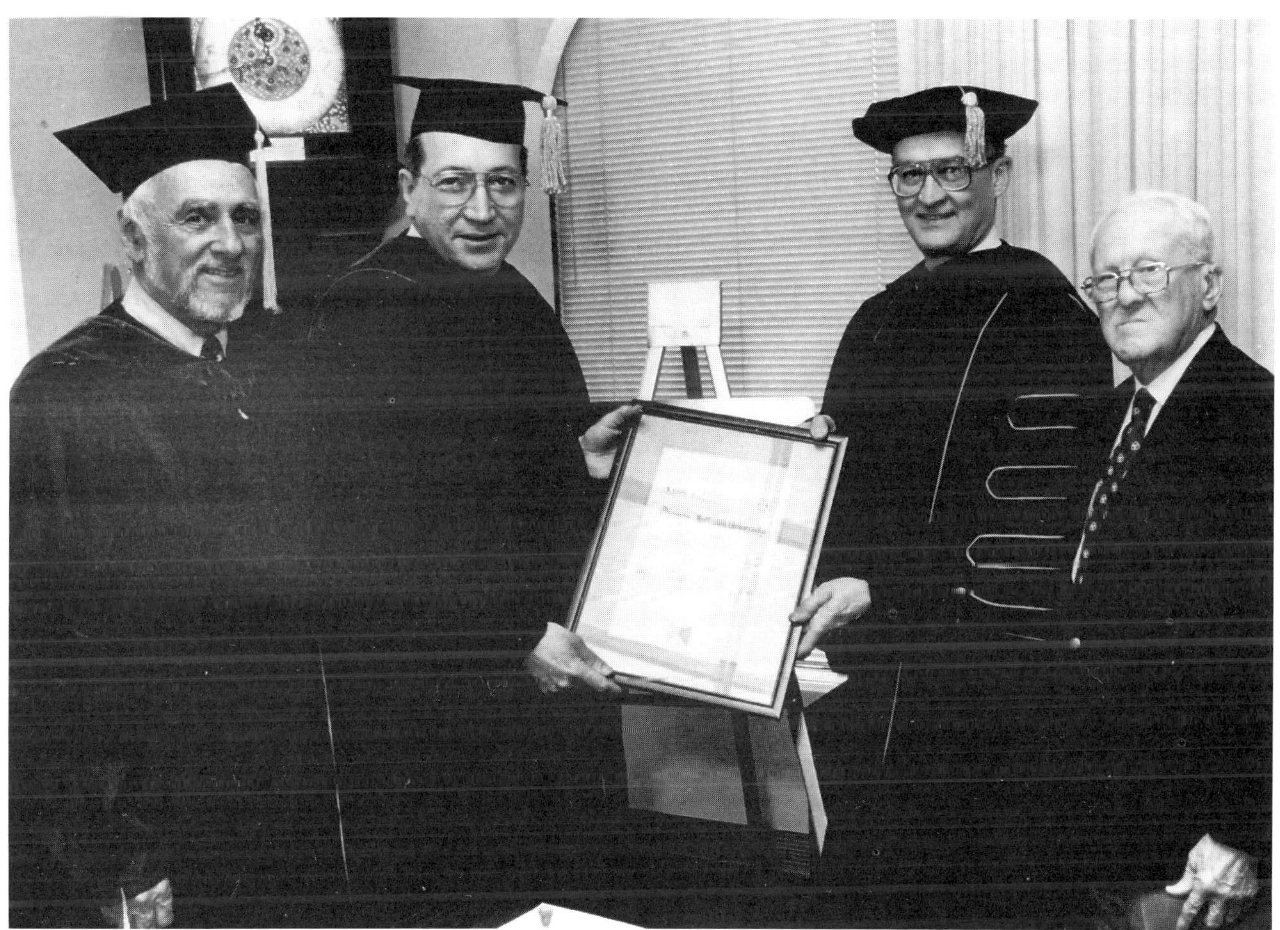

FIG. 25-9. Inauguration of the Michie Professorship of Rehabilitation Medicine on May 8, 1987. Left to right, Daniel B. Michie, Jr., Esq.; John F. Ditunno, M.D.; Lewis W. Bluemle, M.D.; and Clarence B. Michie.

major scientific journal in the field. He also received the honored position of Zeiter Lecturer in 1984. Major contributions to the literature occurred under the guidance of Dr. Herbison. In addition to his skills as teacher and administrator, his laboratory contributed significant papers on exercise and muscle physiology. Dr. Ditunno served as President of the American Academy of Physical Medicine and Rehabilitation and the Association of Academic Physiatrists as well as Chairman of the American Board of Physical Medicine and Rehabilitation. His recognition locally was exemplified by his inauguration in May, 1987, as the first Michie Professor of Rehabilitation Medicine, an endowed Chair provided by a bequest of Jessie B. Michie to Jefferson as a family memorial (Figure 25-9).

By 1988, the Rehabilitation Medicine at Thomas Jefferson University Hospital could not be recognized, at least on the surface, as the offspring of that original facility from the beginning of the century. Research was not a part of the program at that time but the research efforts under Drs. Ditunno and Herbison reached their culmination with a $2.5 million grant from the U.S. Department of Education–National Institute on Disability and Rehabilitation Research for the study of neural recovery in spinal cord injury. Earlier emphasis on electrotherapeutics seemed to be far removed from the modalities used by the new Department. On closer review, however, electricity began to receive focused attention once more. One of the major areas of research involved thrombophlebitis in the spinal cord-injured population, with electrical stimulation of paralyzed lower extremities under study as a preventive measure. Furthermore, in the recovery of upper-extremity functioning in quadriplegics, electricity was being used not only to quantitate muscle strength but also to study neurologic recovery. Indeed the cycle was complete.

Ongoing challenges for the Department involve rehabilitation in congenital disorders, trauma disabilities, and infirmities of an ever-expanding aging population. To improve upon older methods and to develop newer ones remain constant goals of the Department.

References

1. Konkle, B.A., and Henry, F.P., *Standard History of the Medical Profession of Philadelphia.* 2d Ed. New York: AMS Press, 1977, p. 482.
2. Kelly, H.A., and Burrage, W.L., *American Medical Biographies.* New York: Appleton, 1928, p. 64.
3. Bartholow, R., *Medical Electricity: A Practical Treatise on the Applications of Electricity to Medicine and Surgery.* 2d Ed. Philadelphia: H.C. Lea's Son and Co., 1882.
4. McCrae, T., "Memoir of Hobart Amory Hare, M.D.," *Trans. Stud. Coll. Phys. Phila.* 1932, pp. LXVII–LXXV.
5. Gould, G.M., *The Jefferson Medical College of Philadelphia.* Vol. II. Lewis Co., 1904, pp. 44–46.
6. Wagner, F.B., Jr., "The Meigs Medical Association: A Jefferson Tradition," *Jeff. Med. Coll. Al. Bull.* Fall 1983, pp. 20–22.
7. Robison, M.O., *Frank N. Krusen, Pioneer in Physical Medicine.* Minneapolis: T.S. Dennison and Co., Inc., 1963.

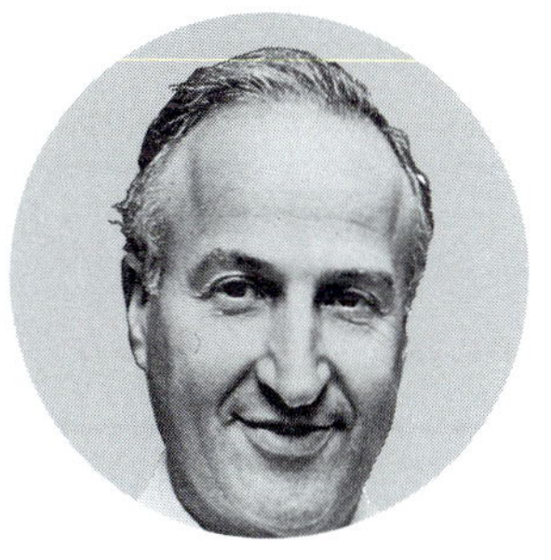

CHAPTER TWENTY-SIX

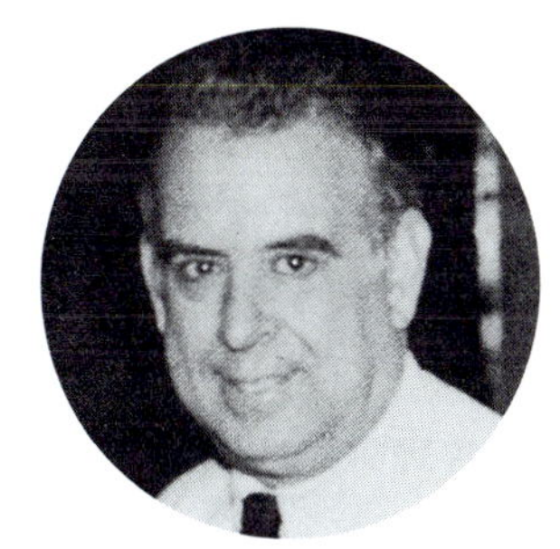

Department of Pediatrics

ROBERT L. BRENT, M.D., PH.D., AND
ARTURO R. HERVADA, M.D.

"Children are not simply micro-adults, but have their own specific problems."

—BELA SCHICK (1877–1967)

THE CONCEPT of a self-governing Department of Pediatrics as it exists today at Jefferson would have seemed unfathomable to eighteenth and nineteenth century physicians, who believed that illnesses of the young were adequately cared for by the same clinicians who treated adults. There was in the United States throughout that time a deplorable attitude toward the welfare of infants and children.[1,2] Medical problems concerning the young were relegated to the midwife, a mother's obstetrician, or the family practitioner, none of whom had broad-based understanding of childhood diseases or the expertise for their treatment. Accordingly, when Jefferson was established in 1824, it was considered unquestionably appropriate that the health care needs of the young come under the auspices of the Department of Obstetrics and Diseases of Children although European medical schools had long since separated child medicine from the care of adult patients.

Jefferson physicians, medical students, and the lay community expressed little concern or interest in this void. Students were indifferent to the poor representation of childhood illnesses within the obstetrics curriculum and were hardly aware that only a few isolated articles on childhood diseases could be found in the scientific literature. Manuscripts usually focused on epidemic topics such as cholera, diphtheritic croup, tuberculous meningitis, and scarlet fever.

In was not until 1825 that the first comprehensive scientific American textbook, *Treatise on the Physical and Medical Treatment of Children,* appeared. It was written by Dr. William Potts Dewees, a fervently loyal alumnus of the University of Pennsylvania. Dr. Samuel D. Gross refers in his *Autobiography* to the competition between the University of Pennsylvania and Jefferson Medical College. When Gross approached Dr. Dewees to review his translation from the French of Hatin's *Manual of Obstetrics,* the latter shunned the request with the statement that "though Gross might be a clever and promising young man, the faculty of the University (of Pennsylvania) could take no notice of anything that emanated from the Jefferson (Medical) School."

The Dewees work was highly regarded and was reprinted eight times. It fostered in other physicians, particularly those practicing in

Philadelphia, an increasingly fervent interest in the study of childhood diseases. Shortly thereafter, Jefferson faculty, including Drs. John Eberle (Professor of Medicine), Charles D. Meigs (Professor of Obstetrics and Diseases of Children), and William Keating (later Professor of Obstetrics and Diseases of Children), added their impressive contributions to children's medical literature.[3–7] Dr. Eberle, already a recognized medical writer, published his *Treatise on the Diseases and Physical Education of Children* in 1833. Eberle's viewpoint differed from that of Dewees; he approached the subject in relation to the practice of medicine, whereas Dewees looked upon the diseases of children as related to obstetrics. An astute observation that placed Eberle's thinking ahead of his time was that children with cholera infantum craved smoked and salted foods. This has a modern counterpart in the correction of hyponatremia in children with acute diarrheal diseases by fluid and electrolyte replacement.

Dr. Charles Delucena Meigs, Professor of Obstetrics and Diseases of Children (1841–1861), published his *Observations on Certain Diseases of Young Children* in 1850. This was an incomplete text that reflected mainly his pediatric lectures of 1849 but exhibited an emphasis on health and diseases of children as a developing discipline.

Pediatrics in the Twentieth Century

It was not until the late nineteenth century that the prevention and treatment of diseases of children as a separate branch of medicine began to emerge. There was a movement toward specialization and subspecialization in all branches of medicine with increasing emphasis on preventive health care. New needs developed, both in educating physicians and in treating patients.

Jefferson responded to the changing times. In 1888 under Dr. J. N. Rhoads an outpatient department for Children's Diseases was established. Dr. Oliver Rex was appointed the first Clinical Lecturer of Diseases of Children.[8] In 1892 Professor Edwin E. Graham (Jefferson, 1887) became Clinical Professor of Children's Diseases. Much credit is due Dr. Graham for his persistence in expanding outpatient services and in developing clinical and didactic sessions for ambulatory and inpatient services. In 1910 he added the didactic pediatric course to the curriculum, and the instructional program was increased to 99 hours for both clinical experience and didactic lectures. This represented a significant achievement for a Medical College in which, only a decade before, the medical uniqueness of children was allocated a minor education role. The Department was titled "Diseases of Children." This designation was retained until 1944, when it became the Department of Pediatrics. The outpatient clinic, however, employed the term "Pediatric Dispensary" beginning in 1909.

Edwin E. Graham, M.D.; First Chairman of Diseases of Children (1908–1926)

Jefferson established an independent Department of Diseases of Children in 1908 and appointed Dr. Edwin E. Graham (Figure 26-1) as its first Chairman.[8] The Department under Dr. Graham's leadership developed its own medical education program and a clinical service of approximately 40 to 50 beds located on the eighth floor of the "Old Main" Hospital. The Pediatric Ambulatory Facility was located in the basement of the main building.

The development of a freestanding Department of Diseases of Children at Jefferson represented a monumental step toward disassociating the care of infants and children from adults and toward satisfying the need for specialty training for physicians who provided health care for the young. In 1916 Dr. Graham authored a major textbook, *Diseases of Children,* published by Lea and Febiger.

Dr. Graham held the Professorship until 1926, at which time he was named Emeritus; he had served his alma mater for 38 years. Physician associates working with him included: Warren H. Johnston, Ralph L. Engle, Eugene Rush, S. Lincoln Baron, Henry Harris Perlman, Howard M. Kuehner, Robert A. Schless, Ralph M. Tyson, Clark O.

Stull, Frank Konzelman, E.A. Harris, Norman M. MacNeill, James C. Harding, Dennis T. Sullivan, John A. Kahler, and John F. Coppolino.[9]

Among these, Dr. Perlman (Jefferson, 1918) had a long career in pediatrics and later was the first board-certified pediatric dermatologist in the United States (Figure 26-2).[10] Dr. John Coppolino (Jefferson, 1922) was for many years the leader in pediatrics among the physicians of South Philadelphia and referred many children to Jefferson's Hospital and Pediatric Clinic. Dr. Ralph M. Tyson (Jefferson, 1915) became Chairman of Pediatrics at Temple University School of Medicine in 1930.

Edward L. Bauer, M.D.; Second Chairman (1926–1954)

Edward L. Bauer, M.D. (Jefferson, 1914) (Figure 26-3) who succeeded Dr. Graham in 1926, represented the seventh in eight generations of sons who became physicians—four generations are recorded as alumni of Jefferson. Dr. Bauer led the crusade against diphtheria in the City of Philadelphia in the early twentieth century and was credited with major public health accomplishments during that period. He had also become Physician to Girard College, a post he was to hold for many years. These accomplishments, especially the diphtheria campaign, impressed Dr. Graham, who favored him as his successor.

Soon after his appointment at Jefferson, Dr. Bauer developed new outpatient programs that included neuropsychiatric services for children in cooperation with Dr. Baldwin L. Keyes. For some years, he arranged for students to rotate through

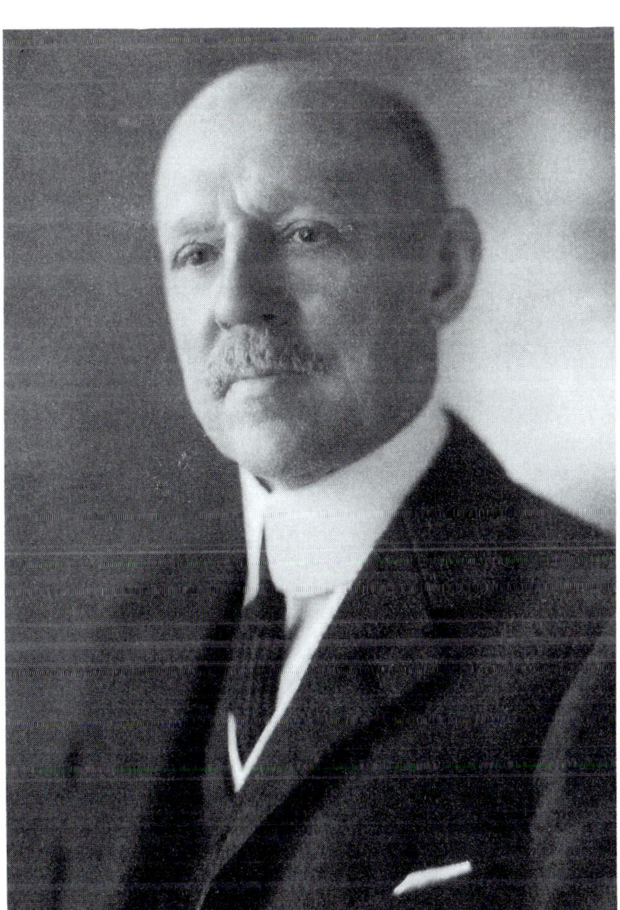

FIG. 26-1. Edwin E. Graham, M.D.; First Chairman (1908–1926).

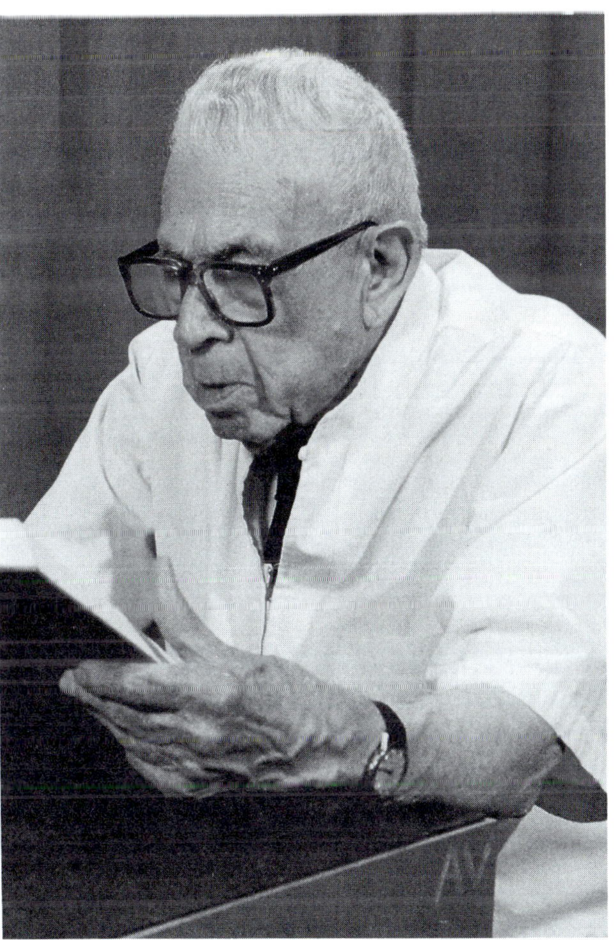

FIG. 26-2. Henry Harris Perlman, M.D., first certified Pediatric Dermatologist.

the Philadelphia Hospital for Contagious Diseases. Although there was little organized research during his tenure, the outpatient program was especially active for students, and the members of the staff were highly respected. Dr. Norman M. MacNeill (Jefferson, 1916) (Figure 26-4) was perhaps the best known by the students. Dr. MacNeill embodied the combination of ideal teacher, humanitarian, Catholic scholar, historian, and role model for two generations of Jefferson students. During the Depression of the 1930s he often paid for medications himself and at times supplied coal for heating homes. He also assisted needy medical students with tuition payments. Following his death in 1965, Dr. Bauer honored his memory with a book, *Profile of a Gentle Man,* published in 1967.

Dr. John Holmes (Jefferson, 1908) was also an able member of the staff at the time, especially known for his diagnostic skills. He had a strong following among patients and physicians in West Philadelphia. Staff members of note during this period included Drs. Edward F. Burt, Aaron Capper, Edward J. Moore, Ruth P. Zager, K. Kalman Faber, LeRoy R. Newman, and Augustin T. Giordano.[12,14] Many of these continued on the staff after Dr. Bauer's retirement.

Medical education consisted mainly of weekly lectures and case presentations by Dr. Bauer or one of his associates, plus experience in the busy outpatient clinic, where 35 to 50 patients were seen each day.[9]

Charles McKhann, M.D.; Third Chairman (1954–1956)

Dr. Charles McKhann (Figure 26-5) came to Jefferson as Chairman of the Department in 1954

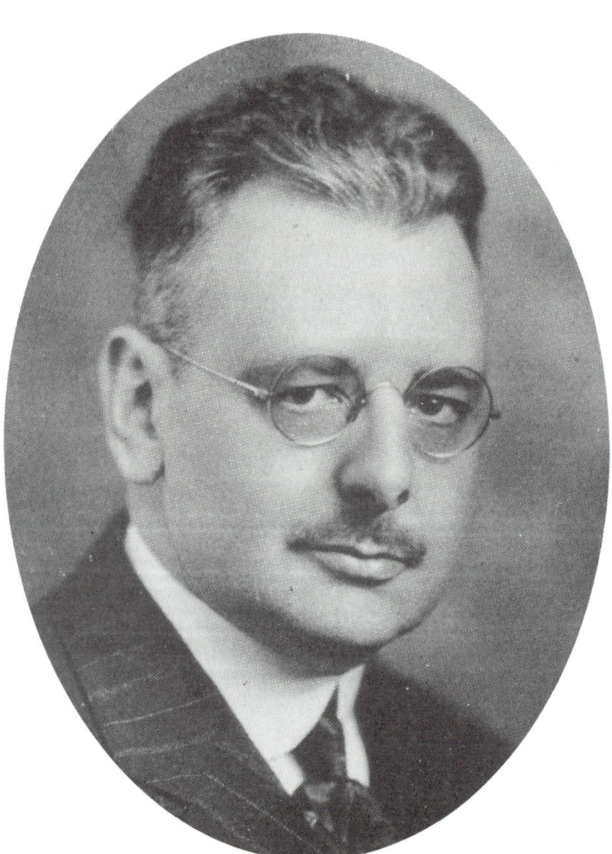

FIG. 26-3. Edward L. Bauer, M.D.; Second Chairman (1926–1954), author and historian.

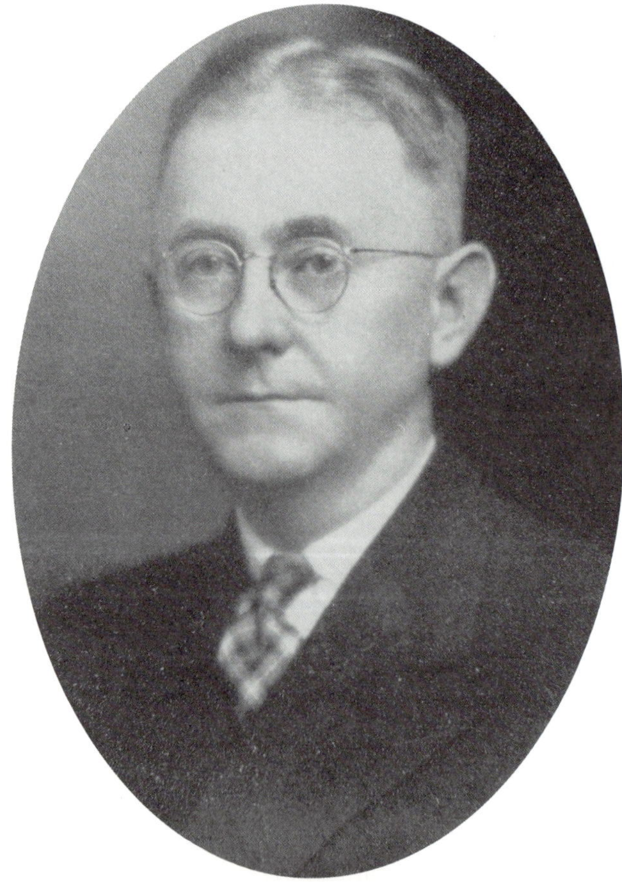

FIG. 26-4. Norman M. MacNeill, M.D., master pediatrician, organizer of outpatient services.

and was hopeful of developing a children's hospital at Broad and Fitzwater Streets, the site of the Barton Division of Jefferson and later the Broad Street Hospital.

Dr. McKhann was a nationally recognized pediatrician who had trained in Boston and became Chairman of Pediatrics at Case-Western Reserve Medical School. He left Western Reserve over the notoriety given a controversial procedure performed in his Department; namely, the anastomosis of the carotid artery and jugular vein for treatment of the mental retardation symptoms present in Down's syndrome. He brought with him an excellent teacher and clinician, Felix Karpinski, Jr., M.D., (Jefferson, S1944).

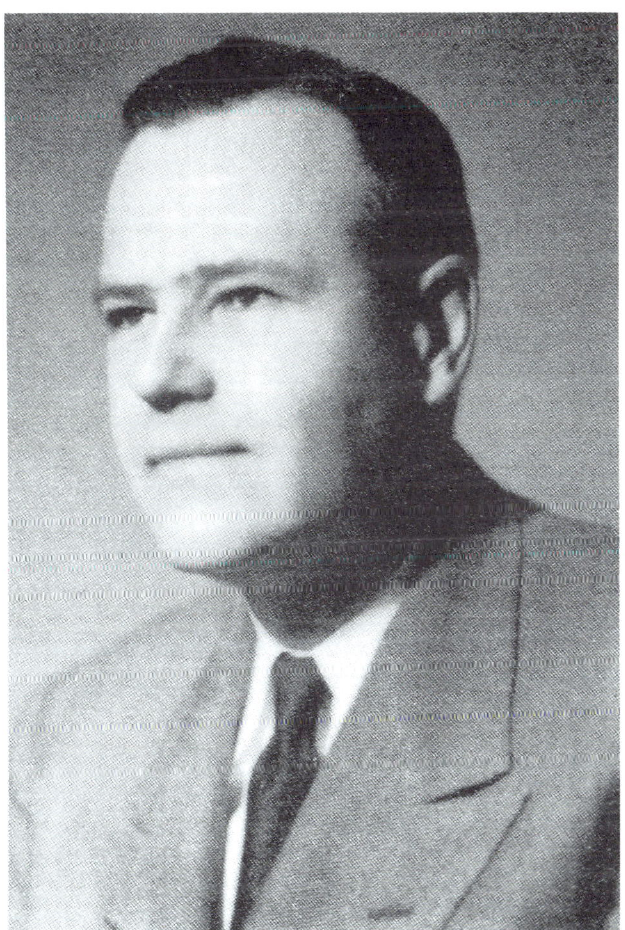

FIG. 26-5. Charles McKhann, M.D.; Third Chairman (1954–1956).

Dr. McKhann left after two years because of outside financial responsibilities and because the children's hospital did not become a reality. He served for some years as President of the American Board of Pediatrics, one of the major appointments in American Medicine.

Dr. Edward Bauer was recalled briefly from retirement to serve as Interim Chairman when Dr. McKhann departed in 1956. He spent his later years researching the history of Jefferson Medical College. These studies led to the publication of *Doctors Made in America* in 1963.[11] A Search Committee was created to recruit a new Chairman, preferably a pediatrician with a strong background in clinical or basic research.

Hans G. Keitel, M.D.; Fourth Chairman (1956–1966)

Dr. Hans G. Keitel (Figure 26-6) came to Jefferson from his research position at the

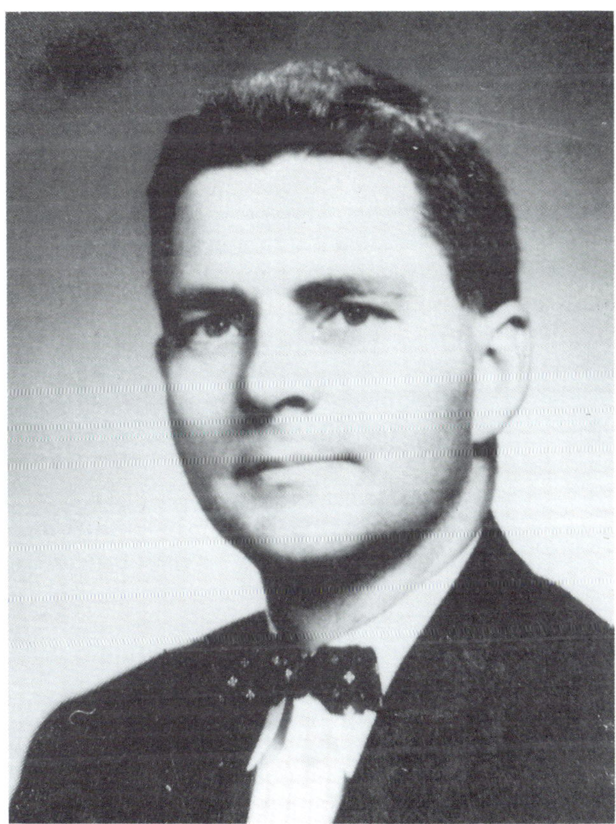

FIG. 26-6. Hans G. Keitel, M.D.; Fourth Chairman (1956–1966).

National Institutes of Health where he made significant contributions in the field of fluid and electrolyte balance. During his Chairmanship he published a book, *The Pathophysiology and Treatment of Body Fluid Disturbances* (1962). He was also the first scientist to recognize the hyposthenuria that is associated with sickle cell disease. Keitel graduated from Columbia University Medical School, received his pediatric training at New York University Department of Pediatrics, then studied endocrinology at the Massachusetts General Hospital. Dr. Keitel trained under some famous American pediatricians: Dr. Rustin McIntosh (Columbia), Dr. Emmett Holt (New York University), and Drs. Allen Butler and Nathan Talbot (Harvard).

When he arrived at Jefferson, Dr. Keitel had the advantage of having the association of Dr. Felix Karpinski (Figure 26-7), a superb pediatrician and teacher. Dr. Karpinski served as the foundation of the clinical and teaching program, which provided Dr. Keitel with time needed for his research, since he was primarily an investigator. Dr. Karpinski proved to be the first to espouse modern pediatric teaching at Jefferson. He was aggressive, devoted, innovative, and able to carry a full teaching load. A master of bedside grand rounds, he evoked the loyalty and admiration of students and house staff and made a lasting contribution to excellence in teaching.

Dr. Keitel proceeded to develop the first full-time faculty. Dr. Henry Kane (Jefferson, 1953), who trained in Pediatric Cardiology with Dr. Helen Taussig at Johns Hopkins, became Jefferson's first pediatric cardiologist. Dr. William McClean from Bowman-Gray and Johns Hopkins became Jefferson's first pediatric neurologist. Dr. Irving Olshin joined the Department in 1961 as a generalist and teacher. Dr. Sumner Root Ziegra from New York University, who was interested in general pediatrics and infectious disease, joined the Department in 1960 and later became Chairman of Pediatrics at the Medical College of Pennsylvania.

Dr. Daniel S. Rowe (Jefferson, 1948) joined the Department in 1960 following a period of general practice and a Residency in Pediatrics at Babies' Hospital in New York City. In 1971 he became Professor of Pediatrics and Public Health at Yale University School of Medicine and Director of Yale University Health Services.

Volunteer faculty members during this period included Drs. Aaron Capper, Kalman Faber, Constantine R. Roscoe (Jefferson, 1938) and James V. Mackell (Jefferson, 1946).[12–14]

Dr. K. Kalman Faber's (Figure 26-8) career at Jefferson began in 1947 as the first Pediatric Resident. His own growth virtually paralleled the development of the Department into a modern pediatric facility. Early in his career he participated in adaptation of specialized technical procedures to infants and children including the opening of the first intensive care nursery. Dr. Faber became a respected member of the Volunteer Faculty, advancing to Clinical Associate Professor. He developed an extensive practice that included the families of many Jefferson colleagues, students, nurses, and hospital employees.

Dr. Aaron Capper was a scholarly, clinically oriented member of the pediatric staff for many years. He was the author of a complete textbook of pediatrics that unfortunately was never published. He advanced to the status of Professor of Clinical Pediatrics.

Dr. Robert L. Brent, destined to become Chairman of the Department nine years later, came to Jefferson in 1957 directly from his position as Chief of Radiation Biology at the Walter Reed Army Institute of Research during the golden years of National Institutes of Health research funding. When Dr. Brent joined the Department, he had already received three research grants from the National Institutes of Health and the Atomic Energy Commission. These research programs in developmental biology and radiation biology were the first funded research programs in the Department of Pediatrics.

The group of faculty members under Dr. Keitel's Chairmanship worked together effectively to provide an excellent pediatric educational program.

Robert L. Brent, M.D., Ph.D.; Chairman (1966–)

The appointment of Robert L. Brent, M.D., Ph.D. (Figure 26-9), to replace Dr. Keitel as Head of the Department and attending

Pediatrician-in-Chief at Jefferson Hospital was announced by Dr. William A. Sodeman, Dean and Vice President for Medical Affairs in 1966. Dr. Brent received degrees at three levels at the University of Rochester in New York. In 1948 he received his A.B. with the Gamma Sigma Award; he received a four-year New York State Professional Scholarship through medical school and graduated in 1953 with honors after being elected to Alpha Omega Alpha; and in 1955 he received his Ph.D. in embryology. Dr. Brent was on the Rochester faculty before entering medical school and continued there until he became a Clinical Fellow of the National Foundation for Infantile Paralysis at the Massachusetts General Hospital (1954–1955). He was then appointed Chief of the Radiobiology Department at Walter Reed Army Medical Center in Washington, D.C., after which he joined the faculty of Jefferson as an Associate Professor of Pediatrics in 1957. He was promoted to Clinical Professor in 1960 and to full Professor in 1961. He has also held full Professorships in Anatomy and Radiology. Dr. Brent was certified by the American Board of Pediatrics, and he clinically subspecialized in pediatric dermatology.

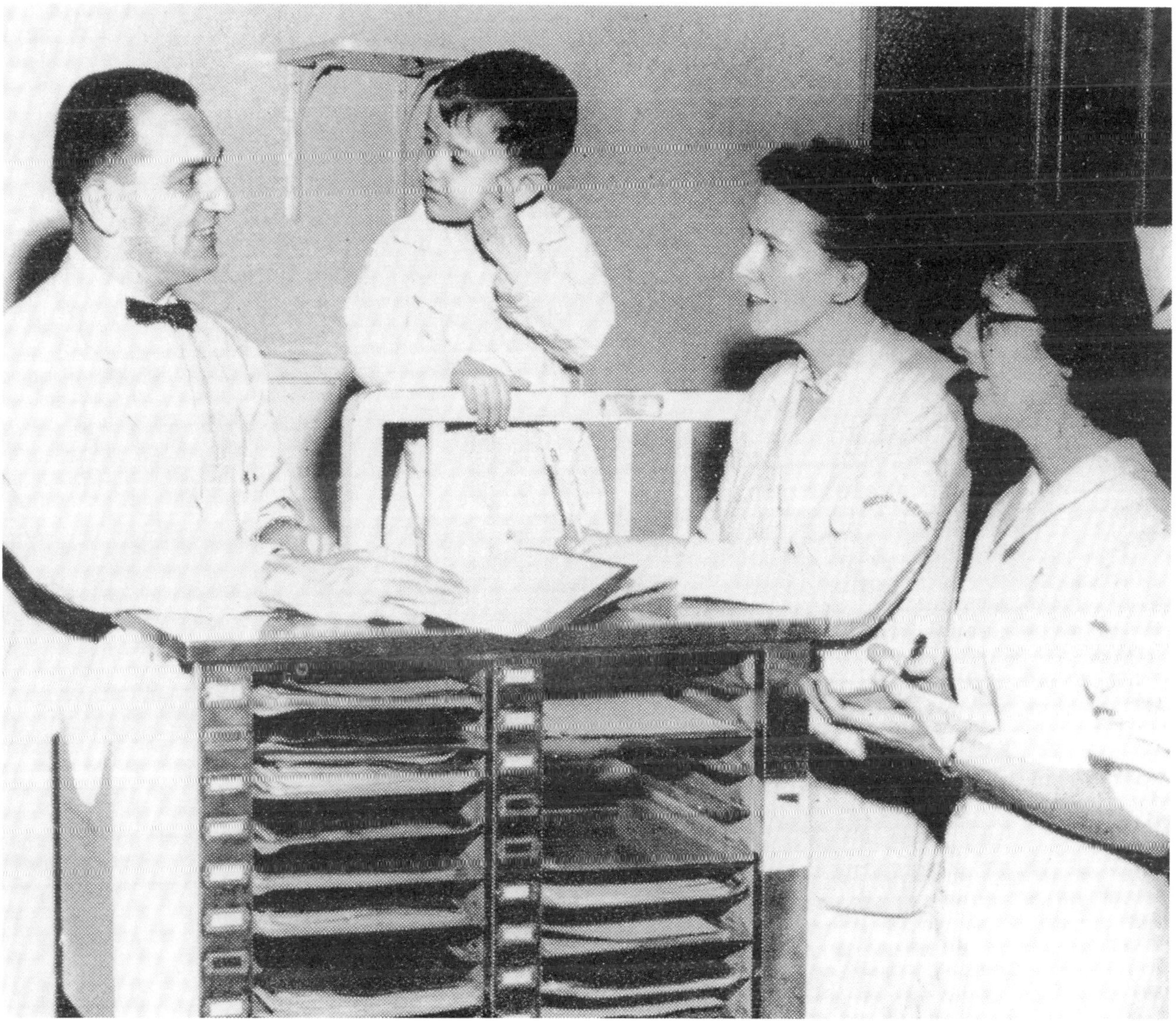

FIG. 26-7. Felix E. Karpinski, M.D., clinician and teacher.

Dr. Irving J. Olshin (Figure 26-10) joined the Department briefly as an Associate in Clinical Pediatrics (1961–1963), then returned to Jefferson in 1967 after various teaching and clinical experiences. In 1968 he became full Professor and Director of Pediatric Education Services. Dr. Olshin has been one of the most admired teachers of Pediatrics in Jefferson's history. A well-rounded physician, scholar, humanist, and historian, he has been able to reflect all these values in his contacts with students, to whom he was always available. His portrait was presented to Jefferson by the graduating Class in 1973.

Dr. Arturo R. Hervada (Medical Faculty of Salamanca University, Spain, 1953), joined the first full-time faculty as Instructor in the early 1960s following training under Drs. Keitel and Karpinski. After several appointments elsewhere, Hervada returned to Jefferson in 1969 as Professor of Pediatrics. At the same time he advanced to the Chairmanship of Pediatrics at Mercy Catholic Medical Center, where he developed one of the first intensive care nurseries in the United States.[15]

At Jefferson Dr. Hervada served as the first Associate Chairman of the Department. He was the only Jefferson faculty member to be President of the Philadelphia Pediatric Society, the second oldest pediatric medical society in the United States. He was also elected an Honorary Member of the Sociedad Catalana de Pediatria of Barcelona, Spain, and of the Alumni Association of Jefferson Medical College.

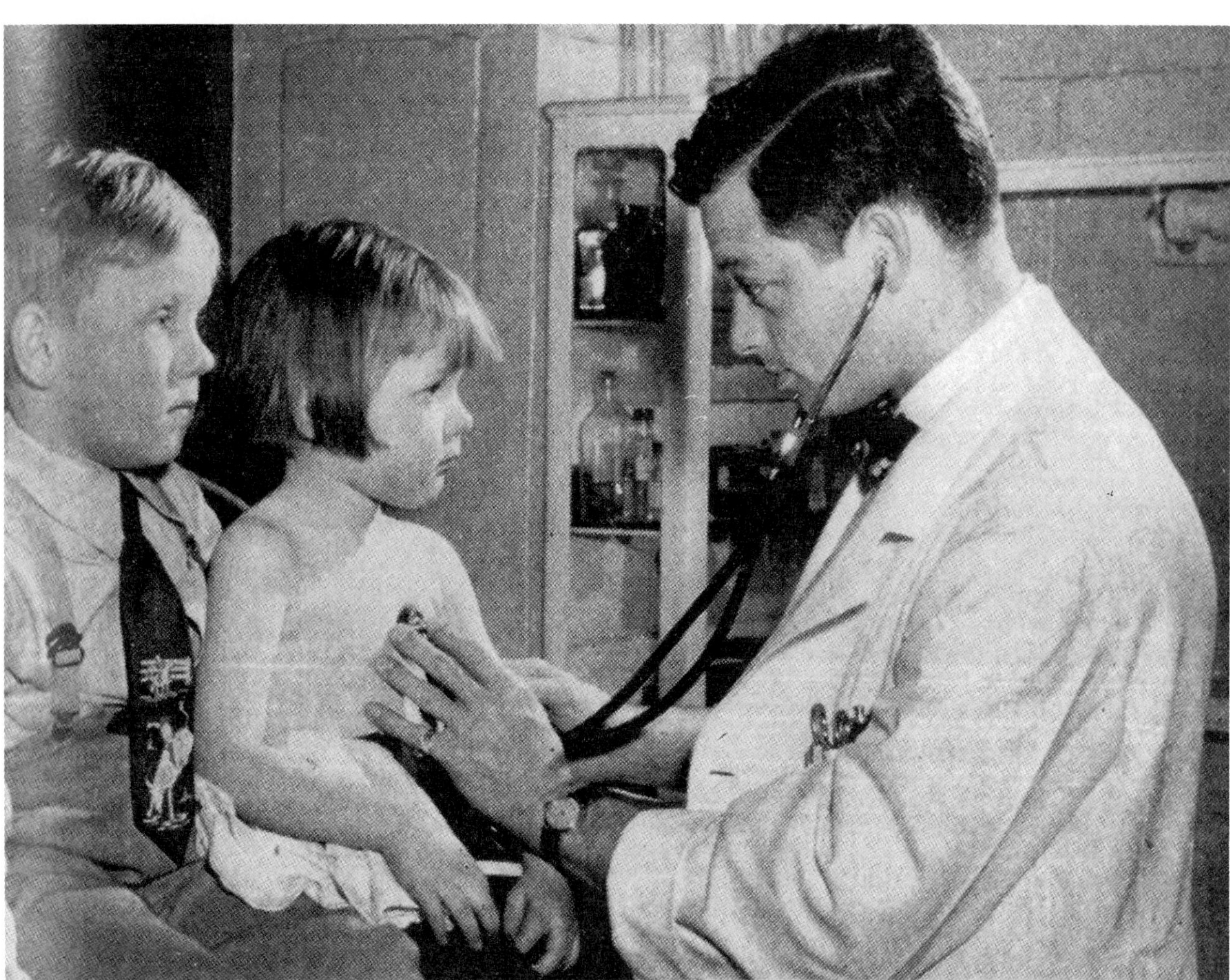

FIG. 26-8. K. Kalman Faber, M.D.; First Pediatric Resident.

Dr. Gary G. Carpenter (Jefferson, 1960) has been an important member of the Department since his return in 1968 as Associate Professor and Director of the Endocrine and Metabolic Division. One of the first to be certified in pediatric endocrinology, he has also been interested in child neurology and neonatology. A humanist, biology student, and gifted artist, his watercolors have been exhibited at Jefferson and in other cities in the United States.

Two Jefferson alumni who have achieved important positions in pediatric education are Drs. Thomas Aceto, Jr., (Jefferson, 1954), Professor and Chairman of the Department of Pediatrics and Adolescent Medicine at St. Louis University School of Medicine; and James Anthony Stockman, III (Jefferson, 1969), Professor and Chairman of Pediatrics at Northwestern University School of Medicine and Children's Memorial Hospital, Chicago. Dr. Stockman is also Coeditor of the *Year Book of Pediatrics*.

Dr. Brent founded the Clinical Teratology and Radiation Biology Division at the Stein Research Center and has served as its Director since 1957. The Stein Center has been supported through the generous efforts of the Louis and Bess Stein Foundation, the Harry Block Charities, and Federal agencies. Under Dr. Brent's direction, Divisional personnel have performed animal studies on the effects of high energy radiation on the developing embryo, placenta transport, embryonic nutrition, developmental immunological studies, biochemical embryology, and various techniques of embryo culture. Outside funding received by the Clinical Teratology and Developmental Biology Division, under Dr. Brent's supervision, represented a significant portion of the ongoing outside support received

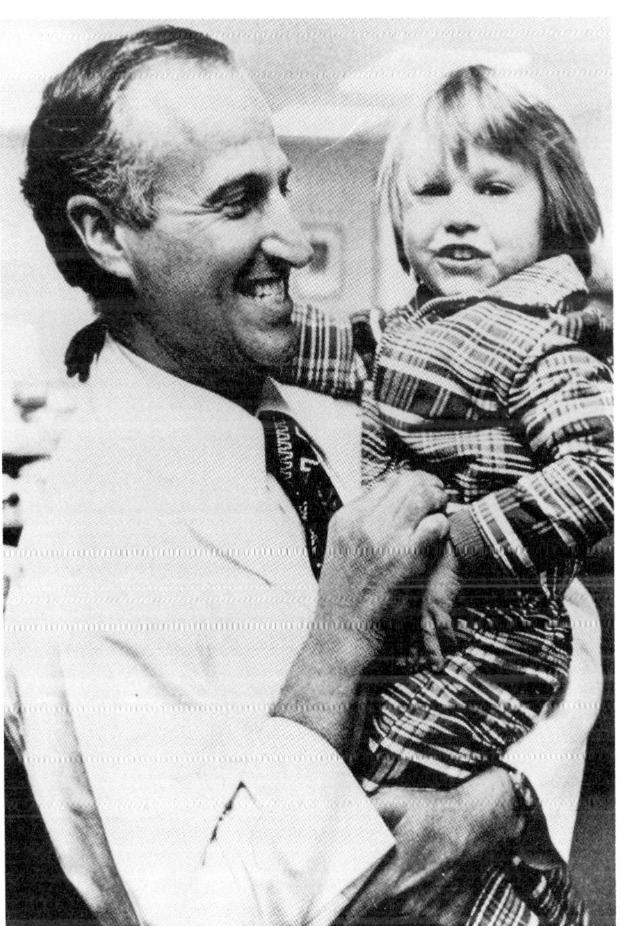

FIG. 26-9. Robert L. Brent, M.D., Ph.D.; Fifth Chairman (1966–), with Professorial appointments in Radiology and Anatomy and Directorship of Stein Research Center.

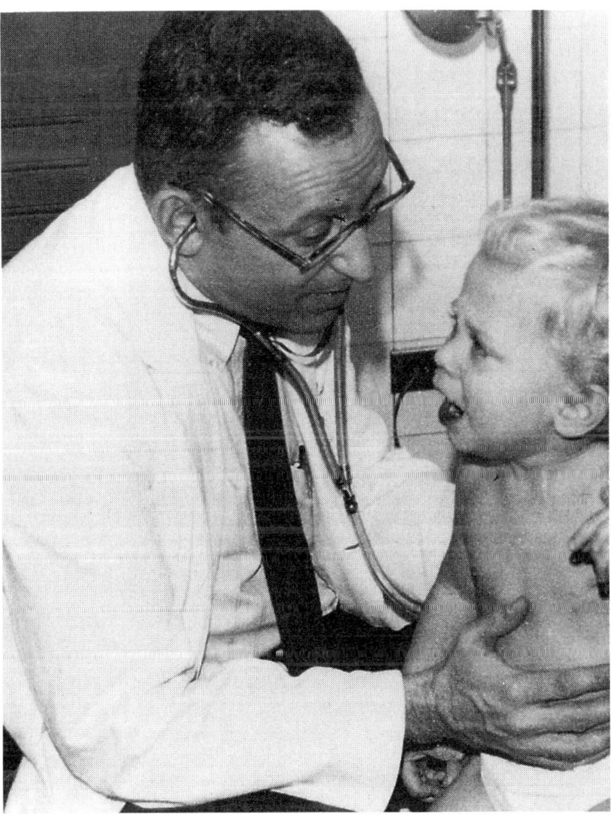

FIG. 26-10. Irving J. Olshin, M.D., Professor and Director of Pediatric Education Services.

by the Department of Pediatrics, which became at this time the second most research-proliferative Department at Jefferson, despite its relatively small size. Before Dr. Brent assumed the Chairmanship, research activities in Pediatrics were minimal, and the development and expansion of the Department's investigative endeavors became largely attributable to his efforts.

In 1985 the Louis and Bess Stein Endowed Professorship in Pediatrics was established by the Stein Foundation. This represented the first Pediatric research endowment at Jefferson, and Dr. Brent was named as the first recipient of the award.

Dr. Brent has an exceptional record of professional accomplishments. In addition to holding Professorships in three Departments at Jefferson, he has contributed over 340 publications to the scientific and medical literature, particularly in the areas of congenital malformations and developmental biology. He is an international authority on the causes of congenital malformations. He has served on the Editorial Boards of *Pediatrics, Teratology,* and *Fetal Medicine,* and has served on numerous committees of the American Academy of Pediatrics, various Federal agencies and professional societies including the American Association of Pediatric Department Chairmen. Dr. Brent's expertise has been used to establish acceptable guidelines for working women of reproductive age relative to the maximum exposure they may receive from radiation or chemicals without significant risk to the embryo.

▪ Pediatric Medical Education

Dr. Brent has maintained an upwardly mobile profile for a Department faced with increasing competition from freestanding children's hospitals, changing patient populations, and burgeoning pressures from prospective payment systems. Under his direction, the pediatric medical education of students and house staff has been improved and broadened. Outstanding patient care programs have been developed in the pediatric subspecialties.

The recent pediatric curriculum consisted of clinical clerkships during which third- and fourth-year students spent six weeks on the pediatric service at the Jefferson Hospital or at one of the affiliates (Mercy Catholic Medical Center in Darby, Our Lady of Lourdes Hospital in Camden, and the Medical Center of Delaware in Wilmington). The students' clinical experience included inpatient, outpatient, and nursery care, and involved formal lectures and teaching sessions as well as hands-on clinical experience. The senior clerkships were available in a variety of subspecialties, offering those students considering pediatrics as their field of endeavor an opportunity to learn about current concepts and methods of treatment in specific areas.

The quality of pediatric teaching under Dr. Brent's Chairmanship is reflected by Lindback Awards for distinguished teaching to three of the leading members of the Department: Dr. Brent himself in 1968, Dr. Olshin in 1969, and Dr. Hervada in 1975.

The Department in its total history reflects changing concepts of the management of health and disease in the first specialty that separated people on the basis of age. It has also responded to increasing needs and opportunities in interdisciplinary research and its adaptation to patient care.

References

1. MacNeill, N.M., "Infant Welfare as Taught in Philadelphia One Hundred Years Ago." *Ann. Med. Hist.* New Series 8, 1936, pp. 36–43.
2. Faber, H., and McIntosh, R., *History of the American Pediatric Society.* New York: McGraw-Hill, 1966.
3. Levinson, A., "The Three Meigs and Their Contribution to Pediatrics." *Ann. Med. Hist.,* 10, 1928, p. 138.
4. Eberle, J., *A Treatise on the Diseases and Physical Education of Children.* Cincinnati: Corey and Fairbank, and Philadelphia: Gregg and Elliot, 1833.
5. Meigs, C.D., *The Philadelphia Practice of Midwifery.* Philadelphia: James Kay, Jr., & Bro., 1838.
6. Meigs, C.D., *Observations on Certain Diseases of Young Children,* Philadelphia: Lea and Blanchard, 1850.
7. Keating, W., *Churchill's Diseases of Children.* Philadelphia: Blanchard and Lea, 1856.
8. Bauer, E.L., "Department of Pediatrics (Historical Review)." *The Clinic, Jeff. Med. Coll.,* 1936.
9. Notes compiled by Mr. Samuel Davis, Director of Special Collections, Scott Memorial Library, August 1986.
10. Perlman, H.H., "History of Jefferson Pediatrics: Recollections in conversations with Dr. Robert Brent," June 1986.
11. Bauer, E.L., *Doctors Made in America.* Philadelphia: J.B. Lippincott, 1963.
12. Roscoe, C., "History of Pediatrics," Recorded recollections, July 1986.
13. Giordano, A.T., "My memories of Jefferson," Recorded recollections, August 1986.
14. *Catalogue, Jeff. Med. Coll.,* 1983–85.
15. Hervada, A.R., and Hartnett, E.M., "Specialized Care for Premature and High Risk Infants." *Hospitals.* 40, October 1, 1966, pp. 54–58.

CHAPTER TWENTY-SEVEN

Department of Dermatology

LAWRENCE C. PARISH, M.D.

"The skin possesses the closest relations with the general economy, as shown by the observation that there are comparatively few so-called general diseases in which it . . . is not at some period involved in a slight or a marked degree."

—LOUIS A. DUHRING (1845–1913)

DERMATOLOGY HAS been an independent Department at Jefferson for eight decades. It has grown from a unit that merely gave lectures and provided clinics for indigent patients to a modern Department fully approved by the American Board of Dermatology for the training of residents. Its clinical facility provides advanced methods of treatment including state-of-the-art lasers, and the faculty has both national and international reputation.

Early Instruction in Treatment of Skin Diseases

Teaching the treatment of skin diseases did not have official recognition at the Medical College until 1866. That year, Jefferson and Bellevue Hospital Medical College of New York both created lectureships on dermatology and venereal disease. Presentations on diseases of the skin had been given in New York as early as 1829, and in 1861 Harvard had established such lectureships. Thus, only two other institutions considered dermatology important enough to offer any instruction before Jefferson did.

Some of the student notebooks of the mid-nineteenth century indicate that skin disease was occasionally included in the course work. For example, T. B. Gibbons in 1854 records that at the Jefferson Medical College Clinic held at Pennsylvania Hospital, diseases of the skin being treated were "erythema, roseola, urticaria, strophulus, lichen, prurigo, herpes zoster, acne, etc." Diagnosis and treatment were extremely rudimentary at that time, and were probably regarded as unworthy of more attention in the curriculum.

When the surgeon Francis F. Maury (Jefferson, 1862) began his series of dermatology lectures for the academic year 1866–1867, a new era began. Dermatology, which had developed in Paris at L 'Hôpital St. Louis earlier in the 1800s and now was flourishing in Vienna under Hebra, was making inroads in America. Specialty medicine, spearheaded by the Civil War, was just beginning to dislodge the notion that a good physician knew all phases of diagnosis and therapeutics. Although Maury (Figure 27-1) died of tuberculosis in 1879, he made a significant contribution to the teaching of dermatology at Jefferson as well as to the entire evolving specialty during his brief career. Jeffersonians, undoubtedly, had more understanding of cutaneous diseases than did other medical students of the era. Maury should also be remembered for having founded the *Photographic Review of Medicine and Surgery,* published for two years beginning in 1871, with Louis A. Duhring, the first Professor of Dermatology at the University of Pennsylvania (1875–1913). That journal was unique in providing practitioners with pictures of interesting cases in color with text that adequately described the problems and treatments of the period.

Samuel W. Gross (Jefferson, 1857), who with his father is intertwined with so much of Jefferson history in the nineteenth century, became the next lecturer. As early as 1839 his father, Samuel D. Gross (Jefferson, 1828), had given the first American description of cutaneous pathology in his textbook *Elements of Pathological Anatomy.* It seemed appropriate when Maury became terminally ill that Samuel W. Gross (Figure 27-2) should take charge of the skin program, giving lectures for the spring session.

In 1884 John V. Shoemaker (Jefferson, 1874), who would become Professor of Dermatology and Dean of the Medico-Chirurgical College (later merged into the Graduate School of Medicine of the University of Pennsylvania), took over the Jefferson lectureships on cutaneous diseases "with practical demonstrations" until 1887. He had distinguished himself by organizing the Pennsylvania Free Dispensary for Skin Diseases, which became the American Hospital for Skin Diseases. Here, the first residency program in dermatology was begun in 1880.

William Joseph Hearn (Jefferson, 1867), from the Department of Surgery, gave the lectures for the next year (1888). He probably was delegated the responsibility because he had been Maury's

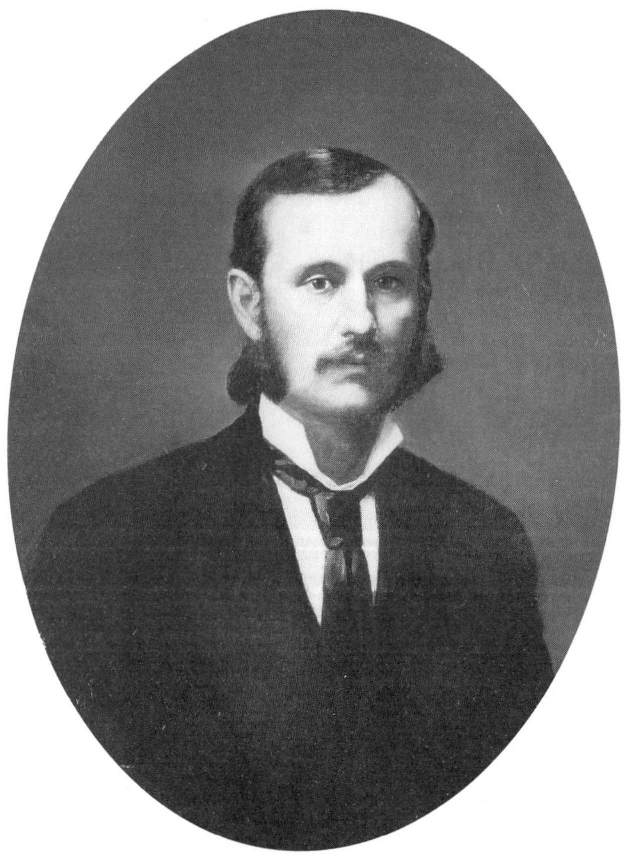

FIG. 27-1. Francis F. Maury (Jefferson, 1862), a surgeon who gave the first lectures on dermatology (1866–1879).

pupil and later Gross's chief of clinic and anesthetizer (depicted by Eakins in *The Gross Clinic*). Hearn (Figure 27-3) had a particular interest in tumors, and his dermatologic career was short-lived.

From 1888 to 1890, one of Duhring's former students, Arthur Van Harlingen, who later would help to found and serve as a Professor at the Philadelphia Polyclinic (merged with the Graduate School of Medicine at the University of Pennsylvania), developed a program for the students. This was a period when the lectures were sometimes an integral part of the course and at other times constituted auxiliary courses of several weeks' duration. Students were given almost no clinical exposure; thus Harlingen's *Handbook of the Diagnosis and Treatment of Skin Diseases* (1884) was useful.

Departmental Status Achieved

When Henry W. Stelwagon (Figure 27-4) was appointed in 1890, a new period in dermatology began. Stelwagon also had been a pupil of Duhring's. In 1892, he became the first Clinical Professor of Dermatology and in 1904 the first full Professor. Stelwagon brought with him a wealth of clinical experience. He was well liked by his colleagues and the students and perhaps is most famous for his textbook, *Treatise on Diseases of the Skin* (1902), which went through nine editions (1921). His lectures were illustrated by hand-painted drawings. Stelwagon also was instrumental in merging the Dispensary for Skin Diseases, founded in 1870, with Jefferson Hospital. This clinic had been founded by Duhring, through his father's financial support, to provide clinic services

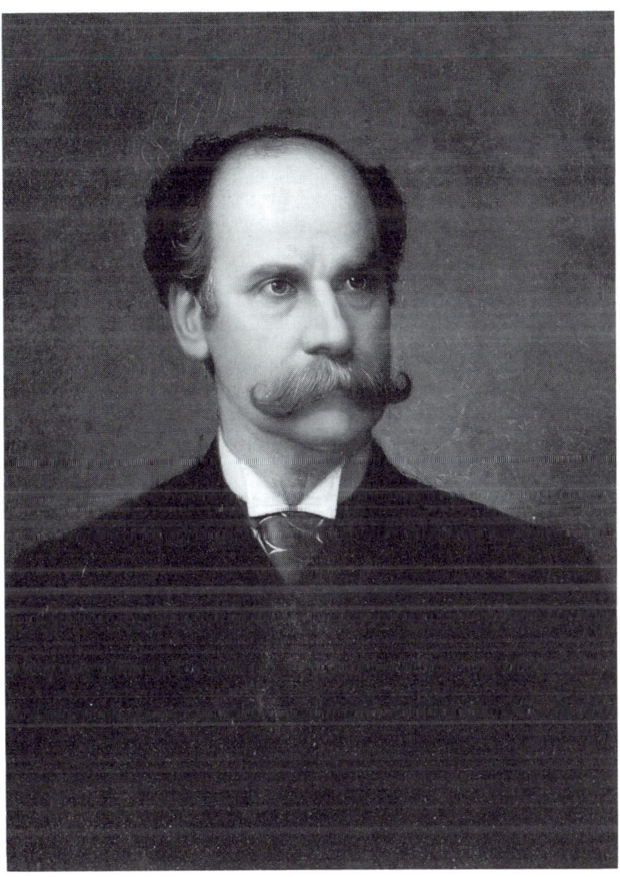

FIG. 27-2. Samuel W. Gross (Jefferson, 1857), the "younger Gross," lectured on dermatology (1880–1884).

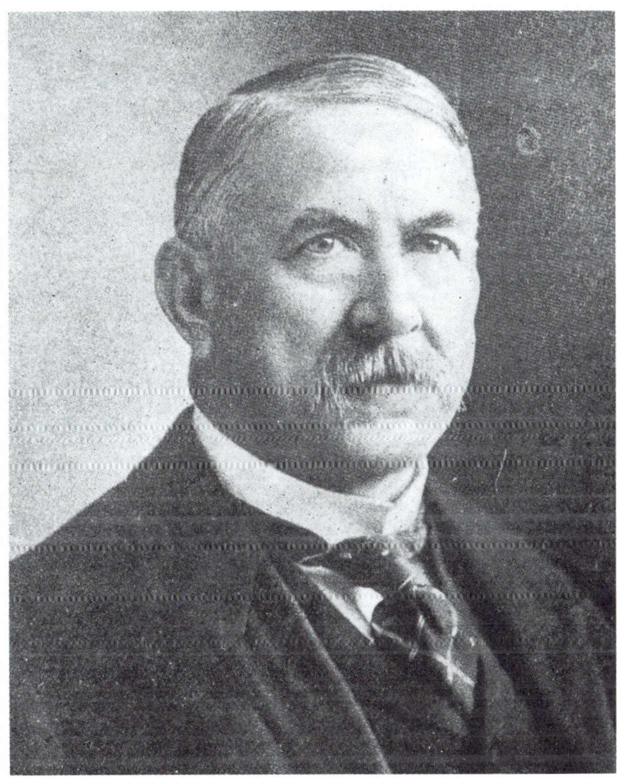

FIG. 27-3. William J. Hearn (Jefferson, 1867) gave dermatology lectures for 1887–1888. He was the anesthetizer in Eakins' *The Gross Clinic*.

for patients with skin disease, something that had been distinctly absent in Philadelphia. Department status was granted to dermatology, as it had been to most of the other clinical departments, in 1906.

Following Stelwagon's resignation in 1918 because of heart disease, Jay Frank Schamberg (Figure 27-5) served as Professor for two years before moving to the Graduate School of Medicine of the University of Pennsylvania, where he would also serve as a Vice-Dean. Schamberg was particularly interested in contagious diseases and wrote two books, *Compend of Diseases of the Skin* (1898) and *Disease of the Skin and the Eruptive Fevers* (1908). In 1917 his Dermatological Research Laboratories had successfully synthesized arsphenamine and neoarsphenamine, making America no longer dependent upon Germany for supplies in the treatment of syphilis.

Frank Grozer Knowles, M.D., Chairman (1920–1946)

In 1920 Frank Crozer Knowles (Figure 27-6) became Professor of Dermatology and was the first to carry the title of Head of the Department. During his tenure, Knowles created a warm atmosphere in dermatology, and the students enjoyed his teaching in the clinic. His textbook *Diseases of the Skin*, first published in 1914, proved to be so popular that it went through four editions (1942). The Class of 1937 dedicated *The Clinic* to him, and students formed the Knowles Dermatology Society. The class of 1939 presented his portrait to the college. When he died of

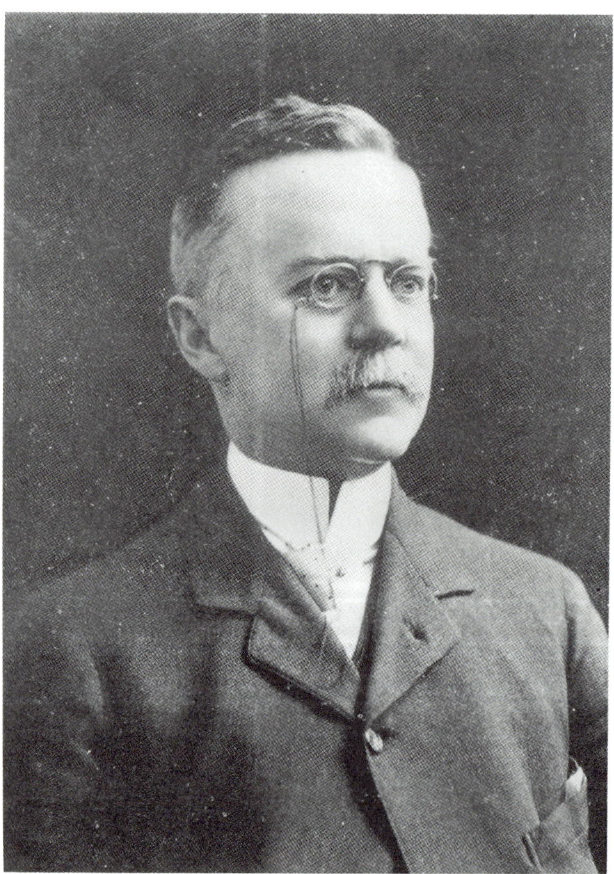

FIG. 27-4. Henry W. Stelwagon, Clinical Professor (1892), full Professor (1904), and First Chairman of the Dermatology Department (1906–1918).

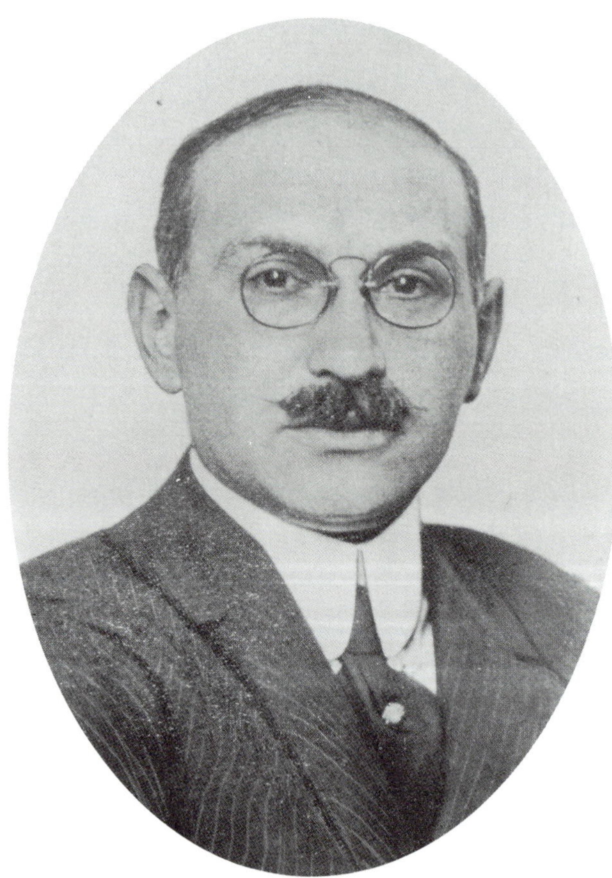

FIG. 27-5. Jay F. Schamberg, Chairman of Dermatology (1918–1920).

multiple myeloma in 1957, Knowles had amassed one of the finest collections of Chinese porcelain in the country.

Subsequent Changes

In 1947 and again in 1949, Edward F. Corson (Figure 27-7) became Head of the Department. He was a good clinician who earned the respect of the students. Clarence S. Livingood (Figure 27-8) assumed the Chairmanship in 1948. A year later, he would move to Galveston, Texas, to become Professor of Dermatology at the University of Texas Medical Branch, and still later, his career would take him to Detroit as Head of Dermatology at Henry Ford Hospital. In his short term at Jefferson, he embarked upon a program to enlarge inpatient service and to effect a temporary affiliation with the Skin and Cancer Hospital, which was then located at Eighth and Pine Streets.

In 1950 Henry B. Decker (Jefferson, 1920) became Chairman of the Department (Figure 27-9). As the size of Jefferson's classes grew, so did the importance of dermatology. Decker conducted several clinics in the famous old Clinic in the Curtis Building. The dermatology clerkship was a required course, with each day's clinical session followed by a "coffee hour" under the auspices of Dr. Decker. He was a student of United States history and particularly that of the State of New Jersey, in which he served as President of the Medical Society. He became Emeritus in the Dermatology Chair in 1958 and died in 1976.

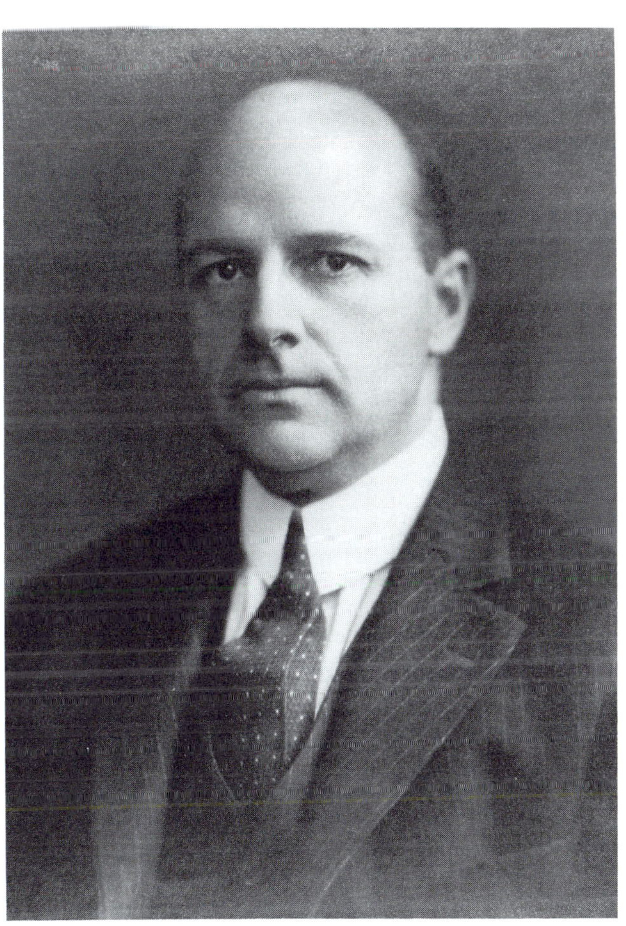

FIG. 27-6. Frank C. Knowles, first to carry title of "Head of Department" (1920–1947).

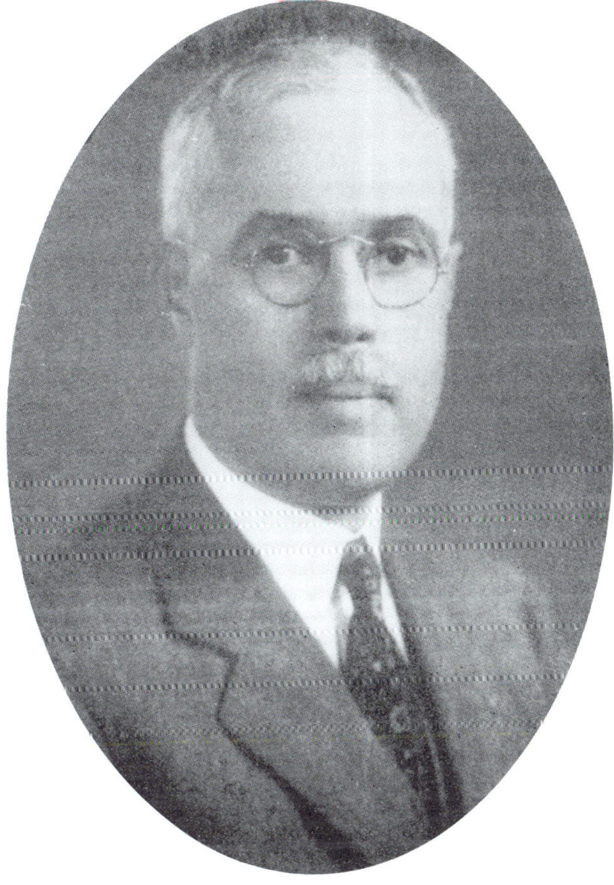

FIG. 27-7. Edward F. Corson, twice Head of the Department (1947 and 1949).

The Luscombe Years (1959–1986)

Herbert A. Luscombe (Figure 27-10) (Jefferson, 1940) assumed the Chairmanship in 1959. During this era, important progress was made in developing a modern Department. Under Luscombe's direction, the Residency was transformed in 1975 into a fully accredited three-year program—until then it had comprised two years at Jefferson and the third year in a didactic course at the Graduate School of Medicine of the University of Pennsylvania. By 1986 more than 35 Residents had been trained; that group constitutes the Luscombe Club, organized in 1983, that meets at the time of the annual convention of the American Academy of Dermatology. In 1973 the clinic moved to the Edison building and in 1978 to the new Hospital. The medical students received the option of electing clinical clerkships in dermatology as part of the specialty rotation.

Dr. Luscombe served as President of the Alumni Association in 1971, and his portrait was presented to the College in 1977. His teaching excellence was recognized nationally when he received the Clark W. Finnerud Award for Teaching from the Dermatology Foundation in 1981. In 1983 the Herbert A. Luscombe Lectureship was established to bring distinguished dermatologists to Jefferson as a way of noting progress in other institutions.

In November, 1986, Dr. Luscombe retired from his position after having served as Chairman at Jefferson for 27 years, the longest term of leadership of any Dermatology Department in the United States. At that time the faculty, in addition to the Chairman, comprised three Professors (Drs. Charles H. Greenbaum, Young Chai Kauh, and Lawrence C. Parish), a Visiting Professor (Dr. Francisco Kerdel-Vegas), and ten other members. Dr. Henry H. Perlman (Jefferson, 1918) deserves special mention for having initiated pediatric

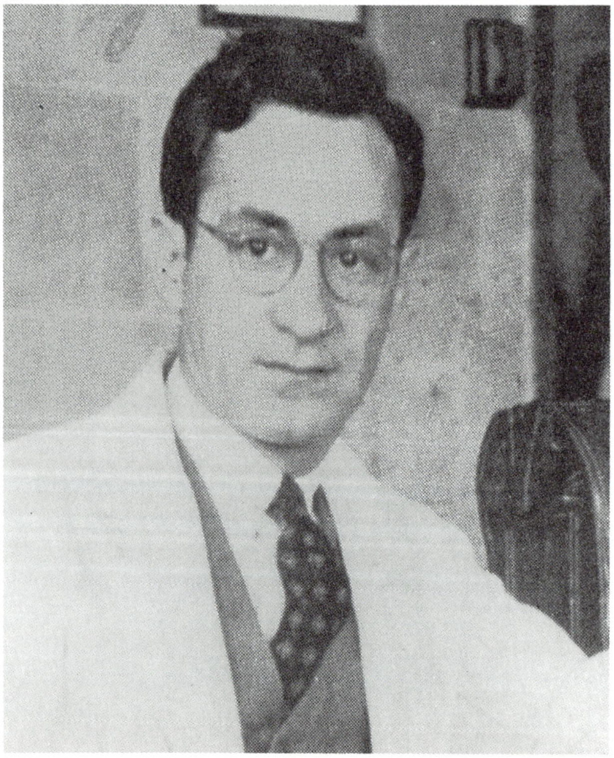

FIG. 27-8. Clarence S. Livingood, Chairman (1948–1949).

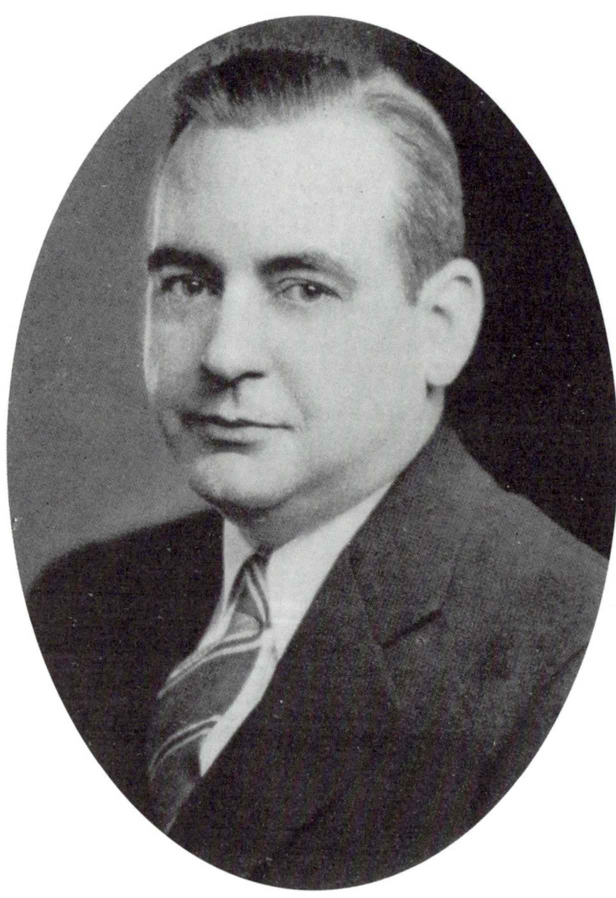

FIG. 27-9. Henry B. Decker (Jefferson, 1920), Chairman (1950–1959).

dermatology as a subspecialty in this country (Figure 27-11). In the early 1980s Perlman was made the first Honorary Member of the Pediatric Dermatology Society.

The Molecular Era Begins: Jouni Uitto, M.D., Ph.D., Chairman (1986–)

Dr. Luscombe was succeeded by Jouni Uitto, M.D., Ph.D., (Figure 27-12), an internationally renowned dermatologist and biochemist

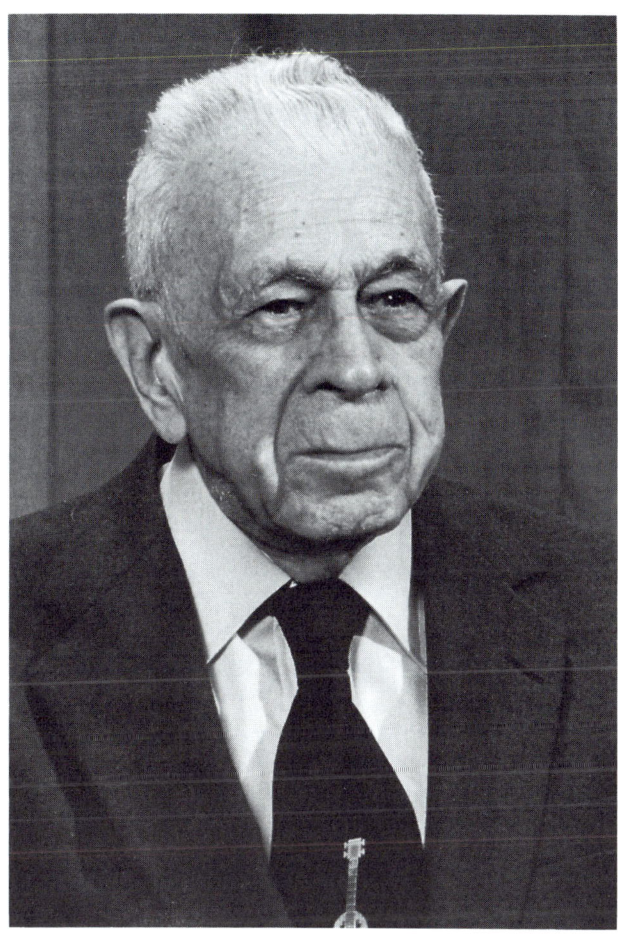

FIG. 27-11. Henry H. Perlman, M.D. (Jefferson, 1918), pioneer Pediatric Dermatologist.

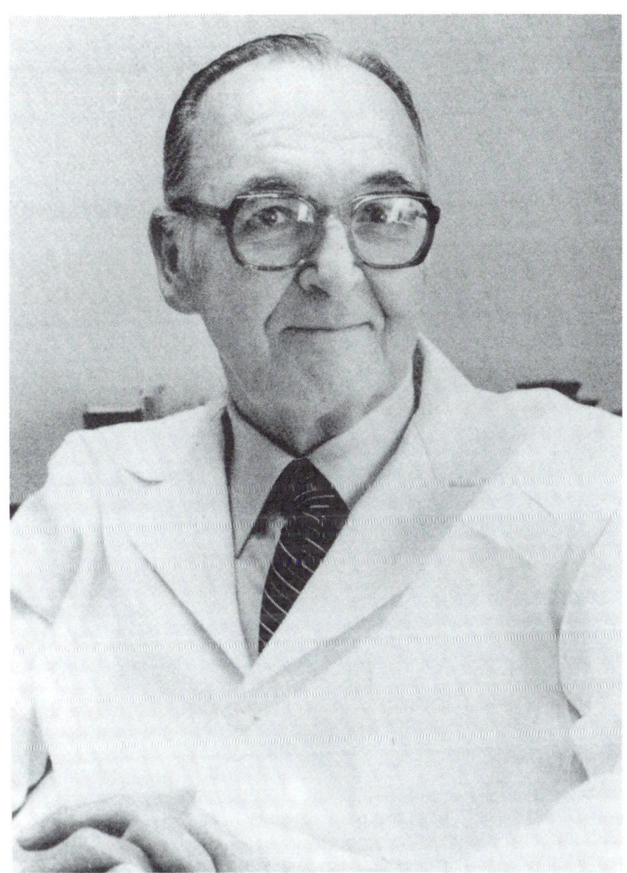

FIG. 27-10. Herbert A. Luscombe (Jefferson, 1940), Chairman (1959–1986).

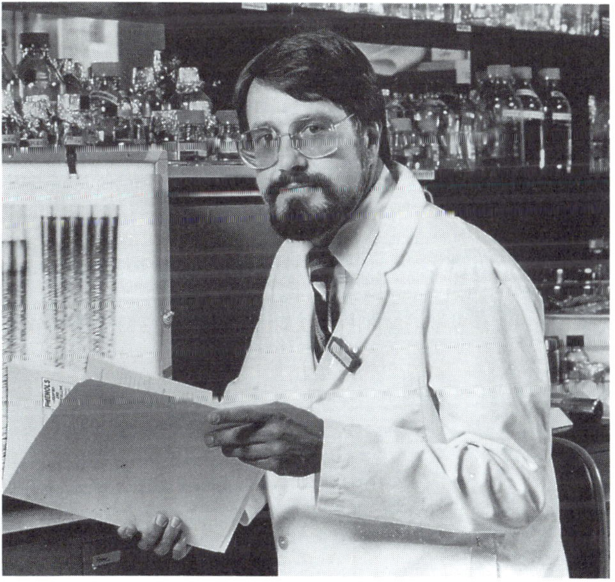

FIG. 27-12. Jouni Uitto, M.D., Ph.D., Chairman (1986–).

recognized for his basic science and clinical research in the field of connective tissue metabolism. Dr. Uitto, a native of Finland, received his degrees from the University of Helsinki and undertook his dermatology training at Washington University School of Medicine in St. Louis. Dr. Uitto came to Jefferson from the University of California (Los Angeles) School of Medicine, where he was Professor of Medicine as well as Associate Chief and Director of Research of the Division of Dermatology at Harbor-UCLA Medical Center. Uitto's previous faculty appointments were at Washington University School of Medicine and the College of Medicine and Dentistry of New Jersey-Rutgers Medical School. Dr. Uitto is a long-time collaborator with Dr. Darwin J. Prockop, currently Chairman of the Department of Biochemistry and Molecular Biology and Director of the newly established Jefferson Institute of Molecular Medicine. This collaboration now continues within this Institute, where dermatology is represented as a Section of Molecular Dermatology.

During the initial year of Dr. Uitto's appointment, the Department grew ever larger, and currently has nine full-time faculty members, including Chief of the Division of Cutaneous Surgery, Dr. Gary P. Lask, and Chief of the Division of Dermapathology, Dr. Richard H. Jacoby. The faculty also includes three Ph.D. members with state-of-the-art expertise in molecular biology.

One of the latest Department developments is the establishment of the Jefferson Center for International Dermatology, under joint Directorship of Drs. Lawrence C. Parish and Jouni Uitto. The Center serves as a catalyst for development of programs in the varied areas of international dermatology, including residency exchange training, faculty development, education in geographic and topical dermatology, and enhancement of investigative dermatology.

The plans for future expansion of the Department call for vigorous development of teaching, research, and patient care activities, to bring Jefferson Dermatology recognition both nationally and internationally as a center of excellence. The Department faces an exciting era in which interdisciplinary involvement will open new frontiers well supported by its rich history.

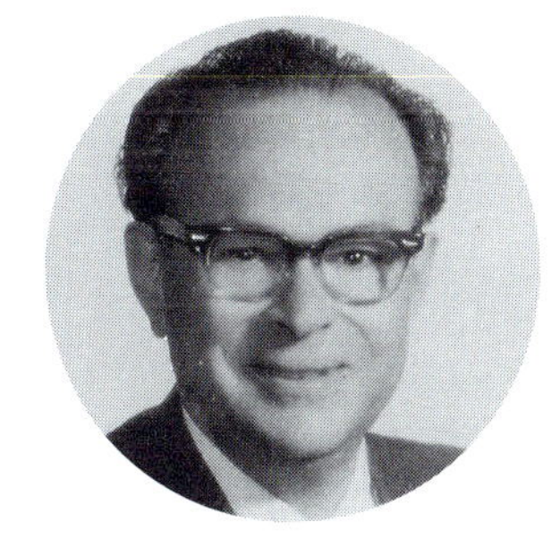

CHAPTER TWENTY-EIGHT

Department of Neurology

NATHAN S. SCHLEZINGER, M.D., SC.D. (MED.)

"As long as our brain is a mystery, the universe, the reflection of the structure of the brain, will also be a mystery."

—SANTIAGO RAMON Y CAJAL (1852–1934).

SOME appreciation of the role of the nervous system as an explanation of the life of human beings existed as far back as Hippocrates[1] around 400 B.C. and, later, at the time of Galen[2] (131-201 A.D.) After the Middle Ages, further interest in neurology was manifested by Leonardo da Vinci[3] near the end of the fifteenth century and by Vesalius[4] in the sixteenth century in their anatomical drawings, and Descartes[5] showed remarkable speculative interest in the neurophysiology of vision.

When the nineteenth century began, neurology engaged the interest of both basic and applied scientists—among physicians active in this movement may be mentioned Charles Bell, Romberg, Erb, Duchenne, Charcot, Marie, Nissl, Alzheimer, Dejerine, Hughlings Jackson, Cajal, and Hortega. In the twentieth century remarkable investigations of the nervous system have continued, and neurology has divided into specialties and again into subspecialties.

Neurology at Jefferson

The scientific approach to neurology in Philadelphia took place at Turner's Lane Hospital during the Civil War with the studies of S. Weir Mitchell (Jefferson, 1850), George R. Morehouse (Jefferson, 1850), and William W. Keen (Jefferson, 1862), resulting in *Gunshot Wounds and Other Injuries of Nerves* (1864). The first neurologic facility in America, The Philadelphia Orthopaedic Hospital and Infirmary for Nervous Diseases, was founded in 1867 and the Philadelphia Neurological Society, in 1884. These developments played a major role in early neurology in this country.

Although neurology as a Department at Jefferson was not established formally until the turn of this century (in 1900), it is appropriate to recall previous members of the Jefferson faculty who were significant contributors during the nineteenth century. John K. Mitchell, Professor of Medicine at Jefferson (1841–1858), published a paper in 1831[6] pertaining to neurology. He was the father of the eminent Silas Weir Mitchell. Robley Dunglison,[7] Professor of Physiology at Jefferson Medical College (1836–1868), first recognized and described chronic degenerative chorea.

Silas Weir Mitchell (Figure 28-1) was born in Philadelphia in 1829 and graduated from Jefferson in 1850. Subsequently, he became a pioneer in neurophysiological research, but was disappointed in his efforts during the 1860s to become Professor of Physiology at Jefferson or the University of Pennsylvania.[8] Considered a genius by his contemporaries, he made classic contributions in neurology[9] and in psychiatry and was regarded just as highly for his novels and poetry. Mitchell is the recognized founder of American neurology; in January, 1884, he was elected first President of the Philadelphia Neurological Society and reelected for five successive years until 1890. He did not accept an offer to become the first President of the American Neurological Association in 1875 but did serve in that position in 1909. In 1886 he received an honorary degree at Harvard's two hundred and fiftieth anniversary and another in 1888 at the University of Bologna on its eight hundredth. He was president of the College of Physicians of Philadelphia for two terms (1886–1888, 1892–1894).

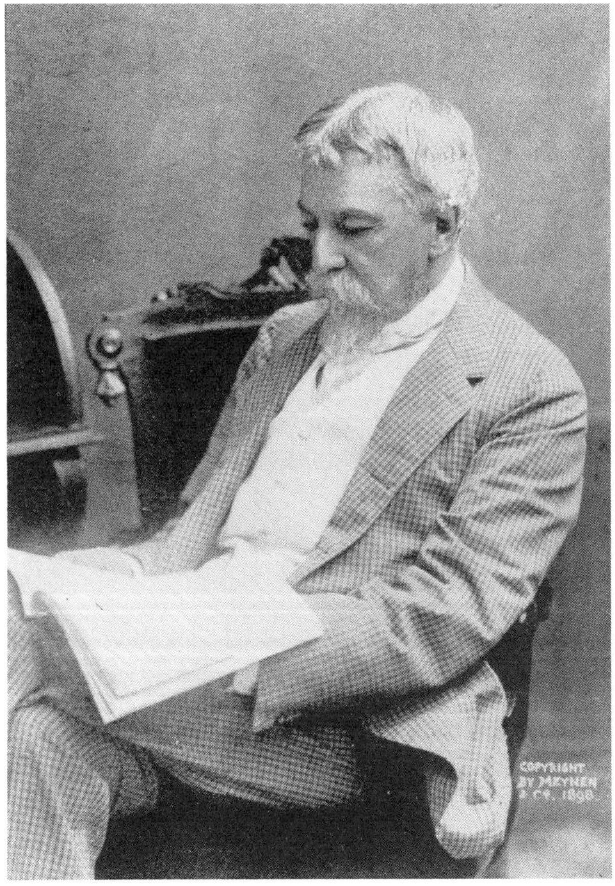

FIG. 28-1. Silas Weir Mitchell, M.D., (Jefferson, 1850), was a pioneer in research and clinical neuropsychiatry as well as a famed novelist.

Dr. James Aitken Meigs[10] was born in Philadelphia in 1829 and graduated from Jefferson Medical College in 1851. In 1869, when he was almost 40, he was appointed the Professor of Institutes of Medicine and Jurisprudence. During his next few years at Jefferson he gave special lectures on "Clinical Studies of Nervous Diseases." His unexpected death occurred on November 9, 1879.

Dr. Roberts Bartholow (1831–1904) held the Chair of Materia Medica and Therapeutics at Jefferson from 1879 to 1893. Well known in his day as a practical physician, Dr. Bartholow was elected President of the American Neurological Association in 1881. He wrote several valuable papers on cerebral localization and function.[11]

Dr. Francis X. Dercum (Figure 28-2) was appointed Clinical Professor of Nervous and Mental Diseases at Jefferson in 1892, thereby first establishing neurology as a special field of interest. Dr. Max Bochroch (Jefferson, 1879) was Chief Clinical Assistant. In the years before 1900 the additions and replacements on the faculty as neurologists included: Drs. T.W. Jackson, Joseph B. Bolton, G.M. Edwards, Albert P. Good, Lucas Henyou, A.F. Torgette, J.O. Arnold, J.B. Conway, W. Jackson, C.A. Hearn, and H.L. Green. Fourth-year students received instruction in neurology at the Philadelphia Hospital, and a weekly clinic was held at Jefferson in nervous and mental diseases, as well as daily instruction in Neurology. Instruction in Insanity was given in the outpatient department or in the wards of the Philadelphia Hospital, which, in addition to its Department for Nervous Diseases, had a large Insane Department. Instruction was provided in class sections in electrotherapy of nervous disorders, and in the Orthopaedic Hospital and Infirmary for Nervous Diseases and the Wills Eye Hospital.

Francis X. Dercum, M.D., Professor of Nervous and Mental Diseases (1900–1925)

In 1900 a separate Department was established, and Dr. Dercum was appointed Professor of Nervous and Mental Diseases. He continued as the Head of the Department until his retirement in 1925, when he became Emeritus Professor. The long and distinguished career of Dr. Dercum at Jefferson marks him as the first giant figure in its history of neurology.

Francis Dercum was born in Philadelphia on October 10, 1856. He received his M.D. degree from the University of Pennsylvania in 1877. His early and sustained interest in biology subsequently manifested as a lively interest in neurology, and he founded the Philadelphia Neurological Society in 1884. His studies led to many publications, including collaboration in a *Textbook on Nervous Diseases by American Authors,* of which he was editor in 1895.[12] Other publications reflected his interest in endocrine disorders and mental diseases. His energy and mental alertness were evident in his teaching, research, publications, and practice. One of his important patients was President Wilson during the years 1919 and 1920.

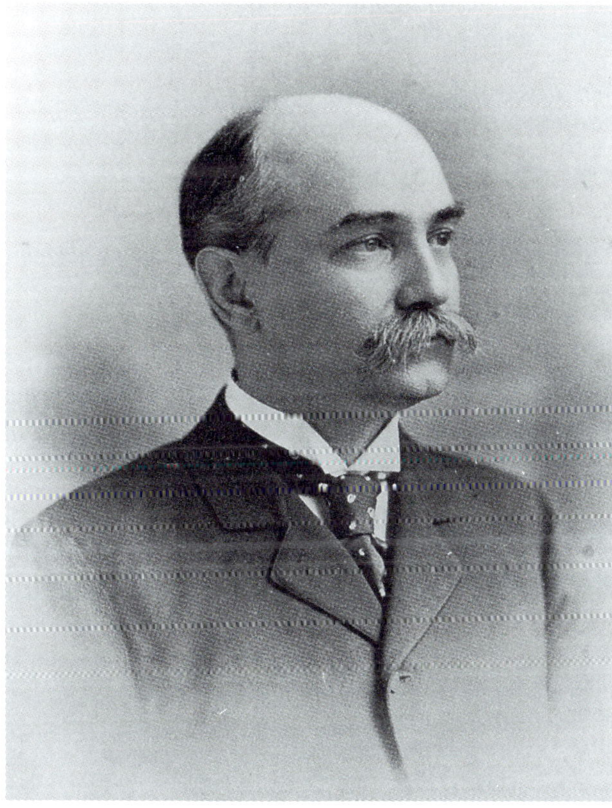

FIG. 28-2. Francis X. Dercum, M.D., Professor of Nervous and Mental Diseases (1900–1925).

Dr. Dercum was President of the American Neurological Association (1886) as well as twice President of the Philadelphia Neurological Society (1892 and 1898). He was elected to membership in foreign neurological societies in Paris, London, and Budapest, and his membership in the Societé de Neurologie of Paris (1908) was a great honor—it had fewer than 50 members from all over the world.

Dr. Dercum was one of those rare physicians in the field of neurology able to achieve recognition by having his name given to a disease that he described in detail in 1897.[13] One aspect of neurology is the discovery and naming of new diseases, and these new diseases often bear unusual names. One of these creations is the disease known as adiposa dolorosa, which, after its description in detail, was called Dercum's disease. Figure 28-3 shows the "lovely" Dolores Adiposa waddling down the corridors of time filled with the joy of new-found life.

At the turn of the century, additions to the faculty included Drs. Alfred Gordon, known subsequently as the originator of the Gordon sign, an upper motor neuron sign; S.F. Gilpin, and Samuel Clark. A clinical neurology prize was established by Dr. Dercum for the best examination in neurology. During the first decade of the twentieth century the Department of Nervous and Mental Diseases expanded under Dr. Dercum with the elevation in faculty ranks of the junior members of the Department. In addition to the instruction in the neurology clinics, the Department in the Jefferson Medical College Hospital was established with Dr. Dercum as Attending Neurologist and Dr. George E. Price as the Assistant Neurologist. In the neurology dispensary, which was held three times weekly, the clinical assistants included Drs. Sherman Gilpin, Michael Burns, and Benjamin Weiss. During the second decade of the twentieth century, Dr. Price was elevated to the position of Associate

Professor, and in the dispensary Dr. S.F. Gilpin was Chief Clinical Assistant, with Drs. Michael Burns, Benjamin Weiss, W.C. Pritchard, G.F. Phillips, P.A. McCarthy, Leon J. Tunitzki, and William L. Clark as Clinical Assistants. Dr. Burns provided additional instruction in neuropathology during the third year. After 1915 Dr. Price provided instruction in mental diseases at the Philadelphia Hospital. In 1918 the Clinical Assistants in the Neurology Dispensary included J.L. Donaghue, Thomas E. Shea, and Thomas Buchanan. After 1920 Dr. Sherman F. Gilpin replaced Dr. Price as Assistant Neurologist in the Jefferson Medical College Hospital, and Dr. C. Fred Becker was added to the group in the dispensary. During the early 1920s the entire senior class began to receive weekly instruction in neurology at the Jefferson Hospital and attend a weekly clinic in mental diseases at the Philadelphia General Hospital. Dr. Gilpin was responsible for the latter clinic.

Dr. Dercum's interest in philosophy resulted in his achievement of a Ph.D. degree, in addition to his M.D., and in 1927 he was elected President of the American Philosophical Society. He died on April 23, 1931, as he was presiding over the two hundred and fortieth Annual Meeting of the Society while seated in the famous "ladder-library chair" made by Benjamin Franklin, the founder of the Society.

Edward A. Strecker, M.D., Professor of Nervous and Mental Diseases (1925–1931)

When Dr. Dercum became Emeritus Professor in 1925, he was replaced by Dr. Edward A. Strecker

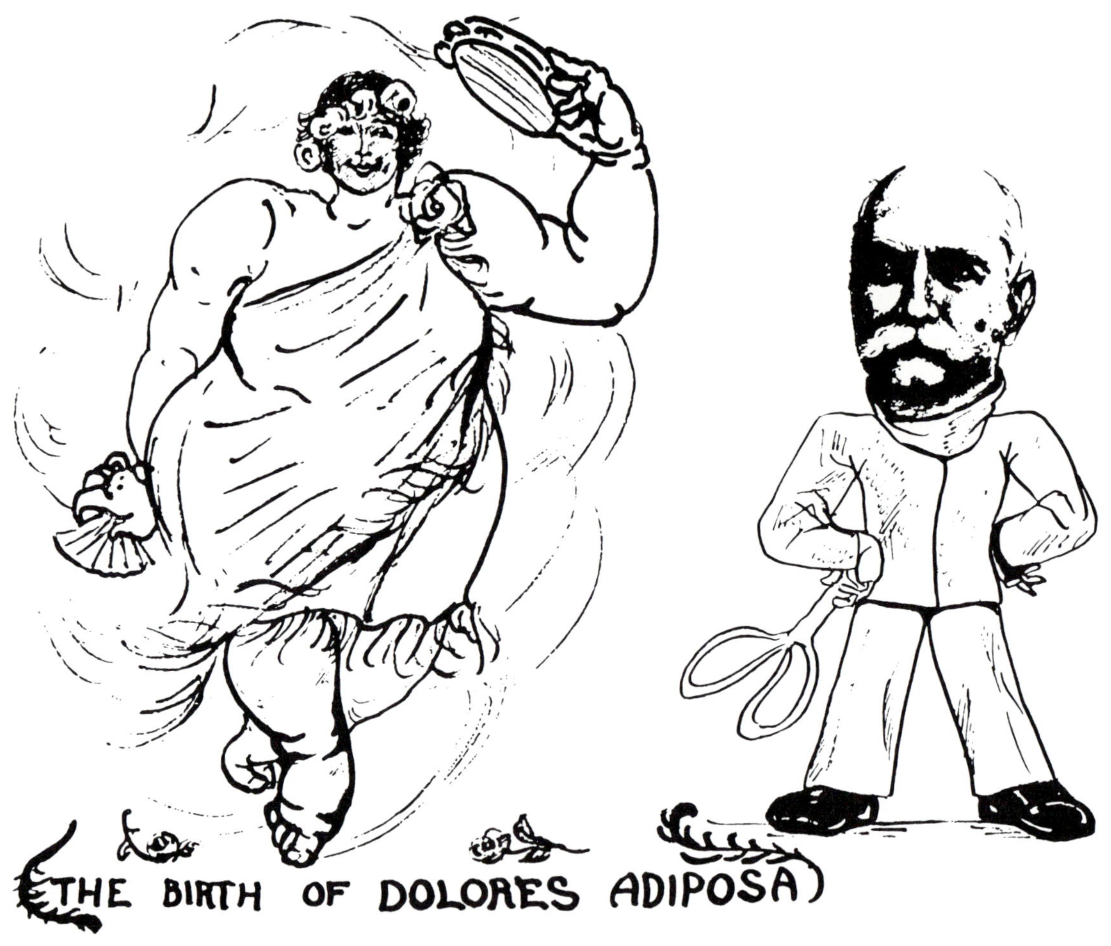

FIG. 28-3. Caricature of adiposa dolorosa, known as Dercum's disease. (Courtesy of Dr. Morton Nathanson.)

(Figure 28-4) as Professor of Nervous and Mental Diseases. Dr. Strecker was a graduate of Jefferson Medical College in 1911 and when a student was taught by Dr. Dercum. In the relatively short period between 1925 and 1931, Dr. Strecker ably maintained the Department. He was Attending Neurologist in the Jefferson Medical College Hospital, and Dr. Gilpin was Assistant Neurologist. The clinical lectures in neurology were provided by both Drs. Strecker and Gilpin, with the clinic of mental diseases at the Philadelphia General Hospital supervised by Dr. Strecker. The latter's weekly clinic there was a "standing-room-only" session. Dr. William H. Schmidt was responsible for teaching electrotherapy, a discipline that was included in the Department.

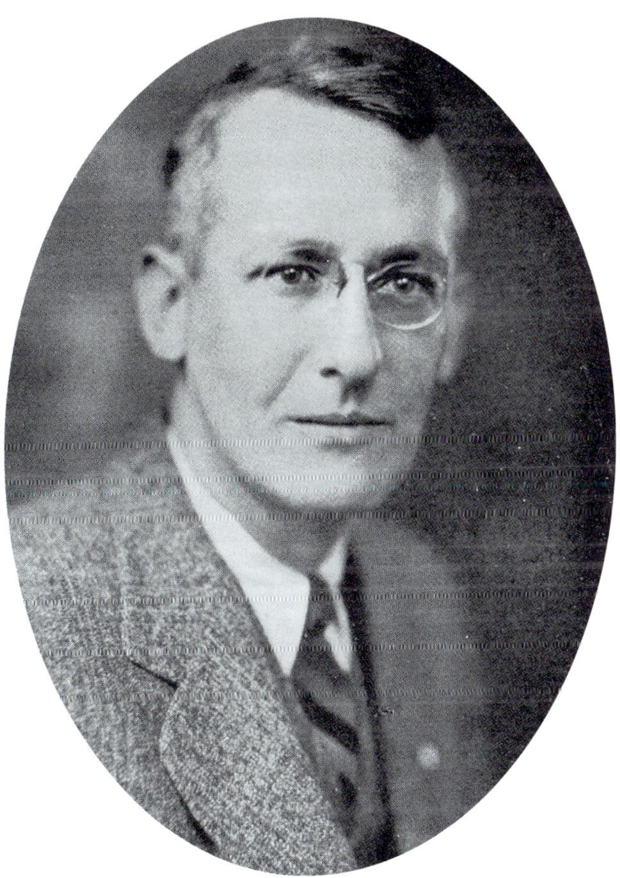

FIG. 28-4. Edward A. Strecker, M.D. (Jefferson, 1911), Professor of Nervous and Mental Diseases (1925–1931).

Dr. Strecker resigned as Professor of Nervous and Mental Diseases at Jefferson in 1931. He went on to enhance his reputation both nationally and internationally[14] in his new position as Professor of Psychiatry at the University of Pennsylvania Medical School. With no replacement for Dr. Strecker at Jefferson for a period of three years, the program of instruction in neurology was maintained under the supervision of Drs. Michael A. Burns, Sherman T. Gilpin, and Benjamin P. Weiss. In 1931 Dr. Baldwin L. Keyes held the title of Demonstrator of Neurology and Dr. Robert A. Matthews began as Instructor, and Drs. Lauren H. Smith as Associate in Nervous and Mental Diseases and Samuel T. Gordy as Assistant joined the Department.

Michael A. Burns, M.D., Chairman (1934–1938)

At a special meeting of the Board of Trustees on May 7, 1934, the faculty position of Professor of Nervous and Mental Diseases was abolished and was replaced by that of Professor of Neurology. At that time, Dr. Michael A. Burns (Figure 28-5) became Professor of Neurology and Head of the Department. Dr. Benjamin P. Weiss continued as an Assistant Professor. Additions to the faculty included Drs. Angelo Erraz, R. Seckell, George L. Stephan, and Ralph L. Drake. In 1936 Dr. William H. Schmidt became Assistant Professor of Physical Therapy. In 1937 Dr. Baldwin L. Keyes became Clinical Professor of Psychiatry and assumed major responsibility for the teaching of psychiatry in the Department of Neurology.

Through the relatively short period of four years before his sudden death on March 7, 1938, Dr. Burns maintained the great interest in neurology that had begun under Dr. Dercum following his graduation from Jefferson in 1907. Burns was in military service during World War I, associated with the Jefferson Unit Base Hospital No. 38. The Department of Neurology showed little change during Dr. Burns' tenure. In addition to the teaching of medical students was the instruction of Interns in the Jefferson Hospital and supervision of both neurological inpatients and outpatients. Dr. Burns was particularly proud of Jefferson and its students, endeavoring always to help them represent the Jeffersonian tradition.

Bernard J. Alpers, M.D., Chairman (1938–1965)

In September 1938, as a replacement for Dr. Burns, Dr. Bernard J. Alpers (Figure 28-6) became the Professor of Neurology. He continued as Head of the Department until his retirement in 1965, when he became Emeritus Professor. Dr. Alpers' long and distinguished career marked him as the second giant figure in Jefferson's history of neurology. He was born in Salem, Massachusetts, on March 14, 1900, the town in which witchcraft was alleged to have been practiced in 1692; was a graduate of the Harvard Medical School in 1923; and achieved the degree of Doctor of Medical Science from the University of Pennsylvania in 1930. Dr. Alpers had extensive training in neuropathology overseas, including four months with Professor A. Jacob in Hamburg, Germany, and a year in Spain, where he had the opportunity to study with Professors Ramon y Cajal and P. del Rio Hortega. He also studied for two months with Professor Charles Sherrington at Oxford. After his return, Alpers continued his research interest in neuropathology and became Director of a Laboratory of Neuropathology at the University of Pennsylvania. Becoming Professor of Neurology at Jefferson in 1938, he also maintained his private practice as a neurologist, a practice that he continued throughout his Chairmanship. Alpers' tremendous energy and interest as a teacher and clinical neurologist enabled him quickly to establish a Residency Program. This major accomplishment permitted the training of many Residents who became distinguished in their subsequent careers throughout the United States. Seven of these became Heads of Departments of Neurology at other institutions, and many

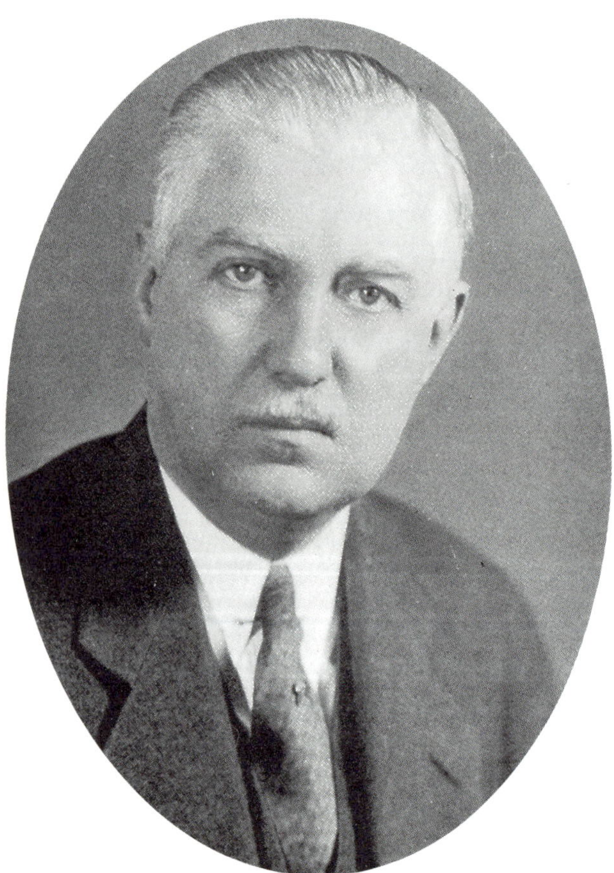

FIG. 28-5. Michael A. Burns, M.D., (Jefferson, 1907), Chairman of Neurology (1934–1938).

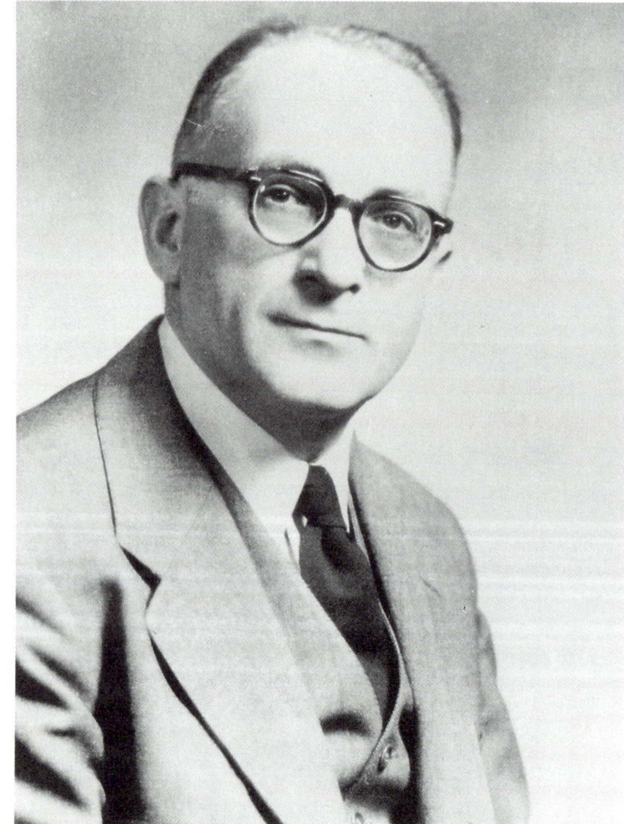

FIG. 28-6. Bernard J. Alpers, M.D., Chairman of the Neurology Department (1938–1965).

Jefferson graduates during Dr. Alpers' Chairmanship selected the field of neurology as their specialty. Within a short time after his arrival, the Department of Neurology expanded considerably through the appointment of physicians who were able to contribute to its growth. In 1939 the Department included Dr. Baldwin L. Keyes as Clinical Professor of Psychiatry and Dr. Benjamin P. Weiss as Associate Professor of Neurology. Dr. William H. Schmidt was Assistant Professor of Physical Therapy and Dr. Robert A. Matthews Assistant Professor of Psychiatry. Other members of the Department included Drs. C. Fred Becker, Samuel T. Gordy, Robert S. Bookhammer, Robert P. Sturr, Robert R. Livingstone, Raphael H. Durante, Thomas K. Rothmell, Nathan S. Schlezinger, R.C. Kell, George L. Stephan, Thomas J. Leichner, Edward C. Britt, and Kenneth C. Corrin. The technical staff increased correspondingly and special Divisions of Neurophysiology, Neurochemistry, Neuropharmacology, and Pediatric Neurology were established. Thus was founded one of the outstanding Departments of Neurology in the United States and, indeed, in the world. Instruction included neuropathology lectures during the second year, clinical neurology lectures in the third year, and clinical lectures and section instruction in neurology during the fourth year. The neurology clinic also was used for instruction and was active three times weekly. In 1940 additional members of the Department included Drs. Eli Marcovitz, Calvin S. Drayer, James J. Ryan, H. Edward Yaskin, and Herbert S. Gaskill. Dr. Gaskill was the first Resident in neurology at Jefferson, and, as many of the Residents, he continued with a Residency in psychiatry. He later became Professor and Head of the Department of Psychiatry at the University of Colorado Medical School.

In 1942 the Department of Psychiatry was established as a separate Department with Dr. Baldwin L. Keyes as Professor and Head. Dr. Bernard J. Alpers continued as Professor of Neurology and Head of the Department. An addition to the members of the Department at that time was Dr. Francis M. Forster as Assistant Professor of Neurology and, subsequently, Associate Professor, until 1950 when he left Jefferson to become Professor of Neurology at Georgetown University Medical School. While there Dr. Forster became Dean of the Medical School in 1953, but in 1958 he left to become Professor of Neurology and Head of the Department at the University of Wisconsin Medical School, where he remained for a period of 20 years before his retirement.

In 1946 Dr. Winslow J. Borkowski (Jefferson, 1943) completed his residency in neurology and joined the Department. Subsequently, over a period of many years, he served as Professor of Neurology with special responsibility for the development of electroencephalography. Dr. Richard G. Berry completed his residency at Jefferson in 1950, left temporarily for additional training in neuropathology, and after his return to Jefferson became for many years the Professor and Director of Neuropathology. Another addition to the Department was Dr. Frederick A. Horner, who was the first member to specialize in Pediatric Neurology. He ultimately achieved distinction as Professor of Pediatric Neurology at the University of Rochester School of Medicine. Dr. Roger Q. Cracco, whose main interest was neurophysiology at Jefferson, subsequently became a Professor and Head of the Department of Neurology at the State University of New York, Downstate Medical Center. In 1958 Dr. Elliott L. Mancall joined the Department and remained until 1965, when he became Professor of Neurology at the Hahnemann Medical College; in 1976 he was named Chairman of the Department there. Dr. Mancall collaborated with Dr. Alpers in the sixth edition of *Clinical Neurology* (1971) and the first edition of *Essentials of the Neurological Examination* (1971). A second edition of the latter text appeared in 1981, and Dr. Mancall began preparing the third edition in 1986.

Among the Residents when Dr. Alpers was Head of the Department were many who achieved distinction as Neurology Department Heads at various hospitals and medical schools. Dr. Rodney A. Farmer (Jefferson, 1941) was Head of Neurology at the Veterans Administration Hospital in Coatesville, Pennsylvania, for many years; Dr. Richard M. Paddison became Professor of Neurology at the Louisiana State University School of Medicine; Dr. Thomas R. Johns became Professor of Neurology at the University of Virginia School of Medicine; Dr. Luis P. Sanchez-

Longo (Jefferson, 1951) became Professor of Neurology at the University of Puerto Rico Medical School; Dr. Leo Madow became Professor of Neurology at the Woman's Medical College and subsequently Professor of Psychiatry at the Medical College of Pennsylvania; Dr. Joseph C. White, Jr., (Jefferson, 1954) occupied the position of Head of Neurology at the Barrow Institute of Neurology in Phoenix, Arizona; and Dr. Alan B. Rubens (Jefferson, 1962) achieved the position of Professor and Head of Neurology at the University of Arizona Medical Center in Tucson.

Included in another group are those neurology residents who remained in the Philadelphia area and became successful: Dr. Martin M. Mandel (Jefferson, 1947), Chief of Neurology at Jeanes Hospital; Dr. Arnold A. Bank, Chief of Neurology at the Northern Division of the Albert Einstein Medical Center; Dr. Edgar J. Kenton, III, Chief of Neurology at the Lankenau Hospital; Dr. Eric J. Freimuth, Chief of Neurology at the Bryn Mawr Hospital; Dr. Albert D. Wagman, Chief of Neurology at the Abington Memorial Hospital; Dr. Lawrence Green (Jefferson, 1964), Chief of Neurology at Crozer-Chester Medical Center; and Dr. Marvin E. Jaffe (Jefferson, 1960), Vice President for Clinical Research with Merck, Sharp and Dohme Research Laboratories.

Residents in neurology also included Drs. Weir M. Tucker, Arnold W. Levine, Harry W. Hogan (Jefferson, 1946), Kalman Frankel (Jefferson, 1943), Peter Machung, Harold L. Baxter, Gustave W. Andersen (Jefferson, 1946), Erwin R. Smarr (Jefferson, 1949), Robert A. Bader, Chester F. Cullen (Jefferson, 1948), Russell S. Bauer, Isaac Silberman, Thomas C. Owens, Richard A. Naef (Jefferson, 1953), Rigoberto Campos, Stephen J. Dutch, James D. Repepi, Morton W. Shrager, Virginia Payne, Edward F. Gonyea, R. Douglas Collins, David M. Geeter (Jefferson, 1958), John Novotny, Joseph Tobia, Stuart B. Brown (Jefferson, 1959), Martin H. Feldman, Austin R. Moody, Erich H.W. Simon, L. Donald Tashjian, Jay Rosenblum, Richard A. Thompson, Theodore W. Wasserman (Jefferson, 1961), Norman J. Schatz, Jack E. Kundin, Gerald J. Quinn (Jefferson, 1962), Charles L. Reese (Jefferson, 1958), Alan B. Rubens (Jefferson, 1962), Morris L. Lorber, Keith A. Roberts, and Harriet Wells.

Deserving of special mention is the establishment of the close connection between the Department of Neurology at the Wills Eye Hospital and the Department at Jefferson. Dr. Nathan S. Schlezinger, soon after his return to Jefferson in October 1938, started at the Wills Eye Hospital under Dr. William Duane for a short time and then under Dr. Alpers as titular Chief of Neurology at Wills until 1957. He became Chief of Neurology and continued as Director of Neuro-ophthalmology until retirement as Consultant Emeritus in 1976. Dr. Schlezinger was a graduate of Jefferson in 1932 and received the degree of Doctor of Medical Science from Columbia University in 1938. As a pioneer in the development of clinical neuro-ophthalmology in Philadelphia, he guided the great expansion of neurology at Wills Eye Hospital and the resultant ever-increasing volume of patients referred to Jefferson for the diagnosis and treatment of their concomitant ailments. Dr. Alpers provided for the support of the expanding program of teaching and research at Wills by the establishment of a regularly scheduled period of four months' rotation at Wills for the Jefferson neurology Residents. This further close relationship between neurology at Wills and at Jefferson was maintained while Dr. Alpers continued as Chairman at Jefferson. Dr. Schlezinger also started the Myasthenia Gravis Clinic at Jefferson, which was continued under his supervision for many years.

The predawn rounds by Dr. Alpers at Jefferson became legendary. He was always known as someone who would never arrive later than 6:00 A.M., and this served to demonstrate the need for the maximum amount of time to do what was required in the course of a day. The warm humor and scholarly attributes of Dr. Alpers were widely known. In 1959 the senior class presented his portrait to the College in a characteristic teaching pose (Figure 28-7).

Dr. Alpers contributed more than 100 papers to the literature during his long career at Jefferson. In 1945 the first edition of his textbook *Clinical Neurology* was published[15]; it continued to be valued by the medical students through five editions (1945–1963). Dr. Alpers also achieved recognition by having named after him a rare disease that he had described in detail.[16]

Dr. Alpers became President of the American

Neurological Association in 1957 and was also President of the American Association of Neuropathology, the Association for Research in Nervous and Mental Diseases, and the American Board of Psychiatry and Neurology. At the 1957 annual meeting of the American Neurological Association, when Dr. Alpers was President, the customary entertainment at the banquet consisted of a creative and original staff presentation by the neurology Residents of Jefferson. This has always been remembered as a measure of their esteem for him.

Dr. Alpers had a life-long interest in religion, especially as a Hebrew scholar. Music and a large personal library were his sources of relaxation, as well as baseball in general and the Boston Red Sox in particular. This exemplary Chairman died on November 2, 1981.

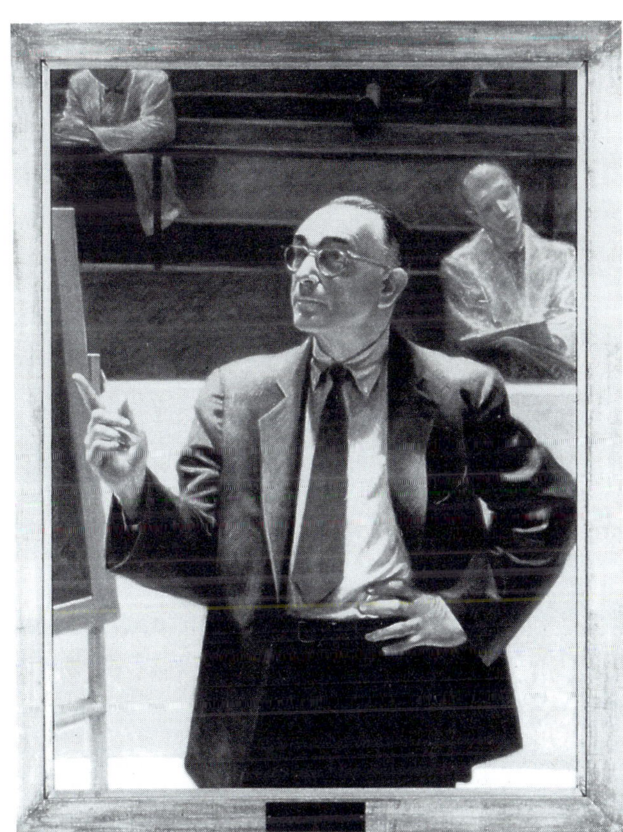

FIG. 28-7. Portrait of Bernard J. Alpers, M.D., in a typical teaching pose (1959).

Richard A. Chambers, M.D., Chairman (1965–1983)

When Dr. Alpers became Emeritus Professor of Neurology in 1965, he was succeeded as Chairman by Dr. Richard A. Chambers (Figure 28-8). Dr. Chambers was born on April 22, 1923, in London, England. He completed his medical education at Oxford University in 1947 and his neurology Residency training at the National Hospital for Nervous Diseases in Queen's Square in London in 1956. He was certified in neurology in 1959 when he was at the Toronto General Hospital, in Canada. Subsequently he joined the Seton Hall College of Medicine and Dentistry, where he became Professor of Neurology before coming to Jefferson in 1965.

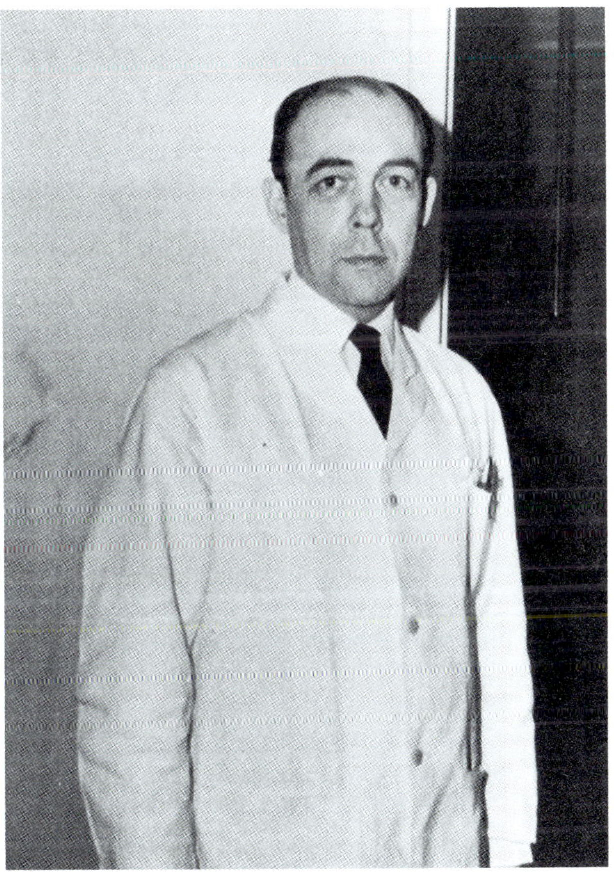

FIG. 28-8. Richard A. Chambers, M.D., Chairman of Neurology (1965–1983).

Dr. Leonard Graziani (Jefferson, 1955) achieved distinction as Professor of Neurology and Pediatrics at Jefferson upon his return in 1966. Dr. Leopold J. Streletz completed his Residency in Neurology at Jefferson in 1973 and was appointed Associate Professor of Neurology at Jefferson with special interest and responsibility in Clinical Neurophysiology as well as becoming Director of the Division of Electrodiagnosis. Recently, Streletz has collaborated with Dr. Graziani to develop a sophisticated monitoring system aimed at investigating the pathological aspects of infant apnea syndrome. Dr. Leonard Katz, after completion of his Residency at Jefferson in 1969, became Clinical Professor of Neurology at Jefferson and Head of Neurology at the Veterans Administration Hospital in Wilmington, Delaware. Dr. Henry F. McFarland, after completion of his Residency at Jefferson in 1970, continued with special training in neuropathology and achieved distinction in recent years in the field of cellular neuroimmunology at the National Institutes of Health, Bethesda, Maryland.

Additional members of the faculty after 1965 were Drs. Donald G. Durencamp, Marius P. Valsamis, Oscar San Martín Marín, Elberto Risdon, and Stephen D. Reznak. Residents in neurology included Drs. Joan Cracco, Robert L. Calmes, Morton Coren, William Haycock, Leonard R. Geiger, Junichiro Kawamura, Chikao Kono, Barbara A. L. Beasley, and Howard J. Kaplan.

After his arrival in Philadelphia, Dr. Chambers was elected President of the Philadelphia Neurological Society (1974). He held membership in the Canadian Neurology Society, the American Association of Neuropathology, the American Academy of Neurology, and the Association for Research in Nervous and Mental Diseases. During the 17 years that Dr. Chambers was Head of the Department, he maintained the quality of teaching and research, as well as supervision of both inpatient and outpatient neurologic patients, and the residency program continued with the aid of other members of the faculty. Gradually some of the valued members of the Department, such as Drs. Mancall and Roger Q. Cracco departed.

Robert J. Schwartzman, M.D., Chairman (1983–)

In 1983 Dr. Chambers was succeeded by Dr. Robert J. Schwartzman (Figure 28-9) as Professor and Head of the Department. Dr. Chambers continued as a member of the Department. Dr. Schwartzman was born in Washington, D.C., on November 28, 1939. He graduated from the University of Pennsylvania Medical School (1965) and completed his residency in neurology in its Hospital (1969). Board certified by the American Board of Internal Medicine (1972) and the American Board of Psychiatry and Neurology (1974), Schwartzman subsequently achieved a faculty position as Associate Professor of Neurology at the University of Miami School of Medicine. He then became Professor of Neurology and Chief of the Division of Neurology in the University of Texas Health Science Center at San Antonio (1978), until he returned to Philadelphia for the Chairmanship at Jefferson.

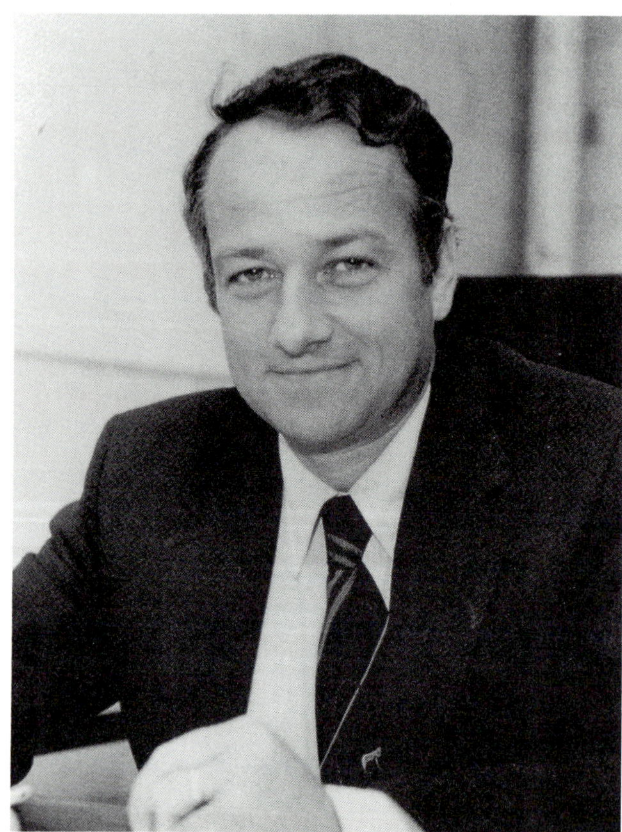

FIG. 28-9. Robert J. Schwartzman, M.D., Chairman of Neurology (1983–).

Since arriving at Jefferson, Dr. Schwartzman has supervised an expansion of the Department with faculty personnel who are active in basic and clinical research. In addition to his major administrative and teaching responsibilities, Dr. Schwartzman has been engaged, in collaboration of Dr. Guillermo Alexander, in a research effort directed toward the study of recovery of the central nervous system after injury. Recent important research is an investigation of the mechanics of neurotoxicity resulting from a drug (MPTP), which induces Parkinsonism in primates and man, in order to discover antidotes.[17]

Dr. Ruggero G. Fariello, Vice Chairman of the Department, attained the position of Professor of Neurology and Professor of Pharmacology as well as Director of Clinical Neurophysiology. His interest in research is concerned with the physiological and pharmacological aspects of convulsive disorders and extrapyramidal disorders. Upon his departure from Jefferson in 1987, he became Professor of Neurology and Chairman of the Department of Neurological Sciences at the Rush Medical College.

Dr. Fred D. Lublin (Jefferson, 1972), following his return from New York, became Professor of Neurology and Professor of Biochemistry as well as Director of the Division of Neuroimmunology and Vice Chairman of the Department. He has been actively engaged in the investigation of the immunological aspects of multiple sclerosis. Dr. Robert Knobler as Associate Professor of Neurology has collaborated in the research investigation of demyelinating diseases from the standpoint of neuroimmunization and neurovirology. Dr. Michael E. Shy, as Assistant Professor of Neurology, has been especially interested in the immune mechanisms of neuromuscular diseases.

Dr. Serge W. Duckett, Professor of Neurology and Director of the Division of Neuropathology, has continued with his interest in electronmicroscopy and the evaluation of various metallic toxic effects on the nervous system. Dr. John M. Bertoni, Associate Professor of Neurology, has been conducting research in central nervous system toxins as well as in the treatment of movement disorders. Dr. Patricio F. Reyes, Associate Professor of Neurology and Pathology, has been engaged in the further investigation of the dementias, including Alzheimer's disease. Dr. George C. Brainard, Assistant Professor of Neurology, has also been actively engaged in the research activities of the Department with a special interest in the effect of light on the nervous system. Dr. Rodney B. Bell has been a recent addition to the faculty as Associate Professor of Neurology and Neurosurgery. He has an active interest in the establishment of a cerebral vascular disease unit within the Department for the further investigation and treatment of these diseases.

Dr. Robert D. Aiken, Assistant Professor of Neurology and a volunteer member of the Department, has maintained his special interest in Neuro-oncology. Dr. Steven Mandel, Clinical Assistant Professor of Neurology, is another active volunteer member of the faculty.

Contributions to the literature from the Department have increased since the arrival of Dr. Schwartzman and his associates, as have presentations at both local and national neurologic meetings. It is anticipated that this activity will be reflected in the increasing importance of the Department in all aspects of patient care, teaching, and investigation of basic causes of neurologic disease.

References

1. Chadwich, John, and Mann, W.N., (translators): *The Medical Works of Hippocrates*. Springfield, Illinois: Charles C. Thomas, 1950, pp. 191–192.
2. Singer, C., "Galen as a Modern," *Proc. Roy. Soc. Med.* 42:563–570, 1949.
3. McMurrick, J.P., *Leonardo da Vinci: The Anatomist*. Baltimore: Williams & Wilkins Co., 1930, p. 206.
4. Singer, C., *Vesalius on the Human Brain*. Oxford University Press, 1952.
5. Descartes, R., "The Passions of the Soul," Part First, Articles XXXI *et seq.*, *The Philosophical Works of Descartes*. Translated by Elizabeth S. Haldane and G.R.T. Ross. Vol. 1, p. 345. Dover Publications, Inc., 1955).
6. Mitchell, J.K., "On a New Practice in Acute and Chronic Rheumatism," *Amer. J. Med. Sci.* 8:55–64, 1831.
7. Dunglison, R., *The Practice of Medicine or a Treatise on Special Pathology and Therapeutics*. Philadelphia: Lea & Blanchard, 1842.
8. Fye, W.B., "S. Weir Mitchell, Philadelphia's 'Lost' Physiologist," *Bull. Hist. Med.* 7(2):188–202. Summer 1983.
9. Mitchell, S.W., *Injuries of Nerves and Their Consequences*. Philadelphia: J.B. Lippincott & Co., 1872.
10. Meigs, J.A., "Observations upon the Form of the Occiput in the Various Races of Men," *Proc. Aca. Nat. Sci. Phila.* 1860, pp. 397–415.
11. Bartholow, R., "Investigations into the Functions of the Human Brain," *Amer. J. Med. Sci.* 67:305–313, 1874.
12. Dercum, F.X. (ed.): *A Textbook of Nervous Diseases by American Authors*. Philadelphia: Lea Brothers, 1895.

13. Dercum, F.X., "Three Cases of an Hitherto Unclassified Affection Resembling in its Grosser Aspects Obesity, but Associated with Special Nervous Symptoms, Adiposa Dolorosa," *Am. J. Med. Sci.* 104:521–535, 1892.
14. Strecker, E.A., "Behavior Problems in Encephalitis: A Clinical Study of the Relationship Between Behavior and the Acute and Chronic Phenomena of Encephalitis," *Arch. Neur. and Psych.* 21:137–144, 1929.
15. Alpers, B.J., *Clinical Neurology.* Philadelphia: F.A. Davis Co., 1945.
16. Alpers, B.J., "Diffuse Progressive Degeneration of the Gray Matter of the Cerebrum," *Arch. Neur. and Psych.* 25:469–505, 1931.
17. Schwartzman, R.J., and Alexander, G.M., "Changes in the Local Cerebral Metabolic Rate for Glucose in the 1-Methyl-4-phenyl-1,2,3,6-tetrahydropyridine (MPTP) Primate Model of Parkinson's Disease," *Brain Research.* 358:137–143, 1985.

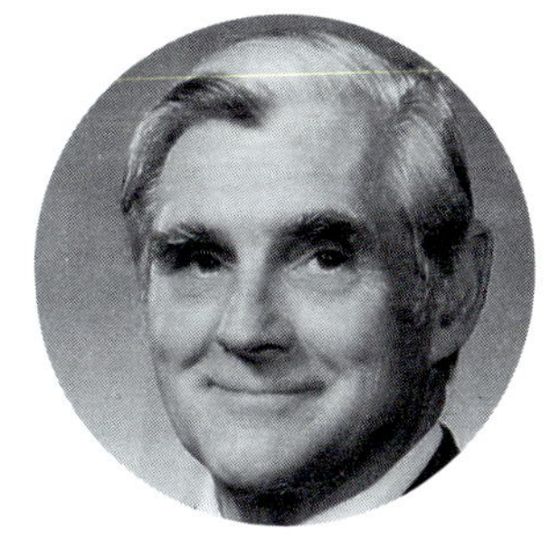

CHAPTER TWENTY-NINE

Department of Psychiatry

John A. Koltes, M.D.

"The more things change, the more they remain the same." —Alphonse Karr (1808–90)

At the beginning of the nineteenth century, it was customary for medical students to go to the great European universities for more advanced theoretical training. America still had very few institutions of higher learning. Numerous Philadelphia physicians, including Benjamin Rush and Phineas Bond, had experience in European universities.[1]

In the eighteenth century, bloodletting was a common procedure for treatment of all kinds of ills, including mental problems. Theories relative to circulation of "humors," toxicity, and the later one of *locus minoris resistentiae* (lessened resistance to invasion by microorganisms and/or their toxins), were the product of speculations relative to cause, and they often led to bizarre treatments. As treatment of mental illness, high colonic irrigations, purges, dental extraction, and removal of tonsils and adenoids each had a vogue that continued into the twentieth century. At one state hospital, as recently as the middle of the current century, a psychiatrist-surgeon practiced this belief by excising long segments of intestine from his patients on the grounds that the colon harbored the site of infection, which led to the development of schizophrenia. Not until the invention of electroshock therapy by Dr. Ugo Cerletti amd Thomas Bini of the University of Rome and introduced in the United States at the Institute of the Pennsylvania Hospital by Dr. Joseph Hughes in 1944 was this method of treatment condemned as ineffective and inappropriate.

Until the latter half of the eighteenth century, mental diseases were thought to be caused by misanthropic theological forces in which God had deserted the mentally ill, who were seen as "possessed" of Satanic forces that obstructed a correct functioning of the mind. The scientific world paid little attention to the psychoneuroses until late in the nineteenth century. Men such as Charcot in Paris, Freud in Vienna, and Maudsley in England began to pay closer attention to the nature of the psychoneurotic process, defining it in terms more consistent with today's concepts. It is therefore interesting that one of the members of the first graduating class of the Jefferson Medical College in 1826, Joel Foster of Vermont, wrote his thesis on "Neuroses."

Early Psychiatric Facilities in Philadelphia

In 1944 a directory of the mental hospitals in Philadelphia was published. It included names of the hospital directors and described their general status.[2] The earliest history belongs to the Philadelphia General Hospital. Founded in 1732, it was located between Third and Fourth and Spruce and Pine Streets, on a site called Almshouse Square, which housed a facility primarily for the care and treatment of indigent and immigrant people. Those in a position to afford private care received it at home. In that period and until recent times, medical care was considered to be an individual matter, whereas it now is considered by many to be a human right. The early settlers in Philadelphia provided facilities only for the care of those totally unable to care for themselves by reason of severe physical illness, mental illness, or poverty. The Almshouse became overcrowded and in 1767 was moved to a tract between Tenth and Eleventh Streets, from Spruce to Pine. In that year 284 inmates were transferred to the new building. Dr. Benjamin Rush, the "Father of American Psychiatry," was on the staff of the infirmary from 1774 to 1777, and George McClellan worked there while a student at the University of Pennsylvania.[3]

Before the turn of the nineteenth century, no facilities existed for the care of insane patients, and those who were violent were housed at the Pennsylvania Hospital at Eighth and Spruce Streets. Evidently this became expensive to the City; to relieve the burden, cells were built in the basement wing of the Almshouse to house ten violent mentally ill people. The basement amounted essentially to an underground prison. The cells were described as "damp, chilly caverns with insufficient light and improper ventilation. They were close to sick and surgical wards and the noise of these creatures bereft of reason exerted an unpleasant influence on the sick." These conditions prevailed until 1834, when 92 insane patients, together with a group from the Almshouse suffering from physical disease, were moved to a farm west of the city in the township of Blockley. This lay across the Schuylkill River, facing the U.S. Naval Hospital at Grays Ferry. The facilities eventually became known as the Philadelphia Hospital and ultimately the Philadelphia General Hospital, one of the great teaching institutions in America, a site that tragically suffered demise at the hands of "progress" in 1977. It is interesting to compare it with the Salpêtrière Hospital in Paris, which has stood on the left bank of the Seine since the middle of the seventeenth century and continues to serve as a public hospital.

In 1859, in an attempt to improve the care of the mentally ill, the insane patients at the Philadelphia Hospital were separated from those suffering from physical disease and were placed under the care of a separate medical officer who received a salary of $1,000 a year. A general program, including activity, outdoor work, and kindness, rather than coercion and imprisonment, was instituted. This must have been a reflection of the work of Dr. Thomas S. Kirkbride, who had founded his mental hospital 20 years earlier in the same general area of West Philadelphia at Forty-fourth and Market Streets.

In 1890 patients with possible mental illness were admitted to wards that treated delinquency and alcoholism. In 1906 similar patients were placed in separate wards with attending physicians. In 1912 the so-called psychopathic wards were established, and Philadelphia General Hospital continued to operate a psychopathic department, separate from neurology and medicine, until the closing of the hospital.

Several psychiatrists were appointed in 1916 to operate this facility. These included Drs. S. DeWitt Ludlum, later to found the Gladwyne Colony and become well known in the treatment of schizophrenia, Sherman F. Gilpin, Sr., A.C. Buckley, and S.T. Ingham. Franklin G. Ebaugh, a graduate of Johns Hopkins in 1919, became the first director of the facility in 1921. He resigned in 1924 to become Professor of Psychiatry at the University of Colorado. He was the junior coauthor, with Dr. Edward A. Strecker, of *Practical Clinical Psychiatry for Students and Practitioners*, published in 1925 and used by Jefferson students for at least two decades.

A six-story building with a capacity of 300 beds for the treatment of the mentally ill was erected in 1931. The admission rate was over 4,000 per year, of which number about 1,500 patients were termed too sick to return to civilian life and were committed to mental hospitals. The importance of the psychopathic wards at the Philadelphia General Hospital with respect to the Jefferson Medical College was its excellent teaching cases for the students. The teaching program was established by Dr. Francis X. Dercum and carried on by Drs. Edward A. Strecker (Jefferson, 1911), Baldwin L. Keyes (Jefferson, 1917), Robert A. Matthews (Jefferson, 1928), and Paul J. Poinsard (Jefferson, 1941) until 1962. These programs were so successful that students would attend the clinics on Saturday afternoon for two hours even when there was a football game at Franklin Field. The interest in mental disorders, the capacity of the professors to demonstrate classical-type cases, and the significance of the care that patients were offered in these facilities could not be overestimated.

The Philadelphia State Hospital for Mental Diseases was established in 1907 and was owned and operated by the City of Philadelphia in conjunction with the Philadelphia General Hospital and the Municipal Hospital for Contagious Diseases at Front and Luzerne Streets. In 1938, when taken over by the State, it contained 96 buildings and occupied 1,100 acres of land in the Byberry section of Northeast Philadelphia at Roosevelt Boulevard and Southampton Road. The total bed capacity was about 6,500, and plans in the 1930s and 1940s suggested the need for a total of at least 10,000 beds. Planners at that time did not have available the potentials for active treatment that were to evolve following World War II. The hospital was staffed in part by graduates of Jefferson and was used as component of Jefferson's teaching program. Dr. Frederick Kramer, a neuropathologist, neuroanatomist, psychiatrist, and Clinical Director of the Hospital, taught Jefferson students through the decades of the 1930s, 1940s, and 1950s.

The Friends Hospital at Roosevelt Boulevard and Adams Avenue, founded in 1813, was the first private psychiatric hospital in America. Through the years it had affiliations with Jefferson as well as the other Philadelphia medical schools. Another facility for the mentally ill was the Philadelphia Psychiatric Hospital, founded in 1937, and located at Ford and Monument Roads.

Among the other outstanding psychiatric facilities in Philadelphia in the nineteenth and twentieth centuries was the Philadelphia Orthopaedic Hospital and Infirmary for Nervous Diseases. This hospital was built in 1867, and in 1870 Dr. S. Weir Mitchell (Jefferson, 1850) joined it, converting it from a specifically orthopaedic hospital into one also treating nervous disorders. Dr. Mitchell had been head of the Turner's Lane Hospital in Philadelphia during the Civil War and had established the "Infirmary for Nervous Diseases" that became incorporated with the Orthopaedic Hospital. The hospital also had a School of Nursing and Physiotherapy, which remained active until the death of Dr. Mitchell in 1914. The Graduate School of Medicine of the University of Pennsylvania became actively involved with the hospital, and in 1938 it was incorporated into the Hospital of the University of Pennsylvania. The final remains of that great neurologic, orthopaedic, and psychiatric institution now exists only as a plaque on the wall of the University Hospital. The former hospital building at Seventeenth and Summer Streets was sold in 1940 to a group of physicians, who changed the name to Doctors' Hospital. They came from St. Agnes Hospital following disagreements between the staff and the nuns who ran St. Agnes at that time.[4]

The Pennsylvania Hospital, with the Department of Mental Diseases, the Department of Sick and Injured, and The Institute, constituted an important element of psychiatric treatment for patients in Philadelphia. Dr. Earl Bond noted that there were four major achievements to the credit of the hospital: the textbook of mental diseases published by Benjamin Rush in 1812; the development of the Department for Mental Diseases at Forty-fourth and Market Streets by Thomas Story Kirkbride in 1841; the outpatient clinic set up by Dr. John B. Chapin in 1885, and the building of the Institute at Forty-ninth and Market Streets in 1930.[5]

The Institute contained facilities for the treatment of psychoneuroses and for the study of neurological disorders by clinical laboratory means. The Rockefeller Foundation maintained a laboratory for biochemical study of brain metabolism, and five Rockefeller Fellows carried on these studies. Dr. Robert A. Matthews, later to become Professor of Psychiatry at Jefferson and

Chairman of the Department, was one of the original Fellows.

In 1925, Dr. Frederick H. Allen started the Philadelphia Child Guidance Clinic at the Children's Hospital at 1711 Fitzwater Street. This facility still exists and is one of the first units of its type in America for the care and treatment of childhood nervous disorders. Before the Child Guidance Clinic opened, however, Dr. Baldwin L. Keyes established an inpatient service for the treatment of nervous disorders at Jefferson Hospital at the request of the Professor of Pediatrics, Dr. Edward L. Bauer. The children's program and its extensive work was an outgrowth of the foundation laid by Dr. Keyes.

All of the medical schools have taught psychiatry for many years. The specialty was independently recognized at Jefferson in 1936, at Temple in 1928, at Hahnemann sometime in about the same era, and at the University of Pennsylvania in the 1920s. Dr. Keyes (Jefferson, 1917) at Jefferson, Max H. Bochroch (Jefferson, 1880) at Temple, John J. Tuller at Hahnemann, Edward A. Strecker (Jefferson, 1911) at the University of Pennsylvania, and Harold D. Palmer at Women's Medical College became the original Heads of specific Departments of Psychiatry in Philadelphia.

The Development of the Department at Jefferson

An independent Department of Psychiatry was not established until 1942, although Dr. Baldwin L. Keyes was appointed Clinical Professor of Psychiatry in 1936 and was responsible for all its teaching. A considerable degree of teaching of psychiatric disorders had existed, however, starting originally with natural philosophy, botany, and anatomy, which peripherally related to mental disturbances as well as physical ones. In the "Summer Courses" of 1870–1872, Dr. Isaac Ray (M.D., Bowdoin, 1827), the distinguished superintendent of the Butler Hospital in Rhode Island, lectured on "Insanity."[6] It was not until 1883, however, that any specific mention was made of a faculty member giving a course in the medical school. This was done by Dr. Jeremiah Thomas Eskridge, a graduate of Jefferson in the Class of 1875.[7] Eskridge was born in Delaware of parents of Scottish descent whose ancestors had come to this country in 1660. The year of his birth marked the year of Germany's 1848 revolution, at which time large numbers of immigrants from Germany fled the strife of their native land only to enter upon military duty within 13 or 14 years at the outbreak of the Civil War in America.

Dr. Eskridge was appointed to the faculty of Jefferson as Assistant Demonstrator of Anatomy in the same year he graduated. In 1879 he was appointed Lecturer on Physical Diagnosis and the following year an Attending Physician at St. Mary's Hospital and Jefferson Medical College Hospital. In 1882 he obtained the position of neurologist to the old Howard Hospital, located at that time at 1518–1520 Lombard Street, and in 1883 he became an Instructor in Mental and Nervous Diseases at Jefferson. It was in this year that he gave his first course (documented in the college announcement), which evidently was an optional part of the curriculum for those interested rather than a required one. In 1884 Dr. Eskridge contracted tuberculosis and abandoned the damp climate of Philadelphia for the higher dryer one of Colorado. Nothing is reported of his activities for the next five years—presumably he was taking the rest cure of that time for his pulmonary disease. In 1889 he surfaced again and was appointed Neurologist of the Arapahoe County, Colorado, Hospital and of St. Luke's Hospital. In 1890 Eskridge became Lecturer in Nervous Diseases at the University of Colorado and by 1892 was named Dean of the medical faculty and Professor of Nervous Diseases and Medical Jurisprudence. He held these positions until 1897. Two years before his resignation he was appointed Commissioner of the Colorado State Insane Asylum and President of the Board of the Asylum, a position that he held until 1902 when he died in Denver of a stroke. He published 60 papers. Dr. Eskridge was the first official faculty member at Jefferson to teach nervous and mental diseases and one of the early Professors of Psychiatry in the country.

Francis X. Dercum, M.D., Ph.D., L.H.D., Sc.D. (1856–1931); Clinical Professor of Nervous and Mental Diseases (1892–1925)

The teaching of psychiatry was not documented as a specific subject following the lectures given by Dr. Eskridge until the advent of Dr. Francis Xavier Dercum[8] (Figure 29-1). Dercum was the first Professor of Nervous Diseases at Jefferson. He was born at Sixth and Market Streets in Philadelphia in 1856, the son of an immigrant Bavarian family prominent in the arts, letters, and professions of Germany; Francis Dercum's father had fled Germany with the outbreak of the Revolution of 1848. Dercum was a graduate of the Central High School of Philadelphia in 1873 and of the Medical School of the University of Pennsylvania in 1877. He subsequently earned a Ph.D. degree at the University. Dr. Dercum studied histology under Dr. George A. Piersol, Professor of Anatomy at the University, and was appointed a Demonstrator in the Laboratory of Physiology. He published articles on the nervous system of fish and wrote other articles on the sensory organs. He also became involved in the pathology laboratory of the State Hospital for the Insane at Norristown. In 1884 he became Chief of the Nervous Clinic at the Hospital of the University of Pennsylvania. While there he studied photographically the movements of horses with Eadweard Muybridge, a pioneer in the photography of motion before the days of motion pictures.

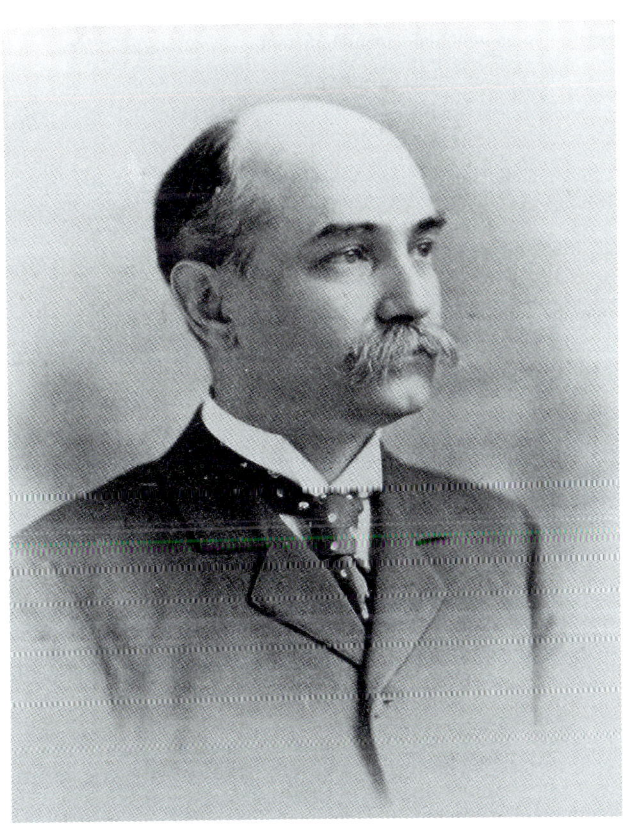

Fig. 29-1. Francis X. Dercum, M.D., Clinical Professor of Nervous and Mental Diseases (1892–1925).

Dr. Dercum, along with Dr. Eskridge, was a founder of the Philadelphia Neurological Society. He became a member in 1885 and President 1896. He was a member of the College of Physicians and appointed Neurologist to the Philadelphia Hospital in 1887, where he remained until 1911. In 1892 he was named Clinical Professor of Nervous and Mental Diseases at Jefferson, a position that he held with distinction until his resignation to become Emeritus in 1925.

Renowned worldwide for his work in the study and treatment of both neurologic and psychiatric disorders, Dr. Dercum was a member of American and European societies, including a Chevalier of the Legion of Honor of France. At the time of his death in 1931 he was President of the American Philosophical Society. In his superb abilities as physician, neuropsychiatrist, scholar, and theorist, Dr. Dercum set the pace for the development of the Department. He was a stout leader who held rank with that of S. Weir Mitchell. He taught admirably in the classroom and laboratory, as well as in his demonstration of cases to the medical students at the Philadelphia General Hospital, and his method of teaching was continued by one of his pupils, Dr. Edward A. Strecker, who succeeded Dr. Dercum as Professor upon the latter's retirement in 1925.

Edward A. Strecker, M.D., Sc.D., Litt.D., LL.D. (1887–1959); Professor of Mental and Nervous Diseases (1925–1931)

Dr. Strecker (Figure 29-2) was among the prominent psychiatrists in Philadelphia who were active in the training of physicians in that specialty, both in the Medical School of the University of Pennsylvania and the Pennsylvania Hospital. He was born in Philadelphia in 1887, graduated from Jefferson in 1911, and was trained in psychiatry at the Pennsylvania Hospital. He continued Dr. Dercum's program of teaching at Jefferson and at the Philadelphia General Hospital in the wards and, on Saturday afternoons, in the amphitheater. He was an outstanding scholar, a brilliant teacher, and a dynamic, forceful physician, who in many ways resembled Franklin Roosevelt in appearance and manner. In 1931 Dr. Strecker left Jefferson to become Professor of Psychiatry at the Medical School of the University of Pennsylvania and was succeeded by Dr. Michael A. Burns. Dr. Strecker continued his activities as teacher, writer, lecturer, and man of national prominence at the University and particularly at the Institute of the Pennsylvania Hospital. He prided himself on being one of the four men (with Drs. Earl Bond, Lauren H. Smith, and Kenneth E. Appel) who trained and placed 29 professors of psychiatry around the country during the tenure of their work there.

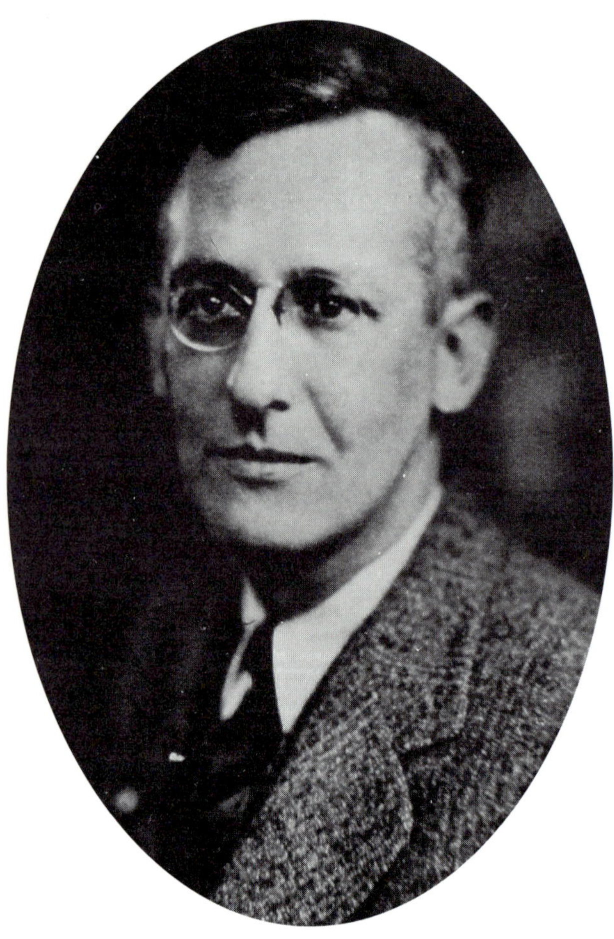

FIG. 29-2. Edward A. Strecker, M.D., Sc.D., Litt.D., LL.D.; Professor of Nervous and Mental Diseases (1925–1931).

Dr. Strecker maintained his office and residence at the Institute. He authored many books and papers; was a pioneer in the treatment of alcoholism; and initiated a therapeutic program with his assistant, Mr. "Dutch" Chambers, that antedated the program of Alcoholics Anonymous.[9] Dr. Strecker died in Jefferson Hospital in 1959 at the age of 72 from lung cancer.

Michael A. Burns, M.D., (1884–1938); Professor of Neurology (1934–1938)

When Dr. Strecker resigned as Professor of Mental and Nervous Diseases in 1931, he was not replaced for a period of three years. The previous programs of instruction were continued under the supervision of Drs. Michael A. Burns, Sherman F. Gilpin, and Benjamin P. Weiss. Some younger men were added to the staff, and the weekly teaching at the Philadelphia General Hospital went on. In 1934 the position of Professor of Nervous and Mental Diseases was abolished and replaced by that of Professor of Neurology. Neurology and psychiatry were lumped together, and the practitioners were neuropsychiatrists. Psychiatry came under the wing of the Department of Neurology, and in that year Dr. Michael A. Burns (Figure 29-3), whose interest was primarily in neurology, was appointed Professor and Head of Neurology (which included psychiatry), succeeding Dr. Strecker.

Dr. Burns was a graduate of Jefferson in the class of 1907 and he, too, was a student of Dr. Dercum. In 1931 the Curtis Clinic was opened and an ever larger number of students showed interest in psychiatric training. Dr. Burns continued teaching students on the wards of Jefferson Hospital and in the amphitheater of the Philadelphia General Hospital on Saturday afternoons. The members of the Department at that time included Drs. Benjamin P. Weiss, N.S. Yawger, R.C. Kell, Baldwin L. Keyes, Robert A. Matthews, George L. Stephen, Samuel T. Gordy, Thomas E. Shea, Angelo M. Perri, William H. Schmidt, B. Ulanski, Henry Golden, S.F. Gilpin, Lauren H. Smith, George F. Phelps, G.M. Tomlinson, Charles F. Becker, Harold D. Palmer, S.F. Gordon, and Walter R. Livingston.[10] Aided by his staff, Dr. Burns continued the work of Drs. Dercum and Strecker in teaching and research. In the 1930s, however, the work load in psychiatry increased disproportionately. Dr. Burns recommended that the Department of Neurology be divided into two separate Departments, one of Psychiatry and the other of Neurology. In 1937 Dr. Baldwin L. Keyes was appointed Clinical Professor of Psychiatry in the Department of Neurology. Psychiatry thus far had evolved from early beginnings as a part of the course in medicine, to part of the Department of Mental and Nervous Diseases, and next to a Division in Neurology. Although not yet recognized as a full Department, it was a separate entity at long last identified as an important aspect of health care.[11]

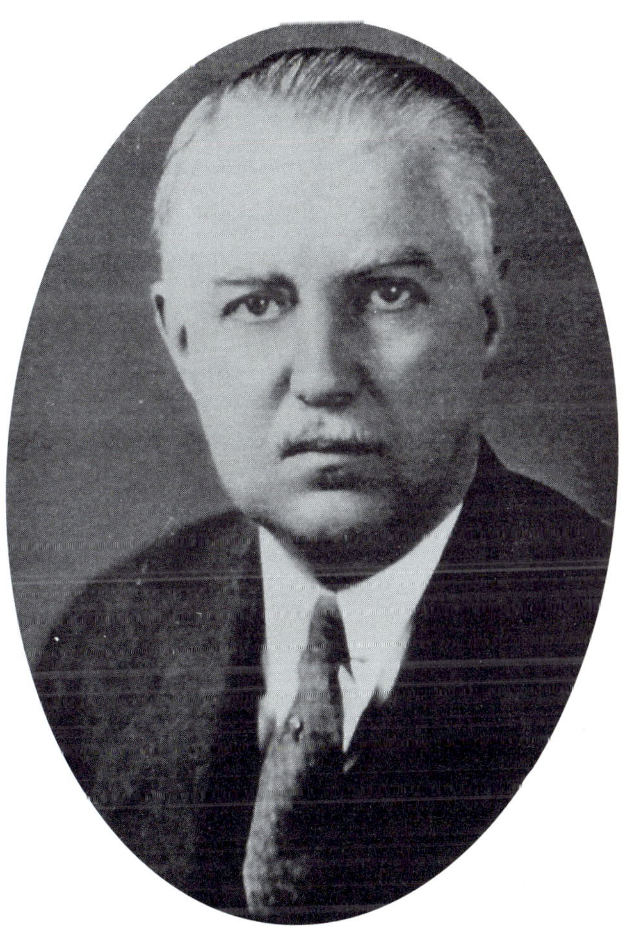

FIG. 29-3. Michael A. Burns, M.D., Professor of Neurology (1934–1938).

■ Growth and Expansion of the Department

In 1934 the Board of Trustees abolished the Department title of "Nervous and Mental Diseases" and established the Department of Neurology with Dr. Burns as Professor and Chairman. At Dr. Burns' request, Dr. Keyes assumed responsibility for teaching psychiatry at Jefferson and at the Philadelphia General Hospital. Dr. Burns died suddenly on March 7, 1938, and was succeeded by Dr. Bernard J. Alpers as Professor of Neurology and Head of the Department.

Baldwin L. Keyes, M.D., D.Sc., LL.D. (1893–); Clinical Professor of Psychiatry (1937–1942), and Professor of Psychiatry and First Chairman of the Department (1942–1959)

A separate Department of Psychiatry was set up under the Directorship of Dr. Baldwin L. Keyes

(Figure 29-4), who in 1937 had been appointed Clinical Professor of Psychiatry in the Department of Neurology and in 1942 was made full Professor and Chairman of the Department of Psychiatry. The establishment of a separate Department of Psychiatry was to have far-ranging effects on the program of instruction at the medical school, symbolizing the changing times, changing attitudes, and the increasing importance and awareness of mental processes as a part of physical disease and as causes of mental disorders. There could not have been a more appropriate choice for Chairman than Dr. Keyes. He served as leader, father figure, scholar, and superb clinician for hundreds of psychiatrists and literally thousands of medical students. He was "a man for all reasons" in his ability to maintain an open mind regarding any reasonable concept of the causes of mental disorders. Throughout a full lifetime of psychiatric practice he preserved a posture of objectivity through a burgeoning set of theoretical positions about mental functioning.

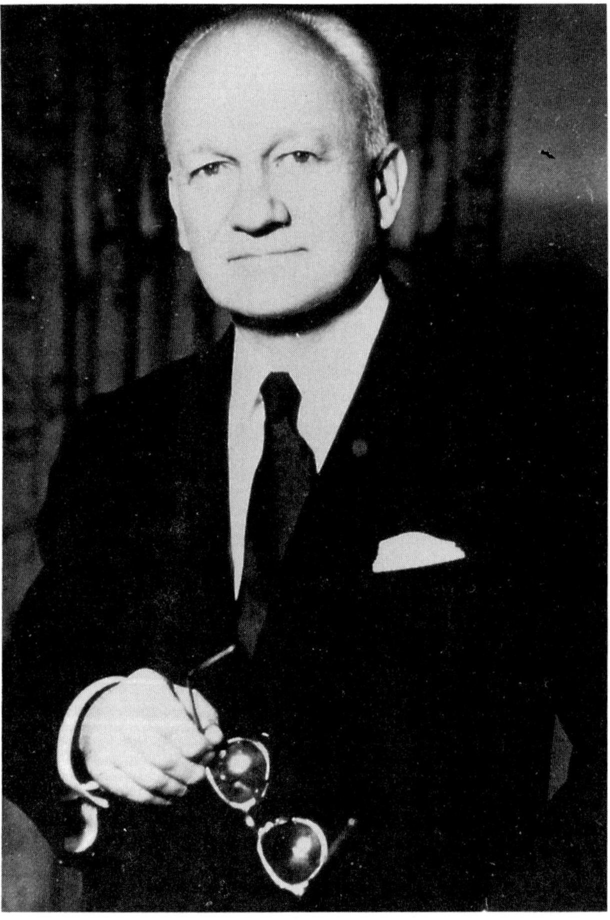

FIG. 29-4. Baldwin L. Keyes, M.D., D.Sc., LL.D., Clinical Professor of Psychiatry (1937–1942) and First Chairman (1942–1959).

Baldwin Keyes, born in Rio de Janeiro in 1893, had a unique childhood. His paternal grandfather, a dentist from Montgomery, Alabama, was a strong supporter of the Confederacy and a close friend of Jefferson Davis. He invested large amounts of money in the secession government, only to lose it in the fortunes of war. He migrated from Alabama to Rio de Janeiro, established a practice in dentistry, and raised his family. His mother, Emily Supplee Longstreth, was from an old Quaker family in Philadelphia. Because of his religious persuasion, her father purchased his way out of the Civil War, which was possible to do at that time, only to learn that the man who took his position for $200 was killed at the battle of Gettysburg. This cast such a heavy burden of depression upon him that he was advised by his physician to take a long sea voyage. Arriving in Rio de Janeiro after much seasickness, he refused to return to Philadelphia and called for his family to join him. Emily Longstreth married Baldwin Keyes' father (also a dentist), and seven children were born of this union. Throughout her life she preserved much of the philosophy of Quakerism, a force that was to have considerable impact on her son Baldwin. The children were raised in an area of Rio in which there was considerable cultural enrichment because much of the diplomatic corps lived nearby. All of the children were registered with the American Embassy as Americans. They learned to speak not only English but also Portuguese, German, French and some Spanish.

After brief education in the schools of Rio to the fourth-grade level, Dr. Keyes was sent to a boarding school in England for six months. He then continued his education in Philadelphia, the home of his maternal grandparents, at Germantown Academy and at Swarthmore Preparatory School, from which he graduated in 1912. Dr. Keyes enrolled in the Dental School of the University of Pennsylvania because of his desire to become an oral surgeon like his father and grandfather. After one year of such study and the ensuing summer in England, he decided to enter medicine. Following additional studies in botany at the University of Pennsylvania he enrolled at Jefferson in 1913 and graduated in 1917. At this time Europe was being ravished by World War I, and Dr. Keyes joined the U.S. Army as a First Lieutenant, Medical Reserve. The United States had declared war on April 6, 1917. The British forces requested 1,000 doctors for combat duty; Dr. Keyes volunteered and was assigned to the Gordon Highlanders in France as a combat surgeon. He was awarded the British Military Cross in 1918 for meritorious service and showing bravery under enemy fire. When the American Expeditionary Forces came to France in 1917, Keyes was recalled to the American Army, where he continued to work as a combat surgeon for a short period. He was then assigned to a hospital for treatment of the sick and wounded from frontline duty at Aix-les-Baines in the French Alps, where he became Hospital Adjunct (second in command) and was promoted to Captain in the Regular Army. He returned home in June, 1919, and transferred his commission to the Army Reserves.

Following World War I, Dr. Keyes entered the Misericordia Hospital on the advice of Dr. Ross V. Patterson, Dean of Jefferson, for completion of an Internship. This had not been done following his graduation from medical school because of immediate war duty. Following this, he entered the Graduate School of the University for the purpose of becoming an oral surgeon. In order to support himself he took the position of assistant to Dr. Edward A. Strecker at the Institute of the Pennsylvania Hospital as a paid physician. This experience led to an interest in neurological and psychiatric disorders, thus terminating his goals in oral surgery. Keyes studied psychiatry instead, at the Department of Nervous and Mental Diseases of the Pennsylvania Hospital under Dr. Earl Bond. He remained on the staff of the Institute of Pennsylvania Hospital as an Assistant in Neurology and Psychiatry from 1921 until 1925.

With interest in psychiatry and neurology firmly established, Dr. Keyes carried out work with Dr. Strecker at the Pennsylvania Institute on ovarian therapy in involutional melancholia. This investigation was reported to the Philadelphia Psychiatric Society in 1922 and published later that year.[12]

Despite an active clinical practice, teaching at Jefferson, serving as Attending Physician to the Pennsylvania Hospital, Roseneath Farms, and as one of the founding members of the Fairmount Farm Hospital, Dr. Keyes again turned his attention to military matters occasioned by World War II. At the outbreak of the war, Governor Arthur H. James appointed Keyes a member of the Selective Service Board. In June, 1940, before the outbreak of the war, the Army Surgeon General promoted him to Colonel and ordered him to organize and command the Jefferson Unit, the Thirty-eighth General Hospital. This hospital was to station in Cairo, Egypt, and serve the African and European theaters of war. From 1942 to 1944, Dr. Keyes served as the Unit's Executive Officer and Commandant in charge of medical affairs, but was then transferred to England as a consultant in neuropsychiatry. He remained in the organized reserves of the United States Army until 1954, when he retired. His last active military post was that of Commandant of the School of Military Neurology and Psychiatry at Mason General Hospital. Following the war he was assigned as a Senior Consultant to the Office of the Surgeon General of the Army and to the Veterans Administration.

On returning to Jefferson after the war, Dr. Keyes became active in the development of the Eastern Pennsylvania Psychiatric Institute, was appointed Psychiatric Consultant to the Municipal Court of the City of Philadelphia, and served on many advisory boards and committees as a part of his sense of civic duty and pride. He was an original member of the Admission Committee of the Medical College. The Jefferson Chapter of Alpha Omega Alpha awarded him an Honorary Membership in 1952. In 1966 he was awarded the Honorary Degree of Doctor of Science from Drexel University, and in 1967 the Doctor of Laws from Jefferson.

A charming man, gifted conversationalist, world traveler, superb photographer, and most of all a man able to influence students through his personal example, Keyes stimulated an interest in more students to enter psychiatry than his predecessor Dr. Strecker was doing at the University. Both continued to teach actively at their individual medical schools and at the Philadelphia General Hospital, but more students went into psychiatry from Jefferson than from the University of Pennsylvania. Indeed, there was more than one occasion when more residents from Jefferson went into psychiatry than into surgery, in spite of the enormous dynamism of the Department of Surgery. When medical students, residents, and staff started to form a Keyes Psychiatric Society, he demurred, recommending that it be called "The Jefferson Psychiatric Forum."

Through the efforts of Dr. Keyes, aided by generous financial support from Mrs. Mabel Pew Myrin, the fourteenth floor of the Thompson Building, a former area of operating rooms, was converted into a Psychiatric Unit opening in November, 1957.[13] This was the first specific unit for the care and treatment of nervous disorders at Jefferson Hospital and one of the first in Philadelphia. There was a bed capacity of 25 with an outstanding corps of nurses under the direction of Mrs. Rachael Clark. The first Director was Dr. John A. Koltes (Jefferson, 1947).

Dr. Koltes was trained in psychiatry at Jefferson, the Friends Hospital, and the Hospital of the University of Pennsylvania. He also received training in psychoanalysis at the Philadelphia Association for Psychoanalysis. In 1955 he studied the operation of certain European mental hospitals at the direction of the Secretary of Welfare.[14] The work of Dr. Maxwell Jones in the Therapeutic Community in London[15] and that of Dr. Manfred Bleuler at the Burgholtzli Hospital of the University at Zürich were the primary sources. Dr. Koltes at that time was Clinical Director of the Eastern Pennsylvania Psychiatric Institute, a facility built in Philadelphia for the purpose of improving the quality of state mental hospital systems by providing training and research for members of the system and for new members to join. Drs. Baldwin Keyes, Robert Matthews, and John Davis, in conjunction with the Secretary of Welfare, were instrumental in the establishment of this program. They visited Dr. Jones in London and several other psychiatrists and hospitals. This latter group was revolutionizing the entire mental hospital system of the country before the days of drug therapy by unlocking the doors and permitting fresh air to enter the dank halls of these large institutions. T.P. Rees at the Warlingham Park Hospital, Surrey, and George Bell at the Dingleton Hospital, Melrose, Scotland, were prime examples of this new approach. The Commonwealth of Pennsylvania published a journal, *Letters from Europe*, by Dr. Koltes outling these programs.

Initially, it was considered feasible to admit patients to the Jefferson psychiatric unit from any ward of the hospital, including patients who were operated upon neurosurgically. It was quickly determined, however, that this was an unsuccessful effort and only patients who were not intensely psychotic or were suffering from severe brain damage could be treated in the inpatient unit. This led ultimately to the recognition that a variety of patients came from sources that had not previously been addressed. They were too sick to be treated as outpatients but not sick enough to be committed to mental hospitals. This work thus led to the establishment of a new perspective about inpatient care of a short-term, intensive nature that previously had not existed. Philadelphia psychiatry had tended to be divided into two groups, private facilities primarily at the Institute of the Pennsylvania Hospital, Friends Hospital, Fairmount Farm, and Roseneath, which together housed 400 to 500 patients, and the public hospitals at Byberry and Norristown, which together housed about 11,000 patients. The psychiatric inpatient service of the general hospital, in contrast, served an entirely new group of people and has continued to do so since its initial establishment.[16,17] Dr. Koltes remained the director of the inpatient unit from 1957 until 1965, when he relinquished the administration to Dr. Howard L. Field (Jefferson, 1954) in order to enter full-time private practice.

In 1958 Dr. Keyes retired by reason of age from Chairmanship of the Department to become Professor Emeritus but continued to practice until July, 1979, when he closed his office at the age of 86. Alumni Association President in 1955, presentation of his portrait to the College by the Class of 1955, recipient of the Jefferson Alumni Achievement Award in 1971, services in the affairs of Jefferson until past the age of 90, brought Dr. Keyes the seldom given title of "Mr. Jefferson."

Robert A. Matthews, M.D. (1903–1961); Second Chairman (1958–1961)

With the retirement of Dr. Keyes in 1958, Dr. Robert A. Matthews (Figure 29-5) assumed the position of Chairman of the Department until he was killed in an automobile accident in 1961. Born in Johnstown, Pennsylvania, Matthews obtained a B.S. degree from the Pennsylvania State College in 1925 and graduated from Jefferson in 1928. He interned at the Philadelphia General Hospital and in 1930 was appointed Chief Resident Physician at the Philadelphia State Hospital (Byberry), where he served for four years as its Clinical Director. At the same time he was named Physician-in-Charge of the Philadelphia Institution for the Feebleminded. He was on the staff of the Nazareth Hospital, where he served as the Director of Neuropsychiatry, and held the same position at the Delaware County Hospital. In addition, he was a consultant to the Veterans Hospital in Coatesville and when in Louisiana in 1950 was Psychiatrist-in-Chief of the Charity Hospital of the Louisiana State University.

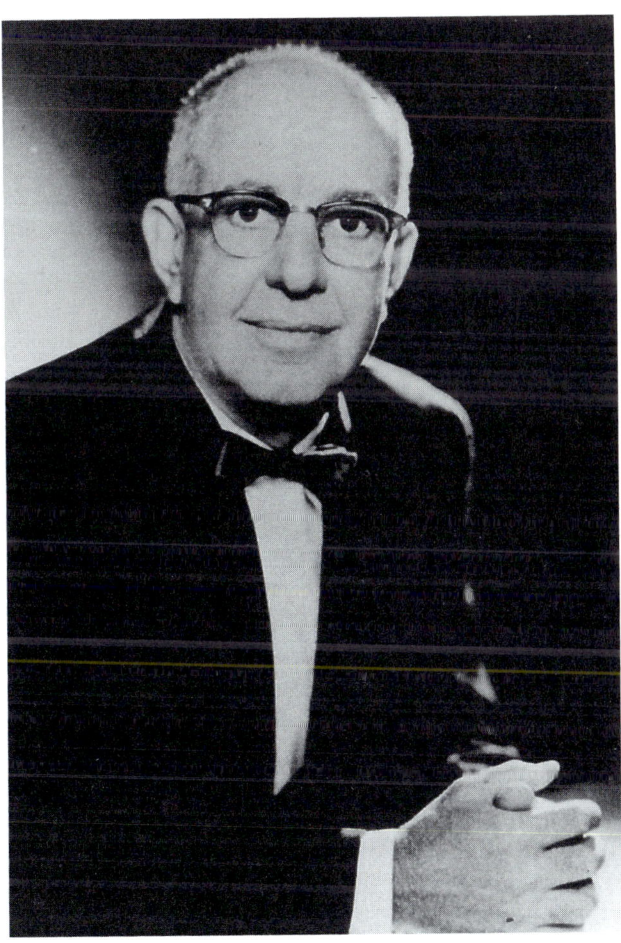

FIG. 29-5. Robert A. Matthews, M.D., Second Chairman (1958–1961).

Dr. Matthews demonstrated great ability to instruct students, residents, and the lay public. He had the capacity to analyze a clinical situation and express it in terms that could be easily understood by those with little knowledge of the principles of mental function. He was a happy man whose hallmark was a perennial smile. One asset that enshrined him as an outstanding teacher was his ability to demonstrate a mental symptom, an unusual gait, or a peculiar habit of a patient that fixed it in the memory of the student. This was not to ridicule or demean the patient but, rather, a teaching device to demonstrate the nucleus of the problem the patient was experiencing so that the student could readily identify, interpret, and thereby incorporate it into his or her own fund of knowledge.

Dr. Matthews continued the clinical teaching lectures at the Medical School and demonstrations from the mental wards on Saturday afternoons at the Philadelphia General Hospital, and his lectures were as popular as those of his predecessors.

Dr. Matthews was the last Chairman who had been trained or in some way affiliated with the Institute of the Pennsylvania Hospital, at which he was a Rockefeller Fellow for 1935–1936. In 1930 Dr. Matthews was appointed Instructor in Nervous and Mental Diseases at Jefferson and was employed as an Attending Physician at the Philadelphia State Hospital. He became an assistant to Dr. Baldwin Keyes, along with Dr. Robert S. Bookhammer (Jefferson, 1928), who also was on the staff of Byberry Hospital. Dr. Matthews rose through the ranks to Assistant Professor of Psychiatry, a position he held from 1939 to 1942. During the war years 1942 to 1946, he was Associate Professor of Psychiatry and Acting Head of the Department during the absence of Dr. Keyes. Upon Dr. Keyes' return, Dr. Matthews was appointed Clinical Professor.

Throughout the war years Dr. Matthews taught neuropsychiatry at the Naval Hospital. In 1950 he accepted the position of Professor of Psychiatry and Head of the Department of Psychiatry and Neurology at the Louisiana State University School of Medicine in New Orleans. This was his first departure from Jefferson in 25 years. In New Orleans he served also as a consultant to the Surgeon General's office of the Army and traveled abroad to the European theater to study the psychiatric facilities of the Army and Air Force hospitals in Europe in the postwar era. He reported his findings to the Office of the Surgeon General and gave a paper on it to the Louisiana Society for Mental Health. Entitled *The Unique Aspects of the Care of the Mentally Ill in Europe*,[18] his paper describes some of the methods of treatment found in European psychiatric centers, including Zürich, London, Tübingen, Munich, and Gheel, the latter a town in Belgium, not far from Antwerp, where mental patients have been taken care of by a small farming community since the year 900. The principles of concern, mercy, and moral support at Gheel are applied as vital factors in the care and treatment of severe mental illness. Interests of this sort led him to further explore the work of Dr. Maxwell Jones, the social psychiatrist from London who had studied at the Institute of the Pennsylvania Hospital in 1939. Dr. Jones became world famous as the developer of the concept of the Therapeutic Community, and Dr. Matthews' interest in the work of Dr. Jones in particular and social psychiatry in general was one of the hallmarks of his later contributions to psychiatry.

Dr. Matthews resigned his position at Louisiana in 1956 and accepted the dual responsibility of Professor of Psychiatry at Jefferson and first Commissioner of Mental Health for the State of Pennsylvania. Newspapers at the time made great note of the fact that he was to receive a salary of $25,000 a year, equal to that of the Governor and $10,000 more than his superior, the Secretary of Welfare. The Mental Health Commissioner position required the Commissioner to supervise 15,000 employees throughout the State's mental health system.

A significant administrative change occurred with Dr. Matthew's tenure as Chairman of the Department. Whereas up to that time the Chairmen had been in full-time private practice and supported themselves by private work, Dr. Matthews became the first Chairman to be a paid Professor in this Department. In 1958 Dr. Thomas Loftus, a former Professor of Psychiatry at West Virginia who had trained in New York, joined the staff as a full-time Professor and as one of the primary academicians in the Department. He contributed actively to the quality of the training programs for undergraduate teaching. During the Matthews administration the subject of Psychiatry was elevated from a minor course in the medical curriculum to a major subject alongside Medicine, Surgery, Obstetrics, and Pediatrics.

Dr. Matthews was successful in his multiple careers as teacher, author, and Commissioner, and in his innumerable lectures to professional and lay groups. He was a pragmatic person, not a dreamer, full of energy, and enthusiastic about life. His contagious sense of well being was easily transmitted to patients and provided a vehicle to carry them toward a state of recovery. His tragic death left an indelible mark upon the minds and perspectives of those who survived him.

One of Dr. Matthews' legacies was the establishment of a strong faculty that resulted in part from his collective work with Dr. Keyes. Physicians were returning from military duty, either to positions formerly held or to new positions, and the Medical School profited by their experience. Dr. John E. Davis, former Clinical Director of the Trenton State Hospital and U.S. Army Colonel, came to Jefferson after the war and in 1951 initiated, within the Department, the Eastern Pennsylvania Psychiatric Institute. The building was dedicated by the Governor in 1955, and Dr. Davis became its first Medical Director. In 1961 he went on to succeed Dr. Matthews as Commissioner of Mental Health, and in 1963 he returned to Jefferson where he worked until his premature death in 1968 from cancer of the lung.

Another distinguished member of the Department was Dr. Robert S. Garber, former military officer, who returned to active teaching at Jefferson. He was also the Clinical Director and later President of the Carrier Clinic in Belle Mead,

New Jersey, and eventually President of the American Psychiatric Association. Both Drs. Garber and Davis had been on the staff of the Trenton State Hospital before the war. Other members of the department who made important contributions to the teaching program were Drs. Frederick Kramer, Milton K. Meyers, Solomon M. Haimes, Louis Kaplan, Albert J. Kaplan, Paul J. Poinsard, William R. O'Brien, Raphael H. Durante, George W. Hager, Jr., John A. Koltes, Wallace B. Hussong, Abraham Freedman, Edgar C. Smith, Coleman W. Kovach, Leopold Potonski, John C. Patterson, George J. Martin, Don Everett Johnson, and Olive J. Morgan (Ph.D., psychology) and Carter Zeleznik (Ph.D., psychology).

In 1957 Zygmunt A. Piotrowski, Ph.D. came to Jefferson as Associate Professor of Psychiatry (Psychology) from New York where he had worked with Dr. Nolan Lewis, the distinguished Professor of Psychiatry at Columbia University and Director of the N.Y. State Psychiatric Institute at Columbia. Dr. Piotrowski had a doctorate from the University of Poznan, Poland, in psychology and the theory of science. His favorite subject as an undergraduate student was algebraic geometry, which influenced his capacity to think in abstract terms. At Jefferson he worked in two primary areas of research—the application of the computer to scoring of the Rorschach test, and the use of psychological tests to differentiate organic from functional mental disorders. In these efforts he was ably assisted by Drs. Barry Bricklin and Carter Zelesnik.

Dr. Piotrowski added a touch of Continental quality to the decorum of the Department as evidenced by his versatility in literature, history, and the arts. His conversations were always intellectually stimulating. With Dr. Albert Biele (Jefferson, 1938) he wrote a book entitled *Dreams: A Key to Self-knowledge* (1986). Dr. Piotrowski retired from Jefferson at age 65 and joined the faculty at Hahnemann, where he continued his research, writing, and teaching until his death in 1986.

Paul J. Poinsard, M.D.; Acting Chairman (1961–1962)

In 1961, following Dr. Matthews' death, Dr. Paul J. Poinsard (Jefferson, 1941) was appointed Acting Chairman of the Department of Psychiatry (Figure 29-6). Dr. Poinsard had served in World War II in the South Pacific as a Flight Surgeon and was the recipient of five battle stars. Following discharge he returned to Philadelphia and matriculated in the Graduate School of Medicine at the University of Pennsylvania in Psychiatry and Neurology. He then entered the Institute of the Pennsylvania Hospital for a three-year residency training program. In conjunction with this, he studied at the Philadelphia Psychoanalytic Society and was trained in both general psychiatry and psychoanalysis. Dr. Poinsard ably administered the

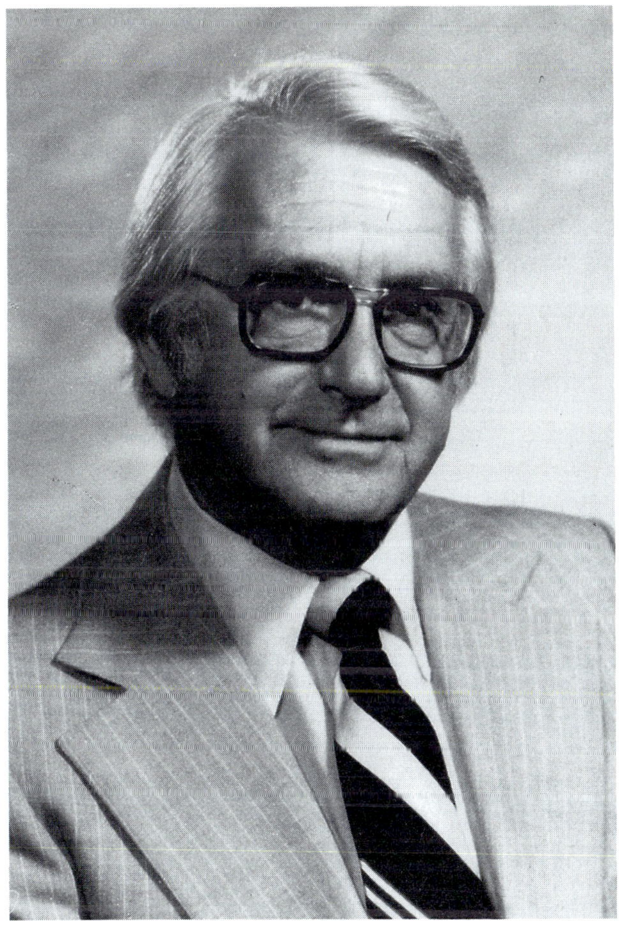

FIG. 29-6. Paul J. Poinsard, M.D., Acting Chairman (1961–1962).

affairs of the department, including its outpatient service, until the appointment of Dr. Floyd S. Cornelison, Jr., in 1962.

Dr. Poinsard was the first psychiatrist to be elected as President of the Thomas Jefferson University Hospital Medical Staff (1979–1981) and served for many years on its Executive Committee. He was elected to the positions of President of the Philadelphia Psychiatric Society, the Pennsylvania Psychiatric Society, the Medical Club of Philadelphia, the Jefferson Alumni Association during the Centennial of its founding in 1970, the Meigs Medical Association, and as the one hundred and twentieth President of the Philadelphia County Medical Society in 1980. He became Emeritus Professor of Psychiatry in 1983 but continued as an active member of the Department, the Hospital, and the Alumni Association.

Although never a member of the Department, Dr. Francis J. Braceland (Jefferson, 1930) achieved great distinction in the field of psychiatry. A graduate of LaSalle College before matriculating at Jefferson, he was trained in psychiatry under Dr. Strecker at the Institute of the Pennsylvania Hospital with continuing experience as a Rockefeller Foundation Fellow in Zürich and London. After a few years as Professor of Psychiatry at Women's Medical College, he was named Professor of Psychiatry and Dean at Loyola University School of Medicine, Chicago. During World War II, Dr. Braceland served as special assistant to the Surgeon General and Chief of Neuropsychiatry for the United States Navy, continuing in the Naval Reserve and retiring in 1962 with the rank of Rear Admiral.

Following the war, Dr. Braceland became Chief of Psychiatry at the Mayo Clinic. In 1951 he moved to Hartford, Connecticut, as Psychiatrist-in-Chief at the Institute of Living and Professor of Psychiatry at Yale University. He served as President of the American Psychiatry Association and Editor of its Journal and as President of the American Board of Psychiatry and Neurology. He was the author of many articles and three books.

Dr. Braceland received seven honorary degrees including one from Jefferson, the Laetere medal of the University of Notre Dame, and was named Knight of St. Gregory the Great by Pope Pius XII. A loyal Jefferson alumnus, he received the Alumni Achievement Award (1967) and served as Alumni representative (1965–1967) on the Board of Trustees.

Floyd S. Cornelison, Jr., M.D. (1918–); Third Chairman (1962–1974)

Floyd Cornelison (Figure 29-7) was born in San Angelo, Texas, in 1918. He attended the public schools there and obtained his B.A. degree from Baylor University in 1939. From 1944 to 1946 he studied at Columbia University and in 1950 graduated from the Medical College of Cornell University. Following graduation he entered psychiatric residency at Boston University, the Massachusetts Memorial Hospital, and the Boston State Hospital. In 1958 he received an M.S. degree from Boston University.

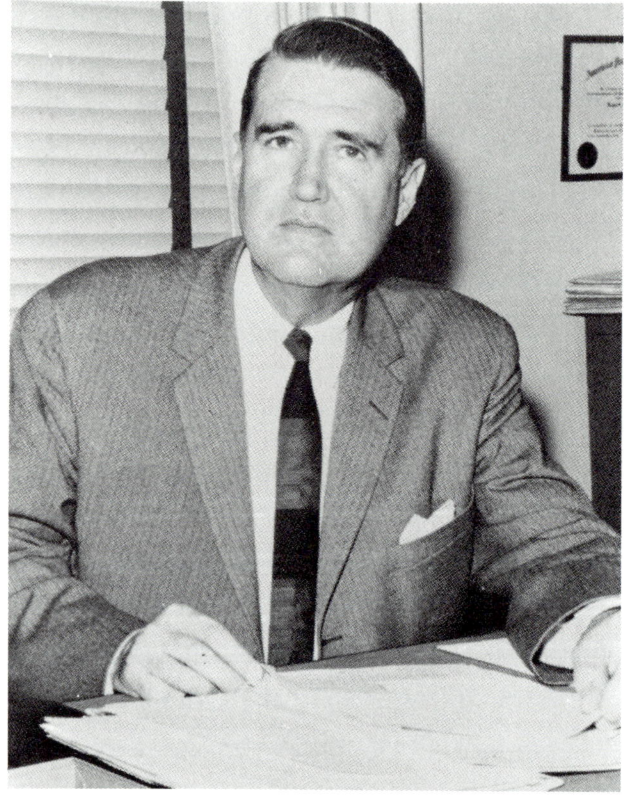

FIG. 29-7. Floyd S. Cornelison, Jr., M.D., Third Chairman (1962–1974).

At the time of Dr. Cornelison's appointment there were 54 members of the faculty and four residents. He requested and followed the sagacious advice of Dr. Braceland regarding the strengths and weaknesses of the Department. At that time only six to ten hours were available for first-year teaching of students, and 19 hours for the second year. Saturday teaching was discontinued as part of a new approach based on the theory that small-group instruction was superior to lectures. Dr. Cornelison brought with him a group of clinicians and researchers who introduced new perspectives into the Department. It was the first time in perhaps 100 years that the Pennsylvania Hospital did not have a direct influence on the teaching and training of members of the faculty of Psychiatry.

Because there were insufficient facilities for the training of students and residents at Jefferson, Dr. Cornelison developed a research and education program at the Delaware State Hospital. This activity was set up with the support of the Governor of Delaware and became known as the Marka DuPont Institute of Human Behavior. He also established an affiliation with the Coatesville Veterans Administration Hospital, which served as a source for much of the Department's research and educational activities.

A man of international reputation, Dr. Robert Waelder was appointed to the faculty as the first Professor of Psychoanalysis. He had received a Ph.D. degree in physics at the University of Vienna at the age of 21 and fled the Nazi tyranny in 1938. His paper, *The Principle of Multiple Function,* identified him among the great thinkers in the world of psychoanalysis.[19] He had been a close colleague of Anna Freud, who in 1964 was invited to give a lecture at Jefferson and receive an honorary degree of Doctor of Science. The daughter of Sigmund Freud, Anna Freud was an eminent child psychoanalyst and director of the Hampstead Child Therapy Clinic of London, England. Appointed with Dr. Waelder as Professor of Psychiatry (Psychoanalysis) was Samuel A. Guttman, M.D., Ph.D., a psychoanalyst who was later to write an important treatise, a *Concordance of the Works of Freud.*[20]

In 1965 Dr. Lawrence S. Kubie was appointed Visiting Professor of Psychiatry. He had been at the Sheppard and Enoch Pratt Hospital in Baltimore and was a nationally famous psychiatrist. In the same year Dr. A. Irving Hallowell, Professor of Anthropology at the University of Pennsylvania, was appointed Professor of Psychiatry. Drs. Edward Gottheil, Alfonso Paredes, Klaus Behnson, Marjorie Bahnson, Ivan Nagy, Robert Clark, and J. Clifford Scott, among many others, were added to the faculty. Miss Theresa Damanski was appointed as the first full-time member of the faculty in social work.

Dr. Kurt Wolff was appointed Associate Professor of Psychiatry to teach undergraduate and graduate students at Coatesville Veterans Hospital. A bus was converted into a "mobile classroom" for lectures or demonstrations to students during the time in which they were commuting from Jefferson to the Coatesville Hospital.

Another important addition to the faculty occurred with the appointment of Dr. Daniel Lieberman on the volunteer staff. He was Commissioner of Mental Health for the State of Delaware between 1964 and 1967. Lieberman taught students at Jefferson and participated in the development of the Jefferson–Delaware affiliation. He was able to obtain Delaware funds to support research by Jefferson personnel. The program between Jefferson and Delaware was greatly strengthened, and eventually Jefferson became the medical school for the State of Delaware with the support of the Delaware Legislature.

Dr. Cornelison had an avid interest in photography, which he applied to his research on "self-image." He was the first to introduce audiovisual tapes into the teaching program. His research on self-image was described in a lecture delivered at the University of Vienna and in similar programs in Milan, Italy, and the University of New South Wales, Australia.

The 1960s witnessed a series of major social upheavals. This was the time of the Vietnam War, when students went on strike, when 56,000 men sacrificed their lives, and when turmoil—economic, social and moral—was on the increase. It was in some respects a post–World War II social revolution following the enormous upheaval of the entire world that had occurred with the deaths of 53 million people during those tragic years from 1939 to 1945. The theories of Maxwell Jones in England, from which he developed the concept of the therapeutic community, were essentially an attempt to deal with the problem of authoritarianism. Jones' work was aimed primarily at "social misfits," people with personality disorders and acting-out disorders who were rebelling against society or who were underachievers. He took the general position that diminishing the role of authority and increasing individual responsibility would aid in the socialization of these people with this type of personality disorder.

At the same time, psychiatry was undergoing tremendous advances in the understanding and therapy of mental disorders. Neuroleptics in the treatment of schizophrenia, lithium in manic-depressive disorders, tricyclic antidepressants in depression, and benzodiazapines for anxiety disorders all contributed to the feeling of optimism about making a major impact, at last, on mental illness in this country. The less effective somatic treatments, such as insulin coma, psychosurgery, and hydrotherapy were discontinued, and electroconvulsive therapy was used in selected cases.

Treatment programs were developing that offered community-based services, particularly to the poor, to augment hospital care. Jefferson decided to increase its mental health services to the community and solicited Dr. Daniel Lieberman, who was completing his work at Delaware, where he had established a Mental Health Department. He came as Professor and Associate Chairman of the Department on a full-time basis and promptly obtained Federal and State funds to construct facilities and acquire staff for this ambitious undertaking. Among the new programs that he initiated were sections on child psychiatry and family therapy, a day hospital, a psychiatric emergency service, a substance-abuse treatment program, consultation services, and additional inpatient and outpatient services. This provided resources for more research and greater clinical education for medical students, and to increase the number of psychiatric residents. When the Community Mental Health Center was discontinued at Jefferson in 1977, these important programs remained as part of the clinical program and thereby provided the resources to increase the number of psychiatric residents from a handful to 32.

The loss of major faculty members, Drs. Robert Waelder, John Davis, and Kurt Wolff, occurred between 1967 and 1970. In the same period Drs. Eli Marcovitz, Maurice Linden, and Gabriel D'Amato were added to the faculty. In 1971 Dr. Terrell Davis, who had been Commissioner of Mental Health for the State of New Jersey, was appointed Professor of Psychiatry. He was later to become Head of the Department of Psychiatry at the Wilmington Medical Center.

An affiliation existed with Friends Hospital, a 200-bed private psychiatric institution founded in 1813, which had a broad range of therapeutic programs and offered a variety of opportunities for the students. This ended in 1970. Other important affiliations that terminated about this time included the Philadelphia General Hospital and the Eastern Pennsylvania Psychiatric Institute.

One of Dr. Cornelison's cherished dreams was the development of a building for treatment and research in psychiatry. He constructed a large model of a building that he hoped to erect on the corner of Eleventh and Walnut Streets. Funds were sought to promote this plan but approval by the President and the Board of Trustees was not forthcoming. Throughout his tenure there was a significant degree of frustration in his not achieving this goal. There is no question, however, that he greatly expanded the interest in research in the Medical School, and he opened a branch of the Department in the old building at the northeast corner of Twelfth and Walnut Streets, formerly the home of Bishop White. There he set up laboratories to develop his interest in photographing patients and replaying the photographs to them during the various phases of their treatment.

By 1974 there were 24 full-time faculty members and 78 part-time members for the education of 800 medical students and ten to 15 residents.[21] Teaching was in small groups rather than the older, more didactic method in the lecture hall. At this time Dr. Cornelison resigned his position as Chairman of the Department and entered full-time private practice in Wilmington, Delaware.

Daniel Lieberman, M.D.; Acting Chairman (1974–1976 and 1983–1988)

Upon the resignation of Dr. Cornelison, Dr. Daniel Lieberman (Figure 29-8) was appointed Acting Chairman, a position he held from 1974 through 1976. He had had considerable administrative experience in the past, including Medical Director of a large mental hospital, Director of the Department of Mental Hygiene in California, and as Delaware's first Commissioner of Mental Health. His establishment of the Community Mental Health Center at Jefferson brought major changes to the Department that increased its budget, faculty, and clinical resources threefold. Lieberman had entered academia for a more scholarly life, but because of his background was called upon continually to provide administrative leadership.

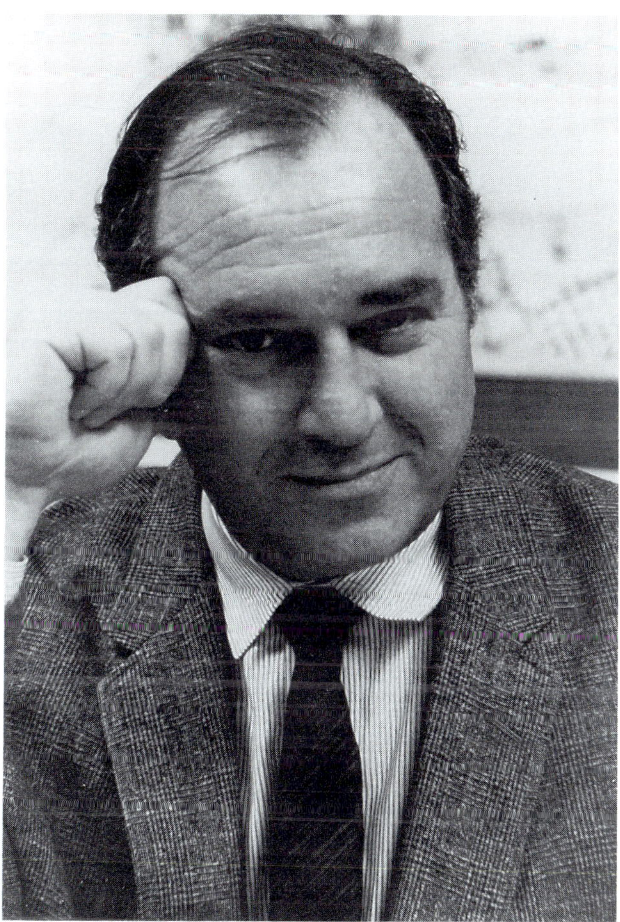

FIG. 29-8. Daniel Lieberman, M.D., Acting Chairman (1974–1976 and 1983–1988).

Dr. Lieberman contributed significantly to the progress of the Department. He brought medical students for their clinical clerkship in psychiatry back to Jefferson. He organized and established a family therapy section, a child psychiatry section, a psychosomatic medicine program, including a biofeedback laboratory, a day hospital, and an additional inpatient unit at Jefferson, together with an expanded outpatient program. A Division of Substance Abuse was developed, and both research and teaching were carried on under the direction of Edward Gottheil, M.D., Ph.D., Professor of Psychiatry, who had come to Jefferson with Dr. Cornelison years earlier.

Dr. Lieberman strengthened the affiliation with the Coatesville Veterans Administration Center and strongly supported the Jefferson–Friends program until that was terminated. At the undergraduate teaching level, he was instrumental in the development of a new program called "Medicine and Society" and was Chairman of the subcommittee of the faculty that developed a two-year program for this curricular change that introduced lectures in psychiatry to the first- and second-year classes.

Additional honors came to Dr. Lieberman during his tenures as Acting Chairman. He was elected President of the Philadelphia Psychiatric Society and Chairman of the Section in Psychiatry of the Philadelphia County Medical Society. In 1987 his portrait was presented to the University by colleagues and friends.

Paul J. Fink, M.D.; Fourth Chairman (1976–1983)

Dr. Paul J. Fink (Figure 29-9) was appointed Chairman in 1976. He was born and raised in Philadelphia and graduated from Temple University, *magna cum laude,* in 1954 and from its Medical School in 1958. He was trained in psychiatry at the Albert Einstein Medical Center, the Philadelphia Psychiatric Center, and by the Philadelphia Association for Psychoanalysis, from which he graduated in 1966. At Hahnemann Medical College from 1962 to 1973 he rose to the rank of Professor of Psychiatry and resigned to become Chairman of the Department of Psychiatry at the Eastern Virginia Medical School in Norfolk.

In directing the Department at Jefferson, Dr. Fink initiated some major changes in the thinking of the faculty and the community of psychiatry in Philadelphia. His views represented a departure from those of his predecessors in their encyclopedic nature and seemed to cover essentially every aspect of medical care from a psychiatric point of view.

Dr. Fink excelled in clinical work, teaching, research, and administration. He was on various councils, associations, and colleges, both national and international, in the field of general psychiatry, psychoanalysis, and sex education for many years. The annual report of the Department for 1982 listed 275 members of the faculty in addition to 20 honorary members and 38 residents. During his tenure until 1983, more than 300 members joined the faculty and almost 200 remained.

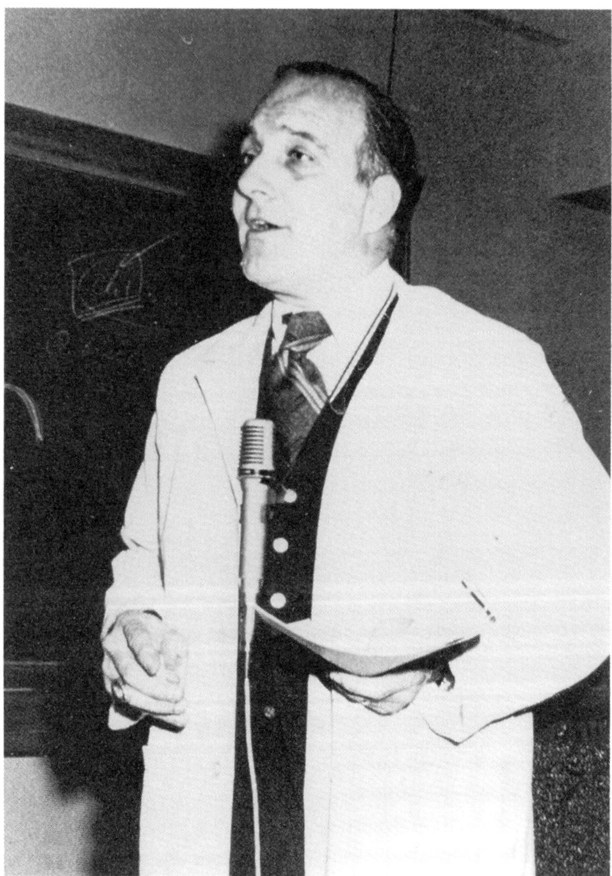

FIG. 29-9. Paul J. Fink, M.D., Fourth Chairman (1976–1983).

Dr. Fink's goal in residency training was to have 40 residents, ten per year in the Jefferson program. He came very close to its achievement. The Residency had started 40 years earlier when Dr. Keyes appointed Dr. John Flummerfelt as the first Resident in Psychiatry in the Jefferson Medical College Hospital. There were no residents during World War II, but Dr. Ivan Bennett was appointed in 1946 and Dr. John Koltes in 1948. Under succeeding Chairmen the numbers gradually rose until a total of 38 were appointed by Dr. Fink, a program fully accredited by the American Board of Psychiatry and Neurology.

Programs in undergraduate and graduate training, clinical treatment, research, and affiliations were expanded. Some of the programs had permanent Directors, whereas others changed as they evolved. A Division of Education was headed by Dr. Roy Clouse, a long-time stalwart member of the Department; the residency training was directed by Dr. Harvey Schwartz, a relatively new member of the Department; a Consultation and Liasion Division was headed by Dr. Lieberman, in the Department now for more than 20 years and ably assisted by Dr. Howard Field. An extensive adult service, both inpatient and outpatient, was maintained, as well as a crisis center; a partial hospital center was headed by Dr. William Dubin; a children's service was directed by Dr. Gabriel J. D'Amato and later Dr. G. Pirooz Sholevar; and a Division of Psychoanalysis was headed by Dr. Harold Kolansky. A program in Behavioral Sciences was headed by Dr. Adrian Copeland; a Geriatrics Section was led by Dr. Sarah Kaye; and alcohol and drug research was conducted by Dr. Edward Gottheil. Other programs included a sleep laboratory, a program for study of impotence, and research in schizophrenia. Several psychologists were added to the staff, and a program of training for psychology interns was developed. The Department expanded so much that additional space had to be obtained in a commercial building at 1015 Chestnut Street.

Affiliations with the Wilmington Medical Center and Coatesville Veterans Hospital, Delaware, were strengthened, and new affiliations with Crozer-Chester Medical Center and the Northwest Institute of Psychiatry were developed. Members of those Hospitals were added to the Faculty of the Medical School. The general size of the Department became so comprehensive that administrative personnel were secured to deal not only with the complexities but with the financing of the extensive programs that evolved. These developments were exciting, provocative, and energetic. The Department of Psychiatry thus became one of the largest of the Medical School. Dr. Fink had the foresight to recognize that psychiatry was moving in new directions and that more research, more education, and wider approaches to fields not often touched by psychiatry in the past were very important.

Dr. Fink resigned the Chairmanship of the Department in 1983 to become Chairman of the Department of Psychiatry of the Albert Einstein Medical Center and Medical Director of the Philadelphia Psychiatric Center. Responsibility for direction of the Department once again fell upon Dr. Lieberman's shoulders.

The period of 1983 to 1988 was one of continuous evaluation, streamlining the operations, upgrading the medical education and research activities, establishing financial and operational stability, and bringing young, enthusiastic faculty to the Department. Dr. Bryce Templeton, a nationally recognized medical educator, became Director of Undergraduate Education. Dr. Kenneth Certa, a former Chief Resident at Jefferson, became head of emergency services in Psychiatry. Several faculty were added to a strengthened inpatient service.

Troy L. Thompson, II, M.D.; Fifth Chairman (1988–)

In March of 1988, Dr. Troy L. Thompson, II (Figure 29-10) became the new Chairman of the Department, arriving from the University of Colorado, where he had headed the Consultation-Liaison Service. He is known nationally for his work at the juncture of psychiatry and medicine, and his challenge is to build upon what has developed thus far so that in the 1990s the Department will remain in the forefront of medical education and research.

In some respects psychiatry at Jefferson has not really changed from the days in the 1880s when it was a one-man lectureship in the Department of Medicine or even a modest Department, of biological psychiatry, under Dr. Dercum. From the golden days of psychodynamic psychiatry under Drs. Keyes, Matthews, Cornelison, and Fink in the 1950s, 1960s, and 1970s, it has redeveloped in the 1980s into a Department of biological psychiatry. Although the contributions of Sigmund Freud to an understanding of normal mental functioning and the nature of the neurotic process still remain the hallmark of psychodynamic psychiatry, the development of technical advances

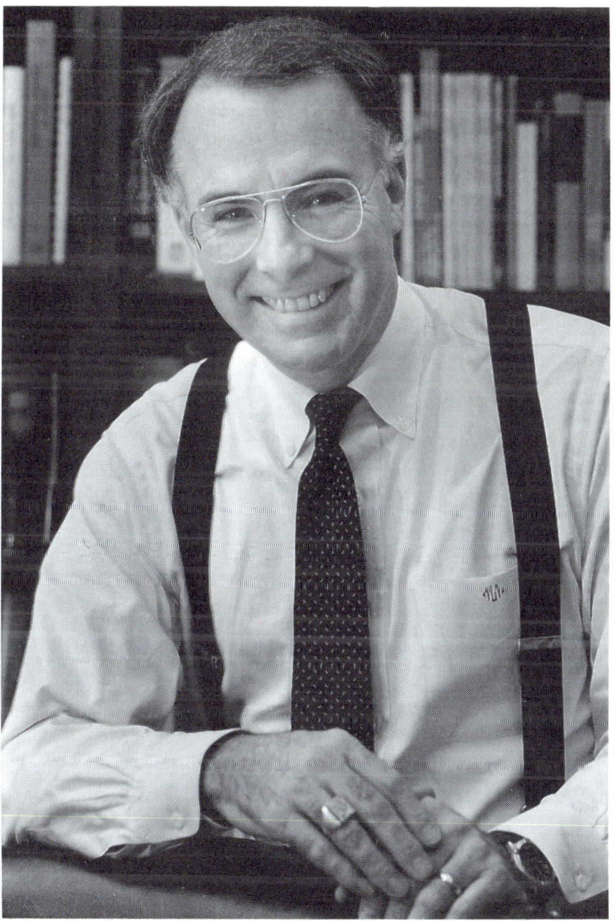

Fig. 29-10. Troy L. Thompson II, M.D., Fifth Chairman (1988–).

in neurochemistry, and the science of the neurotransmitters, microneurosurgery, atomic physiology, and psychopharmacology have once again made biological psychiatry the destination of the science of psychiatry. On the united front—the psychodynamic understanding of mental processes and the contribution of biology—the Department of Psychiatry is prepared to embrace the entire spectrum of mental science teaching, clinical practice, and research, enhancing as never before the great traditions of the faculty of the Jefferson Medical College.

References

1. Packard, F.R., "The Practice of Medicine in Philadelphia in the 18th Century," *Ann. Med. Hist.,* New Series 5, 1933, pp. 135–150.
2. Palmer, H.D., "Philadelphia and Psychiatry," *Amer. Jour. Psychiatry.* 100, 1944, pp. 690–707.
3. Farr, C., "Benjamin Rush and American Psychiatry," *Amer. Jour. of Psychiatry.* 100, 1944, pp. 3–15.
4. Keyes, B.L., Personal communication.
5. Bond, E., "Psychiatry in Philadelphia in 1844," *Amer. Jour. of Psychiatry.* 100, 1944, pp. 16–17.
6. Jefferson Medical College Announcement for 1872.
7. Gould, R.M., *The Jefferson Medical College of Philadelphia.* New York: Lewis, 1904.
8. DaCosta, J.C., "Francis X. Dercum." *The Trials and Triumphs of the Surgeon.* Edited by Frederick Keller. Dorrance & Co., 1944.
9. Strecker, E.A., *Alcohol, One Man's Meat.* New York: Macmillan Co., 1938.
10. College Catalogue, 1931.
11. Keyes, B.L., Personal communication.
12. Strecker, E.A., and Keyes, B.L., "Ovarian Therapy in Involutional Melancholia," *N.Y. Med. Jour.* and *Med. Rec.* July 5, 1922.
13. Keyes, B.L., Personal communication.
14. Koltes, J.A., "Mental Hospitals With Open Doors," *Journal of the A.P.A.* November, 1958.
15. Jones, M., *The Therapeutic Community.* Tavestock Publ. Ltd., 1952.
16. Keyes, B.L., Bookhammer, R.S., and Kaplan, A.J., "Psychiatry in the General Hospital," *Am. Jour. Psych.* Vol. 105, August & November 1948.
17. Koltes, J.A., A Psychiatry Unit in a General Hospital. *Penn. Med. Jour.* 62, 1959, pp. 1671–1674.
18. Matthews, R.A., "The Unique Aspects of the Care of the Mentally Ill in Europe," Lecture to the Louisiana Society for Mental Health, June, 1953, unpublished.
19. Waelder, R.A., "The Principle of Multiple Function," *Psychoanalytic Quarterly,* Vol. 5, 1936.
20. Guttman, S.A., *Concordance to the Student Edition of the Complete Psychological Work of Sigmund Freud.* 6 vols. Int'l. Univ. Press.
21. College Catalogue, 1974.

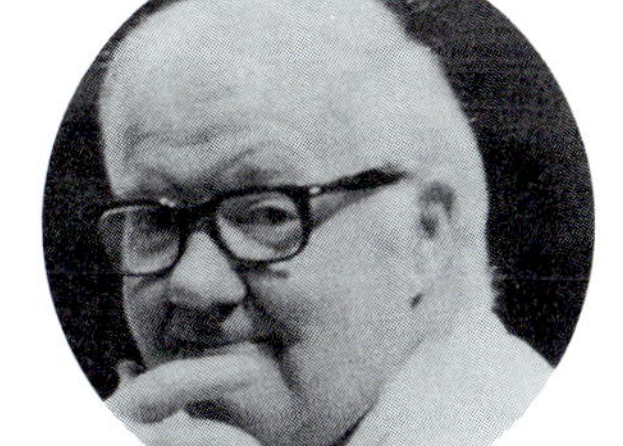

CHAPTER THIRTY

Allergy and Clinical Immunology

Herbert C. Mansmann, Jr., M.D.

"All that wheezes is not Asthma."

—Chevalier Jackson (1865–1958)

An important aspect of medicine—allergy and clinical immunology—has a complex history at Jefferson. For most of the twentieth century, the "specialty" of allergy was not formally organized as a Division of any Department but was related principally to the Department of Medicine until 1982. As a well-functioning Clinic, this in no respect impaired the effectiveness of the discipline.

Historical Background

Numerous references in medicine and literature exist relative to processes now described generally as allergic or that relate to immunologic events. As early as the second century A.D., Aretaeus the Cappadocian described exercise-induced asthma. Moses Maimonides (1135–1204 A.D.) wrote *Treatise on Asthma*. Early awareness of an immunologic process was exemplified by Edward Jenner's 1798 use of vaccine for smallpox prevention. The term "hay fever" was coined by John Bostock in 1819, but identification of pollen as a cause of the problem awaited a description in 1872 by Morrill Wyman. Skin testing and desensitization were attempted as early as 1873 by Charles H. Blackley.

At Jefferson at about the turn of the twentieth century, otolaryngologists in particular showed much interest in this field, and, in addition, Dr. Solomon Solis-Cohen (Jefferson, 1883), later Professor of Clinical Medicine, published a paper entitled *The Use of Adrenal Substance in the Treatment of Asthma* (1900); he also noted vasomotor disturbances as a part of the pathological physiology of common allergic disorders. The increasing role of immune phenomena during the twentieth century is well documented and was not limited to the area of allergy and immunology as it is perceived today. Such areas as transplantation, rheumatology, and nephrology come to mind. The past few decades, however, have seen considerable development in the direct area of allergy and clinical immunology.

Clinical Allergy at Jefferson

The first Allergy Clinic in Philadelphia was established by Dr. J. Alexander Clarke, Jr., (Figure 30-1) in 1921. Dr. Clarke (Jefferson, 1916) interned at Roosevelt Hospital in New York City, where he was attracted to the new and famous allergy clinic there under the pioneer allergist, Robert A. Cooke, M.D. Dr. Cooke was a founding member and first President of the Society for the Study of Asthma and Allied Conditions, of which Dr. Clarke was later President. The Jefferson Clinic was organized under the Jefferson Outpatient Department with Dr. Clarke as Chief Clinical Assistant and Instructor in Medicine. He was soon joined by Drs. George B. Meyer and James S. McLaughlin. The clinic thrived and ultimately developed into one of the largest in the Outpatient Department. Beginning in a small store on Eleventh Street, it was moved to the 1898 College Building at Tenth and Walnut and later to Curtis Clinic. For many years the students were rotated through the clinic.

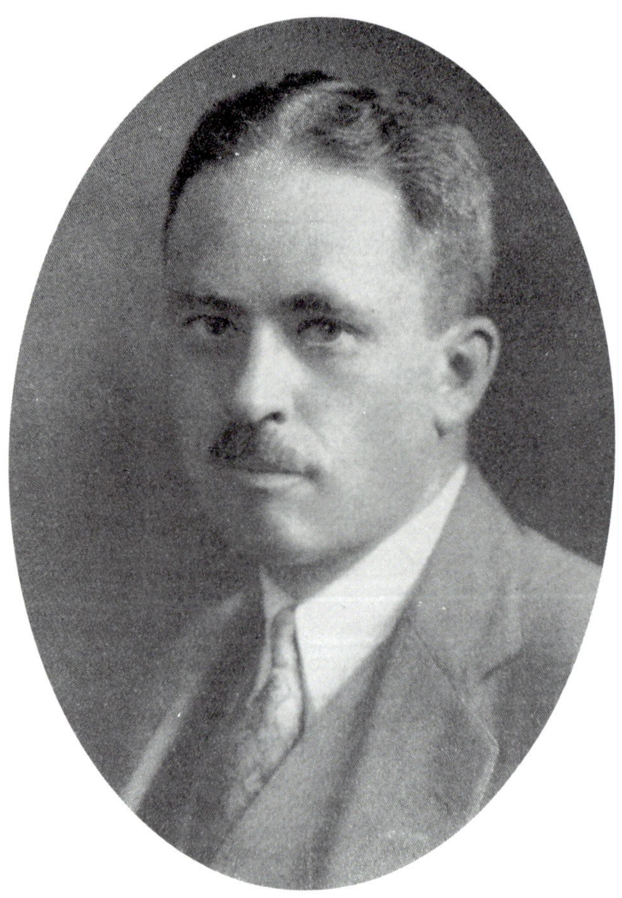

FIG. 30-1. J. Alexander Clarke, Jr., M.D., organizer and early Chief of Allergy Clinic (1921).

Dr. Clarke became a leader in all aspects of his specialty and published numerous articles, but his untimely death prevented publication of the book that was in preparation. Among his early trainees were numerous physicians, who organized allergy clinics in nearby hospitals. For many years the physicians who served in the Jefferson Clinic were volunteers and proved unusually loyal in their attendance at the regular clinic sessions.

During Dr. Clarke's period of activity, he became certified in Internal Medicine with the establishment of the American Board in 1936. In 1942 the subspecialty Board of Allergy was formed and certified him as well.

Harry L. Rogers, M.D., Chief of the Allergy Clinic (1943–1958)

Dr. Clarke became ill during the height of his career and died January 31, 1943, at the age of 52. The Clinic continued under the supervision of Dr. Harry L. Rogers (University of Pennsylvania, 1917) who served as its Head from 1943 to 1958. During this time, the Clinic maintained its previous status as mainly an outpatient enterprise, with only limited hospital association. Dr. Rogers was in charge of all student teaching as well as the laboratory for preparation of antigens for testing and therapy. Among the physicians serving during this period were Drs. James McLaughlin, Howard C. Leopold, Frank J. Gilday, George W. Truitt, Alexander M. Peters, Samuel Rynes, Charles F. Milon, James H. Ruetschlin, and Carl M. High.

Howard C. Leopold, M.D., Chief of Allergy Clinic (1959–1974)

Dr. Leopold (Jefferson, 1932) (Figure 30-2) was appointed Chief of the Allergy Clinic in 1959.

Shortly thereafter, he began a series of lectures to junior students supplementing the Clinic experience. Dr. Leopold, having originally planned a career in pediatrics with residency at Children's Hospital in Philadelphia, interrupted this program to study infections in childhood with Dr. Bela Schick at Mt. Sinai Hospital in New York. Soon thereafter Dr. Schick sent him to the Cooke Clinic in New York, encouraging him to take up studies in allergy. This training resulted in his appointment to Dr. Clarke's Clinic at Jefferson upon his return to Philadelphia in 1936. His activities were widespread, and he was consultant to many regional facilities. During his tenure as Clinic Chief a few clinical research projects were carried out and reported to the American Academy of Allergy. Studies of autoimmunity in chronic bronchial asthma and the detection of antinuclear antibodies in patients with asthma using the fluorescent antibody technique were in progress. During the years of Dr. Leopold's activities, Dr. Robert Wise, Chairman of the Department of Medicine, wanted to develop a full Division of Allergy and Immunology but this did not occur, partly as a result of Dr. Leopold's impending retirement, which was hastened by his illness. He and Dr. Wise had agreed on plans for a full-time Director in 1973, but this was not consummated.

During Dr. Leopold's illness in 1974, Dr. Frank Gilday (Jefferson, 1944) was appointed Acting Director of the Allergy Clinic, and he continued its direction until 1982, when the Clinic was absorbed into the Division of Allergy and

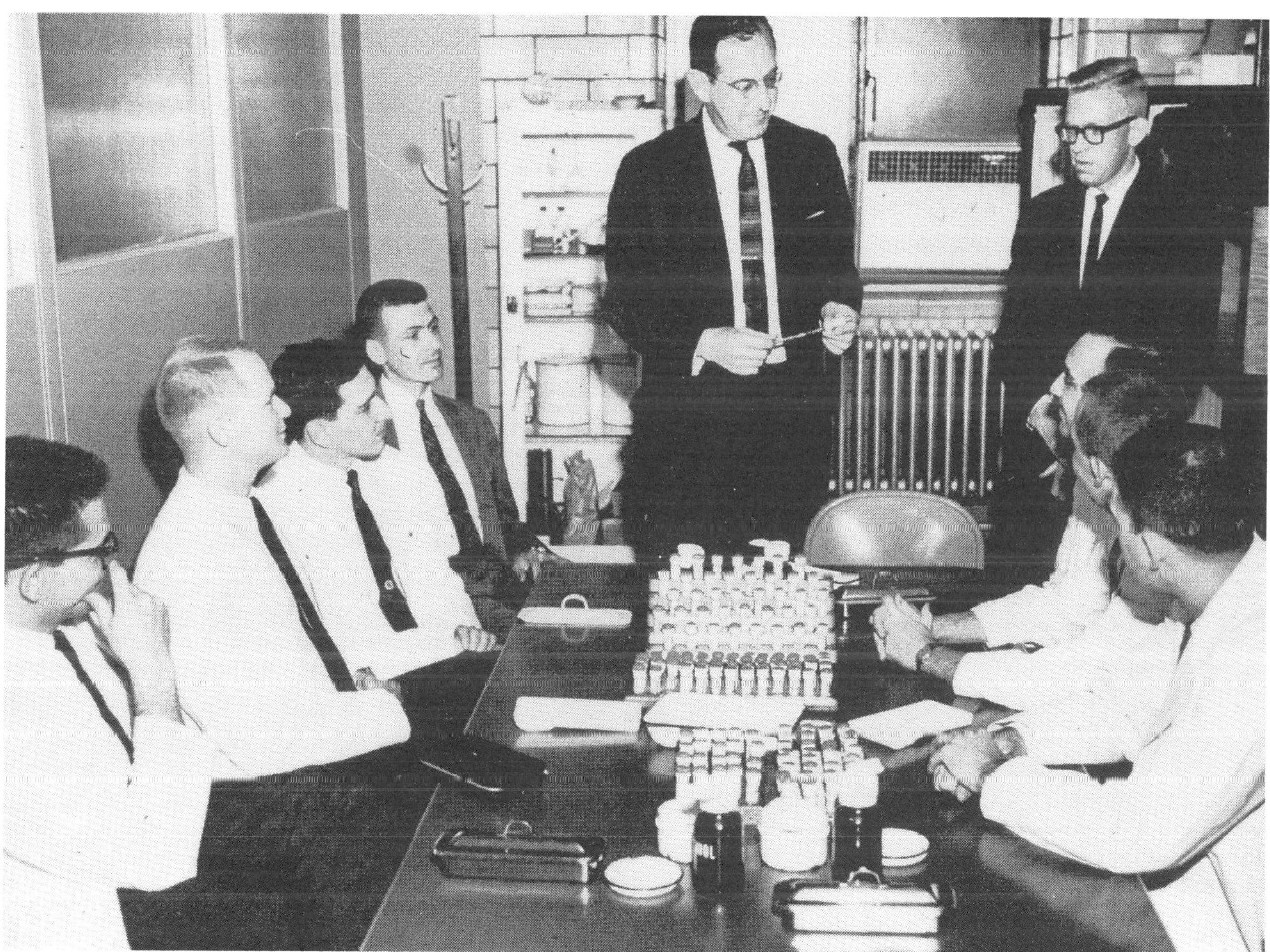

FIG. 30-2. Howard C. Leopold, M.D. (center), Chief of Allergy Clinic (1959–1974).

Immunology of the Department of Pediatrics. Following Dr. Leopold's death, an opportunity was perceived to establish a comprehensive Division of Allergy and Clinical Immunology as a joint facility of the Departments of Medicine and Pediatrics. This was not accomplished but an effective program was nevertheless developed.

Herbert C. Mansmann, Jr., M.D.

Dr. Mansmann (Jefferson, 1951) was appointed Professor of Pediatrics and Associate Professor of Medicine in 1968, having previously been associated at the University of Pittsburgh with Dr. Robert L. Brent, Chairman of Pediatrics, and Dr. Paul H. Maurer, an internationally recognized immunochemist and Chairman of Biochemistry, both of whom came to Jefferson in 1966. All three shared interests and demonstrated skills in immunology. Dr. Mansmann was also made Director of the Division of Allergy and Clinical Immunology in the Department of Pediatrics. The plan was to strengthen the Pediatric Residency program and to develop clinical and research skills in the Department. He was also associated with the Allergy Clinic, which in 1982 was absorbed into his Division.

At the time of his arrival at Jefferson, Dr. Mansmann was already established as a clinician and investigator in the area of pediatric allergy. As a medical student at Jefferson, he had been an allergic patient of Dr. Harry L. Rogers. Following his training in pediatrics at Pittsburgh, he became a Fellow in Allergy in the Department of Medicine at the Massachussetts General Hospital (1955–1956) under Dr. Walter S. Burrage, Director of the Rackemann Clinic. He then served a year at New York University in immunology research, following which he returned to Pittsburgh to begin a research and clinical program.

Dr. Mansmann was certified by the American Board of Pediatrics and its Sub-Board of Pediatric Allergy. In 1968 he became the last Secretary of that Board, and in 1971 became a Founding Member and Secretary of its successor, the American Board of Allergy and Immunology. Since 1974 he has served as Executive Secretary of the Board. He has also been President of numerous professional societies and editor of a new journal, *Pediatric Asthma, Allergy and Immunology*.

The Pediatric Allergy Program

With the interest and support of Dr. Robert Brent, the new program at Jefferson thrived. Training of Residents and Fellows was comprehensive and their response enthusiastic. The policies included subspecialty training, frequently organ systems-oriented. An important special area was that of pulmonary medicine under Dr. Edward Sewall, Professor of Pediatrics and former President of the American Thoracic Society. Dr. Stephen J. McGeady, Associate Professor of Pediatrics with appointments also in Medicine and Biochemistry, joined the program in 1974 after completion of an outstanding training in Allergy and Clinical Immunology at Duke University Medical Center. He headed the Clinical Immunology Laboratory, where research especially into immune cellular functions was conducted. In addition to a laboratory for preparation of testing materials for patient care, there was also a Clinical Pharmacology Laboratory under Dr. Consuelo Saccar, where research into pharmacokinetics and clinical measurements of drug and metabolite levels in body fluids were carried out.

Initially as Medical Director of Children's Heart Hospital (renamed Children's Rehabilitation Hospital in 1986) and continuing as Director of Bronchial Asthma and Pulmonary Diseases, Dr. Mansmann developed successful teaching, research, and service programs. Three allergy and clinical fellows were stationed there to care for the 15 to 20 children with bronchial asthma, chronic lung disease, or immunological diseases. The full facilities of the Department of Pediatrics were available for the care of these children. The laboratories in Curtis and members from the Department of Medicine were also at hand. The Pediatric Pulmonary Function Laboratory, adjacent to the outpatient office in Curtis, saw frequent service.

The Full Program

With respect to adult allergy, which clinically constituted a major proportion of the outpatient activities, the long and successful experiences in the old Allergy Clinic provided a solid base for continuing effort. Newer immunological principles and procedures were responsible for improvement in management and results. Bridging the area between pediatric and adult problems of allergy was no major problem because the mechanisms were similar. In this regard, the staff members from both Pediatrics and Medicine contributed signally to the clinical functions. Drs. John R. Cohn (Jefferson, 1976), Edward S. Schulman (Jefferson, 1975), Bernard W. Godwin, Jr., (Jefferson, 1955), and Charles F. Milon were representative.

Since 1968 there has been an acceleration of achievements, as shown by the numbers of Residents and Fellows who were trained and the continuing interest of the medical students. Sixty Fellows in Allergy and Clinical Immunology completed the program, all but three of them having become board eligible or certified. Twenty-nine were certified by the American Board of Allergy and Immunology and a number of them remained in the educational programs.

The management of allergy at Jefferson has undergone changes consistent with evolving concepts of the nature of immune processes, which in recent decades have become more clearly defined. Allergy has come to include basic science disciplines as well as those related to internal medicine, pediatrics, pulmonary diseases, otolaryngology, and other system-related areas. The program as recently structured has proved effective and progressive. Excellent teaching, research, and clinical capabilities promise further improvements in patient care.

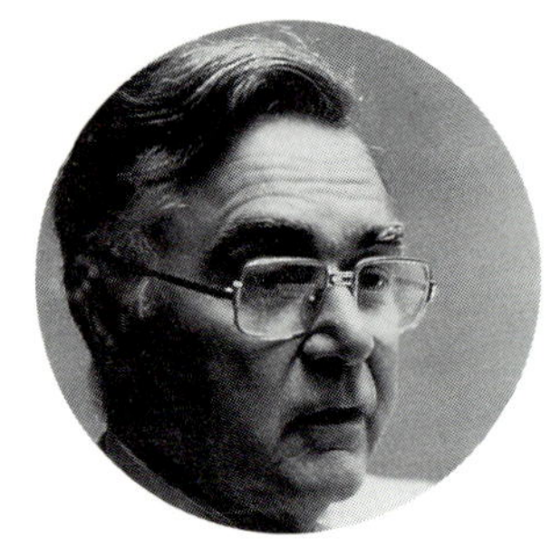

CHAPTER THIRTY-ONE

Geriatrics

John N. Lindquist, M.D.

"Old age, though despised, is coveted by all men."

—Proverb

Perhaps the earliest organized treatment of the elderly at Jefferson began when Dr. J. Chalmers DaCosta was appointed surgeon to the Philadelphia Firemen and Firemen's Pension Fund in 1900, which service he rendered free to the active and retired firemen for 35 years. Final recognition of this service was made in May, 1931, when he was appointed Honorary Deputy Chief of the Philadelphia Fire Department and presented with a diamond-studded badge of office in the clinical ampitheater of the Thompson Annex.

Dr. Louis B. LaPlace (Figure 31-1), Associate Professor of Clinical Medicine, who headed the Cardiac Clinic, constantly reminded the students, interns, and residents of the need for study of care for the aged. The first mention of a Geriatrics Clinic was in the yearly reports of Jefferson Hospital and the Jefferson Medical College Catalogue in 1941. Dr. Louis LaPlace was the Chief Clinical Assistant, and Dr. J. Pancoast Reath (Jefferson, 1937), the Clinical Assistant. In 1942 Dr. Edmund L. Housel (Jefferson, 1935) became Chief Clinical Assistant in the Geriatrics Clinic; in 1946, he became Chief of the Hypertension Clinic. Dr. Housel (Figure 31-2) was assisted by Dr.

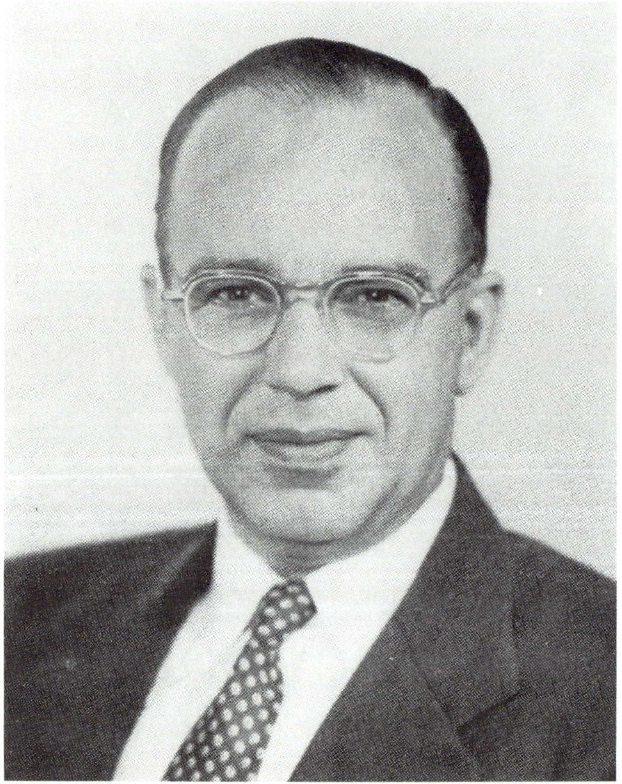

Fig. 31-1. Louis B. LaPlace, M.D., first Chief of the Geriatrics Clinic (1941).

Oscar Wood (Jefferson, 1934) in the Geriatrics Clinic until the latter's untimely death in 1951.

Dr. Housel conducted a study of the use of dexedrine as a stimulant for mildly depressed aged patients and was impressed by its effectiveness in improving their alertness and physical energy. He also conducted a study of the eating habits of the aged.

In 1951 Dr. John N. Lindquist (Jefferson, 1943) became Chief Clinical Assistant of the General Medical Clinic and the Geriatrics Clinic, which he headed until Family Medicine was begun in 1974 (Figure 31-3). He made students aware of the elderly as a special group and stressed the need for their whole care. A mutual referral system developed with the Philadelphia Center for Older People (a day care center for the aged) and the Jefferson Medical and Geriatrics Clinics. Medical care was provided at Jefferson, and social and recreational therapy at the Center.

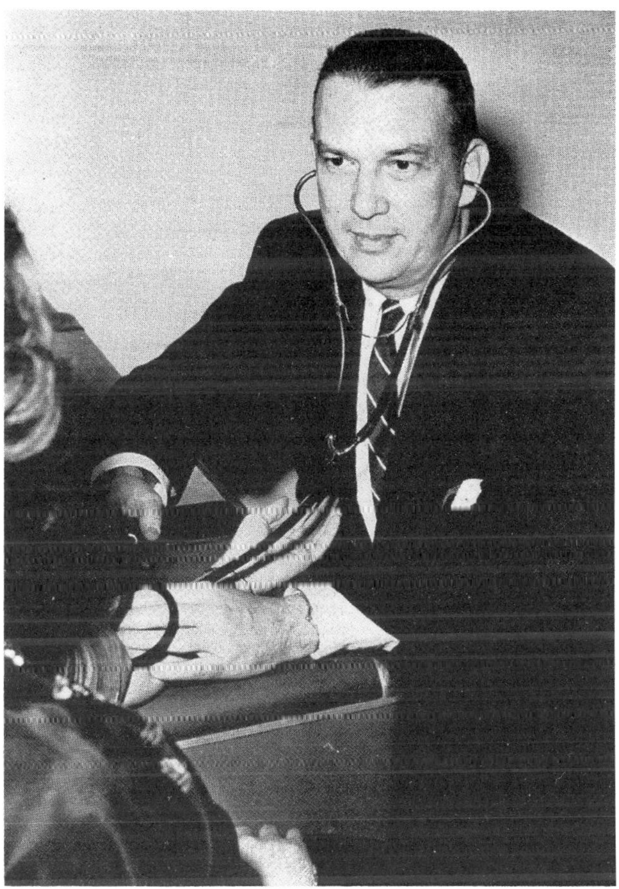

FIG. 31-2. Edmund L. Housel, M.D., Chief of the Geriatrics Clinic (1942) and of the Hypertension Clinic (1946).

From 1965 to 1969 students in the Department of Psychiatry who were sent to Friends Hospital for training were assigned elderly patients and became introduced to the mental problems of the aged. This was an extension of the teaching of geriatrics from the Medical and Geriatrics Clinic. Dr. Lindquist conducted the program with Dr. Kenneth Kool, a psychiatrist. The students presented their aged patients at a weekly seminar attended by the psychiatrist, internist, social worker, nurse, nurse's aide, and recreational therapist. The student was assisted by this team in planning for the patient's immediate and future care.

The current Geropsychiatry Program at Jefferson is headed by Erwin A. Carner, Ed.D., with a staff of 30, whose services are integrated with the Departments of Rehabilitation Medicine, Neurology, Internal Medicine, and Hematology.

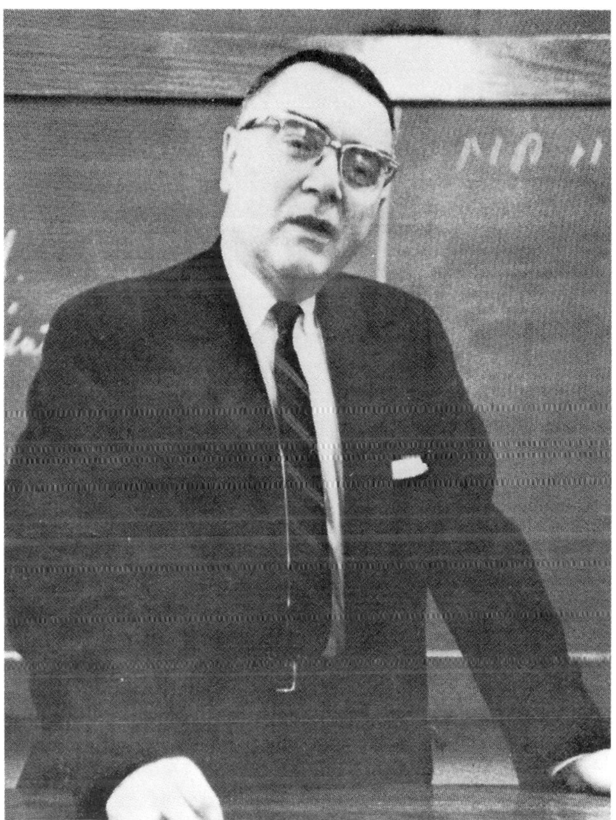

FIG. 31-3. John N. Lindquist, M.D., Chief of the Geriatrics Clinic (1951–1974).

The Center for the Study of Geropsychiatry is a section of the Department of Psychiatry and Human Behavior. Clinically, the Center coordinates the Dementia Evaluation Center, which encompasses the Departments of Neurology, Internal Medicine, and Psychiatry. Patients suspected of having a dementia are evaluated by a team, which includes a neuropsychologist, psychiatrist, neurologist, and a physician who specializes in internal medicine. The Center also operates a geriatric partial hospitalization program for nursing home patients. This program, which has three locations in Philadelphia, serves the mental health requirements of a population greatly in need of such services. The Center has an extensive research program in the areas of Alzheimer's disease, aerobic exercise, and nutrition with nursing home patients and the elderly in emergency rooms. Some of these research projects are grant funded and some are done independently.

An elective in Gerontology exists for Freshman and Sophomore medical students. In this program students work with a well elderly person for two years. The Geropsychiatry Center coordinates a course in the Sophomore Seminar Series as well as constituting a training site for Junior and Senior students.

Over the past four decades there have been sporadic efforts to establish a formal Division of Geriatrics in the Department of Medicine. The interdisciplinary nature of this "specialty" has frustrated such a consolidation. Jefferson's program, in striving for improved approaches to the problems of aging, is comparable to those of similar institutions. Whether ultimately the subject will emerge as a major specialty remains unclear. Despite the diverse aspects of Geriatrics, the care at Jefferson of aged patients in medicine, surgery, and psychiatry has been optimal. Ongoing research promises even greater benefits.

PART III

Clinical Departments and Divisions Continued

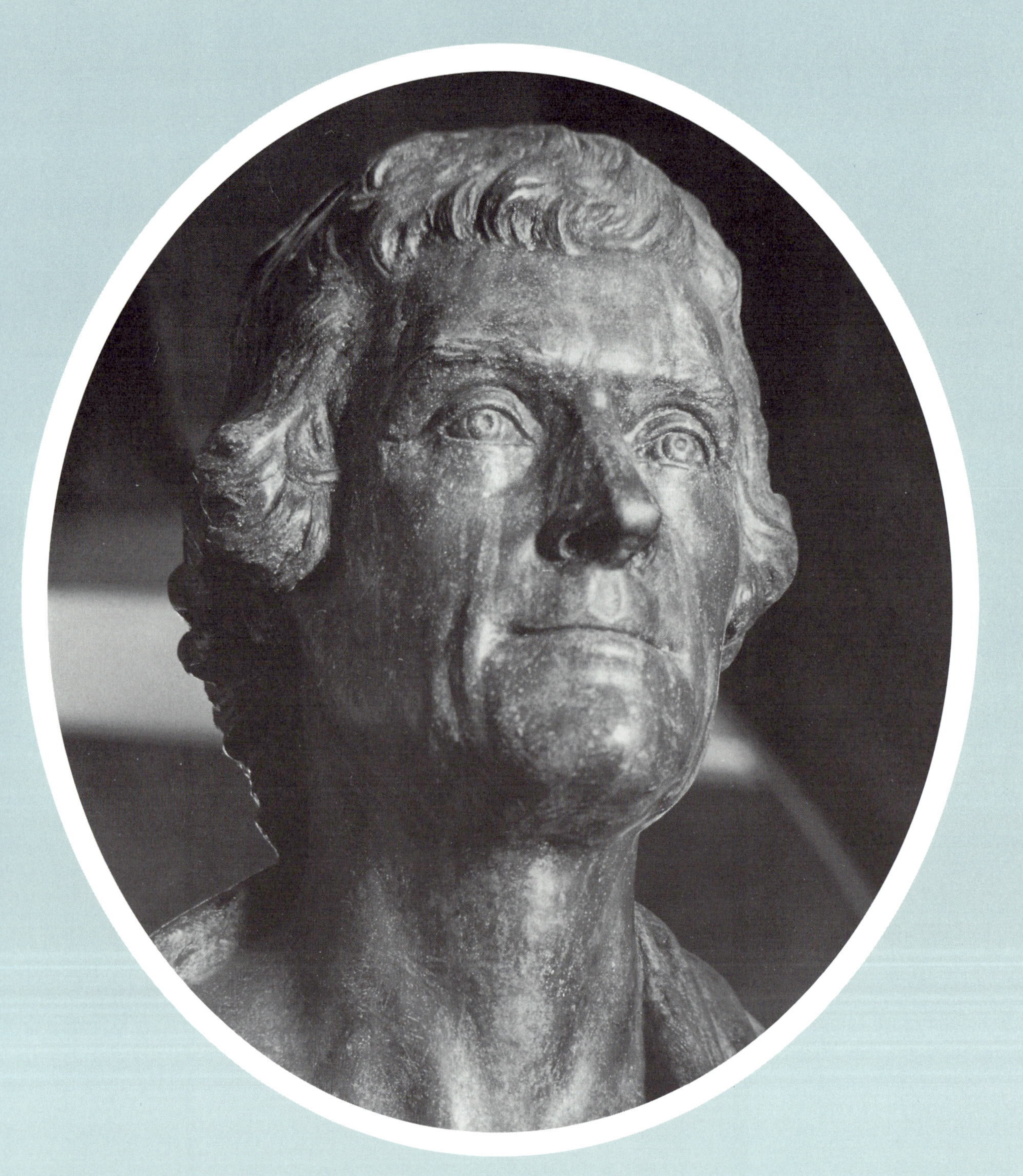

PART III

Clinical Departments and Divisions Continued

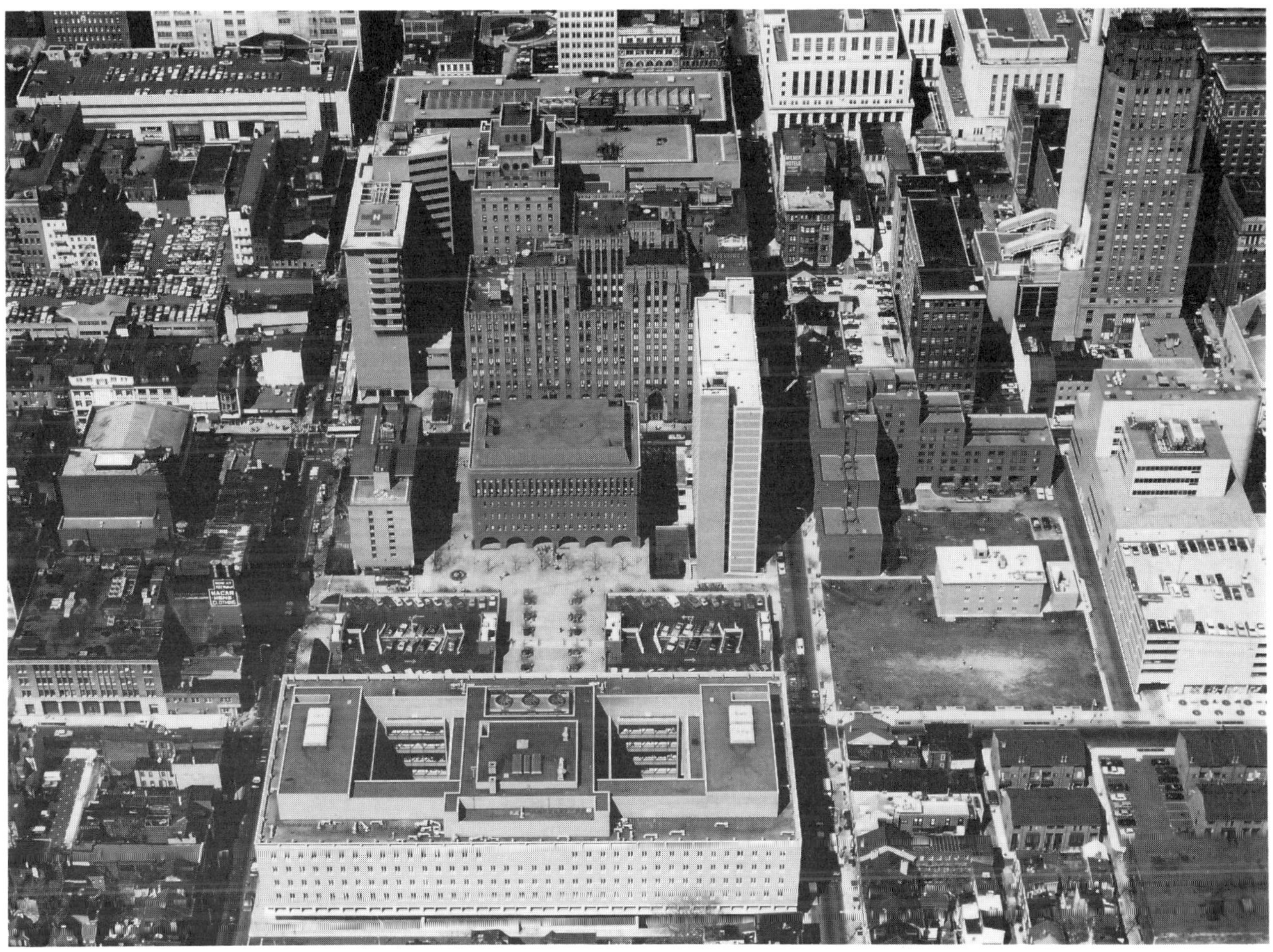

Aerial View of Thomas Jefferson University

← *Opposite page:*
Bust of Thomas Jefferson by
Rudulph Evans

CHAPTER THIRTY-TWO

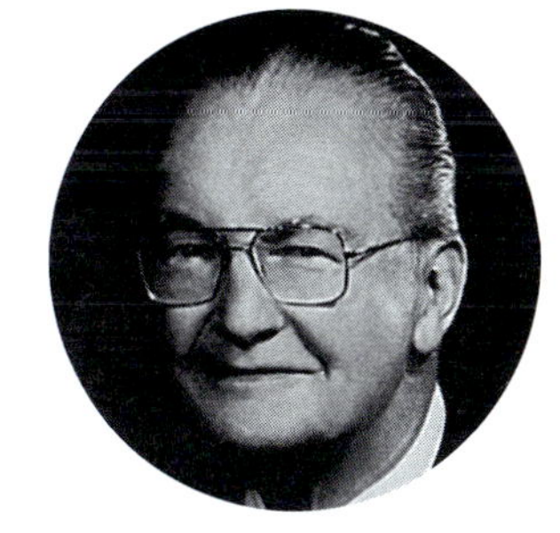

Department of Surgery

Frederick B. Wagner, Jr., M.D.

"No training of the surgeon can be too arduous, no discipline too stern, and none of us may measure our devotion to our cause."

–Sir Berkeley Moynihan (1865–1936)

The Department of Surgery may justly claim its first Professor, George McClellan, as the founder of Jefferson Medical College. It was in 1823 that he first began to consider the founding of a second medical school in Philadelphia that would compete with the University of Pennsylvania, his alma mater (1819). Soon after graduation he had devoted his main attention to anatomy and surgery while conducting an active general practice. With an energy characteristic of his genius he soon attracted large private classes into his office near Sixth and Sansom Streets at a site now occupied by the Public Ledger Building.

Within a few years it was the most successful of the private schools of its kind in the City. He was one of the best teachers in anatomy and surgery, and, while still only in his 20s, was looked upon as the coming man in Philadelphia surgery. At that time, Philadelphia was the focal point of American medicine, with the oldest medical school, the University of Pennsylvania, which had been founded in 1765 and was overcrowded with 550 students. In a daring and seemingly outrageous venture he succeeded in 1824 in establishing Jefferson Medical College of Philadelphia as the Medical Department of Jefferson College at Canonsburg, Pennsylvania.[1]

The genealogy of Jefferson's Surgical Department in terms of its Chairmen is provided in Figure 32-1. In addition to sequence, it graphically demonstrates the division after the retirement of Samuel D. Gross in 1882 and the reunification under John H. Gibbon, Jr. in 1956.

George McClellan, M.D. (1796–1847); First Chairman (1824–1839)

George McClellan (Figure 32-2) was born in Woodstock, Connecticut, on December 23, 1796. He was of Scottish ancestry; his forebears were fighting Highlanders and American Revolutionary patriots. His grandfather, Samuel, had fought in the French and Indian War and served as a Brigadier General under Washington. The military heritage continued under George McClellan's son, General George Brinton McClellan, who was Lincoln's General of the Union Army of the Potomac in the early part of the Civil War.

McClellan received his preliminary education at Woodstock Academy, where his father was Headmaster. He was an excellent student with preference for mathematics and language. In 1812 he attended Yale, from which he graduated in 1815. Both George and his younger brother, Samuel, went on to study medicine and become prominent in the early history of Jefferson Medical College.

George entered the private office of Dr. Thomas Hubbard of Pomfret, Connecticut, under the preceptorship system of the time, in which the aspiring physician would aid his mentor in compounding drugs, running errands, cleaning the office, and by observation learn the art of bloodletting as well as the prescribing of emetics and cathartics for the ill. In the remaining spare time, he would study from the obsolete medical books in the doctor's library. After one year of this George made the important move to Philadelphia, where he became a pupil of the highly respected Professor John Syng Dorsey and entered the Medical School of the University of Pennsylvania.

In the Medical School, McClellan's brilliance as a student was manifested by his extensive reading, hard clinical work, and outstanding interest in

George McClellan, 1824

Joseph Pancoast, 1839

Thomas D. Mütter, 1841

Samuel D. Gross, 1856

Samuel W. Gross, 1882

W.W. Keen, 1889

J. Chalmers DaCosta, 1907
(Gross I, 1910)

Thomas A. Shallow, 1931
(Gross II, 1939)

John H. Brinton, 1882

John H. Gibbon, 1907

Edward J. Klopp, 1931

George P. Muller, 1936
(Grace Revere Osler Professor 1939)

John H. Gibbon, Jr., 1946
(Professor of Clinical and Experimental Surgery)

John H. Gibbon, Jr. (Gross III, 1956)

John Y. Templeton, III (Gross IV, 1967)

Harry S. Goldsmith (Gross V, 1970)

Frederick B. Wagner, Jr., Acting Chairman (1977–1978),
(Grace Revere Osler Professor, 1978)

Francis E. Rosato (Gross VI, 1978)

FIG. 32-1. Genealogy of the Department of Surgery

anatomy and surgery. He also found time to serve as a resident student in the Philadelphia Almshouse at Eleventh and Spruce Streets. There he zealously performed autopsies and operated on cadavers. His colleagues were captivated by his knowledge, skill in dissection, and stimulation of medical discussions. At graduation in 1819 his thesis was *Surgical Anatomy of Arteries.*

McClellan went immediately into practice near Sixth and Walnut Streets and had instant success. So many young men sought him out as a preceptor that he started a private school, which also attracted the aid of several colleagues (John Eberle, Joseph Klapp, and Jacob Green). In 1824, McClellan, joined by these men (Figure 32-3), petitioned Jefferson College at Canonsburg, Pennsylvania, to recognize a Medical Department under their Charter with the State of Pennsylvania as the Jefferson Medical College of Philadelphia (Figure 32-4). This circumvented the opposition of the University of Pennsylvania to the establishment of a second medical college in Philadelphia. McClellan served as the first Professor of Surgery for 15 years and also first Professor of Anatomy (1824–1825) and Interim Professor of Anatomy (1827–1830).

In 1826 Samuel D. Gross came to Philadelphia with a letter for his enrollment from his preceptor, Dr. Swift of Easton, addressed to Drs. Hodge and Dewees of the Medical School of the University of Pennsylvania. So widespread was the reputation of Dr. McClellan and his new school that Gross disregarded Dr. Swift's advice and joined McClellan as a private student as well as a matriculant at Jefferson. Gross became McClellan's most illustrious student. Gross later characterized McClellan as follows:

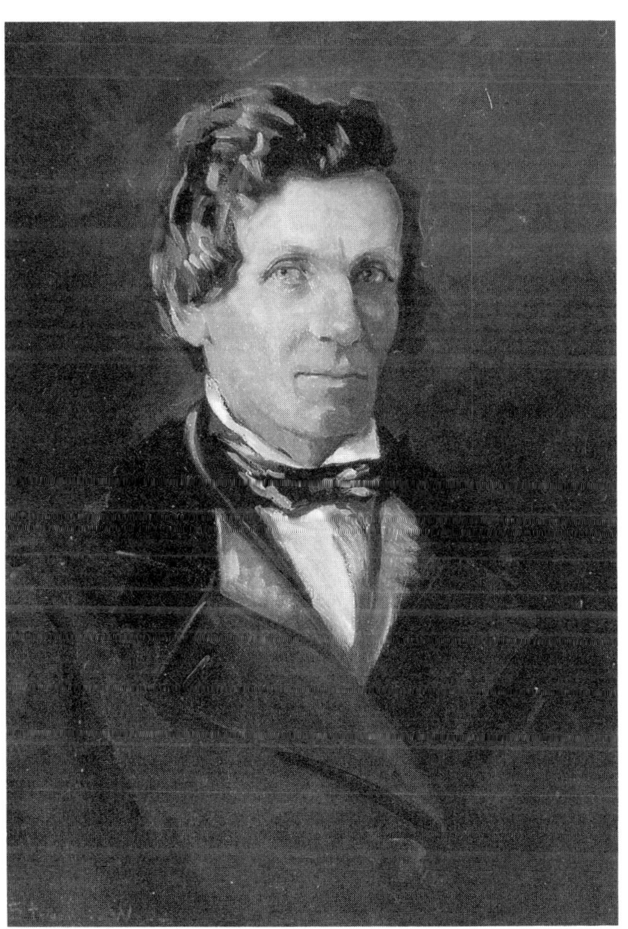

FIG. 32-2. George McClellan, M.D. (1796–1847); First Chairman (1824–1839).

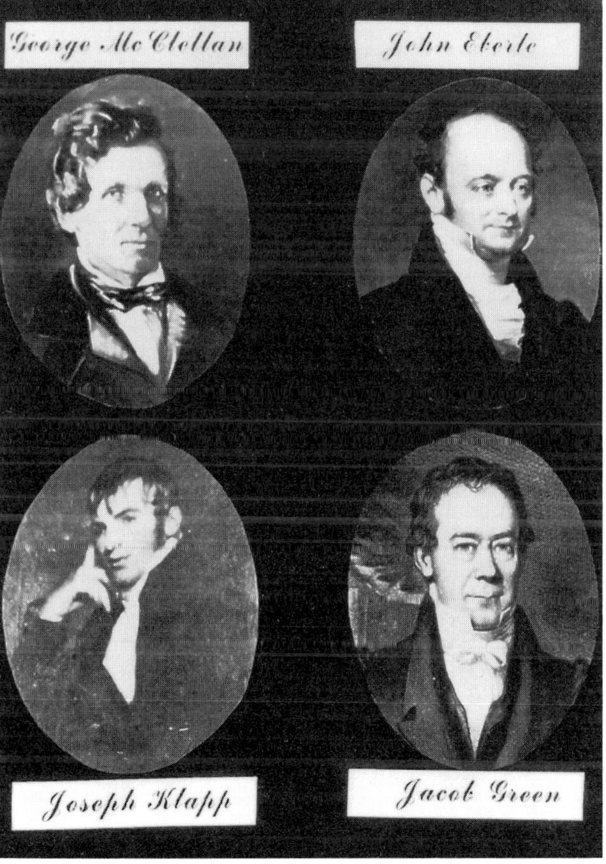

FIG. 32-3. Founders of Jefferson Medical College.

"His impulsive disposition often brought him into trouble; he lacked judgment, talked too much, and made everybody his confidant. Of course the betrayal of his confidence made him many enemies, some of them implacable. He was, moreover, a restless man, always pushing ahead. . . . With many faults, McClellan was unquestionably a man of genius, quick to perceive and prompt to execute. With a better regulated mind he would have accomplished much greater ends and achieved a more lasting fame. Probably no man ever handled a scalpel with more dexterity. . . . His reputation as a surgeon will be in great measure traditional, for he has left no adequate record of his observations and experience. He has, it is true, transmitted to us a small volume on surgery,[2] but it is read by few persons, and it really possesses no conspicuous merit. His fame will rest mainly upon the fact that he was the founder of a school."[3]

Gross apparently overlooked or failed to appreciate McClellan's great innovative contribution to medical education, namely that of practical clinical instruction directly from patients before students in a collegiate setting. In other schools of the time, the teaching was entirely by lectures, and McClellan's method was denigrated as "ineffectual, misleading, and superficial." McClellan's teaching from patients later was adopted in all medical schools and was no better emulated than by Gross in Eakins' portrait, *The Gross Clinic*.

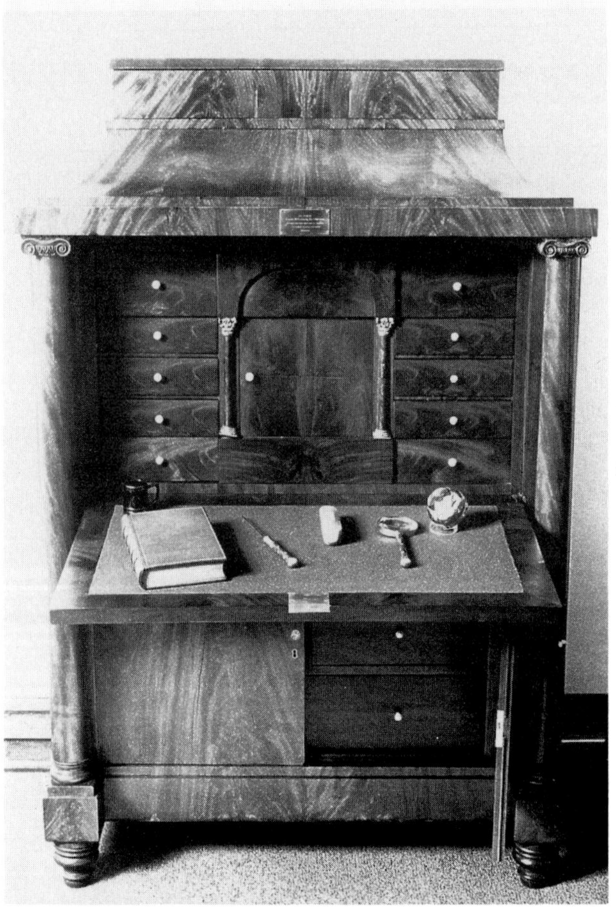

FIG. 32-4. The desk of George McClellan, M.D.

It must be recalled that McClellan throughout his surgical career had to operate without the benefit of anesthesia and that Lister's first paper (1867) on the *Principle of Antisepsis* would not appear until 20 years after his death. His surgery was rapid and crude by today's standards. According to Gross: "As an operator, he was showy, and at times brilliant, yet he lacked the important requisites of a great surgeon—judgment and patience[4]. . . . his saw broke in amputating a poor man's arm; in a moment the limb was bent over his knees and the bone snapped asunder."[5]

McClellan clashed openly with Dr. William Gibson, Professor of Surgery at the University of Pennsylvania, over the feasibility of removal of the parotid gland. McClellan claimed to have accomplished this operation 11 times with only one death. In 1828 McClellan was sued for malpractice for alleged want of skill in removal of a cataract, and a verdict of $500 was rendered against him. The suit had been instigated by professional enemies, of which he had many.

By 1839 McClellan was in open dispute with Jefferson's Board of Trustees, which he denounced publicly. The Board retaliated by dissolving the faculty and balloted for new appointments. In the process Dr. Joseph Pancoast was elected on July 10 by a vote of seven against McClellan's five. The latter's connection with the school he had founded was thus unhappily ended.

The irrepressible McClellan promptly obtained a Charter from the State Legislature for another school in Philadelphia named "The Medical Department of Pennsylvania College" (at Gettysburg). He assembled a good faculty with five associates, including his brother Samuel, and began the first lectures with nearly 100 students in November, 1839. As the result of a quarrel in 1843, McClellan resigned his final Professorship. The school maintained a high rating for two decades, but ceased by attrition during the Civil War because of the exodus of Southern medical students.

Retired from teaching, McClellan spent the remaining four years of his life in practice. He treated all classes of people, but especially among the poor his name was a household word. He died on May 8, 1847, in an attack of acute abdominal pain. His postmortem examination revealed a perforated sigmoid colon.

According to Gross, McClellan died poor. "He bought town lots, built houses, and lost money."[6] He is buried in East Laurel Hill Cemetery, above the East River (Kelly) Drive in Philadelphia, Section L, Lot 46. A well-preserved granite tombstone marks his gravesite with his wife Elizabeth Brinton.

In addition to his military son, General George Brinton McClellan, he had a physician son, Dr. John Hill Brinton McClellan, who graduated from his second medical school. His grandson was Dr. George McClellan, Chairman of Applied and Topographic Anatomy at Jefferson (1905–1913).

Joseph Pancoast, M.D. (1805–1882); Second Chairman (1839–1841)

Joseph Pancoast (Figure 32-5) was born in 1805 in Burlington, New Jersey, the descendant of an Englishman who is reputed to have come to the Philadelphia area under the auspices of William Penn. It was the same year of birth for Samuel D. Gross, who was his senior by only four months. He graduated from the Medical School of the University of Pennsylvania in 1828, also the year that Gross graduated from Jefferson.

Pancoast and Gross became acquainted soon after they settled in practice, the former on North Fourth Street and the latter on the corner of Library and Fifth Streets near the Philadelphia Dispensary. They promptly became warm friends through their mutual interest in a surgical treatise by Bierowski illustrated with beautiful colored plates. Pancoast was able to compete successfully against the better known George McClellan, who was nine years their senior, but Gross barely made a living by translating foreign medical texts. Gross left Philadelphia in 1830, but again became a colleague of Pancoast when he returned in autumn of 1856 as the Fourth Surgery Chairman at Jefferson.[7]

Pancoast had a flair for anatomy, aided by his natural love for dissection. As early as 1831 he offered private courses in anatomy along with his surgical practice. In his large classes of admiring students he made practical applications of anatomy to surgery as well as correlation with diagnosis and treatment of medical disease. In rented obscure rooms he acquired the fame as an excellent clinical teacher that led to his election as Chairman of Surgery at Jefferson in 1839. His hospitals up to that time were the Blockley (Philadelphia General) and its connected Children's Hospital, in which he was Head Physician.

Pancoast was regarded as the equal of George McClellan in the surgery of his day. McClellan

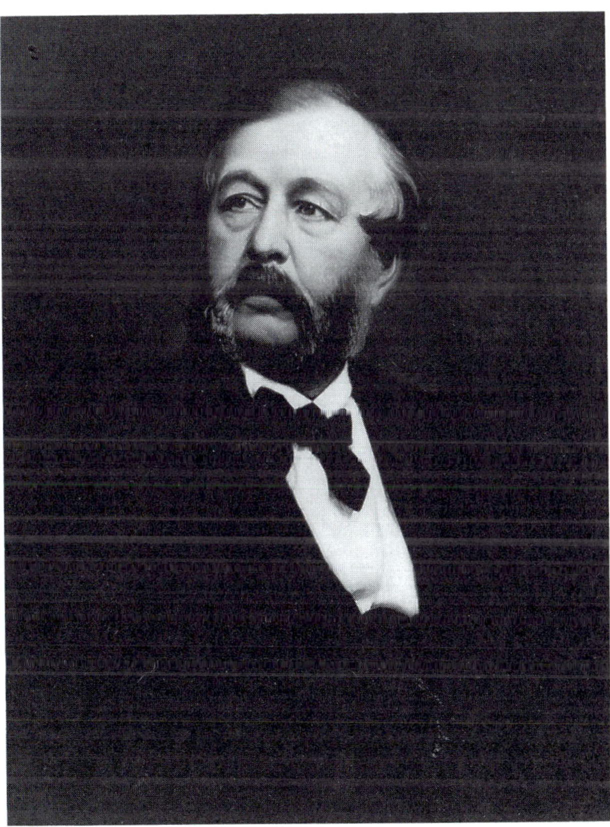

FIG. 32-5. Joseph Pancoast, M.D. (1805–1882); Second Chairman (1839–1841).

held the advantage of nine years' experience and clinical fame before Pancoast graduated. On the other hand, McClellan died relatively young (at age 51), and lacked the advantage of using general anesthesia that Pancoast had for at least two decades.

In contrast to McClellan who preceded him and Mütter who followed him, Pancoast was a prolific writer. In 1831 he published an annotated translation from the Latin of Lobstein's *Treatise on the Structure, Functions and Diseases of the Human Sympathetic Nerve.* In 1844 his chief work was *Treatise on Operative Surgery,* with a third edition in 1852, and a revised edition of Wistar's *System of Anatomy for the Use of Students.* He edited *Manec on the Great Sympathetic Nerve* and on the *Cerebrospinal System in Man,* and *Quain's Anatomical Plates.* He was, as well, a large contributor to the *American Journal of the Medical Sciences, The American Intelligencer,* the *Medical Examiner,* and author of pathological and surgical monographs, essays, and introductory lectures to his classes. He stopped writing during the last 15 years of his life, and, according to Samuel D. Gross, when spoken to on the subject he said he thought he had "done enough of that kind of work."

Pancoast performed diversified operations and developed original ones. He devised a type of rhinoplasty, procedures for soft and mixed cataracts and certain types of strabismus, drainage for empyema of the pleural cavity, use of an ivory tube for obstructed lacrimal drainage, cutting of the posterior muscles of the *velum palati* for unintelligible voice, a lumbar approach for drainage of retrocecal abscesses (probably appendiceal), and invented an abdominal tourniquet for compression of the lower aorta during hip and high thigh amputations. In 1862 he performed his original operation for extrophy of the urinary bladder. The height of his surgical fame was reached when Sir William Ferguson, the leader of English surgery, referred the daughter of Lord Chancellor Lyndhurst to Pancoast for plastic surgery for scars from burns of the face. In the flowery language of that era he was said "to have an eye as quick as a flashing sunbeam and a hand as light as floating perfume." This was despite the fact that Pancoast was portly, with hands that were "large and thick with immense blunt fingers; any other than a hand you would look upon as facile and dextrous, almost beyond belief."

Pancoast was a member of the American Philosophical Society, the Medical Society of Pennsylvania, and other scientific organizations.

In 1841, another reorganization of the faculty was ordered by the Board of Trustees. This became known as the "Famous Faculty of 1841" that lasted without change until 1856. In this setting, Joseph Pancoast was shifted to Chairman of General, Descriptive, and Surgical Anatomy, which position he held until 1874, when he was succeeded by his distinguished son, William Henry Pancoast. The latter became one of the founding fathers of the Philadelphia Academy of Surgery in 1879.

Joseph Pancoast was in all respects a worthy successor to George McClellan. His name is immortalized in operative surgery and anatomical teaching, in both of which he was a giant for more than 40 years (Figure 32-6). He worked harmoniously with his successor, Dr. Thomas Dent Mütter, as a true friend and strong right arm until Mütter's untimely death in 1859. He then continued with Samuel D. Gross until March 7, 1882, when he died, just two years before Gross, who submitted his resignation that same year

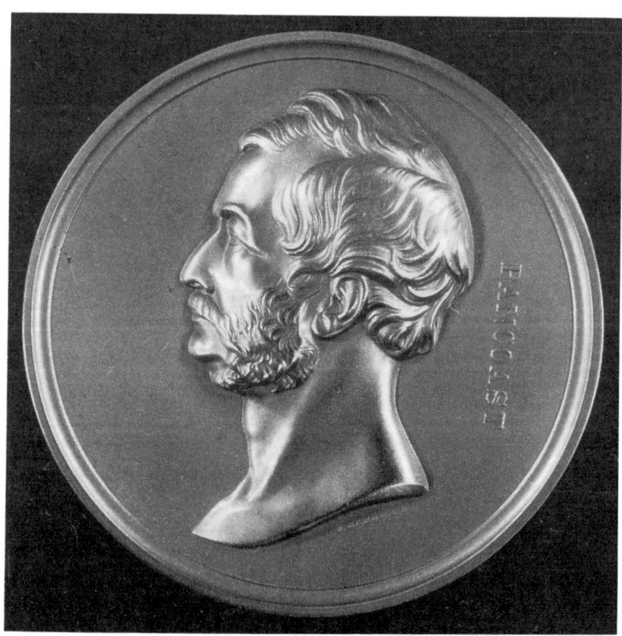

FIG. 32-6. Medal in honor of Joseph Pancoast, M.D., struck by the U.S. Mint in 1870.

because of ill health. Death was ascribed to a perforation of the intestine (most likely a complication of diverticulitis).

Thomas Dent Mütter, M.D., LL.D. (1811–1859); Third Chairman (1841–1856)

Although the Mütter Museum of the College of Physicians of Philadelphia (Figure 32-7) is well known to the scientific community, the Chairmanship for 15 years of Thomas Dent Mütter in Jefferson's famous Faculty of 1841 has remained obscure. The fame of the Museum as well as his surgical contemporaries (McClellan, Pancoast, and Gross) may account to some degree for this oversight.

Mütter (Figure 32-8) was born in Richmond, Virginia, on March 9, 1811, of German and Scottish ancestors who had settled in North Carolina before the Revolution. He was orphaned at the age of eight, but a relative saw to it that he had a good education in preparation for medicine. Like the two preceding Jefferson Surgery Chairmen, he received his M.D. degree from the University of Pennsylvania (1831) at the age of 20. Because of a lung problem he took to sea as a surgeon and subsequently studied in the best clinics of Europe. He became a Francophile for the remainder of his life and, excepting Pancoast, openly declared the superiority of French surgeons. He referred to Dupuytren, Louis, and Liston as his "friends."

Returning to Philadelphia after his year abroad, Mütter devoted himself to surgery and teaching. He achieved renown in the correction of orthopaedic deformities and in plastic surgery. This field included clubfoot, deformities from burns, and numerous other distortions both congenital and acquired. Antisepsis was still not used, but it is likely that a man as impeccable as Mütter was "clean" in his technique.

The honor of Chairman of the Surgery Department at Jefferson was conferred in 1841 on Mütter at the age of 30. Two Chairs of Surgery were considered by the Board of Trustees—Principles of Surgery and Practice of Surgery. Dr. Jacob Randolph of the Pennsylvania Hospital was offered one of the Chairs, but he declined on the basis that he could not accept this concept and did not wish to share a divided Chair. Nevertheless, 41 years later at the resignation of Samuel D. Gross (1882) the Chair did divide.

Mütter has the credit of being the first to introduce the Edinburgh "quizzing" system into this country. One more important first was his use of ethyl ether in Philadelphia, on December 23, 1846, within one month of Morton's announcement of his discovery. This was administered in the upper amphitheater of the Medical College that Gross, his successor, was to make so famous in the *Gross Clinic*. The first Jefferson Hospital was not to be built until 1877.

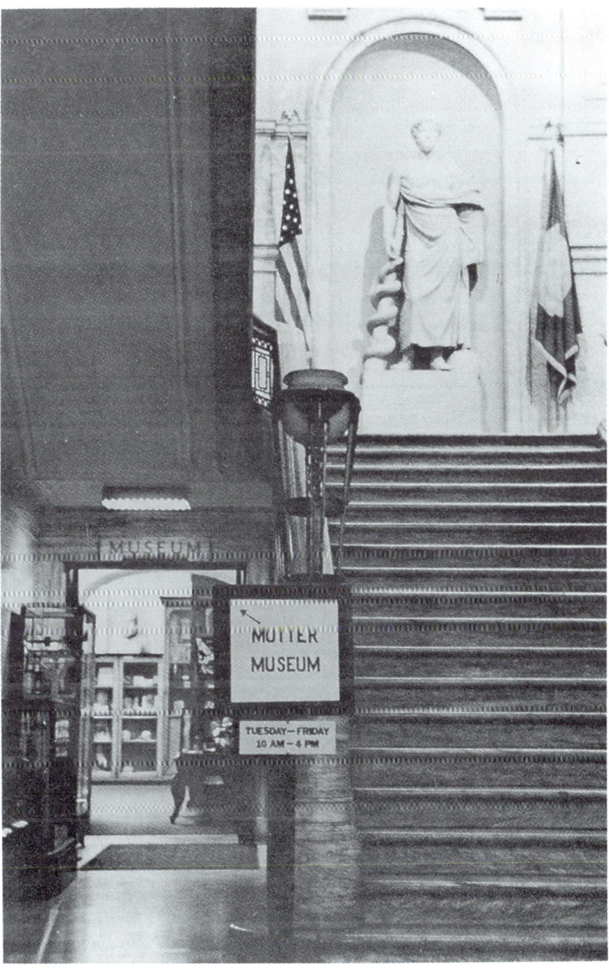

Fig. 32-7. Mütter Museum in the College of Physicians of Philadelphia.

Mütter and his predecessor, Pancoast, worked in perfect harmony, assisting each other in their operations. The association of these two made the "Clinic" so famous that it was usually crowded with practitioners from all parts of the country. The same Sir William Ferguson who had referred the Lord Chancellor's daughter to Pancoast said of Mütter: "The greatest success, before my own views were made public, was achieved by Mütter of Philadelphia, who operated successfully on nineteen out of twenty cases of hare lip."

Mütter, unlike Pancoast who preceded him and Gross who followed him, was not much of a writer. His main works were a monograph of 104 pages on *Club-Foot* (1839) and his editing of Liston's *Operations of Surgery* (1846).

Mütter was forced to resign his Chairmanship in 1856 because of worsening of his old lung trouble, now complicated by gout, but he was made an Emeritus Professor. A winter spent in Nice failed to restore his health. He spent the next winter in Charleston without benefit and died at the age of 48 on March 19, 1859.[8]

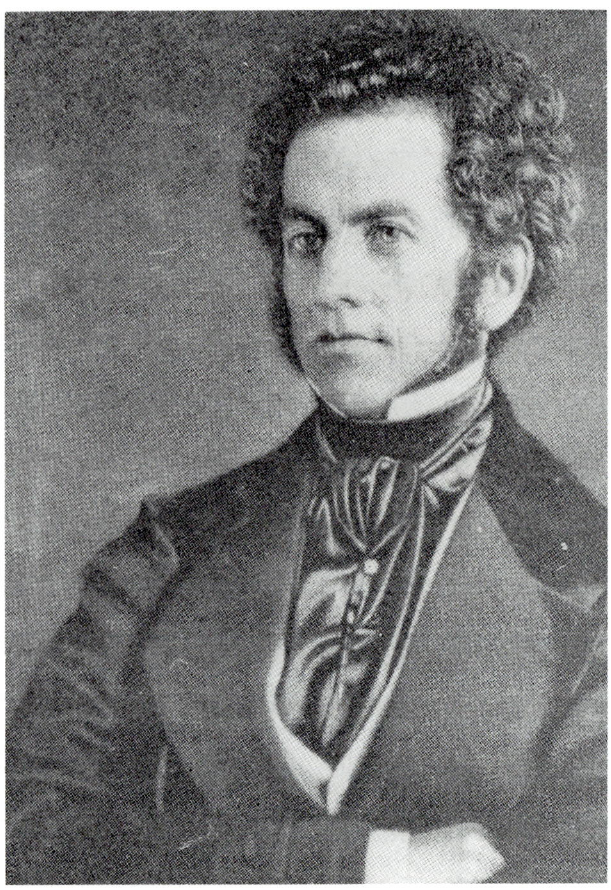

FIG. 32-8. Thomas Dent Mütter, M.D., LL.D. (1811–1859); Third Chairman (1841–1856).

The year before Mütter died he generously bequeathed his Museum to the College of Physicians of Philadelphia with an endowment of $30,000 for maintenance and a Lectureship in connection with it. The Museum is ideally housed for specimens, models, historical instruments, and as archives for unusual memorabilia from throughout the medical world. There is a constant enthusiastic educational activity in the Museum, which has served as his best monument.

Samuel D. Gross, M.D., LL.D., D.C.L. (1805–1884); Fourth Chairman (1856–1882)

The preceding three Chairmen had been graduates of the Medical School of the University of Pennsylvania. Samuel D. Gross (Figure 32-9) graduated from Jefferson Medical College in 1828 and was its first alumnus to be appointed to a Professorship. In succeeding Thomas Dent Mütter in 1856 he was the first replacement in the famous Faculty of 1841 with which his Chairmanship alone would create a new and separate era in Jefferson History. The triumvirate of Gross, Dunglison, and Pancoast gave Jefferson an unsurpassed prestige among medical schools of the time.

Gross was born on July 8, 1805, near Easton, Pennsylvania, on a 200-acre farm. He was the fifth of six children born to Philip and Juliana Gross. His siblings consisted of two sisters and three brothers. It was Pennsylvania Dutch country, where much of the Americanized German patois persists to this day. His great-grandfather had emigrated from the Lower Palatinate of Germany in the seventeenth century. Gross first attended school in a log cabin in which Pennsylvania Dutch was the native language and where both sexes and successive grades were taught in a single room. He first learned English after the age of 12 and carried a slight German accent for the rest of his life. Gross's mother was a devoted Lutheran and one of the brothers became the Reverend Joseph B. Gross of the Lutheran Church. The mother exerted a strong influence on the moral character and discipline of her son Samuel. The father died from a cerebral hemorrhage at the age of 56 when Gross was only nine. His mother lived to be 86 and died during the years at Louisville.

Gross states in his *Autobiography* that his thoughts of studying medicine started at the age of six and he felt himself always to be a "born doctor." As a self-motivated individual, Gross at age 14 became aware of the defects of his public school education. On his own he began to learn correct English, German, and Latin in preparation for apprenticeship to a medical preceptor. At the age of 17 he tried the offices of three physicians, the last being that of Dr. Joseph K. Swift of Easton, who had graduated from the University of Pennsylvania. Again realizing his inadequate education for the study of medicine, Gross made a solemn determination to remedy his ignorance at the highest possible level. This he accomplished by completing an excellent preparatory course at the famous Lawrenceville (New Jersey) Academy. By the age of 19 he had acquired a thorough knowledge of Latin and had studied Greek from a Latin grammar book and, in addition to proper German, learned French well enough to subsequently translate medical texts into English. After further study with Dr. Swift in Easton, he proceeded to Philadelphia in October, 1826, with a letter of recommendation from his mentor to matriculate at the University of Pennsylvania.

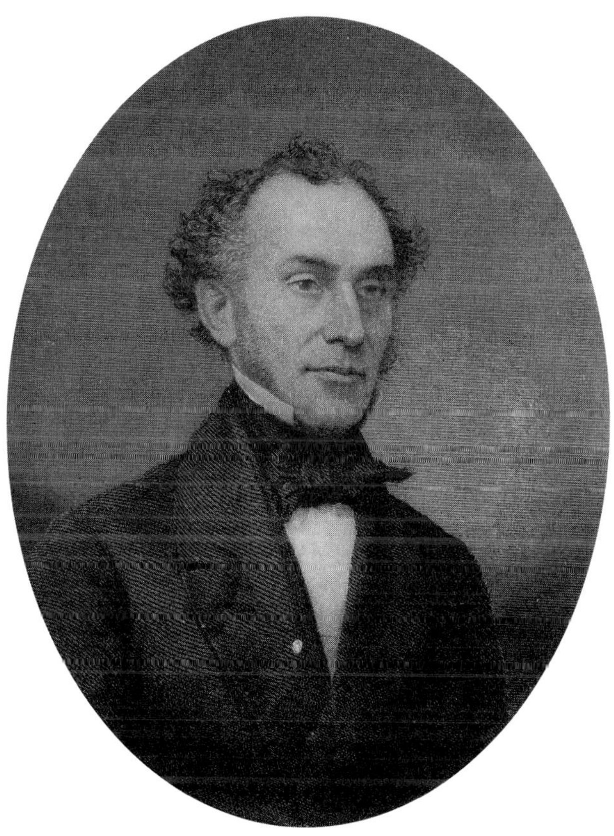

FIG. 32-9. Samuel D. Gross, M.D., LL.D., D.C.L. (1805–1884); Fourth Chairman (1856–1882).

Instead, Gross enrolled as a private student of George McClellan and then matriculated at Jefferson Medical College. He graduated in a class of 27 in 1828 in Jefferson's first Medical Hall, the renovated Tivoli Theater at 518–520 Prune Street (now Locust Walk). His thesis was *The Nature and Treatment of Cataract.* George McClellan delivered the address to the graduates of this third class. As on many other occasions, McClellan was ten minutes late, much to the annoyance of the Reverend Green, President of the Board of Trustees.

The record of Gross's performance as a medical student may be gleaned from his *Autobiography:*

> "I had not only industry, but ambition; my morals and habits were good, and I was a stranger to all amusements. Medicine was the goddess of my idolatry. When, therefore, the time for my examination arrived I had no misgivings in regard to the result. I had planted carefully, and believed that I should ultimately receive the reward of my industry. The thirty-five minutes which I spent in the 'Green Room' of my Alma Mater were amongst the happiest of my life, and I could not help giving expression to my feelings in the presence of my assembled teachers. Such, indeed, was my hilarity that McClellan, my private preceptor, who knew me intimately, was induced to ask me afterwards 'whether I had not been drinking?'—although he was well aware that I was one of the most temperate of youths, and as sober as a judge on the occasion in question. My examination, I had reason to believe, gave entire satisfaction."[9]

After graduation, Gross opened an office on Fifth Street opposite Independence Square, but had difficulty in establishing a private practice. It was mainly through translating foreign textbooks into English that he covered his living expenses. During the first year he translated Bayle and Hollard's *General Anatomy* and Hatin's *Manual of Practical Obstetrics* from the French. The second year he translated Tavernier's *Operative Surgery* from French and Hildenbrand's *Treatise on Contagious Typhus* from German. This experience taught him the writing of textbooks, which he thereafter applied throughout life in prolific contributions to American surgical literature.

This industrious man somehow found time to fall deeply in love and marry a 21-year old widow, Louisa Ann Weissel, the year he graduated. She shared his early financial frustrations and afforded him nearly 48 years of happy family life. Their four surviving children out of eight were endowed with intellectual superiority. Samuel W. (the younger Gross) succeeded his father in surgery at Jefferson, and A. Haller became a successful Philadelphia lawyer. Maria and Louisa were accomplished ladies who married two brothers, both lawyers, from Baltimore. Maria endowed the Gross Professorship in 1910 in honor of her father. It was the first such endowment at Jefferson.

Lack of success in practice forced Gross to move to Easton in 1830. There he promptly gained respect and prominence. In the rear garden of his home he erected a small stone building for experimentation on dogs and cats as well as for dissection of cadavers he obtained from Philadelphia by horse and buggy. Within three months of arrival he completed his first original textbook, *Anatomy, Physiology, and Diseases of the Bones and Joints.* This volume of 400 pages sold 2,000 copies but yielded no remuneration to the author.

Gross encountered debt in Philadelphia and mediocrity in Easton. In the spring of 1833 he contacted his former Professor of Medicine at Jefferson, Dr. John Eberle, who by then was lecturing in the Medical College of Ohio at Cincinnati. Through the latter's recommendation Gross obtained the appointment of Demonstrator of Anatomy, in which capacity he taught for the next two years. In 1835 the school reorganized as the Medical Department of Cincinnati College, and Gross obtained the Chair of Pathological Anatomy. This provided the basis for his next textbook on *Elements of Pathological Anatomy* (1838), which was the first systematic work on this subject on either side of the Atlantic. It won the admiration of Dr. Rudolf Virchow, the famous German pathologist, and eventually led to his honorary membership in the Imperial Royal Society of Vienna.

Gross turned down an offer of the Chair of Anatomy at the University of Louisiana as well as the Professorship of Medicine at the University of Virginia to accept the Professorship of Surgery in 1840 at the Louisville (Kentucky) Medical Institute, later the University of Louisville. At the age of 35 he had attained his ultimate goal.

Gross spent 16 fruitful years at Louisville, from October 1840 to September 1856. Promptly he started his investigations on the nature and treatment of wounds of the intestines and conducted experiments on more than 70 dogs over a period of two years. Gross refers to the irritation felt by some of the faculty members over the numerous fleas on hot autumn days. The Professor of Chemistry had to appear in class with high boots for protection of his legs. This was one of the first exhaustive pieces of animal research for clinical purposes done in the United States. Gross had to obtain his own dogs and pay a caretaker on an income that year of less than $2,000. In 1843 the work was published in a book entitled *Wounds of the Intestines.*

It is well to recall that Gross was also an eminent urologist. An authoritative *Practical Treatise on the Diseases, Injuries, and Malformations of the Urinary Bladder, the Prostate Gland, and the Urethra* was published in 1851. It was an octavo volume of 925 pages with 184 woodcuts. In the Appendix he presented the first attempt in urologic literature to report the prevalence of stone in the bladder and of calculous disorders in the United States, Canada, Europe, and other countries. His operation of lateral lithotomy, for which he was well known, is described thoroughly in the book. A knife with which he performed more than 40 of these procedures is in the Jefferson Archives (Figure 32-10).

The indefatigable Gross never finished one project before starting another. In 1854 he issued his *Practical Treatise on Foreign Bodies in the Air Passages,* which had been two years in the making. It was a pioneer work, attempting to systematize all current knowledge upon this subject. The book, which consisted of 468 pages and 159 woodcuts, gave full reports of 200 cases. It was to be made obsolete by the later work of Chevalier

Jackson to whom Jefferson again lays proud claim.

In 1850 there was a controversy at Louisville regarding the administration of the Medical School. Apparently never without offers, Gross was induced to accept the Chair of Surgery in the University of New York, just vacated by the retirement of the prestigious Valentine Mott, often referred to as "the Father of Modern Vascular Surgery." That winter, relieved of his large private practice, he visited surgical clinics and devoted much time to writing. In reality this turned out to be a sabbatical year. After serving for only one academic session, and before having time to build another private practice, the problem of management in the Louisville school was corrected. He was implored by his old colleagues to return to his former post. His successor, Dr. Paul F. Eve, graciously and gladly stepped aside for him.

The years that Gross spent in Louisville were among the happiest of his life. He found time to cultivate close relations with his fellow Kentuckians despite his large practice, teaching, and literary work. He was beloved, trusted, and popular with patients, colleagues, and nonprofessional friends. His beautiful home provided true Southern hospitality for distinguished men and women both American and foreign. His wife was a charming hostess, who kept an ample table ready at all times for reunions in which "the strains of music mingled with flashes of wit and humor." He had planned to spend the rest of his days in Louisville. Fate was to decree otherwise, for two schools in Philadelphia were about to tempt him to another Professorship.

In 1855 Gross was solicited by Dr. Rene LaRoche, a member of the Board of Trustees of the University of Pennsylvania, to allow his name to be placed as a candidate for the Chair of Surgery vacated by the resignation of Dr. William Gibson, a former bitter rival of Dr. George McClellan. Gross was assured that the entire

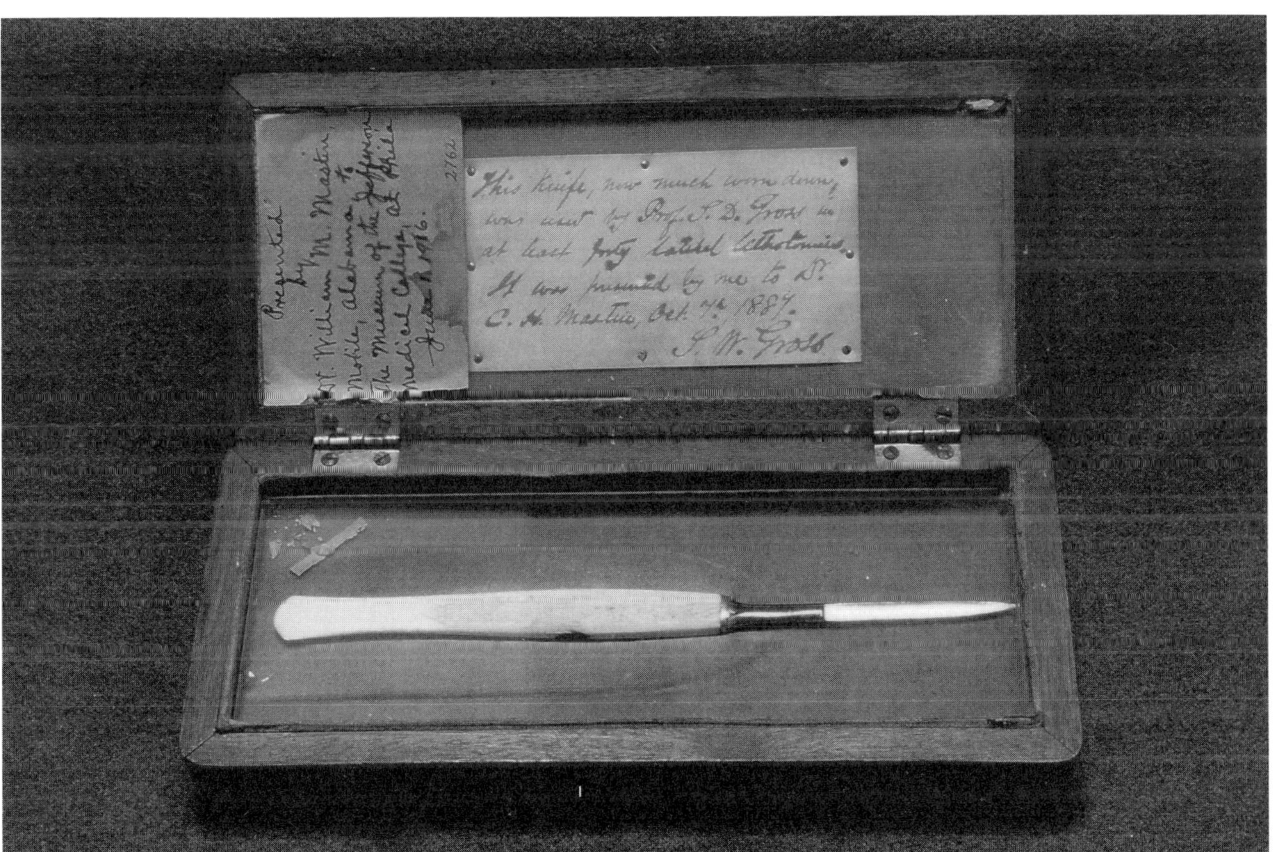

FIG. 32-10. Lateral lithotomy knife of Professor S.D. Gross, authenticated by the younger Gross in 1887.

Medical Faculty, with the exception of Dr. George Bacon Wood, had pledged themselves to support him and would use their best endeavors to secure his election. Various reasons, not the least of which were financial, induced him to decline, and he wrote a warm testimonial in favor of Dr. Henry Hollingsworth Smith, who was elected.

Upon the resignation of the Professorship of Surgery by Dr. Mütter in 1856, Gross received an offer to fill the vacancy. It was an honor from his alma mater that he could not refuse. After a preliminary visit to Philadelphia during which he found Jefferson flourishing, he moved his family in September of that year. For two years he rented Mütter's furniture and house at the southeast corner of Eleventh and Walnut Streets (now the site of the Martin Residence Building) at $2,000 annually. He then purchased the building for $25,000 and added another $2,000 for renovations. During the first winter in Philadelphia (December 24, 1856), Gross was handed a telegram informing him that the University of Louisville had been totally consumed by fire, including all of his books. This amounted to a loss of approximately 2,000 volumes of the finest and most extensive collection of books on the genitourinary organs that had ever been collected in the United States. They had not been insured. Fortunately, another 2,000 of his books had been previously brought to Philadelphia.

In coming to Jefferson as the fourth Chairman, Gross had to compete with the reputation that his idolized predecessor, Mütter, had acquired for charm, teaching, and surgical skill. Gross had visited the Mütter Clinic during his brief Professorship in New York in 1850 and paid it high tribute. Almost immediately, however, Gross became even more popular than Mütter. Students responded with profound respect for his lectures and operations. The growing fame of the Gross Clinic attracted visitors from home and abroad. In 1860 a group of Japanese doctors visited his clinic. It is believed that these were the first ever to visit a clinic in a foreign country.[10]

Several years before leaving Kentucky, Gross started his *System of Surgery,* which was to be the most complete treatise of its kind in the English language. The first edition appeared in 1859 and went through six editions, with updating each time, the last in 1882, only 17 months before his death. The initial work consisted of two octavo volumes to a total of 2,360 pages with 936 wood engravings. Two thousand copies were printed. It was translated into several European languages and spread his fame as well as that of Jefferson throughout the world. The Japanese used the Dutch translation to retranslate the section about the ears for their first reference book on otology. Later, the entire book was translated into Japanese from the German.

In 1861, at the start of the Civil War, Gross wrote a *Manual of Military Surgery* in the incredible period of nine days, with publication two weeks later. For preparation, he visited the battlefield at Shiloh, Tennessee, and examined the wounded on government steamboats at Pittsburg Landing. The book was promptly republished in Richmond in a "pirated edition" for the Confederate Army (Figure 32-11). It became the only mutual communication in the strife between the North and the South. It was retranslated from German into Japanese in 1874.

In the same year (1861), Gross, as a prolific medical historian, edited his *Lives of Eminent American Physicians and Surgeons of the Nineteenth Century.* It contained an account of the life and work of 32 outstanding American physicians and surgeons. His own contribution consisted of sketches of Drs. Ephraim McDowell, Daniel Drake, and John Syng Dorsey. It is an octavo volume of some 800 pages; few copies remain extant, but one can be found in Jefferson's Special Collections of the Scott Library.

Several years later, Gross published *A Full Account of Special Surgery on Diseases and Injuries of Particular Organs, Textures, and Regions,* the fifth edition being issued in 1872. In 1876, for the United States Centennial, he wrote the section on Surgery in the *American Journal of the Medical Sciences* entitled *A Century of American Medicine, 1776–1876.* It is a masterful historical document of 100 pages. Gross, in 1881, at age 76, gave the First Annual Oration of the Philadelphia Academy of Surgery, which he founded in 1879 and of which he was the first President. It was a *Memoir of John Hunter and His Pupils,* published subsequently in book form.

A final gift to posterity and to Jefferson lore was made by Gross in his two-volume autobiography. He began this 1,000-page

Autobiography of Samuel D. Gross, M.D., with Reminiscences of His Times and Contemporaries about 15 years before his death, with the last entry on February 14, 1884. It was published in 1887 by his two sons, Samuel W. and A. Haller, with a memoir by his lifelong friend, Dr. Austin Flint. Gross stated that his reason for writing it was for the gratification of his family and the medical profession. It was his hope that "the devotion which I have shown to my profession may, perhaps, exert a salutary influence upon the conduct of young physicians, and thus serve to inspire them with a desire to excel in good deeds." According to Dr. Flint it remains as a superb portrayal of the life, times, and labors of "one who is declared to have been perhaps the most eminent exponent of medical science that America has yet produced."

In addition to the 14 books that Gross wrote, edited, and translated are more than 1,200 articles and case reports compiled in his bibliography at Jefferson. In them this extraordinary writer revealed his original thinking and vast experience. Generally, he devoted five to eight hours a day to his cherished projects, regardless of what else he had to do. Large portions were composed while riding about the city for his daily professional calls.

With the veneration that we hold for Gross today, it is hard to believe what an abysmal state the practice of medicine and surgery was in during his lifetime. Gross himself was aware of it, tried to improve it, and expressed his expectations for the future. Early in his career physicians bled, administered emetics, purged, and starved their patients. Ether was used at Jefferson shortly after its discovery (1846), but not until Gross was 41 years of age and still at Louisville. At Jefferson,

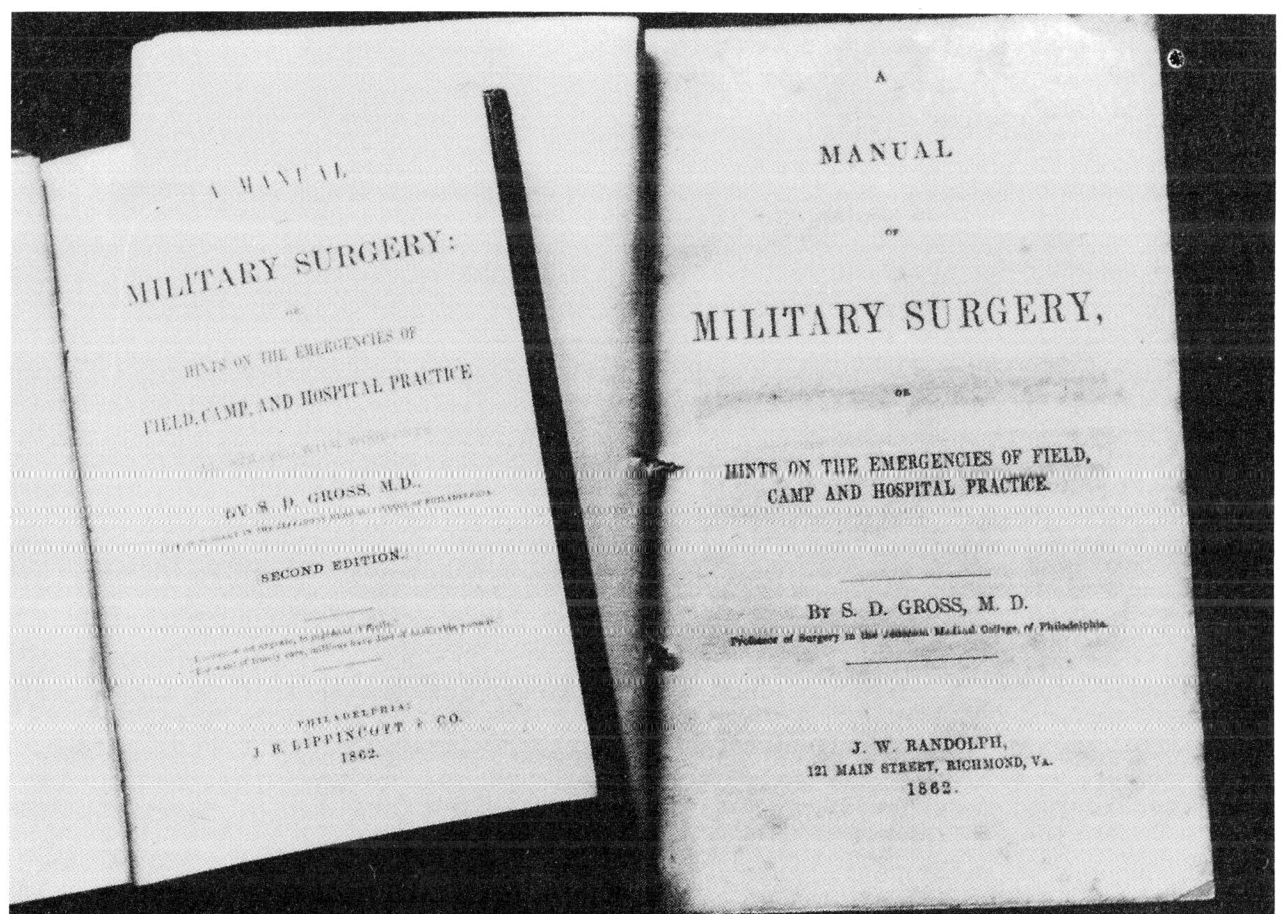

FIG. 32-11. Gross's *Manual of Military Surgery* (1861); the "pirated edition" is at the right.

Gross was often heard to say to his orderly: "Hugh (O'Donnell), get me a tumbler of laudable pus for my lecture tomorrow morning." In the 1860s and 1870s in the miniature College hospital of only 15 beds (before the first detached hospital was built in 1877) pus was always on tap. Its formation was considered as a stage in normal wound healing. One has only to look at Eakins' portrait of the *Gross Clinic* to observe what precautions were not taken against infection.

Gross thought of himself as a physician first and a surgeon second. He enjoyed a large family practice, with much of his consultations of a strictly nonsurgical character. Throughout his long career he met, entertained, or was entertained by six United States Presidents—Jackson, Harrison, Fillmore, Buchanan, Johnson, and Grant. Andrew Jackson consulted him in 1859 for ankylosis of the left elbow. Gross's advice was to leave well enough alone. Gross twice enjoyed private audiences with the widow Polk.

Apart from authorship, Gross made many contributions to surgical technique. Most of these have become so modified through the years that his name is no longer associated with them, while the instruments he devised are now obsolete. Nevertheless, to do justice to his inventive mind, a partial listing of these follows:

- Use of stay sutures to prevent wound dehiscence
- Tracheotomy forceps for extraction of foreign bodies from the air passages
- Wiring the ends of the bones in dislocations of the sternoclavicular and acromioclavicular joints
- Special catheter for draining urine when mixed with blood
- Forceps for arterial compression to arrest hemorrhage from deep-seated vessels
- Tourniquet for compression of vessels of the extremities during amputation
- Instrument for extraction of foreign bodies from the nose and ear (for many years found in doctors' house-call bags throughout the country)
- Modification of Pirogoff's amputation at the ankle joint
- Enterotome for treatment of artificial anus
- Laparotomy for rupture of the urinary bladder
- Direct operation for hernia by suturing the pillars of the external ring
- Operative correction of ingrown toenail
- Use of adhesive plaster for skin traction in treating fractures of the lower extremities
- Treatment of ganglia of the hand or foot by subcutaneous division of the cyst
- Amputation in senile gangrene at a great distance from the process
- Suturing the accidentally divided tendon of the hand

Professor Gross's surgical instruments are shown in Figures 32-12 and 32-13. On March 28, 1882, nearing 77 years of age, Dr. Gross resigned his Chair, whereupon he was unanimously elected Emeritus Professor. He was in full possession of his intellectual powers but now felt the desire to spend his declining years in comparative repose. He had been a widower for the previous six years, his wife Louisa having died after a lingering illness in 1876. Fortunately, his son Samuel W. married Grace Linzee Revere in that same Centennial year and brought this lady into the household at Eleventh and Walnut Streets to continue the tradition of open door and ever-ample table.

Dr. Gross enjoyed a too-short period of good health before his final illness. During the autumn of 1883 he began to experience epigastric distress, swollen feet, and other signs of congestive heart failure. A week's visit to Atlantic City in early April, 1884, was without benefit. Despite the devoted care by Dr. Jacob Mendes DaCosta and Gross's son, Professor Samuel W., aided in consultation by his distinguished friend, Professor Austin Flint, he died on May 6. A postmortem examination performed by Dr. J. M. DaCosta disclosed marked gastric mucosal inflammation, fatty heart, and a large cyst on the right kidney.

Gross was a strong advocate of urn burial, believing cremation to be the most sanitary way of disposing of the body. This was accomplished in Dr. Lemoyne's crematory in Washington, Pennsylvania, one of the few in America at the time. The ashes were placed in the family grave at Woodlands Cemetery in West Philadelphia, next to his wife (Figure 32-14). None of the other Gross relatives underwent cremation.

The "Nestor of American Surgery," who religiously practiced his motto "It is better to wear out than to rust out," published *The Value of Early Operations in Morbid Growths* and *The Best Means of Training Nurses for Rural Districts* in 1883. He wrote until the very end; a paper entitled *Wounds of the Intestines* was read on May 8, 1884, before the American Medical Association two days after he died.

Gross was a master of organization who was deeply involved in membership, founding, and holding office in many societies at all levels. His local societies consisted of the Kentucky State Medical Society (a Founder and President); the Philadelphia Pathological Society (a Founder and first President, 1857); the Medical Jurisprudence Society of Philadelphia (a Founder); the Pennsylvania State Medical Society (President, 1870), the Jefferson Alumni Association (Founder and first President, 1870); and the Philadelphia Academy of Surgery (Founder and first President, 1879).

National societies to which he belonged were the American Medical Association (President, 1867); the American Surgical Association (Founder and first President, 1880); the American Philosophical Society (President); the American Academy of Sciences (President); and the Teacher's Medical Convention, at which he presided in Washington, D.C., in 1870.

Among international societies were the World Medical Congress (President, 1876); the Imperial Medical Society of Vienna; the Medical Society of Christiana of Norway; the Royal Medical and Chirurgical Society of London; the Medical Society of Vienna; the Medical Society of London; the Medico-Chirurgical Society of Edinburgh; the British Medical Association (twice Delegate); and the Royal Society of Medicine of Belgium.

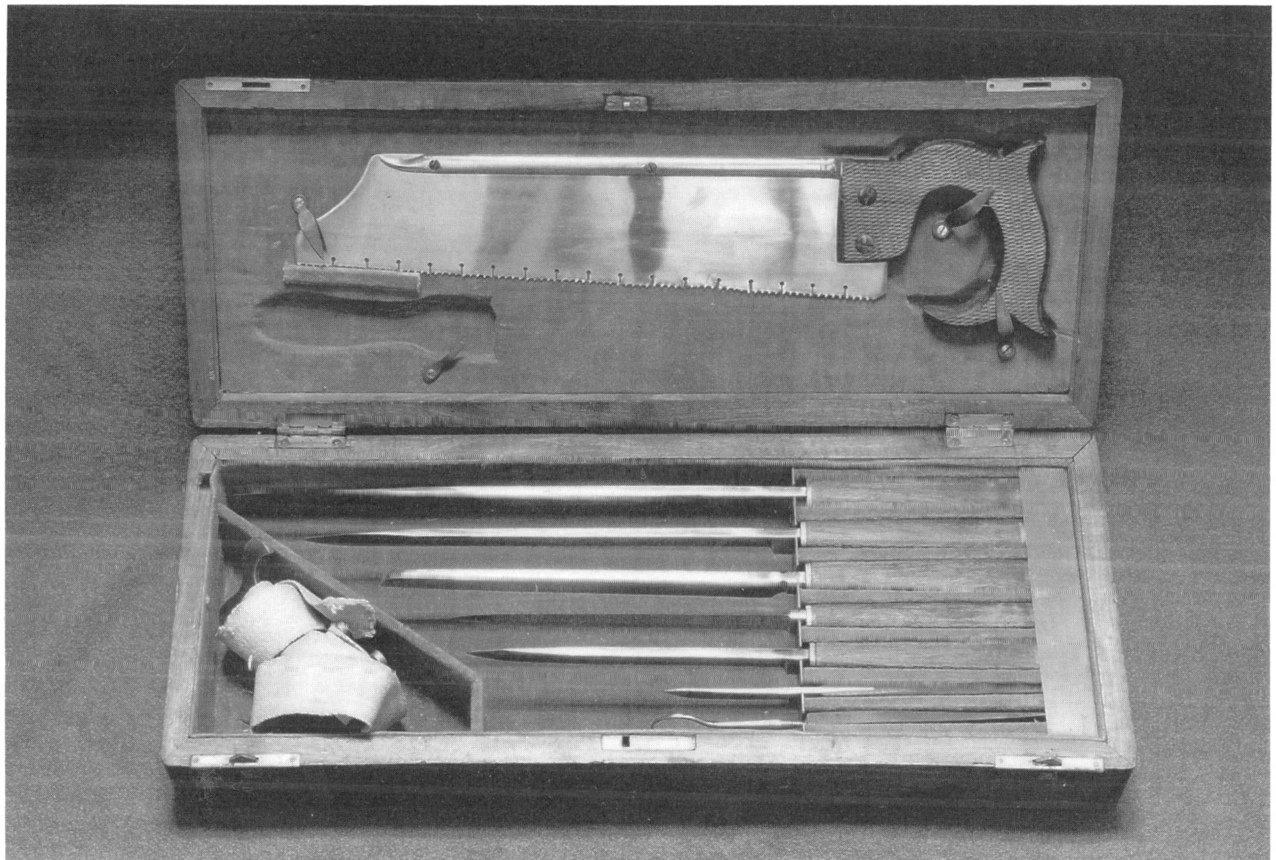

FIG. 32-12. Amputation instruments used by Professor S.D. Gross.

Gross received honors from governments, universities, and societies, both before and after his death. They constitute a formidable list: his portrait by Samuel Bell Waugh (Figure 32-15); the renowned portrait of the *Gross Clinic* by Thomas Eakins (Figure 32-16); his name in mosaic in the ceiling of the Library of Congress (Figure 32-17); a Gross statue (Figures 32-18 and 32-19); honorary degrees (LL.D. in 1861 from Jefferson College at Canonsburg; D.C.L. in 1872 from Oxford; LL.D. in 1880 from Cambridge; LL.D. in 1884 from Edinburgh; and LL.D. in 1884 from the University of Pennsylvania); the Gross Room and Endowed Library in the College of Physicians of Philadelphia; the Gross Prize of the Philadelphia Academy of Surgery; and the Gross Professorship of Surgery at Jefferson endowed by his daughter, Maria Gross Horwitz. Within the Department of Surgery at Jefferson, a Samuel D. Gross Distinguished Service Award was created in 1979, and a Gross Conference Room on the sixth floor of the College was dedicated in 1982.

The Gross College of Medicine

In 1887 the Gross Medical College was started in Denver, Colorado, when a group of doctors united to form a rival medical school to the Denver Medical College of the University of Denver.[11] They chose the name of Gross to honor Jefferson's distinguished Professor of Surgery, Samuel D. Gross (Figures 32-20 and 32-21). The College was moderately successful, and the announcement each year claimed that "few medical colleges in the United States have better facilities for teaching than Gross." It edited a monthly periodical, *The Gross Medical College Bulletin,*

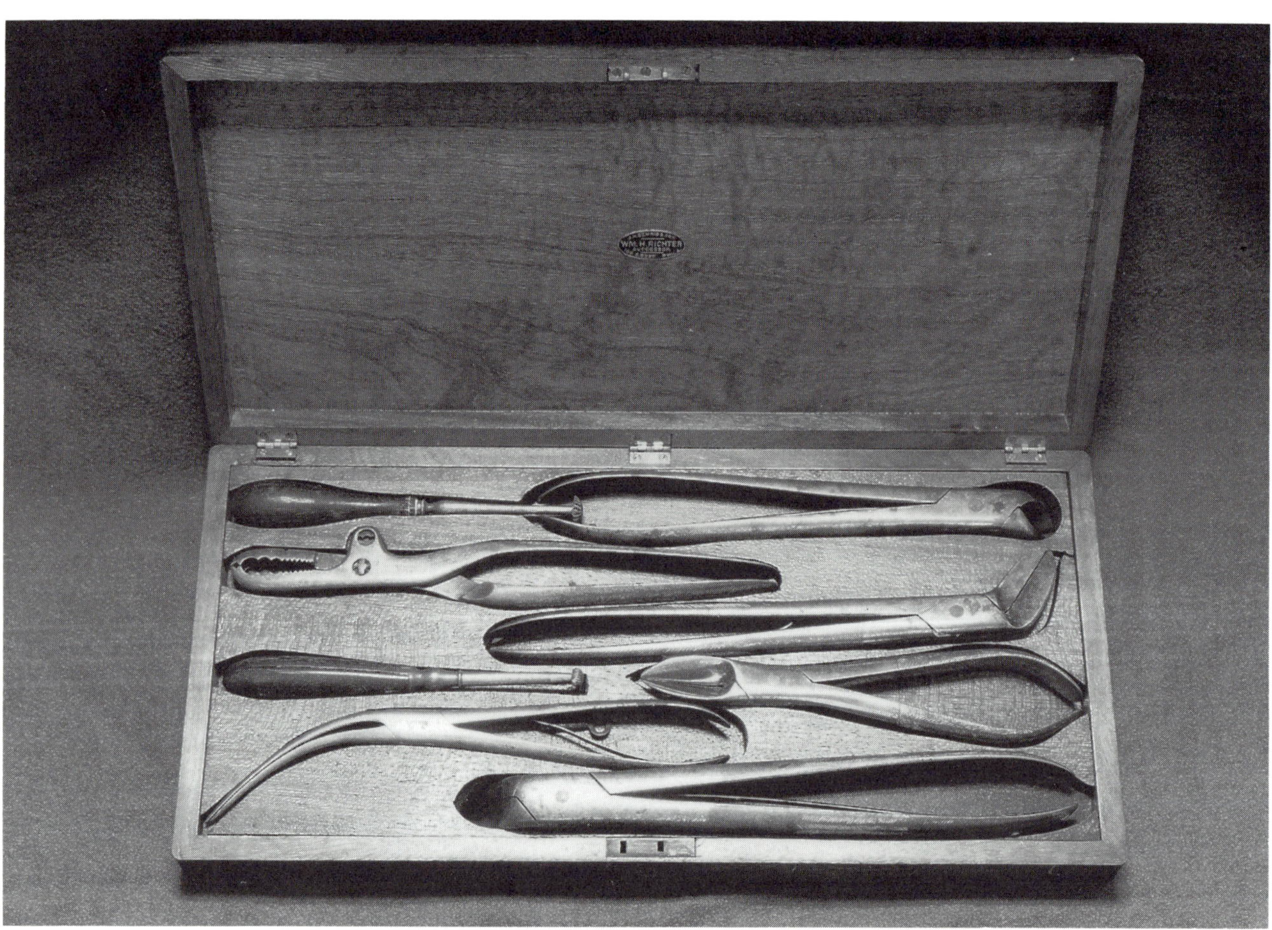

FIG. 32-13. Bone instruments used by Professor S.D. Gross.

which during six annual volumes commented on local medical conditions. In 1902 the Gross College merged with the Denver Medical College, and at the recommendation of the Flexner Report of the Carnegie Foundation for the Advancement of Teaching, the Gross and Denver Colleges in 1910 consolidated with the University of Colorado School of Medicine.

A fitting conclusion may be taken from Dr. J. Chalmers DaCosta, the first Samuel D. Gross Professor, when he wrote that he "beheld the mighty leader a great many times, heard him lecture frequently, and watched him operate, and in him always saw the embodiment of surgical learning, dignity, and distinction, and felt that fifty years of American Surgery were speaking through his lips."[12]

■ The Chair of Surgery Divides (1882–1956)

As early as 1841 the Board of Trustees had approved the concept of splitting the Chair of Surgery into the Principles of Surgery and the Practice of Surgery. At the time of Thomas Dent Mütter's appointment (1841), the second Chair was refused by Dr. Jacob Randolph of the Pennsylvania Hospital because he could not reconcile a difference between principles and practice, along with personal reasons for not wishing to share a divided Chair. The issue remained dormant when Samuel D. Gross was appointed in 1856 but became a reality at his

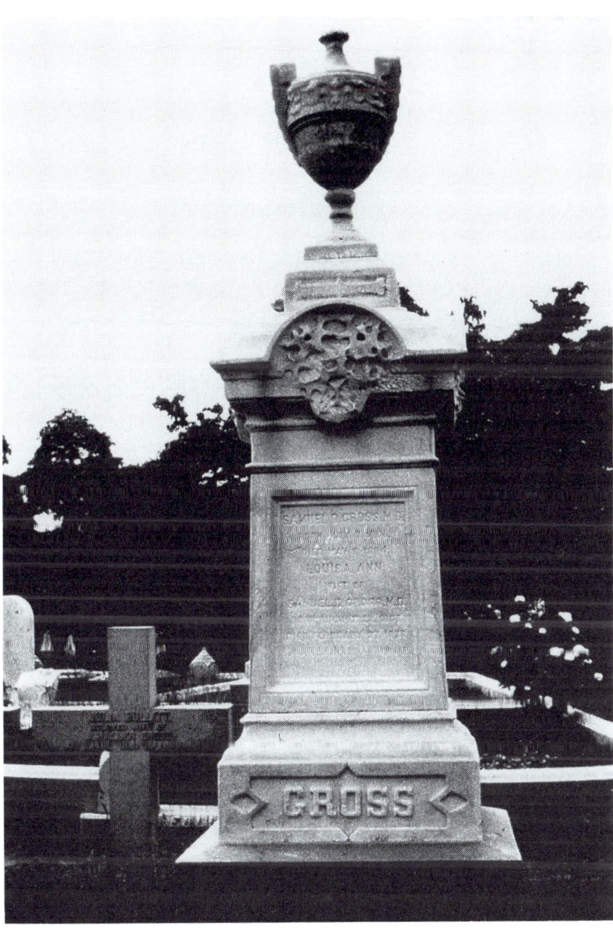

FIG. 32-14. Gross family gravesite in Woodlands Cemetery. (Photograph courtesy of Professor Francis E. Rosato.)

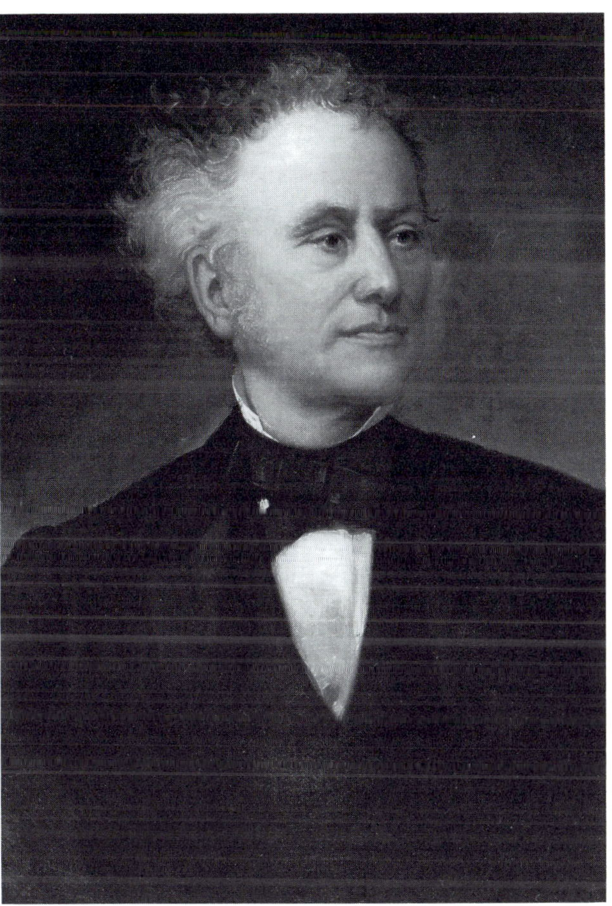

FIG. 32-15. Portrait of Samuel D. Gross, M.D., by Samuel Bell Waugh, commissioned by the Alumni Association in 1874.

retirement in 1882. The Medical College was still proprietary, with fees being paid to the Professors for their individual lectures. This was a transitional period in which science was enhancing the art of medicine and greatly expanding the amount of material to be covered. It was a stark necessity that it required "two pegs to fill one hole." Because each Chair would include Clinical Surgery, there was no need to define the boundaries between principles and practice. Two Jefferson graduates were already on its Hospital Staff and equally well qualified academically and clinically for the posts. In addition, they were boon companions. One was Samuel Weissel Gross (Jefferson, 1857), son of the elder Gross, who was appointed Professor of Principles of Surgery and Clinical Surgery. The other was John Hill Brinton (Jefferson, 1852), who was appointed Professor of Practice of Surgery and Clinical Surgery.

Precedent at Jefferson for son succeeding the father had been set in 1874 when William Henry Pancoast succeeded the eminent Joseph Pancoast as Professor of Anatomy. The succession of the younger Gross to the divided Chair of his world-renowned father raised no cry of political

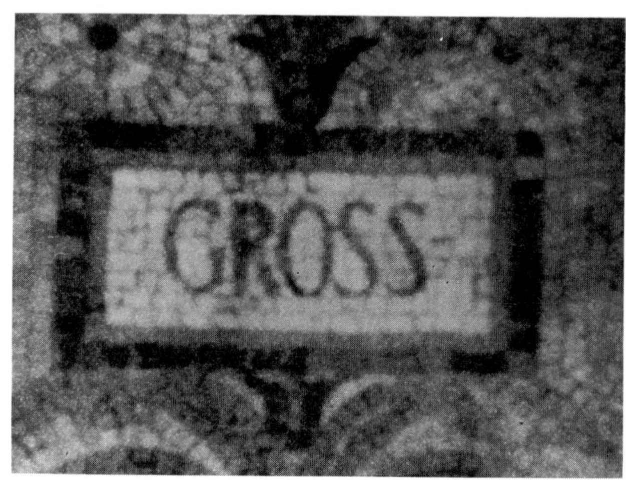

FIG. 32-17. The name of Gross in mosaic in the ceiling of the Library of Congress.

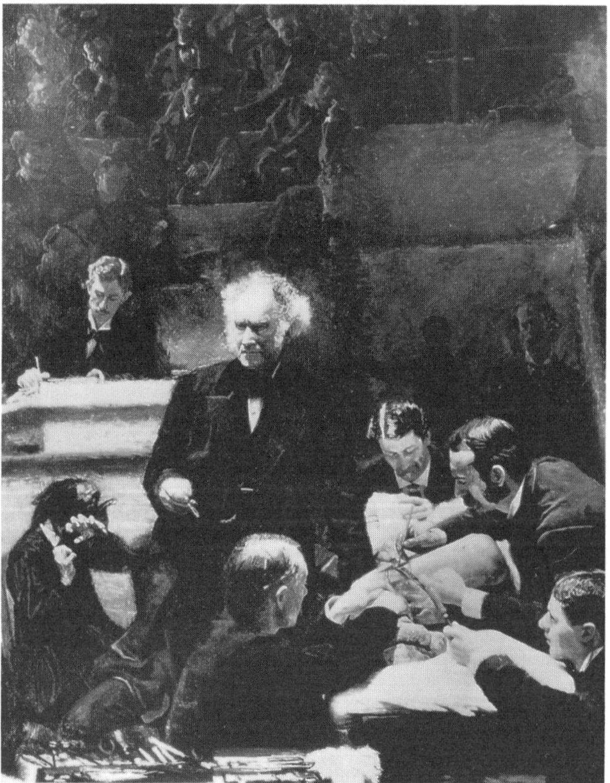

FIG. 32-16. The *Gross Clinic,* painted by Thomas Eakins (1875), considered by many as the greatest masterpiece of American art.

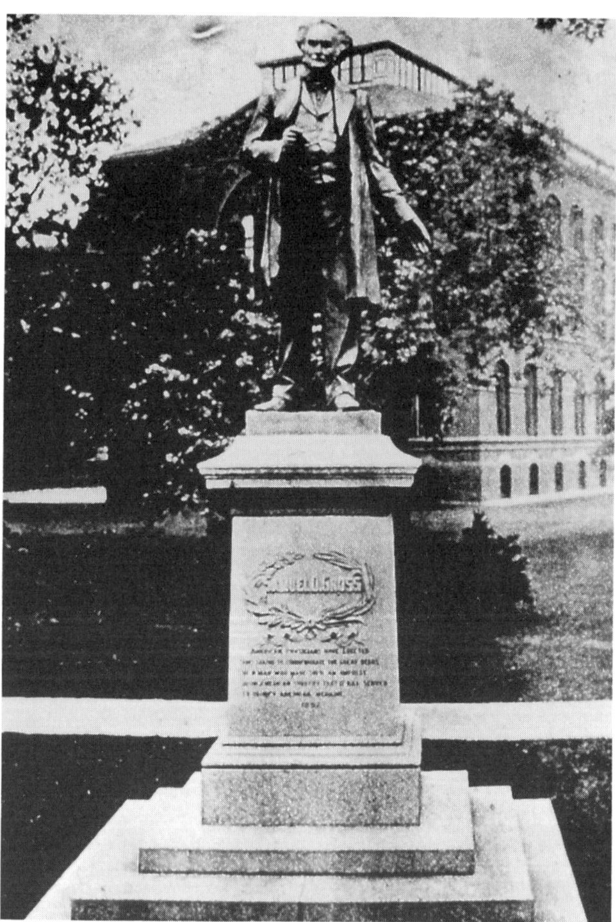

FIG. 32-18. The Gross statue in Smithsonian Park, Washington, D.C., (1897) was moved to Jefferson's Scott Plaza in 1970.

favoritism, and his worthiness remained undoubted. Later Chairmanships of the senior and junior Gibbon proved again that the Board always chose wisely and without interference. It would take 74 years, until 1956, for the divided Chair to once again become unified.

Samuel Weissel Gross, M.D., LL.D. (1837–1889); Fifth Chairmanship (Co-Chairman, 1882–1889)

Samuel W. Gross (Figure 32-22), the eldest son of the famed Samuel D. Gross, was born in Cincinnati, February 4, 1837. He received his preliminary education in Shelby College, Kentucky, and his first year of courses in medicine began in the Medical Department of the University of Louisville, where his father was the Professor of Surgery. When the family moved to Philadelphia, he transferred to Jefferson Medical College, from which he received his M.D. degree in March, 1857.

The younger Gross entered into private practice and under the influence of his father devoted much time to teaching and pathological research. He also aided his father in editing the *North American Medico-Chirurgical Review*. At the outbreak of the Civil War in 1861 he entered the Medical Corps of the Volunteer Service as a Brigade Surgeon with the rank of Major. Most of his duty was as Medical Director in various Military Departments of the country. He was mustered out in June 1865 and the following year received the brevet of Lieutenant-Colonel for his efficient service. The sword he carried may be seen in the College of Physicians of Philadelphia (Figure 32-23). His father dedicated a *Manual of Military Surgery* to him.

At the conclusion of the war, the younger Gross returned to Philadelphia to continue his private practice and to lecture at Jefferson on Genito-Urinary Diseases and General Surgery in the summer courses that started in 1866. Active in clinical surgery, he joined the staff of the Howard Hospital, the Philadelphia Hospital, and the first Hospital Staff of Jefferson in 1877. Early on he evidenced a strong interest in tumors and examined all his own operative specimens under the microscope. He was one of the ten cofounders of the Philadelphia Academy of Surgery in 1879, which today is the oldest of its kind in the United States, and was named the histologist for that organization.

In 1876 the younger Gross at age 39 still found time, in spite of his intense professional activities, to be a "gentleman about town." Greater stability and stimulus to his academic career was added in that year by his marriage to Grace Linzee Revere, the great-granddaughter of the Revolutionary Period patriot. At age 22, and 17 years younger than her husband, she was a welcomed member into the Gross household at Eleventh and Walnut Streets in which Mrs. Samuel D. Gross had died just ten months previously. Grace's Bostonian social and cultural background, coupled with a

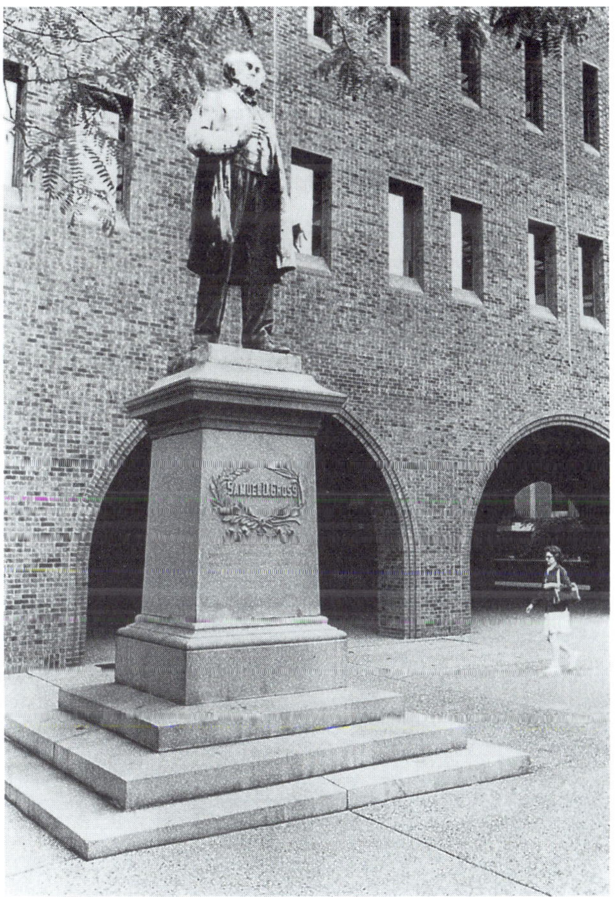

FIG. 32-19. The Gross statue moved to Scott Plaza in 1970.

warm and giving personality, continued the tradition of Gross hospitality. The younger Gross's best literary contributions dated from the time of his marriage: editing of his father's work on *Diseases, Injuries, etc., of the Urinary Bladder* (1876); a *Treatise on Tumors of the Mammary Gland* (1880); *Disorders of the Male Sexual Organs* (1881); and aiding in later editions of his father's *System of Surgery*. He also contributed highly respected editorial articles of a practical nature in the *Medical News*.

In the Professorship of Principles of Surgery and Clinical Surgery of the 1882 divided Chair, Samuel W. Gross immediately commanded the respect and close attention of the students. As an articulate lecturer with a clear strong voice, his opinions were accepted as authoratative. He emphasized to the profession that veins, just as arteries, could be ligated with perfect safety. He was the first American surgeon to advocate extensive operations for cancer of the breast and shares with Halsted the principle of operating for cure. His mastectomy was so wide that he called it "the dinner plate operation," which left a large unclosed wound. At a meeting in which an objection was raised that the granulations in such a large open wound would reproduce cancer, he said: "When oak trees produce polar bears and when fireplugs produce whales, then will granulations produce cancer, and not until then."[13]

Dr. Gross was prominent in local, state and national medical societies. He was President of the Pathological Society of Philadelphia (1879); Vice-President of the Philadelphia Academy of Surgery (1884), which he helped to found; a member of the County and State Medical Societies, as well as the American Medical Association; a Fellow of the College of Physicians of Philadelphia; one of the founders of the American Genito-Urinary Association; and prominent Fellow of the American Surgical Association, which his father had founded in 1880.

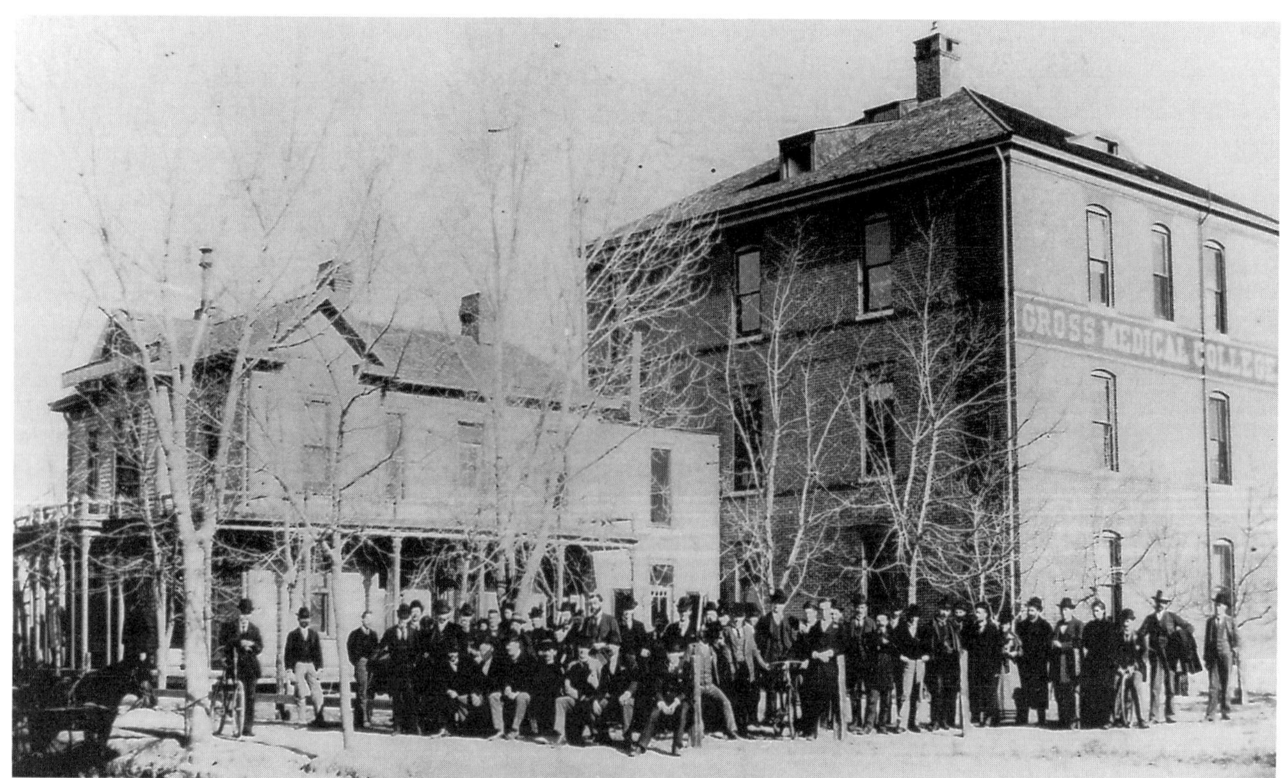

FIG. 32-20. Gross Medical College buildings. The frame building (left) housed the dispensary and administrative offices. The brick building provided lecture rooms, laboratories, and an anatomical dissecting room in the attic. (Courtesy of the University of Colorado.)

Death came to this brilliant surgeon-teacher-investigator at the age of 52, when he was at the height of his contributions to surgical science and art. The event occurred on April 16, 1889, from pneumonia, despite unremitting watch by four of Philadelphia's best doctors—Jacob Mendes DaCosta, William Osler, Orville Horwitz, and Charles Wirgman. On his deathbed Gross extracted a promise from them that they would take care of his wife, Grace. Osler kept his promise by marrying the "Widow Gross" three years later. She never forgot her "first love," for in her will of 1928 she bequeathed £5,000 (roughly $25,000) for the "establishment of a Lectureship in Surgery in Memory of Doctor Samuel W. Gross." This endowment evolved into the Grace Revere Osler Professorship of Surgery at Jefferson.

John Hill Brinton, M.D., LL.D. (1832–1907); Fifth Chairmanship (Co-Chairman, 1882–1906)

Although John H. Brinton was a widely known surgeon, author, and Professor at Jefferson, his name is inadequately remembered. Portraits of all the Surgical Chairmen until 1970 hang on the walls of Jefferson except his, even though he actually was not overlooked, because Thomas Eakins painted his portrait in 1876 (Figure 32-24), a year after he completed the *Gross Clinic.* Jefferson's art collection would be enhanced by this typical Eakins masterpiece, which now is in

In Lecture Room
Gross Med. College
Denver Colo.
Photo. by

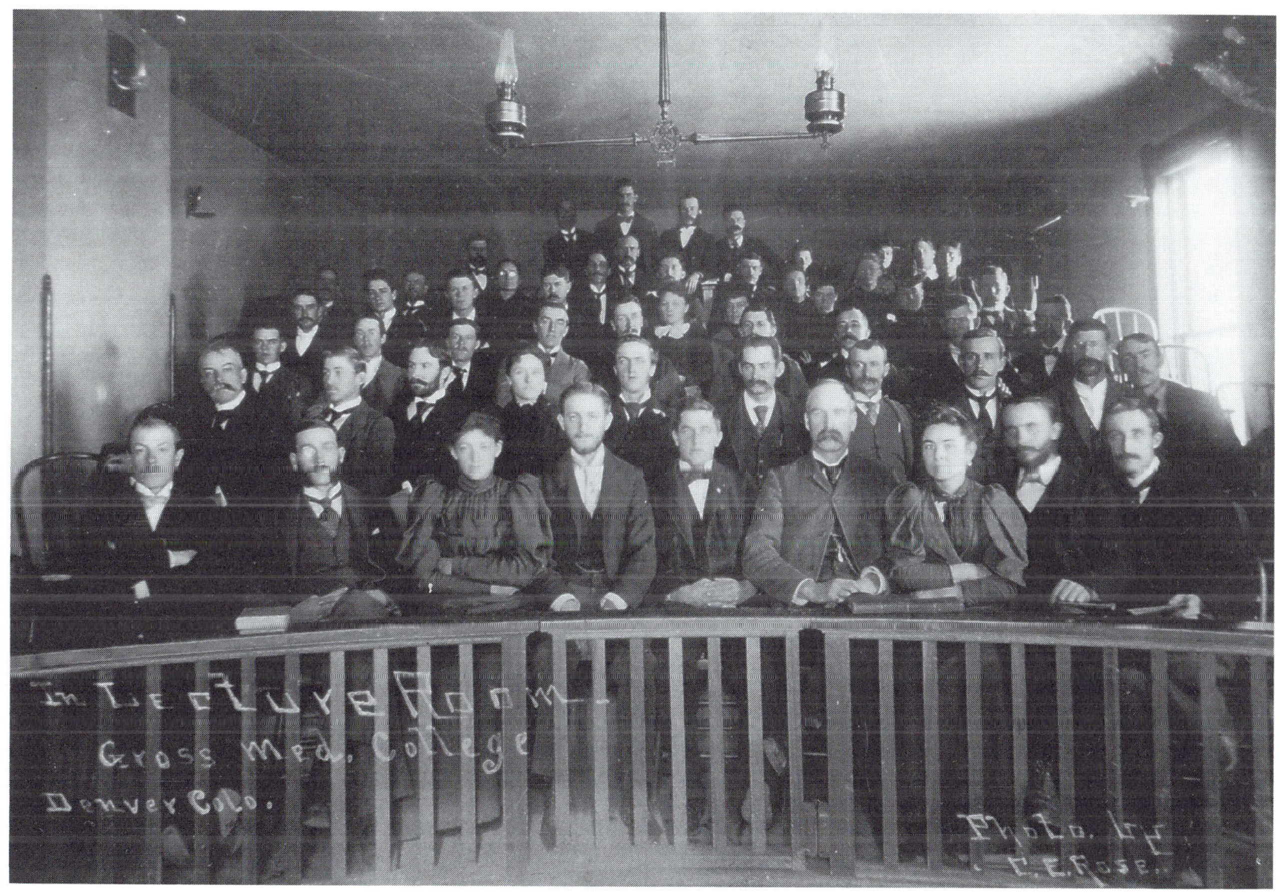

FIG. 32-21. Lecture room of Gross Medical College. Women students were admitted. (Courtesy of University of Colorado.)

the collection of the National Gallery of Art in Washington, D.C. Perhaps to some extent Brinton was overshadowed by the dynamic personality of Samuel W. Gross and the world renowned W. W. Keen, with both of whom he was successively a Co-Chairman. Finally, the strong Quaker influence in his family background may have tended to accentuate the modest, self-effacing quality that marked him as a gentleman in the finest sense.

Dr. Brinton (Figure 32-25) was born on May 21, 1832, at Fifteenth and Chestnut Streets in Philadelphia, the only son of George and Mary Smith Brinton, who also had three daughters. The "Brinton Country" near West Chester, Pennsylvania, is replete with roads, houses, a lake, quarries, a ford, a bridge, a mill, and places of religious worship associated with descendents of the original family. Dr. Brinton's aunt, Elizabeth Sophia Brinton (1800–1889), married George McClellan, M.D. Dr. Brinton was thus the nephew of the Founder of Jefferson Medical College as well as the first cousin of McClellan's two sons, General George Brinton McClellan of Civil War fame and John Hill Brinton McClellan, M.D. By 1962 ten physicians of the McClellan family had graduated from Jefferson. The Brintons, not to be outdone, can lay claim to 11. Milton Brinton attended Jefferson for the session 1826–1827 but died at the age of 21. Ten other Brintons who are Alumni of Jefferson are John B., 1826; John H., 1852; Jeremiah B., 1859; Daniel G.,

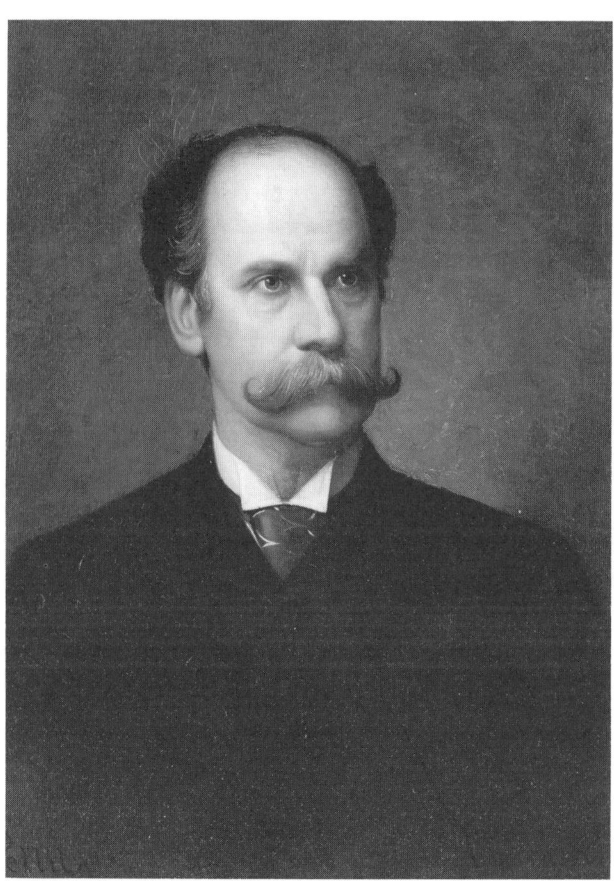

FIG. 32-22. Samuel Weissel Gross, M.D., LL.D. (1837–1889); Fifth Chairmanship (Co-Chairman, 1882–1889).

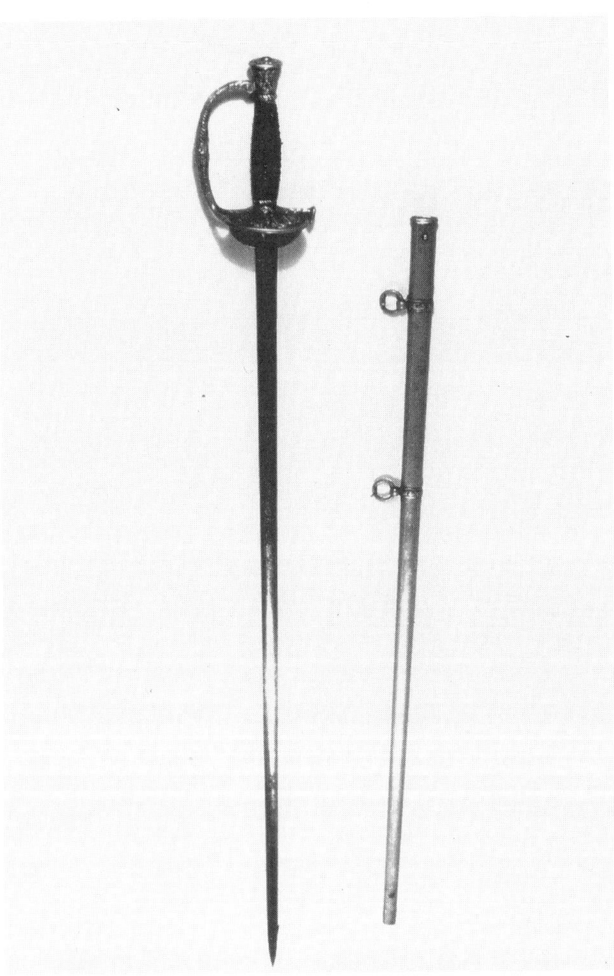

FIG. 32-23. The sword carried by Samuel W. Gross, M.D., during the Civil War. (Courtesy of College of Physicians of Philadelphia, to which it was given by Lady Osler, the widow of S.W. Gross).

1860; William M., 1875; Lewis, 1882; Ward, 1894; William T., 1911; William T., Jr., 1952; and Wilbur M. Pryor, 1971. Dr. Brinton's sister, Sarah Frederica Brinton, married Dr. Jacob Mendes DaCosta, who as a friend and later Professor of Medicine at Jefferson became a brother-in-law.

Brinton enjoyed a superb education from both the cultural and medical standpoints. From the University of Pennsylvania he obtained a B.A. degree in 1850, an M.A. in 1853, and an LL.D. in 1901. He took his medical course at Jefferson and graduated in 1852. His thesis was entitled *Record of Microscopical Observations of One Hundred Tumors.* Well preserved in the archives of Jefferson, beautifully handwritten and bound, the thesis contains sketches and drawings of cellular arrangements that demonstrate the literary ability, academic excellence, and interest in research that were to characterize the rest of his career. William Smith Forbes and Jacob Mendes DaCosta were among his graduation classmates whose portraits were also subsequently painted by Eakins. All three were destined to serve their Alma Mater with distinction in later years as Chairmen in Anatomy, Medicine, and Surgery.

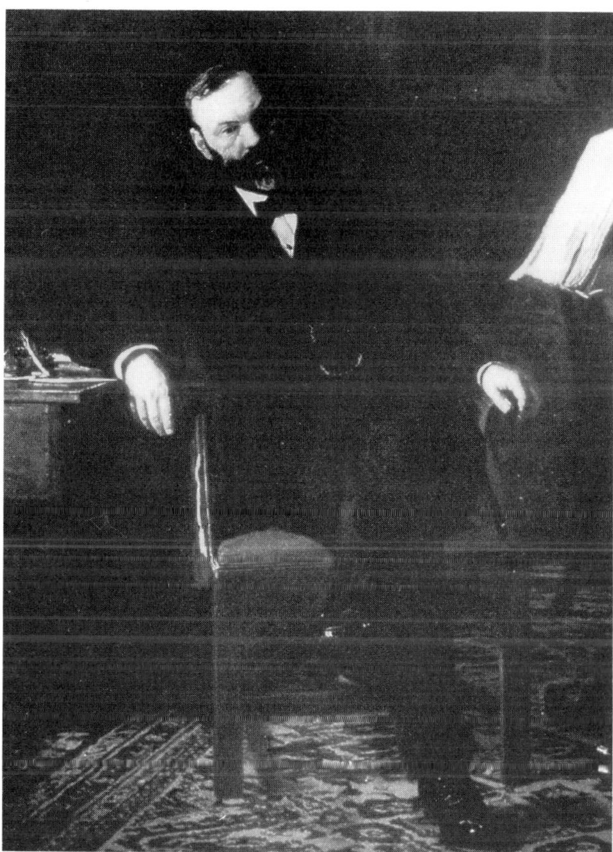

FIG. 32-24. Portrait of John Hill Brinton, M.D., by Thomas Eakins (1876). The book is *Medical and Surgical History of the War of the Rebellion,* to which Brinton was an early contributor.

As was customary for the medical elite of those days, Brinton spent a postgraduate year in Europe. In the company of classmate DaCosta, he first visited Paris, where he most likely met the leaders of French medicine. In Vienna he was influenced by Josef Hyrtl (1810–1894), who was considered the first and greatest teacher of topographic and regional anatomy in the nineteenth century. Brinton thereafter maintained an ongoing interest in research and teaching of anatomy, even aspiring, although unsuccessfully, to the Professorship at Jefferson when it became vacant 20 years later.

On returning to Philadelphia in April, 1853, Brinton entered general practice, but with his

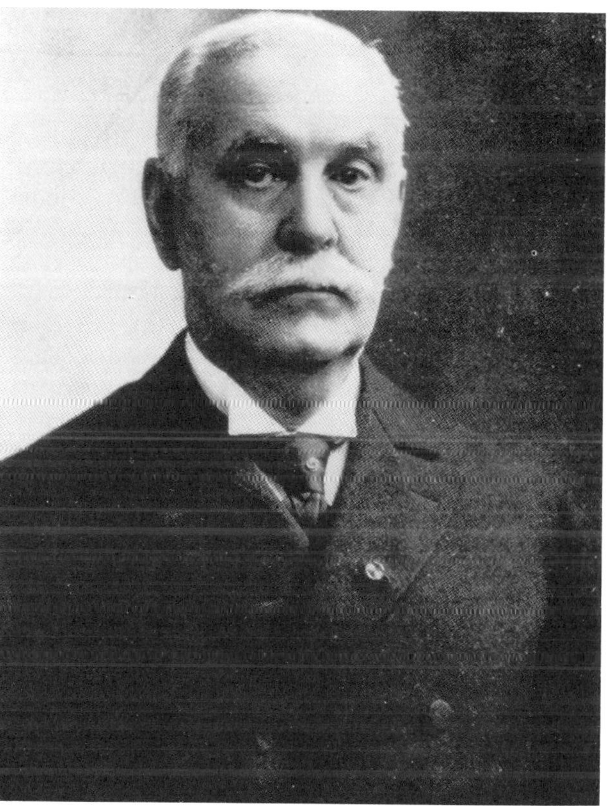

FIG. 32-25. John Hill Brinton, M.D., LL.D. (1832–1907); Fifth Chairmanship (Co-Chairman, 1882–1906).

mind also bent on teaching anatomy and surgery. The combination of self-motivation, tireless energy, lecturing ability, scientific curiosity, and cultural refinement led to his steady rise in the profession. At that time it was almost impossible for an academically inclined young physician to gain a teaching post in one of the Philadelphia Medical Schools, as these were occupied and jealously guarded by men of mature prominence and distinction who had at least one or more textbooks in print. The opportunity and proving ground, however, for future leaders in the profession was provided by the Philadelphia School of Anatomy (1820–1875), the history of which has been thoroughly detailed by Dr. W. W. Keen.[14] It was located on the north side at the upper end of Chant Street, then called College Avenue, behind St. Stephen's Episcopal Church, at or near the site where Benjamin Franklin flew the famous kite that drew lightning from the sky. This area has been absorbed by part of the United States Post Office between Ninth and Tenth Streets and Market and Chestnut. Brinton took full advantage of these facilities for anatomic dissection, experimentation, and lecturing on operative and general surgery.

Working in the third story of the eastern end of the two adjacent anatomic buildings, Brinton repeated Suchet's experiments on tanning muscles after injecting gelatin, and in 1854 developed a method of preserving fresh preparations by applying gutta-percha dissolved in benzole. This work undoubtedly was a factor in his later choice by the United States Surgeon General to be the first Curator of the Army Medical Museum. That same year, only two years out of Medical College, he published an American edition of Erichsen's *Science and Art of Surgery*. In 1856 he reported a previously undescribed valve in the right spermatic vein and suggested its relationship to the lesser frequency of varicocoele on that side. Keen credited this as "one of the few discoveries recorded in macroscopical human anatomy of later years." In addition, he dissected over 100 sternums for his later paper in 1867 on *Luxation of Body of the Sternum*.

Brinton was appointed to the Staff of St. Joseph's Hospital in 1859. He also took time from his increasing clinical practice to give courses on operative surgery as well as general surgical subjects between 1853 and 1861. These lectures were given privately as well as in a Lectureship of the "Summer Association" of the second "Philadelphia Association for Medical Instruction." The "Summer Association" was formed for the purpose of giving lectures during the long recess in the Medical Colleges from March to November, with time off during the hot months of July and August. They were delivered not only in the Philadelphia School of Anatomy but also in a building on Butler Avenue in the rear of Jefferson Medical College, subsequently replaced by the first detached Jefferson Hospital of 1877 (Figures 32-26, 32-27, 32-28, and 32-29). The subjects included surgical anatomy, bandaging and fracture dressings, treatment of hemorrhage, various aspects of trauma, and fractures, all of which laid a firm foundation for the distinguished career awaiting him in the Civil War.

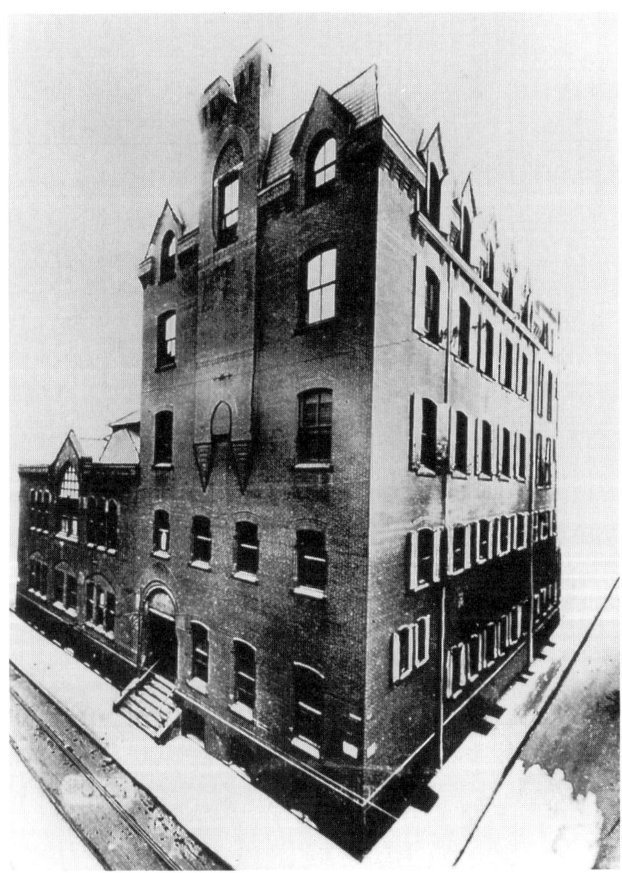

FIG. 32-26. 1877 Hospital on Sansom Street, replaced in 1924 by the Thompson Annex.

At age 29 and only nine years out of Medical School, Brinton was a prime candidate for military service in the Civil War. In July, 1861, he easily passed the examination of the Army Medical Board at Washington, D.C., which was chiefly written and in his words "not very rigid." His commission as Brigade Surgeon of Volunteers was signed by Abraham Lincoln, and the original document is preserved in the archives at Jefferson (Figure 32-30). Indeed, all of his Army orders and communications from Generals Grant, Rosecrans, McPherson and Sheridan, as well as the office of the Surgeon General, are likewise safely kept in a bound volume. His frequent letters home were also collected into two bound volumes. These served him well for his later book on *Personal Memoirs of John H. Brinton, Major and Surgeon, U.S.V., 1861–1865,* completed June 14, 1891, but not published until 1914, seven years after his death. This work in arresting literary aplomb recounts the early chaos in the organization of both the military and medical branches of the Army, insights into the personalities of his commanders, the pitiful plight of the wounded soldiers to which he was committed, the difficulties in setting up hospitals and supplies, the ineptness and inexperience of many of the medical officers, battles as viewed through eyes of a Volunteer Surgeon, his efforts to collect specimens for the Army Medical Museum, service on examining boards, and his collecting statistics for the *Medical and Surgical History of the War of the Rebellion.*

Duly commissioned in August, 1861, Brinton reported to the Department of the West, where he came under the command of General Ulysses S. Grant and was assigned to duty in the office of the Medical Director of the Cairo District of Illinois (Figure 32-31). This marked the beginning of a mutual respect and regard for each other's abilities that extended well beyond the war years. Jefferson's archives contains a letter to Brinton from Mrs. Julia Grant expressing comfort that her husband was under his medical care.

Brinton became an Acting Medical Director and, lacking formal Army medical training, relied upon his native intelligence, initiative, and organizational ability to deal with the confusing and at times chaotic conditions that arose. This

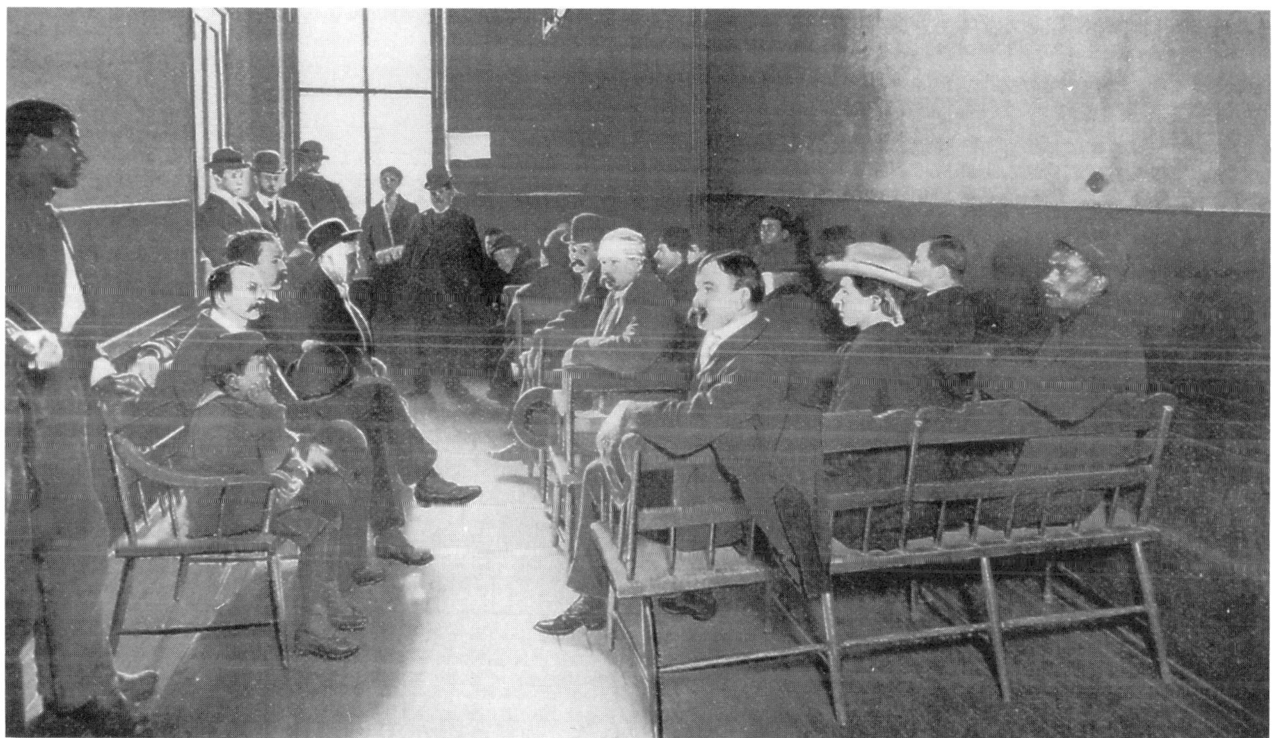

FIG. 32-27. Outpatient surgical clinic men's waiting room of the 1877 Hospital.

could not fail to impress all those with whom he came in contact. His first real test came under General Grant at the Battle of Belmont, Missouri, during which he had the misfortune to lose all of his surgical instruments. Many of these had been brought from Paris, while others had belonged to his old preceptor at Jefferson, Professor Thomas Dent Mütter. In the hurry of leaving for the field at Belmont, Brinton gathered them into a single package, which he entrusted to a young orderly. The latter panicked from the enemy artillery fire and was seen to rush from the open into the woods. The orderly was captured and the instruments fell into the hands of a Mississippi surgeon. General Grant on a flag of truce attempted to barter a captured Arabian pony for the instruments, but the exchange was never consummated.

Brinton was distressed by the inexperience and surgical ignorance of his fellow medical officers. In an effort to remedy this situation he organized the Army Medical and Surgical Society of Cairo, bringing surgeons together chiefly from Illinois, Iowa, Michigan, and Missouri for mutual improvement. The society flourished long after Brinton left Cairo.

The switch from the comforts of a refined home in Philadelphia to the rigors of army life with horseback riding, cramped quarters, tents, filth, sickness, and the many wounded or dead seems to have been made by Brinton without complaint. His description of mince pie that Thanksgiving, however, was unique: "The latter I think was made of dried apples, and the meaty part had a peculiar flavor, suggestive of levee rats and Chinese ideas."[15]

In 1862 Brinton, as Medical Director of the Army of Tennessee, accompanied General Grant in the campaign which captured Forts Henry and Donelson of Nashville, and in the Battle of Shiloh, at Pittsburg Landing, Tennessee. Samuel D. Gross, his fellow Jeffersonian, visited the battlefield at Shiloh and examined the wounded on the government steamboats at Pittsburg Landing for material for his *Manual of Military Surgery,* which was published only two weeks later. Little was Brinton to know at that time that he would succeed the "Emperor of Surgery of the

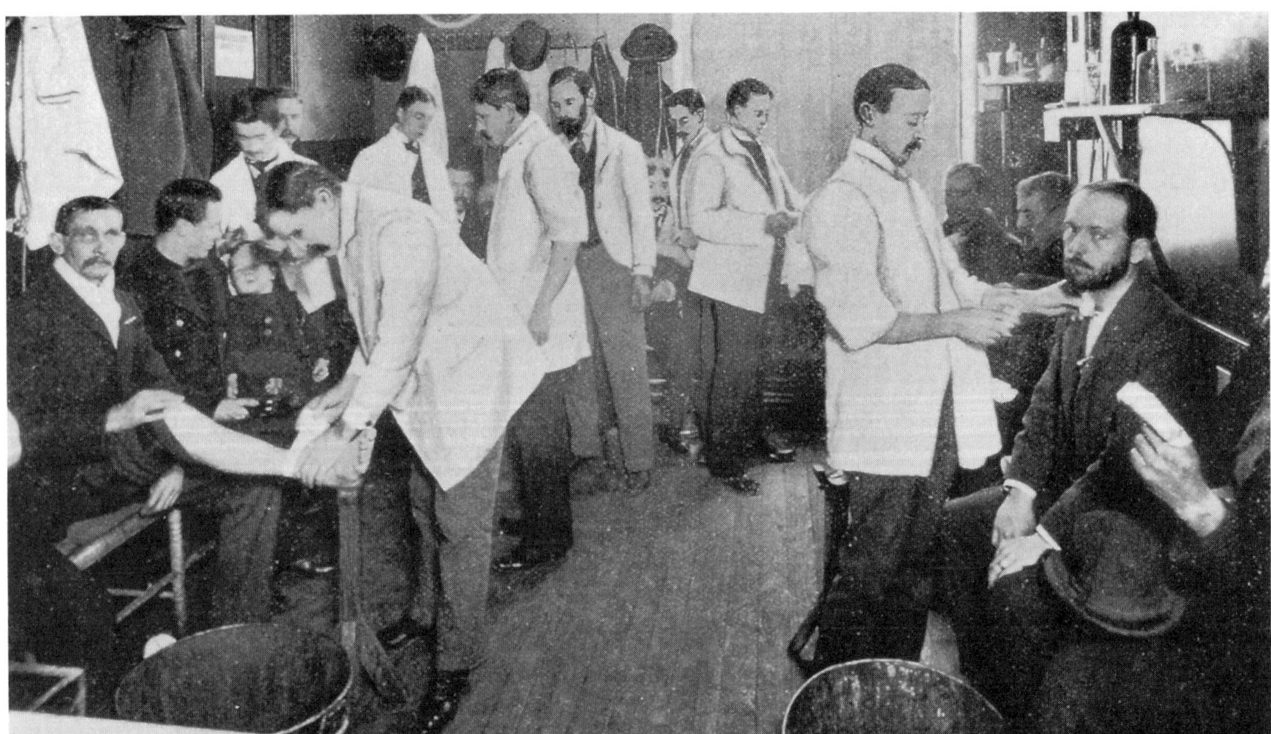

FIG. 32-28. Surgical dressing room for men in the 1877 Hospital.

Nineteenth Century" upon the latter's retirement at Jefferson and share the divided Chair of Surgery with his illustrious son, Samuel W. Gross.

Brinton shortly thereafter was assigned to duty in the office of Surgeon General William H. Hammond in Washington, D.C., and in June, 1862, was ordered to prepare *The Surgical History of the Rebellion*. This was intended to remedy the insufficient and defective statistics on the sick and wounded that became evident in the first year of the war. In August, 1862, he additionally was assigned to collect and arrange all specimens of morbid anatomy that had accumulated in the various hospitals or that might have been retained by any of the medical officers. In carrying out this order, Surgeon Brinton thus established the United States Army Medical Museum. His visits to headquarters of the armies in the field and different hospitals provided data and illustrations for the book and specimens for the museum. The beginning of the museum in that August of 1862 consisted of three dried and varnished specimens placed on a shelf above the ink stand of Brinton's desk. In January, 1863, a preliminary catalogue was printed with brief descriptions of 1,349 objects that had been collected within a five-month period. Of the total, 985 were surgical, 106 medical, 133 missiles, and 125 miscellaneous. By July 1, 1863, Brinton was able to submit a *Consolidated Statement on Gunshot Wounds* for publication by the Surgeon General's Office. It would be misleading and grandiose to give Brinton credit for more than the start of these monumental projects that required additional years and teams of workers, but his name is indelibly linked with them.

One of the great disappointments in Brinton's life was in connection with a proposed Army Medical School that failed to materialize for lack of authorization by the Secretary of War, Edwin N. Stanton. It would have been a postgraduate institution designed to teach medical officers the surgical and medical care as well as the customs of the service under Professors of the Army who were already experienced in these aspects. Lecture rooms, laboratories, and illustrations were arranged in the Army Medical Museum, a curriculum was formulated, a capable faculty was

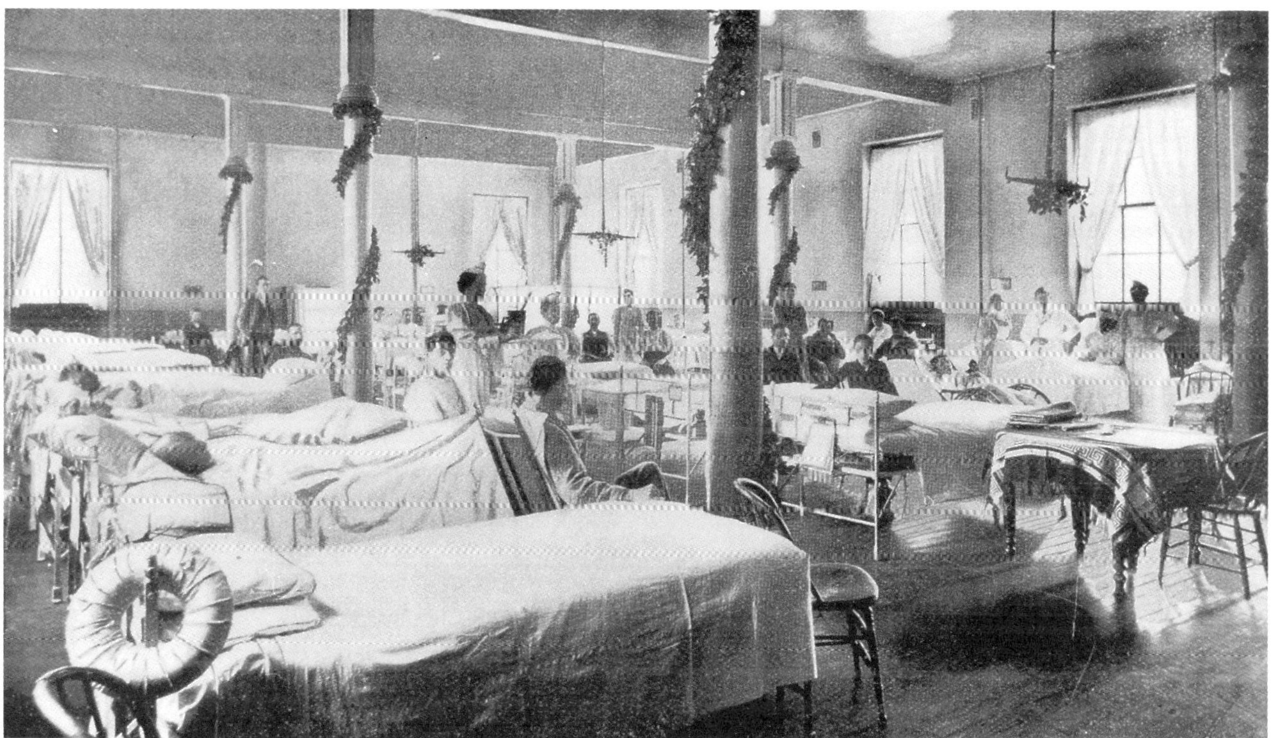

FIG. 32-29. Men's surgical ward of the 1877 Hospital.

available, and Brinton had been instructed to prepare an address for the inauguration of the first military medical course of the United States for the session of 1863–1864. When Mr. Stanton learned the lectures were to be given in the evenings, he dismissed the project with: "They will go to the theater and neglect their duties." A third of a century later, on March 13, 1896, Brinton was gratified to give the Valedictory Address to the second graduating class of the Army Medical School, Washington, D.C., which finally had been established in June, 1893. Brinton's interest in educating physicians committed to a military career reached total fulfillment much later, after his death, by an Act of Congress in 1972, establishing the first Federal Medical School, the Uniformed Services University of the Health Sciences (USUHS) in Bethesda, Maryland, to meet the needs of the Army, Navy, Air Force, and Public Health Service. The first class of 29 physicians received their M.D. degree in May, 1980.

Brinton served on examining boards in Washington on various occasions and was admonished not to be too strict because the need was great for even those of limited knowledge and experience. He was with the Headquarters of the Army of the Potomac in Virginia, at Battles of Antietam, Chancellorsville, Gettysburg, and Grant's march on Richmond through the Wilderness. During his army career he also came to know Generals McPherson, Sheridan, Thomas, and Halleck. Some of these wrote letters on his behalf in later years.

Upon returning to his native Philadelphia, Brinton resumed private practice. He promptly was appointed by the Faculty of Jefferson Medical College as a Lecturer on Operative Surgery in the Summer Course of the School (1866). In 1867, he was elected as one of the Surgeons to the

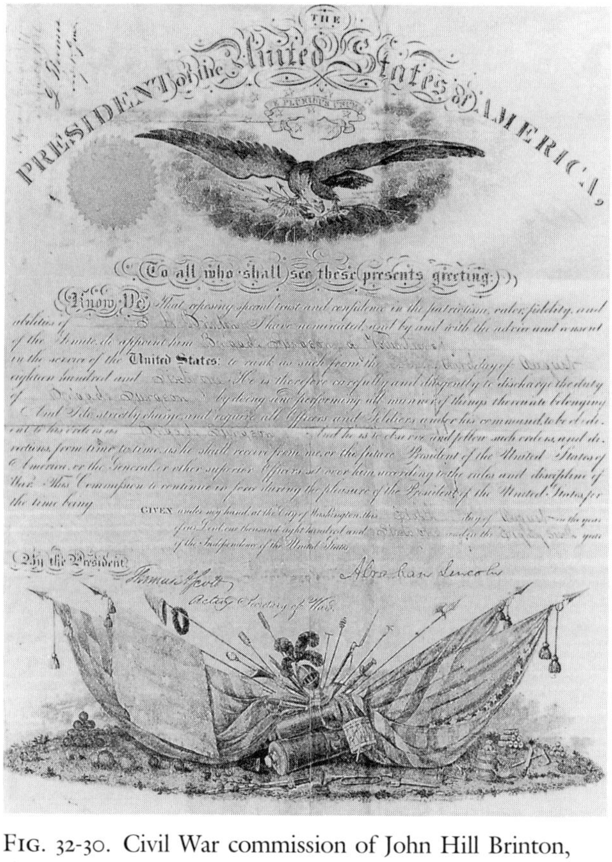

FIG. 32-30. Civil War commission of John Hill Brinton, signed by Abraham Lincoln.

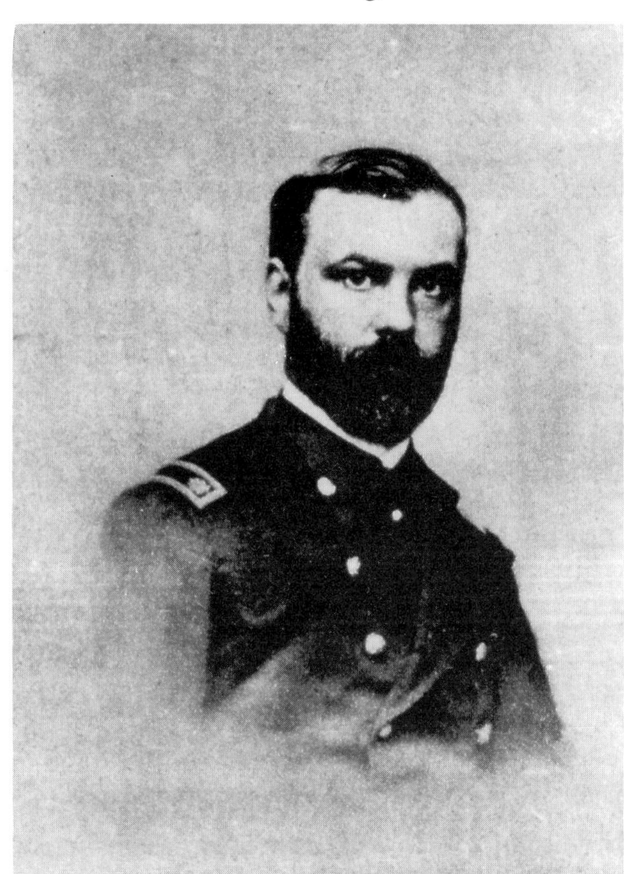

FIG. 32-31. John Hill Brinton, M.D., as Brigade Surgeon of Volunteers in the Civil War.

Philadelphia Hospital. He delivered the Mütter Lecture in 1869 on *Gunshot Injuries, Their Surgery and Pathology* and served as a member of the Committee of the Mütter Museum of the College of Physicians from 1878 for 29 years until his death. During the intermediate years he worked under the inspiration of his Surgical Chief at Jefferson, the immortal Samuel D. Gross, and became a boon companion to his son, Samuel W. Gross. He aided the elder Gross in the founding of the Jefferson Alumni Association in 1870, the Philadelphia Academy of Surgery in 1879, and the American Surgical Association in 1880. When the first detached Jefferson Hospital of 1877 was in the planning stage, Brinton successfully undertook to raise $150,000 through the Alumni. He was elected by the Trustees as one of the Surgeons of the 1877 Jefferson Hospital and served for five years as President of the Staff.

In June, 1873, the famous Dr. Joseph Pancoast resigned as Chairman of the Department of Anatomy at Jefferson, having held the post with great distinction since 1841 and having served as Chairman of Surgery from 1839 to 1841. Initially nine names of candidates were placed in nomination, and that of John Hill Brinton led the list. Four other Jeffersonians were interested, namely William H. Pancoast (the retiring Professor's son), W.W. Keen, William S. Forbes, and Addinell Hewson. Seventeen ballots were taken in succession without any candidate receiving a majority vote. On later balloting in April, 1874, the younger Pancoast obtained a majority. Although Brinton's professorial ambitions in Anatomy were frustrated by William Pancoast at this juncture, the tables turned in 1882 when Brinton was chosen along with Samuel W. Gross for the divided Chair of Surgery of Samuel D. Gross. The younger Pancoast, as a capable surgeon, had been keeping his eye on the forthcoming vacancy, and his disappointment was keen.

Younger Gross had a special interest in tumors, whereas Brinton's was in fractures, but they shared a common interest in genitourinary surgery. With Samuel W. Gross's death in 1889, the Board of Trustees appointed a new Co-Chairman, William Williams Keen, whom Brinton had known and admired for many years.

Brinton continued to write articles until the age of 70. These related to anatomy, general surgery, urology, the military, surgical history, and various introductory and valedictory addresses. He was also the American editor of Ericksen's *Surgery*. His lectures were well prepared, informative, and delivered in a fluent manner that captivated his students.

Brinton had wide-based social and cultural activities. He was one of the earliest members of the Metropolitan Club of Washington, a founder of the Philadelphia Skating Club, and a member of the Philadelphia Club, still considered by many as the most exclusive men's club of the City. He belonged to the American Philosophical Society, the Academy of Natural Sciences, the Sons of the Revolution, the Loyal Legion, the Society of Colonial Wars, and the Historical Society of Pennsylvania.

In May, 1906, Dr. Brinton felt impelled by the weight of advancing years to tender his resignation, which was accepted with Emeritus status. On March 5, 1907, while in his 75th year, he suffered a cerebral hemorrhage. He seemed to be making a recovery, but died suddenly of an exacerbation on March 18 at his residence, 1423 Spruce Street. Buried in Woodlands Cemetery, Philadelphia, are Brinton, his wife, all six children, his parents, and one of his three sisters.

William Williams Keen, Jr., M.D., LL.D., Ph.D., Sc.D. (1837–1932); Fifth Chairmanship (Co-Chairman, 1889–1907)

The younger Gross and his successor, W.W. Keen, Jr. (Figure 32-32), were both born in the same year (1837). Thus, with the premature death of Samuel W. Gross at age 52, the Chairmanship was continued by a man of the same age and professional maturity.[16] As fate would have it, Keen was not only able to complete 18 years of Co-Chairmanship with Brinton but to have 25 more years as Emeritus to the age of 95. His stature in the surgical world was similar to that of the elder Gross, but in company with William

Halsted and Harvey Cushing of Johns Hopkins. "The Emperor of American Surgery" (Samuel D. Gross) was succeeded by three "Marshalls" (Keen, Halsted, and Cushing).

Keen was a descendant of Joran Kyn, an early Swedish settler in Chester, Pennsylvania. He was born in Philadelphia on January 19, 1837, the son of William W. and Susan Budd Keen. After preliminary education at Central High School and Saunders Academy, he entered Brown University at the age of 18 and graduated in 1859 as Class Valedictorian. He then stayed on at Brown for a year of postgraduate study in literature, physics, and chemistry, leading to an A.M. degree (1860). His ties with Brown University persisted throughout his life, during which he was elected a Trustee (1873) and awarded an LL.D. degree (1891). Brown University claims him as proudly as does Jefferson, and many of his memorabilia are contained in their archives.

Keen entered Jefferson Medical College in September, 1860, but after ten months his education was interrupted by the Civil War. Dr. John Hill Brinton, on being asked to select a Surgeon for the Fifth Massachusetts Regiment, chose Keen. In July, 1861, without taking any examination, he was sent to a camp in Alexandria and within two more weeks was at the Battle of Bull Run. There he witnessed the chaos by not receiving a single order, as well as discovering the general ignorance of the surgeons at that time. Shortly after the battle his period of enlistment in the regiment expired and upon being discharged he returned to Jefferson where he graduated in 1862. Two months later he was duly commissioned as Acting Assistant Surgeon in the U.S. Army and put in charge of Eckington General Hospital in Washington. He quickly established a notable reputation by setting up and equipping a hospital within five days. He was put in charge of a hospital at Frederick, Maryland, and subsequently to the Satterlee as well as the Christian Street Hospital in Philadelphia. In 1863 he served with Drs. S. Weir Mitchell (Jefferson, 1850) and George Morehouse (Jefferson, 1850) in the Turner's Lane Army Hospital in an important study upon the injuries of nerves, resulting in their joint authorship of *Gunshot Wounds and Other Injuries of Nerves* (1864). This began Keen's interest in neurologic surgery.

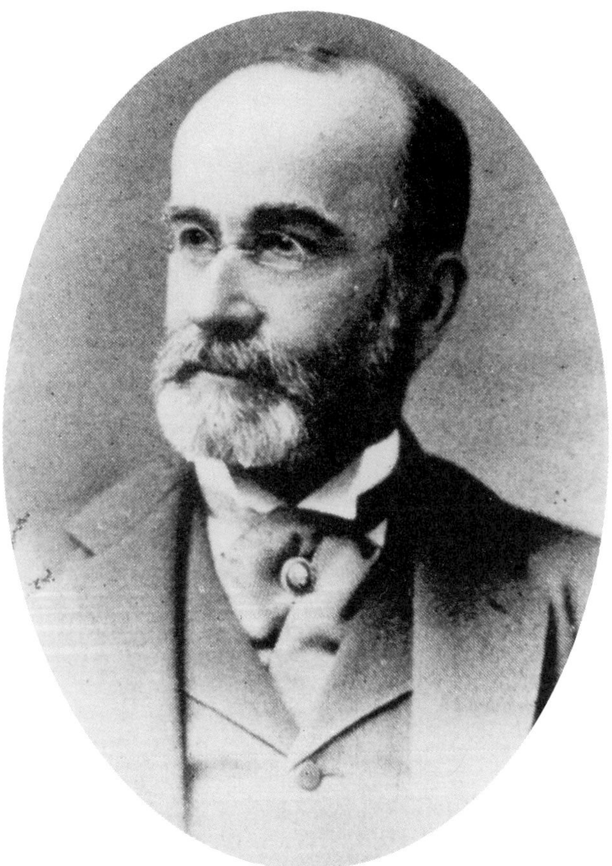

FIG. 32-32. William W. Keen, Jr., M.D., LL.D., Ph.D., Sc.D. (1837–1932); Fifth Chairmanship (Co-Chairman, 1889–1907).

In the grand style of his era, Keen spent two years (1864–1866) in postgraduate study with Duchenne of Paris and in Virchow's laboratory in Berlin. On his return, his lectures in the "Summer Course" at Jefferson (1866–1867) in pathological anatomy were the first ever given in Philadelphia on that subject. Lister's *Principle of Antisepsis* (1867) had not yet been published, let alone accepted, so it was common in the 1860s to come directly from the dissecting room to the surgical clinic to assist in operations. Pancoast and the elder Gross were operating in blood-stained frock coats, "the veterans of a hundred fights." Instruments were not disinfected, and there were no artery forceps. Absorbable catgut sutures were not introduced until 1869. Marine sponges were used, and gauze sponges waited for the 1870s. Fractures of the base of the skull were practically always fatal. Cerebral localization was in its infancy when, in 1874,

Roberts W. Bartholow (later Professor of Materia Medica at Jefferson) first applied electrodes to the human brain. At that time it was generally believed that the brain was of uniform structure, like the liver. The first clinical thermometer that Keen ever saw was a gift from S. Weir Mitchell (Jefferson, 1850), who brought it from London in 1876. Keen in his long life until 1932 would witness the progress of medicine from a time when the physician had little beyond his own fingers, eyes, and ears, to the era of antisepsis, roentgen diagnosis, and the clinical laboratory. Not only would he benefit from these triumphs but would extend their applications to surgery.

In 1866, while already teaching at Jefferson, Keen became the Head of the Philadelphia School of Anatomy until its dissolution in 1875. At that time the courses in the medical schools leading to the M.D. degree were limited to two short terms of didactic lectures. Ambitious students who perhaps could not afford postgraduate study in Europe would supplement their education in these extramural schools that also included clinical teaching. It was through this School of Anatomy that Keen linked his teaching with Jefferson alumni such as Jacob Mendes DaCosta, John Hill Brinton, and S. Weir Mitchell.

In 1875 Keen was appointed Professor of Artistic Anatomy at the Pennsylvania Academy of the Fine Arts (Figure 32-33), a post he held until 1890. It is of interest to note that the famous artist of the *Gross Clinic*, Thomas Eakins, was his chief demonstrator of anatomy at the Academy from 1876 to 1880.

In 1876 Keen was the first in Philadelphia to adopt Lister's principles of antisepsis at the St. Mary's Hospital, and was closely followed by Samuel W. Gross and J. Ewing Mears in the first detached Jefferson Hospital of 1877. In 1884 he was appointed Professor of Surgery in the Woman's Medical College of Pennsylvania, a post he held until called to Jefferson in 1889 to succeed the younger Gross. In 1887 he operated at St. Mary's Hospital on a patient with an accurately localized large meningioma of the brain. It was the first brain tumor successfully removed in America, and the patient lived without recurrence for more than 30 years. The chapter on the Department of Neurosurgery at Jefferson details his pioneer work in this field.

As a surgical teacher Keen was unexcelled. His clinics were crowded, not only by students but by visiting surgeons from throughout the United States and foreign countries (Figures 32-34 and 32-35). According to Dr. John Chalmers DaCosta, who succeeded him: "He had that combination of earnestness and clearness that was absolutely convincing of his own beliefs." DaCosta's opinion of him as a master surgeon was: "He always showed best when the situation was worst. Dr. Keen was always, calmer, quieter, kinder, pleasanter, the worse the surgical situation was, and I never saw it get the best of him. He had a favorite expression when he would finally get hold of the situation and control the hemorrhage. He would say, 'Now we have the whip-hand of it.' It passed into a proverbial expression in the Jefferson Medical College."

In July, 1893, Keen was chosen to assist Dr. John D. Bryant in operating upon President Grover Cleveland for a verrucous carcinoma of the roof of the mouth. It was performed secretly on board a yacht (the *Oneida*) off New York Harbor. Keen fashioned special instruments in preparation for the surgery, which was a complete success. The operation was kept secret in order to prevent possible public panic over a national crisis in silver. Keen published his report on that operation in 1917.[17]

As a prolific writer, Keen was in a rank with Robley Dunglison and Samuel D. Gross. His contributions in anatomical subjects included: Keen's *Clinical Charts* (1870), and *Early History of Practical Anatomy* (1870); and as editor, *Heath's Practical Anatomy* (1870); Flower's *Diagrams of the Nerves of the Human Body* (1872); *History of the Philadelphia School of Anatomy* (1874); Holden's *Medical and Surgical Landmarks* (1881); and *Gray's Anatomy* (1883), with a subsequent second edition (1887).

In 1893, with J. William White, Keen wrote the first compiled American *Text-Book of Surgery*. It was the forerunner of his eight-volume *Keen's System of Surgery*, which became the preeminent text for surgeons of the United States in the first decades of the twentieth century (1906–1921). Other articles related to his academic life included: *Surgical Complications and Sequels of Typhoid Fever* (1898); *Addresses and Other Papers* (1905); *Animal Experimentation and Medical Progress* (1914); *The*

Early Years of Brown University, 1764–1770 (1914); *Ether Day Address* (1916); *Treatment of War Wounds* (1917); Colver Lectures at Brown University on *Medical Research and Human Welfare,* and *Selected Papers and Addresses* (1922).

Keen had deep religious convictions. In 1867 he was appointed Charter Trustee of Crozer (Baptist) Theological Seminary, and in 1898 he wrote the *History of the First Baptist Church of Philadelphia.* Other of his writings in this faith were: *I Beleive in God and in Evolution* (1922) and *Everlasting Life* (1924). He was an ardent Prohibitionist and only once was seen to take one glass of beer.

In 1904 Keen was 67 years old and thinking of retirement. For a successor, he approached Dr. Harvey Cushing at Hopkins, who declined the honor to be considered as a candidate. Keen did retire in 1907 at the age of 70 and was succeeded by Jefferson's incomparable John Chalmers DaCosta.

Keen not only served his country in the Civil War (Figure 32-36) but in 1917, at age 80, he was in uniform as Major in the U.S. Army as a Consultant in the Reserve Corps of World War I (Figure 32-37); his services had been declined as not needed in the Spanish-American War. He was a member of the Founders and Patriots of America, of the Loyal Legion, and of the Medical Veterans of World War I. In addition to his services to President Cleveland in 1893, he was called in consultation to see Franklin D. Roosevelt during his attack of poliomyelitis in 1921.

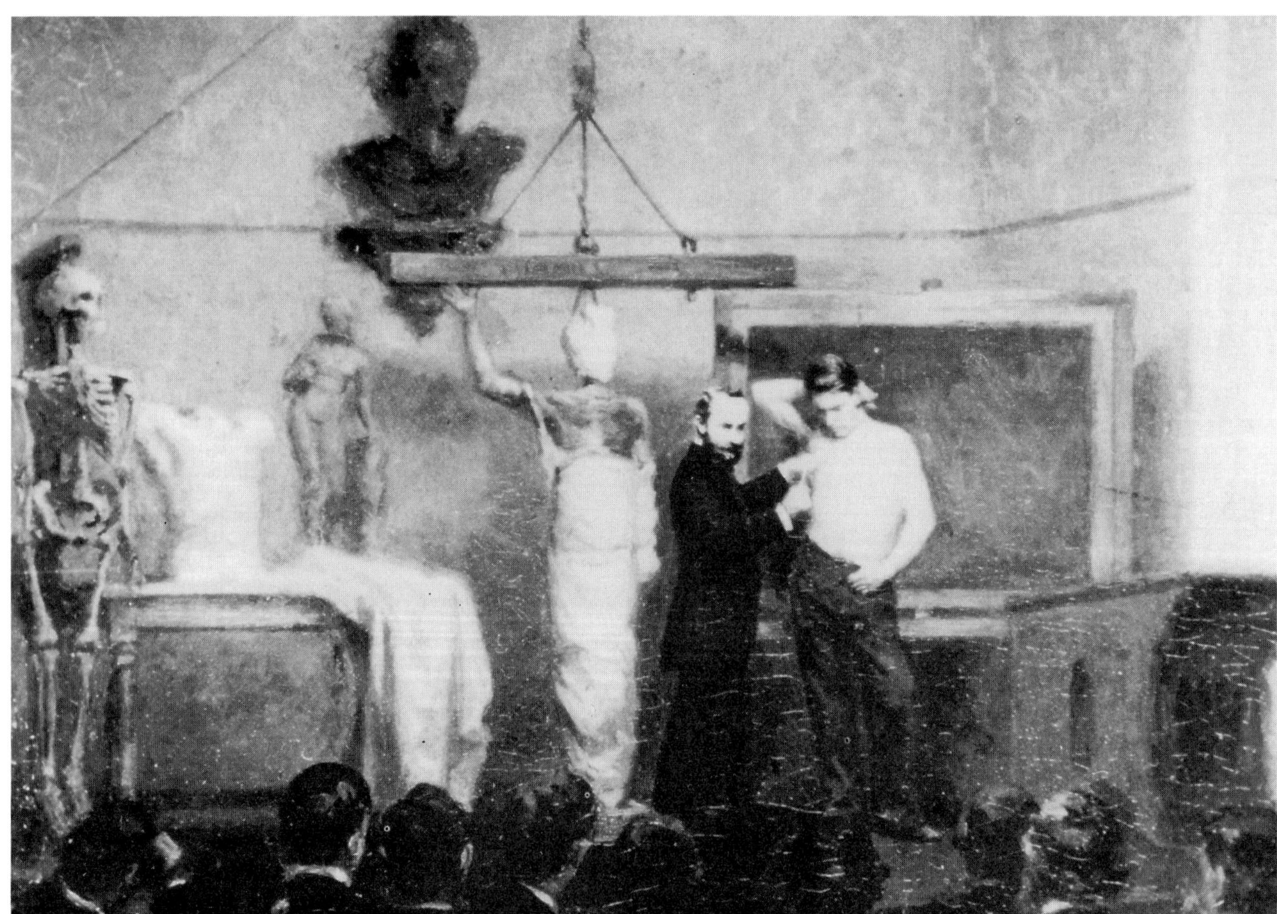

FIG. 32-33. W.W. Keen, M.D., teaching anatomy at the Pennsylvania Academy of the Fine Arts. (Courtesy of Pennsylvania Academy of the Fine Arts).

Keen was active in many societies and received many honorary degrees and awards. He was President of the American Surgical Association (1899), of the American Medical Association (1900), of the College of Physicians of Philadelphia (1900), of the International Congress of Surgery in Paris in 1920 (the first American to hold that office), of the Congress of American Physicians and Surgeons (1903); and of the American Philosophical Society (1907–1917). In 1913 he was the first surgeon in the United States to accept and have conferred upon him an Honorary Fellowship in the American College of Surgeons. He was elected an Honorary Fellow of the Royal College of Surgeons of England, of Edinburgh, and of Ireland, as well as elected to the Italian Surgical Society, the Order of the Crown of Belgium (1920), and Legion d'Honneur of France (1923).

From the Boston Surgical Society he was awarded the Bigelow Gold Medal, and from Brown University the Colver-Rosenberger Medal of Honor. He received LL.D. degrees from Brown University (1891), Northwestern and Toronto (1903), Edinburgh (1905), Yale (1906), St. Andrews of Scotland (1911), and the University of Pennsylvania (1919). Jefferson awarded him the Sc.D. Degree in 1912, and Harvard honored him with the same degree in 1920. The University of Uppsala (Sweden) awarded him a Ph.D. degree in 1907, and in 1923 the University of Paris conferred on him a Doctor, *honoris causa*.

Keen's death occurred on June, 7, 1932. After cremation, his remains were buried in Woodlands Cemetery, Philadelphia, and marked by a modest tombstone (Figure 32-38).

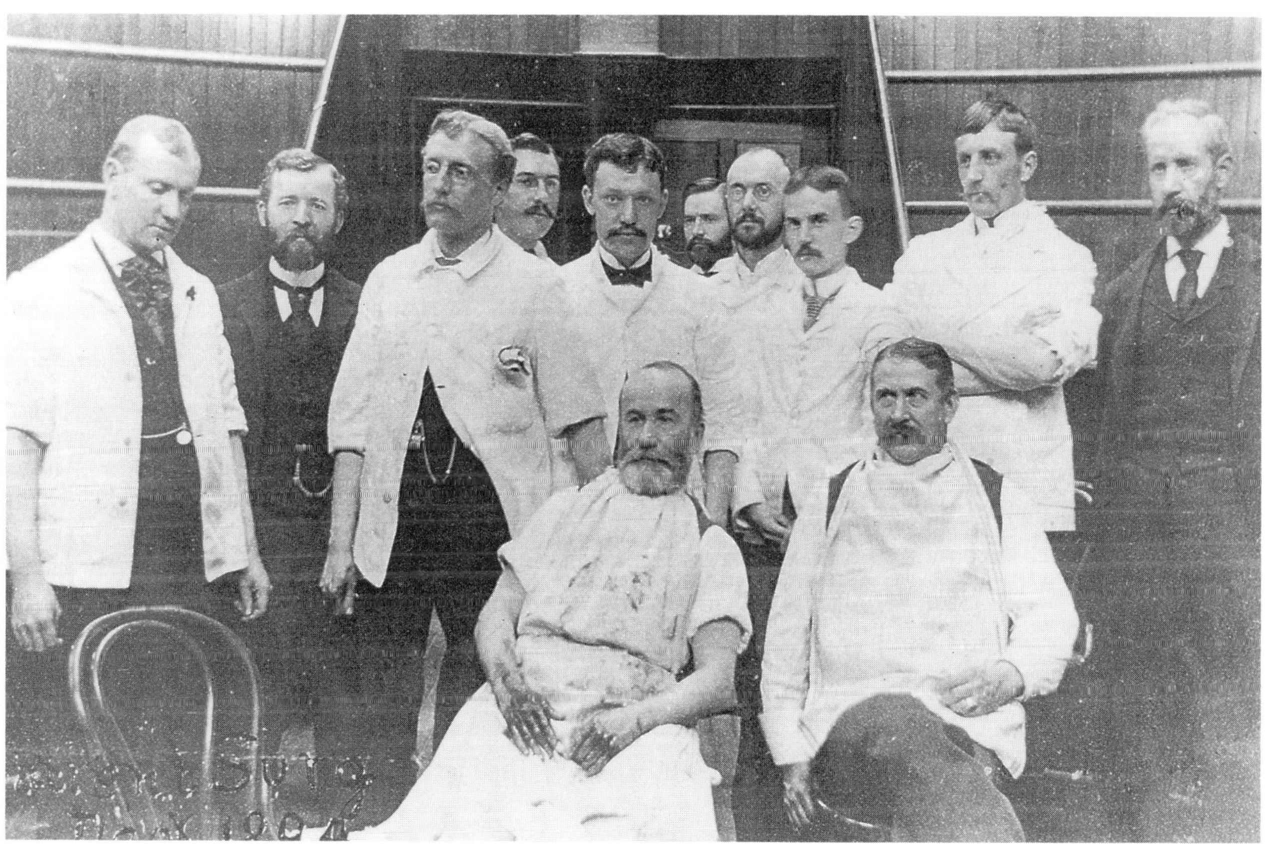

FIG. 32-34. W.W. Keen, M.D., in the amphitheater of the 1877 Hospital (1894). Note the ungloved, bloodstained hands. William J. Hearn, M.D., is seated on the right, and J. Chalmers DaCosta, M.D., is standing to the left and behind Keen.

John Chalmers DaCosta, M.D., LL.D. (1863–1933); Sixth Chairmanship (Co-Chairman, 1907–1931), First Samuel D. Gross Professor (1910–1931)

The successor to W.W. Keen in 1907 was John Chalmers DaCosta (Figure 32-39). Although regarded as a native Philadelphian, he was born in Washington, D.C., on November 15, 1863. His mother, Margaret, was residing there temporarily to be near her husband, George Tallman DaCosta, who was serving in the Army of the Potomac.[18] The DaCosta name was of Spanish ancestry. The Jefferson archives contains a partial genealogy, handwritten by DaCosta, that traces the first identifiable family member to Isaac DaCosta, who migrated from London to Boston in 1697. Some Boston members served during the American Revolution, but the family became established in Philadelphia about a century later.

DaCosta's grandfather had been a cofounder of the Camden and Atlantic Railroad of which his father, George, became President. George's brother (DaCosta's uncle) was Dr. John Chalmers DaCosta (1834–1910), who, after working as an engineer for 20 years, graduated from Jefferson Medical College in 1878 and was a gynecologist on the staff of Jefferson Hospital from 1884 to 1901. This led to a confusing proliferation of John Chalmers DaCostas—not only was the first Gross Professor, John Chalmers DaCosta, named after his uncle, but the uncle had a son named after him as John Chalmers DaCosta, Jr., (1871–1920), who graduated from Jefferson in 1893. The latter taught internal medicine at Jefferson and was called "Black Jack," as opposed to his first cousin, the Surgical Chairman, who was affectionately known as "Jack" DaCosta. The three John Chalmers DaCostas, each a Jefferson graduate and

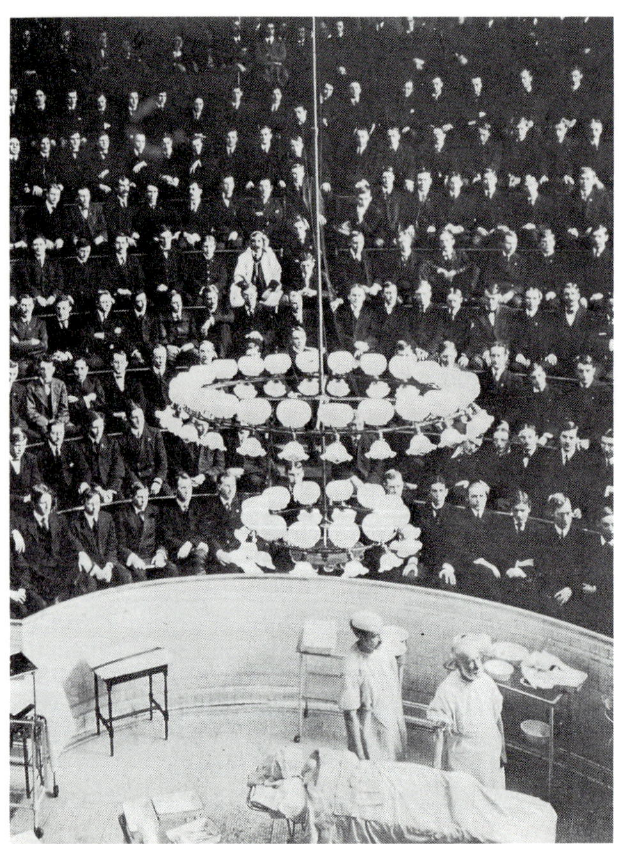

FIG. 32-35. W.W. Keen's Surgical Pit (ca. 1900).

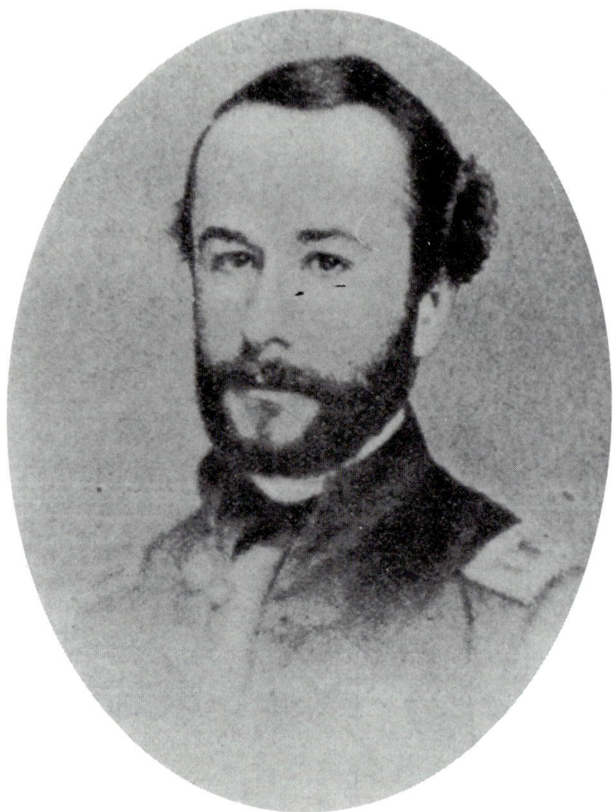

FIG. 32-36. W.W. Keen in the Civil War (1861).

teacher, were not related to Jacob Mendes DaCosta (Jefferson, 1852), Professor of Medicine at Jefferson (1872–1891) whose ancestry was Portuguese.

DaCosta's father, in addition to his railroad responsibilities, was interested in literature and book collecting, which strongly influenced young Jack's impressionable character. His mother taught him much of the history of Elizabethan England by the time he was eight. In this environment he developed an early delight in reciting poetry for the entertainment of his family and friends.

At the age of nine, DaCosta was struck in the right eye by a pine cone, resulting in loss of sight in that eye. Possibly because of the injury, his parents lavished extra concessions upon him, such as letting him ride locomotives to Atlantic City in the cab with the engineer and to occupy the fireman's seat. Friendship with railroad men and joy of riding in locomotives persisted until he became crippled in later years.

When DaCosta was 12, his uncle, Dr. John Chalmers DaCosta, and his father were members of the Volunteer Fire Departments of Haddonfield and Philadelphia. Their associations captured his interest to such an extent that he maintained throughout life an intimate connection with the Philadelphia Fire Department.

Although DaCosta's father wished him to study law, Jack had made the decision to study medicine by the age of 15. He obtained a skull through a medical student and on his own initiative read *Horner's Anatomy*. After receiving his preliminary education at Friends Central and Brown Preparatory School, he entered the University of Pennsylvania (1880) at age 17. While majoring in chemistry, he attended the clinics in the old amphitheater at Blockley (Philadelphia General

FIG. 32-37. W.W. Keen in World War I uniform (1917).

WILLIAM W. KEEN, M.D.
JANUARY 19, 1837,
JUNE 7, 1932.
KEEN

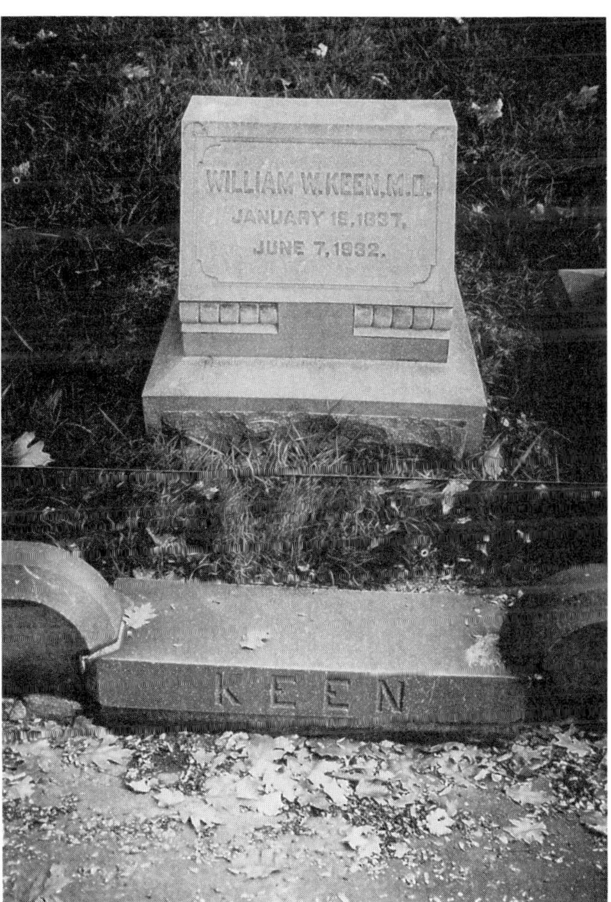

FIG. 32-38. Tombstone of William W. Keen, M.D.

Hospital) to observe the elder Gross and Joseph Pancoast perform surgery. Unfortunately, before completion of his college course, DaCosta's father died and the family experienced financial reversals. Two years of college were more than ample at that time for matriculation at Jefferson Medical College (1882), from which he graduated in 1885 as Class Valedictorian.

After 13 months of residency at the Old Blockley Hospital, DaCosta became Assistant Physician to the Insane Department. His exposure to the antics of the insane drained him emotionally, and when one of the patients committed suicide by hanging he tendered his resignation. In 1887, however, DaCosta was not totally disillusioned, for he became Assistant Physician to the Pennsylvania Hospital for the Insane at forty-fourth and Market Streets, known then as Kirkbride's. His experience with the insane laid the groundwork for his extensive knowledge and prolonged interest in neurology, which later enhanced his diagnostic skill and teaching.

Later in 1887 DaCosta entered private practice but became appointed as Assistant Demonstrator of Anatomy and a Clinical Assistant in the surgical outpatient department of Professor Samuel W. Gross. His office was at 2047 Locust Street, in one room of the first floor of a dressmaking establishment. The first patient not only failed to pay a fee but stole his umbrella.

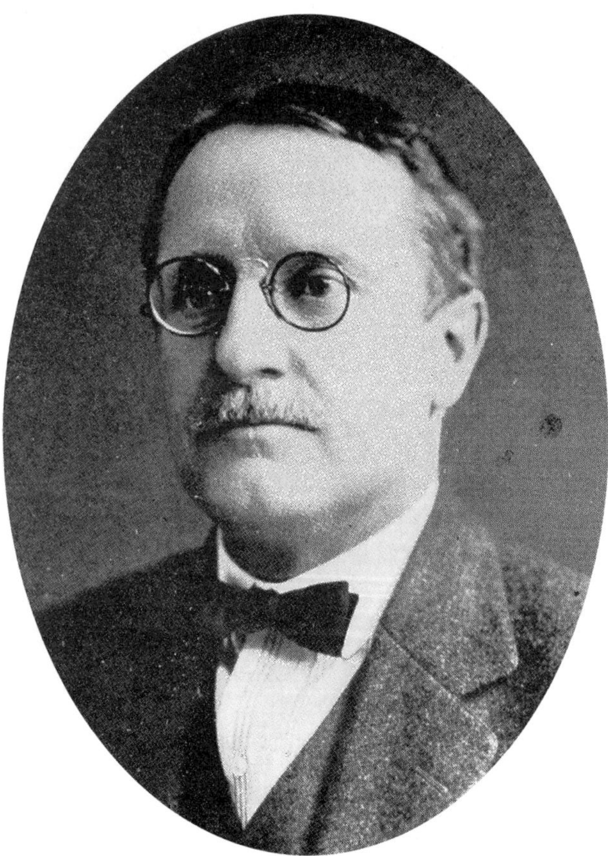

FIG. 32-39. John Chalmers DaCosta, M.D., LL.D. (1863–1933); Sixth Chairmanship (Co-Chairman, 1907–1931), First Samuel D. Gross Professor (1910–1931).

With the unexpected death from pneumonia of Samuel W. Gross in 1889, Dr. W.W. Keen, who succeeded to the Professorship, took on the young and promising DaCosta as an office assistant. The latter had very few patients and was as yet unmarried. He would quip that the name on his office was only "a coffin plate on a dead business." Later he added: "In those days patients regarded the "9 to 1" on my sign as a notice of the odds against them."

DaCosta's spare time away from Jefferson and Dr. Keen's office was spent collaborating on Keating's *Medical Dictionary* and writing his own *Modern Surgery, General and Operative*, first published in 1894 when he was 31 years of age. By the following year, his many articles and prestigious textbook led to his appointment as Clinical Professor of Surgery.

In 1895 Jefferson Medical College was changing from a proprietary school to a nonprofit sharing corporation. Under this situation the full Professors would have to accept fixed salaries for their teaching, and the surplus funds from student's tuition would belong to the School. DaCosta enlisted the Alumni Association at its annual banquet to support this change in a speech entitled *The Professional Jackpot*. This was the beginning of his leadership in the affairs of the Alumni Association (President in 1908), which later would honor him in special ways.

Other medical schools began to offer DaCosta alluring teaching positions. In 1900 the Co-Professors Keen and Brinton agreed to his promotion as a third full Professor in order to hold him at Jefferson. DaCosta, 37 years old, had "arrived."

DaCosta's surgical training was acquired in the system of those times: by serving in the surgical outpatient department, by giving anesthesia, and by acting as office assistant to an established surgeon. His pupil–master relationship had been with the nationally renowned W.W. Keen. In 1907, at Keen's retirement, DaCosta was appointed the successor. With the endowment of the Samuel D. Gross Professorship in 1910 by Maria Gross Horwitz, Gross's daughter, DaCosta was the unopposed and unanimous designate.

The Wednesday afternoon surgical clinic in the amphitheater before the combined junior and senior classes was in its heyday during DaCosta's time and was never surpassed. Edward J. Klopp (Jefferson, 1906), Professor of Surgery from 1931 to 1936, described it as follows:

> "He [DaCosta] loved to teach and his hearers were impressed with his foundation in anatomy, his knowledge of surgery, his familiarity with history, his frequent quotations from literature, and his inimitable manner in presenting a subject. Jack DaCosta always was at his best before a large audience. Only those who saw him before he became incapacitated in 1922 will remember his characteristic attitude while conducting a diagnostic clinic for the students; with amphitheater filled to capacity, the clinic floor and doorway crowded with visiting physicians, confreres, assistants and former students, first standing to one side of the 'pit' with arm resting on the rail and one leg crossed in front of the other, then walking across the floor with body vibrating and knees bending, he spoke, giving clear systematic, unmistakable facts which left an indelible impression. He was the idol of the medical students. Their admiration was spontaneous. He appealed to the imagination, aroused enthusiam, and stimulated effort."

Dr. Benjamin F. Haskell (Jefferson, 1923), later a Clinical Professor of Surgery (Proctology) at Jefferson, remembered as a student the visit to the DaCosta clinic of one of the Mayo brothers in the early 1920s. On being recognized and asked to stand up to make a few remarks, Mayo replied: "In the presence of the greatest teacher of surgery in the United States today, I have nothing to say," and he sat down.

DaCosta served for many years as Surgeon to the Philadelphia General Hospital and later as Consultant to St. Joseph's and Misericordia Hospitals. His thorough knowledge of anatomy and sound surgical judgment were always evident in his operations. His surgical techniques would be considered elementary by today's standards. Anesthesia was administered, usually as open-drop ether, by nurses, interns, or office assistants, with the surgeon in charge as "captain of the ship." Blood transfusions, fluid and electrolyte replacement, and antibiotics were a generation away. Peritonitis was the dreaded complication of abdominal surgery. Primary anastomosis after colon resertion was prohibitive for this reason. Gastroenterostomy was his most complex stomach operation, and he never performed a gastrectomy. Mastectomy, herniorrhaphy, colostomy, hysterectomy, oophorectomy, cholecystectomy, appendectomy, and amputations were the common major operations. It must be recalled that DaCosta was blind in his right eye. His handling of tissues was somewhat rough, and his well-chosen assistants often rescued the situation if bleeding became excessive. Despite this criticism, DaCosta's reputation as a surgeon was always respected by his peers (Figure 32-40). When arthritis struck him, in the early 1920s, DaCosta's "hands" became those of his assistant, Dr. Thomas A. Shallow.

DaCosta's fame as an author rested upon his *Modern Surgery,* which went through ten editions between 1894 and 1931. It was a standard textbook in medical schools throughout the country. He edited an English version of *Zuckerkandl's Operative Surgery* (1898), *Gray's Anatomy* (1905), as well as articles in J.C. Wilson's *Applied Therapeutics*, Hobart A. Hare's *American System of Therapeutics,* Keating's *Encyclopedia of Children's Diseases,* and Wood's *Reference Hand Book*. His medical interests were diversified, encompassing such subjects as osteitis deformans, tumors of the broad ligament, polypharmacy, medical ethics, and medical activities of the Navy. His youthful experiences in neuropsychiatry resulted in articles on surgical treatment of epilepsy, the diagnosis of postoperative insanity, concussion of the brain, suicide, and even the surgery of idiocy and insanity.

In 1903 DaCosta wrote an article on *The Effects of the Inhalation of Smoke and of Irritating and Poisonous Gases of Firemen*. For about 35 years he served without salary as surgeon to the Fireman's Pension Fund. Until his death he had an extension of the Philadelphia fire alarm system installed in his home. It signaled all the first alarms and many of the local calls that emanated from the central station. Wearing his badge, and often his uniform, he would attend all the fires he could, riding on the apparatus drawn by horses. Extinction of fires fascinated him, but his purpose was to render immediate care to injured firemen, care that equaled that given to his private patients. In May, 1931, at one of the Wednesday clinics, DaCosta in his wheelchair was made an Honorary Deputy Chief of the Philadelphia Fire Department, a distinction not previously held by anyone (Figure 32-41). He was presented a diamond-studded badge of office that remains greatly admired in Jefferson's archival treasure trove (Figure 32-42).

Another interest that DaCosta carried into later life was in railroad locomotives. In 1903 he sponsored a free course of illustrated lectures at Jefferson to train employees of the railroads entering Philadelphia in the care of those wounded in wrecks. DaCosta used the railroads in a unique manner to grade the final examination in surgery. He would purchase for $20 a railroad mileage book of 1,000 miles at 2¢ a mile. He would then take a long train ride until all the papers were marked. He also used the train to host fishing parties for his surgical staff and friends at Spidel's Hotel in Atlantic City. In his final days he often wished for just one more train ride to Atlantic City.

In DaCosta's earlier years, his interest in neuropsychiatry, coupled with the necessity to augment his income, led to his appointment as Surgeon to the Eastern Penitentiary. This contact with inmates convinced him that some could be rehabilitated by financial and employment aid. He took the risk of befriending "Split-the-Wind Dunlop," a notorious burglar and safecracker, who had served his prison term, by providing lodging in his own home and obtaining a position for him

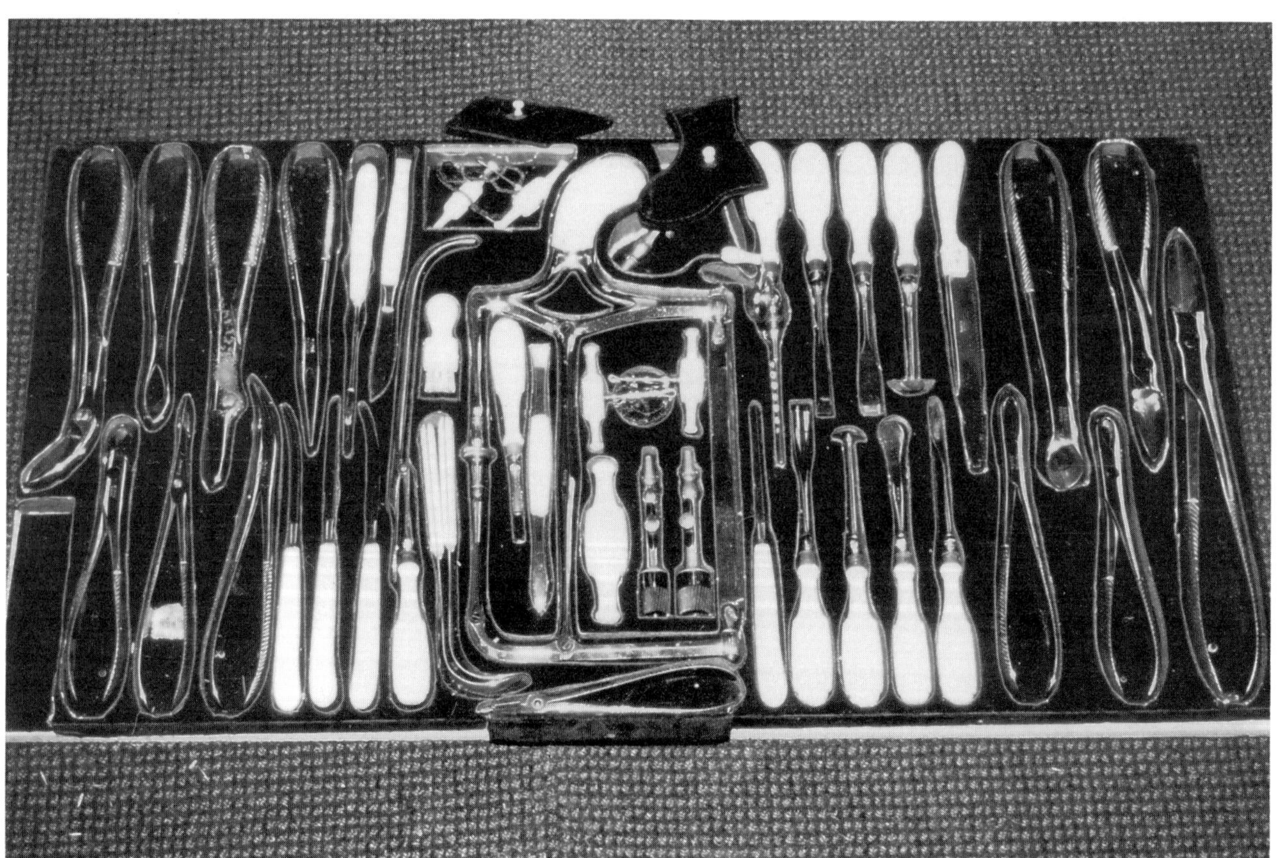

FIG. 32-40. DaCosta's surgical instruments.

as a "Diener" (laboratory helper) in the Anatomy Department at Jefferson. Dunlop became proficient in preparing specimens and was well liked. DaCosta arranged for a private room for Dunlop in 1910, when the latter became seriously ill. He also paid for his burial, to which bunches of flowers were sent by Jefferson friends.

An example of DaCosta's sympathetic nature, belied by his austere demeanor, was his affection for his handyman, Willie Barrett. This black man was occasionally "fired" at the end of the day for the poor performance of a chore. A smile would appear on Willie's face for he knew that on reporting to work the following morning he would receive an extra dollar. When Willie died of coronary thrombosis in the consoling arms of DaCosta, a request for postmortem examination was refused by DaCosta because "Willie would not like it."

Although DaCosta was not a "joiner" in the ordinary sense of the word, he held membership in many societies. These included the American Surgical Association, Society of Clinical Surgery, International Surgical Society, American College of Surgeons (Vice President, 1928–1929), American Philosophical Society, College of Physicians of Philadelphia, Philadelphia Academy of Surgery, Philadelphia Neurological Society, Pathological Society of Philadelphia, Philadelphia County Medical Society, American Medical Association, the U.S. Naval Reserve, and Society of Surgery of Bucharest, Rumania, in which he was an Honorary Fellow.

DaCosta would have qualified as a college professor of English literature or history. His *Selections from the Papers and Speeches of John Chalmers DaCosta, M.D., LL.D.* (1931), dedicated to Dr. Harvey Cushing, are replete with scholarly articles and speeches in these fields, and they are put down in pungent, precise style. Their range and scholarship reveal an encyclopedic mind in historical sketches, biography, political denunciations, critiques of medical trends, and reflections on social dilemmas. He had read all the works of Dickens and could quote some sections from memory. His *Dickens's Doctors* disclosed the low esteem in which the great novelist held the medical profession. In this article DaCosta concluded: "What a pity that he never delineated such a lion-heart as Abernathy's, such a lordly soul as Hunter's, such a noble career as Paget's, or such a helpful life as Gross's. The world will always be poorer because he did not."[19]

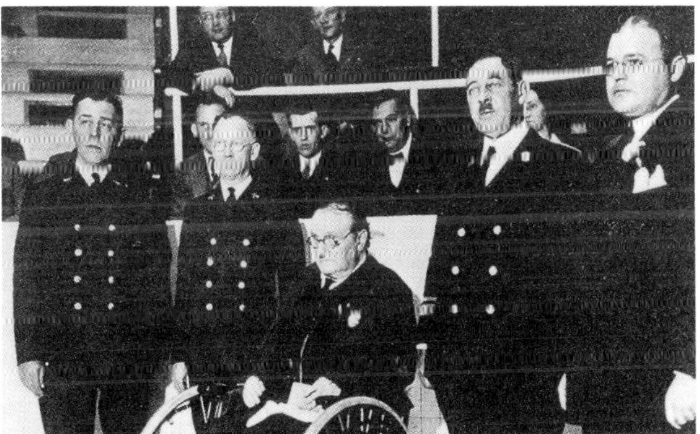

FIG. 32-41. Officials of the Philadelphia Fire Department and City Council present Professor DaCosta with an Honorary Deputy Fire Chief badge at one of his clinics (1931).

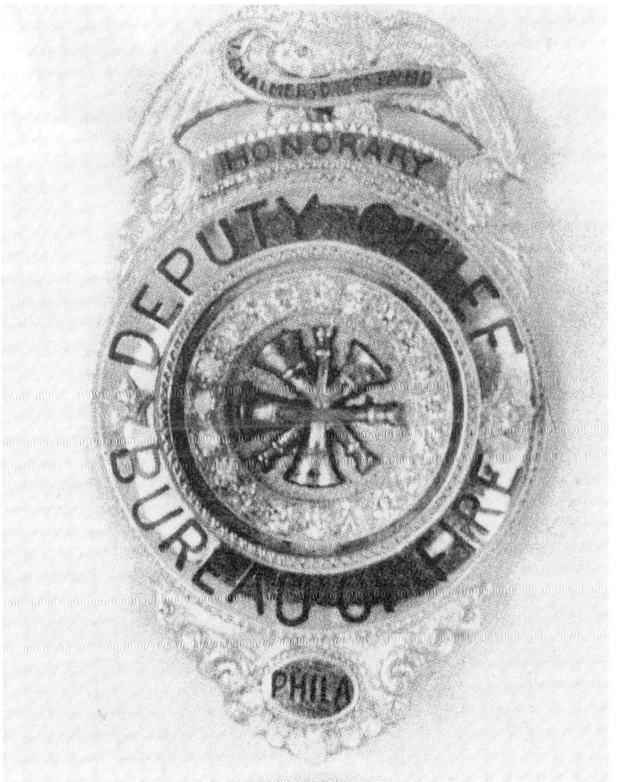

FIG. 32-42. Professor DaCosta's diamond-studded Deputy Fire Chief badge.

One of DaCosta's more tangible acts relating to the appreciation of his alma mater's heritage was his resurrection of the "old operating table." This was the table made in the early 1850s and depicted by Eakins in the *Gross Clinic* painting of 1875. It had served in the upper lecture room of the old Tenth Street Medical College and then in the "pit" of the 1877 Hospital. It had been used for anatomy and obstetrical lectures and for surgical operative clinics. Around 1916 DaCosta wondered what had happened to this venerable table. It was found in the basement holding oil cans and waste material. With his suggestion, the Class of 1916 had it repaired and attached a commemorative plate at one end. The Class of 1917 added a plaque at the other end. It was displayed in the library of the 1025 Walnut Street College for many years and again went into storage. In 1982 it was once more restored and placed in a specially constructed alcove of the Samuel D. Gross Conference Room of the Surgery Department (Figure 32-43). DaCosta's article on *Facts Concerning the Old Operating Table* is a classic.[20]

At the outbreak of World War I, DaCosta served as a Junior Lieutenant in the Navy and was promoted to the rank of Commander (Figure 32-44). In 1919 he sailed on the *George Washington* on a special mission to care for the ailing President Woodrow Wilson while negotiations of the peace treaty and the League of Nations were conducted.

In 1922, at the age of 59, DaCosta became afflicted with progressive rheumatoid arthritis. With tenacity and courage he continued to teach,

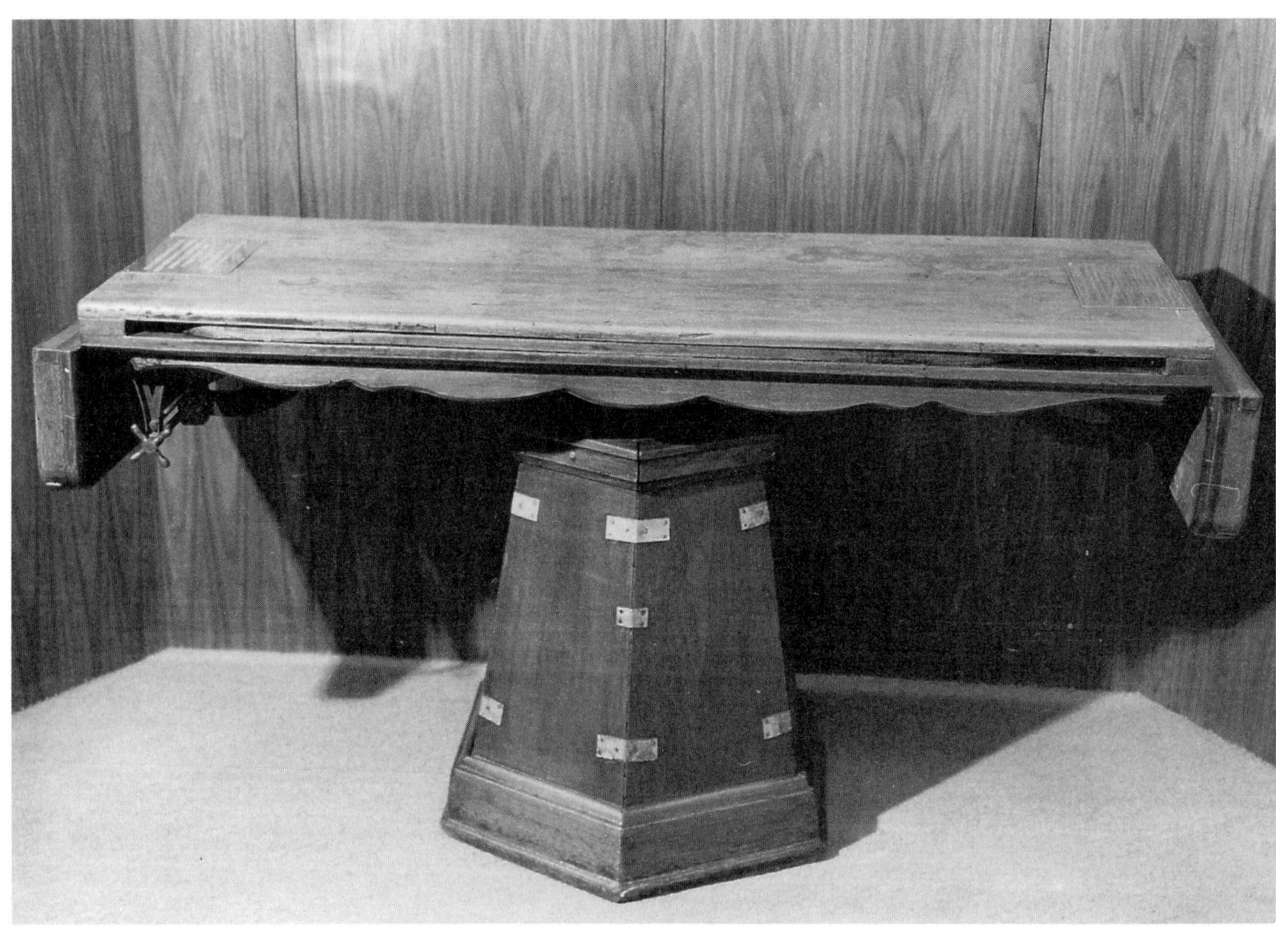

FIG. 32-43. "Old Operating Table" used by Professor Samuel D. Gross and depicted by Eakins in the *Gross Clinic*.

give speeches, write articles, and update his *Modern Surgery*. Two poles placed beneath his wheelchair permitted transport from his home to a waiting automobile. Members of his Staff (Drs. Thomas Shallow, Harvey Righter, and Henry Seelaus) formed a team to ensure his safe passage to and from his Wednesday clinic, which still commanded standing room only.

During this period of deteriorating physical condition, DaCosta's mind remained sharp and active, and he received many well-deserved honors. In 1923 the students' Yearbook was dedicated to him for the second time (the first was in 1906). The Class of 1924 had his portrait painted, depicting him teaching from his wheelchair in the amphitheater. This started the yearly tradition of each class thereafter presenting the portrait of a favorite Professor to the College. The Class of 1902 also presented DaCosta's portrait in 1929, and the Alumni Association commissioned two others. All four portraits are prominently displayed at Jefferson. The Class of 1926 presented him with a gold-headed cane inscribed with his name as the first Samuel D. Gross Professor (Figure 32-45). At its fiftieth reunion in 1976 the same Class endowed a fund in perpetuity to add the name of each succeeding Gross Professor on a separate gold plate. He received the Strittmater Award of the Philadelphia County Medical Society in 1926. The Jefferson Alumni Association, in May, 1927, commissioned a tablet that recorded the gift of $100,000 as a memorial in his honor to the establishment of a Department of Experimental Medicine in the new 1025 Walnut Street Medical College of 1928 (Figure 32-46).

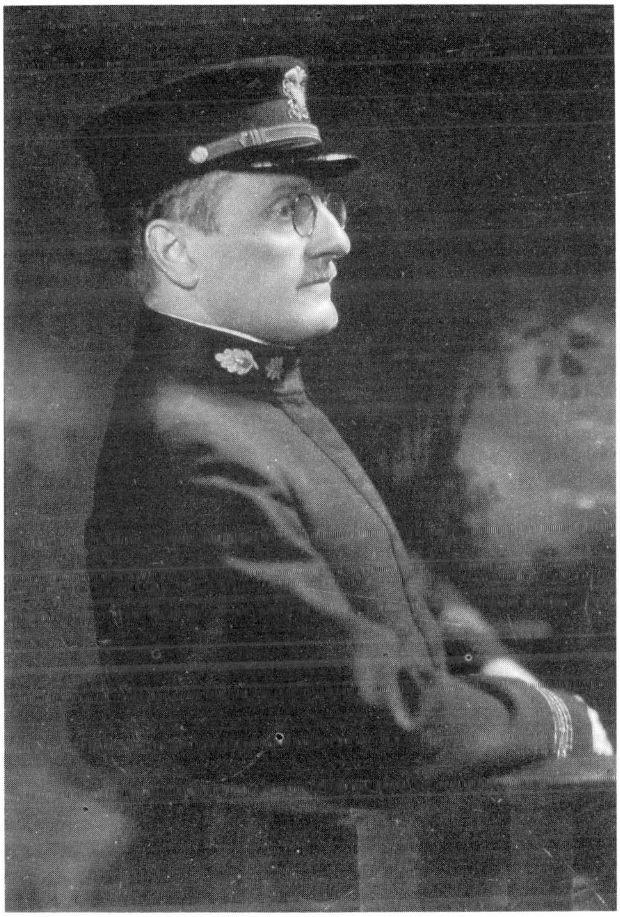

FIG. 32-44. DaCosta as a Commissioned Officer in the Medical Corps in the U.S. Navy in World War I.

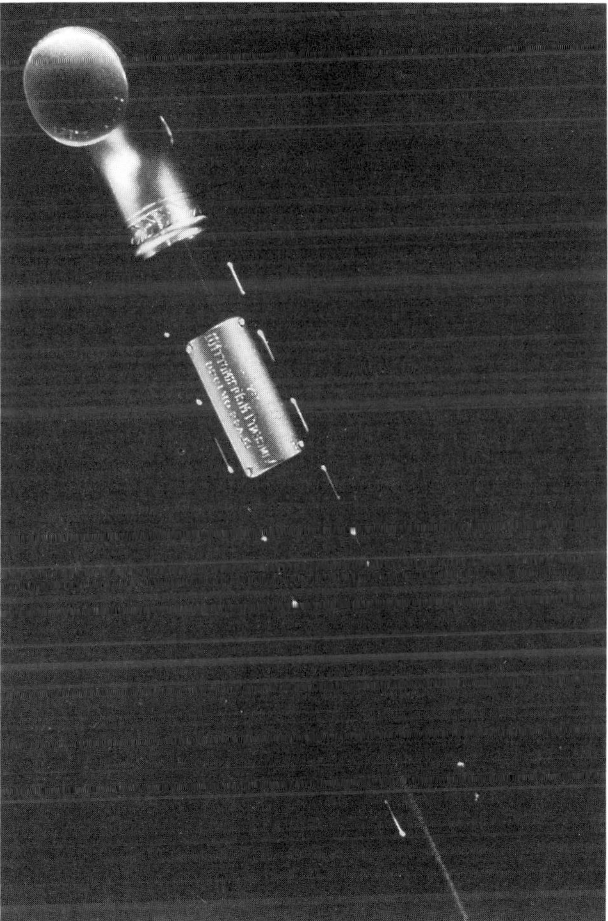

FIG. 32-45. Gold-headed cane of the Samuel D. Gross Professorship.

On April 30, 1930, *The DaCosta Surgical Night* was held under the auspices of the Philadelphia County Medical Society. The purpose was the establishment of the DaCosta Foundation for postgraduate education of members of the Society. Scientific papers were read by Drs. John B. Deaver, Rudolph Matas, and Walter E. Dandy. DaCosta himself gave the second annual oration the following year in a farewell address to the Society. The *Philadelphia Record* reported that "an audience of about 1,000 physicians and their wives alternately shouted with glee and wept as the aged and broken surgeon and teacher denounced and applauded the things he had found good and bad in his profession and in mankind generally."

In his library, where DaCosta had spent the final years of his life on a bed built against the wall, the end came on May 16, 1933. Mrs. DaCosta had provided the last measure of devotion in which she had unselfishly understood and supported him in every endeavor. They had no children. His body was buried in Woodlands Cemetery, Lot 265, Section K, but the man remains as one of Jefferson's immortals (Figure 32-47).

DaCosta wrote poetry that perhaps was more scholarly than inspired. A collection of 27 poems dedicated to his wife was published posthumously in 1942.[21] An appropriate quotation is the following:

> "Give up the play of idle priestly canting,
> Go out among mankind with loaf and cup,
> Without a thought of praying or of chanting,
> Give food and drink and raise the fallen up."

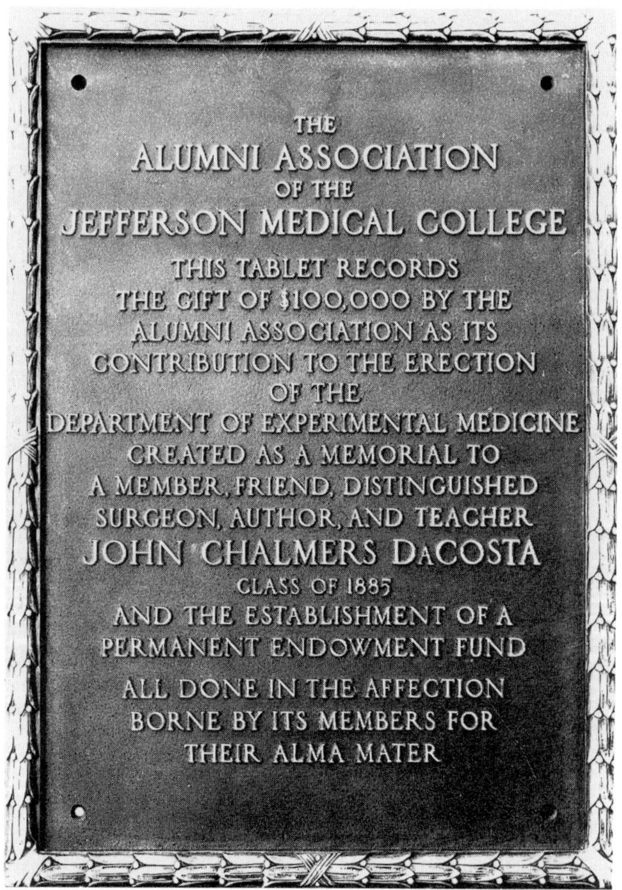

FIG. 32-46. Memorial tablet to Professor John Chalmers DaCosta by the Alumni Association.

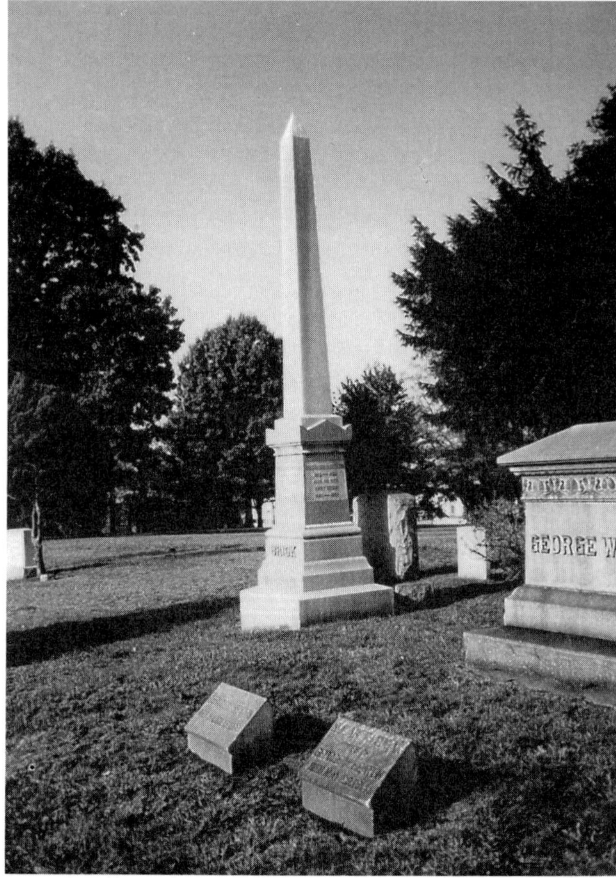

FIG. 32-47. Obelisk marking the gravesite of Professor John Chalmers DaCosta.

John Heysham Gibbon, M.D., Sc.D. (1871–1956); Sixth Chairmanship (Co-Chairman, 1907–1931)

John H. Gibbon (Figure 32-48) succeeded Professor John H. Brinton in 1907 as Professor of Practice of Surgery and Clinical Surgery. Brinton had held his post during the Co-Chairmanship of Samuel W. Gross and William W. Keen in the divided Chair following the retirement of Samuel D. Gross in 1882. Gibbon thus became Co-Chairman with John Chalmers DaCosta, with whom he worked harmoniously in tandem throughout their mutual tenures.

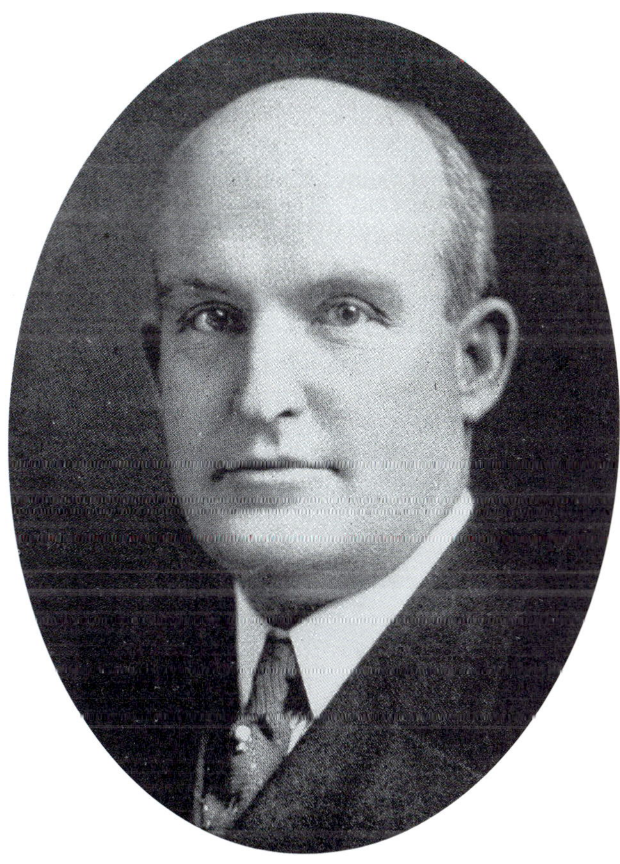

FIG. 32-48. John H. Gibbon, M.D., Sc.D. (1871–1956); Sixth Chairmanship (Co-Chairman, 1907–1931).

Dr. Gibbon was born in Charlotte, North Carolina, on March 16, 1871, with a distinctly medical lineage.[22] His great-grandfather, Dr. John H. Gibbons, was a graduate of the University of Edinburgh in 1786, who lectured privately in Philadelphia on the Theory and Practice of Medicine and became a Charter Member of the College of Physicians of Philadelphia. He died at the early age of 36, leaving one son, also John H., who dropped the "s" from the name. The latter graduated in medicine from the University of Pennsylvania, but instead of practicing devoted himself to scientific interests, especially minerology. He moved in 1838 to Charlotte, where he became the Assayer in the United States Mint. His second son, Robert, was the father of Co-Chairman John Gibbon, and graduated from Jefferson in 1848. Dr. Robert Gibbon had a large surgical practice in Charlotte and was a Brigadier-Surgeon in the Confederate Army during the Civil War. Co-Chairman Gibbon was thus a fourth-generation physician in a direct line. Additionally, his brother, Dr. Robert L. Gibbon, of Charlotte, graduated from Jefferson in 1888 and became a Professor of Surgery in the North Carolina Medical College in 1918. The lineage would extend into a fifth generation in the person of John H. Gibbon, Jr., who would create a new era in cardiac surgery through his heart-lung machine and also, as Samuel D. Gross Professor, would unite the divided Chair of Surgery in 1956.

Dr. Gibbon received his preliminary education at the Macon School in Charlotte, and was graduated from Jefferson in 1891. He served for one year as Resident Physician in the Polyclinic Hospital and subsequently in the Pennsylvania Hospital (1893–1895). Upon beginning practice in Philadelphia he also became an Assistant Demonstrator of Anatomy at Jefferson, with promotion to Demonstrator of Osteology. In 1896 he was appointed a Surgeon in the Outpatient Department of Pennsylvania Hospital. He was elected Chief of the Surgical Clinic at Jefferson Hospital in 1899, a position he held for three years before resigning to become Professor of Surgery at the Philadelphia Polyclinic in 1901. In 1903 Dr. Gibbon was elected Surgeon to the Pennsylvania Hospital to succeed the late Thomas G. Morton. The same year he became an Associate Professor of Surgery at Jefferson until elected to the full Professorship in 1907 as Co-Chairman with Dr. John Chalmers DaCosta.

Dr. Gibbon had a distinguished military record. During the Spanish-American War he served as First Lieutenant and Assistant Surgeon in the Third U.S. Volunteer Engineers. In 1917 he was commissioned as Major in the Medical Reserve Corps of the U.S. Army and attached to Pennsylvania Base Hospital No. 10, which subsequently took over a British General Hospital at LeTreport, France. This unit sailed for France on May 18, 1917, with Dr. Gibbon as Chief of Surgical Services. In October, 1917, he served on detached duty as Surgeon in charge of a Casualty Clearing Station Team in a hospital situated in a small corner of Belgium still held by the Allies. In December of that year he was assigned as Consultant in Surgery to the American Expeditionary Forces. In August, 1918, he became Surgical Consultant to the American Hospitals in England. When his military service was terminated in January, 1919, he held the rank of Colonel (Figure 32-49).

For some years Dr. Gibbon was Surgical Registrar at the Philadelphia General Hospital and had an appointment on the Surgical Dispensary Staff of the Children's Hospital. He also was elected Surgeon to the Bryn Mawr Hospital (1900).

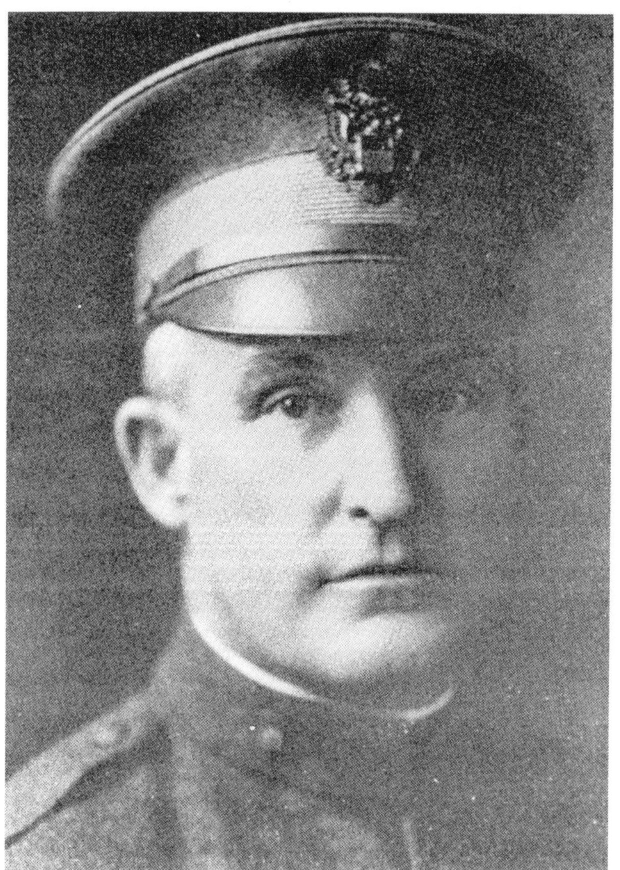

FIG. 32-49. Professor John H. Gibbon in World War I.

Dr. Gibbon wrote more than 60 articles in a diverse range of surgical subjects and several others of historical or philosophical nature. In 1902 he reported the fourth case of penetrating wound of the heart operated upon successfully in the United States. The following year he reported a painless amputation of the leg following the intraneural injection of cocaine. He also became interested in aneurysms, on which subject he wrote several papers. For a number of years he edited the Saunders *Year Book of Surgery* in conjunction with his Co-Chairman, Dr. John Chalmers DaCosta. He wrote the section on "Operative Techniques" in *Keen's Surgery.* His last literary contribution was in 1926 at his Presidential Address of the American Surgical Association on *The Psychology of the Sick Man.*

Through his excellent surgical technique, Dr. Gibbon stressed the importance of gentleness in the handling of tissues. He encouraged those he trained to use local anesthesia in order to acquire this quality. In addition to his clinics at Jefferson, Dr. Gibbon gave a weekly clinic at the Pennsylvania Hospital. Several times a year he presented fractures, in which his interest had dated from his earlier years in teaching osteology. These clinics in the Pennsylvania Hospital were always filled and attracted students from all the medical schools in Philadelphia. His lectures were clear, informative, and interesting.

Dr. Gibbon served as President of the American Surgical Association, the College of Physicians of Philadelphia, and the Philadelphia Academy of Surgery. He was an original member of the Society of Clinical Surgery. In 1948 Jefferson awarded the Honorary Degree of Doctor of Science to Dr. Gibbon because of his significant contributions to the medical profession, to his country, and to humanity.

A strong believer that older men should not wait too long before making way for the younger, Dr. Gibbon resigned his Chairmanship at the age of 60. He timed this to coincide with the resignation in 1931 of his Co-Chairman, Dr. DaCosta, to conclude the Sixth Chairmanship and make way for two new appointees. After retirement, Dr. Gibbon pursued his hobby of carpentry, did much reading, and retained his keen interest in national and world affairs.

Dr. Gibbon had suffered a coronary artery occlusion in 1935 while in Boston for a meeting of the American Surgical Association. He suffered a second one a few years later and a third in December of 1955. On March 13, 1956, he developed sudden pulmonary edema and died within a few hours, at the age of 85. This was the year in which his son, John H. Gibbon, Jr., became appointed the Samuel D. Gross Professor of Surgery and unified the Chair that had been divided for the previous 74 years.

Francis Torrens Stewart, M.D. (1874–1920); Professor of Clinical Surgery (1910–1920)

It is conceded by all Alumni who remember Dr. Francis T. Stewart (Figure 32-50) that he would have been the successor to John Chalmers DaCosta as the second Samuel D. Gross Professor of Surgery. DaCosta himself said that had Stewart lived he would have been the world's greatest surgeon before he was 50. The unfulfilled potential Chairmanship of this brilliant Jefferson surgeon warrants the special place accorded him in this chronicle.

Dr. Stewart, a native Philadelphian, was born in 1874, received his elementary education in the public schools, and graduated from Central High. Following his graduation from Jefferson (1896), he interned at the Polyclinic Hospital (Eighteenth and Lombard Streets), followed by a year as Chief Resident at the Pennsylvania Hospital. During that term he repaired a stab wound of the heart and later added four more successful cases.[23]

As a surgeon, Stewart was phenomenal for his era. His speed in operating (which merited the term "wizard hands") was matched only by his accuracy and sound judgment. It is said that while the intern was closing the skin following a herniorrhaphy, Stewart would totally complete the entire procedure on the contralateral side. His operation for perforation of a typhoid ulcer of the intestine was a matter of minutes. His transverse incision for mastectomy became known as the "Stewart incision." Always in the forefront of advances in surgery, he advocated the more widespread use of lumbar puncture. He also was influential in changing the color of the garb and sheets in the operating room from the traditional white to another color to avoid glare. His personal choice was jet black.

Stewart wrote articles on a diversity of subjects and had the temerity to publish his own *Manual of Surgery* (five editions between 1907 and 1921), despite DaCosta's widely used *Modern Surgery,* which was in its fifth edition, with five more to follow until 1931. This competition with his Chief apparently resulted only in mutual admiration. Among his later papers were those dealing with surgery of the heart and blood vessels; he wrote the section on that subject in the *American Practice of Surgery* (1909).

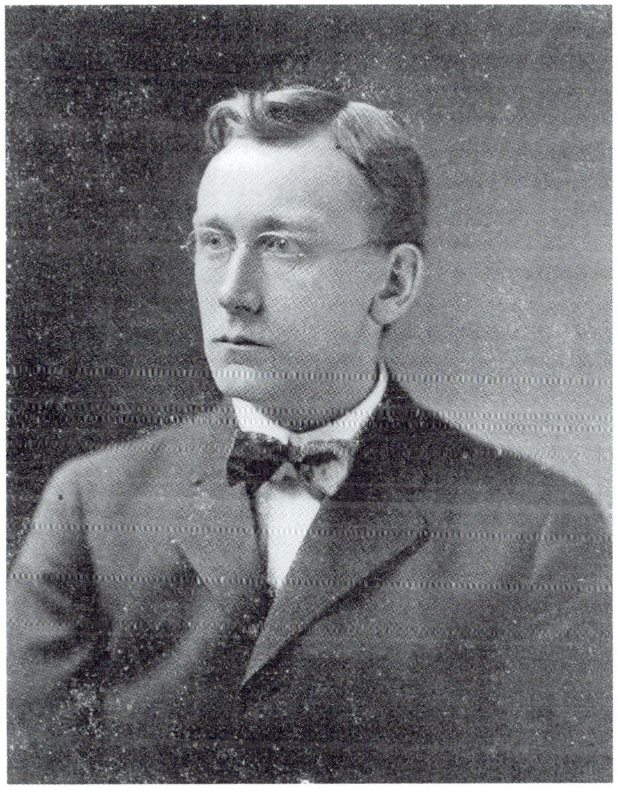

FIG. 32-50. Francis Torrens Stewart, M.D. (1874–1920); Professor of Clinical Surgery (1910–1920).

In 1910 Dr. Stewart succeeded Dr. William Joseph Hearn as Professor of Clinical Surgery. His lectures and clinical demonstrations were greatly admired by the students. Although busy at Jefferson, he was also active on the staffs of the Pennsylvania and Germantown Hospitals. He participated in organized medicine and the important professional societies of his field. On the international level he was a member of the Societé Internationale de Chirurgie. In 1917 he received a letter from William Mayo waiving all formalities of application to unanimous election to the newly formed American College of Surgeons. The same honor at the time was accorded to Drs. DaCosta and Gibbon, Sr.

In 1920 Stewart was found unconscious in his bathtub, and he died of uremia. His death at age 46 was truly a tragic loss to Jefferson. Mathilda Kellar Stewart presented her husband's portrait to the College. She also endowed the Francis Torrens Stewart Research Fellowship to be awarded to graduates of Jefferson of not less than one year or more than ten years for clinical research under the direction of the Professors of that subject.

Thomas Aloysius Shallow, M.D., LL.D. (1886–1955); Seventh Chairmanship (Co-Chairman, 1931–1955), Second Samuel D. Gross Professor (1939–1955)

Professor John Chalmers DaCosta first tendered his resignation in 1929 because of failing health, but it was refused by the Board of Trustees. The Board finally accepted it in 1931, but continued his Samuel D. Gross Professorship until his death in 1933 at an annual salary of $2,400. There was a stipulation that he would oversee the running of the Department of Surgery by two newly appointed Professors, Thomas A. Shallow and Edward J. Klopp.

Shallow was the protégé of DaCosta, and Klopp was the choice of Gibbon. They were of equal and coordinate rank, with Shallow taking responsibility for the seniors and Klopp for the juniors. After the death of DaCosta in 1933, it could have been proper to designate a successor to the Samuel D. Gross Professorship. It seemed at the time, however, that Shallow and Klopp were of equal ability, yet neither had reached a distinction in the profession appropriate to the prestige of the title. It would take six more years and the death of Klopp in 1936 for Shallow to be designated the second Gross Professor in 1939.

Thomas A. Shallow (Figure 32-48) was born on November 26, 1886, in Philadelphia, the city to be the center of activities for all of his 69 years.[24] Of Irish and Scotch-English descent, he was sixth in the family of seven children of Edward F. Shallow, a millwright, and Elizabeth MacQuillan Shallow, both of Pennsylvania. His preliminary education was obtained in the public schools, in which he was outstanding as a student and athlete. At the age of 15 his interest in medicine was already such that he would cut classes at Central High School

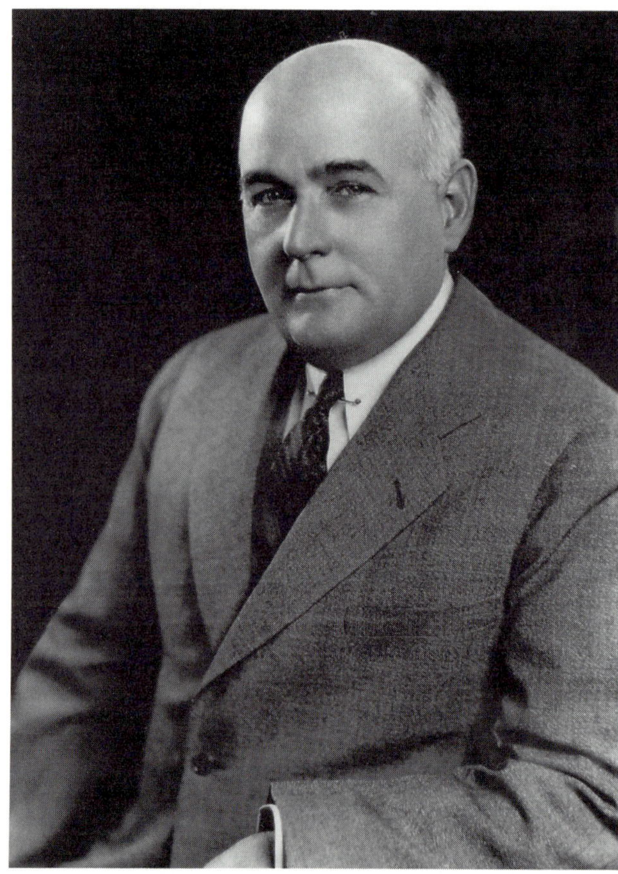

FIG. 32-51. Thomas A. Shallow, M.D., LL.D. (1886–1955); Seventh Chairmanship (Co-Chairman, 1931–1955), Second Samuel D. Gross Professor (1939–1955).

to attend some of the postmortem examinations and teaching clinics at the old Medico-Chi Hospital. In 1907 he matriculated at Jefferson in the 1898 College Building located on the northwest corner of Tenth and Walnut Streets (Figure 32-52). In his sophomore year he was President of the Spitzka Anatomic League and was class historian in his senior year. He also was a prominent member of Jefferson's last track team and last football team. At graduation in 1911 he received the Alumni Prize for the highest general average of the four years as well as several other awards.

After internship in Jefferson Hospital (1911–1913) and during service as Chief Resident Physician (1914), Shallow worked with Drs. Hobart A. Hare in the Department of Experimental Pharmacology and Albert Brubaker as a quiz master in Physiology. Several senior staff members made overtures to him to work as their assistant, but his acceptance was to Professor John Chalmers DaCosta (1914–1925, with exception for military duty).

As a member of Jefferson's faculty, Shallow's career began as Clinical Assistant, with promotion through the ranks to Professor of Surgery in 1931. He reached the zenith of his career in 1939 when he was appointed Samuel D. Gross Professor and Chairman of the Department.

During his earlier years, Shallow served on the staffs of other local hospitals, among which were Philadelphia General, St. Joseph's, Montgomery County, Delaware County, Sacred Heart, and Grand View in Sellersville, Pennsylvania. Later, he

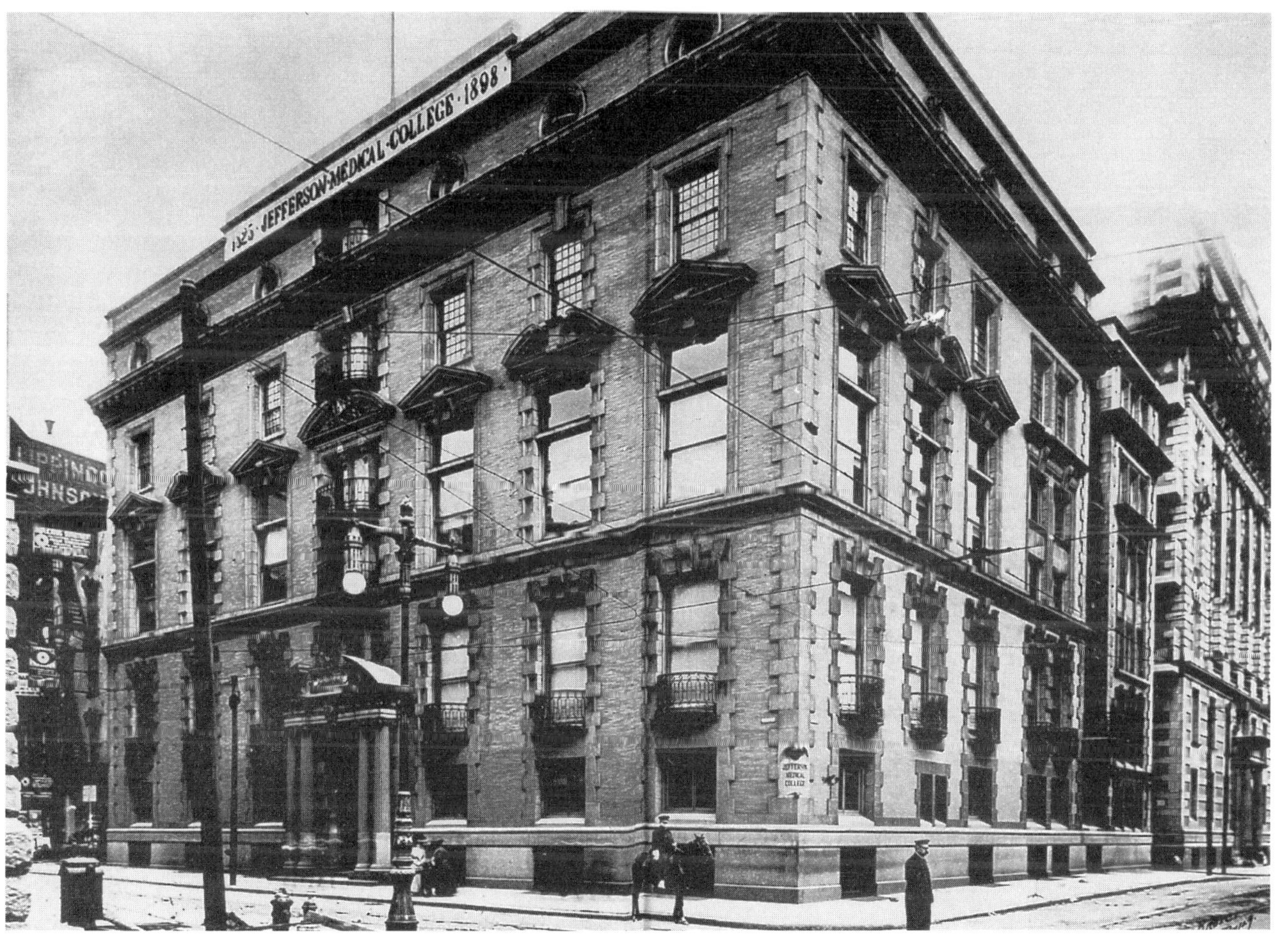

FIG. 32-52. The 1898 Jefferson Medical College Building at the northwest corner of Tenth and Walnut Streets.

restricted his operative work to Jefferson Hospital but remained influential in the affairs of the other institutions.

During World War I (Figure 32-53), Dr. Shallow served as Captain in the Medical Corps (1917–1919). Initially, he was assigned to the Rockefeller Institute, New York, and later acted as Surgeon to Evacuation Hospital Center No. 25 in France. A "trick knee" acquired earlier in his athletic career was quiescent throughout his Army tour of duty but locked as he was leaving the transport ship at the end of the war. Miss Myrtle Luman, who had been DaCosta's operating room nurse, was there to greet him, and they married in 1920.

Dr. Shallow was constitutionally rugged, dynamic, and indefatigable. On the Executive Faculty of the College, his alacrity of thought, coupled with profound knowledge of College and Hospital affairs, aided in his rapid solution of complex administrative problems. His advice was sought and followed by many. In later years he became very influential in recommending deserving young men for staff appointments at Jefferson and elsewhere. He was among the last in the era of the "Geheimrat" and dictatorship in Surgery at Jefferson and other institutions. Known as "the boss," he welcomed being addressed as such.

Dr. Shallow's rough edge made him controversial in academic circles, but in the operating room he was a superb technician with the soundest of judgment (Figure 32-54). His diagnostic acumen was the product of his long association with Dr. DaCosta. His Wednesday afternoon clinics were models of preparation for case presentations in which he would call four students into the "pit" and quiz them as well as

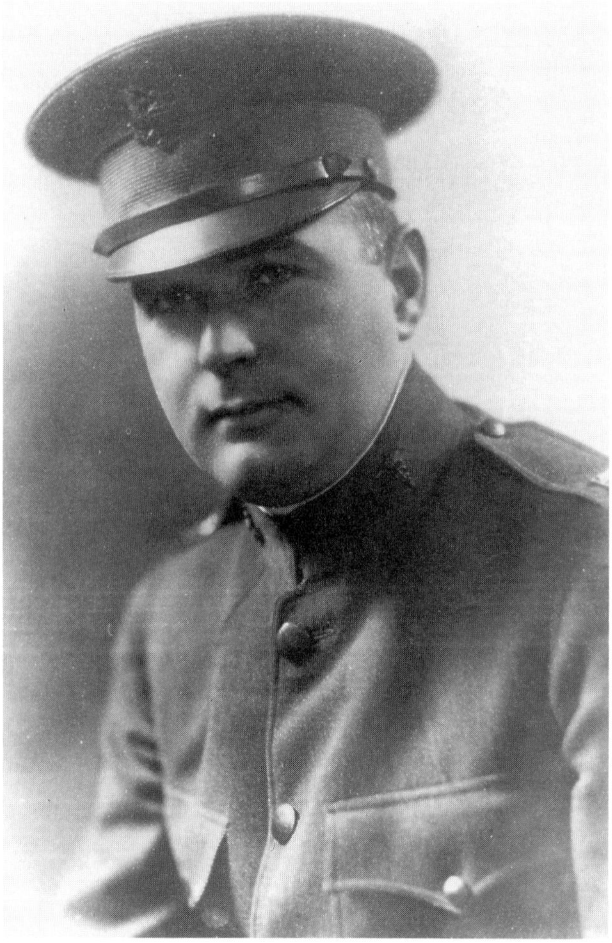

FIG. 32-53. Thomas A. Shallow, M.D., in World War I.

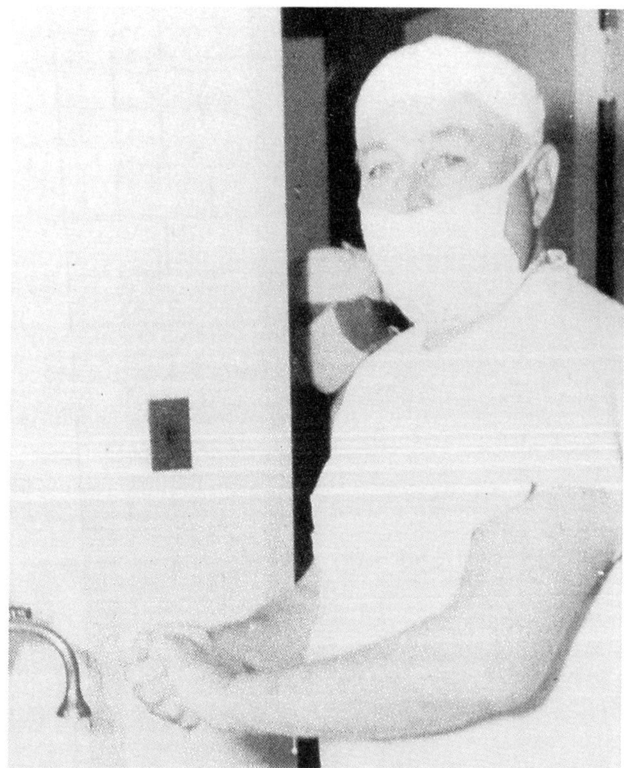

FIG. 32-54. Professor Thomas A. Shallow scrubbing before surgery.

members of his staff, (Figure 32-55). He lacked the literary polish of his old master, DaCosta, but had a flair for sorting out the salient features of a patient's problem and having expert consultants on hand to elucidate the important details. Immediately after the clinic he would perform major surgery before the assembled class, most of whom would remain. It was the last of the type of teaching immortalized in the *Gross Clinic*. Shallow stated that his favorite operation was the one he happened to be doing. It was conceded, however, that his supreme excellence was in surgery of the gastrointestinal tract.

Although not a prolific writer, Shallow contributed more than 80 scientific papers in clinical rather than in laboratory research. He pioneered in the one-stage operation of pharyngeal diverticulectomy, which required the teamwork of surgeon and esophagoscopist. His series of over 400 cases in collaboration with Dr. Louis Clerf at Jefferson was the largest in the country and without a single instance of mediastinitis. He also devised his own operation for gastrostomy and invented an intestinal crushing clamp for extraperitoneal closure of colostomy. His private practice was huge, and his surgical fees were modest—the patients, whether poor or affluent, adored him.

Dr. Shallow spent little time away from Jefferson, but was active in the important societies. He was a President of the Philadelphia Academy of Surgery (founded by Samuel D. Gross in 1879), Fellow of the American College of Surgeons and International College of Surgeons, founder member of the American Board of Surgery, Fellow of the College of Physicians of Philadelphia, member of the County, State, and American Medical Association, the American Association of the History of Medicine, and the American Medical Editors' and Authors' Association. He was active in the Nu Sigma Nu medical fraternity of Jefferson as well as Faculty Adviser for the Alpha Omega Alpha honorary fraternity. He served as President of the Alumni Association in 1938, and his portrait was presented to the College by the Class of 1950 (Figure 32-56). An LL.D. degree from Jefferson Medical College was awarded him in 1953.

Shallow's extramural activities were many and varied. He belonged to the Union League of Philadelphia, Philadelphia Racquet Club, Art Club of Philadelphia, Franklin Institute, and Pennsylvania Scotch-Irish Society. He devoted time to civic affairs and was a member of the Board of City Trusts of Philadelphia, the Board of Directors of Wills Eye Hospital, the Board of Directors of the Municipal Court, Director on the Board of the Old Eagle School (a historical society), and Chairman of the *Philadelphia Inquirer* Hero Award Committee.

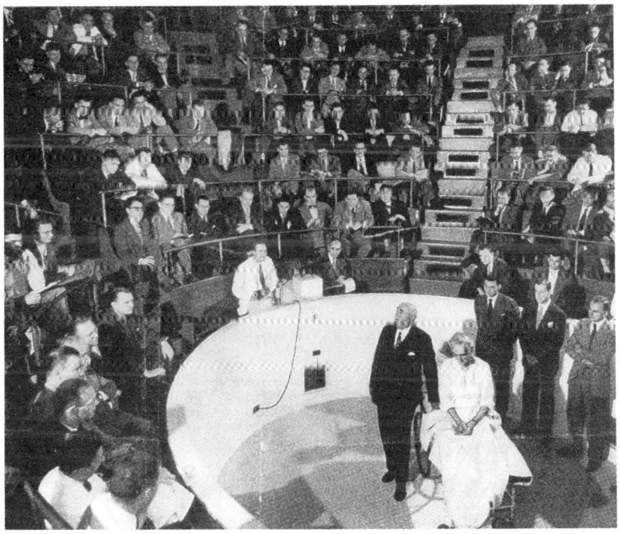

FIG. 32-55. Clinic of Professor Thomas A. Shallow in the "pit" of the Thompson Annex (ca. 1950).

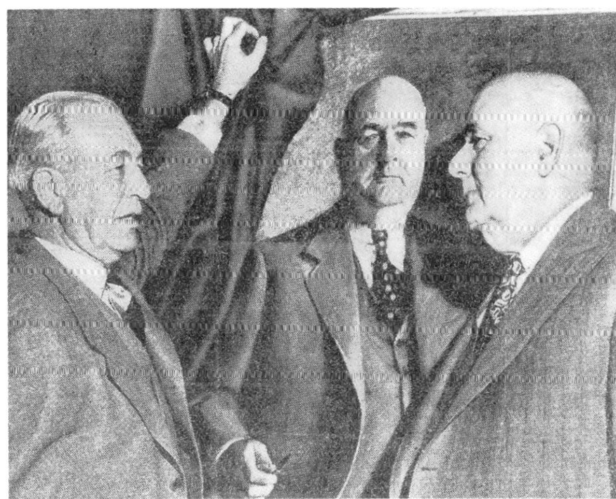

FIG. 32-56. Senior Class (1950) portrait of Professor Thomas A. Shallow, unveiled by Jefferson's President, Vice Admiral James L. Kauffman.

During his last illness from carcinoma of the pharynx, Shallow chose to work despite great discomfort and failing strength. When admitted to Jefferson Hospital for his final days of life, he had four operations on his schedule. On his deathbed he refused to be coddled and maintained his characteristic wit and humor. The end came on December 26, 1955. He was buried in West Laurel Hill Cemetery (Figure 32-57).

Dr. Shallow was the last of the Surgical Chairmen to be nonsalaried. His academic and administrative duties were conducted between operations from a Windsor chair in the surgeon's dressing room on the fourteenth floor of the Thompson Annex. He knew his own faults and advised young men to emulate only his good characteristics. He was truly a man's man, and in his own way was totally devoted to the welfare of Jefferson.

Edward J. Klopp, M.D. (1880–1936); Seventh Chairmanship (Co-Chairman, 1931–1936)

Like the first Co-Chairman, Samuel W. Gross, the life of Edward Klopp was prematurely cut short by an infectious disease. He developed streptococcic endocarditis after extraction of an infected tooth and died at the age of 56. What he might have achieved after five short years of Professorship can only be surmised.

Edward Klopp (Figure 32-58) was born in Sheridan, Pennsylvania, on June 10, 1880.[25] After graduation from the Philadelphia College of Pharmacy and Science (1901) and from Jefferson (1906), he served a two-year internship at Jefferson Hospital, followed by appointment as Chief Resident Physician. The latter supervisory position was an honor accorded to the best of the previous interns.

Klopp began his surgical career in the service of

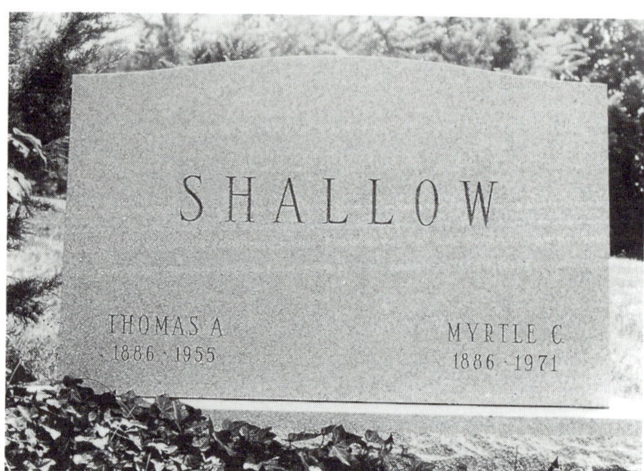

FIG. 32-57. Gravesite of Professor Thomas A. Shallow in West Laurel Hill Cemetery. (Photograph courtesy of Professor Francis E. Rosato.)

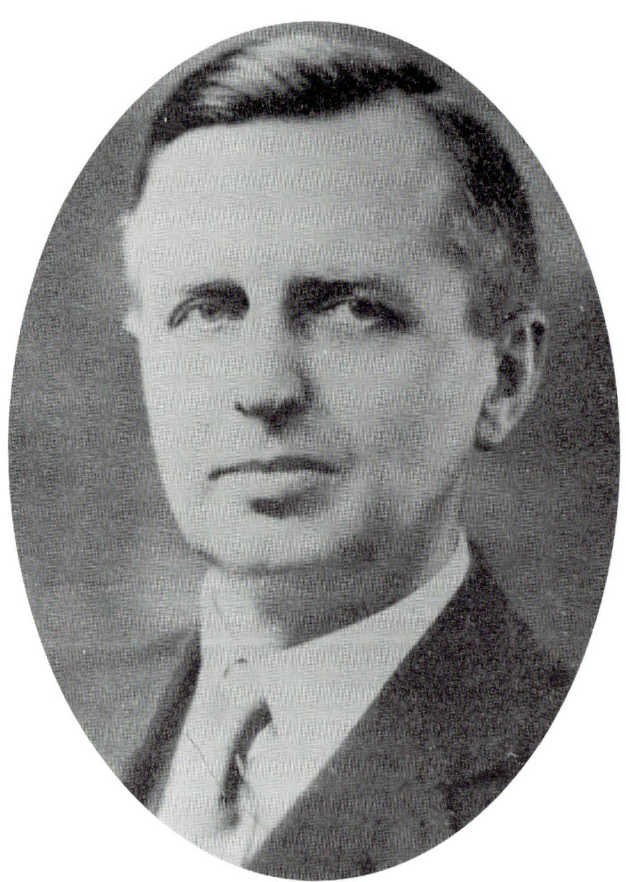

FIG. 32-58. Edward J. Klopp, M.D. (1880–1936); Seventh Chairmanship (Co-Chairman, 1931–1936).

Dr. Francis T. Stewart, Clinical Professor of Surgery at Jefferson, whose brilliant career was also cut short by premature death at age 46 from renal failure in 1920. Through association with Drs. Steward and Gibbon, he acquired staff positions at Jefferson and the Pennsylvania Hospitals, supplemented later as Attending Surgeon to the Memorial and Delaware County Hospitals and Consultant to the Girard College. His surgical technique was characterized by delicacy and dexterity, associated with the calm manner in which he overcame difficulties and complications. His operative skill, coupled with well-developed diagnostic acumen, led to his developing a large surgical practice. He obtained excellent results in an unusually large number of colonic and rectal resections for cancer.

During World War I, Klopp was a member of the Medical Advisory Board of Philadelphia. Although not a large contributor to the surgical literature, he wrote a number of papers on intestinal resection, diseases of the breast, surgery of the thyroid, and blood transfusion. In the various important societies in which he held membership, Klopp kept a low profile but served on many of their committees. He was President of the Alumni Association in 1930.

According to Dr. John H. Gibbon, Sr.: "Although not a brilliant lecturer, he was the best kind of a teacher. He loved his students and was always kind and helpful to them, and in return they exhibited for him a respectful appreciation of his sterling qualities." In 1931 he gave to the junior class the first Grace Revere Osler Lectures that Lady Osler had endowed in honor of her first husband, Samuel W. Gross, for his special interest in tumors. This Lectureship evolved into the Grace Revere Osler Professorship, to which Dr. George P. Muller was the first appointee in 1939.

Dr. Klopp died on September 19, 1936, after an illness of several months in which cerebral emboli complicated his streptococcic endocarditis. The sulfa drugs that became available soon thereafter might have saved or prolonged his life. The Class of 1936 presented his portrait to the College.

George P. Muller, M.D., Sc.D. (1877–1947); Seventh Chairmanship (Co-Chairman, 1936–1946), First Grace Revere Osler Professor (1939–1946)

George P. Muller (Figure 32-59) became Professor of Surgery on November 17, 1936, as the successor to Dr. Edward J. Klopp. He was born on June 29, 1877, in Philadelphia, the son of Philip R. and Francis Hughes Muller.[26] His preliminary education was in the public schools of Philadelphia, with graduation from Central High in 1895. He was a good student, prominent in academic and extracurricular activities.

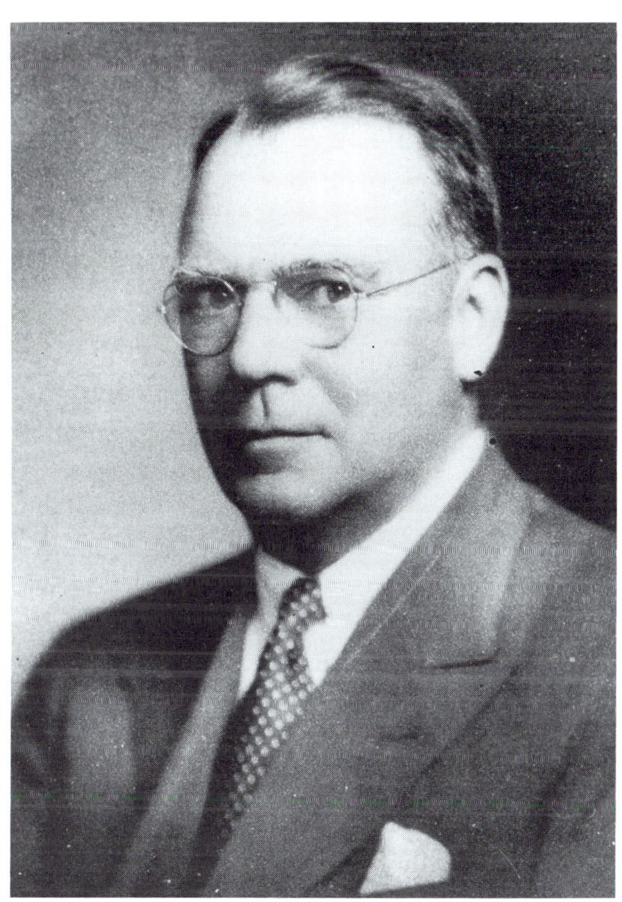

FIG. 32-59. George P. Muller, M.D., Sc.D. (1877–1947); Seventh Chairmanship (Co-Chairman, 1936–1946), First Grace Revere Osler Professor (1939–1946).

Following his graduation in Medicine from the University of Pennsylvania (1899), he interned in the Old German Hospital (Lankenau). While there he became captivated by the diagnostic ability, surgical skill, and dynamic personality of Dr. John B. Deaver (1855–1931). Muller's academic inclinations led to his appointment in a junior teaching position in the Department of Anatomy of the University of Pennsylvania. His depth of knowledge in anatomy coupled with his clinical experience led to his selection to revise Davis's *Applied Anatomy* (1934). This book became a student text in many medical schools throughout the country.

Dr. Muller took his initial surgical training as a junior assistant to Professor Charles H. Frazier, Chairman of Surgery at the University of Pennsylvania. In his rise through the ranks of teaching surgery, he obtained the Chair of Surgery at the Graduate School of Medicine of the University of Pennsylvania from 1918 to 1933, and for several years he was Chairman of the Postgraduate Clinics of Philadelphia. In 1933 he became Professor of Clinical Surgery at the University of Pennsylvania. Following the death of Dr. Deaver in 1931, Dr. Muller returned to Lankenau Hospital as a Senior Surgeon. In addition, he was surgeon to the Misericordia Hospital, Children's Hospital, and the Mary J. Drexel Home, as well as a Consulting Surgeon to several suburban institutions.

On his arrival at Jefferson, Dr. Muller, at 59 years of age, was three years older than his recently deceased predecessor, Dr. Klopp. He was at the height of his prestige, having served as President of the American College of Surgeons, the American Association for Thoracic Surgery, the College of Physicians of Philadelphia, the Philadelphia Academy of Surgery, and the Philadelphia County Medical Society. He ascribed his multiple Presidencies to attending all the business meetings, sitting in the third row, and entering into all the discussions and deliberations.

Shortly after assuming his Chair at Jefferson, Dr. Muller attended a meeting in Chicago to plan with other surgeons the organization of the American Board of Surgery. Its aims sounded very idealistic at that time (1937). He described how a successful candidate would receive a certificate indicating he had passed a qualifying examination. This would not guarantee a hospital or academic appointment.

Muller's background, temperament, and scope were different from those of Klopp. His dynamic qualities were evidenced to their fullest degree in the operating room and in the amphitheater before the entire class. There he was innovative in introducing the use of intravenous fluids to supplant the former use of hypodermoclysis in the thighs and to use the newly available sulfonamide drugs. He was a pioneer in thoracic surgery and in the late 1930s performed many pulmonary resections. Needless to say, the results were not comparable to those one-half century later, and tension and drama could usually be found in his operating theater. Anesthesia, control of hemorrhage, and blood replacement were problems that more commonly led to loss of life on the operating table. His temper was at times immoderate and he was not loathe to throw down an imperfect instrument or demonstrate in physical ways other signs of anger. Some thought he was a prima donna in the operating room, but this was only because of his constant demands on others for perfection. More detail of Dr. Muller's role in the development of the Division of Cardiothoracic Surgery at Jefferson follows in a later section of this history.

Dr. Muller was a prolific writer, who not only edited the Davis textbook of *Applied Anatomy* but contributed many articles, wrote sections in a number of textbooks on surgery, and was a member of the Editorial Board of *Annals of Surgery*. Villanova granted him an Honorary M.S. degree and Muhlenberg College awarded him an Honorary Doctor of Science degree. The Jefferson Class of 1946 commissioned his portrait for the College.

The lectures of Dr. Muller were meticulously prepared and highly informative. He continued the Grace Revere Osler Lectures to the junior class that Dr. Klopp had been giving since 1931. In 1939, when Dr. Shallow was named the second Samuel D. Gross Professor and Head of the Department, Dr. Muller was named the first Grace Revere Osler Professor. The evolution of this second Professorship within the Department of Surgery is of unusual interest.[27]

■ The Grace Revere Osler Professorship of Surgery; the Jefferson Legacy of Lady Osler (1854–1928)

The first husband of Lady Osler (the wife of Sir William Osler) was Samuel W. Gross, whom she married in 1876. The elder Gross (Samuel D.) was her father-in-law, in whose home at Eleventh and Walnut Streets she lived until the great surgeon's death in 1884. She completed the remainder of her 13 years of happy married life at 1112 Walnut Street (present site of the Forrest Theater) until the death of Samuel W. Gross in 1889. The "Widow Gross" then married Dr. William Osler, a close friend of the Gross family, in 1892. Osler, a world-renowned Professor of Medicine at Oxford, died in 1919. Lady Osler (Figure 32-60) never forgot her "first love," Samuel W. Gross. In her last will, signed just four days before her death from a massive stroke on August 31, 1928, she made 42 bequests to eight institutions, 18 relatives, six friends, and ten employees. Jefferson, Hopkins, Oxford, and McGill Medical College were all included in the generosity of this truly gracious lady, whose only son, Revere, had been killed in World War I. The first bequest in her will was to Jefferson, as follows: "To the Jefferson Medical College, Philadelphia, for the establishment of a Lectureship in Surgery in Memory of Doctor Samuel W. Gross, Five Thousand Pounds."

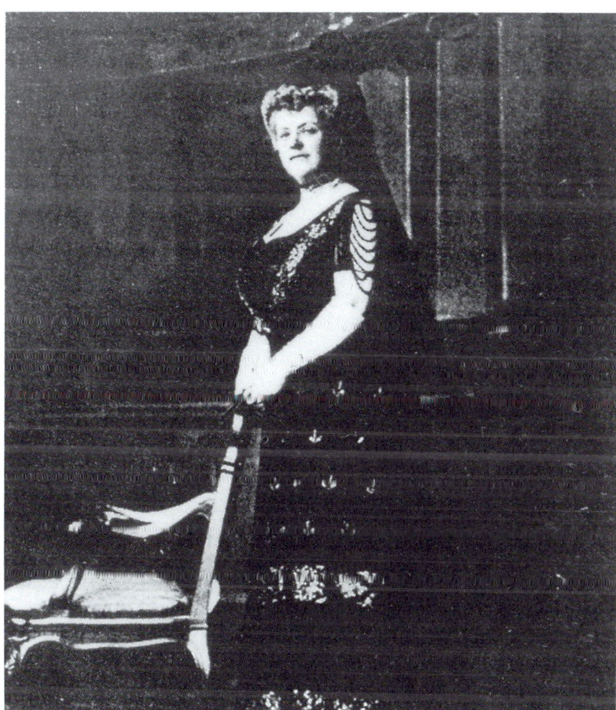

FIG. 32-60. Grace Revere Gross Osler became Lady Osler at the coronation of King George V on June 20, 1911.

On August 26, 1929, a check in the amount of $24,250 was received by the Chairman of the Finance Committee of Jefferson Medical College. The Board of Trustees adopted that the "course of lectures given by the Professor of Surgery to the third year class shall be designated 'The Samuel W. Gross Lecture on Tumors.' At the beginning of the course of lectures the professor giving them shall make a brief statement of the advances made in the knowledge of tumors by Dr. Samuel W. Gross. It was further recommended that the income from the bequest of Lady Osler be used in part payment of the salary of the Professor of Surgery giving the course of lectures."

Samuel W. Gross's special interest in tumors was manifested by the fact that he was among the first surgeons to personally section and examine by microscope all the tumors he removed. In recognition of this, he was designated the pathological histologist for the Philadelphia Academy of Surgery, which he helped his father found in 1879. At the first scientific meeting of this Academy he gave a paper on the treatment of sarcomas.

The Lectureship in Surgery in Memory of Samuel W. Gross first appeared in the Jefferson Medical College catalogue for 1930–1931 and was delivered to the third-year class by Professor Klopp. The Lectureship took on the name of Lady Osler, and alumni of that era recall Dr. Klopp as the first "Grace Revere Osler Lecturer." As already noted, Dr. Muller continued the Lectureship in his capacity as successor to Dr. Klopp. When Dr. Muller was designated the first Grace Revere Osler Professor in 1939, the College catalogue for 1940–41 next listed "The Grace Revere Osler Professorship, a memorial lectureship in surgery established in 1929." The Samuel D. Gross Professorship and Grace Revere Osler Professorship at that time carried an annual stipend of $2,400.

Dr. Muller served until 1946, when he resigned because of ill health. He died on February 18, 1947. With his death the Grace Revere Osler Professorship of Surgery remained vacant until reactivated by Dr. Francis E. Rosato in 1978.

John Heysham Gibbon, Jr., M.D., Sc.D., LL.D., F.R.C.S. (1903–1973); Seventh Chairmanship (Co-Chairman, 1946–1956), Eighth Chairman and Third Samuel D. Gross Professor (1956–1967)

The successor to Dr. George P. Muller, Dr. John H. Gibbon, Jr. (Figure 32-61) entered the Professorship at Jefferson as a lamb in 1946 and left as a lion in 1967. His initial appointment was as Professor of Surgery, Director of Experimental Surgery, and Chief of Hospital Surgical Service

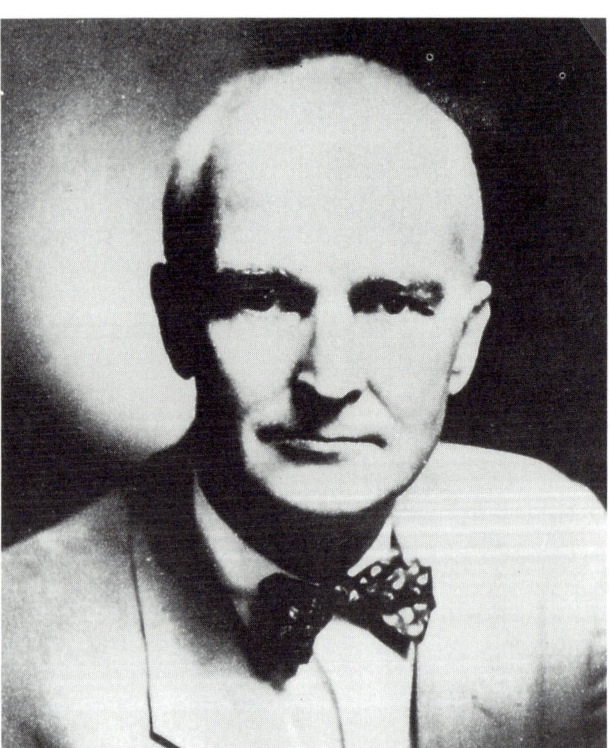

FIG. 32-61. John Heysham Gibbon, Jr., M.D., Sc.D., LL.D., F.R.C.S. (1903–1973); Seventh Chairmanship (Co-Chairman, 1946–1956), Eighth Chairman and Third Samuel D. Gross Professor (1956–1967).

"B." One can only surmise why he was not given the title of Grace Revere Osler Professor held by his predecessor. For one thing, his experimental interest was in surgical aspects of cardiac physiology, although not strictly so, because he performed many operations for lung tumors. As a man of only 43 years, he may justifiably have believed that he would eventually succeed Dr. Shallow, 17 years his senior, as Gross Professor to the Chair, which was the oldest named Chair in the College and the dominant one of the Surgery Department. His eye was on the Gross Chair; he deserved it and bided his time. His genius ranked him with Gross, Keen, and DaCosta. The details of his monumental work in developing the heart-lung machine and its successful application are covered in the chapter on the Division of Cardiothoracic Surgery.

John H. Gibbon, Jr., a fifth-generation physician, was born on September 29, 1903, in Philadelphia.[28] His father (Jefferson, 1891) was Professor of Surgery and Co-Chairman with Dr. John Chalmers DaCosta at Jefferson from 1907 to 1931. The younger Gibbon attended Penn Charter School and graduated from Princeton University (1923). After graduation from Jefferson (1927), he completed his internship at the Pennsylvania Hospital (1929) and accepted a research fellowship in surgery at the Harvard Medical School. In 1930 he conceived the idea of developing an extracorporeal apparatus for temporarily supporting the function of the heart and lungs while taking care of a patient dying of pulmonary embolism. He devoted full time to this project until World War II intervened.

After service in the Army Medical Corps in the Pacific arena (Figure 32-62) and a brief stay at the University of Pennsylvania, Dr. Gibbon continued his ongoing investigations when appointed to Jefferson in 1946. Supported by the International Business Machines Corporation and the National Heart Institute, his invention was proven practical after many successful trials on cats and dogs. It was ready for human surgery in 1953.

On May 6, 1953, Dr. Gibbon successfully repaired an interatrial septal defect in the heart of

18-year-old Cecelia Bavolek of Wilkes-Barre, Pennsylvania. Although the operation lasted only 26 minutes, it represented a major surgical breakthrough. For the first time, a patient's heart and lung functions had been maintained entirely by a machine. This brilliant achievement initiated the era of open heart surgery for repair of congenital and acquired heart defects as well as the transplants of today.

With the death of Dr. Thomas A. Shallow from pharyngeal carcinoma on December 26, 1955, Dr. Gibbon was appointed the third Samuel D. Gross Proffessor and Head of a single unified Surgery Department. Despite his liberality and easygoing nature, old loyalties seemed to persist, and in spirit the Department remained divided between the old regulars of Dr. Shallow and the new, young, "brain trust" that Dr. Gibbon accumulated in his research activities, often referred to as the "combine." Gibbon's brilliance and international reputation brought much pride to the Department and strengthened the residency programs.

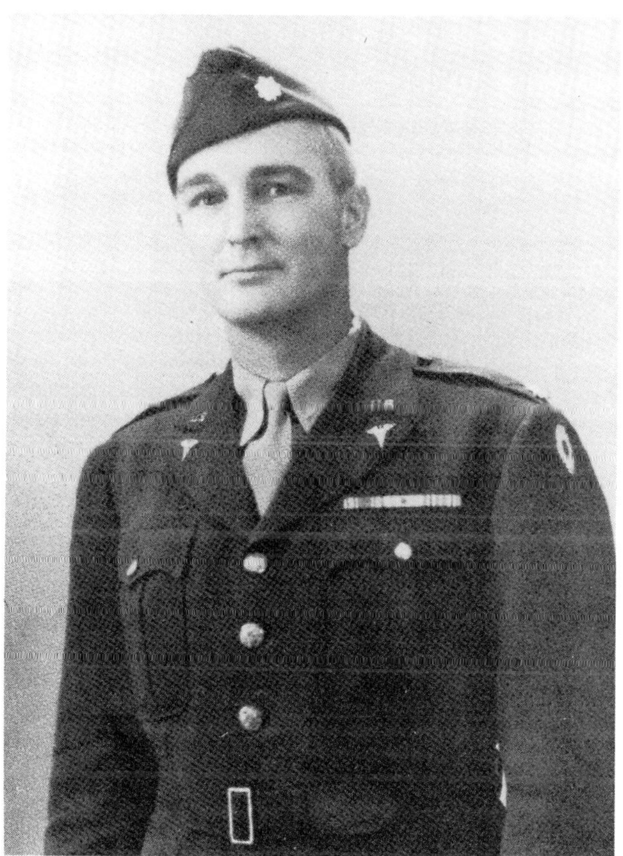
FIG. 32-62. John H. Gibbon, Jr., M.D., in World War II.

Dr. Gibbon was active in matters relating to health, training, teaching, research, professional organizations, and community affairs. He served on the American Board of Surgery, of which he became Vice Chairman, as Chairman of the Conference Committee on Graduate Training in Surgery, the Surgery Study Section of the U.S. Public Health Service, the National Board of Medical Examiners, the Subcommittee on the Cardiovascular System of the National Research Council, the Advisory Committee on Research on the Therapy of Cancer of the American Cancer Society, and the Board of Health of Philadelphia.

He was President of the Philadelphia Academy of Surgery, the College of Physicians of Philadelphia, the Laennec Society of Philadelphia, the Pennsylvania Association of Thoracic Surgery, the Society for Vascular Surgery, the American Association for Thoracic Surgery, and the American Surgical Association. He was a longtime Governor of the American College of Surgeons and served on several of its important committees. Membership was awarded him in the American Academy of Arts and Sciences and the National Academy of Sciences, and Honorary Fellowship in the Society of Thoracic Surgeons of Great Britain and Ireland and in the Royal College of Surgeons of England. He received Honorary Degrees of Doctor of Science from the University of Buffalo (1959), Dickinson College (1967), and Duke University (1970), and the LL.D. Degree from Jefferson (1969). His many other awards of distinction are listed in the chapter on the Division of Cardiothoracic Surgery.

Although best known for his heart-lung machine, Dr. Gibbon's bibliography from 1930 to 1971 lists 93 research and clinical contributions.[29] He was a distinguished editor of *Annals of Surgery* and editor of his textbook *Surgery of the Chest* (1962).

Dr. Gibbon's portrait was presented to the College by the Class of 1963, and his name was inscribed on Jefferson's Winged Ox Column of the 50 most notable physicians in medical history. His name on the Column is preceded by four other immortal Jeffersonians, namely J. Marion Sims, Samuel D. Gross, Carlos Finlay, and Chevalier Jackson. In 1979 a conference room on the second floor of the Medical College Building was named in his honor.

After his prodigious literary output and innumerable honors, Dr. Gibbon entered legend and history by taking early retirement in 1967 at the age of 64. At his home in Media, Pennsylvania (Figure 32-63), he died on February 5, 1973, while playing tennis. This was just before a planned celebration of the twentieth anniversary of his first successful open heart operation and one-half year short of his 70th birthday. An Annual John H. Gibbon, Jr., Lectureship was established at Jefferson in 1987.

John Young Templeton, III M.D., Sc.D., LL.D. (1917–); Ninth Chairman and Fourth Samuel D. Gross Professor (1967–1968)

The Chair vacated by the retirement of John H. Gibbon, Jr., was awarded to his protégé, Dr. John Y. Templeton, III (Figure 32-64), a man of colossal energy, forthrightness, scholastic brilliance, and a pioneer in cardiovascular surgery. His contributions in that field will be detailed in the chapter on the Division of Cardiothoracic Surgery.

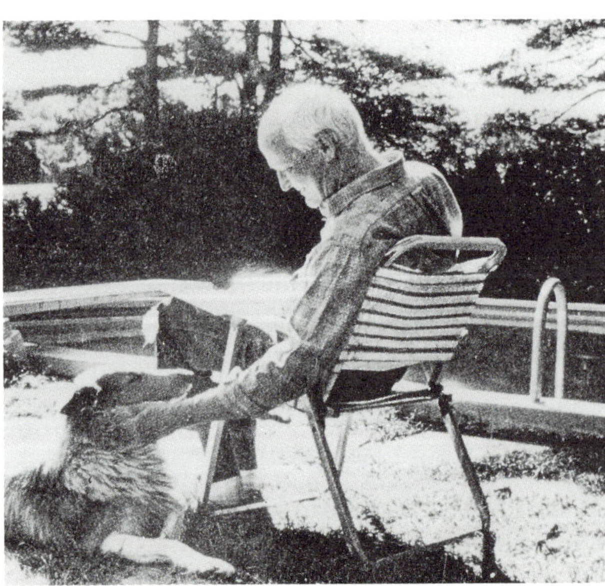

FIG. 32-63. Dr. Gibbon in retirement at his home in Media, Pennsylvania.

John Templeton was born on July 1, 1917, in Virginia but raised in North Carolina, where the roots of his family go back almost to Revolutionary times. His father, John Y. Templeton, Jr., was a Jefferson graduate in the Class of 1913, and his brother, Thomas B., was an Alpha Omega Alpha member of the Class of 1955. Dr. Templeton received his B.S. degree in chemistry from Davidson College, North Carolina, in 1937, and was graduated from Jefferson in 1941 among the top in his class. He was a junior-year member of the Alpha Omega Alpha Honorary Society. After internship at Jefferson, he served four years in World War II (1942–1946), after which his surgical career started.

Templeton began his Residency training under Dr. John Gibbon, Jr., who himself was just starting his Professorship at Jefferson. In this capacity, Dr. Templeton was the first Resident to work with Dr. Gibbon in the laboratory on the heart-lung machine, which at that time was far from perfected. He accompanied Dr. Gibbon to

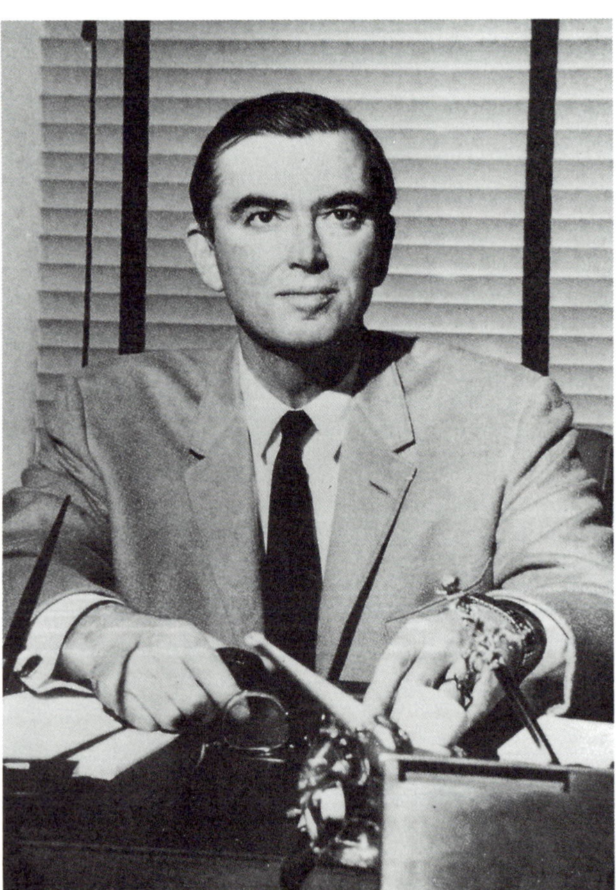

FIG. 32-64. John Y. Templeton, III, M.D., Sc.D., LL.D. (1917–); Ninth Chairman and Fourth Samuel D. Gross Professor (1967–1968).

Endicott, New York, for some of the weekends to consult with the engineers of the International Business Machines Corporation about an experimental model for use in cats and dogs. In 1949, although an adequate method for the extracorporeal maintenance of the circulation in humans was still four years away, he published work on experimental reconstruction of cardiac valves by venous and pericardial grafts.[30] At the completion of his general surgical Residency in 1950, Dr. Templeton continued at Jefferson for two additional years as the American Cancer Society Clinical Fellow and Damon Runyon Fellow.

Dr. Templeton's first faculty appointment at Jefferson was in 1950 as Instructor in Surgery, from which he rose to Clinical Professor by 1957. For ten years of this time he worked closely with Dr. Gibbon both in the laboratory and in clinical practice.

In 1964 Dr. Templeton left Jefferson to become Professor of Surgery in the University of Pennsylvania School of Medicine and the Graduate School as well as Chief of Surgery at the Pennsylvania Hospital. He held these posts until 1967, when appointed Samuel D. Gross Professor and Head of the Department to succeed Dr. Gibbon.

Dr. Templeton's name was engraved on the fourth plate of the gold-headed cane that had been presented to Professor John Chalmers DaCosta by the Class of 1926. There was universal delight within the Department at the well-deserved appointment of Dr. Templeton, matched by equal disappointment when he tendered his resignation "for personal reasons," effective for January 1, 1969. At that time he received the appointment of Professor of Surgery and carried on a prestigious private practice until his retirement on July 1, 1987, the date of his 70th birthday.

The resignation of Dr. Templeton from the Chair came as a shock that could not be related to any dissatisfaction on the part of students, residents, staff, or the administration. His further career was one of uninterrupted increasing prominence in academics, clinical work, professional societies, and organized medicine. He remained admired by students, revered by residents and colleagues, and esteemed by his nursing and cardiac technical staff.

A prolific writer, Dr. Templeton wrote more than 80 articles on subjects pertaining to the lungs, heart, blood vessels, gastrointestinal tract, hypothermia, metabolism, and human resuscitation. His membership in societies numbered more than 50 at the local, national, and international level, with service on the Board of Governors or as Chairman of committees on 14 of them. Among his Presidencies, he treasured most the one of the Philadelphia Academy of Surgery, founded by Samuel D. Gross in 1879. He also served as President of the Jefferson Alumni Association, Pennsylvania Association for Thoracic Surgery, the Laennec Society, the Philadelphia County Medical Society, the Pennsylvania State Medical Society, the Meigs Medical Association, and the Medical Staff of Thomas Jefferson University Hospital.

A portrait of Dr. Templeton was presented to Jefferson in 1980 by residents and colleagues. The John Y. Templeton, III, Annual Lecture in Surgery was first given in May, 1980, by internationally known Dr. Denton Cooley. He received the Alumni Achievement Award (1981) and the Winged Ox Award (1987). His undergraduate alma mater, Davidson College, awarded him the Honorary Degree of Doctor of Science in April, 1987, and Jefferson bestowed upon him the Honorary Degree of Doctor of Laws in September of the same year. Dr. Templeton has been called "a legend in his own time."

Harry Sawyer Goldsmith, M.D. (1929–); Tenth Chairman and Fifth Samuel D. Gross Professor (1970–1977)

The search for a successor to Dr. Templeton extended over the period of a year and one-half, and concluded with the appointment of Dr. Harry S. Goldsmith (Figure 32-65), effective for July 1, 1970. Dr. Goldsmith was born on September 30, 1929, in Newton, Massachusetts. He obtained his A.B. degree from Dartmouth College in 1952 and his M.D. from the Boston University School of Medicine in 1956. During internship and surgical residency at the Boston City Hospital (1956–1961), he was a Research Fellow in the Department of Anesthesia (1959–1960). He then completed a period of military service (1961–1963) as Captain in the U.S. Army Medical Corps, Chief of Surgery in the Seoul Military Hospital, Korea (1961–1962) and Staff Surgeon at Fort Devens, Massachusetts (1962–1963).

While pursuing postgraduate work as Senior Surgical Resident at the Memorial Hospital for Cancer and Allied Diseases (1963–1965), Goldsmith was a Research Fellow in the Sloan-Kettering Institute for Cancer Research (1964–1965). In 1963 he became a Diplomate of the American Board of Surgery.

Dr. Goldsmith's teaching career started as Assistant in Anatomy (1958–1960) at the Boston University Medical School and then as Senior Teaching Fellow in Surgery (1960–1961). He then became an Instructor in Surgery at the Soodo Medical School in Korea (1961–1962). At the Cornell Medical School he rose from Assistant (1964–1965) to Instructor (1965–1967) and to Assistant Professor (1967–1970). From 1968 to June, 1970, he was Director of Surgical Education in the Memorial Hospital for Cancer and Allied Diseases in New York City. At the Memorial Hospital he rose from Clinical Assistant Surgeon in 1965 to Attending Surgeon and Chief of the Gastric and Mixed Tumor Service (1968–1970). In the field of research at the Memorial–Sloan-Kettering Cancer Center he rose from Assistant Director of Surgical Research in 1966 to Associate Member (1968–1970).

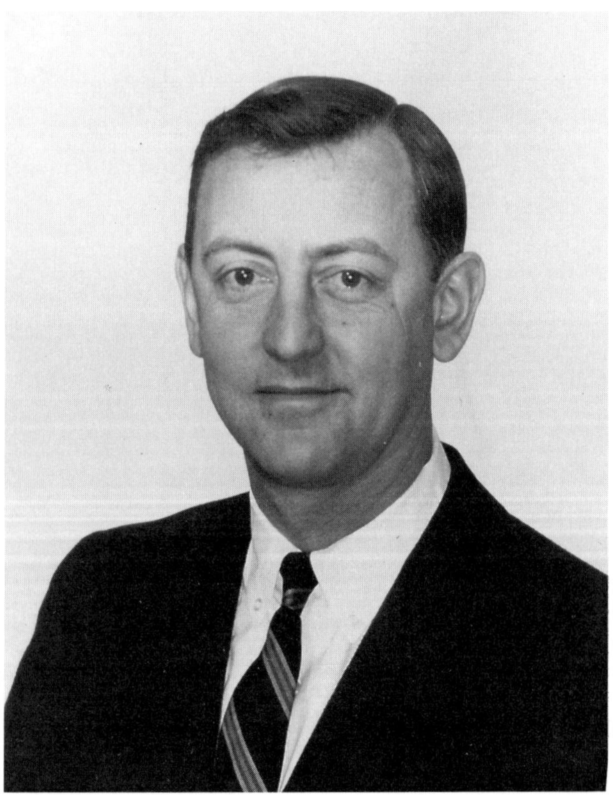

FIG. 32-65. Harry S. Goldsmith, M.D. (1929–); Tenth Chairman and Fifth Samuel D. Gross Professor (1970–1977).

Dr. Goldsmith brought to Jefferson his research and clinical interests in malignant melanoma and revascularization procedures by omental transposition. He also brought new members into the Surgical Staff, which included Drs. Gordon E. Schwartz, with special training in diseases of the breast, Jose Castillo in plastic surgery, Candadai Rangaratham in pediatric surgery, James E. Colberg in renal transplantation, Edgardo S. Alday in gastrointestinal surgery, Louis F. Plzak in cardiovascular surgery, and, subsequently, Stanley K. Brockman as Head of the newly created Division of Cardiothoracic Surgery in 1973.

Dr. Goldsmith's lectures were well organized and appreciated by the students. Saturday morning Grand Round Conferences were instituted and well attended. The first few years of his administration slipped by quietly, but were followed by a period of creeping malaise. Dr. Goldsmith secluded himself in his laboratory, punctuated by long summer sojourns in the Orient as a Visiting Professor. His work in omental transposition for lymphedema, spinal cord injury, and later on for stroke remained controversial. Despite widespread lack of acceptance of his work, Dr. Goldsmith remained productive in scientific papers and in the meetings of his various societies such as the American College of Surgeons, New York Medical Society, Massachusetts Medical Society, New York Surgical Society, James Ewing Society, Society of Sigma Xi, Society for Surgery of the Alimentary Tract, and the Philadelphia Academy of Surgery.

By 1977 Dr. Goldsmith was no longer able to reconcile his personal ideals with the frustrations of his staff, and he resigned. He transferred to

Dartmouth Medical School, Hanover, New Hampshire, as Professor of Surgery. By that time he had written over 140 journal articles and text chapters and took on the editorship of *Practice of Surgery,* published by Harper and Row in twelve loose-leaf volumes.

Dr. Frederick B. Wagner, Jr., Clinical Professor of Surgery in the Department since 1955, was selected by Dean Kellow to serve as Acting Chairman, effective July 1, 1977.

Frederick Balthas Wagner, Jr., M.D. (1916–); Acting Chairman (1977–1978), Second Grace Revere Osler Professor (1978–1982)

Frederick B. Wagner, Jr. (Figure 32-66), a native Philadelphian, was born on January 18, 1916. After graduation from Olney High School in 1933, he received his A.B. degree from the University of Pennsylvania in 1937 (Phi Beta Kappa) and M.D.

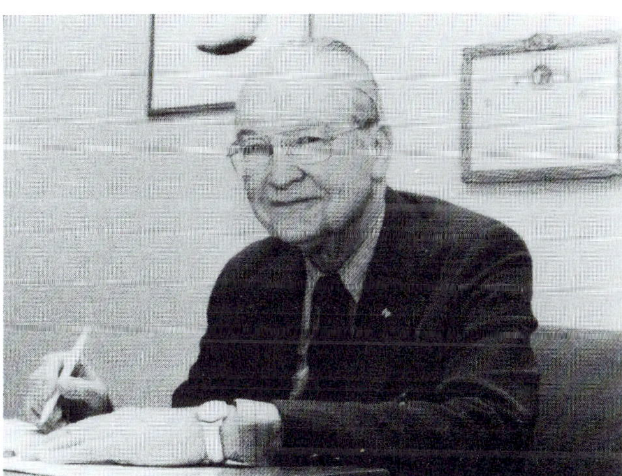

FIG. 32-66. Frederick B. Wagner, Jr., M.D. (1916–); Acting Chairman (1977–1978), Second Grace Revere Osler Professor (1978–1982).

from Jefferson in 1941 (Alpha Omega Alpha). During the last eight of those years he was a church organist, and in 1935 he took a summer course at the University of Heidelberg. Music, languages, and history were to remain pervasive avocations throughout his life.

Following internship at Jefferson (1941–1942) and surgical residency (1942–1945), he was a Ross V. Patterson Research Fellow (1945–1946). Although having taken Reserve Officers' Training throughout medical school, he was honorably discharged as First Lieutenant during World War II on a physical disability that obviously did not shorten his life.

Upon completion of his formal surgical training (Figure 32-67), Dr. Wagner was invited by Dr. Thomas A. Shallow, the Gross Professor of Surgery, to become his private assistant. This honor entailed many duties, which included being present as first assistant at every operation, no matter how small or large, taking care of his emergency surgery after 5 P.M., giving his spinal anesthesias, participating in all his scientific papers and exhibits at meetings, and supervising the residency care of his private patients. The demands of Dr. Shallow were exorbitant but rewarded by Dr. Wagner's advancement from Assistant Demonstrator of Surgery (1943) to Clinical Professor (1955). During this period he authored, or coauthored with Shallow, 45 scientific articles on a diffuse range of general surgical subjects and was a pioneer in arteriography of abdominal blood vessels by translumbar aortography.[31]

With the death of Dr. Shallow, the Chairmanship of a unified Department was assumed by Dr. John H. Gibbon, Jr. in 1956. Dr. Gibbon by then had achieved worldwide fame for the creation of his heart-lung machine that initiated the era of open heart surgery. He became so engulfed in Presidencies of societies, receiving awards, traveling as a Visiting Professor, editing the *Annals of Surgery,* and preparing his large text on *Surgery of the Chest* that he was absent from Jefferson a great deal of the time. Some of his medical students may never have seen him, and he was affectionately known within his own Department as the "Visiting Professor." The weekly staff meetings, which he attended as often as he could, were always highlighted by his inquiring mind that stimulated study and encouraged research. During this period, Dr. Wagner had inherited much of Dr. Shallow's private surgical practice and had little time except for teaching and clinical work. Many of the hospital surgical beds were insidiously absorbed into the rapidly expanding Medical Department, and the busy staff surgeons had to seek outside sources of beds for their patients. In the crunch, Dr. Wagner, although maintaining his home base at Jefferson, became a Consultant in Vascular Surgery to St. Mary's Hospital in Philadelphia (1963–1965) and Director of Surgery at the William B. Kessler Memorial Hospital in Hammonton, New Jersey (1963–1972). For approximately ten years he became associated in practice with Dr. William Bosley Manges (Jefferson, S1944), Clinical Associate Professor in the Department, who also had taken his surgical residency under Dr. Shallow.

Dr. Wagner was startled one day in June, 1977, by an urgent call from Dean Kellow's office to report on "what is going on in the Surgery Department." In the presence of Dean Kellow and Dr. Francis J. Sweeney, Jr., Vice President of the University Hospital, he was given the charge of Acting Chairmanship with the challenge to "heal old wounds and create harmony in the Department."

Dr.Wagner maintained his busy surgical practice while taking on the administrative tasks of a demoralized Department. It was like an innocent swim into the waiting arms of an octopus. The arms were replete with survey forms, committee meetings, conferences, applications, promotion

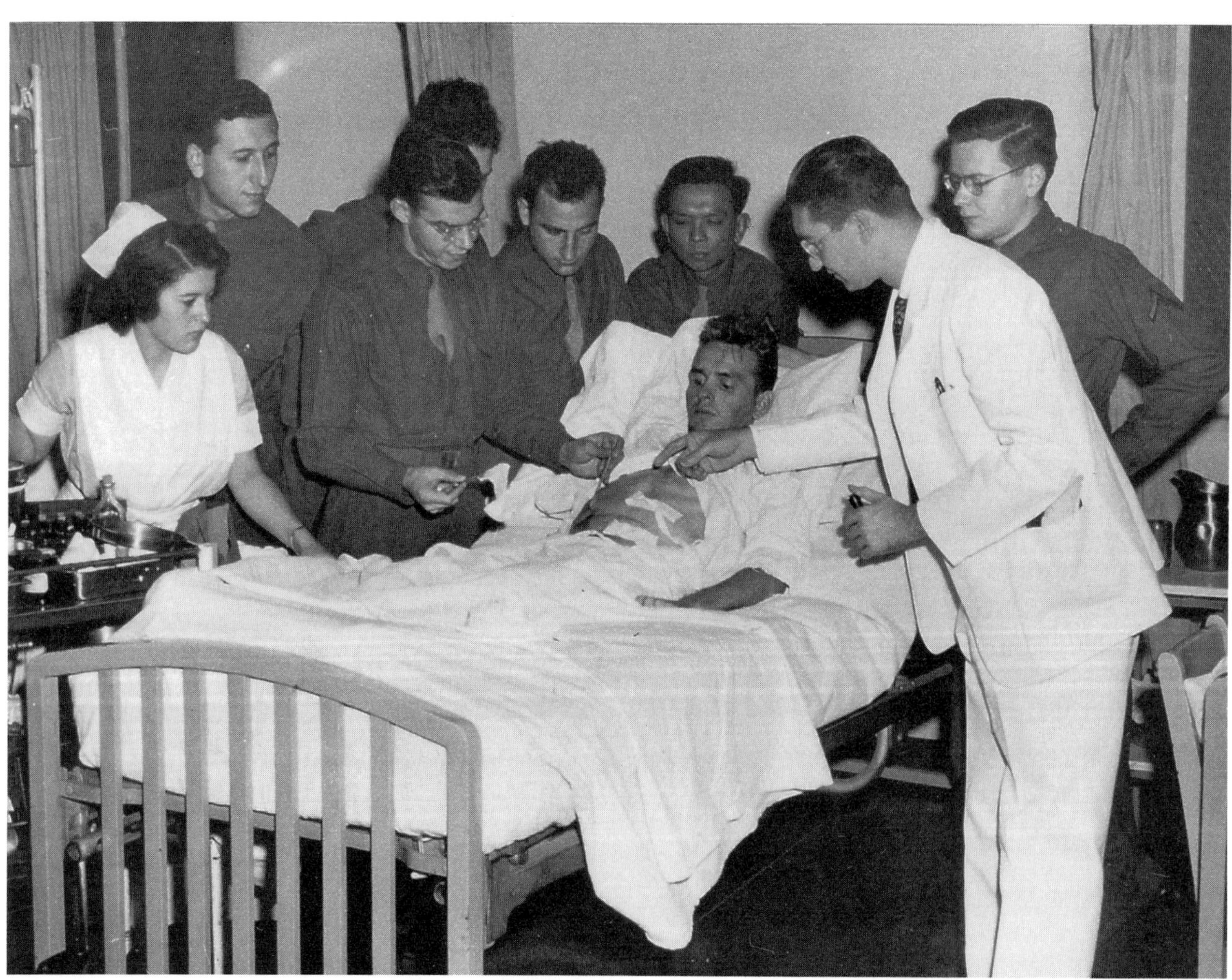

FIG. 32-67. Frederick B. Wagner, Jr., M.D., as Resident in surgery ward with medical students in army uniforms (1944).

papers, students seeking recommendation or advice, operating room problems, emergency room unassigned patients, compensation clinic coverage, medical record delinquencies of the staff, changes in academic programs, departmental self-assay, and endless people dropping by the office for a so-called few minutes. It was a mandate for strong commitment and flexibility to the concerns of students, residents, and staff, and thereby to the Department and Medical School.

Whatever success may have been achieved during the critical year of 1977–1978 must be ascribed to leadership, communication, and teamwork. Carefully selected members of the Department carried out their newly assigned duties in student and resident education and equitable solving of problems through a diligent Surgical Advisory Committee. Research continued in the Division of Cardiothoracic Surgery and on a very limited scale by individual staff members. It was a holding and healing period, while trusting that a newly appointed Samuel D. Gross Professor would consummate the unfulfilled Departmental dreams for the future. This occurred with the selection of Dr. Francis E. Rosato, effective as of August 1, 1978.

Dr. Wagner's portrait was presented to the University by colleagues and friends in 1978. In that year he was also appointed through Dr. Rosato as the second Grace Revere Osler Professor of Surgery and became Emeritus in 1982. On January 1, 1984, he retired from the practice of surgery and started a new career as Jefferson's first University Historian. In 1985 he received the Samuel D. Gross Distinguished Service Award of the Department of Surgery, became an Alumni Representative member of Jefferson's Board of Trustees, and served as President of the Philadelphia Academy of Surgery. The following year a Surgical Library on the seventh floor of the University Hospital was named in his honor by the Residents of the Department. In 1987 he received the Dean's Medal for dedicated service to Jefferson Medical College.

Dr. Wagner coauthored a textbook on *Preoperative and Postoperative Care* (1947) and published *The Twilight Years of Lady Osler* (1985). As a historian he has lectured at Oxford University (1984), the University of Düsseldorf (1986), and at yearly meetings of the American Osler Society. His later writings relate to Jefferson's rich tradition and heritage.

Francis Ernest Rosato, M.D. (1934–); Eleventh Chairman and Sixth Samuel D. Gross Professor (1978–)

Dr. Francis E. Rosato (Figure 32-68) was born in Philadelphia on June 2, 1934. His father was a highly respected general practitioner in the City. After graduating from St. Joseph's College (1955) as a member of Alpha Sigma Nu National Jesuit Honor Society, he became an Alpha Omega Alpha honor graduate of Hahnemann Medical College (1959). His Rotating Internship was taken at the Philadelphia General Hospital (1959–1960) and Residency in General Surgery at the Hospital of the University of Pennsylvania (1961–1964), with Chief Residency (1964–1965). During this time he was also a Postdoctoral Fellow in the Department of Biochemistry of the School of Medicine of the

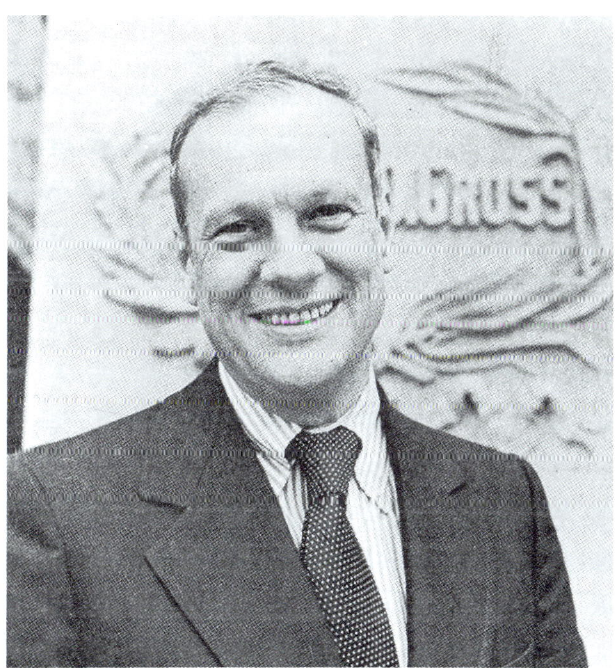

FIG. 32-68. Francis E. Rosato, M.D. (1934–); Eleventh Chairman and Sixth Samuel D. Gross Professor (1978–).

University of Pennsylvania (1962–1963). After becoming board certified in 1966, he took the Radioisotopes Course of the Atomic Energy Commission of the National Science Foundation at the Philadelphia College of Pharmacy (1967).

Dr. Rosato's teaching activities began as Assistant Instructor in Surgery in the School of Medicine of the University of Pennsylvania (1960–1964) and Instructor (1964–65). After one year (1966) as Senior Instructor in Surgery at Hahnemann Medical College, he returned to the University of Pennsylvania and rose to the rank of Professor of Surgery (1972–1975). From 1975 to 1978 he served as Professor and Chairman in the Department of Surgery of the Eastern Virginia Medical School at Norfolk, Virginia.

In the important aspect of clinical experience, Dr. Rosato from 1965 to 1975 held hospital staff appointments at the Hahnemann, Philadelphia General, and University of Pennsylvania Hospitals. He also was a Consultant to the Veterans Administration Hospital of Philadelphia and Chief of the Solid Tumor Program and Co-Director of the Neoplastic Chemotherapy Clinic of the Hospital of the University of Pennsylvania. From 1975 to 1978 he was Director of Surgery in the Norfolk General Hospital, on the Attending Staff of DePaul Hospital in Norfolk, and Consultant in Surgery to the Naval Regional Medical Center, Veterans Administration Hospital and U.S. Public Health Service Hospital of the area.

In basic and clinical surgical research, by the time of his appointment in 1978 at age 44, Dr. Rosato had authored or coauthored more than 125 scientific articles in the prestigious journals of his field. In addition to awards, honors, and research grants, he belonged to a complete array of the important societies of his specialty.

Among the impressive group of candidates for the Samuel D. Gross Chair, Dr. Rosato was the unanimous choice of the search committee, and this situation was capped by his enthusiastic acceptance of the position. He faced the formidable challenge to rejuvenate a major Department that had endured a decade of stasis.

One of Dr. Rosato's top goals on arrival August 1, 1978, was to reactivate surgical investigation. His underlying philosophy was that this activity lends honesty and healthy curiosity to all efforts of surgery. Initially, there was essentially no laboratory work save the skeleton effort of the previous Gross Professor that had been carried out behind locked doors. He recruited Susan P. Lanza-Jacoby, Ph.D., in conjunction with Stephen M. Weiss, M.D., on the clinical side, to begin a basic and clinical nutrition laboratory. Doctor Jacoby established ongoing studies that related primarily to lipid metabolism, which became supported by the National Institutes of Health.

Dr. Rosato was disheartened by the poor quality of the kidney transplant program in which only six had been carried out during his first year as Chairman. He was able to recruit Dr. Bruce E. Jarrell (Jefferson, 1973), who elevated the program to a par with the best in the area and additionally instituted a successful liver transplant program that had been badly needed in the Delaware Valley (Figure 32-69). Dr. Jarrell's outstanding work is detailed in a later section of this Departmental history.

Research work was further enhanced through Dr. Jarrell's interest in endothelial cell culture and its applications to prosthetic graft coverings. The collaboration of Stuart K. Williams, Ph.D., in this effort led to expansion into newly renovated locations in the sixth floor of the College. Dr. Michael Moritz was added for his work on immunologic aspects of cell–cell interaction and cell adherence phenomena, with support from the American Heart Association.

Dr. Richard Edie, who succeeded Dr. Stanley Brockman as Director of the Cardiothoracic Division in 1987, instituted new research studies upon his arrival. He recruited Dr. John Mannion for investigation of *latissimus dorsi* (skeletal muscle) cardiac assist pumps as "holdovers" for end-stage cardiac patients awaiting heart transplantation. Dr. John Francfort was also recruited for basic studies on atherogenesis particularly in deranged metabolic states, starting with diabetes.

Under Dr. Rosato's impetus for research, the laboratories on the sixth floor that had been empty not only filled up but required additional space. A funding of $1.3 million was appropriated by the Dean and Board of Trustees for 1,300 square feet of new research space on the eleventh floor of the Curtis Building and other laboratory renovations in the Department. The effort became supported by $600,000 from outside funds with prospects of increases in subsequent years.

The critical component of trauma planning for patient care and resident training was given strong impetus around 1982 when Dr. Francis J. Sweeney, Jr., Vice President for Health Services and Director of Thomas Jefferson University Hospital, arranged for Emergency Medicine to become an official Division of the Department of Surgery. With involvement of Dr. Jerome J. Vernick (Jefferson, 1962), Jefferson became designated a Level One Trauma Center in 1987.

The Residency Program was rescued during Dr. Wagner's Acting Chairmanship by Dr. Herbert E. Cohn (Jefferson, 1955), but, with the arrival of Dr. Rosato, became highly structured and much sought after. The Department within several years was receiving over 600 residency applications, with interviews of more than 120 to finally select six individuals for full five-year training and four to five additional individuals for one- or two-year training preparatory to moving into other specialties. The pass rate in both written and oral examination for board certification became 95%+, with the goal set at 100%. Dr. Cohn, Professor of Surgery, advanced to become a Vice Chairman of the Department (1985) and President of the Medical Staff (1986–1987).

The undergraduate medical students are the center of the Department entity. The programs for their education have been under the successive direction of Drs. Bruce E. Jarrell, James E. Colberg, and Philip J. Wolfson. In a recent major curriculum review, Surgery came in second only to Pediatrics in terms of student satisfaction. In an American College of Surgeons Long-Range Study, Jefferson across the country became the number two school in contributing students into surgery and surgical specialties. In the years between 1982 and 1987, Drs. Herbert Cohn and Bruce Jarrell

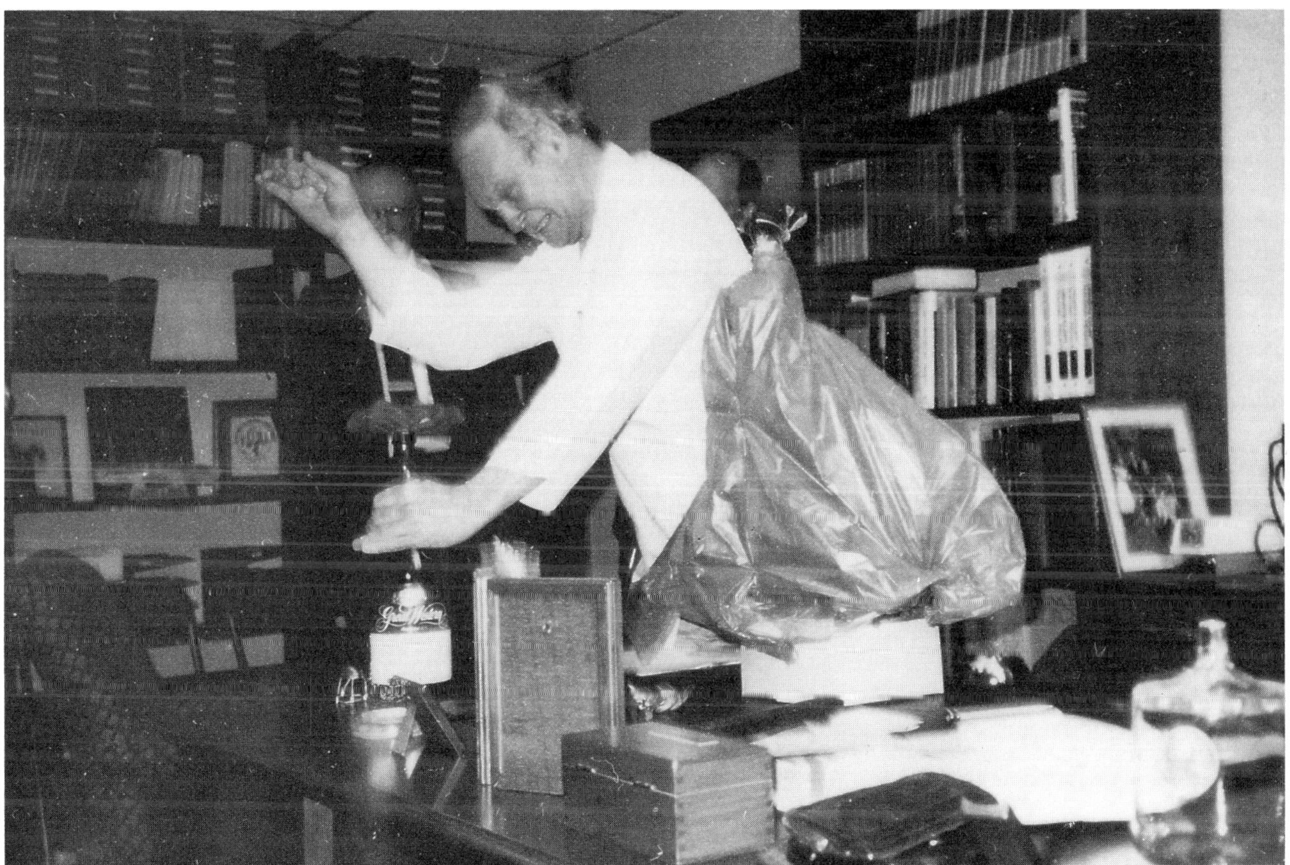

FIG. 32-69. Francis E. Rosato, M.D., jubilantly celebrates his 50th birthday (June 2, 1984) and the first successful liver transplant in Philadelphia (May 31, 1984).

and Chairman Rosato won Lindback Awards for Distinguished Teaching.

The affiliation pattern and philosophy underwent significant changes in which the drive was to bring more of the house officers increasingly within the University and its geographic confines. The eventual hope is to have just one or two strong affiliates that will round out the rather strong and intensive University experience that the residents now receive.

In 1985 a Division of Colorectal Surgery was created in the Department, with Dr. Gerald J. Marks (Jefferson, 1949) as the Director. Dr. Marks also became Chief of the Section of Colorectal Surgery at the Pennsylvania Hospital. He was a founder of the Society of American Gastrointestinal Endoscopic Surgeons, which established an annual "Gerald Marks Honorary Lecture." The Colorectal Surgical Residency at Jefferson became one of the few in the country based in the primary hospital of the academic institution. Within three years it became necessary to recruit two new staff members into the Division, namely Drs. Maryalice Cheney and Scott Goldstein. Dr. Marks, with an international reputation in colorectal surgery, is active in organized medicine and is supervising a series of clinical research projects within the Division.

Organization of two new Divisions is near completion. The first is a Division of Research under Dr. Stuart Williams that will administratively supervise the large research effort and arbitrate issues that relate to shared research space. The other is a Division of Transplantation under Dr. Bruce Jarrell, which will probably be a surgical/medical combined Division.

Over a period of nine years (1978–1987), Dr. Rosato recruited at least 15 new faculty members. This was accomplished not only by improving the morale of the full-time faculty by attracting new people to their ranks, but also by warm acceptance of additional volunteer faculty. The equal interaction and mutual esteem between full-time and volunteer faculty were so effectively united that the goal of a single system was practically at hand.

Dr. Rosato has defied the myth that a Chairman can no longer excel equally in teaching, research, and patient care. In his case one may also add a plaudit in administration. Among recent achievements were his involvement in the performance of the first mesoatrial shunt (anastomosis of mesenteric vein to right atrium of the heart by grafting, for portal hypertension) ever done in this region, involvement in the genesis of a pancreatic cancer program, his strong role in a major liver surgery program that has received acclaim, and coediting with Dr. Jan O. Strombeck of Stockholm, Sweden, a book on *Surgery of the Breast* (1986). He was chosen by *Philadelphia Magazine* as one of the Best General Surgeons in their comprehensive health care survey of June, 1987.

In addition to Chairmanship on prestigious committees of the American College of Surgeons, Rosato served as President of the Philadelphia County Medical Society (1983) and the Philadelphia Academy of Surgery (1986), and as Interim President of the Jefferson Medical Staff (1987). He was recipient of the Shaffrey Award of the Medical Alumni of St. Joseph's College (1981) and Hahnemann's Alumnus of the Year Award (1981). His other civic and scientific society activities constitute a most impressive list.

Samuel D. Gross, who could be considered the patron saint of the Surgery Department, would be astonished and pleased with its renaissance. The spirit of inquiry, the dedication to teaching, and the commitment to patient care have never been stronger.

Other Surgical Faculty Notables and Contributors

The Jefferson Medical College Catalog for 1985–1987 lists 120 members of the Surgical Faculty besides the Chairman: Professors Emeriti, 2; Professors, 21; Associate Professors, 18; Instructors, 60; Assistant Instructors, 2; and Honorary Members, 17. This gamut of talent and dedication, which includes the affiliated hospitals, provides insight into the complexity and advancement of surgical knowledge that have occurred since the founding of the Medical College in 1824. Until the first Summer School Course of 1866, all the lectures were delivered by the one and only Professor. The entire medical course consisted of two years of lectures, with four months in each academic year, with the lectures being the same in each of the two years. The philosophy of repetition was that it would lead in the second year to better comprehension and longer recall. Surgical names that appeared after 1866 were those of Richard J. Levis, John Hill Brinton, Samuel W. Gross, J. Ewing Mears (Figures 32-70 and 32-71), William H. Pancoast, William W. Keen, and William Joseph Hearn (Figure 32-72). It has been noted that with the retirement of Samuel D. Gross in 1882, it took two Professors to conduct the formal required lectures. By 1900 there were still only six surgical names listed in the College Catalog. This increased to 15 by 1910, to 19 by 1920, and to 36 by 1930.

Charles F. Nassau, M.D. (University of Pennsylvania, 1891, and of Jefferson, 1906), LL.D. (Villanova College, 1912), and Sc.D. (St. Joseph's College, 1931), was recruited by Professor John Chalmers DaCosta in 1907. He became a Clinical Professor of Surgery in 1930, President of the Philadelphia County Medical Society in 1932, a founding member of the American Board of Surgery in 1937, appointed Director of the Department of Health of the City of Philadelphia in 1939, and died while in active practice in 1940 at the age of 71. He had studied abroad, written many articles, and was a superb teacher and technical surgeon (Figure 32-73).

Adolph A. Walkling (Figure 32-74), a Jefferson graduate in the Class of 1917, lectured on fractures in the Department before this teaching was transferred to the Orthopaedic Department. He served as Chief of Surgery at the Pennsylvania Hospital and as President of the Alumni Association (1951) and the Philadelphia Academy of Surgery (1958).

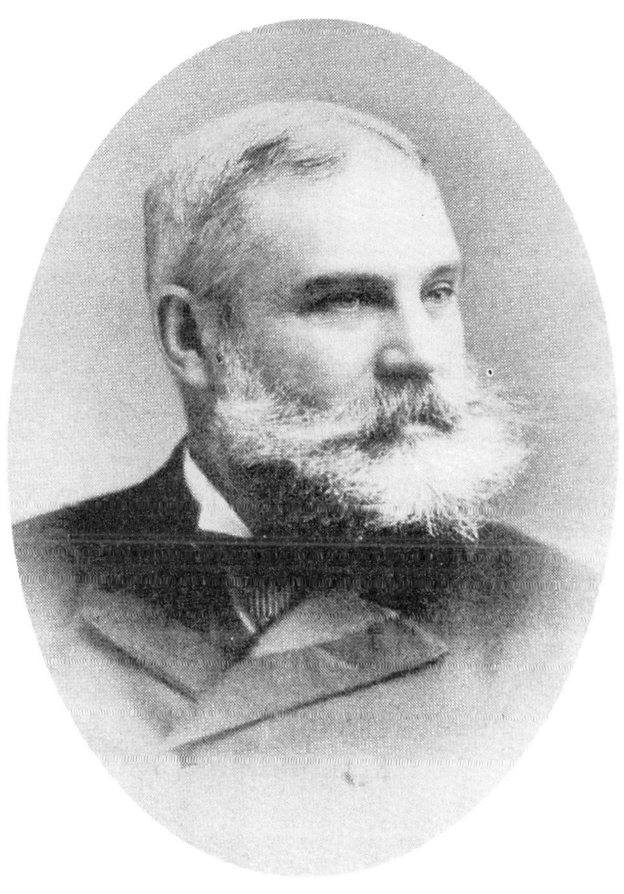

FIG. 32-70. J. Ewing Mears, M.D., LL.D. (1838–1919), gave a course in Operative Surgery, became prominent in gynecologic surgery, and was among the first Philadelphia surgeons to adopt Lister's antiseptic method.

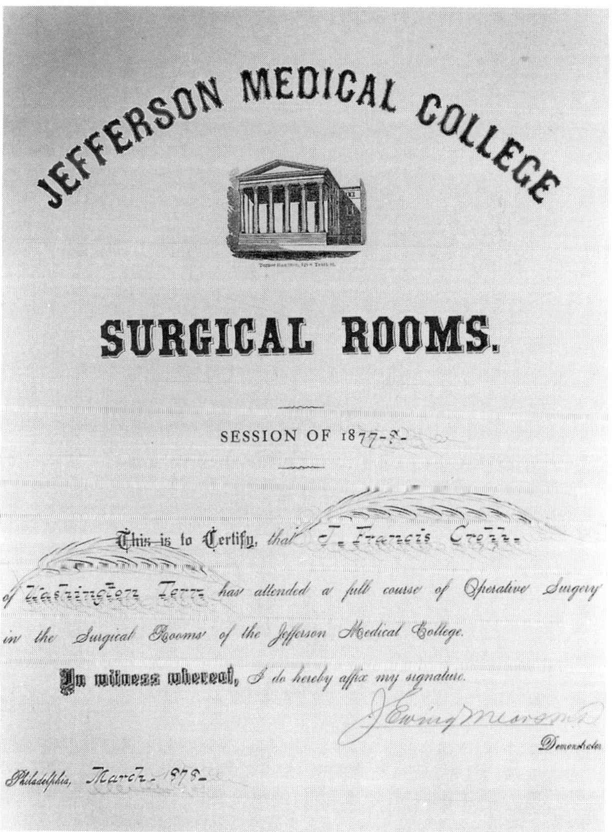

JEFFERSON MEDICAL COLLEGE

SURGICAL ROOMS.

SESSION OF 1877-8-

This is to Certify, that J. Francis Crez[illegible] of Washington Terr. has attended a full course of Operative Surgery in the Surgical Rooms of the Jefferson Medical College.

In witness whereof, I do hereby affix my signature.

J. Ewing Mears M.D.
Demonstrator

Philadelphia, March 1878.

FIG. 32-71. Certificate of Session (1877–1878) from a course in Operative Surgery given by J. Ewing Mears, M.D.

Henry K. Seelaus (Figure 32-75) requires special mention as one who had potential to become a Chairman but whose life was cut short at age 43 by pneumonia in 1937. He was the top man in his Jefferson Class of 1918 and nicknamed "the shark" for his keenness and depth of knowledge. His superbly organized lectures, operative skill, authorship of many papers, and compassion for patients marked him "a coming man in surgery." In the 1918 *Clinic* he was described as "an ordinary-looking individual with the brains of a genius." In the portrait of Professor John Chalmers DaCosta teaching from a wheelchair in the amphitheater, Seelaus is depicted reading the history of the patient.

Two members may be considered surgical martyrs. Duncan L. Despard (Figure 32-76), a Jefferson graduate in the Class of 1901, was shot to death in his office in 1924 at the age of 55 by an insane patient who thought his hernia had been repaired incorrectly. S. Dale Spotts (Jefferson, 1922) was an early victim of excessive x-ray exposure to his hands while reducing fractures under the fluoroscope without protection. He developed a squamous cell carcinoma of the hand that resulted in axillary metastasis, suppuration, and fatal septicemia in 1952. In 1949 Bucknell University had conferred upon Dr. Spotts the honorary degree of Doctor of Science, and in 1950 he was elected a Trustee of that University (Figure 32-77).

William J. Tourish (Jefferson, 1928) performed dedicated service as a Chief in the Outpatient

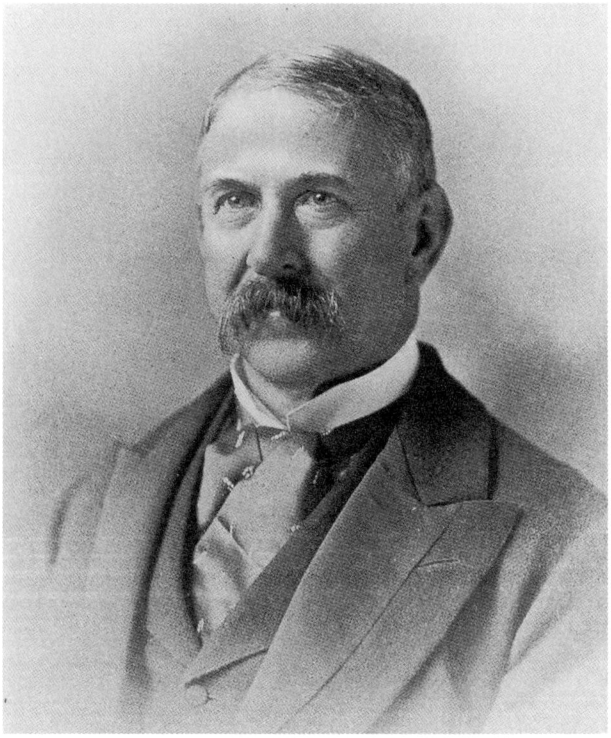

FIG. 32-72. William Joseph Hearn, M.D. (1842–1917), Clinical Professor of Surgery, Anesthetist to Samuel D. Gross, as depicted on Eakins' *Gross Clinic* (1875), and surgeon to many members of the Jefferson Faculty and their families.

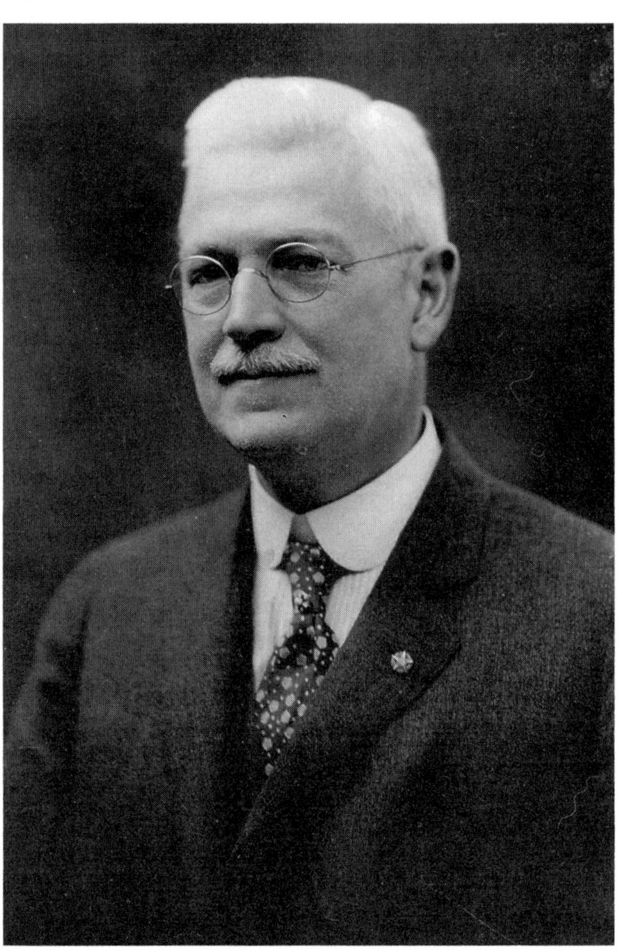

FIG. 32-73. Charles F. Nassau, M.D., LL.D., Sc.D. (1868–1940), was Clinical Professor of Surgery, an eminent teacher, and active in organized medicine and public health.

Clinic during World War II and was active on the Ward Service (Figure 32-78).

Clinical Professor Kenneth E. Fry (Jefferson, 1931) was a role model in his lectures, operative technique, beside teaching of students (Figure 32-79), care of patients, and training of the surgical residents. He served throughout World War II in the Middle East and was very active in Alumni affairs, such as Chairman of Annual Giving and President (1965). He was the first member of the Surgical Department to become board certified (1939).

Additionally, names of those who operated or lectured at Jefferson between the late 1930s to late 1970s with significant impress include: Arthur E. Billings, William T. Lemmon (Figure 32-80), J. Hall Allen (Proctology), William P. Hearn, Patrick A. McCarthy, Sherman A. Eger (Figure 32-81), Hubley R. Owen, Alan P. Parker, Herbert A. Widing, Eli R. Saleeby, Benjamin F. Haskell (whose portrait was presented in 1975), Milton Harrison, Alfred E. Brunswick, Hugh P. Robertson, Paul O. Blake, Lewis C. Manges, Louis K. Collins (Proctology), Ned T. Raker, Thomas B. Mervine, James B. Carty, John J. Cheleden (Proctology), Edward D. Weiss (Proctology), Louis Chodoff, Frederick W. Deardorff, Harry J. Knowles, John D. Allen (Proctology), Benjamin Lipshutz, Herbert Lipshutz, Frederick W. Dasch, Moses Behrend, W. Bosley Manges, Armando F. Goracci, William F. Coghlan, Robert E. Colcher, Harold Rovner

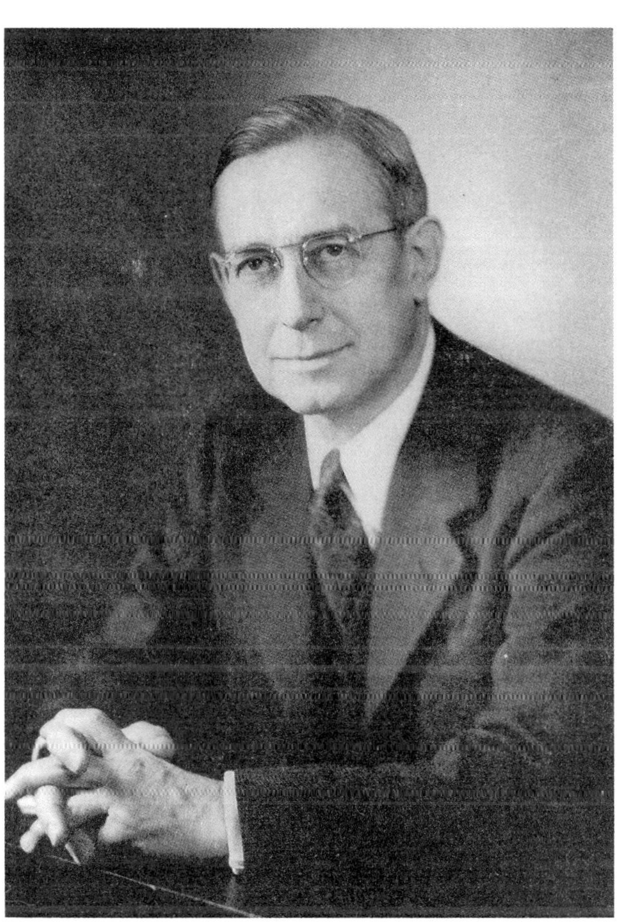

FIG. 32-74. Adolph A. Walkling, M.D. (1895–1966), the last teacher of fractures within the Department of Surgery.

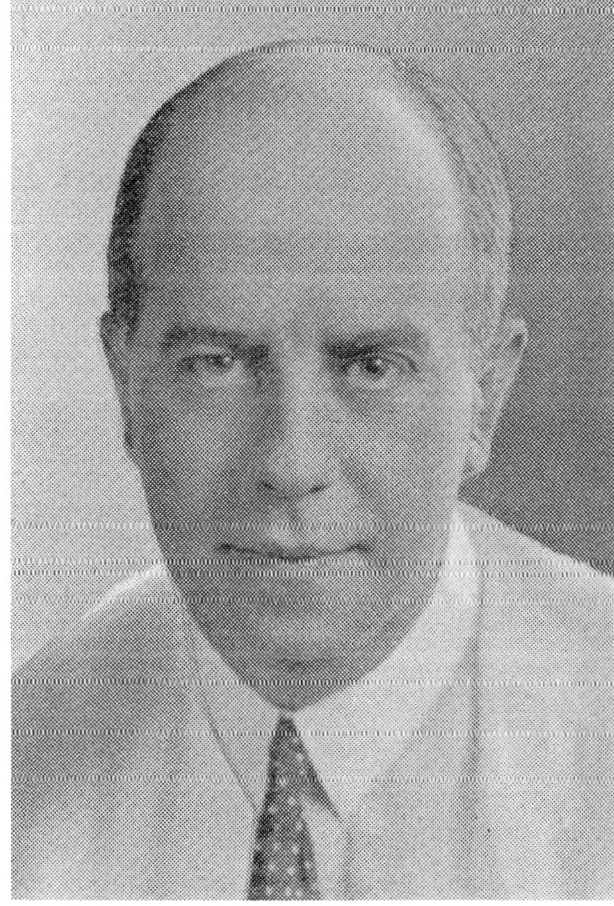

FIG. 32-75. Henry K. Seelaus, M.D. (1894–1937), a brilliant teacher and surgeon, who died prematurely.

(Colorectal), Jose H. Amadeo, William K. Gorham, Henry C. Stofman, Bernard Borkowski, George F. Gowen, Peter S. Liebert (Pediatric Surgery), Edward D. McLaughlin, Stephen Gosin, Norton Hering, Jerry Stiffel, Robert W. Solit, D. Stanton Smullens, Melvin L. Moses, and George S. Nicoll. Many of these were active in clinics and lectures at the Philadelphia General and Pennsylvania Hospital. The services of more than 100 of those unmentioned dedicated staff members connected with the Affiliated Hospitals can only be acknowledged with gratitude.

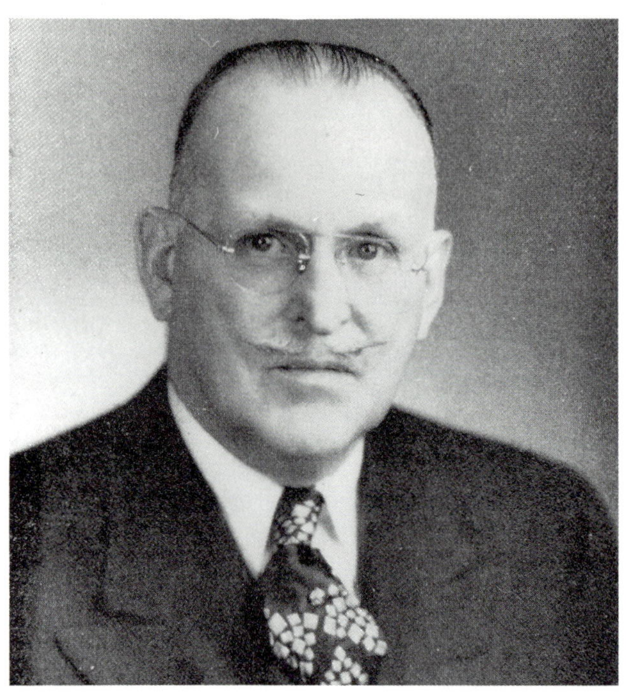

FIG. 32-77. S. Dale Spotts, M.D., Sc.D. (1895–1952), a surgical martyr to early unprotected use of x-rays for reducing fractures.

Surgical Epilogue

In 1879 a dinner was held in honor of Dr. Samuel D. Gross at the St. George Hotel, later to become

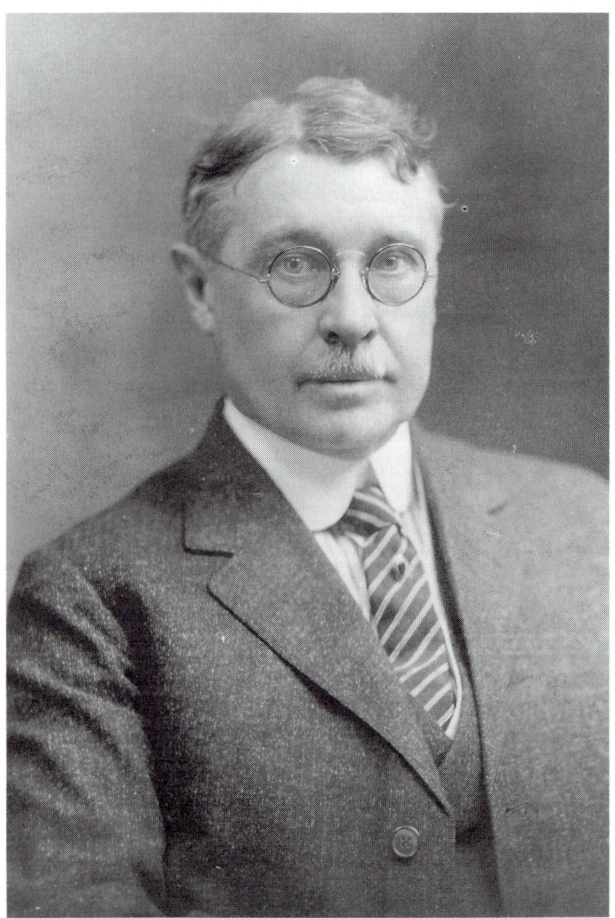

FIG. 32-76. Duncan L. Despard, M.D. (1869–1924), a Surgical Department staff member shot to death in his office by an insane patient.

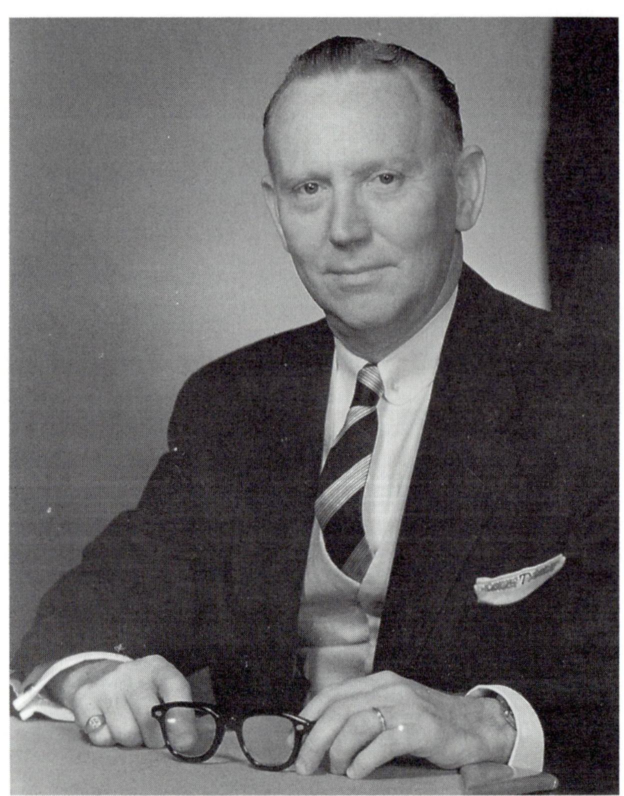

FIG. 32-78. William J. Tourish, M.D., Chief of the Surgery "A" Outpatient Clinic.

the Bellevue Stratford, in Philadelphia. Gross was 74 years old, and the occasion marked the fifty-first anniversary of his entrance into medical practice. D. Hays Agnew, Professor of Surgery at the University of Pennsylvania, as Toastmaster, pinned a jeweled badge, now in the Mütter Museum, on Gross's lapel as a testimonial of esteem from the 105 subscribers. One quote from Gross's acceptance speech expresses the ideals he had cherished: "Oh, for a glance at the profession half a century hence when man, enlightened and refined by education shall reflect more perfectly the image of his Maker!" Gross may have had some insight into the progress to come, but could not possibly have imagined the surgical advances of more than a century. Surgery is never perfected, and new ideas will irrepressibly spring forth from thinking minds.

From 1824 until the Summer Courses of 1866 the Department of Surgery consisted of one person, the Professor. There evolved two Professors when the Chair divided upon the resignation of Gross in 1882. Unthinkable to Gross, the surgical staff of 1987 consisted of a Chairman, 2 Vice-Chairmen, 2 Emeritus Professors, 18 Honorary Members, 16 Professors, 22 Associate Professors, 71 Assistant Professors, and 84 Instructors. This totaled a staff of 212 surgeons in association with 475 faculty members in 13 Divisions of the Department of Medicine (1985).

When Jefferson Medical College changed from a proprietary to a nonprofit status in 1895, the Professors in basic sciences became salaried, and

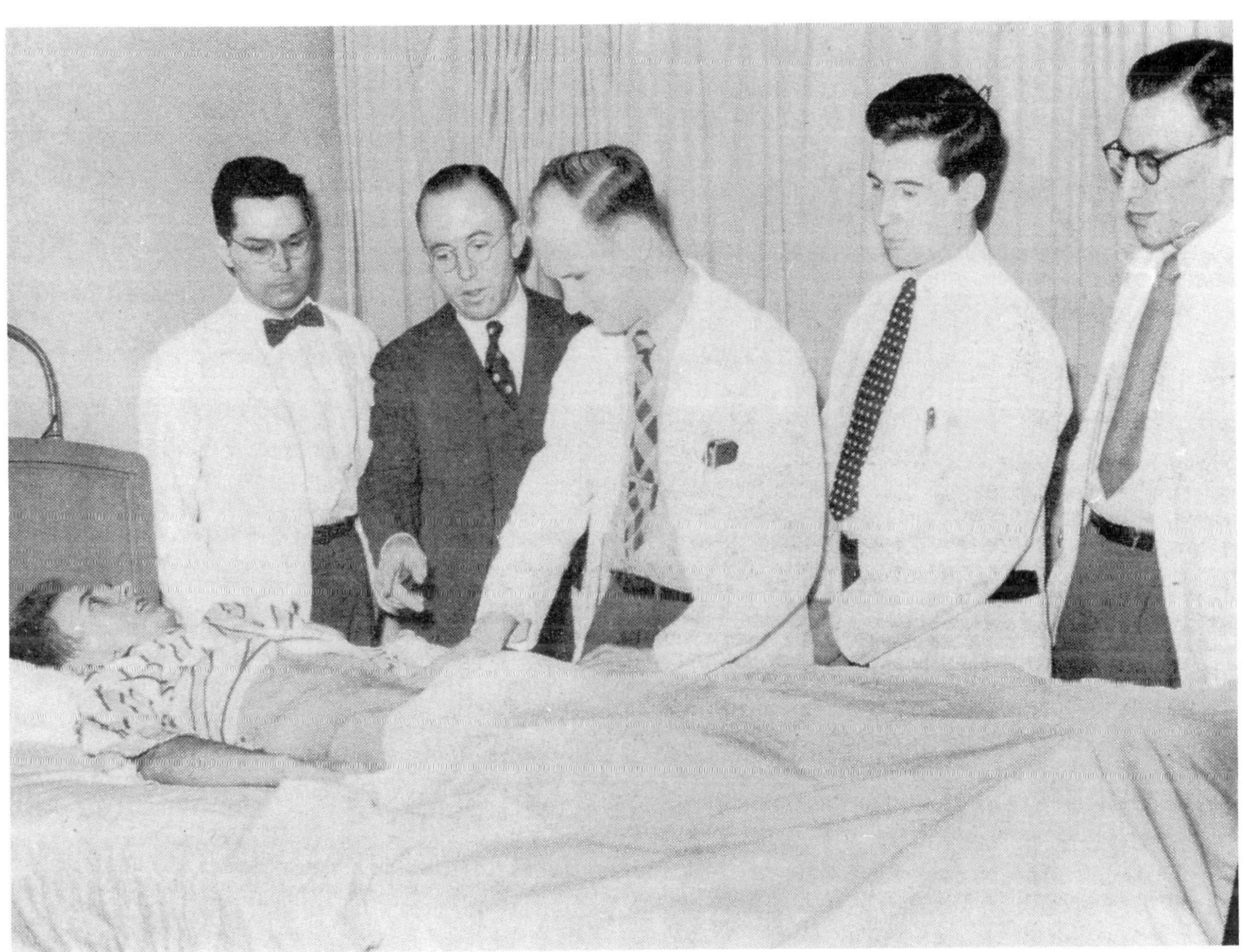

FIG. 32-79. Kenneth E. Fry, M.D., Clinical Professor, outstanding teacher, and surgeon.

the Professors in clinical branches obtained minimal stipends. In the late 1950s and through the 1960s the Clinical Chairmanships became salaried as previous volunteers were phased out. As of 1987 the ratio of full-time fully salaried faculty to volunteers was approximately 50%, but more than 60% of hospital admissions were associated with the full-time faculty. This trend will continue under the influence of complex social, governmental, and health policy changes.

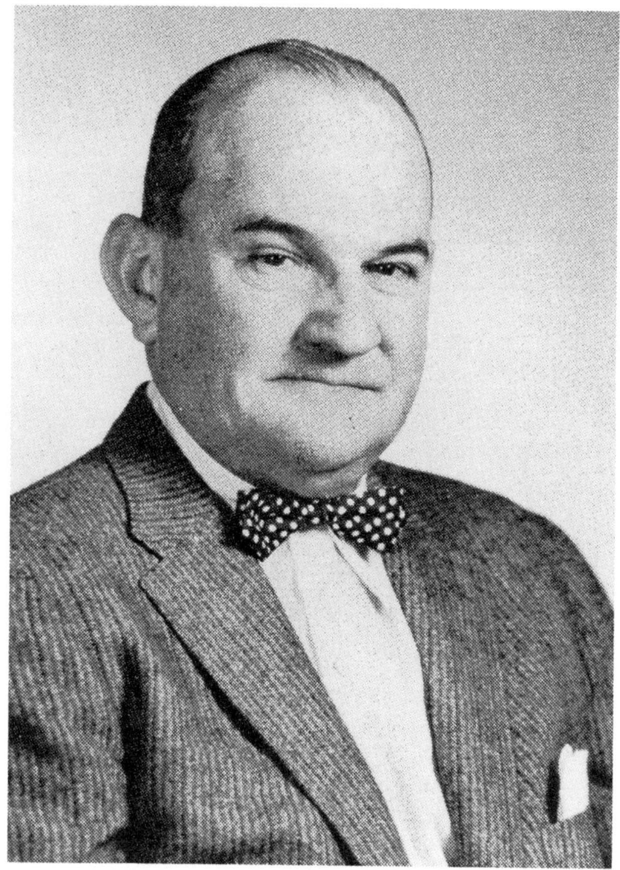

FIG. 32-80. William T. Lemmon, M.D., Clinical Professor, devised continuous spinal anesthesia, was a brilliant anatomist and quizmaster, and was sometimes called "the last of the great general surgeons."

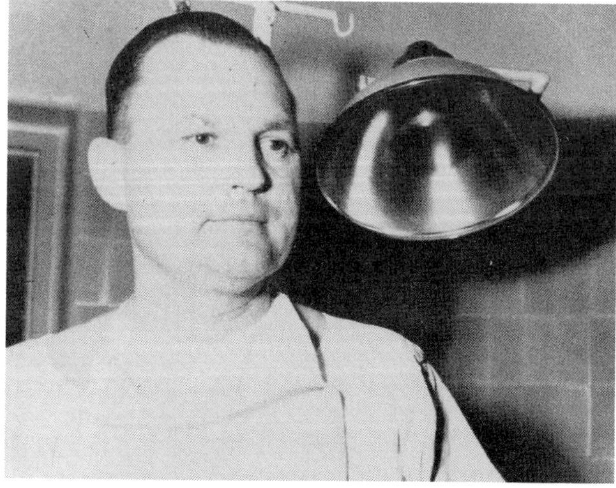

FIG. 32-81. Sherman A. Eger, M.D., Clinical Professor, author, and excellent surgeon.

FIG. 32-82. Books written by Jefferson's surgical faculty.

The Surgical Department's strength has always been in teaching medical students and training highly competent surgeons. Its faculty has contributed significantly to the surgical literature. Samuel D. Gross led the way with 14 textbooks and a bibliography of approximately 1,200 items. Figure 32-82 shows an imposing array of textbooks written entirely by Jefferson surgical faculty. Additionally, the Gibbon heart-lung machine created a new era in surgical history.

While the names of Gross, Keen, DaCosta, and Gibbon shine forth as beacon lights, the others, whether alumni or not, maintain the proud tradition and heritage of the Department.

References

1. Wagner, F.B., Jr., "The Making of a Medical School," *Jeff. Med. Coll. Al. Bull.*, Winter 1980, pp. 16–18.
2. McClellan, G., *The Principles and Practice of Surgery*. Philadelphia: Grigg, Elliott and Co., 1848.
3. Gross, S.D., *Autobiography of Samuel D. Gross, M.D., with Sketches of His Contemporaries*. New York: Arno Press and *The New York Times*, Vol. II, 1972, pp. 251–252.
4. Idem 3, Vol. I., p. 33.
5. Idem 3, Vol. II, p. 251.
6. Idem 3, Vol. II, p. 252.
7. Radbill, S.X., "Joseph Pancost (1805–1882): Jefferson Anatomist and Surgeon and His World," *Trans. Stud. Coll. Phys. Phila.*, Ser. 5, Vol. 8, No. 4, 1986, pp. 233–245.
8. Pancoast, J., *A Discourse Commemorative of the Late Professor T.D. Mütter, M.D., LL.D., Being the Introductory Lecture to the Course of Anatomy in the Jefferson Medical College of Philadelphia, Delivered Oct. 4, 1859*. Philadelphia: Joseph M. Wilson, 1859.
9. Idem 3, Vol. I. p. 39.
10. Wagner, F.B., Jr., "Revisit of Samuel D. Gross, M.D.," *Surg., Gynec. and Obst.*, 152:663–674, 1981.
11. Jobe, W.E., and Hills, D.K., "The History of Medical Education in Colorado," *Rocky Mt. Med. Jour.* 55:68–77, 1958.
12. DaCosta, J.C., "Samuel David Gross," *Surg., Gynec. and Obst.* 35:115, 1922.
13. DaCosta, J.C., "Sketch of Professor Samuel W. Gross, M.D., LL.D.," *Selections from the Papers and Speeches of John Chalmers DaCoasta, M.D., LL.D.* Philadelphia: W.B. Saunders Co., 1931, p. 225.
14. Keen, W.W., *Addresses and Other Papers*. Philadelphia: W.B. Saunders Co., 1905, pp. 41–67.
15. Brinton, J.H., *Personal Memoirs of John H. Brinton*. New York: Neale Pub. Co., 1914, p. 97.
16. Gibbon, J.H., "William Williams Keen," *Ann. Surg.* 97:478–480, 1933.
17. Keen, W.W., *The Surgical Operations on President Cleveland in 1893*. Philadelphia: George W. Jacobs and Co., 1917.
18. Shallow, T.A., "Memoir of John Chalmers DaCosta," *Trans. Stud. Coll. Phys. Phila.*, Ser. 4, Vol. I, No. 2, July–December, 1933, pp. lxx–lxxvi.
19. Idem 13, p. 103.
20. Idem 13, pp. 353–357.
21. *Poems of John Chalmers DaCosta.* Edited by Frederick E. Keller, M.D., Philadelphia: Dorrance and Co., 1942.
22. Flick, J.B., "Memoir of John Heysham Gibbon (1871–1956)," *Trans. Stud. Coll. Phys. Phila.*, Ser. 4, Vol. 25, 1957, pp. 117–118.
23. Goepp, R.M., "Memoir of Francis T. Stewart," *Trans. Stud. Coll. Phys. Phila.*, Ser. 4, Vol. 4, 1936, pp. xxxv–xxxviii.
24. Wagner, F.B., Jr., "Memoir of Thomas A. Shallow (1886–1955)," *Trans. Stud. Coll. Phys. Phila.*, Ser. 4, Vol. 24, 1956, pp. 133–134.
25. Gibbon, J.H., "Memoir of Edward J. Klopp," *Trans. Stud. Coll. Phys. Phila.*, Ser. 4, Vol. 4, 1937, pp. xxix–xxx.
26. Shallow, T.A., "Memoir of George P. Muller," *Trans. Stud. Coll. Phys. Phila.*, Ser. 4, Vol. 15, 1948, pp. 151–152.
27. Wagner, F.B., Jr., *The Twilight Years of Lady Osler*. Science History Publications, 1985, pp. 135–140.
28. Rhoads, J.D., "Memoir of John Heysham Gibbon, Jr., 1903–1973," *Trans. Stud. Coll. Phys. Phila.*, Vol. 42, 1975, pp. 194–197.
29. Shumacker, H.B., Jr., "John Heysham Gibbon, Jr., 1903–1973," *Biographical Memoirs* 53:213–247, 1982.
30. Templeton, J.Y., III, and Gibbon, J. H., Jr., "Experimental Reconstruction of Cardiac Valves by Venous and Pericardial Grafts," *Ann.Surg.* 129:161–176.
31. Wagner, F.B., Jr., "Abdominal Arteriography: Technique and Diagnostic Application," *Am. J. Roent.* 58:591–598, 1947.

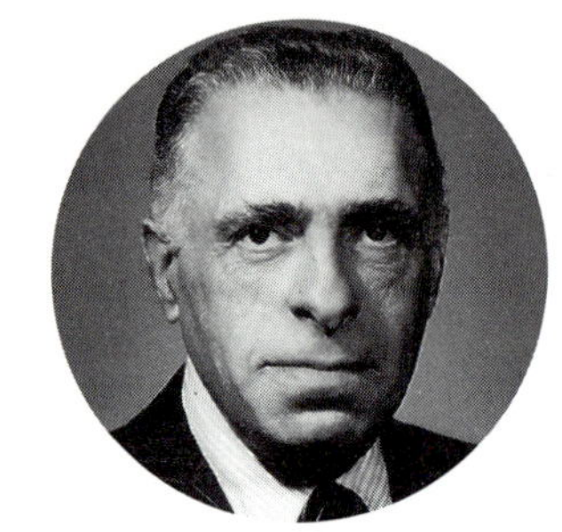

CHAPTER THIRTY-THREE

Division of Cardiothoracic Surgery

BERNARD J. MILLER, M.D., SC.D.

"The only weapon with which the unconscious patient can immediately retaliate upon the incompetent surgeon is hemorrhage." —WILLIAM STEWART HALSTED (1852–1922)

JEFFERSONIANS have made a worldwide impact on the development of cardiothoracic surgery. Perhaps the earliest prediction concerning the future of cardiac surgery was made by John B. Roberts (Jefferson, 1874) who, at a meeting of the American Surgical Association in 1885, suggested that wounds of the heart be repaired by direct suture.[1]

Pioneers

In 1901, again at a meeting of the American Surgical Association, W.W. Keen (Jefferson, 1862) described a new and dramatic operation, the resection of a large portion of the chest wall for sarcoma.[2] A tumor mass measuring 15 × 26 × 7.6 cm. and involving four ribs was removed by wide resection of the associated chest wall. An insufflating apparatus for artificial respiration, a primitive device when compared with present day respirators, did not function satisfactorily, and the lung collapsed. Because of the expertise of the surgeon and the speed of the operation, the patient tolerated the collapsed lung and eventually recovered. The apparatus consisted of a laryngeal tube as used in the treatment of laryngeal edema complicating diptheria and a simple bellows as a source of air pressure.

In 1902 John H. Gibbon, Sr. (Jefferson, 1891), later a full Professor of Surgery at Jefferson (1907–1931), reported the fourth case of a penetrating wound of the heart operated upon in this country.[3]

In 1910 W.W. Keen visited Alexis Carrel at the Rockefeller Institute in New York City and observed him divide the aorta of an experimental animal followed by primary repair. A unique suture technique was employed while respirations were maintained with a Meltzer–Auer apparatus during open thoracotomy. Keen predicted at the time that this method would be applicable to the treatment of aortic disease of man in the future.

Further advances in thoracic surgery were dependent upon the development of a suitable apparatus that could maintain expansion of the lungs and respiration during open thoracotomy under anesthesia. Widely dispersed pioneers such as O'Dwyer, Meltzer, Matas, and Sauerbruch extended the field.[4–7] During the first three decades of the twentieth century thoracic surgery advanced with relation to the treatment of inflammatory diseases of the chest such as empyema, lung abscess, and bronchiectasis.

Surgery for Tuberculosis

Surgery soon became the principal method of treating complicated tuberculosis that did not respond to simple collapse therapy and medical management. Because of the steadily increasing number of cases of tuberculosis, a separate section in the Department of Medicine was established for treatment. In 1913 the Department for Diseases of the Chest was relocated in a private dwelling at 238 Pine Street that had been the Henry Phipps Institute for the treatment of tuberculosis. In 1928 the role of surgery in the treatment of tuberculosis was established, and the Board of Trustees authorized the construction of an annex at adjacent 236 Pine Street. A newly built operating room was used mostly for the establishment and maintenance of pneumothorax until 1938 when closed pneumolysis, phrenicectomy, and thoracoplasty became standard operations in the treatment of complicated cases in which cavitation persisted.

Jefferson's First Thoracic Surgeons

John B. Flick (Figure 33-1) was the first of the group of thoracic surgeons at Jefferson and is credited with the concerted effort to develop a separate Division within the Department. He had received his M.D. degree from Jefferson in 1913 and spent the following year at White Haven Sanatorium in the Poconos, followed by two additional years as an intern at the Pennsylvania Hospital. During 1915 he saw service in the American Ambulance Hospital in Paris and received the rank of First Lieutenant in 1917, with promotion to Captain in 1918. He served as

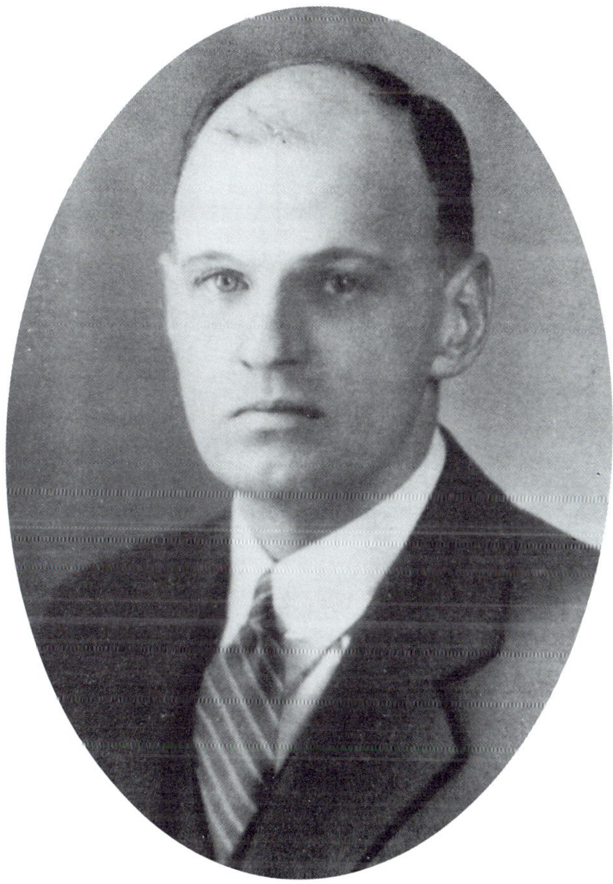

FIG. 33-1. John B. Flick, M.D., pioneer thoracic surgeon at Jefferson (1919–1946), performed the first successful pneumonectomy in Philadelphia.

surgical assistant in a French base hospital and also with a British General Hospital in 1918, followed by duty as medical officer to the British tank reinforcement depot. In 1919 he was admited to the Jefferson faculty. As surgeon to Jefferson, Pennsylvania, and Bryn Mawr Hospitals and White Haven Sanitorium, Flick was noted for his thoroughness, diagnostic ability, careful operative technique, and numerous contributions to the literature.

Dr. Flick performed the first thoracoplasty at Jefferson in 1924. In 1926 he published a paper dealing with the management of 127 cases of lung abscess.[8] Within the following ten years he wrote extensively about techniques and results of thoracoplasty in the treatment of tuberculosis[9] and lobectomy for bronchiectasis. He performed the first successful pneumonectomy in Philadelphia in 1933, soon after Dr. Evarts A. Graham earlier that year reported the first in the world at Washington University in St. Louis. Dr. Flick's was the sixth such operation reported in the literature. Throughout his career he was active in the local and national surgical societies. At Jefferson he was Assistant Professor of Surgery from 1933 to 1935, Associate Professor from 1935 to 1937, and Clinical Professor from 1937 to 1946. He subsequently pursued his distinguished career with teaching affiliations at the University of Pennsylvania. For many years he devoted himself to the care of his invalid wife, and he died in 1979 at the age of 86.

Howard H. Bradshaw (Figure 33-2) succeeded Dr. Flick as the thoracic surgeon at Jefferson. He graduated from Jefferson in 1927 and remained at the Jefferson Hospital until 1929 as an intern. He continued his training during the next five years at Harvard and the Massachusetts General Hospital, where he had the opportunity to serve under Drs. Edward Churchill and Charles Beecher. During that period he published numerous papers with Beecher and Lindskog pertaining to basic research in anesthesia and pulmonary physiology. On his return to Jefferson he activated the thoracic surgical service at the Pine Street Hospital, maintained an active role in clinical thoracic surgery at Jefferson Hospital, lectured to students, and published numerous clinical papers.

Unfortunately for Jefferson, Dr. Bradshaw was frustrated by the limited facilities for basic research at that time. In 1940 his international reputation led to an invitation to the Bowman Gray School of Medicine as Professor of Surgery, where he continued to contribute to the development of thoracic surgery. He died, tragically, of a brain tumor in 1969.

Following the untimely death of Dr. Edward J. Klopp in 1936, Dr. George P. Muller (Figure 33-3) came to Jefferson as Chief of the "B" surgical service and enhanced the existing strength in thoracic surgery. He received his early education in the public schools of Philadelphia and was

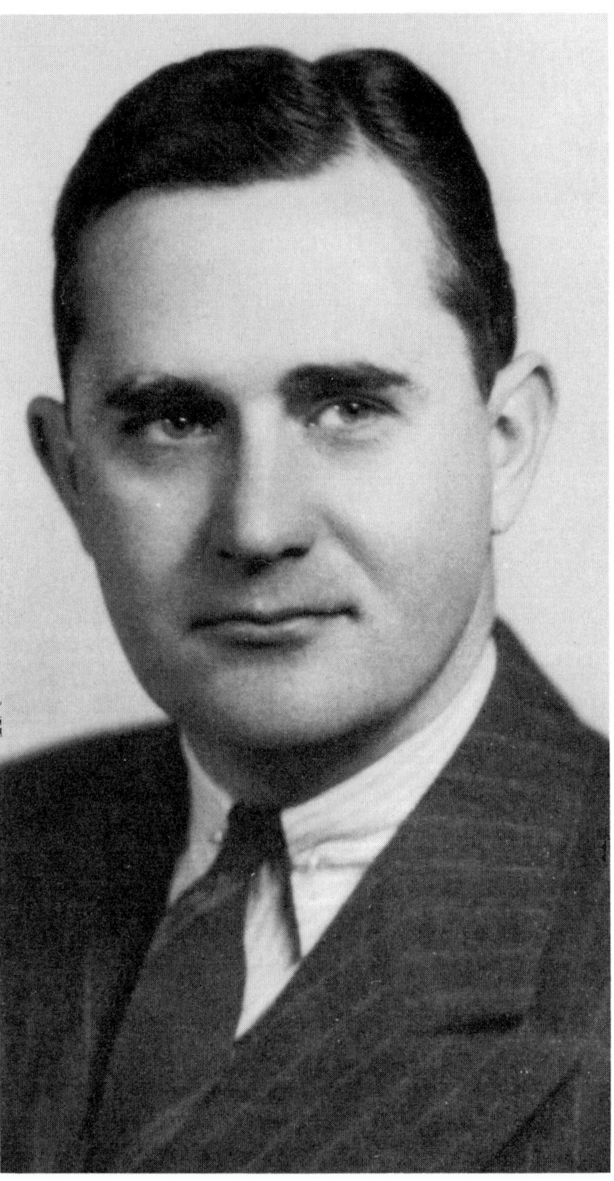

FIG. 33-2. Howard H. Bradshaw, M.D., thoracic surgeon at Jefferson (1934–1940) with special interest in anesthesia and pulmonary physiology.

graduated from Central High in 1895 with an A.B. degree (which was possible to do at that time). He immediately entered the Medical School of the University of Pennsylvania, received his degree in 1899, and served as an intern at the Lankenau Hospital until 1902. Thereafter he became a member of the Department of Surgery at the University of Pennsylvania, where he rapidly advanced to the position of Professor of Clinical Surgery and Professor of Surgery in the Graduate School of Medicine of the University. During the early years at Lankenau he served under John B. Deaver and was next in rank to Charles Frazier at the University. His association with these gifted surgeons aided his rapid national recognition.

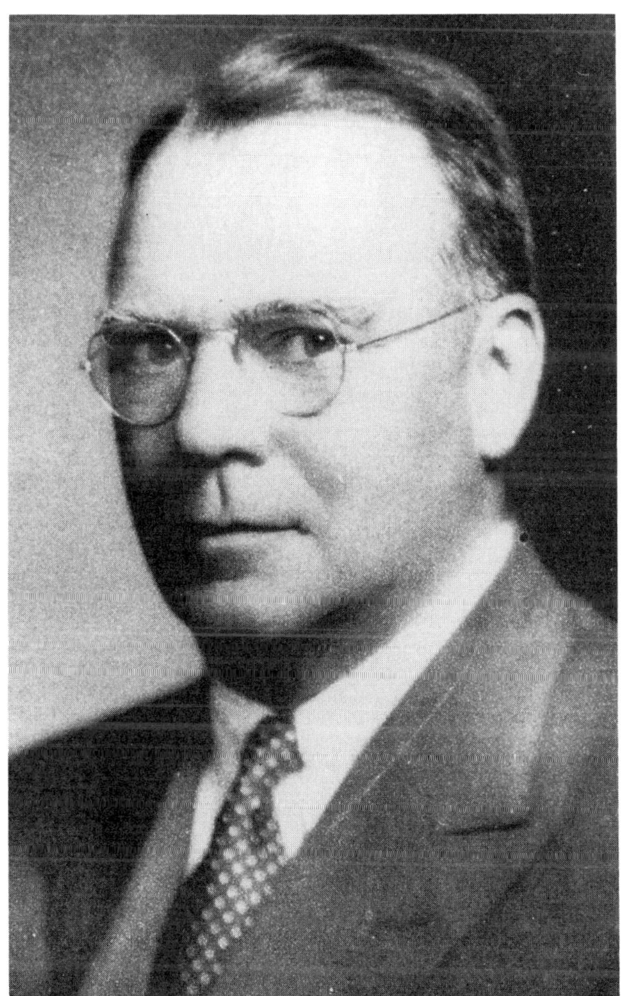

FIG. 33-3. George P. Muller, M.D., Sc.D., Professor of Surgery (1936) and first Grace Revere Osler Professor (1939–1946). He pioneered in the development of thoracic surgery in America.

Dr. Muller was a member of the Founders Group of the American Board of Surgery, President of the American College of Surgeons, the Philadelphia County Medical Society, the Philadelphia Academy of Surgery, the College of Physicians of Philadelphia, and the American Association for Thoracic Surgery, and a member of the American Surgical Association and the Society of Clinical Surgery. He served with distinction in the Armed Forces during World War I. Subsequently he joined the staffs of White Haven Sanitorium, Rush Hospital for Consumption and Allied Diseases, and Lankenau and Misericordia Hospitals. He received honorary degrees from Villanova College in 1926 and Muhlenberg College of Allentown in 1937 and served on the editorial board of *Annals of Surgery*.

Dr. Muller was among the great pioneers in the development of thoracic surgery in America. As early as 1912 he contributed an important article on endotracheal anesthesia and showed at that time a remarkable understanding of the physiology of respiration.[10] He also modified existing endotracheal apparatus. Muller was among the first to describe the removal of foreign bodies from the lung, and he reported such a case (removal of a bullet) in 1918.[11] He was actively involved in the establishment of policies for the treatment of thoracic wounds and the management of empyema in the wounded during World War I. In 1924 he made contributions to the surgical management of carcinoma of the esophagus. He was among the few in Philadelphia actively involved in the surgical management of the complications of uncontrolled active tuberculosis.

With Dr. Muller as Chief, the thoracic surgical section of Jefferson Hospital, in collaboration with Dr. Bradshaw, progressed rapidly. Large numbers of cases were referred for surgical treatment. These for the most part were of intrathoracic inflammatory disease, particularly lung abscess and bronchiectasis, but with an increasing number of cases of pulmonary neoplasms, which were treated by resection. Dr. Muller was among the first in Philadelphia to perform a pneumonectomy for the treatment of lung cancer. He was noted for the vastness of his knowledge, for his quick evaluation of surgical problems, his profound judgment, and a masterful technique. He utilized meticulous sharp dissection and stressed the importance of avoiding contamination of the wound from the skin by the use of wound towels. He forbade the use of large clamps and advocated fine suture material and interrupted sutures. Proper fluid balance by the intravenous route and use of the newly discovered sulfa drugs were taught in his weekly surgical amphitheater presentations. Dr. Muller became the Grace Revere Osler Professor of Surgery in 1939 and Emeritus Professor in 1946. It is believed that this very brilliant man, who died in 1947, developed Alzheimer's disease.

James Miller Surver (Figure 33-4) was born in Altoona, Pennsylvania, in 1905. He attended Franklin and Marshall College and graduated from Jefferson Medical College in 1929. He served his internship at Jefferson from 1929 to 1931, and as Chief Resident Physician from 1931 to 1933. He then went abroad for seven months to visit many of the outstanding clinics in Europe. From November of 1933, he was a private assistant and the protégé of Dr. Edward J. Klopp, Professor of Surgery at that time, until the latter's untimely death in 1936. Starting as a Clinical Assistant in the Surgical Department, Division "B", he rose through the academic ranks to become Assistant Professor of Surgery in 1952. He assisted Dr. George P. Muller, Professor of Surgery and Chief of the "B" Surgical Service, with all the pulmonary surgery and with much of the major abdominal surgery at that time.

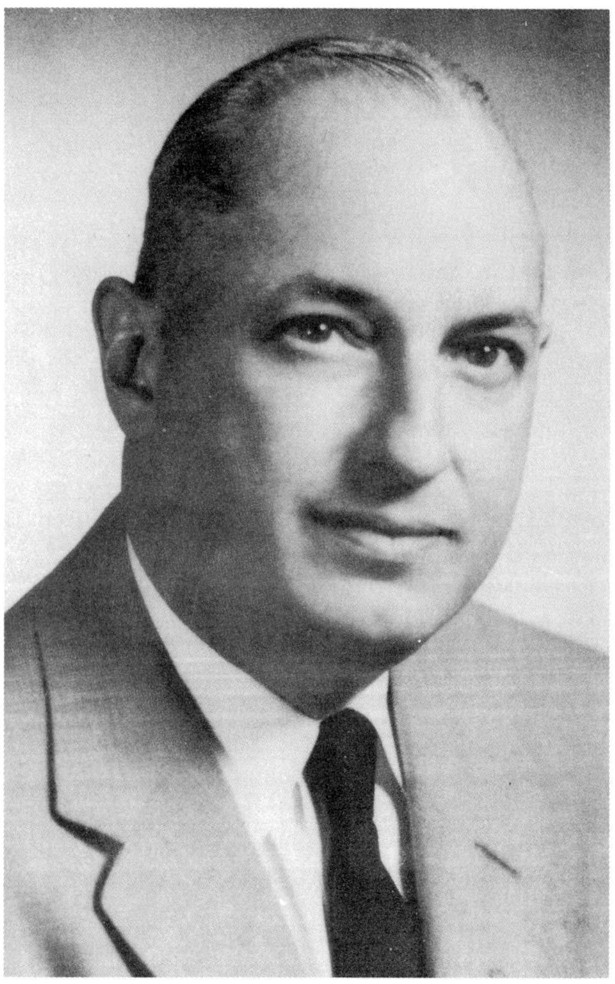

FIG. 33-4. James M. Surver, M.D., thoracic surgeon, teacher, and oncologist (1933–1962).

In the hospital Dr. Surver was always available for assistance to the surgical resident when called, regardless of inconvenience. He lectured on basic principles of surgery in the sophomore year, and on oncology and in the Tumor Clinic during the junior year. He conducted the weekly tumor conferences, which were always well attended by both staff and students. His records were prepared with great detail and delivered with meticulous clarity. The Senior Class of 1954 dedicated its yearbook to him. In addition to general surgery, Dr. Surver was a pioneer in pulmonary surgery and played an important role in the early phases of chest surgery at Jefferson.

Dr. Surver was a Diplomate of the American Board of Surgery, which at that time was a special distinction, and he belonged to the major surgical societies. He published very little but gave many talks on oncology and conducted the Tumor Clinic at Jefferson Hospital for many years. Ill health forced him to resign in 1962, and he died of coronary insufficiency in 1968. To his colleagues he was affectionately known as "Swifty," an opposite attribute, and to his students who held him in highest esteem, he was known as "Shifting Dullness" because of the monotone in which he lectured.

Dr. George J. Willauer (Figure 33-5) was an important participant in the advance of thoracic surgery during this period at Jefferson. He graduated from Franklin and Marshall College in 1917 and enlisted in the U.S. Army, spending two years in the cavalry as a drill sergeant. He entered Jefferson in 1919 and graduated in 1923. Following a year of internship at Jefferson, he studied surgery in Vienna. In addition, he visited a number of other famous surgical centers, particularly Sauerbruch's clinic in Munich. Upon his return to Philadelphia Willauer was admitted to the Jefferson faculty, where he continued his interest in anatomy as Assistant Demonstrator of Operative Surgery in the Daniel Baugh Institute. He then joined with Dr. Bradshaw as a member of the thoracic surgical group, working both in Jefferson Hospital and the Pine Street Division. Some of the principles upon which thoracic surgery is based today were developed by Willauer. He became especially expert in the surgical treatment of tuberculosis and its complications. He was a pioneer in the use of continuous spinal anesthesia for thoracoplasty and devoted much time to teaching students and young staff members. He designed surgical instruments, some of which are in use today. The Willauer modification of the Deaver retractor is invaluable, and the Willauer dissecting clamp has been used worldwide by countless numbers of surgeons. His vividly colorful explanations and descriptions made lasting impressions. With a unique assertiveness, Willauer remained a drill sergeant and taskmaster. He was noted for his great regard for patients and for the extremely high standards he set for himself and others. Willauer saw things in black and white and thus took a strong stand on issues. As an Alumni Association President (1962), fund raiser, and Alumni Trustee on the Board (1968–1971), he could be counted in that select few who from time to time are designated "Mr. Jefferson." His portrait was presented to the College by the Surgical Residents in 1965. This forceful leader died in 1977.

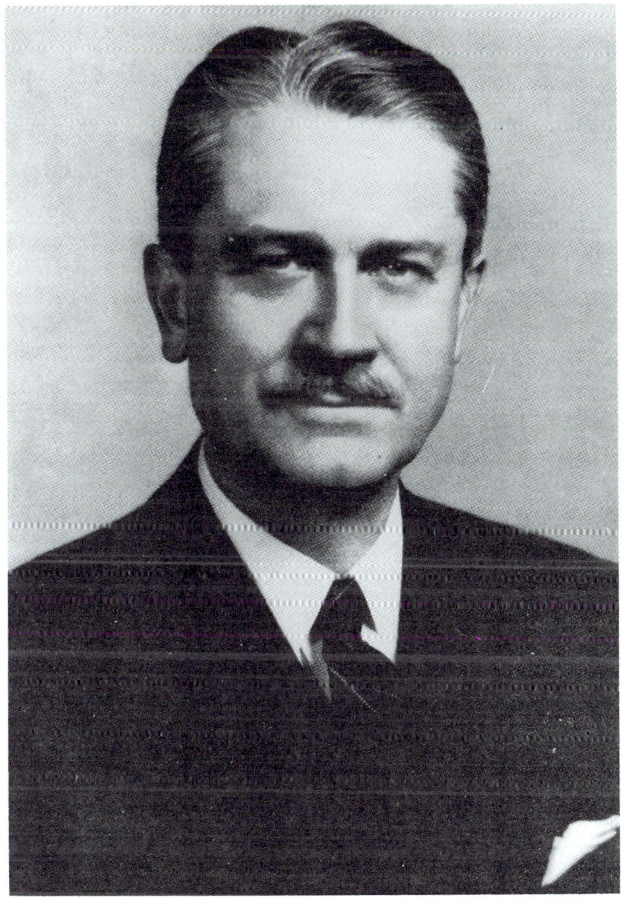

FIG. 33-5. George J. Willauer, M.D., pioneered in the use of continuous spinal anesthesia for thoracoplasty in complicated tuberculosis. He devised surgical instruments currently in worldwide use.

John H. Gibbon, Jr., M.D., Sc.D., LL.D., F.R.C.S.

Dr. John H. Gibbon, Jr. (Figure 33-6) followed Dr. Muller in 1946 with appointment as Professor of Surgery and Director of Experimental Surgery. His arrival at Jefferson initiated a period of rapid development, particularly in the technical and physiological aspects of thoracic surgery. The surgical service became strongly oriented toward research. This period influenced world-wide the treatment of diseases of the chest; under his outstanding leadership the Department of Surgery attracted aspiring young surgeons from great distances for their surgical training. These Residents were stimulated by his knowledge and inquisitiveness. Many of them achieved high academic positions through their contributions to thoracic surgical research. Dr. Gibbon's basic interest was in the development of an extracorporeal circuit containing an aritifical heart and lung. The first heart-lung machine suitable for human use was developed under his direction at Jefferson. In addition to this primary interest, he was concerned with the problems of blood volume changes during thoracic operations and respiratory acidosis during anesthesia.

Dr. Gibbon graduated from Princeton in 1923 with an A.B. degree and from Jefferson in 1927. He served his internship at the Pennsylvania Hospital from 1927 to 1929 and then became a Research Fellow in the Department of Surgery of Harvard Medical College until 1931. Upon returning to Philadelphia he became a Fellow in Medicine at the University of Pennsylvania and also Assistant Surgeon at the Pennsylvania Hospital. In 1933, after two years of clinical practice, he returned to Harvard. It was during this period that he became interested in a heart-lung device. In 1937 he was able with a primitive machine to demonstrate for the first time the feasibility of total maintenance of the cardiorespiratory function during arrest of the circulation in an experimental animal.[12] He returned to Philadelphia in 1936 as Harrison Fellow of Surgical Research at the University of Pennsylvania. It was at this time that the second extracorporeal device was constructed. Additional successful animal experiments provided support for the original notion that the heart-lung machine could be used as a means of maintaining the cardiorespiratory function during arrest of the circulation. Gibbon responded to the call of duty during World War II in 1942, entering the Army as a Major. Promoted to Lieutenant Colonel in 1945, he served as Chief of the Surgical Service at the Mayo General Hospital until his honorable discharge.

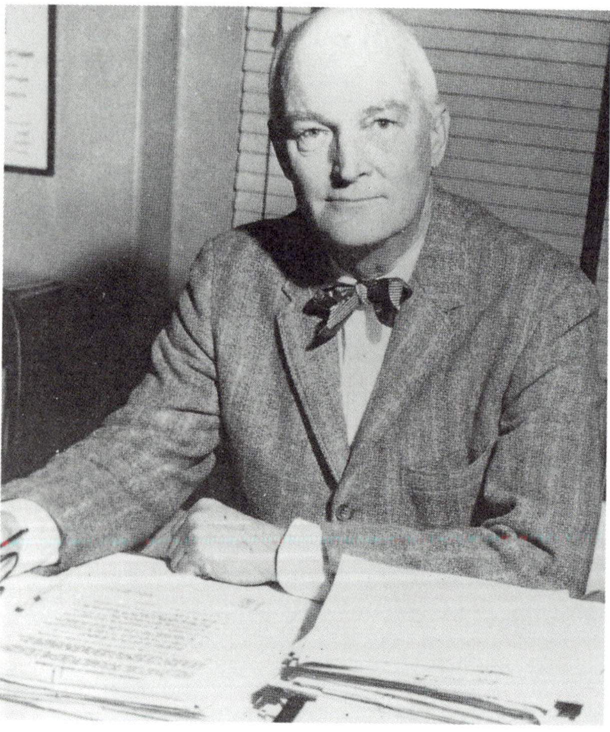

Fig. 33-6. John H. Gibbon, Jr., M.D., Sc.D., LL.D., F.R.C.S; Professor of Surgery and Director of Experimental Surgery (1946–1956), Samuel D. Gross Professor and Chairman (1946–1967), developed the heart-lung machine for the first open heart operation (1953) and initiated a new era in cardiovascular surgery.

The Heart-Lung Machine

Upon arriving at Jefferson in 1946, Dr. Gibbon succeeded in obtaining the services of Mr. Thomas Watson of the International Business Machines Corporation in support of the continued investigation of extracorporeal circuits. A postwar model, similar to the 1933 model in principle, was constructed and placed in the laboratory. The smooth film oxygenator was enlarged to increase its capacity sufficiently to maintain the respiratory function of dogs. In addition, the collecting assembly was improved, and the machine was enclosed in two cabinets. One contained the power supplies and controls and the other contained the oxygenator and pumps. The entire device was temperature controlled. It was at this time that Dr. Gibbon included a period of basic research training in the laboratory as an important addition to the residency training program.

Drs. T. Lane Stokes (Jefferson, 1947) and John B. Flick, Jr., were early Residents to work with the experimental heart-lung machine. Both partial and total perfusion of dogs were studied.[13] The mortality rate was excessively high and a number of serious defects in the first device provided by International Business Machines became apparent (see Figure 33-13). Oxygenation was inadequate. Controls malfunctioned, and hemolysis was excessively high. Stokes and Flick were able to incorporate the principle of turbulence and improve the oxygenation efficiency of the artificial lung.[14] Even with the improved oxygenation it was clearly obvious that the machine was not suitable for maintaining the cardiorespiration of even small dogs. Another period of redesign and experiment was required.

Bernard J. Miller, who had just completed his surgical residency, became Dr. Gibbon's Research Associate in charge of the laboratory. He made critical contributions that led to the eventual perfection and application of the device for human use. The heart-lung machine was stripped to bare essentials (Figure 33-7). A skeleton apparatus was used exclusively for testing of modifications and new components. Another machine, the second IBM model, arrived at Jefferson in 1951, and this initiated the final phase of development (Figure 33-8). On May 6 of 1953, after a period of intense evaluation, the machine was finally used by Dr. Gibbon in the heroic performance of an open cardiotomy for the repair of a congenital interatrial septal defect in a young woman while the cardiorespiratory function was maintained by an extracorporeal circuit (Figure 33-9). An interatrial septal defect was successfully repaired and she was restored to normal health. The operation heralded a new era in thoracic surgery, and cardiac surgery was no longer beset by the barrier which had prevented its advancement.

Dr. Gibbon received many honors. Visiting professorships and lectureships were routine. In 1956 he was the George A. Ball Visiting Professor of Surgery, Indiana University; in 1959 the Taub Visiting Professor of Surgery, Baylor University;

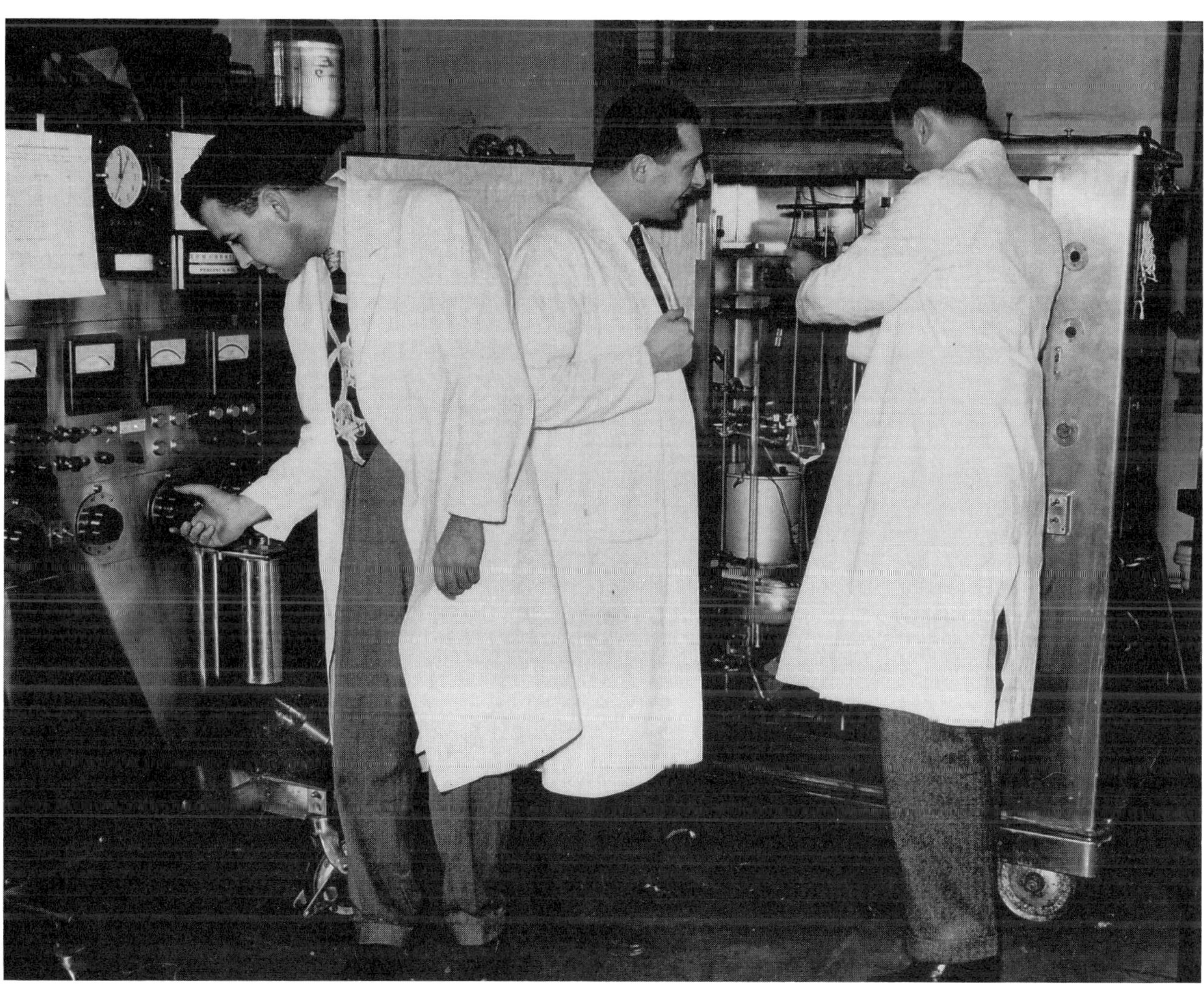

FIG. 33-7. Bernard J. Miller, M.D., Sc.D. (center), Research Associate of Dr. Gibbon, in the laboratory.

in 1960 the Visiting Professor of Surgery, Harvard Medical School; and in 1967 the Barney Brooks Visiting Professor of Surgery, Vanderbilt University. In 1956 he gave the Churchill Lecture, Excelsior Surgical Society; in 1958 the Harvey Lecture at the New York Academy of Medicine; in 1958 the Conner Memorial Lecture of the American Heart Association; in 1962 the Alvarenga Prize and Lectureship of the College of Physicians of Philadelphia; and in 1962 the Arthur Dean Bevan Lectureship at the Chicago Surgical Society. He was away so much of the time that even at Jefferson he was sometimes called "The Visiting Professor."

Dr. Gibbon occupied numerous clinical positions. From 1937 to 1950 he was Surgeon to the Pennsylvania Hospital, and from 1945 to 1946 he was Assistant Professor of Surgery at the University of Pennsylvania. In 1946 he was Attending Surgeon at Jefferson Hospital, and from 1950 to 1967 he was Consultant in General Surgery at the Veterans Administration Hospital in Philadelphia. His appointment as Samuel D. Gross Professor and Chairman of the Department at Jefferson in 1956 unified the Chair that had been split into two divisions since the retirement of the elder Gross in 1882 (Figure 33-10). From 1967 to 1973 he was the Samuel D. Gross Emeritus Professor of Surgery.

The societies to which Dr. Gibbon belonged were: American Association of Arts and Sciences; American Association for Thoracic Surgery, of which he was President from 1960 to 1961; American Cancer Society; American College of Surgeons; Board of Governors of the American College of Surgeons from 1950 to 1964; American Heart Association; American Medical Association; American Medical Writers Association; American Surgical Association, of which he was President in 1954; Association of American Medical Colleges; College of Physicians of Philadelphia, of which he was President from 1964 to 1967; Halsted Society; Heart Association of Pennsylvania; International Surgical Group; J. Aitken Meigs Medical Society; Laennec Society of Philadelphia; Pennsylvania Association for Thoracic Surgery; Pennsylvania Public Health Association; Pennsylvania State Medical Society; Pennsyslvania Trudeau Society; Philadelphia Academy of Surgery, of which he was President from 1956 to 1958; Philadelphia County Medical Society; Pulmonary Neoplasm Research Group of Philadelphia; Society of Clinical Surgery, of which he was President from 1964 to 1965; World Medical Association; and National Academy of Sciences. He was a member of the Board of Directors of City Trusts of Philadelphia. In addition, Gibbon received national honorary memberships, such as the Chicago Surgical Society in 1962 and the Buffalo Surgical Society in 1966,

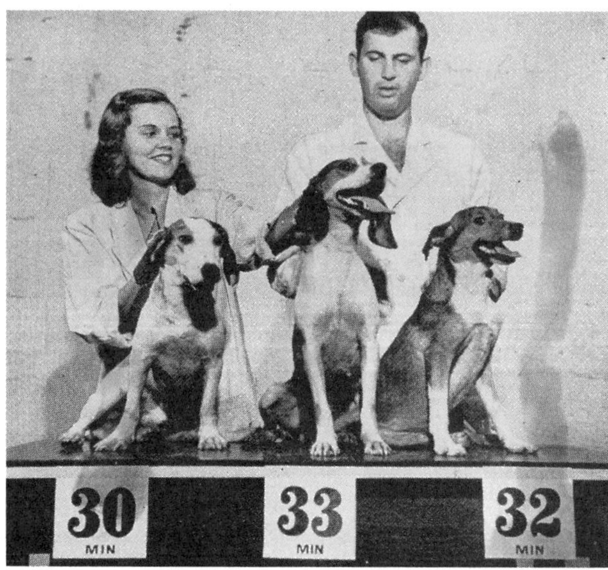

FIG. 33-8. Dogs line up with Dr. John Flick, Jr., Research Assistant, and a laboratory technician. The animals had fully recovered from operations during which their hearts were isolated for 30, 33, and 32 minutes, respectively.

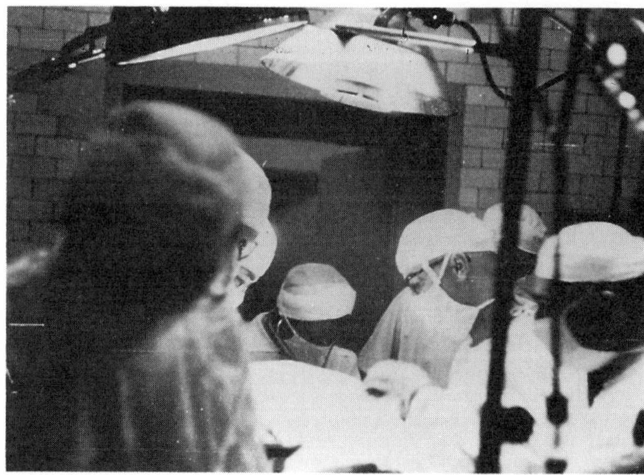

FIG. 33-9. First open heart operation (May 6, 1953) by Dr. Gibbon using the heart-lung machine successfully.

and was initiated into Fellowship of the Royal College of Surgeons of England in 1959 and the Society of Thoracic Surgeons of Great Britain and Ireland in 1961.

Dr. Gibbon served on the editorial board of the *Annals of Surgery* from 1947 to 1973 and on the board of *Circulation Research*. For his accomplishments he received numerous awards, beginning in 1931: the John Scott Award; the Charles Mickle Fellowship (University of Toronto); the Clarence E. Shaffrey Award (St. Joseph's College); the Rudolph Matas Award in Vascular Surgery (Tulane University); the Distinguished Service Award (International Society of Surgery); the Strittmatter Award (Philadelphia County Medical Society); the Distinguished Service Award of the Pennsylvania Medical Society (Figure 33-11); the Philadelphia Award; the Research Achievement Award (American Heart Association); the Roswell Park Medal; the Albert Lasker Clinical Research Award; and the Dixon Prize in Medicine (University of Pennsylvania). Some of the medals associated with these awards are on display in the archives cabinet of the Samuel D. Gross Conference Room. Dr. Gibbon died on his tennis court in 1973.

Residents and Fellows: Improvements in the Heart-Lung Machine

The Residents who received their surgical training in the Gibbon era were John J. DeTuerk, Joseph W. Stayman, Jr., Frederick W. Dash, T. Lane

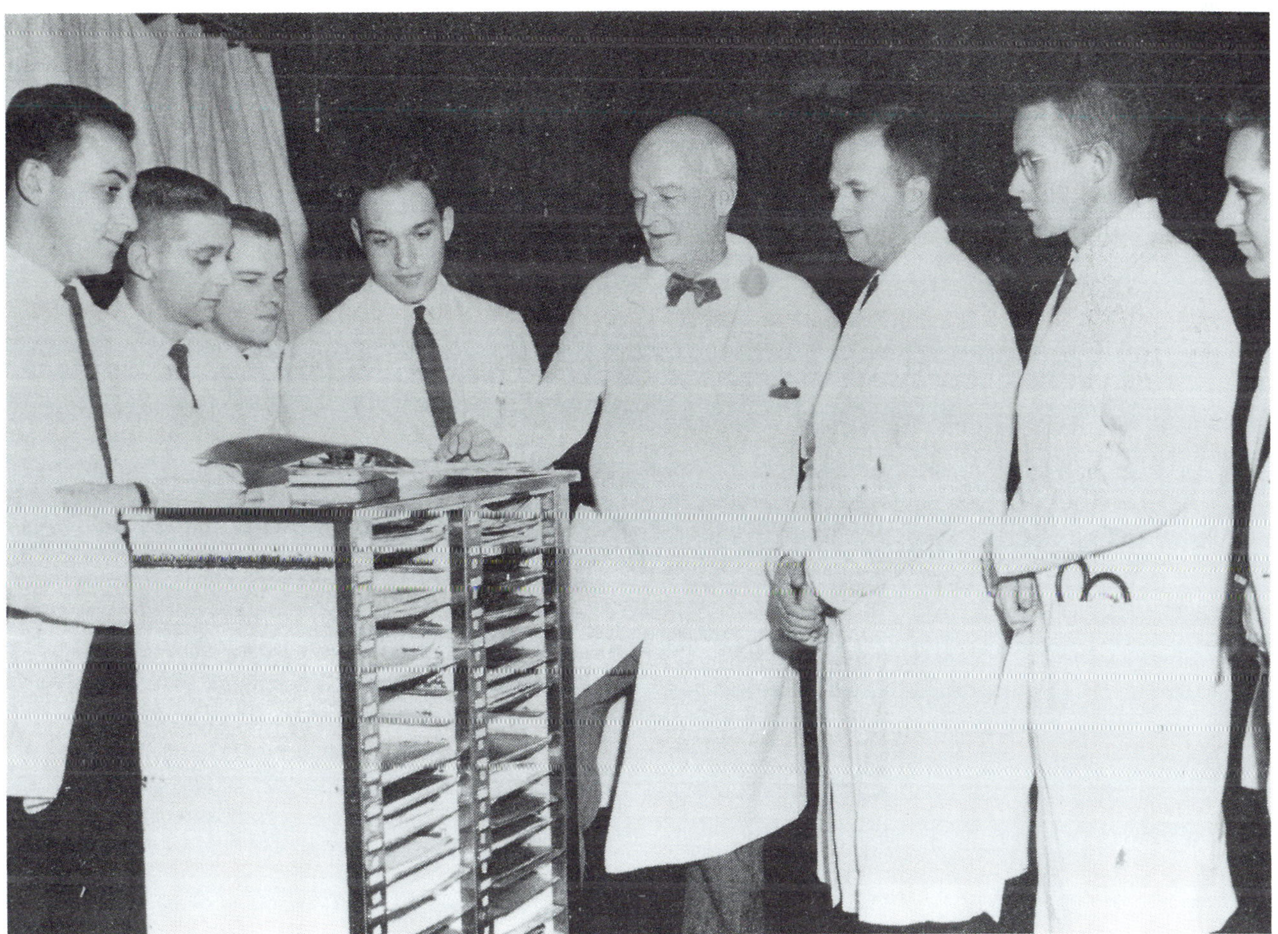

FIG. 33-10. Dr. Gibbon on ward rounds. Dr. Herbert Cohn is at his right.

Stokes, John Flick, Jr., Bernard J. Miller, John Y. Templeton, III, Charles Fineberg, George J. Haupt, Harold C. Cohn, Robert G. Johnson, Thomas F. Nealon, Jr., Anthony Dobell, Robert K. Finley, Jr., Victor J. Greco, John J. McKeown, Jr., Herbert E. Cohn, Rudolph C. Camishion, Leon P. Scicchitano, John R. Prehatny, Henry C. Stofman, Richard Myers, William Milberg, Thomas O'Brien, Martin Snyder, Noel Fishman, Norton Hering, Edward R. Hagopian, William M. Perrige, Antoinette Repepi, David C. Schechter, Benjamin Bacharach, Joseph Hodge, Donald Sokal, Alfred J. Martin, Amy Martin, Francis F. Bartone, Steven C. Sandler, Jerome L. Sandler, Edward J. Baranski, Vincent D. Cuddy, Alfred O. Heath, Joseph S. Brown, Jr., Christopher J. Beetel, Nathaniel P. Ching, William P. Coughlan, Richard Brown, William V. Chase, Michael D. Strong, Paul A. Pupi, John V. Zeok, Allen L. Davies, Anthony M. Padula, Michael G. Christy, Thomas Holder, Bernard B. Borkowski, Harvey J. Sugarman, Robert E. Colcher, Dwight G. Davis, Jr., Robert E. Berry, Stanton N. Smullens, Louis Pierucci, Jose H. Amadeo, Richard T. Padula, Stephen Gosin, Malcolm Herring, Anthony Del Rossi, Victor P. Sencindiver, Robert Swartley, Melvin L. Moses, Russell R. Tyson, and Robert W. Solit (Figure 33-12).

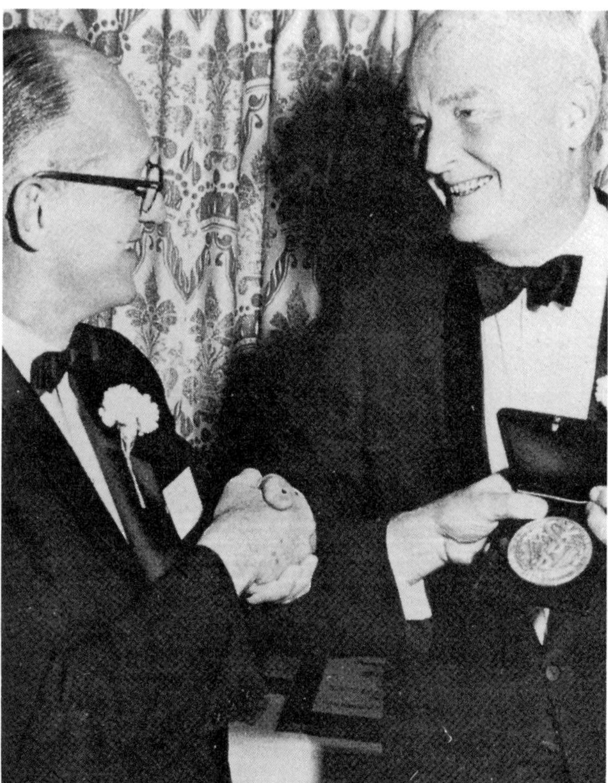

FIG. 33-11. Dr. Gibbon receives the Pennsylvania Medical Society's Distinguished Service Award from President Daniel H. Bee, M.D.

The intense academic environment in the laboratory during the early 1950s provided the stimulus for the staff and residents to engage in both clinical and basic investigation in thoracic surgery. A number of this group were subsequently rewarded by high academic positions on other medical faculties.

Dr. Bernard J. Miller was closely associated with Dr. Gibbon and responsible for the design of electronic and other components within the extracorporeal circuit and conducted the research program that made the heart-lung machine practical for human use. In addition, he demonstrated the important role of expiratory assistance during anesthesia and the method for the avoidance of air embolization during open cardiotomy and total bypass. His vent for the left ventricle remains in standard usage.

Dr. Miller graduated from Villanova College in 1939 with a B.S. degree and from Jefferson in 1943. While an undergraduate at Villanova he engaged in research in embryology and tissue culture at the Research Institute of Lankenau Hospital, which eventually became the Cancer Research Institute at Fox Chase. It was at this period that he was influenced by his first mentor of medicine, Dr. Stanley P. Reimann, Director of the Institute. Dr. Reimann remained his close friend, mentor, and advisor for the following 30 years until his death. During this early period, research in embryology involved the recovery of the first human tubal ova and the first demonstration of induced parthenogenetic activity in the human ovum in vitro. The initial efforts at tissue culture of fertilized rabbit ova using the Carrel–Lindbergh artificial heart took place in the laboratory of the Lankenau Hospital Research Institute. Following this, the effects of some amino acids that had been shown to have selective effects on the various phases of normal cellular growth were studied on fertilized rabbit ova in tissue culture. He worked part-time at the

Institute during his collegiate years and the early part of medical school.

Dr. Miller served his internship at Jefferson Hospital and the early period of his surgical residency from 1944 to 1945 on the "B" surgical service under Dr. George P. Muller. In the Armed Forces he was assigned to the surgical service at Fort Bragg from 1945 to 1947 and then returned to Jefferson to complete the remainder of his surgical residency under Dr. Gibbon, the successor to Dr. Muller. The first assignment during his surgical residency was to study blood volume changes and extracellular fluid losses during major thoracic operations, and the results were presented to the American Thoracic Association in 1948. With completion of his residency in 1950 and appointment as Research Associate to Dr. Gibbon, Miller spearheaded a team effort to improve the heart-lung machine to the point that it could be moved from the experimental laboratory into the operating room for safe use on patients. It has been said of Dr. Gibbon's work that the embryo was planted at Harvard, gestation went on at the University of Pennsylvania, and the birth occurred at Jefferson. A more detailed history of the problems and solutions in the final development of the machine is justified because of the benefit to humanity and the acclaim to Jefferson.

Limitations and defects in the first apparatus built by the International Business Machines Corporation (Figure 33-13) determined that the device could not be used for patients. New data and additional circuits developed in the surgical laboratory were used by the International Business

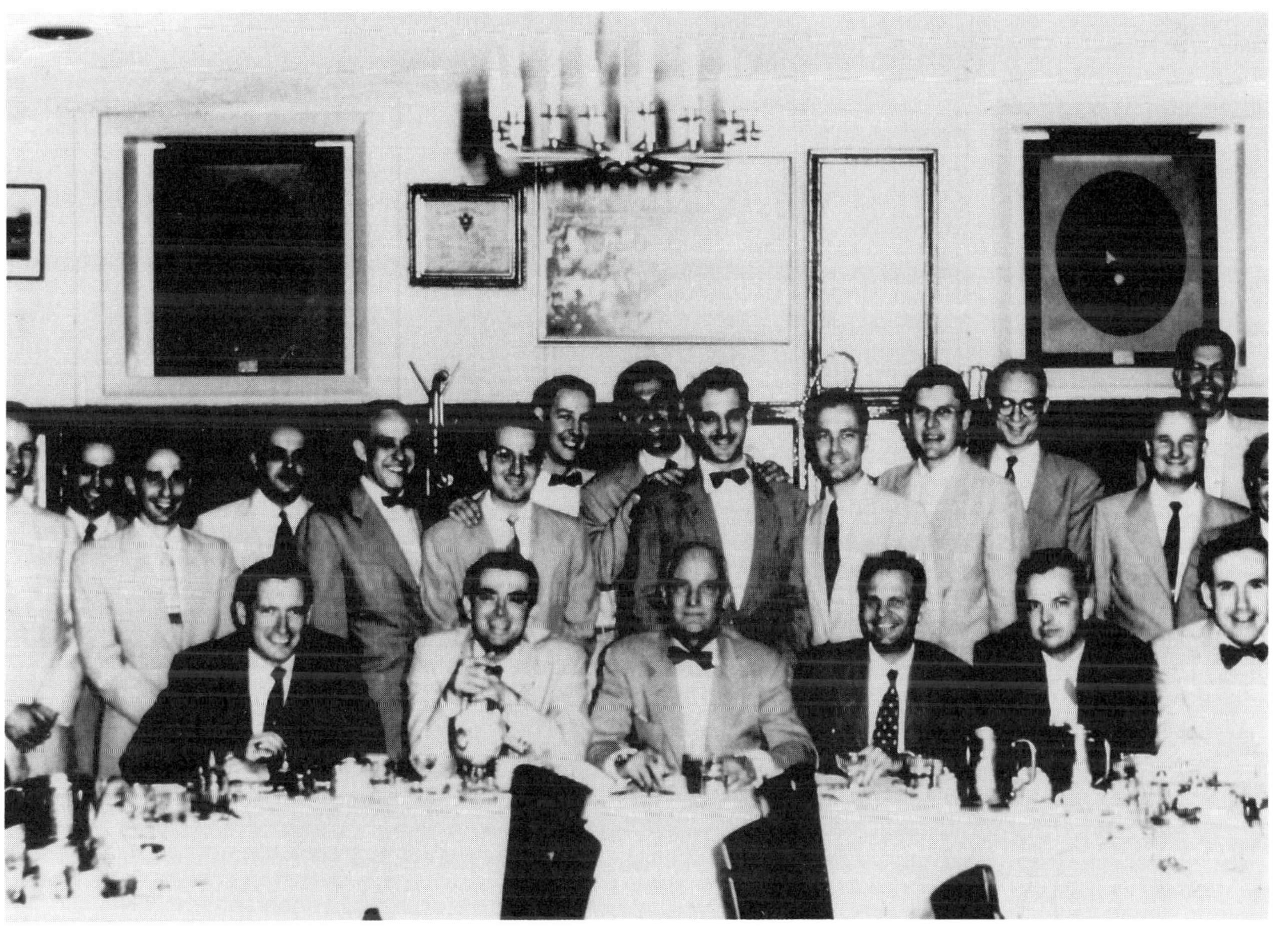

FIG. 33-12. "Rib Crackers" banquet at the Franklin Inn (1954). These Residents had all trained under Dr. Gibbon, and many more were to follow. Seated from left to right: Drs. Thomas F. Nealon, Jr., John Y. Templeton III, John H. Gibbon, Jr., John J. DeTuerk, J. Louis Wilkerson, and John J. McKeown, Jr.

Machines engineers in a second machine (Figures 33-14a and b).[15,16] The oxygenator was redesigned by incorporating the principle of turbulence that Stokes and Flick had demonstrated would enhance oxygenation. In addition, the new oxygenator was no longer cylindrical but consisted of a series of vertical screens suspended from a distributing chamber. The artificial lung, containing six screens, each measuring 30.5 × 45.1 cm., was found to be adequate to maintain the respiratory requirement of large dogs. The electronic control that maintained a constant level of blood at the bottom of the oxygenator was critical for two reasons: first, since the total volume of blood required to fill the apparatus was quite large, it was necessary to reduce to a bare minimum the size of the pool of blood at the bottom of the oxygenator; second, it was imperative to rigidly control this blood level so that air would not be inadvertently pumped by the arterial pump into the subject being perfused. The original photoelectric controls had malfunctioned and were unreliable. A variable capacitor circuit was designed. This control proved to be reliable and was incorporated in the new machine. The new electronic control was also used to sense changes in pressure in the tubes conducting blood from the vena cava to the venous pumps. Occlusion of the vena cava due to high pump rates and resultant high negative pressure was automatically prevented by sensing the changes in the diameter of the tubes conducting venous blood into the machine before complete cessation of blood flow occurred as a result of the caval wall being sucked into the cannula. The capacitor functioned properly in this application. A number of additional controls were incorporated, and a special filter was designed so that fibrin debris could effectively be evacuated during the perfusion.

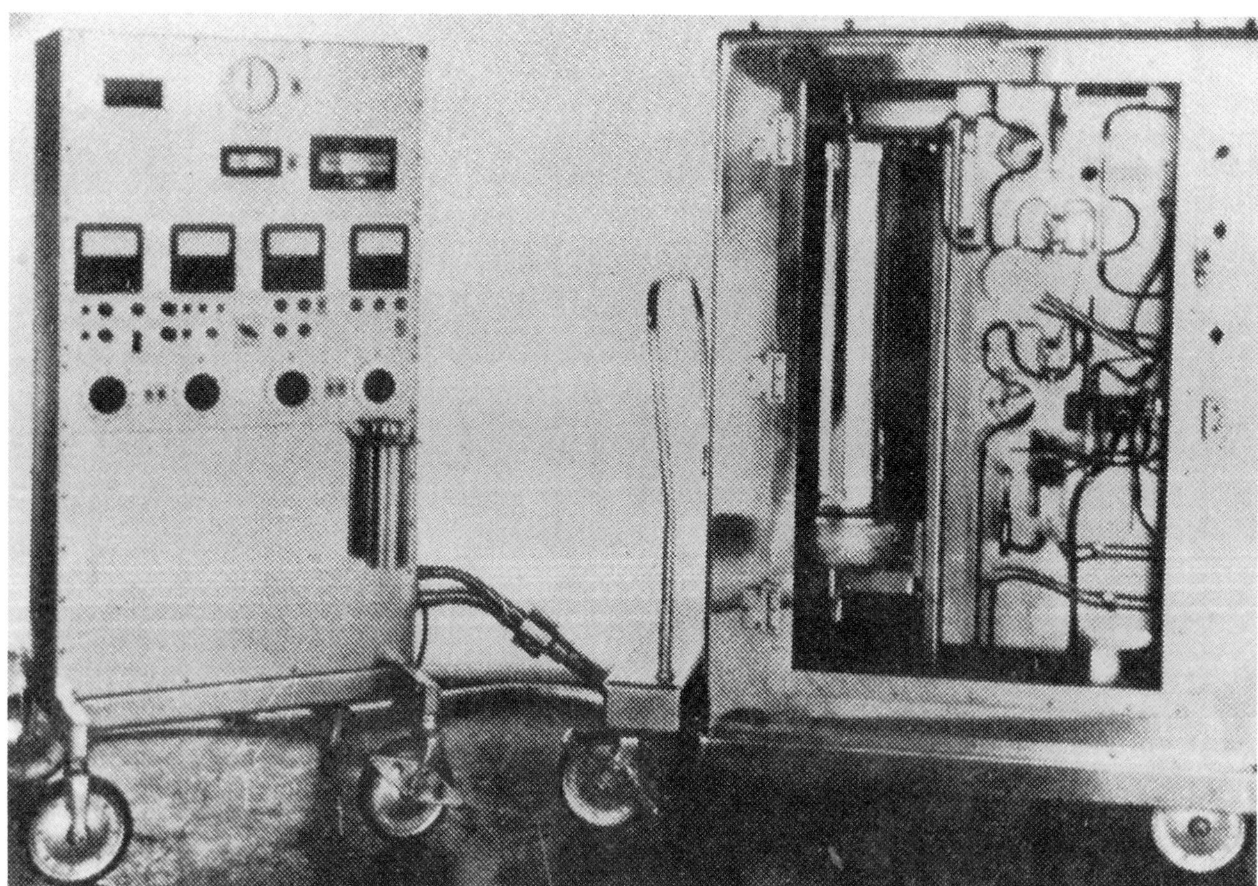

FIG. 33-13. The first heart-lung machine provided by International Business Machines Corporation.

The pH was automatically controlled by utilizing continuous measurement and recording, which in turn automatically controlled the amount of carbon dioxide added to the gas within the oxygenator. The saturation of blood with oxygen was continuously measured and recorded photoelectrically. The temperature of the blood within the extracorporeal circuit was maintained within narrow limits by means of a recording potentiometer. The new machine constructed by International Business Machines in 1951 contained all the new circuits and refinements and was completely enclosed in a hermetically sealed case, containing a small positive pressure of nitrogen. This prevented the possible entry of explosive anesthetic gases from the operating room atmosphere, a potential danger because there was constant sparking in the armature of the arterial pump motor (Figures 33-14a and b).

Beginning in 1951 the new machine (Figure 33-15) was used in a large number of animal experiments in which the systemic venous return to the heart was diverted into the extracorporeal circuit by temporarily occluding the vena cava while arterialized blood from the machine was returned to the animal by means of a cannula placed within the femoral artery. The mortality rate before 1951 was approximately 80%. With the new machine, a markedly reduced mortality rate of approximately 20% was achieved by 1952. The highest mortality occurred in the early bypass experiments. At this point attention was focused on gasometric studies that revealed the development of hypoxia and acidosis during anesthesia with the regular laboratory respirator. The principle of assisting expiration as a means of preventing respiratory acidosis was conceived and incorporated in an apparatus in which suction produced by a Venturi jet was used to rapidly evacuate the tidal gas during expiration.[16–18] The use of negative pressure completely corrected the problem of acidosis. With this new device it was possible to supersaturate arterial blood with oxygen using only room air. In addition, the partial pressure of carbon dioxide in the circulating blood was reduced to the point where the animal would remain apneic for a number of minutes following discontinuance of artificial respiration. This principle was subsequently incorporated into a ventilator known as the "Jefferson Ventilator."

The ultimate goal of this research was to obtain a bloodless cardiac chamber as a means of performing precise surgical operations within the heart while the cardiorespiratory function was maintained by the device. Accordingly, cardiac defects were next made within the interatrial and interventricular septa of dogs and repaired while the cardiorespiratory function was maintained by the heart-lung machine.[18,19] During the first bypass

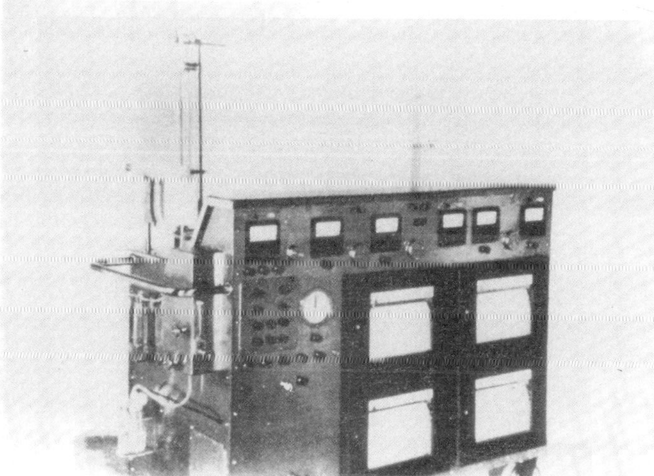

FIG. 33-14a. Front view of the second International Business Machines heart-lung machine used by Dr. Gibbon for repair of an interatrial septal defect in 1953.

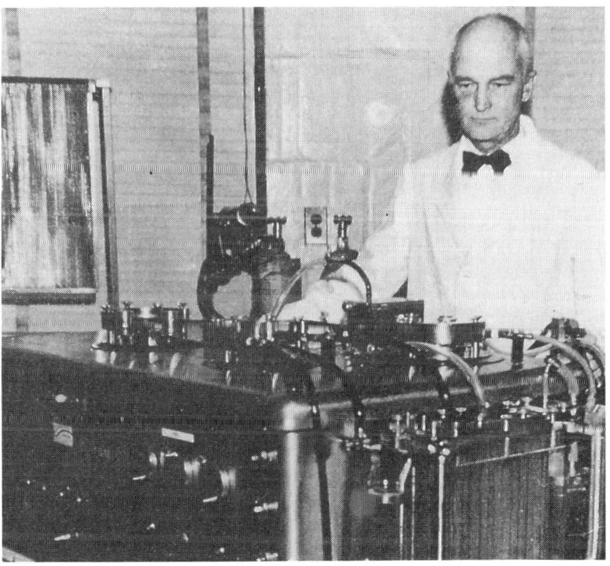

FIG. 33-14b. Dr. John H. Gibbon, Jr. with his successful heart-lung machine of 1953.

and open cardiotomy in an experimental animal the magnitude of cardiac venous blood returning to the right atrium was not fully anticipated. The large volume of blood could not be coped with, and the experiment failed because of uncontrolled blood loss. An additional unforeseen complication also became apparent when experimental interatrial septal defects were produced during bypass. Air entering the left atrium as soon as the interatrial septal defect was produced was trapped beneath the mitral leaflets, and since the heart was still beating, the left ventricle pumped the air into the systemic circulation with resulting embolization to the coronary circulation and other systemic arteries. This was indeed a profound complication, but the solution proved to be simple. A tigon tube was introduced into the left ventricle through a small ventriculotomy at the apex and secured with a purse-string suture.[20] A low-resistance pathway was then provided for the escape of air from the contracting left ventricle with the use of mild suction. A special collecting apparatus was conceived. This collecting chamber received both returning venous blood from the open right atrium and the blood and air aspirated by the left ventricular catheter. Because air was always mixed with the blood, the bubbles were dissipated by the gradual descent of the blood film onto the inner surface of a tall cylinder. In addition, the negative pressure assisted in the dissipation of bubbles. As this blood accumulated in a pool at the bottom of the collecting chamber, the position of the blood level was then sensed by the same variable capacitor circuit used to control the arterial pump. This circuit then energized an additional pump that returned both the cardiac venous blood and the left ventricular blood to the extracorporeal circuit with minimal loss.

Interatrial septal defects produced in dogs under direct vision during total bypass were repaired by a pericardial patch. In some situations the patch was introduced into the right atrium by a stab wound in its mesial wall and remained connected to its base with the aim of providing circulatory support to the graft. In another group of animals, interventricular septal defects were produced during open ventriculotomy and repaired by suture or patch. Because the venous pumps in this new machine were at heart level, a moderate degree of suction was needed to ensure a maximum flow rate from the vena cava. This resulted in frequent occlusions of the cannula at near maximal flow rate. To correct this problem, a further modification was made using low negative pressure. Caval blood was directed into a separate collecting chamber similar to the one used for the collection of cardiac venous blood. Its level was again sensed by a similar circuit, and from there the circuit was as before (Figure 33-16).

In order to initiate total bypass it was merely necessary to remove the clamps from the venous and arterial lines and secure the ligatures about the venae cavae, thus diverting cardiac venous return to the extracorporeal circuit. The extracorporeal

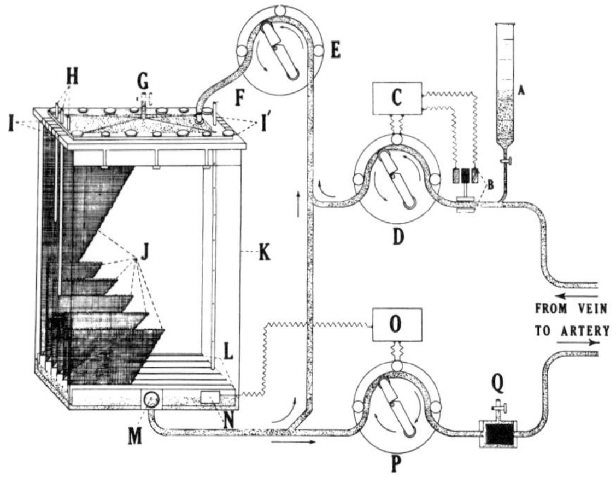

FIG. 33-15. Diagram of extracorporeal blood circuit of the basic 1951 heart-lung machine constructed by International Business Machines Corporation.

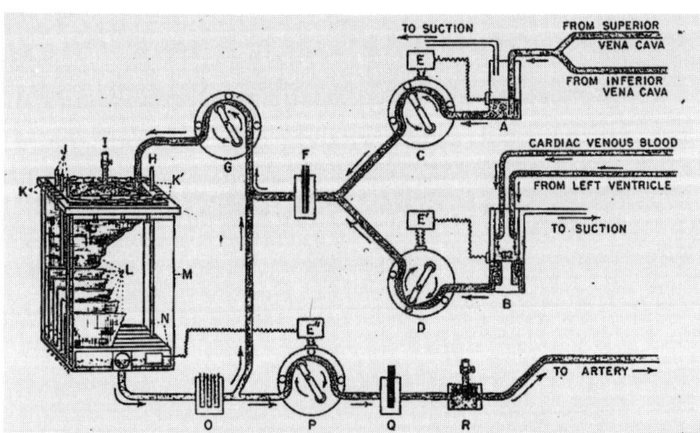

FIG. 33-16. Circuit of the modified 1951 heart-lung machine containing an additional circuit for receiving cardiac venous blood and air from the left ventricle during bypass.

circuit then functioned automatically by continually sensing the flow rate of the diverted venous blood. An occasional adjustment of the negative pressure in the collecting chambers was all that was usually required to maintain ideal perfusion conditions.

A large and successful experimental experience had been achieved by this time. Oxygenation with the new oxygenator was sufficient for a human patient of average size, and all controls functioned optimally (Figures 33-17a and b). There was every indication that the next phase, use of the apparatus in operations on humans, would also be successful. Two children failed to survive for reasons other than failure of the perfusion. Finally, in May of 1953, the first open cardiotomy in a human patient for the repair of an interatrial septal defect was performed by Dr. John H. Gibbon, Jr., assisted by Drs. Frank F. Allbritten, Jr. and Bernard J. Miller. The heart-lung machine was transported from the laboratory on the eighth floor of the College to the hospital operating room (the fourth floor of 1907 "Old Main") along with the newly conceived laboratory device used for collecting both the cardiac venous blood and the blood from the left ventricular vent. After this first successful perfusion of a human, other applications of extracorporeal circuits soon became apparent.

In accord with a long-held interest in anatomy, Dr. Miller joined the staff of the Daniel Baugh Institute, under the Chairmanship of Dr. George Bennett, also Dean of the College. He initiated and maintained an active research program in the Anatomy Department and also developed a private general surgical practice. Miller continued his interest in the further development of extracorporeal circuits and engaged in tumor research; he was a pioneer in the use of a heart-lung machine for segmental perfusion as a method of chemotherapy for inoperable malignant tumors.[21] He designed a completely automatic extracorporeal circuit embodying a single pump and the first hyperbaric oxygenator for this purpose.[22] With this device he was among the first to treat malignant tumors of the extremities, particularly melanomas and sarcomas, by segmental perfusion with the Russian drug sarcolysin[23] and alkylating agents. Miller's work in instrumentation and electronics resulted in five patents.

Dr. Miller was Research Associate to Dr. Gibbon from 1950 to the end of 1954, Chief of Cardiopulmonary Surgery at the St. Mary Franciscan Hospital in Philadelphia from 1951 through 1974, Surgical Consultant to the Philadelphia Naval Hospital from 1971 to 1975, and Chief of the "B" Surgical Service of the Germantown Hospital and Medical Center from 1962 to 1983. He attained the position of Professor of Anatomy at the Daniel Baugh Institute and

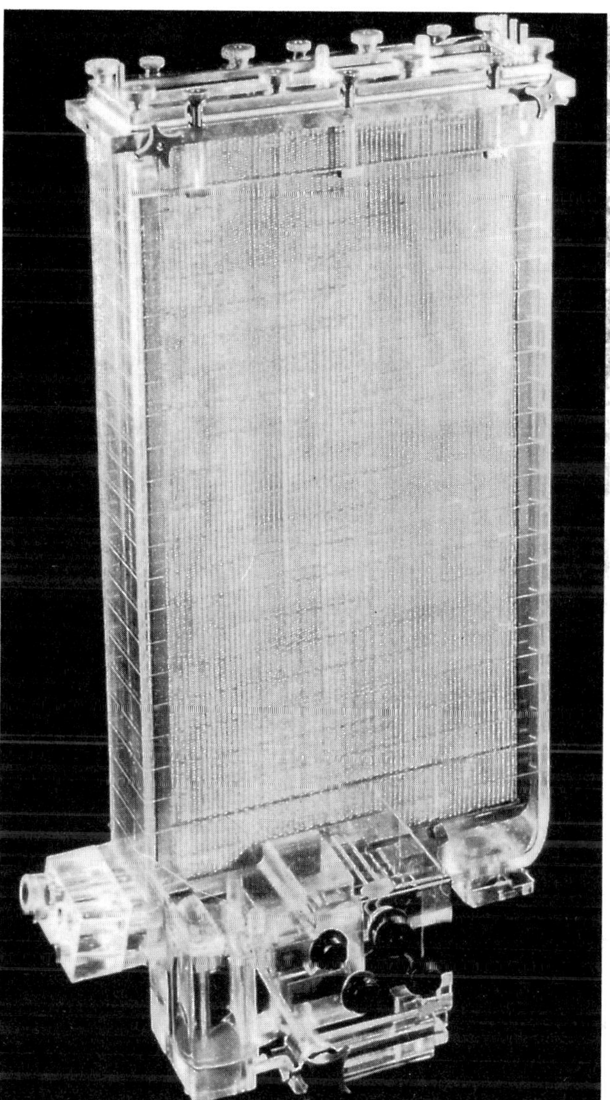

FIG. 33-17a. Enlarged version of the screen oxygenator suitable for human perfusion.

Associate Professor of Surgery. In addition to activity in many local and national societies, Miller was the recipient of the Sheeham Gold Medal in Surgery at his Jefferson graduation, the Samuel D. Gross Distinguished Service Award, and an Honorary Degree of Doctor of Science by his undergraduate alma mater, Villanova University, in 1982.

Frank F. Allbritten, Jr. was an example of Dr. Gibbon's influence on the academic careers of young men. He had graduated from the University of Pennsylvania Medical School in 1939 and served as Intern in the Hospital of the University of Pennsylvania in 1940. After a surgical residency under Dr. Flick at the Pennsylvania Hospital from 1940 to 1943, Allbritten entered the Armed Services during World War II. Upon discharge he assumed the position of Associate to Dr. Gibbon and was also appointed Chief of the Thoracic Surgical Service at the Barton Memorial Division of Jefferson Hospital. His major effort was in clinical thoracic surgery, but he also maintained a peripheral interest in research. With Dr. George Haupt, a Resident at that time, he participated in the investigation of expiratory assistance as a means of improving ventilation and avoiding respiratory acidosis during anesthesia. He made clinical contributions to the treatment of carcinoma of the esophagus, the cardiac end of the stomach, and the lung. In association with Drs. Miller and Gibbon he was involved in studies concerning blood volume loss and extracellular fluid loss during open thoractomy. Allbritten assisted Dr. Gibbon in the historic first open heart operation.

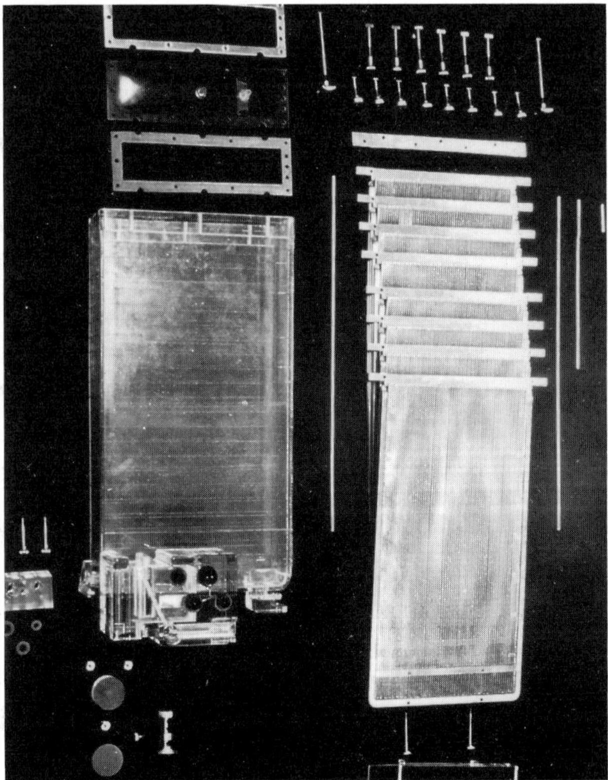

FIG. 33-17b. Components of the adult screen oxygenator.

Dr. Allbritten relinquished his position of Associate Professor of Surgery and Research Assistant at Jefferson to become Professor of Surgery and Chairman of the Department of Surgery at the University of Kansas. There he continued his interest in pulmonary physiology and made additional contributions in general surgery and open heart surgery using both hypothermia and cardiopulmonary bypass. He also served on the editorial board of the *Annals of Surgery*.

John J. DeTuerk (Jefferson, 1938) completed his internship at Jefferson (1940), and began his surgical training as the second Resident on the service of Dr. Thomas A. Shallow (the first Resident was Dr. Ned T. Raker, Jefferson, 1935, who started in July 1939). After serving only one year, he was called from the reserves to active duty (1941) at Camp Lee, Virginia, attached to the Jefferson Unit of the 38th General Hospital. In the summer of 1942 the Jefferson Unit was transferred from Texas to the Middle East near Cairo, Egypt, called "Kilo 13" because it was 13 km. outside of Cairo. He served in the North African theater until 1946. On returning to Jefferson he served for a few months as the last Resident of Dr. George P. Muller. The first Resident on the Muller service had been Dr. James O'Neill (Jefferson, 1936), who started in tandem with Raker in 1939. Dr. John H. Gibbon, Jr., arrived later in 1946, and DeTuerk completed his training (1948) as Gibbon's first Resident. He then entered private practice at both Jefferson and Methodist Hospitals and joined Dr. George Willauer as an Associate. Both men conducted a very active thoracic and general surgical practice. DeTuerk contributed a number of papers to clinical thoracic surgery with

Willauer. He became Chief of Surgery at Methodist Hospital in 1962, occupying this position until 1977. He was President of the Medical Staff and a Trustee at Methodist. The "Annual John J. DeTuerk Lectureship in Surgery" was established at Methodist in 1979.

The major thrust in the establishment of clinical cardiac surgery at Jefferson was the result of the pioneering efforts of Dr. John Young Templeton, III (Figure 33-18), who also was the first resident to work with Dr. Gibbon in the laboratory at Jefferson. He graduated from Jefferson in 1941 and served his internship at Jefferson Hospital. Following service in the Armed Forces, he took his residency under Dr. Gibbon at Jefferson in 1946 and was appointed to the faculty in 1950. While a Fellow of the American Cancer Society and also the Damon Runyon Society, Templeton's major effort was first in surgical research, followed by an outstanding clinical career. As a prolific writer he published more than 80 articles on a wide spectrum of topics related to the heart, lungs, blood vessels, gastrointestinal tract, hypothermia (Figure 33-19), metabolism, and human resuscitation. Among the Residents who assisted him in his investigations were Benjamin Bacharach, George J. Haupt, John Prehatny, John J. McKeown, Jr., Thomas F. Nealon, Jr., Rudolph C. Camishion, Louis Pierucci, and Stanton N. Smullens. His major interest became cardiac surgery, and he worked closely with Dr. Gibbon in the first open heart operations.

With Drs. Bacharach and Smullens, Dr. Templeton continued an active clinical program at the Henry R. Landis Tuberculosis Hospital in Philadelphia, which was a state-operated center for the surgical treatment of this disease. Board certified in thoracic as well as general surgery, he rose in the teaching ranks at Jefferson from Instructor in 1950 to Clinical Professor in 1957. In 1964 he transferred to the University of Pennsylvania as Professor of Surgery and Chief of

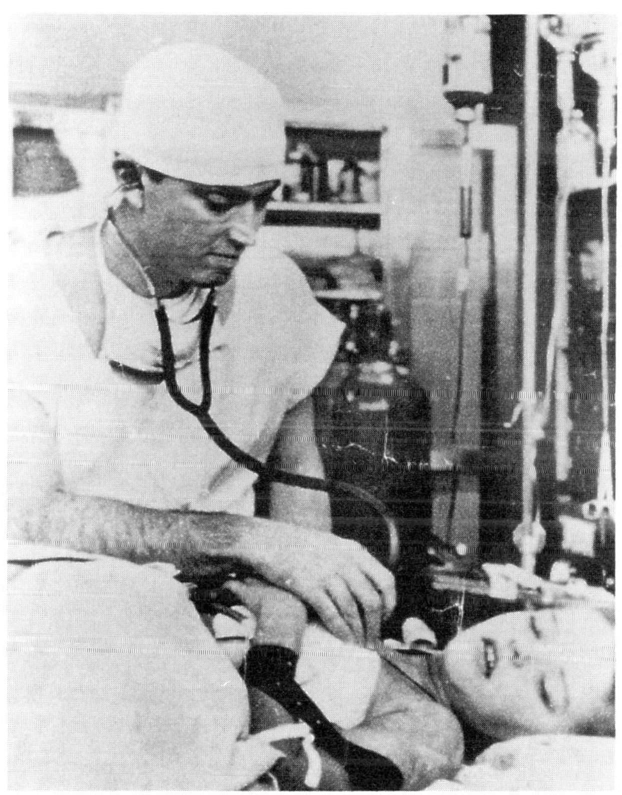

FIG. 33-18. John Y. Templeton, III, M.D., Sc.D., LL.D., a pioneer in open heart surgery.

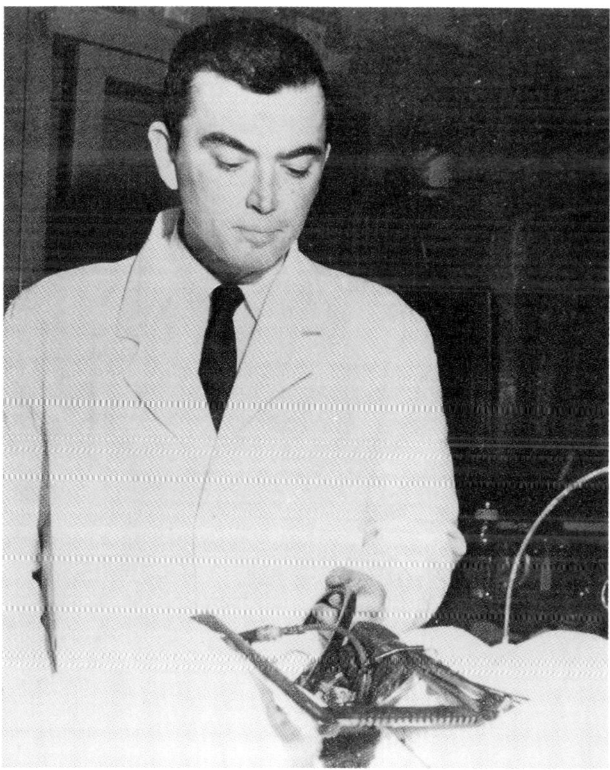

FIG. 33-19. John Y. Templeton, III, M.D., Sc.D., LL.D., examines catheters being used to pump blood to the heat exchanger in a hypothermia experiment.

Surgery at the Pennsylvania Hospital. Templeton's clinical success outside of Jefferson along with his research achievements led to his appointment as the Samuel D. Gross Professor and Chairman of the Department in 1967, as the successor to Dr. Gibbon, who had taken an early retirement. His name was engraved on the fourth plate of the gold-headed cane given to Dr. John Chalmers DaCosta by the Jefferson Class of 1926. In the full bloom of a successful Chairmanship he resigned for personal reasons in January, 1969, and remained as Professor of Surgery.

Dr. Templeton belonged to more than 50 local, national, and international societies and served on the board of governors or as committee chairman in 14 of these. He became President of the Laennec Society, Pennsylvania Association for Thoracic Surgery, Philadelphia Academy of Surgery, Philadelphia County Medical Society, Pennsylvania State Medical Society, and Meigs Medical Association. At Jefferson he served as President of the Medical Staff and the Alumni Association. In 1977 he received the unique award of the "Golden Scalpel" from the Division of Cardiothoracic Surgery, and in 1980 the first Templeton Lecture, established by Dr. and Mrs. Benjamin Bacharach, was given by internationally known Dr. Denton A. Cooley, Surgeon-in-Chief and founder of the Texas Heart Institute. In the same year Templeton's portrait was presented to the College. He received the Jefferson Alumni Achievement Award in 1981. With unanimous respect of his colleagues, he has been idolized by residents, admired by students, and revered by his nursing and technical aides, and has been regarded as "a legend in his own time."

William Wallace Lumpkin Glenn (Jefferson, 1938) completed his internship at the Pennsylvania Hospital in 1940. He was a surgical resident at the Massachusetts General Hospital from 1940 to 1943 and again from 1945 to 1946. A major part of the first period of his residency was spent in the Department of Physiology under the direction of Dr. Cecil Kent Drinker. He was an Associate in Surgery at Jefferson from 1946 to 1948, working exclusively in the research laboratory. He next became associated with Yale University, where he eventually achieved the rank of Professor of Surgery. During the following 30 years at Yale he made many significant contributions in experimental thoracic surgery. His areas of interest encompassed the lymphatic system, the treatment of congenital and acquired heart disease, the use of cardiac prostheses, and the application of phrenic stimulation for the maintenance of respiration. He was the principal author of two texts in thoracic surgery and the chapter on "Cardiac Pacemakers and Heart Block" in Gibbon's *Surgery of the Chest* and received the Jefferson Alumni Achievement Award in 1973.

Joseph W. Stayman, Jr., (Jefferson, 1942) served his internship (1942–1943) and general surgical residency (1943–1945) at Germantown Hospital. He took his Fellowship in thoracic surgery at Jefferson from 1947 to 1948. After appointment as Dr. Gibbon's Associate for the following year he joined the surgical service of the Germantown Hospital in 1949. He played an important role in the teaching of Jefferson surgical residents who were assigned to the Germantown Hospital at that time. After terminating his association with Germantown in 1960 he became Chief of Surgery at the Chestnut Hill Hospital (which became affiliated with Jefferson in 1974) until the time of his retirement in 1980. His teaching was deeply appreciated by the surgical residents on rotation from Jefferson, where he achieved the position of Clinical Professor of Surgery and subsequent Emeritus status.

John J. McKeown, Jr., (Jefferson, 1947) served his internship and a part of his surgical residency at Jefferson Hospital until 1950. Following a period of service with the U.S. Armed Forces (1950–1952) he returned to Jefferson to complete his training (1954). He became Research Associate for experimental and clinical application of extracorporeal circulation in the surgical treatment of congenital and acquired heart disease (1954–1959). A number of his papers dealt with diseases of the chest, the treatment of postinfarction ventricular aneurysm, and studies of the vertical screen oxygenator. He became Consulting Thoracic Surgeon to the Henry R. Landis State Tuberculosis Sanatorium and Attending Surgeon and eventually Chairman of the Department of Surgery of Misericordia Hospital and the Mercy Catholic Medical Center (Figure 33-20). A member of numerous prestigious societies, he attained the rank of Clinical Professor of Surgery at Jefferson (1979).

Robert K. Finley, Jr., (Jefferson, 1948) served his internship at the Lankenau Hospital and obtained his surgical training at Jefferson (1954). He entered the armed services and became Chief of the Department of Surgery in the United States Navy at the submarine base in New London, Connecticut. He then entered private practice in Dayton, Ohio, where he remained. His interests centered mostly about the treatment of severe burns, in which he was among the first to describe their early excision. He was also interested in percutaneous transhepatic cholangiography and published a number of articles on this subject. In addition to appointment as Co-Director of Education and of the Burn Unit at the Miami Valley Hospital, he was appointed Clinical Professor of Surgery at Wright State University School of Medicine.

George J. Haupt (Jefferson, 1948) returned to Jefferson in 1952 as a Resident in surgery, following service in the Armed Forces. He studied respiratory acidosis during anesthesia with Frank Allbritten and developed a mechanical respirator employing the principle of expiratory assistance (Figure 33-21). The patent obtained by him was awarded to Jefferson Medical College. He subsequently became associated with Lankenau Hospital as Chief of Cardiothoracic Surgery and

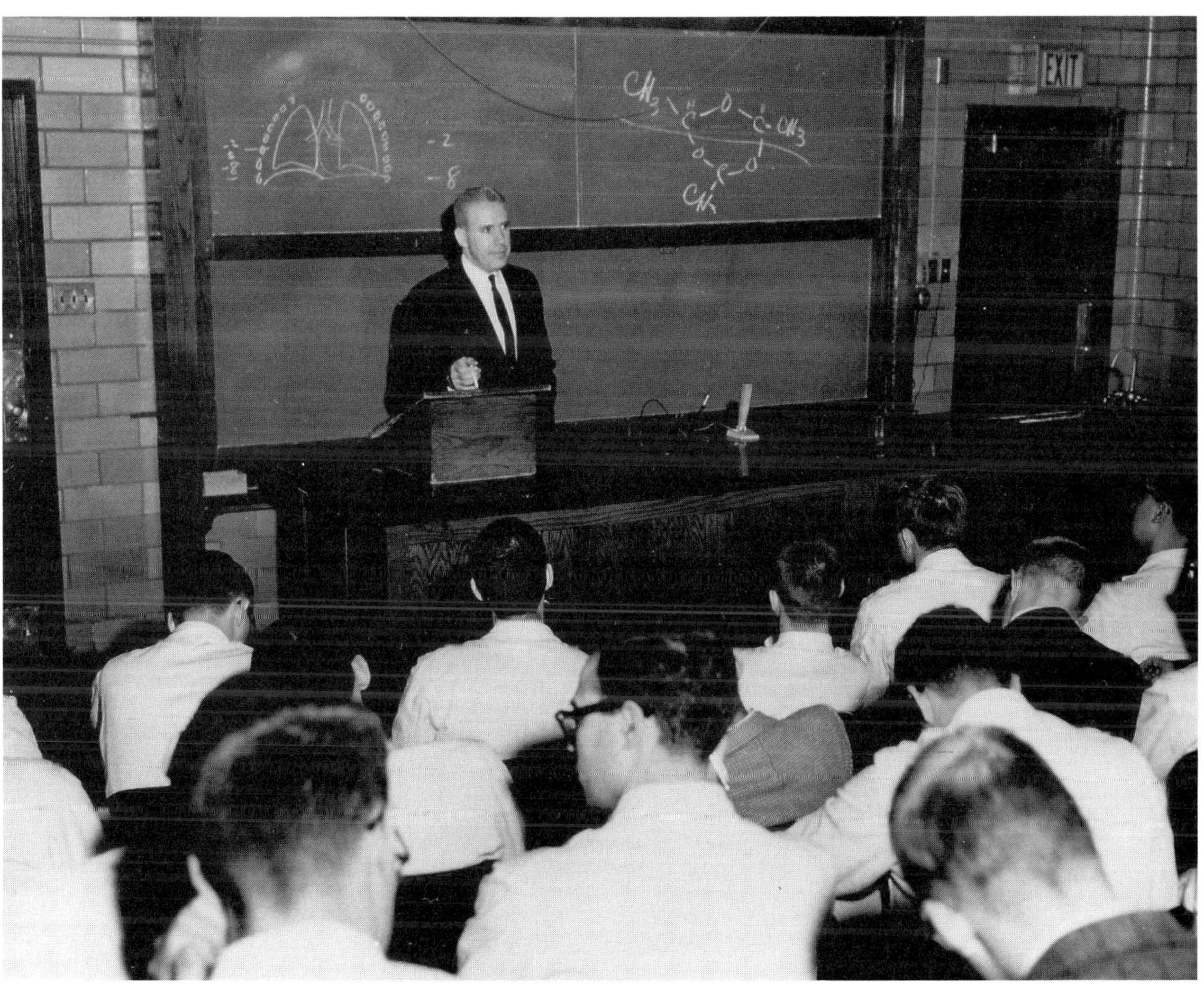

FIG. 33-20. John J. McKeown, Jr., M.D., lectures in the College Auditorium (named The Herbut Auditorium in 1979).

achieved the position of Clinical Professor of Surgery at Jefferson in 1977. At Lankenau Hospital he developed a clinical program in cardiothoracic surgery and became an active investigator in the Lankenau Medical Research Center. Dr. Haupt's contributions to the literature were numerous and of broad scope, including studies of respiratory physiology, especially as they pertained to aerospace science during the 1960s and early 1970s. His widespread activity in cardiothoracic and allied societies paralleled his clinical and research interests.

Harold C. Cohn (Jefferson, 1948) served his internship at St. Joseph's Hospital in Reading and received his surgical training at Jefferson. He participated actively in the laboratory during the period of design and testing of the first successful heart-lung machine. Following the completion of his residency, Cohn returned to Reading and served as a Director of the Vascular Laboratory at the Community General Hospital, of the Vascular Laboratory at the Reading Hospital, and also the Vascular Laboratory at St. Joseph's Hospital. This active practice included bypass grafting for lower-extremity ischemia, treatment of cardiac shock with intraaortic balloon pumping, and wide experience in carotid endarterectomy.

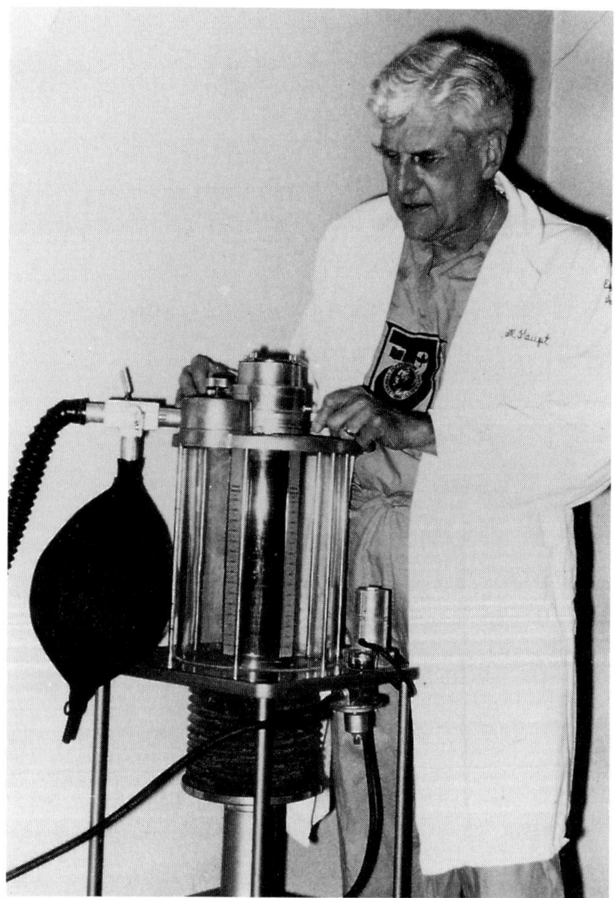

FIG. 33-21. George J. Haupt, M.D., with the "Jefferson Ventilator" employing the principle of expiratory assistance.

Robert G. Johnson (Jefferson, 1949) served his internship and residency at Jefferson. He then continued as a Fellow in Cardiac Surgery and Fellow in Cancer Surgery until 1955. Before coming to Jefferson, Dr. Johnson had a distinguished World War II record in the Armed Forces Second Armored Division under General Patton. He received the Bronze Star, Individual Commendation Award, Purple Heart, Combat Infantry Badge, Presidential Citation, American Defense Medal, ETO medal (five campaigns), Bronze Arrowhead (two campaigns) for invasion landing, Victory Medal, and the Croix de Guerre.

At Jefferson, Dr. Johnson became a Clinical Assistant Professor of Surgery and contributed articles in the field of general surgery. He was among the first to utilize hypothermia in open cardiotomy for the treatment of congenital anomalies of children. He was Chief of the Surgical Outpatient Department at Jefferson and Consultant in Thoracic Surgery at the Methodist Hospital, Veterans Hospital, and Eagleville Tuberculosis Sanatorium. He relocated in Las Vegas, Nevada, in 1971 and pursued private practice.

Thomas F. Nealon, Jr., (Jefferson, S1944) served in the U.S. Naval Hospital and entered Jefferson's surgical residency training program in 1950. He participated in one of the major ongoing problems at that time, namely studies of pulmonary ventilation during anesthesia with the use of expiratory assistance and its effects on cardiac output, the carbon dioxide content, and the saturation of arterial and venous blood with oxygen (Figure 33-22). Following the completion of his residency, Nealon continued an active research program together with clinical surgery and student teaching. He ascended rapidly in academic rank and by 1963 achieved the position of Professor of Surgery. He was appointed Director of Surgery at St. Vincent's Hospital in

New York City and Professor of Surgery at the New York University School of Medicine in 1968. In addition to numerous articles, Dr. Nealon contributed the chapter on "Trauma to the Chest" in Dr. Gibbon's *Surgery of the Chest* and was coauthor with Dr. Gibbon of the chapter on "Neoplasms of the Lungs and Trachea." He was the sole author of *Fundamental Skills in Surgery,* which appeared in 1963 and reached a third edition in 1979, and of *Management of the Patient with Cancer* in 1965, with a third edition in 1986. Along with membership in a host of societies he served as President of the New York Surgical Society and Alumni Trustee on the Board of Jefferson.

One of the outstanding residents serving his period in research training in the laboratory during the early part of this period was Dr. Charles Fineberg (Figure 33-23). He had graduated from Hahnemann Medical College in 1950 and completed his surgical residency at Jefferson in 1955. In addition to work with the extracorporeal circuit, he assisted with studies of the newly designed ventilator, experimental perfusion techniques, and studies of partial perfusion in subjects with experimentally induced pulmonary edema. Following the completion of his residency, he became a member of the Jefferson Hospital staff and the faculty of the College. He also continued active research embracing such projects as experimental myocardial revascularization and various clinical entities in general surgery.

Dr. Fineberg rose through the academic ranks to Professor of Surgery. Among activities in many local and national societies he was Chairman of the Surgical Advisory Committee of the American College of Surgeons, Chairman of the Executive Cancer Committee of Jefferson Hospital, and Director of Thoracic and Vascular Surgery at the Daroff Division of Albert Einstein Medical Center of Philadelphia. His portrait was presented to the College in 1983.

Dr. Anthony R. C. Dobell came to Jefferson in 1952 as Resident in thoracic surgery, after

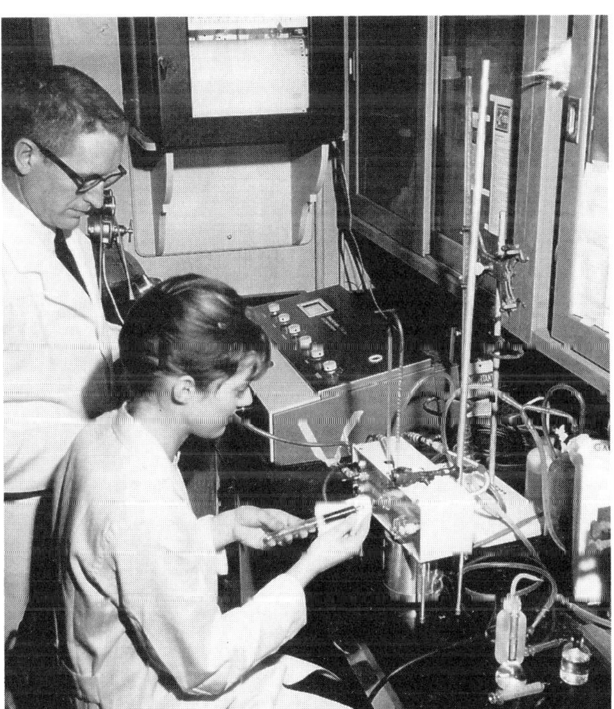

FIG. 33-22. Thomas F. Nealon, Jr., M.D., watches a laboratory technician inject a blood sample into a gas chromatograph that measures concentration of gases.

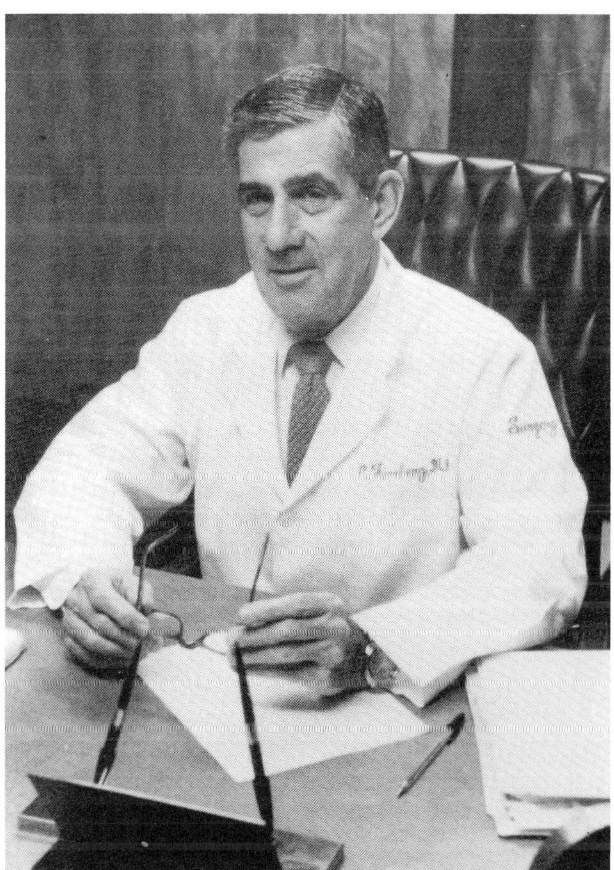

FIG. 33-23. Charles Fineberg, M.D., Professor of Surgery, researcher, and effective teacher.

graduating from McGill University in 1951, and he, too, was among the outstanding group assigned to the heart-lung laboratory. Following the completion of his residency in 1956, he returned to McGill. There he ascended to the position of Professor of Surgery in 1971 and to Director of the Division of Cardiovascular Surgery in 1973. In addition to an active clinical practice in cardiothoracic surgery, he made important contributions to the literature, further advancing the horizons of cardiac surgery, particularly in the treatment of congenital heart disease and in experimental cardiac surgery. He contributed to surgical techniques, studies of heart preservation, and extracorporeal circuits.

Dr. Dobell was appointed to the Montreal Children's Hospital in 1957 and achieved the position of Director of the Cardiovascular Surgical Service in 1968. In 1974 he became Surgeon-in-Chief of the Royal Victoria Hospital. In addition, he served as Senior Surgeon at the Montreal General Hospital and occupied honorary positions at the Santa Cabrini Hospital, the Queen Elizabeth Hospital in Montreal, and the Montreal Chest Hospital Center. He became active in the important cardiothoracic societies of both Canada and the United States.

Jose H. Amadeo (Jefferson, 1952) completed his surgical training at Jefferson, during which time he participated in many of the ongoing problems in the laboratory. In cooperation with members of the surgical staff he published studies of pulmonary ventilation produced by aiding the deflation phase of respiration during anesthesia, the use of a retrosternal route in the placement of the ascending colon for esophageal substitution, the management of spontaneous pneumothorax, and the results of mitral valvulotomy for mitral stenosis.

Amadeo returned to the University of Puerto Rico, where he was involved in studies of infusion chemotherapy for advanced malignancy of the head and neck and the use of adjuvant chemotherapy for the management of carcinoma of the stomach. This led to his appointment as Professor of Surgery and Co-Chairman in the School of Medicine.

Dr. Nicholas Gimbel joined the Department as a Visiting Fellow in May 1953. He had been involved in the development of experimental cardiac surgery and extracorporeal perfusion at the Hospital of the University of Pennsylvania. He subsequently became associated with Wayne University as Professor of Surgery.

Dr. Hans Engel (Figure 33-24) was a Rockefeller Research Associate who came to the surgical laboratory at Jefferson during the period of 1953–1954 when the heart-lung machine was first successfully used on a human being. Dr. Engel had been involved in cardiovascular surgery with Professor Erik Hisbid, the founder of cardiac surgery in Denmark. Following his stay at Jefferson and upon returning to Denmark, Engle participated in the development of the first heart-lung machine in Denmark, where it was used in open heart surgery. He was a member of that operating team and was coauthor of the first published report of the Danish machine in the same year. He became a prominent vascular surgeon in Denmark, founded the Danish Society of Vascular Surgery, and achieved the position of Professor of Surgery at the University of Copenhagen. During Dr. Engel's stay at Jefferson, Dr. Gibbon had provided him with a set of drawings of the heart-lung machine that had been used successfully in the first human case. These plans were subsequently used when a replica of that machine was made in 1982 for permanent display in the College of Physicians of Philadelphia (Figure 33-24).

Rudolph C. Camishion (Jefferson, 1954) served his internship at the Cooper Hospital in Camden, New Jersey, and completed his surgical residency at Jefferson in 1959. He was a National Cancer Institute Fellow until 1962. As a surgical Resident he, too, was assigned to the surgical research laboratory (Figure 33-25), and he investigated myocardial revascularization and methods of inducing hypothermia. After completion of his residency Camishion made important contributions either as a principal investigator or in association with others in studies of carcinoma of the esophagus, use of talc poudrage as a method of controlling malignant pleural effusion, postoperative atelectasis, hydrodynamics of extracorporeal circulation, the technique of cardiopulmonary bypass, and the use of valve prostheses. He rose in the academic ranks at Jefferson to full Professor.

In 1978 Dr. Camishion was appointed Professor

and Head of the Department of Surgery of the University of Medicine and Dentistry of New Jersey, Rutgers Medical School in Camden. In addition to awards and honors, he was active in the local and national societies of his field, including founder membership of the Delaware Valley Vascular Society and the Vascular Society of New Jersey.

Herbert E. Cohn (Jefferson, 1955) served his internship at the Atlantic City Hospital and entered the residency program at Jefferson in 1957 (Figure 33-10). He was appointed to the faculty of Jefferson and to the staff of Albert Einstein, Northern Division. His research experience was related to the various aspects of surgical endocrinology and renal transplantation at Jefferson. His surgical practice emphasized pulmonary disease and the endocrine system. Dr. Cohn achieved the positions of Professor of Surgery, Director of the Residency Training Program, and Vice-Chairman of the Department. He was elected President of the staff of Thomas Jefferson University in 1985.

Louis Pierucci (Jefferson, 1955) served his internship and early residency in the Department of Surgery until 1957. Following a period of duty with the armed forces he completed his residency in 1962. He participated in clinical surgery at Jefferson and continued an active experimental program. In association with Drs. Templeton, Ballinger, and Camishion, he studied experimental profound hypothermia, anaerobic metabolism and metabolic acidosis during cardiopulmonary bypass, the acidosis of hypothermia, and methods of removal of excess lactate in patients during hypothermia and biventricular bypass.

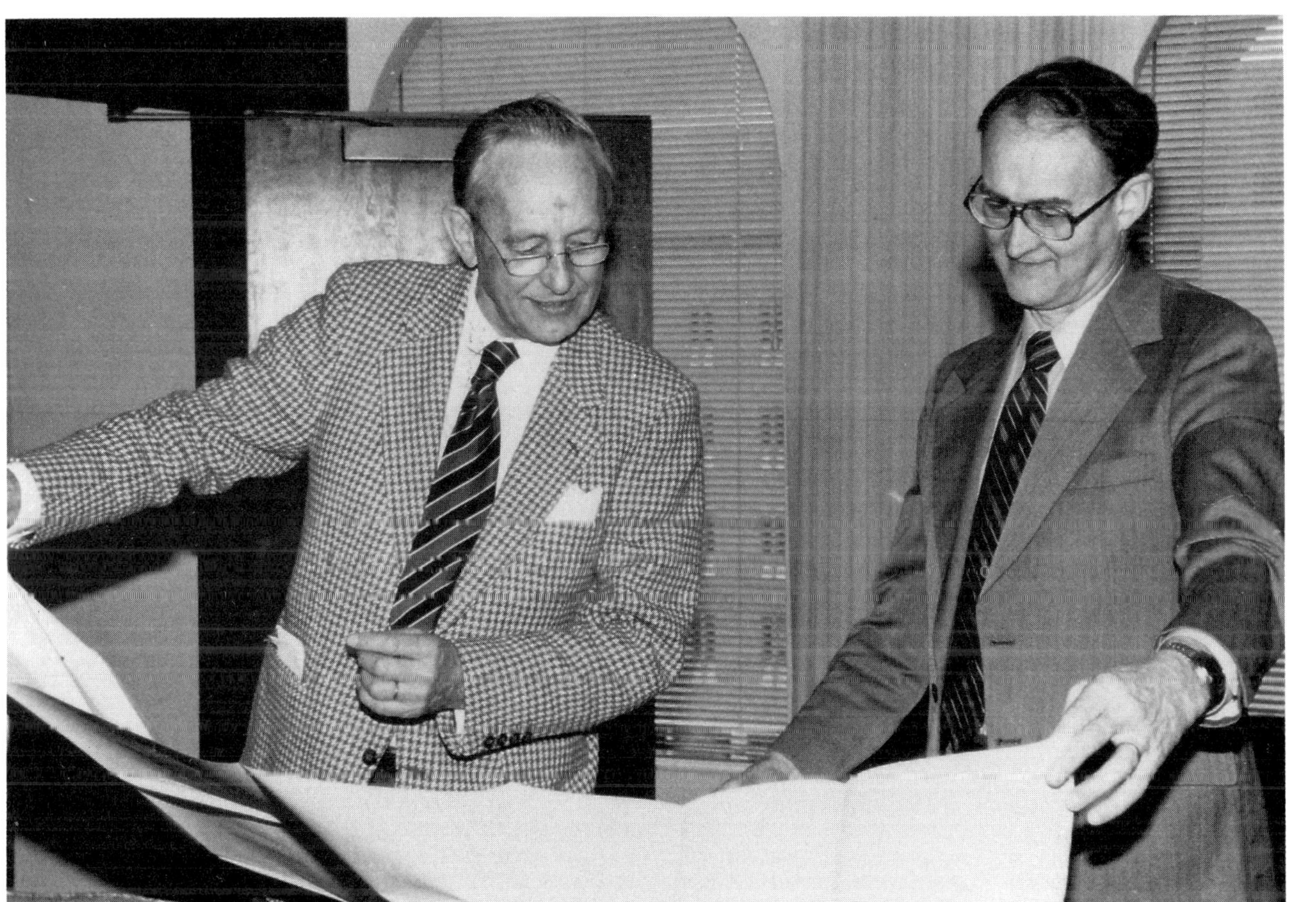

FIG. 33-24. Hans Engel, M.D., with President Lewis W. Bluemle, Jr., in 1982, reviewing plans for a replica of the first successful heart-lung machine, to be on permanent display at the College of Physicians of Philadelphia.

In 1968, Pierucci became the Chief Attending Surgeon of the Cooper Hospital University Medical Center in Camden, New Jersey, and in addition continued an active surgical practice. His interests centered in vascular surgery, of which he made numerous observations concerning the surgical treatment of carotid and vertebral artery insufficiency. He remained an Associate Professor of Surgery at Jefferson while practicing at the Cooper Hospital University Medical Center and other New Jersey Hospitals.

Edward D. McLaughlin (Jefferson, 1956) interned at Jefferson and became a surgery resident at the National Institutes of Health in Bethesda (1957–1959). When at Bethesda he identified a fraction in human blood that appeared to inhibit growth of malignant experimental tumors and received a number of awards for this particular work. He completed his residency training at Jefferson. After an additional six months in England in the Department of Thoracic Surgery at the Hawkmoor Chest Hospital, Bovey Tracey, Devon, he associated with Mercy Catholic Medical Center, Misericordia Division, in Philadelphia as Chairman of Surgery. At Jefferson he ascended the academic ranks to become Professor of Surgery. In 1974 he received the Christian R. and Mary F. Lindbach Award for Distinguished Teaching.

Benjamin Bacharach (Jefferson, 1956) received

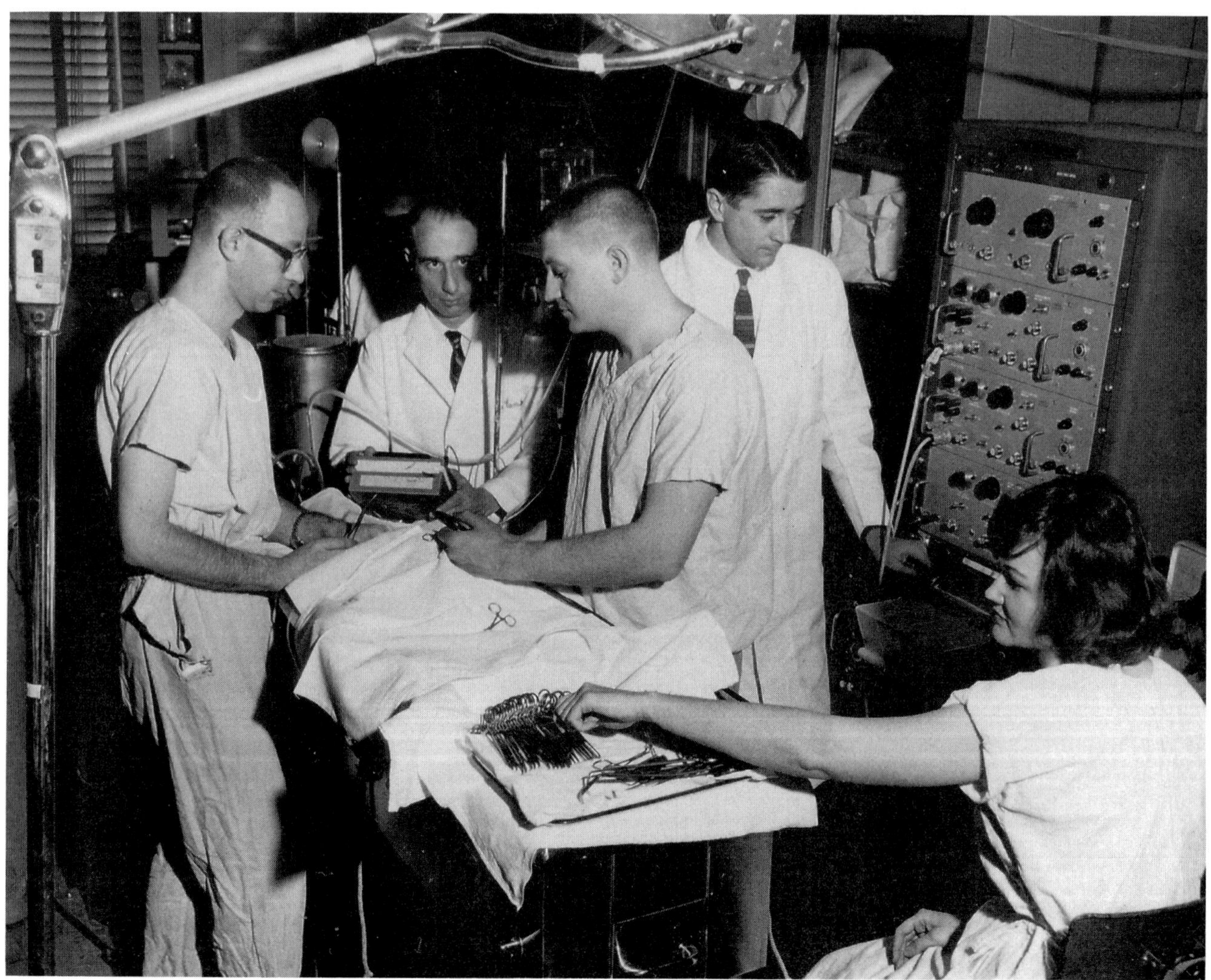

FIG. 33-25. Drs. Leon Scicchitano, Rudolph Camishion, Edward J. Baranski, and Walter Ballinger, with a laboratory technician, studying the effect of the denervation of a lung.

his surgical training at Jefferson (1958–1963) and became a Fellow in cardiothoracic surgery at the Pennsylvania Hospital (1963–1964), following which he associated with Dr. John Y. Templeton in clinical practice.

During his surgical residency he was assigned to the surgical research laboratory to study various oxygenators and methods for inducing profound hypothermia. He was then appointed to the faculty at Jefferson and Attending Physician to the Jefferson Hospital. In the early years of clinical practice, Dr. Bacharach, in association with Drs. Templeton and John McKeown, was responsible for the thoracic surgical service at the Henry B. Landis Tuberculosis Hospital in Philadelphia and operated on most of the cases of complicated tuberculosis during the period of 1962 to 1965. He made extensive studies relating to the inhalation of carbon dioxide and brain cooling during hypothermia, the techniques of induction of profound hypothermia by biventricular bypass, and bilateral carotid sinus nerve stimulation in the treatment of hypertension, as well as some of the early studies of computerized tomography as a diagnostic aid in bronchogenic carcinoma. Dr. Bacharach was President of the Alumni Association in 1981. In 1983 he was advanced to the rank of Clinical Professor of Surgery and also became Associate Dean for Admissions of Jefferson Medical College (Figure 33-26). The following year he was appointed a Vice-Chairman of the Department of Surgery.

David C. Schechter (Jefferson, 56) interned at Jefferson and then continued in the surgical research laboratory. Following a tour of duty with the Armed Forces, he pursued his residency in general surgery at the University of Colorado Medical Center in Denver. He was a recipient of a Fellowship award for postgraduate study and training under Sir Russell Brock at the Institute for Diseases of the Chest at Brompton Hospital in London and Professor Charles Dubost in Paris at the Hospital Broussais. He then associated with the New York Medical College in the Department of Surgery and gradually ascended the academic ranks to become Clinical Professor of Surgery.

Walter Ballinger (Figure 33-25) graduated from the University of Pennsylvania School of Medicine in 1951 and pursued his surgical training at the first Columbia Surgical Division of the Bellevue Hospital in New York. He next joined the Jefferson faculty in 1956 as Assistant in Surgery and in 1964 became Associate Professor of Surgery. He left Jefferson, associated with the Johns Hopkins University School of Medicine as Associate Professor of Surgery, and then became the Bixby Professor of Surgery and Head of the Department at the Washington University School of Medicine until 1978.

Walter Ballinger's interests centered mostly in vascular and endocrine surgery. During his period at Jefferson he was involved in some of the research projects related to the cardiothoracic program (Figure 33-25). He contributed to a number of papers involving the preservation of blood platelets, hepatic physiology and metabolic

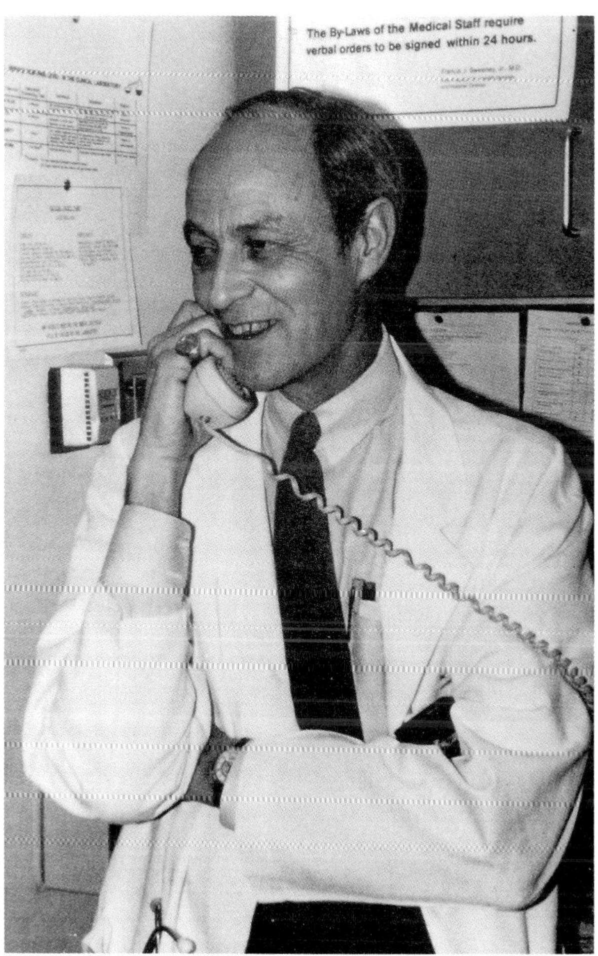

The By-Laws of the Medical Staff require
verbal orders to be signed within 24 hours.
FIG. 33-26. Benjamin Bacharach, M.D., Clinical Professor, Associate Dean for Admissions, and a Vice-Chairman of the Department.

changes during cardiorespiratory bypass, metabolic changes during hypothermia, physiologic changes within the intestine as a result of autotransplantation, methods of small vessel anastomosis, the intestinal effects of vagotomy, and extensive clinical studies of biliary operations and gastric drainage procedures. Dr. Ballinger was named the Markle Scholar in Medical Science from 1961 to 1966 and gave the National Lecture at Sigma Xi. He became concerned with nationwide surgical training programs and served on numerous special committees. In 1971 he was appointed Coeditor-in-chief of *Surgery*. In addition he was Associate Editor of the *Journal of Surgical Research* and also served on the Editorial Board of *Video Surgery*.

John R. Prehatny (Jefferson, 1957) completed his residency training at Jefferson in 1964. He was involved with many of the ongoing problems and participated in a number of studies relating to the oxygen uptake of tissues following profound hypothermia with resulting acidosis, shifts in the partial pressure of carbon dioxide in hypothermia during ventilation with 5% carbon dioxide, the contraindications for the use of biventricular bypass, and the metabolic effects of profound hypothermia and circulatory arrest.

Prehatny became Clinical Professor of Surgery at Jefferson and Chairman of the Department of Surgery of the Methodist Hospital in Philadelphia. Very active in all the affairs of Jefferson, he served as President of the Alumni Association in 1985.

Stanton N. Smullens (Jefferson, 1961), following an internship at the Presbyterian University of Pennsylvania Medical Center in Philadelphia, entered the armed forces for a period of duty. He was Chief of the Outpatient Services, U.S. Army Hospital, Fort Walters, Mineral Wells, Texas. After discharge from the Army, he took his surgical residency at Jefferson in 1964 and in 1965 became a Fellow in cardiothoracic surgery at the Pennsylvania Hospital.

Dr. Smullens associated with Dr. John Y. Templeton and Dr. Benjamin Bacharach in clinical practice. He was appointed Instructor in Surgery at Jefferson and ascended to the position of Associate Professor. He became active in many prestigious societies and was a founding member of the Delaware Valley Vascular Society. His research interests were predominently of a clinical nature. With Dr. Templeton and others, he made studies of the patency of abdominal aortic grafts, describing hypovolemic shock due to massive edema following cardiopulmonary bypass and the surgical management of acute evolving myocardial infarction. His interests centered in the area of vascular surgery, to which he made basic contributions in ultrasonic imaging. He was coinvestigator in the National Institutes of Health contract involved with the assessment of ultrasonic B-scan imaging for detection and quantification of atherosclerotic lesions in the iliofemoral arteries and additional studies concerning prostaglandin (PGE Sub 1) infusion for the treatment of obstructive arterial disease.

Louis F. Plzak, Jr. graduated from the University of Chicago Medical School in 1958. Following his surgical training at the Peter Bent Brigham Hospital, he obtained a pediatric surgical fellowship at the Children's Hospital in Boston. He was appointed the Arthur Cabot Tracy Teaching Fellow at Harvard Medical College. Following two years of military service, he joined the United States Army Medical Research and Development Command within the office of the Surgeon General as Lieutenant Colonel. In this capacity he directed research in shock and trauma and the use of blood and plasma volume expanders. Plzak returned to Harvard in 1970 as Assistant Professor of Surgery in the Department of Cardiothoracic Surgery. In July 1971 he was appointed Professor of Surgery at Jefferson.

Dr. Plzak had an extensive basic research experience beginning during his medical school years in studies related to erythropoiesis and the influence of factor S on red cell production. He published a number of papers during this period and made basic contributions on erythropoietin production. His research interests were next directed toward experimental cardiac surgery, in which he studied the effect of alkalosis on right ventricular hypertrophy in experimentally induced pulmonary hypertension, coronary blood flow and diastolic pressure during prolonged cardiopulmonary bypass, and the amelioration of pulmonary hypertension by metabolic alkalosis. He participated in studies relating to the use of cardiac transplant as a left ventricular assist device.

Dr. Plzak's broad training was evidenced by his versatility in pediatric, general, and cardiothoracic surgery. He belonged to an array of national societies, including charter membership in the American Pediatric Surgical Association. His hospital affiliations, in addition to Jefferson, were at Pennsylvania, the Graduate, and Bryn Mawr.

Division of Cardiothoracic Surgery Established (1973)

Stanley Karl Brockman (Figure 33-27) came to Jefferson in 1973 as Director of the newly created Division of Cardiothoracic Surgery. He had graduated from Boston University School of Medicine in 1955 and was a surgical Resident at the Johns Hopkins Hospital until 1956. He became the Harvey Cushing Fellow in Surgery at Hopkins, followed by an appointment as Senior Assistant Surgeon in the laboratory of cardiovascular physiology in the National Heart Institute at Bethesda until 1959. He completed his surgical training at the Vanderbilt University Hospital in 1963, followed by an immediate appointment as Assistant Professor of Surgery. During 1966–1967 he was on sabbatical leave for a special assignment in clinical cardiac surgery at the Mayo Clinic on the service of Dr. Dwight McGoon. He then became associated with the University of Chicago School of Medicine as Associate Professor of Surgery (1968) and served as Director of the Division of Cardiac and Thoracic Surgery of the Michael Reese Medical Center in Chicago (1968–1973). He rapidly ascended the academic ranks at the University and was appointed Professor of Surgery in 1970.

At Jefferson, Dr. Brockman developed an active clinical program and established the Cardiothoracic Surgical Research Laboratory under the Directorship of J. Yasha Kresh, Ph.D., Research Assistant Professor of Surgery. He made numerous contributions in the areas of experimental open heart surgery with hypothermia, studies of basic physiology of ventricular contraction, the relationship of congestive heart failure and cardiac output in heart block during pacing, valvular replacements, surgical management of cardiogenic shock in acute myocardial infarction, and many studies relating to the use of the pacemaker.

Dr. Brockman promptly commanded respect for his brillance as a teacher and his demands for perfection in the operating room. He sponsored continuing education programs in the form of conferences and symposia with Visiting Professors from the leading cardiothoracic centers of the country. His membership in a host of societies and his training of cardiothoracic fellows further enhanced the reputation of this Division. He resigned from Jefferson in 1986 to direct the cardiothoracic program and service at Hahnemann University.

Richard N. Edie (Figure 33-28) succeeded Dr. Brockman in 1987 as Director of the Division of Cardiothoracic Surgery. He was born in 1937 in Yonkers, New York. After receiving his B.A. degree from Princeton University (1959), he spent

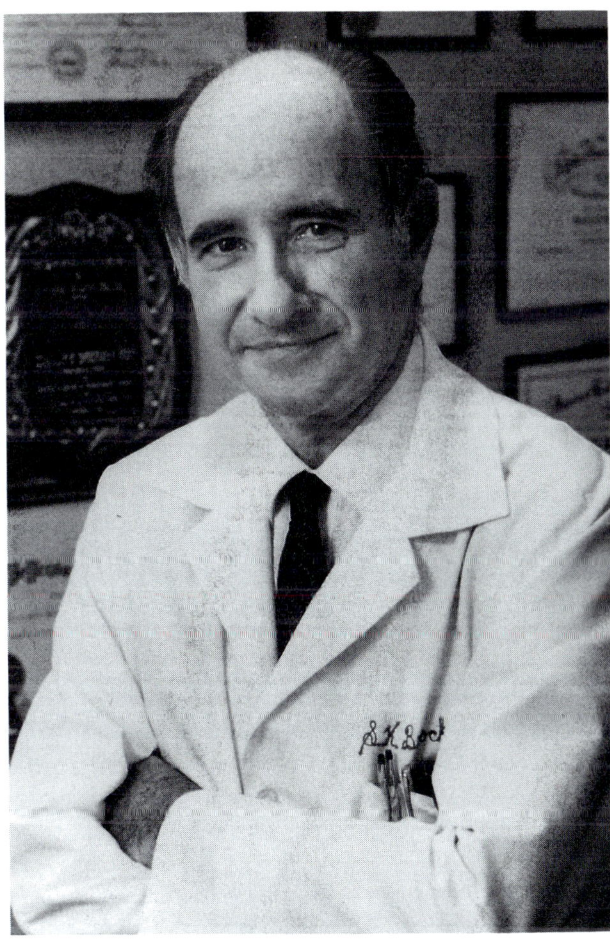

FIG. 33-27. Stanley K. Brockman, M.D., First Director of Division of Cardiothoracic Surgery (1973–1986).

two years in the United States Navy (1959–1961) and earned his M.D. degree at Columbia University College of Physicians and Surgeons (1965), and then interned at Roosevelt Hospital in New York City (1965–1966). He took a residency in General Surgery at the same Hospital (1966–1970) and extended his training at Columbia Presbyterian Medical Center as a resident in Thoracic Surgery (1970–1972). Between 1972 and 1979 he served as Assistant and then Associate Professor of Clinical Surgery in the College of Physicians and Surgeons of Columbia University, while also on the staff of the Presbyterian and the Roosevelt Hospitals. From 1979 to 1987 he was Associate Professor of Surgery at the University of Pennsylvania and on the staff of its Hospital, the Children's Hospital of Philadelphia, and the Presbyterian University of Pennsylvania Medical Center. In 1985 Edie also became an Attending Surgeon at the Pennsylvania Hospital. During this time he had authored or coauthored 34 scientific articles relating to cardiothoracic surgery in the important journals of his field. Certified in general as well as thoracic surgery, he also belonged to the prestigious local and national societies in his specialty.

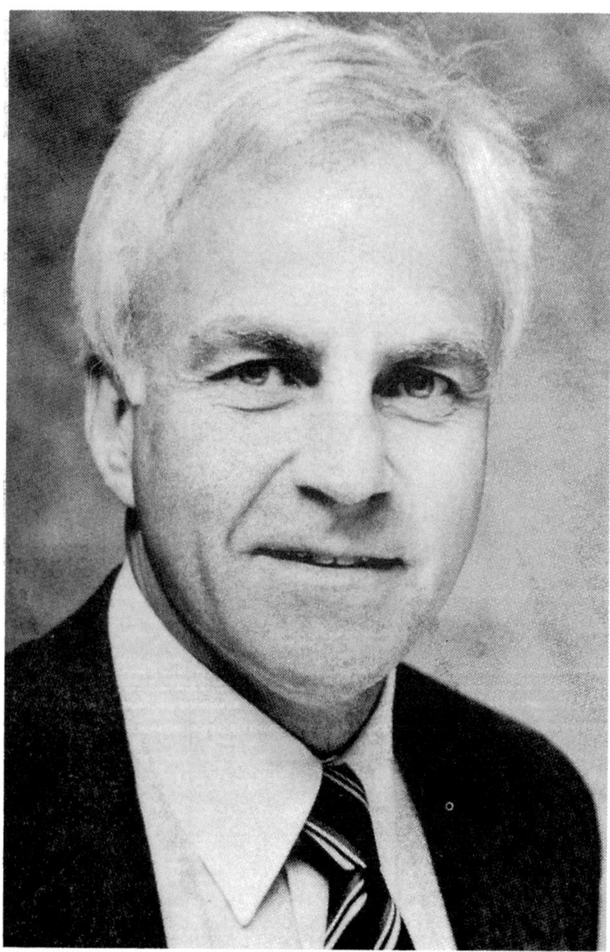

FIG. 33-28. Richard N. Edie, M.D., Director of the Division of Cardiothoracic Surgery (1987–   ).

Dr. Edie brought to Jefferson not only his wealth of experience but an energy to expand the well-established programs in teaching, research, and patient care. Specifically, he has endeavored to interdigitate his Division more closely with that of Cardiology in a cooperative effort for the treatment of acute myocardial infarction and the implantation of ventricular assists of both the autologous and artificial-device types. Another goal is the creation of a unified Thoracic Surgery Service in closer collaboration with pulmonary medicine, radiology, and radiation therapy for even more improved service to patients with lung cancer and other forms of pulmonary disease. His research efforts are directed to development of a corps of clinical scientists who will work with cardiologists in the study of electrophysiology and cardiac drugs.

For more than a century many of the great strides in the growth and development in surgery of the thorax have been made by Jeffersonians at Jefferson itself. From the early attempts at removal of foreign bodies from the heart and lungs to the treatment of inflammatory and neoplastic disease of the lung and to the first great epochal attempt at open heart surgery, Jefferson-trained men have played a leading role. This great contribution to the advancement of the knowledge in thoracic surgery is evidenced by the publication of more than 1,200 scientific papers describing these experiences, both experimental and clinical, appearing worldwide in leading scientific journals.

References

1. Ravitch, M.A., *Century of Surgery.* J.B. Lippincott, 1981, p. 60.
2. Ibid., p. 260.
3. Shumacker, H.B., Jr., *History of the Society of Clinical Surgery.* Indianapolis: Benham Press, 1977, p. 106.
4. O'Dwyer, J., "The O'Dwyer Forcible Respirations Apparatus for Children," *Med. Rec.* 80:576–577, 1911.
5. Meltzer, S.J., and Auer, J., "Continuous Respirations Without Respiratory Movements," *J. Exper. Med.* 11:622–625, 1909.
6. Matas, R., "Artificial Respirations by Direct Intralaryngeal Intubation with a Modified O'Dwyer Tube and a New

Graduated Air Pump in its Application to Medical and Surgical Practice," New Orleans: (*Chez l'auteur*), 1902.
7. Sauerbruck, E.F., "Ueber die pysiologischen und physikalischen Grundlagen bei intrathorakalen Eingriffen in meiner pneumatishen Operationskammer," *Verhandl. d. Deutsch Gesellsch. f. Chir.* 33, pt. 2: 105–115, 1904.
8. Flick, J.B., "Lung Abscess," *Ann. Surg.* 84:323–336, 1926.
9. Flick, J.B. and Gibbon, J.H., Jr.: Applications of thoracoplasy to treatment of pulmonary tuberculosis. *Penn. M.J.* 39:768–772, 1936.
10. Muller, G.P., "Intratracheal Insufflation Anaesthesia," *Internat. Clin.* 22d. ser. 2:175–178, 1912.
11. Muller, G.P., "Bullet Removed from Left Lung," *Ann. Surg.* 68:543–544, 1918.
12. Gibbon, J.H., Jr., "Artificial Maintenance of Circulation During Experimental Occlusions of Pulmonary Artery," *Arch. Surg.* 34:1105–1131, 1937.
13. Stokes, T.L., Jr., "Experimental Maintenance of Life by a Mechanical Heart and Lung During Occlusions of the Venae Cavae Followed by Survival," *Surg. Gynec. & Obstet.* 91:138–156, 1950.
14. Stokes, T.L., and Flick, J.B., Jr., "An Improved Vertical Cylinder Oxygenator," *Proc. Soc. Exper. Biol. & Med.* 73:518–529, 1950.
15. Miller, B.J., Gibbon, J.H., Jr., Gibbon, M.H., "Recent Advances in the Development of a Mechanical Heart and Lung Apparatus," *Ann. Surg.* 134:694–708, 1951.
16. Miller, B.J., Gibbon, J.H., Jr., and Fineberg, C., "An Improved Mechanical Heart and Lung Apparatus and Its Use During Open Cardiotomy in Experimental Animals," *M. Cl. N. Am.* 37:1603–1624, 1953.
17. Miller, B.J., "A Respirator for Laboratory Animals Utilizing Compressed Air and Suction," *Surgery* 44:722–725, 1957.
18. Miller, B.J., Gibbon, J.H., Jr., Greco, V.F., Smith, B.A., Cohn, C.H., and Allbritten, F.F., "The Production and Repair of Interatrial Septal Defects Under Direct Vision with Assistance of an Extracorporeal Pump Oxygenator Circuit," *J. Thor. Surg.* 26:598–616, 1953.
19. Gibbon, J.H., Jr., Miller, B.J., Dobell, A.R., Engell, H.C., and Voigt, G.B., "The Closure of Interventricular Septal Defects in Dogs During Open Cardiotomy with the Maintenance of the Cardiorespiratory Functions by a Pump Oxygenator," *J. Thor. Surg.* 28:235–240, 1954.
20. Miller, B.J., Gibbon, J.H., Jr., Greco, V.F., Cohn, C.H., and Allbritten, F.F., Jr., "The Use of a Vent for the Left Ventricle as a Means of Avoiding Air Embolism to the Systemic Circulation During Open Cardiotomy with the Maintenance of the Cardiorespiratory Function of Animals by a Pump Oxygenator," *Surg. Forum* 4:29–33, 1953.
21. Miller, B.J., and Kistenmacher, J.C., "The Effects of P-Di-(2-Chloroethyl)-Aminophenylalanine on Malignant Tumors." *JAMA* 173:14–21, 1960.
22. Miller, B.J., Talsania, S., and Kistenmacher, J.C., "An Extracorporeal Circuit Containing One Pump and an Oxygenator, Operating at Greater than Atmospheric Pressure." *J. Germantown Hosp.* 2:5–14, 1961.
23. Miller, B.J., Talsania, S., Kistenmacher, J.C., and Masson, N., "Segmental Perfusion of Human Malignant Tumors with P-Di-(2-Chloroethyl)-Aminophenylalanine (Sarcolysin). *J. Germantown Hosp.* 1:5–12, 1960.

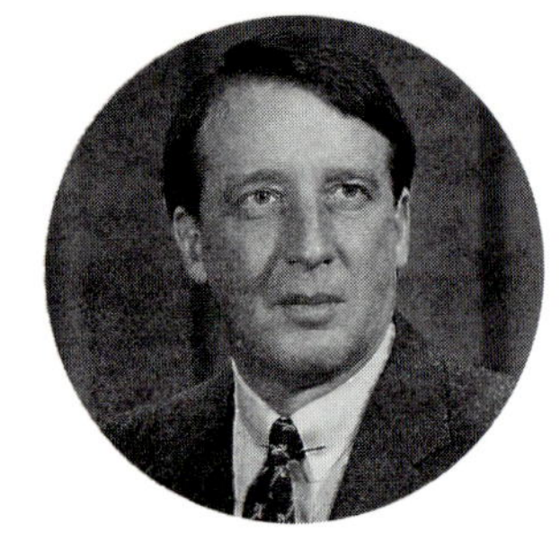

CHAPTER THIRTY-FOUR

Plastic Surgery

James W. Fox, IV, M.D.

"If the world never suspects the face has been lifted, that is the true test of your handicraft."

—Sir Harold Gillies (1882–1960)
and Dr. Ralph Millard, Jr. (1919–)

Plastic surgery denotes a branch of surgery in which shifting or readjustment of tissues is undertaken for the treatment of congenital or acquired deformities and for the improvement of function, comfort, appearance, or contour. Although these words quite adequately describe the creed of plastic surgery as practiced today, they were written by Dr. John Bingham Roberts (Jefferson, 1874) over 100 years ago. The history of plastic and reconstructive surgery at Jefferson actually began with Dr. Joseph Pancoast (Figure 34-1).

Dr. Pancoast, the second Chairman of Surgery at Jefferson (1839–1841), was probably the most prolific American author of articles on plastic procedures of the nineteenth century.[1] He was favorably compared with the European plastic surgical greats of his time, including Dupuytren, Roux, and Velpeau of France, Diffenbach of Germany, and Liston of England. During Pancoast's 35 years of practicing and teaching at Jefferson, he introduced the procedure of rhinoplasty, devised the original dacryo-cysto-rhinostomy for lacrimal duct occlusion and epiphora, described the first myotomies for correction of strabismus, performed the first composite pedicle flap transfer (hair-bearing scalp to replace an eyebrow lost in a fire), developed the first procedure to address velo-pharyngeal incompetence in the cleft palate patient, originated the first genitourinary congenital repair (closure of bladder exstrophy with pedicle flaps), and perfected the procedure of neurotomies in the surgical treatment of facial tics.[2]

Pancoast's greatest contribution is probably his most overlooked. In his famous work, *Treatise on Operative Surgery* (1844), Pancoast describes the procedure of free skin grafting: "In several instances a portion of integument has been entirely detached from the arm or thigh and at once applied on the surface of the open wound." This statement on free skin grafting antedates by 30 years the epochal works of Thiersch published in 1874.

The Third Chairman of Surgery at Jefferson was Dr. Thomas Dent Mütter (1841–1856). Mütter (Figure 34-2), in the words of Pancoast's commemorative lecture of 1859, "had witnessed, while abroad. . . . the great domain in plastic surgery,"[3] which he put to use at Jefferson. He made an exhaustive study of scar formation and the characteristics of burn scar and contracture. Burns were the most common injury at that time because of the always-present open flame used in heating, cooking, and illumination of the house, school, and workplace. The surgical treatment and release of these horrible deformities using rotation and tube pedicle flaps, local Z-plastics, and running W-plastics, as reported by Mütter, entitled him to "claim the merit of having first performed an operation for relief of extensive cicatrices."[4]

Even though possibly Jefferson's greatest surgeon, Dr. Samuel D. Gross, the Fourth Chairman of Surgery at Jefferson (1856–1882), contributed little to the growing specialty of plastic surgery; he did write on refinements in strabismus surgery.

An 1874 Jefferson graduate, Dr. John Bingham Roberts contributed much to the field of plastic surgery. Roberts, a member of the first detached Jefferson Hospital staff from 1877 to 1879, did most of his significant medical writing after leaving Jefferson.[5] His literary output later described septorhinoplasty repair and pin fixation of midface fractures and soft tissue reconstruction of the "tumor, caustic or syphilitically" deformed nose. When at Jefferson, Roberts espoused two principles, one medical and the other philosophic, which were examples of the Jefferson-trained physician. At the time of his award of the Gross Surgery Prize at graduation, he stated that "the devastating effect of physical deformity on the mental attitude of the afflicted individual must always be treated by the tending physician." Later,

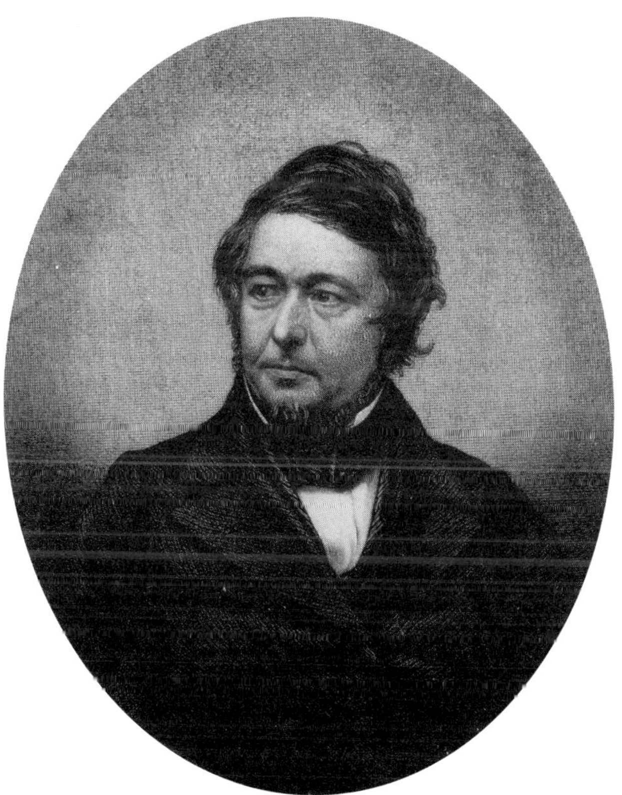

FIG. 34-1. Joseph Pancoast, M.D. (1805–1882); Second Chairman of Surgery (1839–1841), Fifth Chairman of Anatomy (1841–1874), and pioneer in plastic surgery.

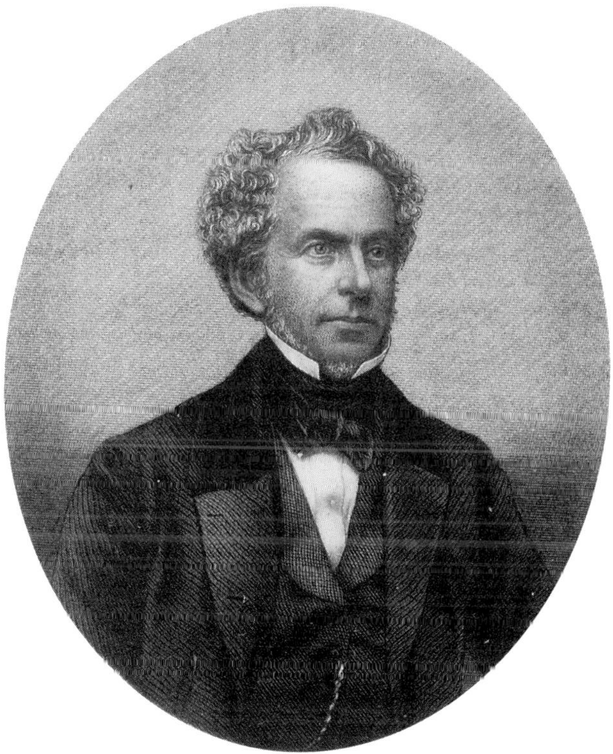

FIG. 34-2. Thomas Dent Mütter, M.D., LL.D. (1811–1859); Third Chairman of Surgery (1841–1856), and pioneer in plastic surgery for burn scars and contractures.

during his two-year period of lecturing to Jefferson students, he suggested that they never forget that "one's birth and social position are merely accidental and that individuals are accepted and valued solely by their merits."

An 1879 Jefferson graduate, Dr. Archimedes Rose of Kentucky, provided a bridge from the early history of plastic surgery at Jefferson of the late nineteenth century to the more organized period beginning in the early twentieth century. Dr. Rose, after completing his education at Jefferson, returned to his Marion County, Kentucky, home to practice. There he crossed paths with Warren B. Davis, a young man raised in Jessamine County, Kentucky, and educated at Kentucky University. Young Davis developed an interest in medicine, matriculated at Jefferson in 1906, and graduated in 1910. When at Jefferson, Davis (Figure 34-3) was elected to Alpha Omega Alpha (an honor medical fraternity) and won the graduation prizes in oral surgery, gynecology, obstetrics, and pediatrics.[6] To the casual observer these various prizes might seem unrelated, but careful consideration reveals that an interest in these subjects could very easily translate into a career caring for the congenital anomalies of the newborn, child, and adolescent patient.

Following an 18-month internship at Jefferson, Warren Davis was awarded the Corinna Borden Keen Research Fellowship and entered the research laboratory of Dr. Ludwig Pick at the University of Berlin. This research effort resulted in a monograph describing the development and anatomy of the nasal accessory sinuses. Upon his return to Philadelphia in 1913, Davis was appointed to the surgical staff by Dr. J. Chalmers DaCosta. He was also appointed to the teaching staff of the Anatomy Department and subsequently held the appointment of Professor of Oral Surgery.[7]

At about this time, Dr. Warren Davis met two other Dr. Roses, neither related to each other nor to the Dr. Rose of Kentucky. Horace Rose (Jefferson, 1903) worked at the Camden Children's Clinic. Dr. Clarence Atwood Rose (Jefferson, 1913) would practice at the Spitzka Anatomic League Children's Dispensary (Blockley Hospital and, subsequently, Philadelphia General Hospital). Dr. Horace Rose first demonstrated cleft palate surgical repair to Warren Davis. Later, Dr. Clarence Rose would provide anatomic data that eventually led to Davis's scholarly approach to congenital anomalies including his published techniques first describing osteoplastic flaps for the repair of cleft palate.

During World War I, Dr. Davis, as a Captain in the Medical Corps, was in charge of the School of Oral and Plastic Surgery at Fort Oglethorpe, Georgia. The major textbook of the period with respect to facial injuries, *War Injuries of the Face*, was published in 1919. The author was none other than the Jefferson graduate of 1874, Dr. John Bingham Roberts.

Dr. Davis returned to Jefferson after the War and went on to be involved at the very inception of development of the surgical subspecialty of

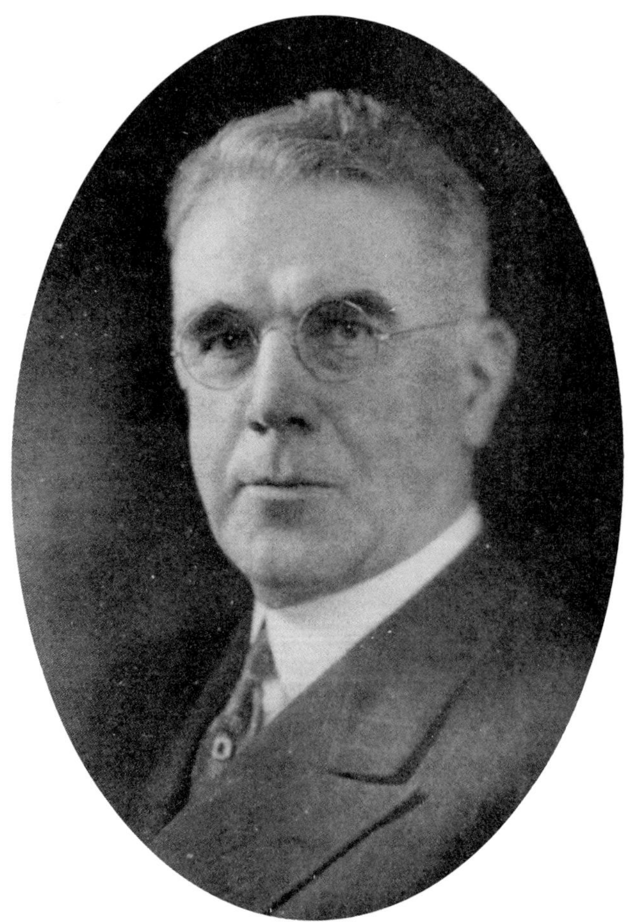

Fig. 34-3. Warren B. Davis, M.D. (1881–1947), Professor of Oral Surgery and pioneer in the repair of congenital facial deformities of children.

plastic and reconstructive surgery. In 1925 he met with 11 other physicians in Philadelphia, most of whom had both medical and dentistry degrees. This led to the incorporation of the American Association of Plastic Surgeons in 1927 in New York, of which Davis became the Senior Trustee in 1935.

Out of this group grew an educational forum, with a goal to spread the principles and techniques of surgeons who confined their practices solely to plastic surgery. Thus another organization, the American Society of Plastic and Reconstructive Surgeons, was born in 1931, with Jefferson's Warren B. Davis as one of the original 12 members. This specialty society was approved by the American Board of Medical Specialists and was made the licensing board for plastic surgery. Davis became its third President (1936–1937).[8]

Because of Davis's early leadership in the Society and his erudite manuscripts in the surgical literature, when the Society instituted its own journal in 1946, *Plastic and Reconstructive Surgery*, Warren Davis was chosen as its first Editor. He held this position until his death in 1947. Because of his stalwart leadership in bringing this publication into being, a fellow plastic surgeon, Dr. Lyndon Peer, wrote that "*Plastic and Reconstructive Surgery* will be a permanent memorial to Dr. Warren B. Davis." Dr. Davis was President of Jefferson's Alumni Association in 1942 and President of the Pennsylvania Society of Plastic Surgeons from 1935 until 1947.

Another plastic surgeon on the staff at Jefferson during this period was Dr. John Gunter, licensed as a medical doctor and also as a dentist. Dr. Gunter worked on the Oral Surgical Staff of Warren Davis from 1919 until 1923.

A 1925 Jefferson graduate, Dr. John D. Reese (Figure 34-4), was an associate of Dr. Davis until 1929, when he entered solo practice. Dr. Reese practiced at Jefferson for 32 years. His famous contribution to the medical world was his skin-graft-harvesting instrument called the "Reese Dermatome." His interests in the surgical physiology of the skin pertaining to its successful transplantation and his early training as a chemist led to his developing this instrument. Reese's unique breakthrough was made possible by his experimentations in rubber chemistry culminating in his technique for "vulcanizing" a synthetic rubber sheathing to a cord supportive layer. This same process was later used in the tire manufacturing industry. Reese's instrument greatly advanced the procedure of skin grafting, as it provided a technique to accurately harvest uniform thicknesses of skin under normal skin tensions.

Another member of the plastic surgical staff at Jefferson was Dr. Charles LaClair. He practiced plastic surgery and otolaryngology at Jefferson from 1932 until 1940, and during World War II he was a member of Jefferson's Base Hospital No. 38.

Dr. John J. Duncan (Jefferson, 1937) practiced at Jefferson from 1939 until 1961, with four years (1941–1945) spent as a medical officer in the China-Burma-India Theater during World War II. He first practiced in association with Dr. Warren B. Davis at Jefferson and subsequently with Dr. Warren Davis's son, Dr. J. Wallace Davis.

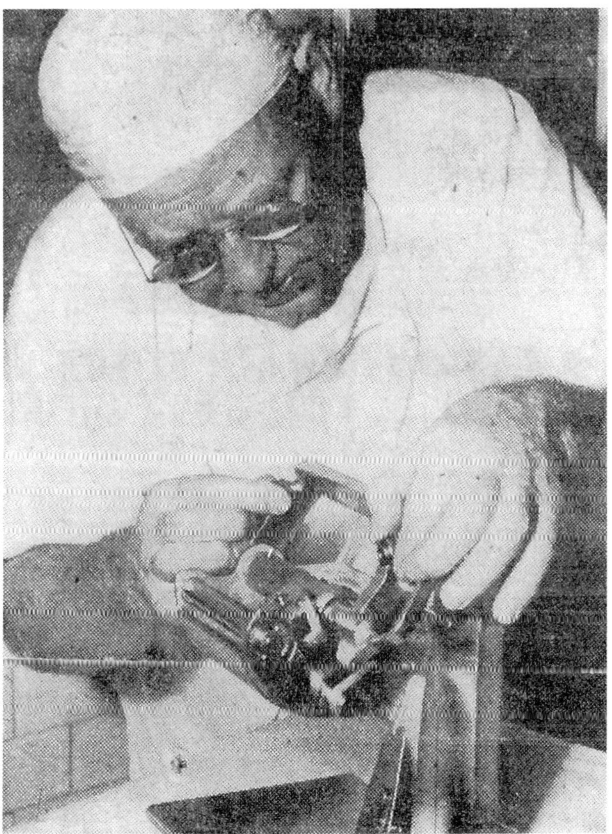

FIG. 34-4. John D. Reese, M.D. (1893–1958), Clinical Professor of Plastic and Reconstructive Surgery and inventor of the "Reese Dermatome."

Dr. J. Wallace Davis (Jefferson, 1942), after spending the years 1943 to 1946 as a Major in the Medical Corps in the China-Burma-India Theater during World War II, returned to Jefferson for training under his father. He subsequently associated in practice with his father and Dr. Duncan. As one of the early pioneers in cosmetic surgery (Figure 34-5), he was one of the original proponents of psychologic good health, considering it to be equally as important as physical good health. Because of his leadership in the field of aesthetic plastic surgery, he gained national recognition in his specialty and served first as an officer and subsequently as a Director and Board Trustee of the American Society of Plastic and Reconstructive Surgery. He also served as the President of all the local and regional Plastic Surgical Societies as well as being Chairman for Alumni Annual Giving at Jefferson for 26 years. He received Jefferson's prestigious Cornerstone Award in 1978.

Dr. Herbert Lipshutz (Jefferson, S1944) returned after World War II and completed his plastic training in 1952 at Jefferson, where he practiced until 1963, at which time he transferred to Pennsylvania Hospital.

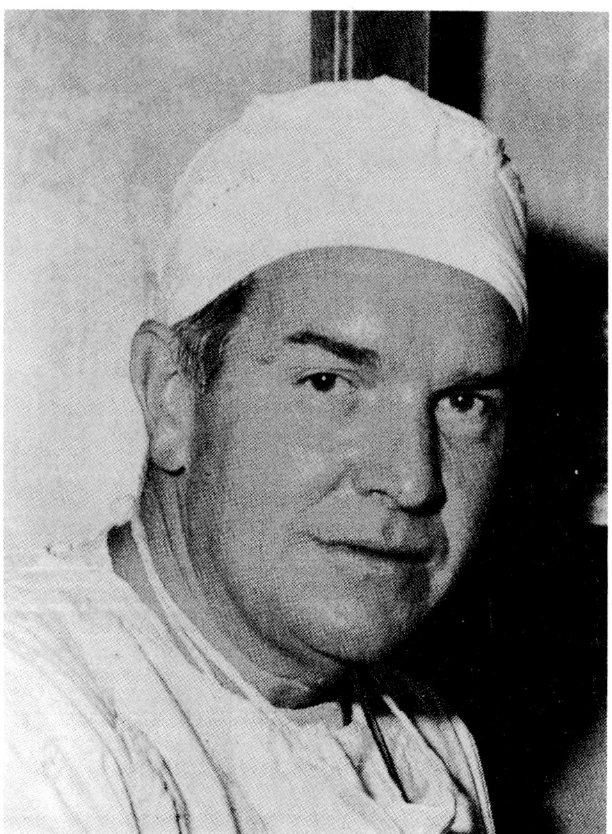

FIG. 34-5. J. Wallace Davis, M.D., an early pioneer in cosmetic surgery.

Dr. Jose Castillo joined the plastic surgical staff in 1970 when Dr. Harry Goldsmith was appointed Chairman of Surgery. Dr. Castillo left in 1974 to enter practice in South New Jersey.

Dr. James W. Fox, IV (Jefferson, 1970) took his general surgical residency at Jefferson (1970–1974) and extended his training into plastic and reconstructive surgery at the University of Virginia, Charlottesville (1974–1976). He then joined the Surgery Department at Jefferson as Assistant Professor in the teaching of his specialty and also joined Dr. J. Wallace Davis in private practice. Dr. Fox's interests have dealt primarily with breast reconstruction, about which he has published 28 scientific articles. He also has been involved in advancement of myocutaneous flap technology and its applications to clinical reconstructions, especially involving the lower extremity.

Plastic and reconstructive surgery at Jefferson has witnessed a rapid explosion of implant technology, the perfection of microvascular surgical techniques, and the never-ending search for further improvements.

References

1. Pancoast, J., *A Treatise of Operative Surgery; Comprising a Description of Various Processes of the Art, Including All the New Operations.* Philadelphia: Carey & Hart, for G.W. Loomis, 1844.
2. Atkinson, W.B., *Physicians and Surgeons of the United States.* Philadelphia: Charles Robson, 1878, pp. 709–711.
3. Pancoast, J., A Discourse Commemorative of the late Prof. T.D. Mütter, M.D., Being the Introductory Lecture to the Course of Anatomy in the Jefferson Medical College of Philadelphia, delivered October 14, 1859.
4. Mütter, T.D., *Cases of Deformity from Burns Successfully Treated by Plastic Operations.* Philadelphia: Merrihew and Thompson, 1843.
5. Shell III, D.H., "John Bingham Roberts: Philadelphia Plastic Surgeon." *Plastic and Reconstructive Surgery* 69:145–154, January 1982.
6. *Jeff. Med. Coll. Al. Bull.,* June 1942, pp. 12–13.
7. Peer, L.A., "In Memoriam: Warren B. Davis," *Plastic & Reconstructive Surgery* 2:505–507, 1947.
8. Paletta, F.X., *History of the American Society of Plastic and Reconstructive Surgery.* Baltimore: Waverly Press, 1963.

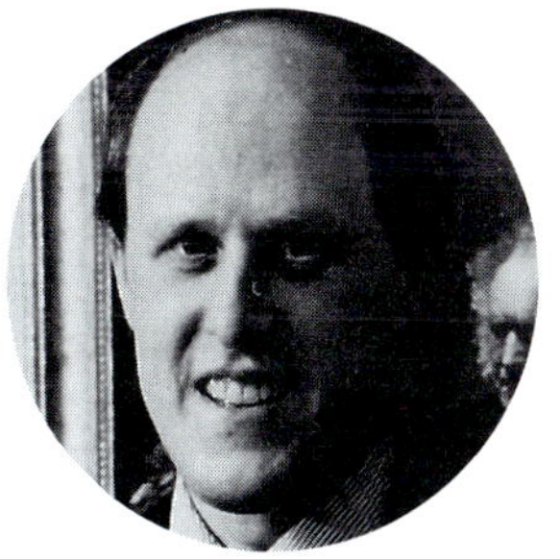

CHAPTER THIRTY-FIVE

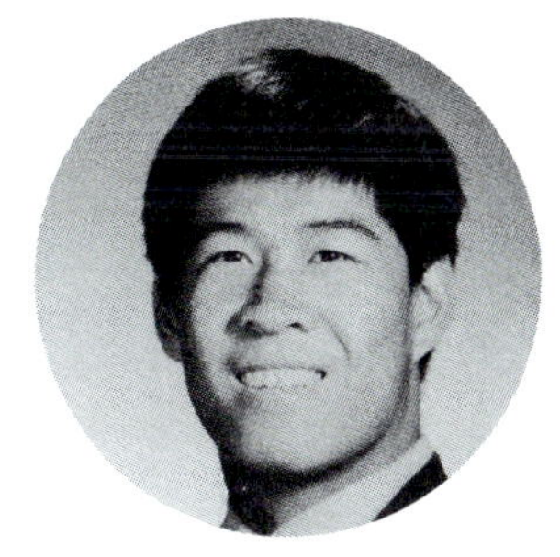

Transplantation

BRUCE E. JARRELL, M.D., AND JONATHAN C. FONG, M.D.

"The solution of the cross-grafting mystery . . . may be as revolutionary as fission of the atom." —SIR HAROLD GILLIES (1882–1960)

THE GROUNDWORK for transplantation capability at Jefferson was laid by Dr. Herbert E. Cohn (Jefferson, 1955) who, as a Jefferson surgical resident, cultivated his interest in nephrology (Figure 35-1). His training completed, Dr. Cohn teamed with Dr. James E. Clark (Jefferson, 1952) to provide renal patients with the most comprehensive surgical and medical care available at the time. The joint effort resulted in a renal dialysis unit affording centralized access for all Delaware Valley kidney patients. Dr. Cohn, after several years of research devoted to improving the methods of dialysis, became increasingly aware of the need for an alternative in the palliation and cure of renal failure. He accepted the challenge of developing the skills needed for kidney transplantation by traveling to well-known transplant centers across the nation. This was rewarded in 1965 when Dr. Cohn ushered in the transplant era at Jefferson with the first transplant of a cadaver kidney. Seven others were done between 1965 and 1968. Dr. Cohn performed the actual transplantation and the care required by the donor, and the recipient was supervised before and after surgery by Dr. Norman Lasker and the Nephrology Division. In 1972, Dr. James F. Burke, Jr., (Jefferson, 1966) joined Dr. Lasker in caring for renal transplant patients. A major contribution was Burke and Lasker's development of a clinical protocol for screening prospective donors and recipients. Their clinical research enhanced the care of renal patients and improved the success rate of the transplants.

From its inception, several obstacles faced the fledgling program. Two major problems were procuring the organs without the support of a regional or national center and gaining the general public acceptance of transplantation as a viable alternative. The underlying cause of the public's rejection of transplantation as a treatment modality was the controversy surrounding the condition of "brain dead" as a classification of clinical death. The objections began to lessen when Dr. Christian Bernard of South Africa successfully completed the first heart transplant in 1967. Literally overnight, transplantation became a household term, and programs began to spread throughout the country.

The modern era of therapeutic transplantation at Jefferson began in 1972. In January of that year Dr. Cohn performed the first successful renal transplant. The kidney came from an identically matched sibling and contined to provide full renal function for the recipient for over ten years.

A major commitment to a full program of renal transplantation was made by the appointment of James E. Colberg, M.D., (Figure 35-2) to establish and direct the Transplantation Service. Dr. Colberg came from Albany Medical College, where he had cofounded and codirected a successful clinical renal transplant program and was director of the tissue-typing laboratory of the Renal Disease Institute of the State of New York.

A major component of the Transplantation Service was the tissue-typing immunology laboratory, which was established with Drs. James Colberg and Steven I. Bulova as codirectors for the proper screening and matching of donors and recipients. Another important emphasis was on cadaver organ procurement for transplantation. Because the whole concept, especially that of brain death, was new, extensive education was necessary in the Jefferson affiliated hospitals. Operative protocols including preoperative care, and immunosuppression for postransplant rejection episodes were developed.

A renal transplant team was established with members from Nephrology, Urology, and Surgery. Drs. Herbert Cohn and Jerome Vernick from the Surgery Department participated in the program. Dr. Colberg performed the first successful non–identically matched renal transplants at Jefferson. On February 16, 1973, he performed the first successful parent and child transplant, and on March 12 of that year, the first successful cadaver donor renal transplant.

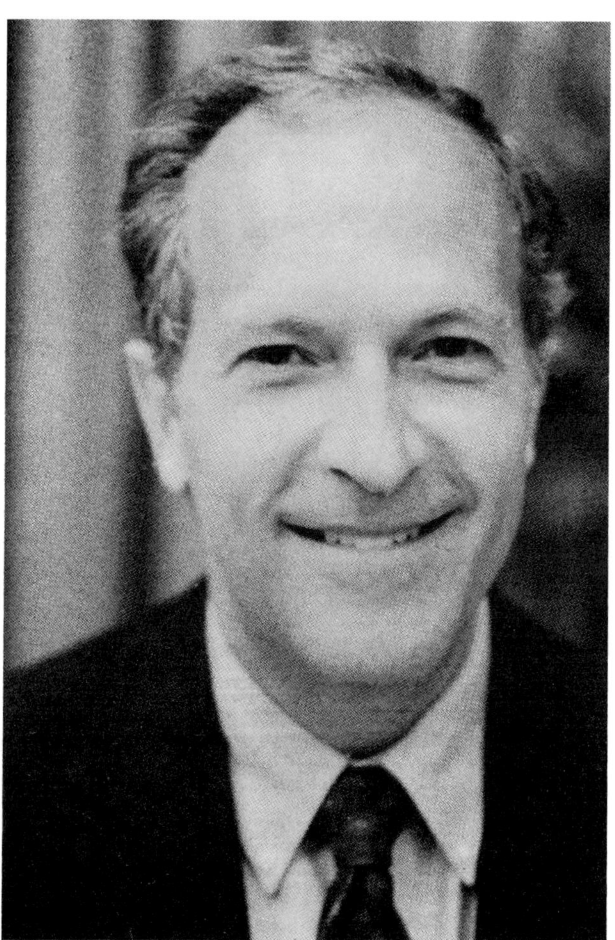

FIG. 35-1. Herbert E. Cohn, M.D., a pioneer in renal transplantation and Vice-Chairman of the Department of Surgery (1985–).

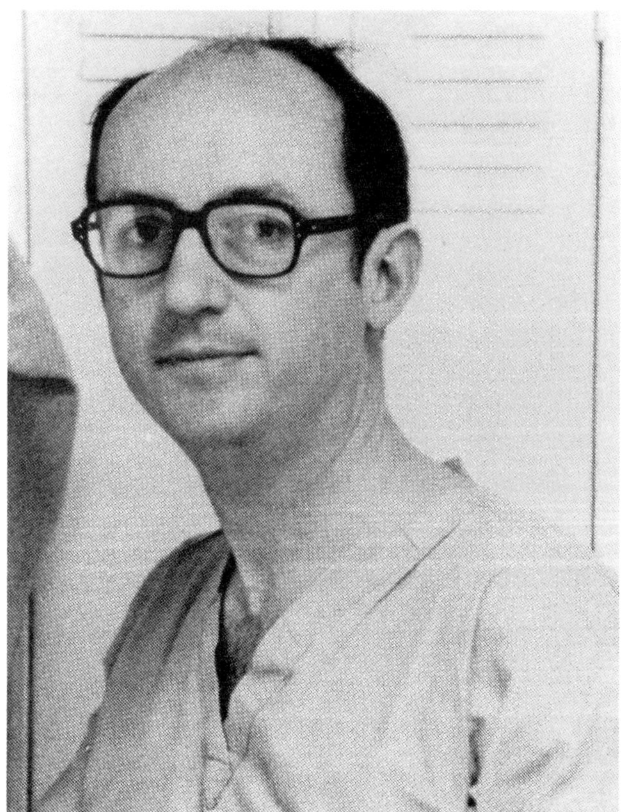

FIG. 35-2. James E. Colberg, M.D., headed the renal transplantation and its ancillary services (1972–1980).

Longer preservation of donor kidneys became necessary. In 1973 Dr. Colberg established a laboratory for preservation of kidneys up to 72 hours.[1] Research programs in renal preservation and immunogenetics were begun, as well as transplant conferences for teaching and patient care.

In 1974, with the encouragement of the Chairman of Surgery, Dr. Harry S. Goldsmith, and the Director of the Dialysis Unit, Dr. Norman Lasker, a coordinated program was established with Our Lady of Lourdes Hospital. After two identical twin transplants were performed there, Our Lady of Lourdes Affiliate decided to develop its own South New Jersey Transplant Program. This resulted in the loss of many potential referrals to the Jefferson Transplant Program.

A very important achievement in these years of intense competition in Philadelphia among Jefferson and the fine, well-established transplant programs of the University of Pennsylvania, Hahnemann, Albert Einstein Northern Division, Lankenau, and Saint Christopher's was the establishment by the Heads of the six programs of the Delaware Valley Transplant Program of a regional procurement agency. It has continued to be one of the largest and most successful in the country.

The Jefferson program in the years 1972–1980 had results equal to those elsewhere, yet it did suffer from a relatively low number of transplants, approximately 15 per year. Cadaver renal transplants, the majority of those done, were at a plateau of results throughout the country of 45% functioning at one year. Nephrologists were somewhat reluctant to refer patients for transplantation due to the results and due to the lack of Federal pressure.

A new clinical research program at Jefferson in collaboration with the University of Minnesota and the National Institutes of Health was begun, using antilymphocyte globulin as a new and less toxic immunosuppressive agent in 1978–1979 in order to improve results.

When Dr. Francis E. Rosato was appointed Chief of Surgery in 1978, one of his plans was to establish a strong transplant service that would have the capability of performing not only kidney transplants but also liver and heart. A successful program was accelerated in 1980 by the appointment of Dr. Bruce E. Jarrell (Jefferson, 1973), whose credentials included previous work with Dr. Lasker in developing the prototype of the peritoneal dialysis machine used in most hospitals today. During his residency and transplantation Fellowship at the Medical College of Virginia, Dr. Jarrell had gained invaluable experience in transplantation with Drs. H.M. Lee and James Wolf. Dr. Jarrell provided a leadership and vision that within five years transformed an ancillary service into one of the largest transplant centers in the country. Among the factors contributing to the success of the program was Jefferson's provision of financial support and long-term commitment. Resurgence of the transplant program was additionally aided by Dr. Jarrell's efforts to increase the patient pool by expanding the area coverage for referrals. This included South Jersey, Delaware, and Central Pennsylvania. At the same time, Dr. Rosato was establishing the necessary contacts to gain the confidence and support of the hospitals in these outlying areas.

Research in the intervening years improved the techniques of transplantation and patient care.[2–4] In addition, the development of cyclosporin, an immunosuppressive agent, allowed more leeway in the matching of disparate donor and recipient tissue. This in turn increased the number of organs available for transplantation. By 1985 Jefferson had the twenty-seventh largest kidney transplant service in the United States, with over 75 transplants per year.

In the spring of 1981, Dr. Willis C. Maddrey was appointed Chairman of the Department of Medicine. He was vitally interested in Jefferson's long-term goal of a liver transplant capability. The following year a visit was made to the foremost liver transplant center at the University of Pittsburgh headed by Dr. Thomas E. Starzl. All those who would be involved in the transplant procedure at Jefferson were represented in this visit. These included Dr. Shuin Yang, who trained under Dr. Starzl during the preceding year, along with Dr. Bruce Jarrell and Dr. R. Anthony Carabasi, III (Jefferson, 1977), who represented the Surgery Department. The Anesthesiology Department, represented by Drs. James Zvargulis and Joseph L. Seltzer (Jefferson, 1971), worked with Dr. Kang of the Pittsburgh team to develop the protocol. Work was begun at Jefferson to establish laboratories needed to hone the technical skills required to perform the complex procedure. Experience with the operation was acquired initially on dogs and pigs. A suitable patient was found in a 30 year-old white male whose only systemic illness was sclerosing cholangitis.

Michael Donahue entered the operating room on May 31, 1984, with no hope for a medical cure and 12 hours later left with a new lease on life. The ease with which the operation was performed and Michael's rapid recovery were a tribute to the careful planning of the first successful liver transplant in Philadelphia.

While kidney transplants continue to dominate the service, a case load of 15 to 20 liver transplants per year is anticipated. Research continues on both endothelial cell seeding of arterial grafts and pancreatic islet cell transplants. In the future, transplantation of other organs is anticipated to establish Jefferson as a complete transplantation center.

References

1. Colberg, J.E., "En Bloc Excision of Cadaver Kidneys for Transplantation," *Arch. Surg.* 115:1238–1241, 1980.
2. Jarrell, B.E., Moritz, M.J., and Radomski, J., "Cyclosporine," in *Transplantation of the Liver,* Maddrey, W.C. (ed.), New York: Elsevier, 1988.
3. Besarab, A., Jarrell, B.E., Hirsch, S., *et al.,* "Use of the Isolated Perfused Kidney Model to Assess Acute Pharmacologic Effects of Cyclosporine and Its Vehicle, Cremophor EL," *Transplantation* 40(6):624–631, 1985.
4. Besarab, A., Wesson, L., Jarrell, B.E., *et al.,* "Effect of Delayed Graft Function and ALG on the Circaseptan (About 7 days) Rhythm of Human Renal Transplantation," *Am. Jour. of Kidney Disease* 35:562–566, 1983.

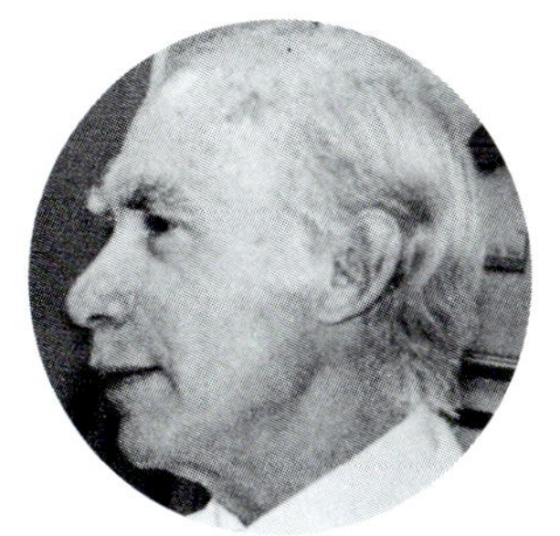

CHAPTER THIRTY-SIX

Division of Colorectal Surgery and the Comprehensive Rectal Cancer Center

GERALD J. MARKS, M.D.

"There is a fundamental principle in medicine, whenever the stool is withheld or is extruded with difficulty, grave illnesses result."

—MISHNEH TORAH

THE ESTABLISHMENT of the Division of Colorectal Surgery followed a period of innovation in colon and rectal surgery. Pioneering efforts occurred in anal sphincter-preservation surgery, in the management of the radiation-injured intestine, and in flexible fiberoptic colonoscopy.[1,2] The latter procedure was launched by a national cooperative study originating at Jefferson. These efforts resulted in national and international attention for this institution. The country's first production-model colonoscope was in use at Jefferson in 1969, and the first colonoscopy symposium held in the world was Jefferson sponsored in 1974.

The success of these activities resulted in encouragement by the American Society of Colon and Rectal Surgeons to establish a university-based colorectal surgical residency program. Dean Joseph Gonnella and Surgical Chairman Francis Rosato authorized the establishment of the Division of Colorectal Surgery in 1984. Dr. Gerald J. Marks (Jefferson, 1949) was appointed Director.

Subsequent American Medical Association approval led to acceptance of Dr. Ignacio Echenique as the first in the residency program in July, 1985. The Division staff was augmented to include Drs. Harold Rovner, Alan M. Resnik, Scott D. Goldstein, and Maryalice Cheney (the second Resident trained).

The Comprehensive Rectal Cancer Center began as a working group of over 20 scientists from a variety of basic science and clinical specialties. This multiinstitutional network of scientists focused on the study and management of rectal cancer based on a program begun in 1975 utilizing sphincter-preservation surgery following full-dose preoperative radiation therapy. The clinical program not only comprised the largest series of full-dose preoperative radiation therapy for rectal cancer and sphincter preservation but also the largest series of sphincter preservation for cancers of the distal six cm. of rectum. The Jefferson experience is cited as a breakthrough in the multimodality management of rectal cancer, in which both the quality of life and survival are enhanced.[3]

Incorporated in the Comprehensive Rectal Cancer Center is a Colorectal Cancer Genetic Center and a Familial Polyposis Registry in collaboration with the Wistar Institute, in which a major grant was awarded by the National Cancer Institute. Joining Dr. Marks are, among others, Drs. Mohammed Mohiuddin, Laird G. Jackson, Harry S. Cooper, Michael Mastrangelo, Harvey Brodovsky, Scott Goldstein, Maryalice Cheney, and Ursula Hahn. The Center, located in the Medical Office Building at 1100 Walnut Street, is viewed as the only one of its kind.

References

1. Marks, G.J., and Moses, M.L., "The Clinical Application of Flexible Fiberoptic Colonoscopy," *Surg. Cl. N. Am.* 43:735, 1973.
2. Marks, G.J., "Flexible Fiberoptic Colonoscopy: A Guide for Its Use in the Management of Diseases of the Colon," *Jour. Am. Med. Assoc.* 228: 1411, 1974.
3. Marks, G.J., Mohiuddin, M., and Borenstein, B.D., "Preoperative Radiation Therapy and Sphincter Preservation by the Combined Abdominotranssacral Technique for Selected Rectal Cancers," *Dis. Col. and Rect.* 28:565–571, August 1985.

CHAPTER THIRTY-SEVEN

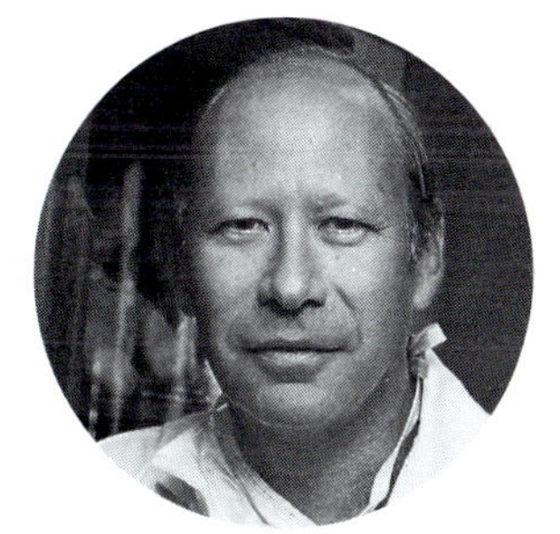

Hospital Trauma Service

JEROME J. VERNICK, M.D.

"A wound heals but the scar remains."

—ENGLISH PROVERB

JEFFERSON HAS produced individuals who contributed to the care of trauma patients over its entire history. In the 30 years between 1877 and 1907, the first detached Jefferson Medical College Hospital at the site of the present Thompson Annex treated nearly 50,000 accident cases (Figure 37-1). From 1907 until opening of the Curtis building in 1931, all accident cases were received on the street level of Old Main Hospital from the entrance on the south side. From 1931 the emergency room on the second floor of the Curtis Clinic was handicapped by a slowly operating elevator. The current emergency department in the Thompson Annex was constructed in the mid-1960s and represented a vast improvement. Plans are now under way for a project for completion in 1990 that will include a state-of-the-art emergency room/trauma center complex occupying the entire first floor of the Main and Thompson buildings.

Trauma training of Residents was recognized as a deficiency in the early 1980s, then overcome by rotating the Residents through trauma programs in Maryland and later at Cooper Hospital in Camden. Jefferson's commitment to trauma increased during this time. The Hospital provided limited funding to start a trauma registry and begin efforts in improving trauma care and training. The advanced trauma life-support course sponsored by the American College of Surgeons became available in 1981. Jefferson was the first institution in Philadelphia to require this course of all house staff in surgery prior to their exposure to the public. This program has now encompassed neurosurgery and orthopaedic surgery as well as other disciplines.

In 1981 Jefferson Hospital began to participate in the major trauma outcome study. This was used as a nucleus for a trauma registry that has now become a sophisticated computer-based data-collection tool, which is an integral part of the Pennsylvania Trauma Systems Foundation's registry and has served as a model for several other trauma programs.

Trauma center designation began with major problems and delays in the mid-1980s. After legislation was obtained through the Commonwealth of Pennsylvania, Jefferson successfully qualified as a Level I regional resource trauma center. This accreditation was renewed in 1987 for two years, the maximum level of approval offered by the State.

The trauma program employs a trauma director on the full-time faculty, a trauma nurse coordinator, a trauma data and research nurse, and an administrative secretary. Efforts are under way to recruit an additional full-time critical care trauma surgeon. The quality assurance department has a full-time trauma quality assurance person, and the social service department is recruiting a full-time trauma social worker. A full-time registered nurse has recently been added to serve as a public educator coordinator. The trauma program has established an outreach trauma prevention program that, in its first year, presented over 50 programs to area schools and provided this service for over 10,000 of its students.

The trauma program depends on advanced trauma life-support-certified attending surgeons, of which there are eight participating in the call roster. Residents, who provide the first line of defense for in-house trauma coverage, will obtain all of their trauma training at Jefferson when commitment to Cooper Hospital expires in 1988. The emergency department has always been an essential part of trauma care, and is a Division in the Department of Surgery.

Active basic research in trauma-related subjects is being carried out by Dr. Allan M. Lefer and his staff in the Physiology Department and by Dr. Susan Jacoby and her staff in the Surgery Department. Clinical research is being conducted by most members of the Trauma Attending Faculty.

Jefferson participates in a helicopter consortium known as Sky-Care, which provides capability to move appropriate patients by air. This has been regarded as a patient-care tool rather than a marketing tool and has helped to maintain a valid perspective in moving patients without incurring unnecessary expenses that are generated by in-house helicopter programs.

Current plans include consideration of a critical care ground transport team, which should provide essential urban environment service. Jefferson's commitment to trauma programs foretells significant contributions in the years to come.

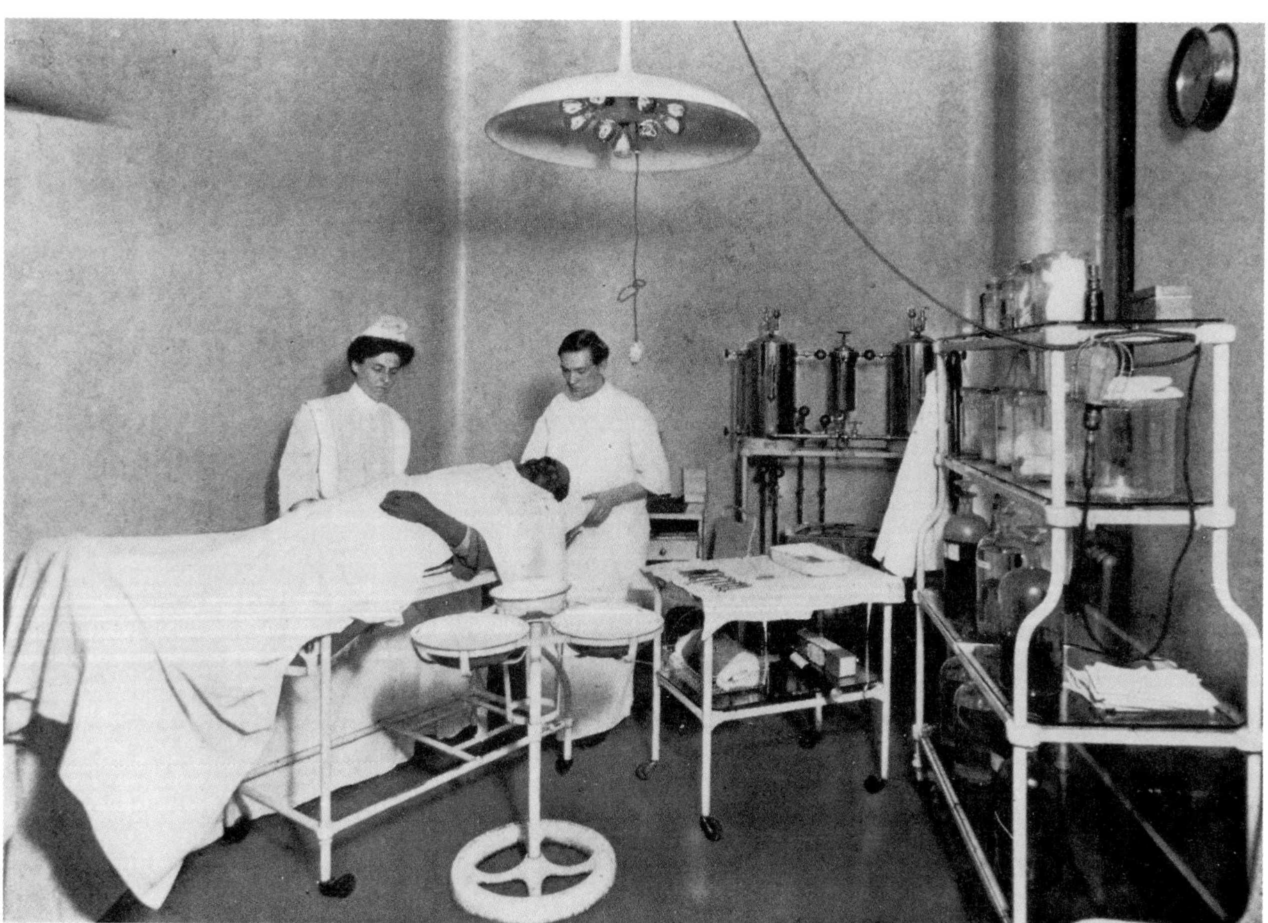

FIG. 37-1. An accident case brought by ambulance to the emergency room of the 1877 Hospital (ca. 1900).

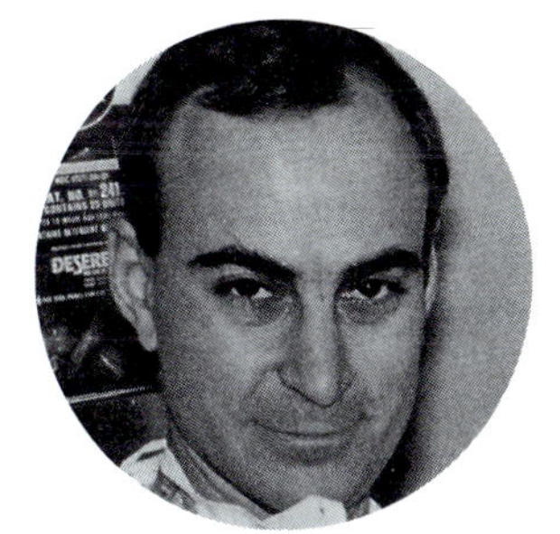

CHAPTER THIRTY-EIGHT

Pediatric Surgery

PHILIP J. WOLFSON, M.D.

"There are few satisfactions that are greater than the operative correction of an anomaly which restores a child to perfect health—a feat which can be accomplished in a surprisingly high percentage of cases." —ROBERT E. GROSS, M.D. (1905–)

AT THE turn of the century little distinction was made between diseases of children and adults. The much higher mortality rates in the young pointed out with increasing emphasis that children could not be considered as diminutive adults. Furthermore, infants and children were subject to types of infections and congenital malformations infrequently encountered in adult life. Surgery in children remained the domain of the general surgeon. In the 1920s, Dr. William E. Ladd at Harvard pioneered in gathering together the special knowledge of the pathology and best procedures required for surgical treatment of children. This culminated in his classical book in 1941, *Abdominal Surgery of Infancy and Childhood,* coauthored by Robert E. Gross, M.D. Ladd became duly regarded as the "Father of Modern Pediatric Surgery." Gross widened the field further in 1953 with publication of his book, *The Surgery of Infancy and Childhood,* which included abnormalities in the thorax and cardiovascular system.

Through the 1940s to most of the 1960s, surgeons at Jefferson operated upon pediatric patients as a routine in their field, not only adopting the technical advances of the time but also the improvements in pre- and postoperative care. The names of Drs. Warren B. Davis, Thomas A. Shallow, William T. Lemmon, Kenneth E. Fry, Frederick B. Wagner, Jr., and Robert G. Johnson are associated with this period. The transition to staff with extra training and interest in pediatric surgery occurred with the appointment of Peter S. Liebert in 1968, Louis F. Plzak, Jr. in 1971, and Candadai S. Rangaratham in 1972. The former two performed cardiothoracic surgery in adults as well, while the latter restricted his activity solely to infants and children. Dr. Rangaratham was regarded as the pediatric surgeon in the Department from 1972 until his resignation in 1979. Despite commendable performance, his progress was frustrated by lack of accreditation by the American Board of Surgery, his passive personality, and the paucity of cases.

In June, 1972, the American Board of Surgery acted "to recognize Pediatric Surgery as an area within Surgery deserving special recognition, to establish requirements for Certification, establish examination procedures and issue Certificates of Special Competence." In 1974, the American Board of Medical Specialties approved the granting of Special Certificates by the American Board of Surgery. The Residency Review Committee for Surgery assumed the responsibility for accreditation of residency programs in this discipline. The first cycle of certifications was completed in 1975.

In 1982 Dr. Philip J. Wolfson was appointed Director of the Section of Pediatric Surgery. A native of the Bronx, New York, he had received his M.D. degree from the Mount Sinai School of Medicine (1974) and served his internship at the Royal Victoria Hospital in Montreal, Quebec (1974–1975). Following a residency in general surgery at the Mount Sinai Medical Center (1975–1979), he took additional training in pediatric surgery at the Montreal Children's Hospital in Quebec (1980–1982). He subsequently became certified by the American Board of Surgery and received the Certificate of Special Competence in Pediatric Surgery.

An inherent problem in building up an adequate Pediatric Surgical Service was the presence of two children's hospitals, Children's Hospital of Philadelphia (founded in 1855) and St. Christopher's Hospital for Children (established in 1875). Jefferson, however, was a high-risk perinatology center with a very sophisticated Intensive Care Nursery. In addition, the relationship with Mercy Catholic Medical Center, a Jefferson affiliate with a very active general pediatric service, was cultivated. Low-risk operations for patients who originated from Fitzgerald Mercy were performed at that institution, whereas infants with surgical conditions requiring tertiary care (such as at a Pediatric Intensive Care Unit) were transferred to Jefferson.

The number of operations performed yearly on children at Jefferson increased steadily from 168 in 1982–1983 to 306 in 1987. Recruitment of a Pediatric Anesthesiologist as well as a Pediatric Intensivist contributed significant expertise in treating very ill pediatric surgical patients.

Antenatal ultrasound has been increasingly successful in identifying congenital structural abnormalities requiring surgical correction shortly after birth. Such early diagnoses have allowed for prenatal parental counseling and usually maternal transport to Jefferson for a planned delivery there. Specific congenital anomalies that have been identified prior to birth and treated successfully at Jefferson include esophageal atresias, duodenal obstructions, jejunal artesias, abdominal wall defects, and neck masses.

Jefferson, as of 1987, is the only institution in the Delaware Valley with an established neonatal Extracorporeal Membrane Oxygenation (ECMO) program. ECMO is the use of a modified heart-lung machine to provide gas exchange for temporary pulmonary support. It has been demonstrated to be lifesaving for a select group of neonates with respiratory failure unresponsive to maximal intensive conventional treatment.[1] In June, 1985, after two years of animal experimentation, a moribund infant was placed on ECMO at Jefferson and survived. Since that time over 40 neonates with predicted mortalities of 90% from respiratory failure have been treated with ECMO; 90% of these babies have survived.

Preliminary research in fetal lambs has investigated the use of ECMO circuit to function as an artificial placenta, providing metabolic needs for the fetus, such as gas exchange, nutrition, and excretory function.

The Section of Pediatric Surgery is strengthening its role in education of the medical students, in the training of residents in general surgery, and in the operative care of this special group of patients.

Reference

1. Bartlett, R.H., Roloff, D.W., Cornell, R.G., Andrews, A.F., Dilon, P.W., and Zwischenberger, J.B., "Extracorporeal Circulation in Neonatal Respiratory Failure: A Prospective Randomized Study," *Pediatrics* 76:479–487, 1985.

CHAPTER THIRTY-NINE

Department of Anesthesiology

JAY J. JACOBY, M.D., PH.D.

"And the Lord God caused a deep sleep to fall upon Adam, and he slept: and he took one of his ribs, and closed up the flesh instead thereof."

—GENESIS 2:21

THE DISCOVERY and development of anesthesia constitute a revolution in the history of medicine. Before the advent of anesthesia surgeons had to be men of steel. They operated upon patients who were screaming, writhing in anguish, and held down by straps, leather belts, and strong men. Lucky patients fainted. The endurance of sick people being limited, the duration of an operation was brief; many were measured in seconds, some in minutes. An operation that lasted an hour was unthinkable. Surgery in the preanesthesia era is vividly described by Thorwald in *The Century of the Surgeon*.[1]

> "The second patient had a tumor of the tongue. As the young man hesitantly sat down, an attendant came up behind him with a portable charcoal burner upon which lay, already glowing white-hot, several surgical cautery irons. The attendant set the burner down where the unfortunate young man could not see it.
>
> "Warren was holding a forceps in his left hand, a scalpel in his right. With his thumb he tested the edge of the blade. One of the resident surgeons, a big, powerful man, stepped up close behind the chair, ready to hold the young man's head. Warren ordered the young man to open his mouth. The patient hesitantly obeyed. As his tongue emerged from the dark opening of his mouth, it was possible to see even at a distance the huge growth that disfigured its tip. Warren's left hand flashed forward and gripped the tongue with the forceps. The young man tried to draw it back, uttering a strangled cry as he did so. But Warren's forceps clamped down hard and drew the tongue further out, while the assistant held the patient's head tightly. Fractions of a second later the knife in Warren's right hand sliced through the tongue with

a single rapid slash. The amputated tip, with the tumor, fell to the ground. Blood gushed out of the stump of the tongue. Warren tossed the scalpel on to the instrument table and stretched his arm out to the side, past the operating chair and far enough so that the attendant could place the handle of a glowing cautery iron into his hand without being seen by the dazed patient. The patient was still uttering gurgling sounds. Warren held the cautery behind his back. With a sudden movement, the resident surgeon covered the patient's eyes with his hands—and Warren pressed the red-hot iron against the bleeding stump of the tongue.

"The patient, struck by frightful pain, tried to jerk his head back. With a mighty effort he pushed himself and the chair several yards across the room. The assistant staggered and barely managed to retain his hold on the patient's head, but Warren followed right after the moving chair. He did not let the tongue go, and kept pressing the iron against the wound. The smell of singed flesh rose up to us. Once the iron slid away and touched the lower lip, but immediately afterward it was again on the wound, cauterizing the last still bleeding remnant of the tongue. Then Warren snapped the forceps open and took a step back. The resident surgeon relaxed his grip. The patient pressed both hands over his mouth. He sprang to his feet, voicing indescribable sounds, and reeled blindly about until two attendants seized him. Warren looked at him coldly, reproaching him for the burned lip and utterly unmoved by the man's torment. 'Well,' he said, 'if you haven't burnt yourself it isn't your fault.' The two attendants led the man out, half tugging, half supporting him."

Considering the horrors of surgery without anesthesia, it is a wonder that anyone was willing to be subjected to an operation. Boiling oil and red hot pokers were in standard use. Most operations that were done then are included in this short list: amputation for fractured or injured limbs (a compound fracture that was not amputated usually meant death from sepsis); incision and drainage of abscess to release "laudable pus"; "cutting for stone" or lithotomy; removal of tumors and bullets; and repair of lacerations. Invasion of body cavities was exceedingly rare. Appendicitis was not even diagnosed in living people, and removal of the inflamed appendix did not begin until after 1886.

The discovery of anesthesia was considered to be the greatest blessing mankind ever received. Since there was no name to describe the phenomenon, scholarly men vied to invent a term to do it justice. Anesthesia being an American discovery, an American finally gave it a name. The famous physician-poet, Oliver Wendell Holmes, put together two Greek words: an = no, and esthesia—sensation. He did not consider the difficulty people would have in pronouncing it and its derivatives. It has also been said that he did not invent the term—he is usually credited with the introduction of the term *anesthetic*, but the word *anesthesia* and adjectives derived from it were in common use throughout the eighteenth century.[2] Because the first successful public administration of anesthesia in the world (October 16, 1846), was done by a dentist, William Morton, at the Massachusetts General Hospital, it was thought that no real knowledge or skill was required to administer it. In America its use was relegated to surgical trainees, medical students, nurses, and sometimes orderlies or family members. For this reason, after its discovery America made no significant contribution to the advancement of the art or science of anesthesia for almost a century.

The Early Years of Anesthesia at Jefferson

When anesthesia was first demonstrated in 1846, Jefferson was already a well-established medical school, and the new discovery was quickly applied. On December 23, 1846, just two months later, the Professor of Surgery, Thomas Dent Mütter, administered the first anesthetic in Philadelphia at his Jefferson Clinic, for removal of a tumor from the cheek. Another physician, Dr. John Kearsley Mitchell, Professor of Medicine, administered ether to a woman in labor at Jefferson, the first obstetrical anesthesia in Philadelphia.

In 1860 a group of Japanese doctors visited the Gross Clinic (Figure 39-1). It is believed that these Japanese were the first ever to visit a clinic in a foreign country. The situation relates to the period of Japan opening its doors to foreign countries. In 1860 the Tokugawa government sent envoys to

Washington, D.C., for the ratification of a Japanese-American Commerce Treaty. The mission stayed in Washington 24 days, and on June 8 began their return journey. On the way, they stopped in Philadelphia. Among the group were three doctors, who with an interpreter, visited the Gross Clinic. The operation being done was for bladder stones, and the anesthetic was administered by none other than the discoverer of ether anesthesia, William Morton, himself. The whole performance was a revelation to the Japanese. They smelled and poured ether on their hands, astonished at the coldness resulting from its evaporation. After the operation, they carefully examined the instruments and showed so much interest that they were invited to visit the College. Among the gifts the group received were medical instruments, an artificial denture on a gold plate, and books on surgery. It can easily be assumed that the Japanese doctors were presented with Dr. Gross's first edition of the *System of Surgery,* which had been published only the year before. It is said that this visit laid the foundation for the modernization of Japanese surgery.[3]

The ether used for the first anesthetics was an impure substance called "letheon" and, later, "sulphuric ether." Dr. Edward R. Squibb (Figure 39-2), a Jefferson graduate of the Class of 1845, invented a continuous process for the manufacture of pure ether in 1852. This was the beginning of the large pharmaceutical organization still prominent today.

News of the discovery of anesthesia was carried like wildfire, as fast as stagecoaches and clipper ships could travel to all parts of the world. An English doctor, who had been present at the demonstration at the Massachusetts General Hospital, raced from Boston to London and introduced anesthesia to Europe. Thereafter, only doctors administered anesthesia in Europe, and virtually all the early work on the understanding and improvement of anesthesia was done in Great Britain.

The first full-time specialist in anesthesia in the world was an English general practitioner, Dr. John Snow. As an astute physician, he also became famous for stopping an epidemic of

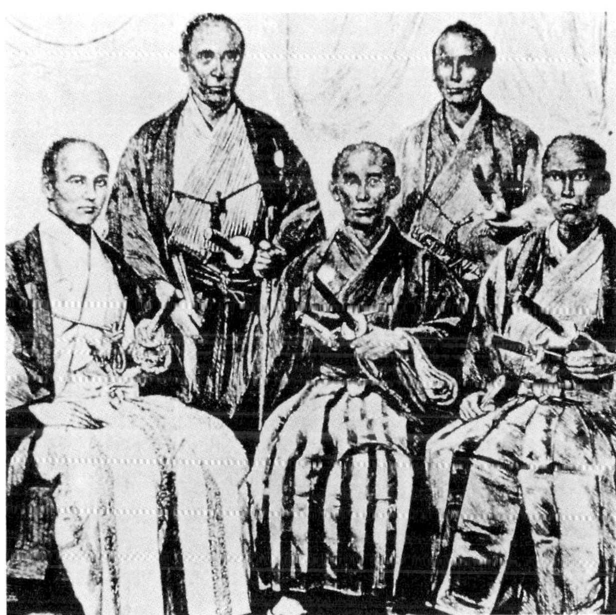

FIG. 39-1. Principal members of Japan's first diplomatic mission to the United States in 1860, wearing formal hakama costumes and swords. (Courtesy of *Nisei: The Quiet Americans* by Bill Hosokawa. N.Y.: 1969, Wm. Morrow & Co.)

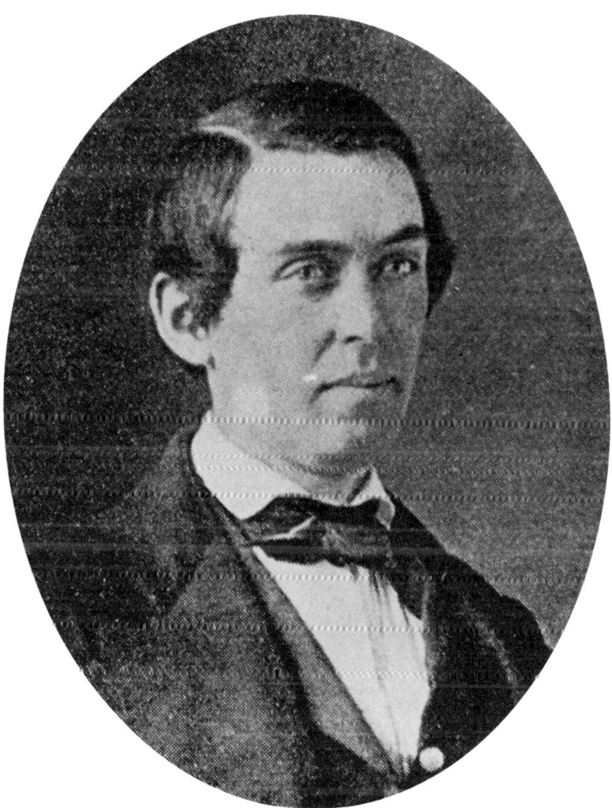

FIG. 39-2. Edward R. Squibb, M.D. (Jefferson, 1845), first manufactured pure ether.

cholera in London in 1854. He noted that the distribution of cases fanned out with diminishing frequency from a particular point. At that hub was a water pump from which the community drew its drinking water. He convinced the police that they should close the pump, and the epidemic was halted. This predated the discovery of germs as the cause of disease. Dr. Snow eventually limited his practice to the administration of anesthetics. He wrote the first two books on this subject: *On the Administration of Ether* and *On the Administration of Chloroform*.

The greatest blessing of mankind was withheld from pregnant women. Clergymen believed that the words of the Bible were to be applied literally. The punishment of Eve when she ate the fruit of the Tree of Knowledge was "In pain shalt thou bear children." Using anesthesia for childbirth was thought to be contrary to the will of the Lord. The first to employ chloroform anesthesia in labor was an Edinburgh obstetrician, Sir James Simpson in 1847. He was denounced by the Scottish clergy for trying to counter the Divine Will.

Queen Victoria was pregnant with the child who was to be Prince Leopold. Having had several children, she was not anxious to experience another childbirth without pain relief. She called in her obstetrician, who informed her that the anesthesia she heard about was forbidden by the Church. As head of the Church of England she declared it proper for herself. Dr. John Snow was called in to administer chloroform for her deliveries in 1853 and 1857. The Ladies-in-Waiting watched this, thought it a miracle, and demanded for themselves "Anesthesia a la Reine," and they were allowed it. This can be called one step forward in the Women's Liberation Movement.

There is no documentation of early anesthetists at Jefferson after Drs. Mütter and Mitchell. Probably the surgical house staff and the operating room nurses provided that service, without training except what they learned from each other. It took many years for surgeons to realize that anesthetics produced less harm if they were administered by trained persons. Surgeons also had very little "training," usually acquired by "walking the wards," or acting as "dressers," or watching from the gallery how the master worked. In the *Gross Clinic* of 1875, Eakins depicted anesthetist Dr. William Joseph Hearn, who regularly gave ether or chloroform for Dr. Gross.+ Physicians aspiring to become surgeons would work in the surgical clinic and give anesthesia for the chief. They were frequently referred to as "etherizers." Through this system Dr. Hearn became a Clinical Professor of Surgery at Jefferson.

Dr. Laurence Turnbull, a fellow graduate with Edward R. Squibb in the Jefferson Class of 1845, was appointed Aural Surgeon to the first Jefferson Hospital in 1877. In 1878 he published the first edition of his textbook *Artificial Anesthesia: A Manual of Anesthetic Agents and their Employment in the Treatment of Diseases.* This treatise of over 500 pages covered all aspects of what was known about anesthesia up to that time and went through four editions.

▪ Era of Nurse Anesthetists

Medical schools had no formal courses in anesthesia, and what little the students learned was taught by the nurse anesthetists. In practice in the small towns of that era, the family doctors administered anesthesia for each other, or showed a family member how to do it, as they operated with the patient on the kitchen table.

The first formal training in anesthesia in the United States occurred in Cleveland, at Lakeside Hospital of Western Reserve University, where a school of nurse anesthetists was founded in 1905. The formal training of nurse anesthetists at Jefferson started around 1926. Miss Louise Graves, a graduate from the Jefferson School of Nursing in the Class of 1920, enrolled in a course in anesthesia at the Cook County Hospital in Chicago. She was engaged by Jefferson as head anesthetist and assigned to train a class of six students, with Dr. Edward Klopp as physician supervisor. The first six months were under strict supervision, with some academic instruction, but the course was mainly practical. During the second six months the students gave anesthesia on their own, except when they required assistance. After one year they received a certificate as "Qualifed Anesthetist" and were eligible to become regular staff anesthetists at Jefferson or elsewhere. Some would become employed as private anesthetists to certain Jefferson surgeons, as, for example, to Drs. Warren B. Davis or Lewis C. Scheffey.

Miss Graves left Jefferson as head anesthetist around 1934 and was followed in succession by Dorothy Brinkman, Isabelle Widing Oaks, and Sylvia Vlam Cole in 1937. The latter instructed until 1947 and was succeeded by Nellie Maloney Moses, who remained in charge until the beginning of anesthesiology under Dr. Lewis Hampton in 1957. After Dr. Klopp's death in 1936, the physician supervisors were Drs. Alan Parker, Howard Bradshaw (Figure 39-3), James Surver, and George J. Willauer.

Dr. Thomas B. Mervine (Jefferson, 1940) was appointed Instructor in Anesthesiology in the Department of Surgery in 1944 and served in that capacity until 1953. He was the first to use intravenous pentothal at Jefferson and to institute routine intravenous infusion at the start of surgery, and he did many of the early endotracheal intubations. He also worked closely with Dr. William T. Lemmon in the early use of continuous spinal anesthesia. Mervine rose through the academic ranks to Clinical Professor of Surgery, became Honorary in 1982, and served as President of the Alumni Association in 1980.

World War II was a milestone in the development of anesthesia practice. Before the war, ether was the common general anesthetic, with nitrous oxide and chloroform also in use. The induction of anesthesia often required half an hour, with a strenuous excitement stage. The physiological abuse was almost unbelievable. There were no intravenous infusions. There was no endotracheal intubation. There were no muscle relaxants. There was no assisted or controlled ventilation. There were no physician anesthesiologists. At Jefferson the task was

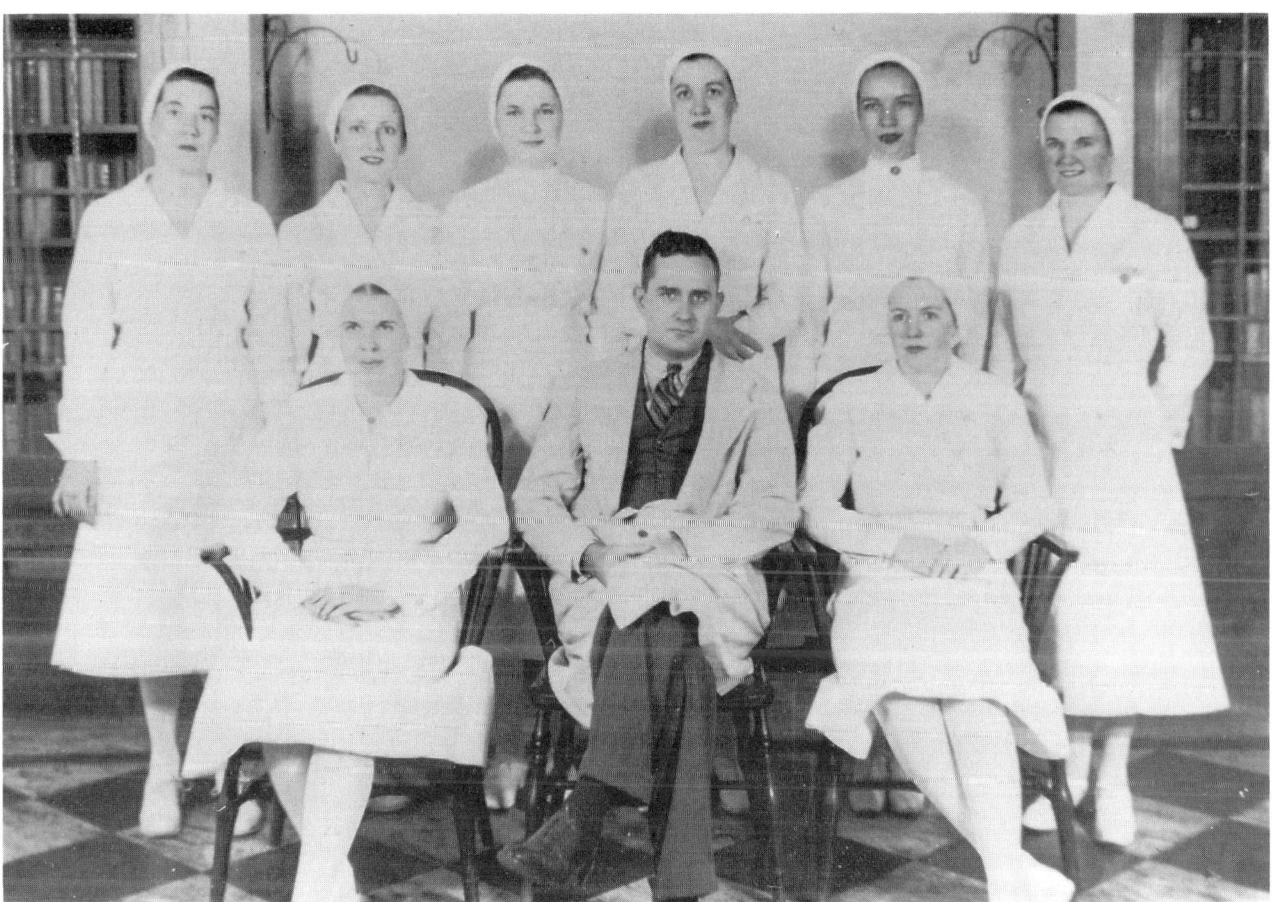

FIG. 39-3. Howard Bradshaw, M.D., and Nurse Anesthetist Staff (1939). Sylvia Vlam Cole, front left; Martha Garver Long, front right, and Nellie Maloney Moses, behind Dr. Bradshaw.

extremely difficult because of the dispersion of the operating rooms in six different locations. Since both ether and cyclopropane are explosive, cumbersome methods were required to avoid sparks, flames, cautery, or other forms of ignition. The Bovie electrocoagulation machine could not be used. Despite these precautions a tragic explosion occurred in 1939 in the fourteenth floor operating room of the Thompson Annex. Dr. Thomas A. Shallow and Louis H. Clerf were performing their operation of combined one-stage pharyngeal diverticulectomy, aided by insertion of the esophagoscope. Nitrous oxide followed by closed circuit ether was being administered when an electric spark set off an explosion. The patient died of internal injuries, the clothing of the nurse anethestist caught fire, and some members of the operating team suffered burns of the face.

After World War II a great deal changed. The pharmacy made intravenous sets and supplied intravenous fluids. Interns and residents learned how to insert intravenous needles that could stay in place. Plastic was not yet available; endotracheal intubation was used for special cases. Intravenous drugs were used to ease inductions, and controlled respiration and muscle relaxants were introduced. Some things had yet to change: Anesthesia for Dr. John H. Gibbon, Jr.'s historic open heart operation with use of the heart-lung machine was administered by a nurse anesthetist as late as May 6, 1953.

Physician Anesthesiologists

The first Medical School Department of Anesthesia in the United States was founded in 1932 at the University of Wisconsin in Madison. It originated through a visit of the Professor of Surgery to Dubuque, Iowa. In the operating room to watch a particularly difficult operation, he was impressed with how easily it was accomplished. He realized that this was due to the excellent anesthesia, and soon he was watching the anesthetist, Dr. Ralph Waters, rather than the surgeon, because Dr. Waters gave a sterling performance. This experience led to Dr. Waters' becoming Professor of Anesthesia at Wisconsin and founding the first residency program in the country. All the rest are his descendants, because his students spread to become professors elsewhere. It took until the 1970s before there was a formal Department of Anesthesia in every medical school of the United States.

Jefferson's most important contribution to anesthesia was made by a surgeon, Dr. William T. Lemmon (Figure 39-4). He was born in South Carolina in 1896 as one of 13 children, three of whom became physicians. After graduation from Clemson College in South Carolina (B.S., 1917) he entered Jefferson Medical College where he received his M.D. degree in 1921. Following his internship at Jefferson Hospital (1921–1923) he began his surgical career by a preceptorship with Dr. Thomas A. Shallow and by teaching gross anatomy at the Daniel Baugh Institute. He maintained an intense interest in anatomy throughout life and was respectfully dubbed "the

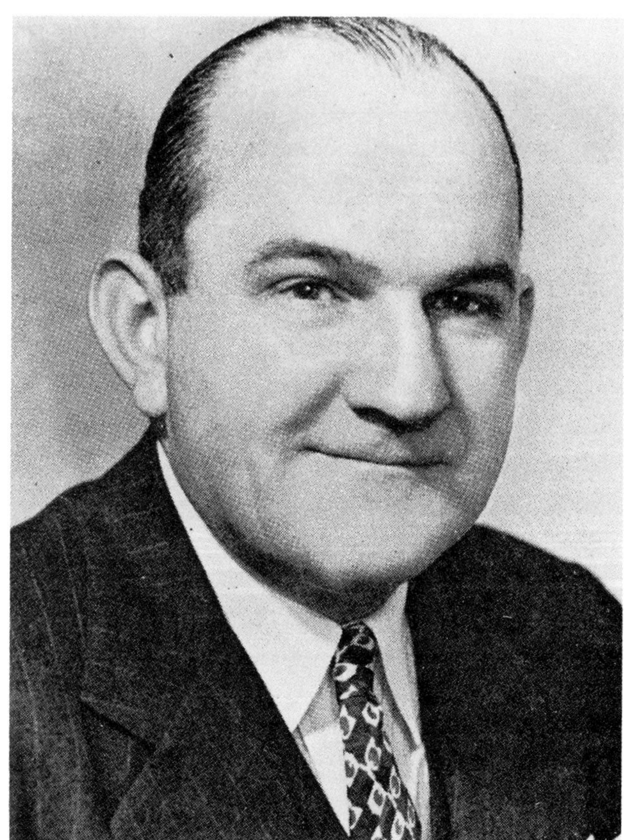

FIG. 39-4. William T. Lemmon, M.D., originator of continuous spinal anesthesia.

last of the great general surgeons" because his operations extended from the brain to the toe. He rose to the rank of Professor of Surgery in 1953.

In 1939 Dr. Lemmon presented to the Philadelphia Academy of Surgery a method of continuous spinal anesthesia that adapted spinal anesthesia for lengthy operations.[5] At this time there were practically no professional physician anesthesiologists. Nurses administered general anesthesia, but surgeons performed their own local anesthesia, nerve blocks, and spinal anesthesias. Surgeons inserted the needles and injected the drug, then left the patient in the care of the nurse while they scrambled to do the operation.

The drug used for local or spinal anesthesia and nerve blocks was procaine. Its duration of action is about 45 minutes. By increasing the concentration and adding epinephrine, the duration can be increased to about 1¼ hours. As surgery became more complex, operations took longer, and sometimes the anesthesia wore off before the operation was finished. The patient then had to be given general anesthesia, considered undesirable to begin with and worse at that point after the patient had gone through an hour of surgery.

Dr. Lemmon thought of a simple but brilliant solution. He left the needle in the spine, attached a rubber tube to it, and attached a syringe to the other end. When the effect of the initial spinal drug started to wear off, he injected more through the tube and needle to reestablish the effectiveness of the anesthesia. Thus was born the concept of "continuous spinal," later extended to continuous epidural and other blocks. The basic principle of the most common and valued technique of anesthesia for childbirth was thus elucidated by a Jefferson surgeon.

Modifications of his technique made it technically easier. These consisted of an operating table with a split mattress, so the protruding needle in the back was not dislodged, and a malleable needle that could be bent to be flush with the skin. Later a plastic catheter was inserted through the needle and provided the flexibility that made it applicable to every case. The millions of women who have painless childbirth every year may thank Dr. Lemmon and Jefferson for this development. His name has been memorialized by his family and son, William T. Lemmon, Jr. (Jefferson, 1960), also a surgeon on the Jefferson staff, who established a prize awarded annually to a senior student who has done original clinical work or writing in the field of anesthesiology.

Jefferson surgeons became experts with spinal anesthesia. The legendary Dr. George J. Willauer, who was nominal head of the nurse anesthesia service for some years, had extraordinary skill with thoracic operations using the Lemmon technique of continuous spinal anesthesia. He or his associate inserted the spinal needle, attached the tubing and syringe, and administered procaine into the intrathecal space. The anesthetic level was advanced until the patient had anesthesia up to the clavicle. Rib resections, thoracoplasties, and sometimes thoracotomies were then performed. The patient breathed spontaneously, with supplementary oxygen, and responded to the surgeon's questions. The operating room nurse would inject more procaine into the spinal canal upon request. The patient's blood pressure usually settled at 70 to 80 systolic, providing induced hypotension and making the surgery relatively bloodless and swift. Willauer reported more than 500 operations done in this way.[6,7] Many subsequent ones were performed in conjunction with Dr. Charles Fineberg, his young assistant, who later became a Professor of Surgery.

A second significant contribution of Jefferson surgeons to anesthesiology consisted in the development of the Jefferson Ventilator (Figure 39-5 and 39-6). The patent obtained by Dr. George J. Haupt (Jefferson, 1945) was assigned by him to Jefferson Medical College. He was aided in this work by Drs. Frank F. Allbritten, Jr. and Jose H. Amadeo (Jefferson, 1952) who co-investigated expiratory assistance as a means of improving ventilation and avoiding respiratory acidosis during anesthesia.[8] Dr. Bernard J. Miller (Jefferson, 1943) had previously conducted research on the important role of expiratory assistance during anesthesia. It was the same Dr. Miller who was closely associated with Dr. Gibbon in the design of electronics and other components for the heart-lung machine.

Throughout the years, artificial respiration was conducted by various methods, mostly ineffective. The iron lung was developed around 1929 by Philip Drinker, a chemical engineer.[9] Although effective, it was a massive, cumbersome machine in which the entire patient, except for the exposed head, was placed. Dr. Clarence Crafoord, a Swedish surgeon, developed a crude positive pressure ventilator. Subsequently, the Jefferson surgeons in the early 1950s created a ventilator that could be used easily and could be adjusted to deliver the desired amount of pulmonary ventilation. The Jefferson Ventilator was the prototype of the thousands of volume ventilators used throughout the world in operating rooms and intensive care units. Untold numbers of patients owe their lives to this development.

Louis J. Hampton, M.D.; First Chairman of Anesthesiology (1955-1964)

The first Chairman of Anesthesiology at Jefferson was Dr. Louis J. Hampton (Figure 39-7), appointed June 20, 1955. A native Pennsylvanian, born in 1909, he obtained his B.S. degree from Franklin and Marshall College in 1929 and his M.D. degree from the University of Pennsylvania in 1933. After internship at the Presbyterian Hospital of Philadelphia (1933–1935), he began private practice on the staff of Monroe County General Hospital (1936–1941) in East Stroudsburg, Pennsylvania, while pursuing special study in cardiology and anesthesiology at the Graduate and University of Pennsylvania Hospitals (1933–1940). He served in the Army in World War II (1941–1945) at Camp Lee, Virginia, at the U.S. Army First Evacuation Hospital and at Walter Reed Hospital. Following a residency in anesthesiology

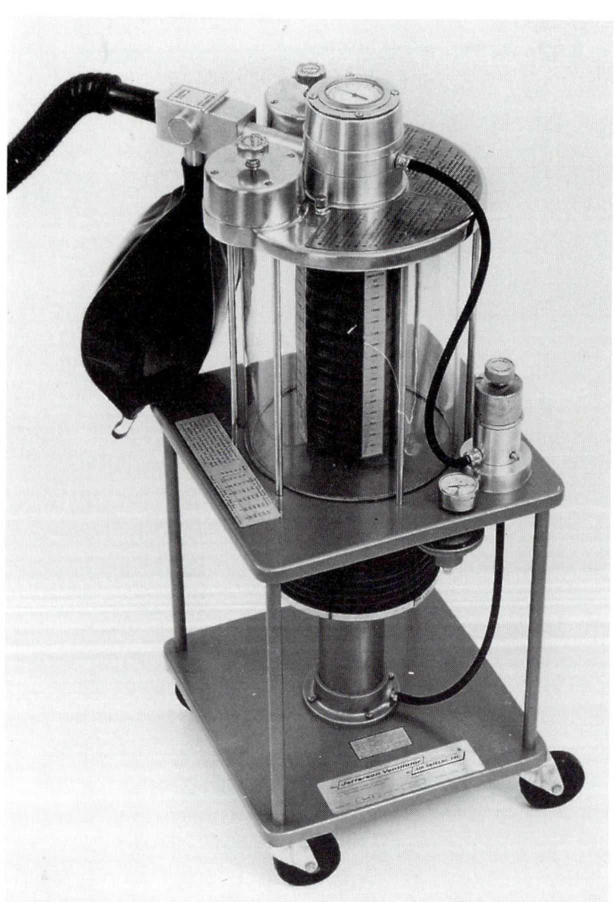

FIG. 39-5. The Jefferson Ventilator.

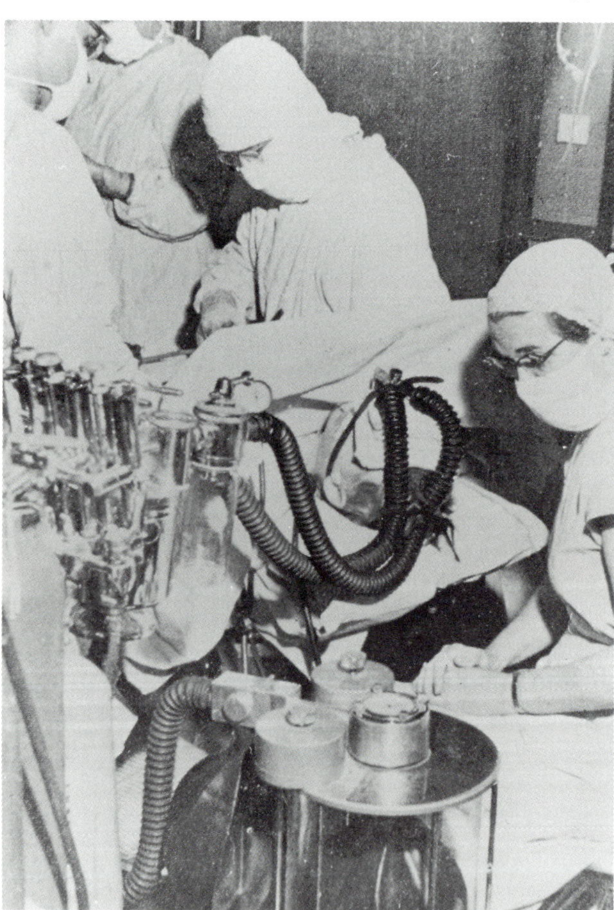

FIG. 39-6. The Jefferson Ventilator being used to assist ventilation of a patient during an operation. George A. Willauer, M.D., surgeon, is in the center, with nurse anesthetist Nellie Maloney Moses at the right.

at the Hartford Hospital (1945–1946), he was certified by the American Board of Anesthesiology in 1947. His academic career in anesthesiology started at Yale University School of Medicine, where between 1946 and 1956 he rose in rank from Instructor to Associate Professor.

Before coming to Jefferson, Dr. Hampton had contributed to the literature of anesthesiology in a broad spectrum of subjects that included his experience with anesthesia in an army hospital in New Guinea, laryngeal edema complicating endotracheal anesthesia in children, sudden death after operation from aspiration after extubation of the endotracheal tube, asphyxia neonatorum, controlled hypotension in anesthesia, anesthesia for surgical correction of cardiorespiratory anomalies, and pharmacologic agents in anesthesia, especially succinylcholine as a muscle relaxant.

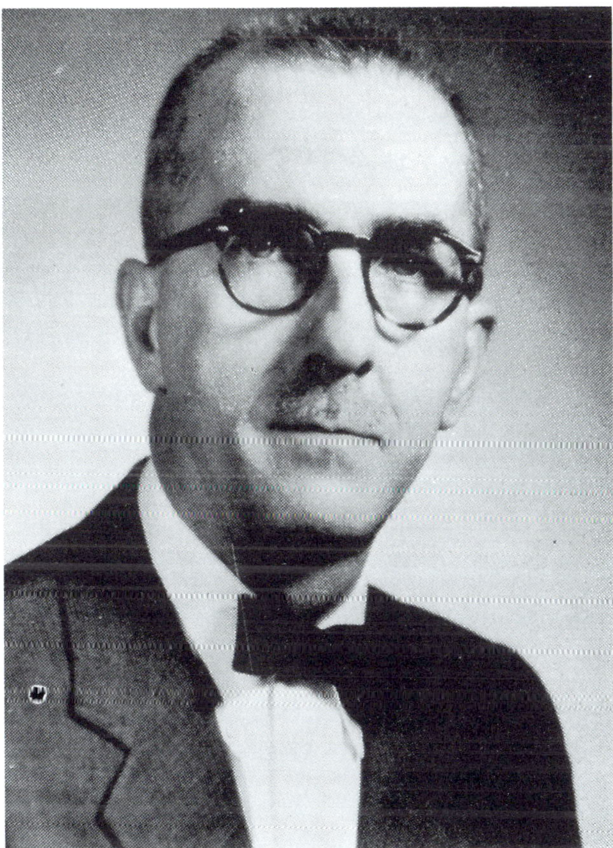

FIG. 39-7. Louis J. Hampton, M.D.; First Chairman of Anesthesiology (1955–1964).

Dr. Hampton's scholarly nature was evidenced by his membership in Phi Beta Kappa, Yale Chapter of Sigma Xi, Connecticut State Society of Anesthesiologists (President, 1948), New England Society of Anesthesiologists, American Society of Anesthesiologists, and International Anesthesia Research Society.

A physician anesthesia staff and resident training program were started at Jefferson by Dr. Hampton. His principal further contribution to anesthesiology was the development of a vaporizer for measured amounts of liquid halothane. This was a unique approach to the problem of accuracy of dosage. Following Dr. Hampton's resignation in 1964, Dr. Jay Joshua Jacoby was recruited for the Chair in 1965.

Jay J. Jacoby, M.D., Ph.D.; Second Chairman of Anesthesiology (1965–1984)

A native of New York City, where he was born in 1917, Dr. Jacoby (Figure 39-8) received his B.S. (1939), M.B. (1940), and M.D. (1941) degrees at the University of Minnesota. Afer internship at Kings County Hospital, New York (1941–1942), he became an anesthetist during World War II in the U.S. Army Medical Corps (1942–1945). After serving as the Surgeon of an air base near the North Pole, he was Anesthetist at the 40th General and 160th General Hospitals in England and France, and then with the 3rd Auxiliary Surgical Group of the First Army, from the Battle of the Bulge to the linking up with the Russian Army in Leipzig. His subsequent military career encompassed lecturer consultant duties for the Navy (1959–1965), the Air Force (1958–1965), and the Army (1966–1984). Upon returning to civilian life he became an Instructor in Anesthesiology at the University of Chicago (1946–1947) and earned a Ph.D. degree in Pharmacology. He then accepted the Directorship of the Department of Anesthesia and title of Associate Professor (1947–1950) and full Professor (1950–1959) at Ohio State University. The next university to beckon Dr. Jacoby was Marquette, where he served as Professor and Director of the Department of Anesthesiology (1959–1965).

Dr. Jacoby became a Diplomate of the American Board of Anesthesiology in 1948, a Fellow of the American College of Anesthesiologists in 1950 (Member, Board of Governors), and a member of the American Association of University Professors, the Association of University Anesthetists, the American Society of Anesthesiologists (Chairman of the Committee on Residencies and member of the Board of Directors), the International Anesthesia Research Society, the Central Surgical Association, the Ohio Society of Anesthetists (President, 1956), the Pennsylvania State Society of Anesthesiologists, and other related, prestigious societies.

In addition to Alpha Omega Alpha (1941) and Sigma Xi (1947), Jacoby was made an honorary member of the Jefferson Alumni Association in 1975, the same year in which the Senior Class commissioned his portrait for the College. He received the Lindback Award for Outstanding Teaching at Jefferson and similar awards at Ohio State and Marquette before his arrival at Jefferson.

Dr. Jacoby's Chairmanship (1965–1984) was an example of aggressive administration. He expanded the staff from four to 17 physician anesthesiologists. The residency program increased from two to 30 participants. The nurses training program was closed, with 11 of the nurse anesthetists remaining as permanent staff members. His continuous tenure as Director and Chairman of Anesthesia Departments in three medical colleges (1947–1984) was among the longest in the United States. He probably attracted as many young people to enter anesthesia, and trained as many Chairmen and Directors of Anesthesia in other institutions, as anyone in the country.

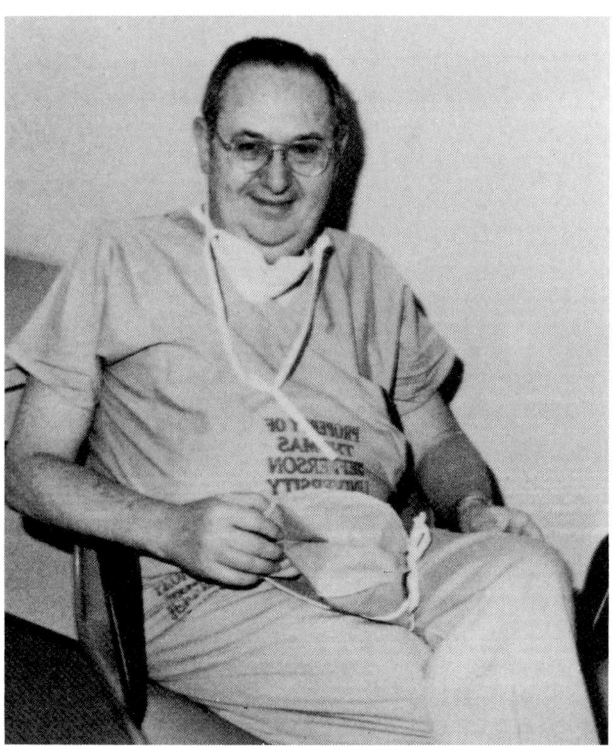

FIG. 39-8. Jay J. Jacoby, M.D., Ph.D.; Second Chairman of Anesthesiology (1965–1984).

Dr. Jacoby's practical expertise in administering anesthesia was legendary. He handled on a daily basis an almost unbelievable number of requests for his personal services to poor-risk patients, physicians and members of their families, students, and prominent people. To a surgeon at Jefferson, happiness was operating with Dr. Jacoby at the head of the table.

A prolific writer, Jacoby authored approximately 100 articles on anesthesia, including chapters in books. He became internationally known for blind nasal intubation to secure an adequate airway, scientifically labeled *Nasal Endotracheal Intubation by an External Visual Technique*. He developed transtracheal resuscitation and did pioneer work on air embolism during surgery. He originated the Code Blue system of resuscitation in hospitals.[10] Another of his contributions was "Jefferson Solution," which contained a balanced mixture of pentothal for induction and maintenance of anesthesia, curare to relax muscles, and morphine for analgesia. This concoction outside of scientific parlance was also known as "Jacoby's Soup." The indefatigable nature of Dr. Jacoby was further demonstrated when, after achieving Emeritus status in 1984, he preferred to continue on the staff as a practicing anesthesiologist.

In 1970 Dr. Arthur B. Tarrow (Figure 39-9) came to Jefferson as Professor and Associate Chairman. Having been a career Air Force officer, he served as Chief Anesthetist of the Air Force, as Commander of the Clark Field Hospital in the Philippines, as Surgeon of the Pacific Theater (18th Air Force) and finally as Inspector General.

His research involved blood transfusions and plasma substitutes, resuscitation, and rescue and recovery of astronauts. At Jefferson he developed the obstetrical anesthesia service and became a highly popular teacher. He retired in 1985.

Others who were prominent members of the Department were Drs. Harold F. Chase, Robert T. McSherry, William E.B. Scott, Ronald L. Clark, James C. Erickson, and Joseph B. Doto, Jr., Nellie Maloney, Virginia Anderson, Isabelle Widing and Elizabeth Phillips remained in the Department as nurse anesthetists for many years. Rose Marie Tomasello acted as a nurse administrator for more than 20 years.

Joseph L. Seltzer, M.D.; Third Chairman of Anesthesiology (1984–)

In 1984 Dr. Joseph Louis Seltzer (Figure 39-10) was appointed Professor and Chairman of the Department of Anesthesiology. Born in Pennsylvania in 1945, Dr. Seltzer received his B.S. degree (1967) from St. Joseph's College and his M.D. (1971) from Jefferson Medical College. After straight surgical internship at the Chandler Medical Center of the University of Kentucky (1971–1972) he took a Residency in general surgery (1972–1973) at Geisinger Medical Center and in anesthesiology (1973–1975) at Jefferson. He became a staff anesthesiologist at Wright-Patterson Air Force Base, Ohio (1975–1977), Assistant Attending Anesthesiologist of State University Hospital, Syracuse (1977–1980), and, in 1980, Attending Anesthesiologist at Jefferson, until his appointment as Chairman of the Department.

In addition to his academic appointments at Wright State University School of Medicine (Dayton, Ohio), University of New York Upstate Medical Center (Syracuse, New York) and Jefferson, Seltzer became a Fellow of the American College of Anesthesiology (1975) and Diplomate of the American Board of Anesthesiology (1976). He is a member of the American Society of Anesthesiologists, Society of Cardiovascular Anesthesiologists, and Association of Anesthesiologists of Great Britain and Ireland.

In less than a decade he authored or coauthored at least 20 articles relating to hazards and safety measures in anesthesia, as well as physiologic and pharmacologic research in the field. He contributed chapters to books, recorded audiotapes, and made many presentations at distant institutions for meetings or as a Visiting Professor.

Dr. Seltzer entered as Chairman of a Department that had matured under the dedication and wisdom of Dr. Jacoby. His youth, teaching, and research interests were challenged to make anesthesia more of a science, to probe its dangers and blessings ever farther, and to enhance the rich heritage of his alma mater.

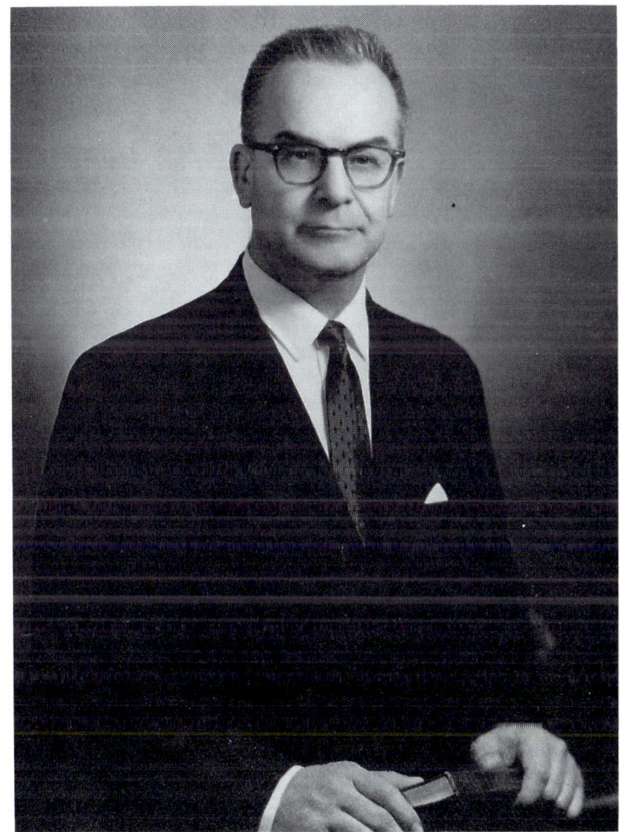

FIG. 39-9. Arthur B. Tarrow, M.D., Professor and Associate Chairman of Anesthesiology (1970–1985).

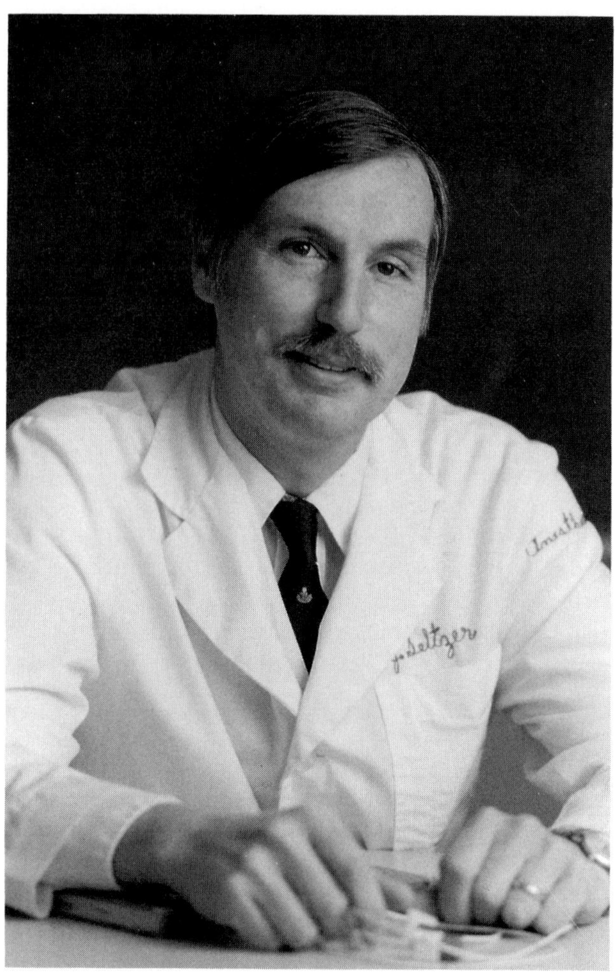

FIG. 39-10. Joseph L. Seltzer, M.D.; Third Chairman of Anesthesiology (1984–)

References

1. Thorwald, J., *The Century of the Surgeon*. Pantheon Books, New York: 1957, pp. 21–23.
2. Mettler, C.C., *History of Medicine*. Philadelphia: Blakiston Co., 1947, p. 220.
3. Wagner, F.B., Jr., "Revisit of Samuel D. Gross, M.D.," *Surg., Gynec. and Obst.,* 1981, Vol. 152, pp. 668–669.
4. Johns, E., *Thomas Eakins: The Heroism of Modern Life*. Princeton, New Jersey: Princeton University Press, 1983, p. 48.
5. Lemmon, W.T., "A Method for Continuous Spinal Anesthesia," *Ann. Surg.* 11:141–144, 1940.
6. Willauer, G., Chodoff, R., and Garcia-Oller, J.L., "Continuous Spinal Anesthesia for Thoracoplasty: A Report of 300 Cases," *J. Thor. Surg.* 16:438–443, 1947.
7. Willauer, G., Gartland, J., and De Tuerk, J.J., "Continuous Spinal Anesthesia for Thoracoplasty: Second Report," *J. Thor. Surg.* 20:296–303, 1950.
8. Allbritten, F.F., Jr., Haupt, G.J., and Amadeo, J.H.: "The Change in Pulmonary Alveolar Ventilation Achieved by Aiding the Deflation Phase of Respiration During Anesthesia for Surgical Operations," *Ann. Surg.* 140:569–582, 1954.
9. Drinker P., and McKhann, C.F., "The Use of a New Apparatus for the Prolonged Administration of Artificial Respiration," *J.A.M.A.* 92:1658–1660, 1929.
10. Ziegler, C.H., and Jacoby, J., "Emergency Service Within the Hospital," *J.A.M.A.* 164:1432, July 27, 1957.

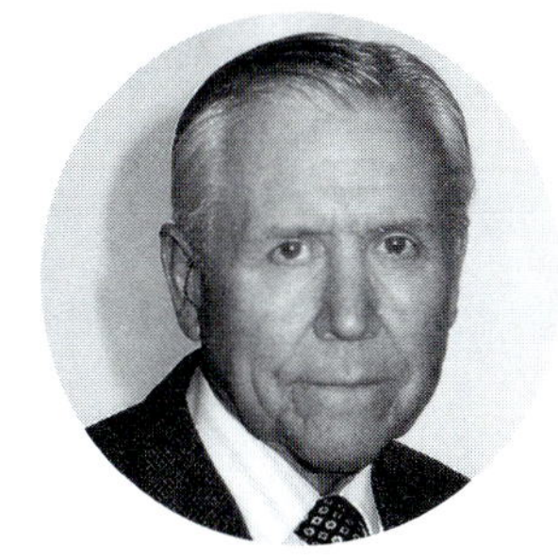

CHAPTER FORTY

Department of Neurosurgery

William H. Whiteley, M.D.

"With all our varied instruments of precision, useful as they are, nothing can replace the watchful eye, the alert ear, the tactful finger, and the logical mind which correlates the facts obtained through all these avenues of information and so reaches an exact diagnosis."

—W.W. Keen (1837–1932)

In order to appreciate the development of neurosurgery at Jefferson one should understand its growth in earlier years and other places. Archeologic evidence of ancient trephined skulls in Egypt and South America tempts the erroneous belief that the oldest form of the practice of medicine was neurosurgery by forgetting that soft tissues do not remain. Old methods persist, as testified to by the Korea of the early part of the twentieth century, where people were still trephining the skull for insertion of a needle to permit the escape of the "evil spirit" causing smallpox.[1]

The evolution of knowledge regarding the functions of the nervous system, its diseases, and particularly its surgical treatment had been relatively slow until the middle of the nineteenth century. Contributions came mainly from Italy, France, Germany, and England. In surgery, the focus was on head injuries, and military surgeons were prominent in the care of them. James Yonge[2] in 1682 collected 60 cases of brain wounds and wrote a book to refute the accusations that "all brain wounds were mortal."[3] Toward the end of the eighteenth century and the first half of the nineteenth, a curious reaction set in with regard to neurosurgical procedures. Surgeons were divided between those who continued to advocate trephining frequently and those who were very conservative.[4] The emphasis had been on the technique, almost as an end in itself, of creating an opening into the skull. Trephination, then craniectomy, and ultimately the modern osteoplastic flap initiated by Durante in Italy (1884) evolved. It is of interest that skull defects were repaired with coconut shells by South Sea Islanders, later by a gold plate (Petronius, 1565), canine bone (into the skull of a Russian monk by J. van Meekren, 1670), and celluloid (Fraenkel, 1890).[5] In 1888 R.F. Weir emphasized the importance of replacing the bone chips after craniectomy and noted that Clarke of Glasgow had already used this technique in 1886 (as had MacEwen since 1873).[6]

Undoubtedly some major innovators and contributors to the art have gone improperly recognized, or not at all. Berlinghieri dictated to a pupil a 488-page manuscript from 1810–1813, never published, detailing his technique for operating for meningiomas by craniectomy.[7] Traditionally, the priority is ascribed to Godlee in London (November 23, 1884) for the first successful removal of an intracranial (brain) tumor, followed by or before Durante's removal of a fibroma of the skull base on June 1, 1884 (1885?).[8] Nevertheless, MacEwen wrote that on about July 22, 1879, he had removed a "whole" intracranial meningeal tumor pressing on the frontal lobe.[9] Moreover, Pecchioli in Italy (1835) removed a meningioma of the right sinciput, and at 30 months there was no clinical evidence of recurrence.[10] In 1856 G. Gioppi in Italy cured a carotid-cavernous fistula by intermittent digital carotid artery compression.[10] It was May 9, 1883, when MacEwen removed a spinal, extradural fibrous neoplasm in a complete transection syndrome with remarkable recovery of the patient. Even Maydle in Vienna (1882) and Morris in New York (1885) had attempted to unite the severed ends of the spinal cord. Finally, Sir Victor Horsley (1857–1916), a giant in the development of neurosurgery in England, was the recorded first to remove an intradural meninigioma of the spinal cord (June 5, 1887).

Early Neurosurgery at Jefferson

Joseph Pancoast, Professor of Surgery at Jefferson (1839–1841) and Anatomy (1841–1874), in *A Treatise on Operative Surgery* (1844), did not include surgery of the nervous system except for a detailed, well-illustrated section on trephination of the skull for trauma. Nevertheless, in 1862 he devised a skillful operation to section the second and third divisions of the trigeminal nerve by transcoronoid approach to the skull base. Likewise, Thomas D. Mütter, Professor of Surgery at Jefferson (1841–1856), wrote extensively on trephination and general care of head injuries in his book on surgery (1846).[11]

In contrast, we find much about neurosurgery in *A System of Surgery* written in 1859 by Samuel D. Gross, Jefferson's esteemed Professor of Surgery from 1856 to 1882. One is struck by the great length of this and other medical texts of those days until one sorts out specifics from an incredible amount of verbosity. Gross wrote in a most detailed manner about diseases of the head and nerves, brain concussion, brain compression (by blood, bone, pus, and foreign body), details of trephination, and chronic hydrocephalus treated by puncture of the skull decades before ventricular puncture was first attributed to Keen in 1888 but actually proposed by Vose of New York and practiced by others before then. He also wrote a section on diseases and injuries of the spinal cord and column that included cord concussion, wounds, lateral curvature, tuberculosis, psoas abscess, and hydrorachitis (meningocele). In a sixth edition in 1882 he discussed tumors of the skull and dura and commented that Grosmann and Pecchioli were able to achieve total extirpation of dural tumors by trephining the skull. One of the earliest textbooks of neurosurgery was *Chirurgie Operatoire du Systeme Nerveux* by A. Chipault (1891). Considering the early state of the art this was quite sophisticated and well illustrated, with each of the two volumes consisting of more than 700 pages.

With so much surgical brilliance in those early days, one wonders why there was such a delay in the development of more modern neurological surgery. The answer lay in three deficits: lack of anesthesia, horrendous surgical sepsis, and the absence of any system of cerebral localization. When these problems were gradually solved by the explosion of medical knowledge and technique in the latter half of the nineteenth century, modern neurosurgery came alive. Ether anesthesia was initiated by Crawford Long, M.D., in 1842 and then "officially" by William Thomas Green Morton, D.D.S., in 1846. Joseph Lister first used carbolic acid for surgical antisepsis in an operation in August, 1865. George W. Corner has pointed to the contrast between the two surgical clinics painted by Thomas Eakins.[12] In the *Gross Clinic* of 1875 there is a pre-Listerian ambience to the scene, whereas a relatively antiseptic atmosphere is depicted in the *Agnew Clinic* of 1889. Lister's *Antiseptic Principle in the Practice of Surgery,* first published in 1867, was accepted very slowly and reluctantly. Lister visited Philadelphia in 1876. W.W. Keen heard him and is said to have been the first surgeon in Philadelphia to have adopted his technique.

The ophthalmoscope was invented by Babbage in 1847, but the idea was dropped until Helmholtz "officially" invented it in 1851. It appeared in neurologic diagnosis in 1860.

The concept of cerebral localization evolved more slowly and over many centuries, generating much controversy, especially when it was demonstrated that both cerebral hemispheres could be removed in a dog that thereafter could still walk. In 1861 Broca gave an autopsy demonstration of softening in the speech center in a man aphasic for 21 years. This led some to denote Broca "The Father of Neurosurgery." Alex Robertson (1866), Hughlings Jackson (1869), Fritsch and Hitzig (1870, cortical electrode stimulation on animals), and Ferrier (1870) provided laboratory and clinical proof to firmly establish the concept of cerebral localization and to permit accurate brain surgery well before the discovery of bone imaging by the X-ray beam in 1895–1896.

To William MacEwen of Glasgow belongs the distinction of chief pioneer of craniocerebral surgery.[13] Even before Rickman Godlee, F. Durante, or Victor Horsley, MacEwen operated successfully for intracranial tumor, abscess, and extramedullary spinal cord tumor.[14]

To William Williams Keen belongs the credit of being America's first brain surgeon. He was a general surgeon like the other pioneers who made great contributions in this field that became established by Harvey Cushing in the twentieth century. That chapter might have been written differently if MacEwen had not rejected the offer of the Chair of Surgery at Johns Hopkins, which went to William Halsted, because the Trustees could not assure him that the supervision and training of nurses would be under his absolute control.[15]

Philadelphia was not only the birthplace of medical education in America but also the focus for the investigation and care of nervous system diseases by Benjamin Rush, John Kearsley Mitchell, W.W. Gerhard, Robley Dunglison, S. Weir Mitchell, W.W. Keen, William Thomson, Roberts Bartholow, William Osler, Charles K. Mills, Francis X. Dercum, Eadwaard Muybridge, and many since then.[16] J. Ewing Mears (Jefferson, 1865), on the Jefferson surgical faculty in 1884, was the first to suggest Gasserian ganglionectomy for tic douloureux.[17]

W.W. Keen was a Philadelphian who, after graduating from Jefferson in 1862, was assigned by the Union Army to the Turner's Lane Army Hospital in Philadelphia to work with another surgeon, George R. Morehouse (Jefferson, 1850), and under S. Weir Mitchell (Jefferson, 1850) to care for war injuries of peripheral nerves. They documented their intensive study of 120 patients in an outstanding 164-page monograph, *Gunshot Wounds and Other Injuries of Nerves* (Lippincott, 1864), one of the most important medical contributions from the Civil War, and enunciated the concept of causalgia and reflex dystrophy. Of interest was a soldier they observed on July 15, 1863, in whom they documented and explained his traumatic Horner's syndrome six years before Horner's description. One is puzzled by the lack of any mention of surgical treatment for those nerve injuries. In 1866 Keen began teaching pathologic anatomy at Jefferson, which he continued for the next nine years. He concurrently directed the Philadelphia School of Anatomy, lecturing upon anatomy and operative surgery to "the largest private class ever assembled in this country."[18] In a historic operation in 1893 he assisted Dr. John Erdmann in the removal of a verrucous carcinoma from the upper jaw of President Grover Cleveland. This was performed in secret aboard the yacht *Oneida* on Long Island Sound.[19] He was a prolific author with a bibliography of at least 405 items. Of these, 249 were papers on medical, surgical, and allied subjects. The largest group, more than 50, were written on diseases of the nervous system.[20] He wrote on intracranial lesions, tapping and irrigating the lateral ventricles (for the first time, 1889), cortical ablation of the hand center for focal epilepsy (1890) utilizing electrical stimulation, and craniectomy for microcephalus in 1890. This was the first patient with this anomaly to be operated upon.[21] Keen also performed linear craniotomy for the same condition. In 1891 he devised and performed a new operation for spasmodic torticollis, namely, division of the upper cervical posterior primary nerve divisions.[22] Finney in 1925 said it was the first really carefully studied, scientific attempt to treat this condition. Keen also reported on Gasserian ganglionectomy, peripheral nerve surgery (including successful nerve grafting), and intracranial tumors. He wrote, edited, or made neurosurgical contributions to many important textbooks.[23–27]

Dr. Keen's most celebrated neurosurgical operation was the removal of an intracranial convexity meningioma from Theodore Daveler on December 15, 1887. This patient survived for more than 30 years. Dr. Aller G. Ellis, a Jefferson pathologist, then went to Lancaster, Pennsylvania, to perform the autopsy and retrieve the brain, which was free of any tumor. This was the first documented successful removal of an intracranial tumor with a proven cure.[28] The tumor specimen and the brain were demonstrated by Dr. William H. Whiteley for surgical neuropathology instruction at Jefferson for more than 15 years until the tumor was apparently thrown out by a careless workman at a bicentennial exhibit in Philadelphia in 1976. Some time later the brain itself also disappeared. Keen's historic operation was performed at Saint Mary's Hospital in Philadelphia, at which time he was Professor of Surgery at Woman's Medical College (1884–1889).

Upon the death of Samuel W. Gross in 1889, Keen became Professor of the Principles of Surgery and Clinical Surgery at Jefferson, occupying that chair until 1907. Dr. Edward L. Bauer noted that "William Williams Keen occupied the center of the surgical stage in America and indeed in the world for many years, even after the days of his Professorship."[29] Dr. John Fulton in his biography of Harvey Cushing identified Keen as "Cushing's principal predecessor in neurosurgery in this country."[30] Dr. Edward Klopp in the 1936 student yearbook remarked that Keen became America's first "Brain Surgeon" and was regarded as the foremost surgeon in the country.[31] Keen also had deep religious convictions and wrote and gave many addresses about theological, devotional, and church missionary matters. He wrote much for the lay press and was an outspoken proponent of vivisection experiments, although he participated very little in such. Dr. John Chalmers DaCosta portrayed him as a "wonderful operator—absolutely fearless—always in a heavenly temper—no superiors as a teacher."[32] It has been suggested that his need to counter the grief from the rather sudden death in 1886 of his wife, who was under the care of Dr. William Osler, drove him therapeutically to an intense level of work, writing, and other accomplishments.[33] Despite that analysis, he had already produced 34 medical papers, six lay papers, and four books before her death. Although Keen retired from practice and teaching in 1907, he continued to be most active and to receive many honorary degrees, honors, and awards until his death in 1932 at the age of 95.

The responsibility for neurosurgery at Jefferson must have been assumed by other general surgeons, although it is difficult to find much concrete evidence of this. In 1907 Alfred Gordon reported on a craniotomy performed by Francis T. Stewart, later Professor of Surgery at Jefferson.[34] John Chalmers DaCosta in 1894 published *A Manual of Modern Surgery,* in which there are three chapters on the surgery of the head, spine, and nerves. These chapters are even more comprehensive, and obviously still personalized, in the tenth edition of 1931. In the 1920s and early 1930s it seems that Dr. Thomas A. Shallow, Professor of Surgery (1931–1955), was responsible for neurosurgery.[35]

The focus of neurosurgery in Philadelphia temporarily shifted to Charles Harrison Frazier (1870–1936), the eminent neurosurgeon and Chairman of the Department of Surgery at the University of Pennsylvania, who was training Fellows in surgery and neurosurgery.

Dr. William Duane, Jr., was the first specific neurosurgeon at Jefferson (Figure 40-1). He was born in 1900, one of four children of William Duane, Ph.D., the illustrious physicist who worked with the Curies in Paris (1907–1913) as

Radium Research Assistant. Duane, Sr. then became Professor of Biophysics at Harvard (1917–1934). It may be significant that his assistant was William T. Bovie, Ph.D., to whom credit has been given for developing the high-frequency electrosurgical "knife" and coagulator in response to impetus from Harvey Cushing. Bovie received the John Scott Medal from the City of Philadelphia in 1928 for his achievement despite the claim by George A. Wyeth, M.D. of New York that he had perfected such an apparatus and presented it to the Surgical Section of the New York State Medical Society in April, 1924, two and a half years before Cushing's initial and famous operation using "the Bovie" on October 1, 1926.[36]

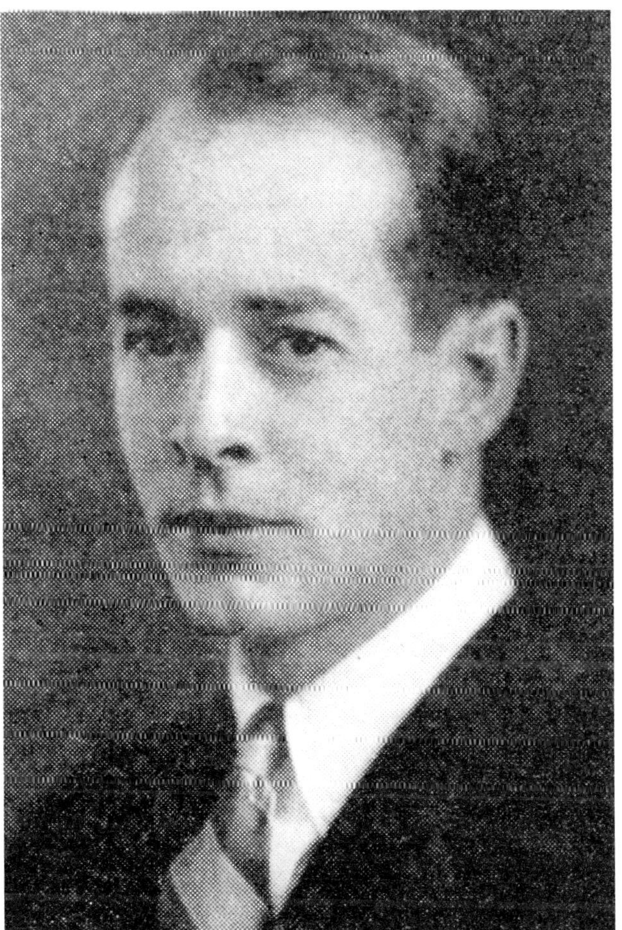

FIG. 40-1. William Duane, Jr., M.D., Jefferson's first specialized neurosurgeon. (Courtesy of Archives of University of Pennsylvania)

Duane, Jr., graduated with an A.B. degree from Harvard in 1923 and most likely was influenced by Bovie's work. He received his M.D. degree from the University of Pennsylvania in 1927 and was a research fellow under Frazier, finally becoming an Instructor in Surgery in Frazier's Department and later under Francis Grant, neurosurgery Chief. He was a neurosurgeon at the Philadelphia General, Mount Sinai, and Graduate Hospitals in Philadelphia when Dr. Thomas Shallow brought him to Jefferson as Demonstrator of Surgery in 1935 to be responsible for neurosurgery. He contributed little to the medical literature but did devise a modification of the McKenzie silver clip and applicator forceps, changing the shape of the clip from a *V* to a *U*.[37] Dr. William H. Whiteley (Jefferson, 1943) assisted Dr. Duane in May, 1943, in an unusual operation upon a man with a massive skull defect. Although Zander in 1940 was the first to use acrylic for cranioplasty, such had not really appeared in this country until Guardjian's as yet unreported case of 1942.[38,39] Duane persuaded an Air Force pilot friend to obtain a broken piece of extremely thick bomber nose which he meticulously and successfully shaped with a coping saw to fill in that skull defect. On October 11, 1943, Duane resigned to enter military service and served in the campaigns in Europe. In 1946 the *Philadelphia Inquirer* reported that he had cared for General Patton for his fatal cervical spine injury in Heidelburg, Germany. Duane abandoned neurosurgery after resuming civilian life, but was appointed Medical Instructor of Anatomy in the Medical School of the University of Pennsylvania (1948–1950). He died September 14, 1963, at the age of 62 after a long and chronic illness.

Jefferson's most important neurosurgical affiliations were with Wills Eye Hospital and the Wilmington Medical Center. Until 1938 neurology and neuro-ophthalmology at Wills were related to the Graduate Hospital and the Graduate School of Medicine of the University of Pennsylvania. Dr. Thomas A. Shallow, who was on the Board of City Trusts, had Dr. Duane appointed to Wills as Chief of the Neurology Service on June 10, 1938. Later he was joined by Dr. Nathan Schlezinger (Jefferson, 1932) who eventually replaced him in that position after a few years of titular command by Professor Bernard J. Alpers. On June 4, 1943, Dr. Duane became chief of the Neurosurgery Service, a consultative position, but only for a few months before entering military service. In the meantime, Dr. Rudolph Jaeger had arrived at Jefferson and shortly became the neurosurgical consultant at Wills, a position he retained for many years. All of this provided a vast number of both medical and surgical neurological/neuro-ophthalmological patients for Jefferson for both treatment and student and resident training. The loss of this pool of important and fascinating cases to another institution after about 1979 was most unfortunate for Jefferson.

John C. McNerney graduated from Jefferson in 1927, spent a year at Jefferson Hospital as Resident Physiological Chemist, and then two years as an Intern. After four years in general practice he became an Instructor in Anatomy at Yale, followed by a year's study in pathology, particularly neuropathology. This led to a year's training in neurosurgery under James G. Gardner at the Crile Clinic in Cleveland. He returned to Jefferson in 1937 to work under Dr. Duane and with him at the Philadelphia General Hospital. These were Jefferson's two neurosurgeons at the time. Dr. McNerney was on the faculty as Assistant Demonstrator of Anatomy (Neuroanatomy), but he left Jefferson in 1941 to become an Instructor in Neurosurgery at Temple University. Shortly thereafter he went into military service in World War II. In 1948 he became Chief of Neurosurgery at the Naval Medical Center at Bethesda, Maryland, for two years, eventually entering private practice in Stamford, Connecticut.

For the first time in the College circular of information of 1938–1939, neurosurgery was mentioned as a teaching discipline in the Department of Surgery, indicative of the slow development of this specialty in this institution. Jefferson's first neurosurgeon at professorial rank was Robert A. Groff.[40] He was a Philadelphian, born in 1903, and graduated from the Medical School of the University of Pennsylvania in 1928. A paternal uncle had graduated from Jefferson in 1898. Groff trained in neurosurgery under Charles Harrison Frazier and Francis Grant at the University of Pennsylvania, under Harvey Cushing in Boston, with Gordon Holmes at Queens Square, London, and with Otfrid Foerster in Breslau, Germany. He became a somewhat itinerant surgeon, working on the staffs of nine hospitals in the Philadelphia area. He was appointed as Assistant Professor of Neurosurgery at Jefferson on February 2, 1942, but served for less than one year, when he entered the army in World War II for four years. He was the first board-certified neurosurgeon (also in neurology) at Jefferson. After the war, he resigned from Jefferson on January 7, 1946, and returned to the Graduate Hospital and the University of Pennsylvania. He became Department Head and Professor of Neurosurgery until 1968 at the University and at the Graduate Hospital until his death in 1975. Groff published many articles, including a book in 1945 entitled *Manual of Diagnosis and Management of Peripheral Nerve Injuries*. Like W.W. Keen did from his Civil War experience, Groff incorporated his learning as a military surgeon. One of his greatest achievements was the training of about 40 neurosurgeons.

The American Board of Neurological Surgery was established in 1940. In 1933 there was only one training program in neurosurgery, at the Medical College of Virginia, with just one position available there. In 1934 there were six training centers in the United States providing nine positions. At the zenith, in 1964, there were 152 training program centers with 522 positions. In 1984, there were 94 programs and 674 positions in existence with 650 filled.[41] In Philadelphia in 1943 the only two training programs in neurosurgery were at the University of Pennsylvania and Temple University. The two cities in Pennsylvania where specific neurosurgical care was available were Pittsburgh and Philadelphia. At Jefferson as late as 1941–1943, Dr. William T. Lemmon, often called "the last of the great general surgeons," did most of the neurosurgery. The time was ripe and long overdue to establish a Department of Neurosurgery.

The Jaeger Years (1945–1961)

J. Rudolph Jaeger (Figure 40-2) was born October 29, 1895, on a farm near Clarksville, Missouri, a small village on the Mississippi River. He attended a one-room schoolhouse before high school, graduated from the University of Missouri, and received his M.D. degree from the University of Pennsylvania in 1920. After internship and chief residency at Denver General Hospital, he joined his uncle in the practice of general surgery in Denver, Colorado. He was also Instructor in Surgery and Neurology at the University of Colorado School of Medicine. He taught anatomy for six years and was in charge of pathology and physiology at the University of Denver School of Dentistry. It is not certain when or how he became interested in neurosurgery, but in 1928 when he foresaw the coming Great Depression, he moved his family to Baltimore and spent nine months with Walter Dandy, the famous neurosurgeon at Johns Hopkins. The totality of his neurosurgical training consisted of observation only, no patient care, and no personal surgical experience. Because neurosurgery was mostly cavitary and more instrumental than manual, he took Dandy's advice and spent much time in the ear, nose, and throat clinic examining cavities and learning to use and modify nasal instruments. He then returned to Denver as a surgical pioneer and became the first neurosurgeon not only there but in all the Rocky Mountain states.

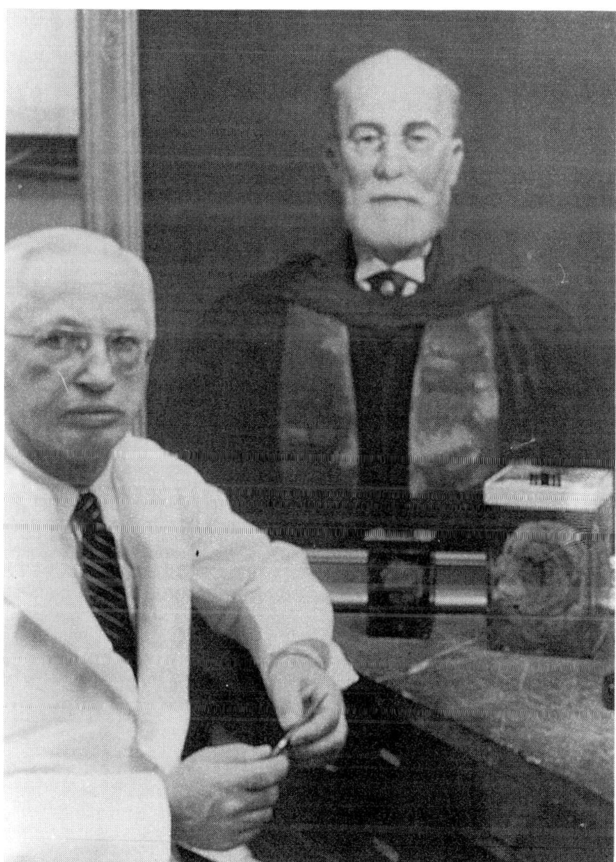

FIG. 40-2. Rudolf Jaeger, M.D., Head of the Division of Neurosurgery (1943–61). The portrait is that of W.W. Keen, Jefferson's pioneer in neurosurgery.

Until 1943 Dr. Jaeger's exceedingly busy professional life included being the only neurosurgeon on the staff of six hospitals and Chief of Neurosurgery at the University of Colorado School of Medicine. He wrote 14 of his eventual 61 scientific papers, and made most of the neurosurgical motion pictures for which he became famous. He spent much time and energy in teaching medical students, and he emphasized to the profession at large the benefits of neurosurgical care, in view of the rather widespread pessimism about it. In fact, as late as the 1960s there was a surgical professor at Jefferson whose routine greeting to this author was "Whiteley, how is your vegetable garden today?" Jaeger's motion pictures were dramatic demonstrations of surgical triumphs, very popular at scientific meetings and conventions. He was the first to show a motion picture at an American Medical Association convention exhibit. By 1959 he and Dr. Whiteley had produced 21 films detailing all the major neurosurgical procedures.

In late 1942 Jaeger was seeking relief from the overwhelming burden of work in Denver. He was also President-Elect of the United States Chapter of the International College of Surgeons, of which Professor Thomas A. Shallow at Jefferson was President. The invitation from Shallow and Dean Harvey Perkins to come to Jefferson, confine his activities to this institution, and initiate and develop a Department of Neurologic Surgery was therefore most welcome. To that time he had not trained Residents and was anxious to do so. Dr. William Whiteley was selected as Jaeger's first Resident after a directive from the Board of Trustees of May 25, 1943, initiated a Division of Neurosurgery in the Department of Surgery. It remained a Division until it obtained Departmental status in July, 1969.

A serious problem in Jaeger's leaving Denver in early 1943 related to the war and the efforts by the government and the medical profession to continue to provide adequate community health care. The other three neurosurgeons had already gone into military service and Jaeger was the only one remaining for a vast geographical area. When the War Manpower Commission heard of his proposed move to Jefferson it raised a great outcry and objection. Of course Jaeger had no intention of leaving until he found his own replacement, which became Olan Hyndman of Iowa City, Iowa.

Jaeger, like other surgeons at Jefferson, had to be in charge of his own anesthesia. When he arrived he brought along his own equipment for administering inhalation anesthesia and for endotracheal intubation, including his suction pump and a blow torch that he had personally modified and transformed into an adapter for giving open-drop ether. Dispersion of operating rooms on the second, third, fourth, sixth, eighth, and fourteenth floors, and in three different buildings, not including the outpatient department, constituted an anesthesiologist's nightmare. It was not until 1955, after the Foerderer Pavilion had been erected (1954), that operating space was concentrated and a Department of Anesthesia begun.

Instrumentation was inadequate and required designing, crafting, modifying, and repairing, all in a special departmental workshop. Innovations in specialized pre- and postoperative care were needed. A neurosurgical art/photography facility for scientific papers, teaching, and scientific exhibits had to be developed. Other demands included teaching medical students, nurses, residents, and the profession at large, conducting neuroradiologic procedures and, finally, developing an experimental research laboratory. Jaeger was not only a skillful surgical technician but mechanically ingenious and an innovator. He devised many neurosurgical instruments and operative techniques, which included an excellent headlight that he eventually manufactured and marketed, aluminum and gold aneurysm clips and applicator forceps, disc removal curettes, forceps and retractors, apparatus and monitoring techniques for safe surgery in the erect position, a method of and instrumentation for continuous spinal drainage during brain surgery, an improved technique for cordotomy with more permanent results, and a catheter technique for intravenous fluid and blood administration, long before any commercial devices were available. He also developed a technique for fractional prefrontal lobotomy using at first electrocoagulation and then hot water injections into the frontal lobes. Especially effective was his method of Gasserian ganglion destruction through percutaneous hot water injection for the relief of tic doloureux and cancer pain. One week before he died he performed that technique on his five hundred twenty-fifth injection patient with tic doloureux.

In those days the neurosurgeon performed all neuroradiology procedures except for some pneumoencephalograms and myelograms, which the medical neurologist shared. In 1949 a neurology Resident, Dan C. Donald, Jr., devised a method of cerebral angiography that was performed by the neurosurgical resident, Stacy L. Rollins, Jr. (Jefferson, J1944).[42] This was the beginning of percutaneous cerebral (carotid) catheter angiography, and it is significant that Jefferson residents took the initiative in originating this now common procedure.[43] Many years later (1972), Dr. Rollins removed the spinal canal bullet from Alabama Governor George Wallace, following the assassination attempt on his life.

Jaeger's varied accomplishments may be ascribed to his high energy level with self-drive, which also drove others as an intense but reasonable disciplinarian. He was a great believer in precept and personal supervision of his Residents. He probably would have delegated much less had he the time to do things himself. He required much from his Residents, but to them he gave much attention. For several years he required that each Resident manufacture his own headlight before certifying the completion of his Residency. He struggled constantly to influence the institution to fulfill its commitments to him. He did succeed, however, largely because of his Prussian background and persistent, insistent attitude. Such persistence often surfaced in his stubborn perseverance at surgery, intent on cure rather than palliation, an attitude he may well have acquired from Walter Dandy in his months at Johns Hopkins.[44] The humorous, generous, and caring side of his personality surfaced periodically at work and routinely at play.

Dr. Jaeger was responsible for the training of 12 Residents and was involved in the training of nine more after he retired as Divisional Chief in 1961. He remained professionally active until about two days before he died on August 16, 1968.

Many of those outstanding Residents had distinguished subsequent careers. The most prestigious of these was Tai Joon Moon (Figure 40-3), Resident in neurosurgery from 1954 through 1957 and also fellow in the Department of Neurology at Jefferson in 1957. He graduated from the College of Medicine, Seoul National University, Seoul, Korea, in 1950, received a doctorate in medical science from Nippon University, Japan, in 1960, and was Chairman and Professor of Neurosurgery at Yonsei University, College of Medicine in Seoul from 1958 to 1966. He pioneered neurosurgery in Korea and established the Korean Board of Neurosurgery to supervise training and certification as in the United States. Many of his Residents later became chairmen of neurosurgical departments in other Korean medical colleges. He became President of the Korean Neurosurgical Society, Korean Medical Association (two consecutive terms), and Confederation of the Medical Associations in Asia and Oceania. He became involved in politics and was elected a Senator in the Korean National Assembly for ten years. He introduced the continuing educational program for Korean physicians, founded the medical malpractice

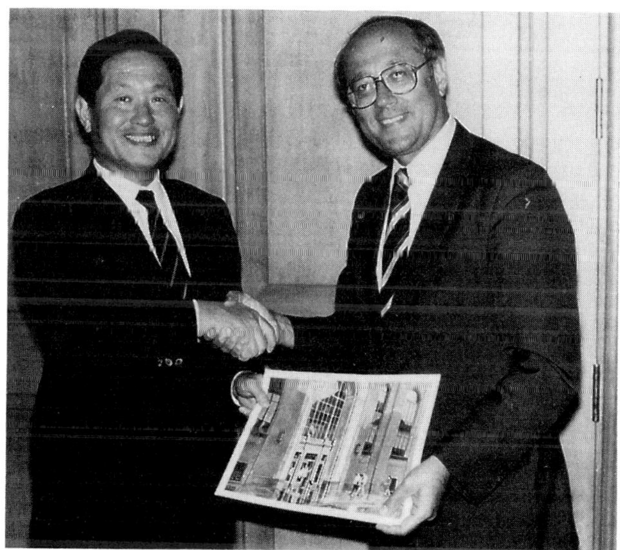

FIG. 40-3. Tai Joon Moon, neurosurgical Resident (1954–1957), shown with Dean Gonnella. Moon was President of the World Medical Association (1985). He received an honorary degree at Jefferson (1987).

insurance program under the Korean Medical Association, and introduced national health insurance for the entire population. He thus had enormous influence upon medical education and upon health care in his own country, to which he returned instead of succumbing to the desire for a medical career in the country of his training. In 1985 he was elected President of the World Medical Association and in 1987 received an honorary degree at Jefferson.

Jaeger's major contributions to the neurosurgical field included hydrothermal prefrontal lobotomy, hydrothermal Gasserian ganglionectomy, surgical demonstration of the spinal cord localization as the site of the injury in brachial plexus avulsion, muscle embolization of carotid-cavernous fistula preceded by distal internal carotid ligation (later known as the "Jaeger maneuver"), and discovery of the irritating effects of emulsified, iodized vegetable oils on the brain and spinal cord. It is a significant reflection of his personality that only eight of his 61 papers had coauthors. Just two of his papers dealt with laboratory subjects, which indicated his clinical rather than laboratory orientation. Nevertheless, he knew the importance of research and would have performed more had he had time to do so. As it was, in the mid-1950s he organized, designed, and set up a laboratory in the college building on Walnut Street and appointed David J. LaFia (Jefferson, 1947), staff neurosurgeon and Instructor in Neurosurgery, as Research Associate in charge of the laboratory under the chief's direction. Their investigations and publications included "The Effects of Renografin as a New Contrast Medium for Cerebral Angiography" and "The Effects of Respiratory Airway Obstruction on the Brain During Craniotomy Under Normothermic and Hypothermic Status." Dr. LaFia went on to publish many clinical, scientific, and literary papers and to develop hospital neurosurgical services elsewhere in Philadelphia, Miami, and California.

Dr. Jaeger had a provincial outlook in organizational medicine, despite his Presidency of the United States Chapter of the International College of Surgeons in 1944, a position he resigned because he could not tolerate the aggressive interference of Dr. Max Thorek, a founder of the International College. This was purposeful, for he believed he should not dissipate his energies at the national level. Thus, he conceived of the Philadelphia Neurosurgical Society, which he formed in 1958 with the help and cooperation of the other academic chiefs of neurosurgery in Philadelphia, namely Robert Groff of the University of Pennsylvania, Axel Olsen of Hahnemann Medical College, and especially Michael Scott (Jefferson, 1932) of Temple University.[45] This society included neurosurgeons not only from Philadelphia but throughout Pennsylvania, New Jersey, Delaware, Maryland, and Washington, D.C. The name was changed to the Mid-Atlantic Neurosurgical Society in 1967. Although its patron saint was Charles Harrison Frazier, it owed its existence to J. Rudolph Jaeger.

During the Jaeger years other staff members at Jefferson included Drs. Stacy L. Rollins, Jr. (Jefferson, J1944), Joseph A. Brady, and Henry Keen Shoemaker (Jefferson, 1949).

The Rovit Years (1961–1965)

Jaeger became 65 in October, 1960, but continued to serve until July 1, 1961, when he was succeeded by Richard L. Rovit (Figure 40-4), who was appointed as Associate Professor of Surgery (Neurosurgery) and Head of the Division of Neurological Surgery. Dr. Rovit was born in 1924, received his undergraduate education at the University of Michigan, and obtained his M.D. from Jefferson in 1950. His postgraduate training in neurosurgery and allied disciplines was in Boston (Beth Israel Hospital, Massachusetts General Hospital, and The Lahey Clinic), in London (The National Hospital, Queens Square), and in Montreal (The Montreal Neurological Institute). Before coming to Jefferson he had research and teaching fellowships at Harvard Medical School and McGill University Medical School and was on the staff of the Montreal Neurological Institute as Assistant Neurosurgeon (1960–1961). During his tenure at Jefferson there was a partial shift from a primarily clinical and technical emphasis to a more academic and research approach. The residency training program was modestly revised in those directions. The Residents were successfully assigned to writing scientific papers as their time permitted. Of the 18 papers produced by Dr. Rovit during or related to his Jefferson years, four were coauthored with Residents. Into 1984 he had written 108 papers, mostly clinical in nature and varied in scope.

Dr. Rovit resigned from Jefferson July 15, 1966, to become Chairman of the Department of Neurological Surgery at Saint Vincent's Hospital and Medical Center in New York City and Professor (1970) of Clinical Neurosurgery at New York University School of Medicine. He became distinguished at local and national levels in clinical, academic, and organizational neurosurgical affairs.

Rovit was instrumental in bringing Dr. Nicholas T. Zervas to Jefferson in 1962. Zervas was born in 1929, received his A.B. from Harvard, and obtained his M.D. from the University of Chicago School of Medicine. He trained at Montreal Neurological Institute, Massachusetts General Hospital, and the University of Paris in

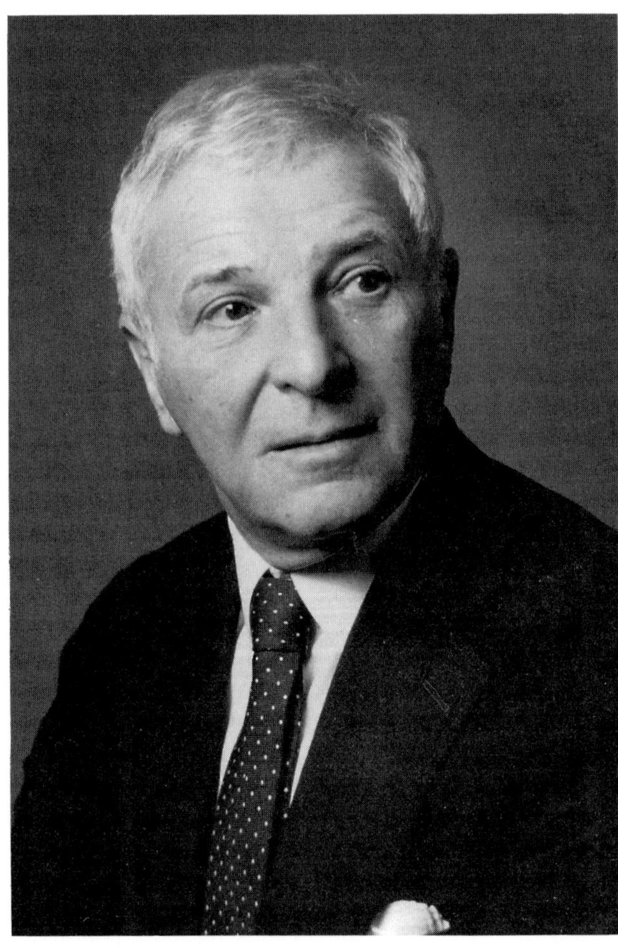

FIG. 40-4. Richard L. Rovit, M.D., Head of the Division of Neurosurgery (1961–1965).

stereotactic cerebral surgery under Dr. Jean Talairach. He came to Jefferson as Associate in Neurosurgery and later became Assistant Professor of Surgery (Neurosurgery). His chief interests were in stereotactic research and surgery as applied to destructive lesions in the thalamus and particularly the cerebellum for movement disorders, and also in thermal, radiofrequency hypophysectomy for breast cancer and diabetic retinopathy. It is of historic interest that these highly successful procedures were eventually supplanted by medical management. Of Zervas's more than 175 scientific papers and abstracts of mixed laboratory and clinical nature, 12 were during or related to his years at Jefferson. He resigned in December, 1967, to become Chief of the Neurosurgical Service at Beth Israel Hospital and Assistant Professor of Surgery (Neurosurgery) at Harvard Medical School. In 1977 he became Chief of the Neurosurgical Service at Massachusetts General Hospital and Professor of Surgery at Harvard Medical School.

The Gordy Years (1965–1973); The Division Under Gordy

Philip D. Gordy (Figure 40-5) was appointed in September, 1965, as Professor of Surgery (Neurosurgery) and Head of that Division of the Department of Surgery. He was born in Southhampton, Pennsylvania, in 1918, and received his A.B. from the University of Michigan and M.D. from its medical school. He trained at New York Hospital and at the University of Michigan. Immediately in 1949 he entered the private practice of neurosurgery in Wilmington, Delaware, until 1962. He then joined the Department of Neurological Surgery at the University of Oregon Medical School, becoming Professor there in 1964. He was a founding member of the Congress of Neurological Surgeons and eventually its President in 1959.

After his arrival Dr. Gordy proceeded to transfer the Division to very large and renovated quarters, formerly occupied by the Department of Pathology on the fifth floor of the Medical College building on Walnut Street. This provided several private offices, a large meeting room, and ample, expanded laboratory space. Laboratory activities, however, were temporarily suspended following Dr. Zervas's departure pending successful acquisition of a research scientist to continue in this area. Twelve Residents were involved in the well-balanced training program during the Gordy years. He enhanced this program by improving communications at the national accrediting level, intensifying the journal club, instigating monthly morbidity/mortality conferences, establishing a joint training venture with the Department of Neurology, and, in particular, creating a teaching affiliation with Wilmington Medical Center. This provided an additional 1,000 beds for residency training and greatly improved Jefferson's accreditation position so that two new Residents were approved for each

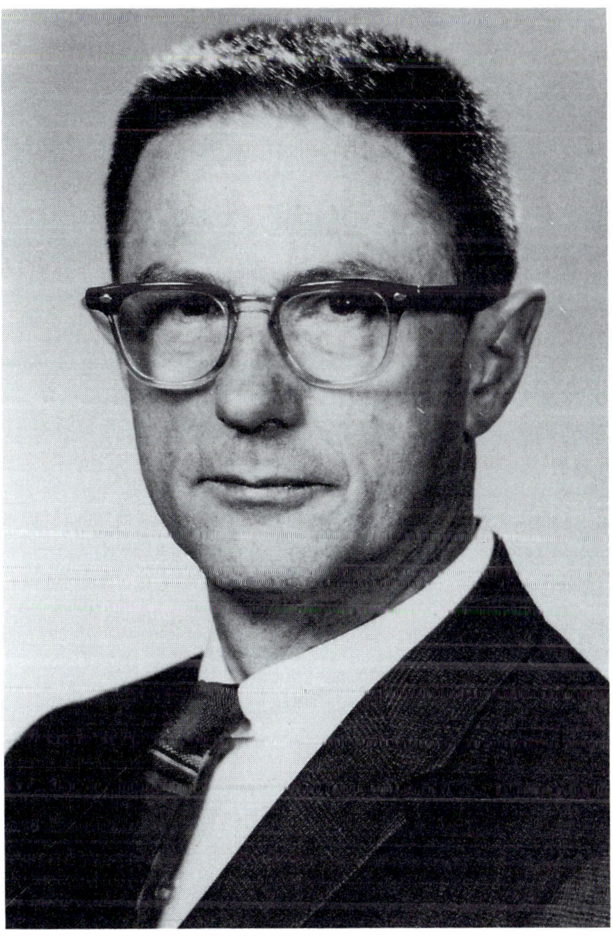

FIG. 40-5. Philip D. Gordy, M.D., Professor of Neurosurgery (1965–1969); Chairman of the Department of Neurosurgery (1969–1973).

year. This affiliation began July 1, 1970, and lasted for 14 pleasant and rewarding years until the accrediting board forced its dissolution on June 30, 1984, because it no longer satisfied more stringent requirements.

There continued to be vigorous teaching of third- and fourth-year medical students during the Gordy years at didactic, bedside, seminar, journal club, and conference levels at Jefferson and affiliated hospitals, including clinical neurosurgery, neurosurgical pathology, and neurophysiology.

Seven neurosurgeons were added to the staff, mostly for teaching purposes at Jefferson or its affiliates: Samuel S. Lyness (Bryn Mawr Hospital), Robert K. Jones and Howard A. Richter (Lankenau Hospital), David A. Yazdan (Jefferson), Livio Olmedo and Martin Gibbs (Wilmington Medical Center), and Harold B. Vogel (Jefferson). In 1974 Harold Haft was appointed from Methodist Hospital and Delaware County Memorial Hospital.

The Division continued to be busy clinically and the Wills Eye neurology affiliation provided a large source of surgical neuro-ophthalmological problems. An operating microscope was obtained soon after microneurosurgery was introduced and this greatly enhanced surgical techniques and teaching.

Stereotactic radiofrequency hypophysectomy continued for diabetic retinopathy and for breast or prostatic cancer. Radiofrequency Gasserian ganglionectomy was begun. Contributions continued to be made to the literature on a variety of clinical topics.

▪ The Neurosurgery Department Established (1969)

One of Dr. Gordy's outstanding accomplishments was the creation of a separate Department of Neurosurgery, converting from its Divisional status in the Department of Surgery on July 1, 1969. This autonomy greatly facilitated Departmental administration, residency training, and budgetary matters.

Another contribution by Gordy was his inauguration of citywide "Grand Rounds," monthly meetings of all the teaching neurosurgical services in Philadelphia for presentations of clinical cases of unusual interest. These meetings were hosted by the various schools, providing a forum for more broad-based discussion of problems and augmenting relationships between the five schools of medicine and their neurosurgeons. Unfortunately, this program ceased after a year or so, probably because of the multiplicity of meetings and obligations.

Harold B. Vogel arrived from the University of Utah College of Medicine on August 25, 1971, to reestablish and direct the laboratory, and was formally appointed Assistant Professor of Neurosurgery on April 3, 1972. He was born in Baltimore in 1932, received his B.A. from Emory University, his M.D. from the Medical College of Virginia, and trained at Albany Medical Center Hospital. Dr. Vogel was interested in brain tumor antigens and proceeded to investigate these by heterotransplantation of normal tissue and human brain tumors on chick chorioallantoic membrane. The focus later shifted to brain tumor tissue cultures after he brought in Debdas Mukerjee, Ph.D., from the M.D. Anderson Hospital in Houston, Texas, as Research Associate Professor. Mukerjee continued his investigations of the viral transformation of fibroblasts. The effect of androsterone and estradiol on cell cultures of human meningiomas was also studied. A.R. Vasantha Kumar, who had trained at the University of California and the University of Vermont, was appointed in 1973 as Clinical Assistant Professor of Neurosurgery. He had studied the effect of procarbazine in the treatment of brain tumors as well as the rate of removal of dead tumor cells from the various body tissues. Another line of investigation, in conjunction with the Department of Neurology, involved the study of spinal cord-evoked potentials in cats and humans in response to a variety of stimulations.

A transitional period occurred when Dr. Gordy requested a leave of absence for reasons of health in January, 1973, to enter private practice in Casper, Wyoming. In 1984 he introduced, developed, and headed a Department of Rehabilitation in the Natrona County Hospital in Casper. Dr. Vogel served as Acting Chairman of the Jefferson Department from June 18, 1973, until August 31, 1974, when he resigned to become Associate Professor in the Division of Neurosurgery at the University of Colorado

Medical School and Chief of Neurosurgery at Denver General Hospital. He continued there in practice and teaching and contributing to the medical literature.

The Osterholm Years (1974–)

Jewell L. Osterholm (Figure 40-6) was appointed Professor and Chairman of the Department of Neurosurgery in October, 1974. He was born in Montana in 1929, attended Montana State University, and received his M.D. from Washington University School of Medicine in 1957. His postgraduate training in neuropathology, neurology, and neurosurgery was at the Montreal Neurologic Institute of McGill University. Immediately thereafter, in 1963, he came to the neurosurgical service at Hahnemann Medical College under Axel Olsen. In 1967 he became Director of the Division of Neurological Surgery there, and soon became Director of the new residency training program, spinal cord injury center, and neurosurgical research laboratories. He came to Jefferson as an experienced administrator with an active research program and a large surgical practice. An efficient administrative organization was promptly established. Departmental offices, conference rooms, and laboratory facilities were all radically renovated and a Departmental library begun and constantly expanded.

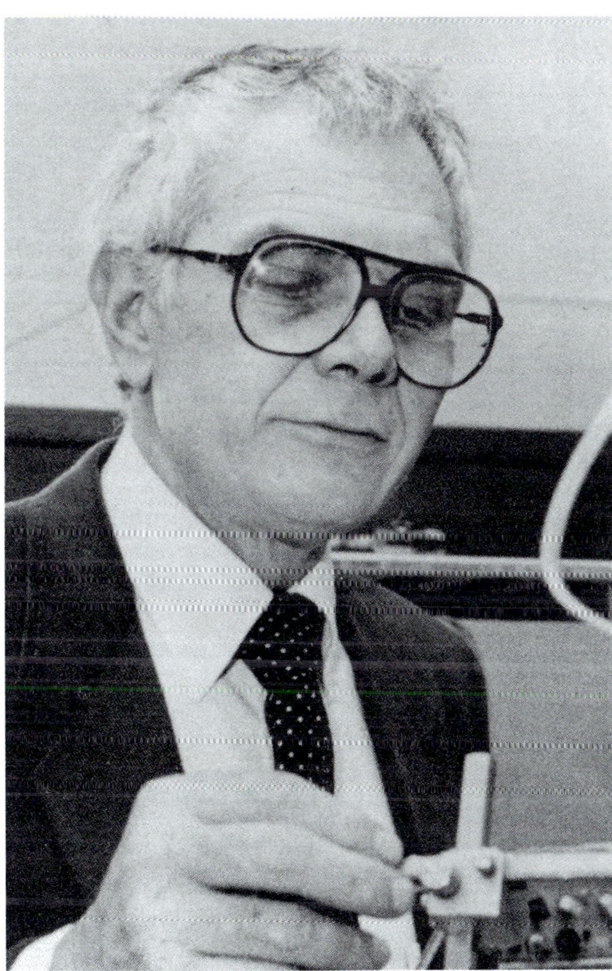

FIG. 40-6. Jewell L. Osterholm, M.D., Chairman of the Department of Neurosurgery (1974–).

Except for a few lectures, the medical student teaching of neurosurgery was abruptly curtailed in June, 1975. It no longer had a core status in the curriculum, and few chose it as an elective in the clinical years. This lack of student exposure to such an important diagnostic and therapeutic discipline in the understanding and management of nervous system diseases was naturally deplored.

On the other hand, residency training greatly accelerated and improved. The number of positions rose to six and as high as eight in 1981–1982. By 1980–1981 the Jefferson/Wilmington program provided more than 1,300 major neurosurgical operations yearly. The disappointment was deep when this relationship had to be terminated in 1984. Although the training program was not crippled in view of the progressively large increase in numbers of both patients and major surgical procedures at Jefferson, there remained optimism about restructuring and resuming the affiliation. By 1983–1984 there were more than 50 applications for each residency position offered yearly. Residency training in both Neurosurgery and Neurology was enhanced, starting in 1982, when an admitting arrangement was developed between these two Departments to provide wider sharing of neurosurgical patients and a more broad-based diagnostic workup. Neurosurgical residents became involved with ancillary disciplines such as the basic neurosciences, neuroradiology, neuropathology, pediatric neurosurgery, medical isotopic diagnosis, electrodiagnosis, and the neurosurgical laboratories. With regard to neuroradiology, a decided change had gradually occurred nationally in the 1970s as this activity, except for some myelography, progressively passed from the hands of neurosurgeons to radiologists. Resident attendance at various local and national conferences became routine. A microneurosurgical laboratory was installed to provide facility in that skill. Board-certification success remained excellent among the Residents.

In the area of patient care, the most modern methods of neurosurgical therapy became routine: very sophisticated monitoring and care in the neurointensive care unit; both radiofrequency rhizotomy and implantation of morphine pumps for intractable pain; television monitoring in surgery as a technical and teaching adjunct; expansion in the use of microsurgery for aneurysms, cranial nerve lesions, transphenoidal pituitary procedures, and spinal cord or intervertebral disc surgery; laser surgery; combined neurosurgery/ear, nose, and throat procedures; extra-intracranial vascular bypass surgery in conjunction with electroencephalogram monitoring and regional blood flow studies; and combined neurosurgical/orthopedic spinal surgery.

This last discipline was an outgrowth of the Regional Spinal Cord Injury Center of Delaware Valley, which was established at Jefferson by the Department of Health, Education and Welfare in October, 1978 (opening on January 1, 1979) under the aegis of the Department of Rehabilitation Medicine in conjunction with the Departments of Neurosurgery and Orthopedic Surgery. In 1983–1984 more than 50% of the neurosurgical service census consisted of spinal cord injury patients and more than 100 such acute patients were admitted to the service yearly.

The progressive intensity of clinical and teaching activity demanded an expansion of the Departmental staff. Lucas Martinez trained in neurosurgery at Hahnemann Medical College and served as a staff neurosurgeon at Jefferson from 1976 to 1980. Bruce E. Northrup came to Jefferson in 1978 as Assistant Professor of Neurosurgery. He was born in Ohio in 1938, was educated at Amherst College and Ohio State University, and received his M.D. from the latter. He trained in neurosurgery at the Johns Hopkins Hospital and came from the University of North Dakota School of Medicine to Jefferson. His special interest was in vascular and spinal disorders.

Donald L. Myers was born in Ithaca, New York, in 1951, attended Pennsylvania State University, received his M.D. from Jefferson in 1975, and trained in neurosurgery at Jefferson. He became Clinical Assistant Professor of Neurosurgery and developed a special interest in the management of intractable pain with morphine pump implantation, and with skull base and acoustic neurinoma surgery. Robert M. Cohen finished his training in neurosurgery at Jefferson in 1971 and entered private practice. He was appointed Instructor in Neurosurgery at Jefferson in 1980 and contributed regularly to the teaching program.

An outstanding feature of the Osterholm years was the intense activity in laboratory research, eventually requiring a move to new, expanded quarters in Alumni Hall. In the early years the research Professors, John L. Alderman, Ph.D., and John D. Irvin, M.D., Ph.D. (who for a time was also a neurosurgical resident), and Mr. Richard Moberg conducted research under Dr. Osterholm. They focused mainly on the reactions of the spinal cord to trauma and its histopathologic, metabolic, neurotransmitter, vascular, and electrophysiologic responses. Numerous grants were obtained, presentations made, and papers published in these areas. Research branched out into the fields of neuroanatomy, neurochemistry, neuropharmacology, histofluorescence, radioautography, and regional blood flow. Interdepartmental collaboration involved anatomy, neuropathology, and pharmacology with contributions by the pharmacologists Anthony Triolo, Ph.D., and C. Paul Bianchi, Ph.D. In 1978 Dr. Osterholm published a book entitled *The Pathophysiology of Spinal Cord Trauma.* Subsequently Madhu Kalia, M.D., came on the research staff as Professor of Neurosurgery and pursued her interests in the neurochemical and morphofunctional features of nerve pathways and nuclei.

In 1977–1978 the research emphasis began to shift gradually to the study of stroke and the relief of cerebral ischemia and cellular anoxia by the unique means of extravascular hyperoxygenation through perfusion of the third circulation with a balanced oxygenated fluorocarbon emulsion. Bikash Bose, who completed his neurosurgical residency training at Jefferson in 1984, was instrumental in establishing a reliable stroke model and in evaluating the effects of the therapeutic perfusion upon regional cerebral ischemia. This project eventually dominated the research program, was well funded, and had most favorable progress. Nine United States patents related to the method were granted to Dr. Osterholm in 1984. In April 1985 he received an award as Inventor of the Year for 1984.

Jefferson, as the birthplace of pioneer neurosurgery in the United States under W.W. Keen, has continued to nurture this rapidly expanding specialty. Increasing momentum in the progressive growth of the Department augurs well for Jefferson's honored position in this field.

References

1. Personal communication, William H. Chrisholm, M.D., missionary surgeon (deceased).
2. Yonge, J., *Wounds of the Brain Proved Curable.* London: H. Fairthorn, 1682.
3. Sachs, E., "The History and Development of Neurologic Surgery," New York: Paul B. Hoeber, 1952, p. 46.
4. Ibid., p. 49.
5. Reeves, D.L., *Cranioplasty.* Springfield, Illinois: Charles C. Thomas, 1950.
6. Weir, R.F., and Sequin, E.C., "Contribution to the Diagnosis and Surgical Treatment of Tumors of the Cerebrum," *Am. J. Med. Sci.* 96:228, September 1888.
7. Bucy, P.C., ed., *Neurosurgical Giants: Feet of Clay and Iron.* New York: Elsevier, 1985.
8. Kirkpatrick, D.B., "The First Primary Brain Tumor Operation," *J. Neurosurg.* 61:809, November 1984.
9. MacEwen, W., "Intracranial lesions," *Lancet* 2:581–582, 1881.
10. Bucy, P.C., ed., *Neurosurgical Giants: Feet of Clay and Iron.* New York: Elsevier, 1985.
11. Liston, R., and Mütter, T.D., *Lectures on the Operations of Surgery.* Philadelphia: Lea and Blanchard, 1846, pp. 71–93.
12. Corner, G.W., *Two Centuries of Medicine.* Philadelphia: Lippincott, 1965, pp. 174–175.
13. Cushing, H., "MacEwen Memorial Lecture on the Meningiomas Arising from the Olfactory Groove," *Lancet* 1:1329–1339, June 25, 1927, p. 1339.
14. MacEwen, W., "On the Surgery of the Brain and Spinal Cord," *Med. News* 53:168, August 18, 1888.
15. Walker, A.E., ed., *A History of Neurological Surgery.* Baltimore: Williams and Wilkins, 1951, p. 178.
16. Rogers, F.B., "Neurology in Philadelphia: Personalities and Events," *Pharos* 23:84–90, 1960.
17. Dercum, F.X., ed., *A Textbook on Nervous Diseases.* Philadelphia: Lea Brothers, 1895, p. 978.
18. Atkinson, W.B., *Physicians and Surgeons of the United States.* Philadelphia: Charles Robson, 1878, p. 74.
19. Keen, W.W., *The Surgical Operations on President Cleveland in 1893.* Philadelphia: George W. Jacobs and Co., 1917.
20. Geist, D.C., "The Writings of William Williams Keen, M.D., Hon. F.R.C.S.: A Selective Annotated Bibliography," *Trans. Stud. Coll. Phys. Phila.* 43:337–371, April 1976.
21. Ibid., p. 345.
22. Keen, W.W., "A New Operation for Spasmodic Wry Neck, Namely, Division and Exsection of the Nerves Supplying the Posterior Rotator Muscles of the Head," *Ann. Surg.* 13:44–47, 1891.
23. Keen, W.W., ed., *Diagnosis of the Nerves of the Human Body* by Flower, W.H., Philadelphia: Turner Hamilton, 1874.
24. Keen, W.W., ed., *Gray's Anatomy, Descriptive and Surgical. A New American Edition from the Eleventh English Edition.* Philadelphia: Lea Brothers and Co., 1887.
25. Keen, W.W., and White, J.W., eds., *An American Textbook of Surgery for Practitioners and Students.* Philadelphia: W.B. Saunders, 1892.
26. Keen, W.W., "Surgery of the Brain, Spinal Cord, and Nerves," in *A Textbook on Nervous Disease,* by Dercum, F.X. Philadelphia: Lea Brothers and Co., 1895.
27. Keen, W.W., ed., *Surgery: Its Principles and Practice.* Philadelphia and London: W.B. Saunders, 1906.
28. Keen, W.W., "Three Cases of Cerebral Surgery," *Am. J. Med. Sci.* 96:329–357 and 452–465, 1888.
29. Bauer, E.L., *Doctors Made in America.* Philadelphia: Lippincott, 1963, p. 228.
30. Fulton, J.F., *Harvey Cushing: A Biography.* Springfield, Illinois: Charles C. Thomas, 1946, p. 330.
31. Klopp, E., *Clinic.* Philadelphia: Jefferson Medical College, 1936, p. 79.
32. DaCosta, J.C., *The Jeffersonian* 8(65):105, April 1907.
33. Geist, D.C., "William Williams Keen, M.D. (1837–1932), Surgeon and Author. (Discussion by Erikson, G.E.)," *Trans. Stud. Coll. Phys. Phila.* 44:192, 1976.
34. Gordon, A., *Publications from the Laboratories of Jefferson Medical College Hospital.* Vol. 4, 1907.
35. Personal communication. John C. McNerney, M.D., January 2, 1985.
36. Wyeth, G.A., "The Evolution and Present Status of Electrosurgery in the Treatment of Cancer," *Radiology* 17: 1028, 1931.
37. Duane, W., Jr., "A Modification of the McKenzie Silver Clip," *J. Neurosurg.* 7:92, 1950.
38. Reeves, D.L., *Cranioplasty.* Springfield, Illinois: Charles C. Thomas, 1950, p. 18.
39. Gurdjian, E.S., Webster, J.E., and Brown, J.C., "Impression Technique for Reconstruction of Large Skull Defects," *Surgery* 14:876, December 1943.
40. Nemir, P., Jr., "Robert Armand Groff," *Trans. Phila. Acad. Surg.* 32:92–94, 1976.
41. Pevenhouse, B.C., "Residency Training in Neurological Surgery: Evolution over 50 Years of Trial and Tribulation," *J. Neurosurgery* 61:999–1004, 1984.
42. Donald D.C., Jr., Kesmodel, K.F., Jr., Rollins, S.L., Jr., and Paddison, R.M., "An Improved Technique for Percutaneous Cerebral Angiography," *Arch. Neurol. and Psych.* 65:508–510, April 1951.
43. Seldinger, S.I., "Catheter Replacement of the Needle in Percutaneous Angiography. A New Technique," *Acta Radiol.* 39:368–376, April 1953.
44. Bucy, *Neurosurgical Giants.* (Ref. 7)
45. Murtaugh, F., Jr., "The Philadelphia Neurosurgical Society," *Trans. Stud. Coll. Phys. Phila.* 37:281–284, 1970.

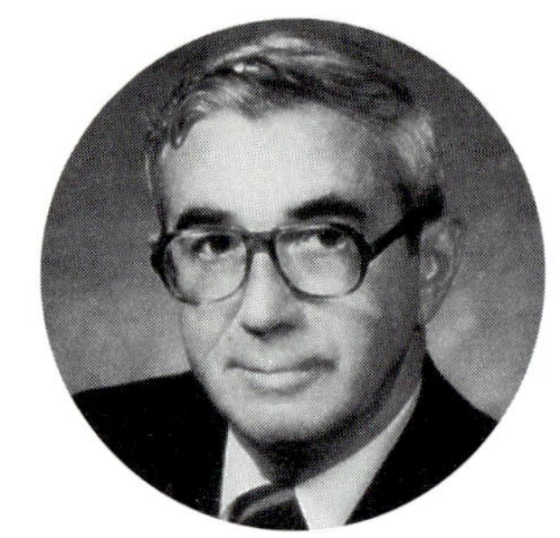

CHAPTER FORTY-ONE

Department of Orthopaedic Surgery

John J. Gartland, M.D.

"The broken bone once set together is stronger than ever."

—John Lyly (1554?–1606)

ALTHOUGH PHYSICIAN involvement with disorders of the musculoskeletal system dates back to medical antiquity, the specialty of orthopaedic surgery was not designated as such until just 83 years before the founding of Jefferson Medical College. Before this formal naming occurred and allowed a specific focus to begin, disorders and injuries of the musculoskeletal system were cared for by that large group of practitioners known simply as surgeons. It is noteworthy that as orthopaedic surgery struggled for its separate identity and began to disassemble from general surgery, Jefferson became one of the first medical schools in the country to recognize the new specialty by founding a Department of Orthopaedic Surgery in 1904.

The term *orthopaedics* was coined in 1741 by Nicholas André, Dean of the Faculty of Medicine of the College de France. He combined two Greek words *orthos*, meaning straight or free of deformity and *paidios*, a child. It called attention to his belief that the prevention of deformed adults lay in the development of straight children. André had no idea that this newly invented word would be later adopted to identify the important medical discipline that concerns itself with the disorders and injuries affecting the musculoskeletal system.

Gradual acceptance of the new term sharpened the focus among those mechanically minded general surgeons of the time who had developed a special interest in the musculoskeletal system. A few of them founded the American Orthopaedic Association in 1887, the first formal orthopaedic organization in the world. Their vision and sense of purpose can be better appreciated when it is noted that the founding of this Association predated the founding of the American College of Surgeons by 26 years.

World War I, with its large volume of musculoskeletal injuries, provided the catalyst for the ultimate emergence of this special field from beneath the mantle of general surgery. By 1935 the American Board of Orthopaedic Surgery had been formed and the American Academy of Orthopaedic Surgeons established. This second national orthopaedic organization was needed to give an organizational home to the hundreds of emerging board-certified orthopaedic surgeons not eligible for membership in the American Orthopaedic Association. The latter organization continued to restrict its membership and be professor-oriented. By 1985 the American Academy of Orthopaedic Surgeons had become the largest orthopaedic organization in the world, with a membership in excess of 11,000 board-certified orthopaedists.

Samuel D. Gross was outstanding in the early American literature relating to the later specialty of orthopaedics. At age 25 and only two years after his graduation from Jefferson in 1828, he published *Anatomy, Physiology and Diseases of Bones and Joints* (1830). This octavo volume of 382 pages sold 2,000 copies in fewer than four years. In 1859 when he was Professor of Surgery at Jefferson, Volume II of his *System of Surgery* contained 253 pages devoted to bone and joint disease, including fractures. Additionally, Eakins' *Gross Clinic,* painted in 1875, depicted Gross removing a sequestrum from the femur.

As early as 1839 Thomas Dent Mütter, Professor of Surgery at Jefferson (1841–1856), published a monograph of 104 pages on clubfoot. In his textbook of *Operations of Surgery* (1846) he devoted four out of 19 chapters to amputations, injuries of muscles and tendons, contractions of the leg and thigh, ankylosis, and clubfoot. Joseph Pancoast, Professor of Surgery from 1839 to 1841 and of Anatomy from 1841 to 1874, wrote extensively on operations for diseases of the bones and joints in his *Operative Surgery* (1844).

The development of orthopaedic surgery at Jefferson closely paralleled the development of the specialty in the country as a whole. Traditionally, formal emergence of the term *orthopaedic surgery* in the curricula and on the faculties of most medical schools can be traced to the identification of a general surgeon with a mechanical turn of mind who evinced interest in disorders of bones and joints. The first such person at Jefferson (after Gross, Mütter, and Pancoast) was Dr. Oscar Huntington Allis, an 1866 graduate of Jefferson (Figure 41-1).

Oscar H. Allis, M.D. (1836–1921); Clinical Lecturer in Orthopaedic Surgery (1888–1891)

Oscar Allis had a great interest in problems of a mechanical nature and devised the Allis forceps, which remains a widely used surgical instrument today. He practiced general surgery in many Philadelphia hospitals and, for a period of about ten years, was a member of the Department of Surgery at Jefferson Hospital. He began giving lectures on orthopaedic surgery at Jefferson, in response to his own interest, during 1879. This interest was formally recognized when he was named Clinical Lecturer of Orthopaedic Surgery in 1888. These lectures were given during the summer courses while he was working in surgery with the younger Gross. He is generally credited with organizing the orthopaedic outpatient clinic at Jefferson in the 1877 Hospital. He focused attention on the mechanical problems encountered

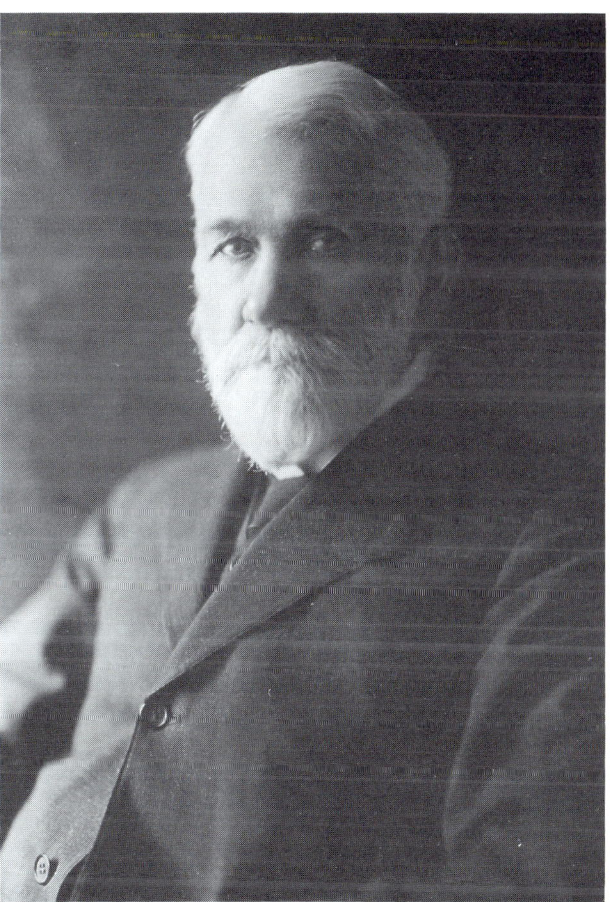

FIG. 41-1. Oscar H. Allis, M.D., Clinical Lecturer in Orthopaedic Surgery (1888–1891).

in surgery, thus preparing the environment for the eventual establishment of a separate Department of Orthopaedic Surgery. He continued to be involved with Jefferson's early interest in orthopaedics until he resigned from the faculty in 1891.

Allis was widely regarded as an authority on fractures and dislocations during his lifetime. He was awarded the Gross Prize of the Philadelphia Academy of Surgery in 1895 for his monograph on *Obstacles to the Reduction of Dislocation of the Hip.* Just before his death in 1921, he completed a work, illustrated with a model, demonstrating the functions of the spinal column with its musculature. He used this device to call attention to the effect of posture on normal spinal curvature and the bad effect of faulty posture. His biographer in *American Medical Biographies* published in 1928 said of Allis: "He shone rather as an investigator of surgical problems and a deviser of useful surgical instruments than as an operator. While he was a man of the finest character, universally respected and trusted, yet he was somewhat dour and set in his opinions."[1] In spite of his early association with orthopaedics at Jefferson, Oscar Allis regarded himself at all times as a general surgeon, and his organizational memberships reflected that distinction. When he left Jefferson, the position of Clinical Lecturer in Orthopaedic Surgery was given to H. Augustus Wilson, an 1879 graduate of Jefferson (Figure 41-2).

H. Augustus Wilson M.D. (1853–1919); Clinical Lecturer in Orthopaedic Surgery (1892–1904) and First Chairman (1904–1918)

Augustus Wilson was promoted to Clinical Professor of Orthopaedic Surgery in 1892. It would seem appropriate to regard this promotion as the exact point in Jefferson history when orthopaedics began the process of ultimate separation from general surgery. Support for this contention comes from Wilson's attitude, since he clearly regarded himself as an orthopaedic surgeon rather than a general surgeon. As early as 1887, he had published an article in the *Proceedings of the Philadelphia County Medical Society* that described a new method for preparing dry gypsum bandages used in the construction of plaster casts.[2] He was invited to join the fledgling American Orthopaedic Association in 1891 and was well regarded by his colleagues in this new organization. He served as Vice President in 1893 and President in 1902. He represented the first Jefferson orthopaedist to hold a major elected office in national orthopaedics. A Jefferson representative was not destined to secure a second major national orthopaedic office until 1979.

A significant reorganization of the Jefferson faculty occurred in 1904. Several disciplines, formerly regarded as part of general surgery, were identified as new and separate Departments. The minutes of the Administrative Committee meeting

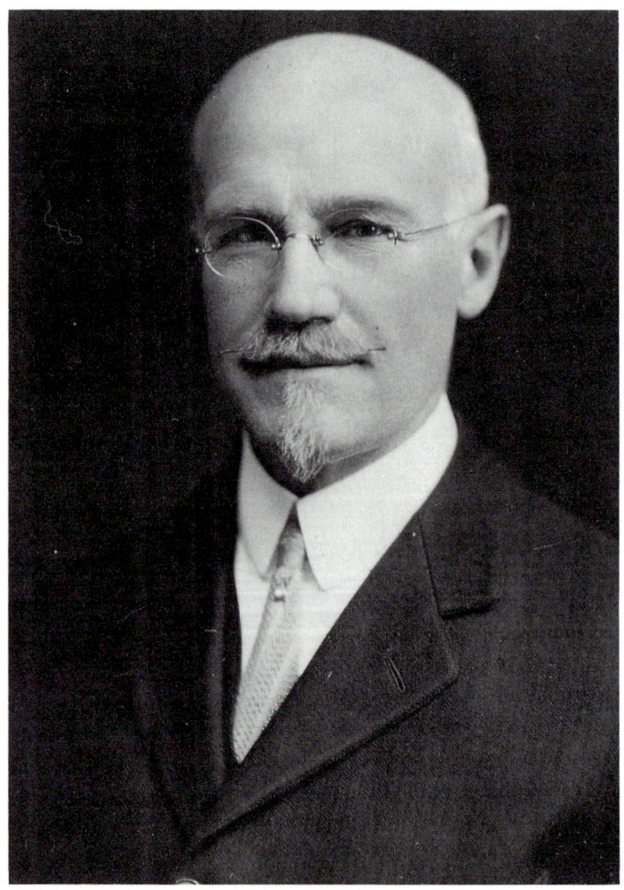

FIG. 41-2. H. Augustus Wilson, M.D., Clinical Professor of Orthopaedic Surgery (1892–1904), and First Chairman (1904–1918).

of November 28, 1904 (forerunner of the Executive Council) state "in view of the fact that the faculty is now composed of Professors who teach and examine in genito-urinary surgery, orthopaedic surgery and laryngology, it is suggested that the Professor of Practice of Surgery and of Clinical Surgery shall be relieved of teaching subjects pertaining to these branches."[3]

Minutes of the Administrative Committee meetings before 1904 do not exist, so one can only guess the reasons for this faculty reorganization. It is probably accurate to surmise that a need was identified to enlarge the major faculty. An interesting question to consider is why Jefferson chose, in 1904, to decrease the responsibility of the Department of Surgery by creating three new Departments out of the fields that were traditionally considered surgical subspecialties. In many, if not most, medical schools, these evolving surgical disciplines were given some separate identity by simply designating them Divisions of General Surgery.

Whatever the reasons happened to be, this action of the Administrative Committee created a Department of Orthopaedic Surgery at Jefferson in 1904 and made H. Augustus Wilson its first Professor and Chairman. Jefferson thus became one of the first medical schools in the country to have a separate Department of Orthopaedic Surgery. It is somewhat ironic to note that despite the suggestion of the Administrative Committee that the Professor of Practice of Surgery and of Clinical Surgery "be relieved of teaching subjects pertaining to these branches," the Department of Surgery continued to dominate the treatment of fractures in Jefferson Hospital and continued to teach fracture principles to Jefferson medical students until about 1948.

Wilson, by all accounts, was a good teacher and an effective Department Chairman. He appointed J. Torrence Rugh (Jefferson, 1892) to serve as Assistant Professor of Orthopaedic Surgery in 1905 and Arthur J. Davidson (Figure 41-3) (Jefferson, 1907) as Instructor of Orthopaedic Surgery in 1908. Both of these men figured prominently in the growth and development of the new Department. Treatment of orthopaedic deformities at this time was given mostly by physical manipulation, mechanical traction devices, and bracing. Not much in the way of open surgery was performed except by a few daring pioneers. References to surgical correction of deformity in the years around 1910 generally referred to the cutting of tight tendons performed through very small incisions. Rugh ultimately succeeded Wilson as Chairman in 1918, and Davidson remained in active teaching in the outpatient clinic until 1954. Arthur Davidson became a recognized expert in the care of foot problems and freely imparted his knowledge to students in the orthopaedic clinic. Unfortunately, he could never be persuaded to put his considerable knowledge into book form.

Writing in the 1936 *Clinic Yearbook,* Rugh made the following comments about these early years of orthopaedics at Jefferson:

> "The outpatient clinic was organized by Dr. Allis and now forms an important part of the student's

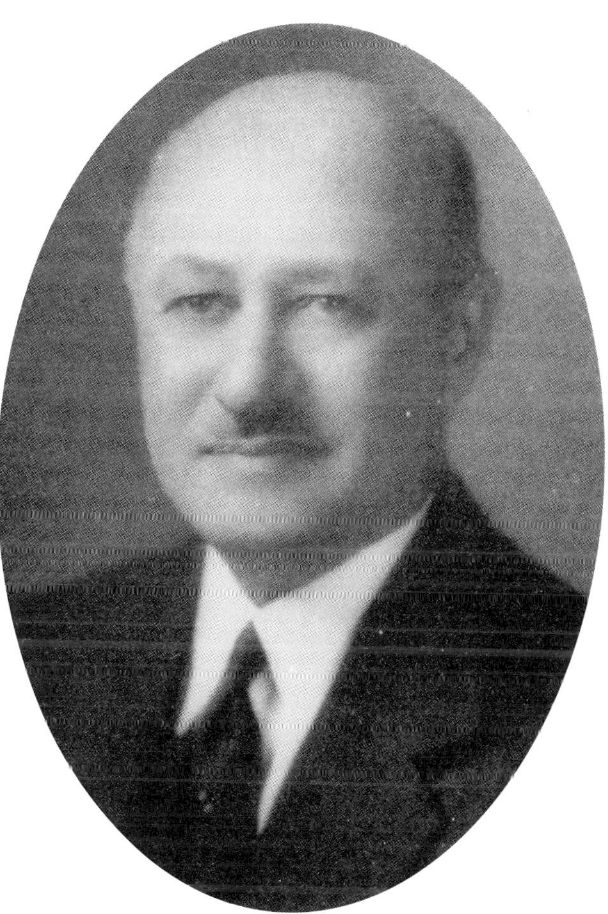

FIG. 41-3. Arthur J. Davidson, M.D., Associate Professor of Orthopaedic Surgery, was especially interested in foot problems.

> instruction. The first dispensary was in the amphitheater of the old hospital. Dr. James Manno of the class of 1887 was chief of clinic and cooperated with Professor Wilson until 1896 when he resigned to accept the orthopaedic professorship in the Medico-Chirugical College. During these years of Dr. Wilson's service, great advances were made in orthopaedics. The surgical phases of the corrective work increased and became more important. New procedures and discoveries regarding the prevention and correction of deformities added greatly to the success of the work in Jefferson."[4]

Professor Wilson resigned the Chairmanship in 1918 and died of uremia on April 16, 1919. He had attained a national reputation in orthopaedic surgery that reflected favorably on Jefferson and its new Department. His obituary was published in 1919 in the *Journal of Orthopaedic Surgery*, forerunner of the present *Journal of Bone and Joint Surgery*. Its author, Dr. R.W. Lovett of Boston, said: "I should say that the man's chief characteristics were earnestness, unselfishness, kind-heartedness and absolute devotion to a cause once undertaken. He was a man of ideas which he never sacrificed, his profession and his family filled his life, and he had few outside interests. He was a most indomitable worker and he had one agreeable trait, that of making the man with whom he talked think more highly of himself than he did before the conversation, for he seemed to look for the best that was in each man and to dwell on that side of his relation to each one."[5]

James T. Rugh, M.D. (1867–1942); Second Chairman (1918–1930) and First James Edwards Professor (1930–1939)

James Torrence Rugh (Jefferson, 1892) succeeded Wilson as Professor of Orthopaedic Surgery in 1918 (Figure 41-4). At the time of his appointment Rugh was on active duty with the Army Medical Corps and did not return to Jefferson until 1919. Originally appointed to the Orthopaedic faculty by Wilson in 1905, Rugh brought extensive clinical experience to the Professorship. He had been the first orthopaedic surgeon appointed to the Methodist Hospital in 1905. He was appointed to the orthopaedic staff of Philadelphia General Hospital in 1912 and in 1914 became Clinical Professor of Orthopaedic Surgery at the Woman's Medical College of Pennsylvania. At one time he was consulting orthopaedic surgeon to six Philadelphia-area hospitals. In addition to these obligations, Rugh worked closely with Wilson at Jefferson during the period 1905 to 1918.

Rugh had gained valuable experience with the surgical treatment of battle casualties during World War I. He rapidly applied these surgical lessons to patient problems at Jefferson. During Rugh's term as Department Chairman the treatment of orthopaedic disabilities gradually shifted from the mechanical methods used by his predecessors to modern open surgical correction. Between 1920

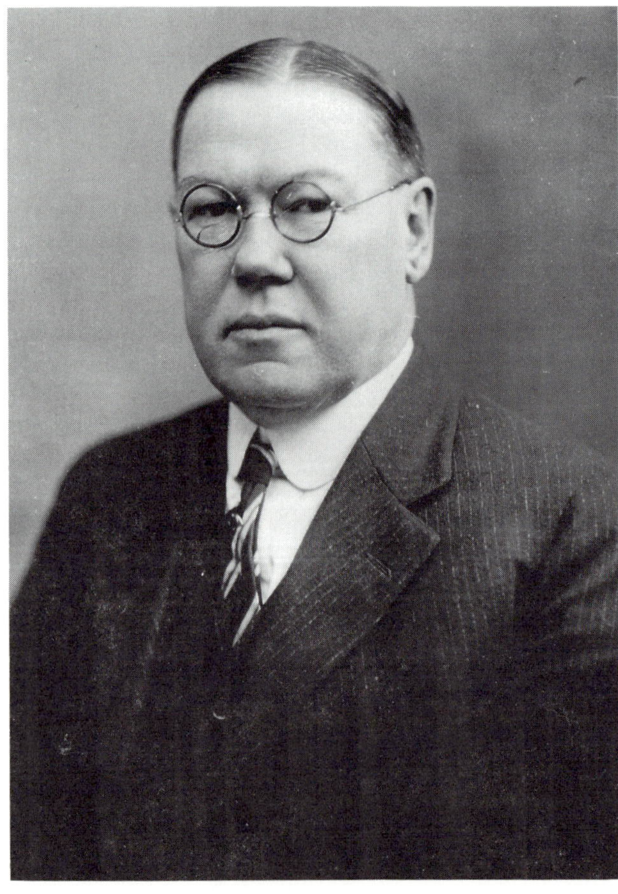

Fig. 41-4. James T. Rugh, M.D., Second Chairman (1918–1939) and First James Edwards Professor (1930–1939).

and 1930, Rugh operated several times at Jefferson on a young boy to correct severe bilateral clubfoot deformity. As fate would have it, this same young patient would grow up to become Chairman of the Department of Orthopaedic Surgery in 1970.

J. Torrence Rugh was an open charismatic man, greatly admired by his colleagues, students, and patients. The Class of 1934 presented his portrait to the Medical College. In making the presentation the students said: "To the students on the benches, Dr. Rugh presents his thoughts with clearness, simplicity and a forceful manner so desirable in teaching and his clinical demonstrations afford a lasting visualization of the principle he sets forth."[6]

Rugh was assisted in his work at Jefferson by Arthur J. Davidson (Jefferson, 1907), an Associate Professor, and James R. Martin (Jefferson, 1910) as Assistant Professor. Martin had served as Chief Resident Physician in Jefferson Hospital before joining the Department of Orthopaedic Surgery. For many years he functioned as Rugh's assistant in the private practice of orthopaedic surgery.

In 1930 the Chair of Orthopaedic Surgery was endowed by a gift of $100,000 in memory of James Edwards, a manufacturer of children's shoes in Philadelphia. Rugh became the first James Edwards Professor of Orthopaedic Surgery and, since 1930, each succeeding Department Chairman has received that title.

An associate of the time described Rugh in these words: "Dr. Rugh is a hard-working, democratic man, strongly conservative by nature, temperate in his habits, always kindly, pleasant and optimistic and with a keen sense of humor. As a teacher, he is practical and straightforward, strongly reliant upon experience and his presentations are clear and concise. He is revered by his staff and associates and beloved by his patients."[7]

Rugh was a frequent contributor to the orthopaedic literature and was well regarded nationally. He was a member of both the American Orthopaedic Association and the American Academy of Orthopaedic Surgeons. He served as Vice President of the American Orthopaedic Association in 1917 and again in 1929. During his time as Chairman both the Thompson Annex and Curtis Clinic buildings were opened. The orthopaedic patient load increased, and the corrective work carried out in the hospital and outpatient clinic developed to a high degree of efficiency. Rugh retired as Chairman in 1939 at the age of 72 years and was succeeded by Dr. James R. Martin. He died in 1942.

James R. Martin, M.D. (1886–1956); Third Chairman and Second James Edwards Professor (1939–1950)

James Martin (Figure 41-5) became a member of the orthopaedic department in 1913 and served originally as Rugh's assistant in private practice. He received several promotions within the Department leading to Assistant Professor and

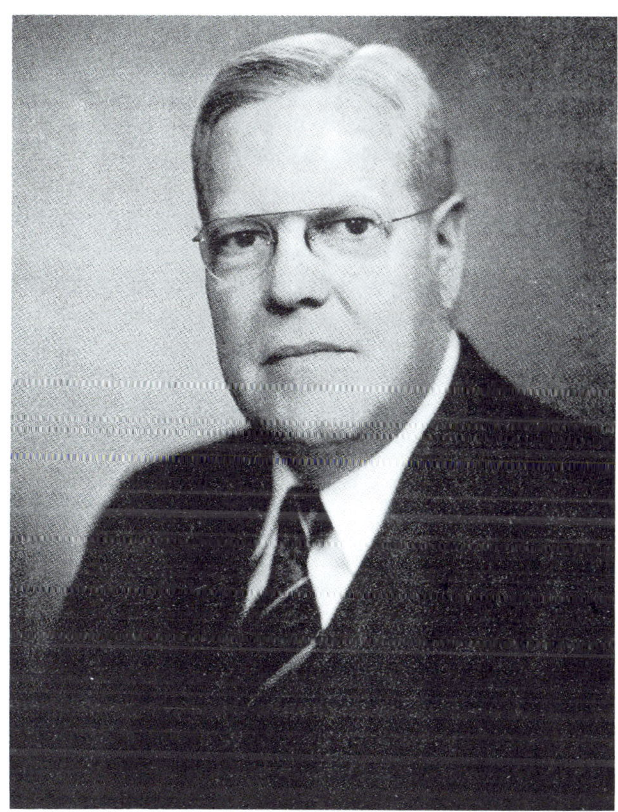

FIG. 41-5. James R. Martin, M.D., Third Chairman and Second James Edwards Professor (1939–1950).

Chief of the Outpatient Clinic by 1938. In that year he resigned to accept appointments as Chief Surgeon at the State Hospital for Crippled Children at Elizabethtown, Pennsylvania, and Director of the Social Security Programs for Crippled Children in Pennsylvania. He was called back to Jefferson in 1939 to become the second James Edwards Professor of Orthopaedic Surgery. In accord with his deep interest in the care of the handicapped child, Martin initiated an association between Jefferson and the State Hospital for Crippled Children. Now known as the Elizabethtown Hospital for Children and Youth, the association begun by Martin has continued to this day. Some Jefferson orthopaedic faculty members still function as active consultants to that institution and some Jefferson orthopaedic Residents receive a part of their education and experience in children's orthopaedics there.

Martin was assisted in his teaching and clinical duties by Drs. Arthur J. Davidson, M. Thomas Horovitz, and Ralph C. Hand. In addition to his duties at Jefferson, Dr. Hand functioned as orthopaedic consultant to Saint Edmund's Home for Crippled Children, now located in Rosemont, Pennsylvania. The association between Jefferson and St. Edmund's Home continued with Dr. John J. Dowling (Jefferson, 1947) assuming the consultant role on Dr. Hand's retirement in 1961. Thomas Horovitz was a bright, energetic orthopaedic surgeon whom many at Jefferson considered to be of professorial caliber. He contributed many fine papers to the orthopaedic literature while in Philadelphia. Unfortunately, Horovitz chose not to return to Philadelphia upon his discharge from World War II service. He relocated in Indianapolis, where he eventually became a full Professor at the University of Indiana Medical School.

James Martin lacked J. Torrence Rugh's background and skill in operative orthopaedics. As a consequence, some of the excitement and forward motion generated clinically by Rugh's introduction of new surgical techniques slowed perceptibly. Davidson and Hand were of the old school and not well versed or comfortable with the new surgical techniques. With Horovitz's decision not to return to Jefferson, none of the remaining orthopaedic faculty had either the skill or the inclination to pursue surgical correction of physical deformities. Gradually, some of the former mechanical treatment methods discarded by Rugh were reintroduced by Martin (Figure 41-6). This reversal occurred at a time when national interest in the surgical correction of physical deformities was in the ascendancy. As a consequence, the students sensed the subtle change, and interest in orthopaedics among students and hospital interns waned.

Martin was a kind and friendly man, dignified, retiring, and unobtrusive. He was quite content with his work and teaching at Jefferson and shunned the national scene. He was a member of the American Academy of Orthopaedic Surgeons but was never invited to join the American Orthopaedic Association. As a consequence of his totally local presence, orthopaedics at Jefferson lost most of the national prominence it had gained under Wilson and Rugh.

The major accomplishment during Martin's Chairmanship was the establishment of the orthopaedic resident education program. It began modestly in 1946 with two Residents appointed yearly and two hospitals, Jefferson and the State Hospital for Crippled Children at Elizabethtown, involved in the clinical experience. Thomas S. Armstrong (Jefferson, 1941) was the first Resident to complete the new program, and he subsequently practiced orthopaedic surgery for many years in Carlisle, Pennsylvania.

By 1945 it had become apparent to faculty leaders at Jefferson that orthopaedic surgery was a Department in a relatively stagnant state compared to other medical schools. A quiet search for an exciting, vigorous figure in orthopaedic surgery led them to the Philadelphia Naval Hospital, where Anthony F. DePalma (Jefferson, 1929), completing the final months of his service commitment, had compiled an enviable surgical record. He was induced in 1946 to come to Jefferson to establish a practice with the understanding he would eventually follow Martin as Department Chairman.

Although Martin continued to function as Department Chairman, DePalma's dynamic, driving style soon stamped him as the leader in everything but name only. James Martin served as President of the Alumni Association in 1948 and formally retired as Chairman in 1950. He then was appointed Associate Dean of Jefferson Medical College and served in this post until his death in 1956. This loyal and devoted Jeffersonian provided funds in his will for the James R. Martin Nurses' Residence, which was built on the southeast corner of Eleventh and Walnut Streets, where Drs. Thomas Dent Mütter and Samuel D. Gross previously had lived.

Anthony F. DePalma, M.D. (1904–); Fourth Chairman and Third James Edwards Professor (1950–1970)

With Martin's retirement in 1950, Anthony F. DePalma (Figure 41-7) was appointed the third James Edwards Professor and Chairman of the Department. Three essential ingredients were in place that could promise further growth and development for orthopaedic surgery at Jefferson. Wilson had provided Departmental status, Rugh pioneered the surgical emphasis for the specialty, and Martin initiated the Residency program. The appointment of a full-time faculty in orthopaedics, however, was still 20 years away. Drs. Wilson, Rugh, Martin, and DePalma all engaged actively in the private practice of their specialty from off-campus offices. They also did their clinical work in other local hospitals in addition to Jefferson Hospital. They contributed time to Jefferson for teaching and managing the administrative details of the Department.

DePalma soon proved himself to be a forceful teacher and a busy clinical orthopaedic surgeon. He was a skillful surgical technician and his practice eventually grew to huge proportions as his reputation spread beyond the confines of Jefferson. A sense of excitement was returned to orthopaedics by DePalma's surgical experience and dynamic teaching style. The students were

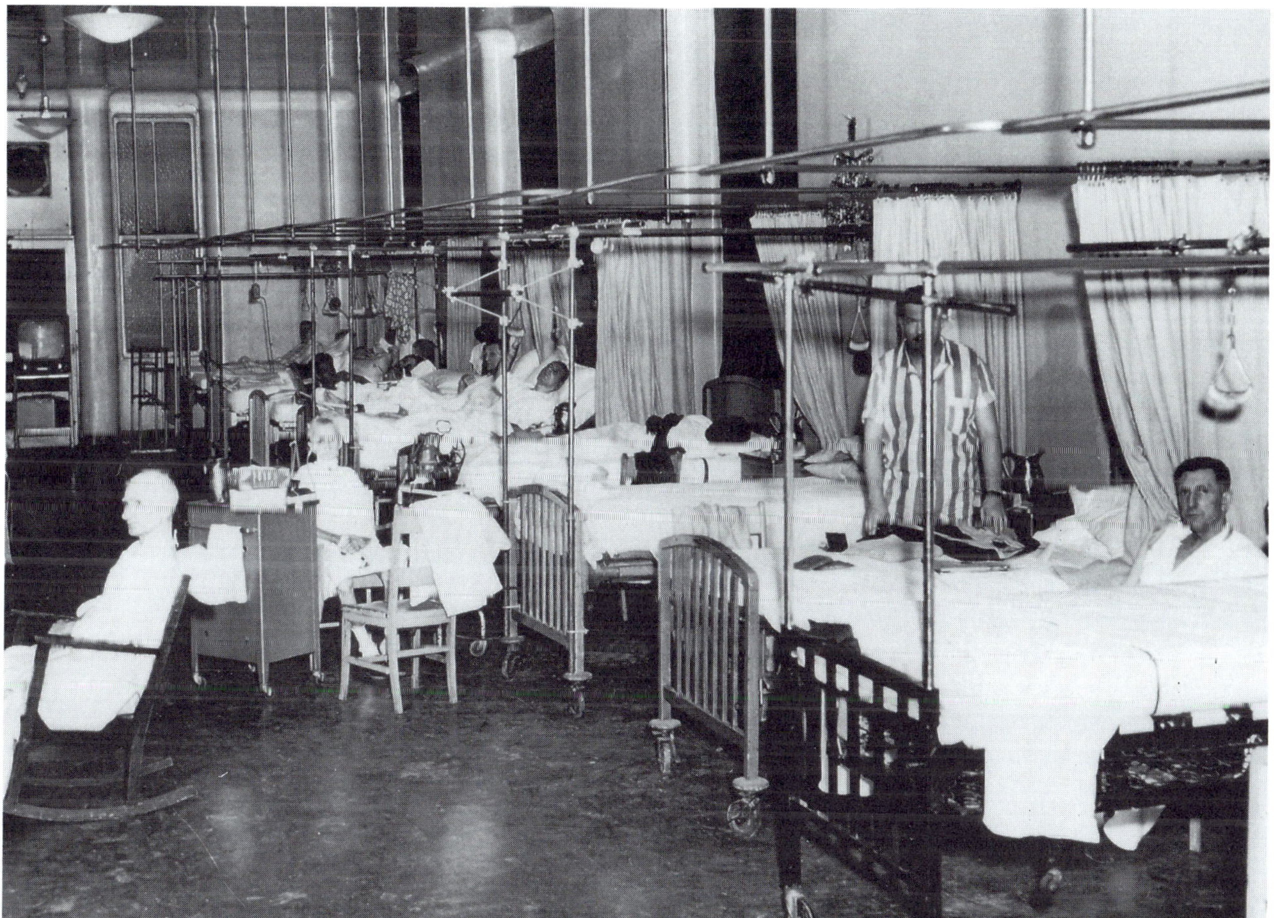

FIG. 41-6. Men's Orthopaedic Ward in Old Main Hospital (ca. 1950).

stimulated, and DePalma influenced many to seek careers in orthopaedic surgery. Many Jefferson students who later held orthopaedic faculty appointments at Jefferson received their graduate orthopaedic education under him. Among the group were Drs. Gerald E. Callery (Jefferson, 1943), John J. Dowling (Jefferson, 1947), Hal E. Snedden (Jefferson, 1950), Jerome M. Cotler (Jefferson, 1952), James M. Hunter (Jefferson, 1953), J. David Hoffman (Jefferson, 1956), Phillip J. Marone (Jefferson, 1957), Richard A. Cautilli (Jefferson, 1958), and John M. Fenlin (Jefferson, 1963).[8] Richard H. Rothman, later destined to become the fifth James Edwards Professor of Orthopaedic Surgery and Chairman of the Department in 1986, completed his orthopaedic residency with DePalma in 1968.

DePalma proved to be a tireless worker both in his own clinical practice and in academic pursuits (Figure 41-8). He was a prolific writer, and his orthopaedic texts are still considered classics. They appeared as follows: *Surgery of the Shoulder* (1950) in three editions; *Diseases of the Knee* (1954); *Degenerative Changes in the Sternoclavicular and Acromioclavicular Joints in Various Decades* (1957); *The Management of Fractures and Dislocations* (1959), in two volumes; and *The Intervertebral Disc,* coauthored with Richard H. Rothman (1970). He also edited *Clinical Orthopaedics,* a series of volumes in symposium form produced under the auspices of the Association of Bone and Joint Surgeons. Because of his constant productivity, Jefferson's national prominence in orthopaedics gradually enlarged.

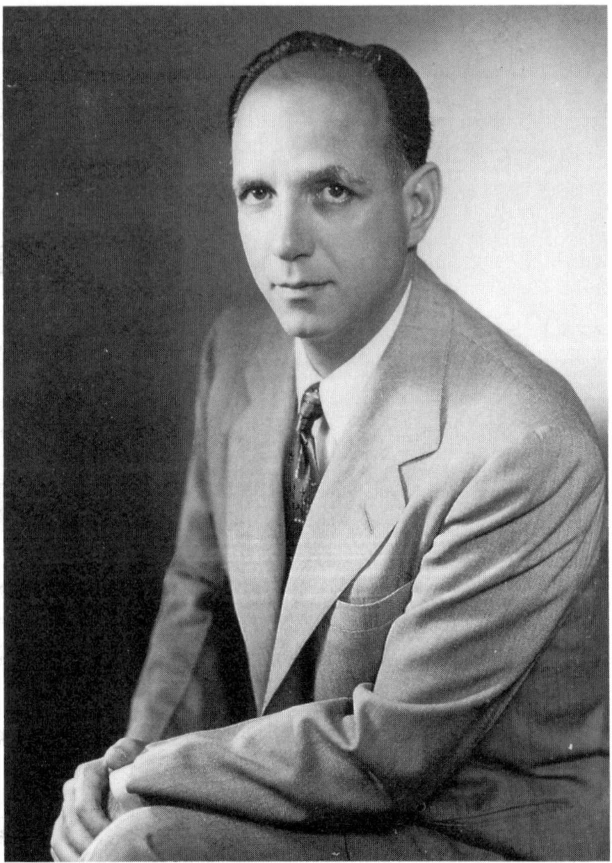

FIG. 41-7. Anthony F. DePalma, M.D., Fourth Chairman and Third James Edwards Professor (1950–1970).

If DePalma had a weak spot, it was his tendency to be too much of a "one-man show." It was difficult for younger faculty members to develop academically and clinically in this environment at Jefferson during those days, and many left to develop their own services elsewhere. DePalma tended to be somewhat arbitrary and brusque when he believed he was correct on a point. As a consequence he did not enjoy a great personal popularity with the other Philadelphia orthopaedic professors. This attitude also tended to hurt him nationally, where he was regarded with respect but, at the same time, considered somewhat controversial. These mixed reviews from his colleagues undoubtedly played some role in delaying his election to membership in the American Orthopaedic Association until 1965.

During his chairmanship, DePalma established an orthopaedic research laboratory in the space formerly occupied by the Department of Pathology on the fifth floor of the College building. In 1953 he became founding editor of *Clinical Orthopaedics,* a respected series of volumes in symposium form still published eight times yearly by J.B. Lippincott Company. The original editorial office for this publication was a small room in the space occupied by the orthopaedic outpatient clinic on the sixth floor of the Curtis Clinic Building. In 1970 this orthopaedic outpatient clinic space was converted into administrative offices for the Department. From 1970 until 1985, this same small room functioned as the administrative office for the senior orthopaedic resident. DePalma founded the Jefferson Orthopaedic Society in 1960, with membership offered to former residents and all Jefferson alumni who had elected careers in orthopaedic surgery. The Society has remained active and holds a two-day scientific meeting on the Jefferson campus yearly. It celebrated its twenty-fifth anniversary with a special meeting in Puerto Rico during November, 1984.

It was also during DePalma's tenure as Chairman that Jefferson developed a specific presence in the important orthopaedic subspecialty of hand surgery. After James M. Hunter (Jefferson, 1953) completed his orthopaedic residency under DePalma, he took a one-year fellowship in hand surgery with Dr. Robert E. Carroll at Columbia-Presbyterian Medical Center in New York. He returned to Jefferson and became the first Philadelphia orthopaedic surgeon to confine his practice totally to surgery of the hand. He originally began practice in association with DePalma but later opened his own office. He was joined by his first associate, Dr. Lawrence H. Schneider, in 1969. As noted previously, Jefferson had no full-time orthopaedic faculty as yet, and all members supported themselves by a private practice conducted in outside offices. From the outset, Hunter (Figure 41-9) was considered Jefferson's hand surgeon, and he responded by keeping his office close to the Jefferson campus and by doing almost all of his surgical work in Jefferson Hospital. Hunter was a hard worker and innovative researcher in both the basic and clinical spheres. His research led, ultimately, to the development of the "Hunter tendon" in 1965, the

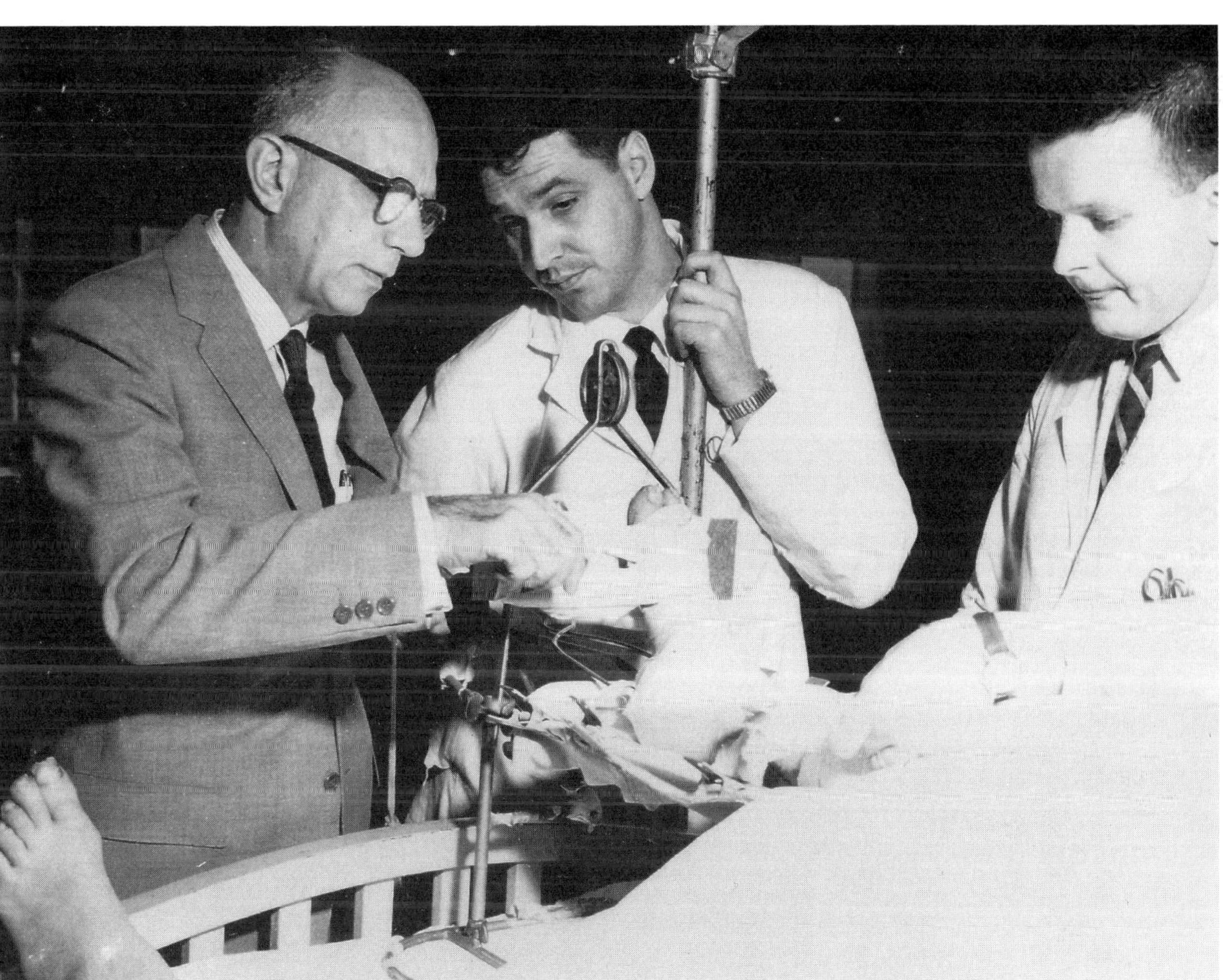

FIG. 41-8. Dr. DePalma instructing in the ward.

first successful artificial tendon for use in reconstructing severely damaged hands.

Hunter's reputation as a hand surgeon grew over the years, progressing from a local to an international stature. In 1978 he coauthored *Rehabilitation of the Hand* with Lawrence H. Schneider, M.D., Evelyn J. Mackin, L.P.T., and Judith A. Bell, O.T.R. A second edition with additional collaborators appeared in 1984. His clinical load grew proportionately, requiring him progressively to increase his professional and support staff. By 1985 this group totalled four hand surgeons, four hand fellows and a support staff of approximately 50 persons, all housed in a building at Ninth and Walnut Streets known as the Hand Rehabilitation Center. Although hand surgery at Jefferson began and remains an essentially private practice, this group officially accepted the designation of Division of Hand Surgery of the Department of Orthopaedic Surgery when the Department was later reorganized by Dr. John J. Gartland, the fourth James Edwards Professor. This reorganization gave administrative structure to hand surgery and allowed participation in the organized educational programs of the Department without forcing a change in their financial arrangements by acceptance of full-time status within the Department.

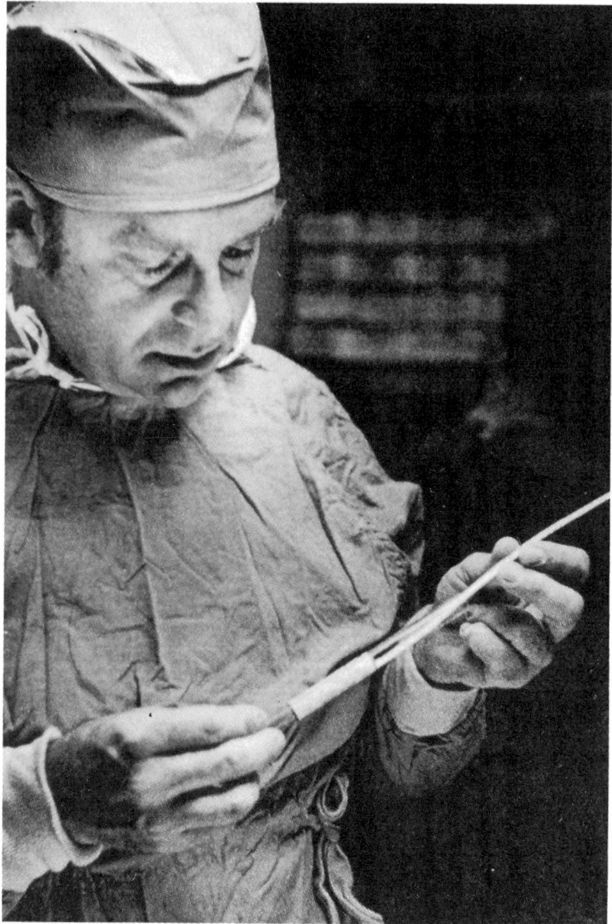

FIG. 41-9. James M. Hunter, M.D., Professor of Orthopaedic Surgery, who developed the first successful artificial tendon for the hand in 1965.

DePalma was the busiest orthopaedic clinician Jefferson ever had or, possibly, ever will have. His clinical practice was enormous, with a huge surgical caseload. As pleasant as this appeared to be to hospital administrators, a price had to be paid. The price was a gradual lessening of the effort put into educational programs for students and residents. Although DePalma tried hard, it was simply impossible for one person to do it all. As a consequence, he delegated much of the responsibility for conducting the educational programs to junior faculty but without giving them authority to make needed changes. At first this seemed to work well, as many young junior faculty appeared stimulated by the challenge to teach. Unfortunately, their enthusiasm waned as they gradually realized there was little chance to develop a clinical practice at Jefferson as long as DePalma remained so busy. He incorporated many of the junior faculty into his office as "Associates" and between 1952 and 1970 there were at least ten such associates. The bulk of responsibility for student teaching fell to Dr. John J. Dowling. He accomplished the assignment so well that the Jefferson Class of 1974 honored him by presenting his portrait to the College. He also served as President of the Alumni Association in 1984.[9]

Between 1950 and 1970 the residency program had been gradually enlarged to a total of 24 Residents basically as a response to the large clinical volume. During this period the hospitals used for resident education in orthopaedics were Jefferson, Philadelphia General, Methodist, and the State Hospital for Crippled Children at Elizabethtown. Unfortunately, the Philadelphia General Hospital was approaching the end of its unique history as a Philadelphia institution, and orthopaedic attending coverage for the residents was sparse. In 1969 the Residency Review Committee for Orthopaedic Surgery noted the imbalance of the Jefferson program toward service demands as compared to educational commitments and strongly suggested the program be reorganized with a larger educational base.

DePalma was a very active participant in Jefferson affairs and chaired many important faculty and medical staff committees. He served as President of the Alumni Association in 1959.[10] He made many lasting and significant contributions to the growth and development of orthopaedic surgery at Jefferson. Although intangible, perhaps, his most important contribution was a legacy of Departmental strength, vitality, and professionalism. He inherited a Department that was admittedly weak in staff members, clinical volume, and faculty influence. His tireless energy and enthusiasm achieved an enlarged clinical volume, enhanced the teaching programs, and commanded faculty respect. He retired as Chairman in 1970 and was followed by Dr. John J. Gartland (Jefferson, S1944) as the fourth James Edwards Professor. At the time of DePalma's retirement, the Department of Orthopaedic Surgery, although still small by most faculty standards, was generally agreed to be one of the stronger Departments of the institution. The Class of 1962 presented his portrait to the College. In 1975, five years after his retirement as Chairman, Dr. DePalma was awarded Jefferson's Alumni Achievement Award.

John J. Gartland, M.D. (1918–); Fifth Chairman and Fourth James Edwards Professor (1970–1985)

Dr. John J. Gartland (Figure 41-10) joined the Department as an Instructor after completing his orthopaedic residency at the Columbia-Presbyterian Medical Center in 1952. DePalma invited him back to Jefferson to become his first associate in practice. This association lasted only one and a half years because of philosophical differences that developed between them. DePalma was primarily a clinician with a huge practice. Gartland, although he also considered himself a clinician, believed a large overwhelming practice stifled academic achievements and took time away from educational pursuits. Their parting was cordial and Gartland retained his faculty appointment, progressively rising through the ranks to be made Associate Professor in 1968. Like other young orthopaedists who followed him on the faculty, Gartland found it difficult to develop much of a clinical practice of his own at Jefferson during those years and did most of his clinical work at other hospitals. He was an attending orthopaedic surgeon at Fitzgerald Mercy Hospital (1954–1960),

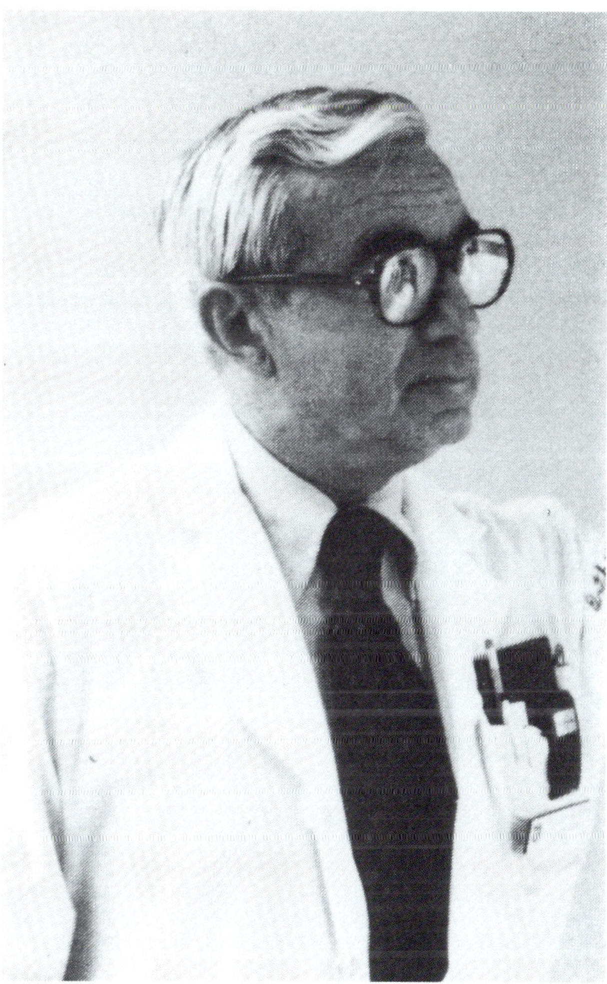

FIG. 41-10. John J. Gartland, M.D., Fifth Chairman, Fourth James Edwards Professor (1970–1985), and first full-time Chairman.

Chief of Orthopaedics at Methodist Hospital (1960–1968) and Chief of Orthopaedics at Lankenau Hospital (1968–1970).

Gartland had a deep interest in orthopaedic education. He wrote *Fundamentals of Orthopaedics,* a textbook for medical students, in 1965, that received national acceptance and by 1986 was in its fourth edition. He was a faculty member in many of the continuing education courses sponsored by the American Academy of Orthopaedic Surgeons and was a frequent contributor to the orthopaedic literature. In 1966 he was invited to become an associate editor of the *Journal of Bone and Joint Surgery,* the official publication of the English-speaking orthopaedic world. He was the first Jeffersonian to be so honored, and he remained active on the editorial board until 1978. Gartland's reputation as an educator grew, and he was elected to membership in the American Orthopaedics Association in 1968.

When Dr. Gartland accepted the Chairmanship in 1970 he became the first full-time Professor of Orthopaedic Surgery and the fourth James Edwards Professor. He saw as his immediate task the need to strengthen the full-time orthopaedic faculty component to complement the volunteer faculty already present and to restructure the residency program to correct the educational imbalance previously noted by the Residency Review Committee for Orthopaedic Surgery. Rather than build an educational structure around the clinical practice of one physician, Gartland believed in a broader based educational program in which the students and residents could be exposed to many teachers, but still one in which the Chairman retained a directing and supervising role.

By 1970 Thomas Jefferson University Hospital had become a sophisticated medical center with a significant level of tertiary care demands. The medical college student body had been enlarged, leading to an increase in the number of affiliated hospitals required for the undergraduate teaching programs. In orthopaedics, specialized care was required for children's orthopaedic problems and for surgery of the hand. The University Hospital was well suited to provide this specialized care. As noted previously, James Hunter's group of hand surgeons was formally incorporated into the department structure as the Division of Hand Surgery. By 1985 this division was supporting four Fellowships in hand surgery yearly and was totally incorporated into the teaching programs of the Department.

Dr. Roshen N. Irani was brought from Children's Hospital in 1972 as the full-time Chief of a Division of Pediatric Orthopaedics within the Department. An affiliation agreement was negotiated with the A.I. Dupont Institute in Wilmington, Delaware, to provide an additional rotation in pediatric orthopaedics for Jefferson residents. In 1982 an additional rotation for Jefferson residents in pediatric orthopaedics was negotiated with Shriner's Hospital of Philadelphia when it became apparent that the Children's Hospital at Elizabethtown might be incorporated into the structure of the new medical school at Hershey, Pennsylvania.

Three men who had trained in orthopaedic surgery at Jefferson under DePalma now headed the orthopaedic services in three of Jefferson's major affiliated hospitals. Phillip J. Marone was Chief at Methodist Hospital, Dr. Hal E. Snedden took over at Bryn Mawr Hospital, and Dr. John J. Dowling replaced Gartland at Lankenau Hospital in 1970 (Figure 41-11).

These affiliated hospitals were incorporated into the newly designed program to provide an experience for the residents in community orthopaedics and trauma. Jefferson's additional agreement with the Wilmington Veterans Hospital allowed orthopaedic resident rotations to that facility for further broadening of the resident educational experience. Cooperative programs were arranged with the Department of Rehabilitation Medicine and the Division of Rheumatology of the Department of Medicine at Jefferson. By 1974 the restructuring of the resident education program was complete and was renamed the Thomas Jefferson University Affiliated Hospitals Program, with a total complement of 24 residents. The new program received full approval from the Residency Review Committee for Orthopaedic Surgery. The restructuring proved successful and gradually developed a national reputation for its excellent clinical and academic background. By 1980 the program was regularly receiving in excess of 350 applications yearly for the six first-year positions from students of the best medical schools in the country.

Gartland viewed himself as orchestrating the best out of all the component parts of the Department. He believed that all the available strengths should be used adequately and fully to provide a well-balanced education for students and residents. He encouraged and supported the development of special clinical interests among his faculty members.

Dr. Jerome M. Cotler became the third full-time member of the orthopaedic faculty in 1973 (Figure 41-12). Cotler had finished his residency under DePalma in 1957 and opened a private practice in Bridgeton, New Jersey. Because of an interest in academic orthopaedics, he gave up private practice to join Gartland as a full-time general orthopaedic surgeon. He proved to be a hardworking and effective member of the faculty, rising eventually to Professor of Orthopaedic Surgery and Vice-Chairman of the Department. He added many clinical strengths, particularly his involvement with the Spinal Cord Injury Center; Thomas Jefferson University Hospital had been designated the regional Spinal Cord Injury Center of the Delaware Valley in 1979. This was a multidisciplinary team effort involving the Departments of Rehabilitation Medicine, Neurosurgery, and Orthopaedic Surgery. Cotler was appointed a CoDirector of this Center and supervised the orthopaedic aspects of the patient care programs.

Cotler was well regarded nationally and served in many important posts, including Chairman of the Board of Councilors of the American Academy of Orthopaedic Surgeons in 1975 and President of the American Board of Orthopaedic Surgery in 1982. He was a frequent contributor to the medical literature and received the Christian R. and Mary F. Lindback Award for Distinguished Teaching in 1979. He remained active in the continuing education activities of the Academy for many years and was elected to membership in the American Orthopaedic Association in 1979.

Gartland turned his attention to reorganizing the orthopaedic research laboratory that had been acquired a decade before, but which had not been

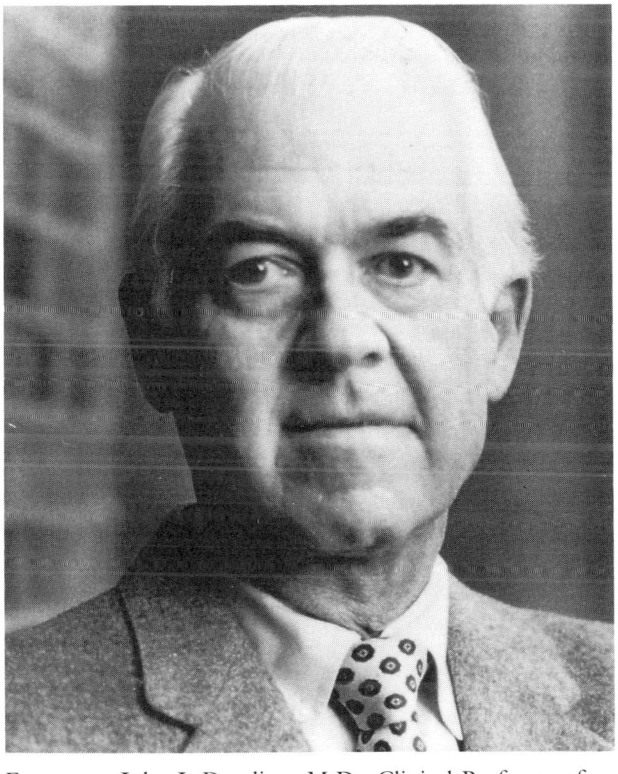

FIG. 41-11. John J. Dowling, M.D., Clinical Professor of Orthopaedic Surgery.

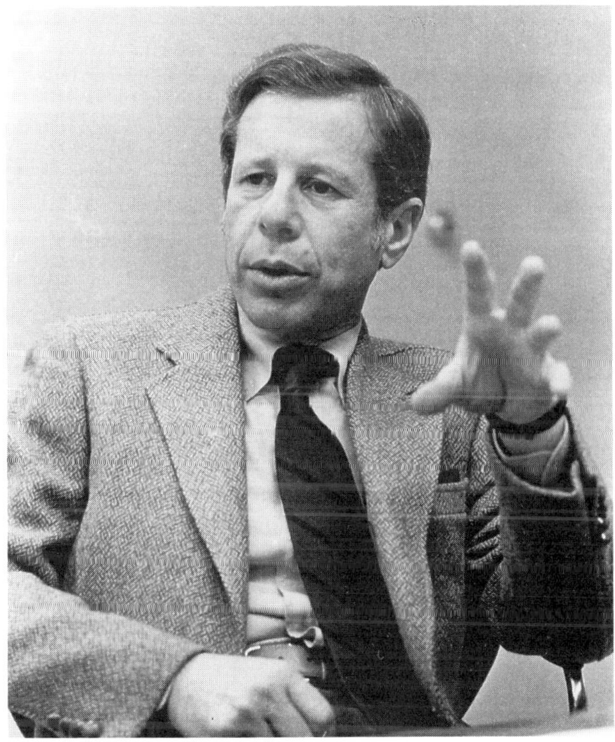

FIG. 41-12. Jerome M. Cotler, M.D., full-time Professor of Orthopaedics, Vice-Chairman of the Department, and Co-Director of the Spinal Cord Injury Center.

effectively utilized in the period 1970–1974. He recruited Peter Frasca, Ph.D., who was a postdoctoral research fellow at Albany Medical College. Frasca's doctorate was in biophysics but his research interest was in bone as a tissue. He joined the Department in 1975 as Research Assistant Professor of Orthopaedic Surgery and Director of the Orthopaedic Research Laboratory. He later obtained a secondary appointment in the Department of Anatomy that enabled him to involve graduate students in his research projects. He was able to obtain National Institutes of Health funding for many of his research efforts and subsequently obtained the first scanning electron microscope on the Jefferson campus.

Podiatry

The care of the feet for such things as the clipping of nails and the trimming of calluses was an area that most physicians were willing to relegate to podiatrists. There had been a question about which of those procedures constituted foot surgery and whether such procedures could be safely and legally performed at Jefferson by podiatrists. Dr. Arthur E. Helfand (Figure 41-13), Professor and Chairman, Department of Community Medicine, Pennsylvania College of Podiatric Medicine, had been providing podiatric services in the hospital and clinics for several years but there was no clearly defined program for him, and therefore his teaching activities were casual. In March of 1977 negotiations were started to integrate him and his work into the Jefferson Medical College and Thomas Jefferson University Hospital Staff. Considerable opposition was met, but because his services and teaching were valuable, particularly to the Division of Endocrinology and Metabolic Diseases, Dr. Gray, Chairman of Medicine, persisted. An arrangement was completed whereby Dr. Helfand received a hospital appointment in the Department of Orthopaedic Surgery in the category of Specified Professional Personnel, to provide consultative services on inpatients and perform minor procedures under local anesthesia at the bedside or in his clinic. His academic appointment was Adjunct Professor of Medicine (Podiatry). His Ambulatory Clinic was established in the area of the Division of General Medicine. Residents in Medicine and students, during their medical clinic clerkship or while on their elective program had the opportunity of working with Dr. Helfand. He authored *Clinical Podogeriatrics* (1981), *Rehabilitation of the Foot* (1984), and *Public Health and Podiatric Medicine* (1987). In March 1985, his appointment was changed to Adjunct Professor of Orthopaedic Surgery (Podiatry).

Further Departmental Expansion

The full-time component of the orthopaedic faculty was raised to four when William C. Hamilton (Jefferson, 1971) became Assistant Professor of Orthopaedic Surgery in 1978. Hamilton had received his orthopaedic education at Jefferson, completing the program in 1976. In the spring of that year he was selected by the American Orthopaedic Association as one of its four North American Traveling Fellows. These

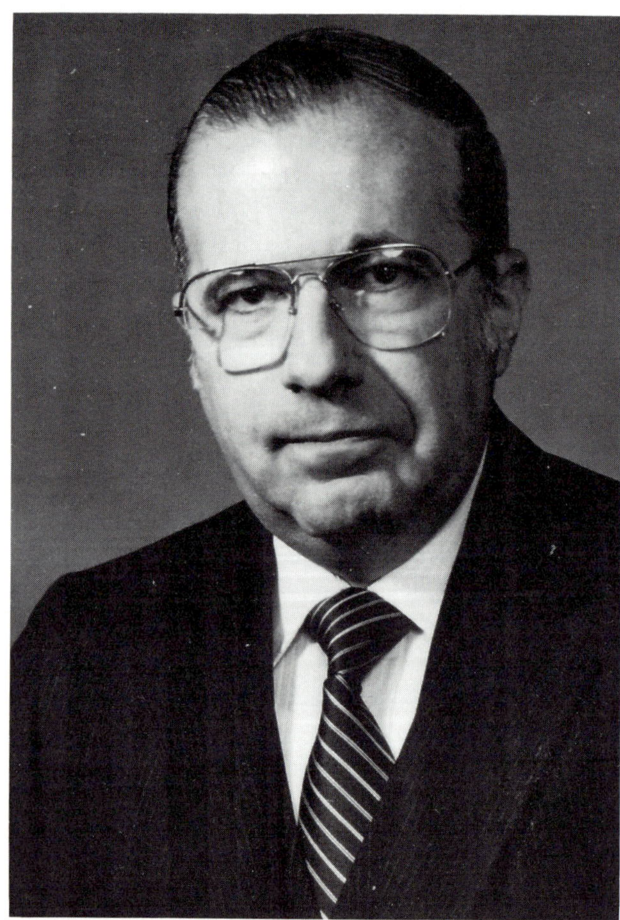

Fig. 41-13. Arthur E. Helfand, D.P.M., Adjunct Professor of Orthopaedic Surgery.

fellowships, sponsored by the American Orthopaedic Association and awarded yearly to senior orthopaedic residents selected by a committee as the best in the country, included a four-week tour of selected orthopaedic centers in North America and Canada. A group of these Traveling Fellows visited Jefferson twice during Gartland's term as Chairman. Hamilton left the full-time faculty in 1982 to go into private practice at Lankenau Hospital but remained active in the Department's teaching activities.

The position of Assistant Professor of Orthopaedics on the full-time faculty was again filled in 1983 with the recruitment of Eric L. Hume. Hume had graduated in medicine from Syracuse but had come to Jefferson to obtain his graduate education in orthopaedic surgery, completing the program in 1983. He proved a happy choice because of his interest in academic orthopaedics. He reorganized the resident teaching program, assisted in teaching biomechanics and psychomotor skills and, in 1985, organized and directed Jefferson's first metabolic bone disease clinic.

Gartland inherited a volunteer group of the orthopaedic faculty who had been working at Jefferson since Dr. DePalma's time. Among them were Drs. John M. Fenlin (Jefferson, 1963), J. David Hoffman (Jefferson, 1956), and Renato J. Nardini. These men joined enthusiastically in the Department restructuring and contributed a great deal of time to the teaching programs. Fenlin developed a special interest in the shoulder joint, including clinical and basic research.

Dr. Scott Jaeger (Jefferson, 1972) joined the Division of Hand Surgery in 1979 after completing his orthopaedic residency at Jefferson and a hand fellowship at the University of Louisville. Dr. Sanford H. Davne, who finished the orthopaedic program at Jefferson, joined the volunteer faculty in 1981 and confined his clinical work to Thomas Jefferson University Hospital. Dr. Mario J. Arena, who finished the Jefferson Residency in 1984, joined Drs. Fenlin and Nardini in practice in 1985, thus further swelling the ranks of the volunteer faculty and contributing to the teaching program and clinical volume.

Physicians involved with teaching orthopaedics to Jefferson students or residents at the affiliated hospitals were offered faculty rank within the Department. A strong and loyal affiliated faculty resulted. By 1985 there were eight affiliated faculty members at Bryn Mawr Hospital, seven at Lankenau Hospital, three each at Methodist Hospital and the A.I. DuPont Institute, and two at the Wilmington Veterans Hospital. Seven of these affiliated faculty members were orthopaedic surgeons who received their orthopaedic education at Jefferson during Gartland's Chairmanship.

In 1971 the senior orthopaedic resident, Dr. S. Terry Canale, now a prominent orthopaedic surgeon in Memphis, Tennessee, persuaded Gartland to undertake the publication of a Department orthopaedic journal as part of the resident's learning process. It was planned that residents would serve as editor and editorial board, negotiate with the printer, plan the layout, and solicit some advertising, with the assistance of a small faculty committee. The idea took hold, and the first issue of the *Jefferson Orthopaedic Journal* appeared in 1972. It has been published yearly since then under the same guidelines. In 1973 the Jefferson Orthopaedic Society adopted the *Journal* as its official publication. Since 1973 the cost of publishing the *Journal* has been divided equally between the Jefferson Orthopaedic Society and the Department. The *Journal* is distributed free to members of the Jefferson Orthopaedic Society and a large group of persons known simply as "Friends of Jefferson." Since the *Jefferson Orthopaedic Journal* has appeared, the Orthopaedic Departments at the University of Iowa and the University of Pennsylvania have begun similar Department journals modeled on the Jefferson publication.

The Jefferson Orthopaedic Society, founded in 1960 by DePalma, had lost most of its forward momentum by 1970. It had deteriorated into a parochial format depending upon orthopaedic residents, Jefferson orthopaedic faculty, and local speakers to put on the yearly program. As a consequence the meetings became less interesting and attendance dropped off alarmingly. Between 1970 and 1974 Gartland and Cotler, because of their national contacts, were able to reverse this trend by the use of an outside invited faculty. The Society membership was persuaded to build its program around a specific orthopaedic theme selected by the Society officers in collaboration with the Chairman. National authorities in the selected area were then invited to come to Jefferson to present their material. Between 1974 and 1985 some of the most prominent orthopaedic surgeons in North America and Canada spoke at the annual Jefferson Orthopaedic Society meetings. Interest in the Society quickened and registrations of 175 to 200 people for the meeting became common. As an additional aid to the resident education program, a Visiting Professor Program started in 1972 was scheduled for the spring of each year. The senior residents chose the Visiting Professor who came for a two-day visit.

In September, 1976, Dr. Everett J. Gordon (Jefferson, 1937), an orthopaedic surgeon then practicing in Washington, D.C., gave the Chairman a significant contribution to establish the Everett J. Gordon Fund for orthopaedic resident education. Proceeds from this fund allowed the orthopaedic faculty to select the "best resident" each year and recognize the selected resident at the annual Jefferson Orthopaedic Society banquet. In addition to this recognition, the selected resident received an appropriate plaque and an expenses-paid trip to the Annual Meeting of the American Academy of Orthopaedic Surgeons.

During 1981 Dr. and Mrs. Thurman Gillespy generously initiated the Gillespy Fund in the Department to be used for special resident educational needs for which no other funds were readily available. Dr. Thurman Gillespy (Jefferson, 1953) completed the orthpaedic residency at Jefferson in 1958 and subsequently practiced in Daytona Beach, Florida.

In 1984 Dr. Richard D. Lackman was recruited to start an adult musculoskeletal tumor service, the first such service in Philadelphia. Lackman had received his orthopaedic education at the University of Pennsylvania followed by a Fellowship in musculoskeletal oncology at the Mayo Clinic. The service flourished, and Jefferson gained additional stature as a center for adult musculoskeletal tumors. Lackman proved a hard worker and enthusiastic teacher.

Gartland was elected President of the Pennsylvania Orthopaedic Society in 1961 and the Philadelphia Orthopaedic Society in 1970. He served as President of the Jefferson Alumni Association in 1974.[11] In 1977 he was elected Second Vice President of the American Academy of Orthopaedic Surgeons, the largest orthopaedic organization in the world. He became First Vice President in 1978 and assumed the Presidency in 1979, considered the key leadership position in American orthopaedics. He was the second Philadelphian and the first Jeffersonian elected to a leadership position in this organization since its founding in 1933.

Gartland represented orthopaedic surgery in the Council of Medical Specialty Societies from 1980 until elected to the Board of Directors of that organization in 1984. From 1980 to 1985 he was a member of the Board of Trustees of the *Journal of Bone and Joint Surgery,* serving as Treasurer (1982–1983) and Chairman of the Board (1984–1985). With these elections and appointments he represented Jefferson in the highest orthopaedic organizational circles. During 1981 his friends and associates at Jefferson presented his portrait to the University. The excess funds were donated to the Philadelphia Orthopaedic Society to support a yearly Gartland Lecture.

The period 1980 to 1985 was an exciting time for orthopaedic surgery at Jefferson and provided visible evidence of the tremendous growth that had occurred in the Department since its founding in 1904. During one four-year period, 1979 to 1982, members of the Jefferson orthopaedic faculty held the three most highly regarded positions in organizational orthopaedics. Gartland was President of the American Academy of Orthopaedic Surgeons in 1979, G. Dean MacEwen (affiliate faculty) was President of the American Orthopaedic Association in 1981, and Jerome Cotler was President of the American Board of Orthopaedic Surgery in 1982.

Dr. Gartland retired on December 31, 1985, to become the James Edwards Professor Emeritus of Orthopaedic Surgery. He then continued his academic career at Jefferson as Director in the Office of Departmental Review.

Richard Harrison Rothman, M.D., Ph.D. (1936–); Sixth Chairman and Fifth James Edwards Professor (1986–)

Dr. Richard H. Rothman (Figure 41-14) became Chairman of the Department on January 1, 1986. Born on December 1, 1936, in Philadelphia, he received his B.A. degree (History) at the University of Pennsylvania and his M.D. in its School of Medicine in 1962. After internship at the Philadelphia General Hospital (1963), he took his residency in Orthopaedic Surgery at Jefferson under Dr. Anthony F. DePalma (1963–1968) and also received his Ph.D. in Anatomy from Jefferson in 1965. He became a member of the Attending Staff of the Children's Hospital of Philadelphia and in 1970 was appointed Director of Orthopaedic Surgery at the Pennsylvania Hospital. On the faculty of the University of Pennsylvania School of Medicine, he rose to Professor of Orthopaedic Surgery in 1979. At the Pennsylvania Hospital, the Rothman Institute was named in his honor in 1984.

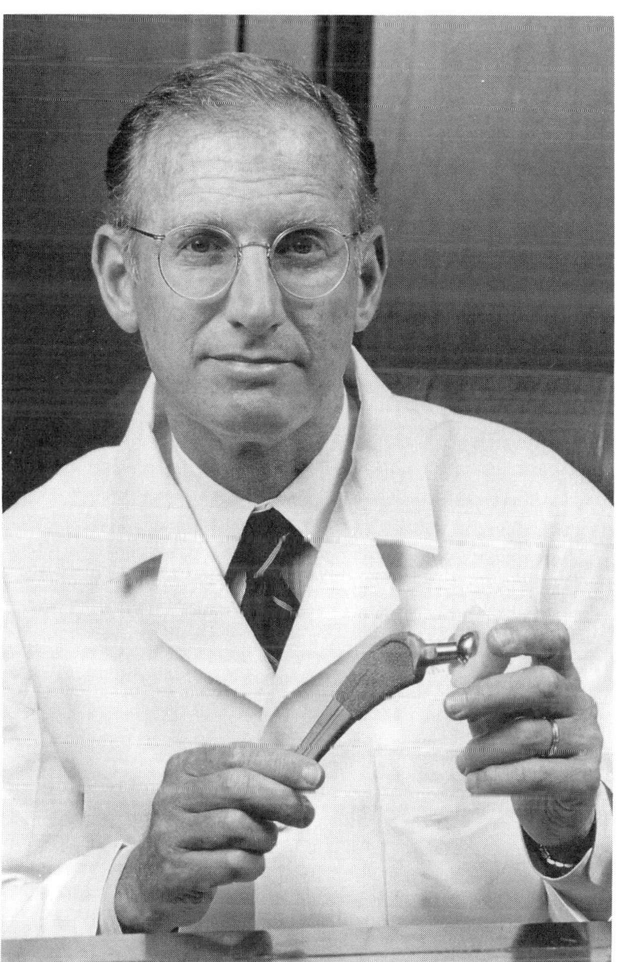

FIG. 41-14. Richard H. Rothman, M.D., Ph.D. (1936–); Sixth Chairman and fifth James Edwards Professor (1986–).

Dr. Rothman brought to Jefferson an impressive experience in administration: Director of the Orthopaedic Research Laboratory of Jefferson Medical College (1969–1970); Vice President of the Philadelphia Orthopaedic Society (1973); Executive Committee, International Society for Study of the Lumbar Spine (1974–1976); President, Jefferson Orthopaedic Society (1976); President, Jefferson Cervical Research Society (1977); Board of Directors of American Academy of Orthopaedic Surgeons; Examiner, American Board of Orthopaedic Surgery; President, Professional Staff of Pennsylvania Hospital (1986); Board Member, Annenberg Institute; Overseer, College of Arts and Sciences of University of Pennsylvania; and Associate Trustee of the University of Pennsylvania.

In addition to memberships in the important societies of his specialty, editorial positions on two journals, and 24 Visiting Professorships, he wrote more than 100 scientific articles and published nine textbooks in orthopaedic subjects.

Dr. Rothman's basic research training and experience were in the study of degenerative changes in connective tissue. He studied the relationship of these changes to blood flow in bone, tendon, and articular cartilage with aging and osteoarthritis. In the realm of clinical research his major emphasis has been on the study of degenerative diseases of the spine, hip, and knee.

On assuming the Chairmanship, Dr. Rothman envisioned his task as one of enriching the Department in terms of its clinical leadership and research productivity. Research both in the basic and clinical realm was an early high order of priority.

The program was modified to expect each Resident and Fellow to be responsible for two major clinical research projects during his or her tenure with the Department that would culminate with manuscripts adequate in quality to be published in national peer review journals. Within two years this was effectively implemented, and 14 original papers were submitted for presentation at the 1988 American Association of Orthopaedic Surgeons' Annual Meeting.

Rothman instituted increased thrust in fundamental research related to the skeletal system. A team was recruited headed by Rocky Tuan, Ph.D., who was appointed as Director of the Orthopaedic Research Laboratories. Dr. Tuan, educated at Rockefeller University, is a nationally recognized investigator in cellular biology with emphasis on the development of the skeletal system and chondrogenesis. He heads a team of five Ph.D. investigators including biochemists and anatomists. His role is not only the development of research related to the skeletal system but education of the Residents and Fellows in terms of contemporary research techniques and to serve as support function to those clinical staff members who wish to participate in fundamental research. His laboratories, funded by Thomas Jefferson University, are modern, 7,000-square-foot facilities on the fifth floor of the Curtis Clinic. His research has attracted substantial ongoing funding from a variety of sources including the National Institutes of Health.

In terms of clinical development, a variety of new resources were brought to the Department to establish regional and national prominence in patient care. First, a partnership was established with the Rothman Institute at Pennsylvania Hospital that immediately brought to the Department the largest unit for hip and knee replacement in the region. Dr. Robert E. Booth, Jr. serves as Chief of the Rothman Institute and is an accomplished surgeon and investigator in the area of total knee replacement. The number of implants performed annually at this Institute approximates 1,000. The Institute also has as one of its key members Dr. Richard Balderston, who heads the Department's Division of Adult Spinal Deformity and acts as Director of Resident Education. Dr. Balderston is acknowledged as an area leader in this complex area of surgical reconstruction.

Dr. Peter Pizzutillo was recruited as Director of Pediatric Orthopaedic Surgery from the Alfred I. DuPont Institute. He has strengthened the Department's Pediatric Division and has built an increasingly strong and sound research and educational program in this area.

Dr. Keith Wapner was recruited as a member of the full-time faculty to develop and head the new Division of Foot and Ankle Surgery. This is the first regional resource geared specifically for reconstruction of the foot and ankle. There has been a geometric growth in the activity of this Division, which is now seen as a unique resource of the University's educational program.

Dr. Phillip Marone, a longtime member of the Professorial Staff of the Department, has recently been appointed as Director of the new Sports Medicine Program. This program, housed in the Edison Building, is yet another important facet of the patient care and educational program of the Department. Dr. Marone plans to coordinate the faculty members engaged in the varied practice of sports medicine and to develop several cooperative interinstitutional programs of research and education in this field.

Dr. Jerome Cotler was appointed in 1987 as Director of Orthopaedic Surgery for the University Hospital. He thereby assumed responsibility for the management of the Hospital Unit as well as serving as Co-Director of the Spinal Cord Injury Unit. His energy and effective management have led to a doubling of the clinical activities between the years 1986 and 1988.

Dr. Rothman sees as his assignment the continued development of the research activities, teaching programs, and clinical patient care within the Department. It is anticipated that under his direction the necessary human resources, financial support, and energies can be brought to the Department to raise each of these areas of activity to increased national prominence.

References

1. Kelley, H.A., and Burrage, W.L., *American Medical Biographies.* New York: Appleton, 1928, pp. 20–21.
2. Wilson, H.A.: "A New Apparatus for Preparing Dry Gypsum Bandages," *Proc. Phila., Co. Med. Soc.,* 8, 1887, pp. 51–52.
3. Minutes, Administrative Committee, Jefferson Medical College, November 28, 1904.
4. J. Torrence Rugh, *Clinic Yearbook, Jeff. Med. Coll.,* 1935, p. 49.
5. Lovett, R.W., "H. Augustus Wilson, M.D., An Appreciation," *J. Orthopaedic Surg.* 1:320, 1919.
6. J. Torrence Rugh, *Clinic Yearbook, Jeff. Med. Coll.,* 1934, p. 214.
7. J. Torrence Rugh, *Clinic Yearbook, Jeff. Med. Coll.,* 1936, p. 48.
8. "The Department of Orthopaedic Surgery." *Jeff. Al. Bull.,* May 1960, pp. 4–16.
9. "The Jefferson Scene," *Jeff. Al. Bull.,* Winter 1984, pp. 12–13.
10. "Alumni President," *Jeff. Al. Bull.,* March 1959, p. 8.
11. "Alumni President," *Jeff. Al. Bull.,* Spring 1974, pp. 28–29.

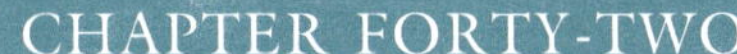

Department of Otolaryngology

William H. Baltzell, M.D. and Louis D. Lowry, M.D.

"Yet it was not possible for me to say to men: speak louder, shout, for I am deaf. Alas! how could I declare the weakness of a sense which in me ought to be more acute than in others—a sense which formerly I possessed in highest perfection, a perfection such as few in my profession enjoy, or ever have enjoyed."

—Ludwig van Beethoven (1770–1827)

The invention of the modern laryngoscope in 1855 by Manuel Garcia, a Spanish singing teacher in London, led to the early development of laryngology as a specialty both abroad and in America. One year earlier, Samuel D. Gross, destined to be the Professor of Surgery at Jefferson in 1856, published *A Practical Treatise on Foreign Bodies in the Air Passages*. It was a pioneer work, two years in the making, which consisted of 468 pages with 159 woodcuts, giving full reports of 200 instances and attempting to systematize all current knowledge upon this subject. It was to be made obsolete by the later work of Chevalier Jackson. It is of further interest that Gross in his *System of Surgery* (1859) devoted 33 pages to diseases of the ear. The Japanese used the Dutch translation to retranslate this section for their first reference book on otology.

The Early Years

The Department of Otolaryngology was not created at Jefferson until 1954. It developed from a fusion of the Departments of Laryngology (1904), Otology (1904), and Bronchoesophagology (1924). This evolution is best understood in terms of the pioneers and early Professors who contributed to Jefferson's stature in this field.

Richard J. Levis, M.D. (1867)

Richard Levis (Figure 42-1) was born in Philadelphia in 1827.[1] The son of Dr. Mahlon Levis, he attended Central High School (the degree at that time was equivalent to that from a Junior College) and graduated from Jefferson in 1848. In 1859 his appointments included Surgeon to Blockley (Philadelphia General Hospital), Pennsylvania Hospital, and Wills Eye Hospital. During the Civil War he volunteered in the Union Army. Upon completion of his military service as Surgeon he was appointed at Jefferson as Clinical Lecturer in Ophthalmology and Aural Surgery in 1867. In 1877 at the opening of the first Jefferson Medical College Hospital on Sansom Street, Levis was promoted to Professor of Aural Surgery.

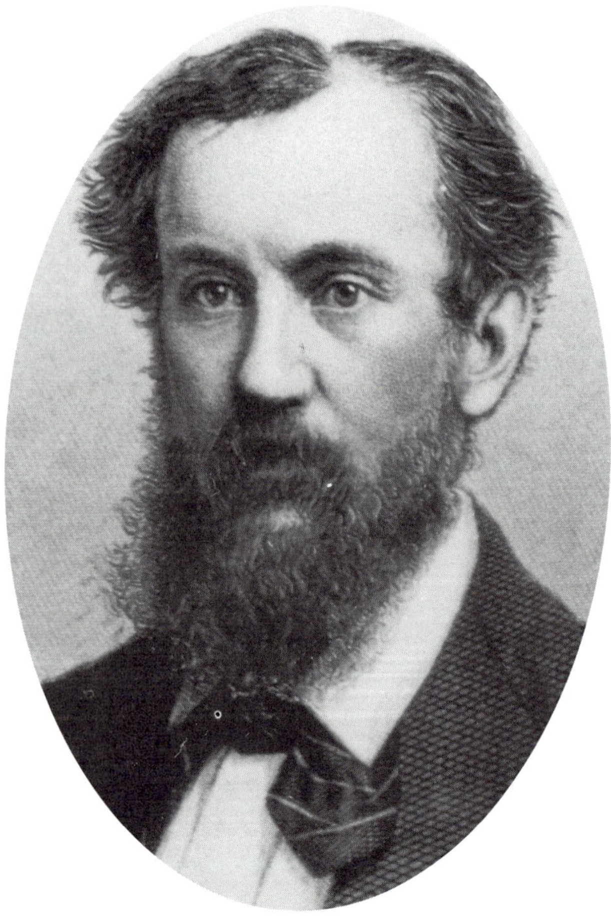

FIG. 42-1. Richard J. Levis (Jefferson, 1848), Clinical Lecturer in Ophthalmology and Aural Surgery (1867), and Professor of Aural Surgery (1877) in the first Jefferson Medical College Hospital.

In addition to his special interest in the eye and ear, Dr. Levis was an outstanding general surgeon. He modified numerous operative procedures and invented surgical instruments and orthopedic appliances. His lectures were "clear and concise,"[2] and he was a prolific writer. In 1879 he aided Dr. Samuel D. Gross in founding the Philadelphia Academy of Surgery and was an original member of the American Surgical Association. His leadership was also manifested in his Presidency of the Philadelphia County Medical Society (1885 and 1886) and of the Pennsylvania Medical Society (1888).

Jacob da Silva Solis-Cohen, M.D. (1868)

One of the most distinguished laryngologists in the nineteenth century was Dr. Jacob Solis-Cohen (Figure 42-2). He was born in New York in 1838 and educated in Philadelphia at the Central High School and the University of Pennsylvania Medical School, where he received his M.D. degree in 1860. After serving as a Surgeon during the Civil War, Dr. Solis-Cohen returned to Philadelphia and became associated with Jefferson. In 1867 he was appointed Lecturer on Electrotherapeutics. In 1869 he became Lecturer on Laryngoscopy and Diseases of the Chest. This was the era of the generalist, and there was much derision of anyone specializing; Samuel D. Gross, in introducing Dr. Solis-Cohen to the class, criticized him for leaving the ranks of legitimate practitioners to become engaged in a narrow specialty: "He devotes most of his time to a cubic inch of the human anatomy. Some day I suppose we will have specialists confining themselves to diseases of the navel."[3]

Like most of his colleagues at Jefferson in the last half of the nineteenth century, Dr. Solis-Cohen wrote many papers and books. In 1867 he published *Inhalation: Its Therapeutics and*

Practice, A Treatise on the Inhalation of Gases, Vapors, Nebulized Fluids, and Powders. His most important book was *Diseases of the Throat and Nasal Passages—A Guide to the Diagnosis and Treatment of Affections of the Pharynx, Esophagus, Trachea, Larynx and Nares* (1872). No other book published in the United States has ever had a greater influence in disseminating a wide and thorough knowledge of laryngology. In 1874 a monograph was published on *Croup in Its Relations to Tracheotomy.* This was based on a study of 5,000 recorded cases.

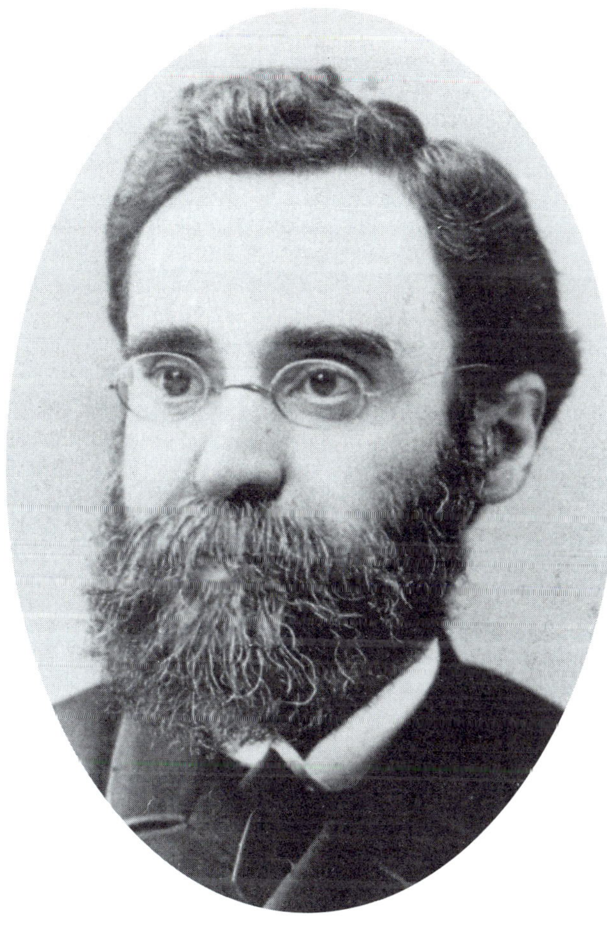

FIG. 42-2. Jacob da Silva Solis-Cohen, Lecturer on Laryngology and Diseases of the Chest (1869); was a pioneer in laryngeal surgery.

Dr. Solis-Cohen considered himself "a physician with a specialty, always stressing the importance of a well-grounded knowledge of general medicine."[4] As a surgeon he was a pioneer and innovator. In 1867 he performed the first successful laryngotomy in the United States for removal of a cancerous growth. In 1892 he performed a closed field laryngectomy, which was successful.

As an organizer and leader, Dr. Solis-Cohen was a founder of the American Laryngological Association in 1878 and the *Archives of Laryngology* in 1880. He was President of the Philadelphia County Medical Society (1887–1888) and also a member of many civil and military organizations. "He was a prime mover, an original investigator, an artist in his specialty. He is one of the brightest stars in the galaxy of American laryngologists."[5] His portrait hangs outside the Solis-Cohen Auditorium in Jefferson Alumni Hall in company with his physician brother Solomon (Jefferson, 1883) and his lawyer nephew, D. Hays Solis-Cohen, a member of Jefferson's Board of Trustees (1951–1970).

▪ Laurence Turnbull, M.D. (1877)

Laurence Turnbull (Figure 42-3), born in Scotland in 1821, emigrated to this country at the age of 17 and was apprenticed to a drug manufacturer, Mr. John Bringhurst. He graduated from the Philadelphia College of Pharmacy and eventually took up the study of medicine in the office of Professor John K. Mitchell.

Soon after graduation from Jefferson in 1845, Turnbull became resident physician at Blockley (Philadelphia General Hospital), and subsequently outdoor physician to the Guardians of the Poor for the district of Moyamensing, as well as vaccination physician for the same district. In 1857 Dr. Turnbull was elected one of the physicians to the Department of Diseases of the Eye and Ear of the old Howard Hospital (at Broad and Catherine Streets). In 1859 he visited Europe, where he studied diseases of the eye and ear. On his return he specialized in aural surgery.

In 1877 Dr. Turnbull was appointed Aural Surgeon and Chief of the Ear Clinic of the newly opened Jefferson Medical College Hospital on Sansom Street. "He was the first surgeon in the United States to perform the operation of perforation of the mastoid for disease in that region."[6] His textbook *A Clinical Manual of the Diseases of the Ear* (1872) went through two editions. *Artificial Anesthesia: A Manual of Anesthetic Agents and Their Employment in the Treatment of Disease* (1878) had four editions. In addition to memberships in various medical societies, he presided over the Section of Otology of the AMA (1880) and the British Medical Association (1881).

Dr. Turnbull had many other interests outside of medicine. He was a member of the St. Andrews Society (a Scottish ethnic organization)[6] from 1842 until his death in 1900. He frequently lectured at the Franklin Institute on such varied topics as *Chemistry Applied to the Arts* and *The Electromagnetic Telegraph*.[6]

Generous with his earnings, Dr. Turnbull was a large contributor to the founding of the 1877 Jefferson Hospital. His pioneer clinical work, teaching, writing, and innovations make him a worthy contender for the title of "Father of American Otology."

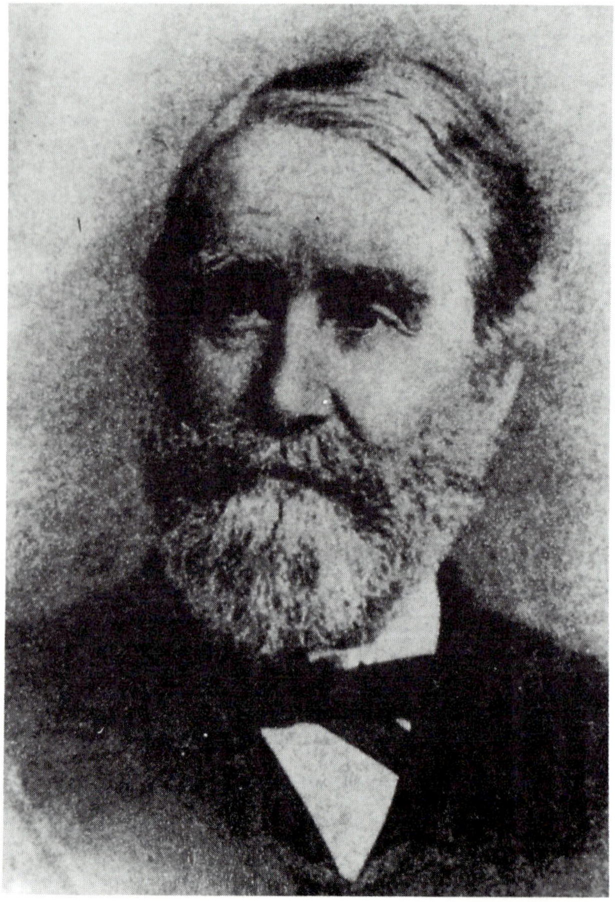

FIG. 42-3. Laurence Turnbull (Jefferson, 1845), Aural Surgeon and Chief of the Ear Clinic in the 1877 Hospital.

David Braden Kyle, M.D.; First Chairman of Laryngology (1904–1916)

As was the fashion in the last half of the nineteenth century, the next Professor of Laryngology, David Braden Kyle (Figure 42-4) had a varied career before entering the practice of otolaryngology. Born in Cadiz, Ohio, in 1863, he graduated from Muskegon College and then from Jefferson in 1891. While at Jefferson he took private courses from Professor William Coplin in bacteriology and pathology, and from Professor John Chalmers DaCosta in nervous diseases,

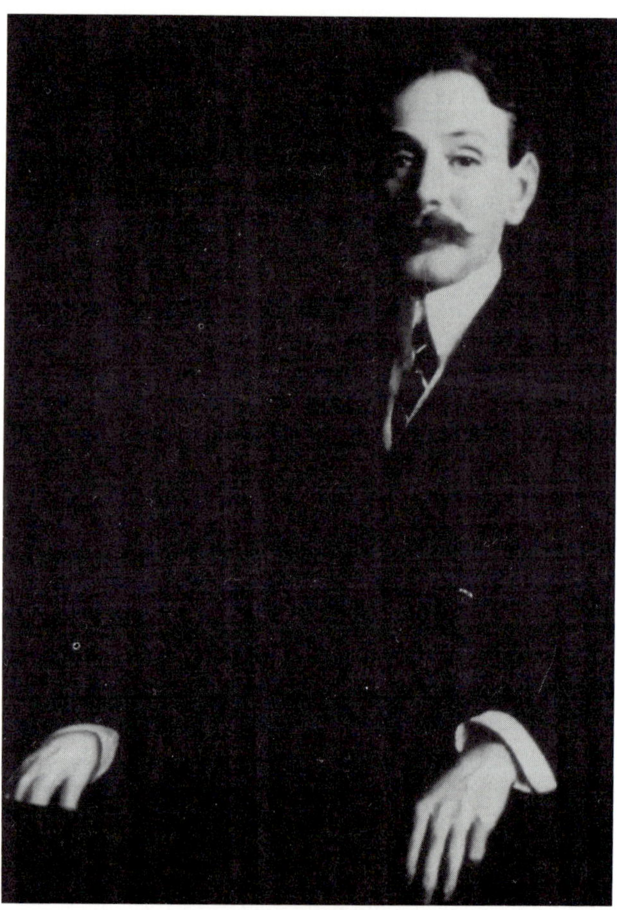

FIG. 42-4. David Braden Kyle (Jefferson, 1891); First Chairman of Laryngology (1904–1916).

anatomy, and surgery. In his senior year he was an office student of Dr. W. Joseph Hearn in surgery. At graduation he was awarded the gold medal by Dr. W.W. Keen for the best essay *The Pathology and Treatment of Tetanus*. He then became Assistant Demonstrator of Pathology. Upon beginning his practice he developed a private laboratory for instruction in clinical microscopy, bacteriology, and pathology. By 1896 Dr. Kyle had developed a practice devoted to diseases of the ear, nose, throat, and chest to such a degree that he was appointed Clinical Professor of Laryngology at Jefferson. He became full Professor in 1904.

Kyle was an active member of many medical organizations and was President of the American Laryngological, Rhinological, and Otological Society in 1900. He was author of *A Textbook on Diseases of the Nose and Throat* published in 1899 with five subsequent editions until 1914. Like most energetic surgeons, Kyle started in the operating room at 6:30 A.M. so that he could personally observe his patients after their surgical procedures. This was a habit following the custom of his predecessor, Dr. Solis-Cohen.

Dr. Kyle died suddenly in 1916 at the age of 53 from an attack of pleuropneumonia.[7]

Seth MacCuen Smith, M.D.; First Chairman of Otology (1904–1929)

Seth Smith (Figure 42-5) was born in Hollidaysburg, Pennsylvania, in 1863. His father, Dr. G. W. Smith, was a physician who obviously inspired his son in the choice of a career. Dr. Smith graduated from Jefferson in 1884 and was resident physician at Germantown Hospital, where he became interested in diseases of the ear, nose, and throat. In 1886 he became Clinical Chief of Otology at Jefferson Hospital under the supervision of Dr. Laurence Turnbull.

Dr. Smith became Clinical Professor in 1894 and full Professor in charge of the Department in 1904. He wrote extensively, mostly on otology. His chapter on diseases of the ear was included in the *Harris System of Practical Therapeutics*. He edited the English translation from the German of the Bruhl-Politzer *Atlas of Otology*. He was on the council of the Triologic Society as well as various other national and international organizations. Upon his death in September, 1929, he left his entire library of over 1,000 volumes to Jefferson.

Chevalier Jackson, M.D.; Second Chairman of Laryngology (1916–1924), First Chairman of Bronchoesophagology (1924–1930)

Chevalier Jackson (Figure 42-6) was born in Pittsburgh in 1865, educated there for his college

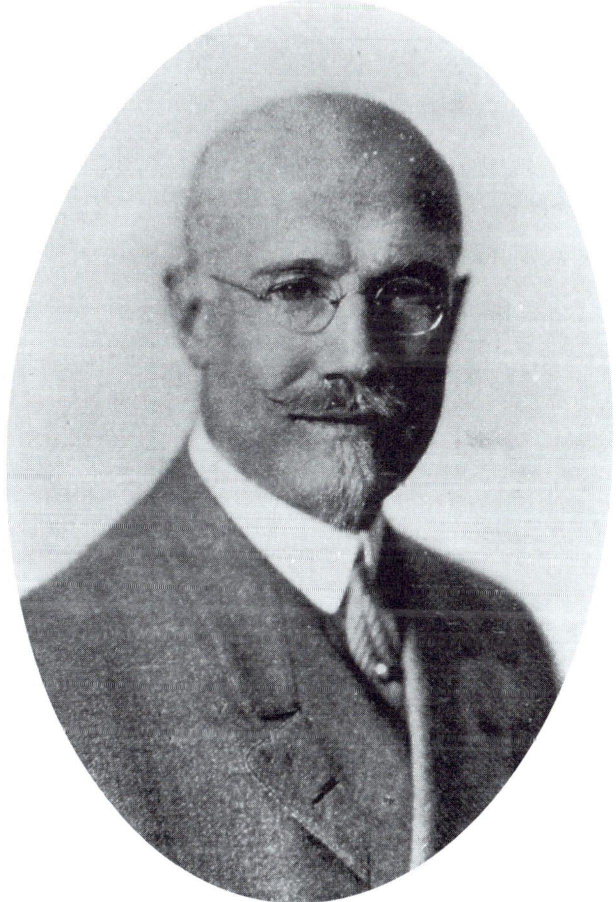

FIG. 42-5. Seth M. Smith (Jefferson, 1884), First Chairman of Otology (1904–1929).

degree, and graduated from Jefferson in 1886, just old enough to get a license to practice. He was much influenced by Professor Jacob Solis-Cohen, and on his return to Pittsburgh he began his practice of laryngology. As most ambitious young men of his time, he studied in Europe, visiting the clinics of Morrell Mackenzie in London and Gustav Killian in Germany. With the development of the tungsten electric light bulb, adequate vision of the esophagus and tracheobronchial tree became possible. Dr. Jackson, as a good mechanic, invented and improved the instruments used for the removal of foreign bodies from the food and air passages. Under skillful management the mortality of these cases was reduced from over 80% to fewer than 5%.[8] In 1916 Dr. Jackson accepted the Chair of Laryngology at Jefferson, and in 1924 a new Department of Bronchoscopy and Esophagoscopy was created for him.

In 1930 Dr. Jackson reached the mandatory age of retirement at Jefferson. He was not ready to retire, so he moved the Jackson Clinic to Temple University while continuing as Professor at Woman's Medical College and the Graduate School of the University of Pennsylvania. One more career lay ahead. He became the President of the Woman's Medical College in 1935 and held that position until 1941.

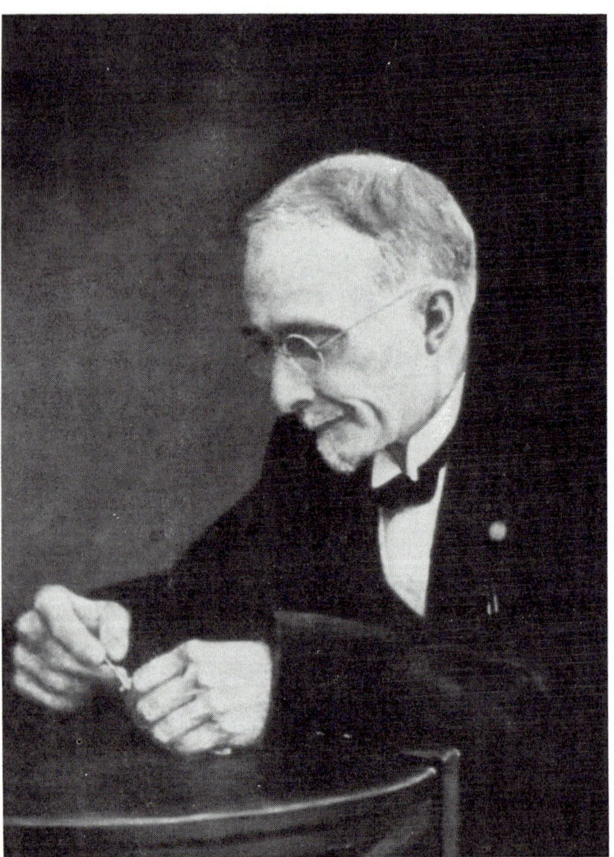

FIG. 42-6. Chevalier Jackson (Jefferson, 1886), Second Chairman of Laryngology (1916–1924), and First Chairman of Bronchoesophagology (1924–1930).

One of Dr. Jackson's greatest contributions to humanity was the passage of a federal caustic poisons law in 1927. He was greatly influenced by the many tragic patients that he treated for lye ingestion. Jackson spent a large amount of time and energy contacting politicians all over the country to ensure the enactment of this legislation.

Dr. Jackson was a prolific writer, contributing hundreds of articles and 12 textbooks that have been translated into five languages. His textbook, *Bronchoscopy and Esophagoscopy: A Manual of Peroral Endoscopy and Laryngeal Surgery* (1922), became a bible in its field. He was at some time the president of every organization having to do with laryngology and a member of a multitude of foreign medical groups, and he was honored with medals and awards throughout the world.

Jackson was delicate in health and small in stature. Most meticulous with details, and never leaving anything to chance, he once stated: "I would be greatly distressed if a situation arose which I had not anticipated and not already provided for."[8] His interest in medicine and people continued until his death on August 16, 1958, at the age of 93.

There is no large medical facility in the world that has not been touched by Dr. Jackson's teachings of the art and science of bronchoesophagoscopy. His name is honored on Jefferson's Winged Ox column, and his portrait was presented to the College in 1956.

Fielding O. Lewis, M.D.; Third Chairman of Laryngology (1924–1934)

Fielding Lewis (Figure 42-7) was born in 1879 in Henderson County, Kentucky. He graduated from the Philadelphia College of Pharmacy in 1901, was President of his graduating class at Jefferson in 1906, and interned there. He became the assistant to Dr. David Braden Kyle and associated with the Philadelphia General Hospital. During World War I he served as a surgeon with the rank of Captain.

Dr. Lewis was appointed Professor of Laryngology in 1924. He unfortunately had a severe "stroke" in 1934, which forced his retirement at the peak of his career. He retired to Chester County where he lived until his death in 1965. It was said that "surgery was done by him with the skill and thoroughness of a master craftsman."[9] He was one of the first in the United States to perform a wide-field laryngectomy.

Among the many organizations to which he belonged were The Triologic Society, American Academy of Ophthalmology and Otolaryngology, and the Philadelphia Laryngological Society. He was the author of over 20 papers including one on President Washington's last illness.[10]

Joseph Clarence Keeler, M.D.; Second Chairman of Otology (1930–1935)

Joseph Keeler (Figure 42-8) was born in Doylestown, Pennsylvania, in 1871 and after college

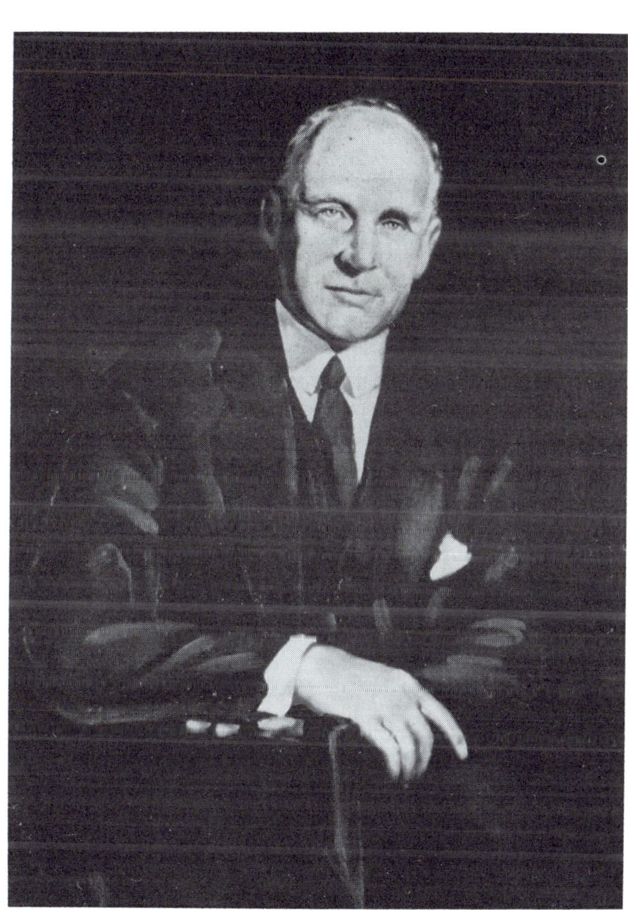

FIG. 42-7. Fielding O. Lewis (Jefferson, 1906), Third Chairman of Laryngology (1924–1934).

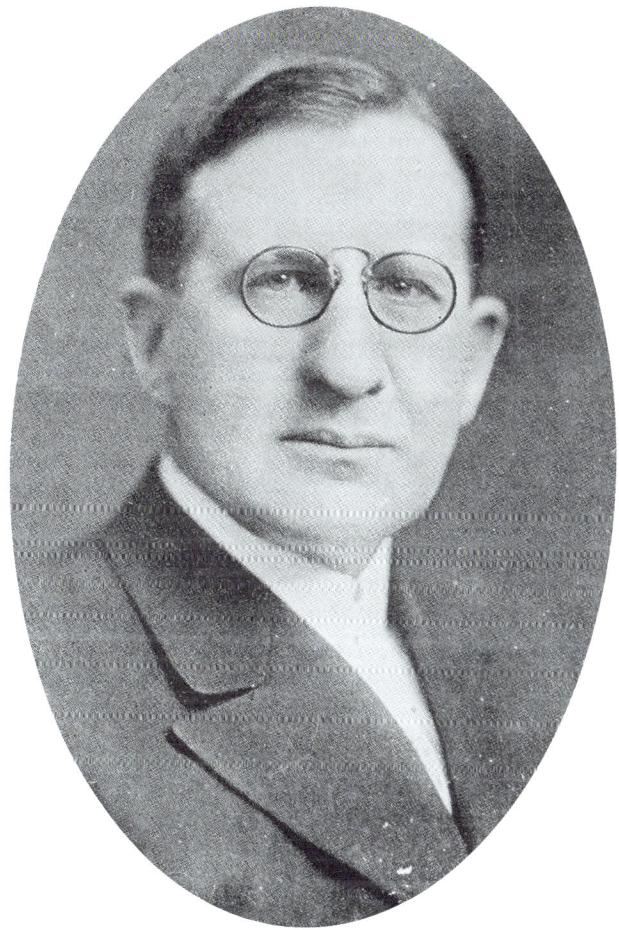

FIG. 42-8. Joseph C. Keeler (Jefferson, 1896), Second Chairman of Otology (1930–1935).

graduated from Jefferson in 1896. Following internship at his alma mater he became the assistant to Dr. S. MacCuen Smith. During World War I he served in the Army Medical Corps. He also was associated with the Germantown Hospital, where he was Chief of Otology.

In 1930 Dr. Keeler was appointed Professor of Otology at Jefferson. He wrote a number of scientific papers including a review of 1,500 cases of mastoid surgery. He was the author of a popular textbook *Modern Otology* (1930), which he dedicated to his mentor, Dr. S. MacCuen Smith. He was a member of the American Otologic Society, the American Laryngological Society, the College of Physicians of Philadelphia, the Philadelphia Laryngology Society, and the American Academy of Ophthalmology and Otolaryngology.

Dr. Keeler was a very caring physician and treated his house staff and personnel with kindness and understanding. He was stricken with a heart attack while performing a mastoidectomy at Jefferson in September, 1935.[11]

Horace J. Williams, M.D.; Third Chairman of Otology (1937–1950)

Horace Williams (Figure 42-9) graduated from Jefferson in the Class of 1912. Following internship there he served in the Army Medical Corps during World War I. On return from military service he became associated with the Children's Hospital and Germantown Hospital, where he worked with Dr. Joseph Keeler. At Jefferson he rose through the ranks to Professor and Chairman of Otology in 1937.

Dr. Williams was a skilled surgeon and excellent teacher. It was said that "to watch him operate with hammer and chisel and curette was to watch a great artist."[12] During most of his career, which preceded the antibiotic era, he often performed five to ten mastoidectomies a week.

Dr. Williams was a member of the American Otologic Society, College of Physicians of Philadelphia, the Philadelphia Laryngological Society, the American College of Surgery, the Triologic Society, and the American Academy of Ophthalmology and Otolaryngology. He died June 5, 1950.

Louis H. Clerf, M.D., LL.D., Sc.D., L.H.D.; Second Chairman of Bronchoesophagology (1930–1954), Fourth Chairman of Laryngology (1936–1954)

Louis Clerf (Figure 42-10) was born in Ellensburg, Washington, in 1889. He always spoke with pleasure of his youth on his father's cattle ranch. After graduating from St. Martin's College in Olympia, Washington, he attended the University of Oregon Medical School. Since most of the

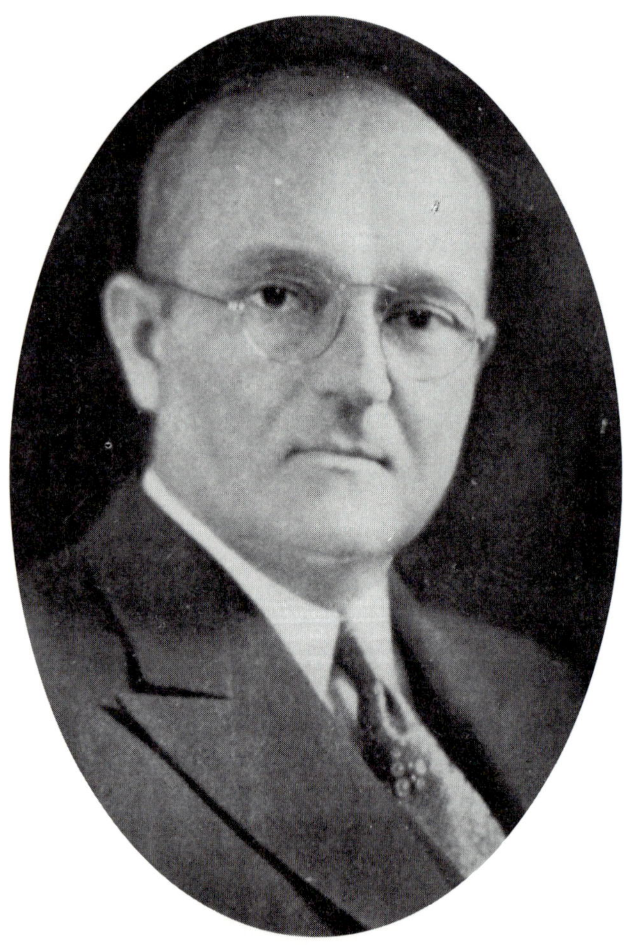

FIG. 42-9. Horace J. Williams (Jefferson, 1912), Third Chairman of Otology (1937–1950).

textbooks he used were written by Jefferson men, he transferred to Jefferson Medical College for his last two years, graduating in the Class of 1912. After two years of internship at Jefferson he became Chief Resident of the Hospital. During World War I he served in the Navy Medical Department, continuing his association in the reserves until he retired with the rank of Captain.

After the War he attended the New York Eye and Ear Infirmary until he returned to Jefferson in 1922 as Instructor in Bronchoesophagoscopy under Dr. Chevalier Jackson. When Dr. Jackson reached mandatory retirement age in 1930, Dr. Clerf was appointed Chairman of Bronchology and Esophagology. In 1936, after the early retirement of Dr. Fielding O. Lewis, Clerf was also appointed Chairman of Laryngology. In 1954 he became Emeritus Professor.[13]

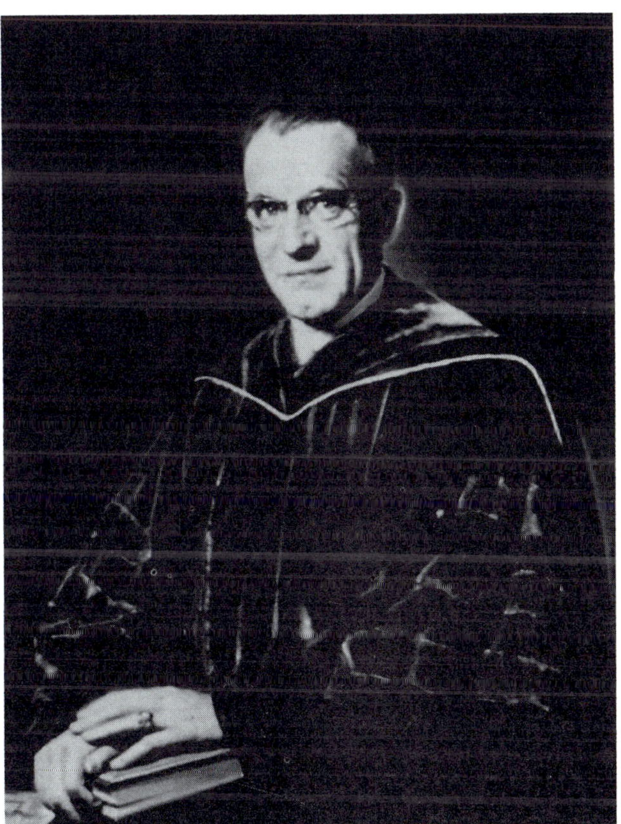

FIG. 42-10. Louis H. Clerf (Jefferson, 1912); Second Chairman of Bronchoesophagology (1930–1954), and Fourth Chairman of Laryngology (1936–1954).

Dr. Clerf gave himself fully to his profession. He was a member of over 25 medical organizations and gave talks in all the 48 states of the Union of his time. He became President of the Philadelphia County Medical Society, American Broncho-Esophageal Association, Philadelphia Laryngological Society, Triological Society, and New York Laryngological Society. He was also on the American Board of Examiners in Otolaryngology and the American Board of Chest Physicians. He received the honorary degrees of Doctor of Laws, Villanova University; Doctor of Science, St. Martin's College; and Doctor of Letters, Jefferson Medical College. In addition to these activities he contributed over 200 papers to the literature. He always carried several pencils, almost too short to use, in his pocket to make notes.

At Jefferson, Dr. Clerf reorganized the Alumni Giving Campaign and headed the Alumni contributions to the Pavilion (Foerderer) Building. His portrait was presented to the College by the Class of 1949, and he was the first recipient of the Alumni Achievement Award in 1964. He was truly one of those recognized as a "Mr. Jefferson."

Fred Harbert, M.D., Sc.D.; Fourth Chairman of Otology (1951–1954), First Chairman of Otolaryngology (1954–1970)

Fred Harbert (Figure 42-11) came to Jefferson as Chairman of Otology in 1951 after an illustrious career in the United States Navy. Born in Detroit in 1905, Harbert received his B.S. degree from Wayne State University in 1928 and within a year his M.D. degree from the same University. After internship at the Philadelphia Naval Hospital he continued on active duty in the Navy until his retirement as Captain in 1954. During his tour of duty he continued his academic career with a year in otolaryngology at the Graduate School of the University of Pennsylvania and received his certification in otolaryngology in 1938. In 1943 he had a residency in ophthalmology at the Illinois Eye and Ear Infirmary and passed his boards in ophthalmology in 1946. He was one of the last eye, ear, nose, and throat specialists.[14,15]

Dr. Harbert succeeded Dr. Williams as Chairman of the Department of Otology in 1951. In 1954, on Dr. Clerf's retirement as Professor of Laryngology and Bronchoesophagoscopy, he was appointed Professor of Otolaryngology and Chairman of the unified Department.

Dr. Harbert's first love was teaching. His lectures were always clear and to the point. The student or resident who came to a session unprepared or who tried to "cover up" was treated in such a manner that it did not occur a second time. Dr. Harbert authored more than 60 scientific papers. He received a Master in Science (Medicine) in 1942 and Doctorate of Science (Medicine) in 1943. He was an examiner for the American Board of Ophthalmology for many years and a member of many national societies. He received the Distinguished Service Citation from Wayne State University.

Following his retirement in 1970 as Emeritus Professor, Dr. Harbert moved to the Eastern Shore of Maryland and remained as a consultant to the Veterans' Administration Hospital in Wilmington, Delaware. His portrait was presented to the College in 1978 by his many friends.

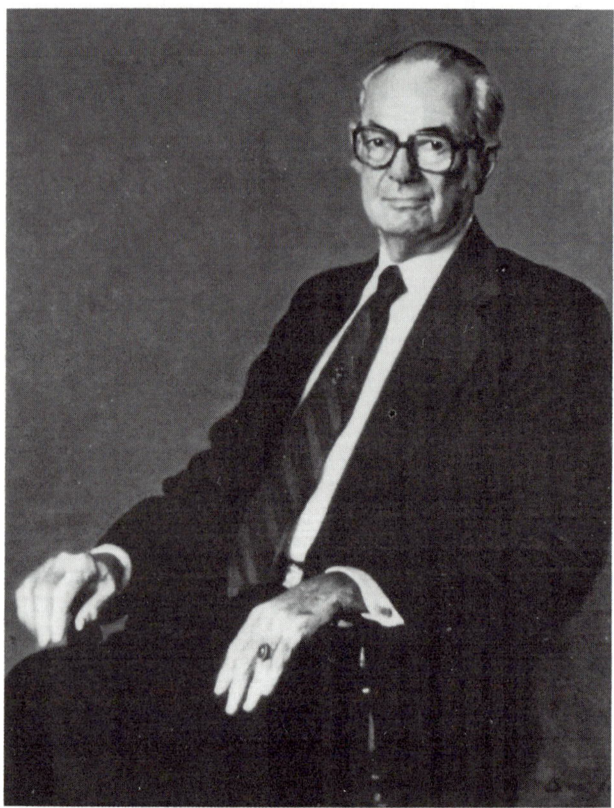

FIG. 42-11. Fred Harbert, M.D.; Fourth Chairman of Otology (1951–1954), and First Chairman of Otolaryngology (1954–1970).

James Robert Leonard, M.D.; Second Chairman of Otolaryngology (1970–1972)

James Leonard was appointed Professor and Chairman of Otolaryngology in 1970. He received his undergraduate education at the University of Iowa, graduating with a B.S. degree in 1955. He graduated from the Medical College of Virginia in 1959. His residency in otolaryngology at Johns Hopkins was completed in 1965. He resigned in October 1972.

John J. O'Keefe, M.D.; Third Chairman of Otolaryngology (1973–1975)

Dr. O'Keefe (Figure 42-12) was a Philadelphian who attended parochial schools and graduated from St. Joseph's College in 1933. Four years later he received his M.D. degree from Jefferson. After two years (1937–1939) in a rotating internship at Jefferson, he received the Ross V. Patterson Fellowship in Bronchoesophagology while acting as assistant to Dr. Louis H. Clerf. His career at Jefferson was then interrupted by three years in the United States Air Force Medical Department during World War II.

Shortly after resuming his career at Jefferson, O'Keefe became a Diplomate of the American Board of Otolaryngology (1946). He also joined the staff of Our Lady of Lourdes and Nazareth Hospitals. At Jefferson he continued through the academic ranks until appointed Acting Chairman upon the resignation of Dr. Leonard in 1972, and Chairman of Otolaryngology in 1973. This position he held until his retirement in 1975.

Dr. O'Keefe was a Fellow of a number of national organizations including the American Academy of Ophthalmology and Otolaryngology;

American Broncho-Esophagological Association; American Laryngology, Rhinology, and Otology Society; American College of Chest Physicians; American Society of ENT Secretaries; American Thoracic Society; Aero-Medical Society; American College of Surgeons, and American Laryngological Association.

His regional organization memberships were legion. He spoke frequently at the national and local societies and was the author of over 50 papers, including one on the development of bronchoscopy at Jefferson.[8] He died from complications of cardiovascular disease on November 9, 1985.

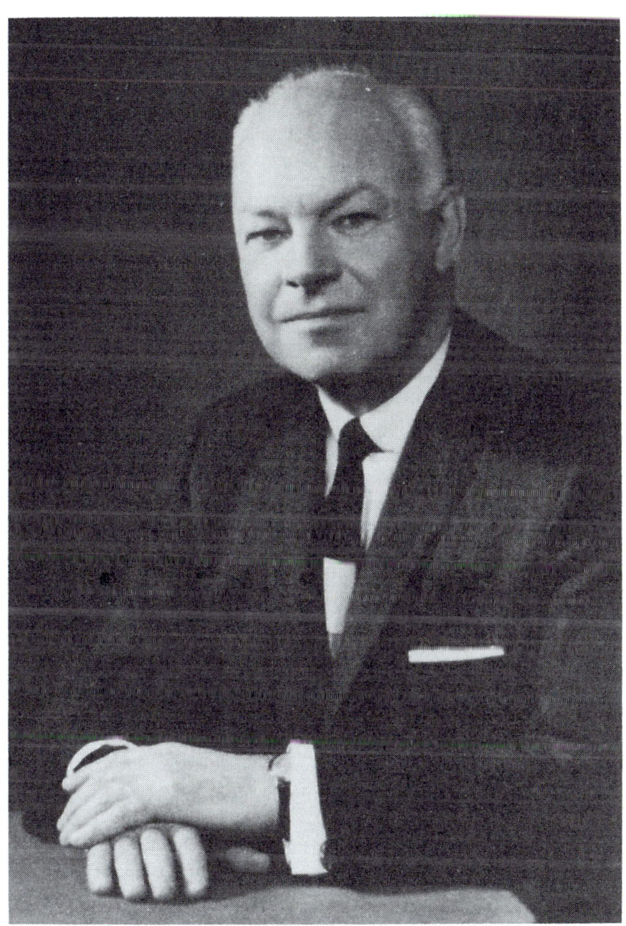

FIG. 42-12. John J. O'Keefe (Jefferson, 1937), Third Chairman of Otolaryngology (1973–1975).

Lindsay L. Pratt, M.D.; Fourth Chairman of Otolaryngology (1975–1977)

Lindsay Pratt (Figure 42-13) was born in 1926. He graduated from Muhlenberg College and received his M.D. degree from Jefferson in 1953. After a residency in otolaryngology at Temple University, he received a Master of Science (Medicine) in 1961. He then became Assistant Professor of Otolaryngology at Washington University School of Medicine in St. Louis.

Dr. Pratt came to Jefferson as Chairman of the Department in 1975. He held memberships in all the important local and national societies of his specialty and had an impressive bibliography. He added strength to the Department through his intense interest and expertise in surgery for cancer of the head and neck. He was well liked and eminently successful as surgeon, teacher, and administrator.

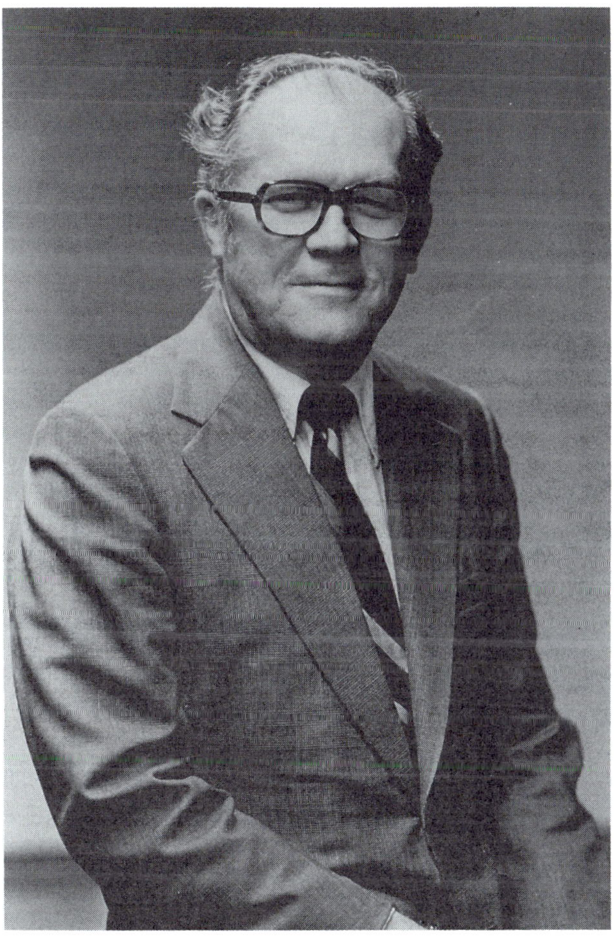

FIG. 42-13. Lindsay L. Pratt, M.D., Fourth Chairman of Otolaryngology (1975–1977).

Unfortunately, limitations on the extent to which Dr. Pratt could be allowed to expand his staff and facilities caused frustrations that led to his resignation in 1977.

Diran O. Mikaelian, M.D.; Acting Chairman of Otolaryngology (1977–1979)

Dr. Mikaelian (Figure 42-14), of Armenian origin, was born in 1938. He received his college (B.S., 1950) and medical (M.D., 1954) degrees at the American University of Beirut, Lebanon. After continuing with an internship (1954–1955) and residency in otolaryngology (1955–1958) at the American University of Beirut, he took a fellowship in otology and laryngology at Johns Hopkins (1962–1965). From 1958 to 1962 and 1965 to 1970 Dr. Mikaelian taught at the American University of Beirut and carried out research in auditory neurophysiology, otoneurology, and problems of laryngo-esophagology. He came to Jefferson in 1970 as Assistant Professor of Otolaryngology and became a full Professor in 1975.

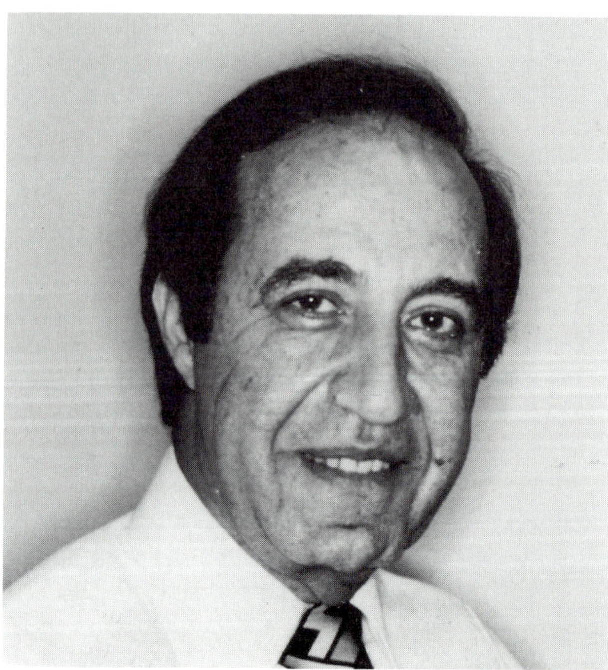

FIG. 42-14. Diran O. Mikaelian, M.D., Acting Chairman of Otolaryngology (1977–1979).

In addition to his clinical expertise, Dr. Mikaelian held memberships in the prestigious societies of his specialty and was a prolific writer in the basic sciences as well as surgical aspects of otolaryngology. In 1978 he was honored with the coveted First Prize of the Fowler Award from the American Otological, Rhinological, and Laryngological Society (Triological Society) for his thesis on *Development and Degeneration of Hearing in the C57*/b*16* Mouse.

With the appointment of Dr. Louis Dale Lowry as Chairman on January 1, 1980, Dr. Mikaelian continued his active professorial role in the Department as clinician, teacher, and researcher.

Louis Dale Lowry, M.D.; Fifth Chairman of Otolaryngology (1980–)

Louis Dale Lowry (Figure 42-15) was born in Fort Scott, Kansas, on March 1, 1937, and was raised in Vernon County, Missouri, on a tenant farm. He received his A.B. in Chemistry (1958) and M.D. (1962) at the University of Missouri. During his internship at the Great Lakes Naval Hospital, he met Dr. George Connor, with whom he had an elective in otolaryngology. At that time Dr. Lowry had planned to become a general practitioner, and since he had had no otolaryngology in his medical school training, he felt that this elective would be important. Dr. Connor's influence became pervasive. Immediately after internship, Dr. Lowry served in the submarine service as a Navy Medical Officer, but upon completing his tour of duty in 1967, Dr. Lowry returned to the University of Chicago for his residency in surgery and otolaryngology. He then became a full-time member of the Department of Otorhinolaryngology at the University of Oklahoma Health Sciences Center in 1971. In 1973 he left Oklahoma for the University of Pennsylvania, where he rose to Associate Professor of Otorhinolaryngology and Human

Communication by 1979. At this time, Dr. Lowry was actively looking at Departments of Otolaryngology for a possible Chairmanship. The appointment at Jefferson was fortuitous in that he did not have to leave Philadelphia. He was appointed in the fall of 1979 and began actively on January 1, 1980.

Dr. Lowry has been on the faculty of the American Board of Otolaryngology and has lectured and taught many courses at national meetings. He has an impressive bibliography of at least 60 articles, along with many presentations at local and national meetings. He belongs to many societies in his field and was President of the Philadelphia Society of Facial Plastic Surgeons (1979–1981). His major contribution has been the development of an artificial larynx by which speech is generated electronically within the oral cavity.

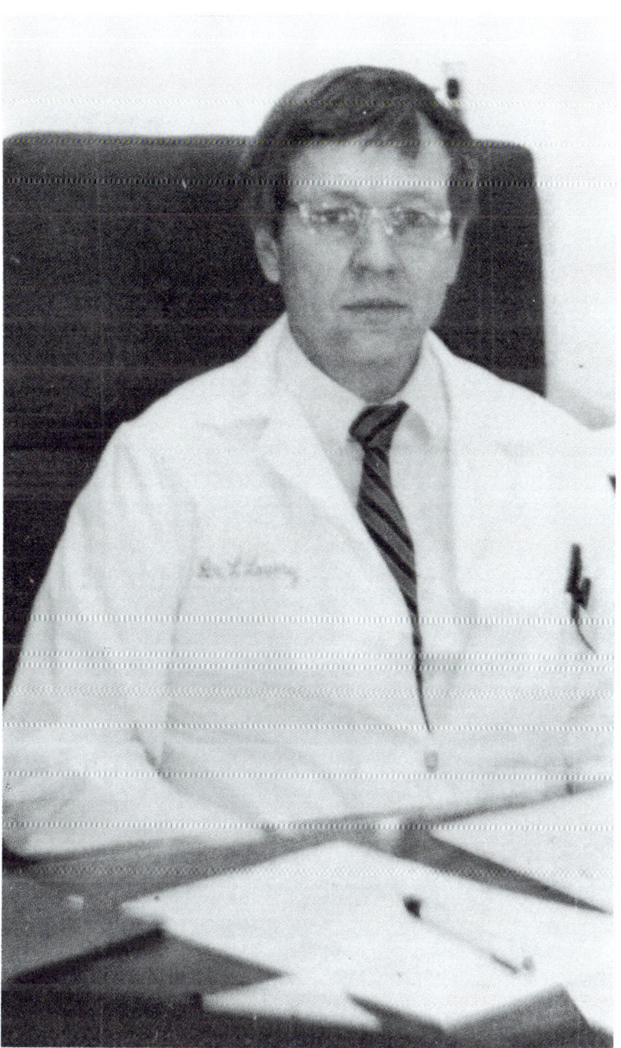

FIG. 42-15. Louis D. Lowry, M.D., Fifth Chairman of Otolaryngology (1980–).

Epilogue

The Department has changed greatly since World War II. Up to that time the professors made their living from their practice and received nothing or only a modest stipend from the College. When residency programs expanded after the War, it became obvious that the Chairman of a Department had many more administrative duties. Until 1950 the number of residents and fellows in the Department was never more than four, usually one or two. This number increased until the mid-1970s when there were 12 residents; in recent years the number has been reduced to nine (three each year). The residency at Jefferson became so well known that at last count there were approximately 140 applicants, 50 of whom were interviewed and three selected.

Although the full-time members shoulder much of the administrative burden, credit must be given to the large number of volunteer otolaryngologists at Lankenau, Bryn Mawr, West Jersey, Methodist, and Veterans (Wilmington) Hospitals who greatly broaden the experience of the residents.

Finally, although this narrative has been limited to the early pioneers and successive Chairmen, there were a large number of superb clinicians and teachers who gave their best to the Hospital and College. Among these were: Austin T. Smith, A. Spencer Kaufman, H. Hunter Lott, Arthur J. Wagers, C. Calvin Fox, Floyd J. Putney, Kelvin A. Kasper, Robert M. Lukens, Davis H. Solo, Joseph Sataloff, Lawrence J. McStravog, Russell J. Brennan, Arthur S. McCallum, Edward C. Britt, William H. Baltzell, Sidney S. Lerner, August P. Ciell, and James E. Brennan. Many others who have worked or trained at Jefferson have gone across the nation and the world to bring honor to the Institution. Internationally known Dr. Jo Ono (Jefferson, 1928) established otolaryngology as a specialty in Japan and received the Alumni Achievement Award in 1976.

Problems in breathing, swallowing, speech, hearing, and cancer still remain. The Department is committed to their better solution.

References

1. "Obituary of Richard J. Levis, M.D.," *Trans. Am. Surg. Assoc.* 9:xxiv, 1891.
2. "Obituary of Richard J. Levis, M.D.," *Boston Med. and Surg. Jour.* 2:123, 1890.
3. Kagan, S.R., "Dr. Jacob da Silva Solis-Cohen," *Leaders of Medicine*. Boston: Medico-Historical Press, 1941, pp. 61–71.
4. Solis-Cohen, M., "The Old Philadelphia Laryngological Society of the Eighteen Eighties," *Ann. Med. Hist.* 3:114–127, 1940.
5. Kelly, H.A., "Jacob da Silva Solis-Cohen," *Encyc. Am. Med. Biog.* Philadelphia: Saunders Co., 1912, pp. lxiii–lxxxi.
6. *Historical Catalogue of the Saint Andrews Society of Philadelphia.* Philadelphia: Longhead and Co., pp. 341–346, 1907.
7. "Memorial of Dr. D. Braden Kyle," *Trans. Am. Clin. and Cl. Assoc.* 32:xxxviii–xli, 1916.
8. O'Keefe, J.J., "The Development of Bronchoscopy at Jefferson," *Trans. Stud. Coll. Phys. Phila.*, April 1965, pp. 171–174.
9. "Memoir of Fielding Otis Lewis," *Trans. Stud. Coll. Phys. Phila.* 36:177–178, 1968.
10. Smith, A. T., *Jeff. Med. Coll. Al. Bull.* 9: March 1955, pp. 8–9.
11. "Obituary of Joseph Clarence Keeler," *Pa. Med. Jour.* 39:186, 1935.
12. "Obituary of Horace J. Williams, M.D.," *Philadelphia Inquirer*, June 5, 1950.
13. Putney, F.J., "Dr. Louis H. Clerf Retires," *Jeff. Med. Coll. Al. Bull.*, 9: March 1955, pp. 10–11.
14. "Harbert Portrait," *Jeff. Med. Coll. Al. Bull.*, 27: Spring 1978, p. 22.
15. "Department of Otolaryngology," *Jeff. Med. Coll. Al. Bull.* 9: May 1956, pp. 6–14.

CHAPTER FORTY-THREE

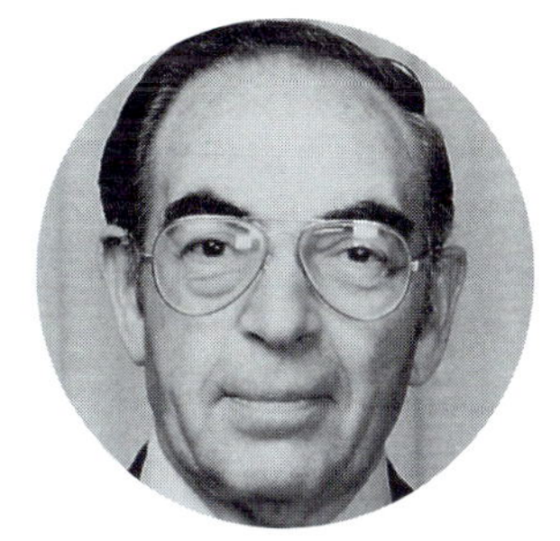

Dentistry and Division of Oral and Maxillofacial Surgery (Otolaryngology)

LIONEL GOLD, D.D.S.

"Every tooth in a man's head is more valuable than a diamond."

—MIGUEL DE CERVANTES (1547–1616)

FROM ITS inception, Jefferson Medical College has had an interesting albeit convoluted relationship with dentistry. A graduate of Jefferson's second class (1827), Samuel S. Fitch, M.D. (Figure 43-1), practiced as a surgeon-dentist and published a *System of Dental Surgery* in 1829 (Figure 43-2).[1] This book, sophisticated for its time, was all the more remarkable because the first College of Dental Surgery was not established in the United States until 1840 in Baltimore, Maryland.

John Hugh McQuillen, M.D., D.D.S., graduated from Jefferson in 1852 while he was also studying dentistry. His D.D.S. degree was honorary. Doctor McQuillen was interested in education, and principally through his efforts a charter was obtained for the Pennsylvania College of Dental Surgery in 1863. He served as Dean and Professor of Physiology at that institution until his death in 1879.[2] Dr. Samuel D. Gross was President of the Board of Trustees of the Pennsylvania College of Dental Surgery from 1880 to 1882. Its building, located at Eleventh and Clinton Streets, became Jefferson's Daniel Baugh Institute of Anatomy in 1911 (Figure 43-3). Dr. Gross included a chapter on *Diseases and Injuries of the Jaws, Teeth and Gums* in his *System of Surgery,* first published in 1859 and expanded it in his final sixth edition (1882).[3]

Another Jefferson graduate, Emile Blaise Gardette, D.D.S., M.D. (Jefferson, 1838), became the fourth President of the Board of Trustees of Jefferson from 1875 to 1888. Dr. Gardette first had been trained in dentistry by his father before beginning his medical training, and he practiced as a surgeon-dentist.

Dentistry at Jefferson Hospital had its official beginning in 1917 with the establishment of a dental clinic under the direction of Joseph Head, D.D.S., M.D. Dr. Head served as Director until 1930, when he was succeeded by Emerson R. Sausser, D.D.S. The dental clinic, located on the second floor of the Thompson Annex, was rebuilt in 1939 through the generosity of the Dietrich Foundation at the solicitation of Dr. Sausser. Serving as clinic staff at that time were Drs. Harry Best, William Bestor, Conrad Hellwege, Aaron Finkelman, Anthony Torre, and Charles Garver, all prominent in Philadelphia dentistry. Mr. Rush Kress, a patient of Dr. Sausser, donated $150,000 through the Samuel Kress Foundation to establish the Emerson Sausser Dental Clinic. This facility was built in 1950 in the Curtis Clinic (Figure 43-4). Its purpose was to give dental treatment to indigent children in a medical setting. Dr. Rodolfo A. Colella (Figure 43-5) was named Director in 1950 and was succeeded by Dr. Edward Cherkas in 1973.

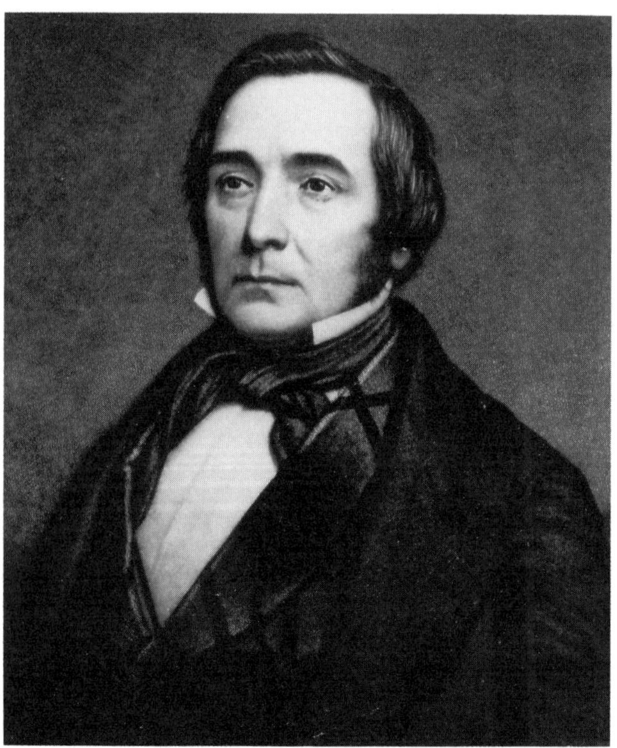

FIG. 43-1. Samuel Sheldon Fitch, M.D. (Jefferson, 1827), a pioneer author in Dental Surgery.

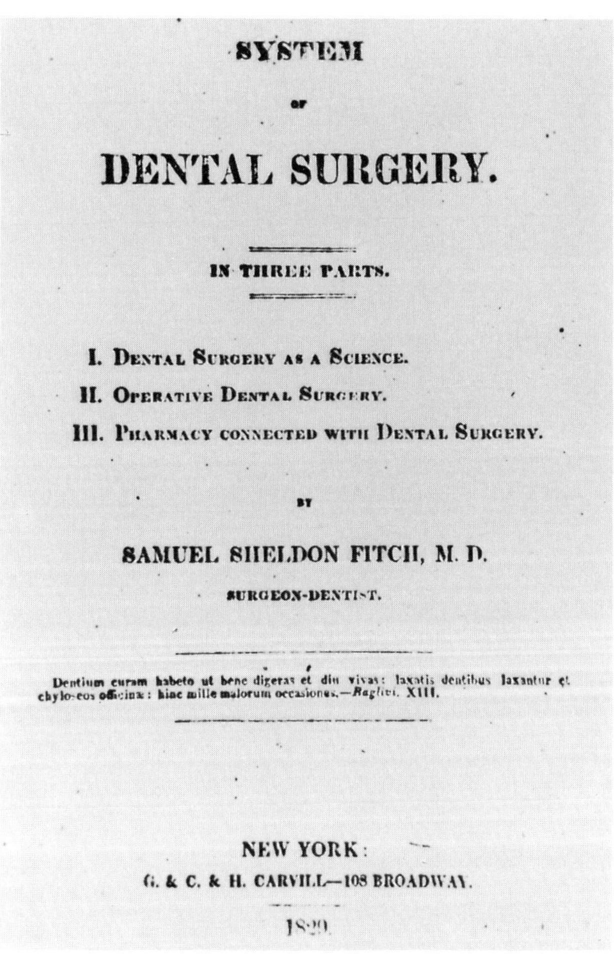

SYSTEM

OF

DENTAL SURGERY.

IN THREE PARTS.

I. DENTAL SURGERY AS A SCIENCE.

II. OPERATIVE DENTAL SURGERY.

III. PHARMACY CONNECTED WITH DENTAL SURGERY.

BY

SAMUEL SHELDON FITCH, M. D.

SURGEON-DENTIST.

Dentium curam habeto ut bene digeras et diu vivas: laxatis dentibus laxantur et chylo-eos officinæ: hinc mille malorum occasiones.—*Baglivi.* XIII.

NEW YORK:

G. & C. & H. CARVILL—108 BROADWAY.

1829.

FIG. 43-2. The title page of *System of Dental Surgery* (1829), by Samuel S. Fitch, M.D.

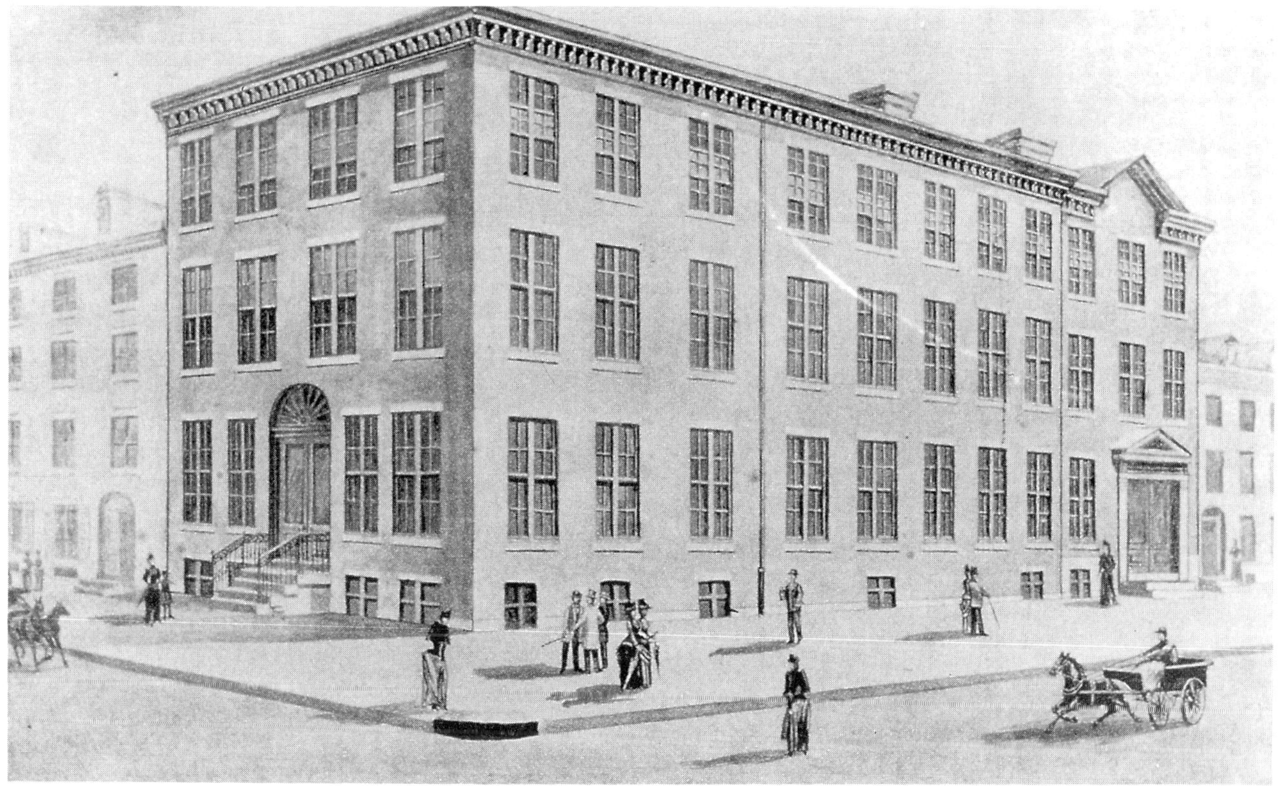

FIG. 43-3. The Pennsylvania College of Dental Surgery, which in 1911 was converted into the Daniel Baugh Institute of Anatomy.

Meanwhile, the Clinic in the Thompson Annex was functioning separately as an oral surgery training facility. Dr. Aaron Finkelman succeeded Dr. Sausser in 1955 as Head of this Clinic. In 1959, the Clinic became the Division of Oral Surgery in the Department of Surgery. Dr. Finkelman invited Dr. Lionel Gold, a young oral surgeon, to join the staff in order to obtain American Dental Association accreditation for the oral surgery training program. This was accomplished in 1960 and a fully accredited graduate program in oral surgery was started (Figure 43-6). In 1961 Dr. Gold was succeeded by Dr. Leonard Reichman. The Division of Oral Surgery was transferred to the Department of Otolaryngology in 1970. Dr. Reichman succeeded Dr. Finkelman in 1972 as Head of the Division.

Earlier in 1969, Jefferson Medical College became a component of Thomas Jefferson University. As part of his plan to make a multicollege health institution, President Peter Herbut with the concurrence of the Board of

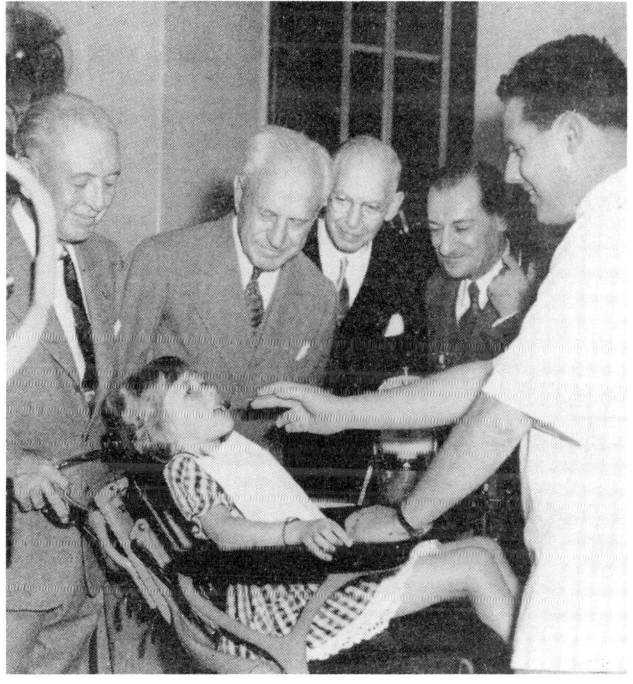

FIG. 43-4. Dedication of The Sausser Clinic (1950). Looking on as the dentist examines the first child patient are (left to right) President Kauffman, Mr. Rush H. Kress, Emerson R. Sausser, D.D.S., and Dr. Rodolfo A. Colella.

Trustees appointed a committee in 1971 to study the feasibility of establishing a college of dental medicine at Thomas Jefferson University. Among those appointed to the committee was Henry S. Brenman, M.S., D.D.S., a practicing periodontist who was also an Associate Professor of Physiology in the Medical College. Dr. Brenman had been a member of the Dental Clinic staff since 1960.

A Department of Dentistry was created in the University Hospital in 1972, and Dr. Brenman was appointed Chairman. Under his guidance, the separately functioning dental and oral surgical units were gathered into one Department. The Department was divided into three subdivisions (oral surgery, orthodontics, and general dentistry) and began operation in the Edison Building in a new facility. The proposed plan to establish a dental school as part of the Thomas Jefferson University was put aside for many practical reasons.[4]

In 1975 Dr. Gold was appointed Chairman of the Division of Oral and Maxillofacial Surgery, which progressed from a two- to a four-year training program. After Dr. Brenman's resignation as Chairman in 1982, Dr. Gold has acted as Chairman of the Hospital Dental Department and Director of Oral and Maxillofacial Surgery.

Oral and maxillofacial surgery, along with

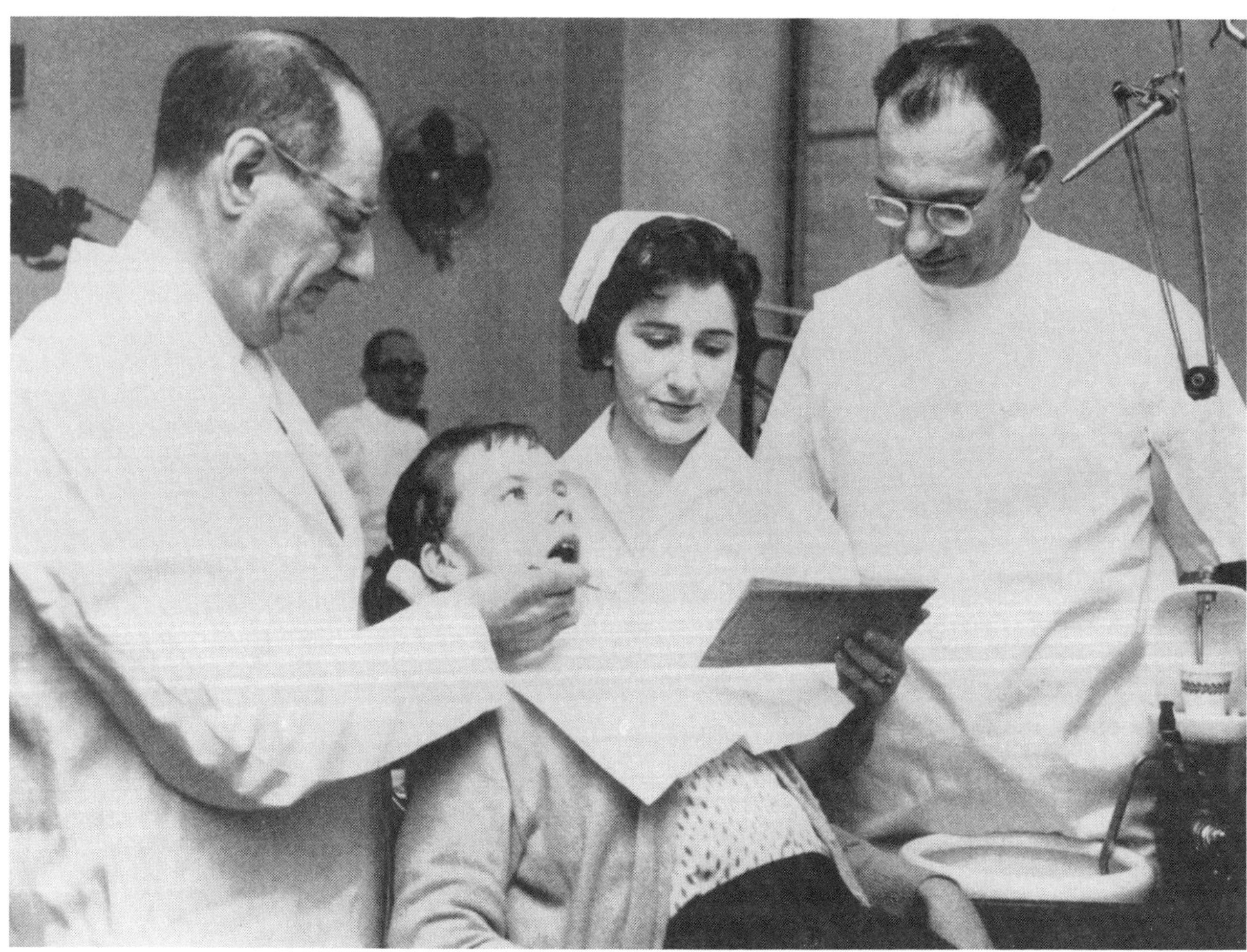

FIG. 43-5. Dr. Rodolfo A. Colella, Director, examines a young patient as Dr. Edward Kerner and Mrs. Harriet Lewis observe.

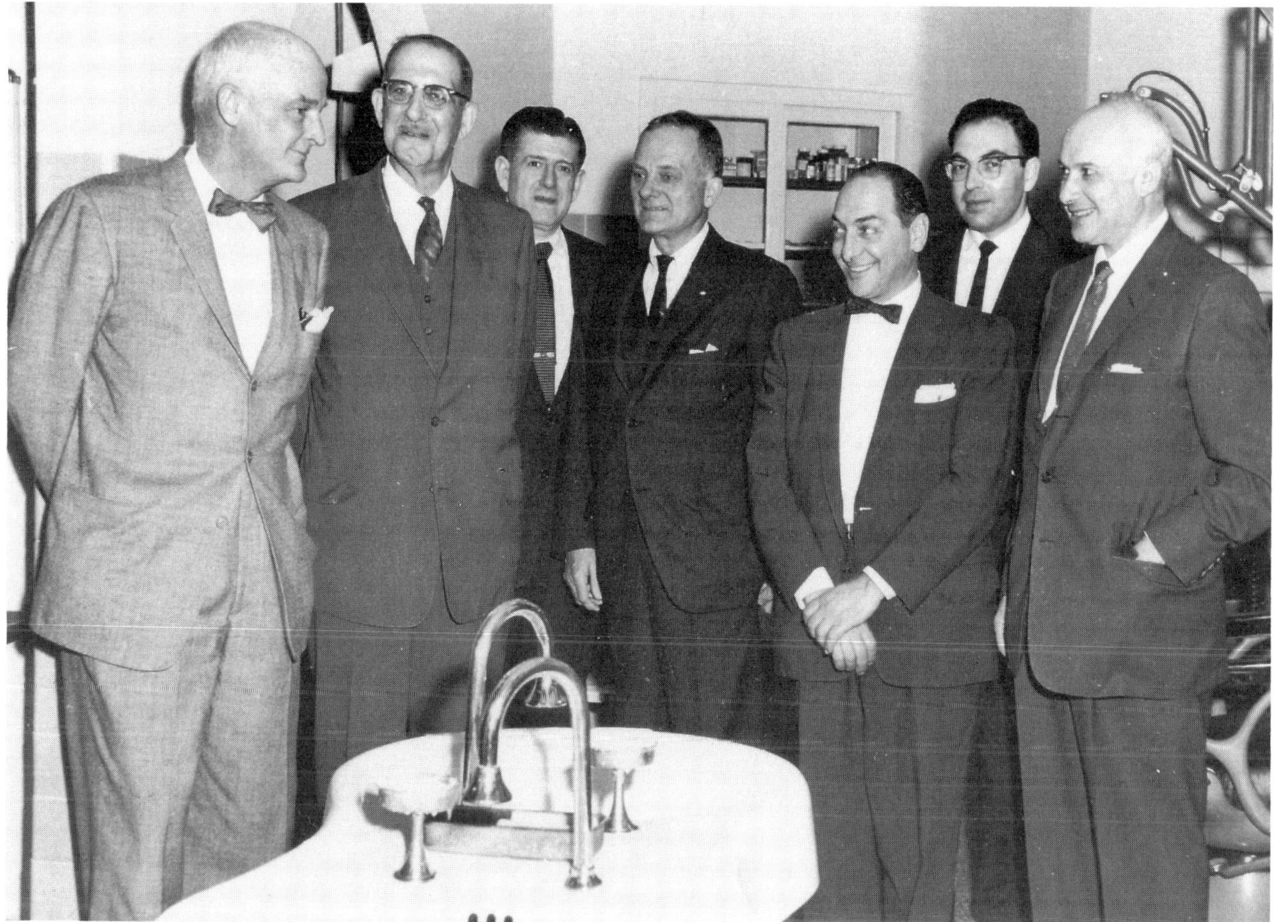

FIG. 43-6. Present at an inspection for accreditation of the Oral Surgery Training Program (1960) are, left to right, Drs. John H. Gibbon, Jr., Franklin Brickman, Anthony Torre, Edward Armbrecht (Inspector for American Society of Oral Surgeons), Frederick Lucchesi, Lionel Gold, and Aaron Finkelman.

dentistry, at Jefferson have served the public well and will play an increasingly important role in the total care of the patient.

References

1. Fitch, S.S., *System of Dental Surgery*. New York: G. & C. H. Carvill, 1829.
2. "Obituary of Professor John H. McQuillen," *Dental Cosmos*. 1879.
3. Gross, S.D., *System of Surgery*. Vol. II. Philadelphia: Blanchard & Lea, 1859 and 1882.
4. *Report on Feasibility of Dental Education at Thomas Jefferson University*, 1973. (In Special Collections of the Library of Thomas Jefferson University.)

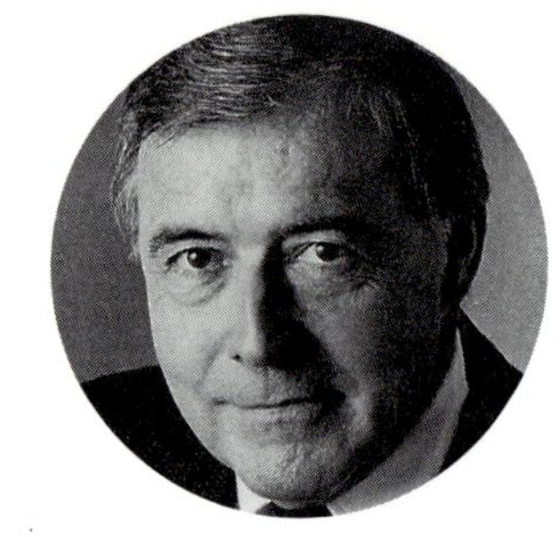

CHAPTER FORTY-FOUR

Department of Ophthalmology

Austin P. Murray, M.D.

"The light of the body is the eye."

—Matthew 6:22

Dr. George McClellan, the acknowledged founder of Jefferson Medical College, was also responsible for masterminding the first eye clinic in Philadelphia. After a few abortive attempts, he was aided by 13 prominent citizens as managers to found the Philadelphia Dispensary for Diseases of the Eye and Ear in March, 1821. On April 14 of that year an advertisement was inserted in the *American Medical Recorder*[1] and in one of the daily "prints" of the city announcing its formation and inviting the poor to partake of its benefits. In the same journal in March, 1822, McClellan published a report of 51 cases for the previous year with his results. It is interesting to note that of 18 cataracts treated, seven were cured, two were "relieved," eight "remained," and one failed. The clinic closed in 1824. Some attributed its demise to the redirection of McClellan's energies to the founding of Jefferson. Several of his colleagues founded the Pennsylvania Infirmary for the Diseases of the Eye and Ear in 1822, but it also had a short life, closing in 1830.

In 1825 a bequest was made to the City of Philadelphia in the will of James Wills, Jr., for the "relief of the indigent blind and lame." Because of a contesting of the will and the time necessary to complete the edifice, the hospital did not open its doors until March 3, 1834.

Early Jefferson Eye Surgeons

The best known general surgeon of that time who practiced ophthalmology was Philip Syng Physick (1768–1837). He trained in London, where he was a favorite of John Hunter, whose influence enabled him to obtain a position on the house staff of St. George's Hospital, where it is said he obtained much of his surgical skill. Physick, "The Father of American Surgery" and a pioneer in American ophthalmology, began his lectures in the Pennsylvania Hospital in 1800 and became Professor of Surgery at the University of Pennsylvania in 1805. He was a skillful eye surgeon who did cataract extractions without the benefit of anesthesia and with both himself and the patient in the sitting position.[2] Among his pupils was George McClellan, who was a graduate of the University in 1819. McClellan very early in his career became keenly interested in eye surgery and usually had excellent results. Unfortunately, one case would forever haunt him. In 1828 McClellan had to face a lawsuit because of a failure in cataract surgery. It arose when Dr. Francis Beattie, a disgruntled former colleague, spread rumors that McClellan had mistreated a Mr. William Davis. The latter had had both eyes operated upon by Dr. Joseph Parrish (1779–1840), with loss of the left eye, and after he developed postoperative complications following surgery on the right eye had been told never to let anyone reoperate. Dr. McClellan did so in the confines of Davis's boardinghouse bedroom and lost the second eye. At the trial Dr. Parrish testified that he had previously only once carried out a cataract procedure similar to the one on Davis and because of the poor result never attempted another of the same nature. Dr. Physick also gave testimony in which he pointed out that Barron Wenzel, a famous German surgeon, had lost a hatful of eyes before he became proficient in the extraction technique. The suit was settled in favor of the plaintiff, and McClellan was fined $500. This was the first eye malpractice suit in Philadelphia and one of the very first judgments levied against a physician in the United States.[3] McClellan's methods[4] were characterized by brilliancy and dash rather than by cool calculation. It was very hard for him to submit to authority or to control the impulses of his ardent temperament. Thus one can easily see why the lawsuit may have been instigated by a colleague. It has also been said that at the time of his death he had virtually no physician friends.

Joseph Pancoast succeeded McClellan as Professor of Surgery from 1839 to 1841 and then became Professor of Anatomy until 1874. In 1844 he published his *Operative Surgery,* in which he devoted 46 pages to operations on the eyeball and its accessory organs. There was very little that he added to the slowly expanding literature on this subject, and he espoused most of the theories and operations of choice that his colleague, Thomas Dent Mütter, promulgated. Nevertheless, the book had many excellent illustrations that emphasized some of the fine points of the surgery.

Thomas Dent Mütter, successor to Pancoast as Professor of Surgery in 1841, devoted 62 pages to eye surgery in his edition of *Liston's Lectures on the Operations of Surgery.* The publication of this book also in 1846 probably accounts for the similarity of hypotheses and modes of treatment. Mütter covered plastic surgery of the lids fairly well, but strabismus was still poorly understood, and knowledge of the anatomy of the eye and its adnexa was spotty. It would not be possible to deal accurately with strabismus until research on the physiology of the eye unlocked its secrets. Both Mütter and Pancoast condemned intracapsular cataract extraction and preferred the couching procedure. This consisted of dislocating the lens into the vitreous. It usually gave immediate visual return if the postoperative inflammation was minimal. Unfortunately, even with good return of vision these patients were prone to glaucoma with later loss of sight.

Even until the latter part of the nineteenth century most surgeons included ophthalmology in their practice. Samuel D. Gross was no exception and excelled in this field. Although he was not personally present at the first International Congress of Ophthalmology in Brussels in 1857, his report on *Ophthalmology in America* was presented.[5] He was one of the first to do strabismus surgery. In his *System of Surgery* he revealed an advanced understanding of the anatomy and function of the extraocular muscles. In the 1859 first edition of this famous book he devoted 110 pages to diseases and injuries of the eye.[6]

Addinell Hewson (Figure 44-1) (Jefferson, 1850) was another general surgeon especially interested in ophthalmology. He was the first member of the Wills Hospital Staff from Jefferson; before 1854 all had been graduates of the University of Pennsylvania. In 1855 he edited Mackenzie's treatise, *Diseases of the Eye,* and was credited with introducing the ophthalmoscope to Wills. He was an unsuccessful candidate for the Chair of Anatomy at Jefferson in 1874; his father, Thomas Tickell Hewson, had been an unsuccessful candidate for the Chair of Surgery in 1839.

Richard J. Levis (Figure 44-2) was appointed Clinical Lecturer in Ophthalmology and Aural

Surgery in 1867. This was the first recognition of ophthalmology as a specialty at Jefferson and presaged the later development of a full-status Department. The invention of the ophthalmoscope by von Helmholtz in 1851 accelerated its development into one of the earliest of the specialties.

Levis, a native Philadelphian, was born in 1827, the son of a physician. He went to Central High School, was an office student of Professor Thomas Dent Mütter, and graduated from Jefferson in 1848. He became prominent as a surgeon, with appointments at Philadelphia, Jefferson, Pennsylvania, Jewish, and Wills Eye Hospitals. During the Civil War he was Surgeon-in-Chief in two U.S. military hospitals in Philadelphia. While at Wills Eye Hospital from 1864 to 1872 he introduced the well-known wire loop used in cataract extraction. He also developed a lacrimal probe that was graduated in caliber from its tip, which dilated stenotic punctae and canaliculi. Variations of both these instruments are used in ophthalmology today. Levis modified numerous operative procedures and devised surgical instruments and orthopedic appliances. On the top floor of his home he maintained a well-equipped workshop for this purpose.

Levis was a fastidious man, extremely well dressed, who would enter the operating room fully clothed even to the tie and French cuffs that were his usual attire. These somehow remained unblemished during his operations. When finished, he washed his hands, bowed to those in attendance, and hastened to greet and treat his private patients, apparently spotless.[7] Always especially considerate of younger physicians, he

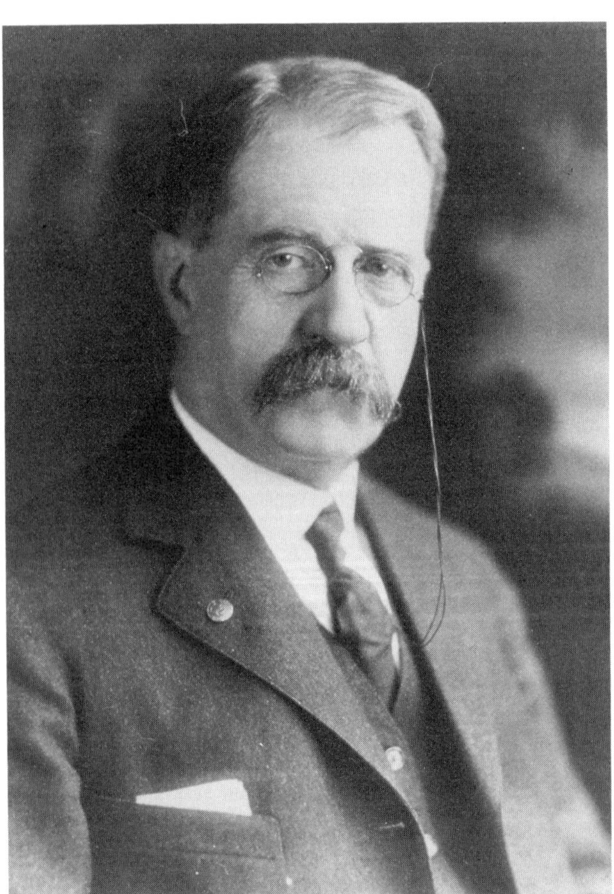

Fig. 44-1. Addinell Hewson, M.D. (1828–1889), introduced the ophthalmoscope to Wills Eye Hospital.

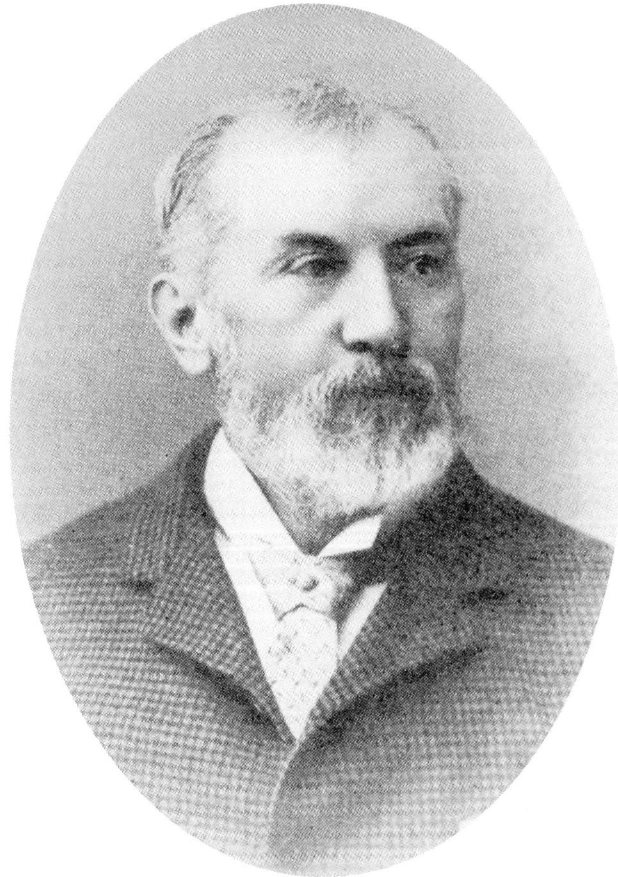

Fig. 44-2. Richard J. Levis, M.D. (1827–1890), the first Clinical Lecturer in Ophthalmology (1867).

claimed he could learn more from them than from older men. Aside from *The Treatment of Fractures of the Patella* and *Traditional Errors in Surgery,* his literary contributions were few. Nevertheless, many of his lectures were recorded by his students and have been preserved in the library of the Pennsylvania Hospital.

Levis resigned his lectureship in ophthalmic and aural surgery at Jefferson in 1875 but continued as an attending physician and lecturer in clinical surgery. He was the first President of the Board of Trustees of the Philadelphia Polyclinic and College for Graduates in Medicine, President of the Philadelphia County and Pennsylvania State Medical Societies, and original member of the American Surgical Association. He aided Samuel D. Gross in the founding of the Philadelphia Academy of Surgery in 1879, the oldest surgical society of its kind in the United States today.

After Dr. Levis's retirement from practice, he traveled in Egypt, where he performed some cataract extractions.[8] It is said that rising early one day to see the sunrise, he met an Arab he had operated upon the day before who was walking around with his head thrown back peering through the crevice between his lids. He also wanted to see the sunrise after his period of blindness. Dr. Levis died at Cedarcroft, Pennsylvania, in 1890 at the age of 63.

William Thomson, M.D. (1833–1907); First Chairman of Ophthalmology (1895–1897)

Dr. William Thomson (Figure 44-3) joined Levis at Jefferson as Lecturer on Diseases of the Eye and Ear in 1874 and succeeded him the following year. This Jefferson graduate of 1855 was destined in 1895 to become the first Chairman of the Department of Ophthalmology we know today.

Dr. Thomson was born in Chambersburg, Pennsylvania, in 1833, a descendant of Scotch-Irish settlers in America from the early eighteenth century. After his preceptorship, six months of study in pharmacy, and obtaining his M.D. degree, he started private practice in a suburb of Philadelphia. In 1861 he began a distinguished military career in the Union Army. He was complimented by President Lincoln for his work at the battle of South Mountain where he took sole charge of 2,500 wounded men. He improved the supply system of field hospitals, reorganized the Douglas Hospital in Washington, and was appointed Inspector of all hospitals of the Washington area. In the newly organized Army Medical Museum, of which Dr. John Hill Brinton (Jefferson, 1852) was the first curator, Thomson contributed largely to the first descriptions of osteomyelitis and wounds of the joints. He aided the establishment of a photographic bureau in the museum that evolved into the Medical Illustration Service of the Armed Forces Institute of Pathology. He took part in experimental photomicrography that led to prints of microscopic fields that could be magnified 15 to 250 times. This work stimulated his interest in

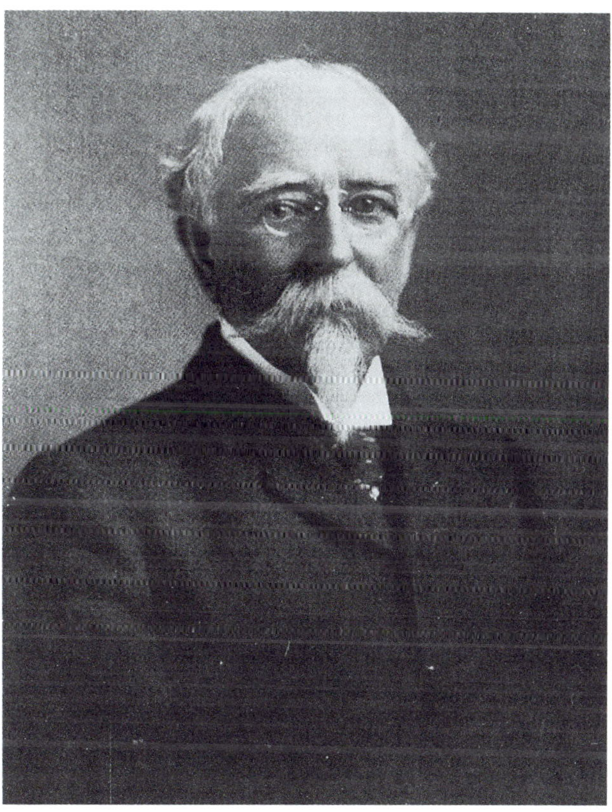

FIG. 44-3. William Thomson, M.D., First Chairman of Ophthalmology (1895–1897).

optics and a medical practice limited to ophthalmology.[9]

On return to civilian life in Philadelphia in 1868, Thomson became an Assistant Surgeon at Wills Eye Hospital and was elevated to full Surgeon in 1872. In the following year he established a daily clinic at Jefferson for diseases of the eye, and then a weekly clinic for instruction of the medical students, which always attracted a full attendance. In 1877, when the first detached Jefferson Hospital was established, he was appointed to the staff as Ophthalmic Surgeon, and in 1880 was advanced to Honorary Professor of Ophthalmology. In that year he also became Ophthalmic Physician to the Pennsylvania Railroad and later the Reading Railroad to apply his method for detection of color blindness by using colored wool and lanterns. This was of importance to the trainman whose ability to see colored signals was vital to railroad safety. He also examined for acuteness of vision and hearing, and his methods were adopted by many other railroads.

As one of the early workers in refractive problems, Thomson designed the ametrometer in 1878, used in diagnosing and correcting ametropia (refractive errors). He wrote on the connection between astigmatism and posterior staphyloma (bulging of the cornea) as well as correction of conical cornea by convex cylindrical glasses. He was among the first to call attention to the hypothesis that headaches could be caused by eyestrain and be corrected by glasses. *The Use of the Ophthalmoscope in the Diagnosis of Intracranial Lesions,* written in collaboration with S. Weir Mitchell, was coupled with *History of the First Brain Tumor Diagnosticated with the Ophthalmoscope in Philadelphia.* Thomson edited the American edition of Nettleship's *Diseases of the Eye,* and revised the chapter on diseases of the eye and ear in the 1872 fifth edition of Samuel D. Gross's *System of Surgery,* as well as "Detection of Color Blindness" in Norris and Oliver's *System of the Diseases of the Eye.*

The College of Physicians of Philadelphia, of which Thomson was a member, houses his ophthalmoscopes, correspondence, 14 volumes of case books, and his portrait by Thomas Eakins in 1907.

Thomson served Jefferson as Professor and Chairman of the Department of Ophthalmology with a seat on the faculty from 1895 to 1897. Upon resigning, he was appointed Emeritus Professor and was succeeded by Dr. George E. de Schweinitz. He died in 1907 at the age of 74.

George Edmund de Schweinitz, M.D. (1858–1938); Second Chairman (1897–1902)

George Edmund de Schweinitz (Figure 44-4) was born in Philadelphia in 1858 of distinguished Huguenot and Silesian ancestry. In 1876 he received an A.B. degree from Moravian College, of which his father was President. For the next two years he taught in the Military Academy of Nazareth, Pennsylvania. He then entered the Medical School of the University of Pennsylvania, from which he graduated in 1881 at the head of his class. After several years as a brilliant and popular quizmaster in therapeutics at the University, he became attracted to anatomy and general surgery. In the pattern of the anatomist-surgeons of that era, he became a Prosector of Anatomy for the

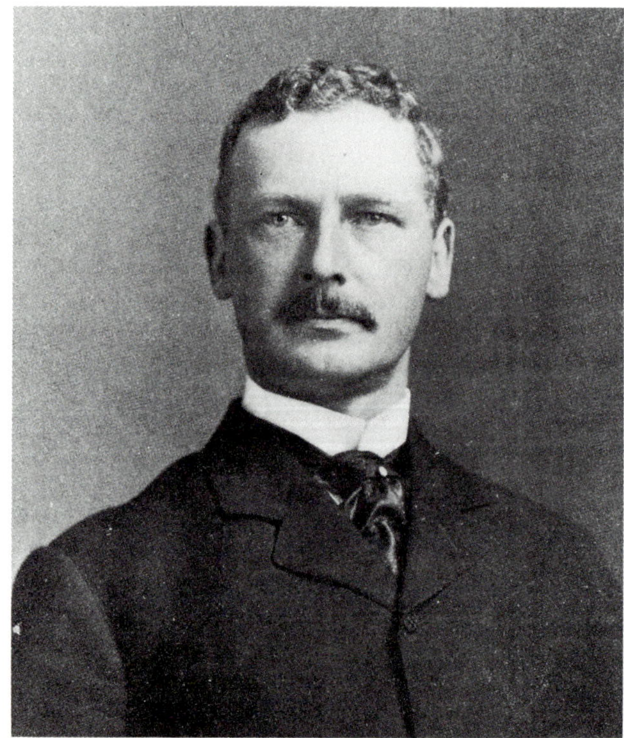

FIG. 44-4. George E. de Schweinitz, M.D., Second Chairman (1897–1902).

internationally famous Joseph Leidy from 1883 to 1885. With acceptance of the position as Assistant to Dr. William F. Norris, Professor of Ophthalmology at the University, he became enamored with the field and devoted the rest of his life to it. Private practice with referral of difficult and unusual cases followed quickly.

Early in his study Dr. de Schweinitz paid particular attention to the effects of systemic diseases upon the eye and how examination of the eye revealed clues to systemic disease. In accord with this habit he required a meticulous general physical and neurologic examination, including examination of the urine, in each new clinic patient. His professional advancement was meteoric, with appointment as Ophthalmic Surgeon to the Children's Hospital, the Philadelphia Hospital, and the Orthopaedic Hospital and Infirmary for Nervous Diseases. He also became Lecturer on Medical Ophthalmology at the University of Pennsylvania and Professor of Ophthalmology in the Philadelphia Polyclinic and College for Graduates in Medicine in 1891. In 1892 he published the first edition of his *Diseases of the Eye,* which was written at the suggestion of his friend, Dr. William Osler, and went through ten editions. Osler in the same year brought out his own magnum opus *The Principles and Practice of Medicine,* in which later editions were carried on by his nephew through marriage, Dr. Thomas McCrae, the first Magee Professor of Medicine at Jefferson.

Dr. de Schweinitz was appointed Clinical Professor of Ophthalmology at Jefferson in 1892 and Professor with a seat on the faculty at the resignation of Thomson in 1897. His Department at Jefferson then embraced Thomson as Emeritus Professor, Howard Hansell, Clinical Professor; Clarence Veasey, Demonstrator; and William Sweet, Assistant Demonstrator. He resigned in 1902 to succeed his former mentor, Dr. William Fisher Norris, at the University of Pennsylvania for the next 22 years.

The career of de Schweinitz continued at the University. In 1902 he was one of the first to list the symptoms common to glaucoma, a disease with multiple subdivisions and aspects, and one of the first to use the tonometer for routine detection of that disease. His interest in pituitary disease began in 1887, culminating in 1923 when he was the first American to deliver the Bowman Lecture in London; he titled it *Ocular Aspects, Especially Field Defects, of Pituitary Body Disorders*. As an ophthalmic surgeon he was described as cautious and thorough, admired for his judgement, but not an impressive technician.[10]

Honors, awards, and degrees were heaped upon de Schweinitz. From 1910 to 1912 he was President of the College of Physicians of Philadelphia, and Sir William Osler at Oxford in 1918 used the auspices of de Schweinitz to present his pomander cane to the collection in the Philadelphia College. He served as President of the American Ophthalmological Society in 1916, the American Medical Association in 1922, and the International Congress of Ophthalmology in the same year. He received honorary degrees from the University of Pennsylvania, Moravian College, the University of Michigan, and Harvard. He belonged to the American Philosophical Society and was on the Board of Trustees of the University of Pennsylvania and the Library Company of Philadelphia. After a period of failing health, he died in 1938 at the age of 79.

Howard F. Hansell, M.D. (1855–1934); Third Chairman (1902–1925)

Howard Forde Hansell (Figure 44-5) succeeded de Schweinitz in 1902. He was born in Philadelphia in 1855 of English lineage. He graduated from Central High School in 1873, from Brown University in 1877, and from Jefferson in 1879. His preceptorship was taken with Dr. James C. Wilson, who in 1891 would occupy the Chair of the Practice of Medicine. Hansell was quiet, reserved and studious. After graduation he joined the medical clinic of Professor Jacob Mendes DaCosta as an Assistant, as well as the ophthalmology clinic of Professor Thomson. Hansell followed the custom of those who sought the ultimate in medical education by going to Europe for additional study. In Germany he took ophthalmologic training under such masters as Hirschberg, Arlt, Fuchs, and Stellway. On return to Philadelphia in 1881 he entered private practice and was given an appointment as Attending Ophthalmologist at the Philadelphia General Hospital, which he held for more than 20 years. As a Professor of Ophthalmology at the Philadelphia Polyclinic Hospital, he was elected President of the faculty for four successive years.

In 1894 Hansell became associated with Jefferson Medical College as Chief Clinical Assistant and the following year was made Clinical Professor of Ophthalmology. He succeeded George de Schweinitz in 1902 and held the Chairmanship until his retirement in 1925, when he was made Emeritus. His lectures were always carefully prepared and well attended by the students. He was an original coeditor of the section on ophthalmology in the *American Year Book of Medicine and Surgery*. Books that he coauthored were: *Clinical Ophthalmology,* with James H. Bell (1892); *Muscular Anomalies of the Eye,* with Wendell Reber (1898); *Diseases of the Eye,* with William Sweet (1903); and *Ocular Muscles,* with Wendell Reber (1912).

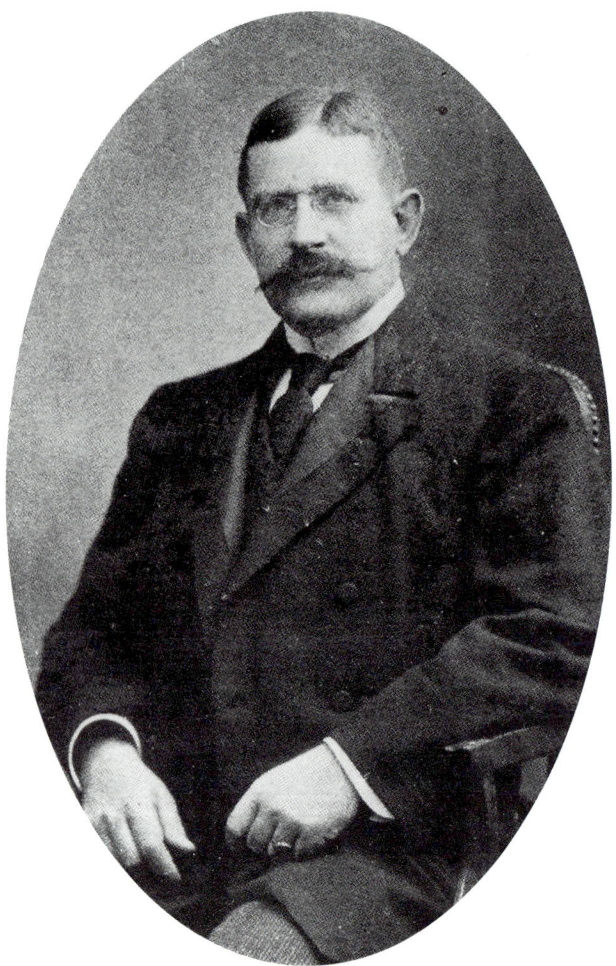

FIG. 44-5. Howard F. Hansell, M.D., Third Chairman (1902–1925).

In the College of Physicians of Philadelphia, Hansell served as Chairman of the Section on Ophthalmology from 1907 to 1908. In 1920 he was a member of the committee appointed by the Section on Ophthalmology of the American Medical Association to report on the selective investigation concerning the extraocular muscles. He was also active in the American Ophthalmologic Society and belonged to other local and national societies. He died in 1934 at age 79 shortly after a return from Europe.[11]

William M. Sweet, M.D. (1860–1926); Fourth Chairman (1925–1926)

The successor to Dr. Hansell in 1925 was Dr. William Merrick Sweet (Figure 44-6). A native Philadelphian, born in 1860, he received his preliminary medical education at Central High School, from which he graduated in 1878. For financial reasons he was unable at first to pursue his ambition to become a physician and obtained employment in an iron and steel company. He also worked for a newspaper and became acquainted with the printing art. Both of these experiences were assets in his later work on foreign bodies in the eye and as editor of the *Transactions of the American Ophthalmological Society*.

Sweet matriculated at Jefferson in 1884 and graduated in 1886. After visiting some of the leading medical centers of Europe he was appointed as Assistant in the eye clinic of Jefferson Hospital and later elected as Ophthalmologist to the Southern Dispensary.

Shortly after Roentgen's paper in 1895 on a new form of light rays, Dr. Sweet began experiments with the rays in an effort to localize intraocular foreign bodies. A description of these experiments and the apparatus employed was reported in 1897 before the Section on Ophthalmology of the College of Physicians of Philadelphia. Some of the pioneer work was done with Dr. Willis F. Manges, later to be the first Professor of Radiology at Jefferson. They worked with biplane x-rays to determine the exact location of opaque foreign bodies in the eye or surrounding structures, permitting their removal by the shortest distance to the surface, especially if they could be drawn out by a magnet. He devised a portable hand electromagnet before 1910 that was successfully used in many of the leading hospitals in the country.

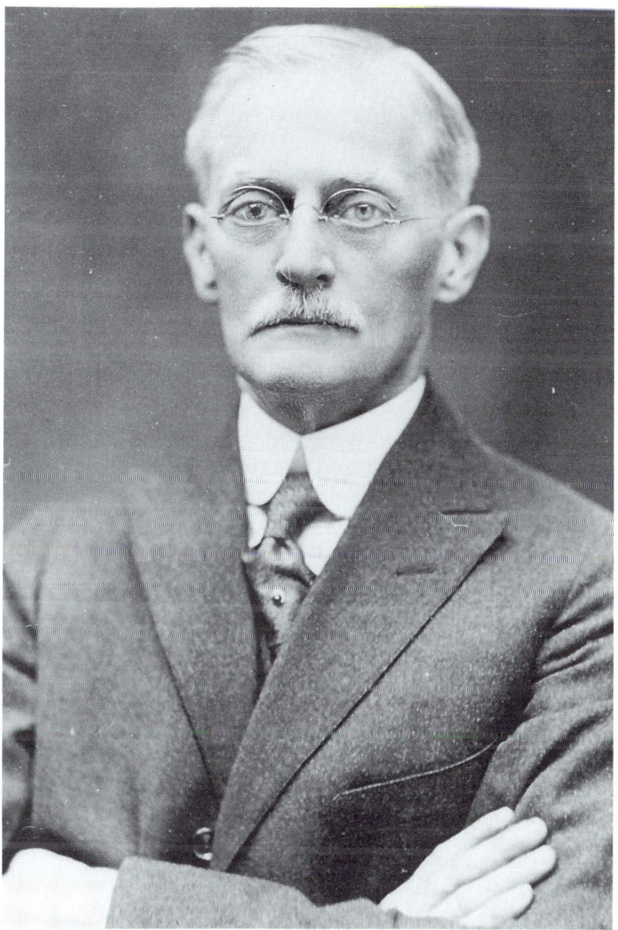

FIG. 44-6. William M. Sweet, M.D., Fourth Chairman (1925–1926).

Sweet was appointed Attending Surgeon in the Wills Eye Hospital in 1911 and served until his resignation in 1919 to become a Consulting Surgeon. From 1914 to 1918 he was the first roentgenologist of that hospital.

The membership of Dr. Sweet in the American Ophthalmological Society was of long duration and benefit to the society. First a member in 1900, he subsequently served as the Secretary-Treasurer from 1908 for ten years, Vice President in 1920, and President in 1921. He edited the *Transactions* and gave most of his papers at the annual meetings.

Dr. Sweet was an able clinician and teacher. In addition to his papers he coauthored *Diseases of the Eye* with Howard Hansell in 1903 and in 1912 edited the second American publication of *Ophthalmic Surgery* by Joseph Meller of Vienna. His appointment as Head of the Department at Jefferson came at the age of 66 and lasted only one and a half years. After a week's illness, lobar pneumonia claimed his life on December 24, 1926.[12,13]

Charles E.G. Shannon, M.D., Sc.D. (1875–1965); Fifth Chairman (1927–1948)

Charles Emery Gould Shannon (Figure 44-7) was appointed Head of the Department in 1927. He was born in Maine in 1875 as one of over 1,000 descendants of Robert Gould, who came to Massachusetts in 1623. His cousin, Dr. George Milbry Gould (Jefferson, 1888) was a noted ophthalmologist, editor of the widely used *Gould Medical Dictionary,* and author of the 1904 two-volume history of *The Jefferson Medical College of Philadelphia*. Shannon received a B.A. degree from Colby College at Waterville, Maine, and in 1902 his M.D. degree from Jefferson.

After an internship at the Pottsville Hospital in Pennsylvania, he pursued postgraduate study in ophthalmology at the Massachusetts Eye and Ear Infirmary. On returning to Philadelphia he became the office assistant to Professor Hansell with an appointment at Jefferson Hospital. In time he was promoted to Chief of the Eye Clinic and Associate in Ophthalmology. In 1911 Shannon was appointed Assistant Ophthalmologist to the Philadelphia General Hospital and Attending Ophthalmologist when Hansell resigned his post in 1919.

Dr. Shannon was a quiet, lovable man and the acme of modesty. He claimed that he was elected to the Chair because he was the only candidate with a college degree, and that the Senior Class of 1948 presented his portrait only because his final examinations were easy. In his lectures he had a way of making the students feel that each topic was a possible examination question and he would clearly indicate the correct answer. By careful study of his notes one could take his examination with a feeling of security but also a balanced knowledge of practical ophthalmology. Although he made no major contributions to operative technique or the literature, he was active in the ophthalmologic societies and commanded the highest respect.

Upon resigning his Chairmanship in 1948 at the age of 73, he moved to Waterville, Maine, where he resumed private practice. Colby College awarded him an honorary degree of Doctor of Science in 1954. He died in 1965, not quite 90 years of age.

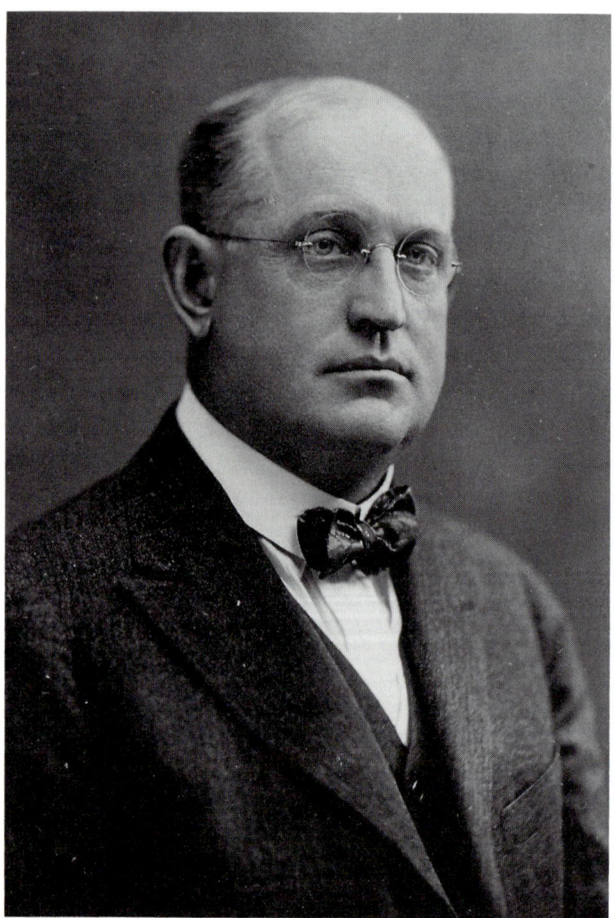

FIG. 44-7. Charles E. G. Shannon, M.D., Fifth Chairman (1927–1948).

Arno E. Town, M.D. (1901–1967); Sixth Chairman (1948–1956)

Arno Emerson Town (Figure 44-8) was appointed Professor and Head of the Department in July 1948. He was born in Ohio in 1901, the youngest of seven children. Despite financial hardships he obtained his undergraduate B.S. from the University of Akron and graduated from Jefferson

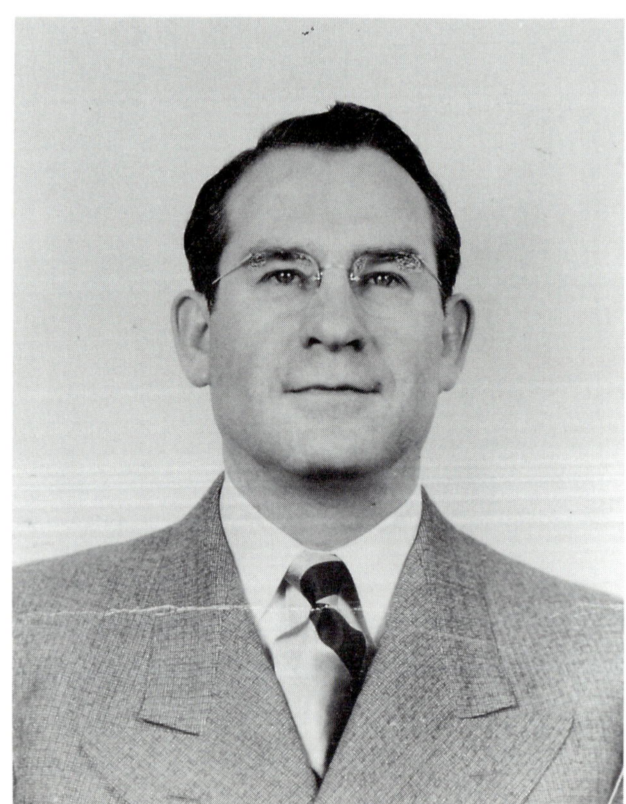

FIG. 44-8. Arno E. Town, M.D., Sixth Chairman (1948–1956).

in 1926. After a one-year internship at St. Mary's Hospital in Philadelphia he earned a Master of Medical Sciences in Ophthalmology at the Graduate School of the University of Pennsylvania in 1929. During the following two years he took a residency in ophthalmology at the Bellevue Hospital in New York City. In 1931 he was appointed to the teaching staff of the New York University College of Medicine and the New York Eye and Ear Infirmary. From 1933 to 1943 he became Chief of Clinic and Assistant Visiting Surgeon at St. Vincent's Hospital, Chief of the New York University Division of Ophthalmology at Welfare Island Hospital, and Ophthalmologist to the City Cancer Hospital and Clinic. Just before World War II he was Acting Chief of Ophthalmology at Bellevue Hospital and Acting Head of the Department at New York University College of Medicine.

During World War II Town entered the Navy, where he achieved the rank of Commander. He was Ophthalmologist at the National Naval Center at Bethesda and also on the Hospital Ship, *U.S.S. Benevolence*. After discharge from the service in 1946 he was appointed Clinical Professor of Ophthalmology at New York University.

While at Jefferson from 1948 to 1956 Town established the first basic research program in ophthalmology in collaboration with the Department of Physiology. He was an excellent clinician and teacher. His contributions to the literature included his thesis on retinitis pigmentosa, bacteriophage in ophthalmology, cyst of the uveal layer of the iris, contact lenses for correction of refractive errors in monocular aphakia, injuries of the eye and eyelids, first aid for eye injuries, a metal eye protector, treatment of various types of conjunctivitis and endophthalmitis with antibiotics, and radioactive phosphorus in the diagnosis of ocular tumors. His textbook, *Ophthalmology,* was published in 1951.

Upon resignation as Chairman and appointment as Emeritus Professor in 1956, Dr. Town retired to private practice in New York City. He retired entirely in 1965 and moved to Florida where he died in 1967 after a long illness.[14,15]

Carrol R. Mullen, M.D. (1901–1961); Seventh Chairman (1956–1961)

Carrol Richard Mullen (Figure 44-9) was born in the same year as his Chairman predecessor, Dr. Town, and was also his Jefferson classmate (Class of 1926). Son of a physician and born in Illinois, he received his B.A. degree from Creighton University in 1922.

Following his internship at the Philadelphia General Hospital, Mullen continued on the ophthalmologic service and became its Chief in 1936. He later resigned this position but remained as an active consultant. He also became associated with Jefferson and Wills Eye Hospital, in which he advanced rapidly. At Wills Eye in 1939 he was appointed the youngest Attending Surgeon and in 1949 the Executive Surgeon. He was the first to occupy the latter position after its reestablishment by the Board of City Trusts.

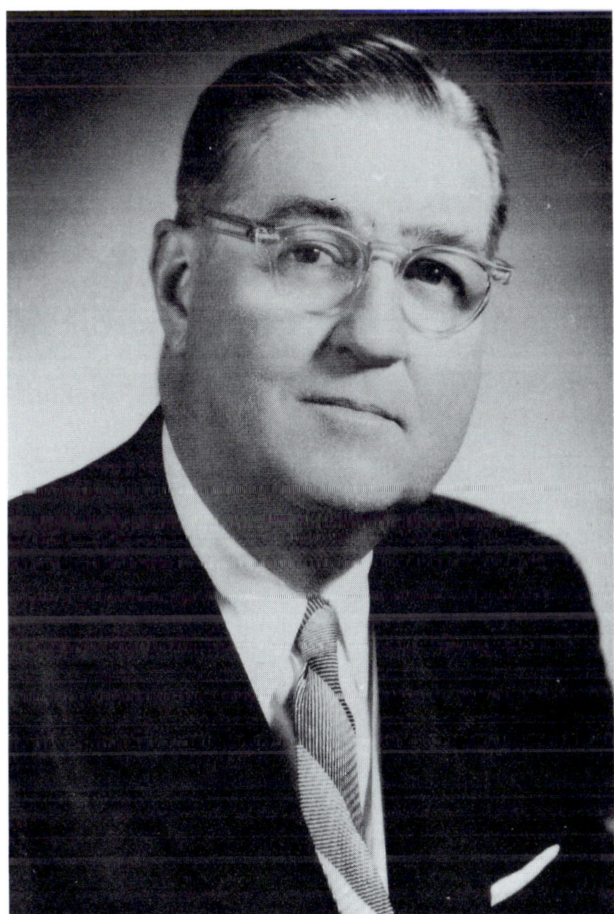

FIG. 44-9. Carrol R. Mullen, M.D., Seventh Chairman (1956–1961).

Dr. Mullen was a charter member of the Fitzgerald Mercy Hospital in 1933 and became Chief of the Ophthalmologic Service. For ten years he was associated with Dr. Charles Heed at Girard College in the Department of Ophthalmology.

While not a prolific writer, Dr. Mullen contributed articles on causes of blindness, infections of the eye and their treatment, "Jaw winking (the Marcus Gunn phenomenon)," and read papers on several occasions in South America. He belonged to all the important local, national, and international ophthalmological societies. In 1960 he received an honor award from the American Academy of Ophthalmology and Otolaryngology for his long service as a teacher. He was President of the Jefferson Alumni Association in 1953–1954 and served as Chairman of the Annual Giving Fund Committee. In the year before his death he conducted the drive that topped all previous records.

Dr. Mullen was the last of the Chairmen of Ophthalmology to have a full-time private practice. It was his unique organizational ability that enabled him to juggle successfully so many "hats." While Chairman he was also Attending and Executive Surgeon at Wills Eye, including the Clinic, and a member of the Board of City Trusts. With boundless energy, diplomacy, and delegation of authority to wisely handpicked associates he faithfully carried out his responsibilities. The brilliant staff that supported him consisted of Gerald M. Shannon, later the Director of the Oculoplastic Service at Wills; Dr. Turgut N. Hamdi, who along with Dr. Warren S. Reese inserted the first intraocular lenses in this country; and Dr. Cyril M. Luce, who was as talented musically as he was surgically. These three men unfortunately died at the peak of their careers. Other members of this distinguished staff were Dr. Joseph Waldman, with special interest in neuro-ophthalmology; Dr. David Naidoff, whose prime involvement was motility; Dr. William T. Hunt, Jr., whose specialty was refraction and whose philanthropy enabled the purchase of one of the early ophthalmic lasers; Dr. Charles G. Steinmetz, III, who was the ophthalmic pathologist and later the interim Acting Head; and Drs. Sidney G. Radbill, William J. Harrison, J. Scott Fritch, Sidney L. Olsho, Albert Merlin, Milton J. Freiwald, Alvin W. Howland, J. Robert Fox, Edward J. Donnelly, and Bernard C. Gettes.

In 1961, with swiftness, acute leukemia claimed Dr. Mullen at the age of 60.[16,17]

Charles G. Steinmetz, III, M.D.; Acting Chairman (1961–1962)

Dr. Charles G. Steinmetz, III was the Acting Head from February 1961 to February 1962. He graduated from Jefferson in 1948, took his internship there until 1950, and completed his Residency at Wills Eye Hospital in 1953. He rose in ranks at Jefferson from Assistant Professor in 1956 to Acting Head in 1961.

Thomas D. Duane, M.D., Ph.D. (1917–); Eighth Chairman (1962–1981)

Thomas David Duane, M.D., Ph.D. (Figure 44-10) assumed the Chair in 1962. Born in Illinois in 1917, he received his B.S. degree from Harvard in 1939 and M.D. from Northwestern in 1943. At the latter institution he developed a deep interest in physiology under the tutelage of Professor Andrew Conway Ivy (1893–1978).

After three years of residency at the University of Iowa he remained there to obtain a Ph.D. degree. His thesis was on metabolism of the cornea. A subsequent private practice in Bethlehem, Pennsylvania, was interrupted by the Korean conflict. Upon entering the Flight Surgeon Program, Duane was assigned to the Naval Air Development Center at Johnsville, Pennsylvania, because of his research interest in physiology. There he did some of the original study of blackout in determining the etiology to be retinal hypoxia rather than cerebral ischemia.

While resuming private practice in Bethlehem, Dr. Duane traveled weekly to Philadelphia for teaching at the Graduate School of the University of Pennsylvania.

One of his first duties upon appointment to the Chair at Jefferson in 1962 was to oversee the construction of a new clinical facility for the Department on the fourth floor of the Curtis

Clinic. The Eye Clinic had remained essentially unchanged since completion of the Curtis Building in 1931. A description of how things were before the major facelift is historically interesting.

The patient entered a central room where the current appointment card was presented to a clerk, and where, upon leaving, the next appointment card would be given (Figure 44-11). In the front of this room to the left of the main door was the lane for visioning of the patients by Mr. James Lavelle, a veteran octogenarian. Immediately behind the visioning lane, further to the left, was a large room with two refracting lanes where the first-year resident refracted the patients every morning (Figure 44-12). In the front right corner of this room was a small room where outpatient surgery and suture removal were carried out. To the right of the main room was the darkroom where fundoscopic examination, indirect retinoscopy, and slit-lamp biomicroscopy were carried out. Further to the right, behind this room, was a conference room. A field room was located to the right of the main room adjacent to the door, directly to the right of the visioning lane. The waiting patients and family members that might be accompanying them sat in the hall on long benches that resembled the sturdy wooden benches that were ever-present in the old railroad stations. At the time of its design it represented the latest and best of everything.

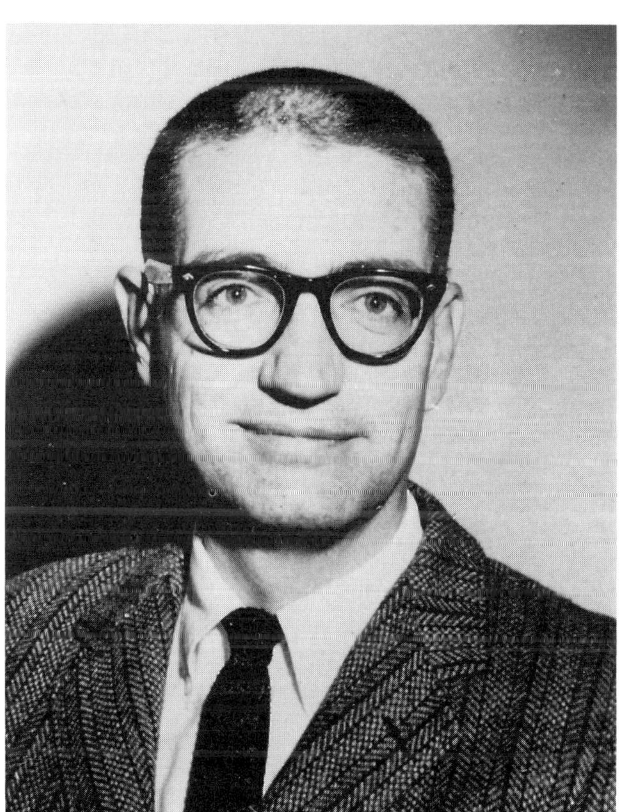

Fig. 44-10. Thomas D. Duane, M.D., Ph.D., Eighth Chairman (1962–1981).

The new clinic incorporated the advances of the previous 30 years, replete with five superbly equipped examining rooms, a room for fundus photography and fluorescin angiography, and a modern library that also served as a conference room. The new quarters were occupied in April 1964.

Dr. Duane's first appointment to his staff was Dr. William C. Frayer, who took charge of Resident teaching. Dr. Frayer received his A.B. degree from Brown University in 1943, his M.D. at the University of Michigan in 1945, and his residency in ophthalmology at the University of Pennsylvania, where he also received the M.M.Sc. in 1952. He was Assistant Professor of Ophthalmology at the University of Pennsylvania when he came to Jefferson in 1962, and was promoted to full professor in 1964.

Dr. Frayer was an excellent surgeon, superb teacher, and productive researcher in ocular pathology. In 1972 he returned to the Scheie Institute of the University of Pennsylvania, where he carried on his multiple activities and served for a time as Acting Head of the Department.

During his first few years at Jefferson, Dr. Duane conducted the first survey of ophthalmic research in the United States. Through the 1970s he served as Secretary of the Section Council on Ophthalmology of the American Medical Association. He was a member of the Board of Directors of the American Academy of Ophthalmology, the American Board of Ophthalmology, Association of University Professors in Ophthalmology, and the National Advisory Eye Council.

Among at least 70 scientific papers, Dr. Duane first described microwave cataracts, the G force origin of blackout, Valsalva retinopathy, and the histopathology of white-centered hemorrhages. He served as editor of *Clinical Ophthalmology* and edited a three-volume set of *Biomedical Foundations of Ophthalmology*. The latter became a standard text.

Dr. Duane, in addition to his Chairmanship at Jefferson, was appointed Ophthalmologist-in-Chief at Wills Eye Hospital in October, 1973. He promptly became involved in plans for a new Wills building that was to be constructed at Ninth and Walnut Streets. In view of the close relationship that existed for many years between the two institutions, eventuating in an affiliation agreement on October 1, 1980, the staffs were amalgamated.

James Wills, Jr., a Quaker merchant, died in 1825 with a legacy of $108,396.35 for the establishment of "The Wills Hospital for the Relief of the Indigent Blind and Lame." When the hospital, located at Nineteenth and Race Streets, opened in 1834, it was the first in the Western Hemisphere especially devoted to the eye. The provision for the lame was carried out only sporadically and the last such case was treated by the late 1870s. The management of the hospital was vested in 1870 in the newly created Board of Directors of City Trusts, which since then has continued its responsibility to guide its destiny.[18]

In 1927 the Board of Trustees of Jefferson was aware of the mutual benefits of an affiliation with the Wills. At a meeting of the Board on June 20 of that year, President Alba B. Johnson stated that he had been in conference with Dr. Hobart A. Hare and Mr. Elmer Greenberg of the Board of City Trusts, relative to advisibility of having the Wills Eye Hospital located in the Curtis Clinic, a nine-story building that was later to open on November 21, 1931. After discussion it was decided that change in the general plan of the new Clinic could not be made at this date, but that it was highly desirable to establish the closest relations

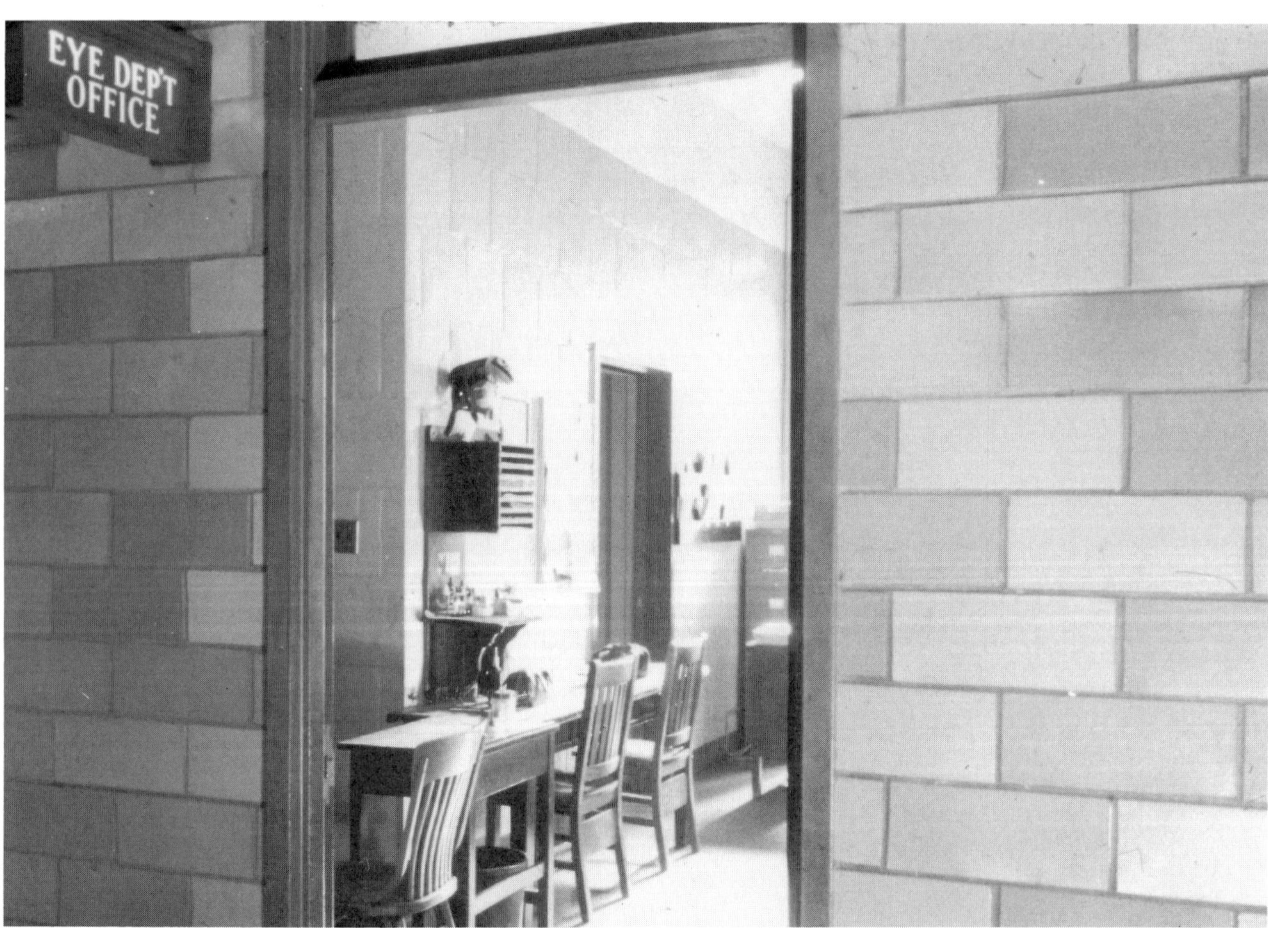

FIG. 44-11. Entrance to the Eye Clinic (ca. 1960).

with Wills Hospital. With increasing demands for more patient space, surgical suites, and laboratories, a new Wills Hospital was opened in 1932 at Sixteenth and Spring Garden Streets. Many Jeffersonians served on the staff not only as ophthalmologists but as consultants for all other conditions that could affect the patients concomitantly.

Again because of growth and scientific progress, another new Wills Eye Hospital was completed and occupied at Ninth and Walnut on April 1, 1980, and dedicated on April 23. It was an architecturally award-winning eight-story structure, nearly doubling the old Spring Garden facility. With 120 inpatient beds it was equipped with such modern equipment as ceiling-mounted microscopes and an audiovisual production center. The ground floor of the 230,000-square-foot building was a reception area and concourse, with a cafeteria in the basement. The first three levels contained the outpatient services, the fourth the laboratories and offices, the fifth the operating suites and ancillary services, and the top three the inpatients. There were eight research laboratories, eight operating rooms, a minor surgery room in the emergency area, and double the previous space for outpatient facilities. Other unique features included the Glaucoma Service Diagnostic Laboratory, the second of its kind in the United States; nuclear medicine and ultrasound testing equipment; and the nation's largest diagnostic photography center for the eye. An audiovisual production center enabled operations to be videotaped and played back simultaneously on television sets in the auditorium and conference rooms for teaching and monitoring purposes. The Lions Eye Bank of Delaware Valley, housed within the Hospital, conducted the collection and

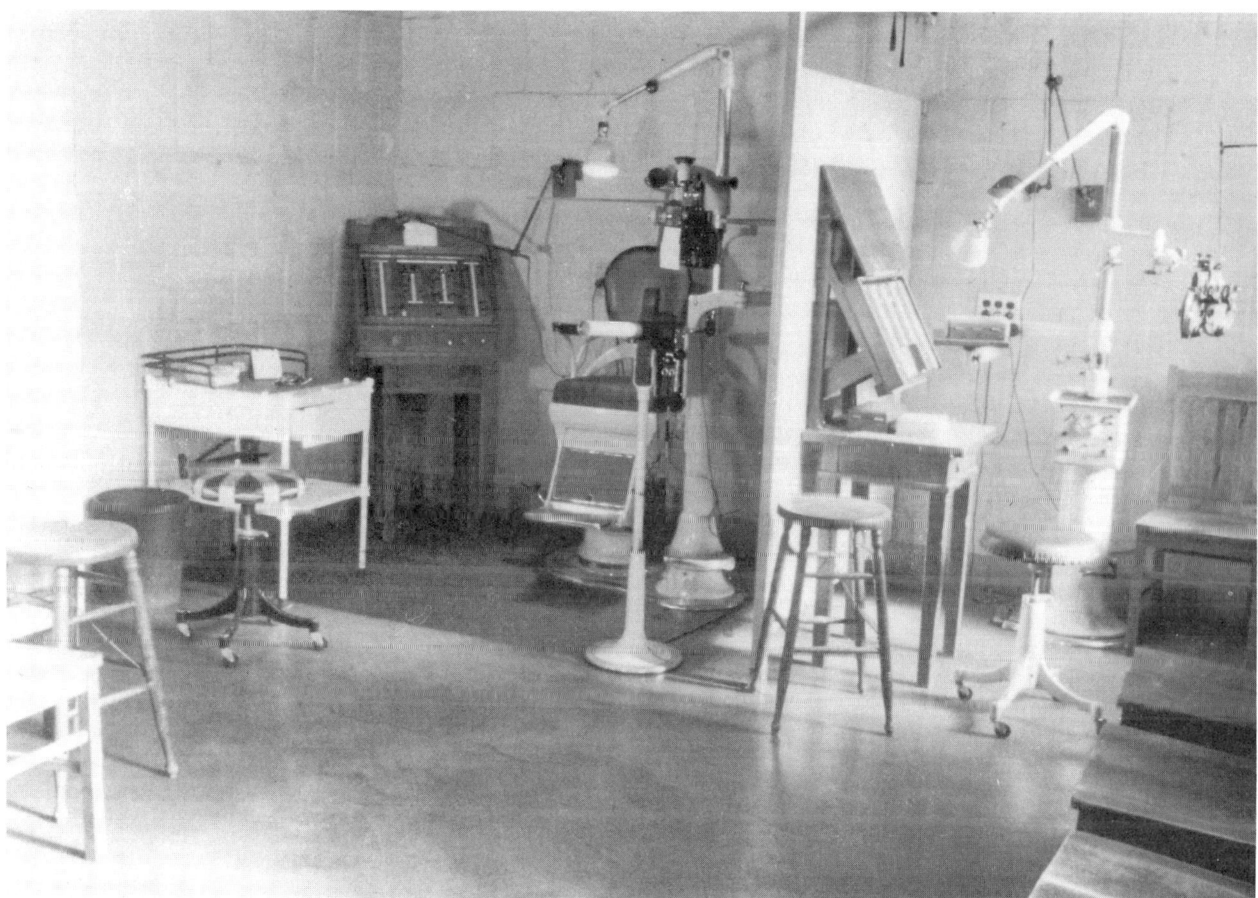

FIG. 44-12. Interior of the Eye Clinic (ca. 1960).

distribution of tissue for corneal transplants for Wills and other area hospitals.

The Wills Day Surgery Unit was expanded, a low-vision center developed, the contact lens service increased, and a center for study of eye movement disorders in children established. Researchers worked in immunology, cell biology, molecular chemistry, biochemistry, oncology, histology, virology, pharmacology, and micromanipulative techniques. The Glaucoma Service Diagnostic Laboratory, as one of only two centers of its kind in the world, was linked with Baylor College of Medicine in Houston as the hub of future worldwide networks.

The affiliation agreement of October 1, 1980, in essence amalgamated both staffs, but with preservation of autonomy and visible identity of each. After the prescribed ten years the agreement would be on a year-to-year basis. The Board of City Trusts still controlled the management of Wills.

Dr. Duane resigned his combined posts at Jefferson and Wills Eye on October 5, 1981, but continued actively in research. His portrait was presented at Wills Eye in 1982.[19] In 1984 he was honored with the American Academy of Ophthalmology's Distinguished Service Award, and on April 12, 1985, the Thomas David Duane Professorship in Ophthalmology was established.

Robert D. Reinecke, M.D. (1929–); Ninth Chairman (1981–1985)

Robert Dale Reinecke (Figure 44-13) was appointed Chairman of the Department at Jefferson and concurrently Ophthalmologist-in-Chief at Wills Eye on October 5, 1981. He was born in Kansas in 1929, the youngest of four children. While attending public high school he became an apprenticed watchmaker. After two years in the United States Army, he attended Kansas State College for two years. He then switched to the Illinois College of Optometry, where he obtained a Doctorate in Optometry in 1949. Returning to the University of Kansas he obtained a B.S. degree in 1955 and M.D. degrees in 1959, followed by internship at the University Medical Center. After a postgraduate course in ophthalmology at Harvard Medical School he took a residency at the Massachusetts Eye and Ear Infirmary from 1961 to 1963. During some of the earlier years he worked in Summer Research Fellowships in the U.S. Public Health Service and Harvard Medical School.

Dr. Reinecke pursued an academic career as a Teaching Fellow at Harvard Medical School (1963–1964) and until 1969 was associated with the Massachusetts Eye and Ear Infirmary, attaining the rank of Assistant Professor. In 1970 he became Chairman of the Department of Ophthalmology at Albany Medical College of Union University until his appointment at Jefferson.

As a prolific writer since 1958, Dr. Reinecke wrote more than 150 articles on a wide spectrum

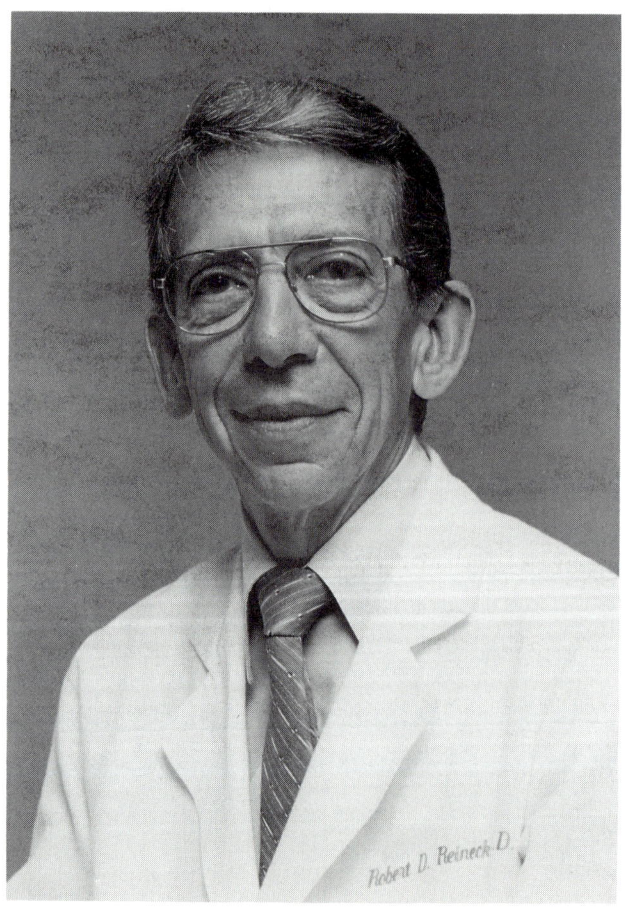

FIG. 44-13. Robert D. Reinecke, M.D., Ninth Chairman (1981–1985).

of eye disorders. One of his outstanding contributions was the report that smooth muscle involvement in temporal arteritis was the initial pathologic change, with fragmentation of the elastic fibers and giant cell reaction being secondary. Another important innovation was his development of the random-dot stereogram for ambylopic (dimness of vision) screening, which was more reliable in the young patient than previous circles tests.

His activities in societies at the administrative and advisory level were numerous. He served as President of the American Association for Pediatric Ophthalmology, Editor for the Internal Strabismological Association, and Co-Chairman of the National Eye Institute's panel on sensory and motor disorders of vision. Dr. Reinecke resigned his dual appointment on June 30, 1985, and became Director of the Foerderer Eye Movement Center for Children at Wills Eye Hospital and Jefferson.

William S. Tasman, M.D. (1929–); Tenth Chairman (1985–)

William Samuel Tasman (Figure 44-14) succeeded Dr. Reinecke as Ophthalmologist-in-Chief at Wills Eye Hospital and Chairman of the Department of Ophthalmology at Jefferson on July 22, 1985. He is a native Philadelphian, born August 9, 1929. He graduated from Germantown Friends School (1947), Haverford College (A.B. degree in 1951), and Temple University School of Medicine (1955). After internship at the Philadelphia General Hospital (1955–1956) and a course in ophthalmology at the Graduate School of the University of Pennsylvania (1956–1957), he served a tour of duty as a Captain in the U.S. Air Force Hospital in Wiesbaden, Germany (1957–1959).

On returning to Philadelphia, Dr. Tasman became a Resident at Wills Eye Hospital (1959–1961) and then took a Fellowship in Retina at the Massachusetts Eye and Ear Hospital (1961–1962) under the tutelage of Dr. Charles L. Schepens, a world-renowned retinal surgeon. Under the stimulating parental influence of Dr. Isaac S. Tasman, who had been an Attending Surgeon at Wills from 1939 to 1960, he initially joined his father in private practice until the latter's failing health necessitated retirement.

In the subspecialty of retinal surgery, Dr. Tasman was appointed Associate Surgeon at Wills Eye Hospital (1962–1974) and Attending Surgeon (1974) and Co-Director of the Retinal Service (1976). He also became Attending Surgeon at Chestnut Hill Hospital (1965) and Consulting Surgeon at the Children's Hospital of Philadelphia (1977).

Dr. Tasman was made Associate Professor at Temple University School of Medicine (1966–1971) and Professor of Ophthalmology and Director of the Department at the Medical College of Pennsylvania (1979–1981). In 1974 he became a Professor of Ophthalmology at Jefferson, a

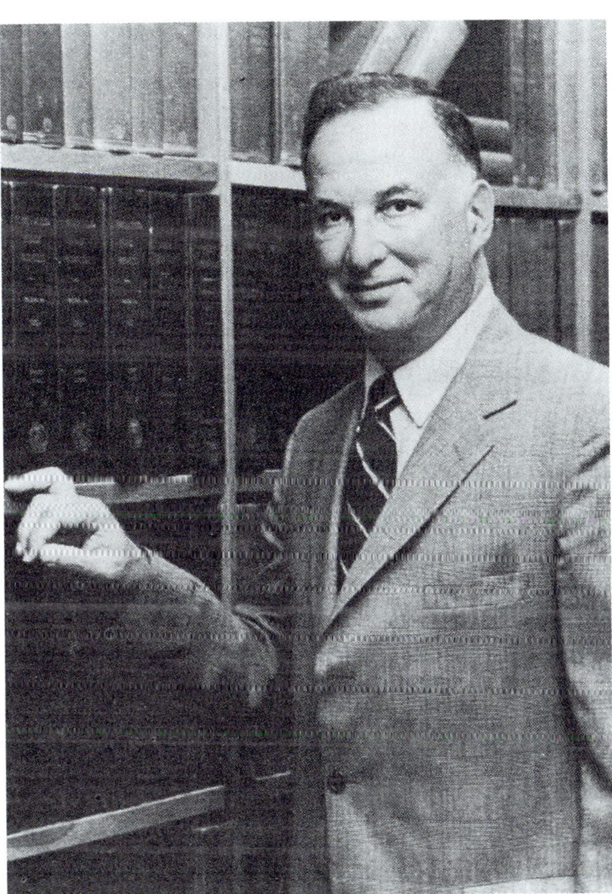

FIG. 44-14. William S. Tasman, M.D., Tenth Chairman (1985–).

position he held until his appointment as Chairman in 1985. He served as member and officer in the numerous local and national organizations in his field and was active in founding the Club Jules Conin Retina Society and was one of the founding members of the Retina Society. His editorial positions include *Survey of Ophthalmology,* since 1971, *AMA Archives of Ophthalmology* (1972–1976), and member of the editorial board of *Ophthalmic Surgery,* since 1983. Over a 14-year period he obtained large grants for retinal clinical research at Wills Eye Hospital and significant contributions to the Retina Research and Development Foundation.

Dr. Tasman has contributed approximately 100 publications as articles or chapters in textbooks, including an authoritative treatise on diabetic retinopathy in conjunction with his partner, Dr. William E. Benson, in *Clinical Ophthalmology.* He was the editor of *Retinal Diseases in Children* (1971), coauthored, with Jerry A. Shields, M.D., *Diseases of the Peripheral Fundus* (1979), and coauthored *Congenital Anomalies of the Optic Disc* (1983), with Gary C. Brown, M.D. In 1980 he published *The History of Wills Eye Hospital.*

The large size and rapid growth of the Department occasioned the omission of many names associated with its progress. From 1946 to 1982, 79 residents were trained. A rough estimate would indicate that over the years perhaps four million eye patients have been treated. In the increasingly sophisticated technology and basic research of ophthalmology, Jefferson is dedicated to retaining a forefront position for the improved eye care of young and old.

References

1. *American Medical Recorder.* 4:402, 1821.
2. Albert, D.M., and Scheie, H.G., *History of Ophthalmology.* Philadelphia: Charles C. Thomas, 1965, pp. 5–17.
3. Tasman, W., *The History of Wills Eye Hospital.* Philadelphia: Harper and Row, 1980, pp. 30–31.
4. Holland, J.W., "A Brief History of Jefferson Medical College." Class Yearbook of 1899. p. 17, 1899.
5. Gross, S.D., "De L'Ophthalmologie en Amerique," Cong. period, internat. d'Ophthal. Compt.-rend 1857. Bruxelles: 1858, pp. 351–354.
6. Gross, S.D., *A System of Surgery: Pathological, Diagnostic, Therapeutic, and Operative.* Vol. II. Philadelphia: Blanchard and Lea, 1859, pp. 329–439.
7. Posey, W.G., and Brown, S.H., *The Wills Hospital of Philadelphia.* Philadelphia: J.B. Lippincott Co., 1931, pp. 81–83.
8. Ibid., p. 83.
9. Zimmerman, L.E., Albert, D.M., and Blumberg, J.M., "William Thomson—Military Surgeon, Pioneer Photomicrographer, Clinical Ophthalmologist, *Am. J. Ophthalmol.* 69:487–497, 1970.
10. Albert, D.M., and Scheie, H.G., *A History of Ophthalmology.* Philadelphia: Charles C. Thomas, 1965, p. 215.
11. Shannon, C.E.G., "Dr. Howard Forde Hansell," *Trans. Am. Ophthal. Soc.* 33:21–23, 1935.
12. Hansell, H.F., "Memoir of William M. Sweet, M.D.," *Trans. Stud. Coll. Phys. Phila.,* Ser. 3, 49:198–201, 1927.
13. Posey and Brown, *Wills Hospital,* pp. 283–285.
14. Harbert, F., "Memoir of Arno E. Town, B.S., M.D., M.Sc. (Med.)," attached to the Executive Faculty Meeting Minutes of January 29, 1968.
15. Radbill, S.G., "Dr. Town Resigns," *Jeff. Med. Coll. Alum. Bull.,* August 1956, p. 53.
16. "Carroll R. Mullen, M.D., Appointed Chairman," *Jeff. Med. Coll. Alum. Bull.,* August 1956, p. 51.
17. Posey and Brown, *Wills Hospital,* pp. 22–26.
18. Steinmetz, C.G., III, "Carroll R. Mullen, M.D.," *Jeff. Med. Coll. Alum. Bull.* March 1961, p. 17.
19. Jaeger, E.A., " T.D. Duane Portrait Presentation," September 28, 1982.

CHAPTER FORTY-FIVE

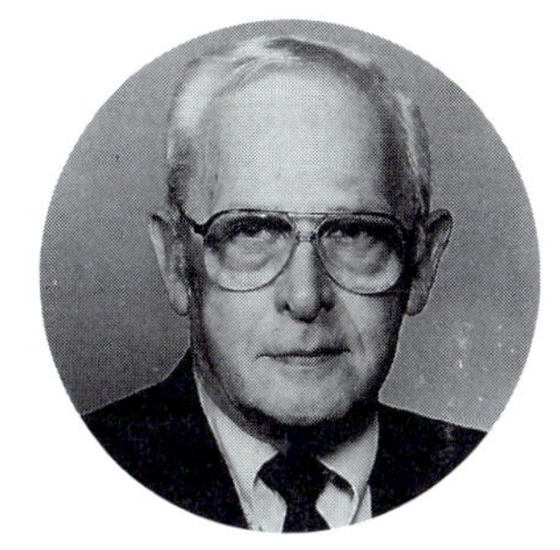

Department of Obstetrics and Gynecology

JAMES H. LEE, JR., M.D.

"The history of man for the nine months preceding his birth would, probably, be far more interesting and contain more events of greater moment than all the three-score and ten years that follow it."

—SAMUEL TAYLOR COLERIDGE (1772–1834)

OBSTETRICS in colonial Philadelphia, as in all of America, was practiced almost entirely by midwives. By the mid eighteenth century, however, a few physicians began to take an interest in obstetrics as a distinct specialty. The first medical school in this country, the Medical Department of the College of Philadelphia, started in 1765 without a Chair of Obstetrics. King's College Medical School in New York opened in 1767 as the second medical school, but it had the first Professor of Midwifery, John V.B. Tennent.[1] It was not until 1791, when the Medical Department of the College of Philadelphia merged with the University of the State of Pennsylvania, that William Shippen, Jr., who was the Professor of Anatomy and Surgery, had "Midwifery" added to his title. Shippen however, had been giving private lectures in midwifery since 1765. The course remained optional until 1813, when it was made obligatory for graduation, according to Scheffey,[2] although Cianfrani[3] says it was not made a requirement until 1831.

In any event, this requirement marked the elevation of obstetrics to a recognized medical science. By the time of Jefferson's founding in 1824, midwifery and diseases of women were becoming of more interest to physicians, and the practice of obstetrics more respectable. Knowledge, based on clinical observation, was increasing slowly, and Ephraim McDowell had performed his first ovariotomy (1809), heralding the development of abdominal surgery. The fetal heart was heard for the first time in 1822. On the other hand, cupping and bleeding were standard treatments for many ailments; purgatives were prescribed in large quantities; ether and chloroform were yet to be used; the hypodermic needle had not been devised; bacteriology was unknown; hemostatic forceps had not been invented; and bleeding in operations was profuse and often fatal. Almost all wounds suppurated.

Instruction was almost entirely didactic. Examination of women, known as the operation of "touching," was performed under covers. While general physicians were expected to have some knowledge of obstetrics, almost none acquired any practical experience in school. Special training required a trip to Europe or an assistantship to a practitioner. A few small lying-in hospitals had been created in the United States and separate wards designated for maternity patients in a few general hospitals. These were intended primarily as asylums for the poor and not for the training of medical students or physicians. Among these were the lying-in wards of the Philadelphia Almshouse, opened in 1802, and the Pennsylvania Hospital, opened in 1803.

The history of the Department of Obstetrics and Gynecology began with the founding of Jefferson Medical College in 1824. At that time a Professorship of Midwifery and Diseases of Women and Children was established. In the early years faculty changes were frequent, and particularly so in the Chair of Midwifery.

Francis S. Beattie, M.D. (1794–1841); First Chairman (1824–1826)

Francis S. Beattie was appointed as the first Professor. He graduated from the University of Pennsylvania in 1821 and spent several years in the Navy before returning to Philadelphia in 1824. Contentious and incompatible with his colleagues, he defaulted on a $20 assessment for the renovation of the Tivoli Theater, Jefferson's first Medical Hall. He was dismissed in October, 1826, after one term. Subsequently, he published a pamphlet claiming persecution by the Faculty and Trustees, which led to a successful libel suit against him by George McClellan.

It is reported[2] that in 1835 Beattie assisted Professor William Gibson in the performance of the first Caesarean section in Philadelphia successful for mother and child. This is of significance, because from 1822 to 1870 only three Caesarean sections had been performed in Philadelphia.

John Barnes, M.D. (1791–?); Second Chairman (1826–1827)

Dr. John Barnes (Figure 45-1) was appointed to fill the Professorship vacated by Dr. Beattie,

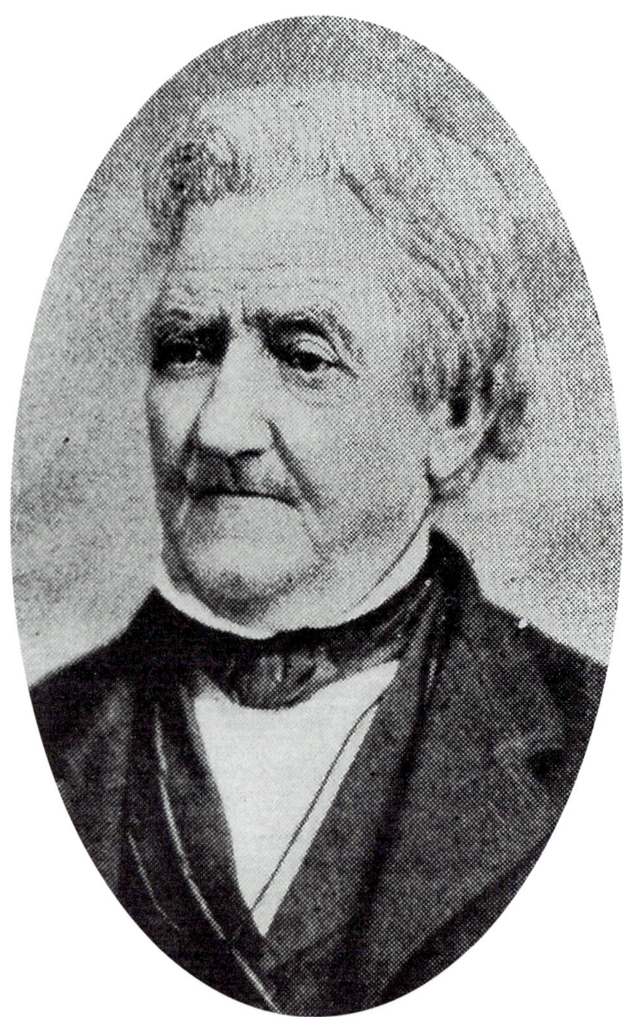

FIG. 45-1. John Barnes, M.D. (1791–?), Second Chairman (1826–1827).

but he, too, was not reappointed the following year. Like Beattie, he published a pamphlet complaining of his treatment by the Trustees and Faculty. According to Samuel D. Gross in his *Autobiography*, "He was the dullest lecturer that it was my lot ever to hear, destitute of all the attributes of a successful teacher."

John Eberle, M.D. (1787–1838); Third Chairman (1828–1831)

Following Dr. Barnes's dismissal, Dr. John Eberle (Figure 45-2), Professor of the Practice of Medicine, was given the additional assignment of Professor of Midwifery, which he held until his departure for Cincinnati, Ohio, in 1831. One of the founders of Jefferson, he had been active in politics and writing, and he was well known both in this country and abroad for his medical writings, although he contributed nothing significant in obstetrics.

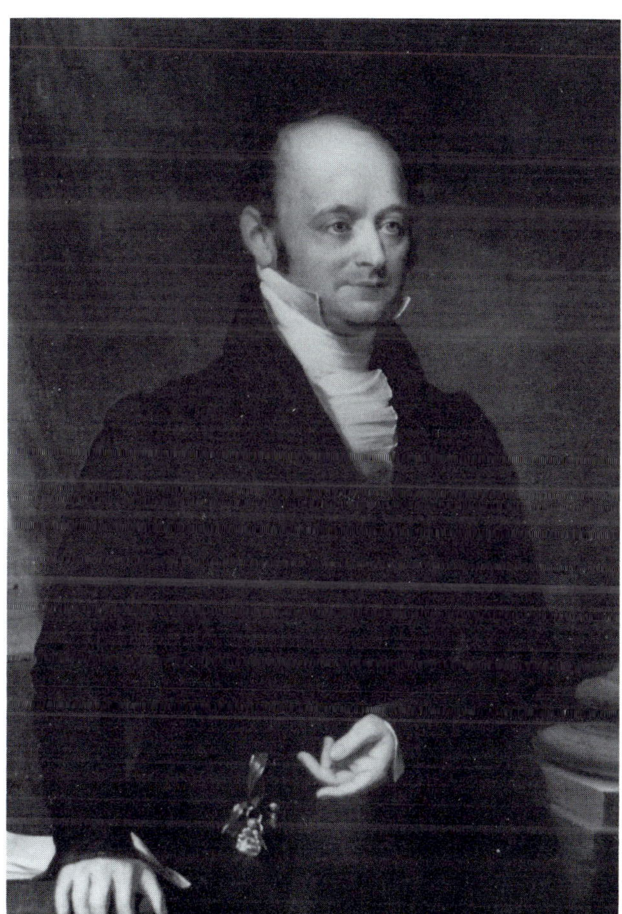

FIG. 45-2. John Eberle, M.D. (1787–1838), Third Chairman (1828–1831).

Usher Parsons, M.D. (1788–1868); Fourth Chairman (1831–1832)

Usher Parsons (Figure 45-3) held the Chair for only one year. A brother-in-law of Oliver Wendell Holmes, he was a former Naval surgeon who was awarded the Congressional Medal of Honor for distinguished service with Perry during the Battle of Lake Erie.

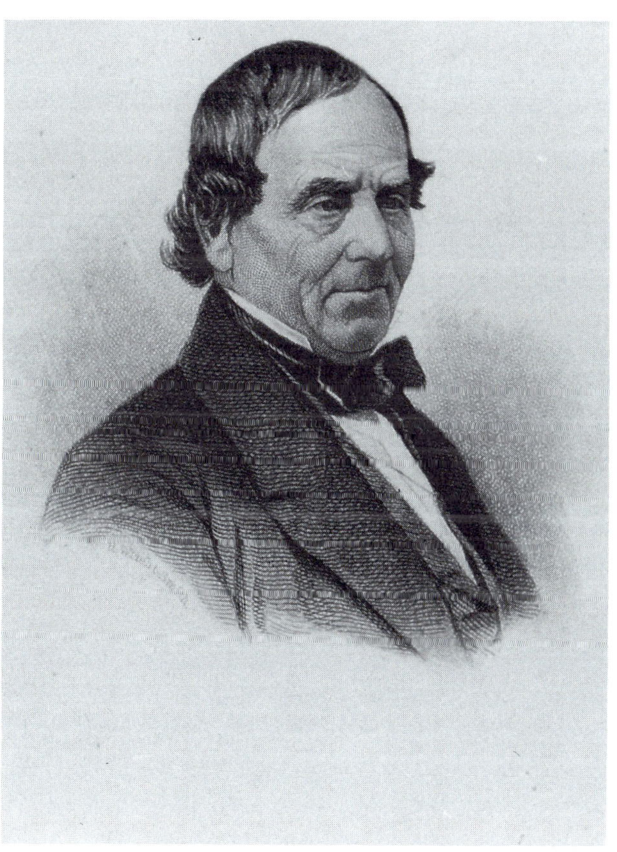

FIG. 45-3. Usher Parsons, M.D. (1788–1868), Fourth Chairman (1831–1832).

Samuel McClellan, M.D. (1800–1854); Fifth Chairman (1832–1839)

Samuel McClellan (Figure 45-4), the younger brother of George, had been a Demonstrator of Anatomy at Jefferson since 1828. He was appointed to the Chair of Midwifery in 1832 and held this position until he resigned in 1839 to join his brother in establishing another medical school.

The bulletins, or catalogues, of Jefferson during this period indicated that the Trustees and Faculty had concerns about the length of the curriculum and did extend it from four months to five. A written examination was also introduced in 1836. Sample questions included: What are the proofs that blood of the mother does or does not pass directly from the uterine vessels to those of the fetus?; From what cause does hemorrhage commonly proceed subsequent to delivery of the child?; Under what conditions can the forceps be safely used?; Under what conditions can ergot be safely given?

The statement also appears in the Bulletin for 1836 that the Professor of Midwifery procures patients from the dispensary for his pupils and these are attended at home by the students under the direction of the Professor. This would seem to indicate that some attempts were being made to provide some practical experience for students.

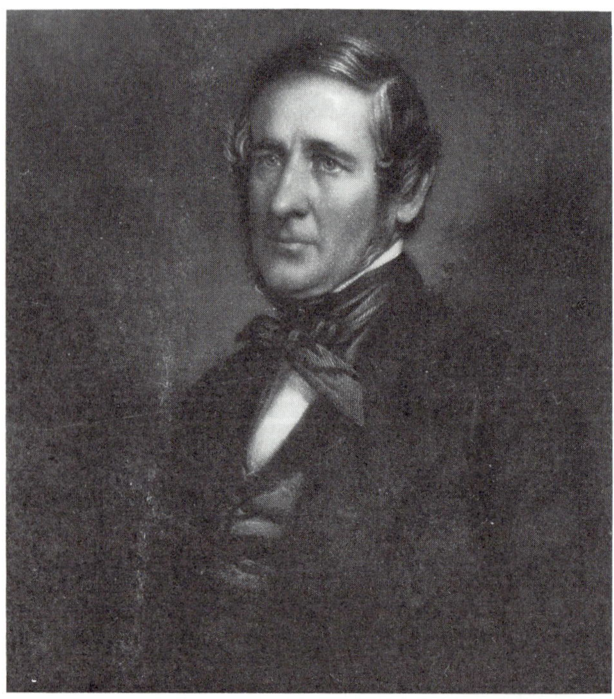

FIG. 45-4. Samuel McClellan, M.D. (1800–1854), Fifth Chairman (1832–1839).

Robert M. Huston, M.D. (1795–1864); Sixth Chairman (1839–1841)

Dr. Robert Huston (Figure 45-5), an 1825 graduate of the University of Pennsylvania, had first been elected to the Chair of Materia Medica but was transferred to the Professorship of Obstetrics and Diseases of Women and Children upon the departure of Samuel McClellan. Although he was better known in Materia Medica and Therapeutics than Midwifery, he is said to have had 20 years of experience as a practitioner of Midwifery. He became Professor of Materia Medica and Dean of the Faculty upon the election of Meigs to the Professorship of Obstetrics in 1841.

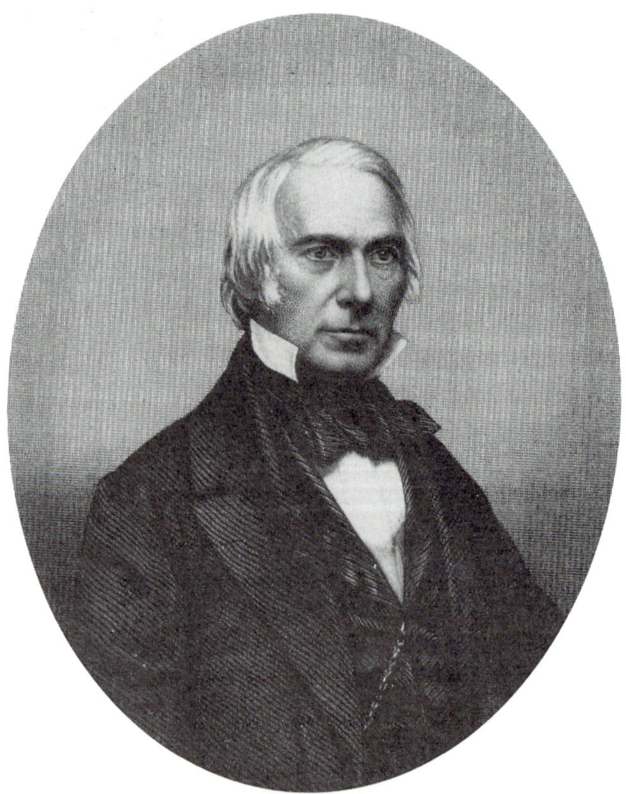

FIG. 45-5. Robert M. Huston, M.D. (1795–1864), Sixth Chairman (1839–1841).

Charles Delucena Meigs, M.D. (1792–1869); Seventh Chairman (1841–1862)

Charles D. Meigs (Figure 45-6), graduated from the University of Georgia in 1809 and then was apprenticed in medicine to Dr. Thomas H.M. Fendall of Augusta. From 1812 to 1815 he took courses at the University of Pennsylvania, receiving his degree in 1817. He practiced for a short time in Augusta, but then returned to Philadelphia. His practice apparently developed slowly, but he soon became intimate with the medical leaders and associated himself with Drs. Hodge, Bache, LaRoche, and others. He was one of the first editors of the *North American Medical and Surgical Journal*. He taught anatomy at the Hewson School from 1822 and from 1830 to 1835 lectured on midwifery in "The Philadelphia Association for Medical Instruction," another private school. In 1835 he contested unsuccessfully with Hugh Hodge for the Chair of Obstetrics at the University of Pennsylvania. In 1837 he was appointed Chairman of the Committee on Midwifery by the College of Physicians to advise the Trustees of the estate of Dr. Jonas Preston, leading to the founding of the Preston Retreat at Twentieth and Hamilton Streets for obstetric care of the deserving poor.

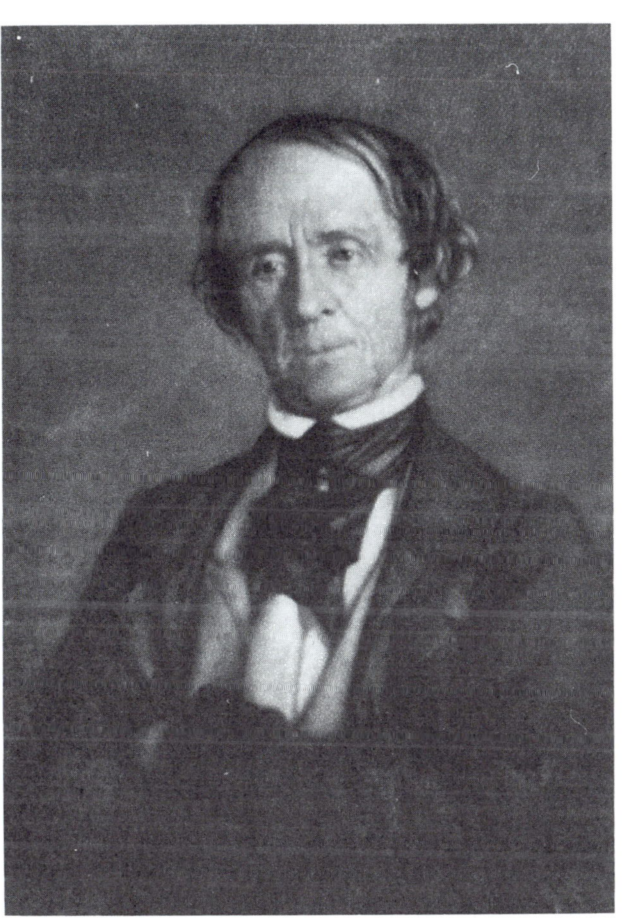

FIG. 45-6. Charles D. Meigs, M.D. (1792–1869), Seventh Chairman (1841–1862).

In 1841 Meigs was appointed Professor of Midwifery and Diseases of Women and Children at Jefferson as part of a major reorganization of the faculty that led to a period of peace and calm in the institution as well as a widening of its influence in medicine and medical teaching.

From the time of his appointment, Meigs became one of the most popular and influential teachers of his time and was recognized throughout the world. He wrote prolifically, including a translation of Velpeau's *Elementary Treatise of Midwifery* (1831); *Philadelphia Practice of Midwifery* (1838); *Woman, Her Diseases and Remedies*(1847); *Obstetrics, The Science and Art* (1849); and many others. For interesting and entertaining reading, his *Letters to His Class* (1847) provide insights into the man and a picture of obstetric and gynecologic practice of the time.

Soon after his appointment there appeared the papers by Oliver Wendell Holmes *On The Contagiousness of Puerperal Fever* (1843) and on *Puerperal Fever as a Private Pestilence* (1855). These aroused widespread controversy. Meigs, with his colleague Hugh L. Hodge at the University of Pennsylvania, strongly opposed the views of Holmes. Meigs wrote often and vigorously over many years in opposition to Holmes and in support of his own thought that puerperal fever resulted from "a strange coincidence of accidents, rather than a peripatetic causation by the doctor." He could not accept the infectious nature of the disease, yet in his report to the College of Physicians on the Preston Retreat he emphasized the importance of cleanliness, adequate ventilation, and rotation of labor rooms to prevent the dissemination of childbed fever.[4]

Meigs also strongly opposed the use of chloroform, primarily on the grounds of safety, and was against the operation of ovariotomy for any reason, saying "that the fact of a surgical operation being necessary in any case, is a reproach to medicine." Likewise, he was also opposed to Caesarean section, a not unreasonable attitude at the time, considering the mortality associated with this operation.

Despite his contentiousness on some subjects, Meigs was erudite and cultured. Widely respected by his students, he undoubtedly elevated the standards of teaching and the practice of obstetrics. He resigned and was made Professor Emeritus in 1861, delivering his farewell address to his class February 27, 1861, but returned to lecture the following year because of the poor health of his successor, William V. Keating. He then retired to his farm where he died on June 22, 1869.

William V. Keating, M.D. (1823–1894); Eighth Chairman (1861–1862)

William Keating was named to replace Dr. Meigs in 1861 but, as already noted, could not complete his course of lectures because of illness.

Ellerslie Wallace, M.D. (1819–1885); Ninth Chairman (1862–1883)

Dr. Ellerslie Wallace (Figure 45-7), a graduate of Jefferson in the Class of 1843, was a Demonstrator of Anatomy for 16 years in his alma mater prior to his appointment as Professor of Obstetrics and Diseases of Women. He held the latter position for 20 years during a period in which great progress occurred in medicine. Advances in anesthesia, pathology, bacteriology chemistry, and asepsis and antisepsis during the second half of the nineteenth century were making medicine a science as well as an art.

During Wallace's tenure, instruction continued to be primarily didactic, although clinical teaching was gradually developing. He was reported to be a brilliant and theatric lecturer. Bland reports that special obstetric clinics were established during his Chairmanship and held almost daily, although they were more of a didactic experience than a clinic as we know it today.

Dr. Wallace was a founding member of the American Gynecologic Society.

Theophilus Parvin, M.D. (1829–1899); Tenth Chairman (1883–1898)

Theophilus Parvin (Figure 45-8) was one of the most brilliant and widely respected physicians to occupy the Chair of Obstetrics at Jefferson. He

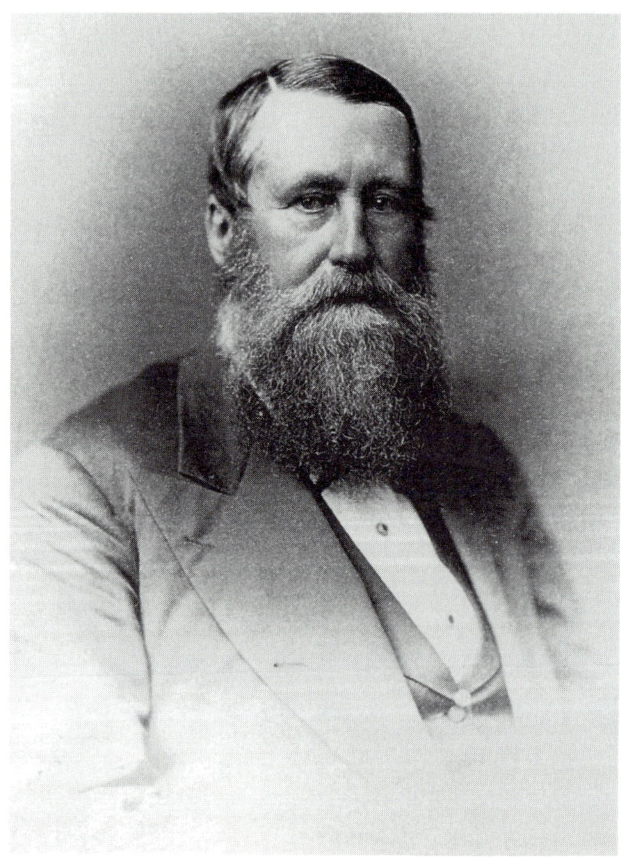

FIG. 45-7. Ellerslie Wallace, M.D. (1819–1885), Ninth Chairman (1862–1883).

was an eloquent speaker, a scholarly writer, and contributed significantly to the development of Obstetrics as a science. In addition, and perhaps most importantly, he pioneered in establishing hospital instruction in obstetrics for medical students in this country and established at Jefferson the first obstetrical clinic in America.

Parvin was born in Buenos Aires in 1829, where his father was a Presbyterian missionary. His mother, the daughter of Caesar Augustus Rodney, who was Attorney General of the United States in the Cabinets of Jefferson and Madison, died when Parvin was only a few weeks old. His father brought him back to this country but died when Parvin was about seven years old. He was then raised by his guardian, the Reverend Dr. Steel, in Abington, Pennsylvania. He received a baccalaureate degree from the University of Indiana in 1847, taught for three years at the Lawrenceville High School in New Jersey while taking courses in Hebrew and Greek at Princeton Theological Seminary; then received a Master's degree in 1850 from the University of Indiana. He next entered the University of Pennsylvania Medical School, receiving his Medical degree in 1852. After internship at Wills Eye Hospital he became a ship's surgeon before returning to Indianapolis to practice. He was appointed to the Chair of Materia Medica in the Ohio Medical College in 1864, resigning that position in 1869 to become Professor of Obstetrics and Diseases of Women at the University of Louisville. In 1876 he accepted a similar Chair at the College of Physicians and Surgeons of Indianapolis. Two years later he became Professor of Obstetrics at the Medical College of Indiana. In 1882 he returned to the Professorship of Obstetrics at the University of Louisville and the following year was appointed Professor of Obstetrics and Diseases of Women and Children at Jefferson.

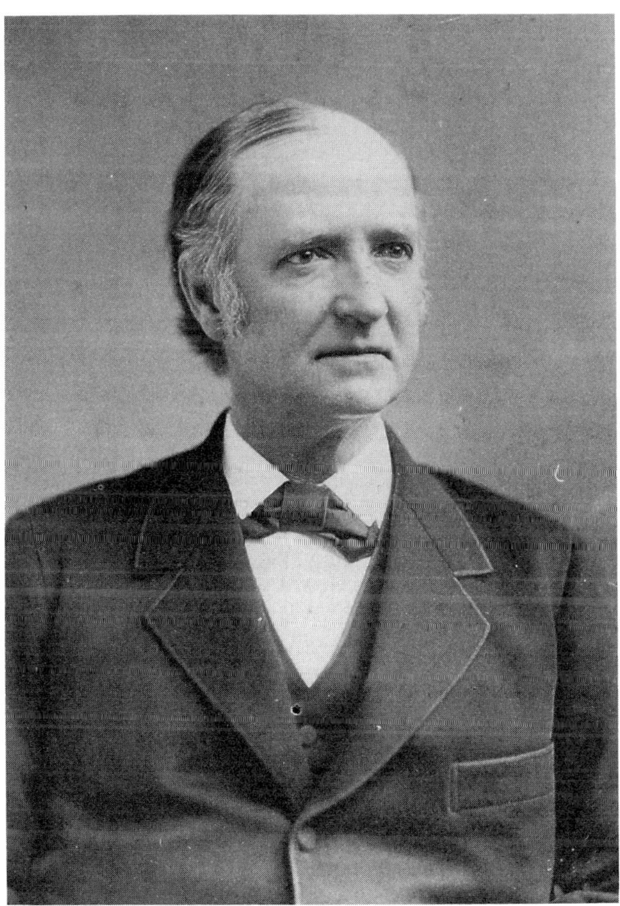

FIG. 45-8. Theophilus Parvin, M.D. (1829–1899), Tenth Chairman (1883–1898).

Parvin was not long at Jefferson before requesting a lying-in unit. In Jefferson's archives is a letter to Dr. Parvin from the Board of Trustees dated November 26, 1885, permitting the use of two rooms on the second floor of the 1877 Hospital for a maternity area and stating that "it being expressly understood that the rooms shall be under the direction and control of the Hospital Committee and the Professor of Obstetrics, who are specially directed to use every reasonable means to keep the rooms in proper condition by use of antiseptics, etc." In 1888 he gave an address before the American Academy of Medicine in New York entitled *The Necessity for Practical Obstetrics in the Course of Instruction Given by Medical Schools*. In this address he pointed out that the vast majority of American medical students were graduated without ever having witnessed, let alone have charge of, a patient in labor. He stated that the practical teaching of obstetrics should be directly associated with its scientific instruction and made a plea that there should be a maternity facility belonging to every medical school in which practical obstetrics should be taught, and any medical school that failed to do so should be condemned. In this address he reported that up to that time in Jefferson's unit, 34 women had been delivered without a maternal death, the ward classes having been instructed by his assistant, Dr. William E. Ashton. Because of lack of room in the Hospital, an outpatient department was established where clinical instruction was also carried out.

Up to that time and, indeed, well into the twentieth century, the majority of women were delivered at home, attended either by midwives or, sometimes, by a physician. Modesty and custom prevented medical students from attending or observing patients in labor. Dr. James S. White, a graduate of Jefferson in the Class of 1834 and the Professor of Obstetrics at the Medical School in Buffalo until his death in 1881, introduced in 1850 the practice of allowing medical students to observe labor and produced a storm of protest and abuse in the medical and lay press, forcing him to bring a suit of libel in self-defense.

On April 4, 1889, the space in the Hospital having been inadequate, the Board of Trustees gave Parvin the authority to "establish a Maternity in accordance with your proposition." The first real Maternity was subsequently established at 327 Pine Street. This building soon became inadequate because of the increasing number of patients applying for care, and a new maternity home was established at 224 West Washington Square in 1894 (Figure 45-9). Here there were greater opportunities for clinical instruction, and students were assigned to study patients antenatally as well as to observe deliveries, both normal and complicated.

Parvin was a prolific writer and editor. His textbook, *The Science and Art of Obstetrics* (1886), went through three editions and was adopted as a text by a number of schools. In it he recommended that the obstetrician should see his patient from time to time, especially in the latter part of pregnancy, and recommended weekly urine testing for albumin during the last two to three months. This was long before the value of prenatal care had been accepted. He also recommended elective Caesarean section, recognized the usefulness of episiotomy, and showed advanced knowledge for his day of the etiology and treatment of puerperal sepsis.

Dr. Parvin received many honors. He was a founder and later President of the American Gynecologic Society, President of the American Medical Association, the American Academy of Medicine, and the Philadelphia Obstetrical Society. He had numerous other honorary memberships and was Honorary President of the Obstetrics Section at the Berlin International Congress in 1890 and of the International Congress of Gynecology and Obstetrics at Brussels in 1892.

Contributions of Nonfaculty Jefferson Graduates to Obstetrics and Gynecology

There were graduates of Jefferson Medical College who, although not associated with Jefferson during their subsequent careers, made significant contributions to the developing science of

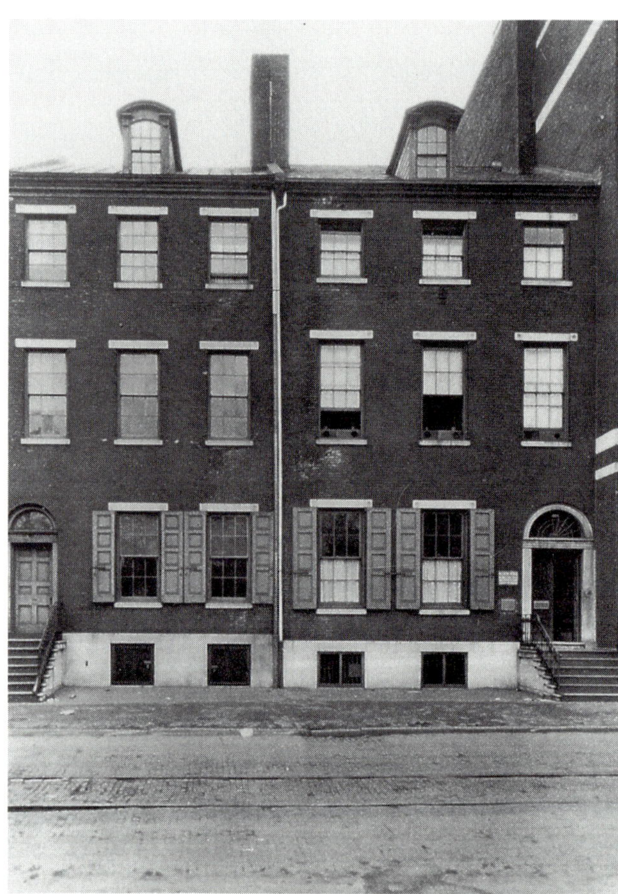

FIG. 45-9. The maternity facility at 224 West Washington Square, established in 1894 for patient care and student instruction.

obstetrics and, particularly, gynecology, during the mid- and late nineteenth century. Those worthy of especial note include Washington L. Atlee, J. Marion Sims, William T. Howard, Thomas A. Emmett, William Goodell, and Robert Battey.

■ Washington L. Atlee, M.D. (1808–1878)

Washington L. Atlee (Figure 45-10) was born in Lancaster, Pennsylvania, graduated from Jefferson Medical College in 1829, and returned to the Lancaster area to practice. He and his brother, John Atlee, who graduated from the University of Pennsylvania in 1820, were instrumental in reviving the operation of ovariotomy, which had been done only sporadically since McDowell's first one in 1809. Washington Atlee did his first ovariotomy on March 29, 1844, and during the next 34 years he performed 387. In 1845 he had returned to Philadelphia to become Professor of Medical Chemistry in the newly formed Pennsylvania College, a position he resigned in 1852 to attend to his surgical and gynecologic practice. The opposition to his work was widespread. He was denounced by many, including Meigs, who wrote that he would be glad to see his procedures prevented by statute. He was honored eventually by his colleagues however, who elected him President of the Philadelphia County Medical Society in 1874. He was a founding member of the American Gynecologic Society and the American Medical Association. In addition to his ovariotomies, he reported the first successful abdominal myomectomy for fibroids in 1845 and additional experience with myomectomy in 1853.

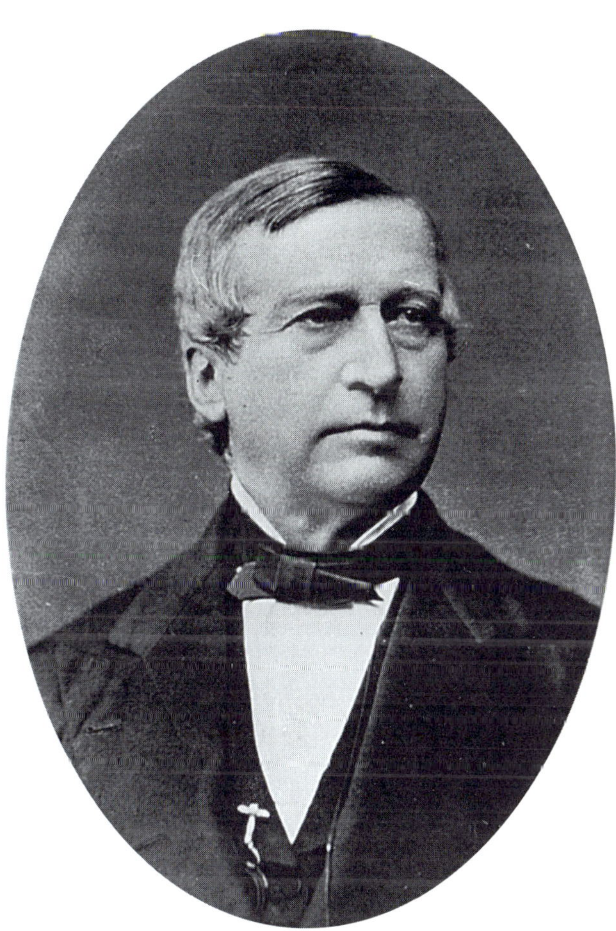

FIG. 45-10. Washington L. Atlee, M.D. (1808–1878), Pioneer in operation of ovariotomy (oophorectomy).

■ J. Marion Sims, M.D. (1813–1883)

James Marion Sims (Figure 45-11), often referred to as the "Father of American Gynecology," was born in Lancaster County, South Carolina, on January 25, 1813. He graduated from South Carolina College in 1832 and returned to Lancaster where he began the study of medicine with a Dr. Churchill Jones. He then took a course of lectures at the Medical College of Charleston before coming to Jefferson, where he graduated in 1835. He returned to Lancaster to practice but soon moved to Alabama, eventually settling in Montgomery in 1840. It was there that he began to develop his reputation as a surgeon, operating successfully for strabismus, clubfoot, harelip and tumors of the jaw.

It was in 1845 that Sims ventured into woman's surgery with the discovery that the knee-chest position permitted much better visualization of the vagina than had been seen before, aided by the speculum he devised that bears his name. The knee-chest position was later modified to the lateral Sims position, which was more comfortable for the patient. His work over the next five years in attempting to repair vesico-vaginal fistulae successfully is well known, during which time he devised instruments and technics, including the use of silver wire sutures. He finally achieved success in a patient he had operated upon 30 times, and soon others were cured of this condition. His results were published in 1852, establishing his fame. Afflicted about this time with a chronic diarrhea, he searched for a healthier climate in which to live and moved to New York in 1853.

After settling in New York his practice and reputation grew rapidly. He had an ambition to establish a gynecologic hospital, and this became a reality with the opening of what was to become the Woman's Hospital of New York in 1855, the first of its kind in America. He functioned as Surgeon-in-Chief until, with the outbreak of the Civil War, he found his position as a southerner in New York difficult. Accordingly, he went to Europe, where for the next six years he practiced in England, France, Germany, and Italy, achieving considerable renown and receiving many decorations and awards. During this period he published his one book, *Clinical Notes on Uterine Surgery* (1866). In 1868 he returned to New York, this time as a Consulting Surgeon to the Woman's Hospital, and resumed his practice, although he continued to commute to Europe. In 1870, during the Franco–Prussian War, he served as Surgeon-in-Chief of the Anglo-American Ambulance Corps.

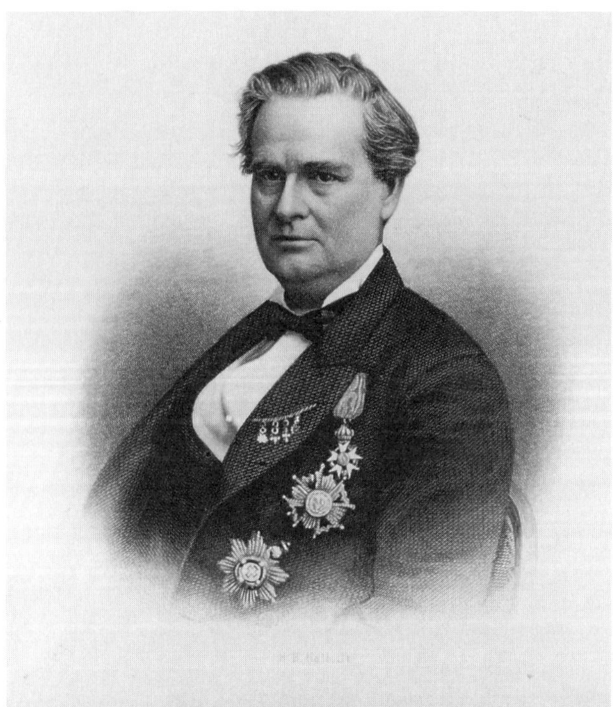

FIG. 45-11. J. Marion Sims, M.D. (1813–1883), the "Father of American Gynecology."

In 1874 Sims resigned from the Woman's Hospital over a conflict with the Board of Managers about their policies of not admitting cancer patients and of limiting the number of visitors at his operative clinics. He perceived a need for a hospital for the care of patients with cancer and his efforts resulted in the opening of a hospital that evolved into the Memorial–Sloan Kettering Cancer Center.

In addition to his foreign awards and decorations, Sims was widely recognized and respected in his own country. He was elected President of the American Medical Association in 1875, and in 1879 he was elected President of the American Gynecologic Society, of which he had been a founding member.

Sims never had an academic appointment. He told the elder Gross that one of his ambitions was to be a teacher of gynecology in some great school, preferably his alma mater. Professor Wallace, who in 1882 was in failing health and realized that his Chair must soon be vacated, spoke to Gross about it. By this time, however, Sims replied, "My health will not permit my acceptance of so onerous a chair." He died November 13, 1883. A statue to Sims's memory stands on Fifth Avenue in New York opposite the New York Academy of Medicine, another in Columbia, South Carolina, and a third in Montgomery, Alabama.

In addition to his contributions to gynecology, Sims performed the first planned operation on the gallbladder, coining the term, "cholecystotomy," and also urged the surgical treatment of gunshot wounds of the abdomen. He promulgated the steps to be carried out and thus opened up another frontier in abdominal surgery. Sims's son, H. Marion Sims, in 1888 reported on the microscopic study of spermatozoa in cervical mucus, the beginning of the Sims–Huhner test used in infertility studies.

scientific, comprehensive work on this subject in English." Like Sims, he was a founding member of the American Gynecologic Society and its President in 1882. He died in 1919.

William T. Howard, M.D. (1821–1902)

William T. Howard, born in Cumberland County, Virginia, in 1821, graduated from Jefferson in 1844. After practicing for a time in North Carolina, he later moved to Baltimore, Maryland. He was Professor of Diseases of Women and Children at the University of Maryland from 1867 to 1897 and was Visiting Surgeon to the Hospital for Women of Maryland and a Consulting Surgeon to the Johns Hopkins Hospital. He also was a founding member of the American Gynecologic Society and was its President in 1884. He died in 1902.

Thomas A. Emmett, M.D. (1828–1891)

Thomas A. Emmett was born in 1828 at the University of Virginia in Charlottesville, where his father was Professor of Materia Medica. After Emmett graduated from Jefferson in 1850 he went to New York where he served as Resident Physician at the Emigrant Refugee Hospital on Wards Island. He joined Dr. Sims in 1855, at which time the latter had opened his Woman's Hospital of New York.

Emmett's relation with Sims was almost like father and son, although they were of different temperaments. Emmett excelled in patience, persistence, and an analytical mind. During their years together they devised or improved many pelvic operations, of which Emmett kept case reports and drawings. He served as Sims's assistant until 1861 when Sims went to Europe, and for the next ten years he carried the responsibility for the work and the Hospital. His biggest achievements were in the field of vesico-vaginal fistula, and in 1868 he published his experience with some 600 cases, of which only three were incurable. He devised numerous instruments including a tenaculum, perineal retractors, curved scissors, needle forceps, and others. His text, *Principles and Practice of Gynecology* (1879), was characterized by Howard A. Kelly as "the first thoroughly

William Goodell, M.D. (1829–1894)

William Goodell was born in Malta, October 17, 1829, the son of missionaries. He was educated at Williams College and graduated from Jefferson in 1854. He practiced in Malta and Constantinople before returning to the United States in 1860. He was selected in 1865 to be the first Physician-in-Charge of the Preston Retreat, which had been established by a bequest of Dr. Jonas Preston in 1835 to create a lying-in hospital for indigent married women.[5] The hospital was completed in 1840, but because of cost and a severe business recession could not be opened for its intended use until 1865. Goodell instituted measures to maintain ventilation and cleanliness, using the four wards in rotation, and insisting on cleanliness of attendants and patients, applying the new principles of asepsis and antisepsis to prevent infection. He resigned in 1887 after having delivered 2,444 women with only six deaths.[6] In 1874 he was appointed Clinical Professor of Diseases of Women and Children at the University of Pennsylvania and held that position until his death in 1894. He, too, was a founding member of the American Gynecology Society and a founder and President of the Philadelphia Obstetrical Society.

Robert Battey, M.D. (1828–1895)

Robert Battey was born in Augusta, Georgia, in 1828. He attended the Philadelphia College of Pharmacy, then graduated from Jefferson in 1857. Following his graduation he studied in Paris from 1858 to 1860, then practiced in Rome, Georgia. He was an eminent gynecologist of his day and was a founding member and President (1888) of the American Gynecologic Society. He was Surgeon-in-Charge of the Gynecological Infirmary in Rome, Georgia, and also Consulting Surgeon of the Martha Battey Hospital, the latter being the gift of Dr. Battey and named after his wife. At the first meeting of the American Gynecologic Society he presented a paper on *Extirpation of the Functionally Active Ovaries for the Remedy of Otherwise Incurable Diseases,* and espoused oophorectomy (he did his first in 1872) for treating sexual disorders, dysmenorrhea, epilepsy, hysteria, and reestablishing good health in general, indications that we know today are mistaken. He did devise an improved operation for fistula and was the originator of iodized phenol. He died in 1895, and a monument stands to his memory in Rome, Georgia.

A Possible Jefferson First: Artificial Insemination

Although assigning "firsts" is always subject to error, there is reported evidence that successful indirect impregnation was first accomplished at Jefferson (1884–1885) by Dr. William H. Pancoast, Professor of Anatomy and a practicing surgeon.[7] Although never claimed by Pancoast (Jefferson, 1856), a member of his student group, Addison Davis Hard, recalled in 1909 that he had witnessed the event.[8] Dr. Pancoast was faced with an infertile couple, a Philadelphia merchant and his wealthy Quaker wife. For reasons not clearly stated or known, Dr. Pancoast obtained semen from one of the students without the knowledge of husband or wife and injected it into the uterus of the anesthetized patient with a hard rubber syrine. A healthy son resulted.[9] Hard stated that Dr. Pancoast later "reluctantly" informed the husband, who to the doctor's relief was pleased but asked that his wife not be told.

In reaction to the report (1909), a number of comments resulted. The only claim to priority, however, involved another Jefferson graduate, Dr. J. Marion Sims (Class of 1835). A Georgia physician claimed that Dr. Sims had inseminated an anesthetized woman with her husband's semen. Sims, however, used semen vaginally obtained following intercourse and actually claimed only one successful pregnancy (lost by miscarriage) in a total of 55 injections in six patients[10] He did not continue his experiments, stating that success would require "greater knowledge of the laws of conception."

It is thus possible that Pancoast's closely guarded "experiment" was actually the first instance of artificial human insemination.

Gynecology Established as a Separate Department (1892)

Since the founding of Jefferson and until 1891, the academic responsibilities included the teaching of Obstetrics and also Diseases of Women and Children. In 1892 a Department of Gynecology was established with Dr. Edward E. Montgomery appointed as Professor of Clinical Gynecology, and in 1892 Dr. Edwin E. Graham was appointed the first Clinical Professor of Diseases of Children. Obstetrics and Gynecology thus became separate Departments, a division that continued until 1945 when they were reunited under a single Chairman (Lewis C. Scheffey, M.D., Sc.D.). Dr. Parvin continued as Professor of Obstetrics until his death in 1898.

Edward Emmet Montgomery, M.D. (1848–1927); First Chairman of Gynecology (1892–1920)

Dr. E.E. Montgomery (Figure 45-12) was born in Newark, Ohio, on May 15, 1848. He was graduated with a B.S. degree from Dennison University in 1871, then taught school and began reading medicine in the office of Dr. J.J. Hamill for a year. He entered Jefferson in 1872 and graduated in 1874 as President of his class. For the next 15 months he was a resident physician at the Philadelphia General Hospital and then began a general practice in the northwestern section of Philadelphia. During this period he taught private classes at Jefferson Medical College for two years in Physiology and two years in Anatomy. In 1878 and 1879 he taught private classes in operative surgery at the Woman's Medical College and was Clinical Surgeon to the Woman's Hospital. In 1878 he was elected to the Obstetric Staff of the Philadelphia General Hospital, a position he held until 1893. In 1879, in that institution, he performed the first successful ovariotomy (oophorectomy) before a public clinic in Philadelphia, the first successful ovariotomy performed at that hospital (although not the first in Philadelphia). In his early years in practice he performed tracheotomy 28 times for diphtheria. He was the first in Philadelphia (August 16, 1887) to intubate the larynx through the mouth for membranous croup (diphtheria), performing this operation more than 70 times with about 45% recoveries. His increasing work in abdominal surgery eventually led to the abandonment of this type of work.

From 1886 to 1892 Dr. Montgomery was Professor of Gynecology in the Medico-Chirurgical College, filling the Chair of Obstetrics and Gynecology the final two years before accepting the appointment at Jefferson. In addition, he was President of the Medical Staff of St. Joseph's Hospital, where for 35 years he was Gynecologist, as well as Consulting Gynecologist to the Kensington, Philadelphia, Lying-In and the Jewish Hospitals.

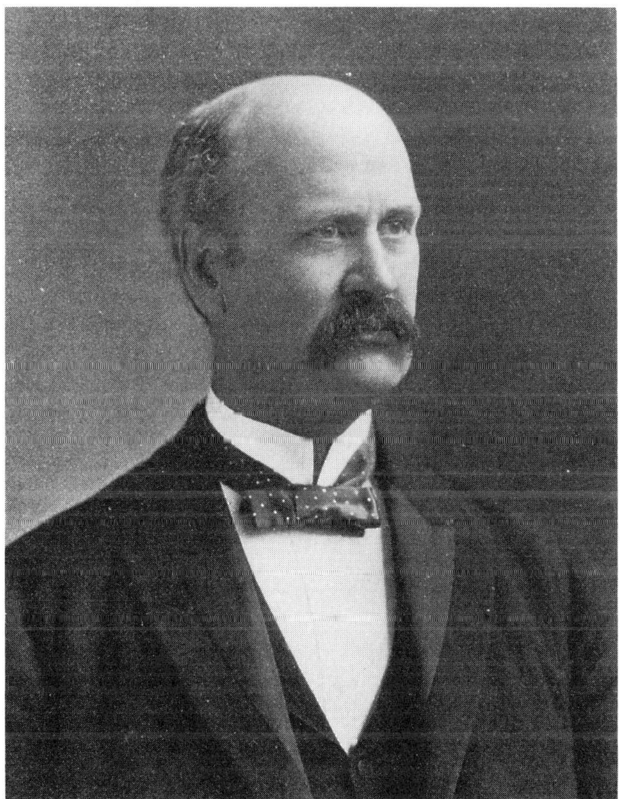

FIG. 45-12. Edward E. Montgomery, M.D. (1848–1927), First Chairman of Gynecology (1892–1920).

He contributed frequently to the medical literature and was the author in 1900 of a well-known textbook, *Practical Gynecology,* that went through four editions. Review of his published papers and case reports provides a picture of the evolutionary advance of abdominal and pelvic surgery as the principles of asepsis and antisepsis were increasingly accepted and knowledge of pathology, physiology, and bacteriology was expanding. In 1898, in a paper read before the Camden Medical Society on the *Early Recognition of Malignant Diseases of the Uterus and the Proper Course of Treatment,* he gave what is by current standards a good description of the physical findings and course of disease, as well as the symptoms of what likely was carcinoma of the cervix. In this paper he indicated that when the diagnosis is in doubt the use of the microscope will make the diagnosis certain but "the more experienced the operator the less frequently will he find it necessary to depend upon the microscope." In the same paper he recommended treatment by vaginal hysterectomy using clamp-forceps that were left on for 36 or more hours and a pack of iodoform gauze for six days, a forerunner of the technique used by James Kennedy (Jefferson, 1899) and for which he was well known.

Dr. Montgomery was active in many medical organizations. He was a founding member and second President of the American Association of Obstetrics and Gynecologists and was the first person to hold membership in both that society and the American Gynecological Society. He was a member of the Board of Trustees of the American Medical Association for 15 years and later its first Vice President in 1910. He also at various times was President of the Philadelphia Obstetrical Society, the Philadelphia County Medical Society, and the Pennsylvania Medical Society, as well as the Jefferson Alumni Association (1895).

After his appointment to the faculty at Jefferson, Montgomery established section demonstrations in the operating room and at the bedside. Students for the first time, under staff supervision, were permitted to examine patients in the clinic. History-taking and clinical instruction became a feature of the curriculum. Lectures to the class in the amphitheater continued, and in that setting patients were brought in for illustration, and operations were also performed (Figure 45-13).

The development and expansion of section teaching on the wards and in the clinics necessitated the appointment of Assistants and

Demonstrators. In this expanded faculty were John M. Fisher, P. Brooke Bland, and F.H. Maier, among others.

By 1903 Dr. Montgomery had included in his staff a professional anesthetist and a pathologist-bacteriologist. The latter was Dr. P. Brooke Bland, later to become the Professor of Obstetrics, who was married to Dr. Montgomery's daughter.

Dr. Montgomery had indicated his intent to resign his professorship in 1917 after 25 years of service. Articles in the newspapers of May 3, 1917, describe his valedictory lecture of that date. His retirement and appointment as Emeritus Professor was nevertheless postponed until 1920, perhaps because of the war. He retired from active practice in 1923 and died on April 17, 1927.

Dr. Thaddeus L. Montgomery, who became a Professor of Obstetrics and Gynecology and Director of the Division of Obstetrics at Jefferson in 1946, was the nephew of Dr. E.E. Montgomery. He states that his uncle after retirement bought a tract of land and financed a housing project. This business venture failed, causing his estate to be in debt.

Edward Parker Davis, M.D. (1856–1937); First Chairman of Obstetrics (1898–1925)

Following the death of Dr. Parvin in 1898, Dr. Edward P. Davis (Figure 45-14), who was Parvin's

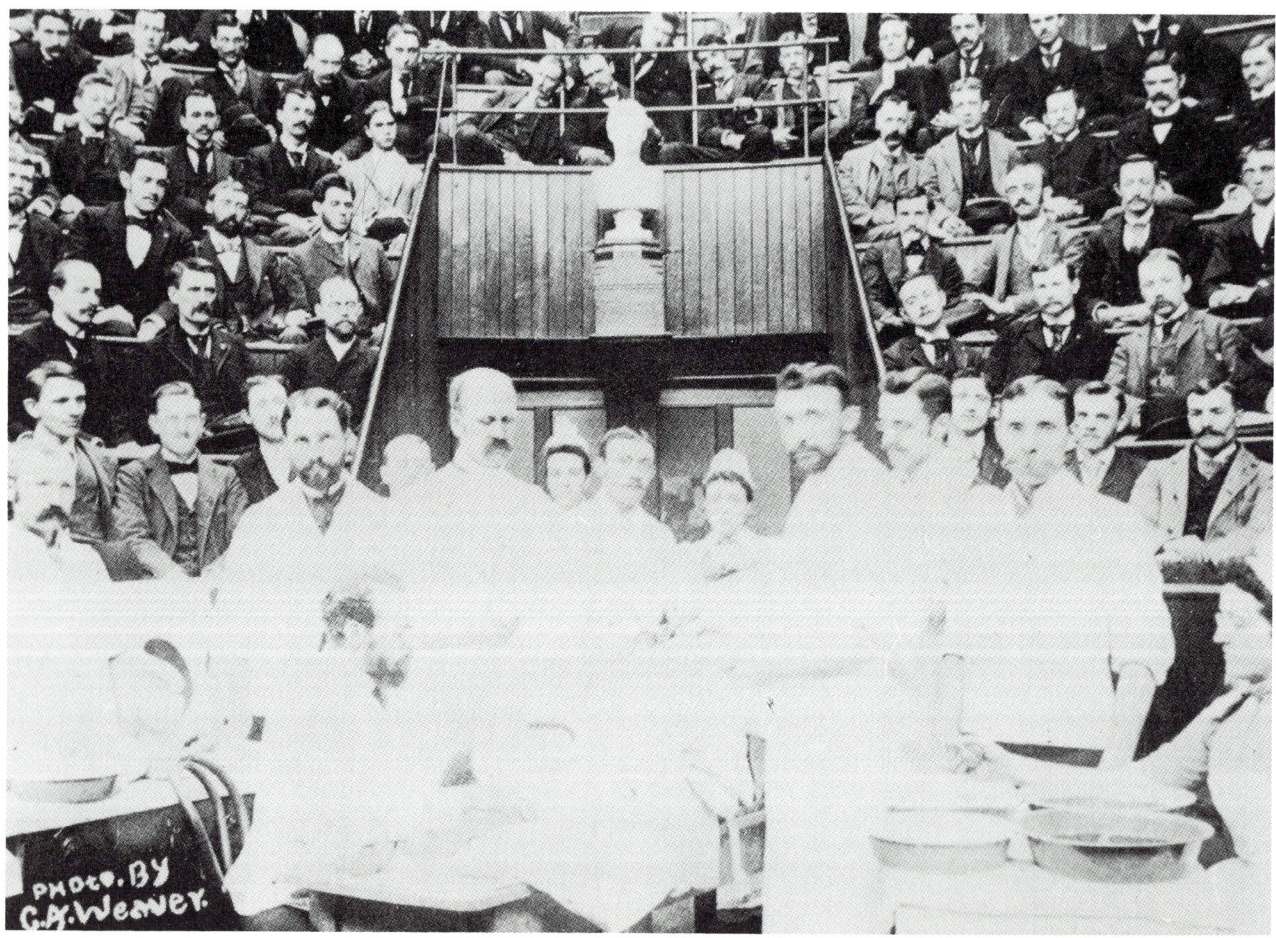

FIG. 45-13. Professor E.E. Montgomery operating in the "pit" in 1898. The surgical team is wearing white coats but no gloves, caps, or masks.

Chief Assistant, was appointed Professor of Obstetrics and filled that position for the next 27 years. During his tenure, increasing facilities for didactic, clinical, and laboratory teaching, both within and without the College, were developed. Clinical instruction was given in the maternity unit at Washington Square and in the amphitheater of the 1877 Hospital. Davis was an interesting and impressive teacher whose lectures were marked by scholarship and a literary quality characteristic of the times. Instruction, in addition to lectures, consisted of manikin courses, weekly quizzes, and case demonstrations in the outpatient clinics and amphitheater. By the early twentieth century, Pennsylvania regulations required that medical students attend 12 obstetric deliveries, so arrangements were made for each student to witness six deliveries in the Maternity Ward and six in patients' homes.

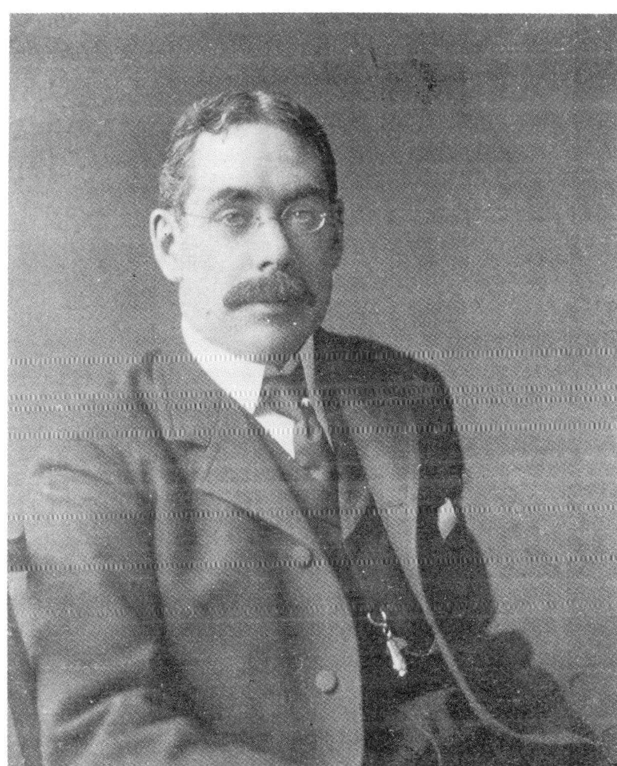

FIG. 45-14. Edward P. Davis, M.D. (1856–1937), First Chairman of Obstetrics (1898–1925).

Dr. Davis held that senior students should have an opportunity to attend a certain number of patients in their homes, believing that this would provide an opportunity to gain insight into the practical phase of obstetrics that could not be acquired elsewhere. This meant that the Department had to provide over 800 full-term maternity patients each year. The Center City Maternity was unable to meet this need, so in 1910 an outpatient department was established at 2545 Wharton Street in anticipation that this neighborhood would provide the necessary patient volume. Here each patient received antenatal supervision and postpartum care, and facilities were provided to accommodate students who were on call for home deliveries. Dr. P. Brooke Bland, describing this facility in the 1928 *Clinic,* noted that in its first 18 years, 6,000 women in confinement were attended by the students with the aid of their supervisors and that "the results with respect to morbidity and mortality compare most favorably with private obstetric practice in general." This dispensary continued to function as an obstetric clinic and a source of patients for home deliveries by students until December, 1946, by which time home deliveries had declined to the point that the facility was no longer needed.

By the time Dr. Davis assumed the Chair of Obstetrics a four-year curriculum had been established in the Medical College. In 1891 the curriculum had been expanded to three years, with basic sciences being taught in the first year. Later, an optional fourth year was offered, and the fourth year became mandatory for those matriculating after June 1, 1895. Obstetrics and Gynecology then, as now, were taught in the third and fourth years.

Edward Davis was born in Baldwinsville, New York, on September 16, 1856, a son of the Reverend Edwin R. and Anna M.D. Parker. He obtained his B.A. (1879) and M.A. (1882) from Princeton. He was graduated from Rush Medical College (now the University of Chicago) in 1882. From 1882 to 1886 he pursued graduate study both in the United States and abroad. After coming to Philadelphia in 1885 he attended classes at Jefferson and graduated in 1887. He then became an assistant to Dr. Parvin and held an appointment as Demonstrator of Obstetrics until 1895, when he was made Clinical Professor of Obstetrics, holding this rank until he was appointed Professor of Obstetrics to succeed Parvin in 1898.

Davis was editor of the *American Journal of Medical Sciences* from 1890 to 1898. His book, *Treatise on Obstetrics for Students and Practitioners,* published in 1896, went through two editions and was a standard text in a number of institutions. He also published a text on *Operative Obstetrics* in 1911 and a number of papers. He first suggested and was one of the first to use x-rays for pelvimetry and the diagnosis of pregnancy. He was known internationally, and in 1910 was a special representative of the United States at a meeting of the International Obstetrical and Gynecological Society in St. Petersburg, Russia. He was President of the American Gynecological Society in 1910, and President of the Obstetrical Society of Philadelphia (1910–1911).

Dr. Davis had been a classmate of Woodrow Wilson at Princeton, and had maintained a friendship with him. He was the Attending Obstetrician at the birth of President Wilson's grandchild, Woodrow Wilson Sayre, at Jefferson Hospital in March, 1919.

Shortly before his retirement, Davis directed the construction and equipment of the maternity wards on the third floor of the new Thompson Annex on Sansom Street. He retired suddenly in 1925 by remarking one afternoon that this was the last time he would visit the Obstetrical Department or meet his students. He then became an Emeritus Professor. Scheffey reports that he gave an address to the Obstetrical Society in 1935 at the age of 80, speaking for an hour without notes. He passed away October 2, 1937. His specific request was that no obituary notice appear in the daily papers, and this was adhered to.

Brooke Melancton Anspach, M.D., Sc.D. (1876–1951); Second Chairman of Gynecology (1921–1940)

Brooke M. Anspach (Figure 45-15) was appointed Professor of Gynecology in 1921, succeeding Dr. E.E. Montgomery, and was the second Head of Gynecology as a separate Department since its separation from Obstetrics in 1892.

Dr. Anspach was born on March 3, 1876, in Reading, Pennsylvania. He entered Lafayette College in 1892 and after one year attended the University of Pennsylvania Medical School, graduating in 1897. He was appointed as a Resident Physician at the University Hospital, serving in that capacity until 1900. Dr. John G. Clark, who had been associated with Dr. Howard Kelly at Johns Hopkins, was appointed to the Chair of Gynecology at the University of Pennsylvania in 1899, and Dr. Anspach was his first Intern. Clark brought the advanced teachings of the Kelly Clinic to Philadelphia, and Anspach eagerly accepted an invitation to join his staff.

After two years of training with Dr. Clark, Dr. Anspach went to Berlin in 1920 and studied with Ludwig Pick, then a leading gynecologic pathologist. After returning to Philadelphia, he continued his association with Dr. Clark at the

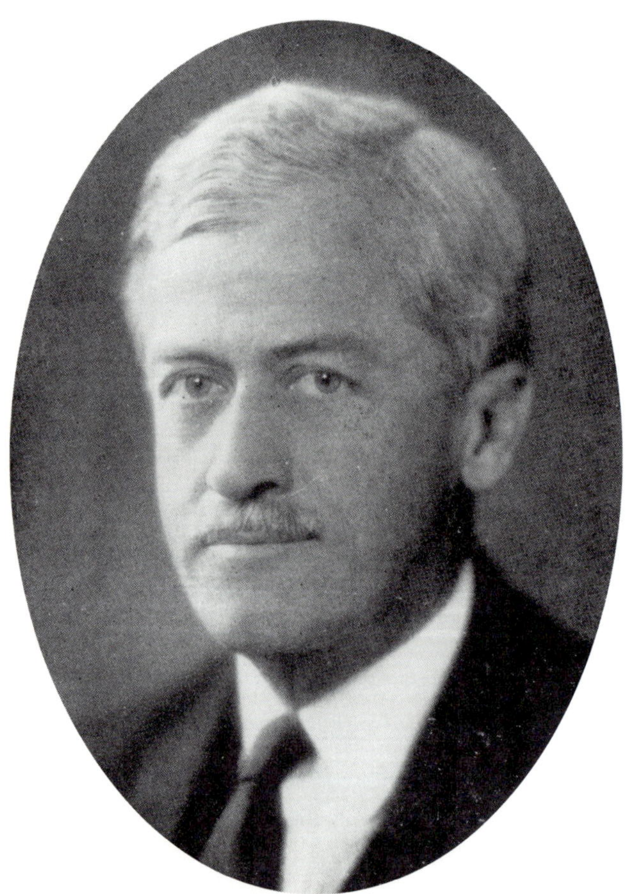

FIG. 45-15. Brooke M. Anspach, M.D., Sc.D. (1876–1951), Second Chairman of Gynecology (1921–1940).

University of Pennsylvania, advancing in rank to Associate in Gynecology at the Medical School and Assistant Gynecologist in the Hospital. During this period he also served as pathologist to the Kensington Hospital for Women (until 1908), and held the positions of Gynecologist and Obstetrician to the Philadelphia General Hospital, Gynecologist to the Stetson Hospital, and Gynecologist to the Bryn Mawr Hospital. He relinquished all of these appointments except Bryn Mawr upon his appointment to the Chair of Gynecology of Jefferson.

Dr. Anspach was a member of the American Gynecological Society and served as its Treasurer from 1916 to 1922 and as President in 1935. He was Secretary from 1910 to 1914 and Chairman in 1914 of the Section on Obstetrics, Gynecology, and Abdominal Surgery of the American Medical Association. In 1925 he was President of the Obstetrical Society of Philadelphia. He was a Fellow of the College of Physicians of Philadelphia and a member of the Board of Governors of the American College of Surgeons.

Dr. Anspach made numerous contributions to gynecologic literature. His textbook on *Gynecology,* first published in 1921, went through its fifth edition in 1934, and he contributed to a number of other texts. His papers included such subjects as studies of elastic tissue in the uterus, the early diagnosis of adnexal cancer, trends in modern obstetrics (in which he criticized Irving Potter's prophylactic internal version operation), the foundation of an endocrine clinic, conservative surgery of the ovaries, treatment of cancer of the uterus, and others.

On coming to Jefferson in 1921, Dr. Anspach inherited some of the members of Dr. Montgomery's staff, bringing with him none of his former associates. The remainder of his staff was developed from Jefferson graduates who had been Residents (Interns) in the Jefferson Hospital. These included Drs. Lewis Scheffey, John Montgomery, Charles Lintgen, and David Farell. He also recruited Drs. Roy Mohler, Thomas Costello, and Jacob Hoffman, who had studied pathology in Berlin.

The plan of teaching inaugurated by Dr. Montgomery was continued by Dr. Anspach. Students were given a course of didactic lectures in the third year. In the fourth year there was section teaching, including demonstrations in the operating room, clinical conferences, and examination and treatment of patients in the clinic. With the erection of the Curtis Clinic in 1931, the facilities for instruction in clinical gynecology were increased, and a research laboratory was provided in the new College building, which expanded the studies in gynecologic endocrinology.

Dr. Anspach was awarded the Honorary Degree of Doctor of Science by Lafayette College in 1936 and by Jefferson Medical College in 1946. His portrait was commissioned to be painted and was presented to the College by the Class of 1938.

Dr. Anspach died July 8, 1951, at the age of 75.

Pascal Brooke Bland, M.D. (1875–1940); Second Chairman of Obstetrics (1925–1937)

Upon the retirement of Dr. Edward P. Davis in 1925, Dr. P. Brooke Bland (Figure 45-16) was appointed Professor of Obstetrics. He accepted this appointment at the urging of Dr. Anspach, although his previous interests had been principally in gynecology.

Born May 9, 1875, in Monocacy, a village near Birdsboro, Pennsylvania, he received his early education in the public and private schools of Berks and Montgomery counties. He graduated from Jefferson Medical College with honors in 1901 and was President of his class in his senior year. After graduation he spent the next 15 months as a Resident Physician in the Jefferson Hospital, part of which time was allocated to the newly created position of Resident Pathologist. Following his internship, Dr. Bland became an Assistant to Dr. E.E. Montgomery and a Demonstrator in the Department of Gynecology, while conducting a general practice in South Philadelphia. He studied in Europe in 1907 and in 1910 to enhance his training, after which he gradually limited his practice to gynecology and obstetrics. He held the rank of Assistant Professor of Gynecology from 1910 to 1925, when he was appointed Professor of Obstetrics and Chief Obstetrician of the Jefferson Hospital.

Dr. Bland took on his new responsibility with industry and enthusiasm, thus strengthening the Department academically and in facilities. He was supported by Drs. Norris W. Vaux and Thaddeus L. Montgomery, both of whom were eventually to succeed him in the Chair. Another staunch supporter was Dr. George A. Ulrich (Jefferson, 1901). Dr. Ulrich rose from Instructor to Clinical Professor of Obstetrics by 1931. He was the author of numerous articles on obstetrical subjects and highly regarded by the students for his manikin demonstrations of the mechanics of delivery. He was the first Clinical Professor to have his portrait presented to the College (by the Class of 1941).

Clinical teaching in Obstetrics continued in the Junior year, with requirements for witnessing deliveries in the maternity wards at Jefferson or at the Philadelphia Lying-In Hospital, as well as attending home deliveries out of the Wharton Street Dispensary. Didactic teaching consisted of lectures to the whole class by the Professor and Senior Associates, manikin courses, and clinical rounds. Graduate education consisted of the rotating internship, 27 months in length, which included a rotation on the obstetric service. The intern's duties were spelled out in detail in a booklet entitled *Rules Governing the Work in the Department of Obstetrics.*

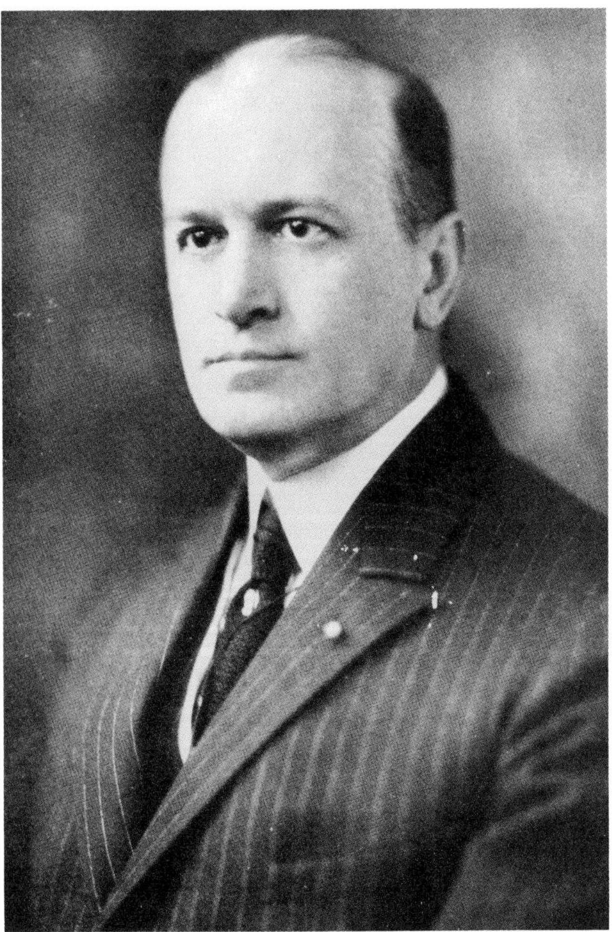

Fig. 45-16. P. Brooke Bland, M.D. (1875–1940), Second Chairman of Obstetrics (1925–1937).

During this period, specialty training in obstetrics and gynecology began to receive increasing attention. Traditionally, one entered general practice following medical school and internship, and received additional training by serving as an assistant to an established specialist. The need for better and more structured training, however, was being recognized, and by 1931, 83 Residency Programs had come into being. The perceived need for guidelines and for criteria of competence resulted in the chartering of the American Board of Obstetrics and Gynecology in 1930. Its first examinations were given in 1931.

Dr. Bland established the first Residency in Obstetrics at Jefferson in 1937, but a combined Residency in Obstetrics and Gynecology was not possible until the Departments were combined in 1946. The first Residents in obstetrics were Drs. John McCormick and Joseph Finn, appointed after completion of their internships, and were paid by Dr. Bland the sum of $100 per month.

Dr. Bland had an illustrious career, serving as Consultant to a number of hospitals in the Delaware Valley area. He held memberships in many societies, including the American Association of Obstetricians, Gynecologists, and Abdominal Surgeons, the American College of Surgeons, and the Royal Society of Medicine in London. He was a Fellow of the College of Physicians of Philadelphia and the Obstetrical Society of Philadelphia, serving as President of the latter in 1928.

He was the author of numerous papers dealing with Obstetrics and Gynecology as well as two major textbooks: *Gynecology: Medical and Surgical,* published by F.A. Davis Co., 1924, which went through three editions; and *Practical Obstetrics for Students and Practitioners,* the first edition in 1932 with the assistance of Dr. Thaddeus L.

Montgomery, followed by two editions in 1934 and 1939 with the coauthorship of Dr. Montgomery. Dr. Bland's interests extended to the history of medicine,[11] resulting in a collection of rare books and valuable historical works. This library, which Dr. Bland bequeathed to Jefferson, formed the nucleus of the Section on Historical Collections, which has become an important part of the Scott Library.

Dr. Bland also bequeathed to the Department of Obstetrics and Gynecology his residuary estate after all direct heirs were deceased. This ultimately amounted to over $1 million and was the largest bequest ever received from an alumnus. The fund has been used to support Fellowship programs in the Department.

Dr. Bland relinquished his Chair to Dr. Norris Vaux in 1937 and became Professor Emeritus. His death on October 31, 1940, at age 65, was an inexplicable suicide.

Norris Wistar Vaux (1881–1958); Third Chairman of Obstetrics (1937–1946)

Norris Wistar Vaux (Figure 45-17) was born on September 1, 1881, in Rosemont, Pennsylvania, the son of Jacob Wahn Vaux and Emily Norris Pepper. His family background was unusual in that the names of Wistar, Pepper, Norris, and Vaux were derived from old, prominent, and distinguished Philadelphia antecedents.[12] During his early undergraduate years at the Delancey School his popularity was evidenced by election to the F.X.I. Fraternity for outstanding ability in the Interacademic Schools. He entered the University of Pennsylvania in 1900 and completed his premedical and medical education by 1905. While in his senior year he was elected to the Sphinx Society as one of the 25 outstanding members of the class, and he rowed on the Varsity crew. After serving his internship at the Pennsylvania Hospital (1905–1907), he completed a year of study in Europe, chiefly in obstetrics at the Rotunda Hospital, Ireland, under Ernest Hastings Tweedy.[13]

Upon returning to the United States to start a general practice at Chestnut Hill, he also started his academic career at Jefferson as Instructor in Obstetrics under Dr. E.P. Davis, where he gave a course in operative obstetrics. This was interrupted by World War I, in which he served from May, 1917, to April 19, 1919. With the American Expeditionary Forces in Base Hospital Unit No. 10 (The Pennsylvania Hospital Unit) and the British General Hospital Unit No. 16, he served overseas for 23 months and was discharged with the rank of Major.[14]

In 1919 Dr. Vaux became a member of the staff of the Philadelphia Lying-in Hospital, Obstetrician to the Chestnut Hill Hospital, and Chief Obstetrician to the Bryn Mawr Hospital (1921–1926). By 1925 he rose to the rank of Clinical Professor of Obstetrics at Jefferson.

Dr. Vaux was highly respected for his teaching of a system of obstetrics that was practical for the

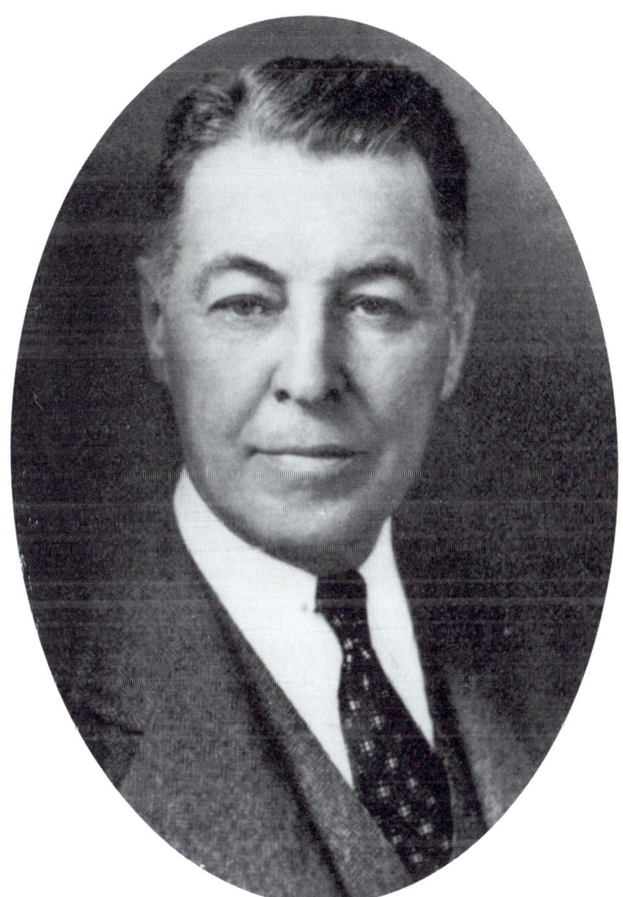

FIG. 45-17. Norris W. Vaux (1881–1958), Third Chairman of Obstetrics (1937–1946).

needs of those going into clinical practice. His lectures were plain, well organized, and interspersed with illustrations and an occasional quiz that demanded only the essential facts of his subject. The important features and common complications associated with pregnancy and delivery were adequately covered. Added to this was his personal warmth, sense of humor, and refinement that marked him as a man "to the manor born." His attention to all aspects of his duty was no better exemplified than in his visits to the ward, the last thing in the evening before going home, to be sure there were no unresolved problems. He was not loath to come in at night to aid in a complicated ward delivery case.

Dr. Vaux was not a prolific writer, but he was editor of *Edgar's Obstetrics* and published numerous papers on eclampsia, antenatal care, pyelitis of pregnancy, placenta praevia, and postpartum hemorrhage. His concern for possible postpartum hemorrhage in certain high-risk cases was accentuated by his demand for the availability of blood for the time of delivery, not a common practice at that time.

In 1937 Dr. Vaux was appointed Chairman of the Department of Obstetrics at Jefferson, a position he held until the end of 1946, at which time he was made Emeritus. In 1938 the Philadelphia Lying-In Hospital merged with the Pennsylvania Hospital, and he became Director of the Department of Obstetrics and Gynecology at that institution also. He was the first Chairman of the Section of Obstetrics and Gynecology of the Pennsylvania State Medical Society in 1936 and President of the American Gynecological Society (1946–1947). The latter position was one of the highest honors in American Gynecology and Obstetrics. The senior class presented his portrait to the College in 1947.

From 1943 to 1947, Dr. Vaux served on the American Board of Obstetrics and Gynecology. He also held membership in the Philadelphia College of Physicians, the Philadelphia Obstetrical Society, the American Committee on Maternal Welfare, and Honorary Membership of the Barton C. Hirst Obstetrical Society and the Washington Gynecological Society. For many years he was Honorary Surgeon to the 1st Troop Philadelphia City Cavalry.

Age the age of 65, Dr. Vaux took the mandatory retirement, effective January 1, 1947, but did not consider his career at an end. On January 21 of that year he became Pennsylvania's ninth Secretary of Health following the inauguration of Governor James H. Duff.[15] His task was to direct an investigation to determine the need for rehabilitation and treatment centers for the assistance of crippled children and adults whose afflictions rendered them useless to society. He served with distinction in this position until 1951, at age 70. Until his death on August 19, 1958, he remained a Consultant in Obstetrics and Gynecology at the Bryn Mawr Hospital.

Lewis Cass Scheffey, M.D. (1894–1965); Third Professor of Gynecology (1940–1946), Eleventh Chairman of Obstetrics and Gynecology, and Director of the Division of Gynecology (1946–1955)

Dr. Lewis C. Scheffey (Figure 45-18) succeeded Dr. Brooke M. Anspach as Professor of Gynecology and Head of the Department upon the latter's retirement in 1940.

Born in Reading, Pennsylvania, in 1894, Scheffey attended the public schools and received his premedical education at the Philadelphia College of Pharmacy and Science, graduating in 1915. He graduated from Jefferson Medical College in 1920 and continued for 27 months as a rotating Intern in the Hospital. Following internship he became Assistant to Dr. Anspach and joined the faculty as an Assistant Demonstrator of Gynecology. He rose steadily through the faculty ranks and was promoted to Clinical Professor of Gynecology in 1938.

Dr. Scheffey had a lifelong interest in pelvic cancer, which led him to establish a Pelvic Cancer Clinic in the gynecology outpatient department in 1928. He continued to direct this Clinic until 1955. Particularly remarkable was its record of complete follow-up studies on nearly 100% of treated patients for over 30 years. He was an early advocate of the value of cervical vaginal cytology and collaborated with George N. Papanicolaou, Joe Vincent Meigs, and others in developing the Inter-Society Cytology Council, serving as President in 1956. He was active in the American Cancer Society and was President of the Philadelphia Division in 1957. He received that Society's gold medal in 1962 in recognition of his contributions to cancer control.

In 1946 upon the retirement of Dr. Norris Vaux as Professor of Obstetrics, the two Departments were reunited with the appointment of Dr. Scheffey as Professor of Obstetrics and Gynecology, Chairman of the Department, and Director of the Division of Gynecology. Dr. Thaddeus L. Montgomery returned then from his Professorship at Temple University to become Professor of Obstetrics and Gynecology and Director of the Division of Obstetrics.

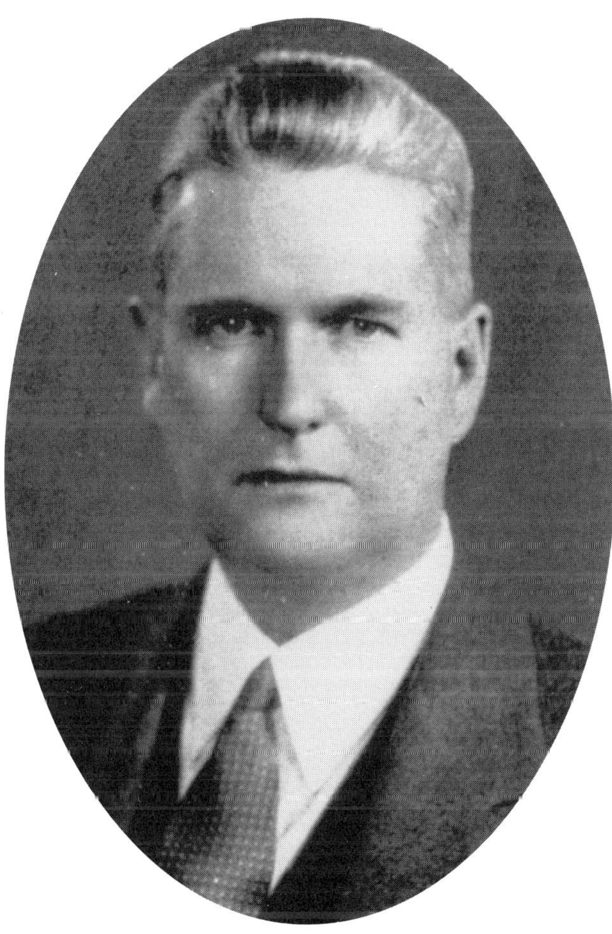

FIG. 45-18. Lewis C. Scheffey, M.D. (1894–1965); Third Chairman of Gynecology (1940–1946), Eleventh Chairman of Obstetrics and Gynecology, and Director of the Division of Gynecology (1946–1955).

The formation of a unified Department permitted the development of a completely integrated program of instruction for medical students as well as the unification of the residency program. The result was the production of a well-rounded teaching program that improved the training of students, residents, and staff.

In 1949 a new maternity wing was opened with seven private and 32 semi-private beds, and facilities for ward patients were expanded. In addition, newborn nursing facilities were provided for care of both full-term and premature babies. The new facilities were equipped with airconditioning and piped-in oxygen. The new rooms were designed to permit "rooming-in" of babies. The Annual Report of 1950 indicated that to that time over 4,500 had been cared for with "rooming-in" in the wards and private rooms at Jefferson, making it a leader in the development of that concept.

By 1953 the teaching facilities consisted of 40 obstetrical ward beds and 32 gynecologic ward beds, as well as the outpatient clinics. In addition, there were affiliations with the Philadelphia General Hospital, Methodist, Cooper, Mt. Sinai, Germantown, and St. Joseph's Hospital.

Dr. Scheffey devoted much attention to bettering the teaching program. As the end of his Chairmanship drew near, the faculty had been augmented to include a number of well-known and able staff members. In the Division of Obstetrics under Professor Thaddeus L. Montgomery, Dr. Abraham E. Rakoff, Clinical Professor, was pursuing his research in gynecologic endocrinology with many publications and presentations that signaled his emergence as a national authority. Drs. J. Bernard Bernstine and Mario A. Castallo were also Clinical Professors and were leaders in student instruction. Assistant Professors included Drs. Arthur First, James F. Carrell, John F. Duggar, Joseph L. Finn, and Warren R. Lang. The Division of Gynecology included Dr. John B. Montgomery, Professor, as well as four Clinical Professors: Drs. Rakoff, I. Charles Lintgen, Roy W. Mohler, and Jacob Hoffman. Assistant Professors were Drs. David M. Farell, George A. Hahn, William J. Thudium, J.

Edward Lynch, George A. Porrecca, and Warren R. Lang.[16]

The Class of 1954 honored Dr. Scheffey by presenting his portrait to the College. He was also active in the Alumni Association and served as its President in 1944. His Society memberships and activities were extensive. In 1958 he was elected President of the American Gynecologic Society. He was also President of the Philadelphia County Medical Society, the Obstetrical Society of Philadelphia, and the College of Physicians of Philadelphia.

Dr. Scheffey retired and became Professor Emeritus of Obstetrics and Gynecology in 1955. He died after a long illness in 1969 at the age of 75.

Thaddeus Lemert Montgomery, M.D., LL.D. (1896–); Twelfth Chairman (1955–1961)

Dr. Thaddeus L. Montgomery (Figure 45-19) was appointed to the Chairmanship in 1955 following the retirement of Dr. Lewis C. Scheffey. He was thus the second Chairman since the reunion of the Departments of Obstetrics and Gynecology in 1946.

Born May 24, 1896, in Macon, Illinois, Dr. Montgomery was educated in the public schools of Decatur, Illinois, and received the A.B. degree from the University of Illinois. He matriculated at Jefferson in 1916 and received his M.D. degree in 1920. Following graduation he interned at Jefferson Hospital.

The internship at that time was a two-year rotating one. Residency programs had not yet been established, and specialty training was by preceptorship or assistantship to a Professor. In this way one acquired judgment and experience, but not much responsibility. There was usually no stipend, and the assistant supported himself by doing general practice.

Following his internship, Dr. Montgomery became an assistant to Dr. E.E. Montgomery, his uncle, who was then the Professor Emeritus of Gynecology. During that period (1922–1925) he held appointments as Instructor in Anatomy and Instructor in Surgery. When Dr. Bland was appointed to the Professorship of Obstetrics in 1925, Dr. Montgomery became his assistant, a position he held until 1935, while maintaining a general practice. In the Department of Obstetrics from 1925 to 1940 he rose through the academic ranks to Clinical Professor of Obstetrics.

In 1940 Dr. Montgomery resigned to become Professor of Obstetrics and Gynecology and Head of the Department at Temple University School of Medicine. His appointment at Temple signaled the combination of the Departments of Obstetrics and Gynecology into a single entity, the first so constituted in Philadelphia.

In 1946 following the retirement of Dr. Norris W. Vaux as Professor of Obstetrics, the Departments of Obstetrics and Gynecology at Jefferson were reunited under the Chairmanship of Dr. Lewis C. Scheffey. Dr. Montgomery then returned to Jefferson as Professor of Obstetrics and Gynecology and Director of the Division of

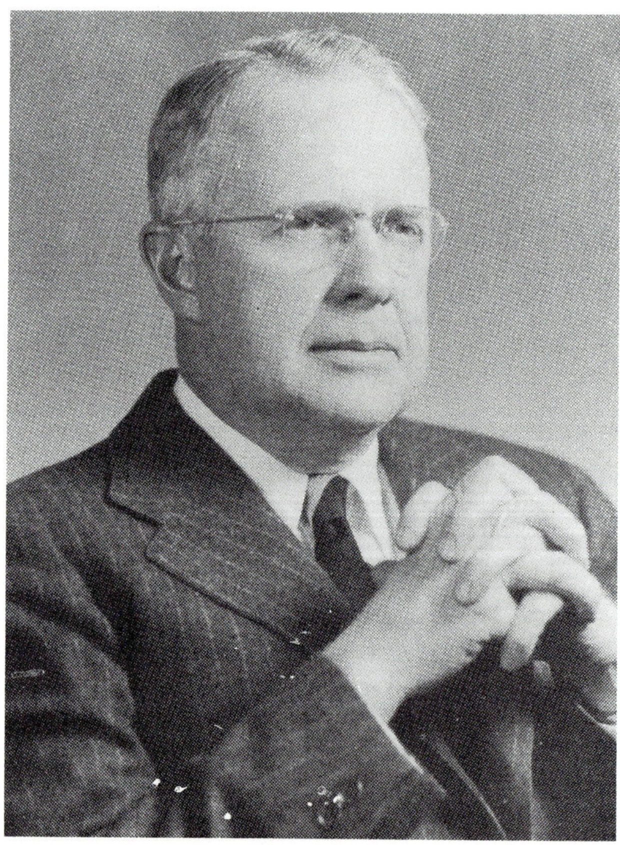

FIG. 45-19. Thaddeus L. Montgomery, M.D. (1896–), Twelfth Chairman (1955–1961).

Obstetrics. He continued in that position until Dr. Scheffey retired in 1955, when he was appointed to succeed Dr. Scheffey as Chairman.

The reunion of the two Departments had contributed to the development of a correlated curriculum that greatly strengthened the undergraduate and graduate teaching programs and encouraged research by members of the Department.

Dr. Montgomery was deeply interested in the "physiologic approach" to childbirth and the establishment of sound physiologic practices in obstetrics. He was concerned about the overuse of operative procedures at delivery and overuse of anesthesia and analgesia and was thus an early proponent of so-called natural childbirth. He was instrumental in introducing "rooming in," allowing the newborn infant to be kept in the room with its mother, as early as 1947 at Jefferson. A stimulus for this practice was concern about the prevention of infection in the newborn nursery. Additionally, he was interested in breast disease and worked to arouse the recognition by obstetricians of their responsibility in the diagnosis of diseases of the breast and to include examination of the breasts in the physical examination.

Additional interests included placental pathology, maternal and prenatal mortality and infection, and in later years, adolescent sexuality and para-marriage (living together as if married, on a trial basis).

He has held memberships in numerous societies, including the Obstetrical Society of Philadelphia (President, 1941–1942), the College of Physicians of Philadelphia, the American Gynecological Society, the Association of Obstetricians, Gynecologists, and Abdominal Surgeons (President, 1955–1956), the American Gynecological Club, the American College of Obstetricians and Gynecologists, and others.

He was editorial assistant to Dr. P. Brooke Bland of a *Textbook of Practical Obstetrics* published in 1932. He was coauthor of two subsequent editions in 1934 and 1939, and the author of a number of papers on the subjects of his interest.

He also served as Chairman of the Obstetrics and Gynecology Section on the National Board of Medical Examiners.

Dr. Montgomery served as President of the Alumni Association (1948–1949) and has remained active in that organization during the subsequent 38 years. In 1963 he was awarded the honorary LL.D. degree at Jefferson's Commencement Exercises.

Dr. and Mrs. Montgomery presented an electric organ to Jefferson in memory of their son, Richard, in 1957. Placed in McClellan Hall, the organ is used for University events.

Dr. Montgomery retired from the Chairmanship and was given the title of Professor Emeritus of Obstetrics and Gynecology on July 1, 1961. Following his retirement as Chairman, he continued in active practice for approximately 20 more years and remains actively engaged in his avocation of painting.

John Barrick Montgomery, M.D., Sc.D., Pd.D. (1900–1987); Thirteenth Chairman (1961–1965)

Dr. John B. Montgomery (Figure 45-20), who had served as Co-Chairman of the Department of Obstetrics and Gynecology from 1955 to 1961 under Dr. T.L. Montgomery, was not a relative. He assumed the Chairmanship when Dr. T.L. Montgomery became Emeritus on July 1, 1961.

Born March 11, 1900, in Lewistown, Pennsylvania, John Montgomery was educated in the public schools of Huntingdon, Pennsylvania, and graduated from Juniata College with the A.B. degree in 1921, followed by a year in graduate school at the University of Pennsylvania. He then entered Jefferson Medical College, where he received his M.D. degree in 1926. He was elected to Alpha Omega Alpha. Following graduation he interned at Jefferson (1926–1928) and then served as a private assistant to Professor Brooke M. Anspach in the Department of Gynecology from 1928 to 1940. During this period he was promoted through the academic ranks, attaining the appointment of Clinical Professor of Gynecology in 1940 and Professor of Obstetrics and Gynecology in 1952. He became Co-Chairman of the Department in 1955.

During his tenure as Chairman, development of the Departmental programs and curriculum continued. The student clerkships were restructured with a six-week block in the third year spent primarily in the clinics, and a five-week block in the fourth year spent on the inpatient services. A core residency of three years was established, and clinical fellowships in Endocrinology were strengthened under the tutelage of Dr. Abraham E. Rakoff. Partly salaried faculty positions, which had been inaugurated during Dr. T.L. Montgomery's Chairmanship, were expanded to strengthen the teaching programs. Drs. Benjamin Kendall and David Farrell were developing techniques in fetal electrocardiography, forerunners of electronic fetal monitoring. Dr. Montgomery was always interested in the progress of the young men in the Department, giving them responsibility and supporting their advancement in other ways. He was always regarded by his students and colleagues as a superb teacher and clinician. This feeling was expressed by the Class of 1965 with presentation of his portrait to the College.

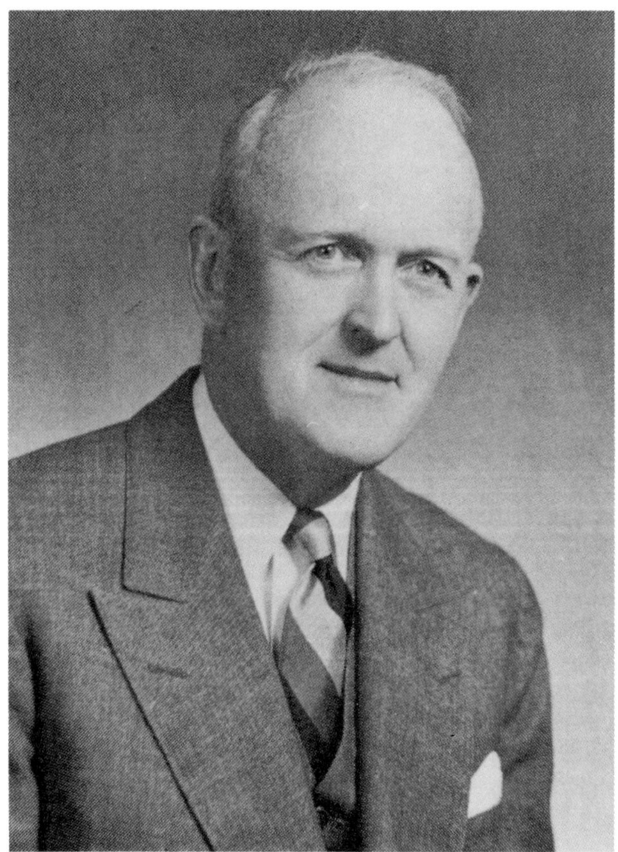

FIG. 45-20. John B. Montgomery, M.D. (1900–1987), Thirteenth Chairman (1961–1965).

Dr. Montgomery was active in local and national medical organizations and held office in several. He served as President of the Obstetrical Society of Philadelphia, and as Vice President of the Philadelphia County Medical Society. In addition, he was a fellow of the American College of Surgeons, the American Gynecological Society, and the American Association of Obstetricians and Gynecologists, among others.

He was also active in civic and social organizations, serving as a Trustee of Juniata College, where he was awarded the honorary degree of Doctor of Science in 1951. He served as President of the Alumni Association (1961–1962). Jefferson awarded him the honorary degree of Doctor of Pedagogy in 1972 and the Alumni Achievement Award in 1979.

The philosophy of his career was based upon his appeal for sympathy and understanding of patients as well as for medical competence. The Jefferson Obstetric and Gynecologic Ex-Resident Society (JOGERS) placed a plaque in the Hospital in 1976 honoring both Drs. John B. Montgomery and T.L. Montgomery for their dedication and teaching efforts.

During these years, a number of members of the staff were performing loyal and dedicated services, contributing to the effectiveness of teaching and advancing the interests of the Department. Among these was Dr. Paul A. Bowers (B.S., Bucknell University, 1933; M.D., Jefferson, 1937) who following Jefferson internship received his specialty training at Chicago Lying-In Hospital (1939–1942). In wartime Army services (1942–1946) he was distinguished by advancement to the rank of Colonel. He joined Dr. Thaddeus L. Montgomery in 1946 and rose academically to full Professorship. As a respected teacher, author of many papers, and an active alumnus, Dr. Bowers' portrait was presented to Jefferson in 1982, and in 1983 he was named Professor Emeritus. He was President of the Alumni Association in 1973 and elected to the first of two terms as Alumni Member of the Board of Trustees in June, 1984. Among many other honors, he received the Winged Ox Award of Thomas Jefferson University in 1985.

Burton L. Wellenbach (Jefferson J1944) joined the staff shortly after World War II and served for many years, advancing to Clinical Professor. In 1983 he served as President of the Almuni Association, and in 1988 he received the Leon A. Peris Award for Distinguished Teaching and Patient Care. Joseph P. Long (Jefferson, 1939) was also a career member of the Department, beginning after military service in 1946 and advancing to Clinical Professor before retiring from Jefferson in 1980. Alvin F. Goldfarb was active in teaching and research, advancing to Professorial rank. Arnold Goldberger (Jefferson, 1933) became Honorary Clinical Professor; Basil J. Giletto (Jefferson, 1937), Assistant Professor; Amos S. Wainer, Assistant Professor; Stewart First (Jefferson, 1956) and Howard First, both Clinical Associate Professors.

Dr. Montgomery died June 30, 1987.

Roy G. Holly, M.D., Ph.D.; Fourteenth Chairman (1965–1974)

According to the rules of the faculty and the Board of Trustees, the date for Dr. John B. Montgomery to relinquish his Chairmanship would ordinarily have been June 30, 1965. The new Chairman, Dr. Roy G. Holly, however, agreed and the Board concurred, that his appointment should begin February 1, 1965. Dr. Montgomery in his characteristic gracious manner, therefore terminated his responsibilities January 31, 1965. He expressed his confidence that the "new regime will bring strength in the areas of weakness and increased vigor and efficiency in the areas where we are strong."[13]

Dr. Holly (Figure 45-21) was born on September 29, 1919, in Waupaca, Wisconsin. He obtained his professional degrees from the University of Minnesota: B.S. (1941), M.B. (1943), M.D. (1944), and Ph.D. (1952). His postdoctoral clinical training was experienced at the University of Minnesota Hospitals: Internship (1943) and Residency in Obstetrics and Gynecology (1944–1946 and 1948–1949). At the University of Minnesota he served on the faculty as Instructor through Associate Professor (1948–1954). Continuing his academic career at the University of Nebraska in the Department of Obstetrics and Gynecology, he was appointed Professor (1954–1956), Professor and Chairman (1956–1961), Dean of the Graduate College (1961–1962), and Vice-Chancellor and Dean (1962–1965). His society memberships encompassed Sigma Xi, American College of Obstetrics and Gynecology, American Gynecological Society, American Association of Obstetricians and Gynecologists, Association of Graduate School Deans, Association of Professors of Gynecology and Obstetrics, Central Association of Obstetricians and Gynecologists, Society for Gynecologic Investigation, and others.

Dr. Holly held positions such as President of the Nebraska State Society of Obstetrics, Associate Examiner of the American Board of Obstetrics and Gynecology, Chairman of the Obstetrics Test Committee of the National Board of Medical Examiners, President of the Association of Professors of Gynecology and Obstetrics, Member of the National Advisory Council of the National Institute of Child Health and Human Development, and Editor-in-Chief of *Gynecology and Obstetrics Guide* of Commerce Clearing House

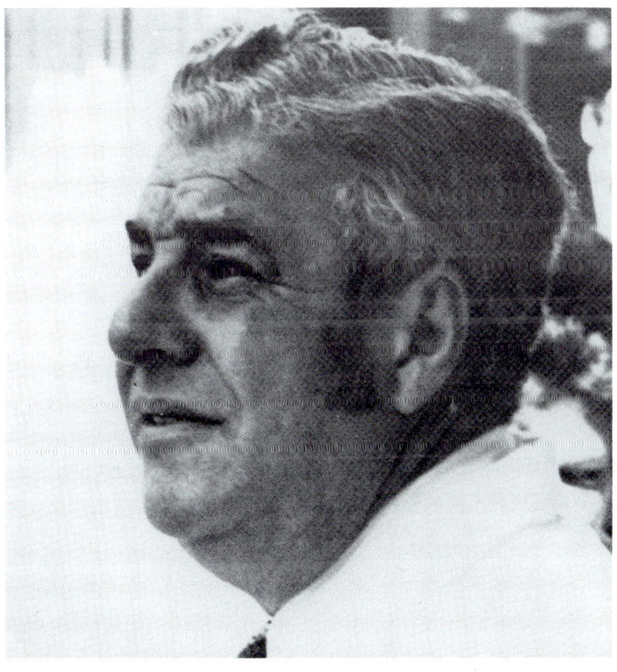

FIG. 45-21. Roy G. Holly, M.D. (1919–), Fourteenth Chairman (1965–1974).

(1963). Between 1946 and 1963 he had published 34 articles in which 24 were devoted to iron metabolism and hematologic disorders of pregnancy. His other research interests were in gynecologic malignancy and endocrinology.

The prime expectation in the appointment of Dr. Holly, who at that time was 45 years of age, was to expand research and develop new strength in that area within the Department. In conjunction with this aspect was Dr. Holly's immediate hope to create at Jefferson a Research Institute in Perinatal Biology. This exciting project had the full endorsement of James M. Large, Chairman of the Board of Trustees, William W. Bodine, Jr., President of the Medical College, William A. Sodeman, Vice President and Dean of the College, and Kenneth R. Erfft, Vice President and Treasurer. It was proposed that the Research Institute be an extension of the National Institute of Child Health and Human Development Direct Operations, funded and operated jointly by Jefferson Medical College and the National Institute of Child Health and Human Development. The proposed Institute was planned to meet the criteria established by the National Institute for the creation of a Research and a Research Training Program with objectives compatible with those of a newly organized Department of Obstetrics and Gynecology at Jefferson under Dr. Holly. This exciting project envisioned research in endocrinology and fertility, maternal and fetal physiology, teratology, genetics, neonatal physiology and development, and neonatal behavior. A second component of the plan was a Training Program in Research and Clinical Aspects of Obstetrics and Gynecology. The third component was one of Communications devoted to Computer Services and a Service Information Center.[18] Unfortunately, this plan with details for administration, space and funding, which had held reasonable promise of consummation, did not materialize and was a keen disappointment.

For several years the Department moved along in its accustomed momentum with a loyal staff, and the two former Chairmen, Drs. Thaddeus L. Montgomery and John B. Montgomery, remained active in the Hospital. It slowly became apparent, however, that a creeping inertia was enveloping the Department. Problems that eventually surfaced involved the Maternal and Infant Care Programs, relationships with the affiliated hospitals, and weak supervision of the financial affairs of the Department. Dr. Holly made attempts to reorganize his Department, but mutual frustration increased between himself and the staff.

A worsening effect on the obstetrical component was the significant decline in the birth rate in the United States. It became socially desirable to have a small family, a goal aided by the widespread use of contraceptive methods and the acceptance of therapeutic abortion. The fertility rate by 1973 fell to its lowest level in the nation's history, with fewer than 2.1 children per completed family required for a one-to-one replacement of the population. A significant number of hospitals were closing their obstetric units or considering such a move in view of the cost of providing staff and facilities for reasonable and improved obstetric care. Jefferson was caught in this crunch, with loss of staff and fewer deliveries, to the extent that a few voiced the notion that perhaps Jefferson should discontinue an obstetrical service altogether and arrange for this function elsewhere. This, of course, was inconceivable for a teaching institution with obligations to instruct students in the Medical and Allied Health Colleges as well as the Hospital's commitment to total health care. In addition, by 1974 plans for a new clinical facility (Thomas Jefferson University Hospital of 1978) were underway, in which a modern viable obstetric and perinatal service was necessary.

Dr. Holly appointed Martin B. Wingate, M.D., as Chairman of a Task Force Committee on the Future of Obstetrics at Jefferson. This Committee met on ten occasions following its inception on September 20, 1973. A report on March 12, 1974, made urgent short-term recommendations for immediate implementation.[19] These were summarized as:

1. Improvement of facilities within the present physical plant to meet the requirements of a regional referral center, with particular emphasis on the immediate acquisition of fetal and maternal monitoring equipment (approximate cost of $150,000).
2. Implementation of an outreach program in

cooperation with the Regional Medical Program Director and the Department of Family Practice.

3. Positive efforts to reattract members of the Jefferson staff who had reduced their obstetric and gynecologic patient commitment to Jefferson.

4. Make personal approaches to individual physicians within a geographic area Jefferson could be considered to serve to encourage them to transfer their affiliation and practice to Jefferson.

5. To minimize costs to patients and to work directly with city health authorities to meet their requirements.

Dr. George J. Andros, in charge of the residency program, was critical of the effectiveness of the program associated with the decline in applications for the residency.

Dr. Holly felt disinclined to cope with these formidable challenges, and tendered his resignation as Chairman on March 18, 1974. He remained a full-time Professor under the Rules and Regulations of the College Practice Plan.

After review of full-time and volunteer members of the Department, it was agreed that a logical choice for Acting Chairman was Dr. James H. Lee, Jr. Dr. Lee was a retired senior naval officer who had had administrative experience as Chairman of the Department at the Naval Hospital, Philadelphia, plus administrative experience at Hahnemann Medical College and Hospital. He was a 1945 graduate of Jefferson Medical College and a full-time member of the faculty.

Dr. Holly resigned his position on the faculty, effective January 1, 1975, to pursue a new position in Wisconsin.

James Harold Lee, Jr., M.D.; Acting Chairman (1974–1975), Fifteenth Chairman (1975–1987)

Following the resignation of Dr. Roy G. Holly from the Chairmanship, Dr. James H. Lee, Jr. (Figure 45-22) was appointed Acting Chairman on March 18, 1974. A search committee was formed that concluded with the appointment of Dr. Lee to the Chair, effective July 1, 1975.

Born in Philadelphia, Pennsylvania, on December 5, 1920, Lee was educated in the public schools of Drexel Hill, Pennsylvania, and Wilmington, Delaware. He was graduated from Dickinson College, Carlisle, Pennsylvania, with the B.A. degree in 1942, and then entered Jefferson Medical College in June of that year. His interest in medicine as a career, as well as the desire to seek admission to Jefferson, had been strongly influenced by his uncle, Arthur R. Gaines (Jefferson, 1916) who had an illustrious career in the U.S. Army and later as Superintendent of the Landis State Hospital in Philadelphia. The class that entered in 1942 was the first to go all the way through medical school in the accelerated program devised to graduate more quickly the physicians needed for the military services during World War II. This was accomplished by maintaining the same curriculum but by eliminating summer vacations and extended holiday breaks, completing the course of instruction in three years rather than four. This year-round program produced some strains and stresses for faculty and students alike. Air-conditioning in the College was nonexistent, and the dress code was modified somewhat by allowing the class to wear long-sleeved white sport

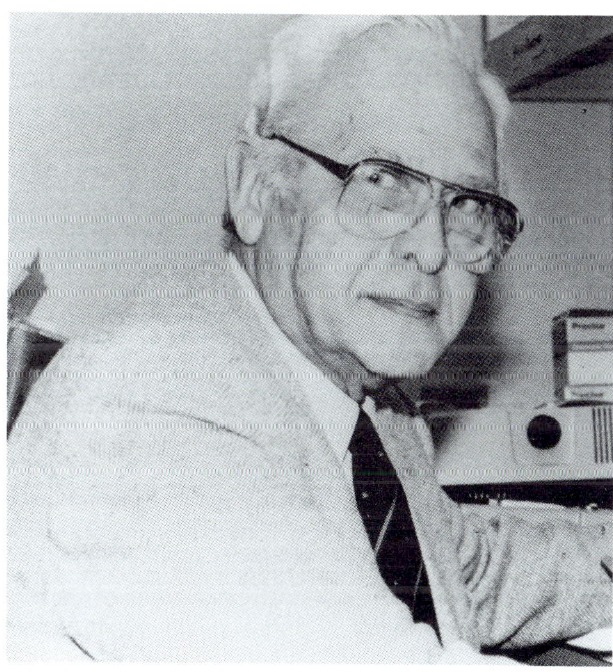

Fig. 45-22. James H. Lee, Jr., M.D., Fifteenth Chairman (1975–1987).

shirts instead of the usual coat and necktie during that first summer. By the next year almost everyone was in uniform as the Army Student Training Program and Navy V-12 Program were instituted, eliminating the problem of deciding what to wear. Despite the increased hardships, the faculty and students managed well through those years. Dr. Lee graduated in the Class of 1945, having served as class President since his sophomore year.

Following graduation Lee served a rotating internship at the U.S. Naval Hospital, Brooklyn, New York, from June 1945 to March 1946. The usual period of one year had been reduced to nine months during the war, but Dr. Lee took an additional four months in obstetrics and gynecology at the same institution. After a tour of duty as Medical Officer aboard the *U.S.S. Amphion* and a few months at the Philadelphia Naval Hospital, he was appointed to the residency program in Obstetrics and Gynecology at the U.S. Naval Hospital, Chelsea, Massachusetts. During graduate training he served as a Fellow in Pathology under Arthur T. Hertia at the Free Hospital for Women, Brookline, Massachusetts (1948–1949). Following residency training in 1951, he served as Chief of Obstetrics and Gynecology at the U.S. Naval Hospital, Beaufort, South Carolina, from 1951 to 1953, and on the staff of Commander, Pacific Service Forces (1953–1954). He resigned from the Navy in 1954 and engaged in the private practice of Obstetrics and Gynecology in Newport News, Virginia, until 1957. During that period he also served as Civilian Consultant to the Army Hospital at Fort Eustis, Virginia. He returned to the Navy in 1957 as Chief of Obstetrics and Gynecology at the U.S. Naval Hospital, Camp Lejeune, North Carolina, until 1961. He then became Chief of Obstetrics and Gynecology at the U.S. Naval Hospital in Philadelphia, a position he held until retirement from the Navy with the rank of Captain on December 31, 1966. While at the Philadelphia Naval Hospital, he was appointed to the Jefferson faculty by Dr. John B. Montgomery and developed an affiliated program for Jefferson students at the Naval Hospital.

In January, 1967, Dr. Lee was appointed to the full-time faculty at Hahnemann Medical College and Hospital as Professor and Co-Chairman of the Department of Obstetrics and Gynecology under Dr. George C. Lewis, Jr., who was the Department Chairman. In July, 1973, he resigned his position at Hahnemann and was appointed to the full-time faculty at Jefferson, as was Dr. Lewis.

Dr. Lee holds memberships in a number of professional societies, including the American College of Obstetricians and Gynecologists, the College of Physicians of Philadelphia, the Obstetrical Society of Philadelphia (Treasurer, 1970–1973; Vice President, 1975–1976), the American Radium Society, Association of Professors of Gynecology and Obstetrics, and Society of Medical Consultants to the Armed Forces, among others. His clinical interests have been in gynecologic oncology and in genital anomalies. He has had a longtime commitment to medical education.

During this period the administrative structure of the Department was reorganized and restructured to make it academically more effective. Considerable effort was directed toward improving communication and integration into Departmental activities of both full-time and volunteer faculty. This in turn contributed to an increase in patient volume in the hospital as a number of volunteer faculty began to concentrate all or most of their practice in the Thomas Jefferson University Hospital. The Department in 1975 assumed responsibility for the outpatient services and integrated these into the practice of the full-time faculty with the objectives of providing high-quality care for patients and improved supervised clinical training for residents and students. This, too, began to increase the number of patients cared for both in the ambulatory setting and in the hospital.

The residency program was restructured and expanded, and affiliations for resident training were developed with Our Lady of Lourdes Medical Center and Bryn Mawr Hospital and expanded with Methodist Hospital.

Undergraduate education received continuous attention with the development of a core clinical clerkship in the third year and an expanded elective program for seniors. Notable among clinical faculty members during these years were Clinical Associate Professors Leon A. Peris (Jefferson, 1955), Leopold S. Loewenberg

(Jefferson, 1956), Marvin R. Hyett (Jefferson, 1963), F. Susan Cowchock (Jefferson, 1968), and David M. Goodner and Ronald E. Traum (Jefferson, 1957). Clinical Assistant Professors included George M. Arnas (Jefferson, 1956), Lorraine C. King, Bruce B. Montgomery (Jefferson, 1960), and Edward M. Podgorski (Jefferson, 1954).

The development and expansion of subspecialty programs in the Department led in turn to the establishment of Departmental Divisions in Endocrinology, Gynecologic Oncology, and Maternal-Fetal Medicine. As these subspecialties received recognition by the American Board of Obstetrics and Gynecology and a certification process was developed, fellowship programs for postresidency training in these areas were organized and accredited. The program in endocrinology under Dr. Abraham Rakoff had been going on for many years. The new Division of Gynecologic Oncology was headed by Dr. George Lewis and strengthened by his appointment as Head of a national cooperative, the Gynecologic Oncology Group. The new Division of Maternal-Fetal Medicine was headed first by Dr. George Andros and later by Dr. Ronald Wapner. This latter program led to development of Jefferson as a major regional referral center for high-risk obstetrical patients. Physical facilities were improved and expanded for the care of patients both in the ambulatory setting and in the hospital to accommodate the changes occurring in patient care.

Dr. Lee retired from the Chairmanship July 1, 1987, but continued his work in the Department as a Professor of Obstetrics and Gynecology.

Oren Richard Depp, III, M.D.: Sixteenth Chairman (1987–)

Dr. Depp (Figure 45-23) was appointed the new Chairman July 1, 1987. Born in Glasgow, Kentucky, in 1938, he received his B.S. (1959) and M.D. (1963) from Tulane University. Following an internship at Charity Hospital (1963–1964), he completed his residency at Tulane-affiliated Southern Baptist Hospital (1964–1967) in New Orleans, he then became Senior Research Fellow in Reproductive Medicine in the Department of Obstetrics and Gynecology at the University of Washington Medical School, Seattle, Washington (1967–1968). There followed a succession of academic appointments at University of Washington School of Medicine, University of Pittsburgh School of Medicine and Northwestern University Medical School, culminating in his advancement to full Professor of Obstetrics and Gynecology at Northwestern in 1981. He was also Director of the Division of Obstetrics at Prentice Women's Hospital and Maternity Center of Northwestern Memorial Hospital.

Dr. Depp became known in the field of perinatology for his research in high-risk obstetrics including the prevention of preterm birth and the

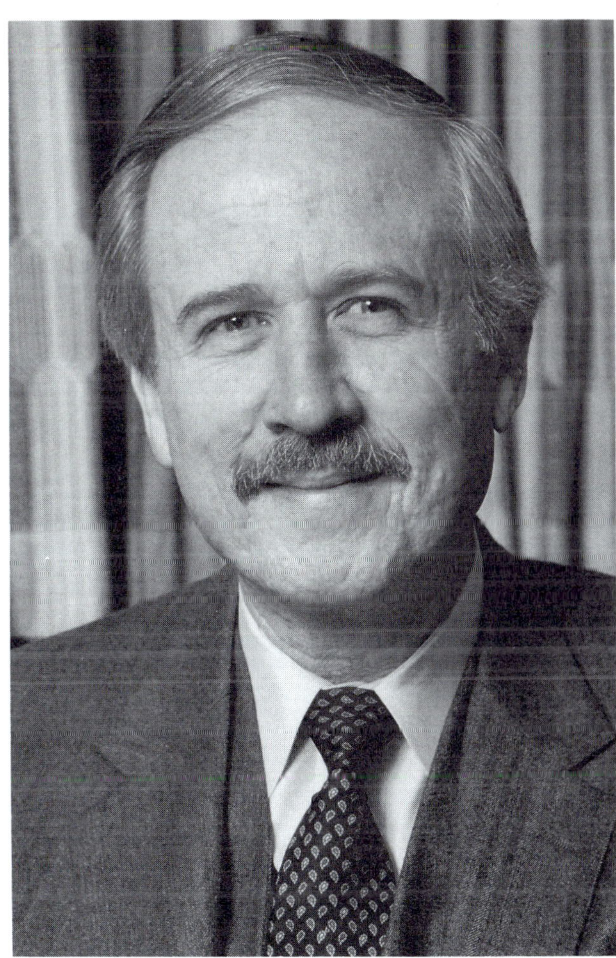

FIG. 45-23. O. Richard Depp, III, M.D., Sixteenth Chairman (1987–).

disorders of fetal growth. Major support was provided by the March of Dimes Birth Defects Foundation, as well as grants for studies on neonatal respiratory disorders, diabetes in pregnancy, and other projects received from the National Institute of Child Health and Development.

He has been a prolific author of medical articles, has served on the editorial board of *Fetal Medicine,* and has been an associate editor and reviewer for other journals. He has also been active in the major societies in his field.

Plans for the Department at Jefferson include the establishment of an Antenatal Evaluation Center where obstetricians together with ultrasound and genetics staff will provide the most advanced services available for the care of the mother, fetus, and newborn. An in-vitro fertilization program is also planned. Reproductive endocrinology and the section on gynecologic oncology will be strengthened. Under the auspices of Dr. Depp, Jefferson has been designated a Center for Maternal Fetal Medicine supported by the National Institute of Child Health and Development.

The Department that began at Jefferson as "Midwifery and Diseases of Women and Children" has segmented into many sophisticated areas involving preventive care, perinatal and genetic diagnosis, and major improvement in the conduct of delivery including fetal monitoring. The associated field of gynecology has witnessed parallel improvement relating not only to surgical technique but also palliation and cure of previously untreatable malignancies. Medical and endocrinological gynecology have expanded the field even further. From the earliest years, the members of the faculty have contributed leading textbooks used throughout the United States (Figure 45-24). It is not too visionary to anticipate even greater changes that will enhance the well-being of mother and fetus in childbirth and improve the treatment of the pelvic structures for all women.

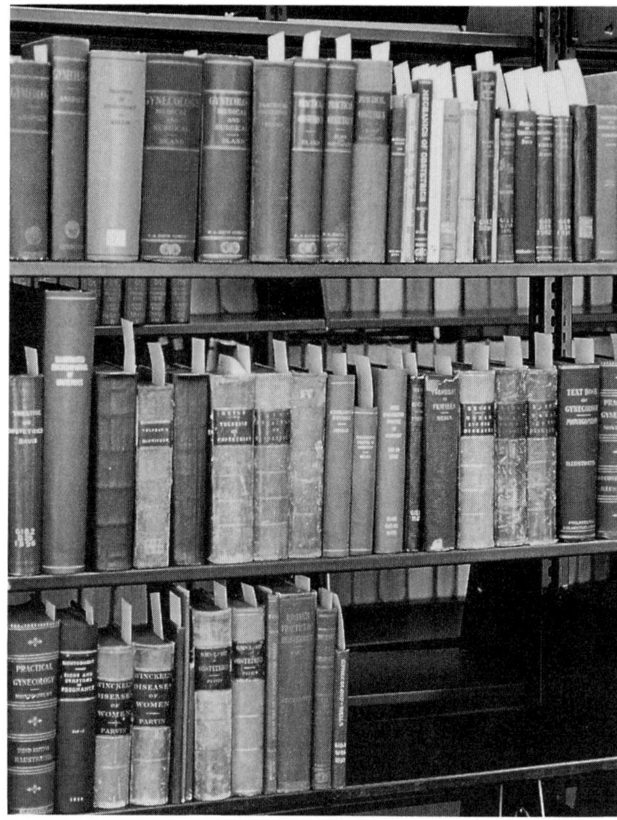

FIG. 45-24. Books published by the Jefferson faculty of Obstetrics and Gynecology.

References

1. Speert, H., *The Sloane Hospital Chronicle.* Philadelphia: F.A. Davis Co., 1963, p. 7.
2. Scheffey, L.C., "The Early History and Transition Period of Obstetrics and Gynecology in Philadelphia," *Ann. Med. Hist.* 32:215, 1940.
3. Cianfrani, T., *A Short History of Obstetrics and Gynecology.* Springfield, Illinois: Charles C. Thomas, 1960.
4. Penman, W.R., "Charles Delucena Meigs, M.D.: An Assessment of His Role in Philadelphia Obstetrics," *Trans. Stud. Coll. Phys. Phila.* Ser. 4, 43:121, 1976.
5. Penman, W.R., "William Goodell and the Preston Retreat," *Trans. Stud. Coll. Phys. Phila.* Ser. 4, 40:112, 1972.
6. Speert, H., "Obstetrics and Gynecology in America, a History," *Am. Coll. Obst and Gynec.* Chicago: 1980.
7. Gregoire, A.T., and Mayer, R.C., "The Impregnators," *Fertility and Sterility* 16:130, 1965.
8. Hard, A.D., "Artificial Impregnation," *Med. World* 27:163, 1909.
9. Hamilton, N.J., "Artificial Impregnation," *Med. World* 27:253, 1909.
10. Sims, J.M., *Clinical Notes on Uterine Surgery.* New York: William Wood & Co., 1869, p. 369.
11. Bland, P.B., "The Department of Obstetrics," *The Clinic Yearbook.* 1936, p. 59.
12. Burt, N., *The Perennial Philadelphians: The Anatomy of an American Aristocracy.* Boston: Little, Brown and Co., 1963.
13. *The Clinic Yearbook.* 1931, p. 11.
14. Stroud, W.D., "Memoir of Norris Wistar Vaux (1881–1958)," *Trans. Stud. Coll. Phys. Phila.,* 26:196, 1958.
15. "Pennsylvania's Health," *Commonwealth of Pennsylvania,* January–March, 1947.
16. Scheffey, L.C., *Jeff. Med. Coll. Al. Bull.,* 8, May 1953.
17. Letter from J.B. Montgomery to Dean William A. Sodeman. Archives of Thomas Jefferson University.
18. "A Research Institute in Perinatal Biology," a position paper in the Archives of Thomas Jefferson University.
19. "Report of the Task Force Committee on the Future of Obstetrics at Jefferson, March 12, 1974," Archives of Thomas Jefferson University.

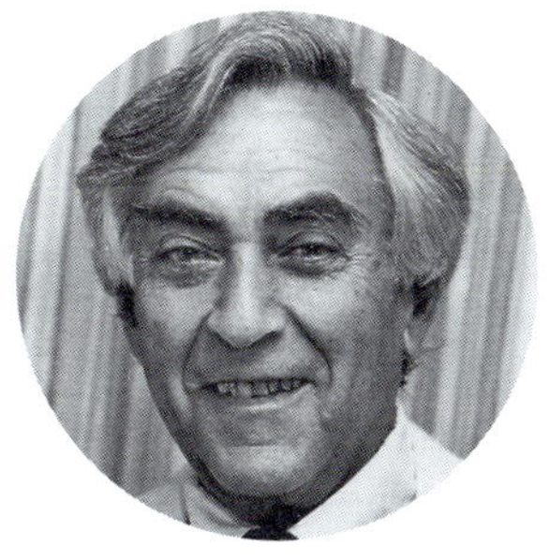

CHAPTER FORTY-SIX

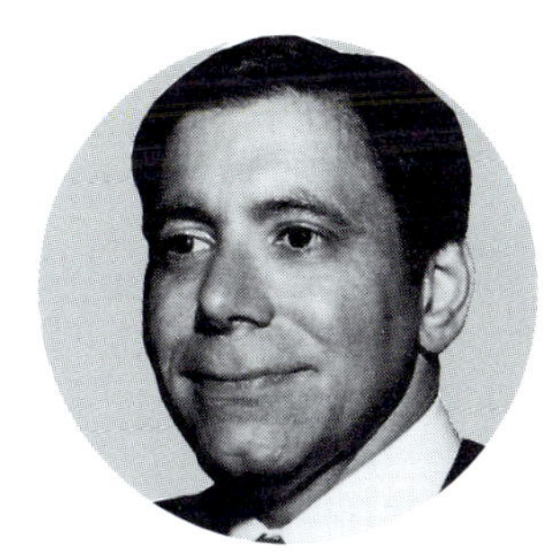

Department of Radiology, Radiation Oncology, and Nuclear Medicine

SIMON KRAMER, M.D., F.F.R. AND ROBERT M. STEINER, M.D.

"If the hand be held between the discharge tube and the fluorescent screen, the darker shadow of the bones is seen within the slightly dark shadow-image of the hand itself. . . . For brevity's sake I shall use the expression rays *and to distinguish them from others of this name, I shall call them* x-rays."

—WILHELM CONRAD ROENTGEN (1845–1923)

WITHIN a year of the astounding discovery of x-rays by Wilhelm Conrad Roentgen in 1895, a Division of Skiagraphy (Radiology) and Photography Laboratory were equipped at Jefferson Medical College Hospital. Dr. L.H. Prince, a member of the Department of Pathology, installed the first equipment under the amphitheater of the old 1877 Hospital. By the end of the first year, 67 x-ray studies and 225 fluoroscopic studies were performed. X-rays or skiagraphs were mainly ordered for metallic foreign bodies or for bony malformations (Figure

46-1). Dr. Prince worked in association with Dr. William L. Coplin, Professor of Pathology, and Dr. Randle C. Rosenberger, later Chairman of the Department of Bacteriology (Figure 46-2). Dr. Thomas J. Buchanan of the Department of Anatomy also took an active role in performing skiagraphy. William S. Newcomet, M.D. (University of Pennsylvania, 1893), who was to become Director of the Lucy B. Henderson Foundation of Radium Therapy at Jefferson in 1915, wrote his pioneer paper on *The Use of X-rays in the Study of the Lung* in 1899.[1]

The growing importance of Radiology was emphasized by John Chalmers DaCosta, Clinical Professor of Surgery, in *Modern Surgery* (1898). In judging the need for experienced radiologists DaCosta wrote: "In order to get the best results, not only must the apparatus be good, but the man who uses it must be expert. Pictures taken by an unskilled man lack clearness of outline and may lead to erroneous conclusions" (Figure 46-3). He further stated that there was "no positive evidence . . . to prove that the Roentgen force is possessed of any therapeutic value."[2]

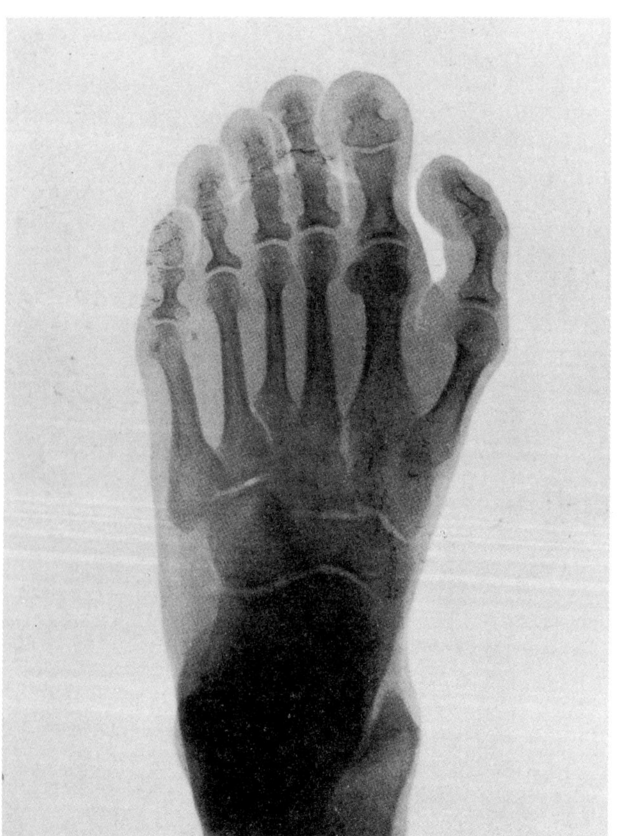

FIG. 46-1. An early "skiagraph" (1904), showing an extra great toe and metatarsal.

Notwithstanding Dr. DaCosta's impression, by 1901 treatment with x-ray radiation was performed for such conditions as cancer, lupus erythematosus, and keloids. During the same year, Dr. William M. Sweet of the Department of Ophthalmology performed skiagraphy of the eye. The Sweet electromagnet for removal of metallic foreign bodies in the orbit was his invention (Figure 46-4).

Roentgenology at Jefferson was relatively unstructured for a number of years following Roentgen's discovery. Dr. Willis F. Manges (Jefferson, 1903) (Figure 46-5) was appointed

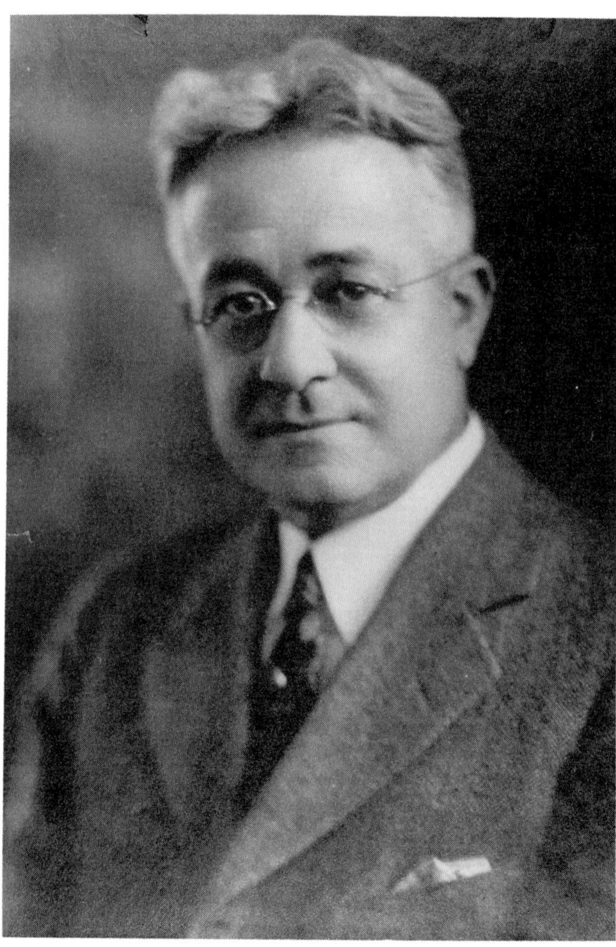

FIG. 46-2. Randle C. Rosenberger, M.D., manifested an early interest in the developing field of radiography. He later became a Professor of Bacteriology.

Assistant Demonstrator of Surgery in 1904, but his activities were directed toward x-ray services almost at once, and an x-ray department was listed among outpatient services of Jefferson with Dr. Manges as Chief as early as 1904. The previous year Dr. S.A.S. Metheny was described in the hospital staff listing as "skiagraphist." Dr. Manges actually served as Head of the Department of Roentgenology from 1904 until his sudden death in 1936.

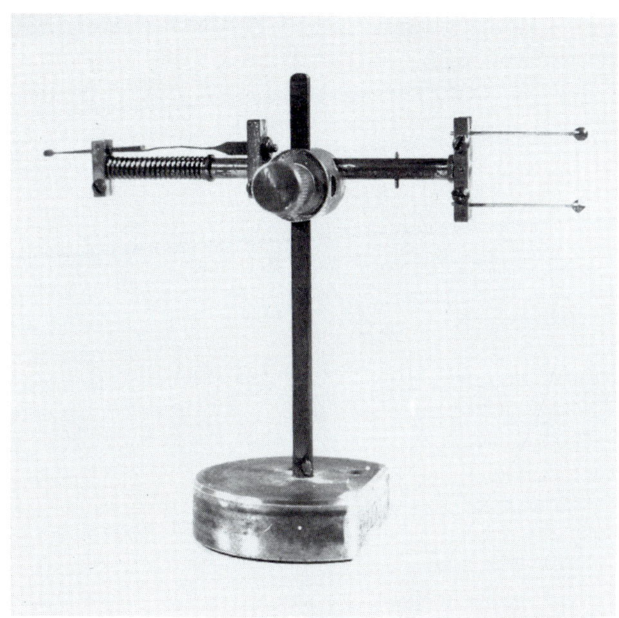

FIG. 46-4. The Sweet device for removal of foreign bodies in the orbit.

The Department of Roentgenology (1904)

Roentgenology grew slowly at Jefferson during the next decade, as illustrated by the Hospital budget of 1911 that showed billings of $592 compared with expenses of $1,700.91 for the

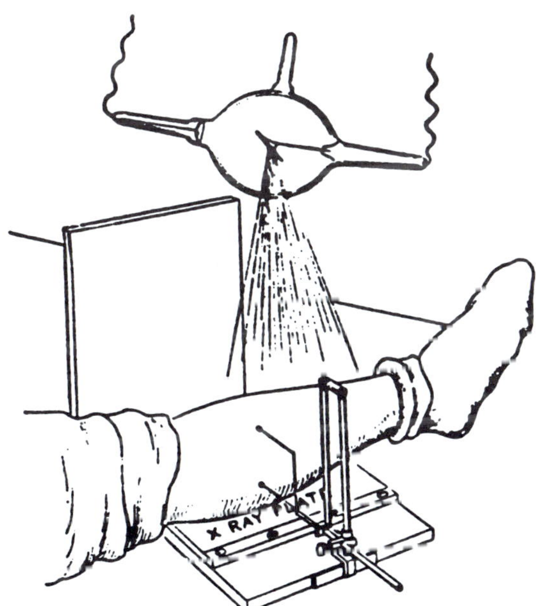

FIG. 46-3. Sweet's x-ray device for locating foreign bodies, as illustrated in John C. DaCosta, *A Manual of Modern Surgery, General and Operative* (Philadelphia: W.B. Saunders, 1898).

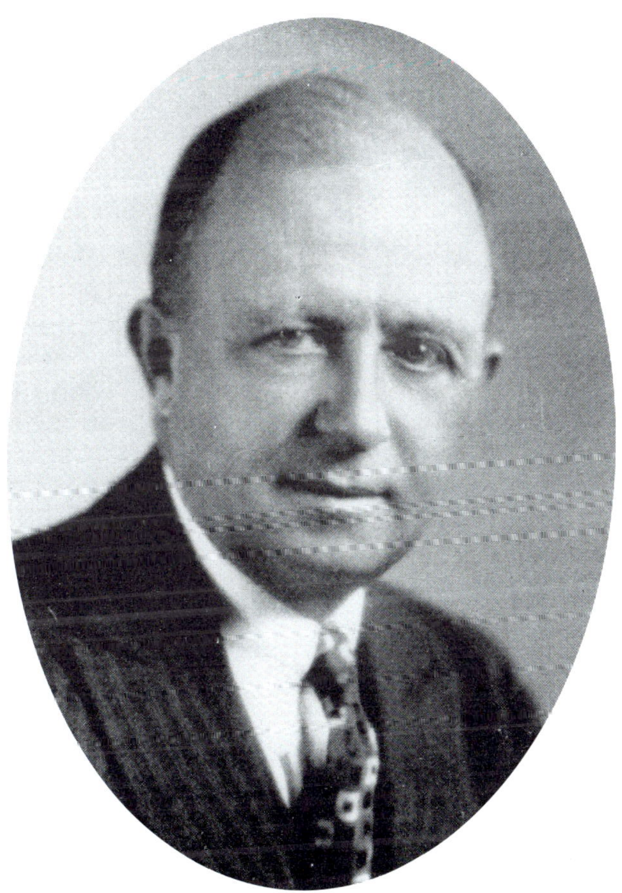

FIG. 46-5. Willis F. Manges, M.D., First Head of Department of Roentgenology (1904–1936).

Roentgenology Department. This is a startling comparison with the current multimillion dollar budgets—Roentgenology was not always a profit-making Division of the Hospital!

Willis F. Manges, M.D.; First Chairman (1928–1936)

In recognition of the growing importance of Roentgenology, Dr. Manges was promoted in 1918 to Clinical Professor of Roentgenology and became full Professor in 1928. He was President of the American Roentgen Ray Society in 1918. In 1920 Dr. Leon Solis-Cohen (Jefferson, 1912) (Figure 46-6) was added to the staff, thus providing an additional member of that illustrious Jefferson-connected family. In 1929 Dr. John T. Farrell, Jr. (Jefferson, 1922), and in 1932 Dr. R. Manges Smith, joined the staff.

By 1932 the Roentgenology Department was heavily involved in its teaching responsibilities. Lectures by Farrell and Smith in fluoroscopy and interpretation of films were given to the sophomore medical students. The juniors were instructed with lantern slides one day a week in both diagnosis and therapy.

John T. Farrell, M.D.; Acting Chairman (1936–1937)

At Dr. Manges' death in 1936,[3] Dr. John T. Farrell (Figure 46-7) was appointed Acting Chairman. Dr. Farrell had considerable experience in chest

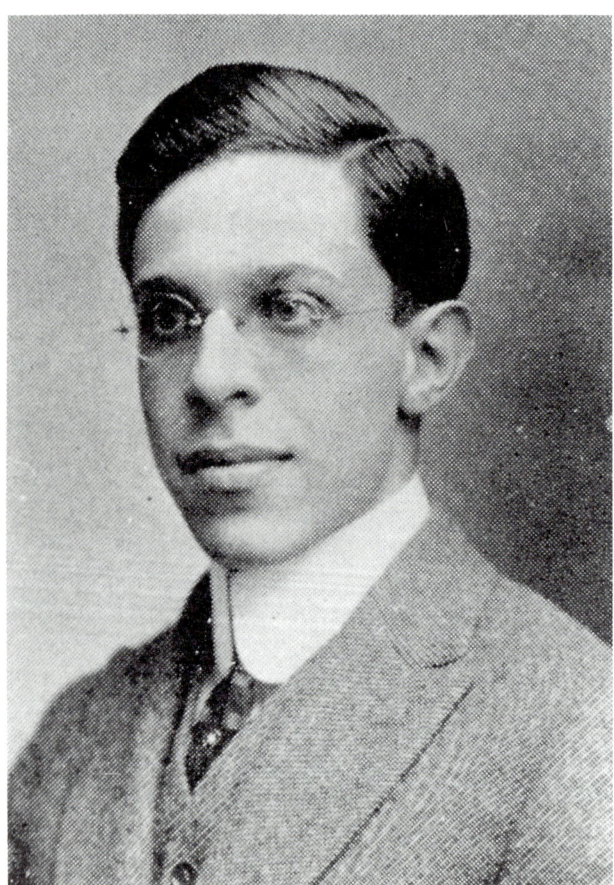

FIG. 46-6. Leon Solis-Cohen, M.D., Jefferson roentgenologist and member of a well-known family of physicians.

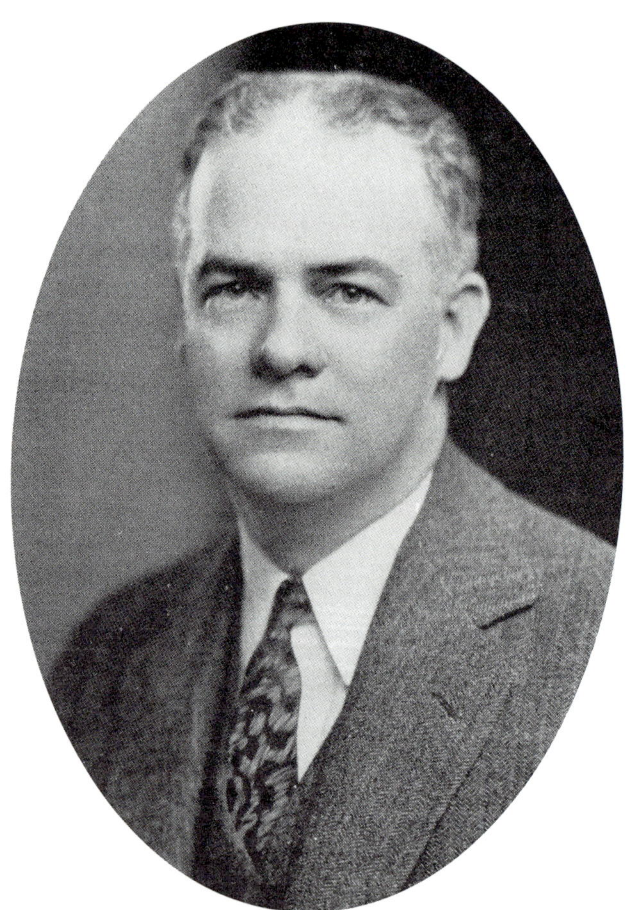

FIG. 46-7. John T. Farrell, Jr., M.D., Acting Chairman (1936).

roentgenology as an active consultant to the White Haven Sanatorium. His work with gastrointestinal roentgen studies later led to the publication of a book, *Roentgen Diagnosis of Diseases of the Gastrointestinal Tract*. His interest in organized medicine was later recognized when he served as President of the Philadelphia County Medical Society (1956) and the Pennsylvania State Medical Society (1958). He was also Vice President of the Radiological Society of North America (1944).

Karl Kornblum, M.D.; Second Chairman (1937–1942)

Dr. Farrell's brief tenure as Acting Chairman was followed by the appointment of Dr. Karl Kornblum (School of Medicine, University of Pennsylvania, 1919) as Chairman in 1937. Dr. Kornblum (Figure 46-8) was recruited from Graduate Hospital, Philadelphia, where he had been Director of Radiology since 1933.

During the World War II years, new members of the staff included Clinical Assistants Herman March and E. Wayne Egbert. In 1942 Dr. J. George Teplick joined the Department as Roentgenologist to the Department of Anatomy and participated actively in teaching. Dr. Teplick later became Professor of Radiology at the Hahnemann Medical College. Dr. Kornblum resigned to join the Radiology Department at the Hospital of the University of Pennsylvania in 1942.

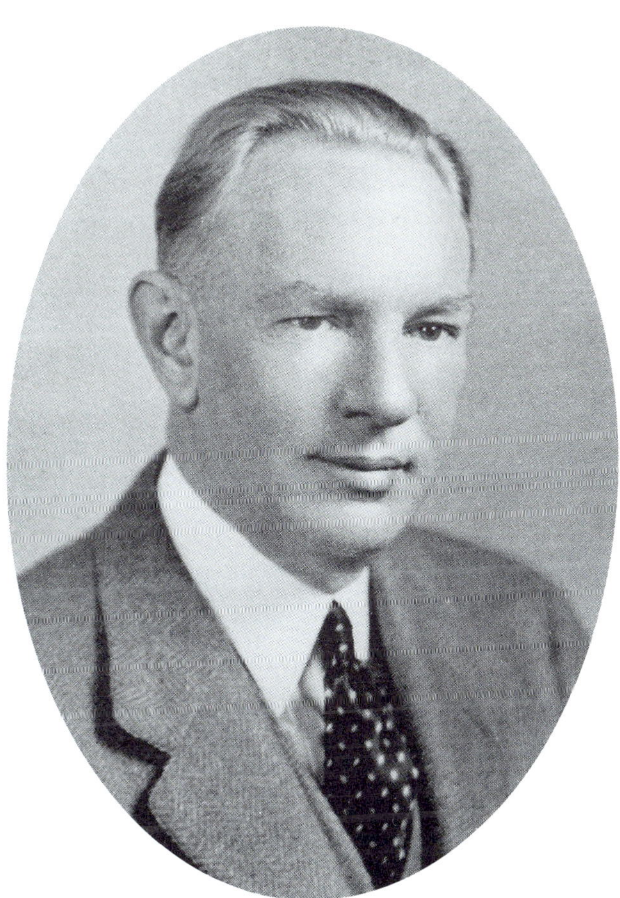

FIG. 46-8. Karl Kornblum, M.D., Chairman (1937–1942).

Paul C. Swenson, M.D.; Third Chairman (1944–1955)

In 1944 Dr. Paul C. Swenson (Figure 46-9) was named Chairman of the Department. Dr. Swenson (University of Minnesota, 1926), a native of Minnesota, was trained in Radiology at the University of Michigan (1928–1930) and at Columbia University, College of Physicians and

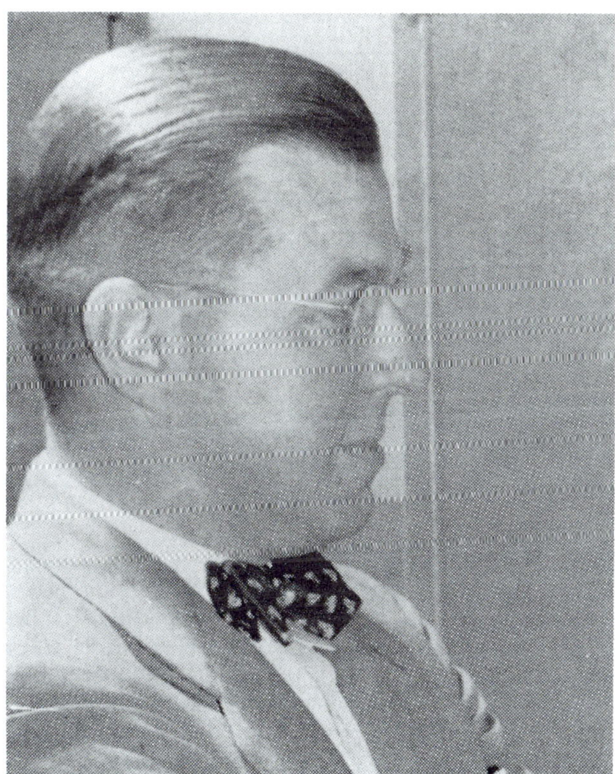

FIG. 46-9. Paul C. Swenson, M.D., Chairman (1944–1955).

Surgeons (1930), where he advanced to Associate Professor of Radiology with many research studies and papers to his credit. His tenure at Jefferson was marked by steady growth of the Department and important staffing changes. New staff members added included Dr. George Hahn, who later became a Professor of Obstetrics and Gynecology, and Willis Manges' son, Willis Manges, Jr. (Jefferson, 1942), who joined the staff in 1945, continuing an established tradition of family involvement in Jefferson radiology.

The Department of Radiology (1946)

The name of the Department was changed from Roentgenology to Radiology in 1946. In that year Dr. Theodore Eberhard was made Director of Radiation Therapy within the Department of Radiology and Assistant Professor of Radiology. Dr. Eberhard (Western Reserve University School of Medicine, 1930) had extensive training and experience in surgery and pathology (Lakeside Hospital, Cleveland, Ohio, and New England Deaconess Hospital, Boston, Massachusetts) in the 1930s before deciding on a career in Radiology. His interest in cancer prompted the change while at Columbia University in 1937. He was certified in Therapeutic Radiology in 1940 by the American Board of Radiology.

By 1947 student teaching became an ever-increasing part of the Department's activities. Classes were taught to the freshmen by Dr. Russell Wigh, and to the sophomores and seniors by Drs. Swenson and Eberhard. In 1949 Dr. William S. Newcomet, Director of the Lucy B. Henderson Foundation for Radium Therapy, retired, and Dr. Eberhard became Director of the Henderson Foundation as a Radium Therapist, thus effectively combining the activities of both Radiation Therapy and Radium Therapy.

Familiar resident physicians who trained during the early 1950s included Dr. Philip Gilbert, later of Cooper Hospital, and Dr. Gerald D. Dodd (Jefferson, 1947), whose distinguished career in American radiology was recognized by the Jefferson Medical College Alumni Association in 1986 with its Alumni Achievement Award. This was only one of many awards and honors he received. Having joined the Jefferson Radiology staff after residency, he became head of diagnostic radiology at the M.D. Anderson Hospital, Houston, Texas, in 1955. After an interval at Jefferson from 1961 to 1966, he was appointed Chairman of Radiology at the Medical School of the University of Texas in 1971 in addition to his former responsibilities as Chief of Diagnostic Radiology at M.D. Anderson. He was also President of the American College of Radiology.

Dr. James Bierly joined the Department as the first Assistant in Radiobiology in the Department and as the Department's first physicist. A Radiation Physics Laboratory was built at that time, "ready to serve any and all individuals who wish to use ionizing radiation clinically or experimentally with a full time physicist and an air conditioned 'hot' laboratory."[4]

Russell L. Nichols, M.D.; Fourth Chairman (1955–1958)

In June, 1955, Dr. Paul Swenson resigned as Chairman following a serious disagreement with Hospital administration over issues of staffing and Departmental policies. The entire professional staff, including all of the Residents, left with him. During this chaotic interregnum, many private radiologists filled the vacuum by accepting hospital patients sent by taxi to their offices in Center City Philadelphia. This tumultuous period ended in August, 1955, when Dr. Russell L. Nichols (Figure 46-10) was appointed as the Professor and Chairman of the Department. Dr. Nichols (University of Chicago School of Medicine, 1938) came to Jefferson from Ogden, Utah, where he was Radiologist at Dee Hospital and Clinical Professor of Radiology at the University of Utah. He was trained in radiology after private practice and Army experience at the University of Chicago, and he joined the staff there in 1947 upon certification by the American Board of Radiology.

In April of 1956 Dr. Simon Kramer (Figure 46-11) was appointed Co-Director of Radiation Therapy with Dr. Joseph Concannon. They assimilated the Lucy B. Henderson Foundation for Radium Therapy into the Department of Radiology. A Radioactive Isotopes Laboratory was organized and staffed by the Division of Radiotherapy under Drs. Kramer and Concannon. Dr. Kramer's training in Radiation Therapy at the Meyerstein Institute of Radiotherapy, Middlesex Hospital, University of London, followed his internship at King's Hospital, London, and British Army Service. He was certified in Radiotherapy in England and in 1954 was appointed Director of Radiotherapy at St. Boniface Hospital, Winnipeg, Canada. His appointment at Jefferson initiated a series of events that would place radiation therapy at Jefferson in a strong position of leadership.

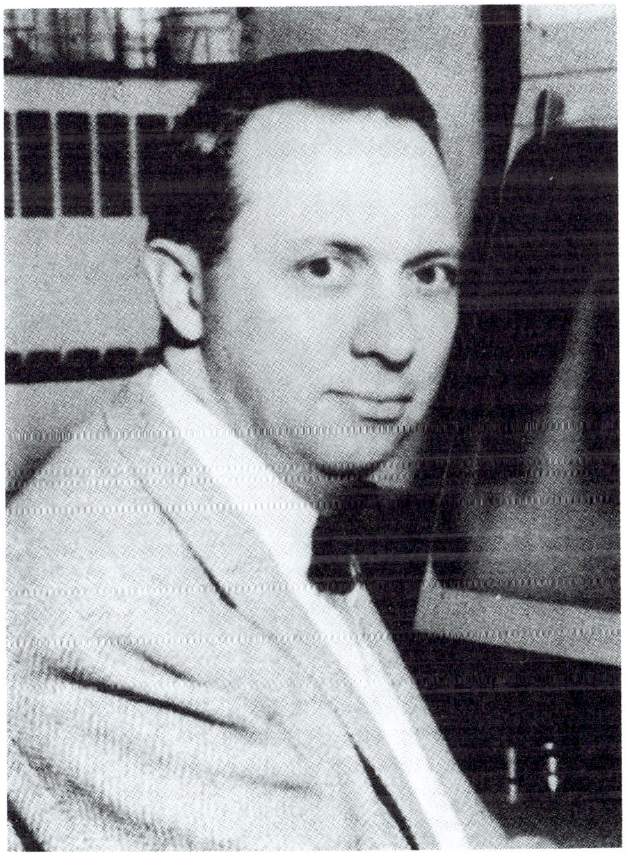

FIG. 46-10. Russell L. Nichols, M.D., Chairman (1955–1958).

Philip J. Hodes, M.D.; Fifth Chairman (1958–1971)

Abruptly in 1958 Dr. Nichols resigned and Dr. Philip J. Hodes (Figure 46-12) came from the University of Pennsylvania as Professor and Chairman of Radiology. Dr. Hodes received all of his education at the University of Pennsylvania following high school in Orange, New Jersey. This included his B.S. (1928), M.D. (1931–1933), and Fellowship in Radiology (1933–1935). He advanced to Professor in the School of Medicine in 1952. A man of many skills and interests, he received such honors as the Gold Medal from the American College of Radiology. He became widely known for his dynamic leadership in teaching, humanitarian pursuits, and radiological research. He brought with him a stellar team of academic radiologists from the University Hospital, including Assistant Professors A. Edward O'Hara (Figure 46-13), Roy Greening, and Jack Edeiken. Dr. O'Hara progressed to major

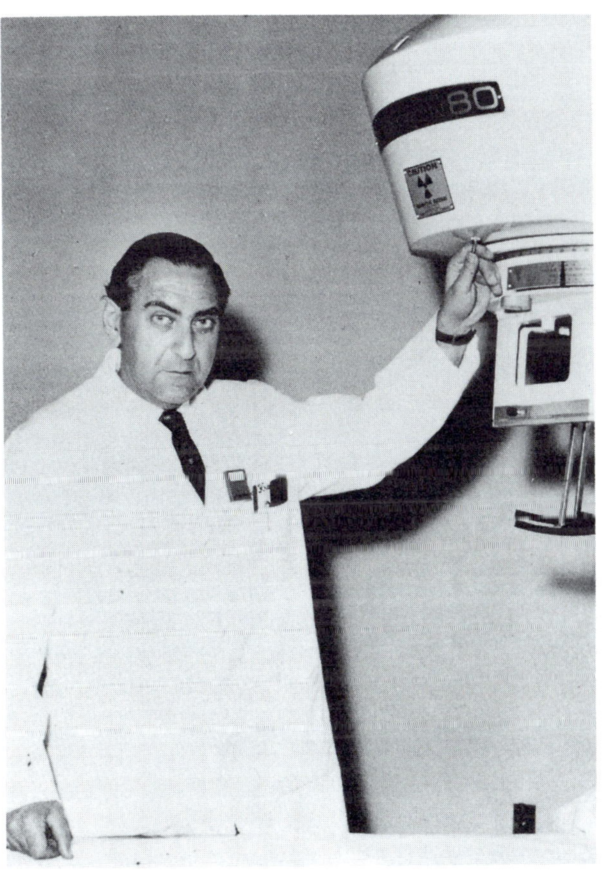
FIG. 46-11. Simon Kramer, M.D., F.F.R., Co-Director of Radiation Therapy (1956) and First Chairman, Department of Radiation Therapy and Nuclear Medicine (1969–1983).

accomplishments in pediatric radiology, Dr. Greening in angiography, and Dr. Edeiken was to succeed to the Chairmanship. Dr. Robert O. Gorson also came to Jefferson at that time as Director of Medical Physics. Residents who trained during that period included Dr. Emanuel Renzi and Dr. Vijay S. Gohel. Dr. Gohel became Associate Professor of Radiology at the University of Pennsylvania Hospital.

By 1960 the Department witnessed a dramatic growth of the Resident program and staff. Residents of that era included Drs. Ronald Clearfield, later President of the Pennsylvania Radiological Society, Renate Soulen, later Professor of Radiology at Johns Hopkins, and Sidney Wallace, Professor of Radiology at M.D. Anderson Hospital in Houston.

Dr. Yen Wang, Professor of Radiology at Jefferson, was a James Picker Fellow in research radiology. Other members of the staff and residents included Dr. Morton Murdock, who entered private practice in Center City Philadelphia, Dr. Mary S. Fisher, later Professor of Radiology at Temple University, and Dr. Irvin Freundlich, who became Professor of Radiology at the University of Arizona, later Director of Radiology at Wellesley-Newton Hospital near Boston and recently joined the staff of Baylor University Hospital, Houston, Texas.

Dynamic growth of the Department occurred under Dr. Hodes. In 1959 there were six staff radiologists. By 1962 there were 22 members of the

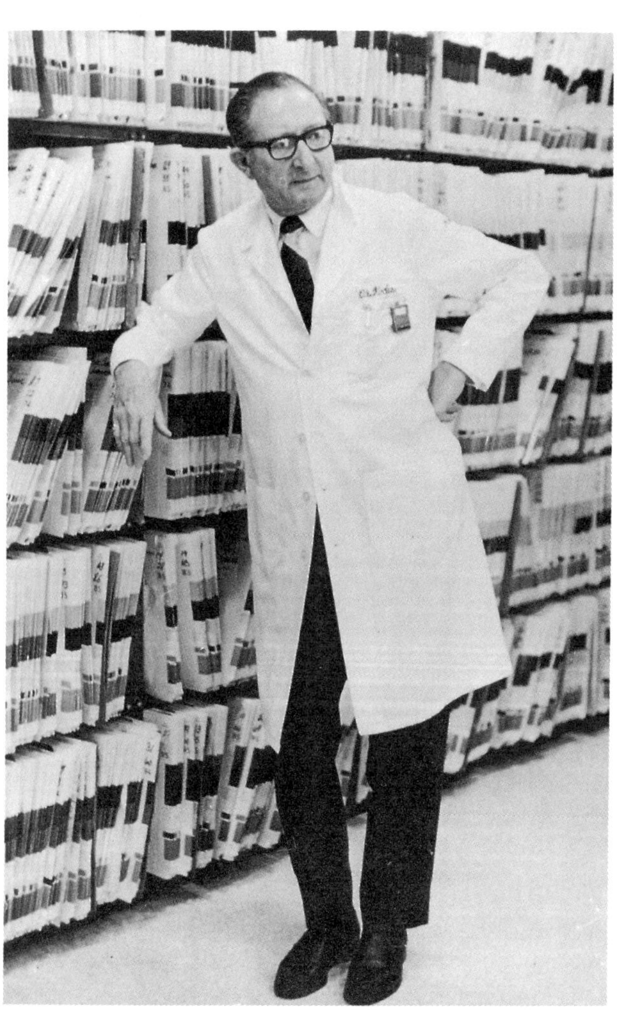

FIG. 46-12. Philip J. Hodes, M.D., Chairman (1958–1971).

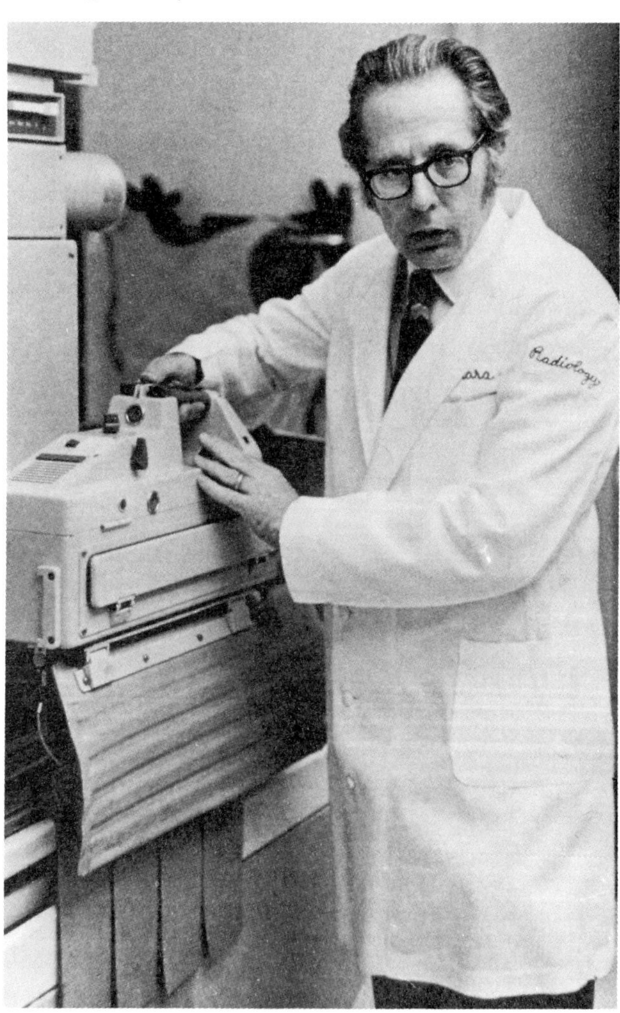

FIG. 46-13. Edward A. O'Hara, M.D., Professor of Radiology and pediatric radiologist.

Department. They included Dr. Robert L. Brent, internationally known expert in Radiation Biology and Chairman of the Department of Pediatrics at Jefferson, and Dr. Carl M. Mansfield, a National Institutes of Health Fellow in Radiation Therapy, who became Chairman of the Jefferson Department of Radiation Therapy and Nuclear Medicine in 1984. Dr. John Harris, who became Professor of Radiology at the University of Texas and is a former President of the American College of Radiology, was also a member of the staff at that time. This was a period of enormous growth in diagnostic imaging. Neuroradiology and interventional vascular radiology became important parts of patient service under Drs. Francis Lee and Koson Kuroda. Mammography, ultrasound, and thermography were in the early stages of development during this period. Jefferson radiologist Dr. Sidney Wallace and Dr. Laird Jackson of the Department of Medicine were pioneers in the development of bipedal lymphangiography. They published several papers in 1961–1962 that influenced the widespread acceptance of this technique.[5,6]

Jefferson Radiology has had close family ties, as exemplified by Beth Edeiken, the daughter of Jack Edeiken, who was a Resident in the early 1970s, and by Jose Landron, a Resident in 1964, whose son Jose Landron, Jr., was a Resident in the early 1980s.

Dr. Gary Shaber, Research Professor of Radiology at Jefferson, Peter Arger, later Professor of Radiology at the University of Pennsylvania, and Herman Libshitz, later Professor of Radiology at M.D. Anderson Hospital, joined the Department in 1964.

Jack Edeiken, M.D.; Sixth Chairman (1971–1985)

Dr. Hodes retired in 1971 after 14 years of distinguished service. His portrait was presented to the College in 1971. He was succeeded by the Chief of Radiologic Diagnosis, Dr. Jack Edeiken (Figure 46-14), international authority on bone radiology and the author of the popular text *Roentgen Diagnosis of Diseases of Bone*. Dr. Edeiken was promoted to full Professor in 1967. He was born in Philadelphia and graduated from Villanova University (B.S., 1943) and from the University of Pennsylvania School of Medicine (1947). In 1958 he came to Jefferson. During his Chairmanship, Dr. Edeiken served as a Visiting Professor at various institutions both in the United States and abroad. He was active as an officer of the American Board of Radiology and numerous national committees.

The Department changed dramatically as Radiology assumed an ever more important role in the medical community.

Diagnostic ultrasonography evolved from a single A mode unit in the Department of Radiation Therapy into the largest and perhaps the finest Division of Ultrasound in the nation under the Directorship of Dr. Barry B. Goldberg (Figure 46-15). Dr. Alfred Kurtz, who trained at Montefiore Hospital in New York, joined the Division. He quickly established an international reputation in genitourinary and abdominal ultrasound.

Mammography, largely developed in Philadelphia by Drs. Gershon-Cohen and Mortimer B. Hermel, also evolved into an important service of the Department of Radiology under the guidance of Dr. Stephen Feig. Dr. Feig (New York University, 1967) came to Jefferson from the School of Medicine, University of Pennsylvania, in 1974. He has carried on research into the benefits and safety of mammography

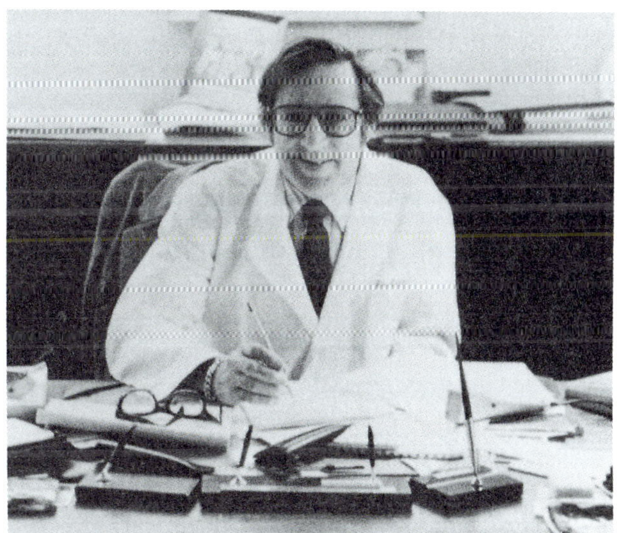

FIG. 46-14. R. Jack Edeiken, M.D., Chairman (1971–1985).

since that time and published 100 papers and chapters including a book, *Breast Carcinoma: Current Diagnosis and Treatment* (1983). He was also one of the authors of a monograph published by the National Council on Radiation Protection: *Mammography, A User's Guide* (1985).

Dr. Esmond Mapp came to Jefferson in 1976 as Chief of the Section of Gastrointestinal Radiology. He served as President of the Radiology Section of the National Medical Association and has been a member of many key committees of the Radiological Society of North America and the American College of Radiology.

Dr. Robert M. Steiner (Jefferson, 1964), Co-Director of General Diagnostic Radiology and Chief of Thoracic Radiology, joined the Department in 1976 and advanced to Professor in 1982. His sabbatical period at the University of Leiden (1983–1984) in magnetic resonance imaging introduced this new technology to the Department.

Dr. Vijay M. Rao, a Resident at Jefferson, rapidly developed an interest in Head and Neck Radiology and spent her sabbatical leave (1985–1986) at the University of Pennsylvania in magnetic resonance imaging to further enhance the Department's expertise in this new technology.

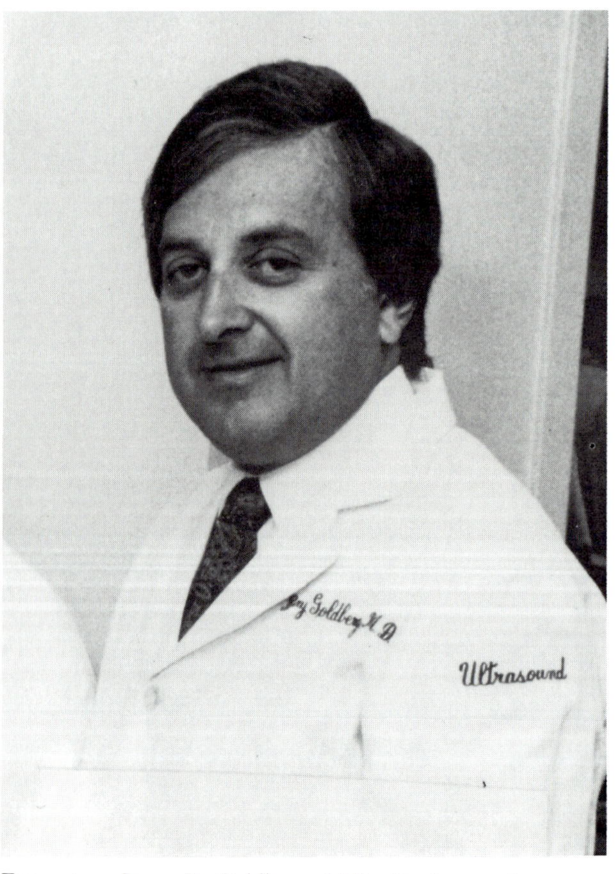

Fig. 46-15. Barry B. Goldberg, M.D., Professor of Radiology and Director of the Division of Ultrasound and Radiologic Imaging.

Dr. Matthew Rifkin joined the Division of Ultrasound and developed an international reputation in the areas of small parts and genitourinary ultrasonography. He became Director of the Division of Magnetic Resonance Imaging in 1986.

David Levin, M.D.; Seventh Chairman (1985–)

In 1985 Dr. Edeiken announced his retirement as Chairman. Dr. David Levin (Figure 46-16), Professor of Radiology at the Harvard Medical School and Director of Cardiovascular Radiology at the Peter Bent Brigham and Women's Hospital, was selected to be the next Professor and Chairman. The Department anticipated a new period of dynamic growth not only in its clinical activities but also in research and teaching responsibilities. The purchase of a high field strength magnetic resonance imaging unit and the establishment of a state-of-the-art cross-sectional imaging center in the new radiology unit in the Thompson Building brought about this new era.

Radiation Therapy

William S. Newcomet, M.D., A Pioneer (1915–1946)

The therapeutic use of ionizing radiation at Jefferson dates back to the turn of the century. Initially, radiologists practiced both diagnostic and therapeutic radiology. Diagnostic radiology joined by Dr. Henry A. Cleaver in 1933. Radiation therapy administered by external beam remained the responsibility of the Department of Roentgenology. Both the training and the practice of roentgenology encompassed diagnostic and therapeutic uses of radiation.

occupied most of their time, and the therapeutic use was empirical, with minimal scientific basis. Radiation therapy by external beam continued to be a minor portion of the work of the Roentgenology Department. In 1915, with funds donated by Lucy B. Henderson, a separate Foundation for Radium Therapy was created. This Foundation was directed by Dr. William S. Newcomet (Figure 46-17), who controlled a good deal of radium, which he used for skin cancers and other superficial lesions both in the hospital and in house calls. By 1917, seventy-eight patients had received 750 individual radium treatments. After working alone for many years, Dr. Newcomet was

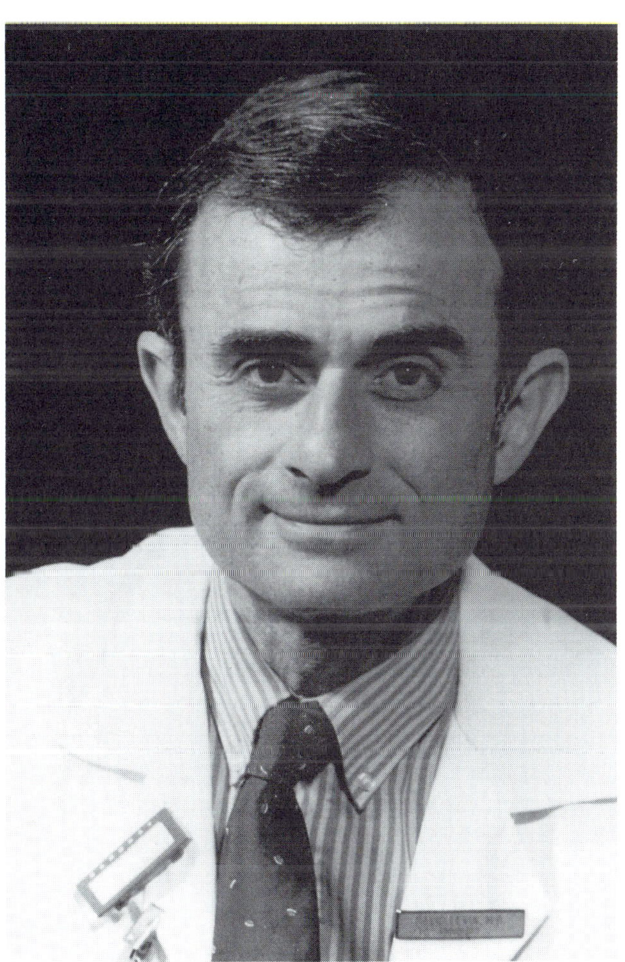

FIG. 46-16. David Levin, M.D., Chairman (1985–).

Theodore P. Eberhard, M.D.; Director, Radiation Therapy and Nuclear Medicine (1946–1956)

It was not until 1946, when Dr. Theodore P. Eberhard (Figure 46-18) joined the Department, that a fully accredited radiation therapist became a member of the staff. Even then Dr. Eberhard had a number of duties to perform in the Diagnostic Division of the Department as well as being Director of the Radiation Therapy Division. In

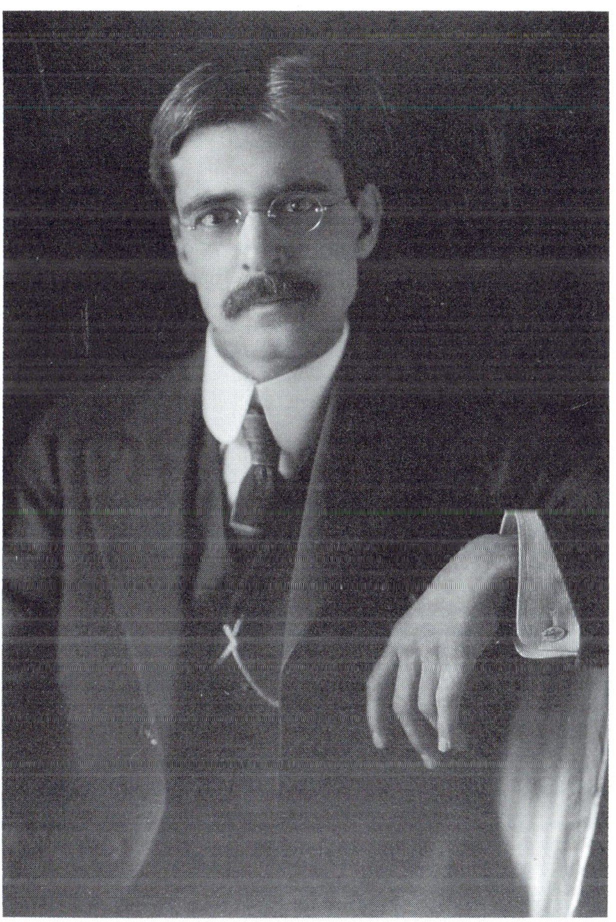

FIG. 46-17. William S. Newcomet, M.D., Director of the Lucy B. Henderson Foundation for Radiation Therapy (1915–1949).

1949 Dr. Newcomet retired as Director of the Lucy B. Henderson Foundation for Radium Therapy and Dr. Eberhard became the Director of the Radium Foundation at the hospital as well. Among the physicians who trained under Dr. Eberhard in the early 1950s were Dr. Luther Brady, later Professor and Chairman of the Department of Radiation Oncology at Hahnemann University in Philadelphia, and Dr. Frank Hendrickson, later Professor and Chairman of the Department of Therapeutic Radiology at Rush-Presbyterian St. Luke's Medical Center in Chicago. The practice of making house calls for the application of radium ceased when Dr. Eberhard took over the Foundation.

Nuclear Medicine

In the early 1950s a Division of Nuclear Medicine was created that, among other things, developed the first mechanical scanner for radioisotopes in Philadelphia. This Division was also directed by Dr. Eberhard while James Bierly became the first physicist to be involved primarily with nuclear medicine. Dr. Bierly was also active in teaching the physics of radiology, both diagnostic and therapeutic. In 1955 Chairman Swenson resigned and took with him all his staff, residents, all but two technologists, and all the records available. His reasons were based on philosophical and financial disagreements with the Hospital administration.

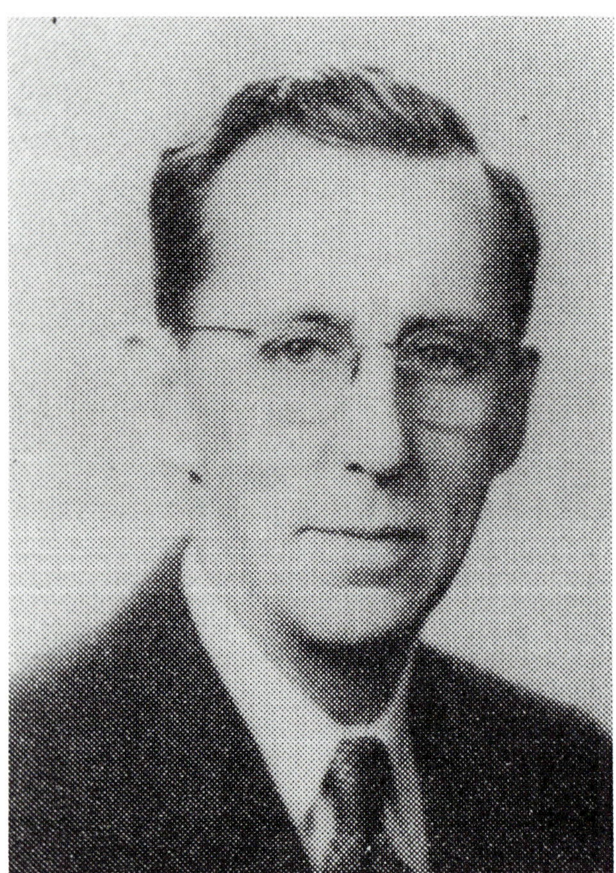

Fig. 46-18. Theodore B. Eberhard, M.D., Director of Radiation and Radium Therapy (1946–1955).

Thus in April, 1956, when Dr. Simon Kramer (Figure 46-11) and Dr. Joseph Concannon were appointed to be Co-Directors of Radiation Therapy, they had to start from scratch. They amalgamated the Lucy B. Henderson Foundation for Radium Therapy into the Department of Radiology and established a new separate Division of Radiation Therapy in separate quarters. Modern equipment was purchased, and modern radiation therapy was established. The Division of Radiation Therapy weathered another difficult period when Dr. Nichols, Chairman of the Radiology Department, resigned in 1958.

More changes took place as Dr. Philip J. Hodes was appointed Professor and Chairman of the Department of Radiology in 1958. Dr. Concannon left to become Director of Radiation Therapy at the Allegheny General Hospital in Pittsburgh. A number of brilliant young physicians came to assist Dr. Kramer. Dr. Stanley Dische stayed at Jefferson for two years and then returned to Britain, from whence he had come, to become the director of a medical research unit at Mt. Vernon Hospital, London. Dr. Ruheri Perez-Tamayo joined the Division for a year and later became the Chairman of the Department of Radiation Therapy at Loyola University in Chicago. In 1962 Dr. Carl M. Mansfield (Figure 46-19) joined the Department as a Fellow in Radiation Therapy and completed his training in radiology. After a year's fellowship in Britain (1963) he returned to join the staff and progressed through the ranks to full Professor. In 1976 he left to become Professor and Chairman of the Department of Radiation Therapy at the University of Kansas.

The Division of Radiation Therapy grew apace. The first cobalt unit had been installed in 1957, and a second unit was installed in 1960. Modern afterloading radium applicators and sources were purchased in keeping with the needs of improved interstitial and intracavity therapy. The Division of Nuclear Medicine continued to flourish as a Division within Radiation Therapy and here, too, modern equipment and expertise were added. In 1964 Dr. Martha Southard (M.D., Ohio State University, College of Medicine, 1947; Figure 46-20) joined Dr. Kramer as Associate Professor of Radiation Therapy and rapidly established a large academic practice. Dr. Southard had an extensive background of hospital training in Columbus and Cincinnati, Ohio, as well as in New York, and further experience as Associate Director of Radiation Therapy at Temple University Hospital, Philadelphia. She was promoted to Professor of Radiation Therapy and Nuclear Medicine at Jefferson in 1969.

The teaching of the Division at that time involved both general radiology residents, residents in radiation therapy, and the medical students. The Division of Physics in Radiology, under the Directorship of Dr. Robert O. Gorson, provided services for diagnostic radiology and radiation therapy.

Later Dr. Gorson was appointed Professor and Director of Medical Physics in the Department of Radiology, and Dr. Nagalingam Suntharalingam held a similar position in the Department of Radiation Therapy, but both held appointments in both Departments.

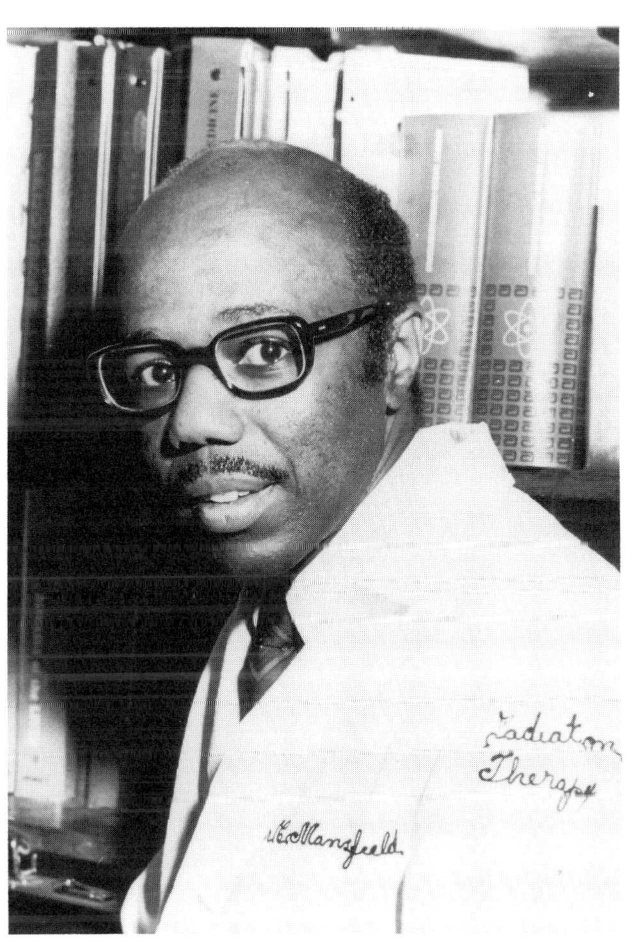

Fig. 46-19. Carl M. Mansfield, M.D., Chairman and Professor of Radiation Therapy and Nuclear Medicine (1984–).

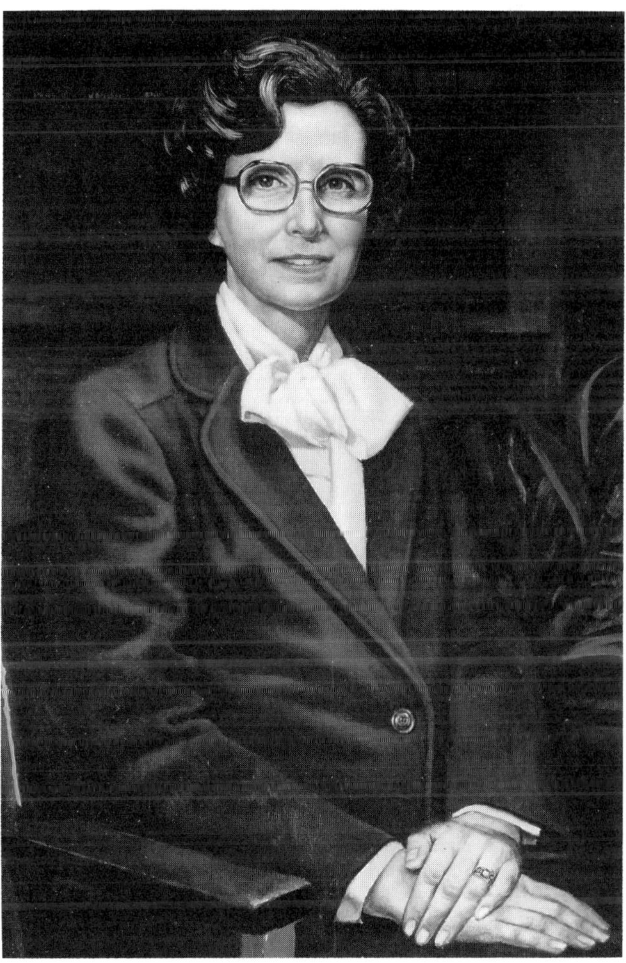

Fig. 46-20. A portrait of Martha Southard, M.D., Professor of Radiation Therapy and Nuclear Medicine.

The Department of Radiation Therapy and Nuclear Medicine (1969)
Simon Kramer, First, M.D., F.F.R.; Chairman (1969–1983)

After 13 years of attempts to establish a separate Department, the Department of Radiation Therapy and Nuclear Medicine was created in 1969 as a distinct entity both in the Medical School and in the Hospital, with Dr. Simon Kramer as the first Chairman. Four Divisions were established in the new Department: a Clinical Division headed by Dr. Martha Southard, a Division of Nuclear Medicine under Dr. Carl M. Mansfield, a Division of Medical Physics under Dr. Nagalingam Suntharalingam, and a Division of Experimental Radiation Therapy under Dr. Dennis Leeper. Considerable development dated from that period. A planning grant for a radiation therapy cancer center was funded by the National Cancer Institute, and shortly thereafter a construction grant was obtained from the National Cancer Institute to totally refurbish and double the size of the Radiation Therapy Department. In 1966 the first radiation therapy simulator in the United States had been developed and was installed at Jefferson.[7] This was later replaced by a commercially manufactured machine. The new Department was equipped with a 45-million-volt Betatron machine capable of the most penetrating x-rays available in the United States, as well as being the first machine capable of electron beams in Philadelphia. A linear accelerator was purchased at that time.

Both basic and clinical research efforts intensified. The extensive experience in the management of pediatric and adult brain tumors was reported. In 1968 the first national randomized study in treating advanced head and neck tumors by radiation therapy and adjuvant chemotherapy was initiated in the Department.[8,9] One year later the Radiation Therapy Oncology Group, a nationwide group of university departments, was created at Thomas Jefferson University Hospital with Dr. Kramer as its first Chairman. Over 10,000 patients have been entered into clinical trials since that time.[10] In 1972 the National Cancer Institute funded a ten-year study to determine the patterns of care in cancer management by radiation therapy. In a "first" in medicine anywhere, this study established national benchmarks and a method of quality assessment for radiation therapy throughout the United States.[11]

Almost all the research done in the Clinical Division, the Division of Nuclear Medicine, the Division of Physics, and the Division of Experimental Radiation Therapy since that time was funded by the National Cancer Institute. Some was also funded from institutional sources. With increase in the academic endeavors there was a commensurate increase in the clinical involvement, with enlargement of the professional and technical staff. By 1983, when Dr. Kramer stepped down from the Chair, there were eight full-time physicians in radiation therapy, three Ph.D.s in radiation biology, five Ph.D.s in radiation physics, and two M.D.s in nuclear medicine. His portrait was presented to the University on the occasion of the First Annual Simon Kramer Lecture and Symposium on November 4, 1983. Dr. Kramer was then honored to become Jefferson's first "Distinguished Professor."

Carl M. Mansfield, M.D.; Second Chairman (1984–)

Plans were developed in 1983 for an entirely new Department of Radiation Therapy and a new and reconditioned area for Nuclear Medicine. Dr. Carl M. Mansfield returned in 1984 as the new Chairman and Professor of Radiation Therapy and Nuclear Medicine. Under his direction the Department of Radiation Therapy and Nuclear Medicine took on added dimensions in the new Thomas Jefferson University Hospital (of 1978), and new techniques of cancer management and research were continued.

The new Department, the Bodine Center for Cancer Treatment (Figures 46-21 and 46-22),

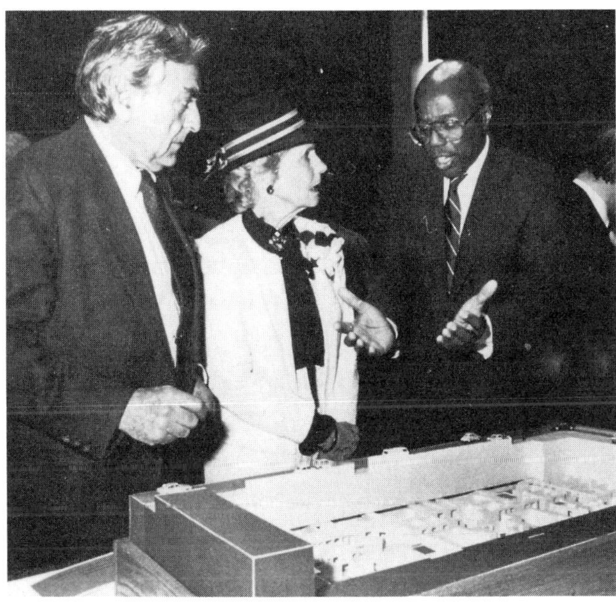

FIG. 46-21. The Bodine Center model; from left to right, Simon Kramer, M.D., F.F.R., Mrs. William Bodine, and Carl M. Mansfield, M.D. (1985).

promised expanded facilities for research in the fields of cancer and radiation biology and clinical research in cancer treatment. The clinical area included new facilities for hyperthermia, intraoperative radiation therapy, a dedicated CT scanner to assist in treatment planning, and four new linear accelerators. Two of the latter are capable of very high energy photon and electron beams. A Day Hospital is provided for patients to receive combined modality therapy or other procedures that do not necessitate inpatient care. In the fall of 1986 Jefferson continued as one of the most up to date facilities in radiation therapy in the United States.

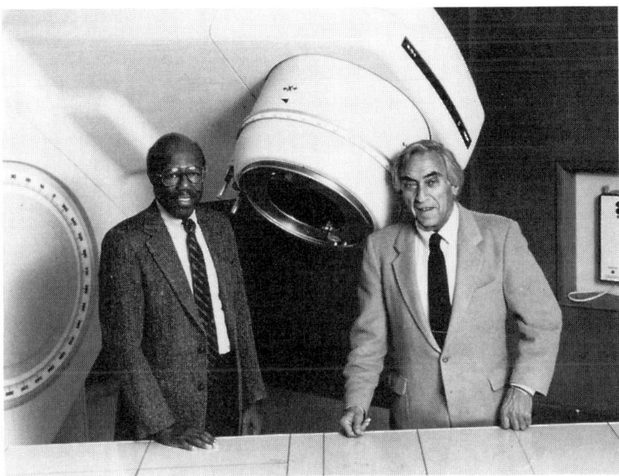

FIG. 46-22. The Bodine Center, 1987; Drs. Carl M. Mansfield (left) and Simon Kramer.

References

1. Newcomet, W.S., "The Use of X-rays in the Study of the Lung," *Proc. Phila. Co. Med. Soc.* 20:277–279, 1899.
2. DaCosta, J.C., *Manual of Modern Surgery* Phila., W.B. Saunders, 1898, p. 878.
3. Farrell, J.T., Jr., "Memoir of Willis F. Manges," *Clinic.* 1937, p. 64.
4. "The Radiation Physics Laboratory." *Jeff. Al. Bull.* December 1951, p. 10.
5. Wallace, S., Jackson, L., and Greening, R.R., "Clinical Applications of Lymphangiography," *Am. Jour. Roentgenology, Radium Therapy and Nuclear Medicine* 88:97–109, 1962.
6. Wallace, S., Jackson, L., Schaeffer, B., Gould, J., Greening, R.R., Weiss, A., and Kramer, S., "Lymphangiograms: Their Diagnostic and Therapeutic Potential," *Radiology* 76:179–199, 1961.
7. Kramer, S., Kusner, D., and Gunn, W., "Clinical Experience with the Jefferson Hospital Radiotherapy Simulator," *Radiology* 87(1):134–136, July 1966.
8. Kramer, S., "Use of Methotrexate and Radiation Therapy for Advanced Cancer of the Head and Neck," *Frontiers of Radiation Therapy and Oncology* 4:116–125. New York: Karger/Basel, 1969.
9. Kramer, S., "Methotrexate and Radiation Therapy in the Treatment of Advanced Squamous Cell Carcinoma of the Oral Cavity, Oropharynx, Supraglottic Larynx, and Hypopharynx," *Can. J. of Otolaryngology* 4(2):213–218, 1975.
10. Davis, L., Gelber, R., Kramer, S., Zelen, M., and Rubin, P., "The Radiation Therapy Oncology Group: A Progress Report," *Cancer Clinical Trials* 1(2):83–88, 1978.
11. Kramer, S., "An Overview of Process and Outcome Data in the Patterns of Care Study," *Int. J. Radiat. Oncol. Biol. Phys.* 7(6):795–800, 1981.

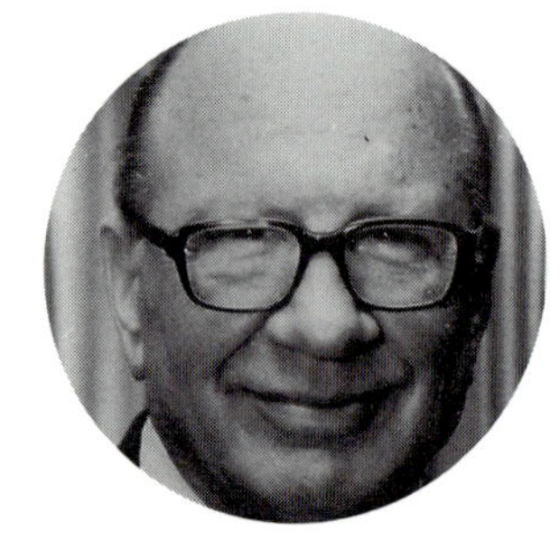

CHAPTER FORTY-SEVEN

Department of Urology

Nicholas R. Varano, M.D.

"As men draw near the common goal
Can anything be sadder
Than he who master of his soul,
Is servant to his bladder?"

—Anonymous

In all probability there has never been a time when diseases of the urinary and sexual organs did not attract the attention of practitioners of the healing art. Among the symptoms were those caused by calculi, retention of urine, painful urination, incontinence of urine, elongation of the prepuce, and venereal infection. For the relief of these conditions, operative procedures were devised such as lithotomy, lithotrity, catheterization, and circumcision. Medical formulae were prepared and administered when operations were not performed.

The Earliest History of the Study of the Urinary Tract

In the *Papyrus of 1550 B.C.*, discovered by Ebers in 1872, the ancient Egyptians recorded concoctions both to increase the flow of urine and to diminish an excessive flow. Circumcision was extensively practiced, but whether for hygienic or religious reasons is uncertain. Cutting for stone was apparently not practiced.

About 1,000 years later the Hindus of India in the *Syurveda of Sucratu* described treatment of strictures by gradual dilatation with sounds of metal and wood, and diseases of the urethra and bladder by injection. Literature of the Persians and Turks described similar conditions and instruments.

Among the Greeks at the time of Hippocrates (460–370 B.C.) passages were recorded referring to painful urination, bloody urine, pus in the kidney, retention of urine, bladder stones, and gout. Treatment was unsatisfactory because of lack of knowledge of anatomy as well as the causes of the conditions. Hippocrates disapproved of operations on the bladder, but did advise cutting into the kidney for the removal of pus. The great Alexandrian anatomist Erasistratus in the fourth century B.C. was one of the originators of human dissection. He left no textbook record, but the work was pieced together out of Galen, the founder of experimental physiology. Erasistratus discovered the exact relations of the urinary organs, especially the anatomy of the prostate gland, and gave it the name it has kept to the present.

Aurelius Cornelius Celsus described Roman medicine during the reign of Tiberius Caesar (14–37 A.D.) as an encyclopedist rather than a physician. The practice was essentially that of the Greeks, and the document was the oldest medical one after the Hippocratic writings. In the excavation of Pompeii (destroyed by the eruption of Mt. Vesuvius in 79 A.D.) there were found many kinds of surgical instruments, among which was a metallic catheter about nine inches in length and with a double curvature. Through a gift of Mr. Daniel Baugh of the Board of Trustees, a reproduction of these instruments was placed in the museum at Jefferson and later transferred for display in the Scott Library. Galen (131–201 A.D.), the greatest Greek physician after Hippocrates, wrote upon incontinence and retention of urine. He described an "S-shaped" or curved catheter for relief of the latter condition.

With the decline of the Roman Empire, most of the advances came to an end and were practically forgotten for some centuries.

Medicine in the eleventh and twelfth centuries was elevated by the School of Salerno, near Naples, from its decline of half a millenium. Arabic medical doctrine was introduced there by Constantinus Africanus (ca. 1020–1087), who imposed Mohammedan modes of thought upon Western European medicine from the twelfth to the seventeenth centuries. During the heyday of the Salernian School, all the physicians were practically urologists, since they depended upon the urine for diagnosis and prognosis. The urinal became the insignia of the physician and the emblem of medicine.

In the beginning of the Middle Ages, urinary tract diseases had been treated medically for 2,000 years, and surgical interference had been practiced sporadically for 1,000 years. The practice of medicine fell into the hands of the monks, and surgery was carried on by barbers and charlatans.

In the latter part of the eighteenth century, there was a decided advance in the analysis of urine. Cotugno in 1764 discovered albumin in the urine of diseased kidneys by boiling that urine, and Rouelle (1773) discovered urea. New forms of catheters were devised for emptying the bladder, sounds for dilating strictures of the urethra, operations on the bladder for relief of urine retention, and external urethrotomy. Around 1762 it was established by Morgagni that enlargement of the prostate was a source of disease of the urinary organs.

At the dawn of the nineteenth century a good basis existed for study of the urine itself as well as treatment of kidney, bladder, and urethral diseases. Tumors of the bladder had been discovered as far back as the seventeenth century. Metabolic experiments yielded many new facts, a few of which were Wollaston's investigation of cystin calculi (1810); Blackall and Wells on albumin in the urine (1812–1814); Marcet's investigation of black urine (1822); F. Rose's biuret tests for albumin (1833); proof by Bouchardat and Peligot that the sugar of diabetic urine is grape sugar (1838); Pettenkofer's test for bile (1844); the quantitative test for sugar in the urine by von Fehling (1848); and Bence-Jones's discovery of a special proteid (albumose) in the urine of patients with softening of the bones (multiple myeloma). Lithotrity, the crushing of bladder stones, was suggested and practiced by French surgeons.

In Philadelphia, which was the medical center of the United States to somewhat beyond the first half of the nineteenth century, Philip Syng Physick (1767–1837) of the University of Pennsylvania became the acknowledged "Father of American Surgery." In 1831, at the age of 63, he performed his famous removal (lithotomy) of about 1,000 calculi from the bladder of Chief Justice John Marshall. This was done without anesthesia, which was still 15 years or more in the future. Marshall, who was 75, survived the operation for some years and died of an entirely different disease. Jefferson's founder, Dr. George McClellan, studied under Physick and was proficient in lithotomy as well as the latest operative procedures of the day. Pancoast (1844) and Mütter (1846), in their textbooks at Jefferson as well as in practice, devoted much attention to the urinary organs. Mütter was the first in Philadelphia (1846) to use ether anesthesia in surgery.

Urology as a distinct branch of general surgery was definitely established in the United States in 1851 by Samuel D. Gross in his authoritative

Practical Treatise on the Diseases, Injuries, and Malformations of the Urinary Bladder, the Prostate Gland, and the Urethra. A second, larger edition appeared in 1855 in an octavo volume of 925 pages with 184 woodcuts. In the appendix he presented the first attempt in urologic literature to report the prevalence of stone in the bladder and of calculous disorders in the United States, Canada, Europe, and other places. His operation of lithotomy for which he was well known is described in his book, and the knife with which he performed more than 70 of these procedures is in the Mütter Museum of the College of Physicians of Philadelphia. Dr. Samuel W. Gross, his son at Jefferson, carried on his father's interest in this field by editing the third edition in 1876 and writing his own treatise on *Impotence, Sterility, and Allied Disorders of the Male Sexual Organs* (1881). Other Jefferson surgeons who wrote or practiced in urologic surgery toward the end of the nineteenth century were John H. Brinton (Jefferson, 1852), W.W. Keen (Jefferson, 1862), J. Ewing Mears (Jefferson, 1865) and W. Joseph Hearn (Jefferson, 1867).

Orville Horwitz, M.D. (1860–1913); Clinical Professor of Genito-Urinary Diseases (1894), First Chairman of Urology (1904–1912)

A Department of Genito-Urinary Diseases was established in the Jefferson Hospital in August 1894. At that time, a body of Clinical Professors in various specialties was instituted but not admitted to full faculty Chairs. Among these was Dr. Orville Horwitz, who was appointed Clinical Professor of Genito-Urinary Diseases (Figure 47-1).

Horwitz was born in Washington, D.C., in June 1860.[1] He came from a distinguished medical family. His father, Phineas J. Horwitz, had been Surgeon-General and Medical Director of the U.S. Navy with special prominence during the Civil War, and his grandfather, Jonathan Horwitz, was an 1811 graduate of the University of Pennsylvania. Through marriage, the two daughters of Dr. Samuel D. Gross (Maria and Louisa) were his aunts. He took his B.S. degree from the University of Pennsylvania (1881) and his M.D. from Jefferson (1883).

After a year of internship at Jefferson Hospital, Horwitz spent three years in resident service at the Pennsylvania Hospital for the Insane and at the Pennsylvania Hospital. Following this he began an uninterrupted service in Jefferson Medical College and Hospital until his resignation in May 1912. His first position was as Demonstrator of Anatomy and subsequently as Demonstrator of Surgery for six years, during which time he worked with Drs. Samuel W. Gross and W.W. Keen.

When Horwitz was appointed Clinical Professor in 1894, he equipped the Department at his own expense. It started with ten cases, and was located

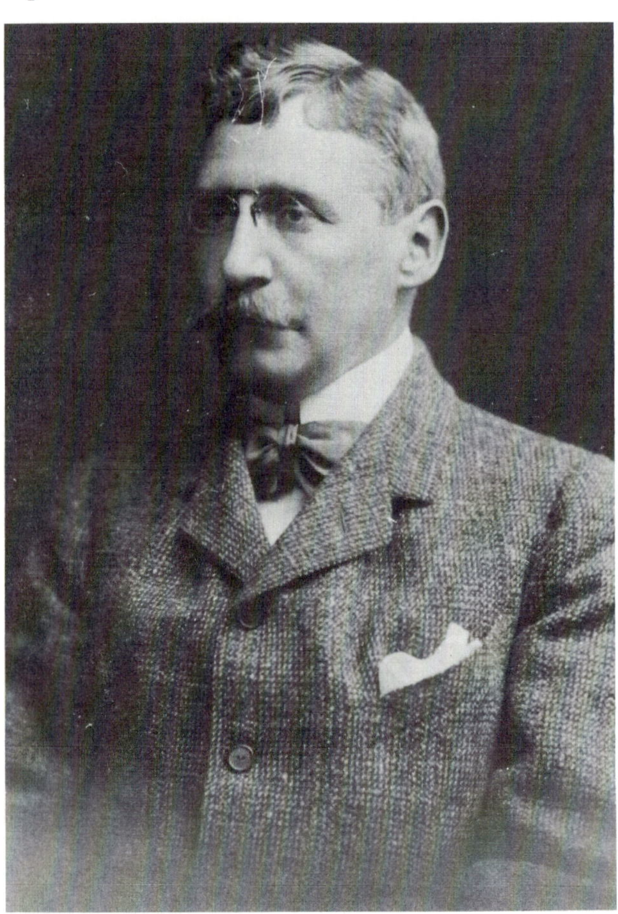

Fig. 47-1. Orville Horwitz, M.D., First Chairman (1904–1912).

on the second floor of the old 1877 Hospital, which has since been replaced by the Samuel Gustine Thompson Annex (1924). For a number of years no outlay was incurred by the Hospital for either equipment or maintenance, since support came from donations of grateful patients. By 1900 the number of new cases for the year was 2,398, and the number of old cases for the year was 21,778, making a total of 24,176. It became one of the largest Departments of the Hospital.

In May 1904, a formal Department in the College was established and Dr. Horwitz was admitted as full Professor to a Faculty Chair. In his short lifespan, cut off prematurely at the age of 53, he contributed many articles to the general surgical and urologic literature and made many presentation at local and national meetings in his field. The lectures of this debonair gentleman were popular among the students for their delivery and content (Figure 47-2). Ill health forced him to resign in May, 1912, and he died at his home, 1721 Walnut Street, January 28, 1913.

Hiram R. Loux, M.D. (1859–1930); Second Chairman (1913–1930)

The successor to Dr. Horwitz, Dr. Hiram Rittenhouse Loux (Figure 47-3), was born in Bucks County, Pennsylvania, in 1859.[2] He received his earliest education in the local schools and at age 13 entered Washington Hall in Trappe, Pennsylvania, from which he graduated in 1876. During the next three years he taught school in Montgomery and Bucks Counties.

Loux matriculated at Jefferson in 1879, where he came under the personal tutelage of Professor Samuel D. Gross. This fortunate circumstance allowed him to observe Gross in his hospital work and to be quizzed in the great surgeon's office at Eleventh and Walnut Streets on Sunday mornings. Gross convinced his protegé to take a three-year course rather than the customary two-year one of that day. Upon graduation with honors in 1882, he also received the Jacob Mendes DaCosta Prize in Medicine for his thesis entitled *High Temperature as a Cause of Heart Disease.*

For the next ten years Dr. Loux practiced general medicine in Souderton, Pennsylvania. An urge toward academic medicine brought him back to Philadelphia in 1892, where he immediately entered the surgical service of Professor W.W. Keen as Assistant in the Surgical Laboratory. A few months later he was appointed a Demonstrator of Surgery and Demonstrator of Fracture Dressings and Bandaging, a position he ably filled for 15 years. In 1894, when the Department of Urology was started in the Hospital, Dr. Loux was appointed Chief Clinical Assistant and Assistant Urologic Surgeon. A few years later he was made Assistant Professor of Urology. Upon the death of Dr. Horwitz in 1913, he was unanimously elected by the Board of Trustees to fill the Chair of Urology.

Dr. Loux was Assistant Surgeon to the Philadelphia General Hospital with Professor Horwitz, and for 18 years he was Senior Surgeon until his resignation from that institution in 1925.

In addition to numerous articles pertaining to general surgical subjects as well as urologic topics, Dr. Loux belonged to the local and national scientific societies in his field. The Class of 1926 dedicated the *Clinic Yearbook* to him and the Class of 1929 presented his portrait to the College. This nationally recognized clinician and surgeon died in February, 1930, while actively in service.

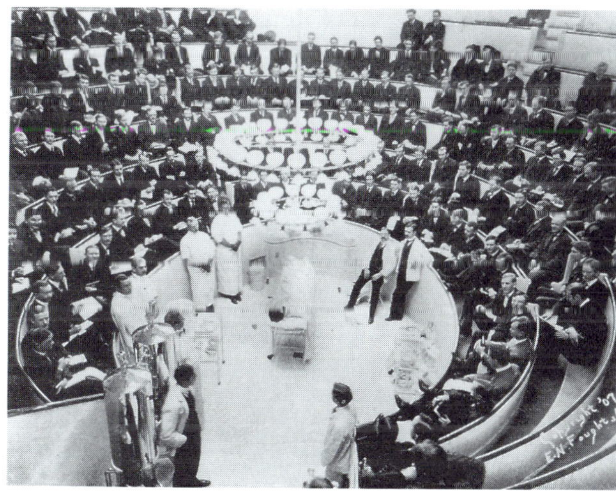

FIG. 47-2. The Clinic of Professor Orville Horwitz, in the pit of the 1877 Hospital (ca. 1907).

Although not directly related to Jefferson history, a major event of urologic importance occurred in the late 1920s. Dr. Moses Swick, Clinical Professor of Urology at the Mount Sinai School of Medicine in New York City, developed intravenous pyelography through his discovery of Uroselectan as a safe contrast medium for the diagnosis of many urologic disorders. This technique was quickly adopted by the Radiology Department at Jefferson and greatly enhanced the care of urologic patients.

Thomas C. Stellwagen, M.D. (1879–1935); Third Chairman (1930–1935)

Dr. Thomas Cooke Stellwagen (Figure 47-4), who succeeded Dr. Loux in 1930, was born in Media, Pennsylvania, in 1879.[3] His ancestors were among the early settlers in Delaware and were distinguished for their service in the U.S. Navy. A graduate of Jefferson in the Class of 1903, Dr. Stellwagen served in World War I first with the British Army and then as a member of Jefferson Base Hospital Unit No. 38. He was sent to the front in charge of a mobile unit and served as a surgeon until the signing of the Armistice agreement.

In addition to his scientific articles, Dr. Stellwagen was a charter member and President of the Genito-Urinary Society and was a member of the Association of Genito-Urinary Surgeons and the American Urological Association. As a surgeon of distinction, he was greatly respected by the students for his teaching. The Class of 1936 barely

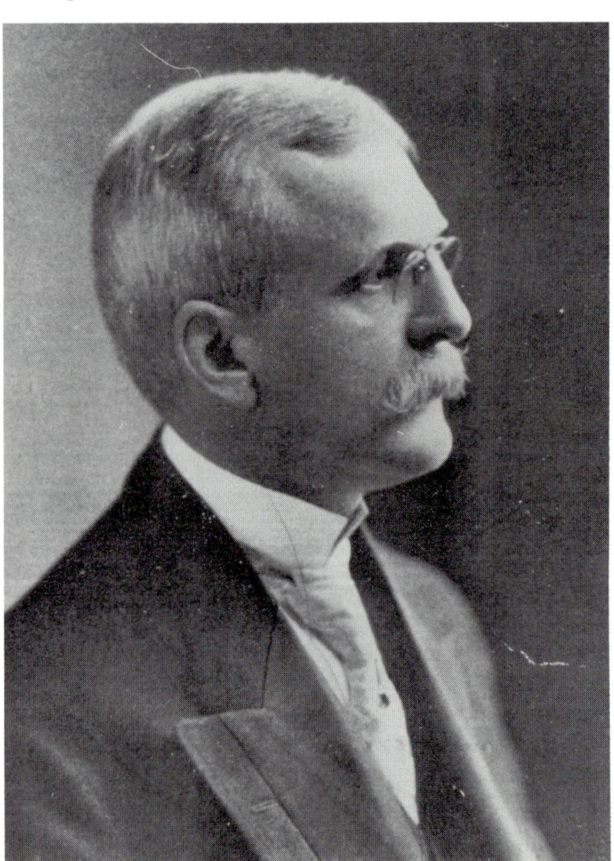

Fig. 47-3. Hiram R. Loux, M.D., Second Chairman (1913–1930).

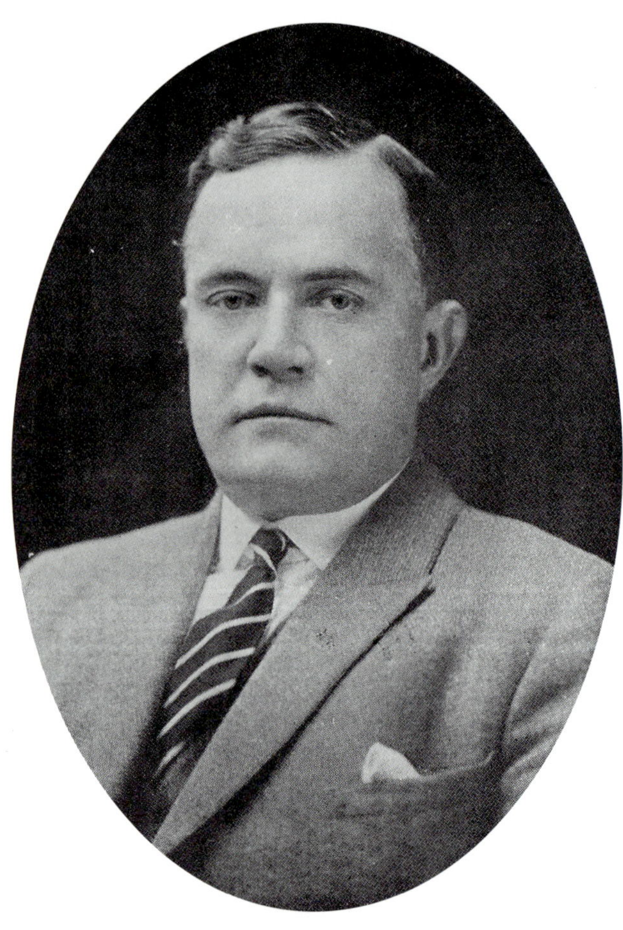

Fig. 47-4. Thomas C. Stellwagen, M.D., Third Chairman (1930–1935).

accomplished the painting of his portrait before his sudden premature death on March 16, 1935, from a heart attack at the age of 56.

David M. Davis, M.D. (1886–1982); Fourth Chairman (1935–1951)

Dr. David Melvin Davis (Figure 47-5) was appointed to succeed Dr. Stellwagen on September 19, 1935.[4,5] Born in Buffalo, New York,

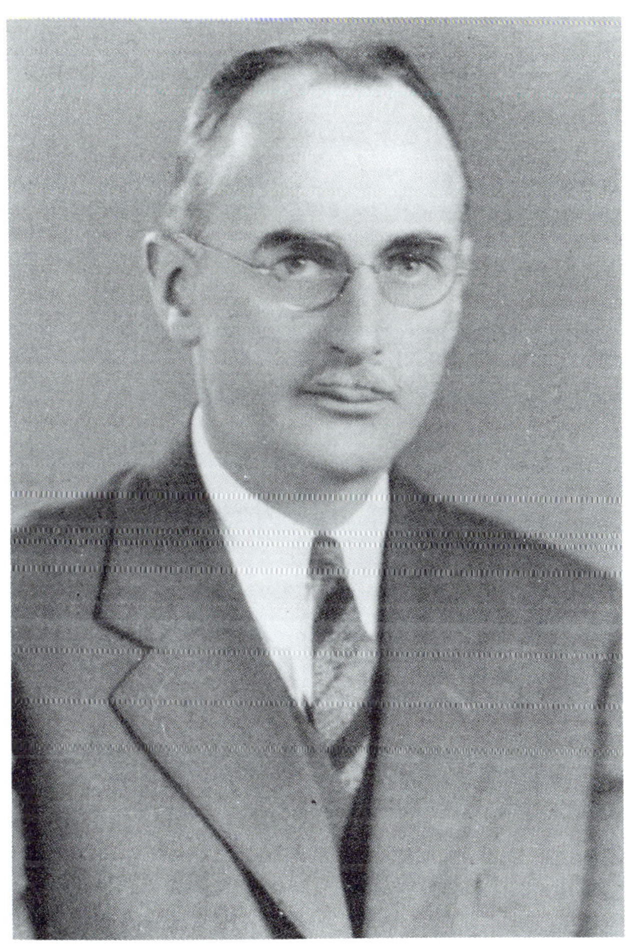

FIG. 47-5. David M. Davis, M.D., Fourth Chairman (1935–1951).

in 1886, he was educated in the public schools there, graduated from Princeton University in 1907, and received his M.D. degree at the Medical School of Johns Hopkins University in 1911. He became a member of Phi Beta Kappa and Alpha Omega Alpha Honorary Societies, respectively, in those institutions. After a year of internship at the Baltimore City Hospital, he became Assistant in Pathology at Hopkins for two years (1913 and 1914), and then Pathologist and Director of Research of the Brady Urological Institute (1914–17). He was made Associate Editor of the *Journal of Urology* at the time of its inception (1917).

At the outbreak of World War I in 1914, Dr. Davis was studying chemistry in Munich. In 1915 he served as Bacteriologist to the American Ambulance Hospital at Neuilly-sur-Seine, France. After attending the Citizens Training Camp at Plattsburg, New York, he was sent abroad as First Lieutenant in the Medical Corps. For those two years he was first attached to the British Army and later with the American Expeditionary Forces, where he rose to the rank of Major.

Back at the Brady Institute of Johns Hopkins, Davis spent a year of research on the gonococcus organism, completed a residency in Urology, and then spent two years preparing the manuscript of *Practice of Urology* as a coauthor with his famous mentor, Dr. Hugh H. Young. In 1924 he was Head of Urology in the new medical school at the University of Rochester, where he organized the Department. In 1928 he resigned to return to Baltimore as an Associate of Dr. Hugh Young. Curiously, in 1930 he went to Phoenix, Arizona, where he abandoned academic urology for private practice.

During the strange interlude (1930–1935) of this brilliant academician in Arizona, he served as Visiting Urologist at the Desert Sanitarium at Tucson. Dean Ross V. Patterson became interested in Dr. Davis as a candidate for the vacant Chair of Urology at Jefferson and received impressive letters of recommendation from Hopkins and the University of Rochester where Dr. Davis had served. Thus followed his appointment to the Chair and the 16 fruitful years at Jefferson.

As an investigator, teacher (Figure 47-6), clinician and authority in urologic surgery, Dr. Davis became known throughout the world. Shortly after his arrival, the Department of Genito-Urinary Diseases changed its name to the Department of Urology. The teaching system was modified by a gradual reduction of didactic lectures and emphasis on small groups with student participation. Dr. Davis was a severe quizmaster with an uncomfortable mixture of invective and cajolery until his point was strongly driven home.

In 1946 a Professorship in Urology was established under the bequest of Henry Reed Hatfield as a memorial to his father, Nathan Lewis Hatfield. Dr. Davis was its first occupant. He was also the first recipient of the Hugh Hampton Young Award of the American Urological Association in 1969. In addition to his memberships in a galaxy of scientific societies, he was President of the Medical and Surgical Association of the Southwest (1934–1935), of the Mid-Atlantic Section of the American Urological Association (1941–1942), and of the Philadelphia Urological Society (1943–1945). He held honorary membership in Urologic Societies of Britain, Greece, Mexico, and Argentina.

Under Dr. Davis's leadership, advanced training in Urology was established. The first residencies at Jefferson started in 1937 in Obstetrics under Dr. P. Brooke Bland, and the Department of Urology established one in 1939. World War II caused a delay in increasing the number of residents, but a second was created in 1946 and a third in 1947. In 1948 an arrangement with Professor John H. Gibbon, Jr., provided a year of training in General Surgery before beginning three years in the Urologic Residency.

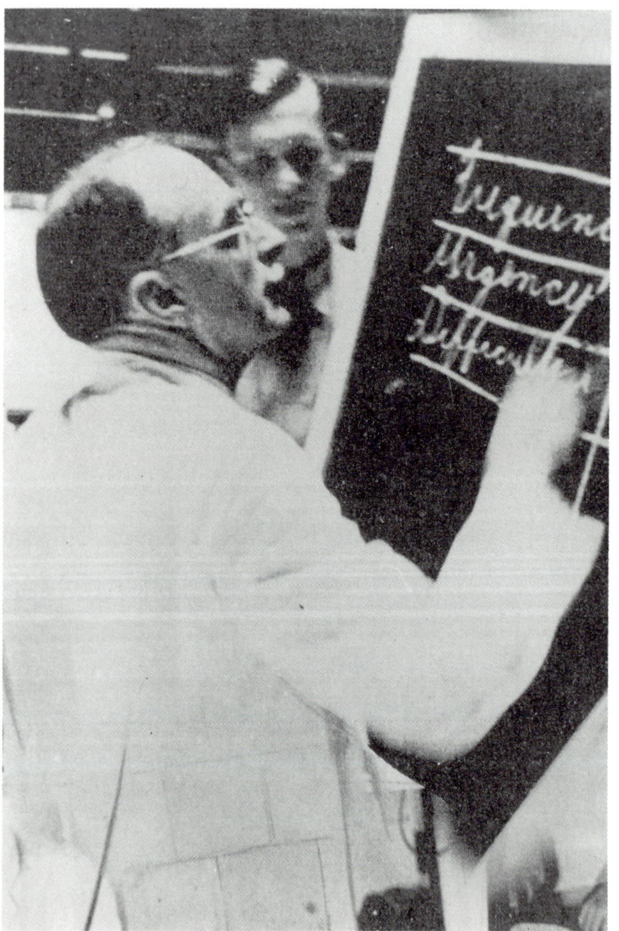

FIG. 47-6. Professor David M. Davis instructing students in the pit of the Thomas Annex (ca. 1948).

Dr. Davis greatly improved the standard of care in the Urology Ward and Curtis Clinic. His teaching staff was strengthened by such members as Theodore R. Fetter, Walter W. Baker, George H. Strong, and Harry Bogaev. Four of these members were certified by the American Board of Urology, four served as Presidents of the Philadelphia Urological Society, and two became Presidents of the Mid-Atlantic Section of the American Urological Association.

In addition to more than 130 journal articles, after academic retirement Dr. Davis wrote a textbook *Mechanisms of Urologic Disease* (1953). He designed a cystoscopic-roentgenographic-fluoroscopic table constructed in Philadelphia by the Franklin X-ray Corporation. On this table the patient rested on a traveling carriage that moved by hydraulic motors back over the X-ray apparatus after the ureteral catheters were in place. His particular interests were in hypospadias, hydronephrosis, and early diagnosis and radical operations for carcinoma of the prostate.

Dr. Davis was most unhappy that the rules of the Board of Trustees caused his compulsory retirement to Emeritus status at age 65 in 1951. The Class of 1952 presented his portrait to the College. He remained active in practice, research, and authorship of articles for another 17 years until December 31, 1968, at which time he was 82 years of age. He died in 1982 at the age of 96.

Theodore R. Fetter, M.D., Sc.D. (1903–1967); Fifth Chairman (1951–1967)

Like Dr. Davis, Dr. Theodore Roosevelt Fetter (Figure 47-7), appointed June 15, 1951, was also to serve as Chairman of Urology for 16 years.[6] Born in Schaefferstown, Pennsylvania, in 1903, he grew up in Atlantic City, New Jersey, where he attended public schools. He took his premedical education at Lafayette College and graduated from Jefferson in the Class of 1926. This was followed by an internship at Jefferson Medical College Hospital for 27 months.

Dr. Fetter promptly chose urology as his lifetime professional interest. In 1929 he was appointed as Assistant in Genito-Urinary Surgery under Professor Hiram R. Loux. He subsequently became the personal assistant to Professor Thomas Stellwagen, who succeeded Dr. Loux. Following the untimely death of Dr. Stellwagen in 1935, Dr. Fetter had the unique opportunity of serving under a third distinguished Professor of Urology, namely Dr. David M. Davis. During these years he worked intensively in the outpatient and on the ward services, where he became especially interested and expert in cystocopy. He also devoted much time to urologic pathology under Dr. Baxter L. Crawford, the Director of Clinical Laboratories in the Hospital.

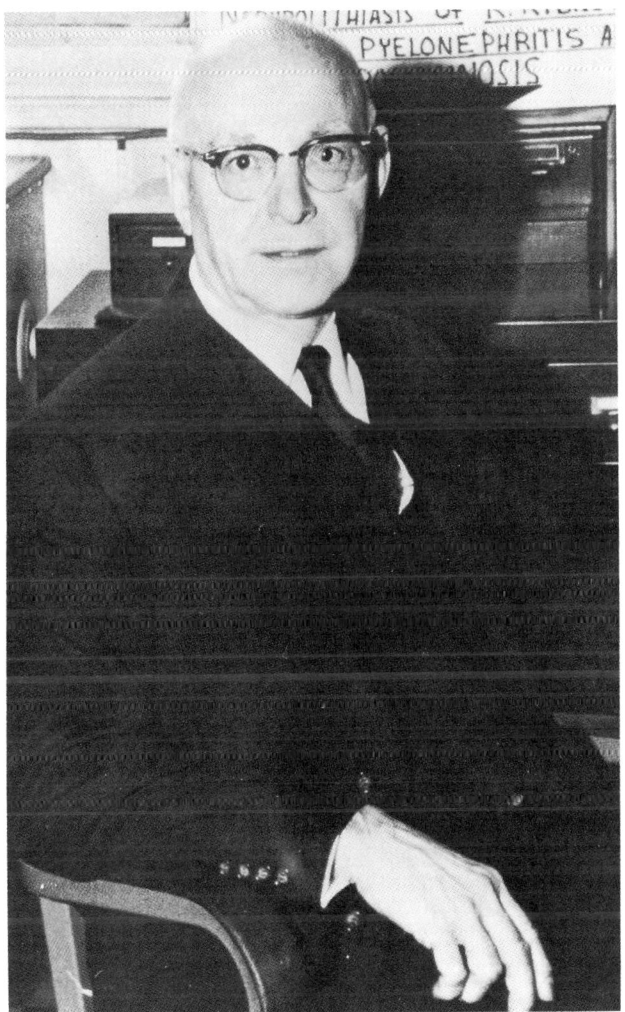

FIG. 47-7. Theodore R. Fetter, M.D., Fifth Chairman (1951–1967).

Modern urology was developing rapidly during these years, based upon newer knowledge of physiology and microbiology. Intravenous pyelography, better cystoscopes, resector-Bovie machines for electric current cutting and coagulation, use of antibiotics, and anesthesia with use of intravenous fluids and blood loss replacement, were all major advances. Dr. Frederick B. Wagner, Jr. (Jefferson, 1941), of the Surgery Department, contributed pioneer work on arteriography in renal diagnosis as related to hypertension, renal artery lesions, and tumors, which was reported in the *Journal of Urology* in 1946.[7] Dr. Davis and his staff, Drs. Charles W. Bonney (Jefferson, 1904), Willard H. Kinney (Jefferson, 1906), James McCahey, Harry Bogaev, and Theodore R. Fetter stayed in the forefront of these advances. Dr. Fetter, as a stellar clinician within the Department, rose through the ranks to Associate Professor and became Chairman upon the retirement of Dr. Davis in 1951. In 1959 Dr. Fetter was named the second Nathan Lewis Hatfield Professor of Urology. In that same year Lebanon Valley College awarded him an Honorary Doctor of Science degree.

In addition to his distinction as a clinician, Professor Fetter contributed nearly 100 articles to the urologic literature on a wide spectrum of topics. These papers were delivered at numerous local and national meetings. He assisted in revising the chapters on genito-urinary disease in the Anspach *Gynecology*.

As a teacher (Figure 47-8), Dr. Fetter was a hard taskmaster and continued Dr. Davis's custom of intimidating the students. His mind was sharp and critical in ward rounds, in which he displayed a broad knowledge of medicine beyond his own specialty. His urologic residents received excellent clinical training under his direct supervision, especially in cystoscopy. To him the giving of the ultimate in the scientific and compassionate care of patients was the most important aspect of medicine.

Although he served as Urologic Consultant to several other hospitals, Fetter's entire career was at Jefferson. He was continually active in the Alumni Association, in which he served as President in 1950. During the fund-raising campaign that started in 1951 in preparation for the "New Pavilion" of 1954 (later named Foerderer in 1962) Dr. Fetter served as Chairman of the Medical Staff Campaign Committee. He rarely missed a faculty meeting or his many committee meetings, and served as President of the Executive Staff of the Hospital for seven years.

From his earliest days in medicine, Dr. Fetter recognized an obligation to organized medicine to which he gave long and devoted service throughout his career. He served as President of the Philadelphia County Medical Society (1948) and the Pennsylvania State Medical Society (1952). He was also President of the Mid-Atlantic Section of the American Urological Association.

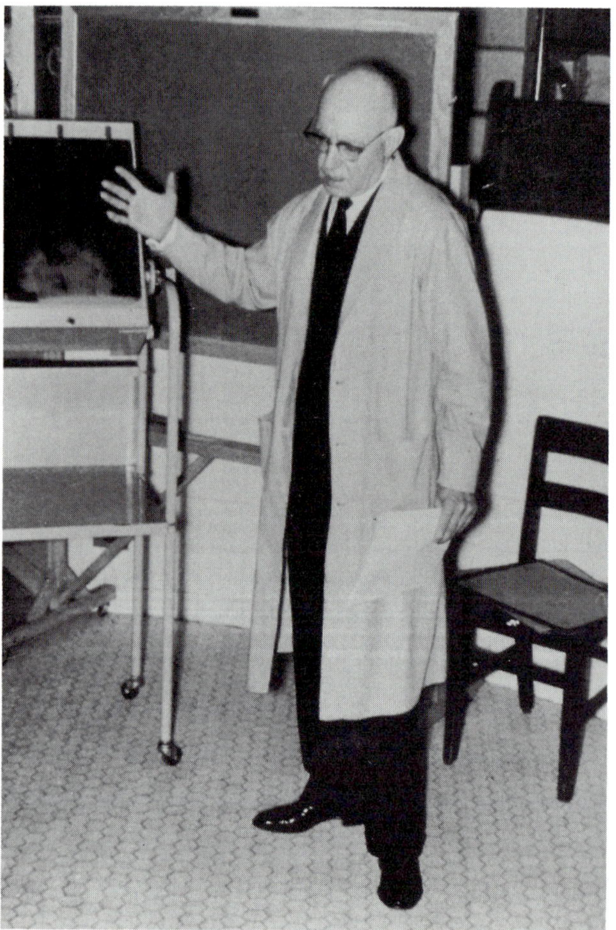

FIG. 47-8. Professor Theodore R. Fetter in the pit of the Thompson Annex (ca. 1960).

Professor Fetter's Chairmanship was still in the era when only the Heads of the Departments in the basic sciences were full-time and fully salaried. He carried on a large private practice in an office outside the Hospital in addition to his many Hospital and College responsibilities. Unexpectedly, he died on January 19, 1967, at age 64 from a heart attack complicated by cerebral emboli. His portrait, given by his family, was accepted by the College in an impressive ceremony on November 8, 1968.

Paul D. Zimskind, M.D., Ph.D. (1931–1976); Sixth Chairman (1967–1976)

Paul Donald Zimskind (Figure 47-9), who succeeded Dr. Fetter in July, 1967, was born in Trenton, New Jersey, in 1931.[8] His father, Dr. Joshua N. Zimskind, graduated from Jefferson in the Class of 1927. After receiving his elementary and high school education in Trenton, he graduated *magna cum laude* from Princeton University in 1953. He was awarded his M.D. degree from Jefferson in 1957. An internship, residency in general surgery for one year, and residency for three years in urology were then completed at Jefferson. With the award of a Postdoctoral Fellowship by the National Institutes of Health, Dr. Zimskind continued as a full-time graduate student in the Department of Physiology, earned his Ph.D. degree in 1964 (Figure 47-10), and maintained an appointment in the Urology Department as Research Associate. His thesis was on *Studies of Urethral Dynamics*. In an academic career in Urology oriented chiefly to research and teaching, he was appointed Assistant Professor at Jefferson in 1964 on a geographic full-time basis and in charge of the Urology Research Laboratories.

In 1966 Dr. Zimskind was selected as one of the 25 Markle Scholars in Academic Medicine out of

68 candidates from throughout the United States and Canada. The John and Mary R. Markle Foundation of New York City provides a total sum of $30,000 at the rate of $6,000 per year for five years to the medical school at which the scholar will teach or do research or administration. This sum is used to supplement salary, aid research, and otherwise assist in the development of the scholar as a teacher or investigator. The committee at Jefferson unanimously proposed Dr. Zimskind as their candidate for this national honor. Little was he to know that during his second year as a Markle Scholar at the age of 36 he would be assuming the Chairmanship of the Department of Urology.

Dr. Zimskind was the natural, undisputed candidate to replace the sudden loss of Dr. Fetter. He became the first full-time, fully salaried Chairman and Nathan Lewis Hatfield Professor of Urology as well as one of the youngest men to reach the status of Executive Faculty. The appointment as Chairman did not interfere with his Markle Scholarship since the combined funds for his salary amounted to a modest $24,000 in 1968.

Dr. Zimskind's accomplishments in education, research, and patient care were commensurate with someone far beyond his years. His Urodynamics Laboratory at Jefferson had an international reputation for its productivity and excellence. He led studies on the dynamics of normal and abnormal urinary conduction using pressure recordings and fluoroscopic motion pictures of urinary tract activity; he evaluated the various laboratory, radiographic, and clinical features in

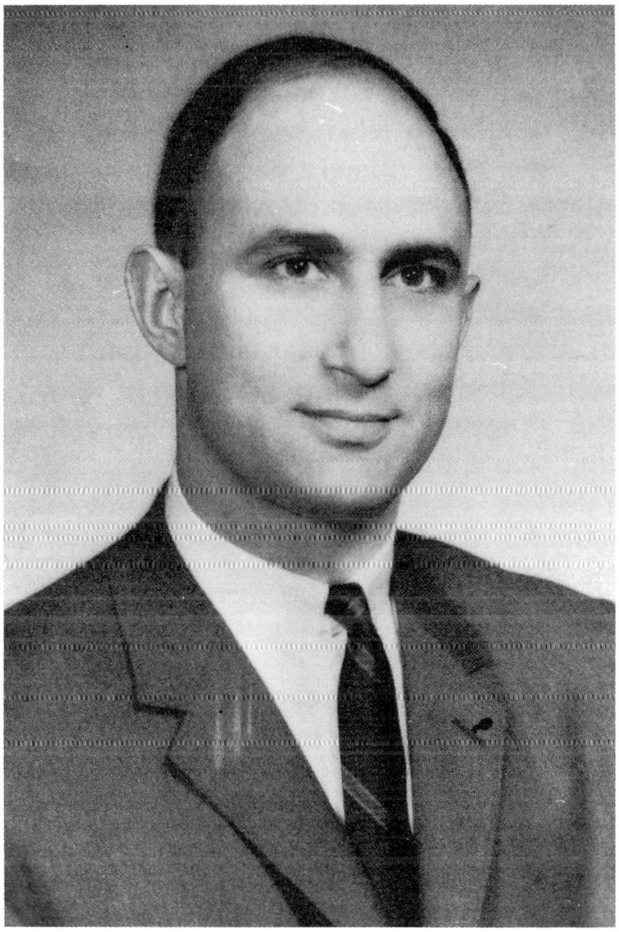

FIG. 47-9. Paul D. Zimskind, M.D., Ph.D., Sixth Chairman (1967–1976).

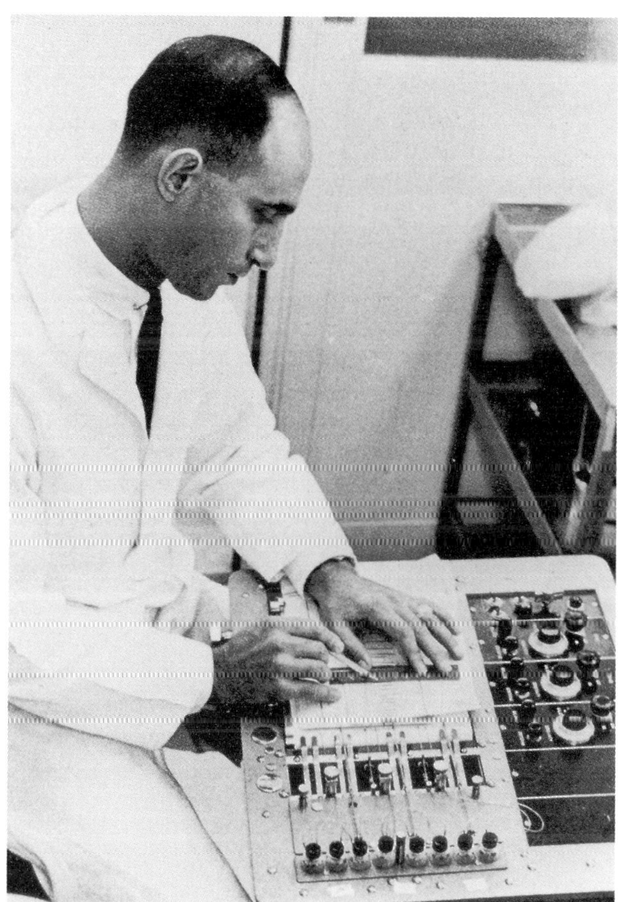

FIG. 47-10. Paul D. Zimskind, M.D., as a research graduate student (ca. 1963).

patients with renovascular hypertension in an effort to establish firm criteria for differentiating potentially correctible versus noncorrectible cases; and he designed projects to discover means of enhancing the preservation of functional renal and ureteral tissues for future organ transplantation.

As a teacher, Dr. Zimskind's lectures to the medical students were models of meticulous organization and clarity, coupled with a most engaging manner of delivery. He stimulated students and his residents in research problems. By the time of his sudden death at age 44, he had written 43 scientific papers and made 77 presentations worldwide.

Beyond his distinction as an educator, researcher, and clinician, Dr. Zimskind was an accomplished violinist who found time to participate in chamber music groups. He had a profound interest in classical and modern theater, accompanied by acting ability, radio experience, and occasional participation as a narrator for documentary motion pictures. In addition to his memberships in the various prestigious urologic societies, he belonged to the Philadelphia Art Museum, the Philadelphia Zoological Society, and was a volunteer in the Philadelphia Council for International Visitors, an organization that provides entertainment of foreign visitors in the home. He was an avid tennis player and photographer.

The entire Jefferson community was shocked by Dr. Zimskind's sudden death on February 29, 1976. This 44-year-old, beloved Chairman was apparently afflicted with an insidious form of Addison's disease that had not previously manifested itself, except, on retrospect, by an unusually dark complexion ascribed easily to his love of the outdoors. Family, colleagues, and friends presented his portrait to the College on April 15, 1983.

Stanford Grant Mulholland, M.D.; Seventh Chairman (1977–)

Jules H. Bogaev, M.D., Clinical Professor of Urology, became Acting Chairman of the Department until the appointment of S. Grant Mulholland as Nathan Lewis Hatfield Professor and Head of the Department on October 1, 1977.

Mulholland (Figure 47-11) was born in Springfield, Ohio, on September 1, 1936. Two years later, his family moved to the Philadelphia area, where he has remained. His father was a prominent Philadelphia urologist who was Professor and Chairman of the Department of Urology at the Medical College of Pennsylvania. After attending Episcopal Academy, Dr. Mulholland received his B.S. Degree from Dickinson College in 1958, his M.D. from Temple University in 1962, and later an M.S. degree from the University of Virginia (1966). His thesis for the latter was *The Effect of Vesical Mucosa on Bacterial Growth.*

With interest in smaller town practice, Dr. Mulholland took his internship at the Reading Hospital in Reading, Pennsylvania. He then chose one year of general surgical training in Florida at the Tampa General Hospital (1963–1964). This was

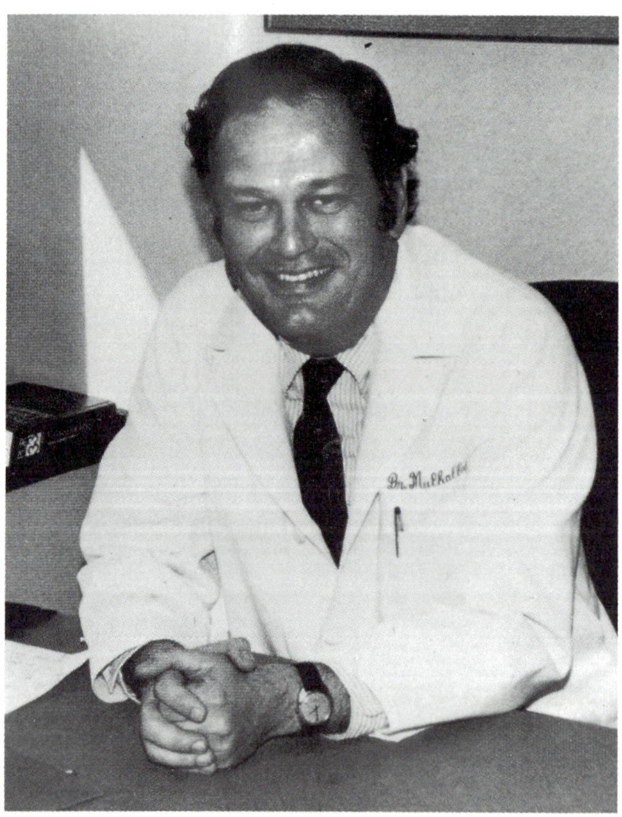

FIG. 47-11. S. Grant Mulholland, M.D., Seventh Chairman (1976–).

followed by residency training in urology at the University of Virginia Hospital, Charlottesville, Virginia (1964–1968). During this period his research interest in urinary tract infection was stimulated and persisted for the ensuing 25 years. Although he became well known for his contributions in this field, his research interests diversified into other areas as well.

After his training at the University of Virginia, Dr. Mulholland entered the U.S. Navy and served at St. Albans Naval Hospital in Queens, New York City (1968–1970). It was during this time that he cared for Vietnam veterans and became interested in urologic trauma. After this tour of duty, Dr. Mulholland secured a position at the University of Pennsylvania as Assistant Professor of Urology (1970–1974) with promotion to Associate Professor (1974–1977). During his seven years there his interest in clinical urology was vastly extended into pediatric urology, surgery for stone disease, and urologic oncology. He served as a Urologist at the Veterans Hospital in West Philadelphia, Children's Hospital, and the Hospital of the University of Pennsylvania. He was also Chief of Urology at the Philadelphia General Hospital through its closure in the mid-1970s.

Dr. Mulholland's immediate goal on arrival at Jefferson was the organization of highest quality teaching for the medical students and residents, which resulted in heightened popularity of the Department. Research was expanded by appointment of Hugh J. Callahan, Ph.D., a biochemist, and three laboratory technicians. The main research interests centered on infection, infertility, and cancer. In 1983, Demetrius H. Bagley, M.D., an international authority on endourology and instrumentation of the entire urinary tract, was added to the staff as Associate Professor in Urology and Radiology. Under Dr. Bagley the Department developed extracorporeal lithotripsy for dissolution of urinary tract stones. Dr. Mulholland also developed the Sexual Function Center, which became well known locally and nationally. Irvin H. Hirsch, M.D., appointed in 1985, added the specialty of infertility and neurourology. This led to activities in sperm banking, artificial insemination, and artificial ejaculation stimulation of spinal cord-injured patients and neurological patients.

Dr. Mulholland has authored nearly 100 scientific articles over the past 25 years. He is a member of the important local, national, and international organizations in his field. Among his many committee activities may be mentioned the Executive Committee of the Philadelphia Urologic Society (President-Elect in 1987) and the Mid-Atlantic Section of the American Urological Association.

In all aspects of modern urology–teaching, research and full-service care, the Department is in a strong competitive stance for continued leadership and productivity.

References

1. *Jeffersonian*, Vol. 14, No. 12, March 1913, p. 17. (In the Archives of Thomas Jefferson University.)
2. "Death of Professor Hiram R. Loux," *Jeff. Med. Coll. Al. Bull.*, Vol. 1, No. 14, May 1930, p. 8.
3. "Sketch of Thomas Cook Stellwagen," *Clinic Yearbook*, 1930, p. 12.
4. Swenson, P.C., "Speech Delivered at Dedication of Portrait of D.M. Davis, April 24, 1952." (In the Archives of Thomas Jefferson University.)
5. "Obituary of David M. Davis, M.D.," *Jeff. Med. Coll. Al. Bull.*, Vol. 31, No. 4, Summer 1982, p. 37.
6. Montgomery, J.B.; "Memoir of Theodore R. Fetter (1903–1967)," *Trans. Stud. Coll. Phys. Phila.*, Ser. 4, Vol. 36, 1968–1969, pp. 174–175.
7. Wagner, F.B., Jr., "Arteriography in Renal Diagnosis: Preliminary Report and Critical Evaluation," *Jour. Urol.* 56:625–635, 1946.
8. Davis, D.M., "Paul D. Zimskind (1931–1976)," *Trans. Stud. Coll. Phys. Phila.*, Vol. 44: 107–108, October 1976.

PART IV

University Components and Activities

CHAPTER FORTY-EIGHT

The Board of Trustees

FREDERICK B. WAGNER, JR., M.D.

"If the Board is to function successfully as a catalyst of University deliberations, it must consist of people of diverse backgrounds."

—FREDERIC L. BALLARD, ESQ. (BOARD CHAIRMAN, 1977–1984)

IN A letter dated June 2, 1824, the Board of Trustees of Jefferson College in Canonsburg, Pennsylvania (Figure 48-1), received a request that their institution be the parent to a Medical Department in Philadelphia. Three physicians and a chemist who signed the letter declared they had formed themselves into a Medical Faculty that would establish thereby a second medical school in Philadelphia. These men were George McClellan, M.D., John Eberle, M.D., Joseph Klapp, M.D., and Jacob Green, Esq. (Figure 48-2).

The guiding genius and undisputed leader was George McClellan. He had conducted a private school in Philadelphia in which his pupils had received good practical medical and surgical instruction. His hands were tied, however, in that he could not complete their education, could not graduate them, and could not grant them an M.D. degree. Along with others before him, he had been unable to obtain a college charter from the State Legislature. His efforts were absolutely refused by the powers at Harrisburg through influential people in medical educational circles of Philadelphia who opposed his plan. Frustrated by his own inability to obtain a charter, McClellan conceived the artful device of looking elsewhere for an institution with the necessary authority to grant diplomas in medicine. The petition to Jefferson College at Canonsburg merely asked their Trustees to assume the nominal guardianship of a medical branch in Philadelphia only to the extent of giving it legal standing with right to confer the degree of Doctor of Medicine.

Within the same month the Board at Canonsburg freely accepted the new trusteeship. They saw no impropriety in establishing a medical branch in a distant city. Although a strict Presbyterian institution, they were not parochial; their goal was to promote general education, and this was just such an opportunity. It is historically germane to indicate that the prompt response might have been aided by the fact that one of the

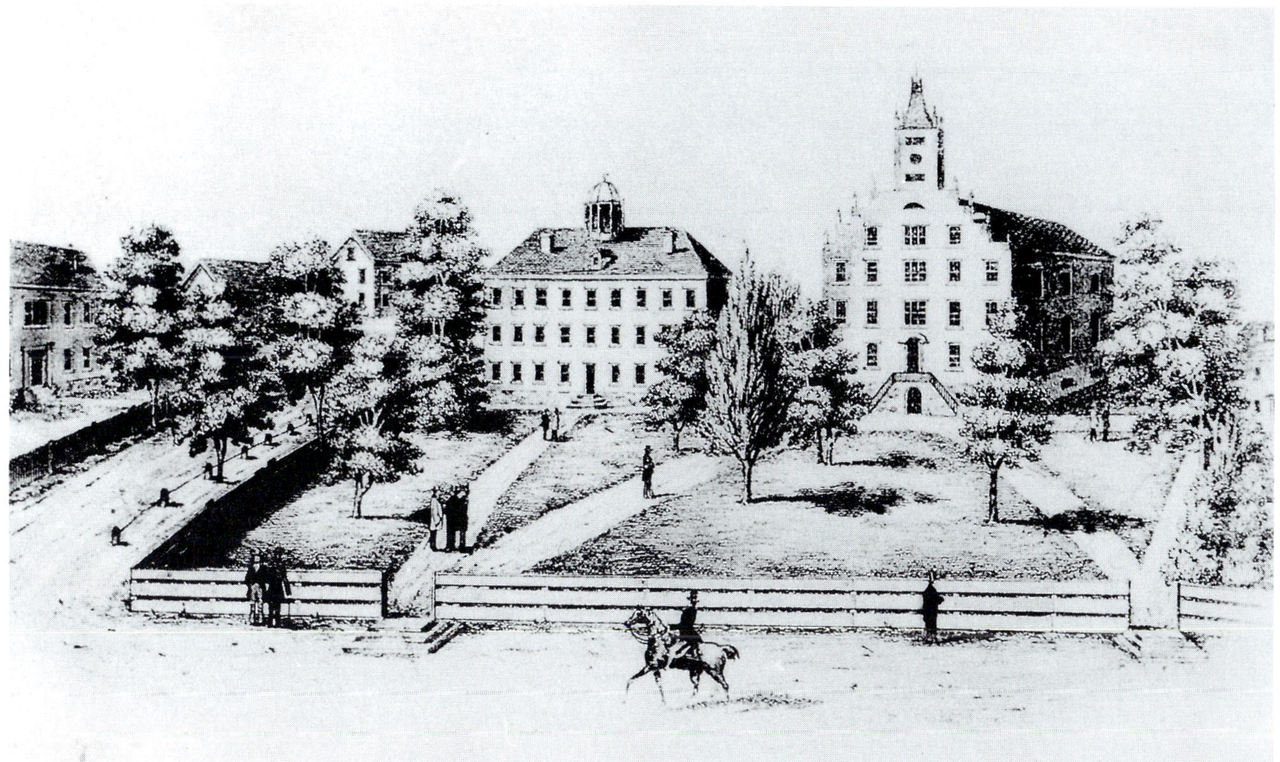

FIG. 48-1. Jefferson College at Canonsburg, 1850. (Courtesy of H.T.W. Coleman, *Banners in the Wilderness*. University of Pittsburgh Press, 1956.)

petitioners, Jacob Green, was the son of a prominent member of the Canonsburg Board, the Reverend Ashbel Green, D.D.

The Canonsburg Trustees of Jefferson Medical College (1824–1838)

The Jefferson College at Canonsburg in western Pennsylvania was chartered in 1802 and named in honor of Thomas Jefferson, who at the time was the third President of the United States. In 1824 the President of the Board was Samuel Ralston, D.D., of Williamsport. Other members from the Presbyterian clergy were F. Herron, D.D.; Robert Johnson; E.P. Swift; Thomas D. Baird; Moses Allen; and William Tiffany (all from Pittsburgh); and the Reverend Ashbel Green, D.D., from Philadelphia. Members from the laity were John McDonald, Benjamin Williams, John Litherman, Craig Ritchie, John Reid, James Carr, William Johnson, John Phillips, Samuel Logan, William Cloaky, and Andrew Monro.

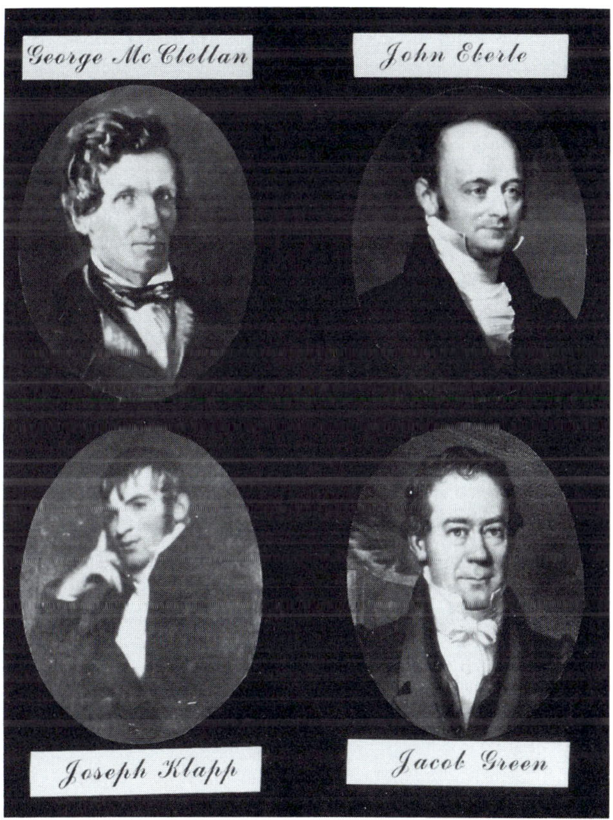

FIG. 48-2. The Founders of Jefferson Medical College.

The Canonsburg Board gave its Medical Department (The Jefferson Medical College of Philadelphia) an existence only, with the sole addition of moral support. In October 1824 they expressly provided in their "Articles of Union" that they would not assume or support any financial obligations but would commend it to students preparing for the medical profession. McClellan promptly assembled a faculty of five professors, rented and had remodeled the Tivoli Theater (Figure 48-3) at 518–520 Prune Street (now Locust), and initiated the formal first academic session of 1825–1826. The University of Pennsylvania thereupon challenged the authority of the "new school" to grant the M.D. degree, with a formal protest on January 30, 1826, that was read in the Pennsylvania Senate.

To settle the issue, the Trustees at Canonsburg engaged in a legal battle before the State Legislature. When McClellan learned that a vote was to be taken on April 7, 1826, he made his legendary ride in horse and sulky, starting the previous day in order to reach Harrisburg for a personal, last-minute plea. So convincing was Dr. McClellan in the Legislature that the bill was passed and signed by Governor J. Andrew Shulze. This allowed the first commencement, which had been postponed from March, to take place on April 14. It was a stunning victory for Jefferson.

The Legislative Act of April 7, 1826, gave the Trustees at Canonsburg the authority to elect ten "Additional Trustees, who may be residents of the city or county of Philadelphia" to superintend Jefferson Medical College.

"Additional Trustees" of Jefferson Medical College (1826–1838)

Ironically, on August 9, 1826, William Tilghman, as Chief Justice of the Supreme Court of Pennsylvania, found it as probably an embarrassing duty to administer the oath of office to the first "Additional Trustee," Edward King, LL.D. Tilghman was also President of the Board of Trustees of the University of Pennsylvania and had written the document in the Senate that opposed Jefferson Medical College as a Medical Department of Canonsburg College. King, who was President Judge of the First District Common Pleas of Philadelphia, in accord with the law, swore in the other nine members, all of whom were outstanding in the religious, legal, military, and business community of Philadelphia: Samuel Badger, James M. Broom, Joel B. Sutherland, Samuel Humphreys, Edward Ingersoll, Charles S. Cox, General William Duncan, the Rev. Ashbel Green, D.D., LL.D., and the Rev. Ezra Stiles Ely, D.D. Thus was established the first Board of Trustees that was directly representative of the Medical College. Their proceedings were subject to approval by the parent Board at Canonsburg and with no voice in the councils related to the mother College.

The new Trustees made regulations governing their own body in the transactions of business and also established rules for authority over the faculty. They required all the Professors to accept these rules and hold their respective Chairs subject to

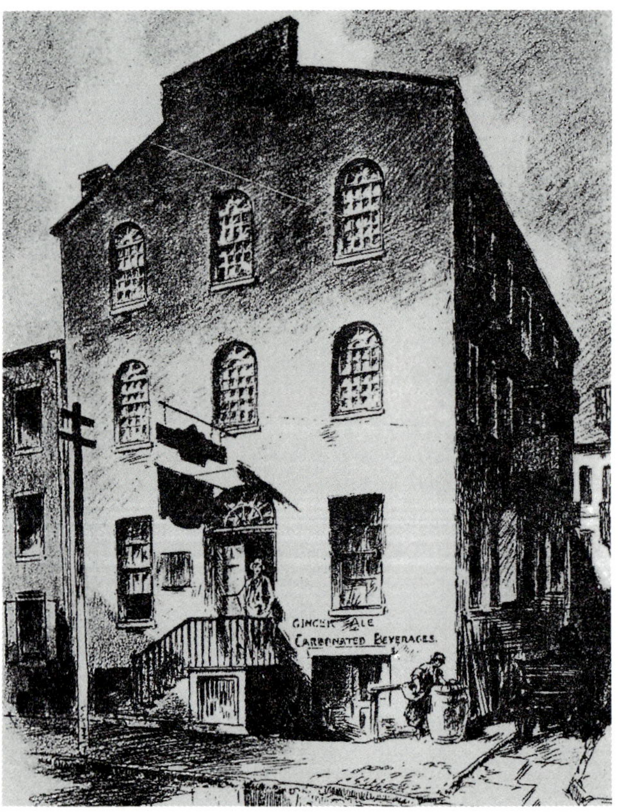

Fig. 48-3. The first Jefferson Medical College Building, the renovated Tivoli Theater at 518–520 Prune Street (now Locust).

them. From the outset the Trustees gave closest scrutiny to the qualifications of new candidates for Professorship or to the disciplining of the old.

The first book of Minutes, handwritten, of the Jefferson Medical College Board of Trustees records the proceedings from August 9, 1826, to February 19, 1840 (Figure 48-4). The first minutes indicated that the Rev. Ashbel Green, D.D., a member of the General Board of Trustees of Jefferson College of Canonsburg, was requested to attend the meeting of August 16 and act as President. On August 31, 1826, only two weeks later, a resolution was communicated to the General Board at Canonsburg that the Chair of Midwifery held by Dr. Francis S. Beattie be vacated. The minutes of September 6 record a resolution "that the committee investigating Dr. Beattie be thanked for their just care of the honor and interests of the school." On September 28, it was recommended that Dr. John Barnes be appointed temporarily to fill the Chair. This was the first decisive action of the Board regarding an "unpleasant inquiry." A more sweeping action was taken in June, 1828, when the Additional Trustees under approval by the General Board vacated all the Chairs and reorganized the faculty. This required "that those gentlemen who were lately Professors in the Medical Faculty of Jefferson Medical College, if they wished to be considered candidates for Professorships, must make application accordingly, or they will not be considered as candidates."

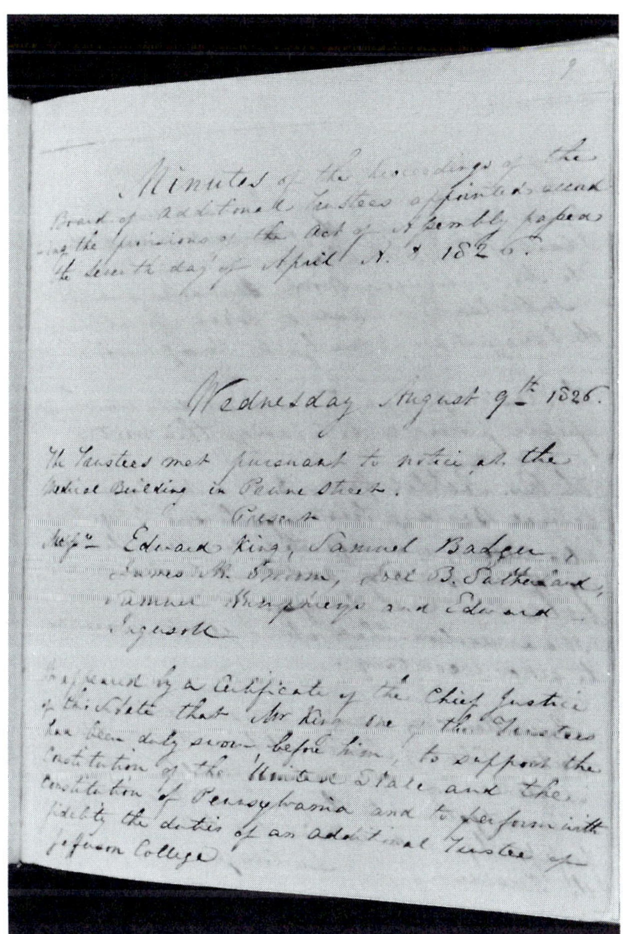

Minutes of the Proceedings of the Board of Additional Trustees appointed according to the provisions of the Act of Assembly passed the seventh day of April A.D. 1826.

Wednesday August 9th 1826.

The Trustees met pursuant to notice at the Medical Building in Prune Street.

Present

Messrs Edward King, Samuel Badger, James R. Brown, Joel B. Sutherland, Samuel Humphreys and Edward Ingersoll

It appeared by a Certificate of the Chief Justice of this State that Mr King one of the Trustees has been duly sworn before him, to support the Constitution of the United States and the Constitution of Pennsylvania and to perform with fidelity the duties of an additional Trustee of Jefferson College

FIG. 48-4. The first page of the Minutes of the "Additional Trustees" of Jefferson Medical College of Philadelphia, dated August 9, 1826.

At first, the General Board at Canonsburg was inclined to hold the Additional Trustees to strict account, but with the actions of the local Philadelphia Trustees showing evidence of watchfulness and control, the General Board virtually regarded the determinations of the locals as conclusive. On the other hand, the Trustees gave the faculty wide latitude in matters of policy. The Professors had founded the school and were responsible for its success and financial survival. The school was proprietary, in that students paid for their individual courses directly to the respective Professors. The Professors in turn paid for rent and maintenance of the building, but kept the profit. The local and general Trustees disclaimed any financial responsibility. Although the Trustees had established early that the faculty was not the supreme power of the College, they became increasingly lax in the performance of their duties and permitted the affairs of the school to be managed almost wholly by the faculty. This eventually led to an unfortunate confrontation in 1838 between George McClellan, founder, and the Board.

The Reverend Ashbel Green, D.D., LL.D.; the First Board President (1826–1848)

Dr. Green's service as President of the Board covered a period of 22 years and was terminated only by his death in 1848. As a member of the Board at Canonsburg he had witnessed the founding of Jefferson Medical College and was interested in its welfare from the beginning. Before the "Additional Trustees" of Philadelphia were constituted, he represented the mother College at Canonsburg with prayer when the Tivoli Theater "Hall of the Jefferson Medical College" was opened on March 8, 1825. By virtue of his relation with the parent institution, but equally by his ripe experience in educational administration, he was the natural choice to lead the Auxiliary Board of the new Medical School. It was fortunate that such a man was at its head to deal with the struggles of the school, the strife among its Professors, and the difficult personality of George McClellan.

Ashbel Green (Figure 48-5) was born in New Jersey in 1762, the son of a Presbyterian pastor, the Rev. Jacob Green. In 1778, at the age of 16, he was already teaching school. That same year he enlisted in the Revolutionary Army and exposed his life to jeopardy at the attack by the British on Elizabethtown Point, New Jersey. He aspired early to collegiate education, in which he received instruction from his father. He entered the junior class in the College of New Jersey (Princeton) in 1782 and graduated the following year as Valedictory Orator of his class. General Washington was present at the commencement.

Immediately following graduation, Green was appointed to a tutorship in his alma mater and two years later was made Professor of Mathematics and Natural Philosophy until 1787. During this time he studied theology and was licensed to preach in 1786. In 1787 he accepted the call to become co-pastor of the Second Presbyterian Church in Philadelphia, and was elected a member of the American Philosophical Society as well.

In 1792, after only six years as a licensed preacher, the Rev. Green was honored with the degree of Doctor of Divinity by the University of Pennsylvania. The same year he was elected Chaplain to Congress in Philadelphia, an office he held for the next eight years until the removal of Congress to Washington. It is said he came to know President Washington well.

In 1812 Dr. Green was chosen President of the College of New Jersey (Princeton) and thus released from his pastoral charge in Philadelphia. In the same year the University of North Carolina conferred upon him the degree of Doctor of Laws. In 1822, after ten years of vigorous labor as President of Princeton and having reached the age of 60, he resigned with a view to lessening his responsibilities, but in returning to Philadelphia he promptly assumed tasks just as demanding.

Green became editor of the *Christian Advocate,* a monthly periodical that he continued until 1834. At the time of his appointment to the Presidency of the Board of Trustees of Jefferson he was 64 years of age. His career had been distinguished as influential in the start of Princeton Theological Seminary and Western Theological Seminary. His

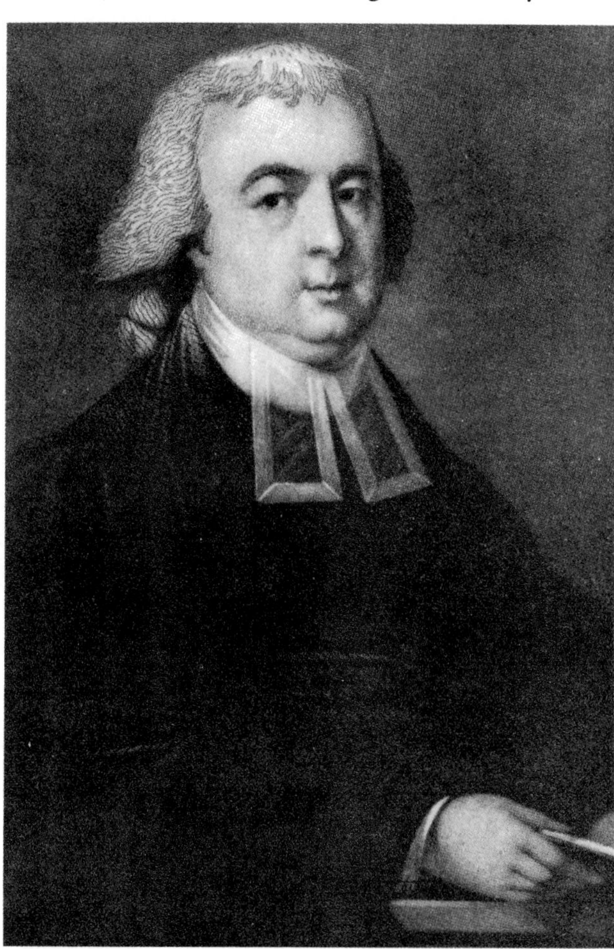

FIG. 48-5. The Reverend Ashbel Green, D.D., LL.D. (1762–1848); First Board President (1826–1848). (Courtesy of the Presbyterian Historical Society of Philadelphia.)

name was the first in Presbyterian history to be associated with organized home missions, for which he served in an administrative capacity for 28 years.

Dr. Green was an eloquent preacher and was additionally impressive because of his large frame, shaggy eyebrows, and gleaming eyes. He wore his clerical wig and queue to the end, which came at the age of 86. He outlived his son, Jacob Green, Professor of Chemistry, by seven years. The latter, often called "old Jaky," died suddenly in 1841 at the age of 51, and was the last of the original Jefferson faculty.

Need for a Permanent College Building

Aside from governing the faculty, setting fees for the Professors' courses, and approving the proper number of lectures to be given, it was evident to the Board that the progress of the College was hindered by the undesirable location of its Tivoli Theater Medical Hall across from the infamous Walnut Street prison. On March 22, 1827, it was "resolved that it is expedient for the Additional Trustees to procure a new and commodious building to be erected before commencement of the next course of lectures for the use of the Professors and students, and to rent the same for a term of years on such conditions as the said Trustees may deem practicable and advantageous." This resolution was a bold one in view of the fact that the General Board at Canonsburg and the Additional Trustees themselves were free of any financial obligations to the College. As constituted, it was the responsibility of the faculty as a proprietary group to raise their own funds. For start-up they had struggled to renovate the Tivoli Theater at 518–520 Prune Street (now Locust), but they lacked the funds for a proper and permanent building. In this deadlocked situation one member of the Board, the Rev. Ezra Stiles Ely, came forward as Jefferson's first benefactor.

Ezra Stiles Ely, D.D., and "N Medical Hall" (Ely Building, 1828)

At a meeting of the Board on May 12, 1827, the Rev. Dr. Ely reported that he had purchased a lot, 56 feet wide by 93 feet deep, on the west side of Tenth Street between Juniper Alley (later called Moravian, running east and west between Tenth and Eleventh) and George Street (later Sansom) for $6,500. He proposed to build a College edifice of brick, the plan of which was displayed and for which the construction and appurtenances would not exceed $10,500. The offer was immediately accepted, along with agreement to pay a $1,200 yearly rental, subject to confirmation by the Canonsburg Board.

The building was completed and opened for the 1828–1829 session (Figure 48-6). Without detracting from the timely philanthropy, it must be understood that Dr. Ely's benefaction was a provision and not a gift. He created shares of Jefferson Medical College Stock for which he was the trustee. Dr. Ely took a risk that most prudent businessmen would have deemed excessive. As later events disclosed, he proved to be a

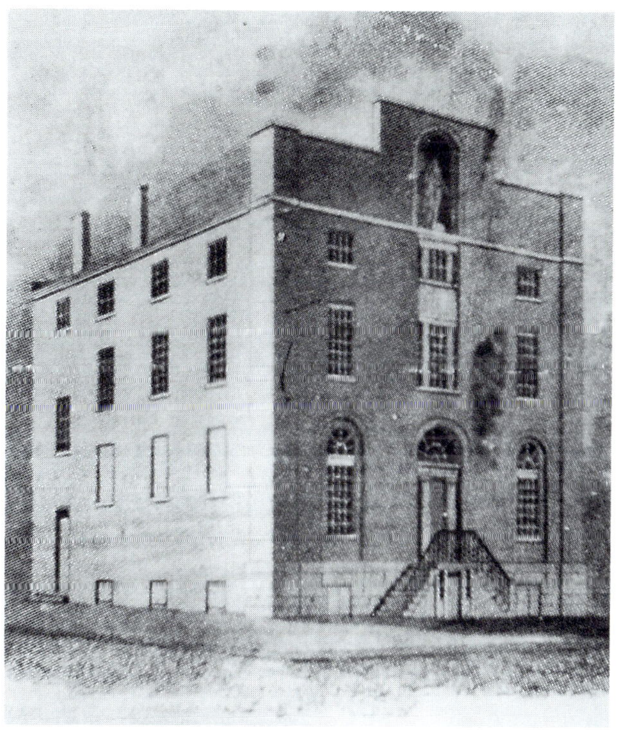

FIG. 48-6. The new Medical Hall (Ely Building of 1828) on Tenth Street.

compulsive entrepreneur, equivalent to a modern wheeler-dealer. His subsequent speculations in land in Missouri were ruinous, leading to bankruptcy, narrow escape from imprisonment, and loss of trusteeship of the Jefferson stock. Fortunately, no one lost money on the Jefferson venture, but it took until 1871 to clear the College of its debt to the Ely family.

In 1847, in a court trial involving his debts, Dr. Ely was cleared of dishonesty or intent to defraud. His integrity as a clergyman was never questioned. For many years, as Secretary of the Board, he kept the minutes in his beautiful handwriting. Later, in 1847, Dr. Ely was elected President pro tempore to fulfill the duties of the venerable Dr. Green, who died the following year.

Independence of Jefferson Medical College (1838)

Three related and sequential events took place during 1838–1839: Jefferson Medical College became independent of Jefferson College at Canonsburg; Medical Hall was renovated; and George McClellan, the founder, was dismissed. The Additional Trustees became aware that Jefferson was in a crisis and losing much of the prestige of the previous six years. The Medical Hall of 1828, which had been erected hastily, was badly in need of enlargement and renovation. Despite the efforts of Dr. Robley Dunglison as a peacemaker among the faculty, petty bickering between two rival camps (George McClellan, Samuel McClellan, and Samuel Colhoun versus Jacob Green, John Revere, and Granville Pattison) went on even as a power struggle between George McClellan and the Board was being voiced outside the institution.

■ The Charter of 1838

An economic problem triggered the necessity for a Charter to free Jefferson Medical College from its mother College. From the very beginning the General Board at Canonsburg proclaimed its freedom from any financial involvement with its Medical Department in Philadelphia. The outlay of money to modernize the existing Medical Hall was not forthcoming from the faculty, and the Rev. Ely was himself in serious financial difficulties in Missouri. The only solution was for the Philadelphia Board to acquire the title to the property still vested in Ezra Stiles Ely. In so doing, the property would belong to the Canonsburg Board and violate the constituted financial agreement. The ultimate solution lay in an independent Jefferson Medical College. The Board, always composed of men of the highest integrity and dedication to the welfare of the College, applied in the spring of 1838 to the State Legislature for an independent charter, to which the Trustees at Canonsburg raised no serious objection. When prompt and favorable action was received from the Legislature, the General Board sent the Trustees of the new College "a warm God-speed and a prayer for continued usefulness and prosperity."

The new Charter was accepted at a last meeting of the Additional Trustees on April 19, 1838, with a resolution "that this board will retain a grateful sense of the kind and fostering care ever exhibited towards them by the parent institution."

Under the 1838 Charter it was stated "that the Medical Department of Jefferson College be and hereby is, created a separate and independent body corporate, under the name, style, and title of 'The Jefferson Medical College of Philadelphia,' with the same powers and restrictions as the University of Pennsylvania . . . to be Trustees of the College created by this Section, with power to increase their number to fifteen." It should be noted that all the members of the General Board at Canonsburg had been Presbyterians as Trustees of a strictly denominational College. Nearly all of the original Additional Trustees were likewise Presbyterian. It is worthy of emphasis, however, that religious preferences were never considered in the choice of Professors, and that after separation from the mother College the Presbyterian element gradually faded out of the Board.

Under its new Charter, the Board of 15 consisted of President Ashbel Green, five other original members (Samuel Badger, the Rev. Ezra Stiles Ely, General William Duncan, the Hon. Edward King, and the Hon. Joel Sutherland), and previously elected or new members (the Rev.

Cornelius C. Cuyler, D.D., Jacob Frick, Esq., the Hon. David Hassinger, U.S. Marine Colonel Samuel Miller, the Hon. John R. Jones, John R. Vodges, the Hon. Jesse Burden, the Hon. Joseph B. Smith, and the Hon. Thomas S. Smith). The new Board promptly began planning for the renovation of Medical Hall.

Renovation of Medical Hall (1838)

The Board accepted an offer from the Rev. Ely, who was in Missouri but kept his position and interest on the Board by correspondence, for a 20-year lease on Medical Hall. Effective as of November 24, 1838, it granted the privilege of paying off the property, then appraised at $29,500, with the annual rent increased to $1,770, which represented a 6% return on the investment to the stockholders.

The plan of renovation of the College building involved extensive interior and exterior remodeling, including an upper and lower lecture room, each with a seating capacity for 450 students. On June 25, 1838, the building committee reported a final estimated cost by the architect, Mr. Thomas Ustick Walter, of $7,500, but the Board approved only $5,000. Despite these obstacles the work commenced promptly, and the building was ready by November for the 1838–1839 session.

The Founder, George McClellan, Dismissed (1839)

With newly acquired independence, an enlarged Board of Trustees, and a renovated Medical Hall, it should have followed that Jefferson was poised for increased prestige. The greatly improved stance of the institution was spoiled by old infighting over policy and fees within the faculty, complicated by conflicts of personalities. On April 2, 1839, Dr. Robley Dunglison, Professor of the Institutes of Medicine, and known as the "peacemaker" because of his neutral position among rival factions, wrote a "Letter of Appeal to the Faculty," which was delivered by the Dean, Dr. John Revere, to the Board. The Board responded immediately by appointing a committee of three "to inquire into the existing state and condition of the Faculty." Although the exact causes for instability among the faculty are undocumented, it is beyond conjecture that Dr. George McClellan was the central figure in the affair. In spite of his professional prestige and popularity with the students, his personality was compulsive, dictatorial, stubborn, volcanic, and even erratic. Tension increased between the forces of faculty domination and supreme authority of the Board. McClellan disgraced himself by publically denouncing the Board as a "parcel of politicians" and "a blackguard Board of Trustees." He proclaimed that the institution was "rotten and going to the dogs" and "with the rascally Board, Jefferson must go down."

On May 2, 1839, the Board "resolved that the present faculty of Jefferson Medical College be dissolved." During eight subsequent meetings of the next three months, debates with balloting settled the new appointments of all the Professors except for Surgery. The Board members were good parliamentarians, and personal attendance was a prerequisite to a voice and a vote in its councils. On July 10, 1839, a vote of seven for Dr. Joseph Pancoast versus five for McClellan gave the Chair of Surgery to Pancoast and the dismissal to McClellan. On September 3, 1839, action was taken that "any property belonging to Dr. McClellan be delivered to him."

Within four months of his dismissal, the undaunted George McClellan, using the same strategy as for the founding of Jefferson, obtained a Charter from the State Legislature for yet another Medical School in Philadelphia called "The Medical Department of Pennsylvania College" at Gettysburg. In November, 1839, the school opened with nearly 100 pupils. It became highly competitive with Jefferson and the University of Pennsylvania, but collapsed in 1861 at the start of the Civil War. As at Jefferson, McClellan became involved in a quarrel and had to resign his professorship in 1843. He spent the next four years—the remaining years of his life—in private practice and died in 1847 at the age of 50. Despite incessant work rewarded with professional success, he ended relatively poor as a result of unwise speculation in real estate.

"The Famous Faculty of 1841"

The radical action of the Board of 1839 resulted in only a temporary suppression of discord among the faculty. The old feeling of discontent arose again in 1841, at which time the Board once more exercised its supreme authority by dissolving the faculty. The disturbing element frequently characterized as "Faculty dissension" was permanently put to rest on this occasion and never again appeared in subsequent Jefferson history.

The Trustees organized the historic faculty of 1841, which consisted of a corps of Professors unsurpassed in any other medical school of the country (Figure 48-7). They excelled in their fields, worked in unbroken harmony for 15 years, and made the name of Jefferson Medical College known throughout the world. Only the resignation of Dr. Thomas Dent Mütter in 1856, because of ill health, broke these ranks, but he was replaced by the great Samuel D. Gross. Henceforth, the Trustees remained the recognized power of the institution, earned by their resolute actions, and they deserved to share the honor of subsequent achievements with the members of the faculty.

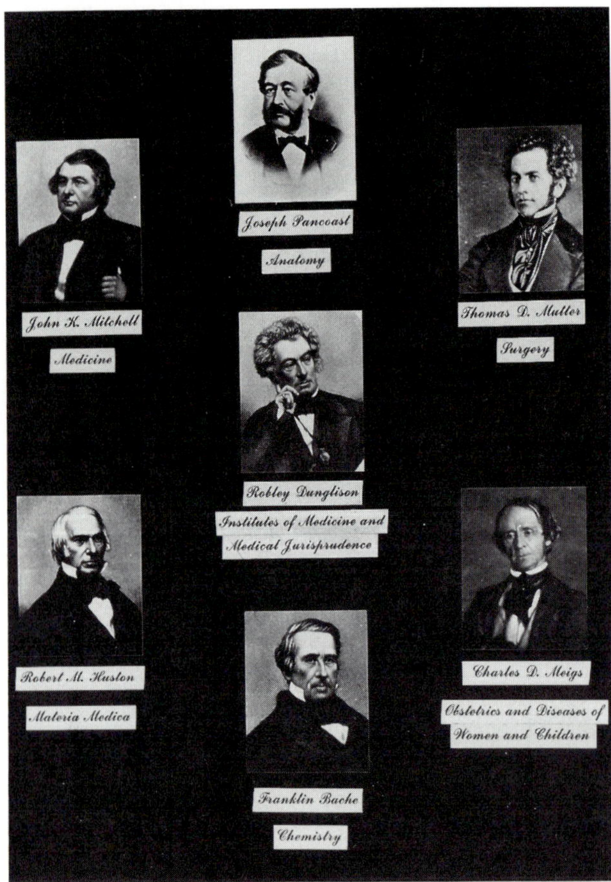

FIG. 48-7. "The Famous Faculty of 1841."

Renovation of Medical Hall (1846)

In 1846 the Ely Building was again renovated (Figure 48-8). The façade was further modified in the form of a Roman temple with six Corinthian columns resting on a base seven feet above the street level. The Building was widened nine feet to the north and extended at the rear. The two lecture rooms were increased to seat 600 students instead of the previous 450. A large dissecting room was provided, and a connection was made into the upper floor of the adjacent store as a miniature hospital ward. The upper lecture hall was the amphitheater, or "pit," in which surgery was performed and in which years later (1875) the *Gross Clinic* by Eakins would be portrayed.

The Reverend Cornelius C. Cuyler, D.D.; The Second Board President (1848–1850)

For the ensuing 25 years the transactions of the Board were mainly of a routine nature. The transfer of the Presidency from the aged Rev. Ashbel Green to the Rev. Cornelius Cuyler in 1848 occurred in a period of tranquility. Dr. Cuyler had been appointed as an Additional Trustee in 1834 for replacement of deceased member the Rev. Gilbert Livingston, D.D. His experience qualified him for the honor of President, but at age 65 he had less than two years to live because of progressive dry gangrene of the lower extremity.

Cornelius C. Cuyler (Figure 48-9) was born in Albany in 1783, a descendant of early American colonists. He graduated from Union College, Schenectady, in 1806. His intention to study law changed to theology, and he was ordained a Presbyterian minister in 1809. He served as pastor of the Reformed Dutch Church in Poughkeepsie until 1833. In 1828 he received from the College of Schenectady the degree of Doctor of Divinity, and another later by Rutgers College at New Brunswick. On transfer to Philadelphia in 1833 he served in the Second Presbyterian Church for which the Rev. Green had been a pastor for 25 years (1787–1812). Dr. Cuyler's life was summarized as "marked by unwearied assiduous and punctual devotedness to his duties."[2] His passing marked the end of Presbyterian tradition on the Board.

The Honorable Edward King, LL.D.; The Third Board President (1850–1873)

The service of Judge King to Jefferson covered a span of 47 years. In 1826, at the age of 32, he was sworn in by Chief Justice Tilghman as the first "Additional Trustee." Judge King then administered the oath of office to his nine co-members. In 1850, after 24 years on the Board, he was elected the President. Like the two preceding Presidents, he kept his office until his death (at age 79) for 23 years.

Edward King (Figure 48-10) was born in the old Southwark district of Philadelphia in 1794. He studied law under Charles Chauncey and was admitted to the Bar in 1816. In 1823, at age 29, he was appointed by Governor J. Andrew Shulze as President Judge of the Court of Common Pleas of the City and County of Philadelphia, and he served until his retirement from the bench in 1851. He was one of the Commissioners appointed to revise the criminal code of Pennsylvania and for two years was connected with the Board of City Trusts.

Judge King had no superiors in his knowledge of common and criminal law and of the principles of equity. As President of the Court of Common Pleas he was "perhaps and best judge that ever occupied that bench, so far as regarded its criminal jurisdiction, and at least equal to any in the civil department of his judicial duties . . . and his written opinions during a period of more than twenty years were indicative of much research, discrimination, and power."[3]

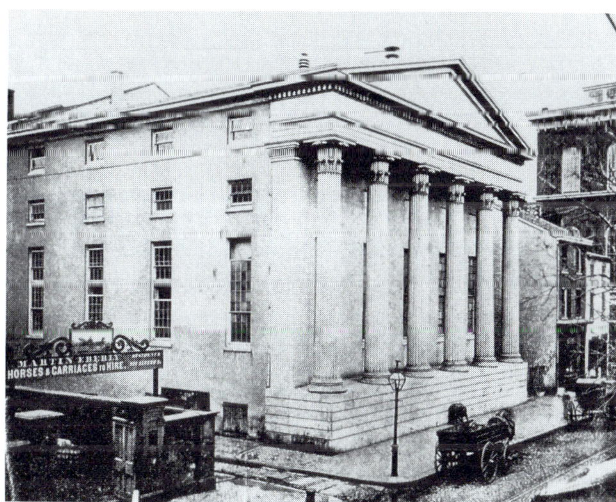

FIG. 48-8. The 1846 renovation of Medical Hall (Ely Building), with the addition of a Grecian façade.

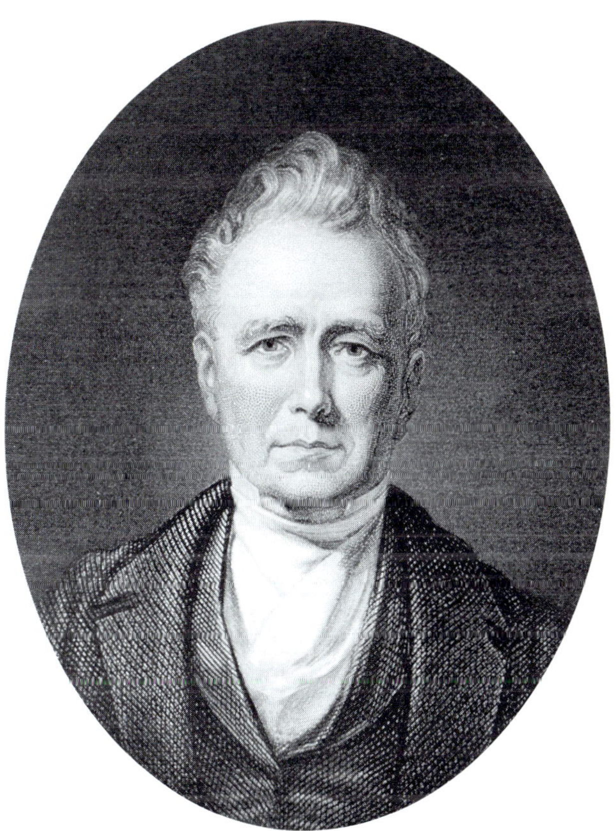

FIG. 48-9. The Reverend Cornelius C. Cuyler, D.D. (1783–1850), Second Board President (1848–1850). (Courtesy of the Presbyterian Historical Society of Philadelphia.)

In 1858 there were 59 total shares of the Capital Stock of the College at $500 each, amounting to $29,500. The College had purchased 23 such shares, amounting to $11,500, leaving 36 shares ($18,000) yet to be acquired. In 1860 the Board resolved to raise the necessary funds "by Bond and Mortgage" to pay the balance due to the stockholders and thus secure the title to the real estate of the College. On November 10, 1870, the treasurer was authorized to pay the interest on outstanding shares of the Jefferson Medical College Stock in gold, and by the following year the entire debt was liquidated. It must be remembered that throughout this period of Jefferson history the school was proprietary, meaning that the Professors kept the profit and paid rent for use of the building. The original rent of $1,200 per year increased to $1,770 and in 1866 was set at $2,500.

Only once during Judge King's Presidency was there any apprehension on the part of the Board with respect to the stability of the College. This occurred just before and during the early years of the Civil War (1861–1865) when Dr. Hunter McGuire led away almost one-half of the students to southern medical schools or to enlist in the Confederate cause. This exodus of southern students also affected the University of Pennsylvania, and was a total disaster for McClellan's second school (the Medical Department of Pennsylvania College at Gettysburg), which closed by attrition in 1861. The loss to Jefferson was only temporary. Its faculty was as competent as any in the country and within a few years restored its previously large enrollment.

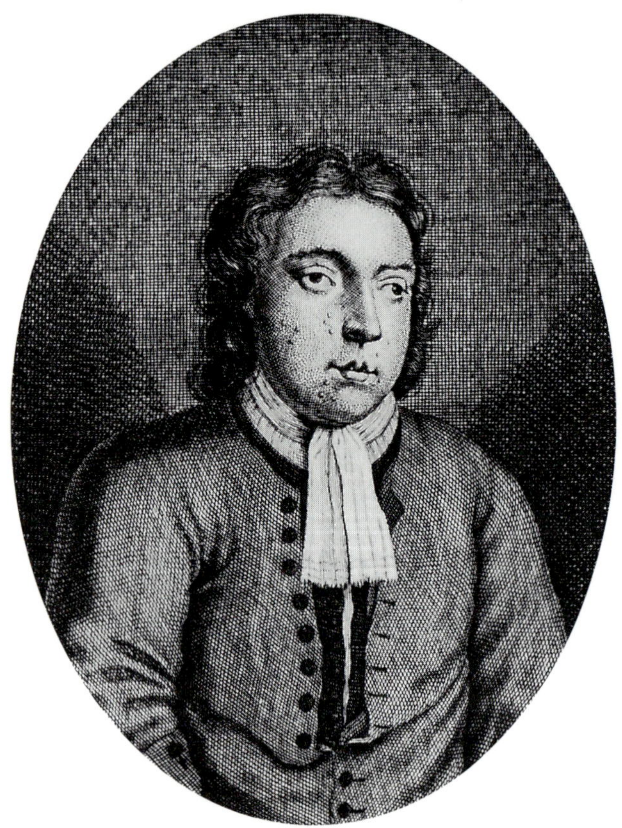

FIG. 48-10. The Honorable Edward King, LL.D. (1794–1873), Third Board President (1850–1873). (Courtesy of the Free Library of Philadelphia.)

The Trustees obtained a faithful ally and dedicated supporter with founding of the Alumni Association by Dr. Samuel D. Gross in 1870. At first the Board was wary of the necessity for such an organization, fearing that it might be a burden rather than a source of help. Mobilization of the graduate forces of the College quickly proved itself a mighty force in counsel and financial assistance. The boost to the Board was enormous, with ready aid in whatever measure was beneficial to the welfare of the school.

The Honorable Jesse R. Burden, M.D.; President, pro tempore (1873–1875)

The Presidency of the Board for its first 25 years was served by two Presbyterian clergymen. The succeeding 23 years were under the good offices of a member of the legal profession. The next 15 years were to be under the aegis of two physicians.

Jesse R. Burden, M.D. (Figure 48-11), a Philadelphian, was born in 1797. It is of singular interest that he obtained his medical degree in 1819 from the University of Pennsylvania as a classmate of Dr. George McClellan, the founder of Jefferson Medical College. In addition to private practice, he served on the Philadelphia Board of Health (1822–1823) and lectured on Materia Medica when the Philadelphia College of Medicine, a fourth medical school, was opened in 1847.

In 1825 Dr. Burden was elected a member of the State Legislature, in which he served faithfully for 15 years. During the latter part of his term he became Speaker of the Senate, where he acquired great reputation as a thorough parliamentarian. After retiring from political life he resumed his medical activities. He served as President of the Board of Prison Inspectors (1835–1855) and for many years was President of the Board of the Guardians of the Poor.

Dr. Burden was appointed to the Board in 1838, at age 40. The following year, when the faculty was dissolved, resulting in the dismissal of George McClellan, Burden with two other Board members had proposed "that the resolution be indefinitely postponed." He was defeated in the voting, but his loyalty to his fellow physician and classmate was documented in the minutes of the Board.

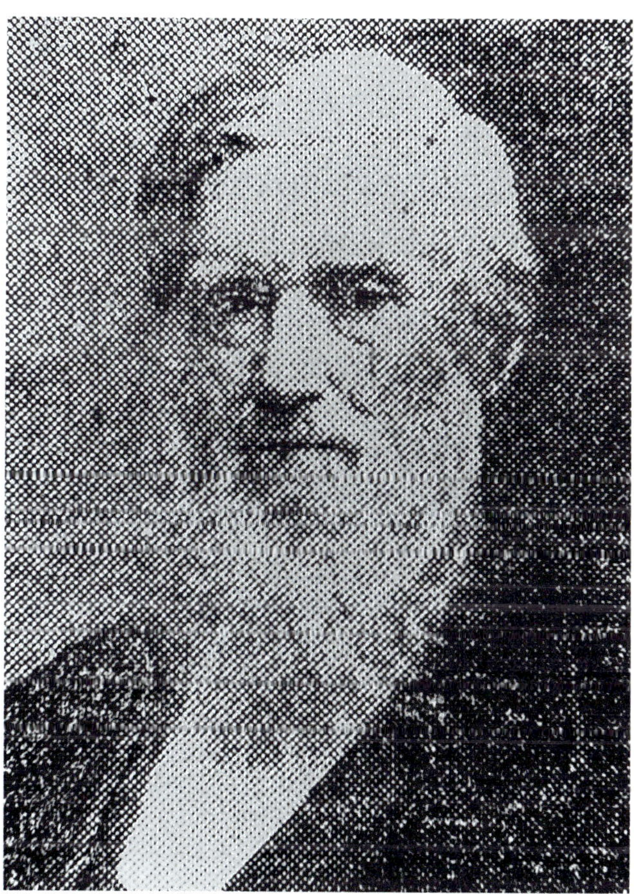

FIG. 48-11. The Honorable Jesse R. Burden, M.D. (1797–1875), President, pro tempore (1873–1875). (Courtesy of the University of Pennsylvania Archives.)

On the death of Judge King in 1873, Dr. Burden was appointed President, pro tempore, at the age of 76. He would serve until his own death on May 2, 1875.[4] This was a time when the faculty, strongly supported by the newly formed Alumni Association, proclaimed the need for a separate hospital facility to take care of the unwieldly patient load that the College had been struggling to house in the adjacent floors of the two stores at the corner of Tenth and Sansom and other nearby buildings. Patients that should have been hospitalized were being taken home in carriages and cared for by the Professors' assistants and students. Cost was a major problem, and the advisability of moving Jefferson's location was another consideration. A possible new site at Broad and Wood was explored and rejected on the basis of price and accessibility. The Board joined forces with the faculty and Alumni Association in an appeal for funds.

In 1873 Dr. Francis Fontaine Maury (Jefferson, 1862) secured an appropriation of $100,000 from the State Legislature toward a separate hospital building, on the basis of matching by a similar sum from the College. Dr. John Hill Brinton, aided by Dr. Samuel D. Gross, undertook to raise $150,000 through the Alumni. The Board rose to the occasion by liquidating all previous debts to the Ely family in connection with the College building, by generous personal contributions, and by a public appeal for funds. The University of Pennsylvania at this time was active with the same problem and were able in 1874 to erect their hospital in West Philadelphia, which was the first in the country to be directly part of a medical school. Jefferson became the second in 1877 when the detached hospital was opened on Sansom Street, between Tenth and Eleventh Streets, where the Thompson Annex now stands.

Emile B. Gardette, M.D.; the Fourth Board President (1875–1888)

Emile Blaise Gardette, M.D. (Figure 48-12) was a unique Board President in that he was a graduate of Jefferson Medical College in the Class of 1838. A native Philadelphian, born in 1803, he was first trained in dentistry by his father, Jacques Gardette (1756–1831), who practiced in Philadelphia for more than 45 years, having started in 1784. The father enjoyed the friendship of many eminent physicians of his day, among whom were Drs. Benjamin Rush, Adam Kuhn, William Shippen, and Caspar Wistar. His son, Emile, was brought up in the professional tradition of dentistry under the preceptorial system. (The first dental school in the world was not founded until 1840 in Baltimore). The father was 47 years old at the time of Emile's birth and died seven years before the latter's graduation from Jefferson. Emile went on to become a celebrated surgeon-dentist.

On becoming a member of the Jefferson Board in 1856, Dr. Gardette took the customary oath before an Alderman of the City of Philadelphia as follows: " . . . who being duly sworn by me on the Holy Evangelist of Almighty God, did depose and say that he would support the Constitution of the United States of America and the Constitution of the Commonwealth of Pennsylvania and that he would perform and execute with fidelity the duties of Trustees of the Jefferson Medical College of Philadelphia." This oath was required by Section two of the State Legislature Act of 1826, which gave Jefferson Medical College the official sanction to grant the M.D. degree. Taking the oath conferred a position on the Board as a "Life Trustee." After July 1, 1969, when Jefferson became a University, the life trusteeship was abolished, and the oath was no longer administered. Members were then elected as Term Trustees for a period of not more than three years but could be subsequently reelected to succeed themselves. Senior members by virtue of long and devoted service could be honored as Emeritus for life but without the right to vote.

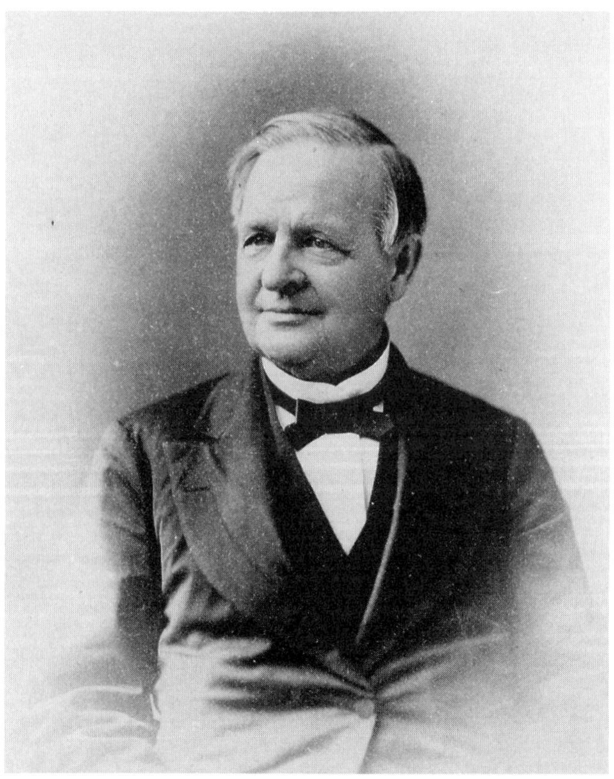

FIG. 48-12. Emile B. Gardette, M.D. (1803–1888), Fourth Board President (1875–1888).

Gardette was a Fellow of the College of Physicians of Philadelphia and a member of the Academy of Natural Sciences, the Historical Society of Pennsylvania, and the French Society of Bienfaisance of Philadelphia. The College of Physicians possesses several of his publications, one of which is *The Professional Education of Dentists* (1852).

Dr. Gardette assumed the Presidency of the Board on May 15, 1875, just one year before the Grand Opening of the Centennial Exposition in Fairmount Park on May 10, 1876. Dr. Samuel D. Gross was unanimously elected President of the International Medical Congress held in connection with the Centennial. For this event Gross also wrote the history of American surgery from 1776 to 1876.

A big accomplishment for the Board was the opening on September 17, 1877, of the first detached Jefferson Medical College Hospital (Figure 48-13). Dr. Joseph Pancoast, already retired for three years and the only survivor of the "Famous Faculty of 1841," gave the address. This hospital was the second in the country to be connected with a medical school for teaching purposes. It was located on Sansom Street behind the old Tenth Street College building where the Thompson Annex now stands. A five-story structure of Gothic design with 125 beds and a large clinical amphitheater (Figure 48-14), it would serve Jefferson's hospital needs until the opening of "Old Main" at Tenth and Sansom in 1907.

During its first year it admitted 441 inpatients and treated 4,649 outpatients.

An event of seemingly minor importance at the time was the purchase by the Alumni Association of Eakins' *Gross Clinic* in 1878 for $200. It was presented to the Board the following year. Eakins had executed this world-famous portrait in 1875 on a voluntary noncommissioned basis as a consequence of his studies in anatomy at Jefferson and his admiration for Dr. Gross. It was rejected for display in the Art Gallery of the Centennial of 1876 but accepted in the Medical Department of the U.S. Government Building at the Exhibition. The Alumni Association had long been interested in acquiring this masterpiece, but all its funds were committed to building the new 1877 Hospital. The preservation of this historic Jefferson scene within its own halls through all the ensuing years has enhanced the name of the institution. In capturing the College's spiritual heritage it became the "holiest of holies," appropriately honored and ultimately handsomely displayed in the special Eakins Gallery, dedicated in 1982.

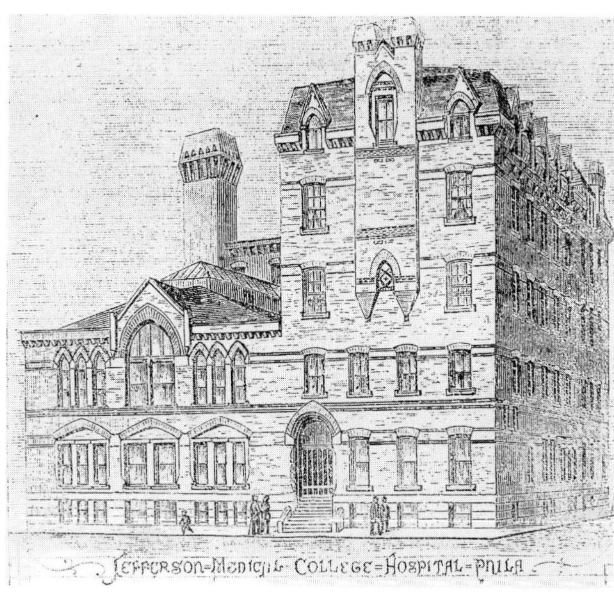

FIG. 48-13. The first detached Jefferson Hospital (1877), on Sansom Street at the present site of the Thompson Annex.

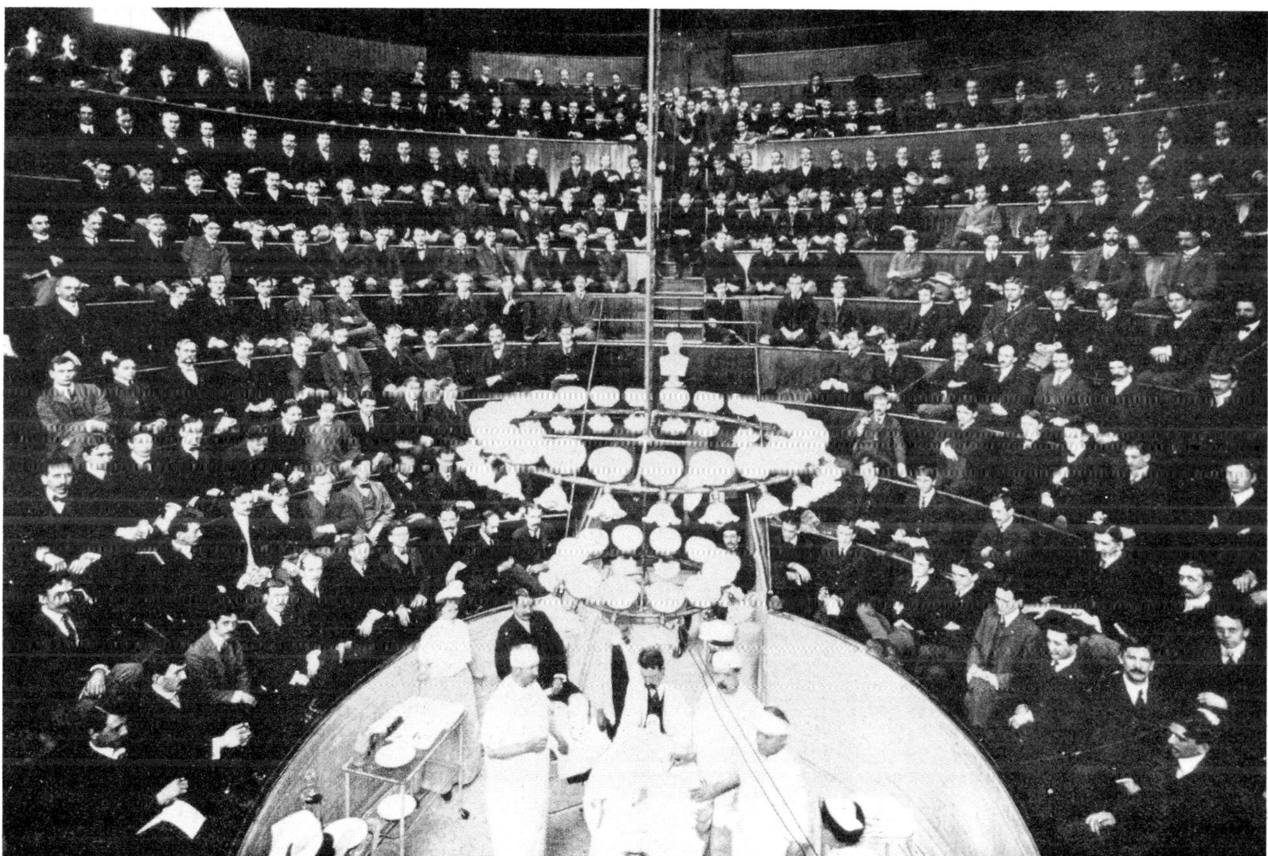

FIG. 48-14. The clinical amphitheater (the "pit") of the first detached Hospital of 1877.

Along with Lister's promulgation of *The Principle of Antisepsis* in 1867 and Darwin's publication of *The Descent of Man* in 1871, a transitional period was developing in which science would enhance the art of medicine. Up to this time at Jefferson the laboratory experience of its students had been limited to anatomy and use of the pathology museum. As an ongoing endeavor after construction of the 1877 Hospital, the Board was able to secure the property at the southwest corner of Tenth and Sansom Streets, adjacent to the College of that time, for construction of facilities for studies in the basic sciences. The new Laboratory Building (Figure 48-15) was completed for the 1879–1880 session. It provided rooms for operative and minor surgery, practical chemistry, microscopy, and physiology.

In 1881 the Grecian façade of the College was replaced by one of Victorian design (Figure 48-16). This allowed an extension of the front by which the seating capacity of the lecture rooms was increased. A new story was added to accommodate extra laboratory rooms.

A complete Maternity Department was organized within the Hospital in 1885, under the immediate charge of the Professor of Obstetrics (Theophilus Parvin, M.D., LL.D.). This afforded clinical experience to the students, whose instruction in that field had previously been limited to the laboratory of practical and manipulative obstetrics of the College.

Dr. Ellwood Wilson, a Jefferson graduate in the Class of 1845, became a member of the Board when Dr. Gardette assumed the Presidency in 1875. He was one of the leading practitioners in Philadelphia in obstetrics and gynecology and President of the Philadelphia Lying-In Charity. He had been one of the most active and foremost of those interested in the construction of Jefferson's 1877 Hospital. Three of his sons graduated from

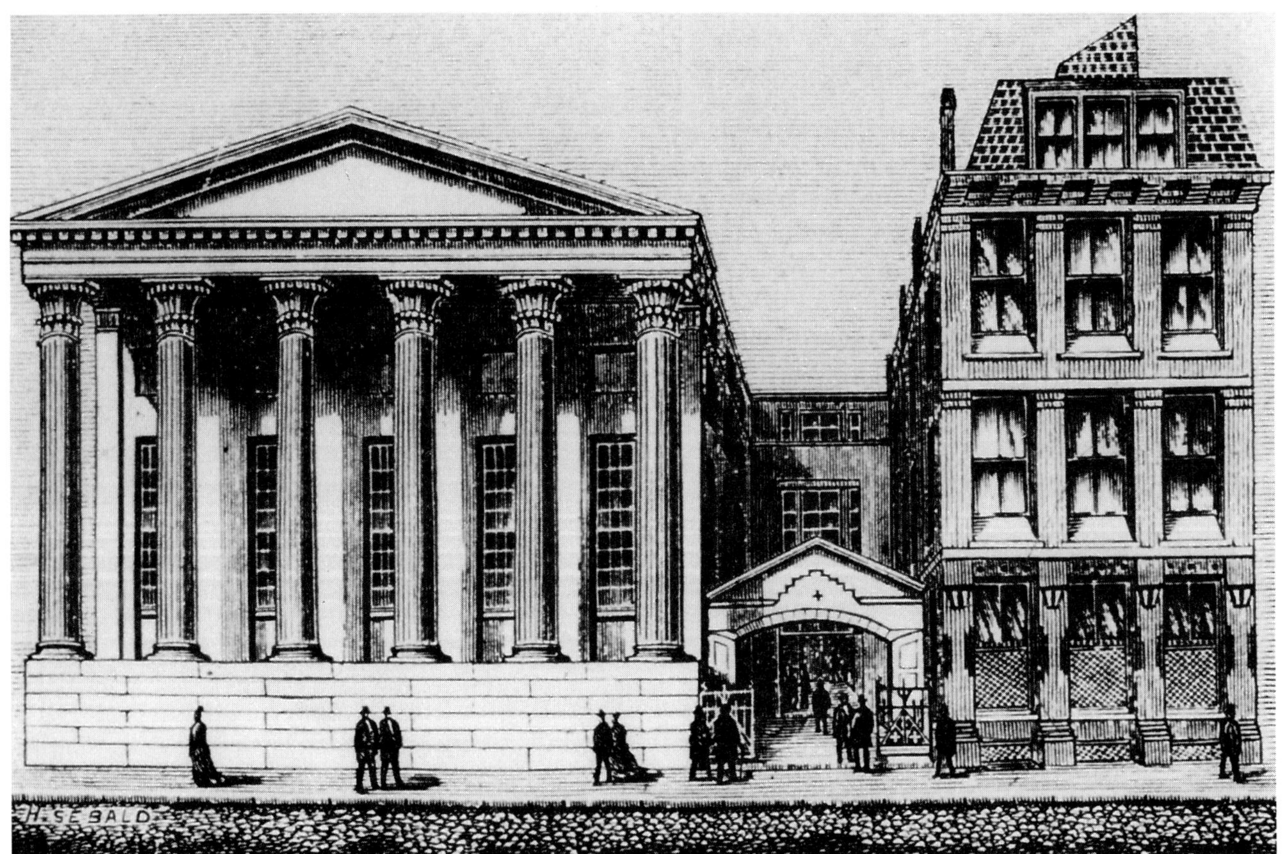

Fig. 48-15. The new Laboratory Building opened in 1879 at the corner of Tenth and Sansom Streets, a space previously occupied by two stores.

Jefferson, one of whom, James Cornelius Wilson (Class of 1869), became the Professor of Medicine in 1891. With the deaths of Dr. Gardette in 1888 and Dr. Wilson in 1889, the Board would not have another member of the medical profession in its ranks until the appointment of Alumni Trustees in 1965.

The Honorable James Campbell; The Fifth Board President (1889–1891)

James Campbell (Figure 48-17) was born in Philadelphia in 1818, the son of a prosperous storekeeper. His parents were Irish and Roman Catholic. His industry and bookish inclinations led him to study law and find recreation in the Philadelphia Library, the Athenaeum, or the debating society. He was admitted to the bar (1833), became school commissioner (1840), and was appointed to the court of common pleas (1842) before he was 30. While on the bench for ten years, he was often called upon to suffer bitter anti-Catholic feeling that dominated the local partisanship of that day. Although not strict in religion, Campbell was loyal to his church and became the best known leader of the Catholic Democrats of Philadelphia. In 1851 he was nominated for Supreme Court Justice but defeated by anti-Catholic prejudice. The following year he was appointed Attorney General of Pennsylvania. In 1853 he became U.S. Postmaster General. While serving in this post for the next four years he attempted to get better rates and more efficient service from the railroad and steamship companies carrying mail. Upon his recommendation the registry system was established, and he laid the foundation for cheaper foreign postage rates. It is of interest that a later Board President, the

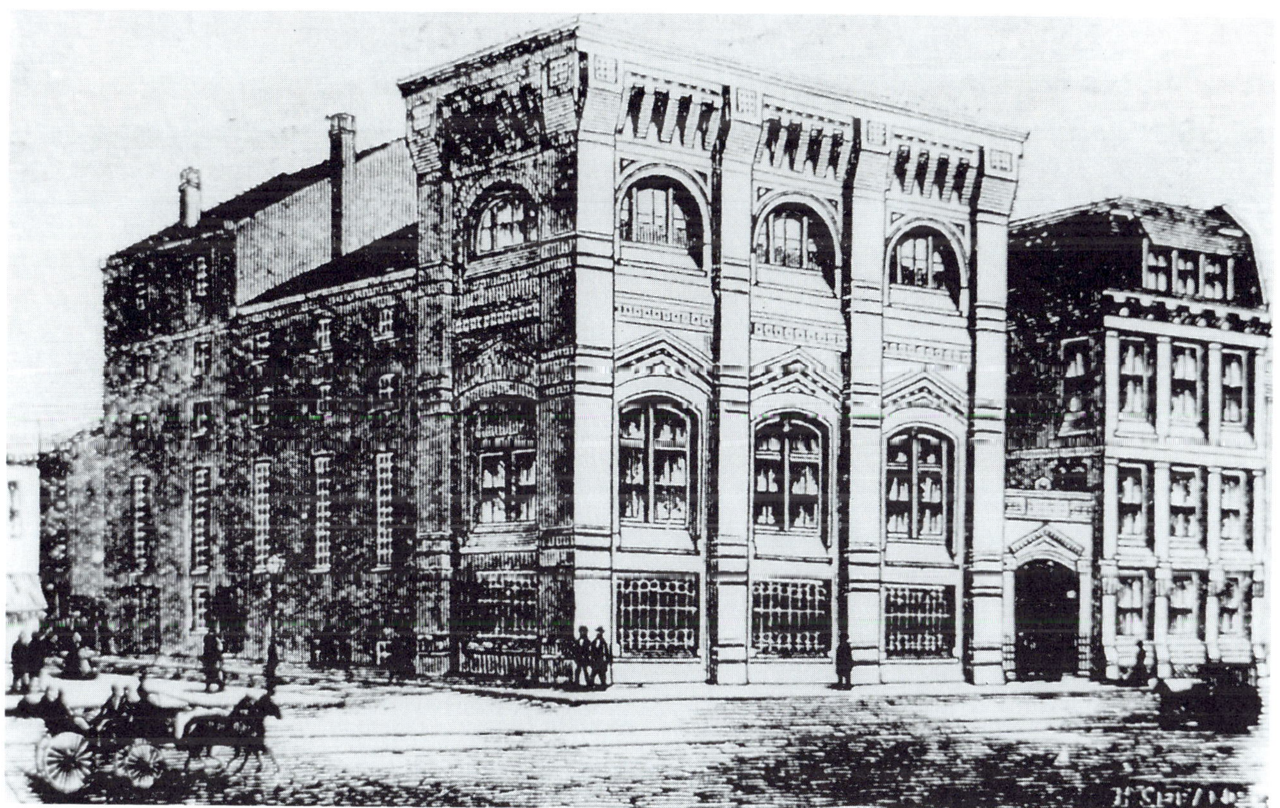

FIG. 48-16. The renovation of Medical Hall (Ely Building) in 1881, replacing the Grecian façade with one in a Victorian style.

illustrious Honorable William Potter, would also be involved in international postage connected with steamship lines.

Although he would nearly be elected to the U.S. Senate during the Civil War, Campbell's return from Washington in 1857 ended his political career. Thereafter he spent his life in the practice of law and as a trustee and director of various charities and institutions. Among these were Girard College and Jefferson Medical College, to the latter of which he was elected to the Board in 1867. His devoted duty and usefulness led to his appointment as President upon the death of Dr. Gardette in 1888. Just as the first two Presidents had exerted no Presbyterian bias, so the question of Campbell's Catholic religion never became an issue on the Board or faculty. Described as "a fat jolly man who tended strictly to business,"[6] he resigned on November 25, 1891, and died on January 27, 1893.

The year 1891 witnessed an important extension of the college curriculum from the traditional two- to a graded three-year course. The entrance requirement was a diploma from a high school or a recognized academy, literary, or scientific school, or a certificate from the examiners of a County Medical Society. In the absence of evidence of satisfactory fitness for entering the study of medicine, an entrance examination was required in English and elementary physics.

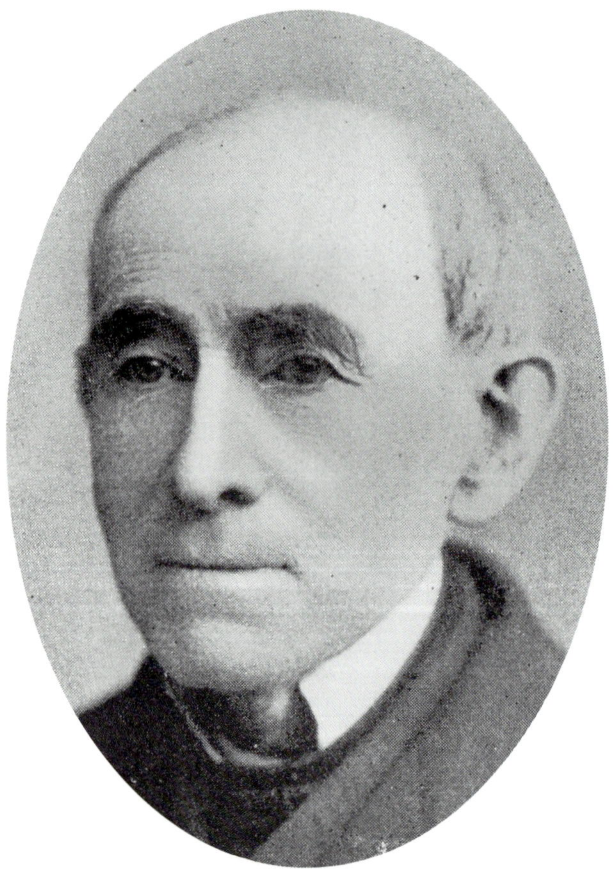

Fig. 48-17. The Honorable James Campbell (1812–1893), Fifth Board President (1889–1891). (Courtesy Historical Society of Pennsylvania.)

The number and variety of lectures were in keeping with the most advanced medical knowledge of that era. The faculty and Hospital staff had greatly enlarged. A Professorship of General Pathology was established to be chaired by Dr. Morris Longstreth. Professor Hobart A. Hare, widely known as teacher, writer, and investigator, was appointed to the Chair of Materia Medica and Therapeutics, which he would hold with distinction for the next 40 years.

The Jefferson Medical College Hospital Training School for Nurses opened its doors in the fall of 1891. This program would last until a final commencement of June 10, 1982, at which time the designation "School of Nursing" ceased and the total number of graduates had reached 5,087.

The Honorable Joseph Allison, LL.D.; the Sixth Board President (1891–1892)

Joseph Allison (Figure 48-18) was a Philadelphian, born in 1819. For over 40 years he was a foremost figure in the history of jurisprudence in Philadelphia and Pennsylvania, and his name in his native city was a household word for nearly half a century. Equity, common law, criminal jurisprudence, trusts, municipal law, and the Orphans court were all in his hands. The system in Philadelphia regulating streets was shaped by him and still constitutes that body of law. He was considered by many as a veritable city father. A distinguished leader of the Bar characterized him as having "the typical qualities of the model

Judge; that he is learned without pedantry; patient without sluggishness; genial without frivolity; suggestive without loquacity; dignified without haughtiness; and firm without harshness."[7]

Judge Allison became a member of the Board in 1874 and served for 18 years, during the last of which he was the President. He resigned on November 23, 1892, and died on February 8, 1896.

In 1892 a voluntary fourth year, not required for the degree, was offered to Jefferson graduates with advanced courses in medicine, surgery, gynecology, dermatology, obstetrics, ophthalmology, and pathology. Within the hospital, Clinical Professorships were established in the specialties of gynecology, dermatology, orthopedics, diseases of children, diseases of the nervous system, and ophthalmology.

As in previous years, classes were available to Jefferson students at the Pennsylvania Hospital, Philadelphia (General) Hospital, St. Agnes's, St. Joseph's, the German (Lankenau), Orthopaedic Hospital and Infirmary for Nervous Diseases, and Wills Eye. These were at that time informal teaching arrangements. During the first half of the twentieth century they became more regularly scheduled but not strictly formalized administratively until the 1960s.

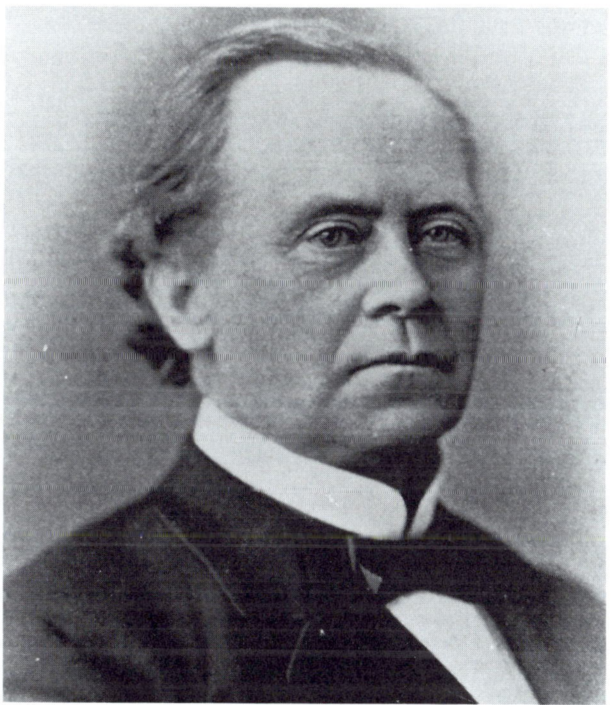

FIG. 48-18. The Honorable Joseph Allison, LL.D. (1819–1896), Sixth Board President (1891–1892). (Courtesy of the Free Library of Philadelphia.)

The Honorable Edwin H. Fitler; the Seventh Board President (1892–1894)

Edwin Henry Fitler (Figure 48-19) was born in Philadelphia in 1825, the son of a prosperous leather merchant and tanner.[8] His academic education was excellent, and he spent four years of legal study in a private law office; mechanical pursuits led him to abandon law and to engage in the cordage business. Through his labor-saving inventions and wise management of employees, his Philadelphia Cordage Works prospered into one of the largest in the United States.

Fitler became one of the best known businessmen of his time, and he was repeatedly

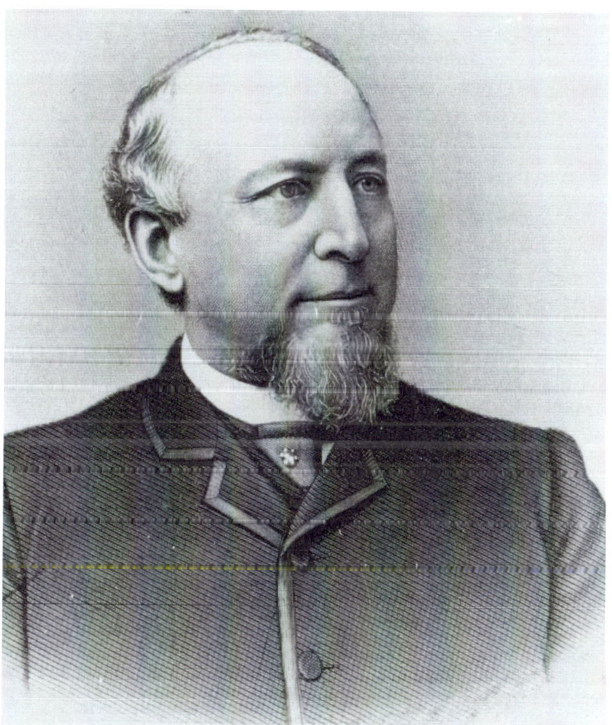

FIG. 48-19. The Honorable Edwin H. Fitler (1825–1896), Seventh Board President (1892–1894). (Courtesy of the Historical Society of Pennsylvania.)

elected President of the American Cordage Manufacturers Association. Intensely patriotic, he sponsored and outfitted a company from his employees for the Union cause in the Civil War. He also served as Vice President and President (1891–1892) of the Union League.

For the Centennial Exposition of 1876 Fitler was a member of its board of finance. He was also one of the founders of the Philadelphia Art Club. In 1887 he was elected the Mayor of Philadelphia with a large majority vote, a position he held until 1891. As the first Mayor under the new city charter he instituted many reforms and improvements in all branches of the city government. At the Republican National Convention of 1888 in Chicago he received the vote of the entire Philadelphia delegation, some parts of Pennsylvania, and a few from other states as their choice for President of the United States.

Fitler was elected to the Jefferson Board in 1891 and became its President on December 5, 1892. He resigned in April, 1894, because of a long illness that claimed his life on May 31, 1896. He is buried in East Laurel Hill Cemetery (listed on the National Register of Historic Places in 1977), where a large monument attests to his prominence.

Fitler joined his fellow Board member, the Honorable Furman Sheppard, along with Professor Hobart A. Hare (newly arrived at Jefferson), in soliciting Dr. William Osler at Hopkins for Jefferson's Chair of Medicine. The letter of May 11, 1891, stated: "A joint committee, consisting of Ex-Mayor Fitler, Professor Hobart A. Hare, and the undersigned (Sheppard), has been appointed by the unanimous action of the Board of Trustees, and of the Faculty of the Jefferson Medical College of the City, to communicate with you with reference to the vacant Chair of Practice of Medicine and Clinical Medicine in that institution. We would be much pleased to have the favour of a personal interview with you, and will gladly come to Baltimore for that purpose . . . ." Osler refused that offer as well as a second one from Harvard Medical School on May 15, 1891. He was engaged in completing his world-renowned textbook on *The Principles and Practice of Medicine* and getting ready to marry Grace Revere Gross, the widow of Samuel W. Gross (the eldest son of Samuel D. Gross, who died in 1889). His actual reason for declining these complimentary offers was his conviction that the newly formed Medical College at Hopkins would further his idealistic goals more effectively.

In 1893 the tuition of the Medical College was $140 for the first year, the same for the second year, and $100 for the third year. The voluntary fourth year also cost $100. There was a matriculation fee of $5, paid only once, and a diploma fee of $30. (The yearly tuition would be more than 100 times greater by 1985, namely $14,100). Students could board comfortably near the College for from $4 to $5 per week with heat and light included. The College Clerk made board arrangements for the students upon their arrival. Every year, five Resident Physicians to the Jefferson Medical College Hospital and five substitutes were elected from the graduating class, chosen from those standing highest in their examination.

In 1894 the Board of Lady Managers (the forerunner of the Women's Board), given approval by the Board as an organization on April 1, 1890, furnished a house at 224 South Seventh Street on Washington Square for maternity patients (Figure 48-20). The Lady Managers paid the annual rent of $1,000, the costs for food, domestic services, and part of the salary for two nurses. The Board of Trustees covered the expenses for fuel, light, medical needs, and the remainder of the nurses' salaries. The purpose of this facility was not only for patient care but for bedside instruction in midwifery to the medical students.

Joseph B. Townsend, Esq.; the Eighth Board President (1894–1896)

Joseph B. Townsend (Figure 48-21), a Philadelphian, was born in 1822.[9] Attracted to law as his life work, he was admitted as an attorney of the Philadelphia courts in December 1842. For more than 50 years he remained active in all branches of legal practice, but lived to be among the last of his associates who could properly be termed "real estate lawyers." He was honored by diplomacy served well to secure more land, to extend the medical curriculum to a mandatory four-year course, and to change Jefferson's proprietary status to a nonprofit sharing corporation. Each of these issues were of major importance and warrant more discussion.

membership on the Board of Examiners for admission to the Bar, and was elected Vice-Chancellor of the Law Association of Philadelphia (1891) and Chancellor (1894), a position dedicated to the maintenance of proper standards of professional learning and honor.

For more than 30 years Townsend was on the Board of Managers of the Western Saving Fund Society. For the same period he was a charter member and charter director of the Union League. His four sons engaged in the active practice of or in allied work connected with the legal profession. One of them, Charles C. Townsend, served on the Jefferson Board from 1899 to 1915.

Townsend was elected a Trustee in 1878 and served as Board President from 1894 until his death in October 1896. His legal talents and expert

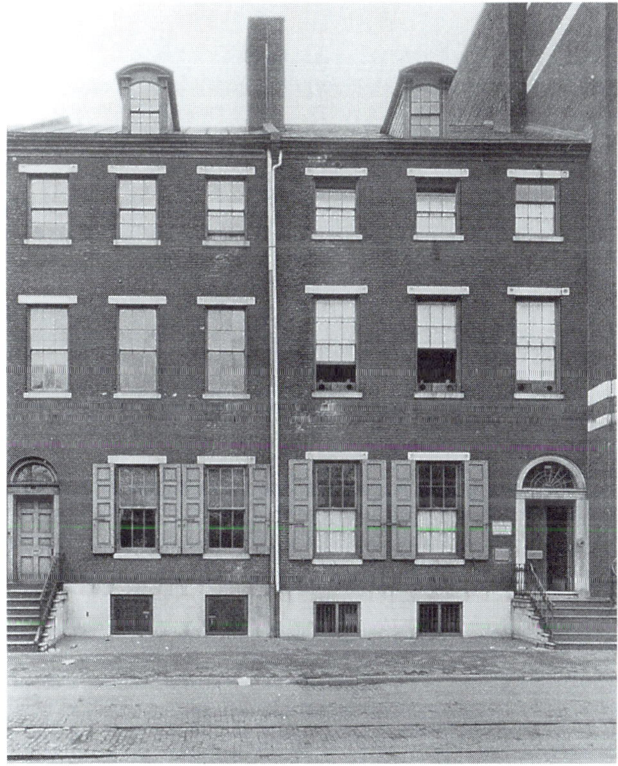

FIG. 48-20. The Maternity facility at 224 West Washington Square, established in 1894 for patient care and student instruction. The adjacent property at 226 was secured in 1895 for lodging Jefferson's student nurses.

Plan for Expansion

Medical Hall, erected as the Ely Building in 1828, had undergone renovations and enlargements in 1838, 1846, 1879, and 1881 that changed its façade from that of a church to a Greek temple, and finally to a florid Victorian style. Around 1894 it was evident to the Faculty and Board that the hodgepodge of College and Laboratory buildings at the corner of Tenth and Sansom Streets was bursting at the seams and that a new Medical College worthy of Jefferson's mission and progress was needed. The Hospital of 1877 was overloaded with inpatients and the dispensaries were greatly overcrowded. The finances of the institution were well in the black, augmented by legacies on ground rents, bonds, and memorials. As on previous occasions, the question of changing Jefferson's location arose, especially critical at this time since the adjacent areas were held by disinterested parties, precluding expansion south or west. Worse still, there was a proposition pending with the Transit Company to build an elevated railroad on Sansom Street that would have rendered operation of a hospital there impossible. New York entrepreneurs had purchased the corner of Eleventh and Walnut

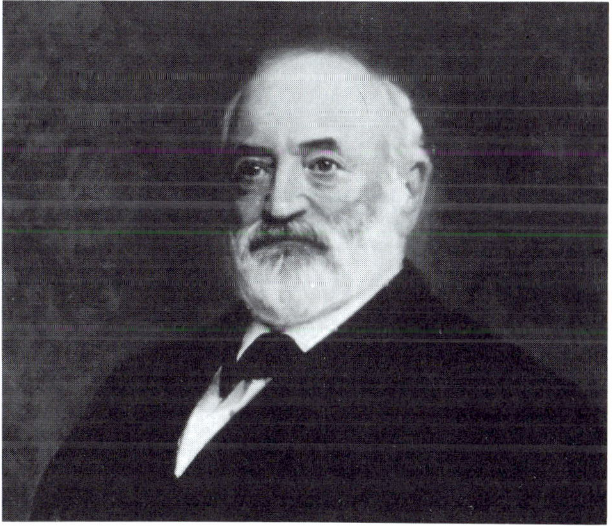

FIG. 48-21. Joseph B. Townsend, Esq. (1822–1896), Eighth Board President (1894–1896).

Streets with a view toward commercial development. A large desirable lot on the northwest corner of Tenth and Walnut Streets had been willed to St. Charles Borromeo Seminary. From this locked-in situation the Trustees purchased land for a reasonable price on the west side of Broad and Christian Streets (about one mile south of City Hall). The faculty, represented by Dean James W. Holland, recommended the Broad Street move. The Board rented out the site in the interim at a profit.

The tide turned in Jefferson's favor when the New York investors lost money and abandoned their project. A protest from the Board to the Philadelphia Council convinced the Transit people of the harm from their "el" on Sansom Street. The owners of property on the north side of Walnut Street saw their land value drop and were willing to sell. The huge Theological Seminary of St. Charles Borromeo, located at Lancaster Pike and City Avenue, had already opened for students of the priesthood in 1871 and had no real need for the land at Tenth and Walnut. The faculty reversed its previous opinion and petitioned the Board to sell the Christian Street property and procure the Walnut Street site. Wisdom prevailed and the Board acted accordingly.

▪ The Four-Year Medical Curriculum

The *70th Annual Announcement for the Session of 1894/95* stated that "all persons beginning their medical studies by matriculation after June 1, 1895, must take four annual courses." This was the culmination of the introduction of science into the art of medicine. Before 1832 the longest term allotted for the year's "Session" of lectures was four months (November through February). In each of the two "Sessions" required for graduation the lectures were identical, the rationale being that the repetition would lead to better understanding and longer remembrance. This was the standard curriculum in the medical colleges of the United States, although in the professional schools of Europe the term was six months. Jefferson took a forward step in 1832 by adding an optional course of two months during April and May for which there was no extra tuition. The M.D. degree still required three years of preceptorship "under the direction of a respectable Practitioner of Medicine," including the two regular "Sessions" of lectures. The candidates had to be at least 21 years of age, pass an oral examination before the Faculty, and submit a satisfactory thesis. In 1849 the regular required "Session" added two weeks by starting in mid-October instead of the first Monday of November. In 1866 the faculty instituted a "Summer Course" with additional staff to reinforce and supplement the regular curriculum. It was actually an added spring and fall session of April, May, and September, with omission of the intolerably hot months of July and August. In 1881 the regular winter session of five months was extended to an obligatory six, with an optional voluntary additional three months. In 1883 a "postgraduate course" was announced for "promoting higher medical education" in medical and surgical specialties for the graduates. This was continued until 1890 as "special instruction for practitioners." A "graded course" was established in 1884, in which students could elect to distribute their lectures over a three-year period instead of the standard two. In 1885 the final oral examination before the faculty was changed to a written one for the Professor in each branch. At the same time the requirement for a written thesis was abolished except in competition for a prize. In 1891 the curriculum became a mandatory three-year course. Requirement for admission to the College was still only a high school diploma or its equivalent. It would be 1914 before the requirement was one year of college. In 1929 it was three years of collegiate work, and in 1940, a bachelor's degree.

The five-year period of 1890–1895 witnessed many other changes in the teaching force that contributed to its variety, thoroughness, and practicality. These improvements placed and maintained Jefferson on a basis equal to any similar institution in the country. Jefferson was among the forefront of medical schools adopting the compulsory four-year course.

In the session of 1894–1895 there were ten Chairs (Professors), two Emeritus Professors, eight Honorary and Clinical Professors, one Adjunct Professor, seven Lecturers, nine Demonstrators, and 36 Instructors and Assistant Demonstrators, an aggregate teaching force of 73. Of the 711 students, 219 were in the first year, 237 in the second, and 229 in the third, with an additional 26 special students. At the 1895 commencement the M.D. degree was conferred on 148 graduates, and the total to that time was 10,398.

Change from Proprietary to Nonprofit Sharing Corporation (1895)

Until 1895 each Professor of the College collected a fee that students paid for the ticket to his lectures. The faculty at this time were paying a rental fee of $3,993 to the Board for use of the College and Hospital. The Board administered the taxes and maintenance costs of the buildings. The profit went to the Professors and was known as "The Professorial Jackpot." Contrary to what might be thought about such profits, the Professors seldom became affluent from this system (Figures 48-22a and b) and at times had to add funds from their own resources to maintain an up-to-date Department. The College was in need of funds for land, new buildings, and laboratory equipment. Public appeals were not appropriate if the Professors were to benefit personally from the donors.

Mr. William Potter, who became a member of the Board in 1894, was a prime mover in negotiations with the faculty to accept fixed salaries as their measure of compensation for services. The surplus funds would thereafter inure to the benefit of the School. This arrangement changed the character of the college from a "proprietary school" to a truly collegiate institution. Harvard Medical College had adopted this policy around 1871, and the University of Pennsylvania followed in 1876. With surprisingly little opposition, there was accord among the College faculty, Hospital staff, and the Alumni Association. The plan of reorganization was adopted by the Board on February 1, 1895, and became effective on June 1 of that year. The Board was now assuming financial responsibility for an integrated College and Hospital.

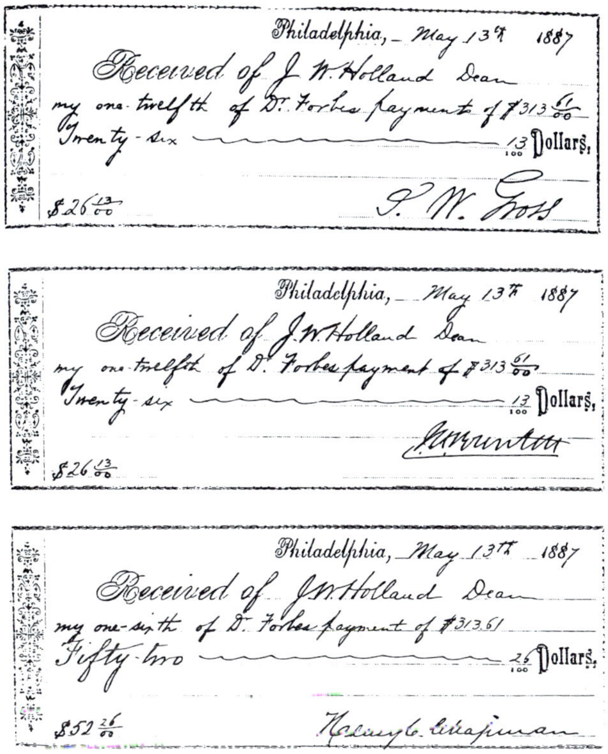

Philadelphia, May 13th 1887
Received of J. W. Holland Dean
my one-twelfth of Dr. Forbes payment of $313 61/00
Twenty-six 13/100 Dollars,
$26 13/00
S. W. Gross

Philadelphia, May 13th 1887
Received of J. W. Holland Dean
my one-twelfth of Dr. Forbes payment of $313 61/00
Twenty-six 13/100 Dollars,
$26 13/00
J. H. Brinton

Philadelphia, May 13th 1887
Received of J. W. Holland Dean
my one-sixth of Dr. Forbes payment of $313.61
Fifty-two 26/100 Dollars,
$52 26/00
Henry C. Chapman

FIG. 48-22a. Receipts (1887) for division of teaching fees to Professors Samuel W. Gross (Surgery) John H. Brinton (Surgery) and Henry C. Chapman (Physiology).

The Honorable William Potter, LL.D.; the Ninth Board President (1896–1926)

William Potter (Figure 48-23) was born in Philadelphia in 1852, the son of a prosperous manufacturer of oilcloth and an eminent citizen. On his maternal side he was a descendant of Brigadier General Bower, who served under Washington in the Revolutionary War. After early education in private schools, Potter entered the University of Pennsylvania in 1874. His father's illness compelled him to leave college to aid in running the firm of Thomas Potter's Sons and Company, and he became a successful director for many years. While engaged in this business for 18 years he studied law and political science. Although admitted to the Bar in 1896, he never indulged in active practice. The University of Pennsylvania granted him a Bachelor of Arts in 1919, and two years later Washington and Jefferson College awarded him a Doctor of Laws.

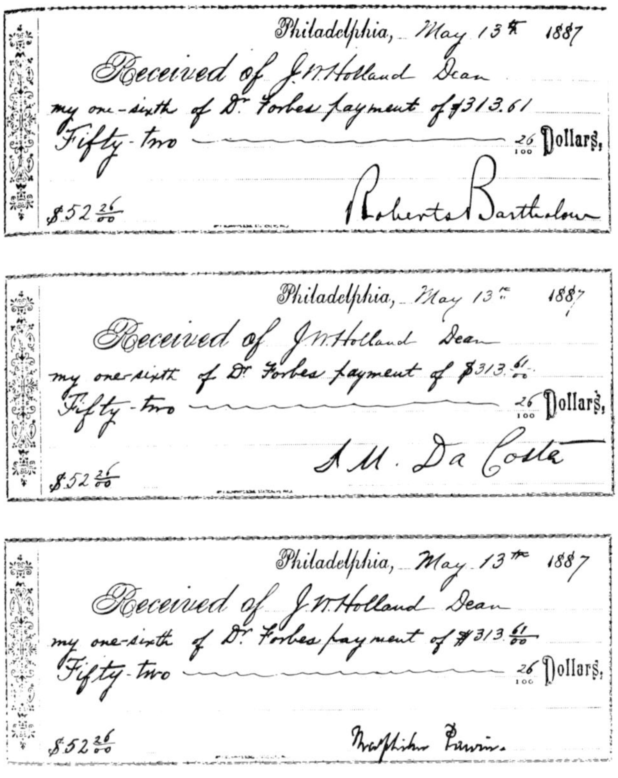

Philadelphia, May 13th 1887
Received of J.W. Holland Dean
my one-sixth of Dr. Forbes payment of $313.61
Fifty-two 26/100 Dollars,
$52 26/100 Roberts Bartholow

Philadelphia, May 13th 1887
Received of J.W. Holland Dean
my one-sixth of Dr. Forbes payment of $313.61
Fifty-two 26/100 Dollars,
$52 26/100 J.M. Da Costa

Philadelphia, May 13th 1887
Received of J.W. Holland Dean
my one-sixth of Dr. Forbes payment of $313.61
Fifty-two 26/100 Dollars,
$52 26/100 Theophilus Parvin

FIG. 48-22b. Receipts (1887) for division of teaching fees to Professors Roberts Bartholow (Materia Medica), Jacob M. DaCosta (Medicine) and Theophilus Parvin (Obstetrics).

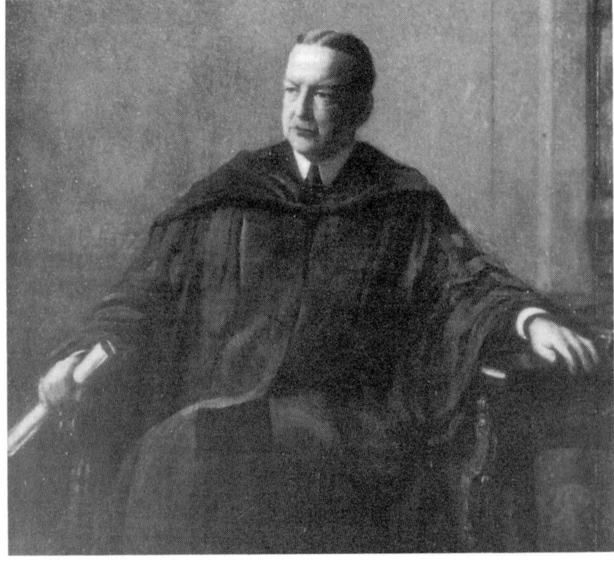

FIG. 48-23. A portrait of the Honorable William Potter, LL.D. (1852–1926), Ninth Board President (1896–1926).

Potter entered politics in 1890 at which time President Harrison appointed him the special commissioner to London, Paris, and Berlin on behalf of the Postal Service to facilitate the handling of transatlantic mail by steamship. The same year he was a delegate to the Postal Union Congress in Vienna and signed a new Postal Treaty. In 1892 he was appointed Minister to Italy, a post he held for two years. He retained a fondness for Italy and its people, enhanced by an interest in archeology. This led to his Vice Presidency of the American and British Archeological Society of Rome and subsequent membership on the Committee of the American Schools at Rome for the Study of Archeology. King Umberto and King Victor Emanuel of Italy both bestowed decorations upon him. In 1896 Potter ran for Mayor of Philadelphia as an antiorganization Republican and was defeated. An invitation by President McKinley in 1897 to be Ambassador to Berlin was declined as well as a later offer to St. Petersburg. His continued interest in civic affairs was manifested by his membership on the Board of City Trusts, Manager of the Pennsylvania Institute for the Deaf and Dumb, membership on the Citizens Permanent Relief Committee, and Chairmanship of the Advisory Board for Philadelphia Mayor Weaver (1905). President Wilson made him Fuel Administrator during World War I to conserve coal and other fuels in Pennsylvania. He became a member of the Board of Directors of the Union League and counselor of the Pennsylvania Historical Society.[10]

In 1894 Potter, at age 42, was elected to the Jefferson Board. With the resignation of Joseph Townsend in 1896 he became President for the next 30 years. His role in Jefferson's change to a nonprofit corporation was only one of many other achievements that marked him as a truly great Board President. Some of these require more detailed review. His son-in-law, Joseph W. Wear (Figure 48-24), served on the Board from 1931 to 1941, and his grandson, William Potter Wear (Figure 48-24), was a distinguished third-generation member from 1941 to 1985.

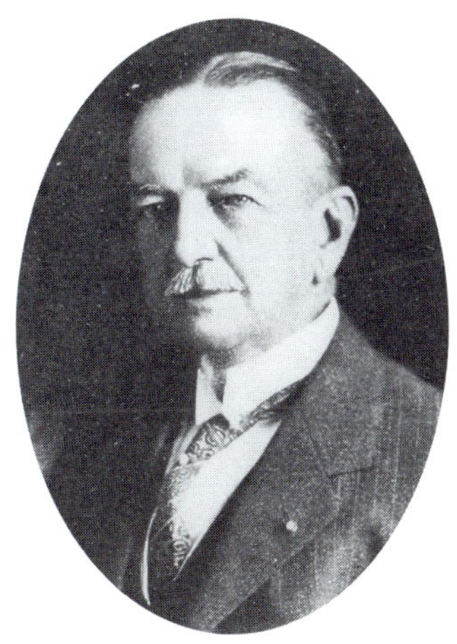

William Potter
Board President (1896–1926)

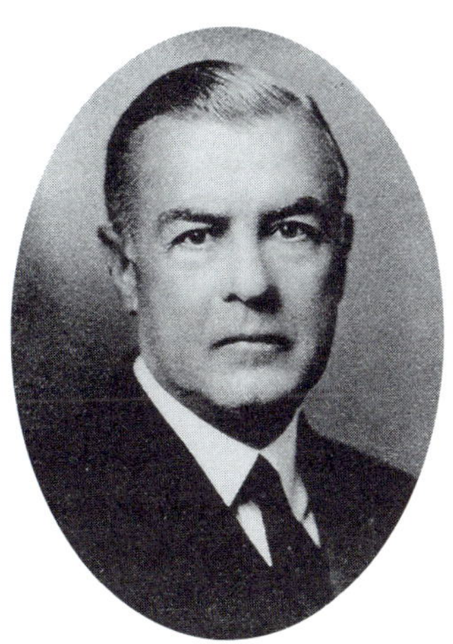

Joseph W. Wear
Son-in-law of William Potter,
Board Member (1931–1941)

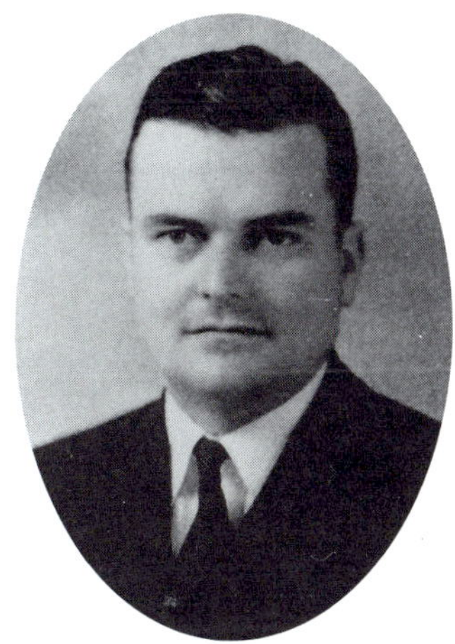

William Potter Wear
Son of Joseph W. Wear,
grandson of William Potter,
Board Member (1941–1985)

Fig. 48-24

On April 24, 1926, Potter was admitted to Jefferson Hospital with a ruptured appendix. In spite of an immediate operation he died four days later. He was buried in East Laurel Hill Cemetery where also lie the remains of George McClellan, the founder, and Robley Dunglison, the "peacemaker," one of Jefferson's greatest deans and personal physician to Thomas Jefferson.

At the suggestion of Dr. Chevalier Jackson, who brought fame to Jefferson for his discoveries in bronchoscopy and esophagoscopy, a William Potter Memorial Lectureship was endowed by his beloved grandson, William Potter Wear. The first was delivered on April 25, 1928, by Sir St. Clair Thomson, M.D., of London, whose topic was *The Strenuous Life of a Physician in the 18th Century*. Mr. Potter in a tribute was called "A man whose life makes a great difference for all. . . . it does not die with him—that is a true estimate of a great life."[11]

Jefferson Medical College Moves to Tenth and Walnut Streets (1898)

Inauguration of the graded four-year course, starting with the 1895–1896 session, created a requirement for new buildings. On the accession of Mr. Potter to the Board Presidency, the Trustees acted on the plans that had been in progress during the previous three years. A commodious College with an adjacent laboratory building was envisioned to comply with the most modern requirements of medical education from both theoretical and practical standpoints. This meant the demolition of the Ely Building at Tenth and Sansom Streets, which had served so admirably for 70 years (1828–1898), and its subsequent replacement by a new hospital ("Old Main" of 1907). The new College and laboratory would locate on the land purchased at Tenth and Walnut.

Jefferson would now extend the entire length of the west side of Tenth Street between Sansom and Walnut, and on Sansom Street from Tenth for about three-fourths of the distance to Eleventh. The street on Jefferson's property running east and west between Sansom and Walnut, which had originally been called Juniper Alley, became Moravian, and then was renamed Medical Street (Philadelphia map of 1885). At present it is the anonymous ambulance and vehicle access between the Curtis Building and "Old Main" Hospital, simply referred to as "the alley."

The new College of 1898 fronted on Walnut Street for 118 feet with a formal English Renaissance facade (Figure 48-25). It had a vertical division of three parts corresponding to the arrangement of the interior. The two lateral parts were symmetrical. The central part began with a classic porch that admitted to a tile-floored vestibule and a lobby for the main stairs and elevator. The basement contained a gymnasium, billiard room, reading room, space for lockers and bicycles, and the Library (Figure 48-26). On the walls of the Library hung the few portraits of Jefferson's infant art collection, but prominently the *Gross Clinic,* which occupied almost all of the space between the floor and the ceiling. The first floor was occupied by administration offices, a recitation room, and the first story of the lower amphitheater. The second floor contained the museum, a laboratory of pathology and the second story of the lower amphitheater. The third floor contained a large west lecture hall. Here also was a small east lecture hall, chemical apparatus room, and a laboratory of physiology. The fourth floor completed the upper part of the two lecture halls and a room for instruction in bandaging and obstetric manipulations, as well as for storage. The fifth floor contained the lower portion of the upper amphitheater, the dissecting room (two stories high), a laboratory of operative surgery, private rooms for professors, and locker rooms for students. The sixth floor housed the upper part of the upper amphitheater, upper part of the dissecting rooms, and an incinerating furnace.

The Tenth Street side of the new College was adjacent to a new laboratory building, by which the two buildings together extended for 108 feet to Moravian Street (Medical Street). Between the two buildings was a large light well. The laboratory building was also six stories high, with ten large laboratories for students and 17 smaller private rooms for individual research. Facilities for pharmacy, medical chemistry, toxicology, physiology, normal and pathological histology, anatomy, bacteriology, research, and recitations were optimal. The laboratories were lighted by windows on three sides, besides incandescent electric lights. There were individual desks equipped by funds partly subscribed by the Alumni. Mr. Louis C. Vanuxem, a Board member from 1895 until his untimely death in 1903 at age 44, at his own expense equipped the physiology laboratory in a manner that placed it in the first rank of such laboratories. Also provided were 150 microscopes of the most recent make for student use, as well as an electric lantern projector, equipment for photography, and other apparatus.

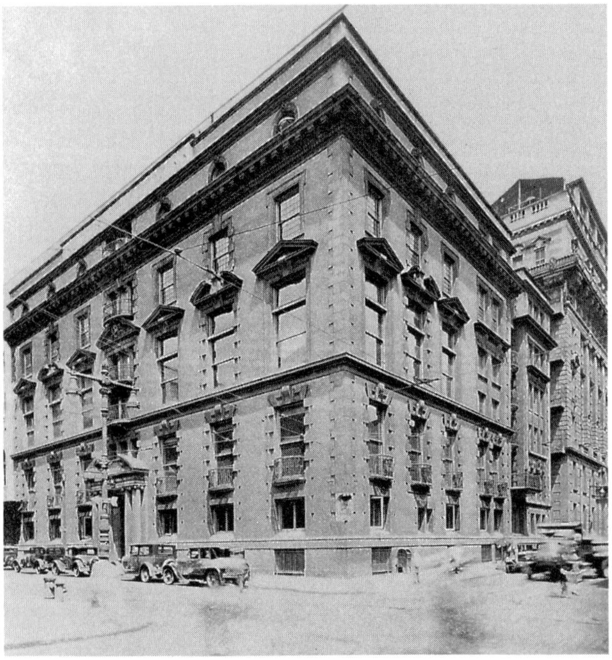

FIG. 48-25. The Jefferson Medical College Building of 1898 at Tenth and Walnut Streets, with the adjoining Laboratory Building at the rear on Tenth Street.

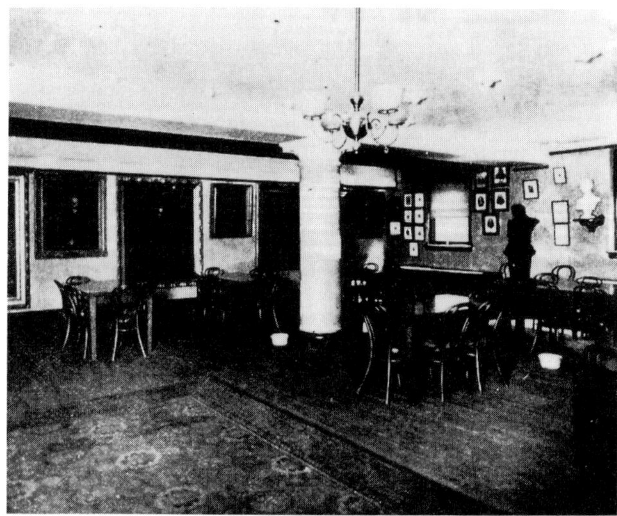

FIG. 48-26. The Library in the basement of the 1898 College. The edge of the *Gross Clinic* is seen at the left.

A committee of the Lady Board of Managers (the future Women's Board) enhanced the amenities of the library, parlor, and clubroom for recreation and student society meetings. They also contributed more than 800 volumes to the library in less than a year.

These new facilities would be among those inspected in 1909 by Abraham Flexner of the Carnegie Foundation for the Advancement of Teaching that contributed to Jefferson's favorable national rating.

The 1907 Hospital ("Old Main")

On completion of the 1898 College and Laboratory Buildings, Mr. Potter and his fellow Trustees turned their attention to improving the medical and educational work of the 1877 Hospital. That first detached hospital provided beds for 140 patients and a clinical amphitheater ("pit") capable of seating 600 students. In 1898, in the outpatient services (Figures 48-27 and 48-28), 75,304 patients were treated for surgical, gynecologic, ophthalmologic, laryngological, aural, genito-urinary, and orthopedic conditions. For medical diseases, including neurological, dermatological, and pediatric, 19,274 were treated. These, added to the 1,783 inpatients, totaled 96,361 for that year. The grand total for the previous 20 years was 1,191,931. Also in 1898, the Maternity Department at 224 South Seventh Street took care of 296 new obstetric cases and 185 babies, providing instruction in midwifery and natal care to each member of the graduating class. By 1907, over a period of 30 years (1877–1907), this hospital would train 5,000 doctors in its halls, care for 2,000,000 patients in wards and dispensaries, treat nearly 50,000 accident cases, and graduate 148 nurses.

By the turn of the century the hospital was antiquated. Beds were insufficient for the demand; the dispensaries were too small for the volume of work; and the building was not fireproof. The Medical School had moved to Tenth and Walnut and by 1902 it was possible to demolish the old Ely Building and Laboratory Building at the corner of Tenth and Sansom for a new hospital. The 1877 Hospital would then be used for education and lodging of nurses, and its clinical amphitheater, one of the largest in the world, would be used until replaced by the Thompson Annex in 1924.

Construction of "Old Main" Hospital at Tenth and Sansom was started in 1903, but slowed down by strikes as well as by drawn out attention to details. It was opened on June 8, 1907, with an impressive ceremony led by the Board President, the Honorable William Potter, and enhanced by an inspired address by Dr. John Chalmers DaCosta (destined to be appointed the first Samuel D. Gross Professor of Surgery in 1910).

Eight stories tall, with ground floor and basement built of steel, concrete, brick, and terra-cotta; floored with tile or other nonflammable material; provided with natural light by three streets; supplied with interior electric lighting; steam heated from an outside plant; cleaned by a vacuum system; and ventilated by a noiseless exhaust system, this ample hospital with more than 300 beds could vie with any of the best in the country. On June 24, 1907, the patients at that time in the "Old Jefferson Hospital" were removed to the new institution (Figure 48-29).

■ The Flexner Report

In 1909 and 1910 Abraham Flexner made a survey of medical education in the United States and Canada on behalf of the Carnegie Foundation for the Advancement of Teaching.[12,13] He personally visited 155 medical schools, of which seven were in Canada. The evaluation, on a state-by-state basis, included the founding, entrance requirements, enrollment, teaching staff, general resources, source of funds, laboratory facilities, clinical facilities, and the date of his visit. His report, *Medical Education in United States and Canada,* appeared in 1910. This document played a sweeping role in changing the course of medical education in America. Even more credit belonged to the American Medical Association, which through its Journal and Council on Medical Education, along with collaboration of the Association of American Medical Colleges, carried out the recommendations. Dr. William H. Welch of Johns Hopkins University and Dr. Simon Flexner (brother of Abraham) of the Rockefeller

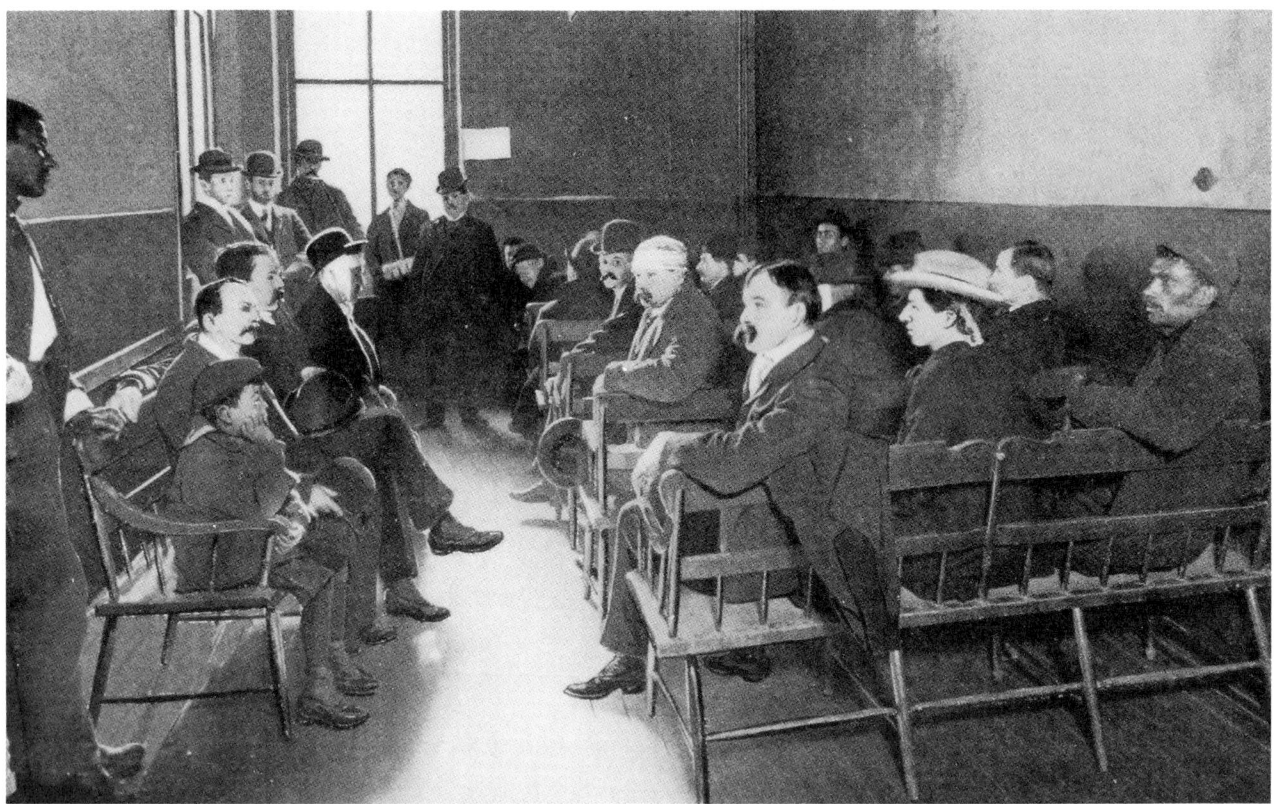

FIG. 48-27. The Men's Waiting Room of the Surgical Clinic of the 1877 Hospital.

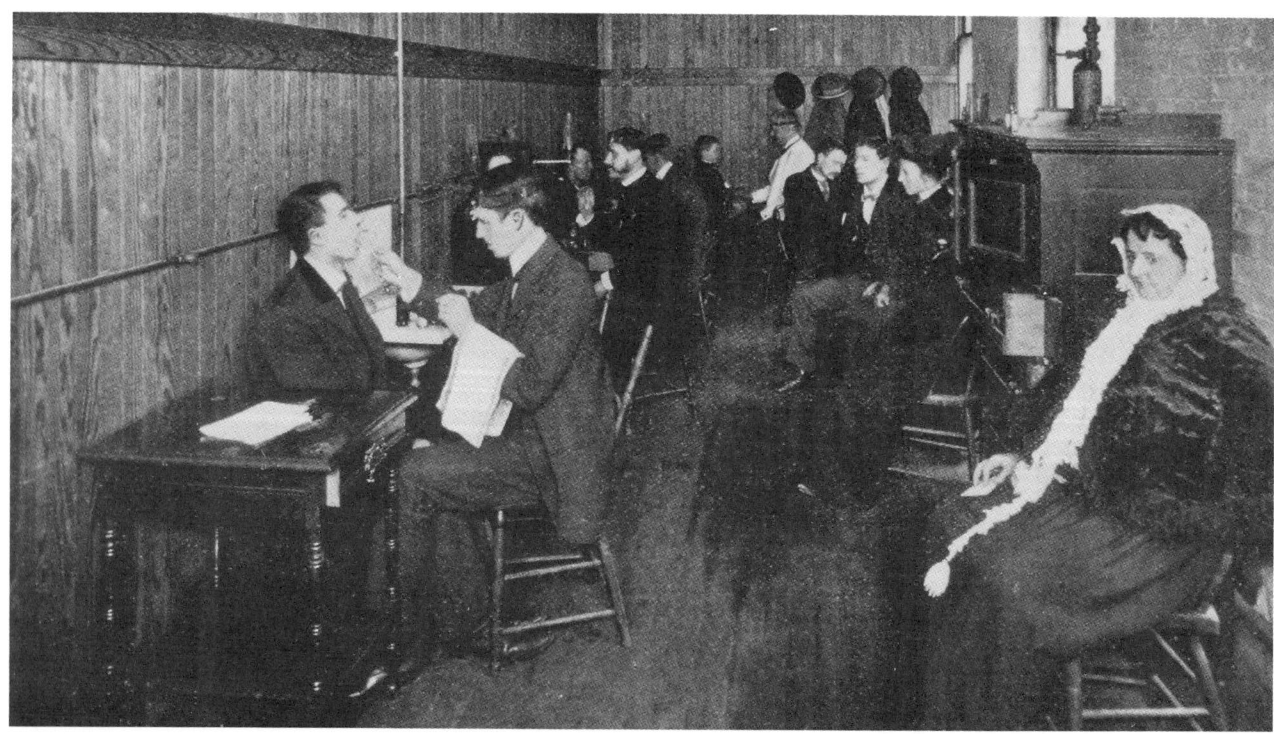

FIG. 48-28. The Clinic of the Ear Department of the 1877 Hospital.

Institute also aided the movement. The result was that 76 medical schools went out of existence between 1906 and 1920 either by ceasing to function or by merging with stronger institutions.[12] Jefferson was visited in March, 1909. Although its rating was favorable, it too would experience an impact from the general suggestions for reform.

The salient features of the report regarding Jefferson were:[13] (1) of all the independent schools outside New York State, Jefferson came nearest to obtaining its published entrance requirements; (2) its enrollment of 591 students was the largest of the eight medical schools, plus one postgraduate school, in Pennsylvania; (3) the teaching staff of 122 included 22 professors and seven instructors who devoted their entire time to the school; (4) student fees amounted to $102,995, of which a part was diverted to paying off building mortgages, while the hospital had independent sources of support; (5) the laboratory building contained separate areas for the various basic sciences with modern and adequate equipment; (6) there was an attractive library, museum, and other teaching accessories; (7) Jefferson Hospital with 223 teaching beds was connected with a dispensary that supplied an abundance of material; and (8) the Maternity Department, with 17 beds, occupied a separate building (224 South Seventh Street). The conclusion was that "the plant of the institution is therefore modern and compact" (Figure 48-30).

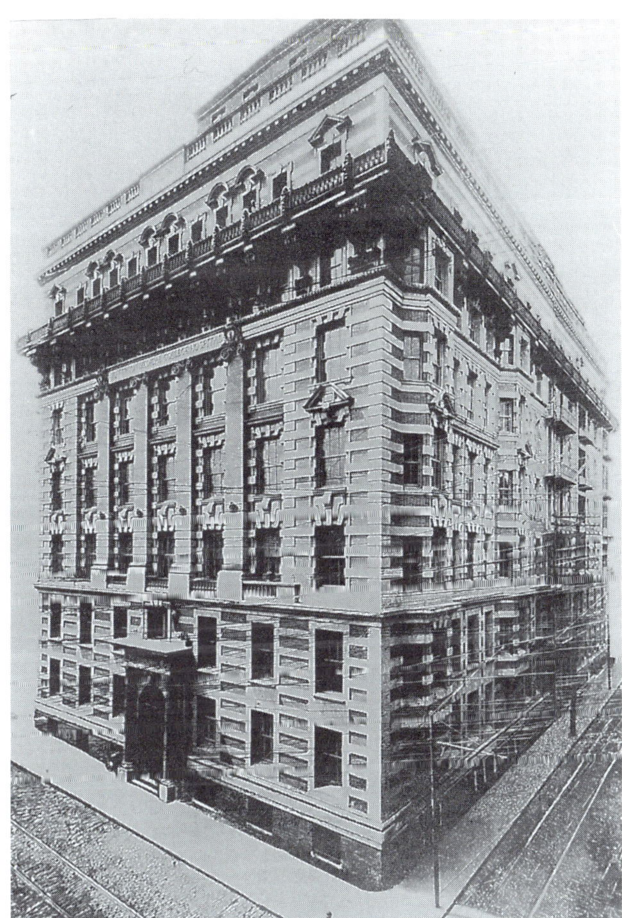

FIG. 48-29. Jefferson Medical College Hospital ("Old Main"), 1907.

On a national basis, the school with the largest enrollment was the University of Louisville, Kentucky, with 600; Jefferson was second with 591; and the University of Pennsylvania was third with 546. For that time the University of Louisville, although the largest of the American schools, was among the worst "which turned out physicians with little regard for their competence."[14] The main thrust of Flexner's overall recommendations was that many of the medical schools should be closed and that others be merged with stronger institutions, preferably universities. He concluded that there should be fewer but better educated medical graduates.

An Invitation from Medico-Chirurgical College to Amalgamate (1910)

The enrollment (480 students) of the Medico-Chirurgical College at the time of Flexner's visit was the third largest in Philadelphia. The entrance requirement was less than a four-year high school education. None of the teaching staff devoted their entire time to medical instruction. The laboratories were well equipped, but with some limitations in anatomy. Except in bacteriology, little or no effort was made to cultivate original scientific activity. The clinical facilities in the hospital and dispensary were adequate, but the library was small. From this setting of a mediocre rating, Mr. Potter received a letter dated January 18, 1910: "Whereas the tendency of medical education is toward elimination of the independent medical school, Resolved that the Board of Trustees of the Jefferson Medical College be invited to confer with the Committee on Amalgamation of the Board of Trustees of the Medico-Chirurgical College upon the subject of affiliation of Medical Colleges." On January 20, 1910, Mr. Potter appointed four other Trustees to constitute with him a committee for joint discussion. No report of the committee appeared in minutes of subsequent meetings of the Jefferson Board, and the matter was apparently aborted.

In 1912 the President of the Board of the Medico-Chirurgical College approached the Provost of the University of Pennsylvania to consider a merger. The school, at Seventeenth and Cherry Streets, was in the path of the proposed Franklin Parkway and would require removal to new buildings. Agreement was reached for the University to absorb the entire teaching staff as well as the dental faculty. The University would acquire all the property and funds of the other school. The latter's pharmacy school was absorbed (1916) by the Philadelphia College of Pharmacy.

In 1917 the Philadelphia Polyclinic and College for Graduates in Medicine, founded in 1883 and located on Lombard Street between Eighteenth and Nineteenth, joined in the University merger. Medico-Chirurgical was combined with the Polyclinic as a single graduate school, which instructed as such in 1919.

■ Osteopathic "Intruders" (1910)

The Flexner Report took note that "The catalogue of the Philadelphia College and Infirmary of

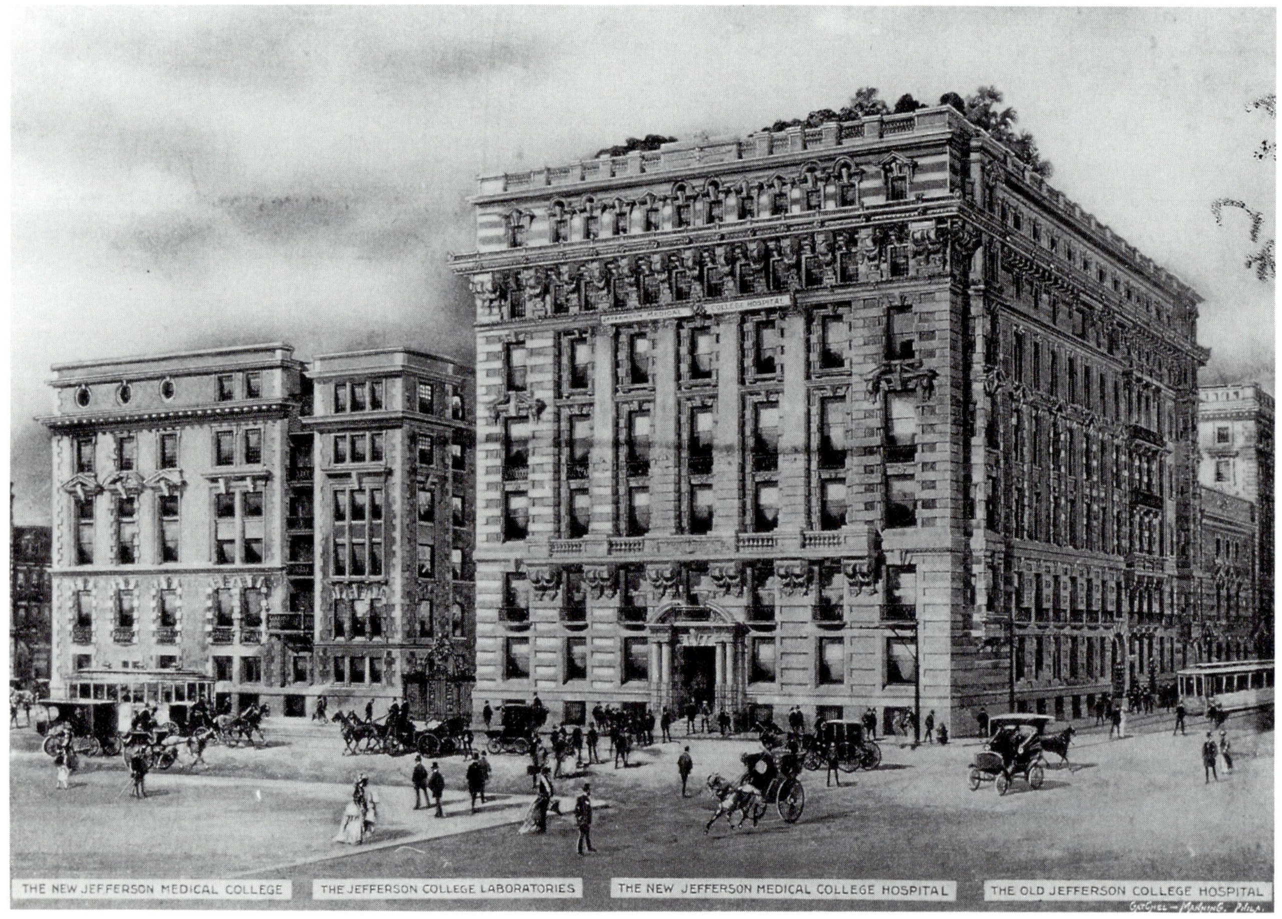

FIG. 48-30. Tenth Street between Walnut and Sansom (ca. 1910). From left to right: the 1898 Medical College; the 1898 Laboratory Building; the 1907 Jefferson Hospital ("Old Main"); and the first Jefferson Hospital, 1877.

Osteopathy announces that its students have the 'privilege of witnessing operations at the University Hospital, Jefferson Hospital, etc.' This is not the case. These students are intruders, without rights or privileges of any description whatsoever."

On February 3, 1910, a resolution from the faculty was read to the Jefferson Board protesting the inclusion of Jefferson's name in the Osteopathic catalogue as "damaging to the ethical standing of the school and libelous." The Board arranged to have its name deleted from the catalogue. The explanation given by the Osteopathic College was that the Jefferson name had been placed by a previous management and "we do not know upon what authority it first was placed there."

■ Offer from Temple University of Union with Jefferson (1910)

At the time of Flexner's report, the Medical School of Temple University was in dire financial straits and its facilities given an unfavorable rating.[13] On February 23, 1910, The Reverend Russell H. Conwell, President of Temple University, wrote a letter to Sub-Dean Ross V. Patterson proposing consideration of a union of Jefferson Medical College with Temple University.

> "It occurs to me that the Jefferson College, with all its honorable history, would secure all its influence for the future if it were connected directly with a University. It may sound absurd on its first suggestion but I think it is a wise measure to meditate upon whether the Jefferson might not be connected with the Temple University and perhaps the Medico-Chi in such a way as to make the greatest medical college in the world. . . . It occurred to me on rather superficial thought that the name of the Temple University could be very easily changed by the State so as to carry the name of the Jefferson University and thus secure not only a venerable name for the University, but in union with Jefferson Medical College, would carry your institution on into the future as a University and give it, and all connected with it, a mightier influence in the future centuries. . . . As the University is now thoroughly established for a great future work, it should have some settled name and the Jefferson College should also have all the rights and dignity of a University. There is no probability that another charter for a University in Philadelphia can ever be obtained, and if ours were used, it carries with it a prestige of 3500 students and its great organized work."[15]

The overture from President Conwell would have greatly benefited Temple University at the time, but Jefferson under its 1838 Charter already had "the same powers and restrictions as the University of Pennsylvania." The long run was more advantageous for Temple, however, in that it solved its own financial crisis, preserved and developed its own excellent Medical School, kept its name, and served well the needs of an expanding Philadelphia.

■ First Endowed Professorship (1910)

In April, 1910, Mrs. Maria Gross Horwitz of Baltimore endowed Jefferson's first Chair, "The Samuel D. Gross Professorship of Surgery," in honor of her father, with a gift of $60,000. On June 2, 1910, Dr. John Chalmers DaCosta (Jefferson, 1885) was unanimously elected as the first Gross Professor of Surgery, "it being understood that he shall not hereafter receive any compensation other than that derived from the fund given by Mrs. Horwitz for that purpose."

A bronze plaque bearing testimony to this endowment is on permanent display in the Samuel D. Gross Conference Room of the College (Figure 48-31).

■ Jefferson's "Medical Preparatory Course" (1913–1916)

The Board of Trustees, upon recommendation of the faculty, advanced the requirements for admission to the medical course, beginning with the academic year 1914–1915, to include one year of college credits in German or French, Chemistry, Physics, and Biology. The arrangement of curricula of most lay colleges would require two years to secure these credits. In order to save a year of a student's time, Jefferson established a preparatory course in which these sciences and language requirements could be met satisfactorily in one year. These courses were established under the provisions of Jefferson's University Charter of 1838. They started on September 24, 1913, so that students planning to matriculate in 1914 could have proper entrance credentials. The preparatory course was parallel in time with the regular medical course. The taking and passing of this course was a secure step in gaining admission to the College medical course, although not so stated in the catalogue.

Jefferson's one-year course in liberal arts lasted three years through the 1915–1916 session. For the session of 1916–1917, two years of study in an approved College of Arts and Sciences, with specified courses in Physics, Chemistry, Biology (with laboratory in each science), and either German or French were required.

■ The A+ Rating of Jefferson by the AMA (1914)

The minutes of the Board for October 18, 1914, recorded the following: "The Jefferson Medical College has finally received tardy justice from the American Medical Association in being placed, the early part of this year, in the A+ Class of American Medical Colleges." A deciding factor in this highest rating was the Daniel Baugh Institute of Anatomy, which increased the basic science facilities.

■ A Proposed Union of Jefferson and University of Pennsylvania (1916)

A situation of serious proportions arose in December, 1915, when Dr. Henry S. Pritchett, President of the Carnegie Foundation, urged

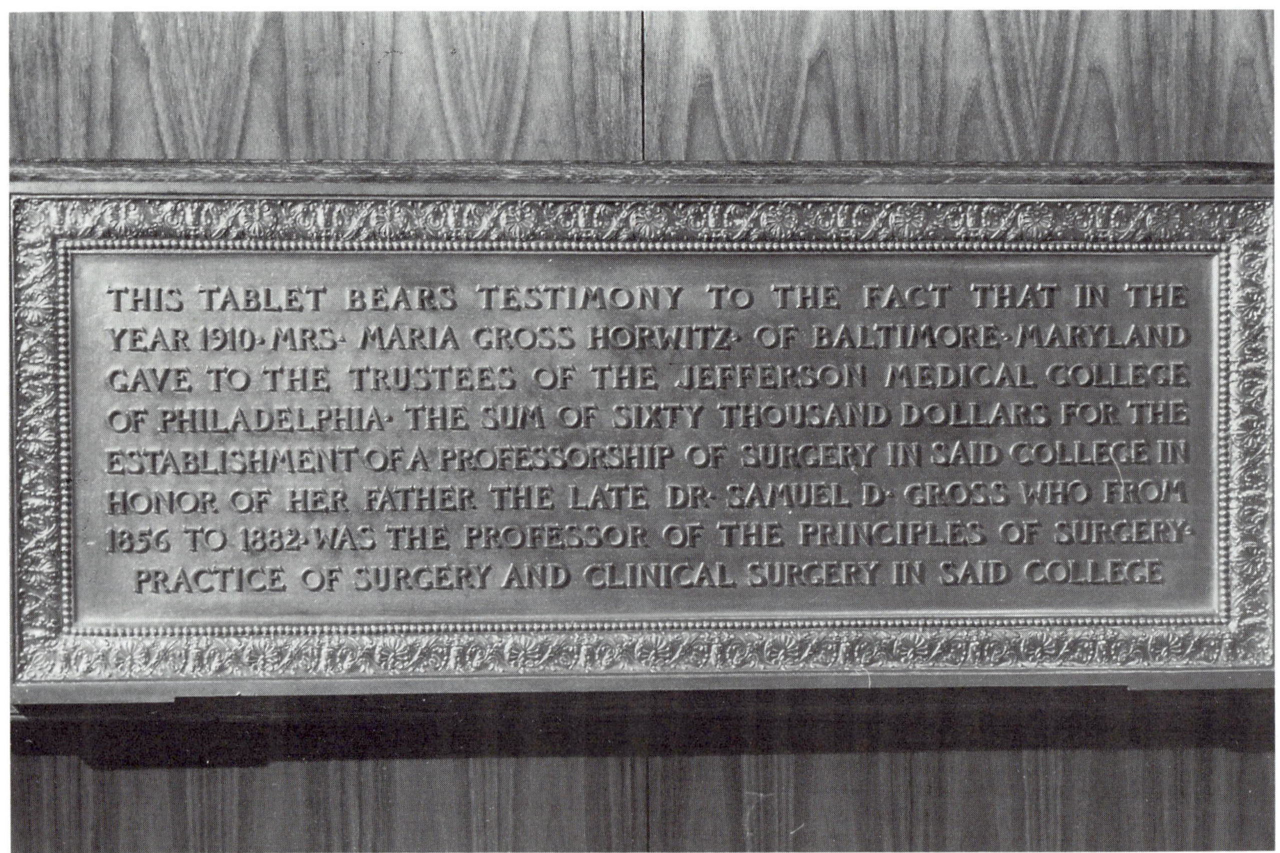

FIG. 48-31. A bronze plaque in the Samuel D. Gross Conference Room, in testimomy to the first Endowed Chair (1910).

Provost Edgar Fahs Smith of the University of Pennsylvania to open conversations with the Jefferson Board of Trustees regarding a possible union of the two institutions. Earlier that year, negotiations of the University with the Medico-Chirurgical College led to considering the idea of including Jefferson Medical College in a possible sweeping merger. This would be a type of union as recommended by the Flexner Report of 1910. Jefferson with 650 students had become the largest medical school in the country. A merger was expected to gain a large financial support from the Carnegie Foundation and perhaps the Rockefeller Foundation.

The year 1916 saw the start and end of the negotiations. Discussions began in January, with enthusiasm on the part of the University and with cautious reserve on the part of Jefferson. In May, a report was approved by a joint committee of three representatives from both institutions. It provided for joint operation under which the combined schools would be called "The Medical School of the University of Pennsylvania and the Jefferson Medical College of Philadelphia." The internal affairs were to remain under the control of their respective Boards, but the combined school would be governed by a committee of eight Trustees, with four from each Board. The Provost of the University would be Chairman. The two faculties were to be combined under a single dean from one institution with a vice-dean from the other. The curriculum, examinations, and current expenses would be administered jointly. Previous endowments would be kept separate. The University's plan to put the united school under its own aegis and Jefferson's understanding to preserve its identity were hardly compatible.

On June 1, 1916, the Boards of the University and Jefferson met separately and voted in favor of the plan. On the same day the Trustees of the Medico-Chirurgical College also agreed to join with the University. The daily press immediately announced both "mergers." On June 7, Provost Smith wrote a letter of congratulation to President Pritchett for what he believed was a consummation of the unions.

At the first meeting of the United Medical Committee of the Trustees, Dr. William Pepper was elected Dean of the combined school and Dr. Ross V. Patterson of Jefferson the Vice-Dean. At a second meeting of the Joint Trustees that summer, while the arrangement still appeared amicable, certain large expenditures were agreed upon. Ongoing discussions revealed more clearly that the University faction assumed that the combined school was part of the University, whereas the Jefferson group viewed it as a new independent school. This meeting adjourned unhappily. At the third meeting that summer the Jefferson Trustees galvanized their stand against University control and insisted on an independent new combined school. Provost Smith wired this basic disagreement to Dr. Pritchett of the Carnegie Foundation, who responded by telegram that the government should rest in the University. Pritchett thereupon wrote letters to the Provost and to Mr. William Potter "that the Carnegie Foundation for the Advancement of Teaching took no interest whatever in any plan not based on University leadership."[16] At a fourth and final meeting that summer it was decided that each school should proceed as in the past, pending a further meeting in the fall. According to Bauer,[17] Mr. Daniel Baugh passed a note to Mr. Potter: "Make no commitment until I talk to you. I pledge my fortune to keep Jefferson independent." To the credit of Mr. Baugh should also be added the influence of the Alumni Association, Dr. Henry K. Mohler, and Dean Ross V. Patterson. There were no further meetings with respect to a University-Jefferson merger.

The Faculty Endorses Coeducation at Jefferson: Overture to the Woman's Medical College (1918)

At a meeting of the Faculty in the College library on November 25, 1918, Dr. Edward P. Davis, Professor of Obstetrics, made a motion that the faculty of Jefferson Medical College approve of coeducation. It was passed unanimously. In demonstrating a willingness to adopt coeducation, it was then voted that a Committee of the faculty be appointed to confer with the faculty of the Woman's Medical College of Pennsylvania, to ascertain what way and to what extent they desired to cooperate with the Jefferson Medical College in the medical education of women. The Committee consisted of Drs. Davis, Albert P. Brubaker, and Ross V. Patterson.

At a meeting held January 13, 1919, there were present from the Women's Medical College: Dr. R. W. Lathrop, Professor of Physiology; Dr. Martha Tracy, Professor of Chemistry and Dean; and Dr. Harry Deaver, Professor of Surgery. The Jefferson Committee, after combined discussion, submitted the following report to the faculty on January 27, 1919.

> "1st. The interchange of teachers and teaching facilities between the Woman's Medical College of Pennsylvania and The Jefferson Medical College of Philadelphia, would not be advantageous or desirable.
>
> 2nd. If affiliation is desirable, it must be complete without the loss of identity, and must secure better teaching for both groups of students with economy of administration. The most obvious economies and advantages may be expected in combining the facilities and personnel in both laboratory and clinical departments in both institutions."

The Jefferson faculty voted to receive this report, upon which no further action was taken and in which no record of these overtures appeared in the minutes of the Board of Trustees. It had been 45 years since John Barclay Biddle, as Dean in 1873, had turned down the application of a woman. It would take another 43 years, until 1961, for women to be accepted as Jefferson medical students.

▪ Alumni Concern About Mergers (1922)

On November 20, 1922, Dr. Elmer H. Funk on the part of the Alumni Association wrote to the Board for expression of its attitude toward a merger of Jefferson with the University of Pennsylvania or any other institution. President Potter responded with a disavowal of the Board "to merge Jefferson Medical College with any other institution of learning, and that such a result could come about only through the failure on the part of the Alumni and friends of Jefferson Medical College to support it in the future."

Daniel Baugh (1836–1921) and His Institute of Anatomy (1911)

The extraordinary commitment and contributions to Jefferson of Daniel Baugh warrant recognition equal to that of any Board President, although in his 25 years as Trustee (1896–1921) he never served in that capacity. The Rev. Ezra Stiles Ely has been designated as "Jefferson's First Benefactor," and Mr. Baugh was named as "Our Greatest Benefactor" in the Memorial Tribute to him in the minutes of the Board at his death in 1921. Board President William Potter characterized him as "the most valuable man ever connected with the Board."

Born in 1836 in Chester County, Pennsylvania, Daniel Baugh (Figure 48-32) was educated in private academies but omitted college to engage in a rapidly enlarging family enterprise of Baugh and Sons Company, manufacturers of chemicals and fertilizers. He continued his own education, however, to such an extent that he was elected to the American Philosophical Society, America's highest ranking learned body.

On joining the Jefferson Board in 1896, Baugh set out to improve its financial base. Through his own generosity and solicitation from others, he raised a great deal of the funds to build the 1907 Hospital ("Old Main") at Tenth and Sansom. By supervising the actual construction he saved $300,000 of the $1,250,000 bid for the project. He donated horse-drawn and electric ambulances (Figure 48-33), the latest x-ray equipment, and many other important items. During the first 12 years of his Trusteeship the assets of the institution increased more than fivefold.

In 1898 it had become necessary to reduce the salary of the "Non-practicing Chairmen" from $5,000 to $3,700. In 1899 that salary was stipulated at $4,000 and continued at this level for several years. Mr. Baugh induced his fellow Trustees to reinstate the $5,000 level by pledging to make up any deficit from his personal funds.

The most recognized of Mr. Baugh's

benefactions was his purchase in 1910 of the building at Eleventh and Clinton Streets (Figure 48-34), recently vacated by the Pennsylvania Dental College. He had it completely renovated, enlarged, and equipped for teaching of anatomy and conduct of research. "The Daniel Baugh Institute of Anatomy" (Figure 48-35), so named by his fellow Trustees, was opened in 1911 with an impressive ceremony. To provide even more space for anatomic research and offices, Mr. Baugh purchased the adjoining building at 1023 Clinton Street. The final cost amounted to $160,000 and rose to $200,000 by the time of his death. The Chairman's title was changed to "Professor of Anatomy, Head of the Department of Anatomy, and Director of the Daniel Baugh Institute." The Institute allowed for expansion of the other basic

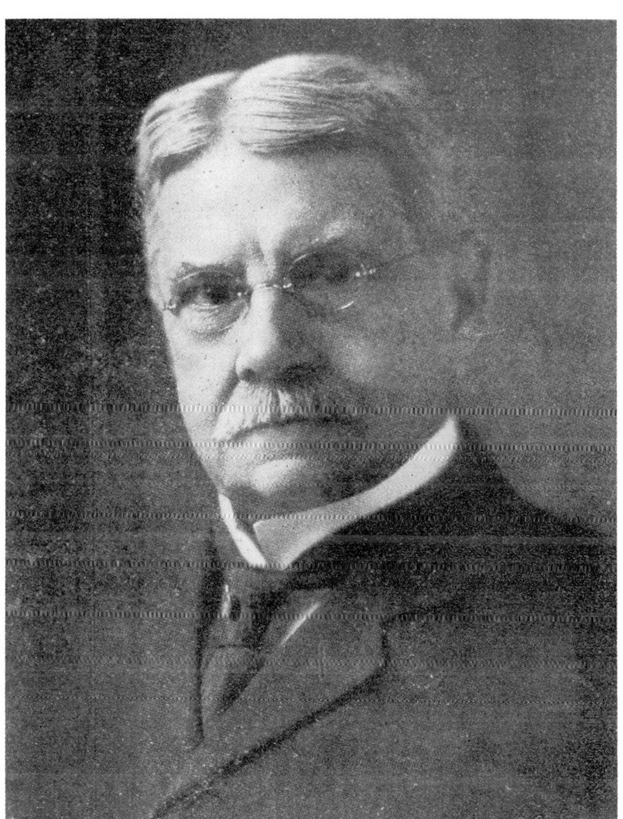

FIG. 48-32. Daniel Baugh (1836–1921), Trustee (1896–1921).

sciences by freeing up two floors of the 1898 College building. When Jefferson Alumni Hall opened in 1968, the Daniel Baugh Institute moved to its fifth floor. The large marble slab acknowledging Mr. Baugh's gift of the Institute to Jefferson was mounted on the wall at the head of the escalator to ensure continued memory of his legacy.

The 1914 Class Yearbook was dedicated to Mr. Baugh, and he was labeled "The Benefactor."

On June 15, 1915, Baugh pledged $100,000 of unrestricted funds to start a general endowment. His stipulation for contribution of an equal amount was matched within one year by his fellow Trustees, faculty, alumni, and friends of the College.

Baugh's will, following his death in 1921, left $150,000 in trust for the salary of the Professor of Anatomy. Actually, he had paid the salary of the Anatomy Professor since 1911. The Chair was in reality endowed one year after the Gross Professorship of 1910, but not officially identified as such until the researches of Dr. Andrew J. Ramsay in 1981 highlighted this benefaction. At a ceremony on September 18, 1981, Dr. Ramsay was named the first Daniel Baugh Professor of Anatomy, and the recently restored portrait of Mr. Baugh with two of his grandsons ("The Three Daniels") was displayed (Figure 48-36). This portrait was then hung at the top of the stairs to the second floor of the College on the wall outside of McClellan Hall where, for so many years, the *Gross Clinic* had hung.

Baugh did not limit his benefactions to Jefferson.[18] He was also a Trustee of Rush Hospital and the Philadelphia Museum; member of the Board of Managers of Howard Hospital and the Permanent Relief Committee of Philadelphia; President of the Sanitarium Association and for 25 years President of the School of Design for Women (later the Moore College of Art); organizer and President for many years of the Philadelphia Art Club; initiator and first President of the Art Federation, which by joining into a Parkway Association, led to completion of the Benjamin Franklin Parkway between City Hall and the Philadelphia Museum of Art. He was a founder of the Archeology and Paleontology Association, serving as one of its Presidents, and gave the address at the presentation of the Museum of Archeology and Paleontology to the University of Pennsylvania. As President of the Philadelphia Medical Publishing

Company he published the highly regarded *Philadelphia Medical Journal* until its merger in 1904 with the *New York Medical Journal.*

The Jefferson Centennial (1924)

When the 1907 Hospital ("Old Main") at Tenth and Sansom was opened, it seemed certain that ample allowance had been made for growth of its services well into the future. By 1917, only ten years later, lack of adequate hospital accommodations resulted in patients being turned away. In March of 1920 the Board received a letter from the Alumni Association stating that 130 patients were waiting for admission to the Hospital and that over 700 applications were received for admission to the freshman class. The Alumni urged the Board to enlarge the institution and pledged to assist in securing funds for extension of the buildings.

Jefferson's education and clinical facilities at that time were as follows:

1. The 1898 Medical College Building and Laboratory, located at the corner of Tenth and Walnut Streets.
2. The Main Hospital (1907) at Tenth and Sansom Streets.
3. A Maternity Hospital and Dispensary at 224–226 South Seventh Street.
4. A Maternity Dispensary at 2545 Wharton Street in South Philadelphia.
5. A Department for Diseases of the Chest at 236–238 Pine Street.
6. Buildings at 1023 to 1029 Walnut Street as an Annex Outpatient Department.
7. A Nurses' Home occupying the four-story buildings at 1012 to 1018 Spruce Street.
8. The original 1877 Hospital on Sansom Street, in which the clinical amphitheater

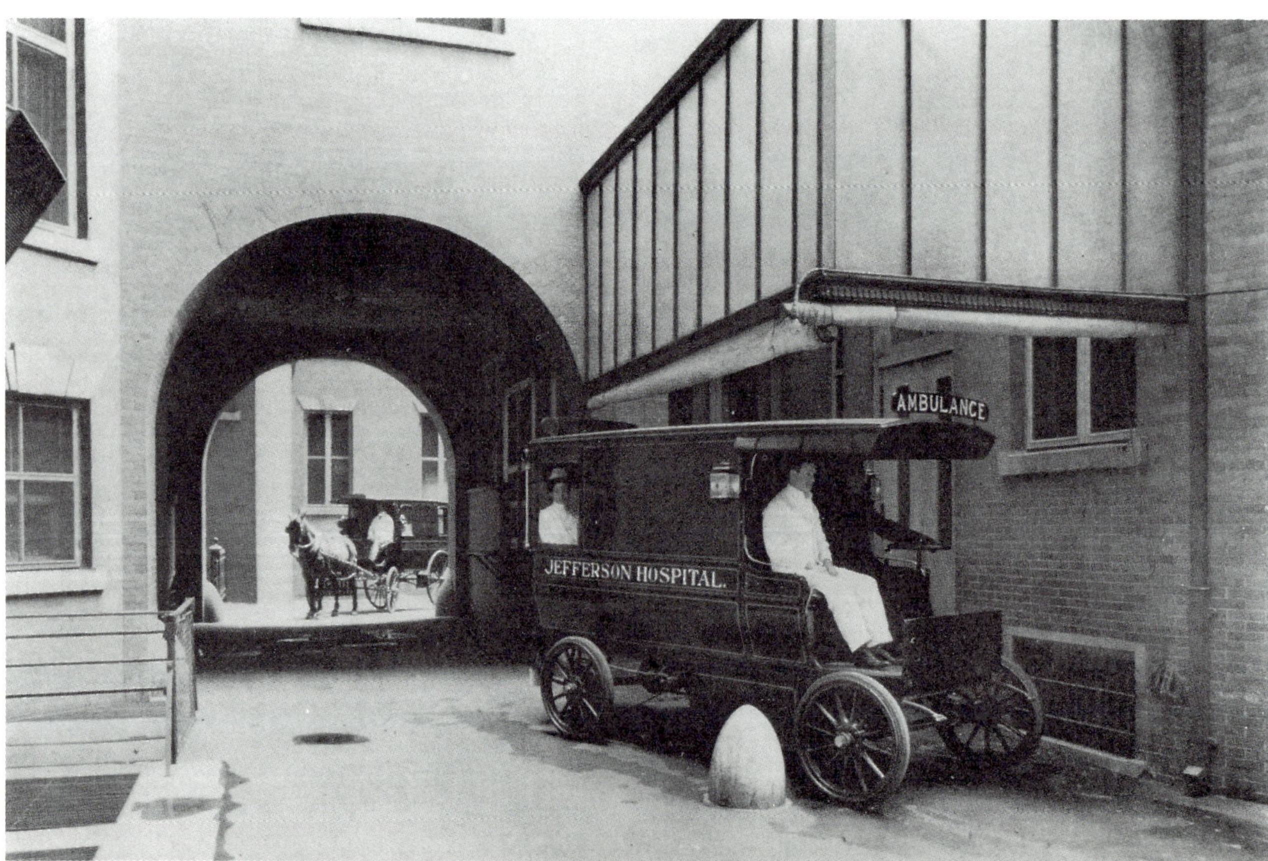

FIG. 48-33. Electric and horse-drawn ambulances of the Emergency Department (ca. 1909).

was still being used and in which the remainder had been converted for nursing education and quarters in 1907.

9. The Ivycroft Farm and Convalescent Home for Men at Wayne, Pennsylvania.

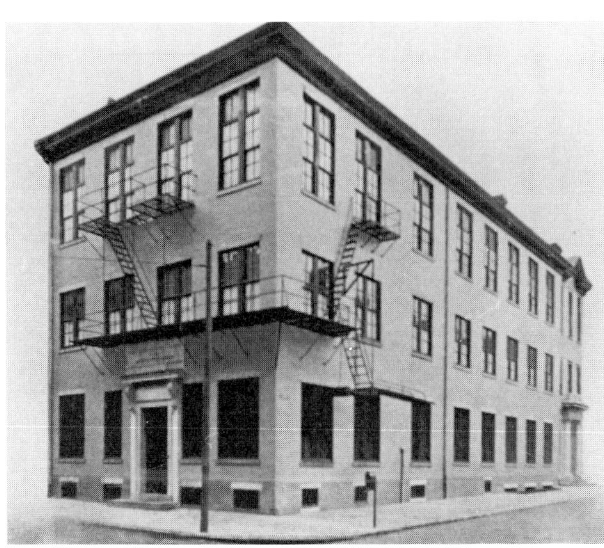

FIG. 48-34. The Daniel Baugh Institute of Anatomy at Eleventh and Clinton Streets.

As the Board under the energetic Presidency of William Potter was considering many plans, an important communication from the Pennsylvania Company was read on January 17, 1921. It stated that the will of Mr. William E. Thompson provided a bequest of $200,000 to the Jefferson Medical College, "paid upon condition that the Jefferson Trustees shall erect an additional building to its hospital property, as a memorial to Samuel Gustine Thompson." Under this impetus it was finally decided in the autumn of 1921 that the most available location for an addition to the 1907 Main Hospital would be the site of the 1877 first Jefferson Hospital on Sansom Street. In July, 1922, demolition was begun to make way for the 16-story Samuel Gustine Thompson Annex. A loan of $1,300,000 was secured from the Philadelphia Saving Fund Society, "payable at the expiration of five years, at the rate of six percent per annum."

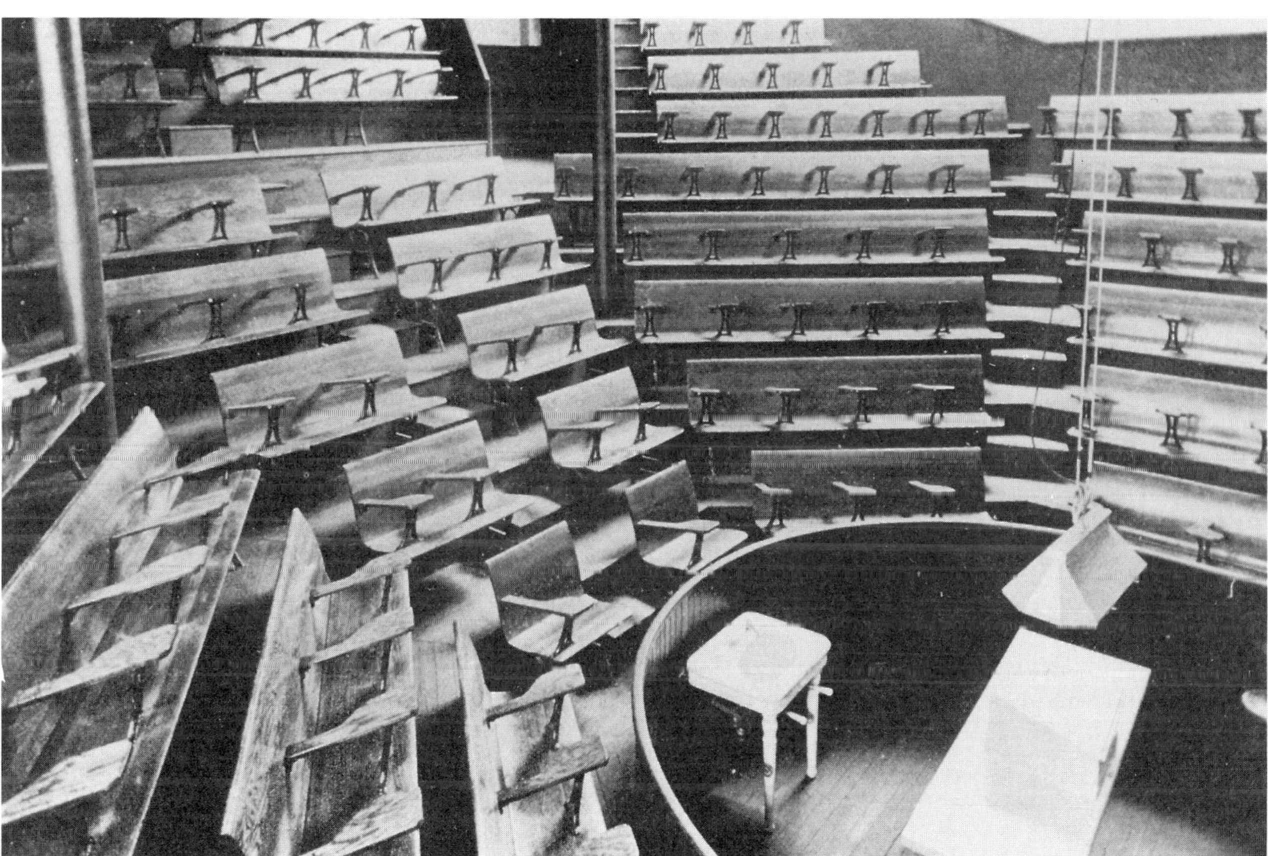

FIG. 48-35. The upper amphitheater of the Daniel Baugh Institute.

Jefferson would observe its Centennial in 1924. Mr. Alba B. Johnson, Chairman of the Hospital Committee, spearheaded the Jefferson Centennial campaign to raise funds for the new hospital annex.

■ The Samuel Gustine Thompson Annex of the Jefferson Hospital

The namesake of the 1924 Annex, the Hon. Samuel Gustine Thompson (Figure 48-37), was appointed a Jefferson Trustee in 1895. His father, the Hon. James Thompson, had also served on the Board (appointed in 1862), had been Speaker of the House of Representatives and a member of Congress for several terms, and had acted for many years as Chief Justice of the Supreme Court of Pennsylvania. The son, Samuel,[19] born in 1837, studied law and became prominent in litigations relating to large financial interests of railroads and corporations. Following in his father's footsteps, he served as Chief Justice of the Supreme Court of Pennsylvania in 1893 and 1903. Judge Thompson's faithful service on the Board was terminated by his death on September 10, 1909, due to "liver obstruction." The minutes of the Board took little note of his passing other than to record on November 30, 1909, that "Mr. J. Percy Keating was nominated for the vacancy in the Board occasioned by the death of Hon. Samuel Gustine Thompson." The name of this Thompson probably would have remained obscure in Jefferson History had it not been for the legacy of his brother, William, which stipulated his memorial.

The new building was dedicated on October 30, 1924, "to the Glory of God, the Relief of Human Suffering, and the Saving of Precious Lives."

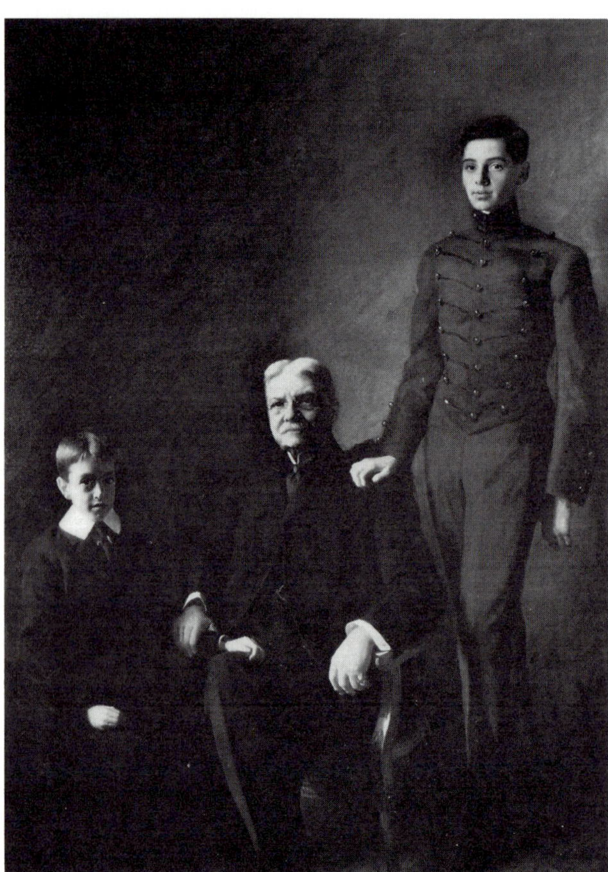

FIG. 48-36. "The Three Daniels"; Daniel Baugh and two of his grandsons.

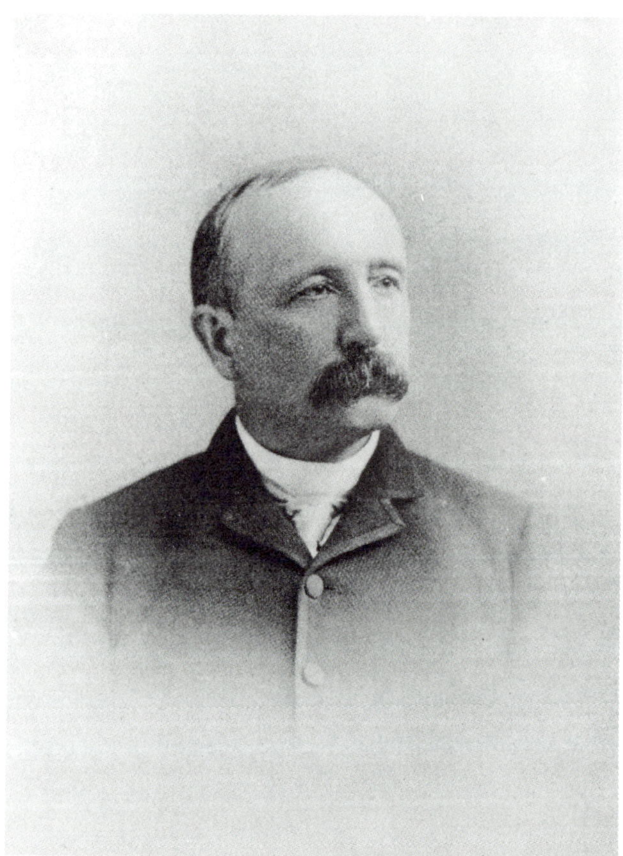

FIG. 48-37. The Hon. Samuel Gustine Thompson (1837–1909), Trustee (1895–1909).

High-ranking members of the three major religious faiths in the city participated in the ceremonies. The opening prayer was offered by the Right Reverend Thomas J. Gartland, D.D., Episcopalian Bishop of the Diocese of Pennsylvania. An address was delivered by the Right Reverend Monsignor Edmond J. FitzMaurice, D.D., Rector of the Philadelphia Theological Seminary of St. Charles Borromeo at Overbrook. An address and benediction by Dr. Abraham A. Neuman, M.A., Litt. H.D., Rabbi of the Congregation of Bnai-Jeshurun, concluded the occasion. There had been remarks by Alba B. Johnson, who presided, an address by President Potter, and an address, written by Dr. William W. Keen, who was confined to his home by illness, was read by Dr. Hobart A. Hare. It was pointed out that in spite of the generous liberality of the Trustees, Alumni, Staff, and a gift of $75,000 from the Jewish community for construction of the Mayer Sulzberger (former Trustee) Pathological Laboratories, there was still a need for $750,000 for the completion and equipment of the Annex. A plea for contributions from the public-spirited citizens of Philadelphia was issued. Only one-half of the Centennial Fund goal of $1,500,000 had been met.

At the time of its construction the Thompson Annex with its 16 floors was the tallest such hospital in the world (Figure 48-38). It connected with the first seven floors of the 1907 Main Building. A clinical amphitheater (Figure 48-39) occupied the southeast portion of the basement, first and second floors, with a seating capacity of 500 as a replacement for the amphitheater ("pit") of the 1877 Hospital. The basement also had an anesthetizing room, surgeon's dressing room, and sterilizing room all on a level with the floor of the amphitheater. The neurological, orthopedic, clinical medicine, and gastroenterological outpatient departments were in the basement. The subbasement contained the storerooms, engine room, and laundry.

The first floor housed the administration and business offices, staff room, social service department, and rooms for occupational therapy. Additional x-ray rooms, the dental clinic, and the bronchoscopic clinic were on the second floor. The third to sixth floors were for temporary lodging of pupil nurses while a nurses' home of six stories (opened for occupancy on May 15, 1925) was being built in the yard space in back of the 1012–1016 Spruce Street buildings. The seventh floor contained a kitchen and dining facilities for nurses. The eighth, ninth, tenth, eleventh, twelfth and star (thirteenth) floors each provided 19 private rooms, a service room, diet kitchen, and nurses' office.

Three surgical operating rooms and two delivery rooms were located on the fourteenth floor. In the adjacent space were the surgeon's dressing room, anesthetizing rooms, nurses' work room, and sterilizing room. The fifteenth floor contained an open roof garden with an enclosed portion for inclement weather. The sixteenth floor surmounted the enclosed portion of the roof garden for the Pathology Laboratories.

The confidence of the Trustees in the support of

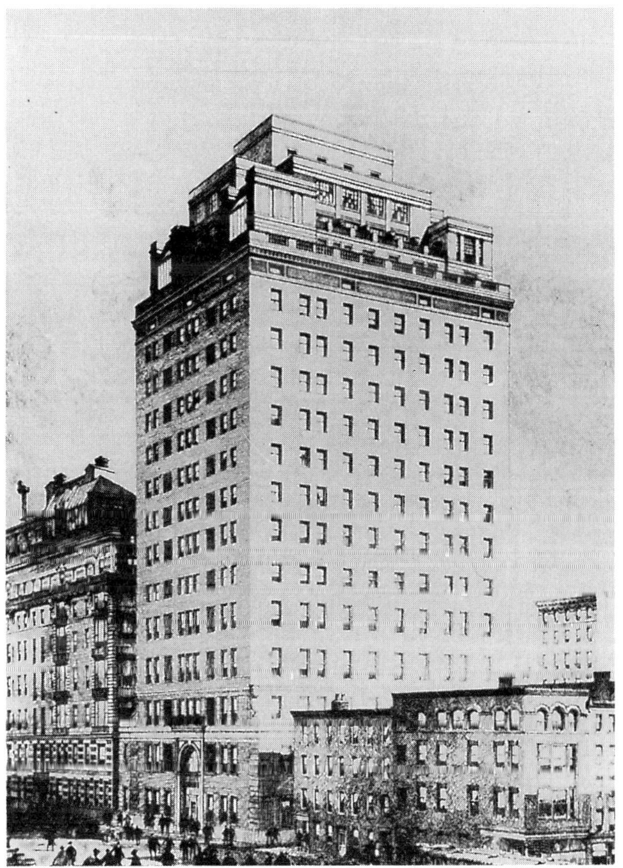

Fig. 48-38. The Samuel Gustine Thompson Annex, on Sansom Street between Tenth and Eleventh, which replaced the site of the 1877 Hospital, opened November 1, 1924.

the Jefferson family, the citizens of Philadelphia, and the State of Pennsylvania, was rewarded by a building that 30 years later would also connect on its west side with an even newer hospital (Foerderer Pavilion, 1954). The Thompson building would serve patients of such outstanding Professors as DaCosta, Bland, McCrae, Reimann, Rehfuss, Mueller, Shallow, Gibbon, Clerf, the Montgomerys, DePalma, and Keyes.

Alba Boardman Johnson, LL.D., the Tenth Board President (1926–1935)

Alba B. Johnson (Figure 48-40) became President of the Board following the death of William Potter. He had previously served as a Trustee since 1904. Born in 1858, he graduated from Central High School in 1876 and found employment in the Baldwin Locomotive Works. He grew with this well-known manufacturing organization and as its President (1911) saw it emerge from comparative obscurity into a leading position in its field.

Johnson brought to Jefferson a rich background of business and administrative experience. His interests were widely dispersed in financial, political, scientific, and charitable organizations. He was a Director of the Federal Reserve Bank in Philadelphia, President of the Pennsylvania State Chamber of Commerce, Director of the

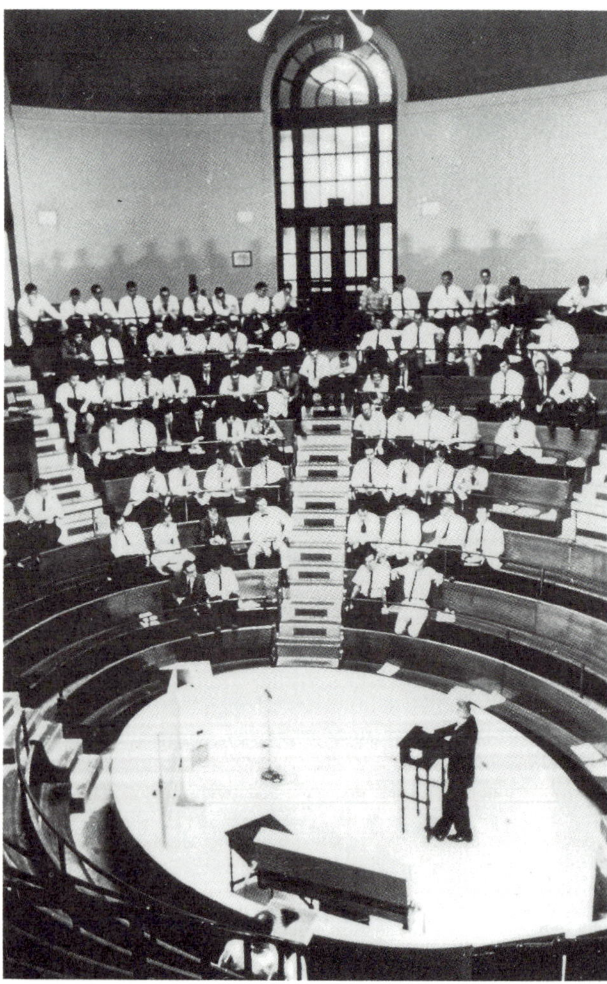

Fig. 48-39. Dr. Robert I. Wise, Magee Professor of Medicine, with students in the clinical amphitheater of Thompson Annex. In 1968 this third and last "pit" was replaced by the Thompson Auditorium and a new Emergency Room.

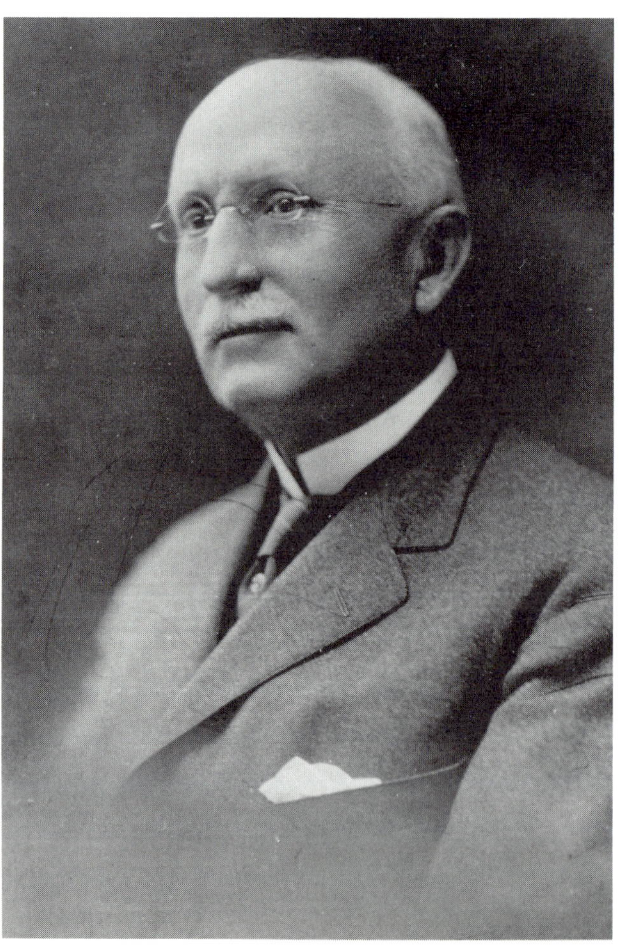

Fig. 48-40. Alba B. Johnson, LL.D. (1858–1935), Tenth Board President (1926–1935)

Philadelphia Art Alliance, and Vice President of the Y.M.C.A. of Philadelphia. His memberships also included the American Philosophical Society, American Academy of Political and Social Science, Union League of Philadelphia, and the University and Manufacturers' Clubs. Johnson was awarded the honorary degree of Doctor of Laws by Ursinus College in 1909. His portrait was presented to the Jefferson Medical College in 1930 at the annual business meeting of the Alumni Association.

During his 30 years on the Board, Johnson witnessed the dedication of the 1907 "Old Main" Hospital, was Chairman of the Hospital Committee for the Centennial Fund (1924) of the Samuel Gustine Thompson Annex, and was President during the opening of the 1025 Walnut Street Medical College (1929) and the Curtis Building (1931). In this expansion of the buildings he gave freely of his time and generously of his means. In addition to the liberal contribution of funds during his lifetime, he bequeathed upon death on January 8, 1935, the sum of $250,000 for the Medical College.

The Ivycroft Farm and Convalescent Home for Men (1917–1948)

The Ivycroft Farm (Figure 48-41) in Wayne, Pennsylvania, was given to Jefferson Hospital by Alba B. Johnson and Mrs. Johnson. Opened on May 5, 1917, as a Convalescent Home for Men, it was the first scientifically conducted institution of its kind in or about Philadelphia. Not only did the Home care for patients convalescing from illness or injury, but also patients not in good health, who, not being sick enough to enter a city hospital, were sent there to receive what was considered "preventive convalescence."

Ivycroft Farm was a pioneer effort in this work in Philadelphia, and was developed under the administration of the Social Service Committee of the Women's Board. Male patients were welcomed from any hospital or physician in Philadelphia or vicinity. The operation started with funding of about $16,000, of which $10,050 was handed to the Trustees for investment as the beginning of an endowment. The remainder was kept as cash flow for running expenses.

In 1927 it was reported that 135 patients had been at Ivycroft during the previous year, of whom 23 were cardiacs. Many rheumatic fever cases were given several months of extended care. Fourteen hospitals and ten other agencies had referred patients. The Farm, with its occupational therapy in a workshop along with recreational facilities (Figure 48-42), had restored healthy nutritional status and allowed men to return to work who would have found that impossible without this aid.

The Farm ceased to operate on December 1, 1948, and in the following year the Department of Preventive Medicine of Jefferson cooperated in the operation of the Fife-Hamill Memorial Health Center at Seventh and Delancey. In this modern outpatient facility Jefferson students received instruction and experience in the conduct of periodic health examinations.

▪ Plans for a New Medical College and Outpatient Building

In November, 1923, Dean Ross V. Patterson reported to the Board that 175 out of 1,900 first-year applications had been accepted. The Alumni Association had approximately $40,000 in its fund and was raising around $5,000 each year. Although the Thompson Annex under construction would keep Jefferson abreast of its clinical needs, this was not true for the College. In April, 1926, a special committee reported that "in order that Jefferson Medical College may retain its high standing among Class A colleges, the committee is of the unanimous opinion that the facilities of the College need to be enlarged and modernized as soon as convenient to the Board of Trustees . . . and suggest that a new Laboratory Building of suitable size be provided and suitably equipped for the accommodation of the fundamental sciences and for special lines of research in connection with clinical departments." William Potter, who, as Board President for the previous 30 years had been so effective in aiding the expansion of the institution, died later that same month. A tablet was erected to his memory in the Thompson Annex.

A campaign goal of $2,000,000 for public solicitation was approved in January, 1927. Alba Johnson, the new President, was empowered to make application to The New York Life Insurance Company for a mortgage loan of $2,000,000 at 5½% interest, maturing in ten years. The plans for the new building called for 12 stories costing about 60¢ per square foot. The upper four floors were to remain unfinished pending future developments. A proposition to have Wills Eye Hospital located in the new College Building was not considered practical at that time. The existing 1898 College Building at Tenth and Walnut was to be altered for outpatient departments and nursing education. In that year (1927) the corporate officers were authorized and directed to pay off all indebtedness of the corporation, matured and unmatured. In addition, the tuition was raised from $300 to $400. It would remain at that level until 1948, when thereafter it pursued an inflationary course.

In October, 1928, Mr. Horace Trumbauer, the architect, informed the Board that the cost of altering the old college building to adapt it for outpatient departments would exceed the cost of a new building. He estimated the cost of a new building at approximately $1,000,000.

At just the right time Mr. Cyrus H. K. Curtis (Figure 48-43), owner of the Curtis Publishing Company, generously offered to contribute $500,000 on behalf of the estimated cost of a new outpatient building, provided the Trustees would agree to subscribe or raise the remainder. The Trustees welcomed this proposition in a letter of resolution to Curtis. The architect was thereupon directed to make such changes in the plans for the college building already under construction as to bring the two into harmony and effect the greatest savings in cost (Figure 48-44).

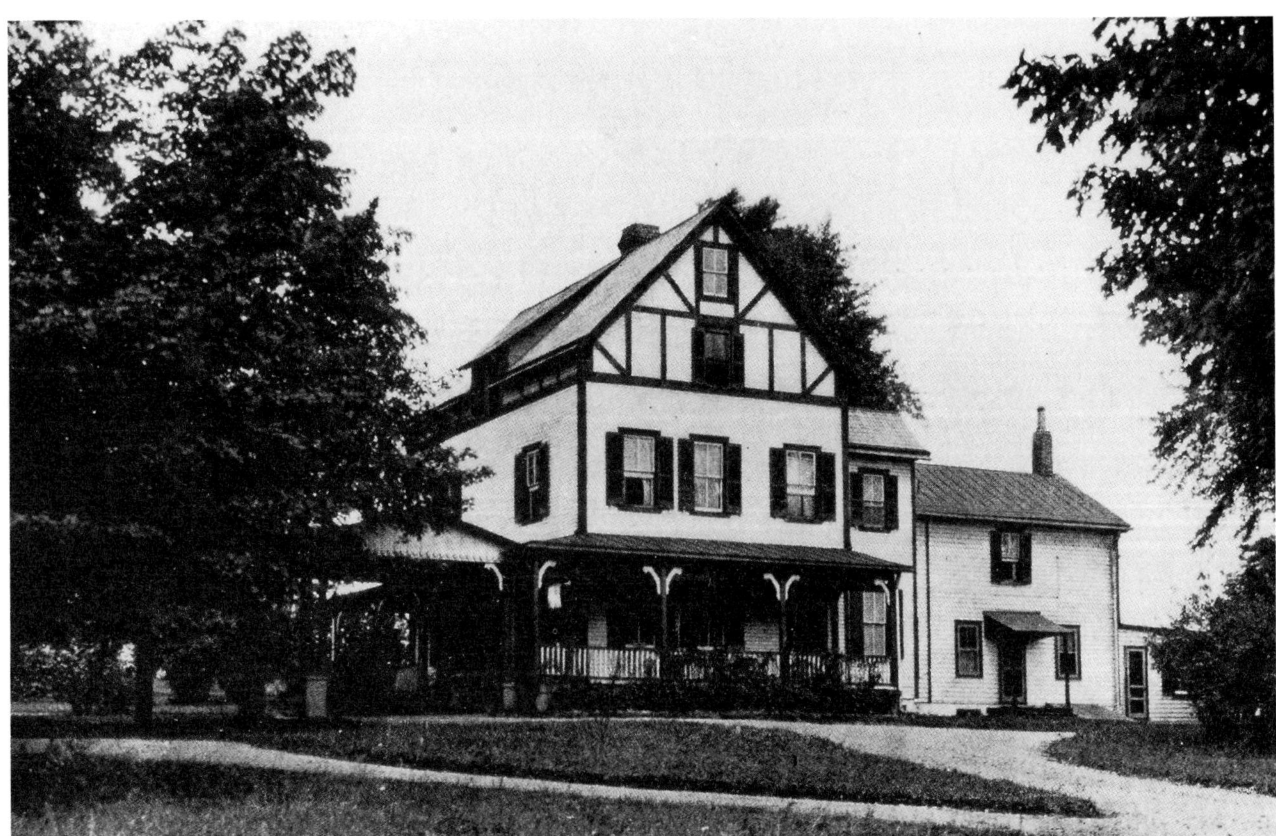

FIG. 48-41. The Ivycroft Farm and Convalescent Home for Men (1917–1948).

▪ The Committee on Research and Research Funds

The Board was increasingly aware that research for advancing the science of medicine in its various branches was an important part of Jefferson's work as a teaching institution. The new College building was being designed to provide facilities for research not hitherto available. The Board accordingly wished to make it known that appropriations from private sources for this purpose were welcomed, but that the use of such money should be under the direction and control of the Trustees, leaving the widest latitude possible to the faculty. On May 23, 1928, it was resolved "that the Chairman of the Faculty be requested to appoint a Committee of three or more of the Faculty to which shall be submitted suggestions or proposals of the subjects for research, who shall estimate the cost of the same and report their recommendations to the Trustees. Acceptance of all gifts or compensation for conducting research must be authorized by them. This does not apply to ordinary departmental research work by staff or students not involving appropriations or donations." Three days later a Research Committee was appointed consisting of Dean Ross V. Patterson, Chairman, Randle C. Rosenberger, Virgil H. Moon, J. Earl Thomas, Elmer H. Funk, and J. Parsons Schaeffer.

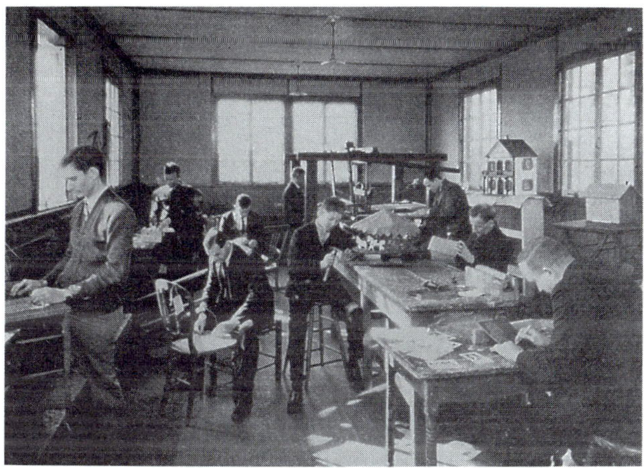

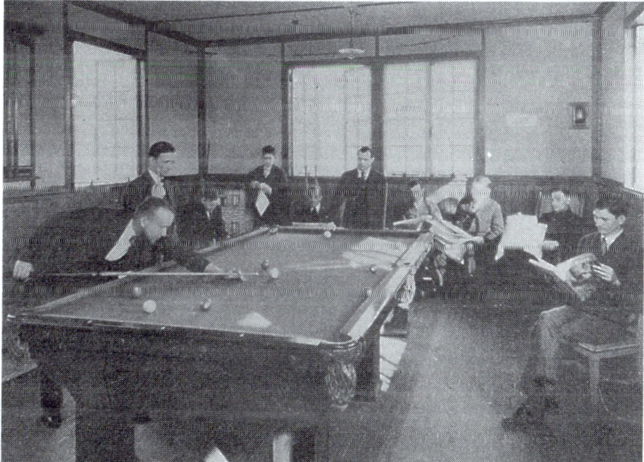

FIG. 48-42. The workshop and recreation room of Ivycroft Farm.

The Medical College (1929) and the Curtis Clinic (1931)

The New Medical College Building at 1025 Walnut Street, completely equipped and furnished, was opened on October 7, 1929. It occupied a plot of ground having a frontage of 158 feet on Walnut Street, east of Clifton Street, and depth of 108 feet to Moravian Street. At that time the 1898 College Building at Tenth and Walnut had been demolished and upon its site an east wing (the Curtis Building) to the new College was under construction. The combined structures occupied a plot of ground valued at $1 million, having a frontage of 276 feet on Walnut Street, and a building cost of $3 million.

The new College of approximately 2,200,000 square feet was of steel frame and was fireproof throughout. The central portion was elevated into a tower to provide for the elevator machinery, tanks, and other accessories. The first eight stories were completed, but the roof was so planned that four additional floors could be added as necessary.

The ground floor contained the students' lockers, a commodious students' lounge, a stack-room for the library, and a large auditorium (later Herbut Auditorium) that extended upward to the main floor and accommodated nearly 200 persons (Figure 48-45).

On the main floor were the executive and administrative offices, the Board Room (Figure 48-46) and the Library (Figure 48-47).

Two large lecture rooms (north and south), a demonstration room (the future Kellow Conference Area), and a large Assembly Hall (the future McClellan Hall) occupied the second floor. Eakins' *Gross Clinic* was hung on the north wall at the top of the stairs and could be seen from Walnut Street through the glass of the main entrance (Figure 48-48).

The Departments of Chemistry and Clinical Medicine were housed on the third floor. Professors' rooms, preparation rooms, workrooms, and a recitation room were winged off from the main laboratory.

The Departments of Physiology and Pharmacology, including a mammalian laboratory, demonstration rooms, preparation rooms, recitation room, and a machine shop occupied the fourth floor.

The fifth floor was devoted to the Department of Pathology. Besides the large students' laboratory there were several smaller laboratories, a recitation room, darkrooms, departmental offices, and the museum of 1500 square feet for the display of study specimens (Figure 48-49).

The Department of Bacteriology was housed on the sixth floor (Figure 48-50). The Alumni Association donated $100,000 for construction of the Department of Experimental Medicine, also on the sixth floor, as a tribute to one of its greatest teachers, Dr. John Chalmers DaCosta. At that time, although disabled from arthritis, he still lectured from a wheelchair as the Samuel D. Gross Professor of Surgery in the Thompson Annex amphitheater (Figure 48-51).

The new College Building was dedicated on February 22, 1930. George B. McClellan, Ph.D., Professor of Economic History at Princeton University (Figure 48-52) gave an inspiring address in which he extolled the character of his great-

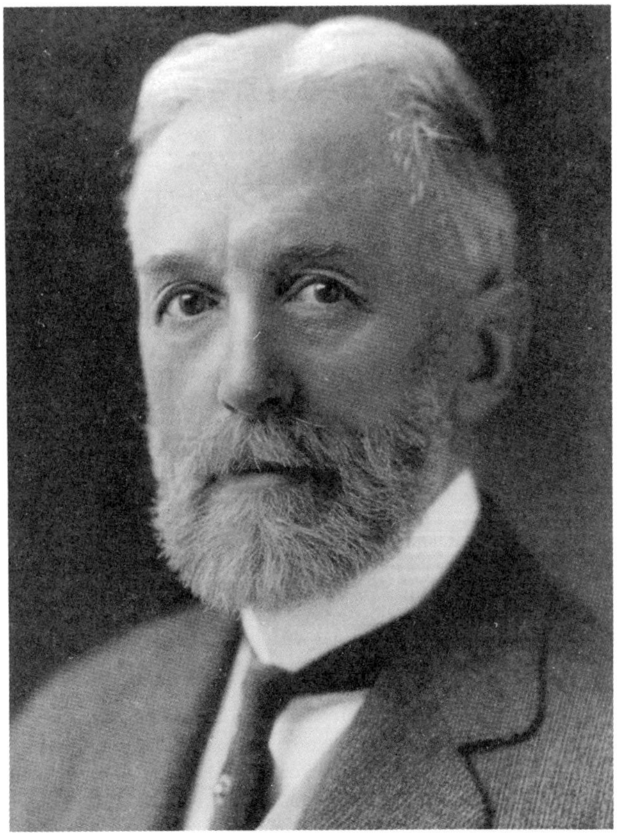

FIG. 48-43. Mr. Cyrus H.K. Curtis, benefactor of the Curtis Building.

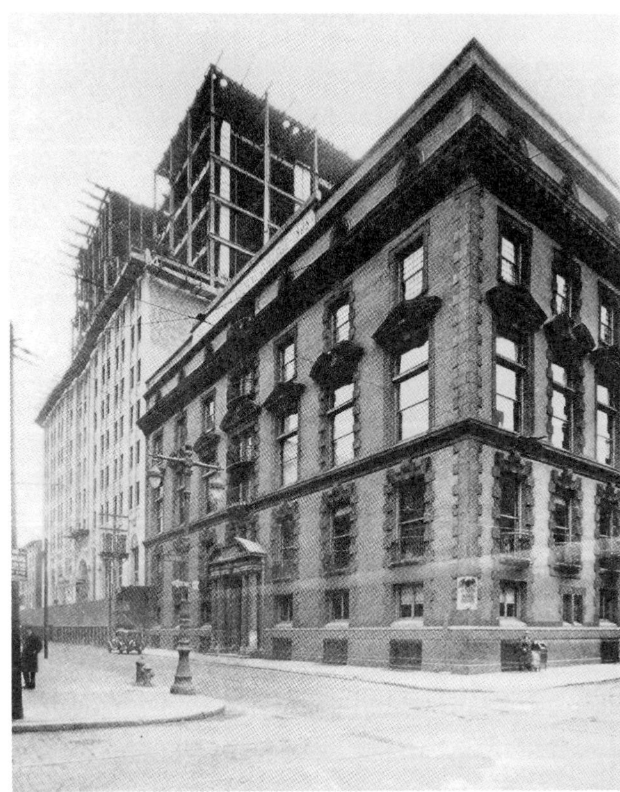

FIG. 48-44. The Medical College of 1898 at Tenth and Walnut, before demolition to become the Curtis Clinic (ca. 1928).

grandfather, George McClellan, the founder of Jefferson and the rich tradition that followed.

On May 20, 1929, it was resolved by the Board that the new building for outpatients, to which Mr. Cyrus H.K. Curtis had contributed one-half million dollars through 4,400 shares of preferred stock in his publishing company, should be designated the "Curtis Clinic of Jefferson Medical College and Hospital."

The Curtis Building of 1015 Walnut Street was completed and opened for treatment of patients on November 21, 1931 (Figure 48-53). Its architecture conformed to that of the completed College Building to which it formed an east L-shaped wing. The first floor contained the admission desks, drugstore, waiting room for new patients, and special examining rooms. An emergency ward was located on the Tenth Street side, first floor, and had a four-bed ward each for men, women, and children, and two operating and treatment rooms. It was accessible from the courtyard that extended from the narrow street (Moravian, later called "the alley") between the Hospital and College.

The second floor had seven offices for the Social Service Department and x-ray facilities for inpatients and outpatients. An overhead passageway connected this floor with the Main Hospital at Tenth and Sansom. A special elevator connected the emergency room of the first floor with the X-ray Department of the second floor, so that patients could be transferred from either area to the general hospital.

The third floor housed the Maternity and

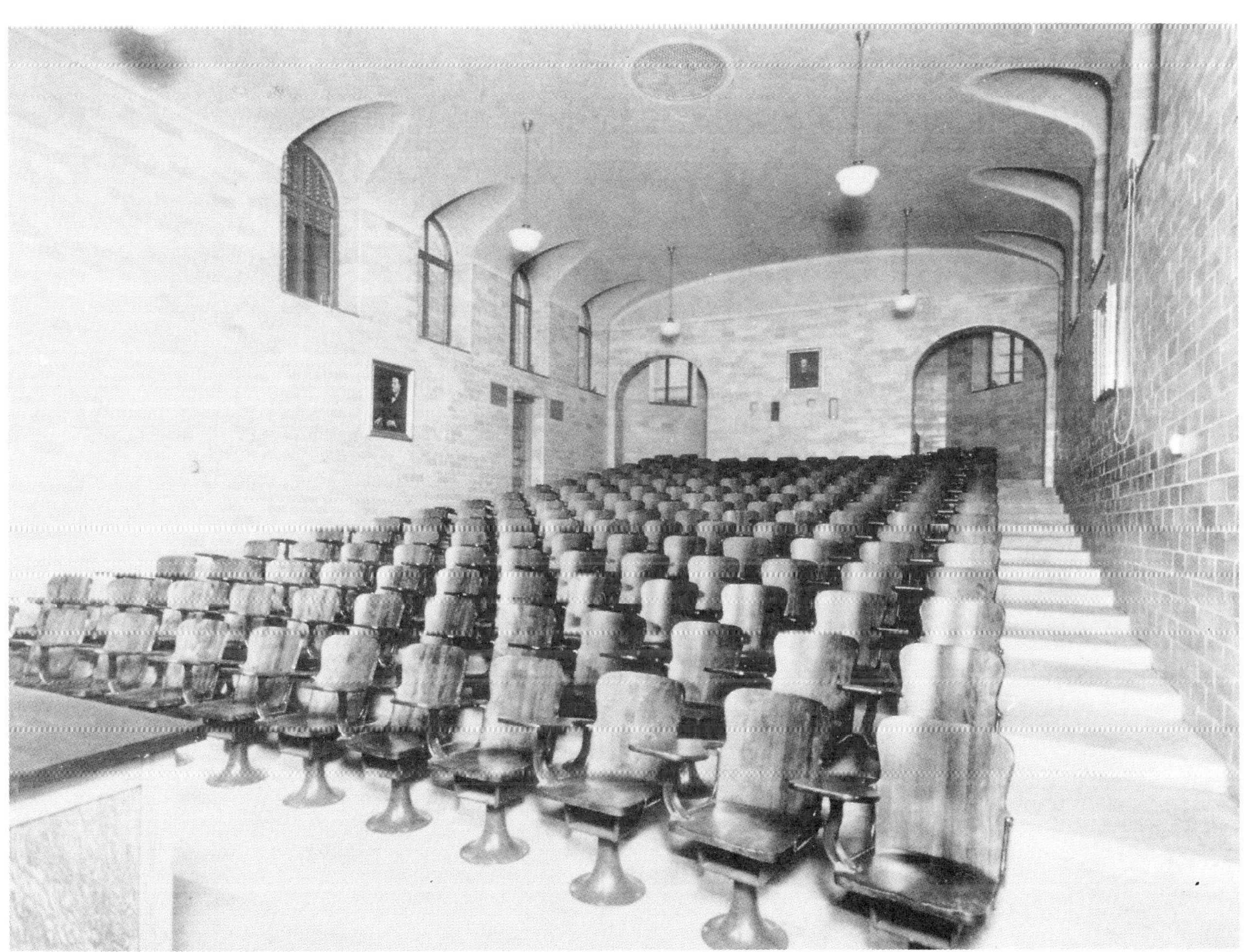

FIG. 48-45. College Auditorium in 1930 (named Peter A. Herbut Auditorium in 1979).

Children's Department; the fourth floor provided Ear, Nose, and Throat, and Ophthalmology quarters; the fifth floor accommodated General Surgery, the Tumor Clinic, and the Gynecologic Department; the sixth floor contained Orthopedic, Neurological, and Immunology areas; the Genito-urinary, Skin Department, and Syphilis Clinic were on the seventh floor; and the eighth floor provided for the Department of Medicine and Clinical Laboratory for the entire building.

The Department of Dentistry occupied the ninth tower floor, which also contained a small apartment for the Medical Director of the Hospital. The tenth, eleventh, and twelfth tower floors were used for the Training School of Nurses. The basement housed the Department of Physical Therapy.

The Curtis Clinic was dedicated on December 17, 1931. Dr. Pascal Brooke Bland on behalf of the Medical Staff presented an oil portrait of Cyrus Curtis to the Board of Trustees, represented by President Alba B. Johnson. The exercises were presided over by James M. Wilcox, Chairman of the Hospital Committee of the Board, who characterized Curtis as a "captain of the victories of peace."

Over the ensuing 50 years the Curtis Clinic, one of the largest in the world, provided treatment for millions of outpatients and maintained its superb structural integrity. As the character of medical care changed and advanced, the building underwent numerous modifications in which expansion of the College Departments and research activities displaced the outpatients into Jefferson's even more sophisticated facilities such as the Edison Building (1974) and the New

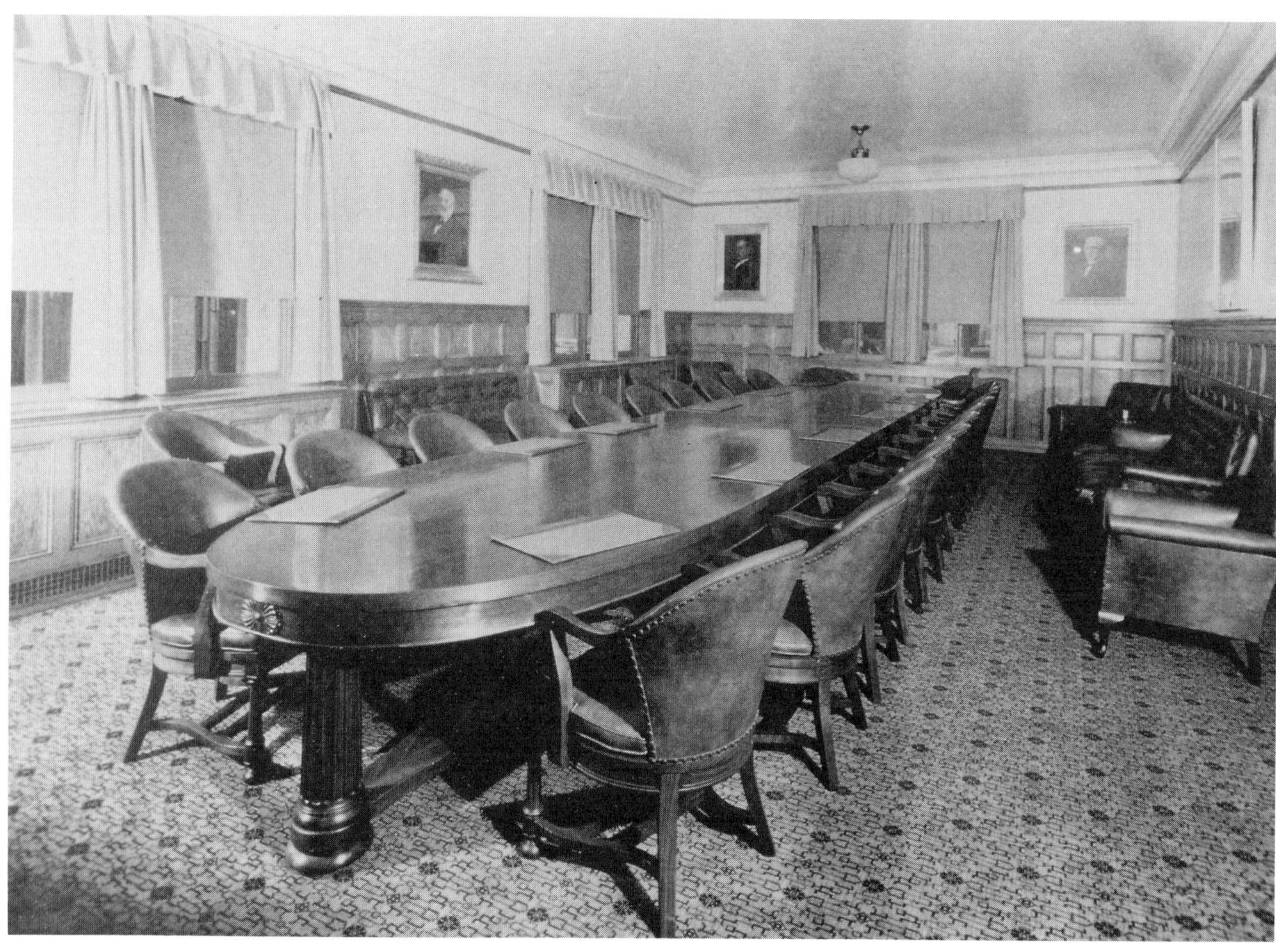

FIG. 48-46. The Board of Trustees' Room in the 1025 Walnut Street College (ca. 1931).

Hospital (1978). Patients who were formerly treated in the clinics received private patient care.

Wilfred Washington Fry, LL.D.; the Eleventh Board President (1935–1936)

Mr. Wilfred W. Fry (Figure 48-54) was elected President at a special meeting of the Board on January 31, 1935. He had been a Trustee since 1931. Born on August 14, 1875, in Mount Vision, New York, he was the son of a Protestant clergyman. This religious influence persisted throughout his life and expanded into a score or more of social welfare, philanthropic, business, educational, and administrative interests. In all these endeavors he was unselfish, untiring, and progressive. His success in the business world was achieved as President of N.W. Ayer and Son, Inc., an advertising organization.

In 1892 Fry entered the Mount Hermon School in Massachusetts but was compelled to leave in his junior year in order to support his widowed mother. Thirty-eight years later, in 1932, he was awarded his bachelor's degree from that school on the same platform with his son's graduating class, the first time this honor had ever been conferred upon a nongraduate.

Immediately upon leaving school, Fry became connected with the Young Men's Christian Association. As general secretary of the Trenton,

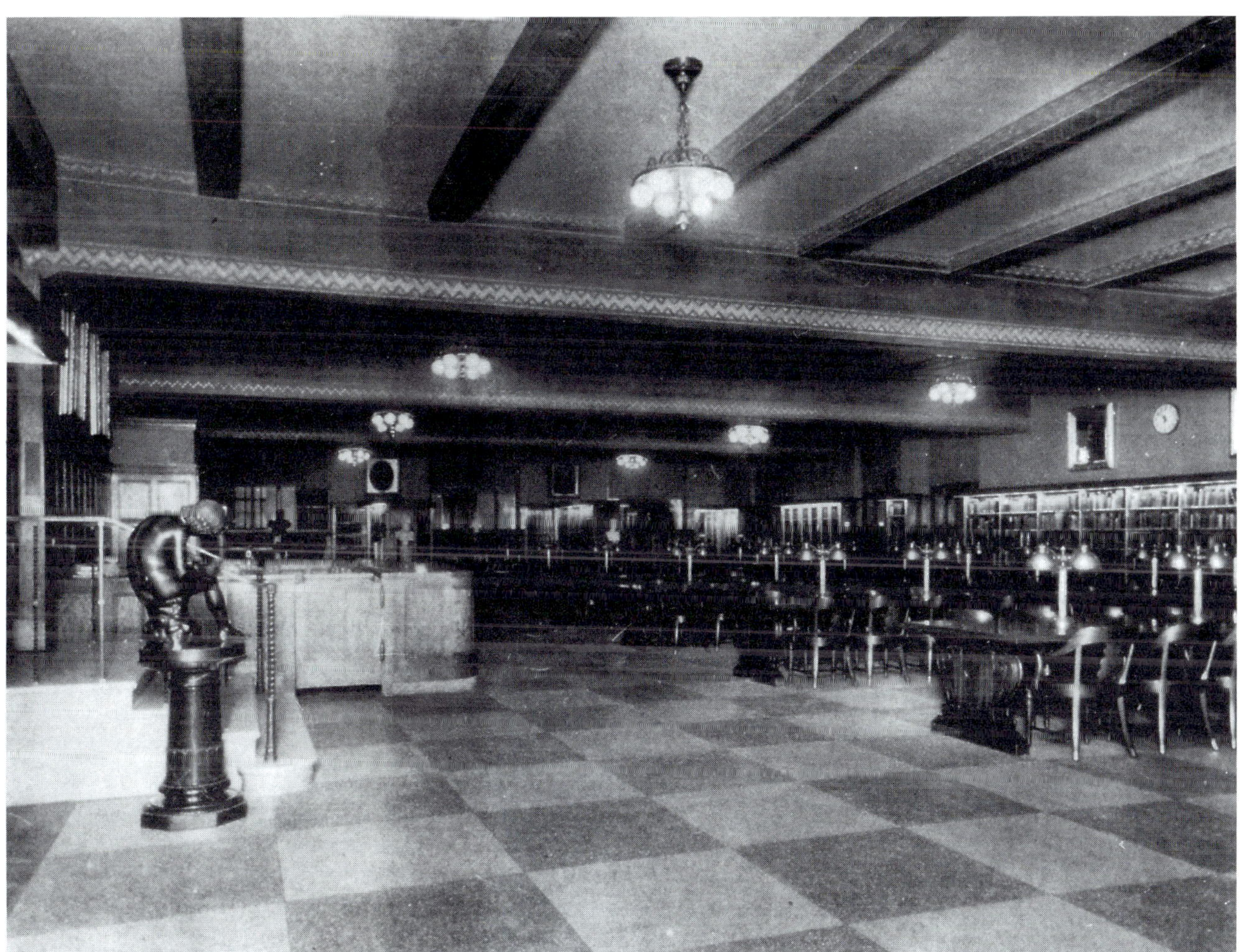

FIG. 48-47. The Library of the 1025 Walnut Street College (1930).

New Jersey, branch he met and married Anna Gilman Ayer, daughter of F. Wayland Ayer, head of the nationally prestigious advertising firm. He started to work for the firm in 1909, became a partner in 1916, and its President in 1929. He also became President of the same firm in Canada, and a governing director of the firm in London.

Fry's business interests diversified into one of the largest Jersey cow breeding establishments in America, accompanied by directorships in banks, insurance companies, and railroads. These business responsibilities failed to lessen his interest in a galaxy of philanthropies especially oriented to youth and education. In 1927 he was awarded the honorary degree of Doctor of Laws by Colgate University. He was also a Trustee of Brown University, Vice President of the Board of Crozer Theological Seminary, and member of the Board of Managers of the Franklin Institute. Playing the organ was one of his hobbies, which led to his becoming an Honorary Associate of the American Guild of Organists in New York, and he served as President of the Musical Art Society of Camden, New Jersey.

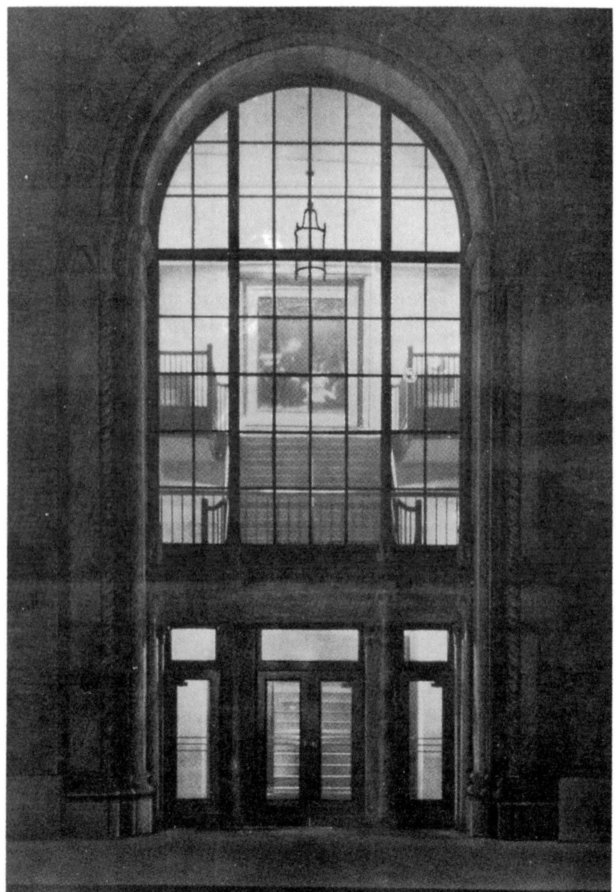

FIG. 48-48. Eakins' *Gross Clinic* on the second floor of the College Building as seen from Walnut Street.

It was most unfortunate that this brilliant, dedicated, and experienced administrator, who took the Jefferson Presidency in apparently good health at age 60, would be fatally stricken after only eight months in the office. He presided at all regular and special meetings of the Board until November 19, 1935, when his absence was recorded as "Fry indisposed." He suffered an attack of influenza that lingered into complications and terminated his life on July 26, 1936. Mr. Robert P. Hooper, who had acted as President pro tempore, was elected to succeed Fry on November 16, 1936.

Robert Poole Hooper, LL.D.; the Twelfth Board President (1936–1949) and the First Board Chairman (1949–1950)

Robert P. Hooper (Figure 48-55) was the natural successor to Fry. As a Trustee since 1920, he was

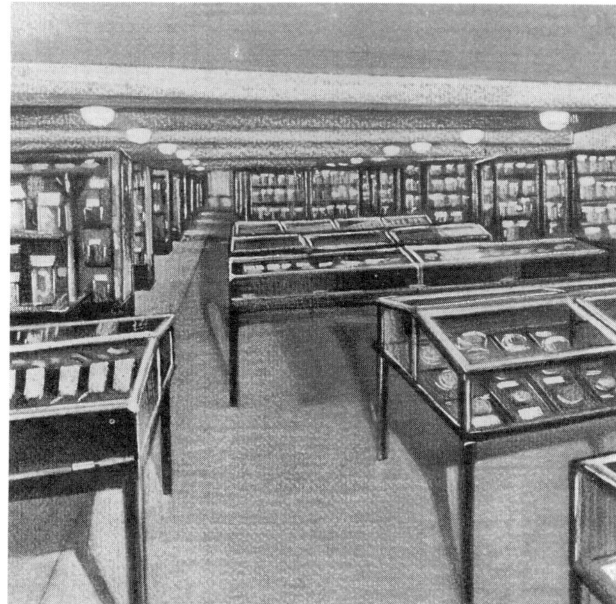

FIG. 48-49. The Pathology Museum on the fifth floor of the College (1930).

the senior member, and had always been active in the affairs of both College and Hospital. He was born in Baltimore, Maryland, on July 15, 1872, a member of a well-to-do family that for three previous generations had been prominent in civic affairs. After private education at the Hill School, he began his business career as a draftsman in the engineering department of the Poole and Hunt Engineering Company in Baltimore. For part of this time he also taught night school at the Maryland Polytechnic Institute.

Hooper became a selling agent in New York for southern manufacturers of cotton products and in 1896 formed a commission house in Philadelphia to handle this business. In 1902 he joined in the organization of Hooper Sons' Manufacturing Company as President and Treasurer. This had been a family business, founded by his great-grandfather in 1800, that originally made sails for clipper ships. Under Robert Hooper's leadership a resistant finish for textiles against fire, water, and mildew was developed. All the canvas used by the Armed Forces during World War I contained this protective coating that Hooper had patented. His business sagacity led further to his membership on the boards of several banks and insurance companies.

As owner of one of the first automobiles in Philadelphia, Mr. Hooper became a pioneer in the promotion of good roads. He was Chairman of the American Automobile Association Good Roads Board in 1906 and its President in 1911 and 1912. President Hoover appointed him a Chairman of the Subcommittee on Parking, Garages, Terminals, and Loading Facilities. While President of the Pennsylvania Motor Federation from 1908 to 1926, the motor clubs within the state became the strongest and largest in the country. He was a member of the Automobile Club of Philadelphia for 50 years and its President for 15.

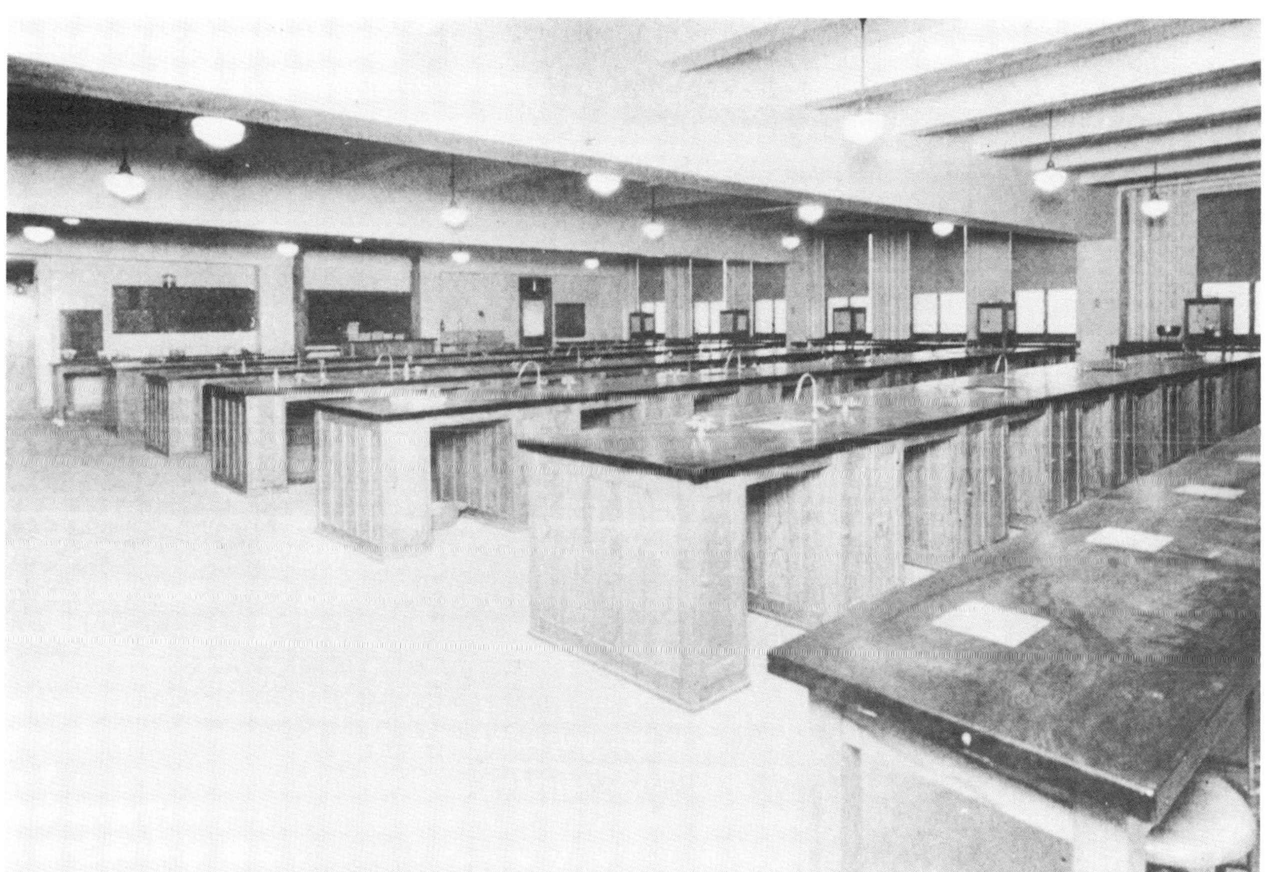

FIG. 48-50. The Bacteriology Laboratory on the sixth floor of the 1025 Walnut Street College (ca. 1931).

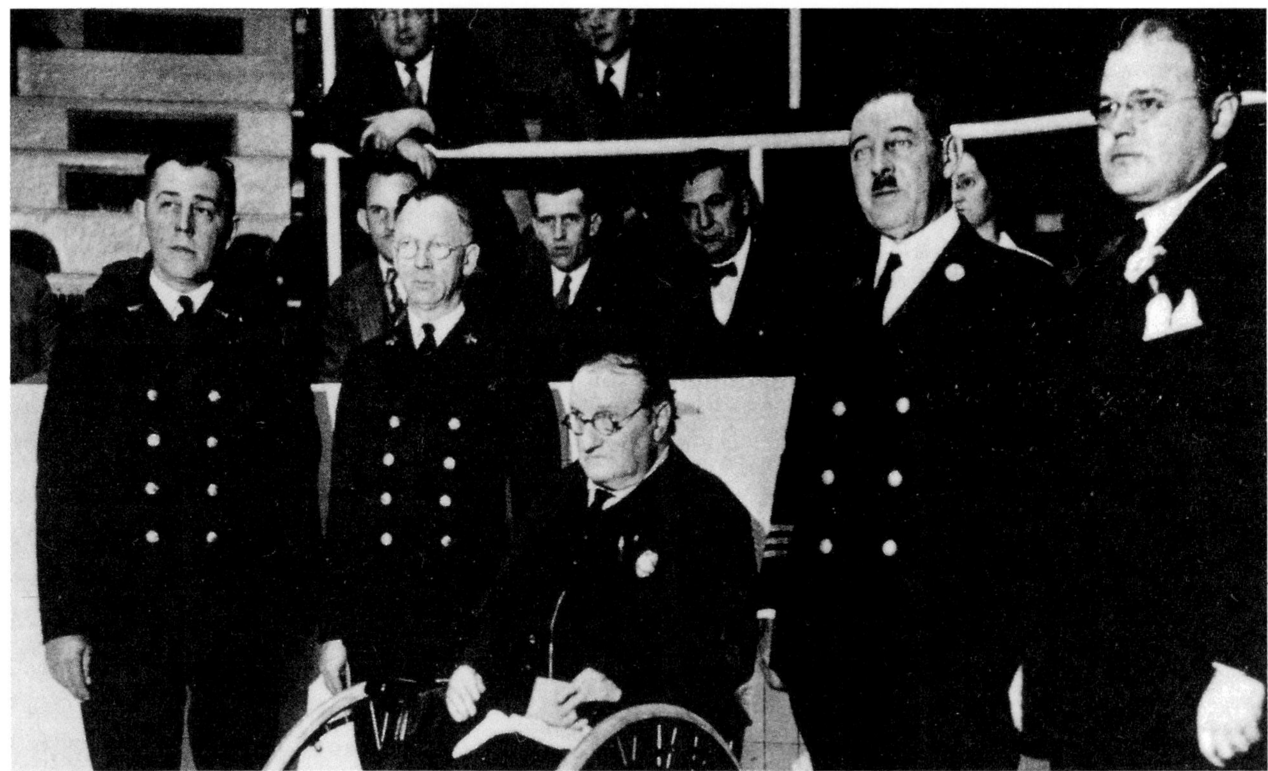

FIG. 48-51. The Clinic of Dr. John Chalmers DaCosta in the "pit" of the Thompson Annex (May 1931). Officials of the Philadelphia Fire Department and members of City Council presented Dacosta with an Honorary Deputy Fire Chief's badge.

In 1947 he received a lifetime appointment as Chairman of its Board.

During Hooper's 13 years as President of the Jefferson Board of Trustees his leadership was outstanding, and his commitment was tireless. He devoted more time to this office than to his business or to other activities. His administration, with force bordering on dictatorship, enabled Jefferson to continue its growth and development during the difficult prewar, war-time, and postwar years.

The Charlotte Drake Cardeza Foundation was organized in 1938 as the Division of Hematology in the Department of Medicine. In 1941 the generosity of Mr. Thomas Drake Cardeza, a Trustee, enabled the Foundation to engage in the study of diseases of the blood and allied conditions. This included a Research Professorship, research laboratories, blood bank, and a biologic photographic unit. In 1946 the Trustees received a bequest from the Pendleton-Barton family that provided funds for the purchase of the former Broad Street Hospital at Broad and Fitzwater Streets. This was designated the Barton Memorial Division of Jefferson Medical College for Diseases of the Chest (Figure 48-56). It provided greatly improved facilities over the previous 236–238 Pine Street building for medical and surgical patient care, nursing care, teaching, and research.

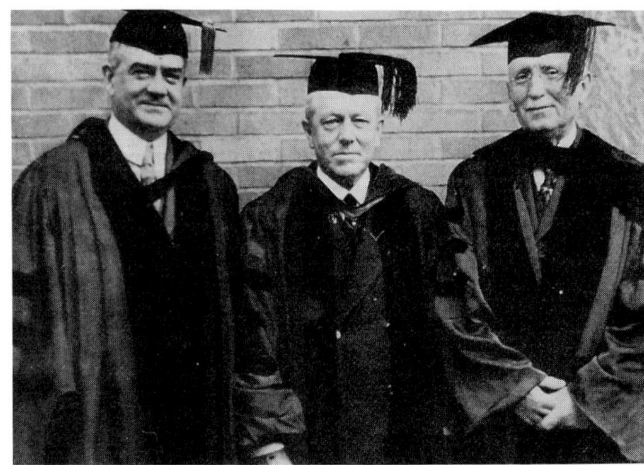

FIG. 48-52. Dr. Ross V. Patterson, George B. McClellan, Ph.D., and Alba B. Johnson at the dedication of the 1025 Walnut Street College (February 22, 1930).

age of 78. The College awarded him an honorary degree of Doctor of Laws in 1940. Despite his busy life he took time to indulge in private clubs and yachting. This loyal leader, who found a place in almost every speech to say "I love Jefferson," died on July 5, 1958, at the age of 86.

■ Reorganization of the Board (1949)

It became evident to Hooper after 13 years as Board President that the business and affairs of Jefferson were so complex that full-time duties were required of its chief officer. The Board concurred that an operating executive of the institution as President should be appointed, and the leadership of the Trustees be under a Chairman. Accordingly, on April 7, 1949, Hooper was elevated to the position of Chairman of the Board and on May 1 of that year Vice Admiral James L. Kauffman, U.S.N. (Ret.), became Jefferson's first full-time President.

Robert Hooper served in the new capacity as Chairman of the Board until March 20, 1950, at which time he was succeeded by Percival E. Foerderer. He had labored for Jefferson until the

James Laurence Kauffman, Vice Admiral, U.S.N. (Ret.); Jefferson's First Full-Time President (1949–1959)

James L. Kauffman was born in Miamisburg, Ohio, in 1887. After attending the Pennsylvania Military Academy he entered the U.S. Naval Academy at Annapolis in 1904 at the age of 17. Following graduation, he was commissioned an Ensign in 1910.

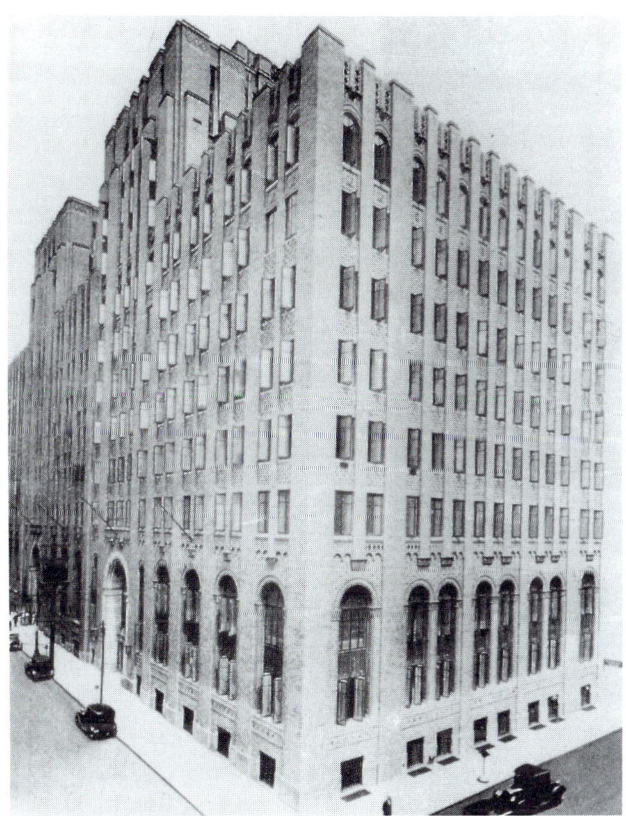

FIG. 48-53. The Curtis Clinic Building (1931).

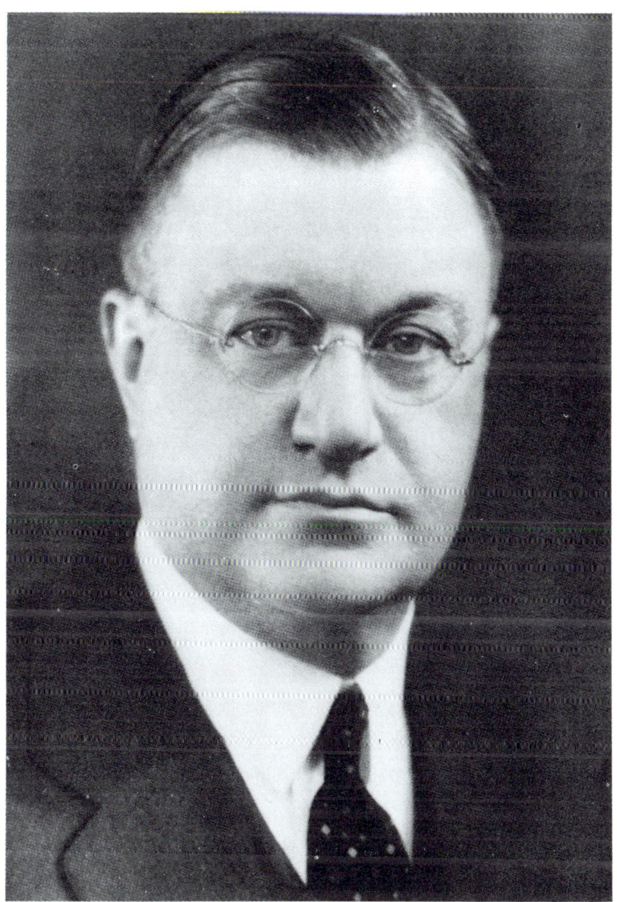

FIG. 48-54. Wilfred W. Fry, LL.D. (1875–1936), Eleventh Board President (1935–1936)

Kauffman became famous as a fighter of enemy submarines in both World Wars. In World War I he was awarded the Navy Cross for distinguished service as commanding officer of the U.S. destroyer *Jenkins* based at Queenstown (now Cobh), Ireland. Between the wars he held assignments at sea and ashore, four years of which were with the U.S. Naval Mission to Brazil. During World War II he continued his antisubmarine service in many parts of the world. He was commander of destroyers of the Support Forces of the Atlantic Fleet during the famous meeting of Churchill and Roosevelt, and established the U.S. Naval Operating Base in Iceland. For his conduct of antisubmarine warfare in the entire Gulf of Mexico and the Caribbean he was awarded the Legion of Merit. For outstanding service as Commander of destroyers and cruisers of the Pacific Fleet, Kauffman received in 1944 the Gold Star in lieu of a Second Legion of Merit. His greatest performance was in the Leyte Gulf operations through which the United States recaptured the Philippines. Following this operation he succeeded Admiral Kincaid as Commander of Naval Operations in the Philippines and received on the recommendation of General MacArthur another Legion of Merit with Army Oak Leaf Cluster. Among other awards were the Order of Leopold II by the Government of Belgium, the Cuban Order of Merit, the Brazilian War Service Medal, The Philippine Distinguished Service Star, and Knight Commander of the Icelandic Falcon.

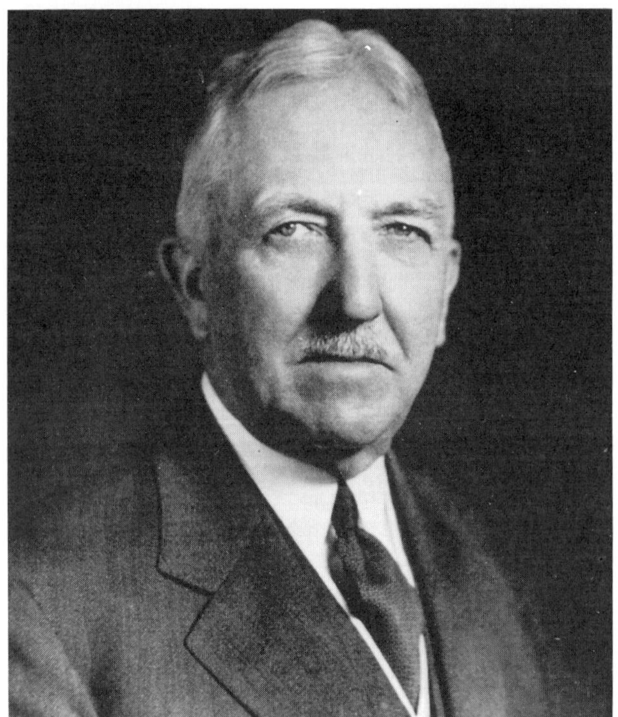

FIG. 48-55. Robert P. Hooper, LL.D. (1872–1958), Twelfth Board President (1936–1949) and First Board Chairman (1949–1950).

From 1946 to 1949 he assumed duty as Commandant of the Fourth Naval District in Philadelphia. Upon retirement at age 62 he accepted the position of first full-time President of Jefferson Medical College under the reorganization plan of Robert Hooper.

As President, Vice Admiral Kauffman served one year under Board Chairman Hooper and the remaining nine with Foerderer. Although capable, distinguished, and respected, Kauffman was somewhat at a disadvantage. His newly created position had ill-defined responsibilities; the Dean (George A. Bennett), Gross Professor of Surgery (Thomas A. Shallow) and Hospital Director (Vice President, Hayward A. Hamrick) were a combine of self-delegated power; and his retired status from the Navy and lack of experience in this specialized position sustained his image as Admiral (Figure 48-57) rather than as President (Figure 48-58). He kept a low profile and few realized that he was dutifully and successfully carrying out his main mission of obtaining yearly increases in the Pennsylvania State appropriation to the College.

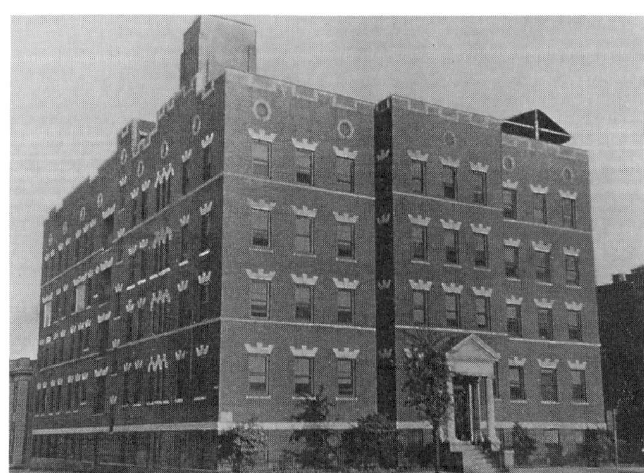

FIG. 48-56. The Barton Memorial Division of Jefferson Medical College Hospital at Broad and Fitzwater Streets, for Diseases of the Chest (1947–1959).

Vice Admiral Kauffman retired from Jefferson in 1959 at the age of 72. He died in 1963 in the Bethesda Naval Hospital following a heart attack.

Percival Edward Foerderer, LL.D.; the Second Board Chairman (1950–1962)

Percival E. Foerderer (Figure 48-59) was born in Philadelphia in 1885, the son of U.S. Congressman Robert H. Foerderer. He was educated at Cheltenham Military Academy, the William Penn Charter School, and the University of Pennsylvania. In 1903 he became Assistant Superintendent of the leather firm established by his grandfather and expanded by his father, that manufactured Vici Kid. From Vice President of the firm in 1906 he advanced to President in 1908. In his further business career Mr. Foerderer became a director of the Land Title Bank and Trust Company, the United States Leather Company, Pennsylvania Forge Company, Philadelphia Park Amusement Company, the Philadelphia Bourse, and Chairman of the Board of Directors of the Pennsylvania Mutual Life Insurance Company.

Foerderer's war-related activities included: Council of National Defense, World War I; and Vice-Chairman of the Employment Management Division and Chief of the Divisional Priorities Section of the War Industries Board; the war service committee of the leather industry; and Chairman, Metropolitan Philadelphia Civilian Aid Committee for the Army Air Corps, World War II. He achieved the rank of Lieutenant-Colonel, Army Specialist Corps, in 1942. His civil activities encompassed directorship in the Philadelphia Chamber of Commerce, Chairman of

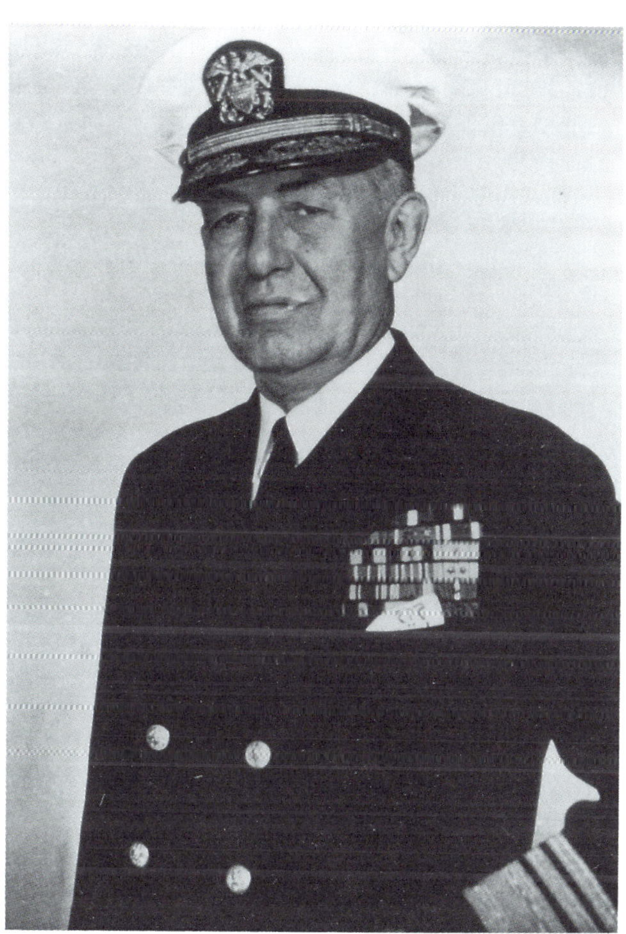

FIG. 48-57. James Laurence Kauffman, Jefferson's first full-time President (1949–1959), in uniform as Vice Admiral, U.S.N.(Ret.).

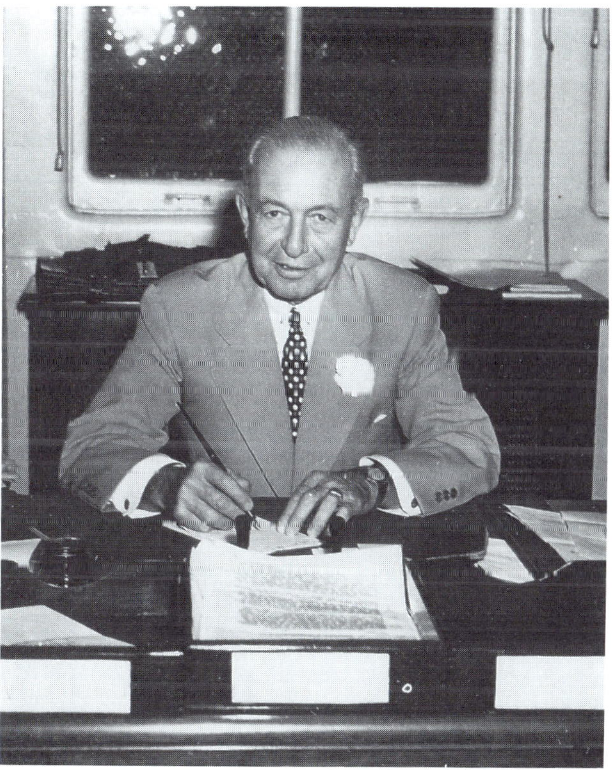

FIG. 48-58. Vice Admiral James L. Kauffman (1887–1963), as President.

the Committee for Economic Development of Philadelphia (1943), Chairman of the Tanner's Council of America, Chairman of the Code Authority for the leather industry (NRA), and Chairman of the Republican Finance Committee of Metropolitan Philadelphia.

Foerderer's service to the Board spanned 33 years. He was elected a Trustee in 1928, became Chairman of the College Committee in 1938, and in 1950 was made the second Chairman of the Board. In the latter capacity he was unusually successful in molding together the four ingredients of an educational institution that must function as a unit: the Board, the administration, the faculty, and the facilities. Under his leadership several floors of the College building were designed to house research facilities for most of the Clinical Departments; the research facilities of the Basic Science Departments were greatly expanded; the "New Pavilion" was opened in 1955; the James R. Martin Nurses' Residence was completed in 1959; the Charlotte Drake Cardeza Laboratories were built at 1015 Sansom Street (Figure 48-60) and opened in 1960 for research; complete rehabilitation of the "Old Main" (1907) Hospital was undertaken; and plans were formulated for a $40,000,000 development program to enlarge Jefferson for occupancy of the area between tenth and eleventh Streets from Sansom to Spruce. In 1957 Foerderer accepted a medal on behalf of the Jefferson Board by the Republic of Cuba in commemoration of the research of Dr. Carlos Finlay (Jefferson, 1855) who in 1881 incriminated the *Aedes aegypti* mosquito as the carrier of yellow fever.

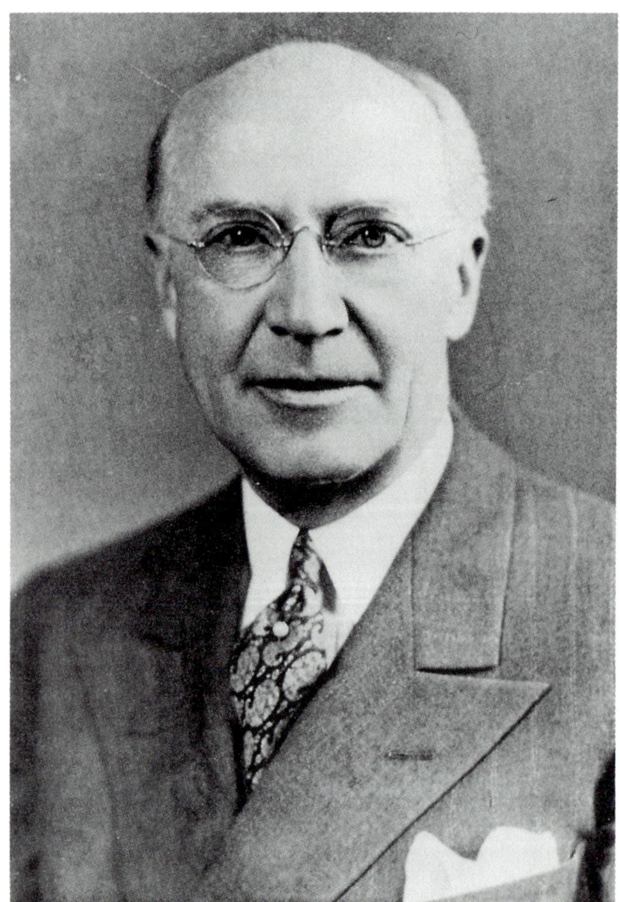

FIG. 48-59. Percival E. Foerderer, LL.D. (1885–1969), Second Board Chairman (1950–1962).

Just as Robert Hooper before him had entertained a close relationship with Dr. Thomas Shallow of the Surgery Department, so Percival Foerderer looked upon Dr. Martin Rehfuss of the Medical Department as a friend and advisor. In 1963 Mr. and Mrs. Foerderer established the Martin E. Rehfuss Lectureship in Internal Medicine, which has continued to attract large audiences.

The modest personality of Mr. Foerderer was disarming and abetted his art of securing cooperation. Always with mastery of teamwork, he spearheaded every venture with an energy that belied his 77 years when he retired to become a Life Trustee on January 1, 1962.

■ The 1954 New Pavilion (Foerderer, 1962)

Despite the combined new Medical College Building (1929) and Curtis Clinic (1931) on Walnut Street, the Board of Trustees with their customary and visionary long-time planning had been assembling for 25 years the adjoining tracts of land for a hospital project expected as inevitable. The decision in 1951 to proceed with a fund-raiser for erection of another hospital (the "New Pavilion") was hastened by the annual patient admissions figure rising from 9,429 in 1924, when the Thompson Annex was opened, to nearly 22,000. The services required for this increase had grown at an even greater rate.

While the prime object of a new wing was to obtain more beds for patients, it also provided for consolidation of laboratories and operating rooms that had spread out in a most inefficient manner. New technical facilities for delivery suites, postoperative recovery rooms, new kitchens, and a modern laundry were planned. The new building was ultimately connected to all but the four top floors of the adjacent Thompson annex.

Ground breaking took place in 1952. Total cost was estimated at $7,500,000 to include extensive revision of technical space in the Thompson Building. Campaign funds provided less than one-half, and financing was completed through limited institutional funds and construction loans. The wing was considered economically feasible because the 300 beds were in the income-producing categories (90% semi-private) in greatest demand due to hospitalization plans for subscribers. It was estimated to accommodate approximately 8,500 additional patients yearly and to enable Jefferson to serve upwards of 30,000 bed patients annually.

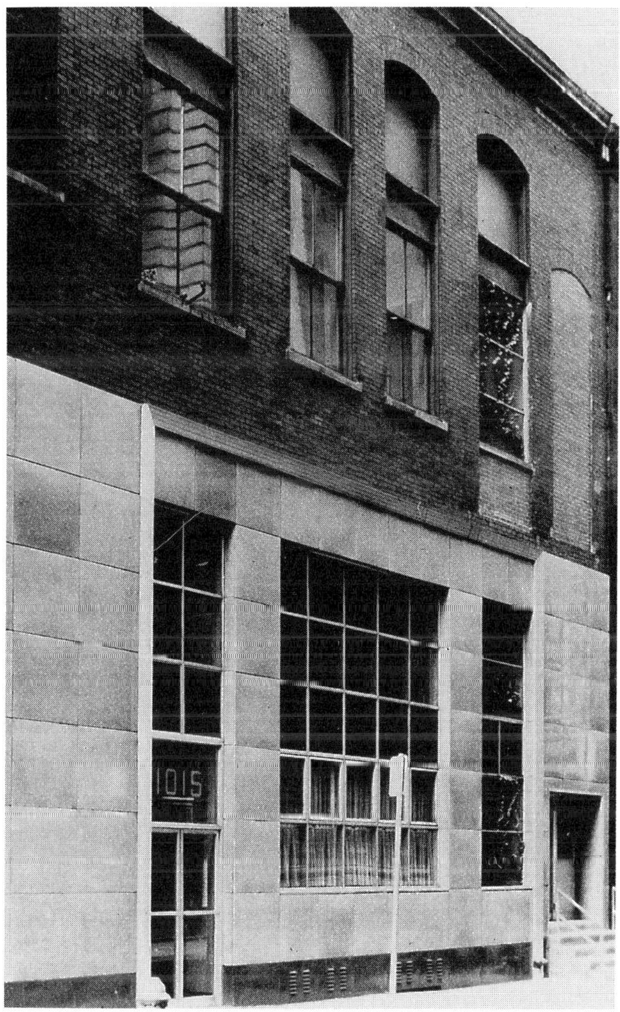

FIG. 48-60. Cardeza Laboratories at 1015 Sansom Street (1960).

The New Pavilion was constructed on the east side of Eleventh Street between Sansom and Walnut according to plans by the architect, Vincent Kling. Shortly before this, Kling had established his reputation with the Lankenau Hospital complex on City Line Avenue. The New Pavilion made many departures from the field of medical philosophy and, like the still-later hospital of 1978, was considered "the hospital of tomorrow." The exterior was of standard salmon brick with strip windows. The first floor was constructed to suggest freestanding pillars, with the walls between the pillars recessed and of glass. The Walnut Street end was open so as to create the illusion that the floors above were "floating." The Walnut Street facade above the open first-floor pillars formed a solid brick wall with top floor balconies that formed an asymmetrical but balanced composition (Figure 48-61). The salient features of the new building follow:

1. The building comprised 254,000 square feet in area in 14 stories above the street as well as two stories below. The support was of fireproof steel and reinforced concrete.
2. The floors were connected to the Thompson Annex so that the adjoining functions were coordinated and unified.
3. The New Pavilion, Thompson Annex, and Old Main Hospital were all connected so as to occupy the entire block of Sansom Street between Tenth and Eleventh. A dual electric service was concentrated in the new subbasement with power adequate for the entire complex.
4. There were seven nursing floors, with one devoted exclusively to maternity patients. Optional "rooming in" maternity service enabled babies to occupy an area adjoining the mother's bed.
5. An attractive hotel decor replaced the usual atmosphere of clinical severity. This was accomplished with good lighting, flat soft colors, and walls finished in nonglazed tile. Draperies,

furniture, and room colors were planned to be bright but restful.

6. Noise was minimized by acoustical sound-absorbing plaster in the ceilings and rubber-tiled floors.

7. The indiscriminate mingling of inpatient traffic with visitor traffic was avoided by using separate lobbies on opposite sides of the elevator system. One lobby serviced visitors in separate cabs while the opposite lobby was used to transport patients with their escorts to surgery, laboratories, or special therapy areas.

8. Every known precaution for safety of patients and employees was incorporated in the structure. This included fire precautions, ventilation, static-arresting floors in the operating rooms, and an off-the-street loading dock.

9. The great majority of the rooms were semiprivate, all with toilet facilities. A few private rooms, at the south end of each floor, had private bathrooms as well. Each bedside had a voice receiver and transmitter for the purpose of contacting the nurses' station. Patient-to-nurse conversation saved many trips to the bedside. Every bedside had a telephone. Flush, in-built storage areas provided for the patient's baggage and assured an orderly room. A piped-in oxygen system was installed in every room.

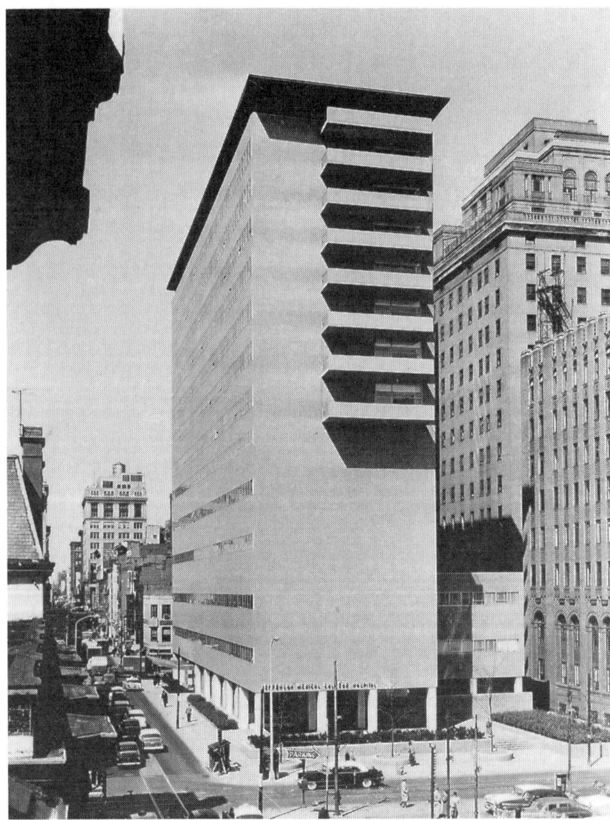

FIG. 48-61. The Walnut Street facade of the Foerderer Pavilion. The College and the Thompson Annex are at the right.

10. A high-speed dumbwaiter system dispatched supplies to the operating rooms and patient areas.

11. The first six floors were completely air-conditioned, and the upper eight floors were power-ventilated and heated with forced hot water.

12. A new kitchen was installed in the Thompson and Old Main Buildings with a capacity for serving 9,000 meals per day.

13. The laundry in the basement, the most modern institutional type of its kind in Philadelphia, handled 25,000 pounds each eight-hour workday. All soiled linen came from the floors through laundry chutes.

14. A glass-enclosed meeting room for the Board of Trustees (Figure 48-62) or important committees was located on the fourteenth floor roof terrace.

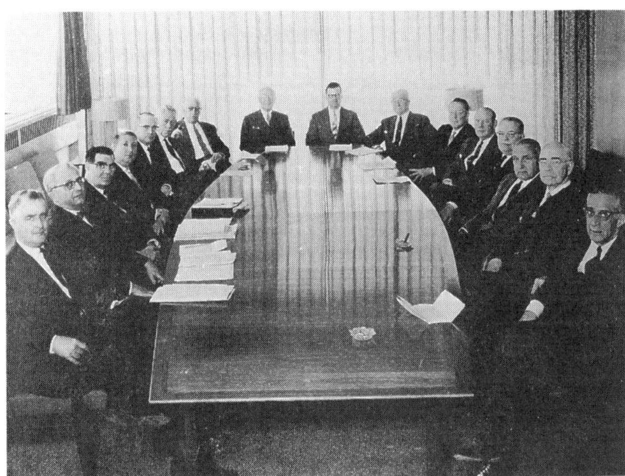

FIG. 48-62. The Board of Trustees (1961) on the fourteenth floor of New Pavilion (named "Foerderer" in 1962). William W. Bodine, Jr. (President), and Percival E. Foerderer (Chairman) are at the head of the table.

15. The Walnut Street entrance was shaded by honey locust trees planted in enclosures surrounded by brick walls capped with limestone.

The formal opening ceremony took place on November 8, 1954, in the lobby, attended by public officials, prominent business leaders and medical authorities. The President, Vice Admiral Kauffman, as master of ceremonies, introduced the principal speaker, Dr. Frank R. Bradley, Superintendent of Barnes Hospital, St. Louis, Missouri, and President of the American Hospital Association. Other speakers were Percival E. Foerderer, Chairman of the Board; Dr. Hayward R. Hamrick, Vice President and Medical Director; and Vincent G. Kling, the architect and supervisor of construction. Mrs. Percival E. Foerderer cut the ribbon across the main entrance lobby. Invocation was given by Reverend Rex S. Clements; prayer was offered by Rabbi Mortimer J. Cohen; and benediction was delivered by Right Reverend Monsignor Ralph G. Cox. A buffet luncheon in McClellan Hall and a building tour followed.

The New Pavilion lived up to expectations and won for its architect, Vincent G. Kling, an American Institute of Architects Gold Medal in 1955. The building did much to enhance the public image of Jefferson in affording not only the finest in professional care, but the comfort of the latest amenities.

At the Board meeting of December 4, 1961, Mr. Foerderer submitted his formal resignation as Chairman to become effective on January 1, 1962. Trustee D. Hays Solis-Cohen read a prepared statement at this meeting: "I wish I could suggest some suitable honor which we, the Trustees, might bestow on him. While I have nothing to offer in that regard, I am very certain that the collective intelligence of the Trustees might be sufficient to accomplish such a discernible objective. I take the liberty to say to his successor, on behalf of all of us, that action to this end is in order."

Much action did indeed ensue at the subsequent meeting of the Board on January 8, 1962. Dr. Peter Herbut, President of the faculty, presented Mr. Foerderer with a silver tray signed by all the members of the Executive Faculty. Mr. Large, on behalf of the Trustees and the Administration, presented to Percival Foerderer an illuminated citation signed by all of the Trustees, President William W. Bodine, Jr., Dean William A. Sodeman, and Medical Director Ellsworth R. Browneller. Mr. Large then stated that it was virtually impossible to find a tangible gift with which to express the appreciation of everyone for Mr. Foerderer's leadership to Jefferson, and thus, it was the unanimous decision of his fellow Trustees that henceforth the Pavilion Building would be known as the "Foerderer Pavilion" in honor of the many contributions to Jefferson made by the entire Foerderer family.

An oil portrait of Mr. Foerderer was hung in the Pavilion lobby bearing a plaque honoring him and his wife, the former Ethel Brown. She was a member of the Women's Board for 51 years (1930–1981) and served as its President for five (1947–1952). In addition to awarding Mr. Foerderer a Doctor of Laws degree in 1951, Jefferson broke precedent in 1964 when the Alumni Association selected him, for the first time choosing a person outside of medicine, for the Alumni Achievement Award.

Percival Foerderer, industrialist, philanthropist, civic leader, and Board Chairman, died on January 22, 1969, at the age of 84. He was one of the rare individuals to whom the term "Mr. Jefferson" is occasionally applied.

The Foerderer Pavilion kept pace with advancing requirements in physical structure and technology. During the early 1980s it underwent a total renovation, culminating on September 17, 1984, in a rededication ceremony. President Lewis W. Bluemle, Jr., who presided on this occasion, stressed "the continued pursuit of excellence in compassionate, humane health care." Members of the Foerderer family and the Foerderer Foundation who had generously provided funds for various of Jefferson's worthy causes toured the updated clinical laboratories where 4,000 to 5,000 diagnostic tests were performed daily. They also viewed the new intensive care nursery that provided the ultimate in monitoring and care of neonatal patients. The ceremony included the addition of the portrait of Ethel Brown Foerderer next to that of her husband on the first-floor lobby wall.

The James R. Martin Nurses' Residence (1959)

In 1959 Jefferson made a major move beyond the boundaries of the block from Sansom to Walnut between Tenth and Eleventh by building a new student nurses' residence across Walnut on the southeast corner at Eleventh, a site that in earlier years was the home of Samuel D. Gross and his predecessor, Thomas Dent Mütter. At a cost of $2,000,000, aided by a bequest in the will of Dr. James Reid Martin, the second James Edwards Professor of Orthopaedics (1939–1950), it was designed by architects at George M. Ewing Company to harmonize with the Pavilion Building. It was not only a significant addition to Jefferson's physical plant but an attraction to qualified women (at that time solely women) interested in professional nursing careers (Figure 48-63).

This completely air-conditioned building had a housing capacity for 336 students, a residence director, and four housemothers in its eight floors of ultramodern facilities. Bathrooms, laundries, and elevators constituted a centralized core area with a corridor on either side. This provided greater privacy for double bedrooms with individual accommodations and outside exposure. Studio beds served as divans during the day and opened full-size for sleeping. Built-in desks and dressers and large closets allowed ample storage space. A lounge and kitchenette on each bedroom floor, a large recreation room on the ground-floor level, and the solarium with a sun deck afforded pleasant recreational facilities. Students could entertain their guests in the first-floor music room and reception lounge.

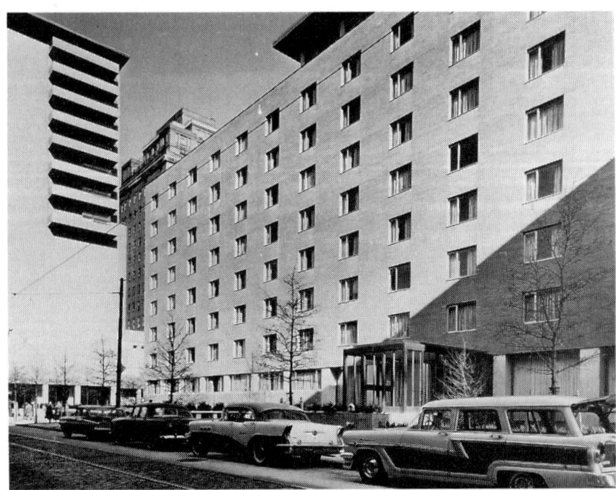

FIG. 48-63. The James R. Martin Nurses' Residence (1959).

The Jefferson Medical College Hospital Training School for Nurses had opened in the fall of 1891 with 13 students, housed in cramped quarters on the upper floors of the 1877 Hospital on Sansom Street. The Board of Trustees in May, 1893, rented quarters at 518 Spruce Street as the first official Nurses' Home. When the enrollment started to spiral, the Trustees in the spring of 1895 moved the trainees to 226 South Seventh Street. This was next door to the Maternity Section of the Hospital, making it convenient for the students to obtain instruction in obstetrical nursing (Figure 48-20).

When the 1907 Hospital was opened on the corner of Tenth and Sansom Streets, there was an immediate increase in the Nursing School from 50 to 90 pupils. The need for larger quarters was solved by renovating the 1877 Hospital (replaced later by the Thompson Annex) as a Nurses' Home. Thereafter the student body expanded to 125.

When the Trustees decided in 1922 to demolish the 1877 Hospital to make way for the Thompson Annex, the displaced nurses were moved to a cluster of residences at 1012–1016 Spruce Street. The yard space in the rear of these buildings was then used to build a new nurses' residence, which opened on May 15, 1925. It had 90 single rooms with hot and cold running water, large closets, and comfortable furnishings. Two floors were added to the original six in 1926 to accommodate 120 students.

With the building of the Martin Nurses' Residence, the properties on Spruce Street were sold and the rear eight-story Nurses' Residence was converted into condominiums. Some of the staff nurses rented or purchased these apartments for long-term occupancy.

On June 10, 1982, the 38 members of the last nursing class graduated. As one of the finest schools of nursing in the nation closed, Jefferson continued its path of excellence in the Department of Nursing within the College of Allied Health Sciences. The Martin Nurses' Residence was then used for administrative offices in its lower floors and for further student housing within the University.

James Mifflin Large, L.H.D., LL.D.; the Third Board Chairman (1962–1970)

James M. Large (Figure 48-64) was born in Philadelphia in 1904. His ancestors included, on one side, General Thomas Mifflin, a delegate to the First Continental Congress, and, on the other side, General George G. Meade, the Union Civil War hero. Large was educated at the Lawrenceville School and Princeton University. A banking career that lasted for 42 years from 1928 led to his presidency of the Tradesmen's National Bank, which through merger became the Provident National.

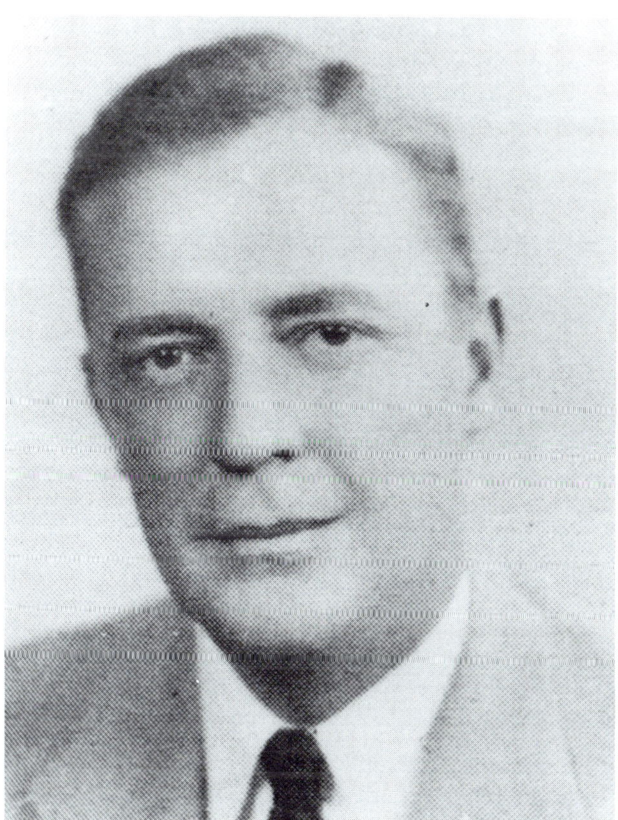

FIG. 48-64. James M. Large, L.H.D., LL.D. (1904–), Third Board Chairman (1962–1970).

Large's talents in the world of finance led to directorships in the Philadelphia Saving Fund Society; Fidelity Mutual Life Insurance Company; Commonwealth Land Title Insurance Company; Horn and Hardart Company of New York; Southco, Inc.; ESB, Inc.; South Chester Tube Company; Chester Tidewater Terminal, Inc.; and Dodge Steel Company.

The civic contributions of James Large were manifested in his co-chairmanship of the 1956 United Community Campaign, the Advisory Board of Philadelphia's Crime Commission, and the Board of the Zoological Society of Philadelphia. He was Vice President and Director of the Pennsylvania Academy of the Fine Arts. The Moore School of Art, in which he served as Chairman of the Board, awarded him the honorary degree of Doctor of Humanities.

Large served in the U.S. Navy with great distinction during World War II. On active duty with the light carrier *USS Princeton,* he experienced nine major combats and was wounded during the sinking of his ship. He subsequently served aboard the second aircraft carrier *USS Princeton.* Awarded the Purple Heart and Silver Star medals, he retired as a Captain, U.S.N.R.

Elected to the Board in 1950, Large became Chairman on January 1, 1962. In this capacity he headed the exciting developments inherited from Mr. Foerderer's administration, which included the $40 million expansion of the physical facilities and the evolution of Jefferson Medical College into the keystone of Thomas Jefferson University (Figure 48-65).

In his eight years as Chairman, James Large participated in every aspect of his obligations beyond the call of duty. He represented the Board at nearly all the College functions, made a tradition of personally presenting awards to the students at Opening Exercises, and maintained close relations with the Alumni Association. At the June Commencement of 1970 he was awarded the honorary degree of Doctor of Laws.

The Stein Research Center (1965)

A basic research arm of the Department of Radiology was developed in 1965 as the Stein

Radiation Biology Research Center (Figure 48-66). It was constructed in a somewhat hidden location at 202 South Hutchinson Street, east of Tenth and south of Walnut. The old building there was reconstructed at a cost of over $600,000 into a striking new edifice named after Louis Stein, who spearheaded the project. Stein, President of Food Fair Stores, Inc., had long been a friend of the Roosevelts and an officer in the Eleanor Roosevelt Cancer Foundation. Recognition of a substantial contribution to the construction was expressed by the designation of three-quarters of the space as "The Eleanor Roosevelt Cancer Research Laboratory." The remaining one-quarter was named "The Harry Bock Memorial Laboratory" for research in prenatal deformities with funds contributed by the Harry Bock Charities. Appropriations from the American Cancer Society and from the federal government through the National Institutes of Health were also received.

An impressive dedication ceremony honoring its benefactors, Mr. and Mrs. Louis Stein, was held on September 20, 1965, in McClellan Hall.

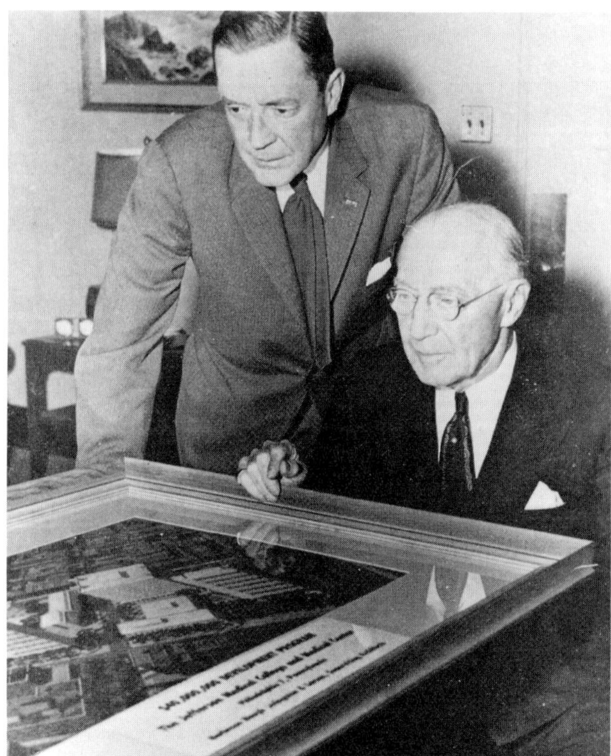

FIG. 48-65. Percival E. Foerderer, just retired as Board Chairman, discussing Jefferson's development plans with James M. Large, who succeeded him (1962).

President of the Medical College, Mr. William W. Bodine, Jr., presided and introduced Mr. James M. Large, Chairman of the Board, who welcomed the guests. He then presented Dr. Philip J. Hodes, Professor of Radiology and Head of the Department, who played a most vital part in the development of the Center. "The Mission of the Stein Research Center," as expounded in his address, was to explore new research frontiers in chromosomes, genetics, tissue cultures, intrauterine life, electron microscopy, radiation physics, and immunity. It was also to prepare young scholars for established professional careers. Dean William A. Sodeman then introduced Mr. Stein, who in modestly accepting the honor expressed his gratitude for the combined effort of the many dedicated people and organizations that aided in the project. Dr. Sodeman, in accepting the Center on behalf of the administration, introduced Dr. Francis L. Schmehl, Chief of the Health Research Facilities Branch of the National Institutes of Health. Dr. Schmehl, in praising Jefferson as an institution "unexcelled in the maturation of medical students," also referred "to the research potential of your College which is increasing at a tremendous rate. . . ."

The keynote speaker was the Honorable James Roosevelt. He referred to the Center as "but the beginning, the first of the major research buildings in a construction program to expand and enrich Jefferson's research facilities." He mentioned his mother's "concern for human suffering, thirst for understanding, and eagerness to engage with the future . . . ," and added, "She would be greatly moved by the naming of the cancer laboratory for her."

Dr. Robert L. Brent, Professor of Pediatrics and Professor of Radiology (Radiation Biology) was named the Director of the Center and of the Roosevelt Laboratory. Dr. Robert O. Gorson, Associate Professor of Radiology (Medical Physics), and Dr. Thomas R. Koszalka, Associate Professor of Radiology (Biochemistry), were appointed as Associate Directors.

house turned publishing office and taken over by Jefferson in 1953, the Stefano Brothers (Cigarette Co.) Building, the Horn and Hardart Commissary, several warehouses, and a row of stores completed the list to be demolished for this section of the expanded Jefferson campus.

Orlowitz Residence Hall (1967)

Through the mechanism of urban development, Jefferson acquired the additional campus area of Walnut to Locust between Tenth and Eleventh. The Martin Nurses' Residence (1959) at Eleventh and Walnut was complemented in 1967 by construction of the Louis B. and Ida K. Orlowitz Residence Hall for students and house staff. It was a regret that the romanesque, massive brown stone Western Savings Fund main office building at the southwest corner of Tenth and Walnut, designed by architect James Windrim in 1877, had to be razed for this purpose. The Mohler Building, a house turned publishing office and taken over by Jefferson in 1953, the Stefano Brothers (Cigarette Co.) Building, the Horn and Hardart Commissary, several warehouses, and a row of stores completed the list to be demolished for this section of the expanded Jefferson campus.

In 1963 Louis Orlowitz donated $250,000 to initiate the Residence that would ultimately cost $4.7 million. Newspapers stated that the gift was in gratitude for the successful surgery and excellent care he had received at Jefferson during a serious illness. Major financing was through a long-term bond issue (1966–2016) under the College Housing Program of the Federal Department of Housing and Urban Development. It constituted an 84% coverage of cost in the amount of $3,925,000 at 3% interest tied to a schedule of rents that would allow repayment in 50 years.

The 20-floor, 239-apartment building of reinforced concrete and brick was designed by the architectural firm of Esbach, Pullinger, Stevens,

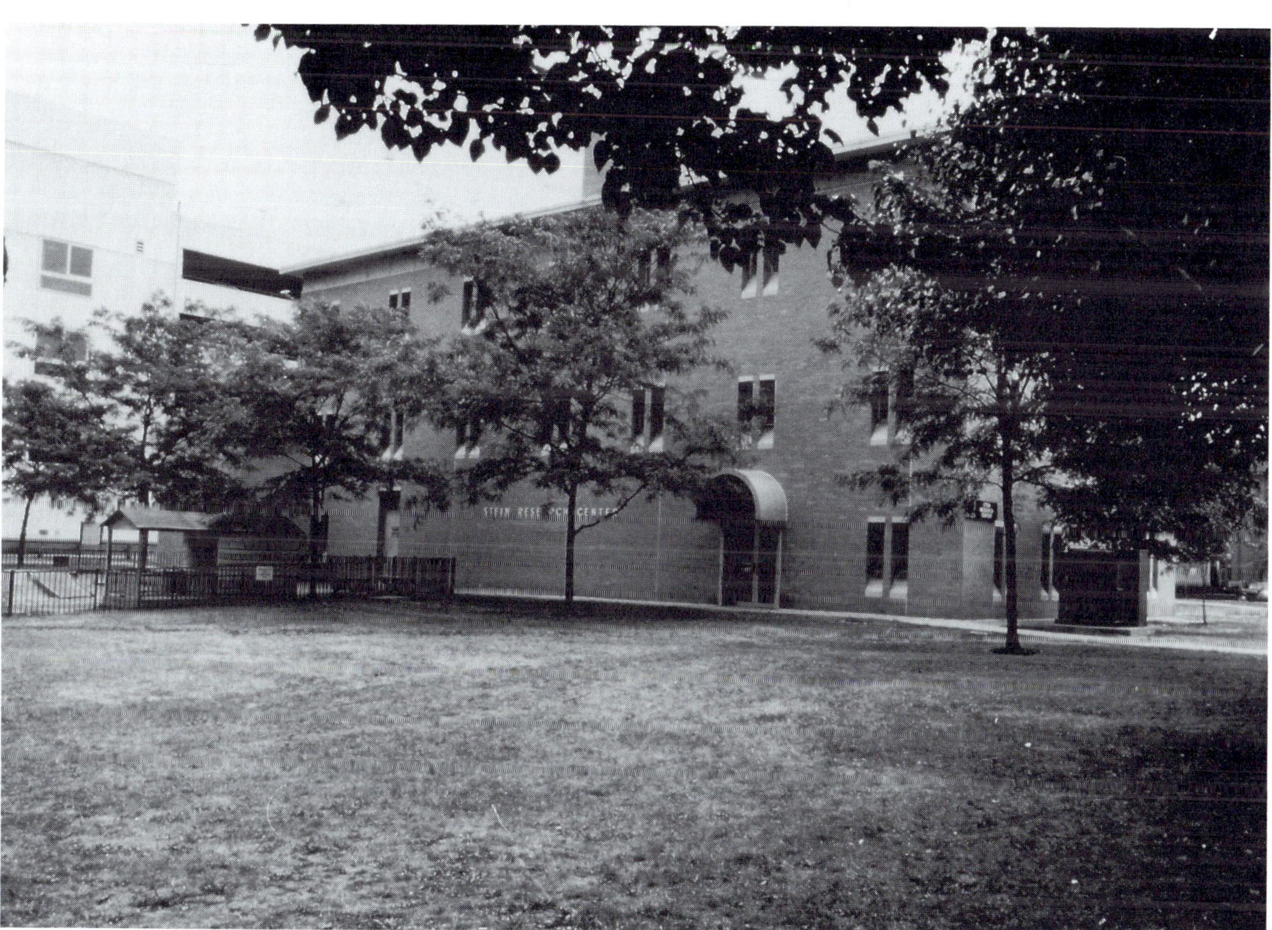

Fig. 48-66. The Stein Research Center (1965).

and Bruder (Figure 48-67). There was a sunken court for sunning or recreation, plus a children's play area with benches, sandbox, and a climbing turtle. A flagstone entrance with planters and benches led to a flagstone lobby with individual mailboxes large enough for journals and magazines. An elevator lobby behind locked doors, opened by signal from the apartments, telephone communication from lobby to apartments, three high-speed automatic passenger elevators, one freight elevator, full air-conditioning, master television antenna system, coin-operated laundry room with 40 washers and dryers, and additional basement storage closet for each apartment were provided. No pets were allowed.

Large windows almost from floor to ceiling made every room bright. Draw drapes were coordinated in color with wall-to-wall carpeting and contemporary lighting fixtures. All-electric kitchens featured a self-defrosting refrigerator, stove, stainless steel sink, formica-faced cabinets and counter tops, exhaust fan, and a vinyl tile floor. Bathrooms had walls of ceramic tile and tub showers. There were 172 one-bedroom apartments, some of which were furnished, 56 unfurnished two-bedroom apartments, and 11 unfurnished with three bedrooms. Each apartment had an ample living room and adequate storage space.

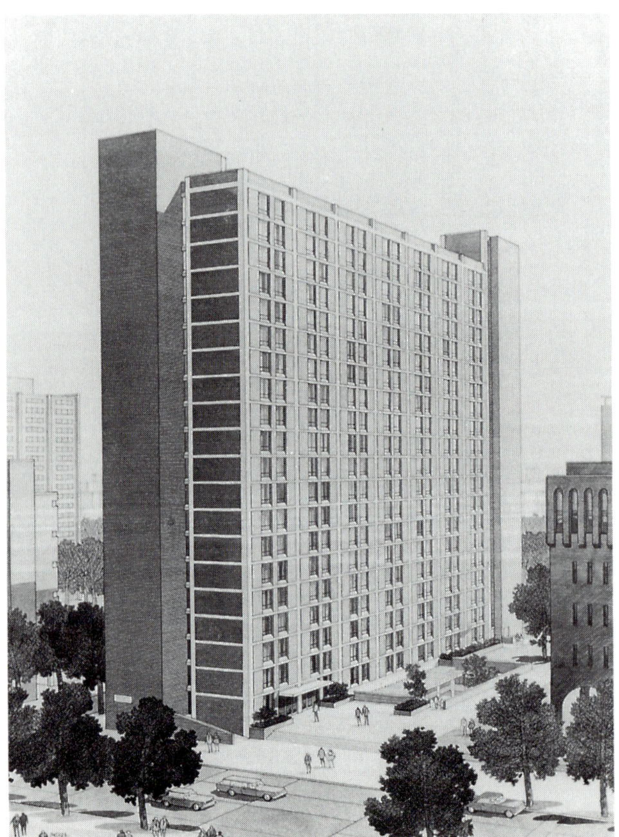

FIG. 48-67. Orlowitz Residence Hall (1967).

Social and professional gatherings for groups up to 100 persons could be accommodated in a 30 by 34-foot meeting room directly accessible from the outdoor sunken patio. It housed an independent cloakroom and kitchen. This facility was available to residents for conferences, private parties, or dances.

Within nine years additional housing space would be provided by the Barringer Residence.

Thomas Jefferson Gains University Status (1969)

The advisability of university status or university affiliation had been raised intermittently at Jefferson for over one-half century. There were flurries of interest in the decade following the Flexner Report of 1910, as already described. In 1953 the issue arose once again on a serious and sustained basis.

Several members of the Executive Faculty (Peter A. Herbut, Kenneth Goodner, and Andrew J. Ramsay) voiced increasing concern about the prospects of a private, independent professional school surviving the increasingly complex demands of an increasingly complex interdependent society—they feared that status quo and academic isolationism could lead toward mediocrity. An inevitable conclusion was reached that Jefferson must seek meaningful university affiliation or itself develop into a university. Both avenues were investigated.

Although gaining university status by metamorphosis was more exciting, the affiliation route would be easier, quicker, and financially more feasible. To explore the latter path, Jefferson considered sixteen schools in Pennsylvania, New Jersey, Delaware, and Maryland.[20] Although geographically separated, Pennsylvania State University emerged as the most appropriate. It had no medical school of its own, and rumors suggested that it was being pressured to acquire a medical school or create one. Furthermore, State-related and -supported Pennsylvania State University would afford Jefferson access to greatly needed Commonwealth funds. The Executive Faculty recommended to the Board that this affiliation meet their approval "providing the identity of our institution be retained and maintained." On June 6, 1960, the Board resolved "That President Bodine be, and he hereby is, authorized to discuss with President Eric A. Walker, of Pennsylvania State University, the possibility of developing an affiliation or association between Jefferson and Pennsylvania State which might enure to the benefit of both of these institutions. . . ." Discussion ensued but was subsequently tabled for "reconsideration at some later date."

In 1963 the Board requested a further study of the problem of university affiliation. On November 4, 1963, the College Committee proposed to the Board "that Jefferson ascertain whether an educational association can be established with Princeton University under terms which would retain Jefferson's autonomy and would provide close academic and research relationships between the two institutions." The Jefferson Board took no action on the recommendation and referred the matter to Chairman Large and President Bodine. Contact was made with Princeton, but Jefferson's consideration of affiliation was not acted upon.

Negotiations with Pennsylvania State University were vigorously renewed, and by the spring of 1966 an affiliation appeared imminent. At the Board meeting of June 6, 1966, it was resolved "that the Jefferson Medical College of Philadelphia ('Jefferson') does hereby approve and adopt the Memorandum of Affiliation between the Jefferson Medical College of Philadelphia and the Pennsylvania State University." On July 25 and August 16, 1966, it became apparent that deep differences existed between the Boards of the two institutions and further negotiations on affiliation collapsed. On September 12, 1966, the Jefferson Board unanimously rescinded the Memorandum of Affiliation. The Penn State–Jefferson relationship was more complicated than these brief facts would indicate, and more detail is warranted.

In 1963, through the efforts of Dean William A. Sodeman, an Accelerated Program was established with Pennsylvania State University whereby exceptional students who made early commitment to the study of medicine could obtain the baccalaureate and medical degrees within a period of five years. This was a response of Jefferson to what appeared at that time to be a national shortage of physicians. The program was later changed to six years when Pennsylvania State University shifted from a quarter to a semester system. Longitudinal studies documented this program to be highly successful. Jefferson has continued this special program and additionally accepts large numbers of Pennsylvania State graduates who pursue the traditional four years of preparation for medicine.

Meanwhile, there was a surprise announcement in the news media on August 23, 1963, that Pennsylvania State University was establishing a new Medical School at Hershey, Pennsylvania. The court had decided that $50 million could be offered from the Milton S. Hershey Foundation to establish and operate a medical school that would have to be located in Derry Township, which included the small town of Hershey. The ongoing dialogue between the two institutions seemed to give the impression that *Jefferson* would be *the* Medical School of Pennsylvania State University. Actually, by November, 1964, Penn State was unilaterally preparing for its own medical school at Hershey, which was 105 miles away from the parent campus.[21] Belatedly, Jefferson was given assurance by their President that the establishment of the Hershey Medical School and Center would not in any way interfere with Jefferson's affiliation proposal or with Jefferson's ongoing programs with Pennsylvania State University in connection with Continuing Medical Education and the Accelerated Medical Programs.[22] As events turned out, it was wiser for Penn State not to have two Medical Schools and for Jefferson to develop university status alone.

At the meeting of September 12, 1966, at which the Affiliation Memorandum was rescinded, the Board authorized the Administration to proceed with plans for the establishment of a proposed School of Allied Health Sciences within Jefferson Medical College. A Graduate School had previously been organized in the six Basic Sciences

Departments in 1949. On January 9, 1967, the Board resolved "That there is hereby established in the Jefferson Medical College of Philadelphia, as a separate department or division, a school to be known as the School of Allied Health Sciences of Jefferson Medical College. . . ." This action immediately opened the door for Jefferson to grow into a University.

At his inauguration, in an impressive ceremony at the Academy of Music on May 3, 1967, President Peter A. Herbut declared that the Jefferson Medical College of Philadelphia would seek university status through the development of a School of Allied Health Sciences. After 14 years of deliberation (1953–1967) the course was set. No one was more qualified or could have worked harder toward this end than Dr. Herbut.[22] It was the crowning achievement of his distinguished career.

On March 31, 1969, President Herbut received a letter from David H. Kurtzman, Superintendent of the Department of Public Instruction in the Commonwealth of Pennsylvania. The first paragraph read: "By the authority given to me under P.L. 137 (amendment to the Nonprofit Corporation Law, Act of May 5, 1933, P.L. 289 as amended), I am pleased to approve the request of the Jefferson Medical College to attain university status and to be designated as Thomas Jefferson University. . . . You and your able staff, as well as the institution generally, are to be commended on the professional accomplishments to date."

The Charter was received in City Hall on May 20, 1969 (Figure 48-68). New members of the Board were no longer required to be sworn into trusteeship. The four Divisions of Thomas Jefferson University, established on a reference date of July 1, 1969, were (1) Jefferson Medical College; (2) College of Graduate Studies; (3) College of Allied Health Sciences; and (4) Thomas Jefferson University Hospital. It was created as a totally health-related, medically oriented University.

Peter A. Herbut, M.D.; Third Medical College President (1966–1969), First University President (1969–1976)

Dr. Peter Herbut (Figure 48–69) succeeded William Bodine as the third full-time President of Jefferson Medical College in 1966 and in 1969 became the first President of Thomas Jefferson University. He served with extraordinary dedication under Board Chairmen Large and Bodine. As Chief Executive Officer for the Board, Herbut masterminded the details of Jefferson's transformation from a Medical College and Hospital into a University. Although not a Jefferson graduate, he distinctly belonged to that group of individuals designated as "Mr. Jefferson." Admired and respected by all for his integrity, methodicalness, and Herculean labor, many regarded him as a genius. This modest man was known affectionately as "Pete."

The ninth of 13 children, Herbut was born in Edson, Alberta, Canada in 1912. After preliminary education in the public schools there, he attended the University of Alberta (1930–1935) and obtained both his M.D. and C.M. (a graduate medical degree) from McGill University in 1937.

After internships in Children's Memorial Hospital, Montreal, and at Wilkes-Barre General Hospital, Pennsylvania, he took his residency at the Medical College of Virginia at Richmond and came to Jefferson in 1939 as an Assistant Demonstrator of Pathology. He became a U.S. citizen in 1942.

Herbut's rise in the Department of Pathology was meteoric, leading to his Professorship and Chairmanship of the Department in 1948, shortly before his thirty-sixth birthday. In 1951 he was named Director of the Clinical Research Laboratories at Jefferson, and in 1952 Chairman of the Department of Pathology at Methodist Hospital. In 1948 he authored *Surgical Pathology* (its second edition appeared in 1954), and subsequently *Urological Pathology* in two volumes (1952), *Gynecological and Obstetrical Pathology* (1953), and *Pathology* (1955 and 1959). His international reputation included his active career in research, concentrated mainly on causes and treatment of cancer. This activity resulted in more than 100 scientific papers. He belonged to 26 societies, five of which were foreign scientific bodies. His portrait was presented to the College by the Class of 1961.

The appointment of Dr. Herbut in 1966 marked the first time in Jefferson's history that a faculty member was advanced to the Presidency. There were those who initially questioned his qualifications for such a position, but all doubts were dispelled by his immediate leadership as well as his integrated teamwork with the Board. The thrust into university status under Chairman Large and the development of additional buildings under Chairman Bodine all dovetailed with President Herbut's ambitions for Jefferson.

On March 31, 1976, President Herbut spoke briefly at a luncheon for volunteers of the Women's Board Pennywise Shop. On return to his home not feeling well in the early afternoon, he died suddenly from a cardiovascular attack. A throng of the shocked and saddened Jefferson community attended his Russian Orthodox memorial service. This giant in Jefferson's history was honored posthumously in 1979 when the College Auditorium was named the "Herbut Auditorium."

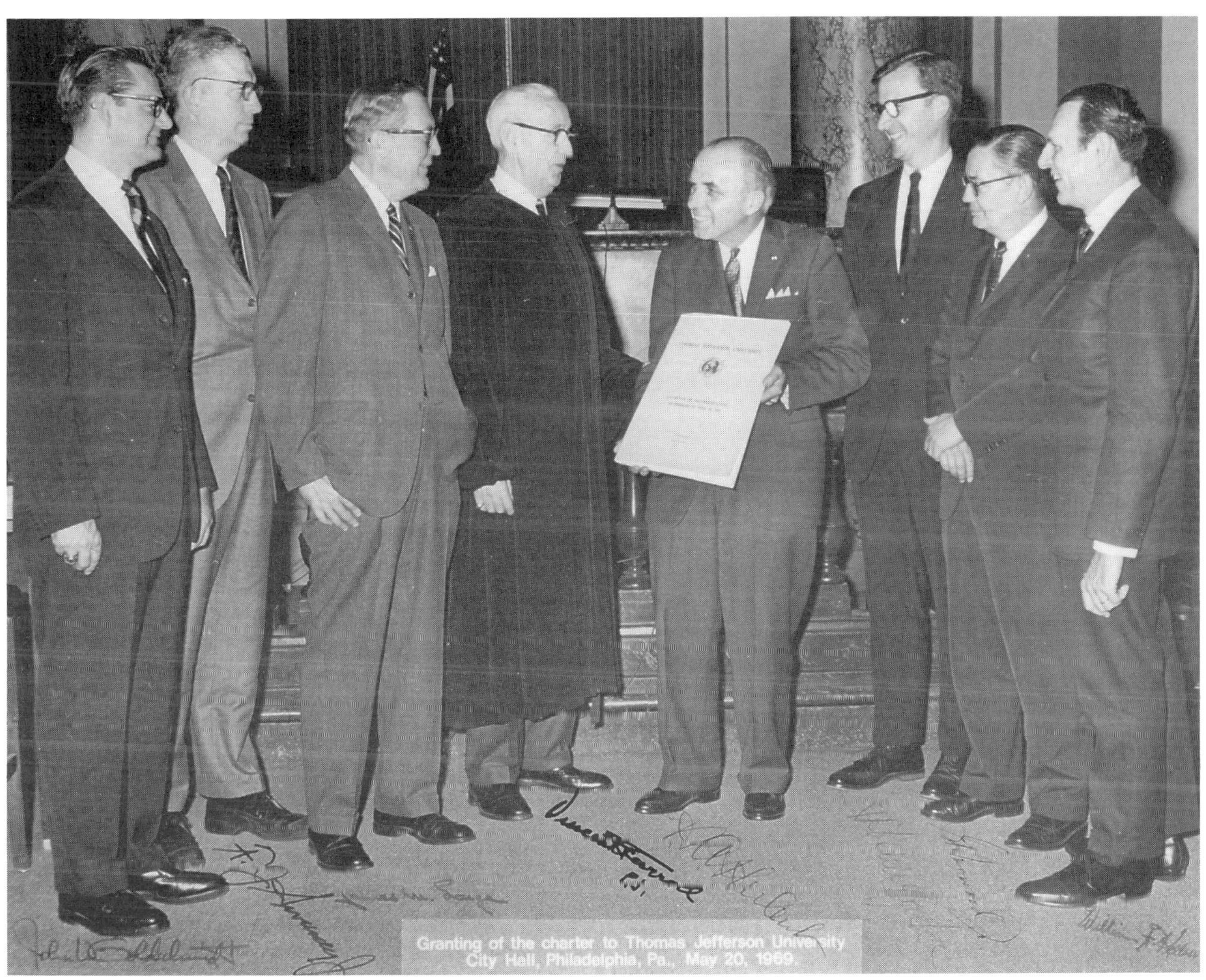

FIG. 48-68. Granting of the Charter to Thomas Jefferson University at City Hall, Philadelphia, May 20, 1969. Left to right: John W. Goldschmidt, M.D. (Dean of College of Allied Health Sciences); Francis J. Sweeney, M.D. (Hospital Director); James M. Large (Chairman of the Board); Judge Vincent Carroll; Peter A. Herbut, M.D. (President); N. Ramsay Pennypacker (Vice President for Development); George M. Norwood (Vice President for Planning); and William F. Kellow, M.D. (Dean).

George M. Norwood, Jr.; Interim President (1976–1977)

At a special meeting of the full Board of Trustees on April 5, 1976, Mr. George ("Mac") Norwood (Figure 48–70) was named University Interim President following the unexpected death of Dr. Herbut the previous week. Norwood had first come to Jefferson in 1965 from the University of North Carolina to serve as Vice President for Business and Finance, and since 1970 had served as Vice President for Planning. In the latter position he had been largely responsible for devising and implementing Jefferson's Master Development Program, aided by the *Report of the Committee for Master Planning* (December 1972, under the Chairmanship of Trustee Frederic L. Ballard). Mr. Norwood also served as a Trustee of the Magee Memorial Rehabilitation Center, and in 1973 as National Chairman of the Planning Coordinators Group of the Association of American Medical Colleges.

During his interim Presidency, Norwood worked assiduously with the Board and with Dr. Francis J. Sweeney, Jr., Vice President for Health Services and Hospital Director, in the complex details of negotiation and construction of the new Thomas Jefferson University Hospital in the city block of Chestnut and Sansom between Tenth and Eleventh. He was honored with the prestigious Alumni Achievement Award in 1978.

After the appointment of Dr. Lewis W. Bluemle, Jr. as the succeeding President, effective on August 1, 1977, Mr. Norwood stepped down to his former position (Vice President) and resigned in March 1979.

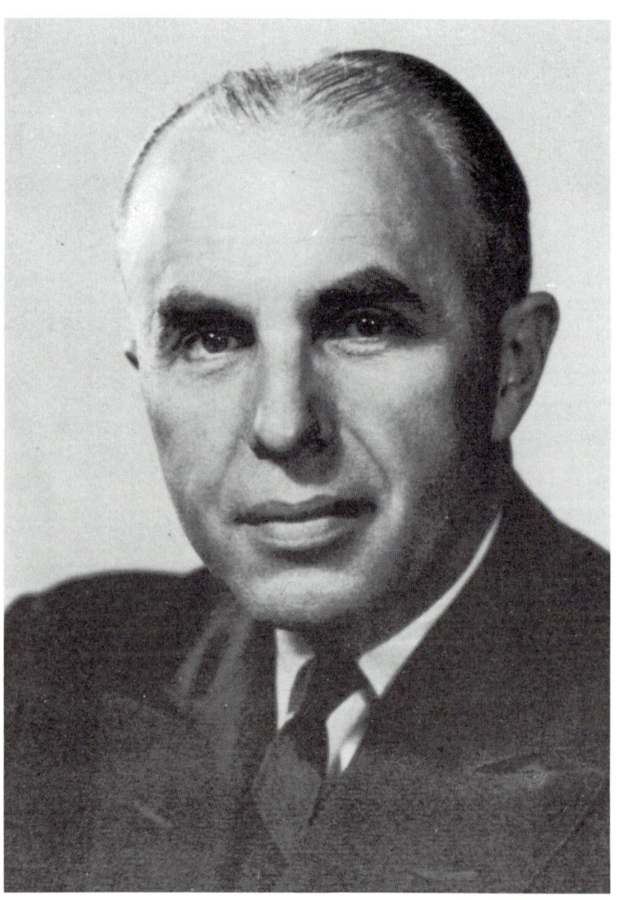

Fig. 48-69. Peter A. Herbut, M.D. (1912–1976), Third Medical College President (1966–1969), First University President (1969–1976).

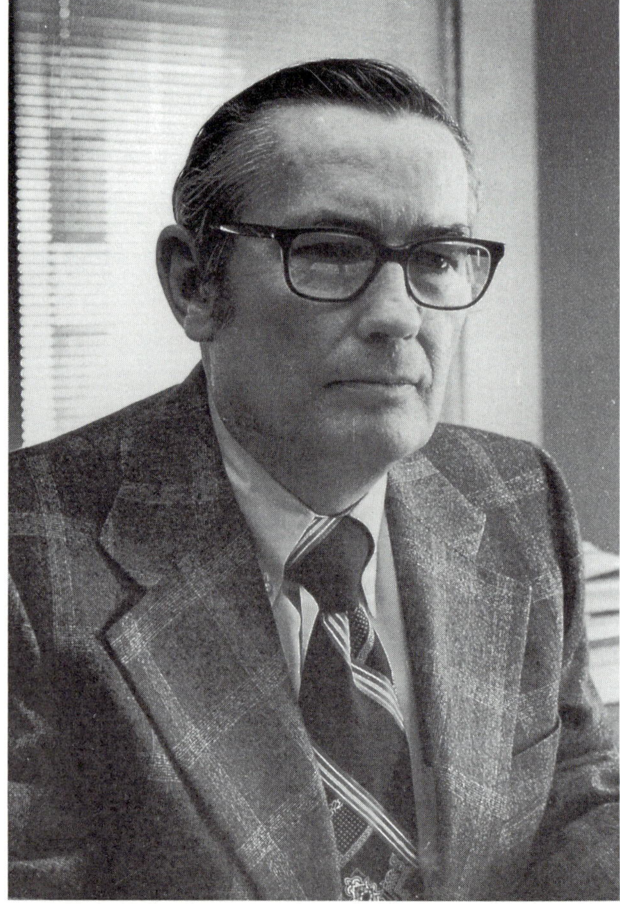

Fig. 48-70. George M. Norwood, Jr. ("Mac"), Interim President (1976–1977).

William Warden Bodine, Jr., L.H.D.; Second President, Jefferson Medical College (1959–1966), and Fourth Board Chairman (1970–1977)

William W. Bodine, Jr. (Figure 48–71) was born in 1918, a descendant of an old Philadelphia family with a tradition of public service. His father, a lawyer, was prominent in the financial world of banking, insurance, and utilities. He set an example for young Bill as president of a series of civic and charitable organizations as well as supporter of political activities. William, Jr. grew in the affluence of the family estate at Villanova and later in youth became a sportsman with preference for polo. His education was provided at Episcopal Academy in Overbrook, at St. Paul's School in Concord, New Hampshire, and at Harvard University. His college career was interrupted by World War II, when he joined the armed forces in 1940. His military career was heroic and extraordinary.

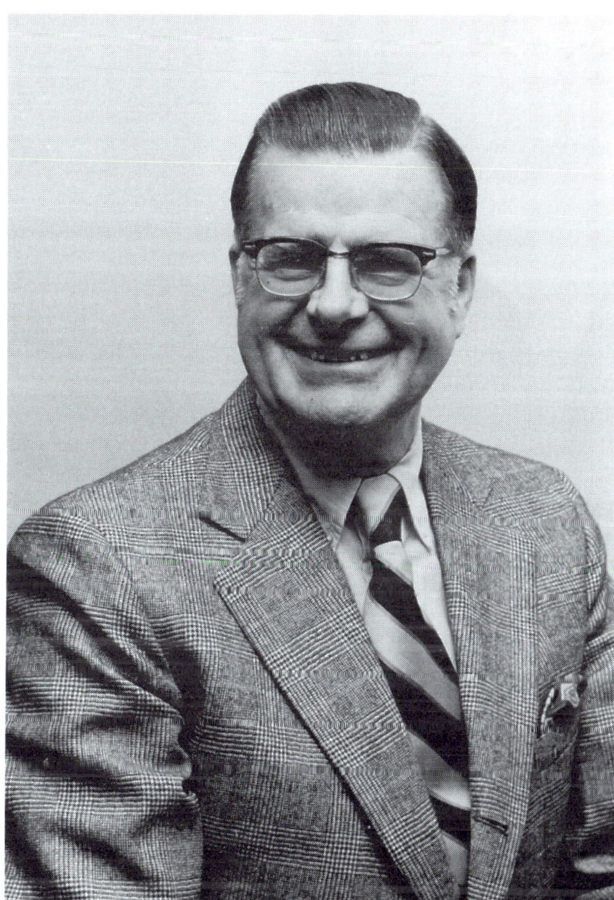

Fig. 48-71. William W. Bodine, Jr., L.H.D. (1918–1983), Second Medical College President (1959–1966), and Fourth Board Chairman (1970–77).

As the commander of a tank destroyer unit he encountered the German Panzers in the Battle of the Bulge. He and many of his men were captured—some were massacred in the Malmedy Woods, but with the survivors he was loaded into a boxcar bound for a prisoner-of-war camp. Although wounded, Bodine escaped to Allied lines where he was hospitalized for five months. As Lt. Col. he was then assigned to Gen. Dwight Eisenhower's staff and awarded the Purple Heart, The Legion of Merit, and the Croix de Guerre with Palm. He emerged from this military experience "tough and driving." On return to the States he became a confirmed Eisenhower Republican and eventually served on the finance committee for the Pennsylvania and National Republican organizations.

In 1959 Mr. Bodine at the age of 41 succeeded Vice Admiral James L. Kauffman, U.S.N. (Ret.) who had served as the first President of Jefferson Medical College for the previous ten years (Figure 48–72). It will be recalled that Mr. Robert Hooper in 1949 reorganized the Board such that the Head would be designated as Chairman, whose function was to determine with fellow Board Members the concepts of what needed to be done; and a President, whose function as operating executive was to carry out what was decided to be done. Mr. Bodine's appointment created an air of excitement, especially among the alumni. Considered an infusion of young blood, he was hailed as a doer, "full of vinegar and other things." He fulfilled all these expectations.

The 24 Bodine years (1959–1983) encompassed Presidency of the College (1959–1966), Life Trustee (1966–1983), and Chairman of the Board (1970–1977). Under his leadership, Jefferson's growth was dramatic. In 1959 the medical center's operating budget was $11 million, and total assets were in excess of $37 million. At his retirement from the Chairmanship in 1977, the University operating budget was over $95 million, and total assets were at $214 million. During the same 16 years the endowment increased from $16 million to $50 million. When he first became President, the clinical, teaching and research functions were carried out in five buildings in 778,000 square feet of space. By 1977 the University had added or renovated ten additional major buildings, which quadrupled the area to three million square feet. Cost of the new buildings was approximately $141.2 million, while additions or renovations of previous structures cost $13.8 million. The total capital expenditure was $155 million. The University's newest hospital (1978) was financed by two major bond issues of which Bodine was instrumental in the success. The first (1975) was for $81.6 million, while the second (1977) was refunded by the sale of an issue totaling $160 million. Although Mr. Bodine's most visible contributions to Jefferson were in the form of buildings, he was ever mindful that the quality of staff was the institution's first priority. He was also mindful that new buildings, to remain cost efficient, required maintenance, complete usage, and endowments. Criticized by some as a "bricks-and-mortar man" and "too bold," the single fact remained that the bottom line was always a balanced budget.

It is difficult to imagine that William Bodine's accomplishments at Jefferson were only a fraction of his staggering array of business, civic, charitable, and political activities. Among the highlights of his distinguished business career were the offices of Assistant Treasurer of Tradesmen's National Bank and Trust Company (now Provident National Bank), Financial Secretary of Penn Mutual Life Insurance Company, and President of Arthur C. Kaufmann and Associates, Inc., a management consulting firm. He was on the board or served as president or chairman of two dozen other organizations, an incomplete list of which were the Free Library of Philadelphia, United Way of Southeastern Pennsylvania, Crime Commission of Philadelphia, Old Philadelphia Development Corporation, YMCA Foundation of Philadelphia and Vicinity, Civilian Aide to the Secretary of the Army of Eastern Pennsylvania, Community Services of Philadelphia, Health and Welfare, Elwyn Institute, Vice-Commander of the Military Order of Foreign Wars of the United States, Wheels for Welfare, the United Nations Association, Eastern Pennsylvania Psychiatric Institute, the Urban Coalition, the Committee of Seventy, the Greater Philadelphia Partnership, and the University Science Center.

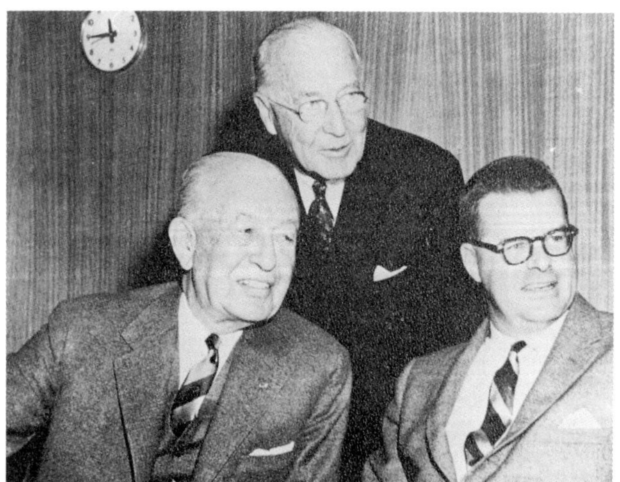

FIG. 48-72. Vice Admiral James L. Kauffman (retiring President), Percival E. Foerderer (Chairman), and William W. Bodine, Jr (incoming President) in 1959.

One of Bodine's activities most widely acclaimed by the general public was the first full-time Presidency as well as Chairmanship of the Board of the World Affairs Council, an organization that he helped shape into a world forum. He won approval, through the Philadelphia public school system, for a school of national affairs, where students could be trained for diplomatic work.

Many honors were bestowed upon William Bodine. In 1950 he was selected Young Man of the Year by the Junior Chamber of Commerce of Greater Philadelphia. In 1962 he received the Good Citizenship Gold Medal of the Philadelphia Continental Chapter of the Sons of the American Revolution. Jefferson Medical College awarded him the Honorary Degree of Doctor of Letters in 1967. In 1978 he received the Achievement Award of Wheels, Inc. Jefferson signally honored him in September 1979 with the dedication of the Bodine Fountain of five frolicking otters on a stone playground (Figure 48–73). The sculptor was Henry Mitchell, who had also created Jefferson's Winged Ox column. Funds for this unique fountain were derived from 1% of the construction costs of the Barringer Residence Hall and the University Parking Garage as an art requirement of Philadelphia's Redevelopment

A rapidly progressive carcinoma of the pancreas claimed the life of this brilliant, dynamic man of colorful personality on August 11, 1983, at the age of 65. He had built with the inspired teamwork of his fellow Board Members the springboard for Jefferson's leap into the twenty-first century.

Authority. A monumental posthumous memorial is the $24 million Bodine Radiation Center (1986) constructed within the 1978 Thomas Jefferson University Hospital.

Bodine strategically timed his retirement for July, 1977, to coincide with appointment of Jefferson's Second University President. Dr. Lewis W. Bluemle, Jr. and the Fifth Board Chairman, Mr. Frederic L. Ballard, Esq. Speaking of Jefferson Presidents at this time, he considered himself as a "fiscal manager," his successor, Dr. Peter A. Herbut (1966–1976) as an "educational reformer," and incoming Dr. Bluemle as "an expert in quality control." Bodine then continued as a Life Trustee.

Jefferson Hall (1968), Jefferson Alumni Hall (1971)

About 1960, new facilities for the teaching of the basic medical sciences as well as facilities for medical student recreation were high on the list of priorities. By 1962 the General State Authority agreed to build what was first planned as two separate buildings, a basic science building with an adjoining commons building. This state agency used the Commonwealth's bond authority to construct buildings for public organizations or those of state benefit. The approved organization

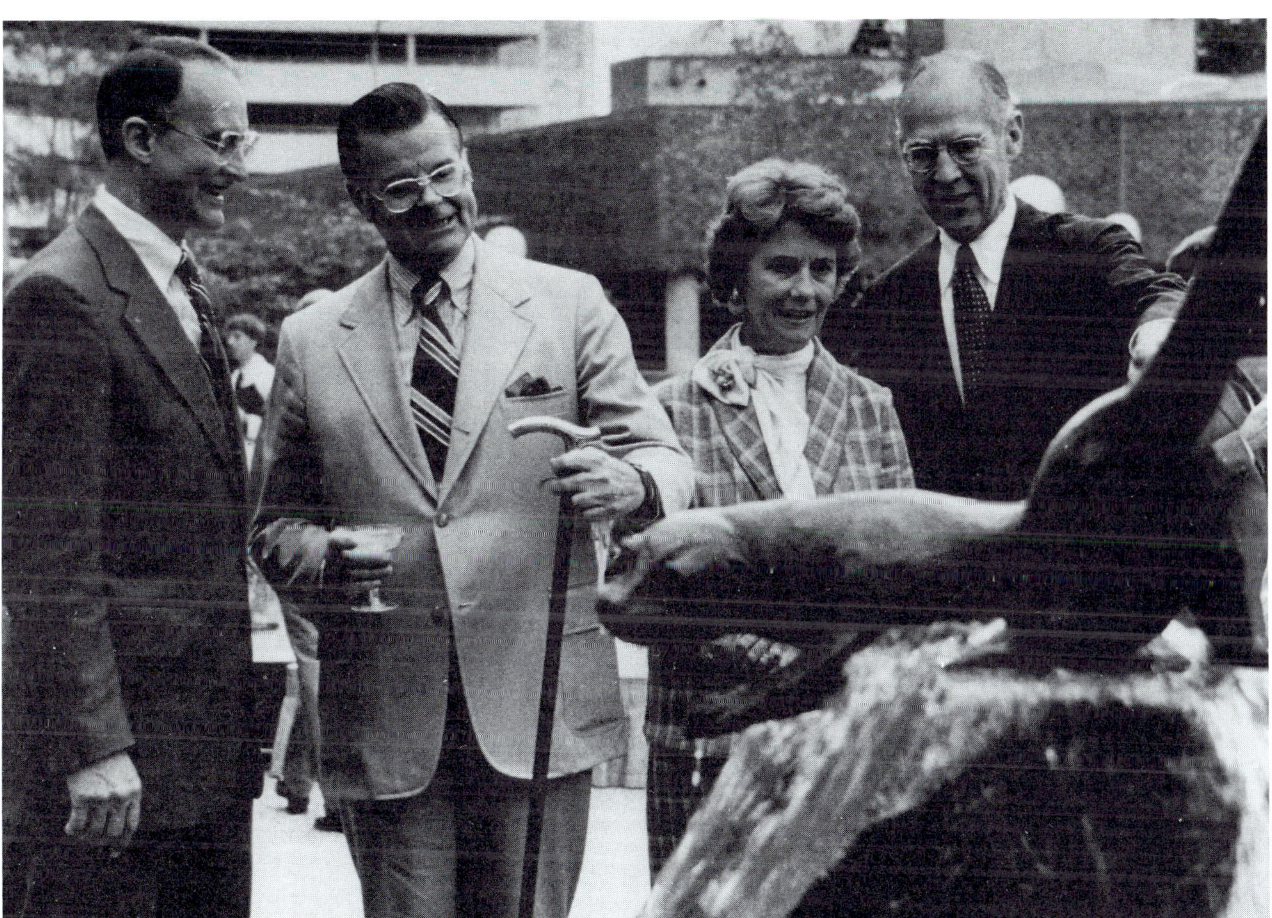

FIG. 48-73. Dedication of the Bodine Fountain (1979); left to right: Dr. Bluemle, Mr. and Mrs. Bodine, and Mr. Ballard.

paid back the State Authority through long-term leases that led eventually to full title ownership. This was Jefferson's first use of this type of state aid.

Jefferson's coordinating architects (Harbeson, Hough, Livingston, and Larson) chose two one-acre sites along the south side of Locust Street between Tenth and Eleventh. At that time Jefferson's total development was planned to extend down to Spruce Street between Tenth and Eleventh. The State Authority chose Vincent Kling and Associates as the architect. Kling's earlier work on the Foerderer Pavilion had won national recognition.

The Board of Trustees was aware of the need for flexibility of construction to allow for a shift to interdisciplinary "team teaching" from the traditional Jefferson separation of disciplines. In the original plan the basic science building required a height of about eight floors, whereas facilities projected for the Commons would require a building of only two floors. (The juxtaposition of a tall with a low building was neither aesthetic nor efficient.) A decision was made to combine the functions of the two buildings within one structure. At the same time the Trustees altered the direction of Jefferson's expansion for this unified building to form the southern boundary for the new campus. Combining the two buildings was estimated to save up to $1½ million, to be more attractive, and to allow more space to be given to the Commons than originally programmed (Figure 48-74).

The Commons facilities were placed on the main and mezzanine floors, with the teaching and laboratory spaces above. Since the longitudinal space on each floor was twice that originally projected, it was possible to place two Departments on a floor. Two interior courts provided placements for two large rooms beneath (the pool and gymnasium), where they reduced structural complexity and expense.

The first floor of the unified building was indented, whereas the mezzanine was extended to the site line. The lower two floors (Commons) thus formed a shelf support suggesting a sense of floating of the basic science upper floors. The top of the building was designed with a coved parapet that masked the utility of the penthouse (the animals' quarters) above the fifth floor (Figure 48–75).

Construction, which began in 1964, was ready for the start of school in September 1968. The dedication was held on March 18, 1969 in the D. Hays Solis-Cohen Auditorium, marked by a basic sciences seminar. This was followed with buffet and guided tours. In 1971, during the Alumni Presidency of Dr. Herbert A. Luscombe, the building was renamed the Jefferson Alumni Hall.

Scott Library and Administrative Building (1970)

Jefferson's first formal library was located as a reading room in the basement of the newly constructed Medical College of 1898 at the corner of Tenth and Walnut Streets. It contained a small collection of volumes supplied by the Women's Auxiliary. By the time of the Flexner Report of 1910 it was rated as "a good library, excellently administered." Charles Frankenberger was appointed Jefferson's first librarian in 1907 and held the position until 1917. Joseph Wilson was the second librarian until 1949.

Samuel Parsons Scott, a lawyer from Hillsboro, Ohio, claimed to have been cured of a chronic respiratory ailment by the prescription of a Jefferson Professor he met accidently during a train ride. The identity of the Professor remains unknown. In his will of November, 1925, Scott bequeathed his personal library of over 8,000 volumes and a substantial endowment, the details of which are covered in Chapter 56 of this volume by Dr. Robert Lentz, Jefferson's third librarian from 1949 to 1975.

In 1929 the library was moved to the College Building at 1025 Walnut Street (Figure 48–76) and in 1931 the name of Scott was added to the library title. It remained the largest and most usable of the medical school libraries in Philadelphia. By the 1960s it was evident that the acute shortage of space could only worsen. A concurrent problem existed—the functions of corporate administration were being carried out in nine different locations scattered throughout various buildings. A central location for major administrative offices under the University status and a much larger library facility were planned for a new building. This culminated in the Scott Library and Administrative Building, which was completed in the fall of 1970 and fully occupied by the end of December (Figure 48–77).

The building was wisely placed at the approximate center of Jefferson's expanding campus. North and south, it was located between the basic science and clinical areas, and flanked on the east and west by Orlowitz Hall and the Martin Nurses' Residence. It replaced the Mohler Building (formerly the Blakiston Publishing Company) and the Stephano Brothers cigarette factory on the south side of Walnut Street between Tenth and Eleventh, across from the Medical College. The architects (Harbeson, Hough, Livingston, and Larson) created what is acknowledged by many to be the "crown jewel" of the campus. The cost of approximately $4.4 million was met by federal funding, $.5 million of accumulated income from the Scott Memorial Library Endowment, and the fund drive as part of Jefferson's $40 million expansion program.

The bold arch motifs with indentation of the first floor areas provided a large loggia for outdoor sheltered festivities and blended in contemporary terms with the earlier buildings across Walnut Street (Figure 48–78). The handsome darker colored brickwork contrasted tastefully with the lighter color of the surrounding structures. The six-story building provided the first four floors for the library and the upper two for administration. The basement was used for storage and also became the center for Jefferson's extensive computer network.

The formal dedication took place on June 9, 1971, to coincide with graduation week, at the north portico of the building (Figure 48–79), and it featured remarks by University President Peter A. Herbut, M.D.; comments by Board Chairman, William W. Bodine, Jr.; an address by the Associate Director for External Programs of the National Library of Medicine, Leroy L. Langley, Ph.D.; and acceptance by Librarian Robert T. Lentz. A reception and tours enhanced the ceremony.

Jefferson Sesquicentennial (1974)

During Jefferson's 150th anniversary a campaign was organized to raise $15 million for the University. Chairman of the Board William Bodine stressed that the objectives fell into four key areas: to educate physicians, to educate

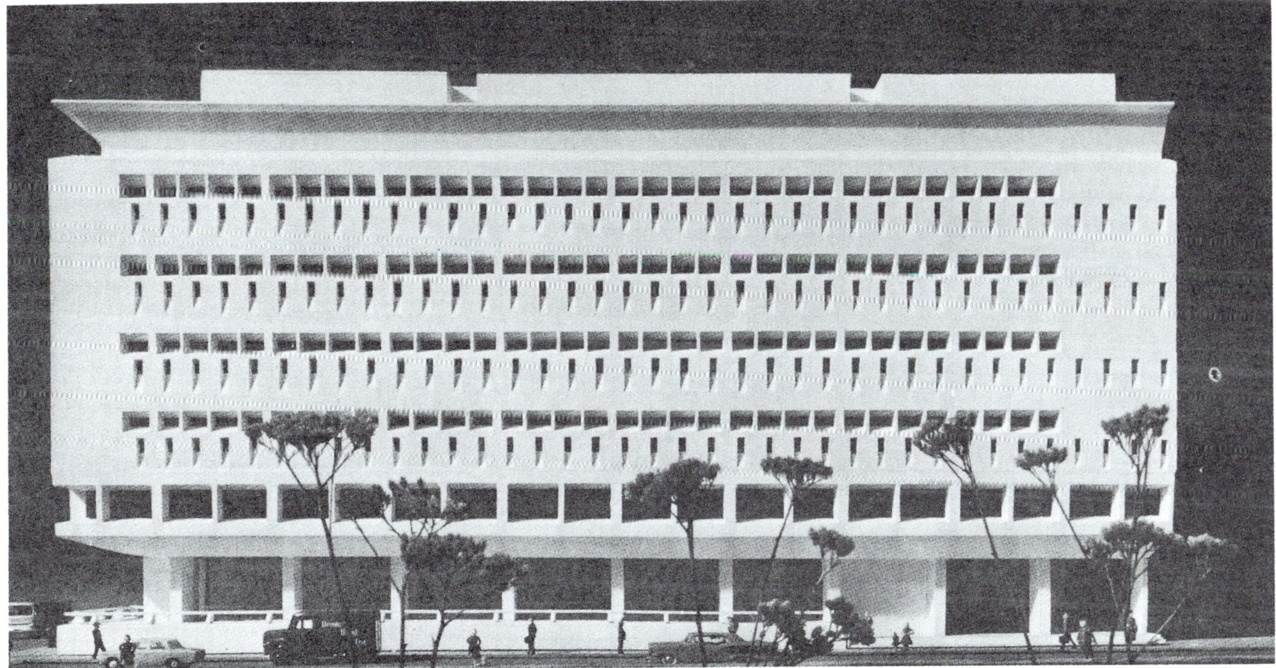

FIG. 48-74. Architect's version of combined Basic Science Building and Commons Building.

paramedical personnel, to produce teachers and investigators in the basic sciences, and to provide outstanding patient care and health services for citizens of the community and of the Commonwealth. Overall Chairman of the drive was Trustee Edward J. Dwyer, and Chairman of the Alumni Phase was Dr. Joe Henry Coley (Jefferson, 1934). By 1975 the Alumni achieved its quota of $4 million, and the total University goal was exceeded by $.75 million from contributions of the Trustees, other members of the Jefferson family, foundations, corporations, and friends.

Throughout 1974 Jefferson commemorated its Sesquicentennial with banquets, symposia, and plans for the future. On March 1, the Alumni Association held its Annual Business Meeting in the Union League at a black tie dinner to which invitations were extended to the teachers and alumni who had brought honor and distinction to their school, as well as to the Emeritus Professors and recipients of the Alumni Achievement Award. A toast was proposed "to the man who made it all possible," George McClellan. Drs. Henry L. Bockus and Francis J. Braceland represented the Alumni Trustees, and President Peter Herbut, the Administration.

On November 15 and 16 the Alumni Association held a weekend gala as a culmination of this commemorative year. On Friday evening, the Royal Swedish Ballet performed for a Jefferson audience at the Philadelphia Academy of Music. Preceding the performance a cocktail party and dinner for 200 was hosted in the Academy Ballroom by Chairman and Mrs. Bodine and President and Mrs. Herbut. A champagne reception was attended by 800 in Jefferson Alumni Hall after the ballet. The evening was highlighted by the premier orchestral performance of the *Jefferson Processional,* written by Philadelphia composer Burle Marx and commissioned by the

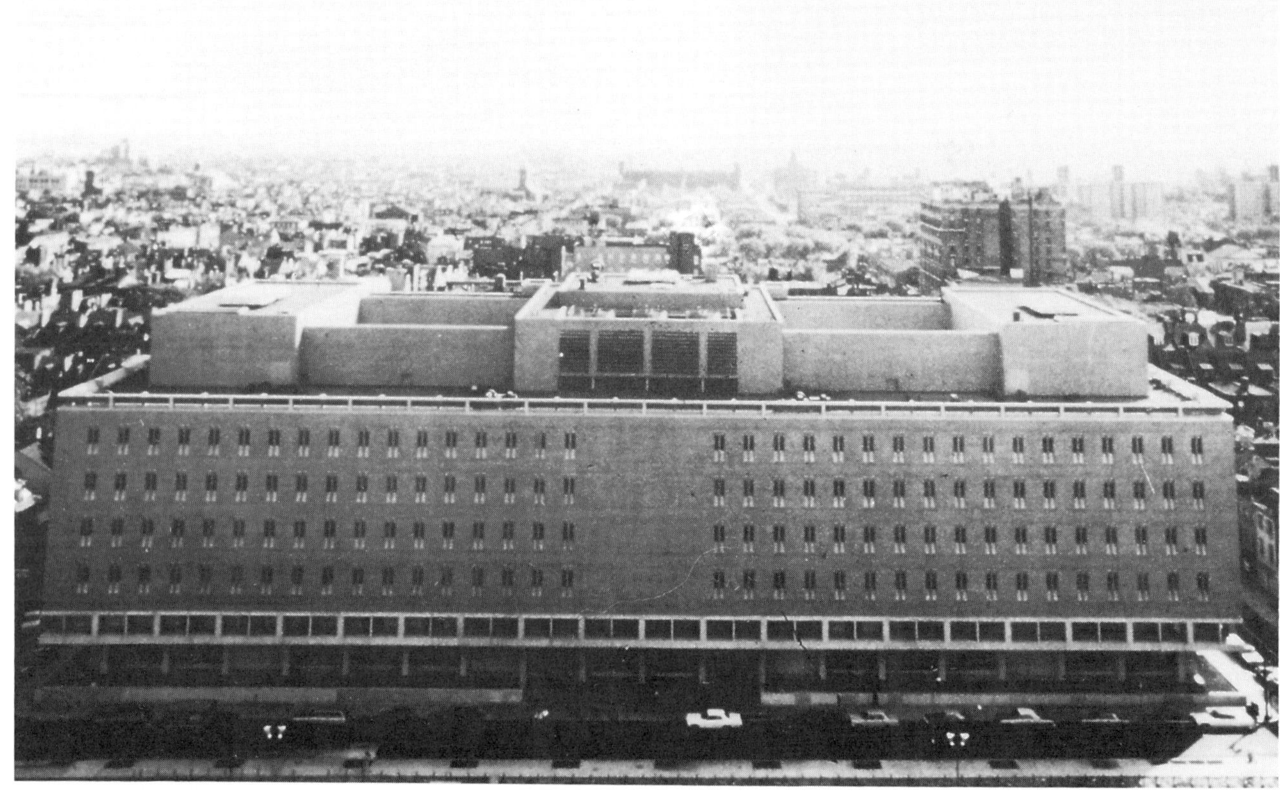

FIG. 48-75. Jefferson Alumni Hall (so named in 1971) and dedicated in March 1969 as Jefferson Hall. Penthouses at the top are the animal quarters.

Alumni Association as its Sesquicentennial gift to Thomas Jefferson University. It has been played at all academic processions of opening exercises and graduations since that time. The following evening the Philadelphia Museum of Art opened its Thomas Eakins galleries to Jefferson alumni and friends, with volunteer guides. Cocktails and hors d'oeuvres were served around the balcony overlooking the grand staircase. It was a successful and festive anniversary year in every respect.

Health Sciences Center (Edison Building, 1974)

The Philadelphia Electric Company built the Edison office building at Ninth and Sansom Streets in the late 1920s. On a lot 100 by 103 feet, it was of fireproof steel construction with masonry walls. Centrally steam heated, air-conditioned, containing two banks of elevators (one with three units and the other with four), this 22-floor building had been kept in excellent condition. When offered for sale in 1972, Jefferson negotiated its purchase at a price of $1.6 million for use as an innovative Ambulatory Care Center, for facilities for the College of Allied Health Sciences, and for physicians' offices. This purchase was part of a package deal that included another multistoried Philadelphia Electric Building at the southwest corner of Tenth and Chestnut Streets in planning for the New Clinical Facility (Hospital) of 1978. For 25 years Mr. Edwin D. Greenbaum, Senior Vice-President of Albert M. Greenfield and Co., Inc. (now Helmsley-Greenfield, Inc.) has acted as Jefferson's real estate agent and consultant for acquisition of most of the properties for the expanding campus. His father, Dr. Sigmund S. Greenbaum, graduated from Jefferson in 1913, and his brother, Dr. Charles H. (Jefferson, 1954), is a Clinical Professor in the Department of Dermatology.

The total volume of outpatient care rendered by the Hospital in 1972, when the plan was formulated, was approximately 160,000 visits per year (90,000 "private" and 70,000 "public" or "service" patients). The "public" patients were lower-income disadvantaged persons whose care was subsidized by government, by higher charges to "private" patients, and by nonoperating income of the Hospital. The Trustees committed themselves to creating a new kind of ambulatory

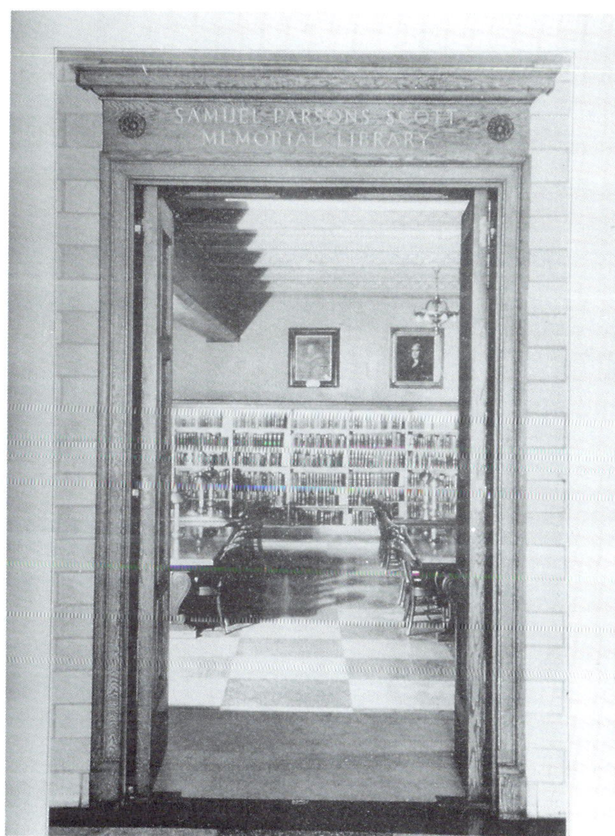

FIG. 48-76. The Scott Library in the 1025 Walnut Street College (ca. 1932).

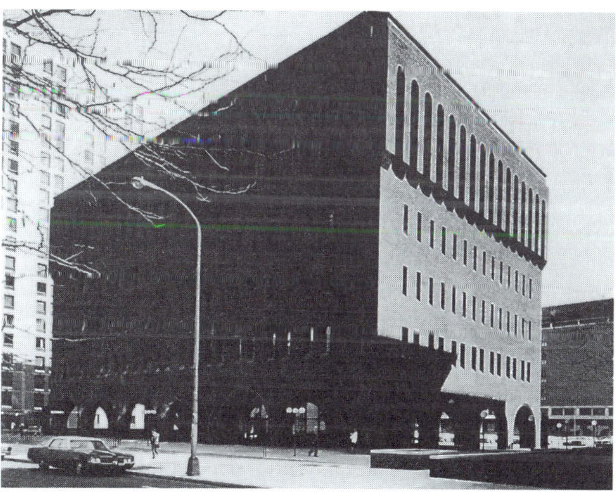

FIG. 48-77. Front view of Scott Library/Administration Building (1970).

center in which all patients would be served equally as private patients, where their care would be as much as possible under a single physician or health team, and where their health care would be comprehensive rather than episodic and symptomatic. All facilities would be private, dignified, and comfortable. All aspects of good medical care, including those for specialty tertiary treatment, would be brought together in one facility and available equitably to all patients, regardless of economic condition, race, or creed. The Ambulatory Patient Care Center represented the implementation of one major recommendation of the Committee for Master Planning in its report of December 1972.

Funds for renovations and equipment required approximately $4.4 million, which, added to the purchase cost, totaled approximately $6 million. The Trustees planned to raise $3 million in the Sesquicentennial campaign for the community services part of the project and to arrange permanent mortgage financing for the remainder to be amortized by the income-producing elements of the building.

Design and demolition work were initiated on January 22, 1973. By June, 1974, the facility was one-third occupied and operating. The total project was fully operative by December, 1974. Members of the Volunteer Faculty were encouraged to move their private offices into this building, and many responded.

The flexibility of this building proved advantageous for adaptation to changing patterns of medical care, education activities of the College of Allied Health Sciences, and private office facilities. When the new Wills Eye Hospital at Ninth and Chestnut Streets began construction in 1978, many of its staff sought office space in this nearby building (Figure 48–80). Jefferson's renal dialysis unit also moved into these quarters.

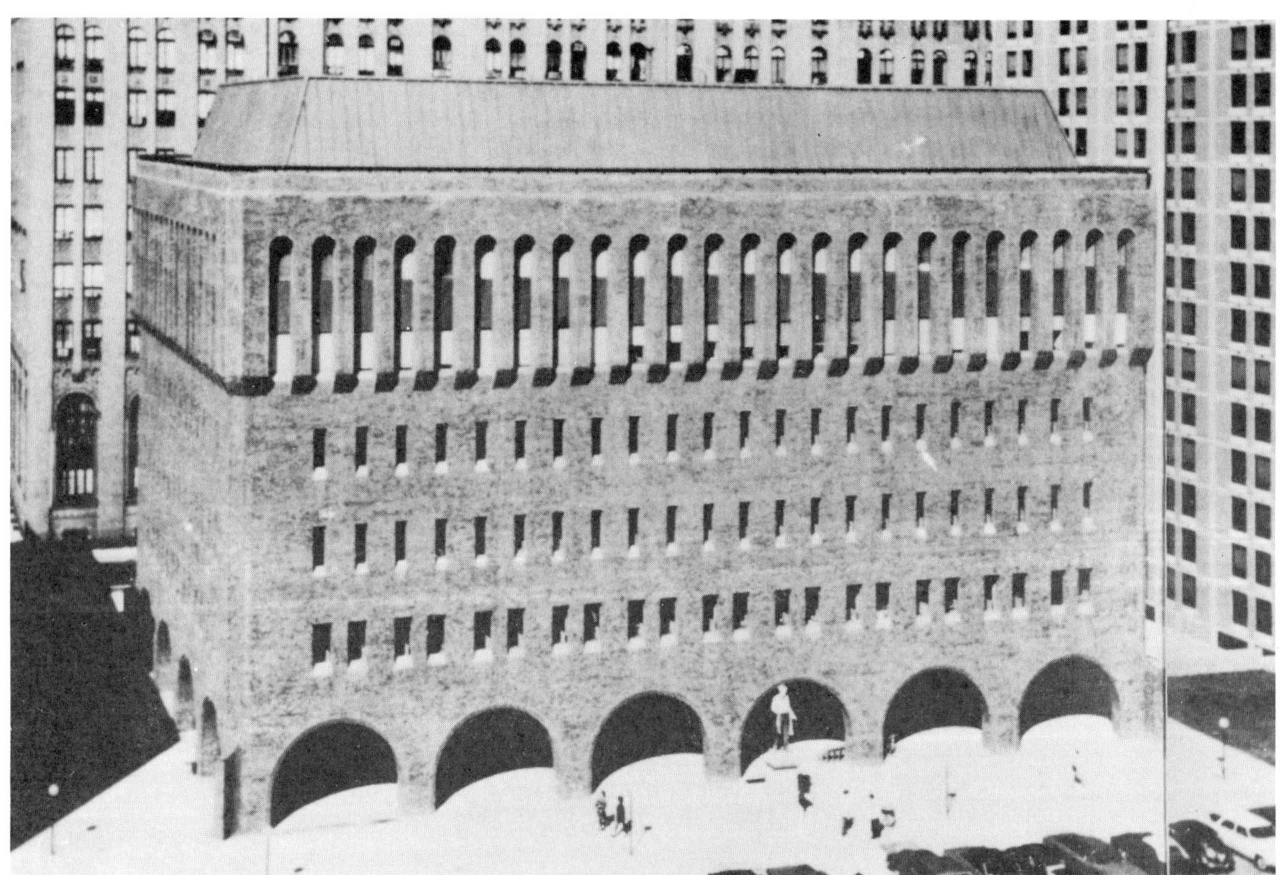

FIG. 48-78. The rear view of the Scott Library/Administration Building (1970).

In a package deal, Jefferson also acquired the Philadelphia Electric Building, at the corner of Tenth and Chestnut Streets, which would undergo demolition as part of the space for the New Clinical Facility (Thomas Jefferson University Hospital, 1978).

The University Parking Garage (1975)

In August, 1974, construction of a 400-car parking facility began on the north side of Locust Street between Tenth and Eleventh, at a cost of approximately $3,725,000. This completed the buildings on the city block allocated by the Redevelopment Authority, between the College and Jefferson Alumni Hall. The Walnut Street buildings consisted of the Martin Nurses' Residence (1959), Orlowitz Residence Hall (1967), and the Scott Library/Administration Building (1970). The architecture of the parking facility was artfully designed to be unobtrusive, with two low-level buildings divided by a wide elevated walkway. It preserved an open area (Scott Plaza) for trees and placement of the Samuel D. Gross statue (Figure 48–81). The four levels of parking (two underground) were opened on October 28, 1975, and dedicated on December 1, 1975. The garage's provision for University personnel, commuters, and visitors eased some of the ever-increasing parking problems.

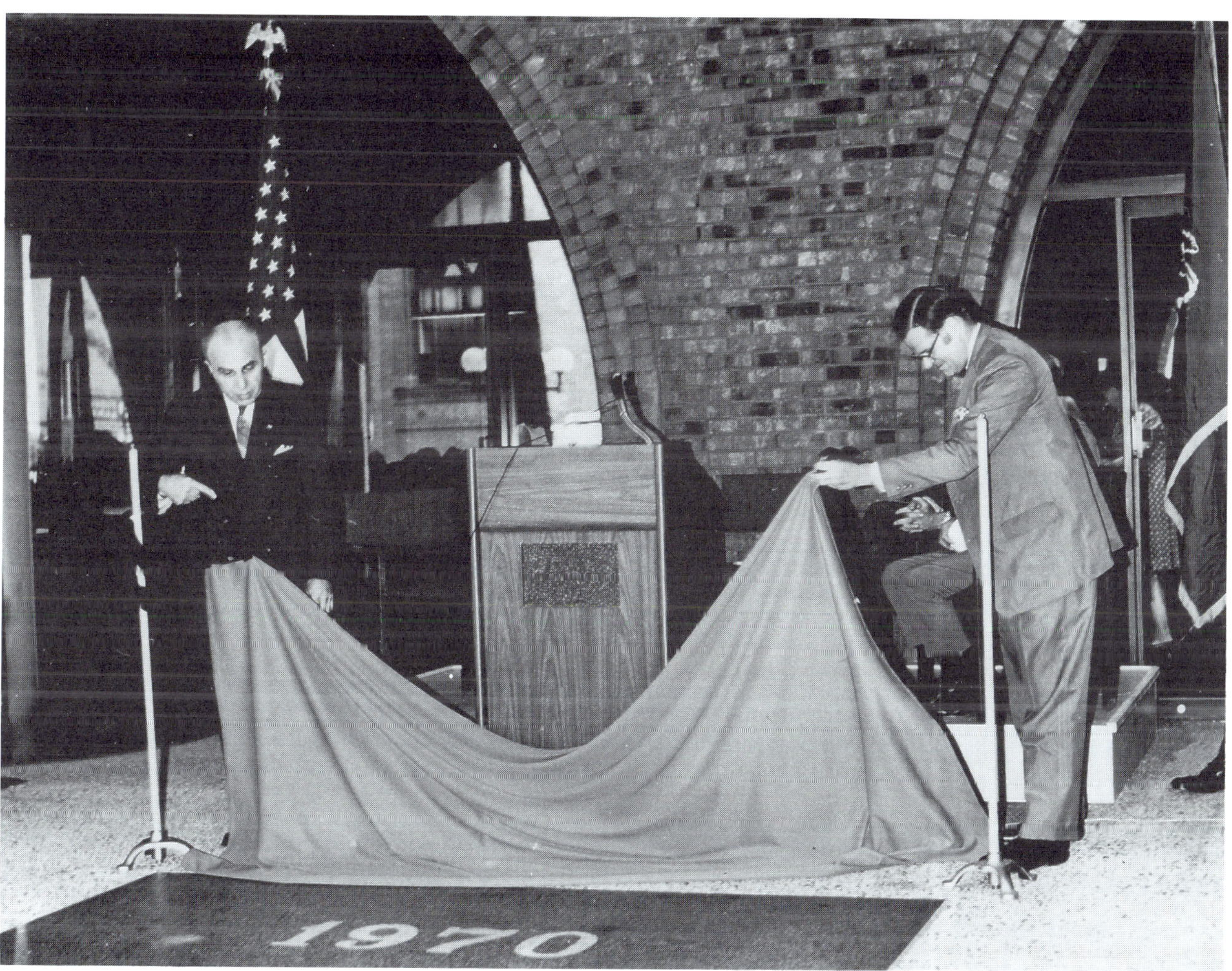

FIG. 48-79. Dedication of the Scott Library/Administration Building; President Peter A. Herbut is on the left, and Board Chairman William W. Bodine, Jr. is on the right.

▪ Barringer Residence Hall (1976)

Jefferson's increase in size for education and health care required additional convenient and comfortable living accommodations at reasonable rents for the University's students and personnel. A site on the southeast corner of Tenth and Walnut, owned by the Philadelphia Redevelopment Authority, was allocated for the building of a residence hall of 138 apartments (12 efficiency, 54 one-bedroom, 63 two-bedroom, and 9 three-bedroom). It would accommodate about 420 occupants, and about one-half of the apartments would be occupied by families. The layouts were based upon those in the Orlowitz Residence, which had proven to be very satisfactory.

The building was L-shaped with extensions along Walnut and Tenth. Each elevation had four-, seven-, and ten-story sections, with the lowest stories at the ends of the one and the highest ones at the vertex. The major entrance was at the vertex (the corner of Tenth and Walnut). The ground floor was constructed for the commercial use of 11 stores, seven of which faced Walnut Street, and additional area assignments of the building included physical plant offices, maintenance facilities, laundry, tenant storage, trash room, meeting room and lobby. Flat dark-brick walls with a regular pattern of identical large windows rose above a colonnade at street level. Storefronts were recessed two and a half feet behind this wall, with the entrance recessed further to create a sheltered space at the corner. The five roof levels provided roof decks for the residents (Figure 48–82).

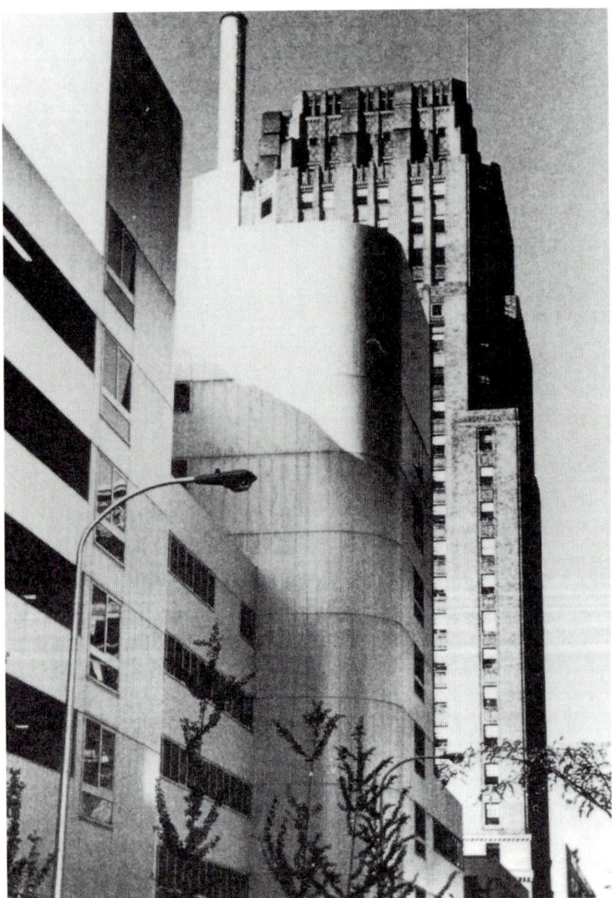

FIG. 48-80. Wills Eye Hospital and the Edison Building (Health Sciences Center) looking north on Ninth Street.

The entire project for ground and construction cost about $6.6 million. It was formally dedicated on November 1, 1976, to honor two generations of Jefferson Trustees. The first was the late Daniel Moreau Barringer, who had served on the Board from 1902 to 1936. The second was his son, Brandon Barringer (Figure 48–83), who had been a Life Trustee and succeeded his father in 1936. Brandon Barringer, as Chairman of the Finance Committee, had skillfully kept Jefferson on a sound financial basis for decades.

Brandon Barringer, in addition to other Board committee appointments at Jefferson, served as Director of the Curtis Publishing Company, the Lehigh Valley Railroad, the Wellington Fund, The Philadelphia Suburban Transportation Company, and the Children's Heart Hospital.

A commemorative plaque for the Barringer Residence Hall read, in part, "in grateful tribute for long, devoted and distinguished service."

Frederic Lyman Ballard, Esq.; the Fifth Board Chairman (1977–1984)

Frederic L. Ballard (Figure 48–84) was born in 1917 in Philadelphia into a family with a history in the legal profession. His grandfather founded and his father was a partner in the firm of Ballard, Spahr, Andrews, and Ingersoll, and Frederic became a senior partner there. Ballard's three brothers also became lawyers. After preliminary education in private schools he received his A.B. degree (1939) and an LL.B. (1942) at the University of Pennsylvania. He began to practice law in 1942 and served with the United States Navy from 1943 to 1946.

Through the years Ballard served as a member of the Executive Committee of the United Way of Southeastern Pennsylvania and the Pennsylvania State Board of Public Welfare, Director of the Greater Philadelphia Movement, and Chairman of the Board of Overseers of the University of Pennsylvania Law School. In the business world he became Director of the Provident National Bank, the Provident Mutual Life Insurance Company, and Pierce Phelps, Inc.

Ballard was elected to the Board in June, 1965, and became the Vice President in 1970. He chaired the prestigious Committee for Master Planning, which, in its 259-page report of December, 1972, "attempted to analyze the institution, its strengths and weaknesses, its challenges and opportunities and the internal and external factors affecting its development." In 1977, when Mr. Bodine decided to step down as Chairman of the Board to become a Life Trustee, Ballard was the unquestioned natural successor.

Ballard's appointment was timed to coincide with that of the new President, Lewis W. Bluemle, Jr., M.D. They both officially started on August 1, 1977. Mr. Ballard saw an opportunity in their starting together to carry out a long-held philosophy of policy to enhance the position of the President to run the University and the Board Chairman, at a lower profile, to preside over the Board meetings and maintain rapport with the administration. Thus, during his seven years as Chairman, he was able as a busy lay person to perform his duties effectively without being totally immersed. In this way he felt justified in deserving

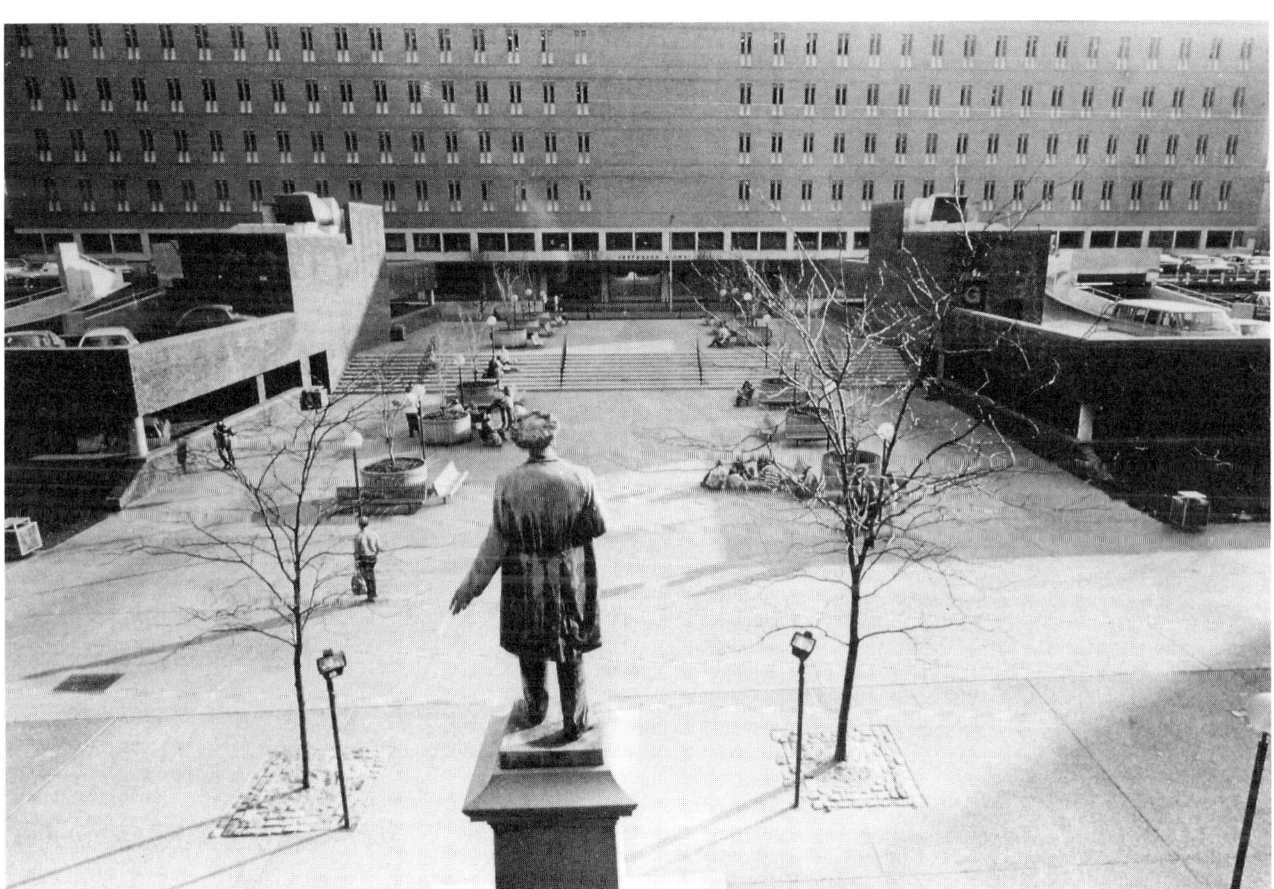

FIG. 48-81. The University Parking Garage and Scott Plaza.

at least a small part of the credit for Dr. Bluemle's many accomplishments.

Frederic Ballard considered his prime achievements as having nothing to do with bricks and mortar, although in his 19 years up to 1984 he was much involved in the teamwork of those activities. In addition to the very compatible working relationship with Dr. Bluemle, he markedly improved all types of communications. He encouraged a freedom of discussion in the Board meetings that improved the quality of the deliberations, dealings, and decisions. Despite much greater fiscal complexity, the reporting and controls were handled with improved clarity.

During the Ballard Chairmanship there was an advance in academic science and research, as noted by comparing the Master Planning Report of 1972 with the one of 1981. The big difference was that by the time of the second report, Jefferson had strengthened its posture enough to talk about scientific standing, academics, research, and the need to upgrade some of the programs. *The real accomplishment was that basic scientific research could be openly analyzed for admission that many of these aspects were not optimal and needed attention.*

At the time of Mr. Ballard's appointment in 1977 the "new clinical facility" (Thomas Jefferson University Hospital) at Eleventh and Chestnut was nearing completion. The official dedication took place on June 9, 1978, in a week of activities planned by a committee chaired by Ballard. In a "Fun Run" for joggers as part of the events, the most notable of the fun runners was Ballard himself.

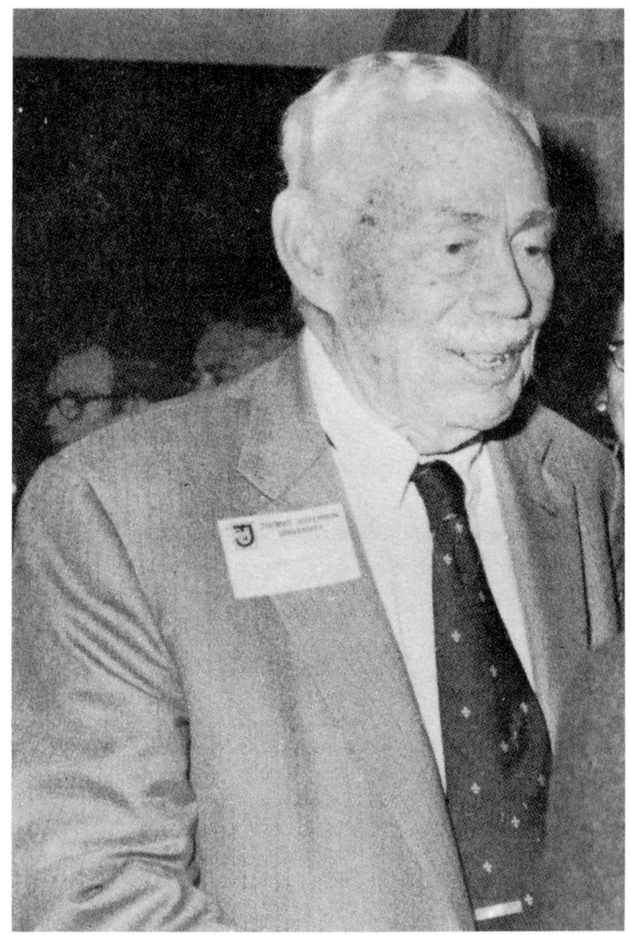

FIG. 48-83. Brandon Barringer, Life Trustee (1936–), who by 1986, had served on the Board for 50 years.

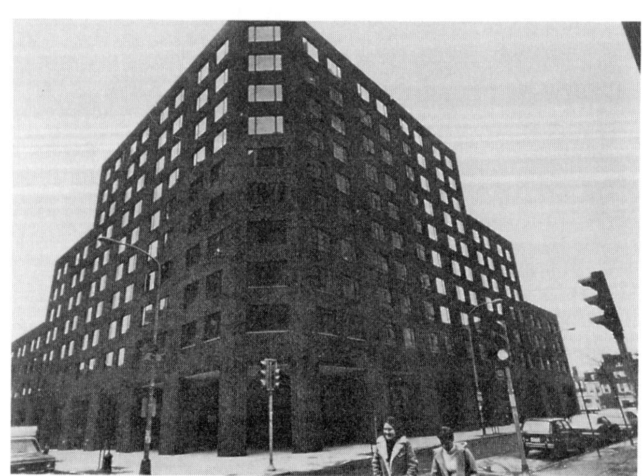

FIG. 48-82. Barringer Residence Hall (1976).

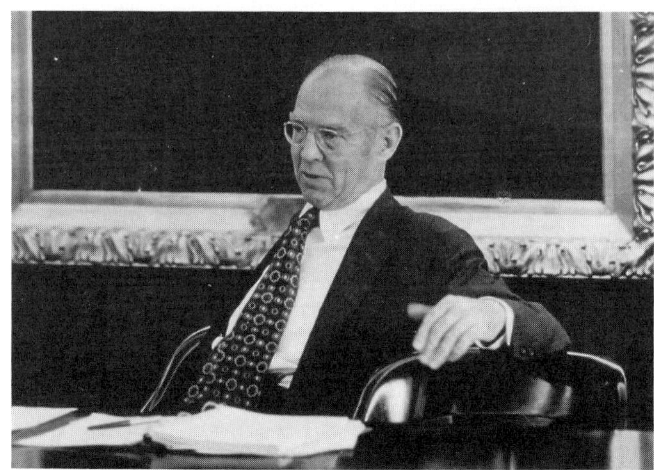

FIG. 48-84. Frederic L. Ballard, Esq., Fifth Board Chairman (1977–1984).

▪ The New Clinical Facility (1978)

The "Hospital of Tomorrow" (Figure 48–85), located along Chestnut and Sansom Streets between Tenth and Eleventh, was built at a cost of $51.5 million. Funding was through a bond issue that in a sense placed ownership of the Hospital in the hands of the public. Two major innovations in design were developed to effect greater ease of movement: the mini-hospital concept, in which four of the nine floors functioned as self-contained miniature hospitals, each with approximately 100 beds; and the exchange cart system. The preponderance of single-patient rooms emphasized Jefferson's pluralistic approach to health care delivery at a level that preserved the dignity of all patients regardless of ethnic origin, race, color, or economic status. It was a far cry from Jefferson's first Hospital (1877), 100 years earlier, when care was predominantly for the poor. At that time the hospital was the last resort, even for the poor, and regarded as a place where people died. Those who could afford to be treated privately preferred to stay at home.

The new facility provided 411 acute care beds, 110 physicians' offices, and most of the Hospital's diagnostic, therapeutic, and support services, replacing many of the inpatient functions of the previous buildings. Glass-enclosed bridges connected the third to ninth floors with the Foerderer Pavilion (Figure 48–86). East and west sky-lit atria allowed natural light either from the interior or from the street to each inpatient room (Figure 48–87). A cafeteria on the second floor of

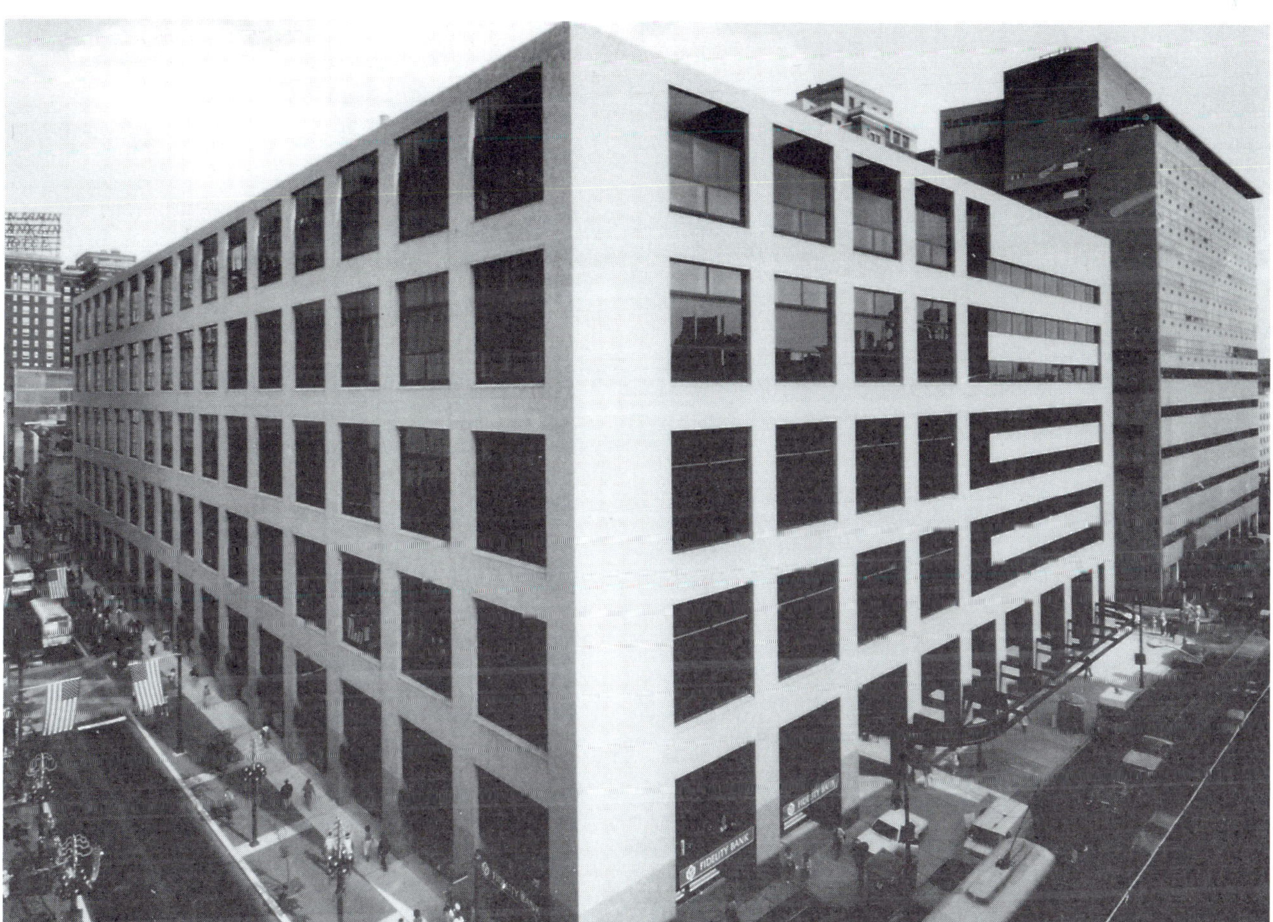

FIG. 48-85. The new clinical facility (1978), Thomas Jefferson University Hospital, looking east (left) on Chestnut Street and south (right) on Eleventh.

each atrium had the humanizing effect of providing good quality food services and pleasant atmosphere to visitors, staff, and employees (Figure 48–88). Each of the hospital floors (3, 5, 7, and 9) focused on the treatment of a particular group of patients. The patients were grouped in an "E" pattern around the two atria. The back of the "E" flanked Chestnut Street, and ancillary services most directly related to floor-care programs were located on the Sansom Street side. Physicians' offices were located on even-numbered floors (4, 6, and 8). These ambulatory floors were integrated in a fashion to allow physicians in a particular specialty to see their outpatients in one area, with their inpatients housed in an immediately adjacent floor above or below. This provided an economy of time for the physicians, their staffs, and particularly their outpatients to be close to ancillary services required for their particular illnesses. The prototype for all this was in the Edison Building, and most of the physicians moved from there to the new Hospital.

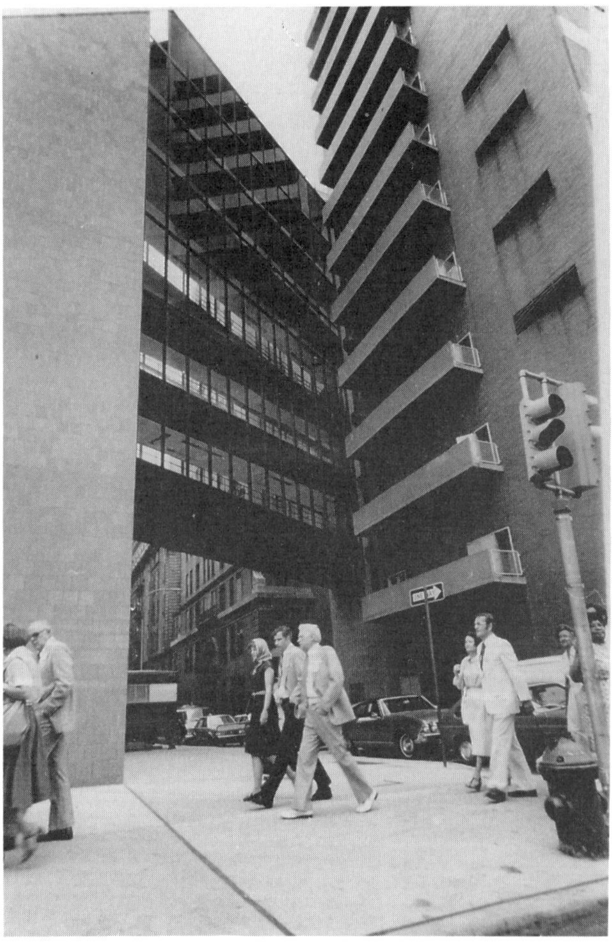

FIG. 48-86. Bridges connecting Foerderer Pavilion with the new Thomas Jefferson University Hospital.

The first floor along the Chestnut Street side was leased for commercial purposes. The third floor housed the Medical Care programs (general medicine, infectious diseases, gastroenterology, hematology, endocrinology, family medicine, and dermatology). The fifth floor contained both medical and surgical facilities for cardio-pulmonary care, and the seventh floor was for the Surgical Care programs. The ninth floor was for Neurosensory-Musculoskeletal Care. Each of the patient floors had intensive care units related to the appropriate specialities.

At the heart of the supply system were the exchange carts (Figure 48–89), case carts, and three pneumatically driven lifts that accelerated materials to the relevant floors. It took 26 seconds for a "Supply, Processing, and Distribution" cart (5 feet high, 5 feet deep and 2½ feet wide) to go from the second to the ninth floor. It was tagged so that a mechanism on the lift read the proper destination and ejected the cart accordingly. Distribution of patient care materials, food, and operating room instruments was very rapid.

The Hospital kept pace with latest developments in computer technology as applied to all aspects of data collection, statistics, billing, laboratory, and patient information. More than 400 computers were assembled into an integrated system.

The proposition to have Wills Eye Hospital located in the 1025 Walnut Street Medical College Building of 1928 was not considered practical at the time. On a second occasion, around 1974 in the planning of the new Hospital, consideration was given to putting on two extra floors as a condominium for the Wills Eye Hospital. This was turned down by the Wills Eye Medical Staff.

As occurred with the previous buildings, the "Hospital of Tomorrow" reached "Tomorrow" very swiftly. The interior had been constructed so as to allow renovations for updating of services at least expense. One exception was the new Bodine Radiation Center, which at a cost of $23.5 million would bring the latest features of nuclear medicine into the Hospital by late 1986. This required extensive reexcavation and renovation. The same year would witness the opening of yet another building, the eight-story Jefferson Surgical Center at the southwest corner of Eleventh and Walnut Streets.

Lewis William Bluemle, Jr., M.D., D.Sc., L.H.D., F.R.C.P. (Edinburgh); Second University President (1977–)

Dr. Lewis W. Bluemle, Jr. (Figure 48–90) was born in Williamsport, Pennsylvania, in 1921. He obtained his A.B. degree (1943) at the Johns Hopkins University as a Phi Beta Kappa student and his M.D. (1946) in its School of Medicine with similar distinction of election to Alpha Omega Alpha Honorary Society. From 1946 to 1968 his career continued at the University of Pennsylvania as Intern, through Resident in internal medicine, to Associate Professor of Medicine. During some of these years he was also Assistant Director, Army Hepatic and Metabolic Unit, Valley Forge Army Hospital (1948–1950), Fellow in the Chemical Section of the Department of Medicine of the University (1950–1951), and from 1959–1961 was Assistant Director, and from 1961–1968, Director, Clinical Research Center, Hospital of the University of Pennsylvania. His interest in administration was evidenced by his also serving as Associate Dean in the School of Medicine of that University (1966–1968).

Dr. Bluemle was especially interested in diseases of the kidney, and he became a pioneer in the treatment of renal failure by use of the artificial kidney. He authored or coauthored more than 60 scientific articles in this field. As a clinician he was Chief of the Dialysis Unit (1951–1968) at the

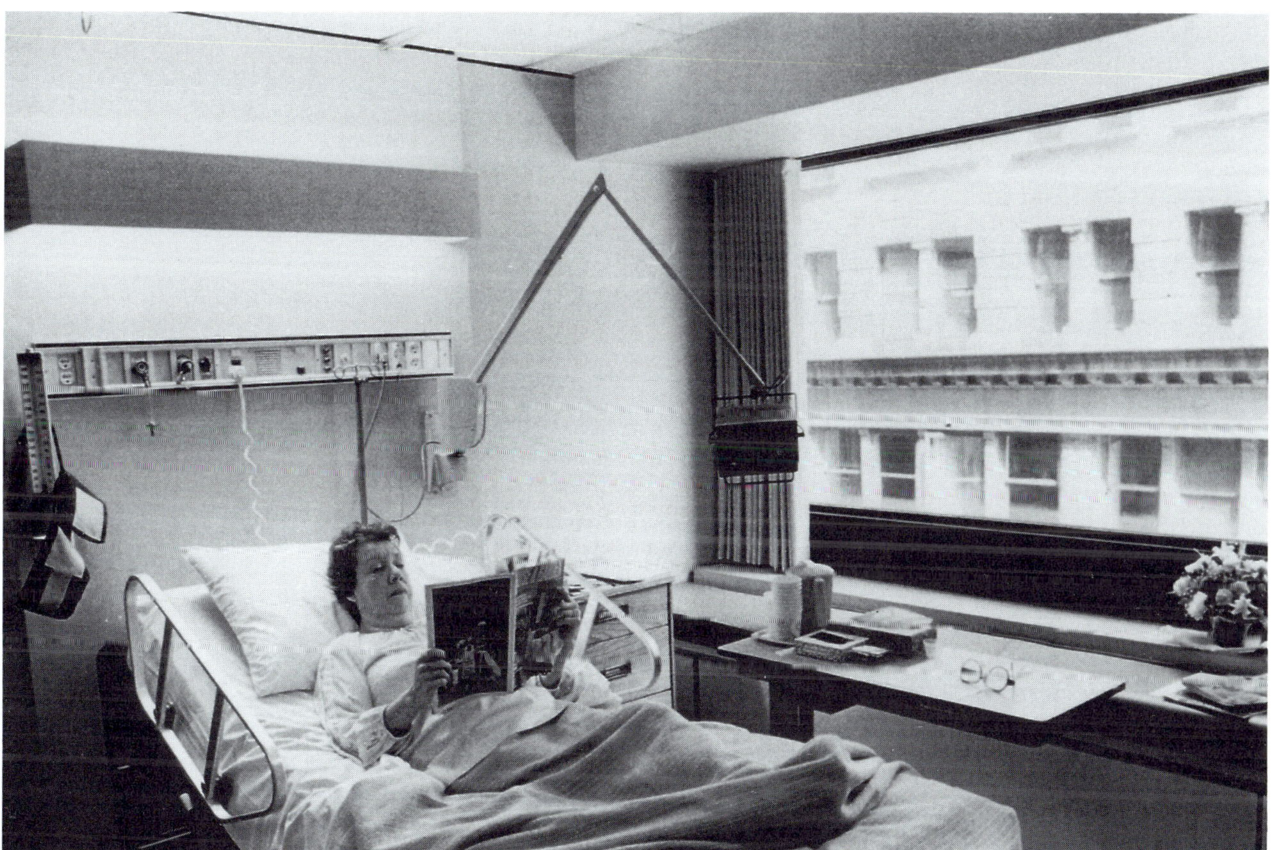

FIG. 48-87. A room in the new clinical facility, showing natural lighting from Chestnut Street.

Hospital of the University of Pennsylvania; Attending Physician at the Veterans Administration Hospital in Philadelphia (1953–1967); and Consulting Physician at Bryn Mawr Hospital (1963–1968).

In 1968 Dr. Bluemle accepted an appointment as President of the Upstate Medical Center (Syracuse) of the State University of New York, a position he held until 1974. From 1974 to 1977 he served as President of the University of Oregon Health Sciences Center in Portland, Oregon.

The appointment of a new President to replace the prestigious Dr. Herbut in 1976 was considered very seriously by the Board. It was felt that a small search committee might be slanted or biased in one direction or another and lead to recriminations at a later date if a poor choice were made. To circumvent the problem, the Board decided to use the former Committee for Master Planning (of 13 members), which had been formed some years earlier when the appointment of a President was not a consideration. Thus, this was the largest search committee ever previously organized by Jefferson for appointment to a post. There was input from many sectors, including the Alumni Association. The plan worked well and resulted in an acceptance by Dr. Bluemle to start August 1, 1977.

The performance of President Bluemle is sequentially documented in his "Triennial Report to the Trustees" from 1977 to 1980, 1980 to 1983, and 1983 to 1986. These three self-analyses are models of candor, insight, initiative, and dedication to implementation of the "Strategic Plan for the Eighties." As classics in clarity and scholarship, they delve into sensitive and complex issues requiring confidence, diplomacy, as well as trust.

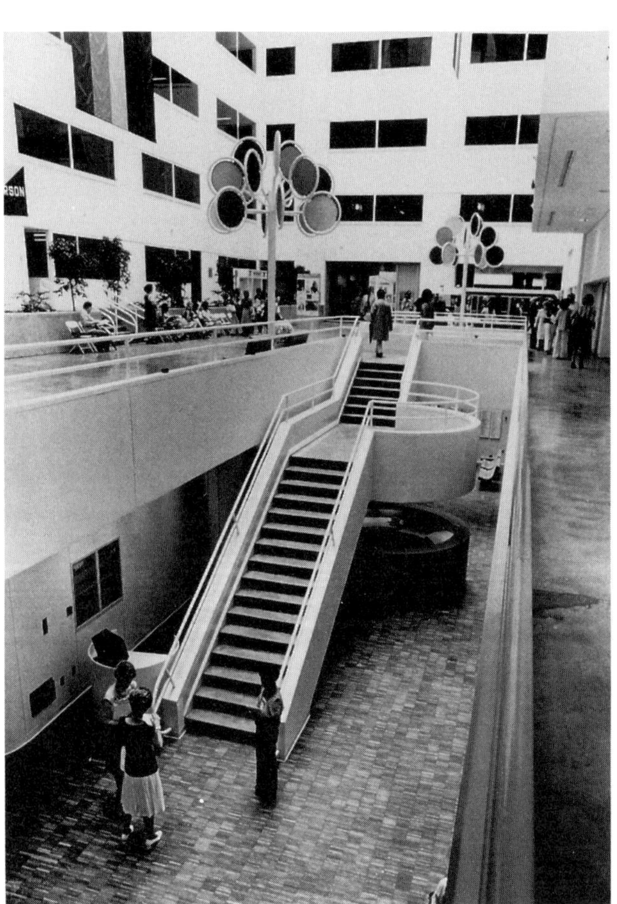

FIG. 48-88. The entrance to the west atrium and cafeteria.

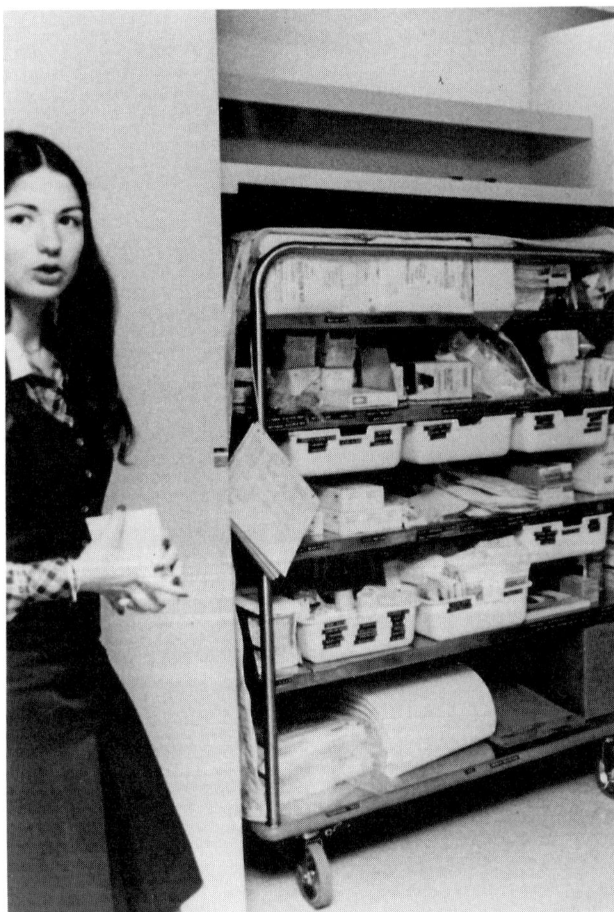

FIG. 48-89. An exchange cart.

President Bluemle's leadership influenced improvements in administrative organization, choice of new senior officers, strengthening of the three deanships, developing of faculty and programs that led to increased research, changes in legal counsel, and fostering a closer relationship between the Trustees and major constituents of the University.

In addition to his many scientific articles, President Bluemle published a stream of papers relating to medical education and health care. His professional appointments, civic activities, and memberships on boards of directors of associations and business organizations have earned him universal respect. He has not only been active on the committees of a host of medical organizations but has served as President of the American Society for Artificial Organs (1967–1968) and the College of Physicians of Philadelphia (1980–82). His honors and awards include: Markle Scholar in Academic Medicine (1955–1960), Lindback Award for Distinguished Teaching (1966), Honorary Degree of Doctor of Science from the Philadelphia College of Pharmacy and Science (1980), Honorary Degree of Doctor of Humane Letters from Washington and Jefferson College (1981), and Fellowship in the Royal College of Physicians of Edinburgh (1981).

In suggesting that thought for the 1990s and beyond should include plans for his successor, President Bluemle states that "Jefferson needs a president whose inner joy derives from helping good people achieve their own goals in broadly, but not precisely, coordinated pathways." As such a President himself, he has been eminently successful.

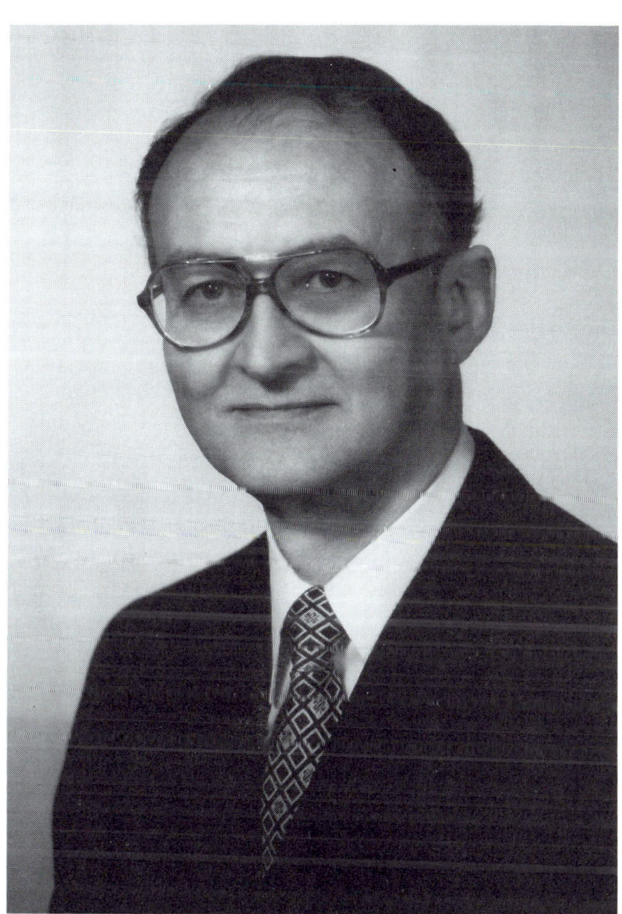

FIG. 48-90. Lewis W. Bluemle, Jr., M.D.; Second University President (1977–).

Strategic Plan for the 1980s

In the summer of 1978 a task force of 29 members from various sectors of the University was organized into six committees: University Relations, Cooperative Programs, Academic Affairs and Research, Management and Organization, Health Services, and Finance and Resources. The purpose was to accomplish a comprehensive overview of significant issues and problems relevant to preparation of the University for the forthcoming decade. Frederic Ballard, who had chaired the Committee for Master Planning (which reported in December, 1972) and was now Chairman of the Board, presided over the combined meetings of the various committees.

Thirty-eight Task Force recommendations were documented in a report of April, 1981. Five basic beliefs constituted the foundation of the plan, as follows:

1. That Jefferson's future should be built on its many strengths as an academic health center rather than on previous aspirations to become a comprehensive University with non-health-oriented components.
2. That a better balance between patient care, education, and research will be sought by giving greater emphasis to the scientific pursuit of new knowledge.

3. That Jefferson's financial and organizational stability should not be jeopardized by unnecessary growth during a period of change in health professional education, research and patient care.

4. That the University's resources should be invested primarily in improving the quality of its existing programs through limited well-planned innovation, and

5. That future planning must be oriented to perceived needs and capabilities in the private sector as tax-based support for education, health care and research diminish.

▪ The Decade Fund of the Eighties

Fund raising at Jefferson in an organized drive first started in 1873. In that year a committee for public appeal was formed from five members of the Board, two from the faculty, and two from the alumni. Dr. Francis Fontaine Maury (Jefferson, 1862) obtained an appropriation of $100,000 from the Pennsylvania State Legislature on condition that it be matched by a similar sum. Dr. John Hill Brinton (Jefferson, 1852) undertook to raise $150,000 from the Alumni. Aided by Dr. Samuel D. Gross (Jefferson, 1828), the Trustees, and friends of the school, the 1877 Hospital and grounds were funded at a cost of $186,000. Even though the Medical College was proprietary at that time, the detached Hospital was financially controlled by the Board on a nonprofit basis. This drive was at Jefferson's one-half century of existence, but no one seemed to think of it in terms of a particular milestone.

At Jefferson's Centennial in 1924, Alba B. Johnson, Chairman of the Hospital Committee, spearheaded a campaign to raise funds for a New Hospital Annex. A bequest of $200,000 had been made in 1921 in the will of Mr. William Thompson on condition that the Annex be named for his brother, Samuel Gustine Thompson. The Trustees, Alumni, staff, and public swelled the fund to $750,000, which represented only one-half of the goal of $1.5 million when the building was opened in 1924. The remaining required funds subsequently filtered in.

A gift of $100,000 was made by the Alumni Association toward construction of the Department of Experimental Medicine in the 1025 Walnut Street College (1929), and Mr. Cyrus H.K. Curtis contributed $.5 million to the Curtis Building (1931), but these and other sporadic gifts were not part of organized drives.

The third organized fund raising campaign started in 1951 in preparation for the "New Pavilion" of 1954 which would be named "Foerderer" in 1962. The estimated cost was $7.5 million. The campaign funds amounted to less than one-half of the cost, and the financing was completed through institutional funds and loans.

The fourth drive was the Sesquicentennial Fund of 1974, which attained its goal of $20 million. The Alumni Association's quota of $4 million was completed by 1976. Additionally needed funds for Jefferson's expansion of the campus were obtained through bond issues that sold readily.

For the decade of the 1980s it was realized that large-scale giving was more essential than ever, even though the bricks-and-mortar stage had essentially passed. Funds were needed to attract the best possible new faculty leadership, to encourage research, and to offset imminent decreasing external support by government and third-party payors through cost containment and large-scale contractual arrangements in a competitive market. Endowments and spendable gifts were also sought for student aid, as tuition costs crept steadily higher. The spirit of regular giving by Trustees, Alumni, and all segments of the Jefferson family had become so traditional that yearly increments of 10% seemed reasonable to expect. A goal of $65 million for the 1980s was deemed appropriate and attainable. The mystique of "the Spirit of Jefferson," which is the wonderment of Alumni of other institutions, expressed itself so visibly that by 1986 the amount subscribed, aided substantially by foundations and corporations, reached the $60 million mark. Just as peace and prosperity are the basic goals of all Americans, so progress in its missions and a balanced budget are Jefferson's hallmarks.

Edward Carroll Driscoll; the Sixth Board Chairman (1984–)

Edward C. Driscoll (Figure 48–91) became Chairman of the Board on October 1, 1984, as the successor to Frederic Ballard. First elected as a Trustee in June, 1974, he subsequently chaired the finance committee and health affairs committee. He was a member of the capital projects committee that was responsible for the renovations of the Foerderer Pavilion and Thompson Annex. Prior to assuming the Chairmanship he had served as Vice-Chairman of the Board.

A native Philadelphian, born on Christmas, 1929, Driscoll graduated from the University of Pennsylvania with an A.B. degree in 1951. He then served in the U.S. Navy (1951–1954) during the Korean Conflict in the Amphibious Forces of both the Atlantic and Pacific fleets. Following this experience he entered the construction field, in which he became Secretary of the L.F. Driscoll Company in 1964 and its President in 1967. His firm has constructed hospitals, schools, hotels, condominiums, and office and research buildings in the Delaware Valley.

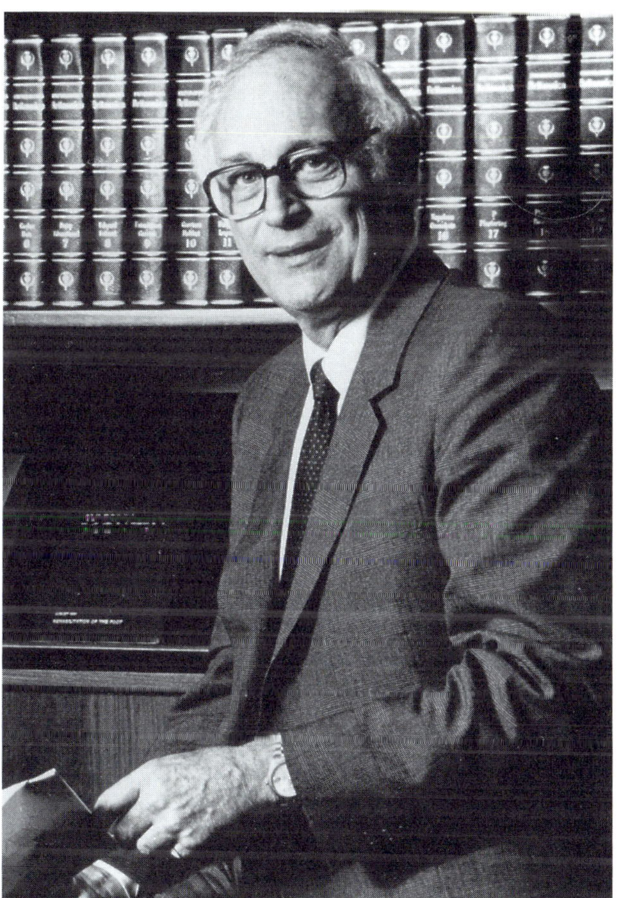

FIG. 48-91. Edward C. Driscoll (1929–), Sixth Board Chairman (1984–).

Driscoll has been active in civic and educational affairs such as the Young Presidents' Organization, the Chief Executives' Organization, and the Center for the Study of Aging at the University of Pennsylvania, and he is also Director of the Provident Bank and the International House of Philadelphia.

The new Chairman states that his major challenge in the 1980s "will be to see that Jefferson is able to adapt to and grow in the rapidly changing climate created by government's active involvement and announced intention to control and reduce costs in the interrelated fields of health care and medical education."

The New Medical Office Building (1986)

The Jefferson campus was extended further with the erection of the new Medical Office Building on the southwest corner of Eleventh and Walnut Streets, adjacent to the Forrest Theater (Figure 48–92). A century earlier the younger Professor Gross (Samuel W.) and his wife had lived at 1112 Walnut Street, and even as long ago as that had paid $39,000 for this choice location of property.

The building at a total cost of $12 million was dedicated on July 29, 1986. The $2.5 million cost of the Surgicenter component was financed with University funds (Hospital surplus). The remaining $9.5 million was financed through a tax-exempt bond issue for $8.7 million through the Philadelphia Industrial Development Corporation (PIDC), and the difference through University funds.

The eight-story building was planned for an organized variety of outpatient departments, along with physicians' offices supplementing those in the Edison Building (1974) and the new Thomas Jefferson University Hospital (1978). The lower level was reserved for a Breast Imaging Center.

The main lobby was provided with a pharmacy, support facility for the Surgicenter, and a loading dock that would also be available to the Forrest Theater. The second-floor Surgicenter was equipped to care for the 38% outpatient load of surgical cases, which by 1990 is estimated to constitute 50% of all surgery. The upper six floors

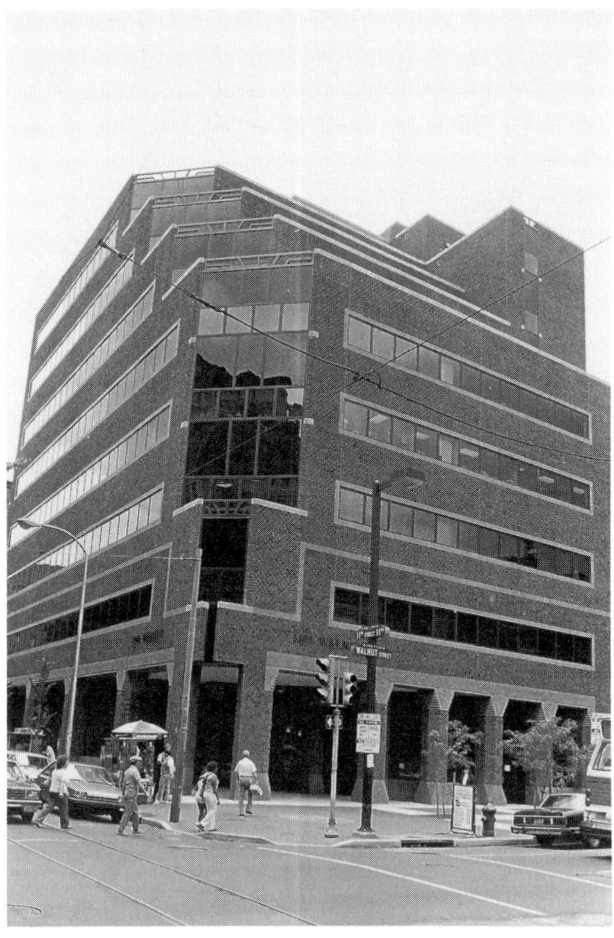

Fig. 48-92. The new Medical Office Building and Surgicenter (1986).

were distributed for outpatient otolaryngology, facial plastic surgery, allergy problems, medical genetics, family medicine, a rectal cancer center, and for clinical pharmacology.

This most recent of the Jefferson buildings embodies the latest in automatic temperature control, fire protection, security, and computer access at the phone connections. With inevitable progress in medical care, education, and research, Jefferson must anticipate and plan for further expansions of the campus.

The members of the Board have individually earned distinction and honor in various aspects of philanthropy, business, law, civic affairs, administration, and academia. From the founding of Jefferson, they have collectively constituted a leadership community indispensable to the success of this large, independent, and influential University (Figure 48–93). Through their continued diverse associations and accumulated public experience, through their wisdom in

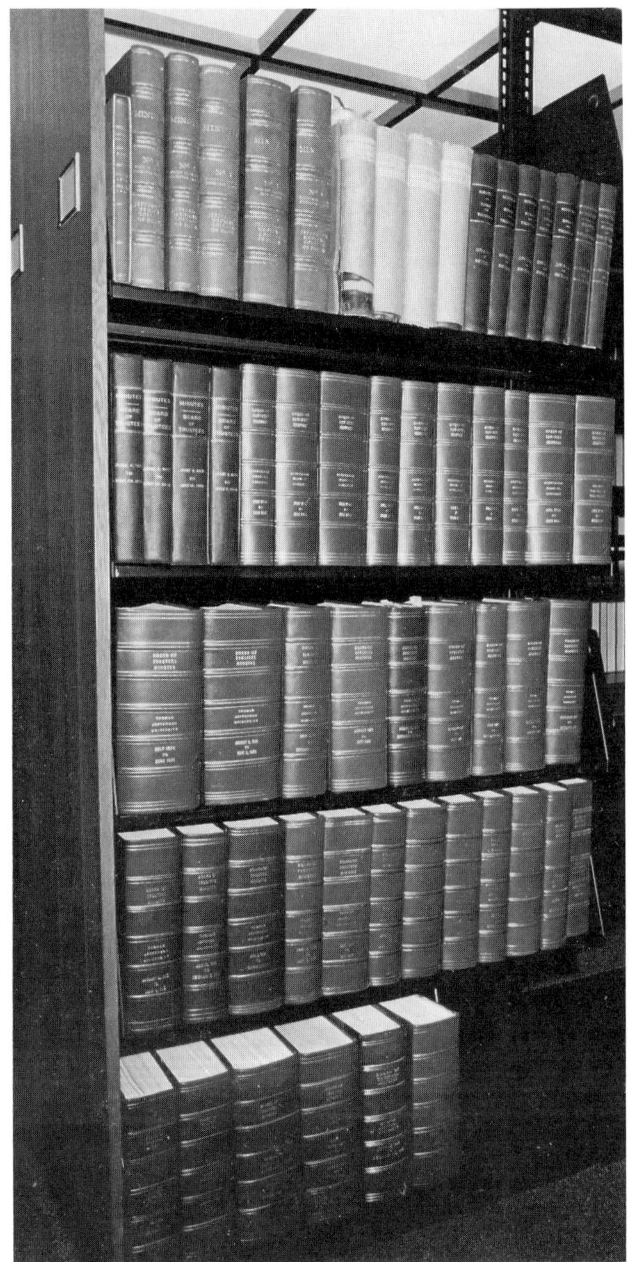

Fig. 48-93. The bound Minutes of the Board of Trustees (58 volumes) from August 9, 1826, to June 4, 1984.

management and choice of faculty, and through their dedication to excellence, the foreseeable future of Jefferson in the advance of medical education, biomedical research, and quality health care is assured.

References

1. Ashbel Green, D.D., LL.D., *Presbyterian Reunion Volume.* Presbyterian Historical Society of Philadelphia, p. 103.
2. Jones, J.H., "A Discourse Commemorative of the Life and Character of the Rev. Cornelius C. Cuyler, D.D., Phila., 1850," Presbyterian Historical Society of Philadelphia.
3. Scharf, J.T., and Wescott, T., *History of Philadelphia, 1609 to 1884.* Vol. II. Philadelphia: L.H. Everts and Co., 1884, p. 1538.
4. "Obituary of Jesse R. Burden, M.D.," *The Philadelphia Inquirer.* May 3, 1875
5. "Obituary of Emile B. Gardette, M.D.," *Dunglison's College and Clinical Records,* Vol. 9, July 1888, p. 182.
6. "James Campbell," *Dict. Am. Biog.* Vol. II. New York: Chas. Scribner Sons, 1958, pp. 454–455.
7. "Joseph Allison," *The Legal Intelligencer.* Vol. 53, No. 7, February 14, 1897.
8. "Edwin Henry Fitler," *Dict. Am. Biog.* Vol. III. pp. 431–432.
9. "Joseph B. Townsend, Esq., "*The Legal Intelligencer.* October 23, 1896, pp. 423–424.
10. "Sketch of the Life of William Potter," *Jeff. Al. Bull.* Vol. I, No. 6, May 1926, pp. 2–3.
11. A Tribute: Hon. William Potter, President of the Board of Trustees; *Jeff. Al. Bull.,* Vol I., No. 4, Feb. 1925, p. 7.
12. Bordley, J. and Harvey, A.M., *Two Centuries of American Medicine.* Philadelphia: W.B. Saunders Co., 1976, p. 164.
13. Flexner, A., "Medical Education in the United States and Canada. A Report to the Carnegie Foundation for the Advancement of Teaching," *Bull. No. 4, 576.* New York: 1910, p. 294.
14. Bordley and Harvey, *Two Centuries of American Medicine,* p. 163.
15. Letter from Russell H. Conwell, February 22, 1910. Jefferson Archives, Special Collections in the Scott Library.
16. Corner, G., *Two Centuries of Medicine.* Philadelphia: J.B. Lippincott Co., 1965, p. 255.
17. Bauer, E.L.. *Doctors Made in America.* Philadelphia: J.B. Lippincott Co., 1963, p. 318.
18. Ramsay, A.J., "Daniel Baugh: Benefactor," *Jeff. Al. Bull.,* Fall 1981, pp. 18–21.
19. "Hon. Samuel Gustine Thompson," *The Legal Intelligencer.* Vol. 60, December 4, 1903, p. 502.
20. Herbut, P.A., *Thomas Jefferson University: Creation,* Vols. I and II.
21. Harrell, G.T.: "Humanities in Medical Education: A Career Experience." *Perspectives in Biol. and Med.* 28, 3. Spring, 1985, p. 392.
22. Herbut, P.A.: Thomas Jefferson University: Position Paper. Sept. 15, 1967.

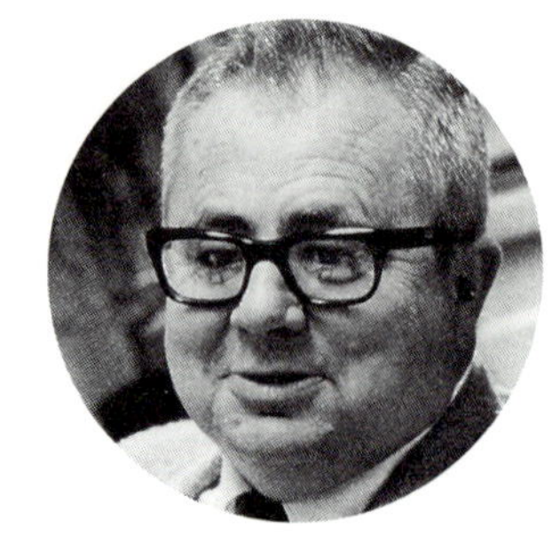

CHAPTER FORTY-NINE

The Medical College Deanship

Samuel S. Conly, Jr., M.D.

"I will teach you, and guide you in the way you should go. I will keep you under my eye."

—Psalms 32:8

At the first regular meeting of the faculty of Jefferson Medical College held on December 20, 1824, Dr. Benjamin Rush Rhees, who was serving as Secretary, was appointed Dean of the Faculty, the first Dean of this new medical school. Just six months previously, Jefferson had come into existence as the Medical Department in Philadelphia of Jefferson College located in Canonsburg, Pennsylvania.

From 1824 through 1986, Jefferson Medical College has had 22 Deans, one Interim Dean, one Acting Dean (who became the Dean), and numerous Associate Deans, Assistant Deans, and Assistants to the Dean. The Deans are listed in Table 49-1, their Associates in Table 49-3.

While the average tenure of a Dean of a United States medical school is given as 3.5 years, the Deans at Jefferson Medical College remained in office longer, averaging 7.4 years, with a range from one (Eberle, Barton, Dickson, Lowenstein) to 29 years (Holland). One Dean served for 13 years (Huston), two for 14 years (Dunglison, Kellow), and one for 22 years (Patterson). The average age of Jefferson Deans at the time of appointment was 47, in a range from 27 (Rhees) to 70 (Dickson). Only one of the 22 Jefferson Deans was a woman (Lowenstein, 1982–1983). All had the M.D. degree, and one (Lowenstein) a D.Phil. degree. Many were granted special academic recognition by the award of honorary degrees. All held the rank of Professor in various Departments of the College: 18 in clinical fields (Medicine, Therapeutics, Materia Medica, Obstetrics, and Preventive Medicine); three in preclinical fields (Chemistry, Toxicology, and Anatomy); one in both (Medicine and Biochemistry).

Table 49-1 Deans of Jefferson Medical College

Name	*Tenure*	*Medical Degree From*	*Age When Appointed Dean*	*Professorship at Jefferson*
Benjamin Rush Rhees	1824–27	University of Pennsylvania	27	Institutes of Medicine and Medical Jurisprudence
John Eberle	1827–28	University of Pennsylvania	40	Medicine
William P.C. Barton	1828–29	University of Pennsylvania	42	Materia Medica and Botany
Samuel McClellan	1830–34	Yale University	30	Anatomy and Midwifery and Diseases of Children
Samuel Colhoun	1835–39	University of Pennsylvania	48	Materia Medica and Medical Jurisprudence
John Revere	1839–41	University of Edinburgh	52	Theory and Practice of Medicine
Robert M. Huston	1841–54	University of Pennsylvania	46	Materia Medica and General Therapeutics
Robley Dunglison	1854–68	Erlangen	56	Institutes of Medicine
Samuel H. Dickson	1868–69	University of Pennsylvania	70	Practice of Medicine
Benjamin Howard Rand	1869–73	Jefferson	42	Chemistry
John Barclay Biddle	1873–79	University of Pennsylvania	58	Materia Medica and General Therapeutics
Ellerslie Wallace	1879–83	Jefferson	60	Obstetrics and Diseases of Women and Children
Roberts Bartholow	1883–87	University of Maryland	52	Materia Medica, General Therapeutics and Hygiene
James W. Holland	1887–1916	Jefferson	38	Medical Chemistry and Toxicology
Ross V. Patterson	1916–38	Jefferson	39	Therapeutics
Henry K. Mohler	1938–41	Jefferson	51	Therapeutics
William Harvey Perkins	1941–50	Jefferson	47	Preventive Medicine
George Allen Bennett	1950–58	University of Munich	46	Anatomy
William A. Sodeman	1958–67	University of Michigan	52	Medicine
William F. Kellow	1967–81	Georgetown School of Medicine	45	Medicine
Leah Lowenstein	1982–83	University of Wisconsin	51	Medicine and Biochemistry
Joseph S. Gonnella	1984–	Harvard University	50	Medicine

It is interesting that the word Dean comes from the Latin *decanus* meaning "one set over ten." The word evolved through a series of meanings: a head, chief, or commander of a division of ten (1483); head of the chapter in a collegiate or cathedral church (Middle English); the registrar or secretary of the faculty (1524); ten officers in the colleges of Oxford and Cambridge appointed to supervise the conduct and discipline of the junior members (1577); head of ten monks in a monastery (1641); a presbyter invested with jurisdiction over a division of an archdeaconry (1647); the president of a faculty or department of study in a university; or the president, chief, or senior member of any body.

Typically, a Dean is the administrative head of a college and reports directly, or through a Vice President, to the President, who is responsible in turn to the Board of Trustees, the governing body. Each college of a university usually has its own Dean. Thomas Jefferson University has three Deans, one for Jefferson Medical College, one for the College of Graduate Studies, and one for the College of Allied Health Sciences. Before Jefferson Medical College became a university in 1969 there was but one Dean who supervised the Medical School and also the early days of the Graduate School. Before 1949 the Chairman of the Board of Trustees was also President, and the Dean functioned under his supervision. In reporting to the President, the Dean was reporting directly to a member of the Board, the Chairman. Since 1949, the President of the Corporation and later the President of the University did not have membership on the Board, and the Dean no longer reported directly to a Board member. Since 1962 the Dean's title has also included the title of Vice President.

The Dean is the chief executive officer of Jefferson Medical College and has the responsibility for developing and managing the administrative officers, academic programs, and research in this college. He or she should be a competent supervisor who by training, experience, and personal attributes is qualified and has the authority to interpret and implement high standards in medical education. The Dean should have the respect and support of the faculty, the President, other officials, and the Board of Trustees.

The Dean directly or indirectly supervises or influences the following:

1. Students (recruitment, admission requirements, selection, evaluation, counseling, financial aid, organizations, discipline, academic and nonacademic programs, attitudes and conduct, records, government, publications, societies, services, graduation, health, facilities, and rights and privacy protection);
2. Faculty (recruitment, selection, evaluation, teaching methods, research activities, advancement, compensation, facilities, support, tenure, discipline, and student–faculty relationships);
3. Curriculum (objectives, control, implementation, and evaluation);
4. Research (facilities, support, and evaluation);
5. Budget (sources, distribution, and adequacy of finances);
6. Facilities (adequacy, maintenance, expansion, and utilization);
7. Continuing Medical Education (objectives, implementation, sponsorship, control, policies, and funding);
8. Graduate Medical Education (selection of house staff, teaching by house staff, program, and evaluation);
9. Alumni (supplying information, speakers at meetings, accessibility, and maintenance of good relationships); and
10. Affiliated Hospitals (teaching and program, evaluation, student assignments, and affiliation agreements).

The Deanship is thus a position of power, but with accountability.

The increasing responsibility and complexity of the Dean's Office is illustrated by the financial activities for the period 1961–1986. (Table 49-2).

Biographical data relative to the first 17 Deans of Jefferson (Rhees through Perkins) are located in the Office of the Dean. The remaining five Deans (Bennett through Gonnella) were personally known by the present author who worked with each one in the Dean's Office. Their biographies include his own observations and reaction.

Table 49-2 Jefferson Medical College Financial Activity for Fiscal Years 1961–1986

Fiscal Year	*Medical College Operation*	*Sponsored Programs*	*Medical Practice*		*Total*
1960/61	$ 2,807,332	$ 663,709	$ -0-	=	$ 3,471,041
1965/66	4,064,138	3,897,621	-0-	=	$ 7,961,759
1970/71	8,801,904	7,391,170	320,000	=	$16,513,074
1975/76	15,009,582	10,648,334	3,024,993	=	$28,682,909
1980/81	20,942,686	10,863,324	9,051,202	=	$40,857,212
1985/86	33,283,688	13,358,947	23,724,932	=	$70,367,567

In late 1824, the same year as its founding, Jefferson Medical College had its first Dean, but it was not until more than 100 years later, in 1931, that the office of Assistant Dean was created. The varied activities of the Dean's Office increased in number and complexity as the years went by, and additional help was necessary to carry the burden. By the year 1987, there were two Senior Associate Deans and four Associate Deans (a fifth Associate Dean recently died) aiding the Dean in his heavy and diverse responsibilities. Supporting the office functions are a long procession of secretaries, clerks, financial aid officers, business managers, registrars, librarians, supervisors of facilities and space planning, and directors of sponsored programs, development, and alumni affairs.

The following list contains only the names of the Assistants to the Dean, Assistant Deans, and Associate Deans arranged in the order of their appearance on the scene.

Table 49-3 Associates of the Dean

Dean's Assistant	*Faculty Rank*	*Dean's Office Titles*	*Dates*	*Deans*
Joseph O. Crider, M.D.	Professor of Physiology	Assistant Dean	1931–49	Patterson, Mohler, Perkins
W. Paul Havens, M.D.	Associate Professor of Preventive Medicine	Assistant to the Dean	1949–50	Perkins
James R. Martin, M.D.	Professor of Orthopaedic Surgery	Associate Dean	1951–56	Bennett
Robert Bruce Nye, M.D.	Assistant Professor of Medicine	Assistant Dean	1951–60	Bennett,
		Associate Dean	1960–66	Sodeman
Samuel S. Conly, Jr., M.D.	Associate Professor of Physiology	Assistant to the Dean	1956–60	Bennett, Sodeman
		Assistant Dean	1960–65	Sodeman
		Associate Dean	1965–67	Sodeman, Kellow
		Associate Dean and Director of Admissions	1967–82	Kellow, Lowenstein
Robert P. Gilbert, M.D	Associate Professor of Medicine	Associate Dean	1965–70	Sodeman,
		Associate Dean and		Kellow
		Director of Extramural Programs	1970–72	Kellow
John H. Killough, Ph.D., M.D.	Associate Professor of Medicine	Assistant Dean for Continuing Ed.	1965–68	Sodeman, Kellow
		Associate Dean for Continuing Ed.	1968–70	Kellow
		Associate Dean and Director of Cont. Ed.	1970–77	
		Associate Dean and Director of Affiliation Programs and Continuing Education	1977–81	Kellow
Joseph S. Gonnella, M.D.	Professor of Medicine	Assistant Dean	1967–68	Kellow
		Associate Dean	1968–70	
		Associate Dean and Director of Academic Programs	1970–83	Kellow, Lowenstein
		Acting Dean, Dean for Educational Programs and	1983–84	

Table 49-3 Associates of the Dean (continued)

Dean's Assistant	*Faculty Rank*	*Dean's Office Titles*	*Dates*	*Deans*
		Director of the Center of Research in Medical Education and Health Care		
Carl L. Hansen, M.D., Ph.D.	Professor of Radiology	Associate Dean and Director of the Regional Therapy and Nuclear Medicine Medical Program	1968–72	Kellow
Robert C. Mackowiak, M.D.	Clinical Professor of Medicine	Assistant Dean and Director of Student Affairs	1972–75	Kellow
		Associate Dean and Director of Student Affairs	1975–81	
		Associate Dean and Director of Allied Programs and Continuing Education	1981–83	Kellow, Lowenstein
James H. Robinson, M.D.	Clinical Professor of Surgery	Associate Dean and Director of Minority Affairs	1975–81	Kellow
		Associate Dean and Director of Student Affairs	1981–84	Kellow, Lowenstein
Jussi J. Saukkonen, M.D.	Professor of Microbiology	Dean of Scientific and Faculty Affairs	1983–84	Gonnella
		Senior Associate Dean of Scientific and Faculty Affairs	1984–	Gonnella
Benjamin Bachrach, M.D.	Clinical Professor of Surgery	Associate Dean for Admissions	1983–84	
		Associate Dean, Admissions	1984–	Gonnella
Joseph R. Sherwin, Ph.D.	Associate Professor of Physiology	Assistant Dean of Scientific Affairs	1983–84	
		Assistant Dean Scientific Affairs	1984–85	Gonnella
		Associate Dean, Scientific Affairs	1985–	Gonnella
Robert Blacklow, M.D.	Professor of Medicine	Senior Associate Dean	1984–	Gonnella
Carla E. Goepp, M.D.	Clinical Associate Professor of Medicine	Associate Dean, Student Affairs, Student Counseling and Career Planning	1984–	Gonnella
Joseph F. Rodgers, M.D.	Clinical Associate Professor of Medicine	Associate Dean, Affiliations and Residency Programs	1984–	Gonnella
Clara Callahan, M.D.	Clinical Assistant Professor of Pediatrics	Assistant Dean for Student Affairs	1987–	Gonnella
George Alexander, M.D.	Assistant Professor of Radiation Therapy and Nuclear Medicine	Assistant Dean for Student Affairs	1987–	Gonnella
Peter Chodoff	Professor of Anesthesiology	Assistant Dean; Director of Education and Research Medicine, Medical Center of Delaware	1987–	Gonnella
James B. Erdmann, Ph.D.		Associate Dean for Administration and Special Projects	1987–	Gonnella

charming gentleman, abounding in Christian charities, in varied information, in biblical and classical lore, and in all the amenities which adorn the domestic and social circle. Had his life been spared to an advanced age, he would have earned an enviable reputation as a teacher and practitioner, if not also as an author."

Benjamin Rush Rhees, M.D.; First Dean (1824–1827)

The first regular meeting of the Jefferson Medical College Faculty was held December 20, 1824, with Dr. Eberle in the Chair and Dr. Rhees as Secretary. On motion, Dr. Rhees was appointed Dean. It may be noted that the office of Dean carried little weight in the early years, and for a time the Deanship could not be held by the same incumbent even for two successive years. Dr. Rhees was Professor of the Institutes of Medicine and Medical Jurisprudence.

Benjamin Rush Rhees (Figure 49-1) was a native of Pennsylvania, born in 1798, and was educated in the University of Pennsylvania. His medical preceptor was Dr. James Rush. For a time Rhees was resident physician to the City Hospital, and later, after a period of foreign travel and study, he settled in practice in Philadelphia, where he also gave private instruction. One of his pupils was Henry D. Smith, the first matriculate of the Jefferson Medical College. In the College, Rhees taught several subjects at various times, as emergency required, until his death. He was a man of varied accomplishments, a careful, conscientious teacher, and a patient student of classical literature and theology, qualities not often found in medical men of those times. His example and influence in early Jefferson Medical College history were beneficial to the institution and to the graduates who left its halls during the period of his Professorship. In speaking of Professor Rhees' qualities as an instructor, Gross said:

> "His discourses were always written out at full length, and it was evident that he availed himself freely in their composition of the works of Bostock and Beck, at the time the great standard treatises upon three respective branches of medicine. Although his voice was naturally feeble, it possessed uncommon sweetness and there was an earnestness in his manner and delivery that made him one of the most captivating and agreeable lecturers I ever listened to. Besides, he was a

Dr. Rhees died of tuberculosis in 1831 at age 33.

It was during Rhees' attendance as a student at the University of Pennsylvania that an incident occurred that exerted no ordinary influence upon his future. As early as 1818 an effort had been made to obtain a charter for a new Medical College. The friends of the University, fearing that the attempt, if successful, would be prejudicial to its interests, deemed it proper to organize a counter movement. Among other expedients was the appointment of a committee of the class that

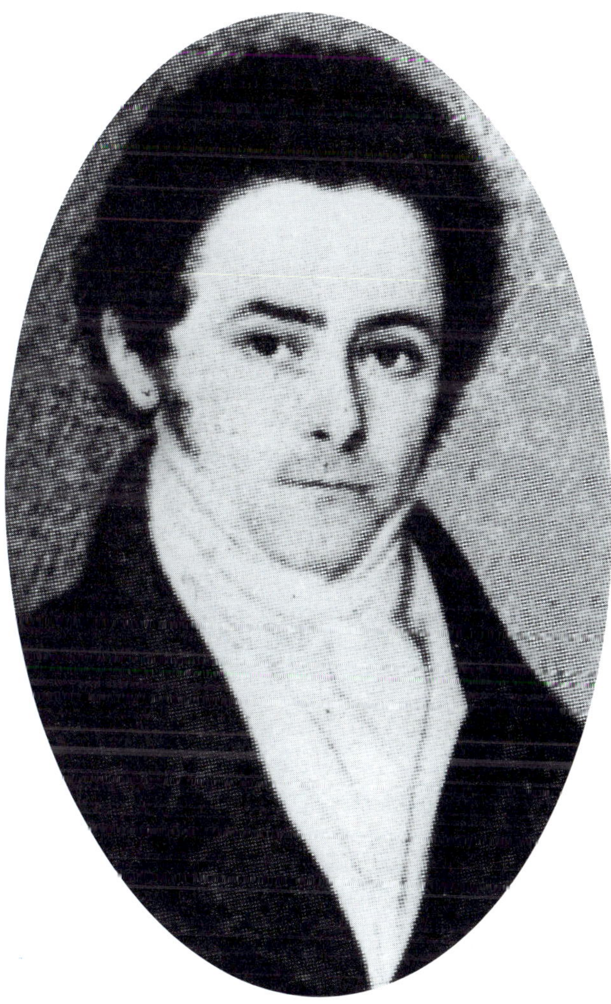

Fig. 49-1. Benjamin Rush Rhees, M.D., First Dean (1824–1827).

reported a series of resolutions strongly adverse to the scheme. A unanimous approval of these resolutions had been anticipated, and the presiding officer was about to put the question, when suddenly and unexpectedly a tremulous voice was heard in the back part of the hall, addressing the chair and requesting to offer a few remarks.

> "All eyes were turned in the direction of the speaker, and considerable commotion for a time prevailed. Order being restored, and the speaker, in the meantime having ascended one of the back benches of the amphitheatre, was found to be a gentleman of slender frame, somewhat diminutive in stature, and quite juvenile in appearance. With considerable embarrassment of manner, but with the great force of reasoning, he attacked the positions of the committee, disputed their premises, and in a lucid argument combated their conclusions, and argued the importance and necessity of a second Medical College. This man was Benjamin Rush Rhees."

John Eberle, M.D.; Second Dean (1827–1828)

Dr. John Eberle (Figure 49-2) was born of German parents in 1788 and was graduated in medicine from the University of Pennsylvania in 1809. He early displayed ability as a writer on political subjects. In 1818 he edited the *Recorder*. Soon afterward he issued *Materia Medica and Therapeutics,* and later, *The Diseases and Physical Education of Children*. He joined McClellan in his School of Medicine, and was his earnest friend and fellow worker for many years. He was a man of learning and filled satisfactorily the important Chair of Theory and Practice when the first faculty was completed. In 1831 he went to Cincinnati, Ohio, and continued his career as a lecturer, but he died in 1838. Dr. Eberle was a factor for good in the early history of the College and helped to lay the foundation for its subsequent prosperity. Dr. Gross, in an address on the first faculty, said that John Eberle was in many respects a remarkable man, that he came from an obscure Pennsylvania family, had no early educational advantages, but that he rose by force of his own native ability, industry, and perseverance to high rank in the profession. His work on *Materia Medica* and his treatise, *The Practice of Medicine,* were standard productions in their day, and created for him a wide reputation both at home and abroad. The former, soon after its publication, was honored with a German translation and secured for him a membership in the Medical Society of Berlin. Eberle was a devoted student and in the truest sense a "bookworm." In consequence of his secluded habits, he never enjoyed a large practice, the public foolishly assuming that a man who wrote so many books could not have much time to attend to the sick.

On September 26, 1827, Dr. Eberle was elected Dean and served until 1828, when he was

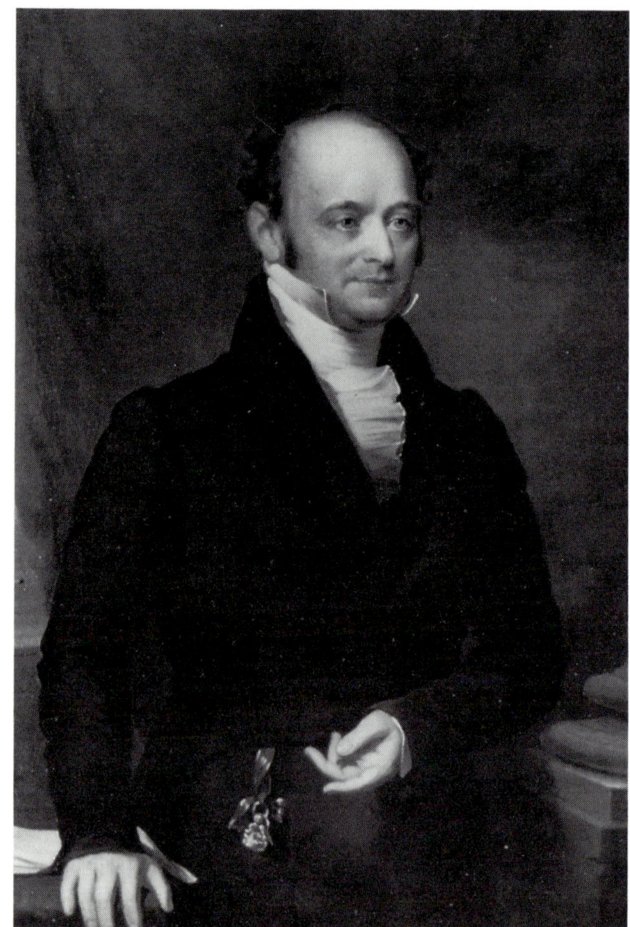

Fig. 49-2. John Eberle, M.D., Second Dean (1827–1828).

succeeded by Dr. William P.C. Barton. Dr. Eberle, Professor of Medicine, resigned from the faculty in 1830, subsequently to join Dr. Daniel Drake in Cincinnati. His portrait along with that of his wife, Salome, are highly regarded in Jefferson's art collection.

William Paul Crillon Barton, M.D.; Third Dean (1828–1829)

Dr. Barton (Figure 49-3), a Navy surgeon, was born November 17, 1786, into a distinguished family of Philadelphia physicians. He received his A.B. degree from the College of New Jersey (Princeton) in 1805 and his M.D. degree from the University of Pennsylvania in 1808.

Dr. Barton was a man of untiring energy, with a high sense of duty, to whom the Medical Department of the Navy owes some valuable reforms. He was also a writer of ability and a noted botanist. Among his more outstanding writings may be mentioned: *A Treatise Containing a Plan for the Organization and Government of Marine Hospitals* (1814); *Vegetable Materia Medica of the United States* (1818); *Compendium Florae Philadelphicae* (1818); and *A Flora of North America*, with colored plates (1821).

He held the position of Professor of Botany in the University of Pennsylvania from 1816 to 1828 and was Professor of Materia Medica and Botany at Jefferson from 1828 to 1830. Previously, he had also been a member of the Medical Staff of the Philadelphia Hospital from 1821 to 1822.

Dr. Barton was Dean of Jefferson Medical College from 1828 to 1829. In 1830 he was called to active duty in the Navy. There he rapidly advanced in rank to become Chief of the Naval Bureau of Medicine and Surgery in 1842, which position he held until retirement in 1844. Dr. Barton died in Philadelphia, February 28, 1856, and was buried with military honors in East Laurel Hill Cemetery. His life-size bust is displayed in the Army Medical Museum at Washington, D.C.

Samuel McClellan, M.D.; Fourth Dean (1830–1834)

Samuel McClellan (Figure 49-4) was born in Woodstock, Connecticut, in 1800. The early years of his life were devoted to agricultural pursuits on his father's farm. In 1819, however, he commenced the study of anatomy with Dr. Daniel Lyman, a respectable physician of his native town, with whom he remained one year.

In 1820 he entered the office of his brother, Dr. George McClellan, in Philadelphia, and for the next two years also attended lectures at the Philadelphia Almshouse, the Pennsylvania Hospital, and the University of Pennsylvania.

In March 1823, he graduated in Medicine at Yale College and, intending to locate in South America, he obtained both from the faculty of that College and from the Board of Examiners the

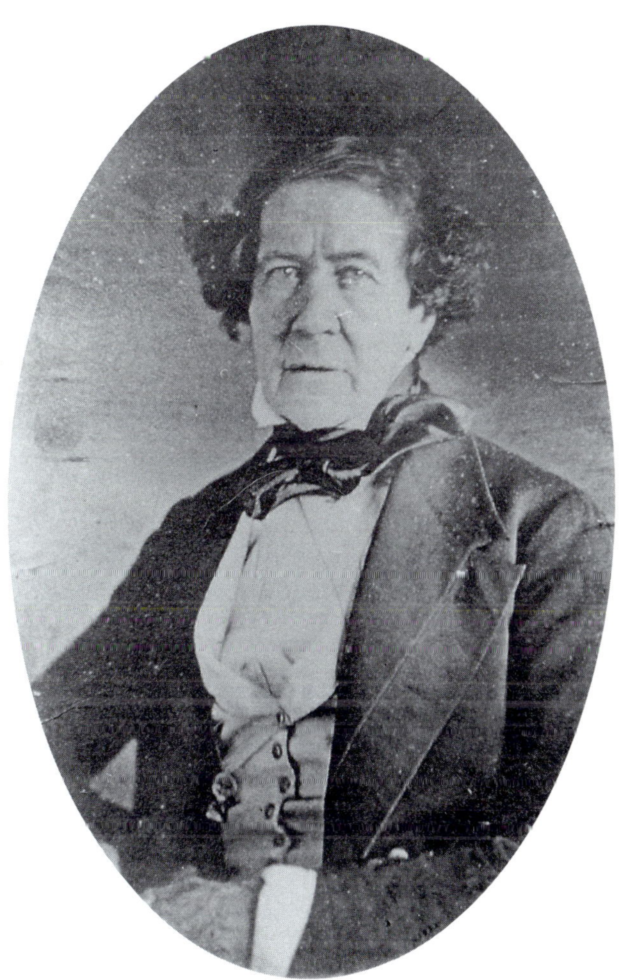

Fig. 49-3. William P. C. Barton, M.D., Third Dean (1828–1829).

most satisfactory letters as to his qualifications for the practice of his profession.

The next three years of Dr. McClellan's life were spent traveling through Mexico in company with a noted English naturalist. At this time his attention was particularly directed to the diseases of the eye, in the treatment of which he was signally successful. At last, tiring of a foreign climate, he returned to Pennsylvania and settled in the town of Bristol.

In 1828, at the solicitation of his brother, McClellan removed to Philadelphia and became Assistant Demonstrator of Anatomy at Jefferson. In 1829 he was appointed Adjunct Professor of Anatomy, and in January, 1830, Professor of Anatomy. This Chair he held until the close of the session of 1832, when he resigned in favor of Dr. Granville S. Pattison. In March of the same year he was elected to the Chair of Institutes, Medical Jurisprudence, and Midwifery. He held this post until June 24, 1836, at which time the Institutes of Medicine and Medical Jurisprudence was made a separate Chair given to Dr. Robley Dunglison. Dr. McClellan served as Dean from 1830 to 1834, a time when reputations depended more upon performance as Professors than as Deans. From mid-June, 1836, until 1839 he held the Chair of Obstetrics and Diseases of Females: developing the foundation of his future reputation in the practice of this branch of his profession. In the latter year, the faculty of Jefferson was dissolved and all the Chairs vacated. Upon the appointment of a new faculty, Dr. McClellan was again elected to the Chair of Obstetrics and Diseases of Women. In September of the same year, however, he resigned.

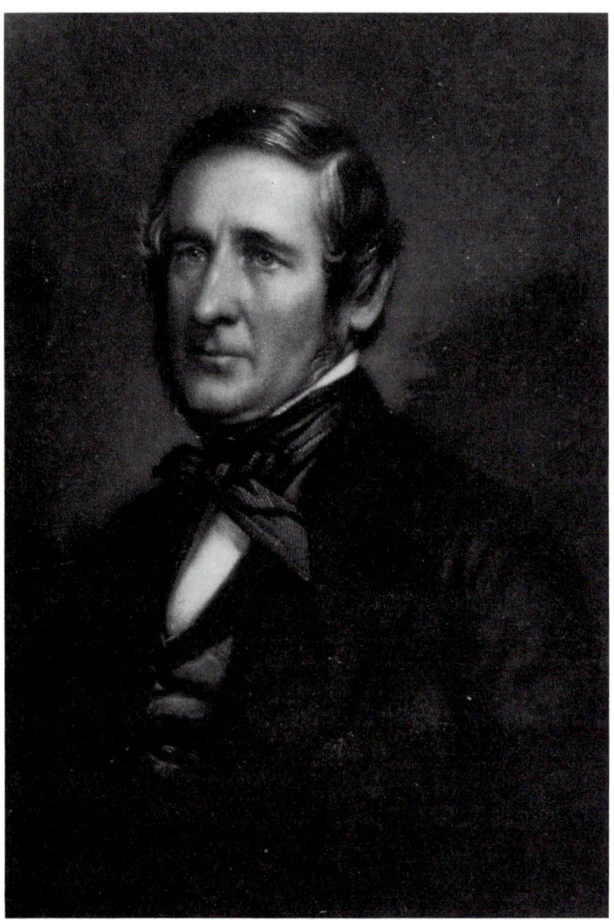

Fig. 49-4. Samuel McClellan, M.D., Fourth Dean (1830–1834).

Dr. Samuel McClellan was a quiet, unassuming man who shrank from rather than sought applause. He was noted among his friends for his remarkable memory. His mind grasped and never forgot the most minute details of his studies. The last 20 years of his life were devoted to private practice, in the discharge of the duties of which he was conscientious and kind, but unyielding. In January, 1854, after a short but painful illness aggravated by excessive application to his studies, he died as he had lived, beloved by all who knew him.

Samuel Colhoun, M.D.; Fifth Dean (1835–1839)

Samuel Colhoun (Figure 49-5) was born in Chambersburg, Pennsylvania, in 1787, and graduated from Princeton in 1804 and from the University of Pennsylvania Medical School in 1808. During his nine years as a member of the Jefferson faculty he was Professor of Materia Medica and Medical Jurisprudence and also served as Dean (1835–1839). He was a faithful friend of George McClellan and, after the latter was dismissed, joined him in the third medical school. Colhoun was a bachelor, a learned man and of a genial, generous nature. He died in 1841 at the age of 54.

John Revere, M.D.; Sixth Dean (1839–1840)

Another conspicuous figure in faculty circles was Dr. John Revere (Figure 49-6), who in 1831 was appointed to the Chair of Theory and Practice of Physick. He was born in 1787, graduated from Harvard in 1807, and four years later received his medical degree in Edinburgh. His professional career was begun in Baltimore, from which city he came to Philadelphia and to the Chair of Medicine at Jefferson. He served as Dean for the 1839–1840 term. "Here," says one writer, "his excellent qualities as a physician and lecturer added greatly to the strength of the Faculty during his ten years of service. He and Dr. Pattison both resigned in 1841 to take Chairs in the University of New York."

Dr. Revere died in New York at the age of 60. He was the son of the Revolutionary War patriot, Paul Revere, and was the paternal grand-uncle of Grace Linzee Revere. Grace Revere married Samuel W. Gross (1876) and after his death became the wife of Dr. William Osler (1892). She endowed a Professorship in Surgery (1929) at Jefferson in honor of her first husband for his interest in tumors.

Robert M. Huston, M.D.; Seventh Dean (1841–1854)

Dr. Huston (Figure 49-7) was a Virginian, born in 1794. He served as Assistant Surgeon during the War of 1812 and afterward settled in Philadelphia, where he practiced medicine many years before he identified himself with the Jefferson Medical College. In 1838 he was appointed to the Chair of Obstetrics, and in 1841, upon the reorganization of the faculty, he was retained and assigned to the Chair of Materia Medica and Therapeutics. In the

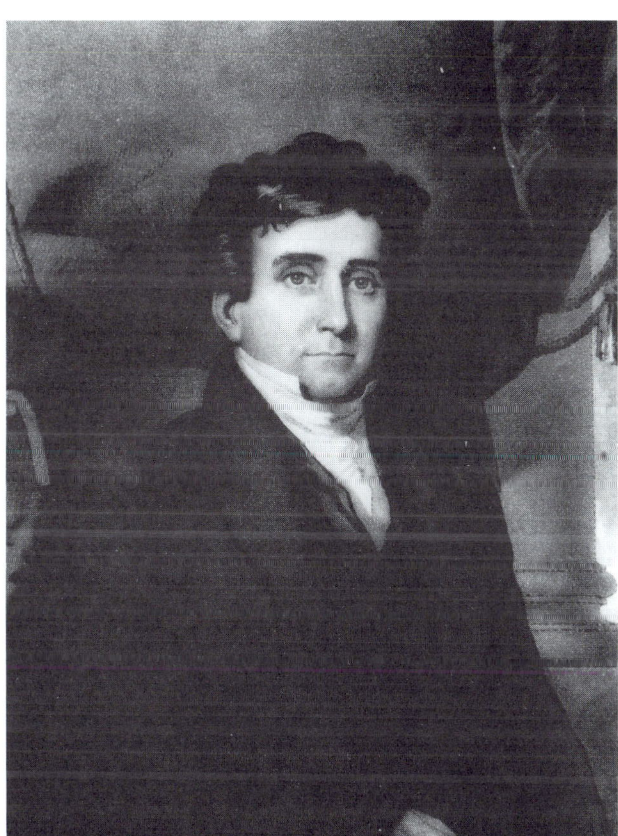

FIG. 49-5. Samuel Colhoun, M.D., Fifth Dean (1835–1839).

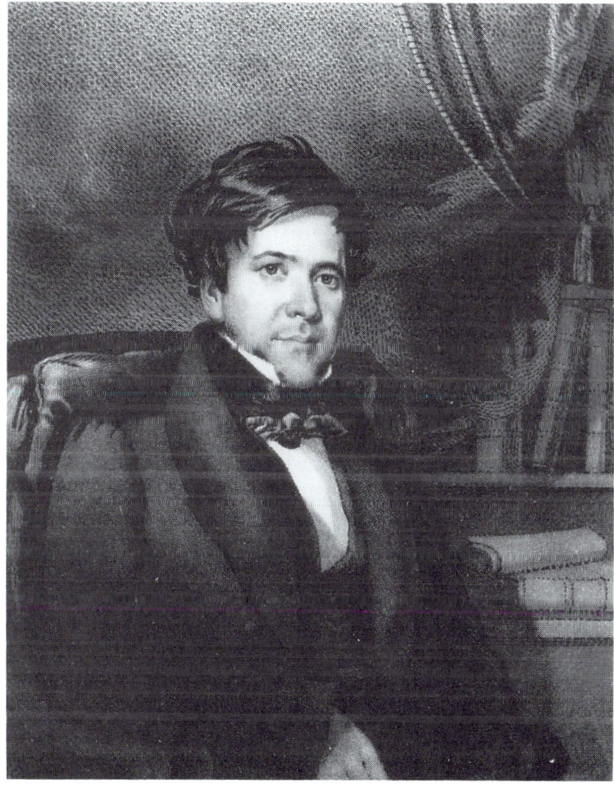

FIG. 49-6. John Revere, M.D., Sixth Dean (1839–1840).

same year he was made Dean of the Faculty and served in that capacity until 1854. In the next year he resigned his Chair and was made Emeritus.

Dr. Huston's lectures were delivered from manuscript and were marked by honesty and faithfulness in their teaching. He dwelt much upon therapeutics, a subject more to his taste than obstetrics, which he formerly taught. In whatever capacity he was called to serve, he always acquitted himself well and to the credit of the school. In addition to his qualifications as a teacher, Dr. Huston possessed excellent business ability. This was shown during his incumbency of the Deanship, where his services contributed far more than ever was publicly known to the advancement of the College and the placement of its affairs upon a solid financial basis.

Upon Dr. Huston devolved the double duty of attending to the business affairs of the College, such as usually were put upon the Dean, and also the active work of an important Chair. He was a constant toiler, with an abundance of nervous energy, yet his manifold duties never appeared to worry him. One of his best traits was his perfect simplicity, a quality that showed itself in his lectures, his everyday conversation, his personal habits, and his methods of business. Dr. Huston died in 1864, and the loss of his counsel was deeply felt in College and professional circles.

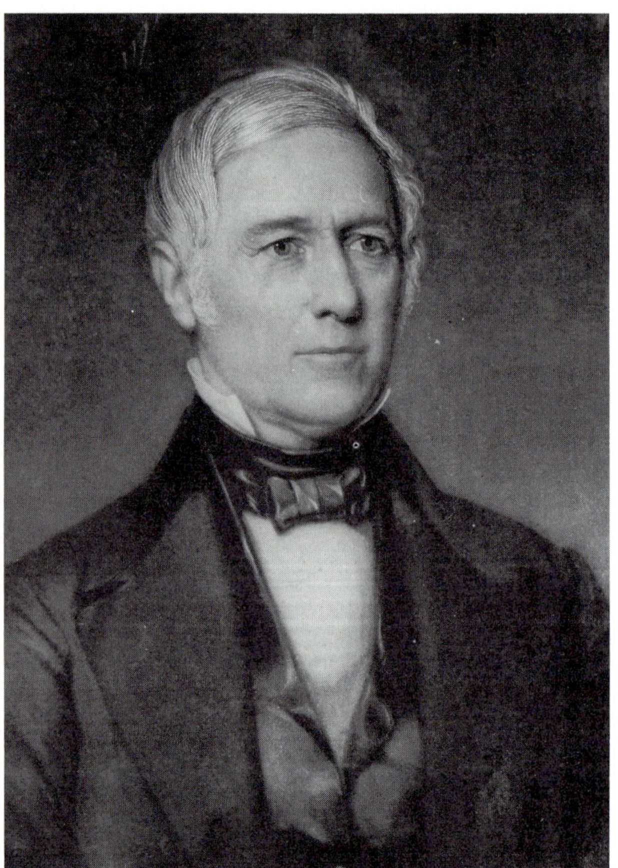

FIG. 49-7. Robert M. Huston, M.D., Seventh Dean (1841–1854).

Robley Dunglison, M.D., LL.D.; Eighth Dean (1854–1868)

Robley Dunglison's career at Jefferson began with his appointment as Professor of the Institutes of Medicine in 1836. In 1854 he succeeded Dr. Huston as Dean and served in that additional capacity until 1868.

Dr. Dunglison (Figure 49-8) was born January

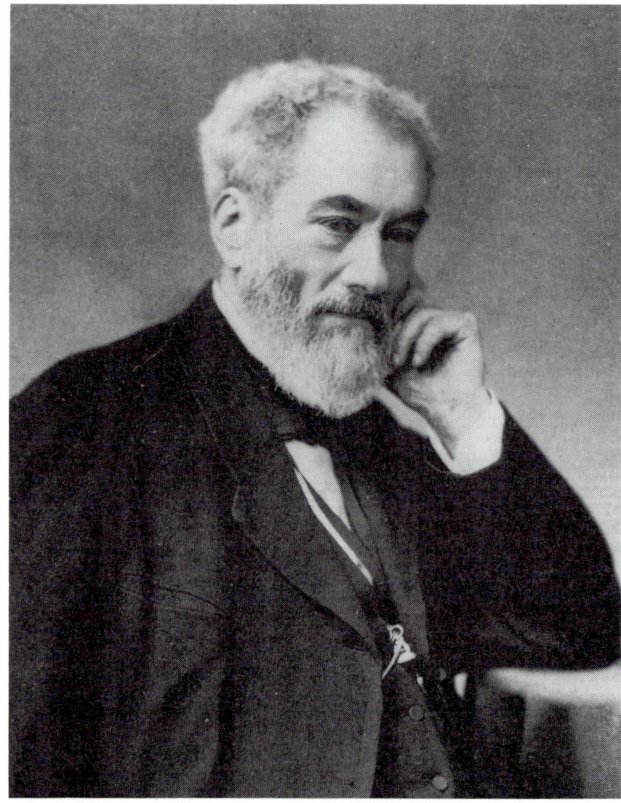

FIG. 49-8. Robley Dunglison, M.D., LL.D., Eighth Dean (1854–1868).

4, 1798, at Keswick, in Cumberland, the beautiful lake country in the north of England. In his seventeenth year he began the study of medicine in Cumberland, and afterward went to London. He subsequently attended one course of lectures at the University of Edinburgh, visited Paris, and, having returned to London, passed his examinations at the Royal College of Surgeons and at Apothecaries Hall. He began practice in London in 1819 and obtained his medical degree from Erlangen, Germany, in 1824.

At first Dr. Dunglison intended to restrict himself to medical and obstetrical practice, especially the latter, and had announced a course of lectures on midwifery for the fall of 1824. He had also begun his career as an author, and was about to associate himself with Dr. Copeland, writer of a well-known dictionary. Just at this time he received from ex-President Jefferson, Rector of the University of Virginia, the offer of a comprehensive Chair in that institution. He accepted the position and remained nine years at the University, winning fame as a lecturer and building up his reputation as an author and man of letters. He became the personal physician to Thomas Jefferson and attended him at death.

In 1833 Dr. Dunglison became Professor of Therapeutics, Materia Medica, Hygiene, and Medical Jurisprudence in the University of Maryland. In June 1836 he was elected to the Chair of Institutes of Medicine at Jefferson, which he filled until the early part of 1868. Thus, for more than a third of a century he was a Professor at this school. In 1854, after an absence of 30 years, he revisited England. Late in the same year he returned to America, at the urging of Dean Huston who was relinquishing his Deanship.

Dr. Dunglison was an extraordinary man, a man of learning in the highest sense of the term, familiar alike with the classics of medicine and with the medical literature of his day. No professional topic escaped his keen observation. He was cognizant of all theories but was not carried away by any of them. The bent of his mind was eminently judicial. He listened patiently to all arguments, sifted all evidence, rejected the false and held fast to the true, and his decision, once reached, was in the end almost always correct. He was not an enthusiast nor an ardent investigator in the modern sense of the term. He preferred rather to analyze the research of others and to base his conclusions upon accumulated evidence.

As a writer on medical subjects, Dr. Dunglison early won repute with the profession, but his literary efforts carried him into fields other than those of purely medical character. His *Practice of Medicine, Therapeutics, and Materia Medica; New Remedies; Physiology;* and also his *Medical Dictionary,* were for many years an enduring monument to his professional and literary genius. His best works, the textbooks and the dictionary, passed through many editions, and some of them were found on the tables of nearly every practitioner in the land. His qualities as a writer gave him a stronghold on the medical profession, and it is not surprising that medical students pursuing their preliminary courses in physicians' offices should seek to place themselves under the personal instruction of a man of such distinguished ability.

Dunglison's appreciation of character was remarkable. His judgment of the moral attributes of men was rarely at fault. As a friend to young men, no one could be more true, and no advice was more to be depended upon than his. His knowledge of the world and of the motives that impelled men's actions was accurate. In the expression of his opinion he was cautious and guarded, qualities he endeavored to inculcate in others.

Dr. Dunglison was a fluent speaker. His language was lucid and elegant. He never wanted for a word, and every word was well chosen. His diction was Johnsonian, and his lectures, always extemporaneous, never failed to command the attention of his class. He stood before the world as an exemplar of medical science, and the honors heaped upon him from so many lands in memberships in more than 100 scientific bodies testified to the esteem in which he was universally held.

In 1868, after 32 years of active service, Dr. Dunglison was compelled by failing health to resign the Chair of Institutes of Medicine (1836–1868), and also the important office of Dean (1854–1868). His colleagues were reluctant to part with their faithful co-worker, whom they regarded as the balance wheel of the College and whose counsel and influence always were for its best interests; but the worthy senior member of the faculty was now broken in health and bowed with infirmities of age, having passed the allotted three score and ten years. He had earned retirement, but his continued association with faculty work was desirable, hence his appointment as Emeritus Professor of Institutes of Medicine and Medical Jurisprudence. His death, in April, 1869, was a serious loss not only to Jefferson but to the great community of scholars and to the medical profession at large.

Samuel H. Dickson, M.D.; Ninth Dean (1868–1869)

Samuel H. Dickson (Figure 49-9) was born in Charleston, South Carolina, in 1798, and was graduated from Yale in 1814, at the age of 16. In 1819 he was graduated from the Medical Department of the University of Pennsylvania, and five years later (1824) joined with Ramsay and Frost in founding the Medical College of South Carolina, he taking the Chair of Institutes and Practice. After 22 years of experience and faithful service in this institution, Dickson was called in 1847 to the University of New York to succeed John Revere. In 1850 he returned to his former position and remained there eight years more. The degree of LL.D. was conferred by the University of New York in appreciation of his splendid character and service while a member of the faculty of that institution.

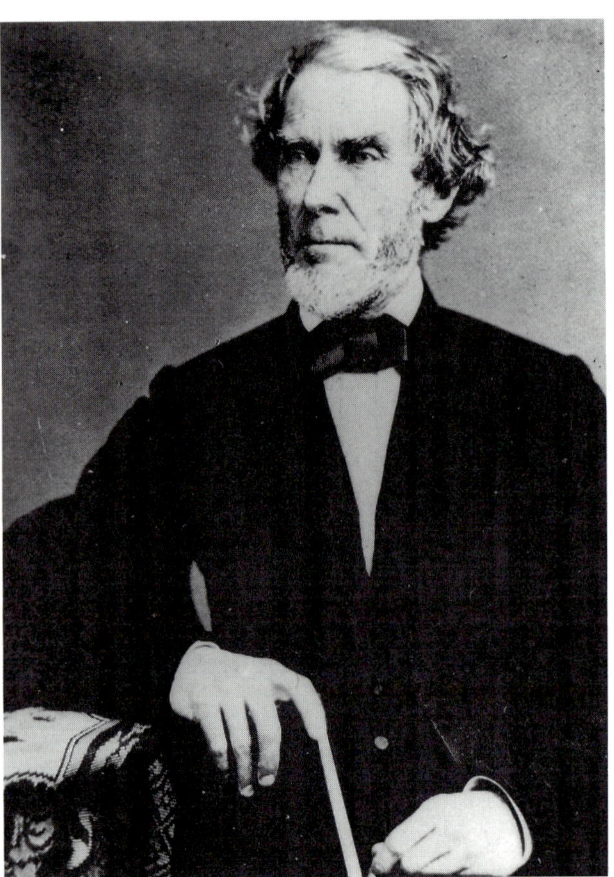

FIG. 49-9. Samuel H. Dickson, M.D., Ninth Dean (1868–1869).

In 1858 Professor Dickson was called to the Chair of Practice of Medicine at Jefferson. He spent the remaining 14 years of his life in that position and served as Dean from 1868 to 1869.

Both Dickson and Thomas D. Mitchell were well advanced in years when they accepted their Chairs at Jefferson. Dickson's office during this period must be associated with his successor, Jacob Mendes DaCosta, who had been for several years an influential teacher in the school, and who during the four closing years of this period (1872–1876) gave abundant evidence of the exceptional ability that always marked his teachings.

Benjamin Howard Rand, M.D.; Tenth Dean (1869–1873)

When Professor of Chemistry Dr. Franklin Bache died it was with considerable satisfaction that the faculty announced the appointment of B. Howard Rand (Figure 49–10), a native Philadelphian. Bache's successor would have to be a teacher of unquestioned strength, for he was to replace one of the model faculty of 1841. Rand had been tried and proved. Born in 1827, he had studied medicine under Huston, and for two years as a Jefferson student he had been Clinical Assistant to Mütter and Pancoast. Following graduation in 1848, Rand was connected with the Academy of Natural Sciences, at one time was its Secretary, and also was Lecturer on Chemistry at the Franklin

Institute and at the Philadelphia College of Medicine until that institution passed out of existence at the outbreak of the Civil War. Rand's *Medical Chemistry,* published in 1865, was for several years a popular reference and textbook. Rand was elected in 1864 and was one of the faculty for 13 years, until 1877, when ill health compelled him to resign. On the basis of his business ability he was appointed Dean of the Faculty and served creditably in that capacity four years (1869–1873). There were many changes during this time, and responsible duties devolved to the Dean. He died in 1883 at the age of 56. His portrait was painted by Thomas Eakins in 1874 and remains one of Jefferson's art treasures.

John Barclay Biddle, M.D.; Eleventh Dean (1873–1879)

John Barclay Biddle (Figure 49–11) was born in Philadelphia in 1815. He received an excellent elementary training and classical education, having been graduated from St. Mary's College, Baltimore. He took up the study of law, but changed his determination and became a student of medicine under Nathaniel Chapman. He was graduated from the University of Pennsylvania School of Medicine in 1836. He then spent a year or more in Europe, chiefly in France, pursuing his medical studies. Upon his return he began his professional career in Philadelphia. In 1838, with Dr. Meredith Clymer, he founded *The Medical Examiner,* an early, popular, and very successful medical publication. In 1846 he joined with Rogers, Van Wick, Tucker, Clymer, and Leidy to found the Franklin Medical College. There he took the Chair of Materia Medica, which he held for a few years until the institution closed its doors.

Biddle was a graceful and forceful writer, especially on medical topics, but he excelled as a teacher. His address was pleasing, his language clear and pertinent. His monographs won him popularity with the profession, and when he issued *Biddle's Materia Medica* the work was regarded as authoritative. It was published in 1852 and was a reference book for several years. His success as a teacher and writer made Biddle the natural successor to Thomas D. Mitchell (1865). He held the Chair of Materia Medica for 13 years until failing health made him retire. During the last six years of that period (1873–1879) he served as Dean and was one of the most earnest supporters of the first Jefferson Hospital, which was erected during his time (1877). Dr. Biddle died in January 1879 at 64 years of age.

Ellerslie Wallace, M.D.; Twelfth Dean (1879–1883)

Ellerslie Wallace (Figure 49–12) was a native of Philadelphia, born in 1813, and was of Scotch

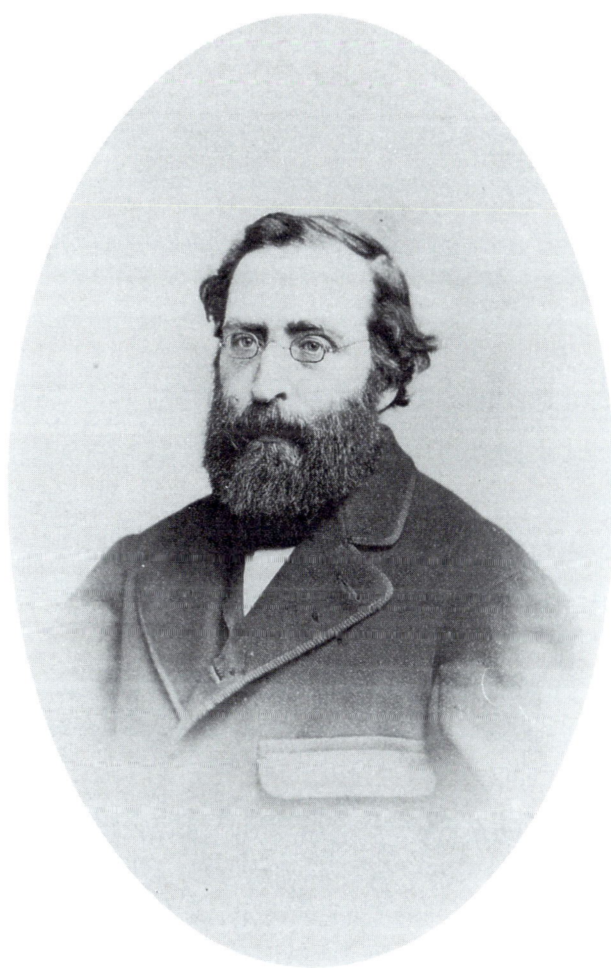

FIG. 49-10. Benjamin Howard Rand, M.D., Tenth Dean (1869–1873).

ancestry. He was educated at Bristol for civil engineering but was attracted to medicine by his brother, Dr. Joshua Wallace, then Demonstrator of Anatomy at Jefferson. He matriculated there in 1841 and received his degree in 1843. His professional career was begun in Philadelphia, where he was soon appointed Resident Physician at the Pennsylvania Hospital.

In 1846 Wallace resigned his position at the Pennsylvania Hospital in order to become Demonstrator of Anatomy at Jefferson. For the next 16 years he was an efficient teacher. When it was found that Professor Keating would not be able to perform the arduous duties of the Chair of Obstetrics, Wallace was called upon to take his place for the remainder of the session, was then appointed to succeed him, and for more than 20 years afterward was recognized as one of the leaders in the faculty. With his ability as a teacher he combined excellent business qualities, as was shown by his four years' incumbency in the office of Dean from 1879 to 1883.

After the close of the session of 1882–1883, Professor Wallace was forced by failing health to resign the Chair of Obstetrics and the Deanship, but he had no inclination to sever all connections with the College. He was given the honorary title of Professor Emeritus, which he held for two sessions. Death ended his useful career in 1885.

Roberts Bartholow, M.D.; Thirteenth Dean (1883–1887)

A graduate in arts from Calvert College, Roberts Bartholow (Figure 49–13) received his degree in medicine from the University of Maryland in 1852 in his twenty-first year. From 1857 to 1864 he was

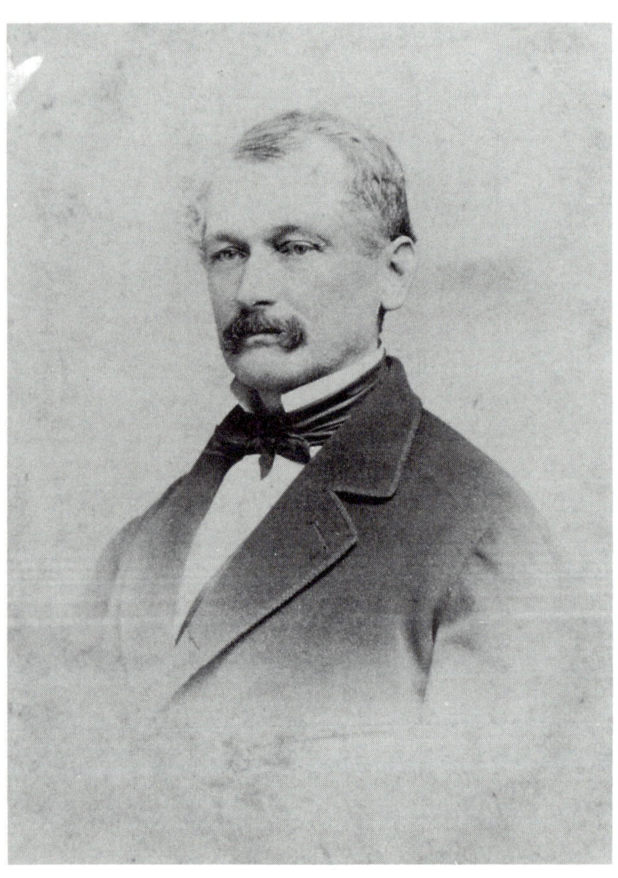

FIG. 49-11. John Barclay Biddle, M.D., Eleventh Dean (1873–1879).

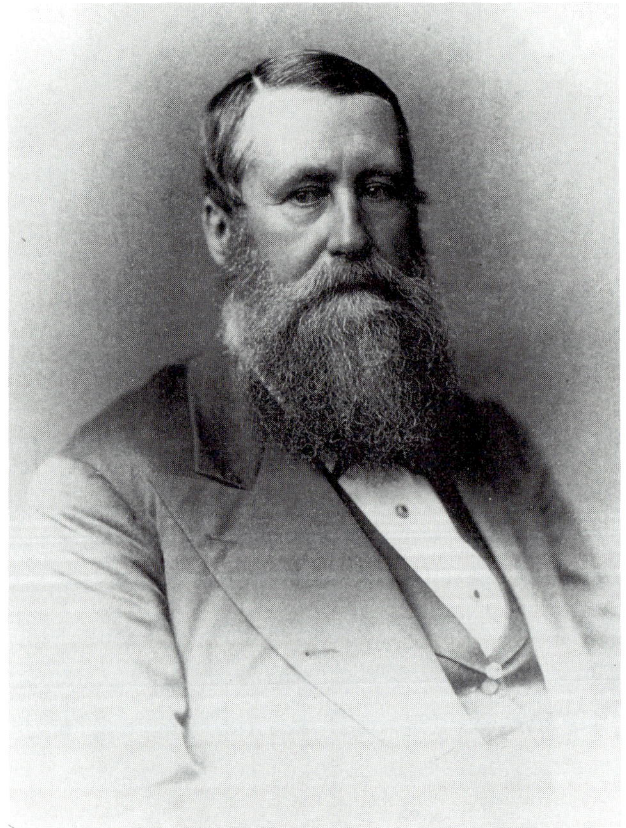

FIG. 49-12. Ellerslie Wallace, M.D., Twelfth Dean (1879–1883).

a surgeon in the United States Army and resigned in the latter year to take the Chair of Theory and Practice of Medicine, and later the Deanship, in the Ohio Medical College at Cincinnati. In 1879 he resigned to become Professor of Materia Medica and Therapeutics at Jefferson. He was chosen Dean in 1883. In 1887 he resigned that position to resume his work as a Professor, in which he continued until he was made Emeritus in 1893. Bartholow was the author of several medical works; among the best known were *Hypodermic Medication, Treatise on Therapeutics and Materia Medica,* and *Practice of Medicine,* the last of which was translated into Japanese. He was a member of the Royal Medical Society of Edinburgh and the Société Medicale Pratique of Paris, as well as an active member of leading American professional bodies. His portrait is in the Jefferson art collection.

James W. Holland, M.D.; Fourteenth Dean (1887–1916)

Dr. James W. Holland (Figure 49–14) was born in Louisville, Kentucky, April 24, 1849, the son of Dr. Robert and Elizabeth (Turner) Holland. Dr. Holland received his collegiate education at the University of Louisville, from which he was graduated with the B.A. degree in 1865 and M.A. in 1868. He became acquainted with Professor J. Lawrence Smith, one of the most brilliant and distinguished of American chemists. Professor Smith had studied abroad under Orfila, Dumas, Desprez, Becquerel, Dufrency, and Liebig. The benefits derived from such an acquaintance were reflected in his accomplishments as a teacher of chemistry.

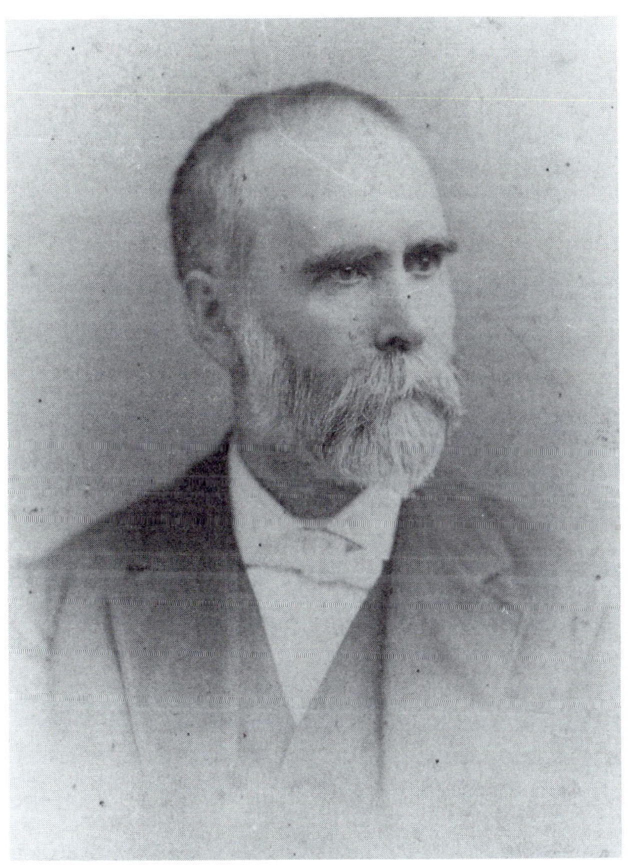

Fig. 49-13. Roberts Bartholow, M.D., Thirteenth Dean (1883–1887).

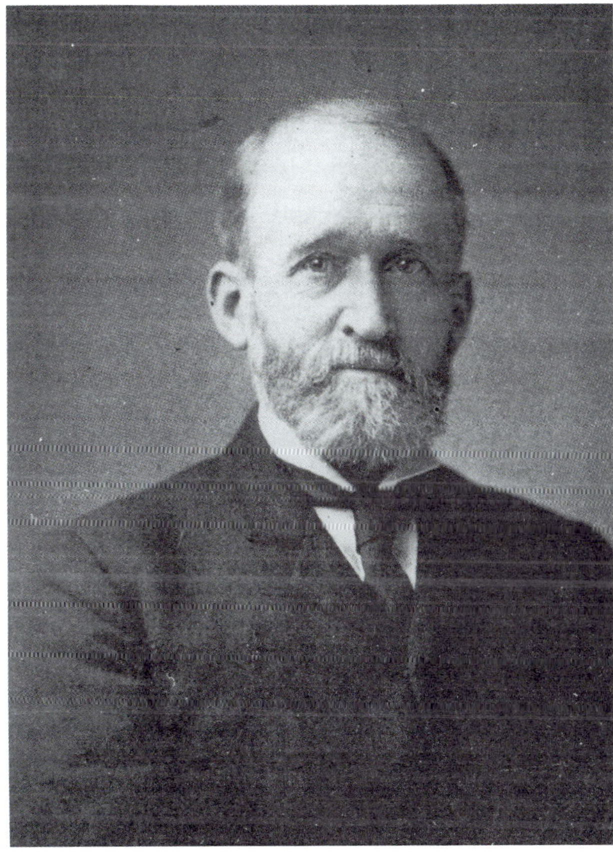

Fig. 49-14. James W. Holland, M.D., Fourteenth Dean (1887–1916).

Dr. Holland received his medical training at Jefferson. Upon graduation in 1868 he returned to Louisville and engaged in practice. In 1872 he was elected to the Chair of Practice of Medicine and Clinical Medicine, University of Louisville, where he served for 13 years. In 1885 he was called to the Chair of Medical Chemistry and Toxicology at Jefferson. He was chosen Dean of the Faculty in 1887, in which capacity he served for 29 years until 1916. After a service of 27 years as Professor of Chemistry, he resigned and was elected Emeritus (1912). In 1913 Holland was honored with the Sc.D. degree.

His course of lectures was remarkable for the freshness and thoroughness of his chemical knowledge. He appeared fully abreast and even in advance of the general status of the science. He spoke as a master. His experiments and illustrations were often novel, spectacular, and generally successful, owing to the fact that every experiment of any moment was tried out immediately preceding its presentation. Attention was always directed toward the practical side of his subject and its relation to medicine.

His constant admonition to his associates in his Department was to teach "chemistry as applied to medicine," and not as a chemical profession. His enunciation was clear, his words well chosen and forcibly expressed, and his presentation such that he could easily and at all times hold the attention of his classes. His lectures on toxicology were fascinating. In them was reflected the advantage of his acquaintance with Professor Smith. Orfila, who was Professor Smith's master in toxicology, was the foremost authority on toxicology of his day. Temperamentally, Dr. Holland was tranquil, and during most trying moments he gave no outward evidence of displeasure. He had many rare preserved specimens and toxicological preparations, some of which were 50 years old.

During his incumbency he had the pleasure of directing the development of the teaching in the chemical laboratory from a most elementary to a very respected clinical and physiological course. At the end of his final lecture in chemistry, the Class of 1915 presented him with a token of remembrance in the form of a magnificent facsimile of the original "Victoire de Pompei," symbolic of the "Crowning Glory" of a long and useful career.

Dr. Holland served as editor of the *Medical News*. He was a member of the College of Physicians of Philadelphia, the American Philosophical Society, and the Council of Medicine of the American Medical Association from 1907 to 1916.

Among his writings were the following: *Diet for the Sick; Common Poisons and the Urine; Inorganic Poisons; Medical Chemistry and Toxicology;* and many papers and contributions on medical subjects. A portrait of Holland hangs in the Dean's office suite, but the famous one by Thomas Eakins, called *The Roll Call* (1899), belongs to the Boston Museum of Art. A copy of the latter hangs in Jefferson's Eakin Gallery.

Ross V. Patterson, M.D., Sc.D., LL.D.; Fifteenth Dean (1916–1938)

Dr. Ross Vernet Patterson (Figure 49–15), Dean of Jefferson and Assistant Professor of Medicine, was born in New Orleans, Louisiana, October 5, 1877. His mother was Marguerite Jeanne Vernet, whose maternal ancestry was Scottish and paternal inheritance was French, the Vernet family having included artists and soldiers who sought refuge in Louisiana during the French Revolution. Patterson's father was John Harrison Patterson of Illinois, whose lineage went back to the Colonial period of American history. Ross Patterson's childhood and early life were spent in the South and West (Louisiana, Illinois, Missouri, Kansas, and Colorado). On the Western plains, as a small boy, he saw the Wild West disappear: the cattle trails fade, the cowboys ride away, and the buffalo vanish. Early in life he had decided to study medicine—a great-grandfather had practiced in New York City. His preliminary education was obtained in various schools—common school courses in Colorado Springs, college preparatory work begun in Central College, Missouri, and completed in Chenet's Institute, New Orleans, Louisiana. He then entered Washington University in St. Louis and completed two years, after which he matriculated at Jefferson and graduated as Class

Orator in 1904. During his preparatory studies he played on the football and tennis teams and was captain of the baseball team.

Two years following graduation were spent in residence at the Philadelphia Hospital, in which he served as Intern, Assistant Physician to the Department for the Insane, and Assistant Chief Resident Physician.

Dr. Patterson was appointed Subdean at Jefferson in 1906 and Dean in 1916, serving until his death in 1938. He taught in the Department of Medicine from 1906 to 1927, and was Physician in Charge of the Department of Electrocardiography. In May 1934 he was appointed Sutherland M. Prevost Professor of Therapeutics.

Dr. Patterson served as President of the Medical Society of the State of Pennsylvania (1930–1931) and President of the Association of American Medical Colleges (1933–1935). Although the Presidency of the Jefferson Alumni Association is ordinarily for a term of one year, Dr. Patterson served for three (1923–1925). His portrait was presented to the College by Alumni in 1930. He was awarded Sc.D. degrees by LaSalle College (1931) and Colgate University (1932), and LL.D. degrees were bestowed by Ursinus College (1935) and Wake Forest College (1937). A strong, often uncompromising administrator, his term as Dean covered World War I, the Great Depression, and a period of great change in the teaching and practice of medicine. He left his estate to Jefferson to establish Ross V. Patterson Fellowships in Research.

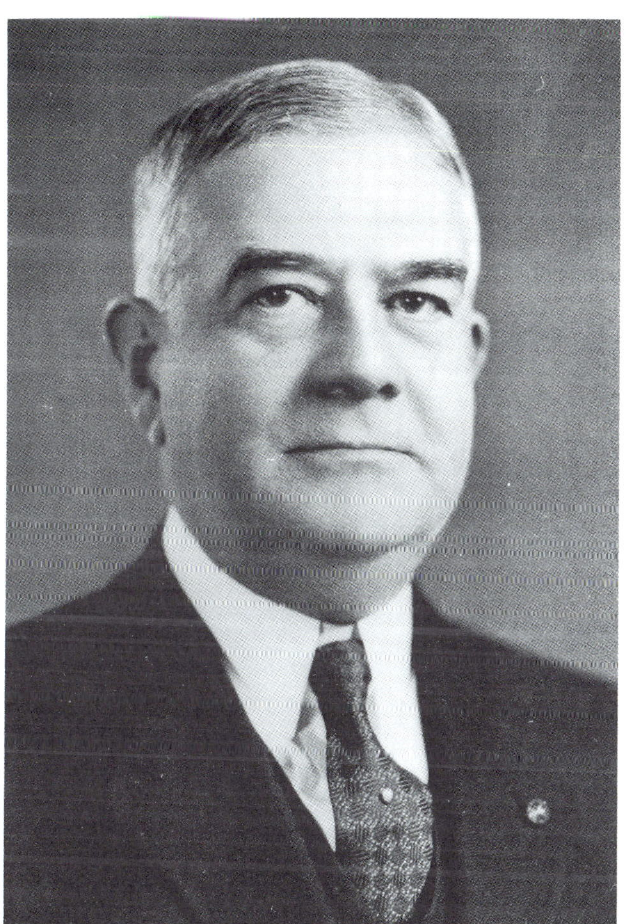

FIG. 49-15. Ross V. Patterson, M.D., Sc.D., LL.D., Fifteenth Dean (1916–1938).

Henry Keller Mohler, M.D., Sc.D.; Sixteenth Dean (1938–1941)

Henry Keller Mohler (Figure 49–16) was born April 2, 1887, in Ephrata, Pennsylvania. He attended the public schools and was graduated from the Ephrata High School in 1904. That same year he entered the Philadelphia College of Pharmacy, from which he received a Pharm.D. degree in 1907 and stood as first man in his class. Next he entered Jefferson and received his degree in 1912. He was President of his senior class and was voted its "most popular man."

After serving his internship in Jefferson Hospital, Dr. Mohler was placed in charge of the Laboratory of Clinical Medicine until 1914 and while still on that post was named Instructor in Medicine. He rose through the ranks to Clinical Professor of Medicine in 1936. In June 1938 he was elevated to the position of Sutherland M. Prevost Professor of Therapeutics. In 1939 he served as President of Jefferson Alumni Association. An Honorary degree, Doctor of Science, was conferred on him by LaSalle College.

Dr. Mohler served as Medical Director of the Jefferson Hospital from 1914 to 1938, during which time he was in immediate contact with the affairs of both College and Hospital. In 1918 he served as

Lieutenant-Colonel in World War I in France with U.S. Base Hospital No. 38. He returned in 1919.

He was elected Dean of Jefferson Medical College on August 1, 1938, and served in this capacity until his death on May 16, 1941.

William Harvey Perkins, M.D., Sc.D., LL.D.; Seventeenth Dean (1941–1950)

Dean Perkins (Figure 49–17) was born in Philadelphia on October 21, 1894. He was a graduate of Central High School and received his M.D. from Jefferson in 1917. After an internship in Jefferson Medical College Hospital, he went to France in 1918 as First Lieutenant, Medical Corps, U.S. Army, Base Hospital No. 120, Tours, France.

Dr. Perkins held a Fellowship in the Rockefeller Foundation (1924–1926), and went to Siam (now Thailand) in 1926 as Professor of Medicine at Chulalangkarana University, Bangkok. At the same time he was physician to the Siamese Government and in 1930 received the Order of the White Elephant from the King of Siam. He then returned to the United States and was appointed Instructor in Medicine at Tulane University. From 1931 he held the Chair of Preventive Medicine at Tulane.

Perkins' specialty was Preventive Medicine, and he held the following offices: President, Tuberculosis and Public Health Association of Louisiana; Chairman, New Orleans Mental Hygiene Association; President, Louisiana Mental Hygiene Association; Chairman, Health Division of the Council of Social Agencies of New Orleans; Representative Director of the National Tuberculosis Association; Chairman, Social Hygiene Section, Louisiana Parent Teachers Association; and Past Vice-Chairman of the Section of Public Health of the American Medical Association (1933). He was a member of the New Orleans Academy of Sciences, the Synthesis Club (philosophical), and Theta Kappa Psi and Alpha

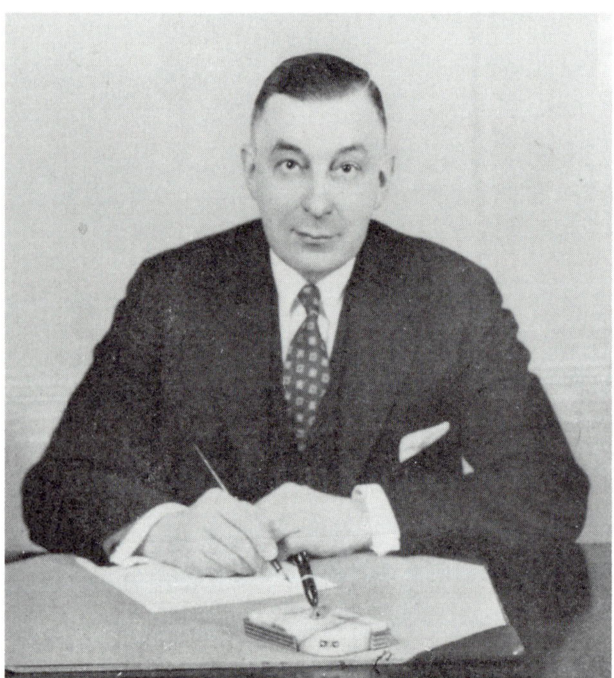

FIG. 49-16. Henry K. Mohler, M.D., Sc.D., Sixteenth Dean (1938–1941).

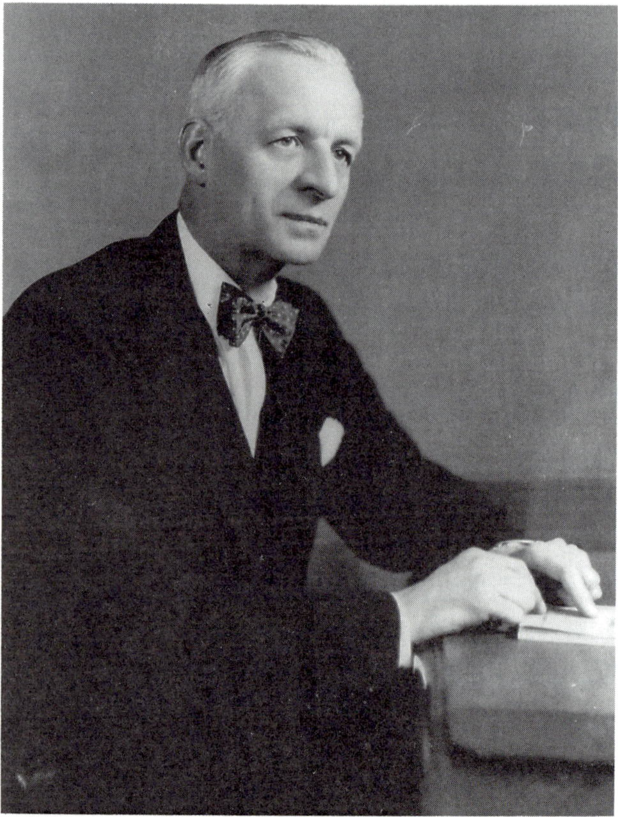

FIG. 49-17. William Harvey Perkins, M.D., Sc.D., LL.D., Seventeenth Dean (1941–1950).

Omega Alpha Fraternities. He came to Jefferson as Dean and Professor of Preventive Medicine in September, 1941, serving during the difficult years of World War II. Due to illness, he retired as Dean on November 6, 1950.

Dr. Perkins authored numerous papers on public health problems and preventive medicine, and a book, published in 1938, entitled *Cause and Prevention of Disease*. He served as President of the Alumni Association in 1945. His Class of 1917 presented his portrait to the College in 1951. He was awarded the Sc.D. degree from Franklin and Marshall College and the LL.D. degree from Dickinson College. One of the rooms in the Kellow Conference Area (on the second floor of the College Building) was named in his honor in 1977.

George Allen Bennett, M.D., Sc.D., LL.D.; Eighteenth Dean (1950–1958)

There is uniform agreement among the students instructed by George Allen Bennett (Figure 49–18) as teacher of anatomy in the amphitheaters and dissecting room of the Daniel Baugh Institute of Anatomy at Eleventh and Clinton Streets that this Professor was among the best teachers they had ever had. Not only was he effective in making the material clearly understandable, but his booming voice carried to all corners of the largest room. He was perceived as being committed, dedicated, very bright, well prepared, insistent, courteous, and a strong motivator. His phenomenal memory is cited frequently and ranks highly among anecdotes shared at Jefferson alumni reunions. He memorized the names, schools, and selected personal history of each member of the entering class in association with their pictures supplied with the entrance papers. He never referred to notes, and when he called on a student he addressed him by name and could even remember where he had sat the previous day. He would remember names years later when graduates returned for visits. When he became Dean, Jefferson lost one of its finest teachers. Dr. Bennett's educational background was unusual for his time, reflecting his own avid search for knowledge and his later skill in inspiring students. A Phi Beta Kappa graduate of Wabash College in Indiana, a Ben Hur Scholarship took him to the University of Athens, Greece (1923), and then to the University of Zürich, where he studied ancient history and archaeology. This was followed by a five-year study of philosophy and medicine at the University of Munich. In 1928 he received the rank of Artzt (physician). After fellowships at Baylor University College of Medicine and Harvard University, he returned to Munich for six more months in anatomic research in 1929. In 1930 he was appointed Professor of Histology at Georgetown Medical School, also serving for a time as Acting Head of the Department of Biology at Georgetown University. In 1934 he returned to Munich, where he conducted research

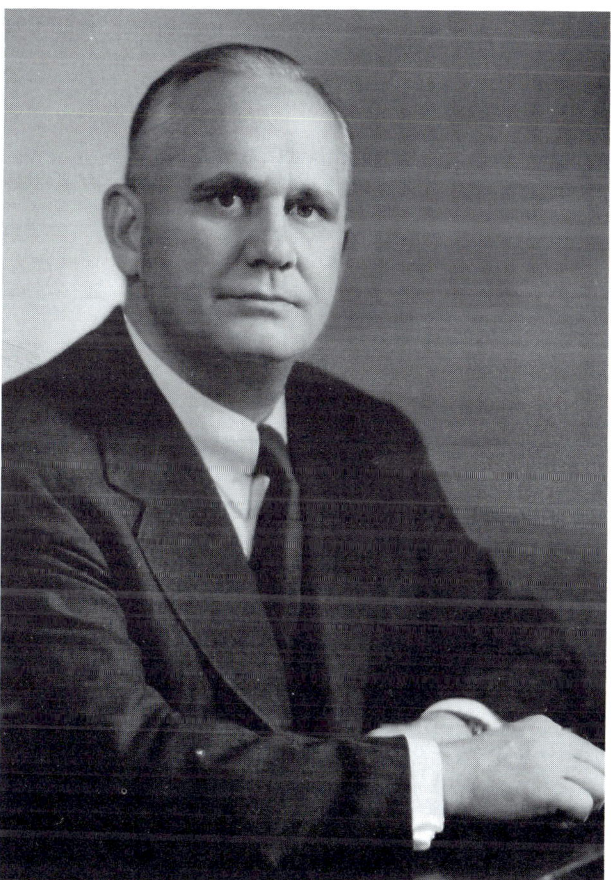

FIG. 49-18. George Allen Bennett, M.D., Sc.D., LL.D., Eighteenth Dean (1950–1958).

and multiple studies in dermatology, anatomy, and thoracic surgery. Lifelong interest in the musculature of the tongue followed. His thesis in 1937 resulted in the award of the degree of Doctor of Medicine *summa cum laude* from the University of Munich. He joined the Department of Anatomy at Jefferson in 1939.

Dr. Bennett quickly demonstrated his superb teaching skills and was promoted in rank until he succeeded Dr. J. Parsons Schaeffer as Chairman of Anatomy in 1948. The students dedicated their yearbook to him in 1944. For 15 years he taught applied and surgical anatomy to the medical officers of the Army and Navy, for which he received the "Consultant's Certificate of Merit" from the Armed Forces of the United States. He undertook many research projects including muscle-shoulder joint studies, for which he received (with Drs. Anthony F. DePalma and Gerald E. Callery) the gold medal of the American Academy of Orthopaedic Surgery in 1948.

Succeeding Dr. Perkins as Dean in 1950, Doctor Bennett displayed exceptional competence, sagacity, and determination. In recognition of his academic stature and accomplishments, he received honors and degrees, including the Doctor of Science from St. Joseph's College (1951), Doctor of Laws from Temple University (1951), and Doctor of Science from Dickinson College (1955) and Grove City College (1956). A bronze medal, "The Order of Carlos Finlay" was presented to him by the government of Cuba in recognition and appreciation of his role in the Centennial celebrations (1955) of the graduation of Carlos Finlay from Jefferson. The Wabash College Alumni Award of Merit was given to Doctor Bennett in 1951. Through his premature death, however, he failed to receive an honorary degree that he would have cherished—this was scheduled for presentation on June 11, 1958, by Wabash College, but he died February 27, 1958, at age 53 while attending the meeting of the Council on Medical Education and Licensure in Chicago. His portrait was presented to the College by the Board of Trustees in 1959.

William Anthony Sodeman, M.D., Sc.D., L.H.D.; Nineteenth Dean (1958–1967)

Dr. William A. Sodeman (Figure 49–19) came to Jefferson as Chairman of the Department of Medicine in 1957 but served only one year before succeeding Dr. Bennett as Dean. He brought exceptional talents to his new tasks, and his accomplishments during the next nine years reflected his breadth of concept, medical knowledge, analytical skills, and ability to arrive at balanced decisions quickly. He had been acquainted with Dr. Perkins at Tulane and succeeded him as Professor of Preventive Medicine there in 1941.

Dr. Sodeman was a native of Charleroi, Pennsylvania, and received his B.S. and M.D. degrees from the University of Michigan. His experience at Tulane began in 1932 following internship at St. Vincent's Hospital, Toledo, Ohio. He progressed in Medicine, Public Health, and Tropical Medicine to Chairman of Tropical Medicine and Public Health (1946–1953). From

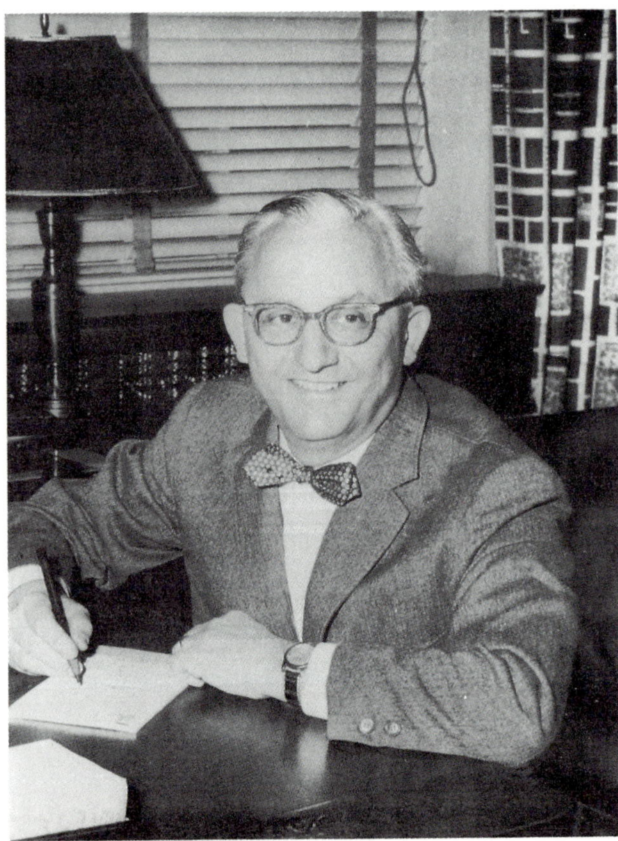

FIG. 49-19. William A. Sodeman, M.D., Sc.D., L.H.D., Nineteenth Dean (1956–1967).

1953 to 1957 he served as Chairman of the Department of Internal Medicine at the School of Medicine, University of Missouri.

Upon assuming the Jefferson Deanship, Dr. Sodeman had already become an internationally recognized medical educator. During his early career he had developed into a well-rounded internist and consultant beginning with fellowships in New Orleans and at the University of Michigan during the 1930s that encompassed cardiology, tropical medicine, and preventive medicine. He became Senior Visiting Physician at Charity Hospital and in 1951–1952 was Visiting Professor of Medical Sciences at Calcutta School of Tropical Medicine. Later he was Consultant to the United States Public Health Service Hospital, Carville, Louisiana, and to the Bureau of Special Services, U.S. Public Health Service, Washington, D.C. He was also an official examiner for the American Board of Internal Medicine.

Sodeman served on several Boards of Trustees and had membership in numerous medical societies. He published over 200 articles in the medical literature and was author of the textbook *Pathologic Physiology,* which was translated into several foreign languages. He belonged to several prestigious clubs and the following fraternities: Phi Beta Pi, Phi Beta Kappa, Alpha Omega Alpha, and Delta Omega. He was on the editorial boards of the American Journal of Cardiology (1964–1970) and the Journal of Laboratory and Clinical Medicine (1957–1960). He received the Shaffrey Medal at St. Joseph's College of Philadelphia for Distinguished Contribution to Medical Science (1962) and the University of Michigan Sesquicentennial Award (1967). Villanova University awarded him the Honorary Degree of Doctor of Science in 1959, and Jefferson bestowed the Doctor of Humane Letters Degree in 1967.

Dean Sodeman felt that faculty *esprit* needed strengthening and arranged several faculty retreats off campus where in-depth discussions took place on such matters as curriculum changes, student evaluation, graduate school development, hospital activities relating to academics, and relationships with affiliated hospitals. Resolution of differences and a team approach carried over into regular meetings. The faculty felt a new sense of direction and greater participation in final decision making.

National board examinations were introduced as an aid in evaluating Jefferson students and comparing their performance with medical students in other schools. A solid program of continuing medical education was begun for practicing physicians, at first in conjunction with Pennsylvania State University, which had continuing education offices across the Commonwealth. Later, Jefferson alone conducted programs in Delaware and at home. A medical accelerated program was initiated with Penn State whereby highly selected high school graduates could in five calendar years obtain the B.S. and M.D. degrees, thereby shortening the usual process by three years. This program became very successful.

Women medical students were admitted to Jefferson for the first time in 1961. Alumni of Jefferson Medical College were given memberships on the Board of Trustees. Research was encouraged and increased. Jefferson began receiving more national attention both as a result of its programs and because Dean Sodeman was prominent in major medical educational activities. He served for ten years on the Council on Medical Education, and for four years (two years as Chairman) on the medical school accreditation body (the Liaison Committee on Medical Education). The size of Jefferson's first-year class rose from 175 in 1958 to 192 in 1967. Curricular changes involved large blocks of elective time while still requiring a core of basic studies. Under Dean Sodeman's vision and leadership, Jefferson enhanced its image.

William Francis Kellow, M.D., D.Sc., L.H.D.; Twentieth Dean (1967–1981)

Dean Kellow (Figure 49–20) arrived at Jefferson after having been Dean at Hahnemann Medical College for six years. His tenure at Jefferson lasted for 14 years and would undoubtedly have lasted longer if serious illness had not forced his retirement. Only two Jefferson Deans were in office longer (Holland, 29 years, and Patterson, 22 years) and one (Dunglison) served for the same length of time as Dean Kellow.

Dean Kellow was a well-organized and hard

worker. It seemed that no matter how early his assistants arrived at their desks he was already in his office. He jealously guarded the hours before the normal workday began and used this time for uninterrupted concentration and accomplishment. He was serious, sensitive, kind, orderly, dedicated, systematic, gentlemanly, humble, and self-restrained. His demeanor suggested patience and calm, but on occasion he could become visibly annoyed and insistent. He was often heard to say that some causes are worth dying for, some not. He had excellent ability at a meeting in maintaining order and stimulating productivity. As a strong administrator, he knew how to delegate responsibility, monitor unobtrusively, and give back-up support.

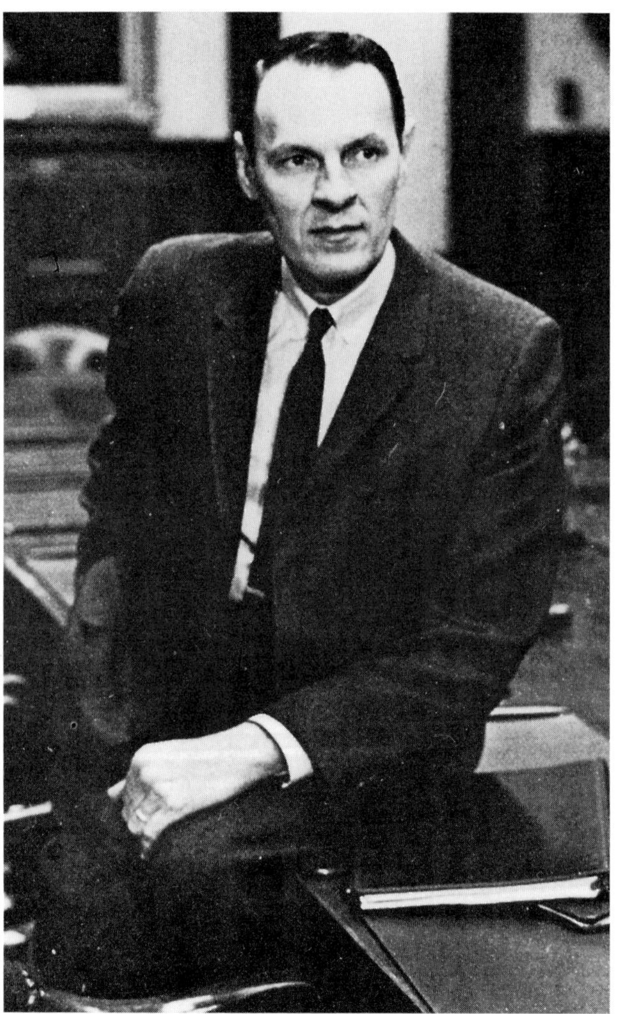

FIG. 49-20. William F. Kellow, M.D., D.Sc., L.H.D., Twentieth Dean (1967–1981).

Born in Geneva, New York, on March 14, 1922, Kellow received the B.S. degree from the University of Notre Dame in 1943 and the M.D. degree from Georgetown School of Medicine in 1946. Honorary degrees included the D.Sc. from St. Joseph's University in Philadelphia (1967) and from Georgetown School of Medicine (1979), and Doctor of Humane Letters from Hahnemann Medical College (1978).

His postgraduate training was mostly at the District of Columbia General Hospital: Intern (1946–1947), Assistant Medical Resident (1947–1948), Senior Medical Resident (1949–1950), and Chief Resident in Pulmonary Diseases (1950–1951). He was Assistant Surgical Resident at Georgetown Hospital (1948–1949) and a Captain in the U.S. Air Force Medical Corps (1951–1953).

At Georgetown School of Medicine, Dr. Kellow was Clinical Instructor in Surgery (1947–1948) and Clinical Instructor in Medicine (1948–1953). At the University of Illinois College of Medicine he was Clinical Instructor in Medicine (1953–1955), Assistant Professor of Medicine (1955–1959), Assistant Dean (1955–1959), Associate Professor of Medicine (1959–1961), and Associate Dean (1959–1961). He was Dean and Professor of Medicine at Hahnemann Medical College (1961–1967) and Dean and Professor of Medicine at Jefferson Medical College (1967–1981).

Some of his awards and honors included: Centennial of Science Award, University of Notre Dame, 1965; Mastership, Alpha Omega Alpha, Jefferson Medical College, 1978; first recipient, Winged Ox of St. Luke Award for Distinguished Service, Thomas Jefferson University, 1981; and Alumni Achievement Award, Jefferson Medical College, 1981. His portrait was commissioned both by the Hahnemann Medical College and Alumni Association of Jefferson Medical College (1978). He belonged to many medical and scientific societies and participated in several influential local and national extramural professional activities. Some of these included: Board of Trustees, Eastern Pennsylvania Psychiatric Institute (1962–1969); Regional Comprehensive Health Planning Committee, City of Philadelphia (1969–1971);

Board of Trustees, Educational Commission for Foreign Medical Graduates, Philadelphia (1970–1980); General Research Support Program Advisory Committee, National Institutes of Health (1971–1974); Board of Regents, American College of Physicians (1970–1976); Advisory Committee on Undergraduate Medical Education, American Medical Association (1974–1980, and Chairman, 1977–1980); Liaison Committee on Medical Education, American Medical Association and Association of American Medical Colleges (1974–1981, and Chairman, 1981); and Council on Medical Education, American Medical Association (1979–1981).

Dean Kellow had outstanding managerial skills; in particular, he was proficient in handling fiscal matters. He kept a tight rein on the College budget, avoided deficit spending, and proportioned funding wisely and prudently to maintain and improve programs and to support new activities. Financial facility assumed even greater importance when, two years after his Deanship began, Thomas Jefferson University was formed and Jefferson Medical College became one of the component parts.

Kellow gave the faculty a feeling of greater democracy by providing increased opportunities for faculty participation in decision making, both in existing procedures and in developing new directions. He formed a General Faculty and Professorial Faculty to create a forum where individuals could be heard. A set of bylaws was developed that for the first time allowed membership on committees by the faculty at large; previously, only Chairmen of Departments could sit on most committees of the College. An Annual Report from the Dean's Office was prepared and given wide distribution, making quickly available current information on the functioning of the various aspects of the Medical College. With the help of the faculty he developed a Medical Practice Plan that allowed a balance between private practice and academic responsibilities.

Many changes and new programs developed during Dean Kellow's long tenure. The size of the entering first-year class rose from 192 to 223. This continued to qualify for federal per capita appropriations and also helped to increase the output of physicians in order to lessen the threat of a physician shortage in the country. To aid in the better distribution of future physicians, a Physician Shortage Area Program was begun in affiliation with Indiana University of Pennsylvania. Particular attention for a limited number of places in the class was paid to applicants from physician shortage communities in Pennsylvania who stated their desire to return to these areas and gave promise of doing so.

In order to increase heterogeneity of the student body and provide greater opportunity for underrepresented groups in medicine to gain admission and receive counseling as students, an Office of Minority Affairs was created, and a black Associate Dean (James H. Robinson, M.D.) was appointed to supervise this activity.

A Department of Family Medicine was created in 1973, and all students were required to spend a segment of their curricular time in this discipline. Two hospitals with strength in Family Medicine located in rural Pennsylvania were added as affiliates: Franklin Hospital in Franklin and Latrobe Area Hospital in Latrobe.

In partnership with the Delaware Institute of Medical Education and Research, the University of Delaware and Wilmington Medical Center, Jefferson established a program in 1970 funded by the legislature of Delaware to provide each year access of up to 20 qualified residents of Delaware to Jefferson's first-year class. Delaware had determined that it was too small to establish its own medical school but recognized the problem its residents had in gaining admission to medical schools since most schools received state appropriations and had to limit the number of out-of-state places in their classes.

He established an Office of Medical Education in 1968, as he had done while Associate Dean at the University of Illinois College of Medicine. The Jefferson office instituted a longitudinal study of Jefferson students that has attracted national attention and this made a significant contribution to medical education.

On December 4, 1981, the illness that the previous month had forced his retirement, took his life. At the time he left Jefferson a suite of rooms on the second floor of the College building was designated the Kellow Conference Center. Each of the six rooms was named after a Jefferson physician who had made an outstanding contribution to medical education.

Frank W. Gray, Jr., M.D.; Interim Dean (1981–1982)

To fill the vacancy in the Dean's Office, Dr. Frank W. Gray, Jr., Magee Professor and Chairman of the Department of Medicine, was named Interim Dean (Figure 49–21). Dr. Gray's administrative experience served well during the period from Nov., 1981 to July, 1982 while the search for a new Dean was in process.

Leah Lowenstein, M.D., D.Phil.; Twenty-first Dean (1982–1983)

The first women medical students matriculated at Jefferson in September, 1961. Jefferson thereby became the last all-male Medical School to become coeducational. Dr. Lowenstein (Figure 49–22) was the first woman to become a Dean at Jefferson and the first woman Dean of a coeducational medical school in the United States; during her tenure she was the only woman Dean of a medical school in this country. Her Deanship lasted from July 1, 1982, to September 1, 1983, when she resigned for health reasons. She died of cancer on March 6, 1984, at age 53.

A native of Milwaukee, Wisconsin, Dr. Lowenstein received her M.D. degree from the University of Wisconsin in 1954 and completed an internship at the University of Wisconsin

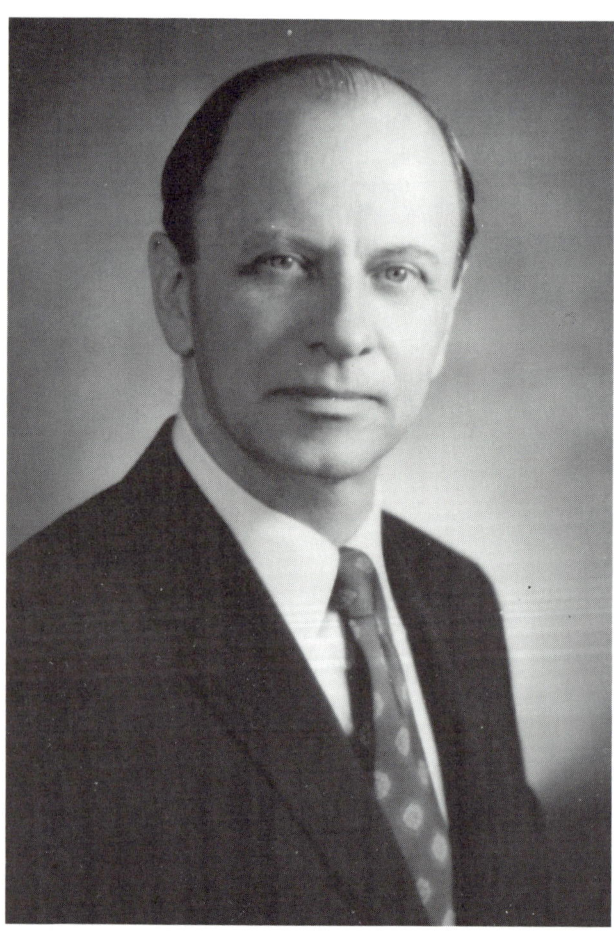

FIG. 49-21. Frank W. Gray, Jr., M.D., Interim Dean (1981–1982).

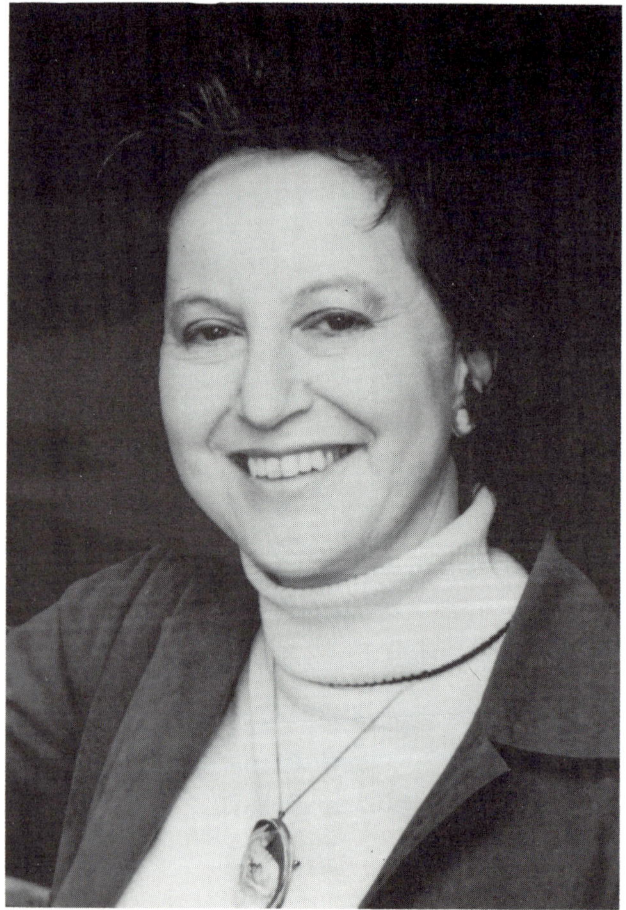

FIG. 49-22. Leah Lowenstein, M.D., D.Phil., Twenty-first Dean (1982–1983).

Hospital. For three years she was a research associate in the Department of Anatomy (Biophysics) at Oxford University in England and received her D.Phil. degree through Summerville College in 1958. Returning to the United States, she completed a residency in Internal Medicine at Beth Israel Hospital of the Harvard Medical School and a fellowship in renal and metabolic diseases at the Veterans Administration Hospital, Tufts University School of Medicine. She served on the faculty of Tufts and Thorndike Memorial Laboratories at Harvard Medical School. In 1968 she was appointed Assistant Professor of Medicine at Boston University School of Medicine and, at the time of her selection as Dean of Jefferson, was Professor of Medicine and Biochemistry and Associate Dean at this school.

Dr. Lowenstein held several key hospital appointments in Boston including Attending Physician at University Hospital, Boston University School of Medicine; Physician-in-Chief, Medical Service, Boston City Hospital; Medical Director of the Alcohol Research Unit of Harvard Medical School and Boston City Hospital; and Director of Basic and Clinical Sciences of the Gerontology Center and Director of the Unit of Metabolic Nephrology at Boston University School of Medicine. She was also medical advisor in the Office of the Assistant Secretary for Health of the former Department of Health, Education and Welfare (1978–1979).

Lowenstein was a member of the Academy of Sciences and a Fellow of the American Association for the Advancement of Science. A member of Phi Beta Kappa and Alpha Omega Alpha, she was honored at her alma mater, the University of Wisconsin, in 1983 with an award recognizing her "outstanding service to medicine and medical education."

Dr. Lowenstein published extensively on kidney and metabolic disorders and lectured throughout the nation and abroad. She was coeditor of *Becoming a Physician: Development of Values and Attitudes in Medicine* and coeditor and coauthor of *Mammalian Models for Research on Aging*.

Selected for the Deanship after a nationwide search that included 177 nominees, Lowenstein was identified as an experienced administrator and teacher and was highly respected as a superb investigator in the field of kidney disease. It was felt that she would continue Jefferson's traditional commitment to excellence in medical education, research, and patient care. Her background, accomplishments, and outgoing personality gave great promise. Unfortunately, health problems shortened her tenure to but one year and little can be accomplished in such a short span of time. She believed that Jefferson needed strengthening in the quality and quantity of its research and wanted the institution to become more successful in competing for the limited amounts of extramural support in this area.

Joseph S. Gonnella, M.D.; Twenty-second Dean (1984–)

Joseph Salvatore Gonnella, M.D. (Figure 49–23) became the Dean of Jefferson Medical College on May 7, 1984. He had been Acting Dean since September 1 of the previous year, Associate Dean from 1969 to 1983, and Assistant Dean from 1967 to 1969. He was the first member of the Dean's office staff to rise through the ranks to full Dean.

Born on April 5, 1934, in Pescopagano, Italy, Gonnella moved to this country at age 12 with his family. His early education was in his hometown in Italy, then in public schools in Westfield, New Jersey. His undergraduate college was Dartmouth (B.A., 1956, *summa cum laude,* Phi Beta Kappa) and for his medical education he attended Dartmouth Medical School (1955–1957) and Harvard Medical School (1959, Alpha Omega Alpha). Postgraduate training as an Intern and Resident in Internal Medicine took place at the University of Illinois Research and Educational Hospitals (1959–1961 and 1963–1965). It is interesting that during the first phase of his residency he became acquainted with the Attending Physician there, Dr. William F. Kellow, who became Jefferson's twentieth Dean in 1967; a mutual regard was a determining factor in the direction of Dr. Gonnella's professional career. Dr. Gonnella's residency was interrupted for two years (1961–1963) when he served as Captain in the Medical Corps of the U.S. Army. In the first year of this period he was assigned to a medical detachment in Korea, where he met his wife,

Margaret Linda Rapp, who was serving there with the Red Cross. In 1963 he returned as Resident in Internal Medicine at the University of Illinois Research and Education Hospitals and was Chief Resident the next year (1964–1965).

The year following his residency (1965–1966), Dr. Gonnella became a Fellow and Research Associate in the Office of Research in Medical Education, University of Illinois College of Medicine. The very next year he was appointed Assistant Dean at Hahnemann Medical College, Philadelphia, under Dr. Kellow, who had become Dean in 1961. The same year, upon Dr. Kellow's appointment as Dean at Jefferson, Dr. Gonnella joined him as Assistant Dean and Assistant Professor of Medicine. The Department of Medicine quickly recognized his teaching talents as he progressed to Professor of Medicine. In the Dean's Office, he advanced from Assistant Dean, through Associate Dean, Acting Dean, and finally Dean and Vice President in 1984. In addition, he had been since 1969 Director of the Office of Medical Education (now Center for Research in Medical Education and Health Care), which has been conducting an impressive longitudinal study of Jefferson students, as well as other significant studies. He has taught medical students and house staff, been counselor and financial aid officer to medical students, been responsible for curriculum evaluation and development and for guidance and letters of recommendation for Jefferson students for postgraduate training, served on and chaired many faculty committees, and has been prominent in extramural, local, national, and international activities. For years he had been highly visible to Jefferson's Board of Trustees, Senior Officers, Department Chairmen and other faculty, nonprofessional personnel, and students. Gonnella's proven competence generated enthusiasm widely, but particularly among the faculty, at the time of his candidacy for the Deanship. He was identified as being a "known quantity" and was selected with confidence.

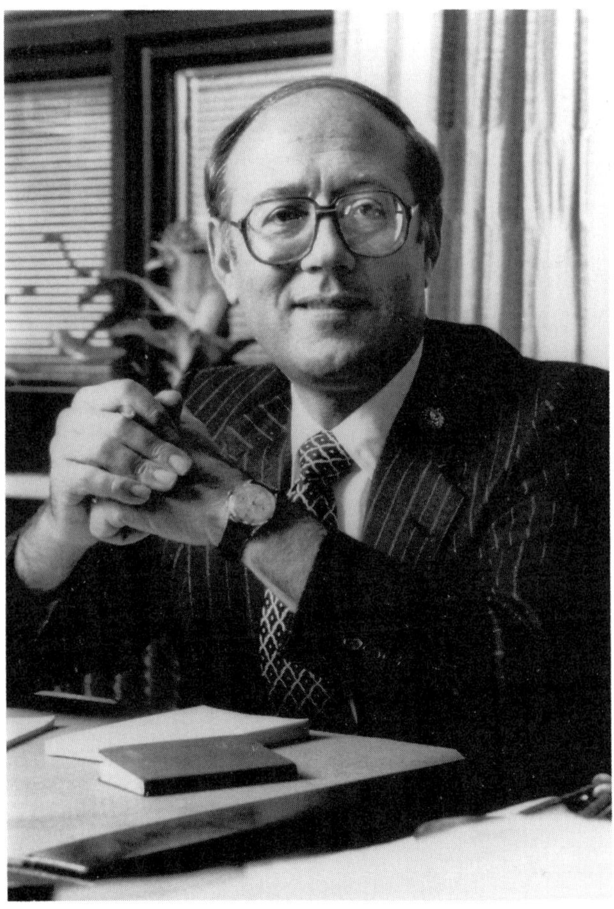

FIG. 49-23. Joseph S. Gonnella, M.D., Twenty-second Dean (1984–).

Dr. Gonnella's extramural professional activities have been extensive and include advisory, consultant, membership, and chairmanship duties in the following: Alliance for Continuing Medical Education, American Board of Medical Specialties, American Medical Association, Association of American Medical Colleges, Department of Health and Human Services, Educational Commission for Foreign Medical Graduates, Institute of Continuing Biomedical Education, Joint Commission on Accreditation of Hospitals, Ministry of Health (People's Republic of China), National Board of Medical Examiners, Philadelphia College of Physicians, Philadelphia Professional Standards Review Organization, State of California's Department of Health and the World Health Organization (Certificate of Appreciation); University of Chieti, Italy (Honorary Degree of Medicine), and Australasian and New Zealand Association for Medical Education (Guest Speaker). He is a member of a number of prestigious professional societies.

Dean Gonnella, in pursuing the goal of excellence, clearly recognizes that the objective of advancing Jefferson Medical College in its role of educating competent physicians requires careful handling of varied activities. As Dean he has responsibility for the administrative affairs of Jefferson Medical College, and as Vice President he has staff responsibility for many University service areas. Important among these is establishing criteria for selection of students that emphasize humane, caring attributes as well as academic qualifications—attention to student development regarding the social aspects of medicine, professional ethics, and skills in patient care is vital. Faculty matters relate to recruitment and development of superior teachers and assuring adequate time and facilities for both basic and clinical research. Also important is the maintenance of an appropriate balance among teaching, patient care, research, and administration on the part of faculty members. Dr. Gonnella has pursued these objectives effectively in his 20 years (1967–1987) and has contributed impressively to the institution's prestige. His relative youth is the potential for fruitful years that lie ahead.

Jefferson Medical College takes justifiable pride in the choice of its Deans and their accomplishments.

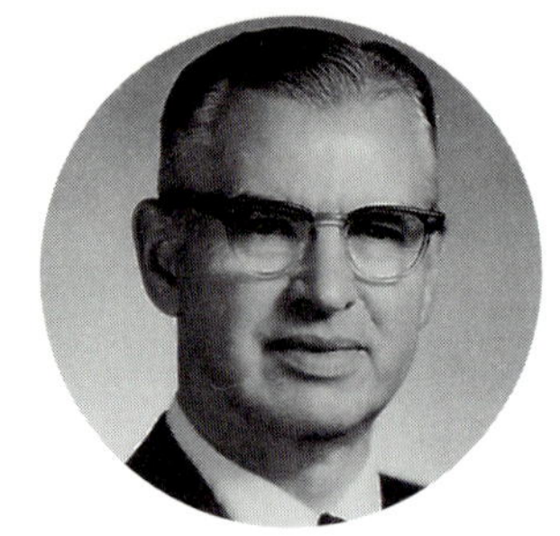

CHAPTER FIFTY

Hospital Administration

J. Woodrow Savacool, M.D.

"Hospitals are the outcome of the innate tenderness that marks all noble souls in whatever land they dwell and in whatever creed they are received."

—Sir Henry Burdett (1847–1920)

Hospitals have always existed in one form or another. Whether known by the name *hospital* or not, there have been places for the sick, poor, aged, and disabled since history was recorded. The origin of the hospital is credited by historians not to medical science but to religion. The Christian Church played a large part in the development of hospitals early in the Christian era, and, being associated with churches, administration became largely the responsibility of ecclesiastical personnel. From the sixteenth century the functions of hospitals expanded, and physicians came to be more intimately involved in such services and responsibilities. The hope for cure of disease as a reason for hospitals' existence is relatively recent. They began mainly to isolate infectious persons or for custodial and domiciliary care of the mentally ill and the chronically disabled. Physician administrators became more frequent during the nineteenth century, and by the beginning of the twentieth century they dominated the scene. The increasing complexity of services performed in hospitals, however, resulted in a need for delegated responsibilities, with eventual transfer of major duties to lay administrators.

At the time of the founding of Jefferson Medical College in 1824, there was no perceived need for a hospital as a component of the teaching process for medical students. The medical school functioned as a didactic teaching facility with instruction by lectures to which medical students added preceptorial experience. No American medical school had an affiliated hospital—the Hospital of the University of Pennsylvania, the first associated with a medical school, was not founded until 1874. (There were seven hospitals in all the United States in 1800 and only 87 in 1850).[1] From the beginning, however, Jefferson students experienced patient care through an outpatient dispensary for medical and surgical cases, which was George McClellan's radical and innovative contribution to medical education. To be sure, the Pennsylvania Hospital (founded in 1751) was available for certain aspects of teaching. Students of medicine were accommodated there by arrangement with their preceptors plus the payment of an annual fee, which in 1751 was £1. Hospital management at Pennsylvania was geared to care of the poor, the Board of Directors from the beginning having been elected by the contributors. The Directors were immediately responsible for management.[2] During the mid-nineteenth century, hospital practice slowly changed from almshouse and domiciliary care to accommodation of injured patients and surgical patients, although most surgery was still done in the home.

Jefferson patients were at first cared for only in the dispensary (the Tivoli Theater building and its successors) but soon the need for short-term admissions led to makeshift hospital facilities, mainly for the poor. A historical summary in the 1912 Hospital report states: "As the classes grew and demands for advance in methods became more evident, the facilities were extended until ten and later twenty patients could be temporarily housed, resting often on cots of the most temporary kind, and in quarters having no semblance to what now would be called a hospital. The nursing care was by volunteer assistants, mostly from the student body."[3] At the time, patients were being operated upon by distinguished surgeons connected with the College, and the custom was that those unable to reach their residences in other ways were taken home in the doctor's carriage. Some were cared for near the operating room by unpaid nurses and attendants, and food was obtained from a nearby restaurant or brought from the kitchens of the attending surgeons. It is obvious that during this period virtually no administration was required, and presumably the attending physicians and surgeons were totally responsible. Partly related to Civil War experiences was the gradually increasing awareness of the need for organized facilities. Action was taken at the instigation of the Alumni Association and the faculty during the early 1870s, and the first Jefferson Medical College Hospital building was opened in 1877 on Sansom Street between Tenth and Eleventh (the present site of Thompson Annex).

First Hospital Management (1877)

Administration of the first Hospital appears to have been the responsibility of the Board of Trustees with major delegation to the Medical Staff. The earliest report of the Trustees to the contributors to the Jefferson Medical College Hospital, dated 1881,[4] indicates an administrative arrangement whereby the Trustees had hospital committees designated for each month. At the time, the President of the Trustees was a physician, Emile Blaise Gardette, M.D. (Jefferson, 1838) and the first election of the Hospital Staff was made by the Board, March 28, 1877. In that report no hospital directors or administrators are listed. There was a steward, a housekeeper, and an engineer. These were responsible to the Board of Trustees. The close supervision of the Hospital by the Board continued into the 1890s, as noted in an 1891 publication of Rules and Regulations.[5] The Hospital Committee of three members was required to "visit the Hospital at least once every week . . . and receive reports of its condition, requirements, receipts and expenditures." The booklet also defines the status and duties of a Superintendent, although the identity of the Superintendent is not stated.

Some of the earlier functions of the Trustees appear to have been taken over by the Dean of the Medical College in the latter part of the century. The Hospital Report for the year ending September 30, 1893, includes a "Dean's Annual Report." At that time, administrative changes occurred with more management functions assumed by the faculty. Dr. Edward E. Montgomery, Professor of Gynecology, was named Superintendent and under him a layperson, George Bailey, Jr., was designated Assistant Superintendent. The same report describes the inauguration of the Training School for Nurses, established in 1891, with Miss Effie Darlene as Director. The title of Superintendent was replaced in 1894 when Dr. James C. Wilson (Jefferson, 1869), Professor of Medicine, was made Medical Director (Figure 50-1). George Bailey, Jr., continued his post as Assistant Superintendent. This administrative arrangement appears to have continued for the next few years, but in 1895 Dr. Joseph S. Neff was made Medical Director, and in 1897 George Bailey, Jr., was named Superintendent.

Joseph S. Neff, M.D.; Medical Director (1895)

Dr. Joseph S. Neff (Jefferson, 1875) may be described as a prototype of the modern hospital administrator, his areas of responsibility having extended well beyond those of the period (Figure 50-2). Educated at the University of Pennsylvania (B.A., 1873; M.A., 1877) and in Vienna with a year at the Allgemeines Krankenhaus, he was appointed Attending Physician at Jefferson in 1881. He was named to the same post at Philadelphia General Hospital in 1882. Impaired health caused his resignation from practice and hospital appointments in 1889. A year later he joined the firm of L.C. Vanuxem and Co. in a business appointment, during which time he appears to have developed his management skills. His medical career was resumed a few years later, and in 1895 he was made Medical Director of Jefferson Hospital. Dr. Neff made major contributions to the planning of the 1907 hospital, sharing committee duties with Trustees William Potter and Alba B. Johnson without the employment of a

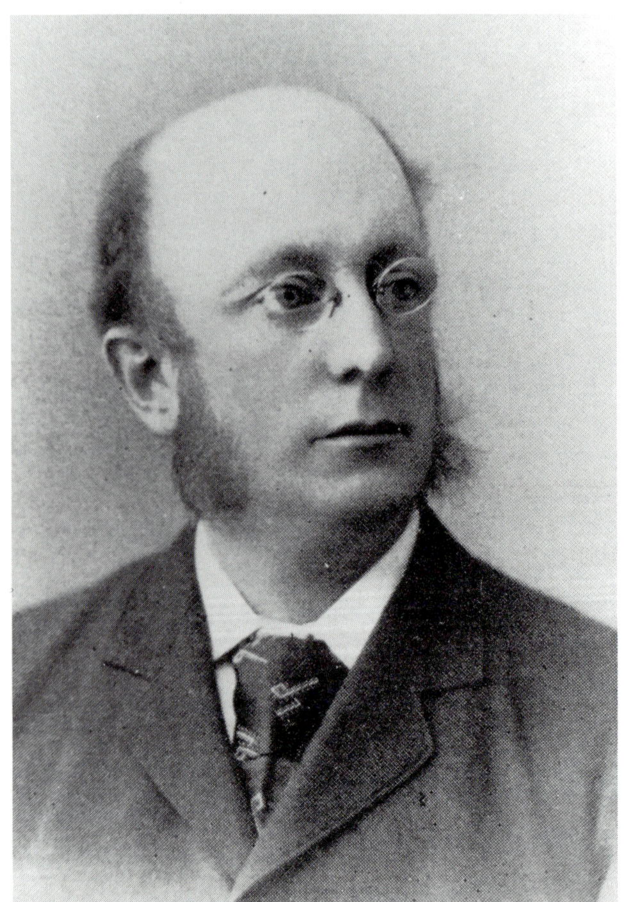

FIG. 50-1. James C. Wilson, M.D. (1847–1938), First Medical Director (1894–1895).

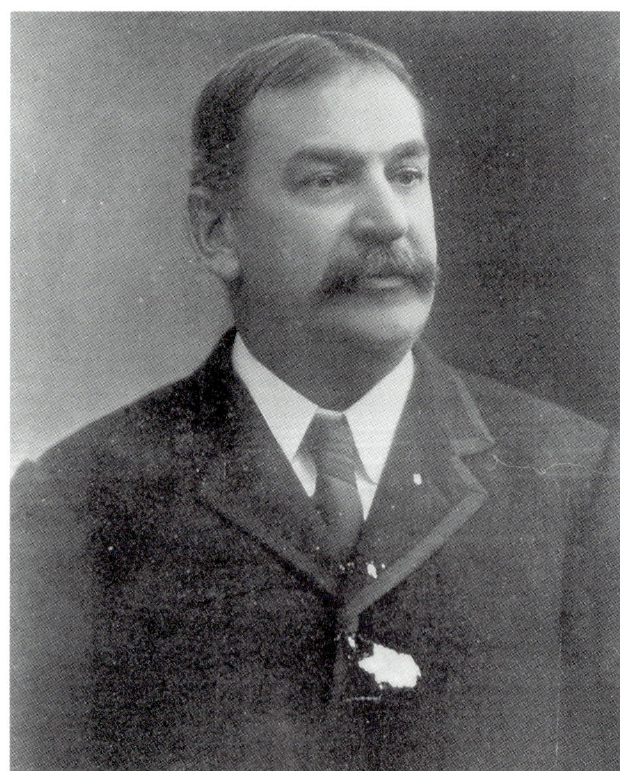

FIG. 50-2. Joseph S. Neff, M.A., M.D. (1854–1930), Medical Director (1895–1907).

(Jefferson, 1906), later to become Professor of Surgery (1930–1936), was made Chief Resident in 1908.

general contractor. His career changed again with his appointment as Director of the Department of Public Health and Charities of the City of Philadelphia in 1907, and he was named Emeritus Physician by the Jefferson Board of Trustees in 1909. Dr. Neff served as President of the Hospital Staff as well as Medical Director.

In 1900, during Dr. Neff's administration, a fire occurred in the 1877 Hospital building as a result of an explosion across the street. Dr. W.W. Keen reported in the *Philadelphia Medical Journal* the "Heroism of Nurses and Physicians in the Path of Duty." He described the excellent discipline that prevented fire-associated injury to any hospital patients and was highly complimentary, especially of the nurses' behavior.

William M.L. Coplin, M.D.; Medical Director (1907–1912)

The post of Medical Director continued as a part-time one until midcentury. Dr. Neff was succeeded in 1907 by Dr. William M.L. Coplin, Professor of Pathology since 1896 (Figure 50-3). Dr. Coplin was an able successor whose managerial skills had been proven by his recent experience as Director of the Department of Public Health and Charities for the City of Philadelphia. The first few weeks of his administration in the latter position (1905) had been marked by major exposure of neglect and graft in the operations of Philadelphia General Hospital. Increasing administrative responsibilities and decisions relative to the opening of the new Hospital in June 1907 (Old Main) were met with determination and success by Dr. Coplin, who continued his teaching and research in pathology without interruption and also served as President of the Medical Staff from 1908. The increased patient load also required increased numbers of resident physicians and new definition of their responsibilities. Previously numbering seven, 15 were now appointed. Dr. Edward J. Klopp

The Twentieth Century

The administrative pattern changed under Dr. Coplin. No Superintendent was named, but in 1909 John M. Smith was listed as Steward, later to be succeeded by Joseph W. Mott, who was in turn replaced by F.E. Jacob and, in 1913, by F.W. Sellick. This post was filled in 1914 by a Mr. D. Adams, who served for a number of years. Dr. Elmer H. Funk (Jefferson, 1908), who was Chief Resident Physician in 1910, became Acting Medical Director in 1912 (Figure 50-4), succeeding Dr. Coplin until Dr. McCrae appointed him Director of the new Department for Diseases of the Chest in 1913. In the latter post he was responsible to Dr. McCrae as Attending Physician and to the Board of Trustees for administration. Dr. Coplin continued as President of the Medical Staff until

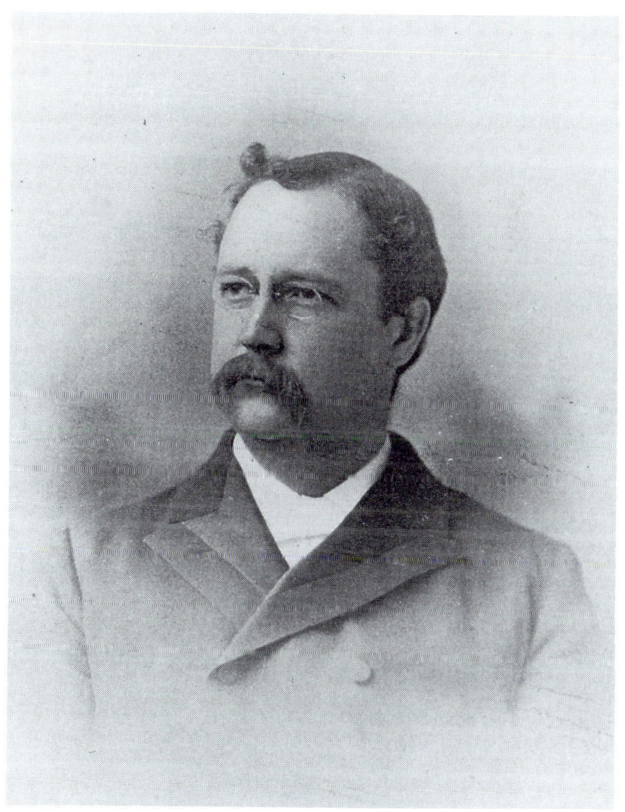

FIG. 50-3. William M.L. Coplin, M.D. (1864–1928), Medical Director (1907–1912).

1922, when he was replaced by Dr. Hobart A. Hare. Dr. Henry K. Mohler succeeded Dr. Funk as Acting Medical Director in 1914 and was named Medical Director the following year, serving in that capacity for many years.

Hospital administrative duties during the early decades of the twentieth century underwent some changes, although not nearly as remarkable as those that occurred after 1930. Primary responsibility continued to be vested in the Board of Trustees, and the operation of the Hospital was delegated largely to the Medical Director and his appointees, whereas the affairs of the Medical College were in the hands of the Dean whose responsibilities to medical students and faculty complemented the duties of the Hospital Medical Director in the provision of medical care.

There was a brief wartime period (1918–1919) when Dr. Elmer Funk was again called upon to serve as Medical Director, while Dr. Mohler was on active military duty as Lieutenant Colonel and Chief of Medical Services, U.S. Army General Hospital No. 38 in France.

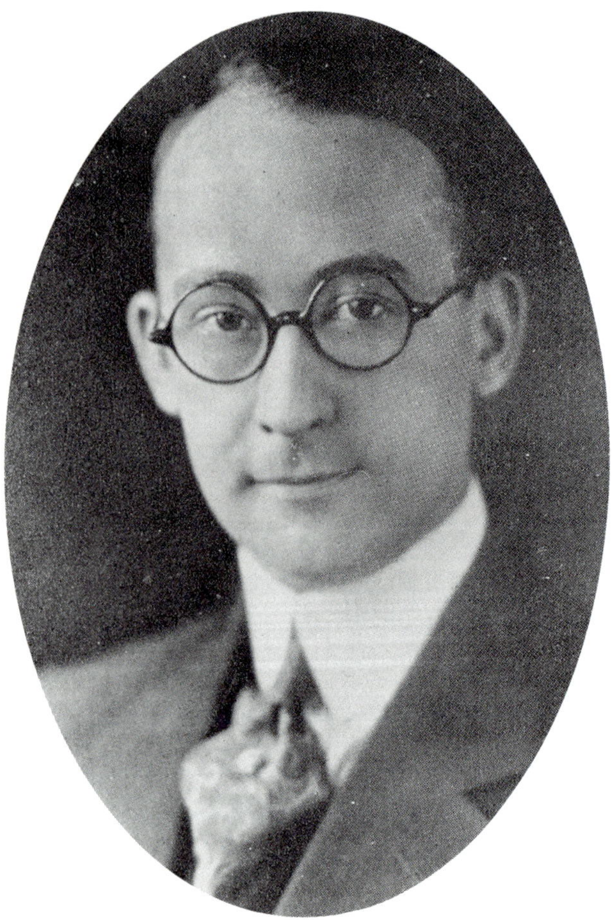

FIG. 50-4. Elmer H. Funk, M.D. (1886–1932), Acting Medical Director (1912–1914).

The Mohler Years (1914–1938)

Dr. Henry K. Mohler (Figure 50-5), a Jefferson honor graduate of 1912, soon demonstrated his leadership qualities as he assumed the post of Director, continuing in that capacity until he succeeded Ross V. Patterson as Dean in 1938. At the same time he advanced in the Departments of Medicine and Therapeutics, and as Dean he also was made Professor of Therapeutics in 1938. During his Directorship there was a rapid increase in the diversity of problems relative to hospital management which he coordinated well with his clinical career even while dealing with the strong medical personalities of the Jefferson Staff. There was perhaps no one who was as familiar with Jefferson affairs for three decades as Dr. Mohler. He was a charter member and Fellow of the American College of Hospital Administrators, a member of the American Hospital Association, and belonged to many local and national societies. He received an Honorary degree of Doctor of

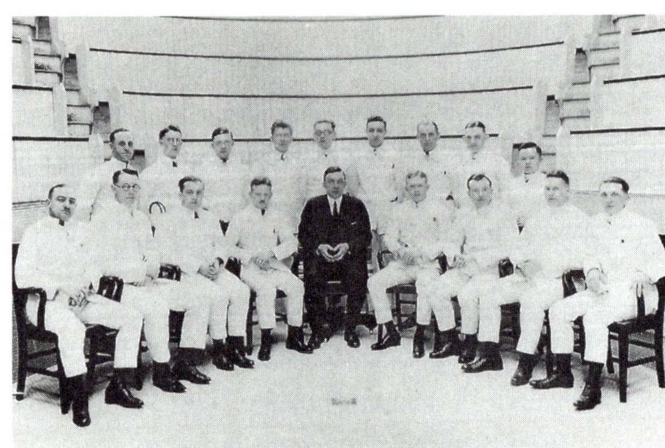

FIG. 50-5. Henry K. Mohler, M.D., D.Sc. (1885–1941), as Medical Director (1914–1938) with Interns in the amphitheater of the 1877 Hospital (ca. 1920).

Science from LaSalle College in 1939. The Class of 1940 presented his portrait to the College. His career as Dean was brief, ending with his sudden death in 1941.

The construction of the Thompson Annex in 1924 and the opening of the new College building and Curtis Clinic in 1931 provided many new challenges and experiences in administration. Dr. Mohler's continuity as Director during these changes proved useful. When the Curtis Clinic, Jefferson's new outpatient facility opened in 1931, it was directed at the outset by another bright, youthful clinician, Dr. Robert Bruce Nye (Jefferson, 1927). Dr. Nye (Figure 50-6) quickly adapted to the challenge of administrative duties, his success in the post resulting in his appointment to succeed Dr. Mohler as Medical Director of the Hospital in 1938 when the latter became Dean. His tenure was interrupted by World War II when Dr. Nye served as Lieutenant Colonel with the 38th General Hospital from 1942 to 1945.

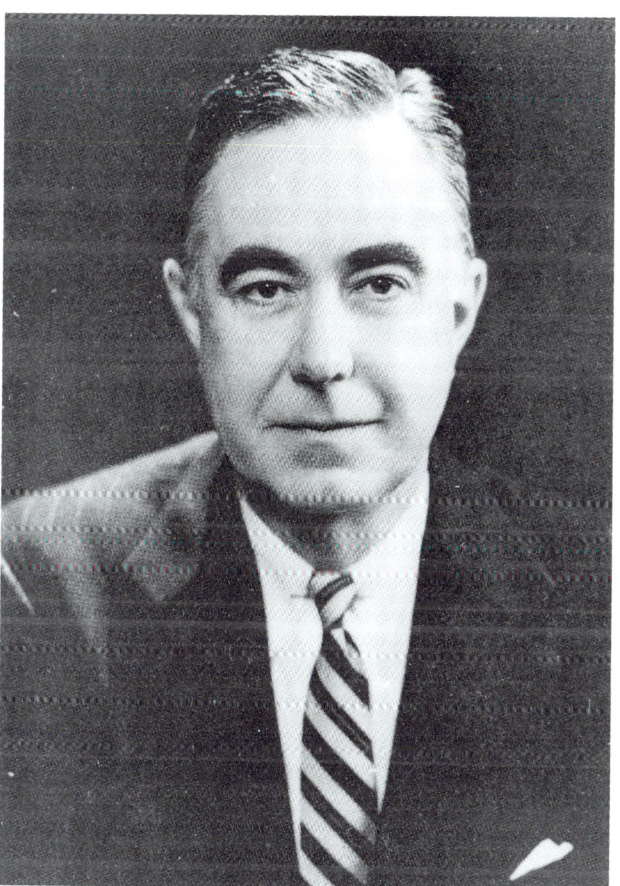

FIG. 50-6. Robert Bruce Nye (1905–1966), Curtis Clinic Director (1931–1942) and Hospital Medical Director (1938–1942).

World War II Changes

Dr. Hayward R. Hamrick (Jefferson, 1935) who had succeeded Nye as Curtis Clinic Director in 1938, was appointed Acting Medical Director in 1942. In 1943 he became Medical Director of the Hospital and Director of the Curtis Clinic (Figure 50-7). Dr. Nye returned to his teaching post in the Department of Medicine in 1946 and in 1951 became Assistant Dean. He was promoted to Associate Dean in 1960 and until his sudden death in October, 1966, he was intimately concerned with medical school admissions.

Dr. Hamrick followed the pattern of

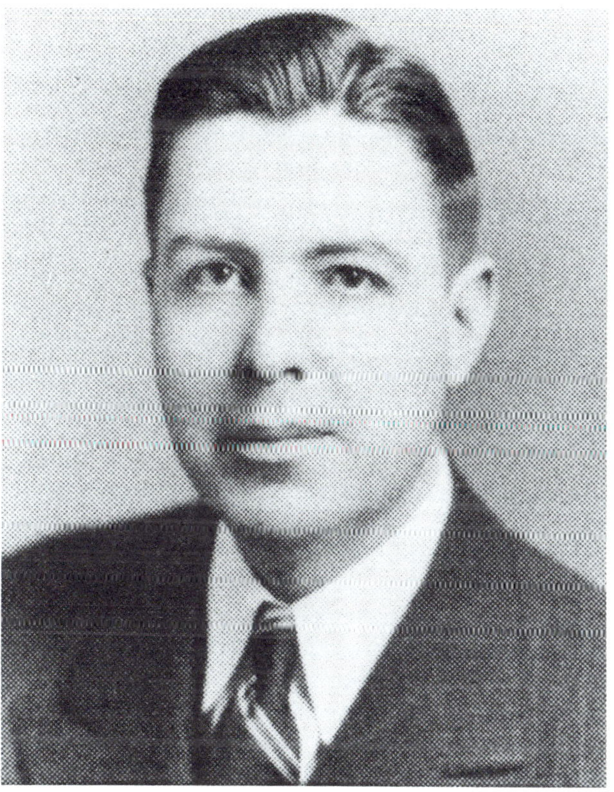

FIG. 50-7. Hayward R. Hamrick (1907–1957), Curtis Clinic Director (1938–1957) and Medical Director (1942–1957).

administrators drawn from the Departments of Medicine and Therapeutics established through Drs. Patterson, Funk, Mohler, and Nye. His experience began as Chief Resident Physician (1937–1938), and his appointment as Curtis Clinic Director directly thereafter prepared him further for the succession to Medical Director of the Hospital. His familiarity with all the aspects of Jefferson affairs was enhanced by his appointment as Acting Secretary and, in 1943, Secretary of the Board of Trustees, which post he held until his death. Special wartime challenges and subsequent postwar expansion caused his appointment to amount to a virtually full-time one, supplemented only by his continuing interest in cardiology and electrocardiography. He quickly mastered the power structure of the institution and wielded his responsibilities effectively. Membership in the American College of Hospital Administrators and the American Hospital Association broadened his perspective. In 1948 the Board of Trustees recognized his accomplishments by electing him to a newly created position of Vice President of the Corporation.

Middle Twentieth Century

In company with the postwar burgeoning of industry, research, and development, medical and health-related matters underwent major mid-century changes. The age of medical technology and increasing awareness on the part of the public of the curative role of hospitals resulted in major expansion of their responsibilities. Patterns of administration changed. In many instances the specialized functions of administrators demanded educational preparation not usually associated with physicians' training. Organizationally, the American Hospital Association, founded in 1906, provided a forum mainly for physician directors. Gradually, lay administrators came to be frequently seen, and in 1933 the American College of Hospital Administrators was founded. The need for specialized education was recognized as early as 1913, when a committee of the American Hospital Association reported on the "desirability of university training of hospital administrators."[6] In 1924, Marquette University established a College of Hospital Administrators for training of executives, technicians, dieticians, and other hospital specialists. Other universities followed with degree courses, and in 1934 the University of Chicago established the first graduate program in hospital administration.[7] An increasing proportion of nonphysician hospital directors was already a trend between 1930 and 1950, but by 1952 only one-third of hospital heads were physicians. By 1962 only one-fifth were medical graduates,[6] even though Faxon in 1952,[1] in describing the attributes of a successful administrator, stated that "physicians are most appropriate for 'larger' hospitals."

The administrative process at Jefferson underwent a change in 1949 when the Board of Trustees elected James Laurence Kauffman, Vice Admiral, U.S.N. (Ret.) as President of the Corporation, and the title of the Head of the Board of Trustees was changed to Chairman. This brought about little immediate change in the responsibilities of the Medical Director but presaged an ongoing process of increasing administrative change. Dr. Hamrick soon became involved in planning for the new Foerderer Pavilion that was built in 1954, thereby increasing the administrative burdens. It was his fate not to survive very long to share in the realization of the fruits of the building program. He died on January 21, 1957.

Professional Administration Begins

As a successor to Dr. Hamrick, the Board appointed Dr. Ellsworth R. Browneller (Jefferson, 1948) as the first administrator to have had formal postgraduate training (Figure 50-8). Following U.S. Naval service from 1948 to 1954, he enrolled at the School of Public Health and Administrative Medicine at Columbia University and was awarded an M.S. degree in Medical Administration. He served an administrative residency under Dr. Robin C. Buerki at Henry Ford Hospital in Detroit, Michigan. He joined the administrative staff at Jefferson immediately upon completion of his educational program in June

1956, and was designated Acting Medical Director on January 25, 1957, directly following Dr. Hamrick's death. Later the same year he was made Medical Director. His administration was featured by many new programs, some of which were introduced after 1959, when Admiral Kauffman was succeeded by William W. Bodine, Jr. as President. Dr. Browneller was responsible for the introduction and institutionalization of professional management principles.

By midcentury the increasing complexity of hospital management resulted in further changes in administration. Procedures varied in different institutions, some hospitals retaining a physician as the executive. In others the chief administrator became designated as President or as Hospital Director. Larger institutions developed sectional administrative heads as local needs dictated.

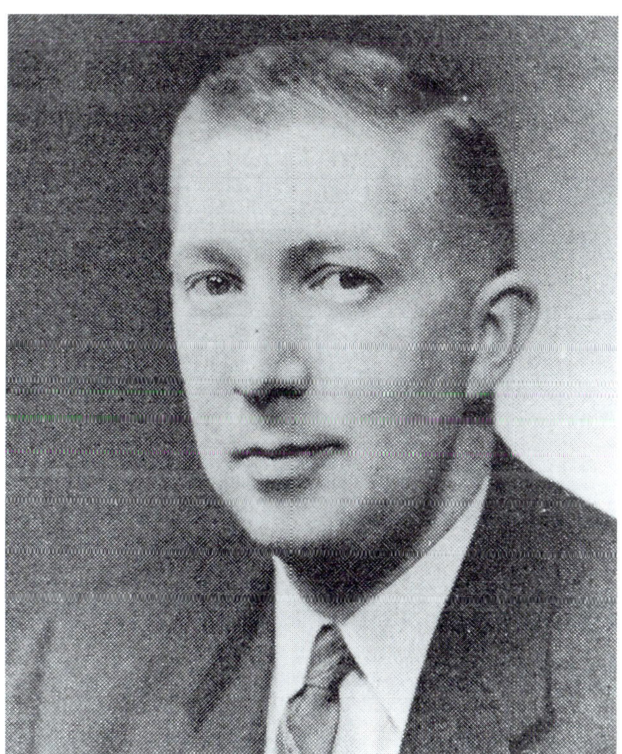

FIG. 50-8. Ellsworth R. Browneller, M.S., M.D. (1923–), Medical Director (1956–1962).

Insurance, legal, financial and ethical problems assumed new importance, and full-time associate personnel were required. Jefferson developed the team approach under Dr. Browneller. During the 1950s, two assistant directors and two administrative assistants were recruited. These included Mabel C. Prevost, R.N., M.S., who was first appointed as Administrative Assistant in 1958 and promoted to Assistant Administrator in 1959. She had served as Director of the School of Nursing and Nursing Services since 1953, the last to hold that position.

In 1959 the first administrative resident was accepted from the School of Public Health and Administrative Medicine at Columbia University. This training program escalated during the next two decades so that by 1985, up to four or five administrative residents were being accepted annually. A number of these trainees went on to important posts at Jefferson and elsewhere. Under Dr. Browneller regular administrative conferences were developed as all aspects of hospital management came under organized supervision.

Dr. Browneller resigned on March 9, 1962. His successor, Maurice P. Coffee, Jr. (Figure 50-9), was appointed Acting Director, and on July 18, 1962, his appointment as Director of Jefferson Medical College Hospital was confirmed by the Board of Trustees. Coffee had pursued a management career from the beginning (B.S. in Institutional and Hotel Administration, Pennsylvania State University, 1955; M.S. in Hospital Administration, Northwestern University, 1957). He came to Jefferson as Associate Director January 1, 1961, following residency experience at Lankanau Hospital in Philadelphia and an appointment as Assistant Administrator at Shadyside Hospital, in Pittsburgh, from 1958 to 1961. Coffee's term at Jefferson was marked by new experiences, especially related to the implementation of the National Medicare Program in 1966. He resigned on August 31, 1967, to join a new health management firm as Vice President.

Francis J. Sweeney, Jr., M.D. (1967–1984)

Having followed the principle of appointing a lay person as executive during Coffee's tenure, the Trustees once more went back to recruiting a physician to succeed him. Dr. Francis J. Sweeney,

Jr. (Jefferson, 1951) was appointed Director in 1967 and served Jefferson with devotion until 1984 (Figure 50-10). Dr. Sweeney, whose academic background included teaching and research in the Department of Medicine (infectious diseases) and a four-month study of cholera in Thailand, served as Attending Physician and Chief of Medicine on the Jefferson Service at Philadelphia General Hospital (1966–1967). His medical background and administrative abilities merged admirably as his career progressed, although his medical role gradually diminished under the weight of increasing management responsibilities. Nevertheless, he advanced in the American College of Physicians governing councils to ultimately become Governor for the Pennsylvania Chapter in 1969 and Chairman of the organization's Board of Regents in 1982.

Dr. Sweeney quickly mastered the organizational aspects of his new duties and established a position of authority as Director. It was a time characterized by increasing health and hospital costs as well as problems of insurance and government regulations. He became influential in local and national hospital groups including the Delaware Valley Hospital Council, serving as its Chairman for 1973–1974. A director of the National Health Council in 1976, he represented the American Hospital Association on the same Council in 1978. He was a Trustee of the Hospital Association of Pennsylvania the same year.

Upon the succession of Dr. Sweeney, the administrative structure was well in place with associate and assistant administrators in each established area of responsibility. He was,

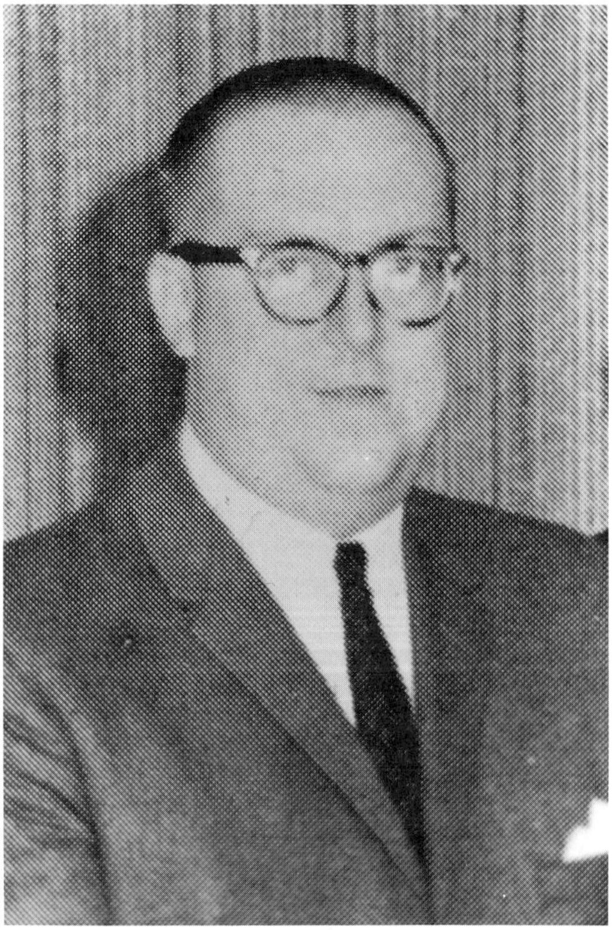

FIG. 50-9. Maurice P. Coffee, Jr., M.S. (1931–), Hospital Director (1962–1967).

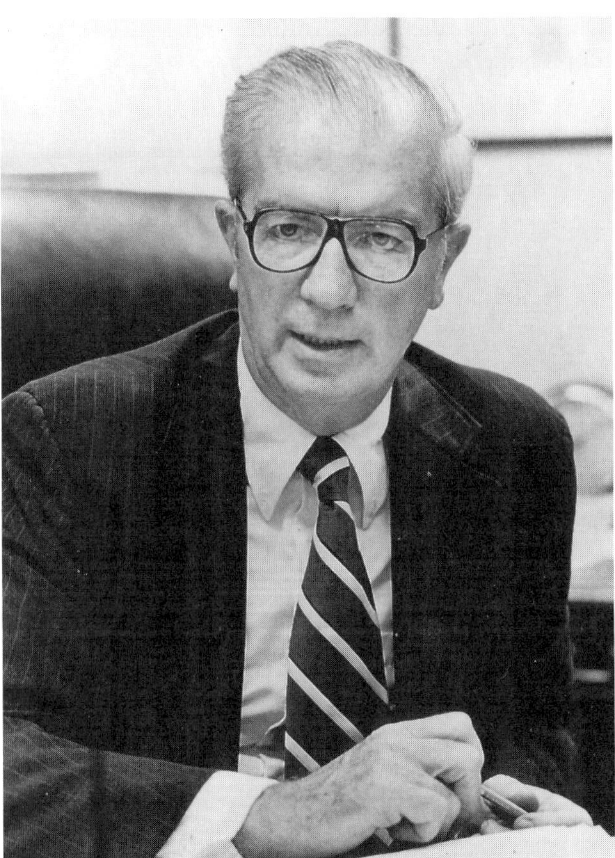

FIG. 50-10. Francis J. Sweeney, Jr., M.D. (1925–), Medical Director (1967–1984) and Vice President for Health Services (1972–1984).

however, faced with some challenges new to the process, especially with respect to Medicare and third-party payment programs, which caused major changes in hospital experience generally. The handling of cost reimbursement proved successful, especially as good relations with Blue Cross management eased some of the problems that accompanied the new programs.

Almost at once the need for expansion of hospital facilities and changes in methods of provision of hospital care became apparent. The adoption of the policy of "one level of care" would eliminate the long-established ward–private differential. At the same time the total number of beds had to be decreased as a reaction to the new and anticipated realities. It proved totally impractical and cost ineffective to renovate existing buildings, so a new hospital structure was decided upon. Dr. Sweeney began with planning in the early 1970s, and in 1972 he was appointed Vice President for Health Services. To free him from routine executive duties Edwin J. Taylor was brought in as Chief Executive Officer of the Hospital. Following completion of the basic planning for a block-long hospital building, many meetings were held to present and discuss the innovative plans with the Medical Staff and other involved persons. By 1976 the design was completed and construction was under way.

Edwin J. Taylor, M.S., M.H.A. (Figure 50-11), the new Hospital Director, came to Jefferson with a background of long experience in health care administration. His service (Captain) in the administrative corps of the U.S. Army was followed by graduate training at Columbia University, leading to the degree of M.H.A. in 1948. From 1948 to 1972 he served as Director of the Graduate Hospital of the University of Pennsylvania. Taylor's experience and business skills were quickly recognized at Jefferson, and in 1976 he was appointed University Vice President for Business Affairs. At that time, Dr. Sweeney resumed the duties of Hospital Director.

The opening of the New Hospital required many administrative adaptations and increased personnel. One of the major new changes related to patient care programs. Six were developed, each under an Associate Administrator. Renovation of the Foerderer Pavilion was a part of this process, and planning proceeded immediately upon occupancy of the New Hospital. Psychiatry and maternity care programs were then located in Foerderer. Major expansion and modernization of the Clinical Laboratories in Foerderer proceeded at the same time.

Michael J. Bradley (1984-   )

In 1984 Dr. Sweeney resigned to accept a new appointment as Vice President for the Health Sciences Center of Temple University. He was succeeded by Michael J. Bradley, M.S., C.P.A., who had served as Vice President for Finance of Thomas Jefferson University since 1979 (Figure 50-12). Bradley's career following graduation from Drexel University in 1969 included a four-year

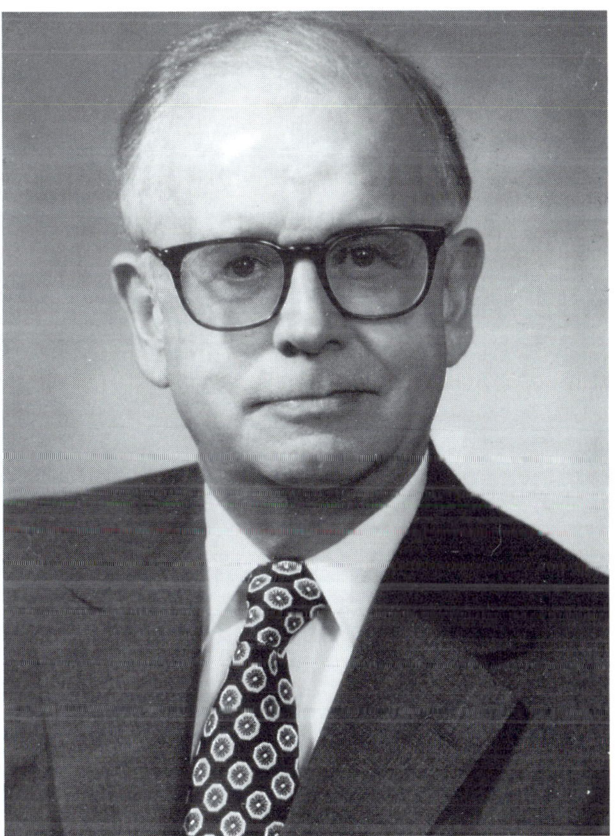

FIG. 50-11. Edwin J. Taylor, M.S., M.H.A. (1919–), Hospital Director (1972–1976) and Vice President for Business Affairs (1976–1983).

experience in accounting and finance with Touche Ross & Co. He joined the Jefferson staff in 1973 as Chief Financial Officer of the Hospital Division and quickly manifested skills in management and finance, resulting in his 1979 promotion. He was well poised to assume the full duties of Vice President for Health Services and Executive Hospital Director.

Hospital administration has become a major process in recent years, and Jefferson's experience is a prime example. In addition to the numbers of personnel and the multiplicity of programs to be administered, entirely new challenges have developed. The pattern of organization of administrative services under Bradley is far removed from the simple arrangements that worked well at the turn of the twentieth century. In 1987 there were four Associate Executive Directors and 11 Assistant Directors, with many divisions and programs under each one. The training program continued with administrative residents. Bradley's strong financial management and highly regarded organizational skills have contributed greatly to the stability of Jefferson's increasingly complex administrative requirements.

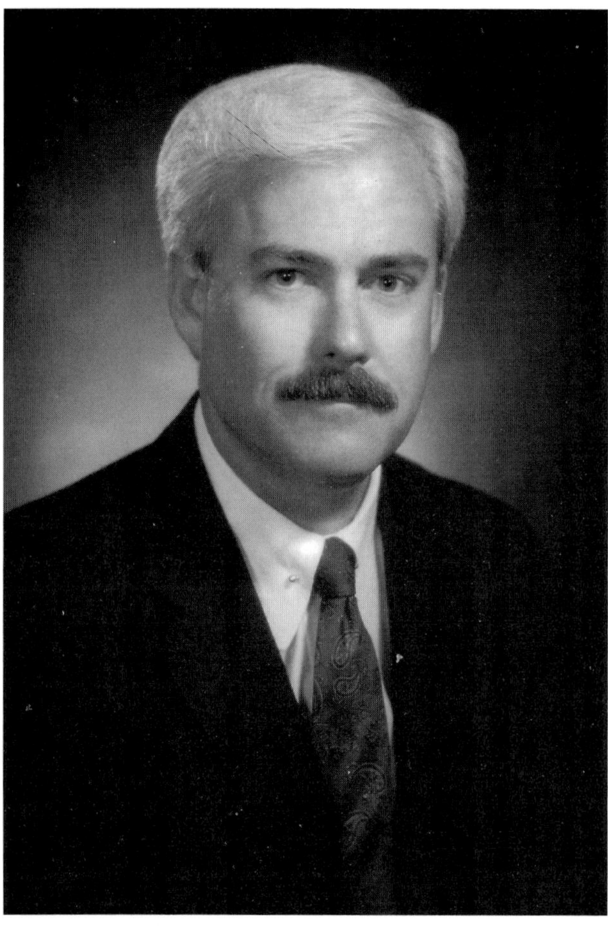

FIG. 50-12. Michael J. Bradley, M.S., C.P.A. (1944–), Vice President for Health Services and Executive Hospital Director (1984–).

The modern hospital, in addition to its service commitments, must deal with conflicts in health policy, governmental agencies, corporate medicine, uncontrollable inflation, and legal surveillance, which mandate a highly accountable administrative process, often referred to as a bureaucracy. At the same time the hospital must manage the fundamental leveling and unchanging experiences of birth, disease, accident, and death. The challenge is not so much to emphasize advances in technology but to humanize the mystical powers of the healing within the hospital walls.

References

1. Faxon, N.W., "Hospital Administration," *New Eng. Jour. Med.*, 247:127–130, 1952.
2. Morton, T.G., and Woodbury F., *History of the Pennsylvania Hospital, 1751–1895*. Philadelphia: Times Printing House, 1895.
3. Jefferson Hospital Reports, 1912.
4. Ibid, 1881.
5. *Jefferson Medical College Hospital, Rules and Regulations*. Philadelphia: MacCalla and Co., 1891. (Located in the Jefferson Archives.)
6. Letourneau, C.V., *The Hospital Administrator*. Chicago: Starling Publications, 1969.
7. Rakich, J.S. and Darr, K., *Hospital Organization and Management*, Third Ed. New York and London: Medical and Scientific Books, 1983.

CHAPTER FIFTY-ONE

The School of Nursing (1891–1982)

Doris E. Bowman, R.N., M.S. (Ed.)

"The trained nurse has become one of the great blessings of humanity, taking a place beside the physician and the priest, and not inferior to either in her mission."

—Sir William Oser (1849–1919)

Although the history of the School of Nursing has been documented in a separate book, *A Commitment to Excellence*[1] (1982), the highlights in the development of a school that grew to make a significant contribution not only to Jefferson but to society must be revisited. The School of Nursing formed a sound base for the development of the College of Allied Health Sciences and the Baccalaureate Program in nursing. The graduates continue to serve at Jefferson as well as throughout the world.

Jefferson Hospital Training School for Nurses opened in 1891 with 13 students. Ella Benson was Director of the new School. Applicants had to be between 21 and 35 years of age, be of "superior education, culture, and refinement," and present certificates of good health. A 30-day probationary period was required before final acceptance into the School. Students worked a 14-hour day, including classes that covered general medical, surgical, gynecological, and obstetrical nursing, plus dietetics. In the second year, students were given an opportunity to gain experience in private homes under the supervision of the attending physician.

Ella Benson was succeeded by Katherine Darling as Director. During her tenure the first graduation exercises were held (November 23, 1893), and diplomas were awarded to five of the original 13 students who survived the two-year courses. The program was soon extended to three years, and enrollment steadily increased (Figure 51-1). The living accommodations were moved from the Hospital to rented quarters at 518

Spruce Street, and later to 226 South Seventh Street.

In 1894 Susan C. Hearle (Figure 51-2) succeeded Katherine Darling. Miss Hearle, a graduate of Philadelphia General Hospital Nursing School, received her early training in Great Britain under Florence Nightingale. During her time as Director, several new courses were added to the already expanding curriculum. These included nursing in diseases of children, nursing in diseases of the eye and ear, bandaging, therapeutics, and massage. Miss Hearle was also influential in establishing the Nurses Alumnae Association (1895).

New Hospital (1877): New Challenge

The 1877 first detached Jefferson Medical College Hospital was subsequently well served by founding of the School of Nursing in 1891. By the time of the 1907 opening of Old Main Hospital, 148 nurses had graduated (Figures 51-3, 51-4, and 51-5).

Dedication to service and response to need have consistently characterized "Jeff" nurses. As early as 1898, they helped in the typhoid epidemic, and in 1900 they rendered aid to the sick and injured during the Galveston flood.

In 1908 Hearle was succeeded by Anna E. Laughlin, the first graduate of the School to serve as Director. Physicians continued to do most of the teaching, with the Director of Nurses and her Assistant responsible for "recitations from assigned lessons" and demonstrations in massage and dietetics. Students no longer were assigned to experience in the home, and they remained in the Hospital for the three-year period.

In 1909 the first bill regulating the practice of nursing was passed in Pennsylvania, and it subsequently provided for a Board of Examiners, consisting of five professional nurses. The first list of approved schools in Pennsylvania was published in 1918, and Jefferson was among them.

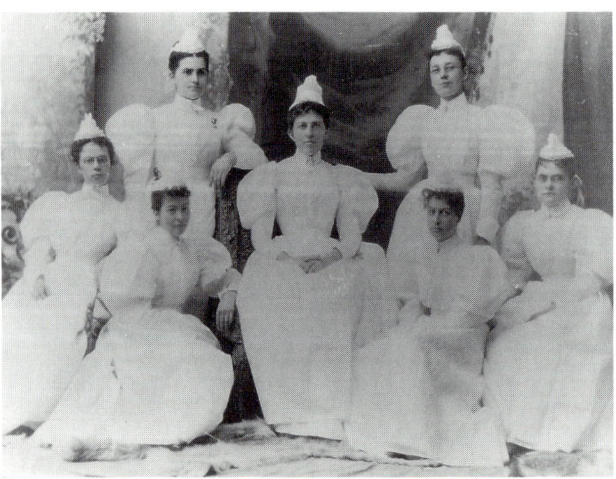

FIG. 51-1. The Graduating Class of 1893–1894.

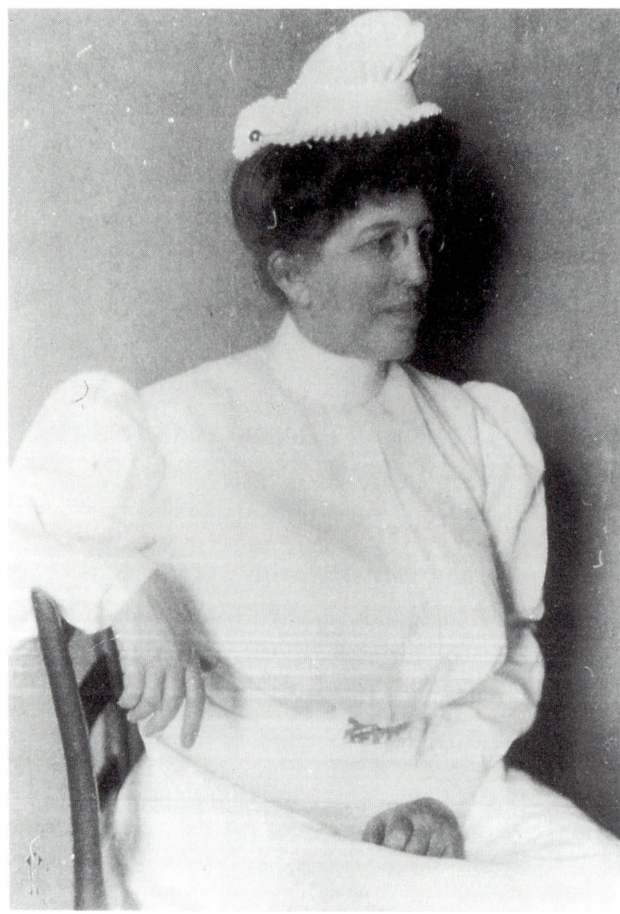

FIG. 51-2. Miss Susan C. Hearle, an early Director (1894–1908), received training in Great Britain under Florence Nightingale.

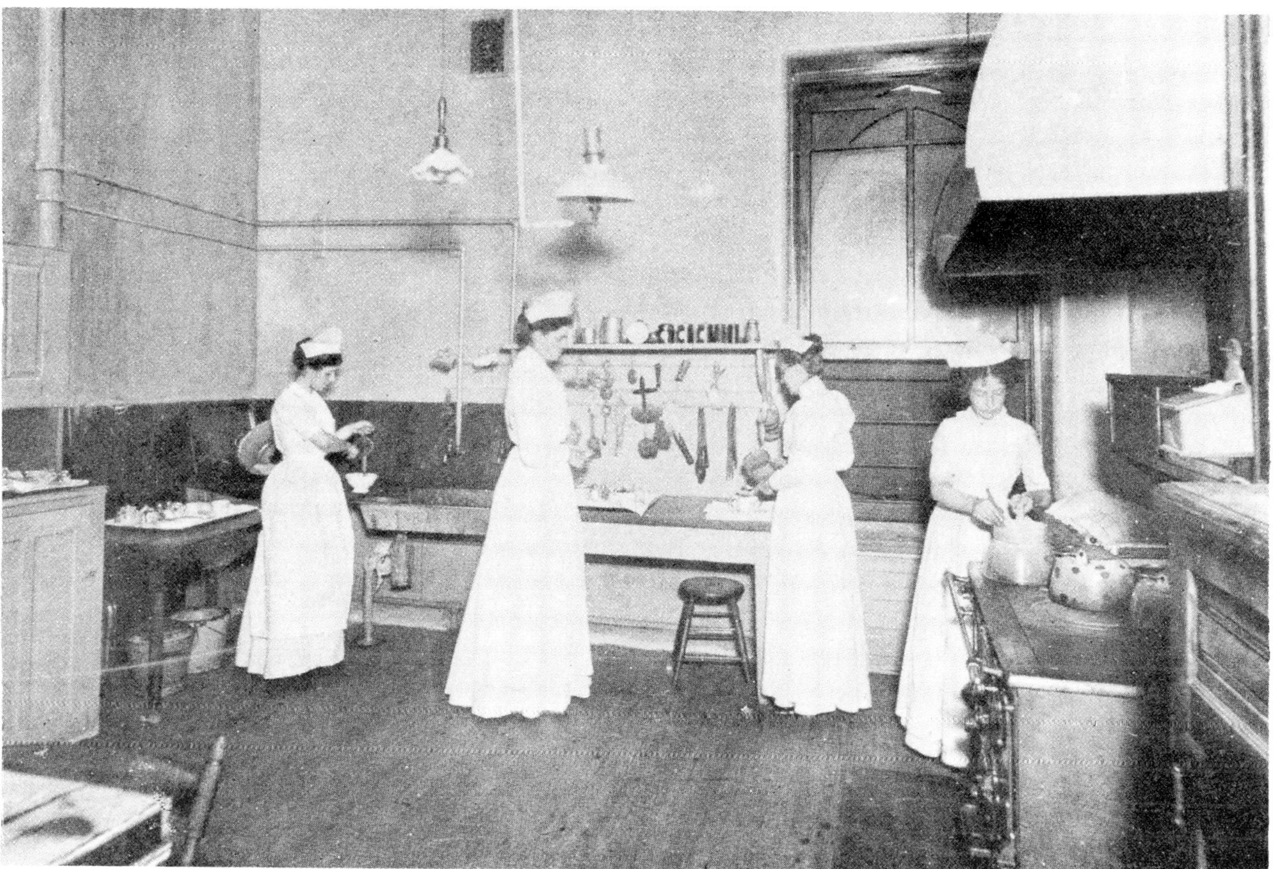

FIG. 51-3. The Teaching Kitchen for student nurses in the 1877 Hospital.

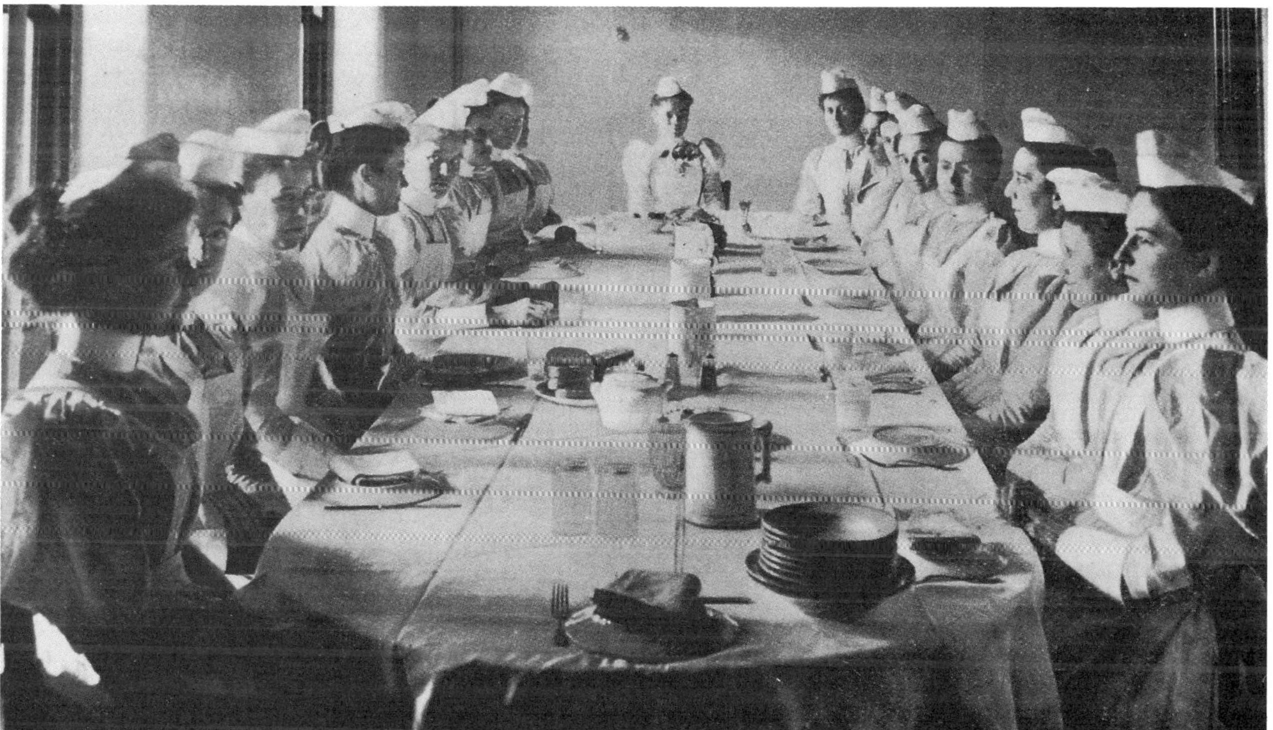

FIG. 51-4. The third relay for dinner in the 1877 Hospital.

Legislation was passed later, making this a mandatory type of approval; accreditation by the National League for Nursing, which followed at a much later date, was a voluntary approval process.

Clara E. Melville, R.N.; Director of Nursing (1915–1937)

The second graduate of the School to become Director of Nursing was Clara Melville (Class of 1910), who left an unforgettable aura that lingered with many throughout the School's history (Figure 51-6). Her struggle to achieve excellence and her concept of what was "right" was shared by Anna Shafer (Figure 51-7) the Night Supervisor, and Adele Lewis (Figure 51-8), Head Nurse on the sixth floor. These as well as earlier leaders established the foundation and traits that characterized the School throughout its history.

Members of the Class of 1909 were the first to receive a school pin in addition to the diploma. The original gold pin bore a replica of the head of Florence Nightingale, surrounded by the name of the School. In 1910 the pin was changed to a type of gold scroll containing a blue cross, surrounded by black enamel. The lettering of Jefferson Hospital was later changed to Thomas Jefferson University (Figure 51-9).

As early as 1910, classroom space was limited and classes were held wherever space could be found near the ward areas. The doctors who taught classes usually held oral examinations for the students in their offices.

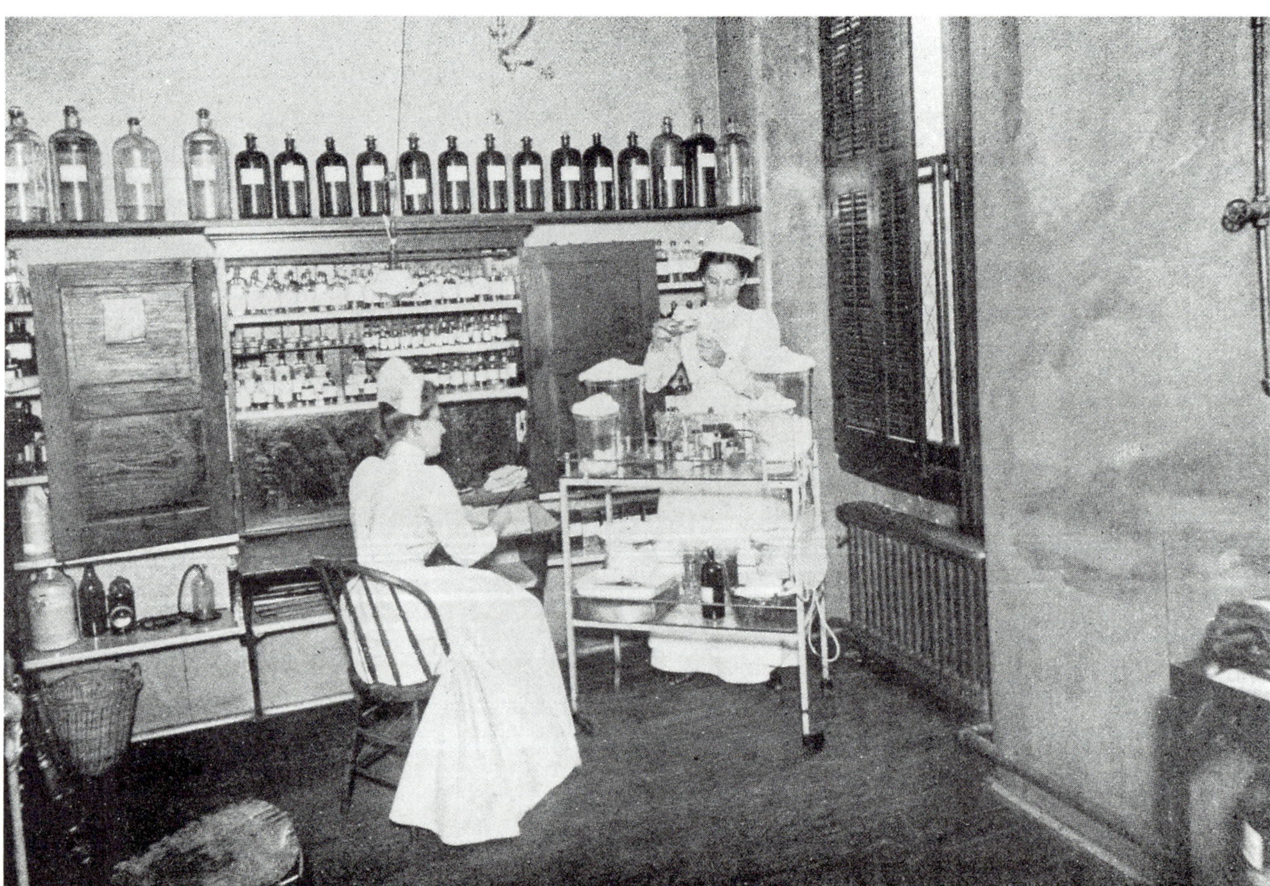

FIG. 51-5. Nurses' offices on the fifth floor of the 1877 Hospital.

edge. This basic uniform was replaced in summer by a slightly lighter material with a lawn kerchief around the neck instead of a collar. By 1915 the puffed sleeves had been replaced by more tailored ones, and the bishop's collar was replaced by a regular-style stiff collar (Figure 51-10).

The "Pinky" Uniform

While the Jefferson uniform was always pink and the cap white organdy or lawn, changes in style and length occurred as fashions in general changed. The first uniform was floor length and made of solid pink cotton material with buttons down the front and a high bishop's collar. Balloon sleeves fastened tightly at the wrist and had cuffs that reached halfway to the elbow. The bib and apron were combined and made of a white lawn material. The cap was of a white lawn or organdy with a wide band turned back and a ruffle on the

World War I and the 38th General Hospital

In answer to the need for medical care for soldiers overseas during World War I, the 38th General Hospital was formed with Dr. William Coplin in command and Clara Melville as Chief Nurse. The unit, with 100 nurses joining the medical staff, left New York on May 10, 1918, on the Army transport *Saturnia*. They arrived in England eight days later

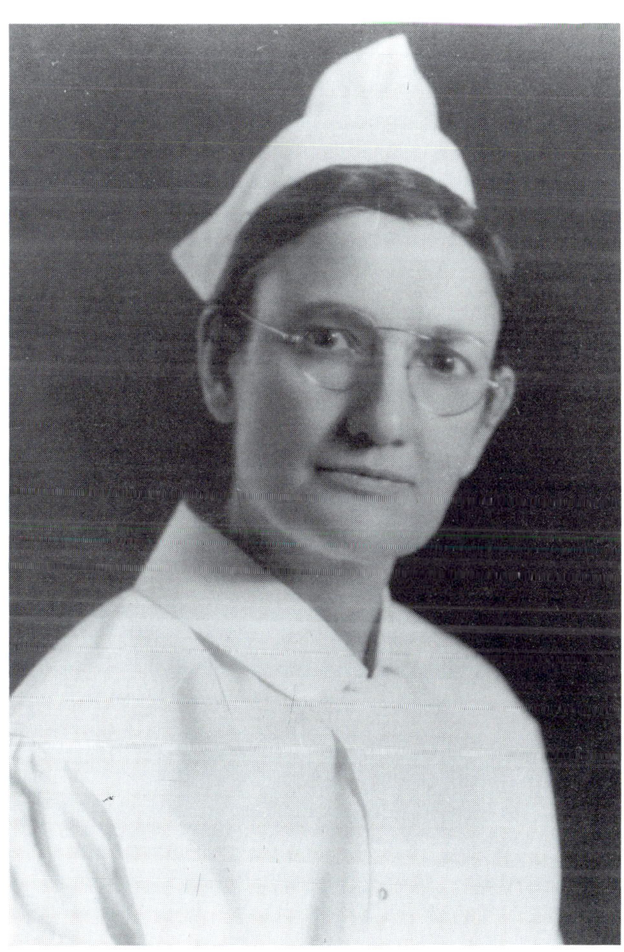

FIG. 51-6. Miss Clara E. Melville, Director (1915–1937).

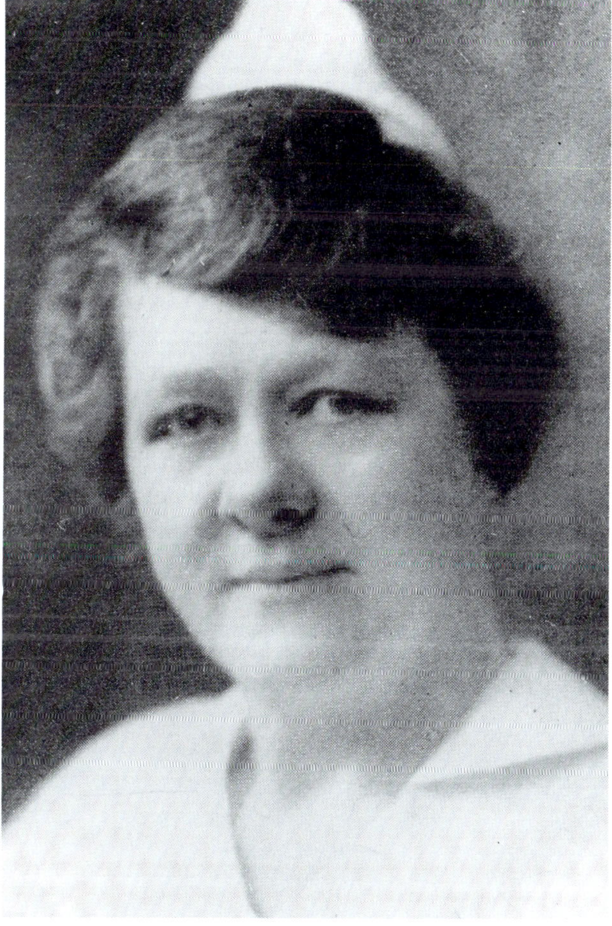

FIG. 51-7. Miss Anna ("Annie") Shafer (Class of 1910), a legendary Night Supervisor.

and then proceded to Nantes, France, on June 6, 1918. Because of a desperate need at front-line medical stations, many of the nurses were sent to other posts in France. Miss Melville was left with seven nurses and six civilians to staff Base Hospital No. 38.

In Miss Melville's absence, Nora E. Shoemaker was Acting Director of Nursing. She not only had the problems in staffing caused by the exodus of the nurses who were serving with the 38th, but those caused by the relentless epidemic of influenza in the autumn of 1918. Upon Miss Melville's return in 1919, Miss Shoemaker resigned to join the American Red Cross for relief work in Siberia.

Post World War I Expansion

When the original Hospital Building was demolished in 1922 to make way for the Samuel Gustine Thompson Annex, student nurses who had been housed there underwent several temporary housing changes, eventually settling into a cluster of residences at 1012, 1014, and 1016 Spruce Street. The space in back of these buildings was the site for a new nurses' residence, which opened in May, 1925. By 1926, the "new building" housed 120 students.

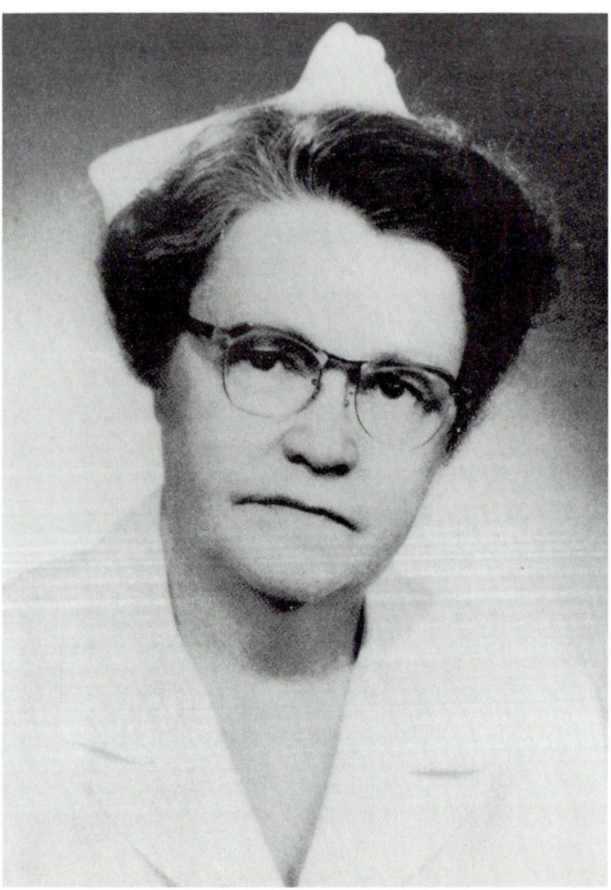

FIG. 51-8. Miss Adele Lewis (Class of 1915), for many years the Head Nurse on the sixth floor of "Old Main."

During this period, teaching facilities were upgraded with expanded classroom space and the addition of two new laboratories (dietetics and chemistry). Nora E. Shoemaker was appointed Assistant to Miss Melville, as the first Educational Director in September, 1924. Prior to this time, the education of the student nurses was the responsibility of the Director of Nursing.

From its inception, discipline, hard work, and excellence were synonymous with the School's training. Residence rules were strict and a student five minutes late from a monthly pass that ended at midnight was subject to punishment. Classroom and practice hours added up to 12 to 14 hours per day. In addition to caring for patients, students were expected to sweep the floors, clean the bedside tables, and "carbolize" bedpans and urinals. If the "bedline" was not straight by the time the chief made rounds about 9 A.M., the student in charge was likely to be severely reprimanded.

By 1925 the uniform skirt had risen to five inches above the floor, revealing that other part of the uniform that endured much to the chagrin of students—black stockings and black oxfords.

A tradition lasting until the close of the School in 1982 was begun in 1928 by Dr. Harvey Righter. He presented each graduating student with a red rose that became the beginning of the "Rose Arch" concluding Commencement ceremonies until 1982 (Figure 51-11).

When the Curtis Clinic opened in 1931, the upper three floors were delegated to the Education Department of the Nurses' Training School. Offices, a small classroom and a dietetics laboratory were located on the tenth floor; a nursing arts laboratory and a chemistry library on the eleventh floor; and a large classroom for 175 students with an adjacent classroom for 25 on the twelfth floor. The probationary period became

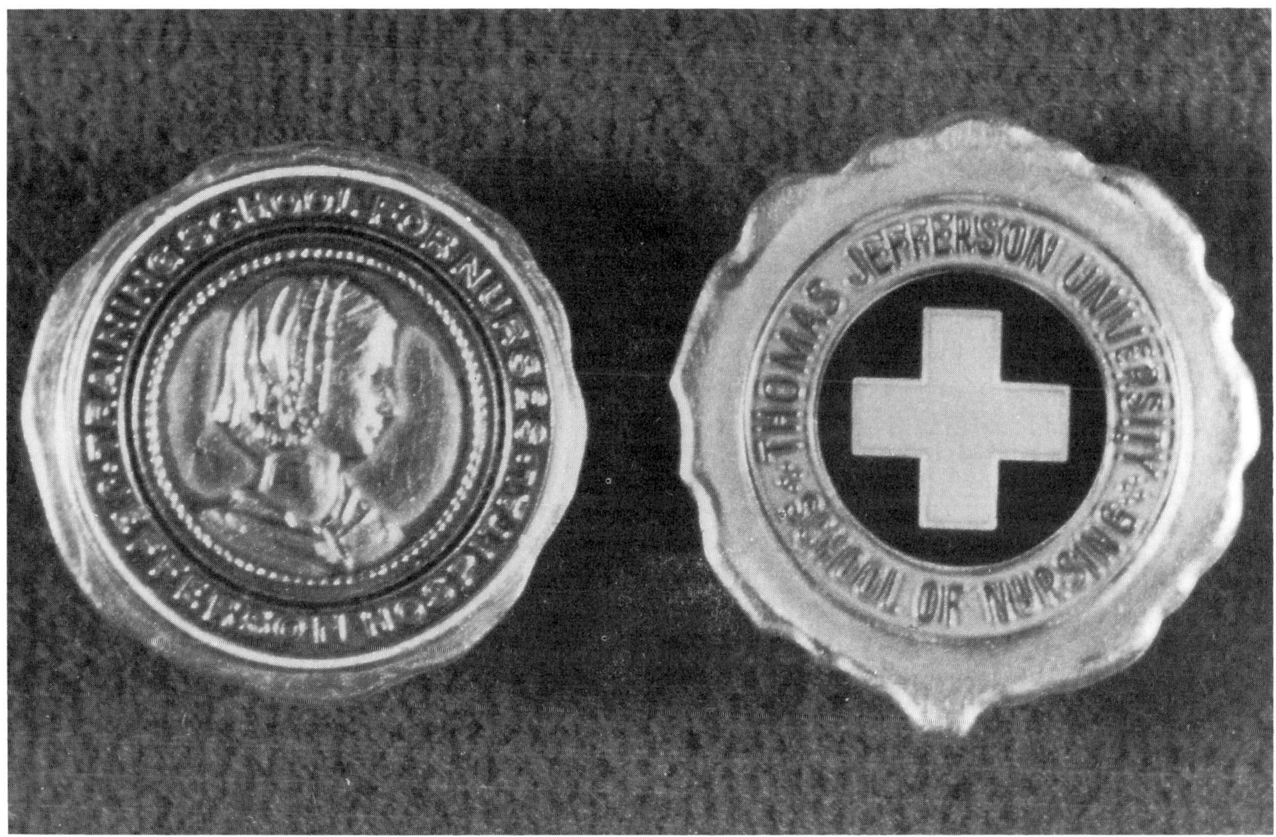

FIG. 51-9. Class pins. The pin on the left, replaced in 1910 by the pin on the right, featured Florence Nightingale.

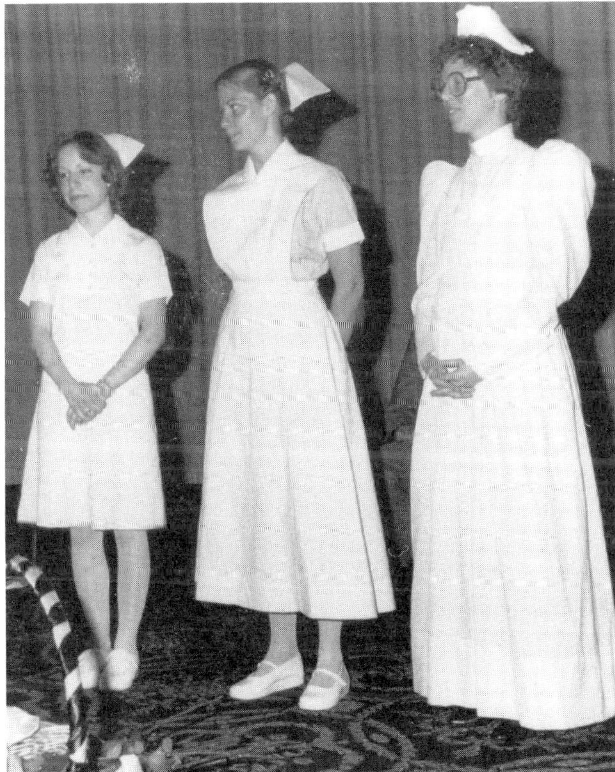

FIG. 51-10. Major changes (right to left) in the student nurses' uniforms from 1891 to 1982.

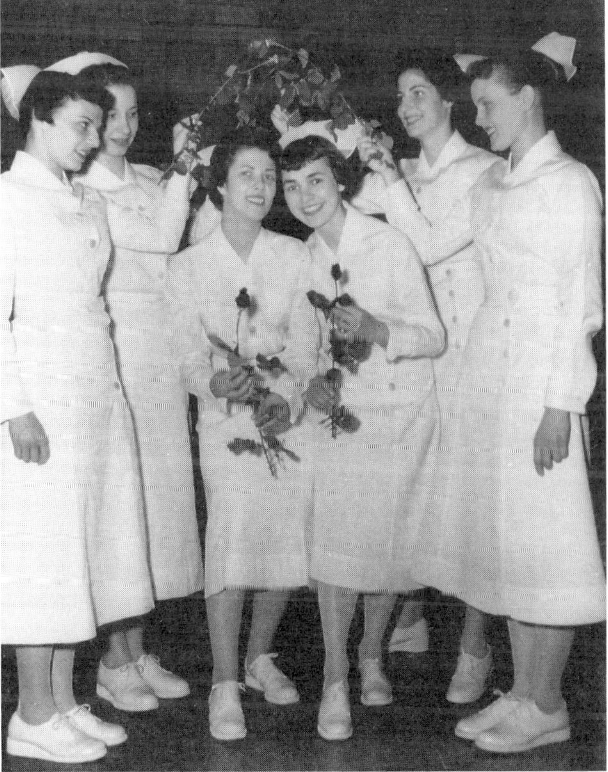

FIG. 51-11. The Traditional Arch of Roses at Commencement.

four months, and theoretical instructions covered 763 hours of classroom work plus long hours of clinical practice.

In 1935 a reference library of 1,200 volumes was presented to the Nurses' Home by Ross V. Patterson, Dean of Jefferson Medical College (1916–1938). This was the beginning of a much-needed library for students. Two rooms of the first floor at 1012 Spruce Street were set aside for a library. That same year the Jefferson Choral Club was organized, and it put on its first annual minstrel show in 1938.

The first official Alumni Day was held on April 21, 1933, and became an annual event. That same year, the student yearbook, previously published under different titles, was permanently named *Nosokomos* (of Latin origin, meaning "attendant on the sick").

Commissioned by the Alumni Association in recognition of Miss Melville's 20 years of service, a portrait was presented on May 4, 1935. This assumed an honored position in Jefferson's art collection. Miss Melville died in 1937 and was succeeded by her Assistant, Nora E. Shoemaker (Figure 51-12). During her six years (1937–1943), a social sciences course was added, a recreational program was set up, and an affiliation with the Pennsylvania Hospital for Mental and Nervous Diseases was initiated.

Back in 1933 a pink-and-white finely checked uniform had been introduced to be worn the first year and one-half, with a solid pink for the last year and one-half. In 1936 short sleeves with separate cuffs were added. Later (1959) the bib and apron became obsolete and the three-piece uniform was replaced by a one-piece pink, pin-stripe pinfeather material.

During the 1930s, enrollment in the School averaged 230 to 240 students. Its already high admission standards were reinforced by a 1935 Pennsylvania State Law requiring a high school education and proof of citizenship for registration at "schools of nursing." Jefferson's curriculum included 35 subjects covering basic sciences and all aspects of practical and specialty nursing. Extensive on-the-job training was provided in all areas of the Hospital and the Chest Unit at Pine Street.

World War II: 38th General Hospital Reactivated

Early in the 1940's Jefferson again answered the call to a growing national emergency, and Base Hospital No. 38 was reactivated. Baldwin L. Keyes, M.D., having been appointed Medical Chief of the Unit, recruited doctors and nurses to staff a 1,000 bed hospital. On the afternoon of the Pearl Harbor attack (December 7, 1941), he reported that the Jefferson Unit was ready for active duty. On May 15, 1942, a special train pulled out of Broad Street Station for Camp Bowie, Texas, with a group of 90 nurses and 60 doctors. Thirty to 40 more nurses were added later in Texas.

After about six weeks of training on the hot and dusty Texas plains, the 38th left Camp Bowie for an unknown destination. Speculation was rampant. After stops at Charleston, South Carolina, and

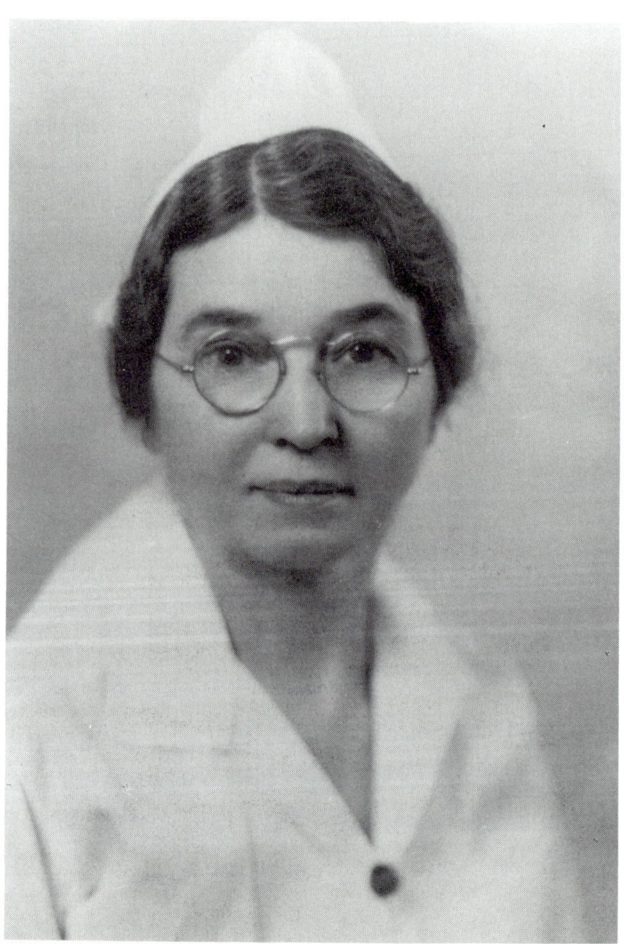

FIG. 51-12. Nora E. Shoemaker (1908), Director of Nursing (1937–1943).

Camp Kilmer, New Jersey, the 38th embarked September 21, 1942, on the converted British Liner *Aquitania,* at Staten Island. Accommodations were less than luxurious and food less than tasty, mutton being the main dish nearly every day. Staterooms were crowded with bunk beds and little air. One canteen of water per day served both for daily bathing and laundry. The ship was without convoy, so followed a tedious zigzag pattern in an effort to foil any German U-boats. After a stop in Rio to pick up supplies, the *Aquitania* landed in Capetown, South Africa. It was a welcome relief finally to set foot on land. After an overnight stay, the ship headed up the coast of Africa through the Indian Ocean to the Red Sea and through the Suez Canal. On October 24 the Equator was crossed for a second time, with arrival at Teufik a week later. At the time of landing, bombs could be heard in the distance, and later it was learned that Rommel was fleeing across the desert, never to be seen in the Cairo area again.

After an overnight stay in tents, the group was transported to the final destination, the desert about 13 kilometers from Cairo. Only a few buildings were completed, and the nurses were housed in barracks, while the doctors were assigned to tents (Figure 51-13). The beds were cots of rope, and the furniture consisted of any box available. There were not only bedbugs, sand fleas, and kangaroo mice to deal with, but intense heat and sand storms to endure. By Christmas, furniture arrived and life became somewhat more comfortable. The Hospital opened on Armistice Day (now called Veterans' Day), 1942, and again there was much improvising of supplies and equipment. Willie L. Alder, 1931, who was originally in charge of the nurses, left to take

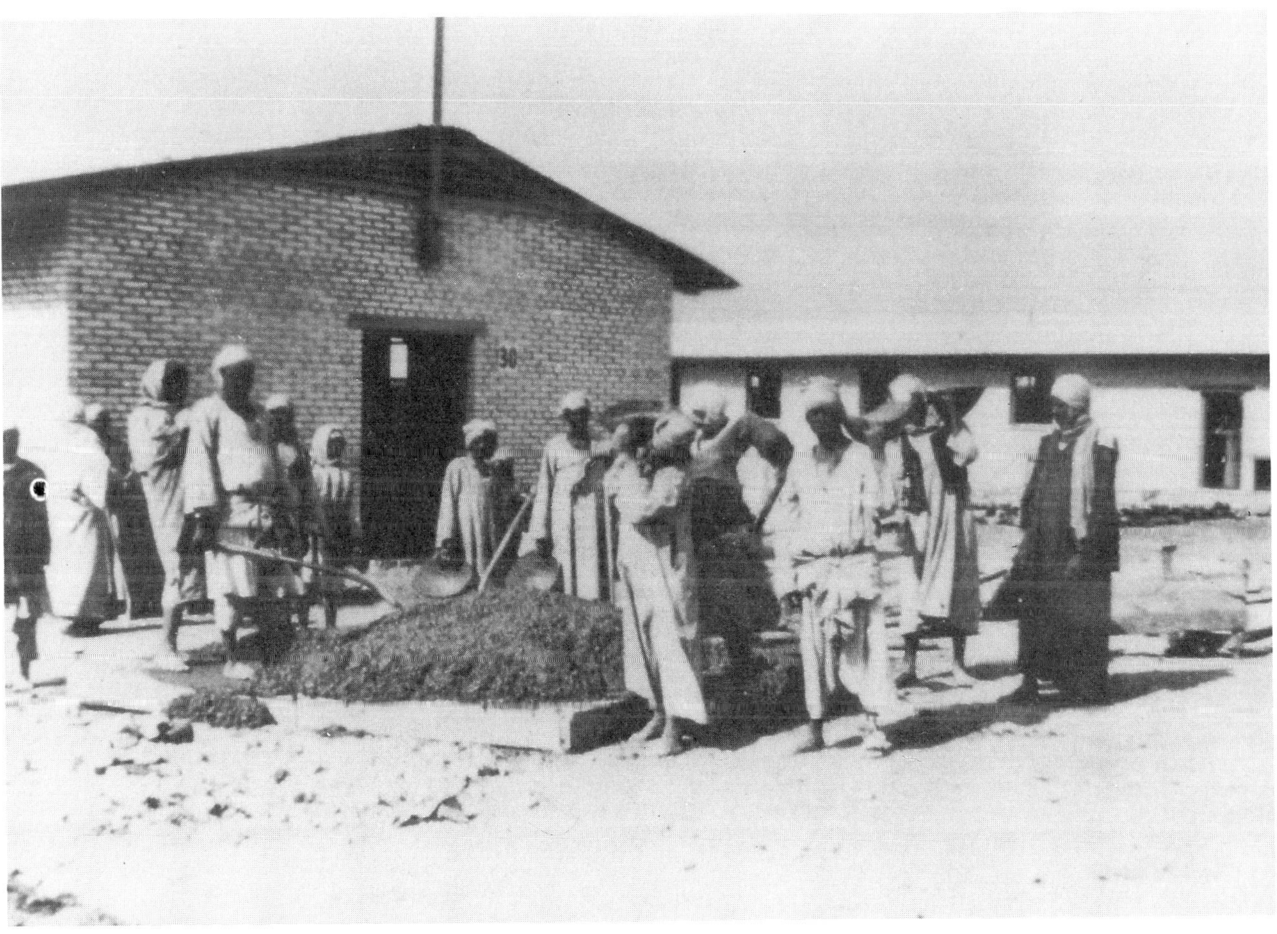

FIG. 51-13. Setting up barracks for Jefferson nurses at Base Hospital No. 38.

over nursing services for the whole Middle East Theater. She was succeeded by Edna Scott, 1928, as Chief Nurse at the Hospital, now designated as Camp Huckstep.

For a time the 38th was busy with casualties from the 9th Air Force raids on the Ploesti oil fields as well as other areas, plus a stream of victims of sandfly fever and malaria. As the fighting moved northward into Europe, the 38th was gradually reduced to a 500-bed hospital.

Many other nurses from Jefferson served valiantly in other areas of combat throughout the world, not only in World War II but, later, in South Vietnam.

The Home Front (1942)

With the exodus of so many nurses into war duty, staffing of the Jefferson Hospital at home was a most difficult task, and much of the burden for nursing care fell upon the shoulders of the student nurses. There were several changes of Nursing Directorship during the period. Nora Shoemaker was replaced in 1943 by Ethel Hopkins, formerly Educational Director. She was succeeded by Miss Margaret Jackson in 1944. Student enrollment had increased to 347 by 1945, related largely to creation of the Cadet Nurse Corps by Congress in June, 1943.

Student government was organized early in 1945. It soon persuaded the School Administration to grant more time off, with a late pass until midnight one night each week, providing that work was satisfactory. Another progressive step initiated by the Class of 1946 was permission to wear white shoes and stockings rather than the black.

New Personnel: New Directions

The *Curriculum Guide for Schools of Nursing*, published in 1937 by the National League for Nursing, became the model for curriculum changes of the 1940s. It emphasized the social, psychological, and public health aspects of nursing. These subjects were added to the curriculum, and a closer correlation between class and clinical teaching was attempted.

In July, 1947, Katherine Childs was appointed Director of Nursing. During her time, classes were divided into two sections. While one group was on clinical practice, the other was in class. Four days a week students were assigned to clinical practice and two days to class, with one day off. The basketball team was organized in 1947 and continued to be one of the most popular student activities almost until the School closed in 1982. The team as well as the cheerleaders won many championships (Figure 51-14). The scope of other

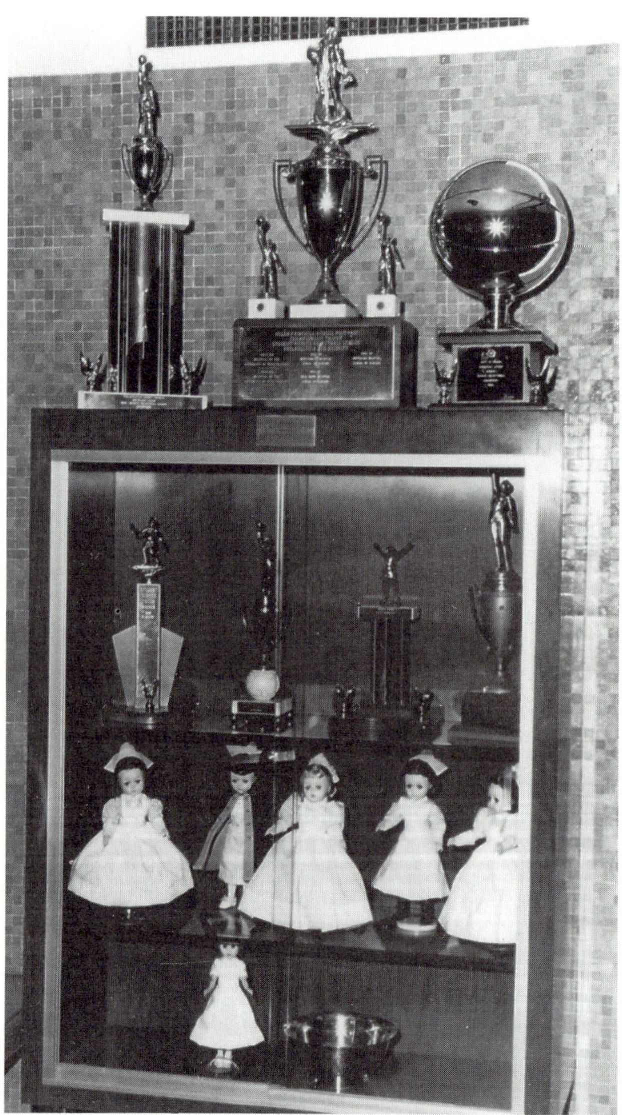

FIG. 51-14. Championship trophies (at top) and dolls dressed in period student nurses' uniforms.

social activities was expanded under the Student Council.

When Barton Memorial Division opened in 1946, students received a clinical experience in pulmonary disease there rather than at Pine Street. The affiliation with Pennsylvania Hospital for Mental and Nervous Diseases continued, and a second affiliation was arranged with Sheppard and Enoch Pratt so that all students could receive an experience in caring for the mentally disturbed.

Following the resignation of Katherine Childs in 1953, Mabel C. Prevost (Figure 51-15) was appointed Director of Nursing. During her administration, the School continued to grow through rigorous recruitment efforts. A campaign was waged for a more modern nurses' residence, and more aggressive steps were taken to secure accreditation from the National League for Nursing (a voluntary type of accreditation that was rapidly becoming mandatory). Additional classroom and faculty office spaces were secured in the Hospital so that instructors could be closer to the clinical practice areas to which the students were assigned.

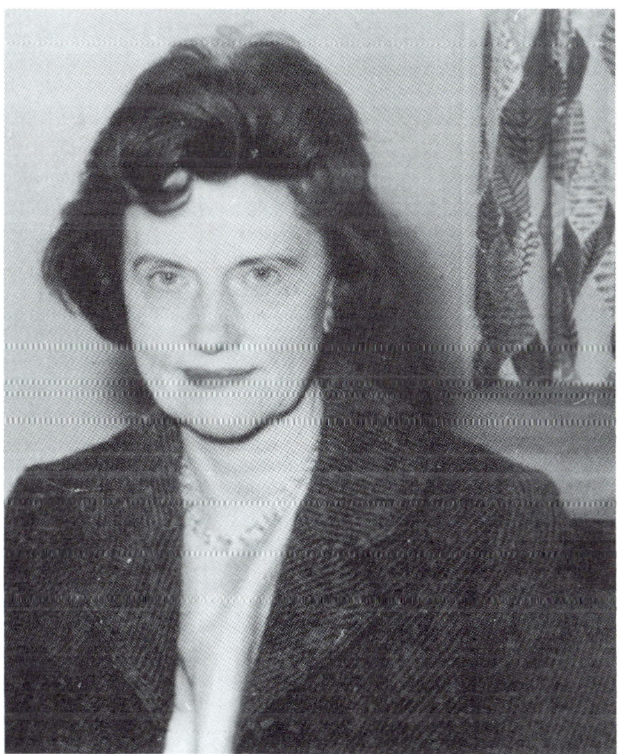

FIG. 51-15. Mabel C. Prevost (1929), Director of Nursing (1953–1958) and Assistant Hospital Director (1958–1974).

A long-awaited dream became a reality in 1959 with the opening of the James R. Martin Residence for student nurses (Figure 51-16). For the first time in many years all the students could be housed under one roof. The $2 million, eight-story, air-conditioned building at the corner of Eleventh and Walnut Streets had beds for 336 students and appropriate accommodations for four housemothers. On this site was once the house owned by Thomas Dent Mütter and subsequently by Samuel D. Gross, both eminent Professors of Surgery at Jefferson.

Nursing Education in Evolution

In 1958 a significant change in the organization of the Department of Nursing occurred. Miss Prevost was promoted to Hospital Administration as Assistant Director, and two positions for a Director of Nursing were created, one as Director of the School of Nursing and the other as Director of Nursing Service. Being given her choice, Doris E. Bowman, then Associate Director of Nursing, elected the School and became the Director of the School of Nursing in January, 1958.

An Advisory Committee to the School was formed in 1958. Its membership included representatives from the Board of Trustees, Medical Staff, Hospital Administration, and Nurses' Alumnae Association, a clergyman, general educators, and the Director of the School. Dr. Baldwin L. Keyes chaired the committee. Its purpose was to advise and assist the School in promoting its programs, especially as they related to financial aid, endowment funds, scholarships, and recruitment. The committee served meaningfully until phased out in 1973.

The Burt-Melville Department, formerly the Nurses' Home Committee of the Women's Board formed in 1908, continued to provide additional amenities for the students and the School as years passed. Especially helpful during the final decade of the School's existence was the financial support they gave to the Faculty In-Service Program.

Consistent with changes in nursing and nursing education, the curriculum of the School evolved from six courses in 1891, taught mainly by physicians, to 30 courses in 1960, taught mainly by nurse educators. In addition, a concerted effort was made to have concurrent classes and clinical practice with the same instructors teaching. Basic nursing techniques were first taught via closed-circuit television in 1964.

In 1962 the "Miss Jefferson" contest was launched under the sponsorship of the student newspaper, *Caps and Capes*. Candidates were nominated by the students, screened by the faculty, and judged by the Nursing Staff, Physicians, and Faculty on the basis of appearance in uniform, nursing care, personality, school spirit, talent, and residence deportment. The winner received a blue sash with the title and year, a gold bracelet with a charm, and a bouquet of roses. During its eight years run, the show drew an enthusiastic crowd. Robert J. Mandle, Ph.D., and Milton Toporek, Ph.D. served faithfully as masters of ceremonies.

Students also wrote and staged a smash hit show in 1962, *Showboat,* which was rerun in 1963 and followed each year by an equally rewarding performance of other plays.

The basketball team, inspired by cheerleaders

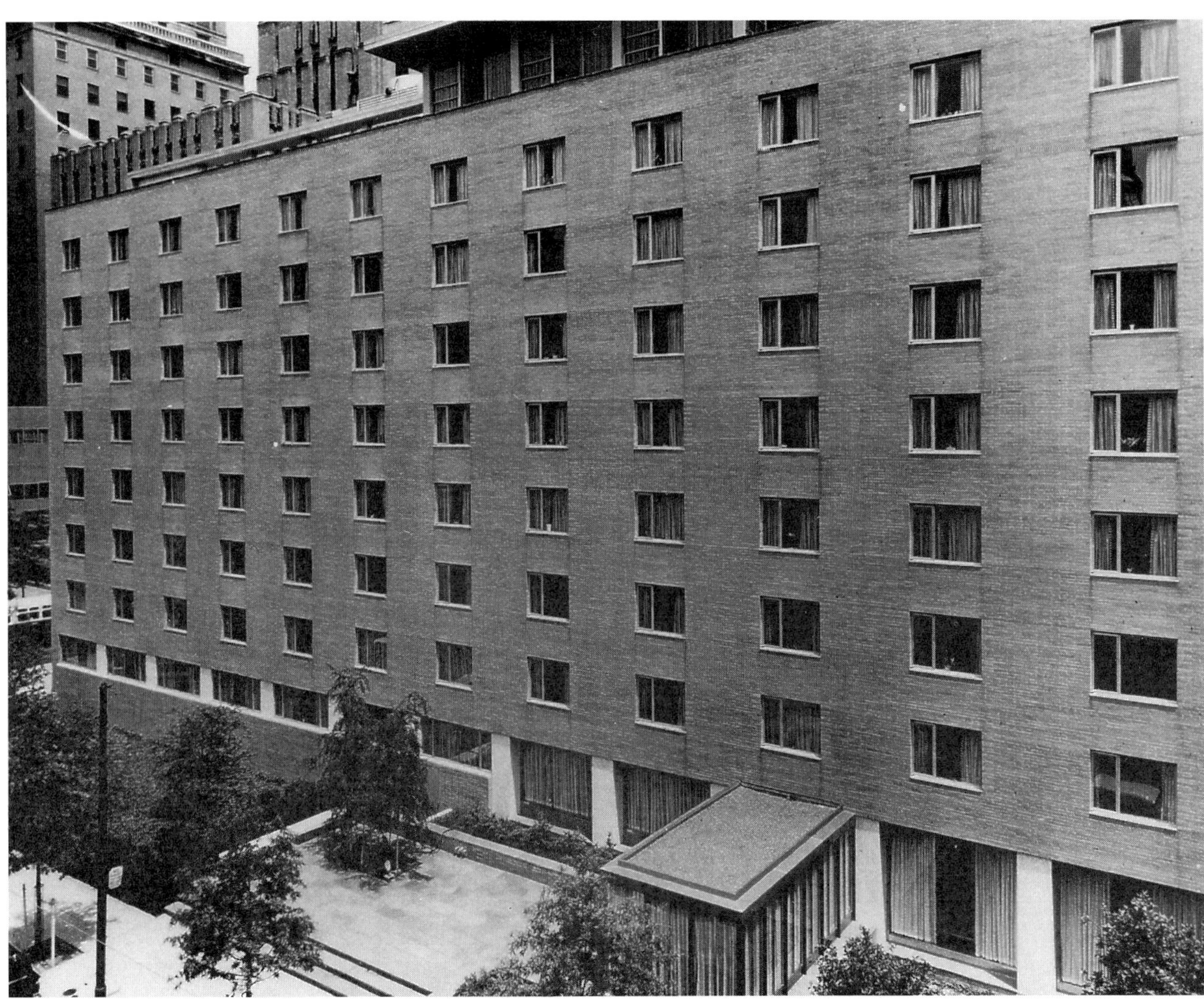

FIG. 51-16. The James R. Martin Residence for student nurses (1959).

and student audiences, continued to make impressive showings and eventually filled two cabinets with their trophies. Students also won their share of prizes in competitions staged by the Area No. 1 Chapter of the Student Nurses' Association of Pennsylvania (SNAP).

The School of Nursing marked its Seventy-fifth Anniversary in 1966, at which time there were 4,000 graduates. Total enrollment in the 1960s ranged from 300 to 322. By 1969 there were 33 full-time faculty members in the School, and Members of the Medical College taught the basic sciences (Figure 51-17).

In 1968 the School of Nursing became a part of a newly organized School of Allied Health Sciences. Allied Health became a "College" in 1969, and the Director of the School reported to its Dean rather than to Hospital Administration. That same year, the College Entrance Board Examination became an admission requirement.

Jefferson Alumni Hall opened in 1968, greatly enriching the students' recreational facilities, and their basic science courses were taught in the basic science classrooms.

Professional Nursing Upgraded

In December 1965 the American Nurses' Association (ANA) published a document that had far-reaching effects on nursing and nursing education not only at Jefferson but throughout the

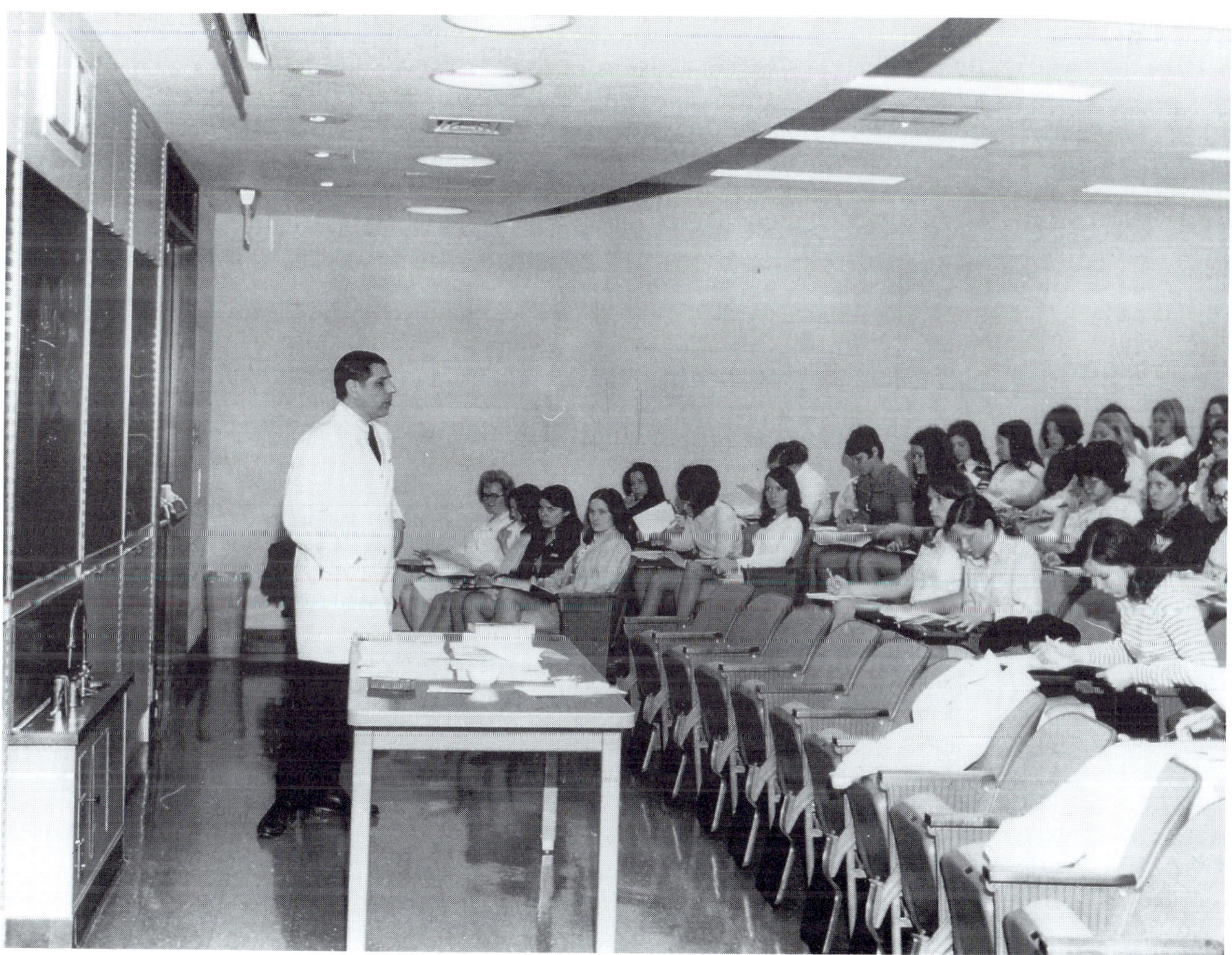

FIG. 51-17. Anthony J. Triolo, Ph.D., from the Department of Pharmacology, teaching student nurses.

country. This later became known as the "ANA Position Paper." It stated that by 1985 basic professional nurse education should take place in institutions of higher learning and lead to a baccalaureate degree. Protests, student unrest, disillusionment, and counterproposals were heard nationally. Each convention (ANA as well as NLN) was riddled with debate, controversy, and open hostility. The position taken by the Professional Nurses' Organization, however, rode out the storm.

By the end of the decade, many diploma schools had either closed or shortened their programs. Of the 501 diploma programs accredited by the National League for Nursing, only 58 continued to have the traditional three-year program. The average program length was 121 weeks, exclusive of vacations. Without sacrificing the quality of the Jefferson program, approval was granted by the State Board to reduce the program to 33 months. College credit courses in psychology and sociology were added and additional college credit courses were added at a later date to a total of 20 credits.

With the opening of the Baccalaureate Program in Nursing in 1972 and the existing Practical Nursing Program, hospital facilities for clinical practice experience became overburdened. The School of Nursing, therefore, cooperated with these two programs to plan experiences that would minimize conflict. Each program scheduled class and clinical days accordingly.

In the 1970s a policy was adopted in favor of accepting married students, and the first male students were admitted in 1973. Beginning in 1974–1975, the curriculum was reorganized to provide 11-week quarter sessions for the junior and senior year, and the affiliation in Psychiatric Nursing was changed from Philadelphia State Hospital to the Philadelphia Psychiatric Center.

The morale of the School's Administration Staff and Faculty rose in August, 1975, with a move to newly renovated and more spacious offices in the Health Sciences Building (Edison) from its former cramped offices in the Martin Residence. Classrooms were also transferred, and the three previously occupied floors in the Curtis Clinic were assigned to other departments. Also in the same year, since students from other programs within the University occupied the Martin Residence, responsibility for its supervision was transferred from the Director of the School of Nursing to the Director of Housing of the University.

Phaseout of Diploma Program

From 1976 there was a consistent decline in enrollment. Recruitment efforts were stepped up, and the School Counselor visited many of the better high schools in an effort to attract students. After much soul-searching and efforts to consider all aspects of the School relative to its present status and future, the Faculty on March 22, 1979,

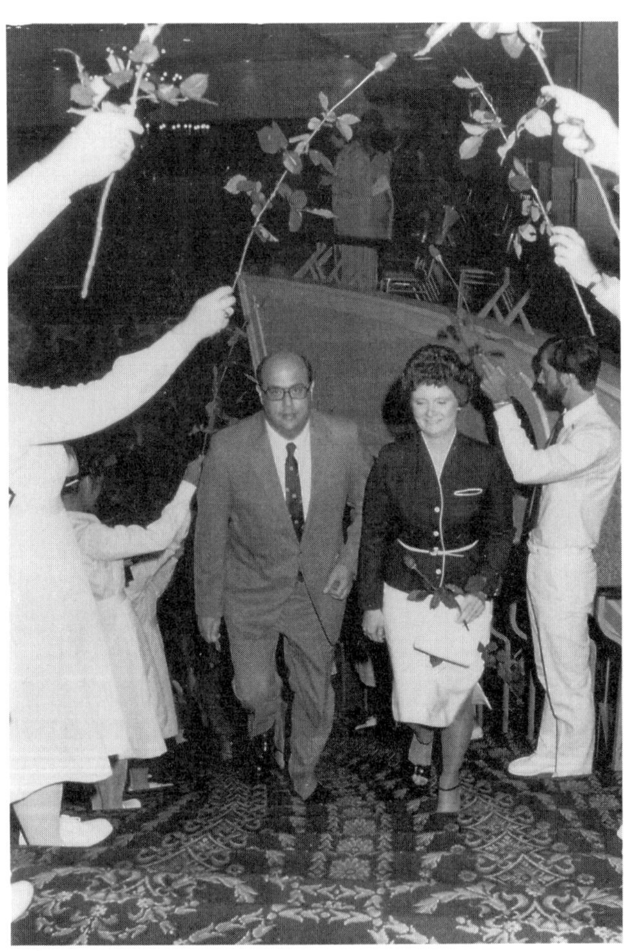

FIG. 51-18. Lawrence Abrams, Ed.D., Dean of College of Allied Health Sciences, walks through Arch of Roses with Kathleen A. Carlson, R.N. (1968), Assistant Executive Director, Pennsylvania Nurses' Association, who gave the last Commencement address (1982).

resolved by consensus to recommend to the Dean of the College of Allied Health Sciences that the School be phased out over a three-year period, with the last class to be graduated in June, 1982. Dean Abrams accepted the proposal, and it was later endorsed by the University Board of Trustees.

During the three-year phaseout, a loyal Faculty and Staff struggled to maintain the same high standards that had characterized the School since its inception in 1891. On June 10, 1982, the last class (38 members) wound its way under the traditional Arch of Roses to join over 5,000 previous graduates (Figure 51-18). The joy of this occasion was somewhat marred by the realization that this was the end of one of the finest Schools of Nursing in the country. Doris E. Bowman, who had served for 24 years as Director, retired later that year and became Emeritus Professor of Nursing. The Class of 1980 honored her with a presentation of her portrait to the University. Also, the history of the School of Nursing, *A Commitment to Excellence* (1982), was dedicated to her.

The "spirit" lives on and is destined to survive for many years. It is rewarding to hear from graduates and to converse with the over 300 who faithfully return each year to the Annual Alumni Luncheon. They all sing the praises of "Dear Old Jefferson" and the deep respect they have for the program they experienced—a program always committed to excellence.

Reference

1. Shearer, A.W., *A Commitment to Excellence*. Wynnewood, PA: Heyden-Livingston, Inc., 1982.

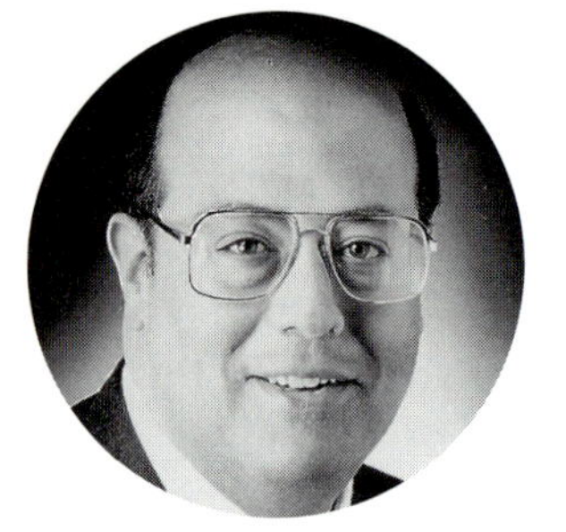

CHAPTER FIFTY-TWO

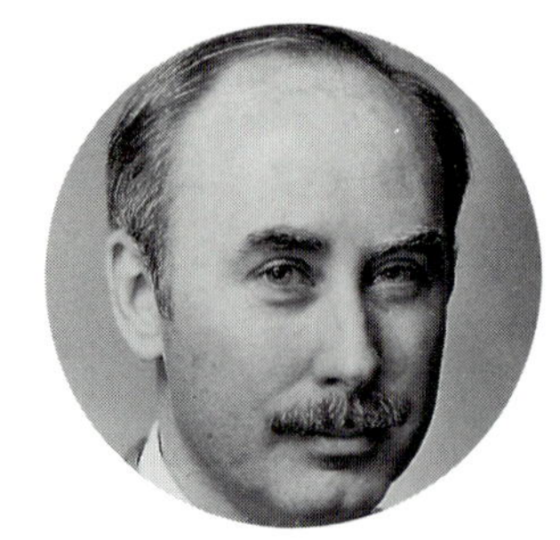

The College of Allied Health Sciences

LAWRENCE ABRAMS, ED.D. AND JOSEPH W. DONOVAN, M.A.

"An allied health professional is someone who is an ally of the patient as well as an ally of the other members of the health care team. . . . They are not ancillary members of the health care team. They are the people we depend on for the bulk of our health care services."

—LEWIS W. BLUEMLE, JR., M.D., PRESIDENT, THOMAS JEFFERSON UNIVERSITY

IT WAS AT the landmark September 9, 1968, meeting of Jefferson's Board of Trustees that the name "College of Allied Health Sciences" was approved to be effective July 1, 1969. The new name was to replace the School of Allied Health Sciences, which had been created in 1967.

That same meeting produced another significant name change, from Jefferson Medical College of Philadelphia to Thomas Jefferson University. Jefferson Medical College and the College of Allied Health Sciences were joined by the newly named College of Graduate Studies and by Jefferson Hospital, thereby forming the new University Health Science Center. Each Division was organizationally parallel, with a separate administration directly responsible to the President under the overall control of the Board of Trustees.

Roots of the College

The roots of the College extended much deeper than the 1967 School of Allied Health Sciences. Education of nurses at Jefferson, which ultimately would come under the jurisdiction of the College, had begun in 1891. Over the years, the Hospital had been active in training programs in a variety of allied health areas: medical technology since 1929; radiologic technology since 1935; and cytotechnology since 1953.

Plans for the College had their origins in 1952 when key members of the Executive Faculty of Jefferson Medical College discussed the development and expansion of teaching in the paramedical field. In 1953 several members of the Executive Faculty also raised the question of University status, either by affiliation or on its own.

Among those members was Peter A. Herbut, M.D., Professor and Chairman of the Department of Pathology and Director of the Clinical Laboratories, who would later become President of Jefferson Medical College and Medical Center and then of the University in 1969.

In April, 1964, a meeting of the Executive Faculty of the Medical College in Hershey, Pennsylvania, identified a need for an academic program in the allied medical fields.

The School of Allied Health Sciences

By April, 1966, the Special Committee on Paramedical Studies, which had been formed in 1965 and was chaired by Peter A. Herbut, M.D., delivered its report that recommended the establishment of a School of Allied Health Sciences. The recommendation, which noted that it was "a golden opportunity to take the lead in the field of health professions and occupations," was endorsed by the Executive Faculty.

The first School of Allied Medical Professions had been established at the University of Pennsylvania in 1950, and it had become the prototype of such schools in subsequent years. It was the Allied Health Professions Act of 1966 that prompted a rapid increase in organized allied health education.

After negotiations held over the summer of 1966 with the Pennsylvania State University regarding an affiliation agreement collapsed, Dr. Herbut, then President, appointed the School of Allied Health Sciences Committee in October and also a Subcommittee for Planning. He chaired both the Committee and the Subcommittee. Joining Dr. Herbut on the Subcommittee for Planning were William A. Sodeman, M.D., John W. Goldschmidt, M.D., and Mr. Lawrence Abrams.

Jefferson's Board of Trustees, on January 9, 1967, made a resolution to establish the School of Allied Health Sciences of Jefferson Medical College and to appoint John William Goldschmidt, M.D. as the first Dean.

Dean John W. Goldschmidt, M.D. (1967–1975)

John W. Goldschmidt, M.D. (Figure 52-1) spent almost 25 years at Jefferson, first as a medical student following his 1950 graduation from Villanova University, until his resignation in December of 1975 when he left, in his words, "to

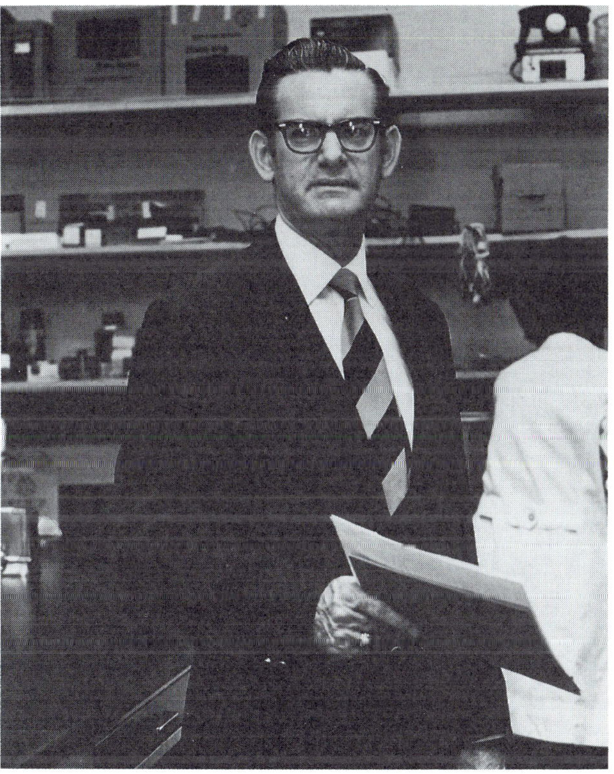

FIG. 52-1. John W. Goldschmidt, M.D., First Dean, School of Allied Health Sciences, (1967–1969), College of Allied Health Sciences (1969–1975).

return to practice of my medical specialty." Dr. Goldschmidt joined the Medical Faculty in 1959, and in 1961 he was presented the coveted Lindback Foundation Award for Distinguished Teaching.

Dr. Goldschmidt became a nationally recognized leader in the field of rehabilitation medicine. He designed and developed the Rehabilitation Center at Jefferson, which served as a model for many other such facilities throughout the country. He also served as Director of Physical Medicine and Rehabilitation at Jefferson Medical College.

Dr. Goldschmidt's eight-year tenure as Dean of the School of Allied Health Sciences, and later the College of Allied Health Sciences, witnessed the evolution of the new Division into an organized College.

In his 1971 "Plan for the College of Allied Health Sciences," Dr. Goldschmidt addressed the need for Jefferson to take the initiative in solving the nation's health care crisis, which included serious shortages of health care personnel. He noted too that "health professionals must be educated to be both scientists and humanists."

A believer in the concept of teamwork for health professionals, Dr. Goldschmidt wrote in 1975, in the first issue of the *Allied Health Review,* a publication for College alumni and friends: "A basic skill to be learned by all of us in the College of Allied Health Sciences is the skill of interpersonal collaboration. . . . A basic premise of the College is that if we have learned together and shared experience and responsibility together, we will learn to work collaboratively."

▪ Early Programs

When the School of Allied Health Sciences was founded in 1967, it represented the first provision for undergraduate college education at Jefferson under the charter of 1838 granting full University rights and privileges to Jefferson Medical College. The early programs, including nursing, medical technology, histotechnology, cytotechnology, and radiologic technology, were transferred from the Hospital to the academic and administrative structure of the School of Allied Health Sciences.

It was during this time that Lawrence Abrams, a member of the original planning committee while Coordinator of the Education Office in the Department of Rehabilitation Medicine, became the Coordinator of the Office of Program Planning and Director of Admissions and Registrar for the School. This appointment proved to be the first in a string of promotions and broadening responsibilities that would culminate in his becoming Dean of the College in 1978.

The Office of Program Planning and the administrative offices for the School were established at 1008 Chestnut Street on February 5, 1968. Its neighbors were the Philadelphia Electric Building at the corner of Tenth and Chestnut streets with its courtyard on one side and Pearson's Sporting Goods store on the other side.

▪ Health Careers Guidance Clinics

In June, 1968, the School received a grant from United Health Services and Heart Association of Southeastern Pennsylvania for "Demonstration of Function and Effectiveness of a Health Careers Guidance Clinic." What ultimately developed from that grant was a more than 20-year commitment to a public service activity sponsored by the College of Allied Health Sciences.

By August, 1968, Mrs. Dorothy Grieb was appointed Project Coordinator for the Health Careers Guidance Clinic, a program "designed to provide individualized and personalizing guidance and counseling to students and others who have an interest in or can be motivated toward a health career."

Designed to fill gaps in recruiting and counseling services of both the educational and employment systems, the Clinics featured separate programs for guidance counselors, high school students, and college students. During its first year of operation, 1968–1969, the project serviced 533 students, representing 93 area schools, including seven local colleges and universities. The tradition of service continued over the years, and by the 1986–1987 academic year over 5,000 students had been served by the Clinics (Figure 52-2). An independent consultant evaluating the Clinics in 1983 noted that the concept had been "farsighted in determining the need" and that the "Thomas Jefferson model is worthy of recognition."

Another component of the program, the *Health Careers Guidance Manual,* a reference book with in-depth descriptions of health careers, educational opportunities, and related material, gained recognition well beyond the Delaware Valley.

The *Manual,* compiled and edited by Lawrence Abrams and Dorothy Grieb, was published periodically throughout the years. By the time of its eighth edition in 1985, it had attracted widespread recognition and was believed to be the only publication of its kind in the United States.

Much of the success of the Health Careers Guidance Clinic program was attributed to continuity, not only to Lawrence Abrams and Dorothy Grieb, who stayed involved over 20 years, but also to the educational counselors, Dr. Mozelle McKay, Phyllis Neill, Karen Brubaker, Gwen Joyner, and Joseph Dorsanio, who had long tenures with the Clinics. Their expertise and dedication were noted by many participants.

The College of Allied Health Sciences

By the time the change of name from the School of Allied Health Sciences to the College of Allied Health Sciences was made effective in July, 1969,

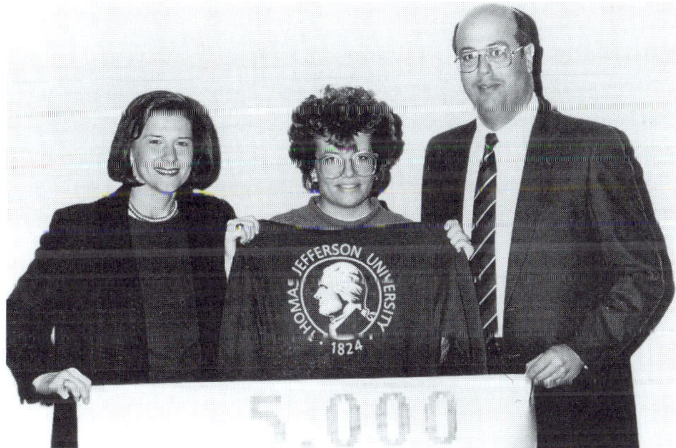

FIG. 52-2. The College-sponsored Health Careers Guidance Clinics had served 5,000 students by 1986. Clinic Project Coordinator Dorothy Grieb and Dean Lawrence Abrams flanked high school participant Tricia Neal to acknowledge the occasion.

the transition from the Hospital-based programs had been completed, and undergraduate college-level courses in general studies were instituted in cooperation with the Philadelphia College of Pharmacy and Science.

The pattern of development in the College at that time was to begin to upgrade certificate programs to baccalaureate degree programs, as well as to add new programs at the baccalaureate level. Medical technology became the first baccalaureate degree program of the College. Implemented as an upper-division program, the junior and senior years, it enrolled its first ten students in the fall of 1970, and in the spring of 1972 these students were the first to receive Bachelor of Science degrees from the College.

By December, 1970, the College's administrative offices had moved from 1008 Chestnut Street to the second floor of Jefferson Alumni Hall, and the administration had expanded to serve the growing student body.

By fall of 1971 enrollment in all programs of the College had reached 671 students. Dean Goldschmidt in a report that same year wrote: "The development of the College has progressed encouragingly and much valuable groundwork has been laid. Most disappointing has been the failure of federal and state financial support to materialize."

Shortly after Dean Goldschmidt wrote his report, however, the first grant proposal to the Bureau of Health Manpower Education, National Institutes of Health, U.S. Department of Health, Education and Welfare, was approved and funded in the amount of $10,237 as a Basic Improvement Grant for the baccalaureate program in medical technology.

At this time, Dean Goldschmidt wrote that budgetary support for the College was "provided principally by allocation from the Hospital, based on historic practice and formulae of valuation of service rendered by students in training." Administrative income was derived 30% from a Hospital allocation for administration of the various training programs and 70% from the Thomas Jefferson University Founders Association for planning and development functions.

In 1971 the College comprised four schools: the School of Nursing, a three-year diploma program; the School of Practical Nursing, a one-year certificate program and a 21-month work-study program; the School of Radiologic Technology, a two-year certificate program; and the School of Medical Technology with three programs, a one-year certificate in histologic technology, a third-year certificate program in cytotechnology, and the third- and fourth-year baccalaureate degree program in medical technology.

Instructional activities took place in existing areas throughout a variety of campus buildings, and much discussion took place at this time about the possibility of consolidating College facilities into one building, including consideration of the S.S. White Building, the Edison Building of the Philadelphia Electric Company, and the possibility of a new building designed specifically for the College.

The Department of Baccalaureate Nursing accepted its first class, 46 students, in September, 1972. During the 1972–1973 academic year, the College administration included Dean Goldschmidt; Lawrence Abrams as Associate Dean, (after serving one year as Assistant Dean) and Director of Student Affairs and Services; Dorothy Grieb as Assistant Director of Student Affairs and Services; John E. Andrews as Director of Admissions and Financial Aid; Robert D. Bailey as Registrar; and Carl R. Adams as Director of Business Administration. College enrollment stood at 454 full-time students, with 82 in degree programs and 372 in nondegree programs. The faculty numbered 52 full-time and 51 part-time.

▪ The Mid-1970s

In November, 1974, Dean Goldschmidt, who had continued his role as Associate Professor of Rehabilitation Medicine at Jefferson Medical College, was installed as President of the American Congress of Rehabilitation Medicine. His interest in returning to his medical specialty led him to accept a position at the Rehabilitation Institute of Chicago and Northwestern University. Upon Dean Goldschmidt's resignation, effective December 31, 1975, Lawrence Abrams, Associate Dean and Director of Student Affairs, was appointed Acting Dean by President Herbut until the appointment of Marten M. Kernis, Ph.D., effective September 1, 1976, as the second Dean of the College.

Dean Marten M. Kernis, Ph.D. (1976–1978)

Dr. Kernis came to Jefferson from the University of Illinois, where he was Associate Dean of the School of Basic Medical Sciences in the College of Medicine. He was also Associate Professor of Anatomy and Obstetrics and Gynecology. He had received his doctorate in anatomical sciences from the University of Florida.

As Dean Kernis' tenure began, he witnessed the Departments of Cytotechnology and Radiologic Technology, newly organized as upper-division baccalaureate degree programs, accept their first degree students in the fall of 1976, and saw the formal establishment of the Department of General Studies that same year.

The Department of Dental Hygiene's upper-division baccalaureate program began in September, 1977, and ribbon-cutting ceremonies were held on November 9, marking the opening of the Department's new clinical facility on the eighteenth floor of the Edison Building, also known as the Health Sciences Center, as well as the administrative offices on the twenty-second floor. Dean Kernis welcomed the guests, and remarks were made by Lewis W. Bluemle, Jr., M.D., who had been inaugurated President of Thomas Jefferson University at Opening Exercises two months earlier, and by Linda Kraemer, Chairman of the Department of Dental Hygiene (Figure 52-3).

At the age of ten, the College showed many signs of growth and maturity. In that 1977–1978 academic year, the College was educating and providing clinical training for 602 students. The first College catalog, covering the years 1975–1977, had been published. The first College yearbook was started in 1976 by seniors in medical technology and baccalaureate nursing. The yearbook was named *Karyon,* the winning entry in a name contest, which had been submitted by Susan Barbuto, a junior baccalaureate nursing student.

Dorothy Grieb, Assistant Director of Student Affairs and Services, who was instrumental in the publication of the catalog and who served as advisor to the yearbook, left her full-time position in October, 1976, but continued in her role as Project Coordinator of the Health Careers Guidance Clinics through the late 1980s.

The College's student life areas continued to develop. A class ring designed by senior radiologic technology students was approved in 1976. The College hosted active Orientation Day programs for incoming students each year.

The first annual College of Allied Health Sciences Achievement Award for Student Life was presented at the 1977 Opening Exercises. The award was given to Bonnie L. Dymek, a senior in the Department of Radiologic Technology, who qualified academically and who had made contributions to student life. Among other activities, she had served as coeditor of the College yearbook and had been on the Search Committee for the University's President.

After her graduation, Bonnie Dymek was appointed Admissions Counselor in the Office of Admissions, Records, and Financial Aid. Subsequently she married, became Bonnie L. Behm, and assumed the position of Coordinator, and later Director, of Financial Aid, positions she held through the late 1980s.

The College had begun to accumulate an impressive record for quality education and preparedness for employment. A Placement Survey of 1976 Graduates, typical of other surveys, showed 100% passing rates on the state board licensure or the national registry examination in five of the College's six programs. The remaining program was 98%. The number of graduates employed at the time of the survey was 96%.

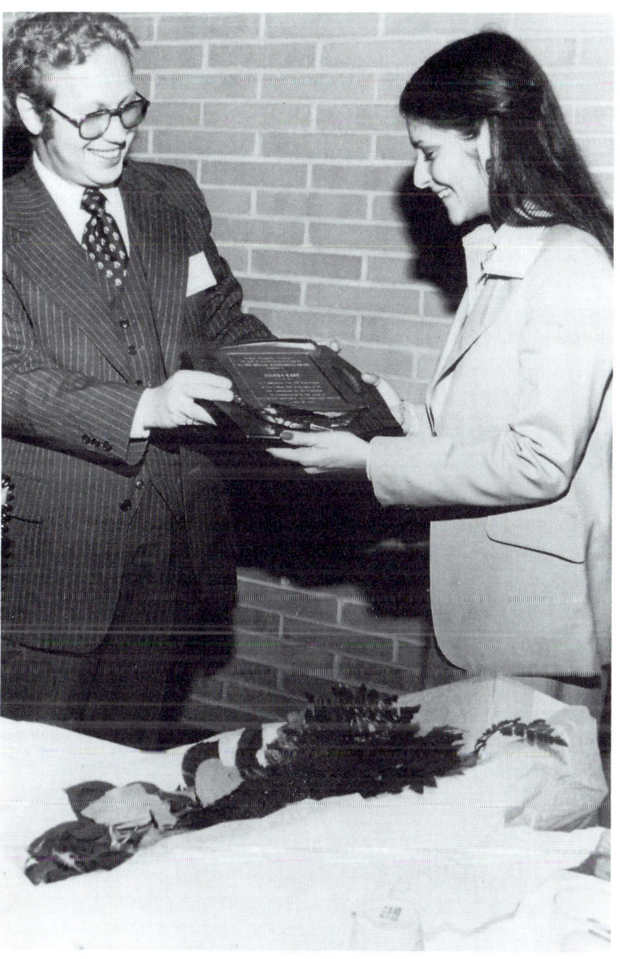

FIG. 52-3. In 1977, Marten M. Kernis, Ph.D., Second Dean of the College of Allied Health Sciences, presented Rhonda Karp, Ed.D., then Chairman and Professor, Department of Cytotechnology, with the College's first Alumni Achievement Award.

■ The Late 1970s

The late 1970's brought a change of leadership to the College of Allied Health Sciences when Dean Kernis decided to return to the University of Illinois College of Medicine to become Deputy Executive Dean. Upon his resignation, effective June 16, 1978, Associate Dean and Director of Student Affairs and Services Lawrence Abrams accepted President Bluemle's nomination to serve as Dean pro tempore.

A Search Committee was formed, and named Lawrence Abrams the third Dean of the College effective December 4. Upon his appointment, President Bluemle said, "We are fortunate that Larry Abrams will be the new Dean of the College of Allied Health Sciences. He has been associated with the College for a decade in very responsible positions. He is young, energetic, and brings to the position broad experience he has gained in the other positions he has held at Jefferson."

Dean Lawrence Abrams, Ed.D. (1978–)

A 1961 graduate of the Pennsylvania State University, where he was an active student leader and earned a Bachelor of Science degree in Business Administration, Lawrence Abrams continued his education at Temple University, receiving his Master of Education degree in Counseling Psychology in 1964.

From Coordinator of the Office of Program Planning for the College in 1968, Abrams moved steadily up the administrative ladder for the next ten years, serving subsequently as Director of Admissions and Registrar (1968–1971), Assistant Dean and Director of Student Affairs and Services (1971–1972), and Associate Dean and Director of Student Affairs and Services (1972–1978), as well as holding the Acting Deanship (1976) and Deanship pro tempore (1978) during Search Committee activities.

In 1978 he earned his Doctor of Education degree in higher education at Nova University in Fort Lauderdale, Florida. By that time Dr. Abrams had become a member of many professional organizations including the American Association of University Administrators and the American Society of Allied Health Professions.

He had been Co-Principal Investigator of the Health Careers Guidance Clinic project (1968–1970) and had been a consultant to the Department of University Affairs of the Brazilian Ministry of Education and Culture and for the U.S. Department of State's Agency for International Development in recommending appropriate allied health educational programs to meet that country's needs.

At the time of his appointment as Dean, Dr. Abrams was also Principal Investigator in a U.S. Department of Health, Education and Welfare project entitled "Women's Alternative Center: A Residential Treatment Program for Female-Headed Households with Serious Problems."

Over the next decade, Dean Abrams led the growth and development of the College as it moved into a position of national prominence among allied health institutions in the 1980s.

▪ Program Growth

When the Advanced Placement Program for Registered Nurses who wished to earn a baccalaureate degree was added in 1978, it brought the total number of College programs to ten. Over the next ten years, the number of programs doubled. Pressures for college-educated nurses and for the baccalaureate degree in particular by nursing associations led to the phaseout of the Practical Nursing program (1980) and the Diploma Nursing program (1982; Figure 52-4).

The Practical Nursing program, under the direction of Elizabeth Sweeney, B.S., M.Ed., had, since 1964, graduated 665 licensed practical nurses. The final graduating class was the largest, with 66 students. The long and distinguished history of the Diploma Nursing program is recounted in Chapter 51.

While the two nursing programs were phased out, new programs were being added. In 1980 the Department of Dental Hygiene added a Post-Certificate Program for licensed dental hygienists wishing to earn the baccalaureate degree.

The Occupational Therapy and Physical Therapy Departments opened in 1983, and in that same year the Department of Radiologic Technology expanded its offerings to include an Advanced Placement Program and a new program in Diagnostic Medical Sonography (Ultrasound). By 1985 the Department of Cytotechnology had added a Post-Certificate Program.

In 1986, the College of Allied Health Sciences, after years of planning and discussion, and with the cooperation of the College of Graduate Studies, introduced graduate education in nursing with a Master of Science in Nursing degree, specializing in rehabilitation nursing. The following year, the two Colleges combined efforts again to offer a Master of Science degree in occupational therapy.

When three new programs in the laboratory sciences area, comprising a Cytogenetic Technology Certificate Program, a combined Cytotechnology/Cytogenetics Program, and an Advanced Placement Program for medical laboratory technicians, were formed in 1987, it brought to 20 the number of programs offered by the College, twice what was offered in 1978.

Throughout these years, the College and its individual programs were accredited or reaccredited by the appropriate external agencies, typically for the longest allowable times for each program and frequently with commendations about program quality.

▪ Development in the Early 1980s

By 1980 the growth of the College was reflected in part by renovations and location changes of both administrative and academic departmental offices.

The Department of Baccalaureate Nursing and the Department of Radiologic Technology had already established themselves in the Edison Building. Work had begun on the second floor of Jefferson Alumni Hall in July, 1979, to make changes to increase office space to accommodate new staff positions. This provided for Dean Abrams and his staff, the Office of Admissions, the faculty offices for the Department of Cytotechnology, and those of the Department of Medical Technology.

Among the recent additions to the administrative staff at that time was the appointment of Rhonda Karp, Ed.D., as Assistant Dean, a newly created position. Dr. Karp had originally come to Jefferson as a student and was a 1971 graduate of the School of Cytotechnology. She became the School's Education Coordinator in 1975, and eventually Professor and Chairman of the Department of Cytotechnology. Dr. Karp had been appointed Special Assistant to the Dean in January, 1979, and Assistant Dean on July 1 of that year. Her appointment made her the first woman officer in the College's history.

Dr. Karp was promoted to Associate Dean in 1982 and held that post until 1987, when she became the Executive Associate to the University President, Lewis W. Bluemle, Jr. During her term as Associate Dean, Dr. Karp was able to make substantial contributions to the administration of the College while maintaining a foothold in her original field of cytotechnology.

A Temple University alumna three times over, with a B.S. in education in 1971, an M.S. in pathology in 1975, and an Ed.D. in adult and continuing education in 1978, Dr. Karp was the College of Allied Health Sciences' first recipient of its Alumni Achievement Award in 1977.

In the field of cytotechnology, she published and served as editor of *The Cytotechnologist's Bulletin* (1981–1986) and was named "Cytotechnologist of the Year" by the American Society of Cytology in 1987. Named an

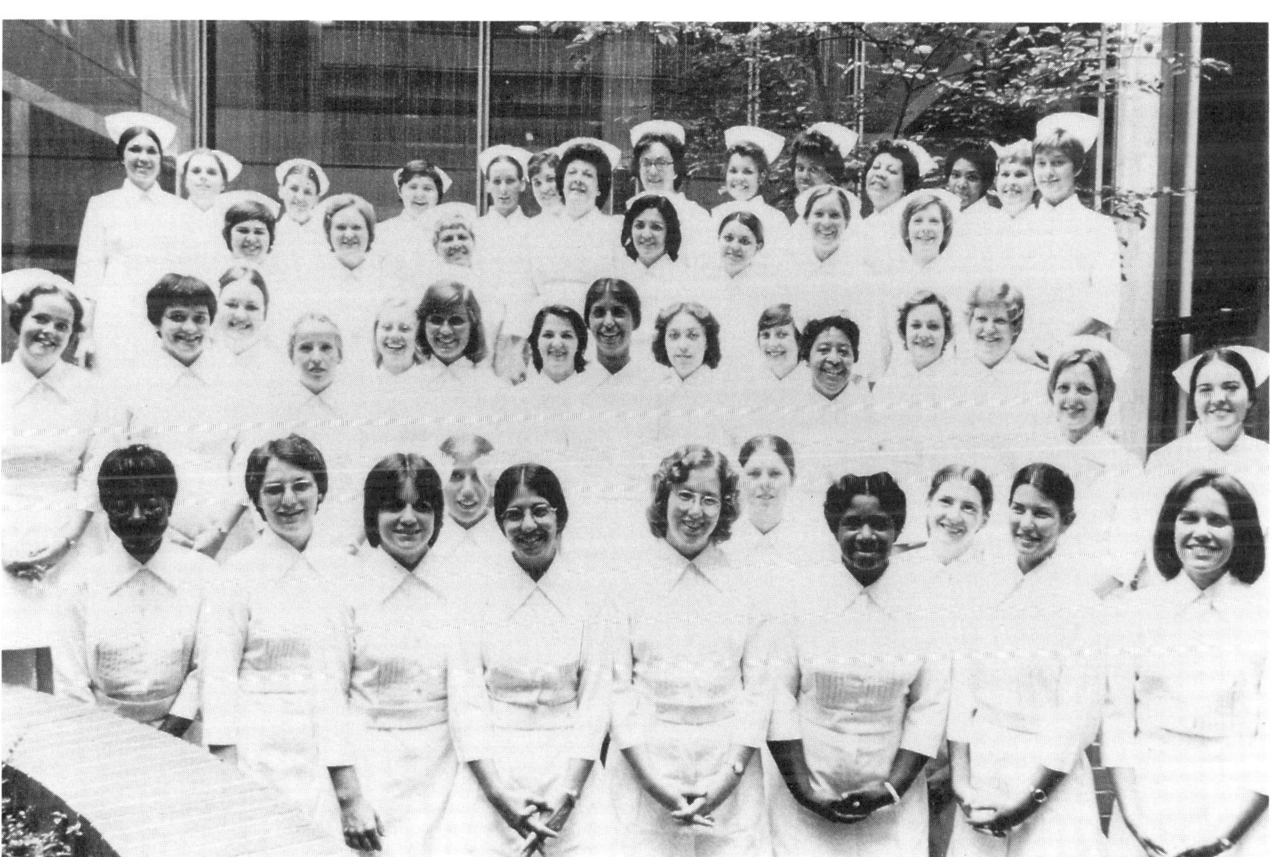

FIG. 52-4. The Class of 1975, School of Practical Nursing.

"Outstanding Young Leader in Allied Health" by the American Society of Allied Health Professions in 1984, Dr. Karp was awarded a Fulbright Lectureship in Quito, Equador, that same year. Her national role in allied health education was underscored in 1985 when she was elected to the Board of Directors of the American Society of Allied Health Professions and to the Committee of Allied Health Education and Accreditation of the American Medical Association in 1987.

The College of Allied Health Sciences Commencement Exercises in 1980 were noteworthy. Since its first graduating class in 1972, the College had shared the same graduation ceremony with Jefferson Medical College and the College of Graduate Studies at Jefferson's traditional commencement site, the Philadelphia Academy of Music. The location remained the same, but the College's ceremony in 1980 was held separately for the first time. It was significant, too, because one of the three honorary degree recipients was the College's founding Dean, John W. Goldschmidt, M.D., who received an honorary Doctor of Science degree from Dean Abrams.

Seven years later, at the recommendation of President Bluemle, the College was able to have its own Grand Marshal, Linda G. Kraemer, R.D.H., Ph.D., Chairman and Associate Professor, Department of Dental Hygiene. Dr. Kraemer first marched as Grand Marshal with the University mace in the 1987 Commencement Exercises (Figure 52-5).

The early 1980s saw the formation of a chapter of the Alpha Eta Society at Jefferson. A national honor society under the auspices of the American Society of Allied Health Professions, Jefferson's Alpha Eta chapter became the twenty-second nationwide when established in 1982.

Commencement exercises in June, 1983, featured a standing ovation for baccalaureate nursing graduate Peter J. Leporati, the winner of the College's Student Life Award. Leporati, a former Philadelphia policeman who decided to change his career path to nursing, had become a well-known and popular figure on campus. Leporati was President of the Nursing Student Government and Vice President of Jefferson's chapter of the Student Nurses' Association of Pennsylvania, among his many student activities. In addition, the story of his unusual career change, particularly for a man in nursing, gained local media coverage.

In September, 1983, at the one hundred and sixtieth Opening Exercises ceremony of the University, President Bluemle presented Dean Abrams with a "Citation for Distinguished Service," citing the "remarkable progress the College has been making under your guidance for the past five years." Also worthy of noting about that September were the 354 entering juniors, the largest College of Allied Health Sciences class to that date. The students came from colleges and universities in 27 states and ten foreign countries.

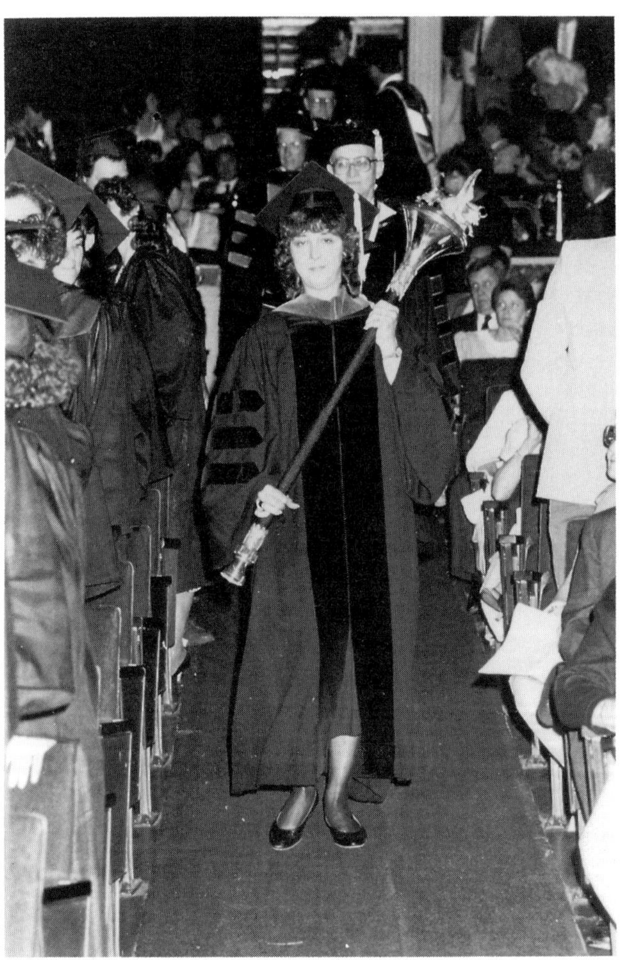

FIG. 52-5. The College of Allied Health Sciences' first Grand Marshal, Linda G. Kraemer, R.D.H., Ph.D., at the 1987 Commencement exercises.

The Mid 1980s

By the 1984–1985 academic year, Kevin J. Lyons, Ph.D. already had one year behind him on the staff of the Dean's office with Drs. Abrams and Karp. Dr. Lyons had been named Assistant to the Dean and Director of Continuing Education. Before coming to Jefferson, Dr. Lyons was Director of off-campus programs in the Graduate School of Education at the University of Pennsylvania. He had earned his doctoral degree in educational administration at the University of Maryland in 1975.

Dr. Lyons' responsibilities included the cultivation of research activities among College faculty and administration. Dean Abrams had made research a priority in 1979 in his "Report to the University Planning Task Force Committee on Academic Affairs and Research in the College of Allied Health Sciences." Dr. Abrams had written: "Quality research is vitally important in allied health as in other health-related disciplines in order to continue to provide the best education and the best patient care possible in light of new developments in science and technology."

Dr. Lyons, who was promoted to Assistant Dean in 1985 and to Associate Dean in 1986, also served as liaison to the College of Graduate Studies as the two Colleges worked together on joint graduate education programs.

Among the administrative staff in 1984–1985 were Bonnie Lee Behm, B.S., R.T., as Coordinator of Financial Aid, later named director of Financial Aid, Theodore M. Bross, M.A., Acting Director of Admissions, later named Director of Admissions; Joseph J. Collins, B.S., CPA, Director of Business Administration, who had been chief of general accounting in the University's Controller's office until coming to the College in 1979; Joseph W. Donovan, M.A., in the newly established position of Coordinator of Public Relations for the College; Michael J. Paquet, M.A., Registrar, who had served in the Registrar's Office in the Medical College until 1980; and William Thygeson, M.Ed., Director of Student Affairs and Services since coming to Jefferson in 1979 from his post as Associate Dean of Admissions and Freshman at Muhlenberg College.

By this time, the Office of Student Affairs and Services had an active program of academic support services, including reading and study skills workshops and individual counseling. A Leadership Development Retreat for selected students from each department proved highly successful and was made an annual event. The Office sponsored other annual events such as Orientation Day for new students, as well as Parents' Day, later renamed Family Day. A Student Advisory Committee gave student representatives from each academic department a forum for exchanging views with College Administration.

Organized social events for students were usually centered in Jefferson Alumni Hall, whose cafeteria served for years as the scene of an annual dance, known as the Winter Social, held in February. "Jeff Hall," as it was more informally identified, was also the site of most Class Night activities, which became an annual tradition of departmental acknowledgements of the end of the year for graduating seniors. Held the night before Commencement Exercises, with each Department in its own room or auditorium depending on the size of the class, programs featured the pinning of seniors, awards, and sometimes humorous presentations made by students to the faculty. Families were invited to attend, and a collegewide reception followed, held on Scott Plaza, weather permitting.

Jefferson Alumni Hall was also the home of the "Commons," where students of all three Colleges of the University enjoyed membership privileges for recreational use and for programs sponsored by the Student Activities Office, ranging from lunchtime entertainment to intramural sports programs. In 1985 Dean Abrams was appointed Student Affairs Officer for the University with responsibility for the Commons, among other areas of student life.

The Mid-1980s and Beyond

By 1985 the College of Allied Health Sciences had emerged as a national leader in allied health education. In the previous year, Dean Abrams had been made a Fellow of the American Society of Allied Health Professions (ASAHP), and an article in the University's monthly publication *Directions* quoted the President of ASAHP, Edmund J.

McTernan, Ed.D., Dean of the School of Allied Health Professions, State University of New York at Stony Brook, as saying that Jefferson's College of Allied Health Sciences "ranks as one of the top half dozen in the country." The Executive Director of ASAHP, Carolyn M. DelPolito, Ph.D., said "the people at Jefferson are having an impact at the national level." The opportunity to expand that impact would come three years later when Dean Abrams would assume the Presidency of ASAHP. The emphasis that the College had placed on research years earlier became evident as faculty, administrators, and students increased dramatically the quantity and quality of research-based publications and presentations.

The evolution of the College continued in 1987–1988 when its administrative offices and the Department of Laboratory Sciences moved from Jefferson Alumni Hall to the Edison Building, thus bringing about the geographical consolidation of the College of Allied Health Sciences that had long been sought (Figure 52-6).

As the decade of the 1980s was coming to a close, the issue of shortages of health care personnel that had been the impetus for the founding of the College of Allied Health Sciences had once again surfaced at the national level. This time, however, a matured institution stood ready with a Task Force to plan the focus of the College for the 1990s with the goal of planning education programs that would meet the needs of the public and professional communities and ultimately contribute to the health of the nation.

Department of Medical Technology

Education in medical technology, in one form or another, has been part of Jefferson since the inception of the Hospital's first laboratories. In 1929, for the first time, first-year students of technology were taught in all disciplines of the Hospital's laboratories, including chemistry, endocrinology, hematology, histology, immunohematology, microbiology, parasitology, serology, and urinalysis. The medical technology program during those early years lasted 12 months and consisted almost entirely of one-on-one instruction by a laboratory technologist. While they learned, students were tested orally on a continuous basis by the technologist. At the end of the year-long program, an oral examination was conducted by the pathologist in charge of the laboratory. On average, two or three students were accepted into the program each year. During the beginning years of the program, no tuition was charged, and the students were provided with lunch, the laundering of their uniforms, and free hospital care.

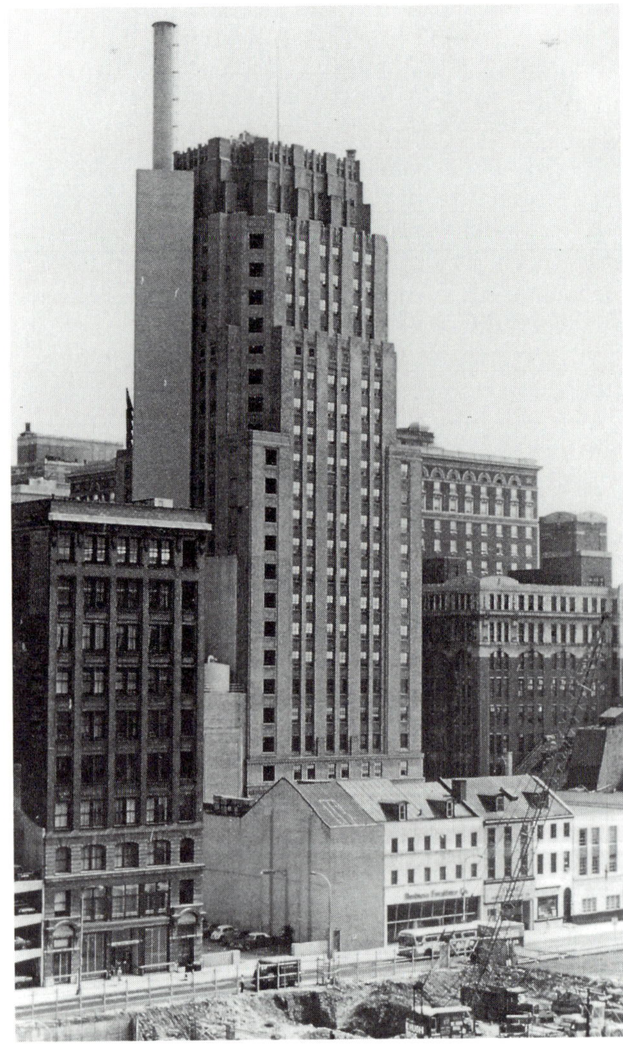

Fig. 52-6. The Edison Building at Ninth and Sansom Streets (shown here in a photograph taken in the mid-1970s) eventually became the home of a consolidated College of Allied Health Sciences in 1988.

The 1930s

In the early 1930s, an informal arrangement with Ursinus College allowed students from that institution to pursue their medical technology laboratory education at Jefferson. By this time, the program was extended to 18 months, with students spending two months in each of the Hospital's nine laboratories.

In 1936 a Board of Registry was established by the American Society of Clinical Pathologists (ASCP) to maintain the competency of technologists employed in clinical laboratories. About four years later, the Board of Registry required medical technology professionals to pass a test in order to be classified as registered. Technician candidates had to be graduates of an education program approved by the Board of Schools (a committee established by the ASCP to review education programs in medical technology) and employed by a laboratory affiliated with ASCP.

Formation of a Program

In September of 1941, the first formal class of four students was accepted at Jefferson. These students rotated through all the Hospital laboratories and worked side by side with paid employees. At that time, the laboratories were located on the top floor of the Thompson Annex. In 1942 Jefferson's medical technology program was extended to include formal lectures, given on an irregular schedule by Hospital personnel. By 1950 the medical technology program was accredited for 15 students.

In 1952 the program was reduced to a 12-month period. Students worked in the Hospital 44 hours a week, and written, oral, and practical examinations were required. Tuition was $100, plus a breakage fee of $5. The Medical Technology School at Jefferson was reaccredited in 1953, in 1963, and again in 1968. In each instance, the accreditation was conferred with distinction.

Until the program was incorporated into the School of Allied Health Sciences in 1967, the medical technology program had no budget of its own and was funded through Jefferson Hospital's laboratory. Likewise, the faculty members for the program were employees of Jefferson Hospital's clinical laboratories who added the responsibility of teaching the students to their schedule of activities.

Toward a New Identity

In the mid-1960s, the faculty of the medical technology program recognized the need for an increase in the number of lectures and student laboratory experiences. In 1968 the curriculum was revised and divided into two segments. The first was a four-month period, during which students spent their time in lectures and the student laboratories. The remaining eight months the students spent "at the bench" of the hospital laboratory for more practical experience. During this time lectures were limited to those that would enrich the students' bench experience.

In 1969 medical technology students were the first accepted into Jefferson's newly organized College of Allied Health Sciences, created at the same time as Thomas Jefferson University. To reflect this major change in status, the curriculum was redesigned, extended to 24 months, and consisted of courses in each of the content areas that awarded academic credit. To follow in the tradition of practical experience, during one-third of the curriculum, the students worked at the bench in the Hospital laboratory in clinical rotation.

Upon the successful completion of the curriculum, graduates were awarded the degree of Bachelor of Science in Medical Technology and were then eligible to take the certification examination of their choice. This program was reaccredited in 1970 on a two-year academic-basis in the College of Allied Health Sciences (Figure 52–7).

The Nontraditional Program

Under the leadership of Elizabeth A. Turner, Ph.D., who had been appointed the Department's Education Coordinator in 1971 and Chairman in 1973, the Department was granted five-year funding for the Nontraditional Interinstitutional Academic Program (NIAP) in Medical Technology by the Department of Health, Education and Welfare of over $2 million.

This program, begun in 1976, was created to offer an alternative to the traditional academic one for earning the Bachelor of Science Degree in Medical Technology. It was designed as a weekend alternative for currently employed medical laboratory personnel who could utilize their employers' facilities to perform clinical assignments. The program also included autotutorial instruction where the student was "tutored" individually by means of mediated study materials.

The plan was a consortial one with the University of Pennsylvania and Temple University. This arrangement allowed the student to earn a degree at the University of Pennsylvania as well as at Thomas Jefferson University, since both institutions accepted NIAP course credits as meeting major program and residency requirements. The student was subject to regular admission at the place of degree choice.

■ The 1980s

With the 1980s came a challenge for the Department of Medical Technology as the numbers of applicants and matriculants began to decline, a problem that occurred in programs throughout the country, attributed in part to the decrease in the college-age population and the increase in the availability of other professions for women. To address the enrollment problem, the College of Allied Health Sciences increased its student recruitment efforts, and the department moved to create an Advanced Placement Program for registered medical laboratory technologists (MLTs) who sought a baccalaureate degree.

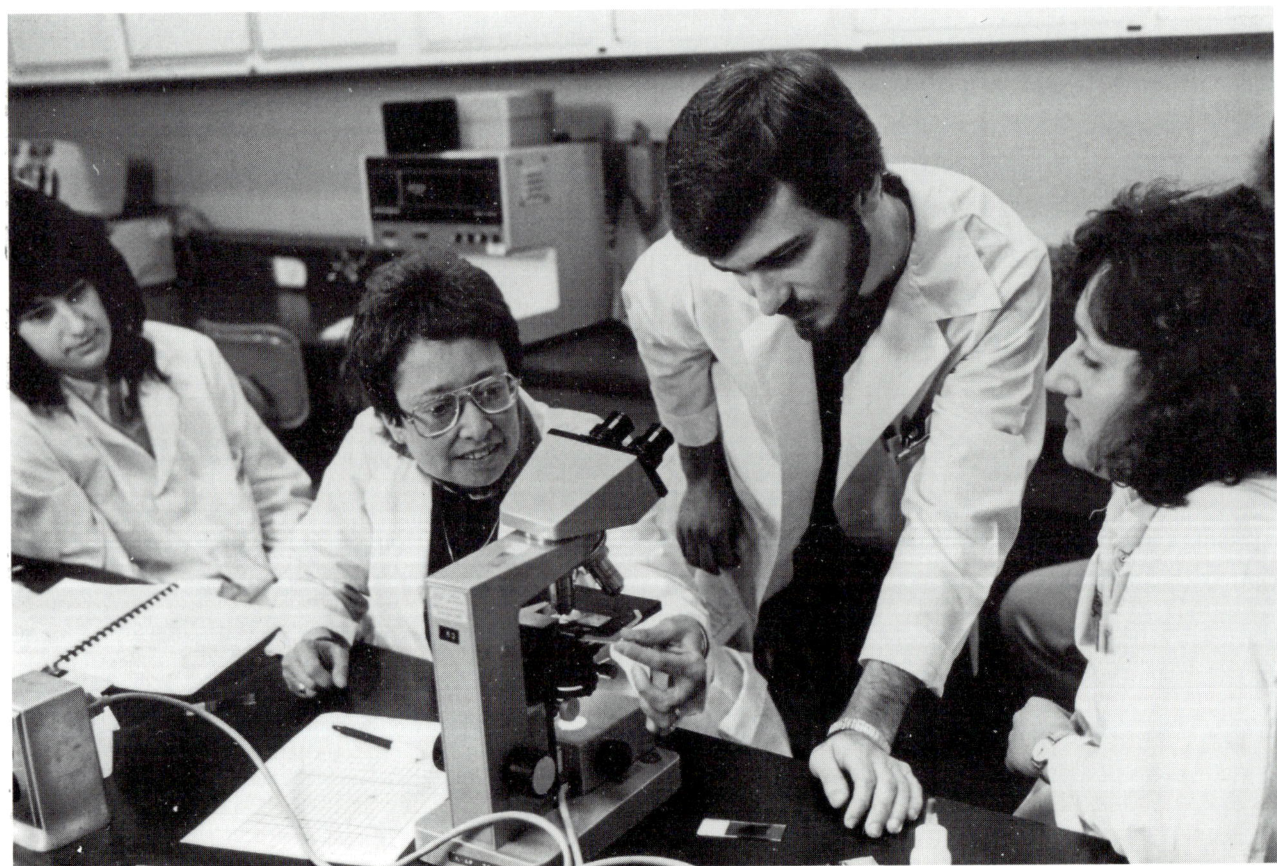

FIG. 52-7. Medical technology students worked closely with faculty members in the laboratory.

The department also had plans to offer degrees in a variety of specialties allied with laboratory analyses, as well as a generalist degree. New attention in the curriculum was directed to the application of computers (Figure 52–8).

Not only its long history at Jefferson but also its past and current record of educational excellence within the field of medical technology ensures a solid future for this Department.

Department of Nursing

Although the decision to establish a Bachelor of Science in Nursing degree program was made by Thomas Jefferson University's Board of Trustees on November 2, 1970, nursing education had already been a major part of Jefferson Medical College since the end of the nineteenth century. Starting as a two-year course in 1891, it became a three-year Diploma Nursing School in 1894.

The decision to initiate a collegiate nursing program was a result of the University's commitment to assume a leadership role in educating nurses and allied health professionals. In 1971, Charlotte Voss, R.N., Ed.D. was selected as the first Chairman of Jefferson's Department of Baccalaureate Nursing. Dr. Voss developed a curriculum encompassing a broad base in the natural and social sciences, arts and humanities, which included emphasis on episodic care (care of the ill) and distributive care (care of the healthy). Dr. Voss was also instrumental in obtaining a special project grant of over $94,000 from the United States Department of Health, Education and Welfare, Division of Nursing for the purpose of paying for consultation fees, physical space costs, and learning resource equipment, and in recruiting faculty members from major specialty areas.

The Initiation of Baccalaureate Nursing

From its planning stages, the undergraduate nursing program at Jefferson placed great emphasis on excellence in clinical education and the study of professional nursing. The curriculum-planning design was innovative and one of the first in the Philadelphia region to adopt a framework to teach nursing concepts. In addition to the traditional acquisition of knowledge and skills necessary to care for hospitalized patients, Jefferson also offered learning experiences in health promotion and disease prevention. Students had the opportunity to care for individuals in a variety of settings, ranging from schools and senior citizen centers to ambulatory health care facilities to acute care institutions. Emphasis was placed on utilizing the best clinical agencies as resources for clinical learning experiences (Figure 52–9).

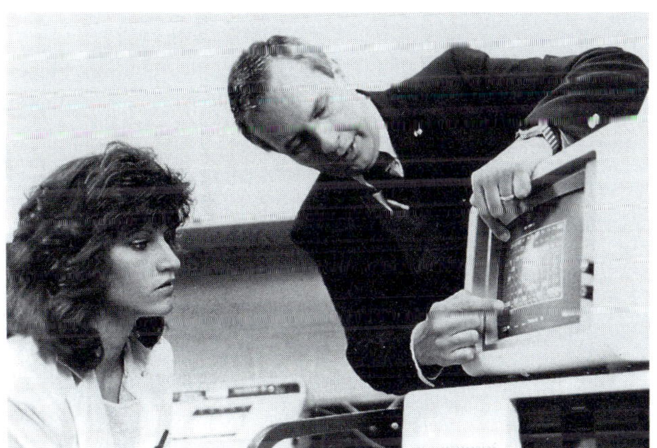

FIG. 52-8. The role of computers in medical technology gained importance in the 1980s.

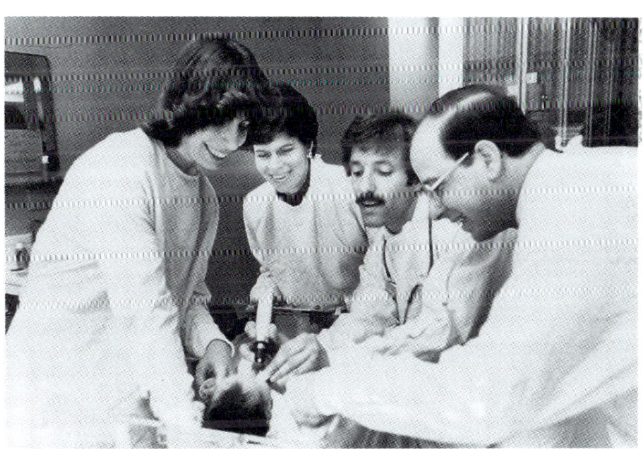

FIG. 52-9. Excellence in clinical skills was regarded as a hallmark of the Jefferson nursing program.

With approval of the Commonwealth of Pennsylvania State Board of Nurse Examiners, the baccalaureate nursing program in the College of Allied Health Sciences admitted its first class of 46 students, hailing from a wide range of educational and social backgrounds, into the two-year, upper-division (junior and senior years) program in September of 1972. Of these students, 40 had completed requirements for the Bachelor of Science in Nursing degree by 1976, and 39 were successful in passing the examination for licensure.

From its inception, the Department's activities were organized to provide maximum opportunity for faculty and students to participate. Committees, including academic affairs, curriculum, educational resources, evaluation, faculty affairs, advanced standing, and continuing education, were established.

In December of 1974 the department received full approval from the Commonwealth of Pennsylvania State Board of Nurse Examiners. The next year the University was involved in the Middle States Association of College and Secondary Schools accreditation process. The Middle States team notified the University of its formal accreditation in February of 1976. In April of that same year, the Department of Baccalaureate Nursing received accreditation for the maximum eight years from the National League for Nursing, Department of Baccalaureate and Higher Degree Programs.

■ The Growing Years

Following a self-study process and the achievement of full accreditation status, the last half of the 1970s was a period of stability and refinement for the Department. During this time, the American Nurses' Association and the National League for Nursing firmly supported the baccalaureate degree as entry-level into the nursing profession. In 1978 the first registered nurse students were admitted into the Department's Advanced Placement Program, which was designed to enable registered nurses to capitalize on their educational and practical experience in order to earn a Bachelor of Science in Nursing degree in two years of study.

The Department's continuing education activities became more extensive and formalized during this period, with programs offered both on campus and at satellite locations. The faculty also began to engage in a number of scholarly activities, including the publication of texts and articles in nursing journals and participation in professional organizations. That same year, the Department was approved for a chapter of Sigma Theta Tau, the international nursing honor society.

■ The 1980s

Mary D. Naylor, R.N., Ph.D. became the second chairman of the Department of Baccalaureate Nursing in September, 1980. While the emphasis on academic and clinical excellence continued, the goals of the Department broadened to include leadership, scholarship, faculty practice, and community service. Faculty members presented papers at international, national, and regional meetings of nurses and other disciplines and published major clinical texts, research articles, and scholarly articles in nursing and related-discipline journals. One of the texts authored by Elizabeth J. Forbes, R.N., Ed.D. received the *American Journal of Nursing* Book of the Year Award in 1982. Faculty members also functioned as consultants for the White House Conference on Aging, the Division of Nursing.

In response to an increased need for professional nurses and in the presence of a large pool of qualified applicants, the Department experienced a period of expansion from 1980 through 1983. During that time, the Department maintained an approximate enrollment of 140 generic and 40 registered nurse students in each class. The Department was successful in consistently recruiting skilled and knowledgeable students from colleges and universities throughout the United States. Among these students were former teachers, social workers, psychologists, musicians, and artists. Commensurate with the growth in the student population was an increase in the number of faculty, from 18 full-time members in 1980 to 37 in 1984.

In 1981 and 1982 multiple faculty workshops culminated in the development of a comprehensive philosophical statement, a conceptual framework, and program objectives that guided the refinement of existing courses as well as the development of new course offerings. On April 3, 1984, the Department of Baccalaureate Nursing received full reaccreditation from the National League for Nursing for eight years. The accreditation body commended the Department's opportunities for independent learning and guided individualized studies, including the ability of students to study nursing throughout the United States and all continents of the world.

A visit from representatives of the Commonwealth of Pennsylvania State Board of Nurse Examiners resulted in continued full approval status for the Department in 1980 and again in 1982. During the latter visit, the site visitor commented on the consistently strong performance of Jefferson nursing students on licensing examinations.

In 1982 the Star (thirteenth) floor of the Edison Building was renovated in order to build the department's Learning Resource Center. The Center contained three clinical simulation areas, three audiovisual rooms, and a reception area (Figure 52–10). A five-year plan to develop and implement computer technology into the nursing curriculum was formed in 1982, and a nursing elective course, "Computers in Nursing," was developed and introduced in 1985. By the academic year 1983–1984, faculty offices were housed on the tenth, twelfth, thirteenth, and fifteenth floors of the Edison Building. The main office space on the twelfth floor was renovated to provide a reception and waiting area.

In 1984 two additional program options were offered to registered nurse students, including a

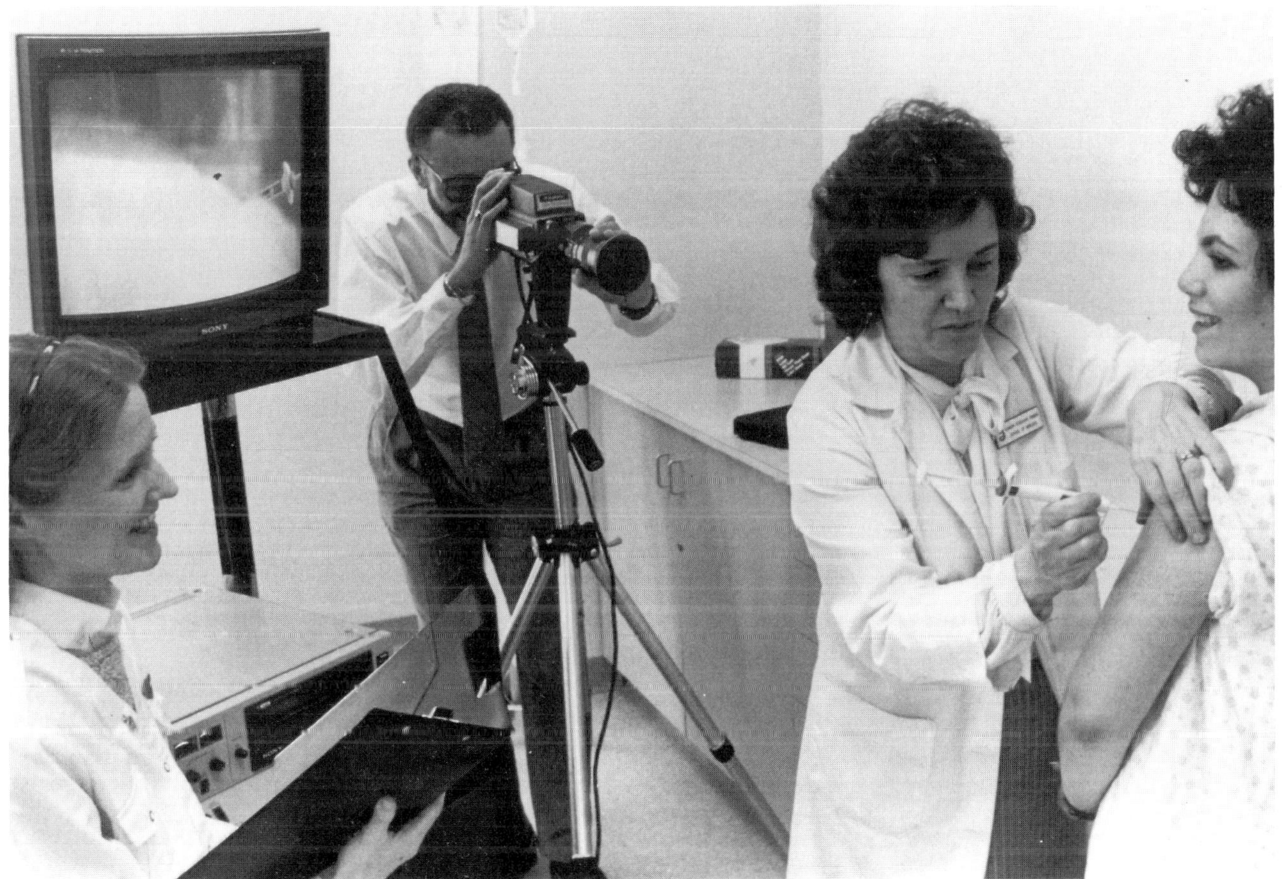

FIG. 52-10. Videotaping of procedures in the Learning Resource Center enabled students to review educational materials on an independent basis.

part-time evening program and a satellite part-time program in Harrisburg. Consistent with the directions evolving in health care, with an increased emphasis on ambulatory care, home health care, and long-term health care, student placements were obtained in agencies that provided these learning opportunities. In order to support the faculty's efforts to offer a full range of educational opportunities including both undergraduate and graduate programs, the name of the Department was officially changed to the Department of Nursing in the spring of 1984.

New Visions for Nursing

In August of 1985 a Plan for Preeminence was submitted by the faculty to Lawrence Abrams, Ed.D., Dean of the College of Allied Health Sciences. Using a quality undergraduate program as its base, the faculty sought the addition of educational programs including a Master of Science in Nursing (M.S.N.) program and a Doctor of Philosophy Program in Nursing. By 1986 the M.S.N. degree program had been approved, and the first class began in September of that year.

Since the early 1980s, the nursing leadership in the Department recognized that its efforts to earn a regional and national reputation as a center for excellence in clinical nursing depended to a large degree on the scholarly productivity of Jefferson researchers. The department accordingly proposed the establishment of a Clinical Nursing Research Center. In the mid-1980s the Department also took several measures to strengthen its recruitment efforts in wake of the shrinking applicant pool for nursing. It demonstrated flexibility in meeting the needs of a changing market by developing a part-time option for its generic students in 1985.

During this time, the Department of Nursing emphasized teaching strategies designed to promote critical thinking and independent decision making. Also emphasized were the development of independent study modules, small group seminars, and interdisciplinary learning experiences. While reflecting on almost 100 years of nursing education at Jefferson, the Department of Nursing was looking toward the next century with the pride and anticipation of creating yet a new tradition in nursing excellence.

Department of Cytotechnology

Cytotechnology has been practiced and taught at Jefferson since the early 1940s. It was then that researchers discovered uterine cancer could be detected by examining cells. Across the nation and at Jefferson, where Dr. Abraham Rakoff was studying the potential diagnostic applications of cytology, the need for the development of training facilities was recognized. As a result, Jefferson became one of 15 AMA-approved institutions to offer American Cancer Society–funded fellowships to support physicians in their study of cytology. As the concept of "mass screening" became a reality, the need for technical assistance to handle the increasing specimen volume became apparent.

Through the years, Dr. Rakoff organized material to be utilized in a formal cytology training program at Jefferson. On September 21, 1957, Norma Ermler, a medical technologist, became the first student in Jefferson's formal cytology program. The American Cancer Society, along with the Cancer Control Program of the United States Public Health Service, contributed funds for support of students and teaching staff, as well as for the purchase of equipment and educational materials.

In the beginning, the one-year program attracted an average of five students per year. In 1960 it acquired accredited status according to requirements established by "The Essentials of an Acceptable School of Cytotechnology," the first set of standards established for cytology schools, which were later accepted by the American Medical Association. Jefferson's program emphasized a student's proficiency in preparing cytologic specimens for microscopic analysis and in distinguishing between benign and malignant cells of the body's systems.

The 1960s

Student enrollment remained steady throughout the 1960s during which time approximately 108 students were accepted into the program and 81 graduated. The program was under the administration of Dr. Peter Herbut, Director of Clinical Laboratories, who became the third full-time President of Jefferson Medical College in 1966 and in 1969 became the first President of Thomas Jefferson University. In 1966 Dr. Gonzalo E. Aponte succeeded Dr. Herbut as Director and continued the strong tradition of leadership.

During this time, students spent a total of 40 hours per week in the classroom/laboratory located on the third floor of the Foerderer Pavilion. Philadelphia-area physicians donated specimens from their laboratories, which helped increase the students' practical experience and developed their abilities to make critical differential diagnoses.

The need for cytotechnologists during the 1960s was great, accounting for the fact that the most consistent recruiters for the program were area pathologists who sent members of their technical laboratory staffs to receive cytology training. It was also during this time that cytotechnology began to increase its professional status nationwide and create improved employment opportunities.

In 1968 the cytology laboratory was granted independent status within the clinical laboratories, and Dr. Misao Takeda was appointed Director. Along with this distinction came a move from the third floor of Foerderer Pavilion to the second floor of Jefferson Alumni Hall.

Changes in the 1970s

By 1970 cytology education at Jefferson and elsewhere was on the verge of a major transformation when the United States Public Health Service funds were terminated. Although 13 schools closed, Jefferson's cytology school battled financial difficulties by charging tuition for the first time in its history. The fee was fixed at $50 per student for the six-month course. This provided funding for the students but the teaching/supervisory position had lost its support. The program turned to the College of Allied Health Sciences in hope of assistance. Dean Goldschmidt gave his approval to bring the supervisor's position into the College. Thus the Jefferson program survived the transition in funding sources and grew closer to its goal of becoming fully integrated with the College and enhancing the likelihood of a degree program.

At this time educators were beginning to consider seriously the establishment of degree programs in cytotechnology. This issue proved to be a controversial one, creating a flurry of views and comments from cytotechnologists and pathologists across the country. Jefferson was one that aspired to offer such a degree program. Through the early 1970s the groundwork that would lead to departmental status in the College of Allied Health Sciences was established. A decision was made to increase the training to a 12-month period, and in 1974 the first seven students graduated.

To begin active planning for a bachelor's degree program and to make revisions in order to convert the curriculum, Rhonda Karp joined the faculty in July of 1975 as Educator Coordinator. Karp, a cytotechnologist and Jefferson graduate, had recently received a master's degree in pathology from Temple University.

In 1976, under the direction of Chairman Karp, the School of Cytotechnology became the Department of Cytotechnology within the College of Allied Health Sciences, the first in the nation to offer a two-year, upper-division degree program.

Sixteen students were enrolled as juniors in the first class in September of 1976. The program was reviewed by the American Society of Cytology's Programs Review Committee, received a favorable report, and was awarded a five-year accreditation status. The new department acquired additional space in Jefferson Alumni Hall, and a television microscopy unit was purchased, allowing the instructor to demonstrate cellular changes to an entire class via a television monitor (Figure 52–11). Revisions in the curriculum and increased laboratory skills broadened the educational background of the students during the 1970s.

Also during that decade, the Department of Cytotechnology increased its participation in continuing education activities and faculty involvement in professional organizations, especially the Inter-Society Cytology Council (whose founding members included Drs. Abraham Rakoff and Peter Herbut). It is known today as the American Society of Cytology. Other activities included development of microscopic workshops, sessions, and lectures, and the publication of numerous articles concerning cytology education and research.

Chairman Karp, who became Dr. Karp in 1978, having earned an Ed.D. at Temple University, chaired the department until June 1979, when she was appointed Assistant Dean of the College and Professor of Cytotechnology. Subsequently, she became Associate Dean in 1982 but continued to contribute to her field, including active participation in the American Society of Cytology and editorship of *The Cytotechnologist's Bulletin*, 1981–1986.

■ The 1980s

In the early 1980s, Marilyn McHenry became Department Chairman and Dr. Warren Lang became Medical Director. Through a project of McHenry, supported by the National Institutes of Health and the United States Department of Health, Education and Welfare, faculty members were given the opportunity to attend professional workshops on methods for the incorporation of the humanities into a technical curriculum. Dr. Lang, a pathologist and a gynecologist, had the ability to add an extensive clinical dimension to his teaching of female genital tract cytology. Dr. Lang served as President of the American Society of Cytology in 1984 and at the 1985 annual meeting in Atlanta was presented with the Papanicolaou Award, recognizing his many contributions to the organization and profession. Both Drs. Lang and Takeda, as primary and collaborative authors, published numerous articles as a further contribution to cytology education and research.

In 1984 Shirley E. Greening, CFIAC, M.S.,

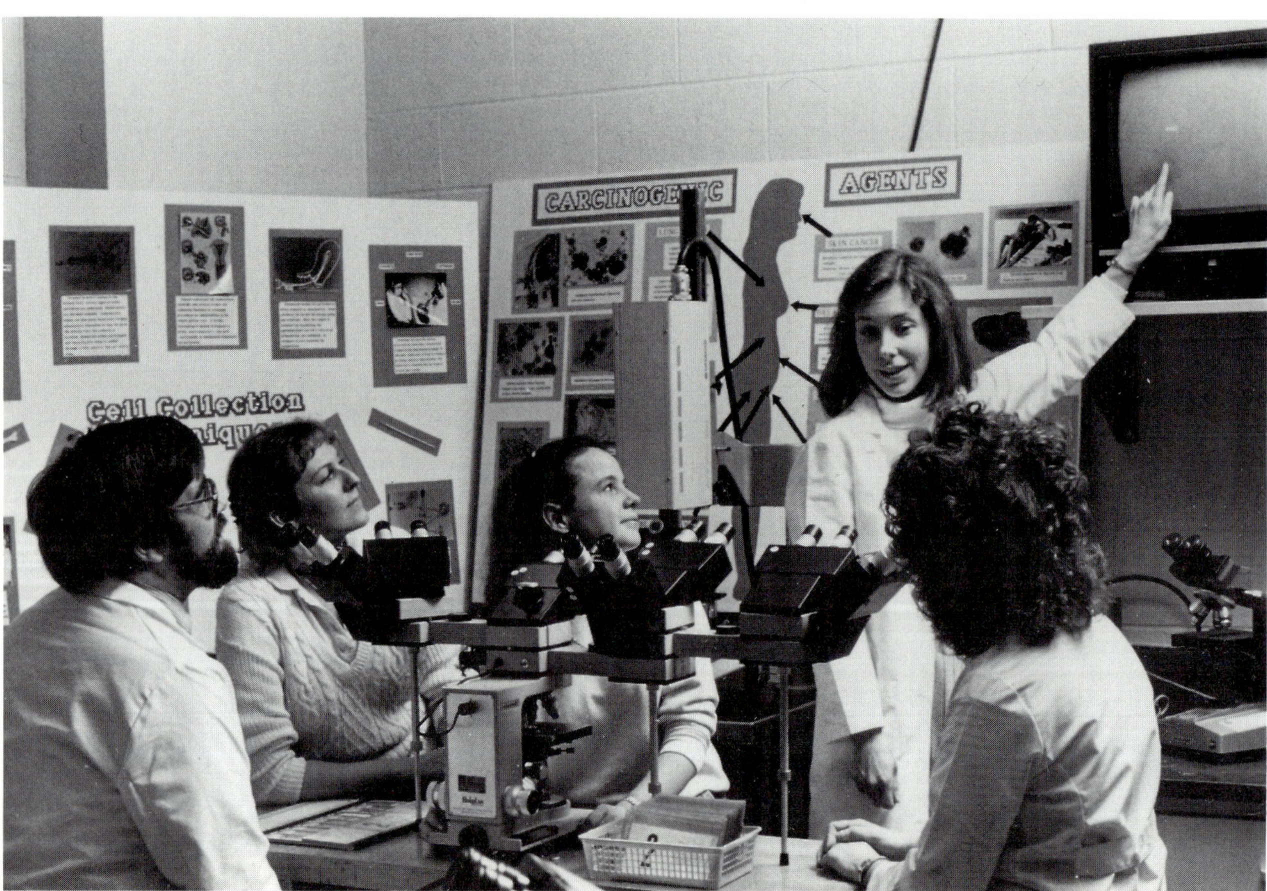

FIG. 52-11. The College's cytotechnology program featured state-of-the-art technology.

from the University of Miami School of Medicine, became Chairman, sparking a new period of development in the Department (Figure 52–12). Ms. Greening developed a Post-Certificate program for cytotechnologists who held a professional certificate and who wanted to earn a bachelor's degree. In the fall of 1985, the first students were accepted into the program.

Ms. Greening also reorganized the curriculum, focusing first on female genital tract cytology, then nongynecologic cytology, and finally, advanced courses studying diseases and their cellular manifestations. This change allowed students to concentrate on one major area at a time and gain competency in that area before moving on.

Greening also recruited ten new clinical affiliate sites in order to expose students to a wide variety of cytologic specimens, laboratory settings, and case volumes. In 1985, as President of the American Society for Cytotechnology (ASCT), she hosted that organization's annual meeting in conjunction with the Department and the American Cancer Society. That same year, National Cytotechnology Week was cited in Philadelphia by Mayor W. Wilson Goode. During this time, Greening's contributions to the College of Allied Health Sciences cytotechnology program were matched only by her contributions to her profession. Active in everything from continuing education to research, publications to professional standards, workshops to political and legal issues affecting the profession, Greening proved to be a true leader.

In 1987 faculty member Carol M. Trew,

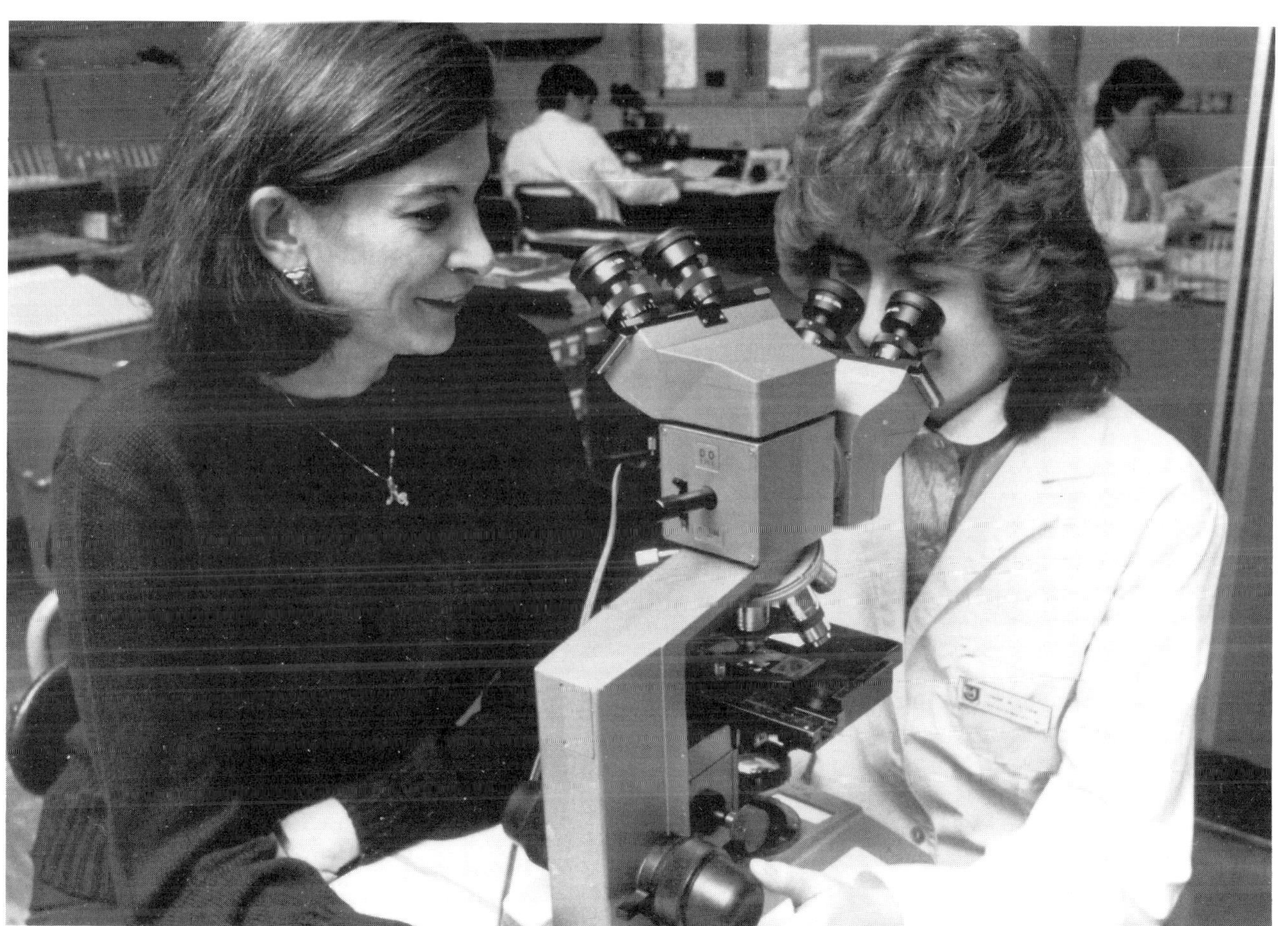

FIG. 52-12. Department Head Shirley E. Greening, CFIAC, M.S. (left), served as President of the American Society of Cytotechnology in 1985.

CT(ASCP), CMIAC, B.S., became President of the American Society for Cytotechnology, continuing the Department's tradition of leadership in the field.

The 1980s brought great changes for cytotechnologists. It took years before cytotechnologists were able to move from "technician" to "technologist" status and to be recognized for the health-preserving role they play in being responsible for the detection of malignant or abnormal cells. As testing became more selective and restricted, however, cytology specimens shifted from hospital laboratories to large independent commercial laboratories. As a result of these diminishing volumes, many hospital laboratories as well as cytotechnology schools were forced to close, making the future uncertain for many in the profession.

Jefferson's Department of Cytotechnology braced itself to battle that problem with increased student recruitment, the expansion of the post-certificate program, the development of histotechnology and cytogenetics curriculum tracks, and the establishment of basic cytology education on a part-time basis. By increasing the avenues by which a bachelor's degree in cytology may be obtained, Jefferson began addressing itself to new audiences that included the older student, the working professional, and the second-career individual.

In the late 1980s, the Department stood ready to face the challenge of the future as it had in the past in the tradition of leadership not only at Jefferson but also in the field of cytotechnology, a field where Jeffersonians have labored to develop, promote, and nurture its growth.

Department of Diagnostic Imaging

One of the first x-ray technician training programs in the United States was founded at Jefferson Hospital in 1934. A year after it opened its doors, the program was accredited in the American College of Radiology's (ACR) first roster of approved schools. Since that initial formal nod, Jefferson has continuously featured a fully accredited program of radiologic technology.

In its early years, Jefferson's x-ray technology curriculum was very practice-oriented and served as an apprenticeship for the students, who worked alongside technicians during the hospital workday. Like most hospital-based radiology programs of that time, Jefferson's school of x-ray technology focused primarily on patient care. Rather than classroom-based training, instruction leaned more toward informal, one-on-one practice at x-ray machines. During this time period, Jefferson's graduates were highly successful when taking their national certifying examinations.

From 1934 to 1974 the direction and methods of the hospital-based program at Jefferson were remarkably stable. In March of 1966, the ACR noted that Jefferson had "a general excellent program," and in June of that year the program received the approval of the Council on Medical Education (CME) of the American Medical Association (AMA) for its 24-month program. During its first 30 years in operation, the program remained faithful to the objective stated in one of its earliest brochures: " . . . to prepare men and women for a challenging and rewarding career in the health services." During these decades, Jefferson's radiology program provided entry-level practitioners in radiography to hospitals in Philadelphia and the Delaware Valley. In March of 1969, the CME of the AMA gave "unqualified continuing approval" to the program and raised the approved number of students to 44.

■ Major Changes in the 1970s

By 1971, with 48 new students enrolled in the program, Jefferson's radiography program listed 472 graduates in its roster. The program employed 12 part-time faculty members, mostly employees of the Radiology Department, with an annual operating budget of $55,000.

It was in 1971 that Peter Dure-Smith, M.D., the Medical Director of the program, set in motion a series of sweeping changes that would transmute the hospital-based radiology program into the Department of Radiologic Technology. Dr. Dure-Smith sought this change after much research and documentation concerning the state of x-ray technology. After a thorough review of documents and reports, and considering the long-range career prospects of Jefferson's radiology students, he decided that the use of professional educators would be both efficient and cost-effective, and he communicated this to Dean Goldschmidt of the College of Allied Health Sciences.

That year, George McArdle, representing the Radiology Department, and Lawrence Abrams, Assistant Dean and Director of Student Affairs and Services of the College of Allied Health Sciences, representing the College, met to arrange several carefully planned stages that would implement the transplant of the hospital-based program into the College of Allied Health Sciences (Figure 52–13).

From 1973 until 1975 the graduates in radiologic technology were awarded the traditional diplomas. In September of 1974, of the 91 applicants, 26 students were admitted to the class to graduate in 1976. During this same period, the College of Allied Health Sciences assumed full management of the curriculum and the administration of student recruitment. The affiliation with the College allowed radiology students, for the first time, access to student services, including professional advisement, student housing, and financial aid.

The core of the two-year, upper-division baccalaureate degree program was designed by Anthony D. Gilkey, the first Chairman of the College of Allied Health Sciences' Department of Radiologic Technology, and Loretta C. Tate, the program's first clinical instructor.

Officially, the School of Radiologic Technology was organized as an upper-division baccalaureate

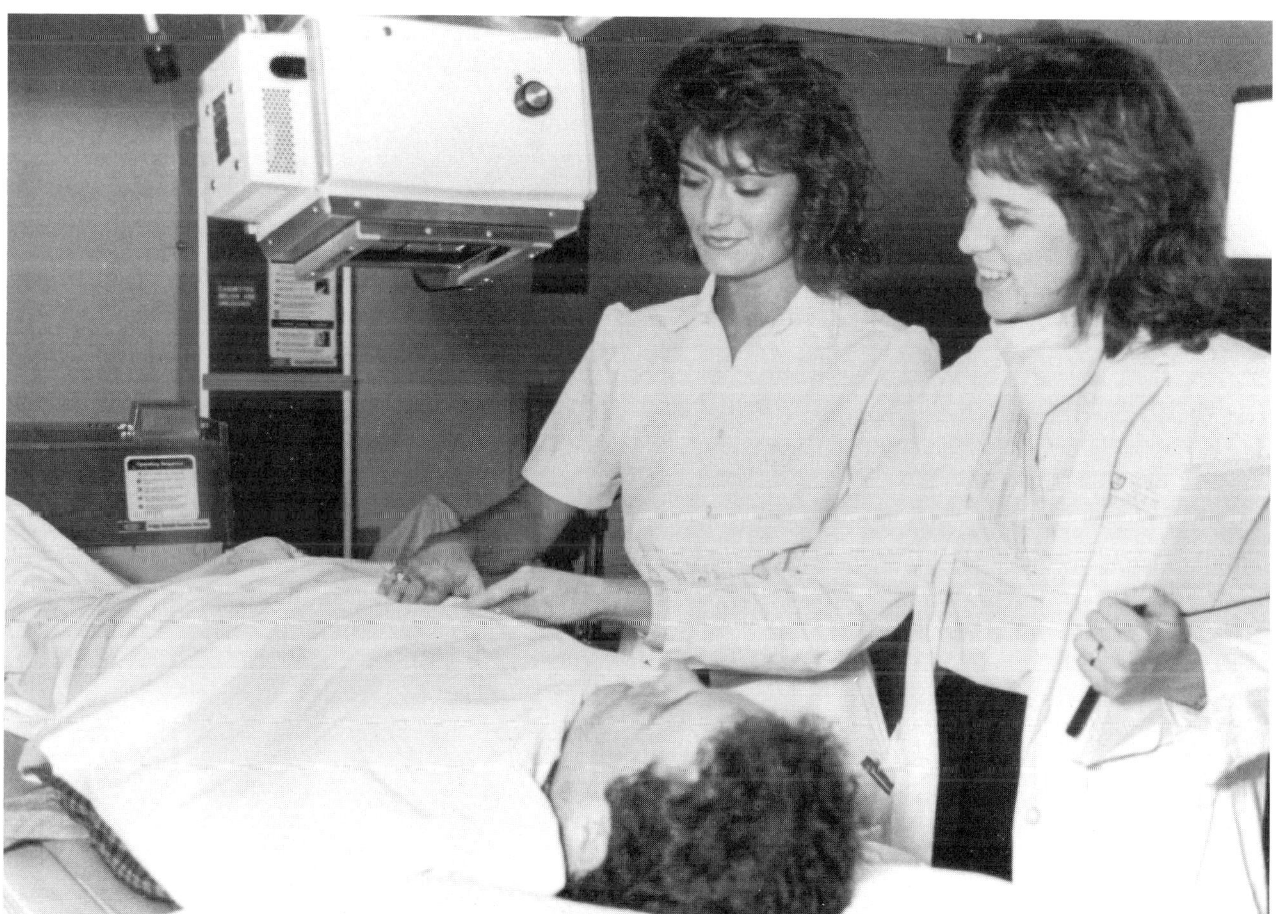

FIG. 52-13. The College's close relationships with the Hospital provided students excellent clinical opportunities.

degree department within the College on July 1, 1976. The Joint Review Committee on Education in Radiologic Technology of the American College of Radiology and the American Society of Radiologic Technologists notified Jefferson on January 26, 1977, that the Thomas Jefferson Hospital Program "will be discontinued as of September 1, 1977, in favor of an affiliation with Thomas Jefferson University."

In September of 1977, the second baccalaureate degree class began with ten students. Classes were held on the second and sixth floors of Jefferson Alumni Hall, the energized laboratory of the Central Animal Facility. In 1978 the class that was admitted in September of 1976 became the first to receive the Baccalaureate Degree in Radiologic Technology. At this time, Anthony Gilkey left the Department and was succeeded by Lawrence W. Walker, who expanded the efforts of the Department nationally. Under Walker's direction, the Department managed two educational programs funded by the Allied Health Training Institutes, which were attended by radiologic technologists from all over the country.

Development in 1980s

Lawrence Walker also originated Pilot Project 21, an innovative curriculum change that condensed the time frame of the degree program from 24 months to 21. In 1980, when Walker left Jefferson for government service, Loretta Tate assumed the duties of Department Chairman. During her tenure, Pilot Project 21 was approved and implemented. Tate's initiatives included the development of the Advanced Placement Program, for graduates of certificate and associate degree radiologic technology programs who wanted to earn a baccalaureate degree.

A major development for the Department had its roots in 1983 when the College of Allied Health Sciences began negotiations with Jefferson Hospital's Division of Ultrasound for the purpose of incorporating the ultrasound program into the College's Department of Radiologic Technology.

Ultrasound, or diagnostic medical sonography, training had been a part of Jefferson since February of 1977 when Barry B. Goldberg, M.D., brought his Ultrasound Department from Episcopal Hospital in Philadelphia. By then, Dr. Goldberg had established an international reputation in the ultrasound field.

At its inception in 1977, the ultrasound certificate program offered two options, a six-month program and a twelve-month program. Each option had three students under Program Director Sandra Hagan-Ansert, B.S., R.D.M.S., with Dr. Goldberg as Medical Director.

Later that year, the six-month option was eliminated, and in July six students were accepted. Thereafter, new students were admitted every six months, in January and in July, into the year-long program.

In July of 1978, Joseph Darby, B.S., R.D.M.S., a Jefferson certificate graduate of the 1977 class, was named Program Director. Until this time, the program had functioned in an on-the-job training model. Recognizing the desirability of more formal preparation in the theoretical aspects of ultrasound, Mr. Darby initiated didactic coursework in 1979, moving the program closer to an academic model. The 12-month program continued for several years more with student enrollment that grew to eight per session.

By 1983 the Strategic Plan of the College of Allied Health Sciences, approved by the Board of Trustees, had pointed the direction for years ahead by planning to absorb hospital-based allied health programs into the College as the demands of the profession required additional academic background.

The dialogue of 1983 led to the application in January, 1985, for initial accreditation of a baccalaureate degree ultrasound program by the Joint Review Committee on Education in Diagnostic Medical Sonography of the Committee on Allied Health Education and Accreditation of the American Medical Association.

Christine H. Rhoda served briefly as Acting Chairman after Loretta Tate's resignation early in 1985. In August of that year, Albert D. Herbert, Jr., R.T., L.R.T.(R), M.S., was named Acting Chairman of the Department; he was made Chairman the following year. Before his appointment at Jefferson, Mr. Herbert was Division Director of Medical Imaging and Radiation Therapy and Associate Professor in the School of Community and Allied Health at the University of Alabama at Birmingham.

Mr. Herbert expanded the Department's research and service components and developed a thorough review of the Department's curriculum as well as an assessment of the long-range demand for a multiplicity of diagnostic imaging services (Figure 52–14).

▪ Changes for the Future

In 1986 the Department was renamed the Department of Diagnostic Imaging to better reflect the contemporary and future functions of its faculty and graduates. As the variety of imaging modalities increased, the Department moved to keep pace. Plans to include magnetic resonance imaging and to move toward multicompetency of the graduates were being made as the Department looked to the future.

Department of Dental Hygiene

The Department of Dental Hygiene had its beginning in 1973 when the Report on Feasibility of Dental Education, after two and one half years of study, recommended to the Board of Trustees that the University "plan, develop, and implement a comprehensive series of innovative programs in dental education and training."

Early in 1976 Linda G. Kraemer, R.D.H., B.A., M.S., a graduate of Columbia University's master of science degree program in dental hygiene, was appointed to implement planning activities and gain institutional, professional, and dental hygiene education approval for an upper-division

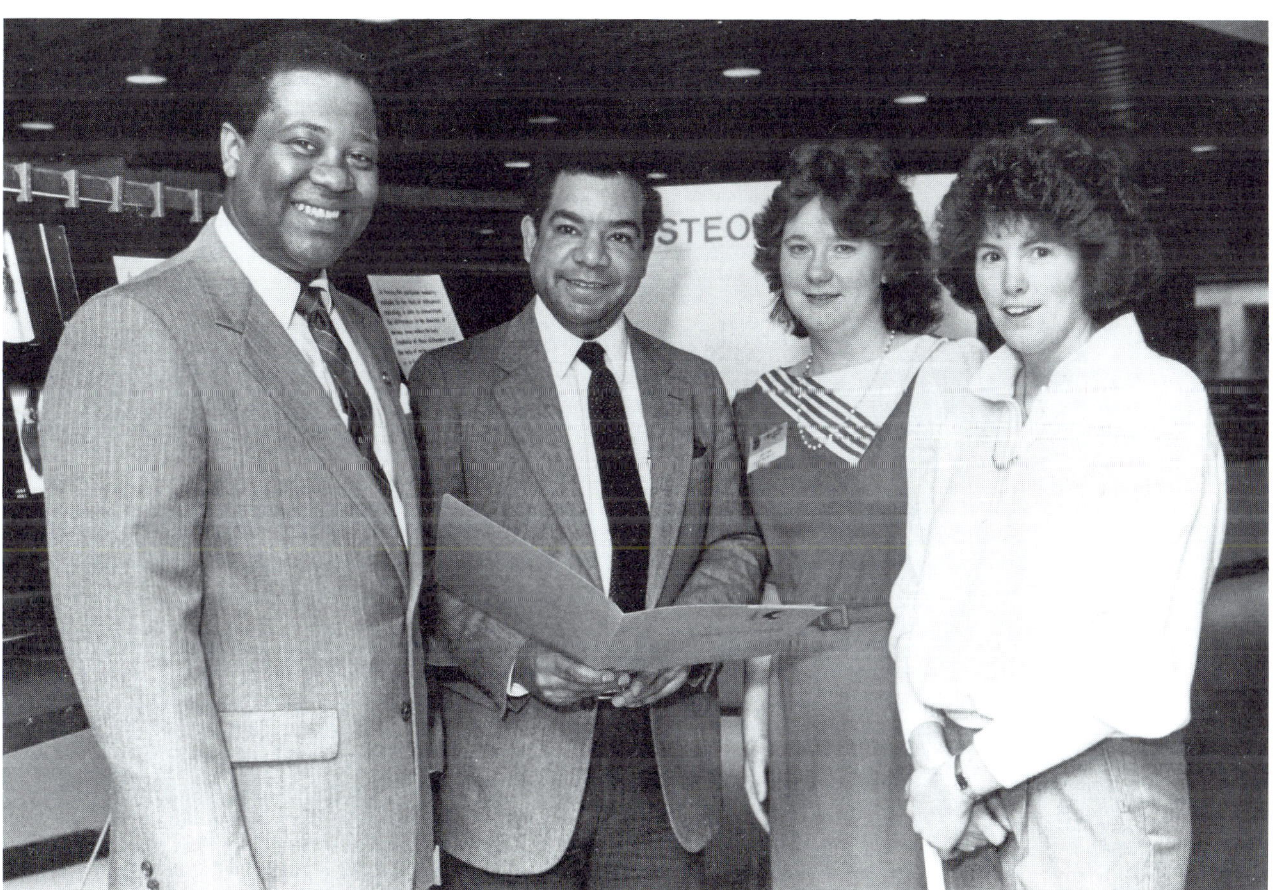

FIG. 52-14. Department Chairman Albert D. Herbert, Jr., R.T., L.R.T. (R), M.S. (left) with participants at the Department's annual Roentgen Memorial Day of Learning in 1987.

baccalaureate degree program in the College of Allied Health Sciences. Kraemer and Associate Dean Lawrence Abrams made numerous site visits and attended national meetings to compile and evaluate various trends in dental hygiene education. A feasibility study documented the need for dental hygienists on both the national and state levels. The study indicated that Jefferson's new program was unique because it combined clinical skills, liberal arts, basic sciences, and knowledge in a selected elective specialty area.

The administrators agreed to emphasize the development of learning experiences for the professional growth of the students and to concentrate on career alternatives for graduates. In keeping with this philosophy and to prepare graduates with multiple career options and avenues for advanced study, the curriculum was designed to include 24 hours of elective specialization so that students could combine clinical training with selected areas including education, public health, and health management.

On April 15, 1976, the College of Allied Health Sciences Committee of the Board of Trustees approved the recommendation to establish a Department of Dental Hygiene in the College of Allied Health Sciences effective July 1, 1976, and to recruit students for a September, 1977, entering class. On May 20, 1976, the full Board of Trustees met and approved the recommendations.

▪ Construction Begins

Beginning July 1, 1976, all space for the Department of Dental Hygiene, including faculty and administrative offices, classrooms, laboratories, radiology facilities, and the dental hygiene clinic was assigned to floors 18 and 22 of the Health Sciences Center Building (Edison Building) at Ninth and Sansom Streets. In October of 1976, the Board of Trustees approved plans for construction of the dental hygiene facilities. Work began in April of the following year and the construction was completed by the end of August, 1977. The eighteenth floor, which comprised 5,130 square feet, housed the teaching and patient care facilities, including the dental hygiene clinic with 24 teaching stations, a classroom laboratory, dental radiography operatories, a wet laboratory, darkrooms, a plaque control room, a special-procedures/audiovisual room, a sterile supply area, and a patient reception area. The twenty-second floor, which consisted of 3,020 square feet, housed offices for the Chairman, faculty, and administrative support personnel, a conference room, and a student locker and lounge area. A total of $176,175 of the Health Sciences Center renovation fund was used to construct the dental hygiene facilities (Figure 52–15).

▪ Dental Program Begins

In October of 1976, Kraemer was promoted to Chairman and Associate Professor in the Department of Dental Hygiene. She and a new faculty member, Mary Burns, R.D.H., M.S., were instrumental in developing an "accreditation-eligible" application, which was submitted to the American Dental Association's Commission on Accreditation of Dental and Auxiliary Dental Educational Programs in November of 1976. After on-site evaluation the Commission adopted a resolution to grant "accreditation-eligible" status to Jefferson's dental hygiene program in May of 1977.

Recruitment efforts for the first class included hundreds of direct-mail letters, newspaper advertisements, visits to local schools, and meetings with high school counselors. On September 6, 1977, when the department officially opened its doors, ten students were enrolled.

The following academic year, the Department was one of only 20 dental auxiliary programs selected nationwide by the American Dental Association's Commission of Accreditation of Dental and Dental Auxiliary Educational Programs to pilot test a new self-study accreditation manual. In May of 1979, the Commission granted full accreditation status to the dental hygiene program. That same year, the Department received almost $90,000 in grants for program development and for national workshops for dental hygiene educators.

Sixteen new students had matriculated into the program in September, 1978, and in June of 1979 seven of the original ten students were graduated from the program. The seven took the National

Board Dental Hygiene Examination and the Northeast Regional Board Examination and passed with scores well above the national and regional averages.

Faculty members began publishing articles in professional journals, presenting papers at professional meetings, and holding offices in local, state, and national organizations. The Department's petition to establish a chapter in Sigma Phi Alpha, the national dental hygiene honor society, was approved by the organization's Executive Board in November, 1979. In 1980 the department received national recognition when it was selected by the American Dental Hygienists Association as one of four dental hygiene programs to develop and test geriatric curriculum modules in dental hygiene education, supported by the United States Department of Health, Education and Welfare in order to sensitize hygienists to the needs of the aged. All 16 students who graduated in the class of 1980 passed their examination boards.

Post-Certificate Program

In 1980–1981, twenty students entered the Department's first Post-Certificate Program in dental hygiene, designed for dental hygienists who already possessed a certificate or an associate's degree in dental hygiene. It became the only dental hygiene Post-Certificate Program in Pennsylvania and the largest one of its kind in the country. Mary Burns Sheridan, who had planned the program and served as the first Post-Certificate Coordinator, resigned from this position on June 1, 1981, and transferred to the Office of the Dean in the College of Allied Health Sciences. Her position was assumed by Marcia Brand, R.D.H., M.S., who came from the dental hygiene faculty at Old Dominion University.

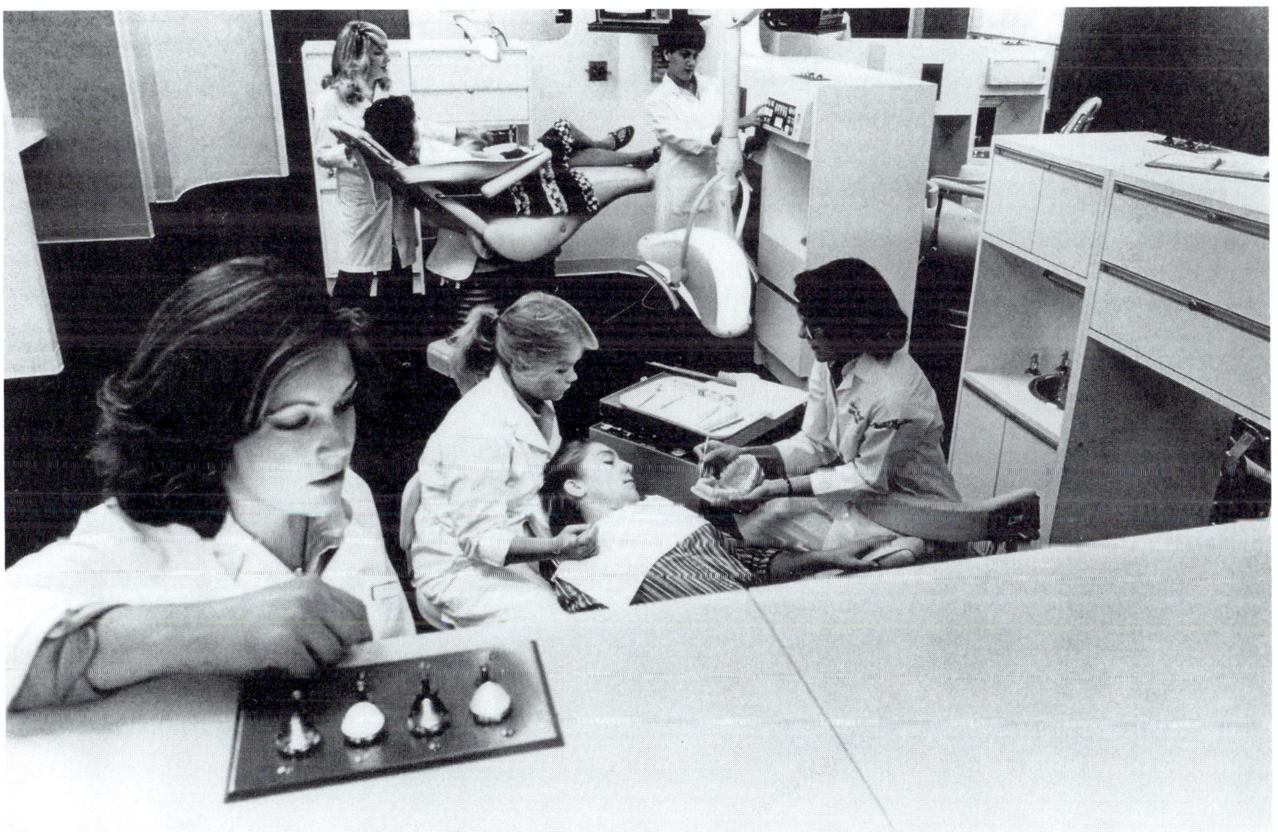

FIG. 52-15. A typical scene in the Department of Dental Hygiene's Clinic located on the eighteenth floor of the Edison Building.

Students

The 13 graduates of the class of 1981 all passed their national and regional board examinations. In 1982 a total of 29 senior students graduated, making this the largest graduating class. In 1983 twenty students graduated, including 11 from the Post-Certificate Program. Twenty-six students matriculated in the junior class in September, 1983 and in June, 1984, eight generic and 11 post-certificate seniors graduated. While some students entered graduate programs, other graduates secured positions not only in clinical practice but in teaching, management, and public health.

The largest post-certificate class matriculated in September, 1984, with a total of 23 juniors. This enrollment indicated a rebound from the slumps in 1981 and 1982 that were evident not only at Jefferson but also nationally. The graduating class of 1985 consisted of 11 students from the Generic Program and 12 from the Post-Certificate Program. The fact that Jefferson continued as the only dental hygiene baccalaureate program in Pennsylvania, Delaware and Southern New Jersey helped many of the graduates to line up jobs before graduation. Enrollment in 1985 dipped, however, with only seven juniors and 13 post-certificate juniors entering the Department.

Scholarship

By June of 1983, faculty and students had published four manuscripts in major dental hygiene journals and presented abstracts at professional meetings, including the American Society of Allied Health Professions, American Association of Dental Schools, and the Ninth International Symposium on Dental Hygiene.

Faculty and students initiated nine research projects in 1984 in areas such as gerontology, nutrition, public health, periodontology, and attitudes about dental hygiene practice and education. Faculty members continued to work toward and receive their doctoral degrees.

During the 1984–1985 academic year, the Department again offered continuing education courses and initiated seven research projects. Responding to increased demands for scholarship by the College, reflected in revised criteria for appointment and promotion, the faculty devoted more time to this activity, publishing eight manuscripts in seven publications: *Dental Hygiene, Educational Directions, RDH, Education Update, Update, Journal of Dental Education,* and *Journal of Allied Health.*

Students, encouraged and directed by the faculty, prepared and submitted 23 manuscripts to dental hygiene journals and developed a reference textbook in hospital dental hygiene and an annotated bibliography on geriatrics in publishable form. Of the nine abstracts submitted by faculty for presentation at professional meetings, all were accepted and presented at national and state meetings. The faculty also continued to hold leadership positions in national organizations, including the American Association of Dental Schools, American Dental Hygienists' Association, and the American Association of Hospital Dentists.

The Mid-1980s

The 1985–1986 academic year began with the submission of the Interim Review accreditation report to the American Dental Association's Commission on Dental Accreditation. On December 12, 1985, the Commission on Dental Accreditation informed Dr. Lewis Bluemle, President of the University, that the Department of Dental Hygiene was granted full approval.

For the first time ever, a week in September, 1985, was designated "National Dental Hygiene Week." To celebrate, faculty and students provided a variety of programs to increase the public's awareness of the role of the dental hygienist. The department received local and national attention in the dental hygiene community when the Mayor of Philadelphia, W. Wilson Goode, attended a ceremony held in the dental hygiene clinic and issued a proclamation (Figure 52–16).

Philosophy

The Department of Dental Hygiene's history reflects an educational philosophy that promotes student inquiry. The faculty served as the major barometers of the program's growth, innovation, and development. The overall curriculum, both for Generic and Post-Certificate Programs, remained consistent with the original plans, although modifications were made based on changing goals of the profession, employment and enrollment patterns, and financial conditions. In 1983, for example, a new elective specialty tract in hospital dental hygiene was developed and introduced because of growing employment opportunities and student interest in this area. Jefferson was one of the first, if not the first, Department of Dental Hygiene in the country to offer this course of specialized instruction.

▪ Looking Ahead

As the Department of Dental Hygiene looked to the future decade, the goals included plans to offer graduate education in dental hygiene, either at the master's or doctoral level, and to develop a national center for dental hygiene research. More immediate needs included increasing funding opportunities and planning national conferences on issues in dental hygiene education, practice, and research.

With those goals and contributions by enthusiastic faculty and students, the Department of Dental Hygiene looked to remain in the position that it had established for itself—locally, regionally, and nationally recognized for excellence and innovation, leadership, and scholarship.

Department of Physical Therapy

By the late 1970s, the profession of physical therapy was growing nationwide at an astonishing rate. A 1978 study by the American Physical Therapy Association concluded that a "conservative estimate of the need for physical therapists is probably somewhere around twice the number now employed full-time and part-time."

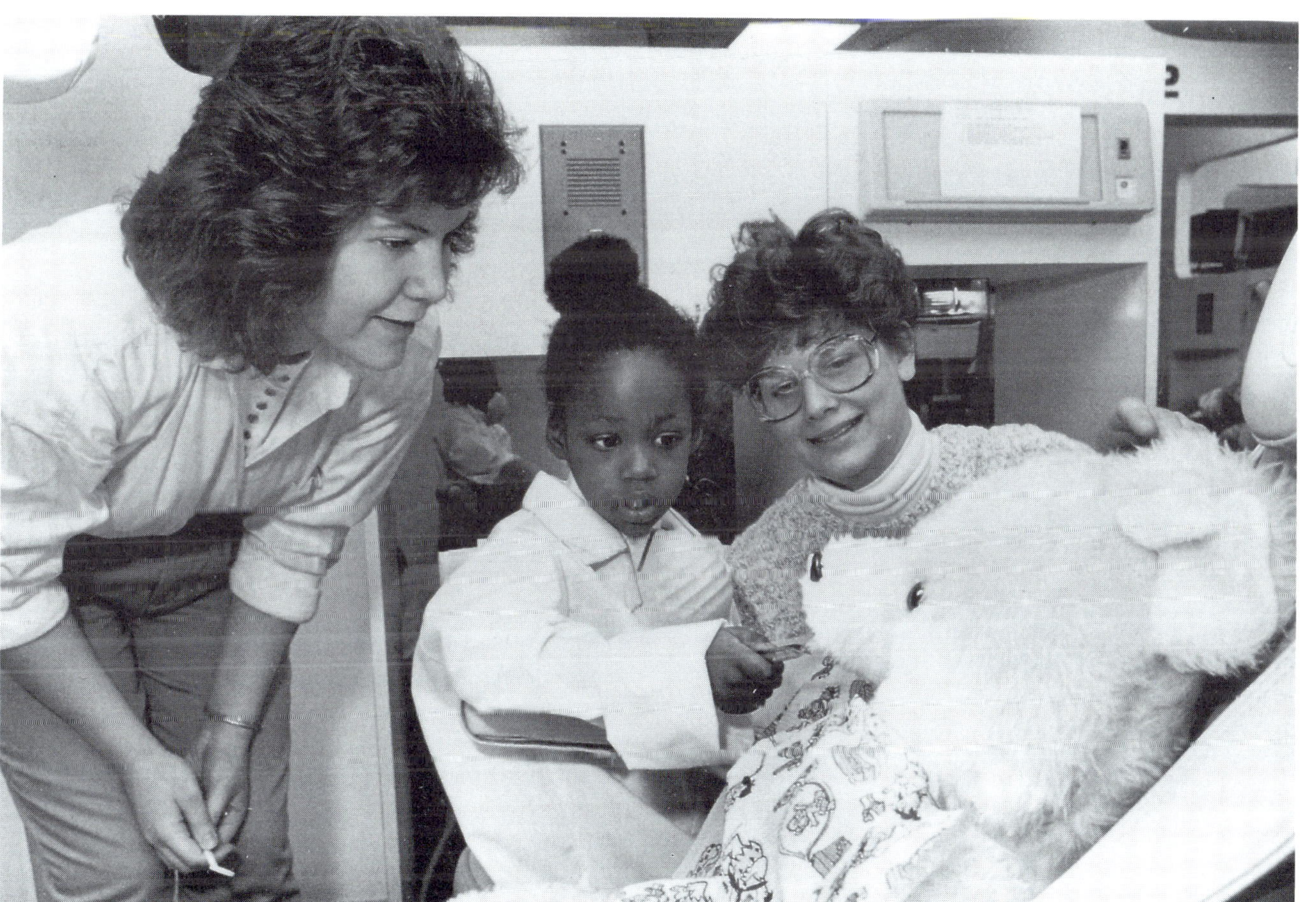

FIG. 52-16. Dental Hygiene faculty and students used "Teddy Bear/Baby Doll Clinics" as part of their community outreach efforts in the 1980s.

In the Philadelphia area, the number of graduates from various physical therapy programs was insufficient to meet local demand. Statistics for the area, issued by the Pennsylvania Bureau of Labor Security, confirmed the need for therapists.

In 1979 an initial planning document established the need to develop a Department of Physical Therapy in Thomas Jefferson University's College of Allied Health Sciences. The final proposal was submitted to the Board of Trustees to continue planning activities for a Department of Physical Therapy, pending adequate funding. The financial support for the Department was confirmed in October of 1981, and on November 2 of that year the Board of Trustees gave their approval for the formal establishment of the Department.

In May of 1983, Jeffrey Rothman, P.T., Ed.D. was appointed Chairman and Associate Professor of the Department. Dr. Rothman had originally been a program planning consultant in 1982. Through discussions with national physical therapy educators and a close review of physical therapy literature, Dr. Rothman, with the assistance of Dr. Rhonda Karp, Associate Dean of the College of Allied Health Sciences, developed a unique program for Jefferson based upon problem solving in health and wellness.

The program planning report stated that physical therapy students and faculty at Jefferson would have the benefit of an excellent acute care facility for their core clinical experiences as well as learning opportunities at facilities affiliated with Jefferson, including the Hand Rehabilitation Center, Magee Rehabilitation Center, and the Children's Heart Hospital (subsequently called Children's Rehabilitation Hospital).

The report also indicated that about 50% of the hospitals surveyed anticipated the need for additional physical therapists within three years. In addition, the 1980–1981 edition of the *Occupational Outlook Handbook,* published by the U.S. Department of Labor, had reported that "employment of physical therapists is expected to grow much faster than the average for all occupations through the mid-1980s because of increased public recognition of the importance of rehabilitation."

▪ Early Development

It was the eventual construction of an innovative physical therapy curriculum that brought Jefferson to the forefront in preparing physical therapists to assume a leadership role in preventive health care. Contributing to the curriculum development were the first faculty members of the Department of Physical Therapy: Phyllis Brust, Clinical Education Coordinator; Holly Cintas, Assistant Professor; Ruth Badyrka, Assistant Professor, and John Barbis, Assistant Professor.

In September of 1983, the first physical therapy students entered Jefferson's two-year, upper-division program leading to a bachelor of science degree, and on June 15, 1985, the first class of 49 physical therapy graduates participated in the University's commencement ceremonies. In September, 1985, 59 seniors and 60 juniors, representing a wide and interesting diversity of backgrounds and experience, enrolled in the program.

Throughout the 1980s, sixty students were admitted to the program each year. Many had earned baccalaureate degrees in other fields. During this time, admission was highly competitive, with applications numbering in the 400 range annually.

The eighth floor of the University's Edison Building housed the Department's faculty and secretarial offices. On the ninth floor, the Clinical Performance Laboratories provided space for teaching, student practicums, and patient care simulations, as well as research and continuing education areas (Figure 52–17).

The teaching philosophy of the Department emphasized the role physical therapists play in programs of health promotion and disease prevention, and studies were structured to develop a broad knowledge base for the physical therapy students. Clinical skills were designed as an integral part of the curriculum, encouraging students to identify potential health problems through health care screening as well as through traditional physical therapy evaluation procedures. Consumer education and the encouragement of wellness through proper nutrition, exercise, and stress management were emphasized for both the student and client. Integration of a holistic model of health and wellness with clinical problem-solving methodologies was carefully structured to allow students to respond to professional and social changes within the health care delivery system.

Because of the unique nature of Jefferson's physical therapy curriculum, the Department received national recognition in the physical therapy community. This was noted at both the 1984 Annual Conference of the American Physical Therapy Association and the 1985 Annual Conference of the American Society of Allied Health Professions, where Jefferson's physical therapy curriculum and research findings were presented and praised by many of the nation's leading educators.

When the Department of Physical Therapy received full accreditation in May, 1985, from the American Physical Therapy Association, the final accreditation report described five major strengths of the program: administration, faculty, University and community support, students, and curriculum. The report commended the Department's curriculum as an innovative, futuristic, and progressive model for allied health and physical therapy education. It also noted that the students seemed to have internalized the importance of holistic health and wellness for themselves as individuals, as well as for their future practice in physical therapy.

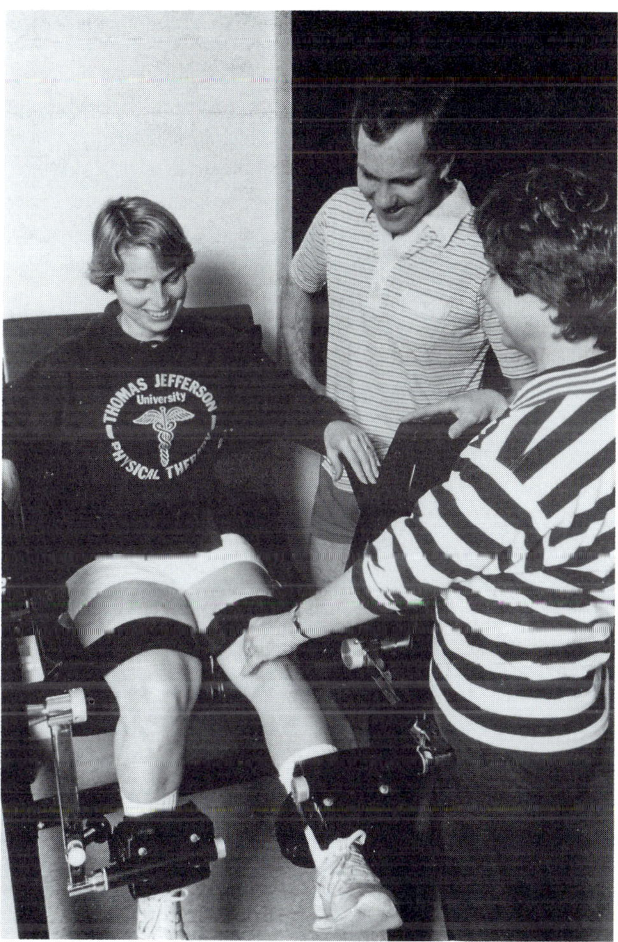

FIG. 52-17. Students using the Department of Physical Therapy's well-equipped Clinical Performance Laboratories on the ninth floor of the Edison Building.

Clinical Resources and Affiliations

The Department benefitted by its association with the Division of Physical Therapy, Department of Rehabilitation Medicine at Thomas Jefferson University Hospital. Besides acute care and general rehabilitative services, the Department of Rehabilitation Medicine served as the regional acute care spinal cord center, thereby providing unique clinical opportunities for the students.

During the mid-1980s over 150 clinical facilities signed contractual affiliation agreements with the College's Department of Physical Therapy. They represented some of the leading rehabilitation institutions and private practice facilities in the United States and in England. Jefferson's physical therapy students had the opportunity to affiliate with these institutions in areas such as pediatrics, sports medicine, pain management, geriatrics, and cancer and cardiac rehabilitation.

Physical Therapy Students

The Department of Physical Therapy supported projects that provided the students with firsthand experience designed to further their knowledge of their future patients. An annual tradition was a Handicapped and Barrier Awareness Day, when junior students went out into the community simulating a physical disability (in wheelchairs, leg braces, darkened glasses, or other handicaps) in order to better understand the physical, psychological, and social barriers that had to be confronted by handicapped individuals (Figure 52–18).

Also employed was an Aging Simulation

Exercise that demonstrated to students the losses inherent in the aging process. The goal of the exercise was to increase the students' understanding of and sensitivity to the elderly.

The Department held a Health Fair annually that provided an opportunity for senior students to display their projects. Held in Jefferson Alumni Hall and open to the public, the Health Fair included projects such as a guide to exercise and diet for patients in a heart attack recovery program, a videotape about prevention of back injuries, a stress management workshop, and a program of "mall walking" for senior citizens.

During the mid-1980s physical therapy students also organized dance marathons for charitable causes.

As the American Physical Therapy Association endorsed the concept of having a master's degree in physical therapy become the standard for an entry-level position in the field, the College's Department of Physical Therapy responded by proposing such a program in 1987.

At the close of the 1980s, prospects for the Master's Degree Program, like the prospects for physical therapy graduates, looked promising.

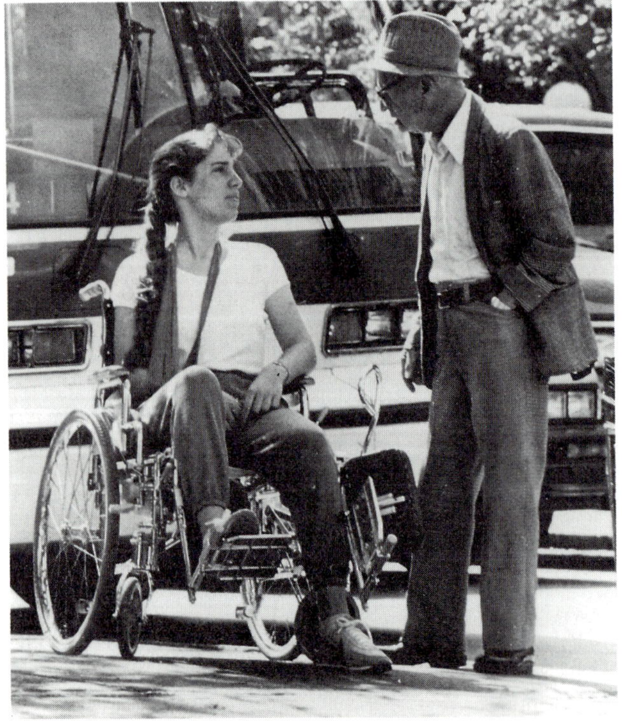

FIG. 52-18. The annual Handicapped and Barrier Awareness Day took physical therapy students into the community.

Department of Occupational Therapy

At the end of the nineteenth century, occupational therapy developed in scattered institutions throughout the United States as a way of providing psychiatric patients with specific, directed activities such as handicrafts. By the end of World War I, occupational therapy was used to help returning disabled soldiers adapt to their physical disabilities and return to some sort of rewarding occupation or activity.

Nearly a century after its inception, occupational therapy had mushroomed into a highly specialized therapeutic field. By the 1970s occupational therapy had become a therapy in which the occupational therapy professional taught handicapped or convalescing individuals skills for daily life activities and for specific occupations, with the goal of providing recreation and exercise and maximizing the capabilities of the person.

As medical advances extended life expectancy and saved increasing numbers of accident victims in the latter half of the twentieth century, the need for occupational therapy services increased.

▪ Jefferson Enters the Field

Aware of both state and local shortages of qualified occupational therapists, Lawrence Abrams, Ed.D., Dean of the College of Allied Health Sciences, initiated a study in the late 1970s to review the situation. The study indicated a substantial need for an additional occupational therapy program in the Philadelphia area, based on the growing need for hand rehabilitation, home care, and other health services. As a result, a preliminary document, outlining the College's plans for an occupational therapy department, was completed in 1979. By November, 1981, the University's Board of Trustees gave its official approval for the formal establishment of Jefferson's Department of Occupational Therapy.

Planning and Curriculum Development

Initial planning activities for the Department were carried out by Dean Abrams and Rhonda Karp, Ed.D., Associate Dean. Early in 1982 Dawn Sousangelis Papougenis, M.B.A., O.T.R., was appointed as Physical Therapy/Occupational Therapy Program Planning Coordinator/Instructor.

Curriculum development began shortly afterwards, when Ruth Ellen Levine, OTR/L, Ed.D., joined the staff as a part-time program planning consultant. In July of 1982, Roseann C. Schaaf, OTR/L, M.Ed., was engaged as a consultant for the development of the basic science and neurodevelopmental curriculum. In the fall of 1982 Ellen L. Kolodner, OTR/L, M.S.S., FOATA, joined the occupational therapy faculty as an Assistant Professor and helped plan courses in psychological dysfunction and other areas.

After consulting with experts in the field, the team of planners chose a holistic occupational behavioral model for Jefferson's curriculum. It was based on the concept of occupation, defined by occupational therapy theorists as "goal-directed activity which fulfills a human need." Planners for the Department felt that the occupational behavioral model was exceptional because it focused on attainment and maintenance of health, organized the occupational therapy knowledge base, and utilized the theory and skills required to analyze and solve health problems based on a biopsychosocial perspective.

Facilities

In the summer of 1982, Associate Dean Rhonda Karp and representatives of the space management office for the University joined with the faculty to plan space renovations for the Department. Parts of the eighth and ninth floors of the Edison Building were renovated for the occupational therapy program and its administrative offices, conference room, library, photoreproduction area, and classrooms.

For the special needs of the Department, a developmental laboratory with a one-way evaluation/observation area, a modalities laboratory with power tools and activities supplies, and a wheelchair-accessible kitchen with training facilities for daily living were installed (Figure 52–19). Space was also allocated for evaluation instruments, a small printing press, and brain and nerve models. The Department also made room for a splint cart and computer for the use of patients, faculty, and students.

Faculty

At the outset, development of the occupational therapy faculty was shaped to consist of a Chairman and three full-time and two half-time faculty members. Dr. Ruth Ellen Levine, one of the consultants responsible for the development of the occupational therapy program, was named Chairman of the Department. An occupational therapy graduate of the University of Pennsylvania, Dr. Levine had earned her master's and doctoral degrees in education at Temple University and had served as an Associate Professor of occupational therapy there before coming to Jefferson.

Ellen Kolodner and Roseann Schaaf, who also served as consultants, joined the full-time faculty, along with Assistant Professor Elizabeth DePoy, OTR/L, M.S.S., an expert in therapy for head trauma victims.

Nancy Strub, OTR/L, B.S., chief occupational therapist in Thomas Jefferson University Hospital's Department of Rehabilitation Medicine, served as Clinical Assistant Professor and worked closely with the occupational therapy faculty in planning, teaching, clinical education, and research.

Scholarly activity was a priority for the faculty from the beginning. In 1983 all faculty members presented papers at the annual meetings of both the Pennsylvania Occupational Therapy Association and the American Occupational Therapy Association. The tradition continued through the 1980s as the College of Allied Health Sciences made scholarly research a higher priority.

Recognition of contributions to and leadership in the field began in 1984 when Dr. Levine was given the outstanding achievement award by the Pennsylvania Occupational Therapy Association (POTA) and Ellen Kolodner earned the same honor in 1985. Dr. Levine became President of POTA in 1987.

■ The Program Develops

Jefferson's first occupational therapy students, numbering 30, began classes in September of 1983. Some students entered the two-year, upper-division, baccalaureate program as juniors. Other students, who had already earned bachelor's degrees, entered the Department's Certificate Program, which required 18 months of accelerated work. Forty new juniors joined 28 remaining seniors to constitute the occupational therapy student body in 1984. Thereafter, through the 1980s the program operated at capacity because of the demand for occupational therapists and the reputation of the program.

In January of 1985, the Department received its official accreditation notification from the Committee on Allied Health Education and Accreditation of the American Medical Association in collaboration with the American Occupational Therapy Association. The accreditation, granted for the maximum possible five years, identified the program as having nearly a dozen major strengths, including the comment that it "provided a quality occupational therapy education focused towards professional excellence and leadership."

The College of Allied Health Sciences' Commencement exercises in June 1985 marked the first time that Jefferson occupational therapy graduates marched down the aisle of the Academy of Music. The Department's effectiveness was demonstrated shortly after Commencement when all of the 1985 graduates who sat for the National Certification Examination in occupational therapy

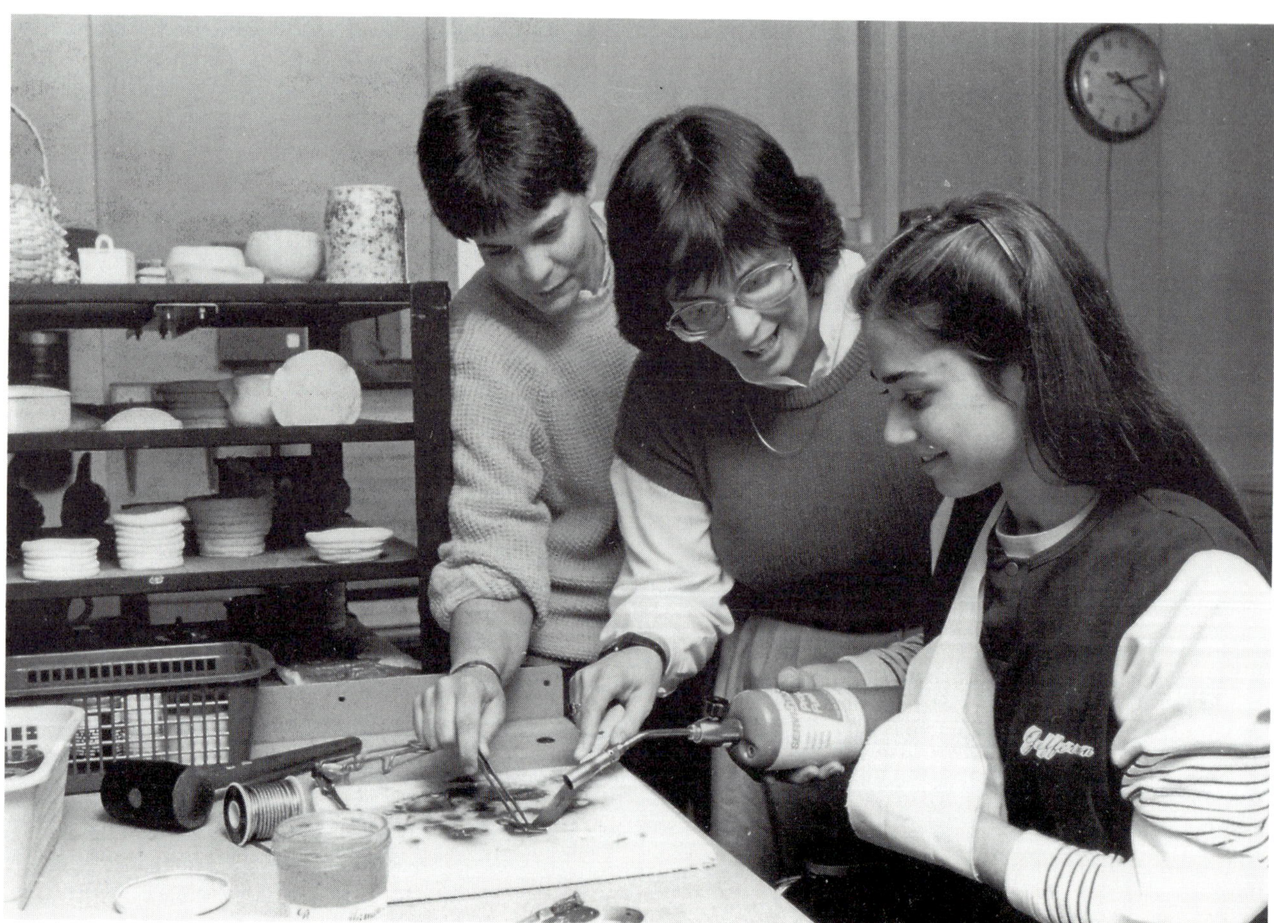

FIG. 52-19. The Department of Occupational Therapy's modalities laboratory.

passed. The 100% passing rate also continued for the Classes of 1986 and 1987.

By the mid-1980s, the Department had established over 200 clinical affiliations for its students, including major hospitals, rehabilitation facilities, mental health institutions, and unconventional settings like the City of Philadelphia's Anti-Graffiti Network, where new applications of occupational therapy were tested (Figure 52–20).

Each spring the Department hosted a "Clinical Council Day" to which representatives from the clinical affiliations were invited. The event served to solidify the relationship between the Department and affiliates while providing a forum for the discussion of current issues in the field and a current practice update. In addition to Clinical Council Days, the Department annually sponsored continuing education programs and workshops for area practitioners.

In an effort to reach out to the occupational therapy community in yet another direction, the Department proposed a Master of Science Degree Program designed to enhance the leadership, management, and research skills of licensed occupational therapists. Approved by the University's Board of Trustees in February, 1987, the program opened its doors that September with eight matriculating students and 21 others taking selected courses.

As the decade of the 1980s was coming to a close, the College's Department of Occupational Therapy, in a relatively short time, had built a solid educational and clinical reputation in the region and had set its sights on national recognition.

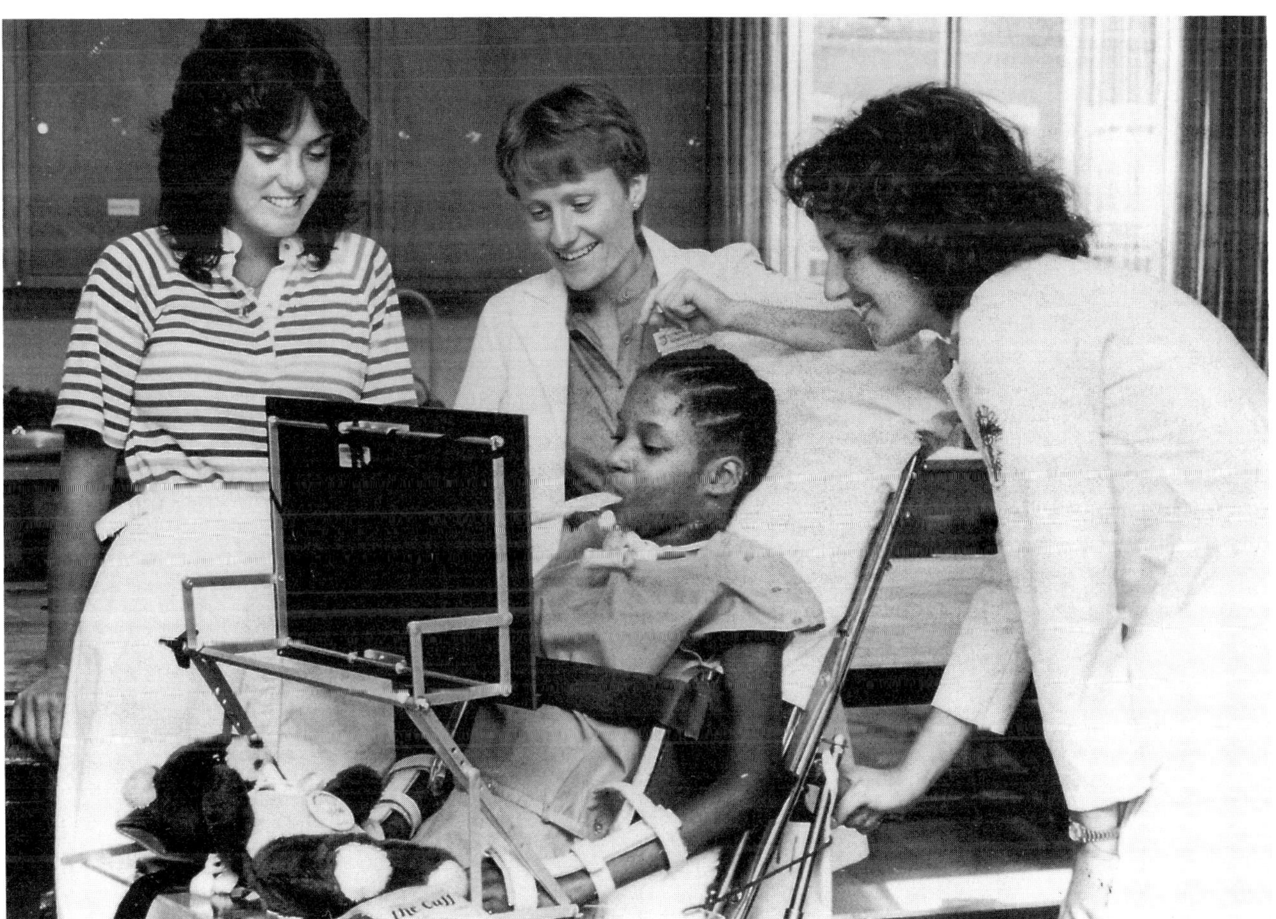

FIG. 52-20. A wide variety of clinical settings gave occupational therapy students a broad range of experience.

The Department of General Studies

The General Studies Program was established in the fall of 1968 as an opportunity for students in the School of Nursing, students in other allied health programs, and all employees and other members of the University community to begin or continue working toward an associate or baccalaureate degree in courses of study leading to advancement in the allied health professions and occupations. The establishment of this program was one of the many changes that occurred during the late 1960s as Jefferson moved from hospital-based allied health courses to degree programs in allied health.

The General Studies Program included courses in the humanities, the social sciences, and the natural sciences. Instruction in certain basic science courses was provided at the Philadelphia College of Pharmacy and Science. This was made possible through an affiliation agreement signed by the College and the Philadelphia College of Pharmacy and Science on April 10, 1968. Part-time faculty from this affiliated institution and other colleges and universities provided the instruction for the other General Studies courses as well. Approval of these courses leading to an Associate degree was received from the Pennsylvania Department of Public Instruction.

Arrangements were made for students from the Schools of Nursing at Lankenau and Pennsylvania Hospitals to begin taking General Studies courses as part of their nursing curriculum in the fall of 1969 and 1970, respectively.

Beginning July 1, 1972, as part of the institutional fringe benefit program, all full-time, nonbargaining employees of Jefferson became eligible to participate in a tuition reimbursement program for course work taken in the General Studies Program. While this benefit clearly encouraged the full-time employees to pursue coursework at their own campus, another plan to augment the enrollment of the General Studies Program was underway. Approval was sought and granted by the Board of Trustees to extend the opportunity to take courses to community residents from the Washington Square West Civic Association and the Society Hill Civic Association beginning in the 1973–1974 academic year.

■ Leadership and Other Changes

Initially the General Studies Program was managed by Lawrence Abrams, who also served as the Director of Admissions and Registrar, and Coordinator, Office of Program Planning. However, as the program and the Collegewide responsibilities of Mr. Abrams continued to grow, it became evident that it was no longer feasible for one person to manage the program as part of a larger set of responsibilities. Thus, on September 18, 1975, Fred R. Petrone, Ed.D., was appointed the Director of the General Studies Program. Lawrence Abrams subsequently became Dean of the College of Allied Health Sciences.

In the 1976 Commencement Exercises, two employees who were enrolled in the General Studies Program received Jefferson's first Associate in Arts Degrees. Another important event occurred in 1976 when the General Studies Program became the Department of General Studies and the Director's title changed to Chairman. Under Dr. Petrone's leadership, and during the 1976–1977 academic year, the Department of General Studies offered evening courses in the basic laboratory sciences for the first time.

In response to a Middle States' recommendation during this same time period, a General Studies Evaluation Committee comprising University faculty was convened. Monthly meetings were held from April 28, 1976, through June 29, 1977, when a final report was issued. Recommendations included the development of an information bulletin and a manual of information for lecturers.

■ The 1980s

Dr. Petrone resigned from the Chairmanship of the Department of General Studies on June 30, 1980. In his place, Rhonda Karp, Ed.D., Assistant Dean, was appointed Acting Chairman until a new Chairman could be appointed. Dr. Karp served as the Acting Chairman through June 30, 1981. As

Acting Chairman, Dr. Karp implemented the plans begun by Dr. Petrone to offer college-credit courses to students enrolled in the Bryn Mawr Hospital School of Nursing.

Dr. Karp also requested that an internal audit be conducted of various operations that generated revenue and expenses within the Department. In their final report, the auditors noted that the procedures in effect within the Department of General Studies were adequate. In addition, Dr. Karp commissioned Kenneth A. Miller, Ed.D., to conduct a survey of enrolled students and supervisory personnel of Thomas Jefferson University. Many suggestions were generated from the results of the two surveys, including arranging the schedule so that the students could take two classes in two nights during the same quarter and advertising the services that were offered to students.

Following Dr. Karp's Acting Chairmanship, the Department of General Studies was administered by Karen R. Stubaus until she left the University on August 14, 1981. At that point, Dr. Abrams assumed responsibility for the administration of the Department until a new Chairman could be named.

In September of 1981, Thomas K. McElhinney, Ph.D. was appointed Acting Chairman of the Department of General Studies. Within months of his appointment, he proposed and received approval to implement a semester calendar for the evening program. The adoption of the semester calendar in 1982–1983 stimulated an increase in evening enrollment.

The Task Force on Liberal Arts

The Task Force on Ethics, the Humanities, and Human Values was convened by President Bluemle to undertake a thorough analysis of the Department of General Studies and formulate recommendations for the future direction of the Department within the College and University. The Task Force was composed of representatives from all four divisions of the University and was chaired by Dr. McElhinney. The Task Force engaged in a number of activities, including development of position statements and statements of premises and principles; collection of information from other schools; assessment of the Department's extension of input within the University, and the identification of a consultant.

Dr. McElhinney served as the Acting Chairman until June 30, 1984. He was succeeded by Raymond W. Campbell, Ph.D. Dr. Campbell served as Acting Chairman from July 1, 1984, to February 3, 1986, when he was named permanent Chairman.

Through the mid-1980s the Department of General Studies continued to offer lower-division and upper-division courses in the humanities, the social sciences, and the natural sciences. The Department also served Jefferson employees and local community residents through an evening program, provided courses for the day programs within the College, and conducted an extension program at the Bryn Mawr Hospital School of Nursing until May 1986, when that hospital decided to close its School.

The Evening Program

For the evening program, the valued ingredient of the Department was its emphasis on flexibility. With the aid of an advisor (the Chairman of the Department), a student was able to plan courses to be taken at a self-determined pace. These courses were designed to meet the particular needs, interests, and goals of the nontraditional student who desired to fulfill the requirements for the Associate Degree in Arts or Science, to make up course deficiencies in the liberal arts and basic sciences, to pursue a second career, or to seek professional advancement or personal enrichment (Figure 52–21).

By fall, 1985, enrollment consisted of 301 part-time students, and by then 22 associate degrees had been awarded. Several graduates had continued their education toward the baccalaureate degree at other universities.

The Day Program

During the day, the Department provided an opportunity for students enrolled in baccalaureate degree programs of the College to meet graduation requirements, or to broaden their educational experience through selection of electives. These offerings included such courses as Principles of Management, Statistics and Research Methods, Introduction to Physics, Introduction to Group Dynamics, Educational Psychology, and Methods of Teaching.

Faculty and Personnel

Day and evening courses offered by the Department were taught predominantly by part-time persons who held full-time faculty appointments in neighboring academic institutions such as Drexel University, University of Pennsylvania, West Chester University, Villanova University, and Delaware County Community College. A few courses were taught by selected professional personnel from Jefferson and the local area, in addition to the basic science courses taught by full-time Jefferson faculty of the various Departments of the Medical College and the College of Graduate Studies.

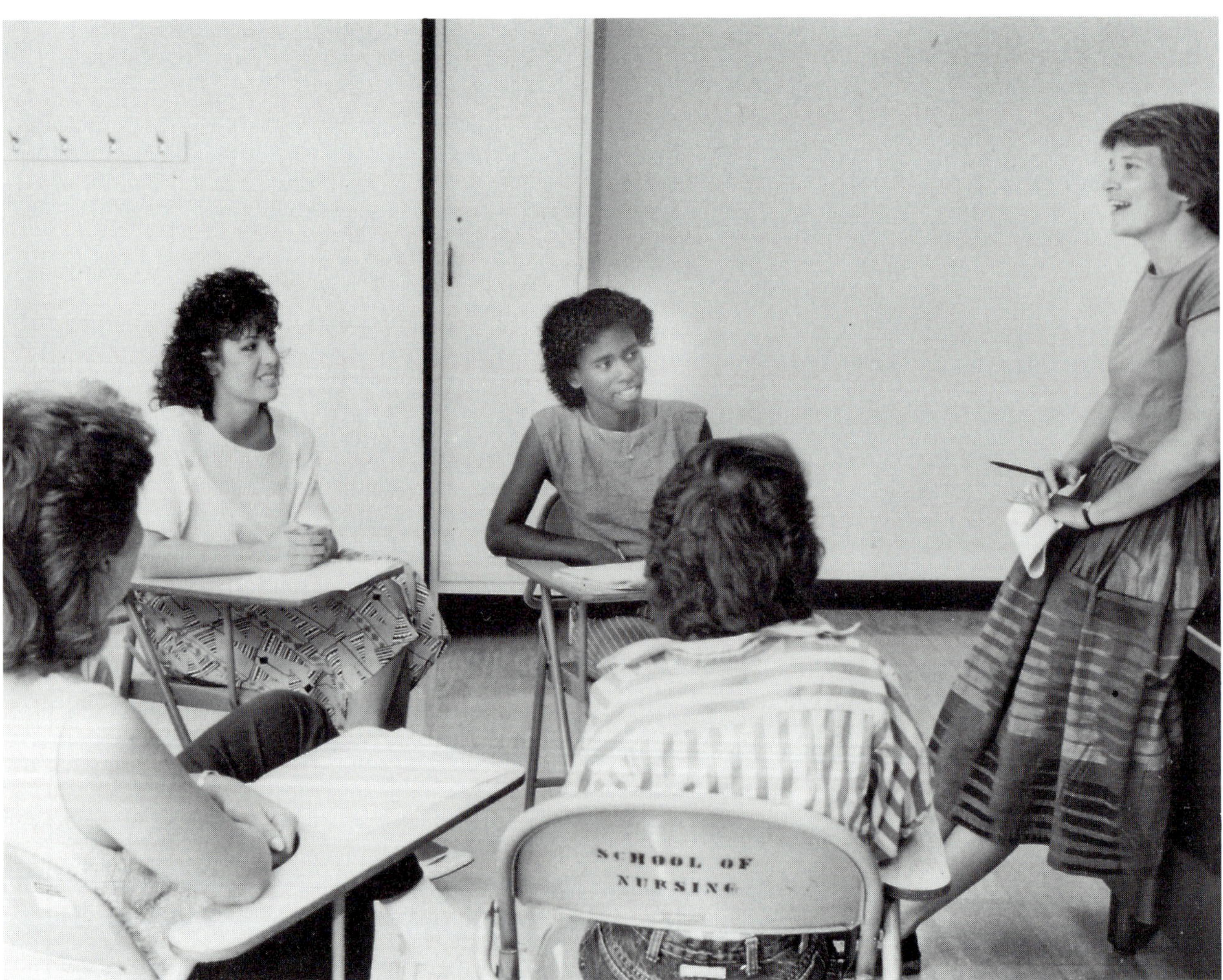

FIG. 52-21. General Studies courses such as Interpersonal Communications met the needs of degree-seeking students as well as those seeking personal enrichment.

■ The Role of the Department

Under the leadership of Dr. Campbell, the Department's role within the College was reaffirmed in 1987 for inclusion in the College of Allied Health Sciences' 1987–1988 edition of the Catalogue:

> "In recognition of the commitment to balanced degree programs in terms of professional courses and liberal arts courses, the College of Allied Health Sciences, through its Department of General Studies, offers upper-division and graduate courses in the Humanities, the Social Sciences, and the Physical Sciences to the daytime and evening students majoring in one of the professional programs. The Department also offers selected introductory courses in these same areas for Jefferson employees, and city residents and workers, to begin or continue working toward an associate or baccalaureate degree."

As the decade of the 1980s was coming to the end, the Department of General Studies continued to examine ways that it could support and enhance the College's professional programs, from leading the effort to establish an integrated course for all College of Allied Health Sciences students, to implementing strategies for improving the quality of teaching and conducting feasibility studies for new ventures.

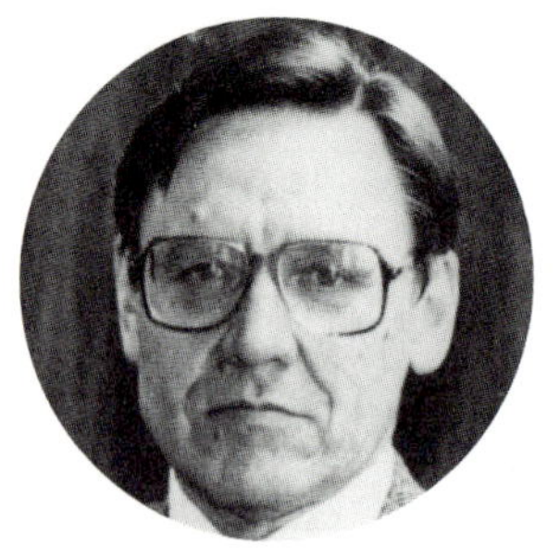
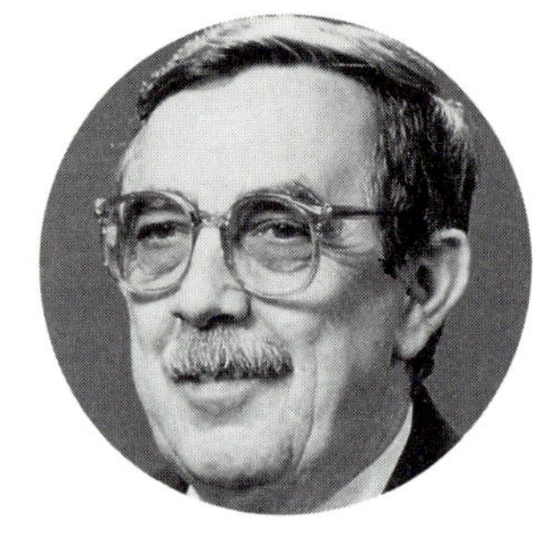
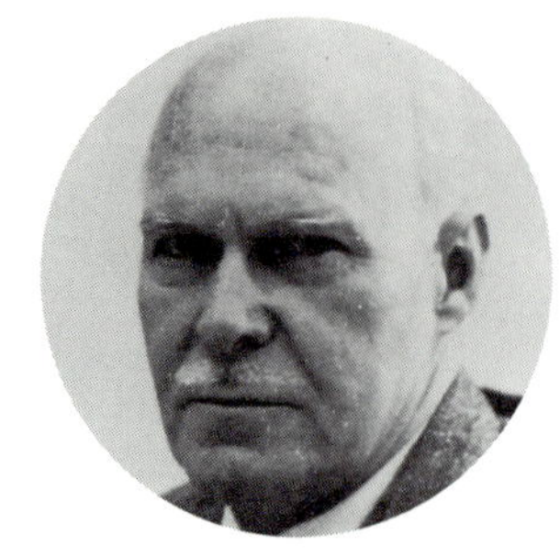

CHAPTER FIFTY-THREE

College of Graduate Studies

Jussi J. Saukkonen, M.D., Harry L. Smith, Jr., Ph.D., and Andrew J. Ramsay, Ph.D., Sc.D.

"That man can interrogate as well as observe nature, was a lesson slowly learned in his evolution."

—Sir William Osler (1849–1919)

Graduate programs leading to advanced degrees other than that of the Doctor of Medicine have a long history at Thomas Jefferson University. Since the early 1900s, interest in other forms of postgraduate education went along with the interest of faculty members in clinical and basic science research, and with the need to train interested people in these areas. From an historical perspective, the development of the College of Graduate Studies proceeded through three periods.

The First Period (1912–1923)

The first period of development was initiated by Philip Bovier Hawk, Ph.D. (Figure 53-1). On succeeding James W. Holland, M.D. as Head of the Department of Physiological Chemistry in 1912, Dr. Hawk found the academic environment to be devoted entirely to the education of medical students. No research of consequence was being conducted in the basic sciences, as contrasted to

Hawk's experience at Illinois, University of Pennsylvania, and other places where he had been on the faculty. To address this matter, Dr. Hawk proposed to the faculty that a course of studies be instituted that would lead to master and doctoral degrees in Physiologic Chemistry. This was approved by the faculty and by the Board of Trustees under the University charter granted to the institution in 1838.

The rules and regulations for this program were established, stipulating the formation of a five-member Committee of Postgraduate Education.

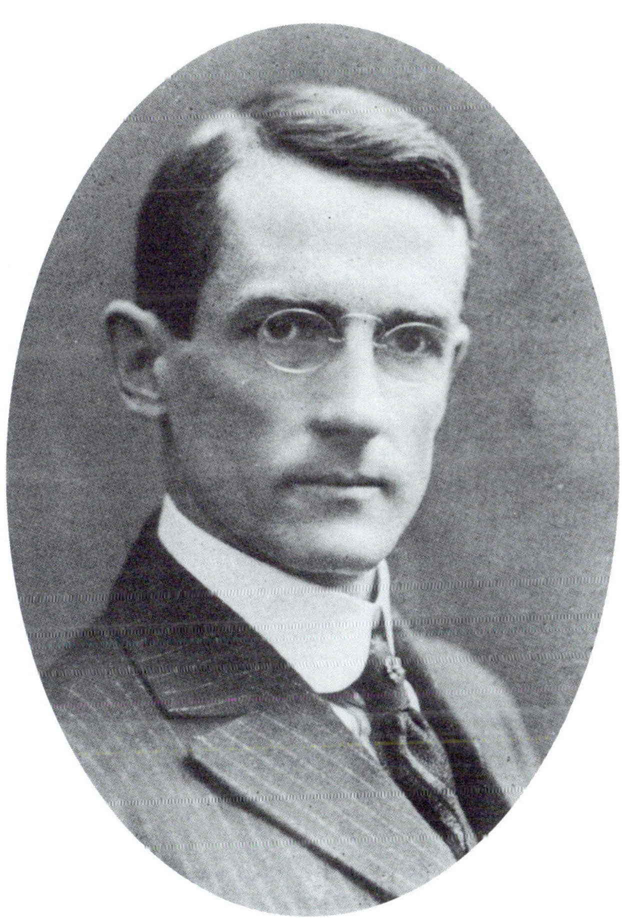

FIG. 53-1. Philip B. Hawk, Ph.D., Professor and Head of the Department of Physiological Chemistry (1912–1923), who first instituted courses leading to master and doctoral degrees.

The document described the requirements for residency on the campus, tuition (matriculation fees only), and an examination by an appropriate committee before a degree could be conferred by the Board of Trustees. There was no mention about required course work, not unusual at the time, reflecting the traditions of the old European preceptor system.

The program appeared to start well. Fifteen degrees (eight M.S., four Ph.D., and three Sc.D.) were awarded in the next ten years. In December, 1923, however, the Administration of the Medical College received communications from alumni that the good name of their alma mater and those of some of its faculty were seen in advertisements for such products as Postum and Fleischman's Yeast.

On December 11, 1923, the Board of Trustees requested an investigation into the matter by the Dean and faculty. Dr. Hawk was called before the Executive Faculty to give his side of the story before any action was taken.

Dr. Hawk, under questioning, revealed that he had had a long association with certain food companies who provided monies to him in return for analyses of their products and a permission to use the results with the names of the faculty members in their advertisements. He used these funds to support the research in his Department, including that done by graduate students and other faculty members. No one else in the Department knew the source of the funds, for Dr. Hawk thought it would be unethical for them knowingly to do such work. Dr. Hawk felt that he had not done anything unethical and had not violated any College rules. The Faculty reacted that he had indeed violated general understanding and unwritten rules. On December 18, 1923, the Board of Trustees severed all ties of Jefferson Medical College with Dr. Hawk. He departed immediately, and the graduate program ceased for the next 26 years.

The Second Period (1949–1967)

The second period, represented by the Board for the Regulation of Graduate Studies, began in 1949. At the Executive Faculty meeting of the Jefferson Medical College on January 31, 1949, Dr. Kenneth Goodner proposed the establishment of graduate courses leading to M.S. and Ph.D. degrees in Anatomy, Bacteriology-Immunology,

Biochemistry, Pathology, Pharmacology-Toxicology (Figure 53-2) and Physiology. This proposal was promptly approved by the Faculty and the Board of Trustees. The Board for Regulation of Graduate Studies was created, composed of the Chairmen of Departments, namely: George Bennett (Anatomy), Kenneth Goodner (Bacteriology), Abraham Cantarow (Biochemistry), Peter Herbut (Pathology), Charles Gruber (Pharmacology), and Earl Thomas (Physiology). In addition, the Dean of the Medical College, Dr. W. Harvey Perkins, was also appointed. Rules and regulations were formulated and approved by the Faculty and the Board of Trustees. They included not only the appointment of the Medical College Dean to the Board regulating these programs, but also a limitation on the number of students who could enroll in the programs. A stipulation was also made that this was not an alternate route for a student to gain admission to the Medical College. A $500 tuition was established.

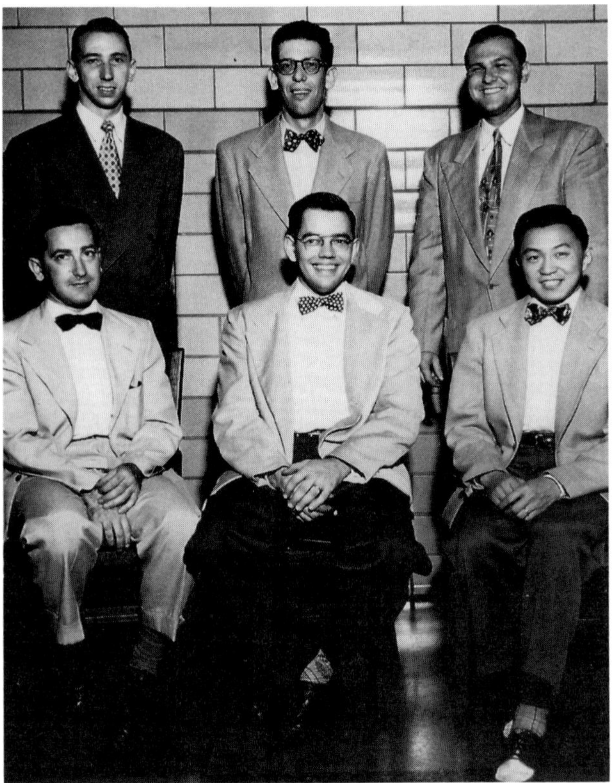

FIG. 53-2. Graduate students in the Department of Pharmacology (1951); standing, from left to right: Mr. Richard Matthews, Jr., Mr. Melvyn I. Gluckman, and Mr. Walter W. Baker. Sitting, from left to right: Dr. Thomas C. Aschner, Mr. Max A. Heinrich, Jr., and Mr. James Inashima.

Dr. Goodner was elected first Chairman of the Board and Dr. William G. Sawitz was appointed Secretary. The first application was from Sonia Schorr, and the first Ph.D. was given to Russell Miller in Bacteriology in 1951.

The members of the Graduate Board were strong personalities with unique characteristics, but sharing the common characteristic of being short on patience. Dr. Sawitz, as Secretary for the Board, was responsible for maintaining records and scheduling. Although not a voting member he helped the Board in his quiet diplomatic manner to calm individual members when their pet projects were threatened. Within an environment in which the conditions for improvement were not easily attained in these early years, much time was spent in debating programs and in experimenting with the educational process.

The limitation on the number of students permitted in the program was removed in 1959. Graduate students were recognized as giving more to the education of medical students than they were receiving. It appears that the Executive Faculty had first been concerned that graduate education might interfere with the prime responsibility of the school to educate medical students. With graduate students being teaching assistants in the basic science courses, however, they helped to improve the student–instructor ratio and thus facilitated a more individualized education for medical students. In addition, graduate instructors were of the same age as the medical students and a good rapport was easier to establish.

The Third Period (1967–)

Under the initiative of Dr. Peter A. Herbut in December, 1967, the third period of graduate studies began. Although no Department of Physics existed at the College, arrangements were made with the Bartol Research Foundation of the Franklin Institute Department of Physics to have it recognized as the Department of Physics at Jefferson. This provided a mechanism for this group to offer a graduate program, the degrees being granted by Jefferson under the regulations established for the basic science Departments. Approval was received in late spring of 1968. This program continued until June 30, 1977, when, because of the move of the Bartol physics laboratory from its original location in Swarthmore to the University of Delaware, the faculty shifted their appointments to the latter University.

This is an example of one of the formal arrangements that had been made by the Graduate Board with sister institutions in and around Philadelphia. A program, begun in 1967 and still functioning, is the cooperative program in basic sciences with Hahnemann University, Temple University, and Medical College of Pennsylvania (formerly Woman's Medical College). More recently a Cooperative Program has also been initiated with the Philadelphia College of Pharmacy and Science. The expertise in a variety of areas is shared so that each member of the group does not need to duplicate efforts.

Some earlier efforts to broaden the scope of graduate programs did not succeed. Programs in biomedical engineering and in nutrition with another University in the city never progressed beyond the planning stage.

Robert C. Baldridge, Ph.D.; First Dean (1970–1981)

When Thomas Jefferson University was established in 1969, the College of Graduate Studies replaced the Board for the Regulation of Graduate Studies. In accord with the new designation, Dr. Robert C. Baldridge (Figure 53-3) was appointed the first Dean. Born on January 9, 1921, in Herington, Kansas, Dr. Baldridge obtained his B.S. degree (Chemistry) at Kansas State University (1943), an M.S. (Biological Chemistry) at the University of Michigan (1948), and a Ph.D. (Biological Chemistry) also from the latter institution (1951). After teaching biological chemistry at the University of Michigan (1951–1953), he transferred to Temple University School of Medicine (1953–1970) where he rose to Professor of Biochemistry and Associate Dean of the Graduate School (1966–1970). His Deanship at Jefferson in 1970 included a Professorship in Biochemistry.

Dean Baldridge undertook the responsibility of having the new College recognized as an accredited Graduate School. Initially there was the task of formation of a Graduate Council that was, in part, representative of members of the faculty other than the Department Chairmen. This was a delicate situation. It was decided that three Department Chairmen would sit on the Council and that three additional members were to be elected from Departments whose Chairmen were not sitting. All members had a two-year term, and the Department Chairmen rotated through their

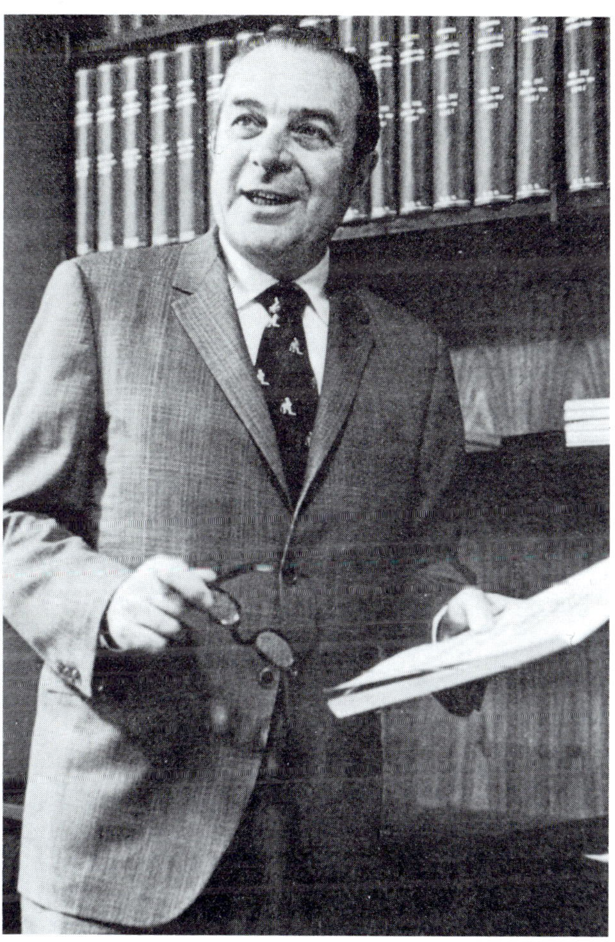

FIG. 53-3. Robert C. Baldridge, Ph.D.; First Dean (1970–1981).

terms. The Dean of the College of Graduate Studies presided at Council meetings, and the President of the University was an ex-officio member.

After more than a decade of fruitful service, Dr. Baldridge resigned in 1981 to pursue his earlier interest in teaching and research. His investigations continued in inborn errors of metabolism as related to biochemical genetics. From July 1, 1985, to April 1, 1986, he served as Acting Chairman of the Department of Biochemistry and retired on June 30, 1986.

Jussi J. Saukkonen, M.D.; Second Dean (1981–)

Jussi J. Saukkonen (Figure 53-4) was born on October 10, 1930, in Helsinki, Finland. He became Candidate of Medicine (bachelor's degree) at the Helsinki University School of Medicine (1951); Research Fellow, Institute for Experimental Cancer Research, University of Heidelberg, and Institute for Physiological Chemistry, Philipps University, Marburg/Lahn, West Germany (1954–1956); Licentiate of Medicine (M.D.), Helsinki University School of Medicine (1955); Doctor of Medicine and Surgery (thesis), Helsinki University (1956); and Postdoctoral Fellow, Cell Chemistry Laboratory, College of Physicians and Surgeons, Columbia University (1957–1959). He conducted a general practice of medicine in Helsinki (1959–1962); became Head of the Biochemistry Laboratory of the Central Public Health Laboratory (1959–1965); and was Director of the Department of Biochemistry in the latter agency (1966–69). From 1962 to 1970 he was Lecturer in Medical Chemistry (part-time) at the Helsinki University School of Medicine.

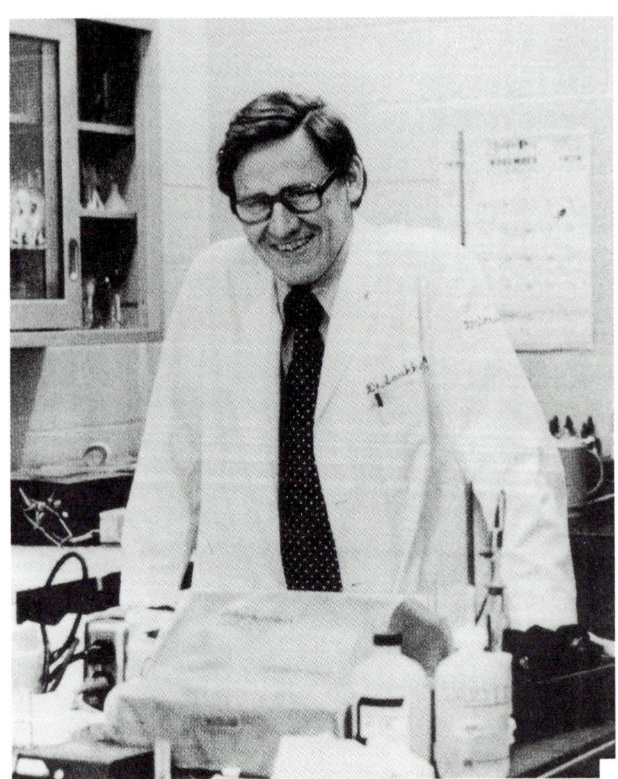

FIG. 53-4. Jussi J. Saukkonen, M.D.; Second Dean (1981–).

Dr. Saukkonen came to Jefferson in 1969 as Associate Professor of Microbiology and rose to full Professor in 1972. His teaching has been in aspects of microbial physiology and genetics. He lectures to the medical students on bacterial infections and to the graduate students on molecular biology.

On July 1, 1981, Dr. Saukkonen assumed the Deanship of the College of Graduate Studies, in which capacity he continues to serve along with his Professorship in Microbiology. In 1983 he additionally became Senior Associate Dean for Scientific and Faculty Affairs in the Medical College. He has served on local, national, and international editorial boards and chaired important committees in planning, accreditation, and graduate programs in academic health centers.

Two Assistant Deans were appointed in 1981: Robert M. Greene, Ph.D., from the Department of Anatomy, primarily to oversee recruitment and admissions, and Joseph R. Sherwin, Ph.D., with primary responsibility for curriculum development and student affairs.

Three new programs were added under the Baldridge and Saukkonen Deanships. A Master of Science in Clinical Microbiology began in 1974. Its purpose was to enhance the training of clinical microbiologists in management skills while increasing their knowledge in the basics of the disciplines that make up microbiology. A Master's Program in Toxicology was established in the Department of Pharmacology in 1978. It received funding from federal sources and was intended to train individuals holding doctoral degrees in other disciplines to qualify as toxicologists. In 1986 a Master of Science degree program in Rehabilitation Nursing was begun. The latter was the initial step in establishing professional graduate programs in areas in which the faculty strength extended into the College of Allied Health Sciences.

Since graduate students are generally supported by stipends, there have been determined efforts to provide scholarship funds to help recruit the best possible graduate students. The Deans have initiated several projects that provide such funds. In the mid-1970s, a tutorial program was established in conjunction with the College of Allied Health Sciences. Substantial sums of money provided by the Foerderer Foundation have supported a number of students. The Smith Scholarship Fund provides continuing support for a student over his or her course of study. The Rocco Fund provides tuition support for Master's degree students in Clinical Microbiology.

It is well established that graduate students can play a substantial role in the day-to-day conduct of research (Figures 53-5 and 53-6). The growth in the College of Graduate Studies between 1969 and the present time has paralleled the growth in interest in biomedical research at the University. In 1969 the basic science Departments in which the graduate programs were housed received slightly less than $1.4 million to support research. By 1986 this had risen to over $5.5 million per year. Moreover, the number of federally funded predoctoral training programs rose to three: one in developmental biology, one in cardiovascular physiology, and one in experimental pathology. With a major commitment to reserach during the decade of the 1980s, future growth should be equally impressive.

Prizes have been established for outstanding students as evidenced by their research theses. The Charles W. LaBelle Prize was awarded from 1965 to 1977. This was replaced in 1980 by the Alumni Prize.

Tables 53-1 and 53-2 indicate the yearly graduates since 1950 as well as the distribution of degrees among the various disciplines. In an era of ever-increasing sophistication in technology and research, the College of Graduate Studies is in appropriate balance with the prestige of the other components of Thomas Jefferson University. It offers the same high-quality programs and potential for growth that have been the hallmark of Jefferson since its inception more than a century and one-half ago.

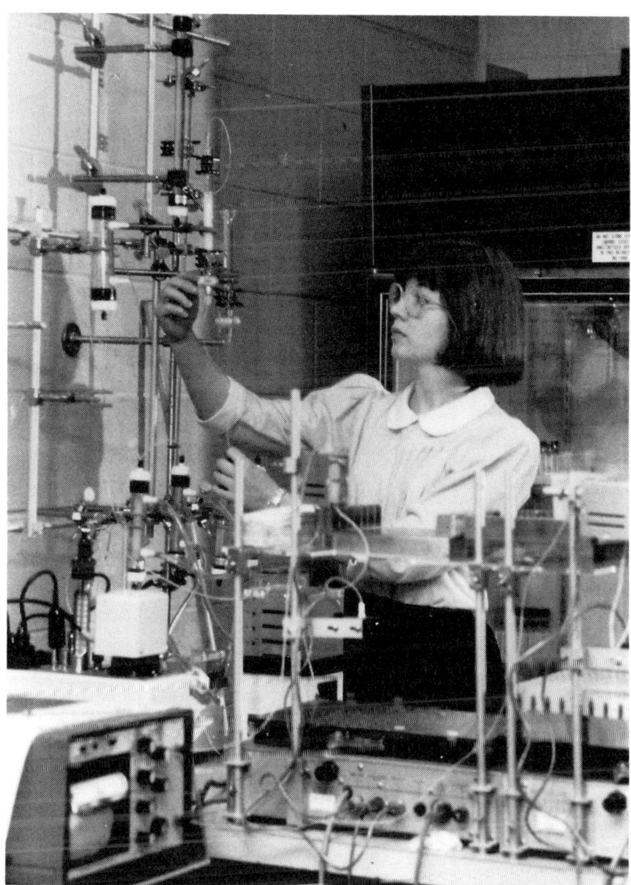

FIG. 53-5. Jo Lynda Jones, graduate student in anatomy (1986).

Table 53-1 Yearly Graduates Since 1950

Yr.	*Anat*	*Biochem*	*Med*	*Micro-biol*	*Clin Microbiol (M.S.)*	*Path*	*Pharm*	*Physics*	*Physiol*	*Toxicol*	*Total*
1950				1							1
1951	4			3			1				8
1952	0			1			2		1		4
1953	0			3			3		0		6
1954	2			3			3		1		9
1955	0	1		0			2		1		4
1956	0	0		0			4		1		5
1957	0	0		1			2		2		5
1958	0	0		0			0		1		1
1959	0	0		2			2		2		6
1960	0	1		1			1		1		4
1961	1	0	2	1			0		3		7
1962	0	0	0	5			3		1		9
1963	2	0	1	2			5		3		13
1964	1	0	1	0		5	5		6		18
1965	2	0	0	5		0	0	1	1		9
1966	1	1	0	3		1	0	1	4		11
1967	0	0	1	1		0	5	0	7		14
1968	1	0	0	4		2	2	1	5		15
1969	2	2	0	1		2	1	0	5		13
1970	2	1	0	1		1	5	0	2		12
1971	2	3	0	1		0	1	0	2		9
1972	3	1	2	4		0	4	1	5		20
1973	1	2	2	2		2	3	1	4		17
1974	1	1	0	3	11	0	5	3	7		31
1975	4	0	0	2	2	0	2	1	4		15
1976	1	3	0	1	8	1	2	0	5		21
1977	1	2	0	0	13	0	5	2	4		27
1978	1	1	0	4	11	0	4	0	3		24
1979	4	0	1	5	15	1	4	0	2		32
1980	2	1	0	2	12	4	7	0	1		29
1981	1	0	0	4	7	0	2	0	2	5	21
1982	1	2	0	3	12	0	5	0	4	0	27
1983	1	3	0	3	4	0	5	0	1	0	17
1984	1	2	0	2	6	2	1	0	2	1	17
1985	2	0	0	2	8	0	6	0	1	1	20
1986	2	1	0	2	2	0	3	0	2	1	13
1987	1	1	0	0	3	1	3	0	1	0	10
Total	47	29	10	78	114	22	108	11	97	8	524

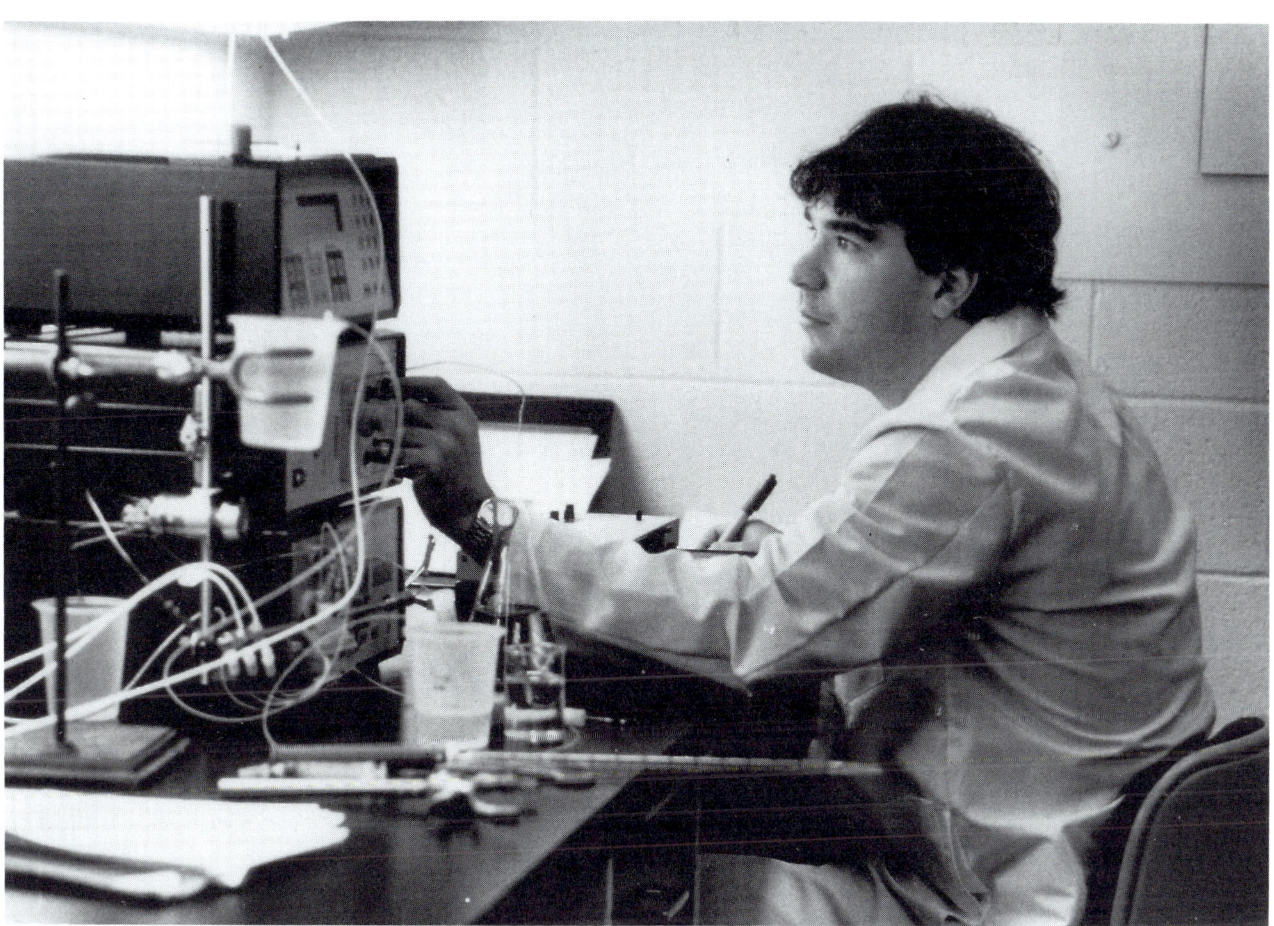

FIG. 53-6. Brian Learn, graduate student in microbiology (1986).

Table 53-2 Distribution of Degrees Among Individual Disciplines

Department	*Total No. Degrees*	*Total No. People*	*M.S.*	*Ph.D.*	*M.S. and Ph.D.*
Anatomy	47	45	14	33	2
Biochemistry	29	29	3	26	0
Medicine	10	10	10	0	0
Microbiology	192	183	144	48	9
Pathology	22	22	1	21	0
Pharmacology	108	103	17	91	5
Physics	11	10	3	8	1
Physiology	97	95	22	75	2
Toxicology	8	8	8	0	0
TOTAL	524	505	222	302	19

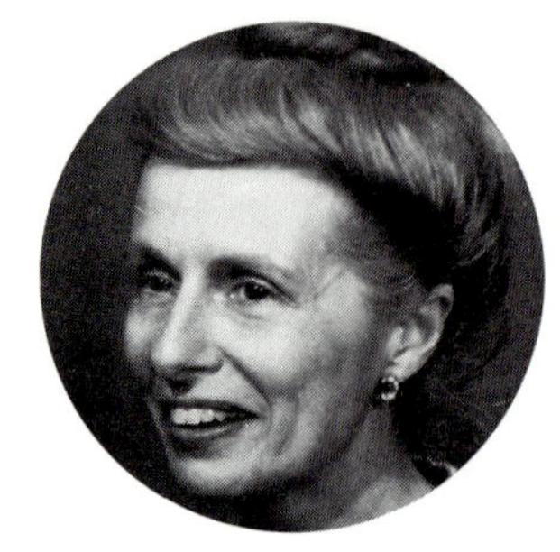

CHAPTER FIFTY-FOUR

Jefferson Affiliations

Carla E. Goepp, M.D.

"Particles of science are often very widely scattered." —Samuel Johnson (1709–1784)

A significant proportion of the excellent clinical training of Jefferson students and house staff has been received at the hospitals affiliated with Jefferson. Indeed, since the increase in the size of each medical school class to 223 in the early 1970s, more than one-half of the clinical instruction has been given at the Affiliates. In the overall history of Jefferson, this process has evolved into a most important aspect of student teaching and house staff training. Opportunities for clinical experience were provided Jefferson students from the early days, but during the nineteenth century such opportunities were loosely structured. Beginning near the turn of the twentieth century, with student visits to Philadelphia General and Pennsylvania Hospital, the volume and diversity of clinical material there proved increasingly valuable. Building upon this experience, student assignments were formalized, and the teaching became more effective. Appointments of Jefferson physicians to other hospital services provided the link in this process. Reciprocal service and teaching relationships with Jefferson house staff rotating through the Affiliated Hospitals was a natural outgrowth of the earlier arrangement. A salient affirmation of the critical importance of the Affiliated Hospitals was the appointment on April 1, 1986, of Dr. Joseph F. Rodgers as Associate Dean of Affiliations and Residency Program Coordinator.

Philadelphia General Hospital (Blockley)

As early as 1818, Jefferson's founder, Dr. George McClellan, while a student was elected "Resident Physician" to the Philadelphia Almshouse, then situated at Tenth and Spruce Streets. Its successor, Philadelphia (General) Hospital, as a public institution attracted academic physicians as volunteers to positions that commanded increasing prestige later in the nineteenth century. Students were gradually involved in informal teaching arrangements and attended "clinics" conducted by service chiefs who also held Jefferson appointments.[1] At the turn of the century, teaching became more formalized with students joining in rounds and teaching conferences on a scheduled basis. Medicine and Surgery were primarily involved, but other Departments including Ophthalmology, Urology, Obstetrics-Gynecology, Pathology, Neurology-Psychiatry, and Otolaryngology followed. All teaching related to inpatients, because Philadelphia General had no outpatient service until 1919. Among the early people who served were Drs. Solomon Solis-Cohen and R. Max Goepp in Medicine, Dr. J. Chalmers DaCosta in Surgery, and Dr. Orville Horwitz in Genito-Urinary Surgery. Jefferson physicians later included Drs. Samuel A. Loewenberg and Harold L. Goldburgh in Medicine and Dr. William Lemmon in Surgery.

During the three decades following 1920, the affiliation program was greatly expanded and strengthened. Gradually the medical schools of Philadelphia assumed a more specifically defined role in the clinical activities. Ultimately the departments were separated along medical school lines. As student teaching and house staff rotation were organized, Dr. Francis J. Sweeney, Jr. was appointed Director of Medical Services in 1966. Sophomore, junior, and senior students went to Philadelphia General for clinical experience. This arrangement ended in 1971, and the hospital closed in 1977.

Pennsylvania Hospital

From the time of the founding of Jefferson, students were encouraged to supplement their lectures with clinical observation. Pennsylvania Hospital during the nineteenth century was a free source of patients and more or less formal clinics were conducted by Jefferson Professors with Pennsylvania appointments. Policies relative to teaching students of medicine were in place from the founding of the Hospital in 1751, even before a medical school existed.[2] Early Jefferson physicians included Dr. John Kearsley Mitchell in Medicine (1827–1834); Dr. Charles D. Meigs, who served in the Lying-In Department (1838–1849); Dr. Joseph Pancoast in Surgery (1854–1864); Dr. James Aitken Meigs in Medicine (1868–1879); Dr. Richard Levis in Surgery (1871–1887); and Dr. Morris Longstreth as Pathologist and Curator (1870–1890). The teaching arrangements became incorporated into the regular curriculum as time went on, with assignment of students to ward rounds and to demonstrations and lectures held in the old Clinical Amphitheater at Pennsylvania.[3] Physicians prominent during the period before World War II included Drs. Thomas McCrae and Garfield Duncan in Medicine, Dr. Adolph Walkling in Surgery, and Drs. Norris W. Vaux and P. Brooke Bland in Obstetrics.

It is clear that the long-standing relationship between Jefferson and Pennsylvania Hospital with its established commitment to medical education was a great benefit to the students before the era of clinical clerkships. Upon affiliation of the Hospital with the University of Pennsylvania in 1957, this program ended.

Lankenau Hospital

Jefferson physicians had been staff members at Lankenau since its early days as the German Hospital, and some teaching had been carried out since 1949. A formal teaching arrangement was developed in 1966, after which time students have profited greatly from their experience in this hospital. Although primarily a community hospital, research and academic activities have long complemented its clinical facilities. Lankenau has also maintained a hospice service offering care for terminally ill patients at home and in the hospital. Since 1966, students were assigned to rotate through Lankenau as clinical clerks in Medicine, Obstetrics-Gynecology, and Surgery, as well as receiving instruction in many of the other Departments. Joint residencies in Orthopaedics, Otolaryngology, Ophthalmology, and Neurology have been developed.

Our Lady of Lourdes Hospital, Camden, New Jersey

This institution had an exceptionally strong tie, since many of its Medical Staff received student, residency, and fellowship training at Jefferson. An affiliation agreement was reached in 1972 through the efforts of Associate Dean John Killough and Our Lady of Lourdes officials. This was extended to include rotation of students and house staff in Medicine, Pediatrics, Surgery, Urology, and Orthopaedics.

Bryn Mawr Hospital

This long-established suburban community hospital of 402 beds became a major affiliate of Jefferson in 1972. In recent years sophisticated programs such as the Imaging Center, the Center for Radiation Oncology, and the Alcohol and Drug Intervention Unit have been added to its traditional medical and surgical functions. The clinical educational program has involved medical students in Medicine, Surgery, Obstetrics-Gynecology, Urology, and Family Medicine. Jefferson residents have rotated through Surgery, Urology, Otolaryngology, Orthopaedics, and Obstetrics-Gynecology.

Chestnut Hill Hospital

In 1974 informal teaching relationships that had existed for some years were firmed into an agreement of affiliation that has proved beneficial to both parties. The initial link was through the Department of Family Medicine. A well-financed community hospital with 220 beds and a strong Surgery Department, Chestnut Hill has provided teaching of medical students and a Transitional Residency program that have broadened the base of the educational experience. Affiliations were developed for both junior and senior students in Family Medicine. Other Departments with teaching arrangements have been those of Surgery, Pediatrics, Urology, Orthopaedics, and Anesthesiology.

Methodist Hospital

Because of the long association of South Philadelphia with Jefferson graduates and faculty, Methodist Hospital with its large accident and outpatient services was easily accommodated into a closer relationship during the few years following World War II. Informal affiliation in General Surgery developed about 1950 and later in the decade extended to Medicine and Obstetrics-Gynecology. In the 1960s the still informal arrangement included students and residents rotating in Surgery and students in Orthopaedics. In 1971, the formal agreement of affiliation was signed to permit rotation of students and residents in Medicine, Surgery, and Obstetrics-Gynecology. Rotation of residents in Otolaryngology and Emergency Medicine occurred later.

Mercy Catholic Medical Center

This general medical center of 800 beds and large emergency and outpatient services became affiliated with Jefferson Medical College in 1969. The timing coincided with the merger of Misericordia and Fitzgerald-Mercy Hospitals to form the largest Catholic medical complex in the Delaware Valley serving a widely divergent population. Jefferson teachers had previously been active in both hospitals. The affiliation included clinical instruction in Medicine, Obstetrics-Gynecology, Surgery, and Pediatrics.

Wills Eye Hospital

Wills Eye Hospital, the nation's oldest and largest hospital devoted to the prevention and cure of eye disease, has been affiliated with Jefferson since 1972. Physicians at Wills became the Ophthalmology Department for Jefferson Medical College and Thomas Jefferson University Hospital. Traditionally, Wills receives more eye trauma cases than any other institution in the Delaware Valley. Wills' specialized medical staff, strong research program, and high technology permit unique handling of full needs relating to ophthalmology. Wills' resources became available for both elective and core rotations for Jefferson's students in their clinical years. Jefferson students participated in firsthand observation not only of the patients in the hospital's trauma center but also have received training in preventive eye care and retinal, corneal, oculoplastic, and oncologic problems.

Children's Rehabilitation Hospital of Philadelphia

Children's Rehabilitation Hospital was a successor (1986) to Children's Heart Hospital, a facility founded in 1927 by businessman William M. Anderson for convalescent care of children with heart disease, usually of rheumatic fever origin. Antibiotic treatment and prophylaxis of streptococcal infection diminished the need for such long-term care, and admission of children with a variety of chronic illnesses followed.

In 1970 the Hospital became related to Jefferson at the request of Children's Heart Hospital Trustees. Jefferson assumed operational and clinical responsibility, and the hospital has been operated through a committee of the Board of Trustees. Many children with intractable asthma and bronchopulmonary diseases have been treated there. The services have also included children with developmental disabilities such as spina bifida, cerebral palsy, and Down's syndrome, as well as acquired disabilities.

Research, education, and patient care have come into balance. Junior students have rotated for periods of one day to two weeks, and an elective for seniors in the care of chronically ill children became available. Second-year Pediatrics Residents were involved, and the services were coordinated with specialized procedures in the Departments of Pediatrics and Rehabilitation Medicine at Jefferson.

The Magee Rehabilitation Hospital

Anna J. Magee, a center-city philanthropist and a grateful patient of Dr. J.C. Wilson, died in 1923 leaving a bequest for the establishment of the hospital, which finally opened in 1958. She also provided funds for the endowment of the Magee Chair of Medicine at Jefferson. She specified in her will that the Board of Directors of Magee Hospital should include a representative from Jefferson.

Almost from the beginning, the Magee Hospital developed an affiliation with the Department of Internal Medicine of Jefferson Medical College and Hospital, thus enhancing the monitoring of patients with multiple disabilities. The affiliation also provided an opportunity for residents in internal medicine to participate in the procedures of rehabilitation and to observe the responses and tolerance of the patients.

The close association with training programs at Jefferson was moved forward in 1977 when Dr. William E. Stass (Jefferson, 1962), Professor of Rehabilitation Medicine, became President and Medical Director at Magee. The affiliation agreement was reached in 1975, and residents began rotations in 1977. Subsequently, Residents in Family Medicine as well as Rehabilitation Medicine rotated at Magee. Teaching there has included second-year students in the physical diagnosis course as well as third- and fourth-year students for a two-week clinical rotation.

Veterans Administration Medical Center, Coatesville, Pennsylvania

Veterans Administration Medical Center, Coatesville, Pennsylvania, supplies a key service to the veterans who occupy its 1,494 beds and utilize its many outpatient facilities. This affiliate became linked for instruction with the Department of Psychiatry and Human Behavior in 1967 for training students and residents in psychiatry and neurology. Training was jointly supervised by the Office of the Associate Chief of Staff for Education at the Medical Center and the Dean's Committee at Jefferson, which included faculty in Psychiatry and Neurology. This Center also conducts training in clinical psychology, social work, nursing, dietetics, dental, and occupational speech therapy.

Latrobe Area Hospital

This semirural hospital has served an area where Jefferson graduates have traditionally been strong. In recent years, however, Latrobe has shared with similar regions the problem of attracting physicians. At the same time, the new policy developing at Jefferson to train physicians for underserved areas led to talks between the Dean's Office and Latrobe Hospital officials in 1973 during which the benefits of affiliation soon became obvious. The timing coincided with the beginning of the Department of Family Medicine under Dr. Paul C. Brucker in 1974, and an agreement permitted the first class of Residents to begin in July and the first students in August. The agreement included monthly visits by a Visiting Professor to participate in rounds, conferences, and lectures.

The program provided for six junior students in Family Medicine each six weeks for purely outpatient service. Later a senior program was added for one to four students to include 50% inpatient service. The relationship has proved cordial in every respect. Almost all the local faculty and 70% of the hospital residents have been Jefferson graduates.

The Jefferson–Delaware Medical Education Program

Medical Center of Delaware (formerly Wilmington Medical Center) became affiliated with Jefferson in 1970; at that time the Center was composed of three separate hospitals. Part of the plan was to link all of the smaller hospitals in Delaware into a special Continuing Medical Education network; Dr. Wayne Martz spearheaded and directed the program until 1986. The original link was through the Department of Family Medicine. The newest part of the Medical complex was developed in Christiana, where the 1,050-bed hospital has offered clinical opportunities in Medicine, Surgery, Pediatrics, Obstetrics-Gynecology, Neurology, Anesthesiology, Orthopaedics, Urology, Neurosurgery, Family Medicine, Radiology, and Psychiatry and Human Behavior.

Since 1970 Jefferson has been the designated Medical School for the State of Delaware, providing for up to 20 places for qualified residents of Delaware for each first-year class under the Delaware Institute of Medical Education and Research program.

Eligible applicants must have met Jefferson's premedical requirements at an accredited college or university. Participants in the joint program were expected to serve major portions of their clinical clerkships at Delaware Hospitals affiliated with Jefferson.

Dr. Peter Chodoff (Jefferson, 1951), Director of Medical Education and Research at the Medical Center of Delaware, was appointed Assistant Dean of Jefferson Medical College on July 1, 1987.

Veterans Administration Medical Center, Wilmington, Delaware

The Veterans Administration Medical Center has been part of the V.A. Medical and Regional Office Center, Wilmington, Delaware, and has served veterans of the Eastern Shore of Maryland, Southern New Jersey, Pennsylvania, and Delaware. This affiliation with Jefferson has been managed by a Dean's Committee since 1980. The Center includes a 336-bed acute medical and surgical hospital, a modern research facility, and a 60-bed nursing home.

Recently, student and house staff instruction has been available in Internal Medicine, Pulmonary Diseases, Gastroenterology, Cardiology, Hematology/Oncology, Rheumatology, Nephrology, General Surgery, Otolaryngology, Urology, Orthopaedic Surgery, and acute Neurology. There is also a unique Maxillofacial Prosthodontia Program at the Wilmington V.A. Hospital.

were required to begin the intensive course early in June. Successful students were granted a B.S. by Penn State after completion of the second year at Jefferson. Despite the intensity of the course, this program has been successful in reducing the total time for medical education of a limited number of qualified students. Several other medical schools have developed programs similar to this one pioneered by Jefferson and Penn State.

Delaware State Hospital

The Delaware State Hospital (at Farnhurst) and Jefferson signed a special affiliation agreement in 1975. This cooperative venture related primarily to the academic program of mental health education and research in the Department of Psychiatry and Human Behavior, and at this facility provided third-year clinical clerkships in psychiatry for Jefferson students. Resources available to the program included inpatient and outpatient facilities and psychiatric emergency services. Child, adolescent, geriatric, forensic, and community psychiatry comprised the required clerkship as well as the student electives. Many faculty are Jefferson graduates or graduates of the psychiatric residency program at Delaware State Hospital.

Bryn Mawr Rehabilitation Hospital

This 92-bed hospital, known for special concerns in trauma therapy and rehabilitation, became affiliated with Jefferson in 1982. Common goals for joint programs in Rehabilitation Medicine were developed. In addition, plans include promoting continuing medical education and research. Residents in Rehabilitation Medicine have been rotating through Bryn Mawr every three months, and student electives are planned.

The Penn State-Jefferson Cooperative Program

In 1963 an exploratory B.S.-M.D. program for gifted students was developed jointly by Pennsylvania State University and Jefferson Medical College. At first a five-year program, it was extended to six years in 1983. Students were selected during the last year of high school and

A.I. DuPont Institute, Wilmington, Delaware

A special affiliation was developed between DuPont Institute and Jefferson in 1970. This provided for one year of training of two Jefferson residents annually in pediatric orthopaedics.

Albert Einstein Medical Center—Daroff Division

This hospital of 250 beds affiliated with Jefferson in 1971, offering instruction in Medicine, Surgery, Obstetrics-Gynecology, Anesthesiology, Orthopaedics, and Urology. The programs were discontinued in 1987.

Underwood Memorial Hospital

This 330-bed community hospital in New Jersey became an affiliate of Jefferson for clinical experience in Family Medicine in 1980.

Geisinger Medical Center

Geisinger, founded in Danville, Pennsylvania, as a regional medical center in 1915, is a multi-institutional system of health care. Its full-time staff of 391 physicians serves the Geisinger Medical Center of 649 inpatient beds, the Geisinger Clinic, the Geisinger Wyoming Valley Medical Center of 250 beds, as well as 43 satellite clinics and 34 communities in Northeastern and Central

Pennsylvania with a population of over 2,000,000 people. During its 73-year history, Geisinger has been a model for comprehensive patient care and more recently has entered into the field of research.

The formal Jefferson–Geisinger affiliation began in July of 1988. Sophomore students were sent for their miniclerkships and junior students were sent in Internal Medicine, Surgery, Obstetrics-Gynecology, Pediatrics, and Family Medicine. This will be expanded to include more students in more Departments as well as to initiate mutual programs in clinical research and exchange of residents and fellows. The affiliation will provide the students with a different view–an experience slanted more toward ambulatory care, which is one of the growing needs in medical education.

Other Affiliations

Through the years, reciprocal teaching and service arrangements, always emphasizing the bilaterality of the relationship, have been made with numerous other hospitals and institutions. Many of these have been of limited duration or for specific stated purposes. Affiliations no longer in effect have included Veterans Hospital of Philadelphia, Hunterdon Medical Center, Henry R. Landis State Hospital, U.S. Naval Hospital, Cooper Hospital of Camden, Germantown Hospital, and Atlantic City Hospital.

In addition to the Medical College, the College of Allied Health Sciences has developed a broad network of affiliations with more than 200 hospitals and related facilities throughout the United States and other countries. These affiliates have cooperated in the teaching of technicians, laboratory managers, physical therapists, and other technical trainees. Such institutions as Drexel University and the Franklin Institute of Pennsylvania have also been affiliated for special purposes.

References

1. Croskey, John W., *History of Blockley*. Philadelphia: F.A. Davis Co., 1929.
2. Morton, Thomas G., *The History of the Pennsylvania Hospital, 1751–1895*. Philadelphia: Times Printing House, 1895.
3. Packard, Francis R., *Some Account of the Pennsylvania Hospital of Philadelphia*. Philadelphia: Pennsylvania Hospital, 1956.

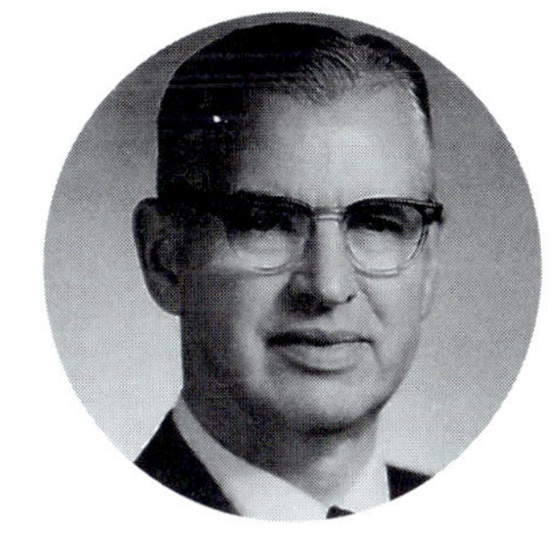

CHAPTER FIFTY-FIVE

The Volunteer Faculty

J. Woodrow Savacool, M.D.

"The only places where American medicine can fully live up to its possibilities are the teaching hospitals."

—Bernard De Voto (1897–1955)

Jefferson Medical College has for generations been an institution for the training of clinically oriented physicians. Late in the nineteenth century, when practical teaching effectively supplemented lectures, Jefferson developed a program of faculty appointments of physicians who wished to contribute teaching of medical students in return for hospital privileges and an academic association. Voluntary faculty positions became popular during those years and led to contributions of note by many teachers and professors whose main reward was an academic position. The title of "Professor" was generally reserved for the department heads but sufficient prestige attached to Clinical Professor, Associate and Assistant Professor to attract important clinicians to the faculty. Young graduates often enhanced their clinical training by working in the outpatient department where diversity of clinical material was always superb, then advancing to hospital appointment and academic status and acquiring proficiency in certain areas of medicine that created a demand for their services. A voluntary teaching appointment was therefore a valued and valuable educational tool. In fact, the major portion of clinical teaching was the responsibility of voluntary faculty members.

As time went on and American schools of medicine gradually joined the trend toward full-time teaching, Jefferson's volunteer program continued strong. The involvement of physicians in practice, however, remained an important factor in the development of good and complete physicians to practice medicine. Even when other medical faculties in Philadelphia became closed as full-time entities, the well-established Jefferson plan resisted the change. The involvement also affected setting of hospital policies, since a large number of beds were occupied by patients on the services of volunteers. At midcentury, when research was assuming an increasing role in medical education, the responsibilities of volunteers in patient care were perceived to be somewhat at variance with the teaching functions of full-time faculty members. Especially was this true at the level of teaching of Residents and the availability of teachers for small-group-section instruction on the clinical floors. Complaints were at times voiced by Residents and their chiefs that volunteers were interested only in the services provided by Interns and Residents and were not devoting time for clinical teaching. While it was acknowledged that such complaints had some validity, it was generally agreed that most volunteer faculty members were indeed contributing a great deal to teaching of medical students and house staff.

A number of forces came into play in the 1950s and 1960s that had an impact on the volunteer process. Besides increased emphasis on research, these included the intrusion of government and insurance controls into hospital services and practices, technological advances and their impact on medical care, and changes in the nature of illnesses brought about by medical progress. The strong traditional commitment of Jefferson physicians to clinical skills and concern for the patients aided in slowing the trend toward full-time faculty. Resistance to change and cost factors were also of consequence.

With the arrival of Dean Kellow in 1967, the previous efforts of Dean Sodeman to provide for research and funding were more aggressively pursued. The Dean instituted a "practice plan" whereby each full-time faculty member would be on salary and his income from fees for patient care would be shared among the College, the Department to which he was attached, and the faculty member. The inauguration of this plan was not graciously accepted by many longtime volunteer faculty members and added to the reasons for the organization of the Volunteer Faculty Association of Jefferson Medical College.

The Volunteer Faculty Association

In the latter part of 1970, informal discussions of these matters plus concerns about power structures and decision making led to the formation of an organization to address the perceived problems. The prestige of early leaders lent authenticity to the group, and their respected judgment in general led to an ability to contribute some balance to the process, as opposed to the occasionally heard criticism that its interests were limited to those of a pressure group. Among the leaders were Drs. Abraham E. Rakoff and Benjamin Haskell, both of professorial rank. Dr. Rakoff was elected the first President. A set of bylaws was promptly developed, the procedural authority being vested in a Board of Governors (Figure 55-1). By March 4, 1971, the Association was well established, and the meeting of the Board of Governors gave evidence of a structure already functioning with committees to address specific issues. Among the goals and objectives as stated in the bylaws were the support of the Medical School and University, academically and economically; the protection of the private practice of medicine; equal access of all faculty to medical and teaching opportunities; the identification and correction of inequities "that are perpetrated because of volunteer or full-time status"; efforts to increase representation of the Volunteer Faculty Members on the University's decision-making bodies; and the assurance of recognition by the Administration and community of the importance and function of the Volunteer Faculty Association.

The organization prospered, and the recognition desired was promptly forthcoming from President Herbut and Dean Kellow, both of whom were guests at stated meetings of the Association. Space was provided, staff engaged, and numerous issues were addressed, the mere discussion of which often defused them. Retired Dean Sodeman, a speaker in 1975, made a cogent observation regarding increasing emphasis on ambulatory care and the need for voluntary teachers including internists as providers of primary care. Some of the issues related to efforts to obtain more hospital and faculty appointments for volunteers, especially recent residents, allocation of unassigned emergency room and clinic patients to volunteers, and representation on faculty policy and research committees. A constant problem was the shortage of hospital beds and their allocation.

Before long, efforts to obtain an authoritative voice in hospital affairs led to the candidacy of volunteers for positions on the Executive Committee of the Hospital Staff and, for some years, domination of the officers elected to that body. For a time, the Association also endeavored to obtain a position for one of its members on the University Board of Trustees. Although this was not accomplished, in 1981 a manner of representation was acknowledged because the President of the Hospital Medical Staff was attending the meetings of the Hospital Committee of the Board.

Having become established and functioning effectively, the Association Board of Governors met with Dean Kellow on June 24, 1976, with special reference to the Full-time Practice Plan, but also addressing the usual issues of full-time-volunteer relationships. The Dean pointed out that budgetary problems had become acute with the loss of federal and state funds for medical education and ancillary programs such as those related to minority groups, underserved areas, and family medicine. The practice plan was one of the sources of new funds to replace those lost. He indicated that one of the objects of the plan was to restrict the practices of full-time faculty so that their research, teaching, and administrative functions could be carried out effectively. Also discussed was the matter of tenure for volunteers as compared with full-time faculty. The meeting proved cordial.

The opening of the New Hospital in 1978 changed but did not eliminate problems of relationships between volunteers and full-time faculty and the allocation of hospital beds. Gradually, however, the perception of a teaching hospital as a tertiary care facility resulted in more subspecialty patients being referred to full-time members. Also the change to virtually full-time status of new department and division heads gradually diminished the number of volunteers receiving referrals. In this process, the proportion of hospital patients on the services of full-time members increased by 1987 to 64%.

The Association discussed the matter of the clinical teaching in the affiliated hospitals and

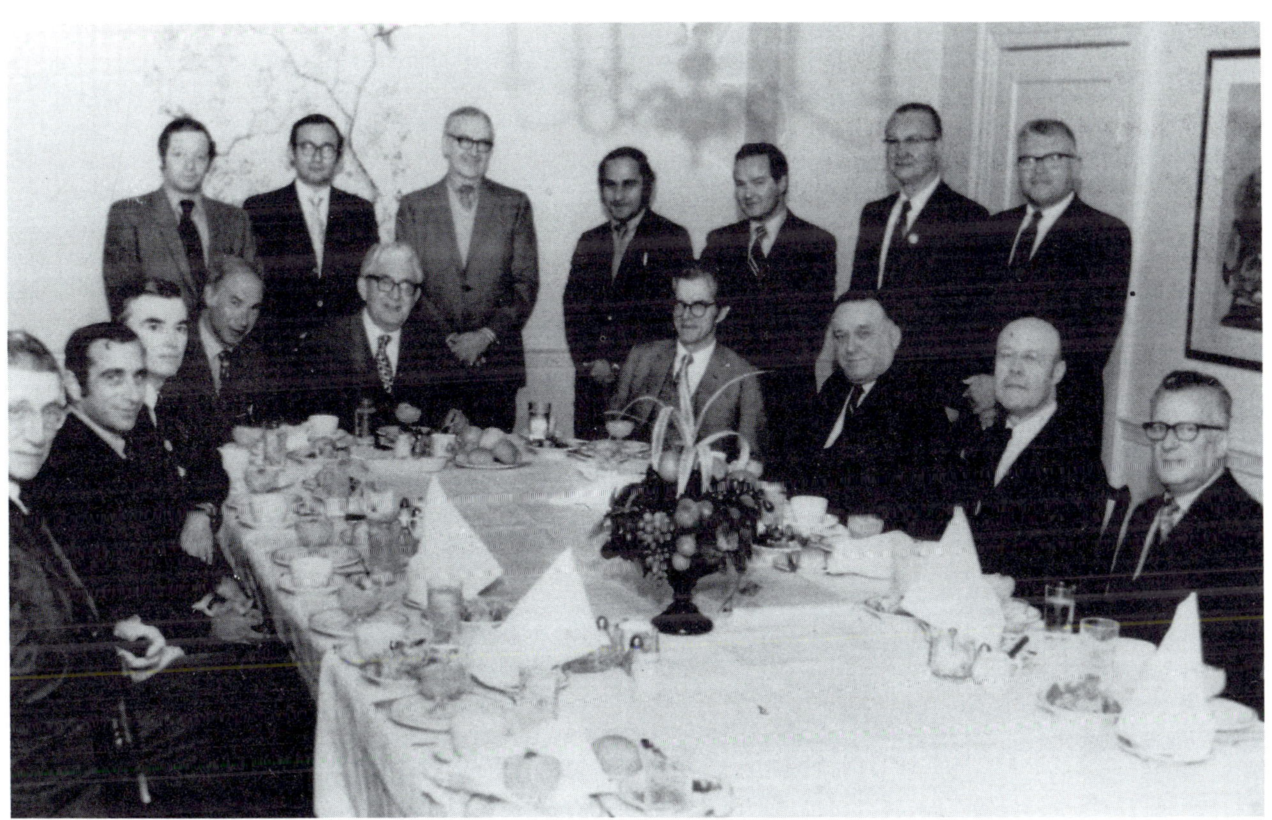

FIG. 55-1. The Board of Governors of the Volunteer Faculty Association (1971). Seated, left to right: Drs. Benjamin Haskell, Leopold Loewenberg, John Templeton, Gerald Marks, Abraham Rakoff, William Baltzell, John Reddy, George Strong, and Joseph Medoff. Standing, left to right: Drs. Kalman Faber, Philip Bralow, Paul Poinsard, Norman Schatz, Joseph Rogers, Frederick Wagner, and Jules Bogaev.

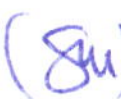

some effort was made to include in the Association those appointed to the affiliated volunteer staff. This proved impractical in view of the distances involved. During the late 1970s and the 1980s the Association also examined nursing care of hospital patients as well as the ancillary services for patients. A general meeting was addressed by Dr. Laura Merker, Associate Hospital Director for Nursing Services, on November 8, 1979, and these concerns were discussed. This type of interaction was useful in promoting understanding between the Association and the power structures to the benefit of the Medical School and the University.

The Association has continued its functions but changes in recent years have resulted in a leveling off of the problems originally faced. A number of earlier members have joined the full-time staff, and the volunteers generally have organized into groups. Hospital practice in the foreseeable future will no doubt be further influenced by collective organizations such as Health Maintenance Organizations. Increasing reliance on affiliated hospitals for the teaching of primary care medicine will no doubt influence the need for voluntary teaching for some time to come. The teaching of outpatient medicine, recently of increasing importance, will probably also depend upon community hospitals and practices, a trend that has escalated with the advent of Family Medicine as a Clinical Department.

Despite the changes and uncertainties, the Volunteer Faculty Association continues to fulfill its mission of achieving harmony in its integral role in the welfare of the College and Hospital.

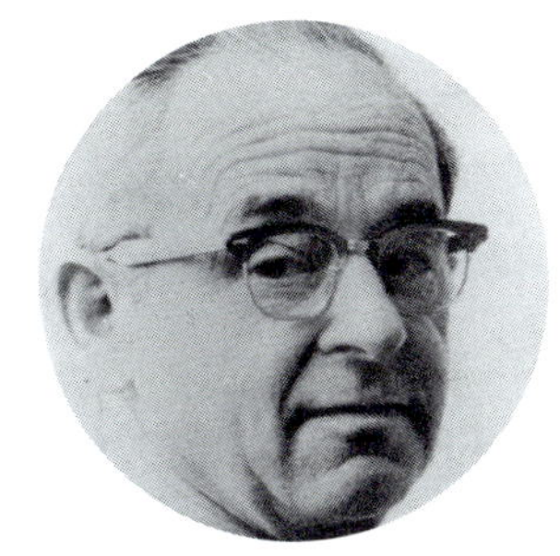

CHAPTER FIFTY-SIX

The Samuel Parsons Scott Memorial Library

Robert T. Lentz, M.S., Sc.D. (Hon.)

"Libraries are successively the cradles and the sepulchres of the human mind."

—Santiago Ramon y Cajal (1852–1934)

As one cannot judge a book by its cover and one cannot judge an institution by its early efforts alone, so one should not judge the Samuel Parsons Scott Memorial Library by its humble beginnings. Although there were certainly collections of books in the various Professors' offices and suites, there is no record of a central library for students' use before 1894.

Early in the fall of 1894 the rooms on the second floor of a building at the southeast corner of Tenth and Walnut Streets were rented by the recently organized Jefferson YMCA. Certain rooms were designated as student reading rooms and were comfortably furnished with reading tables, chairs, and bookcases. The tables, according to an item in the *Jeffersonian*, "were constantly covered with the best magazines, newspapers, medical journals and other current literature. A large bookcase was filled with a medical reference library. The annual expense of maintaining these rooms was nearly $800.00."[1]

During 1895 the Ladies Auxiliary of Jefferson Medical College was organized. This auxiliary, composed of wives and daughters of trustees and faculty members and friends of the college occasionally gave teas and receptions to the students. In the fall of 1895 the reading rooms and library were turned over to the management of the Ladies Auxiliary. The library remained in the YMCA rooms through 1896.

Late in 1896 the Board of Trustees bought the Hamilton and Diesinger Building at the southwest corner of Tenth and Medical Streets to be fitted as the laboratory to the new College building then being planned (Figure 56-1). When the building was readied, the Jefferson Student's Reading Rooms were moved into this laboratory building. As the *Jeffersonian* reported this move:

> "The library now comprises 700 volumes of standard medical books, which are accessible to students without expense, as the librarian is provided by the managers. The rooms provide a place in which the meetings of the various students' societies are held in the evenings, while in the daytime they are used as reading and study rooms. The recreation room is now used as a poolroom, a small charge being made to assist in defraying the expenses of a janitor and repairs to

the tables. The Bureau of Information investigates boarding houses, and endeavors to provide newly arriving students with suitable places. Receptions are held three or four times during the college sessions."[2]

When the College building on the northwest corner of Tenth and Walnut Streets was opened in 1899, the Auxiliary (which had become the Board of Managers) was fortunate to have increased space and much finer facilities (Figure 56-2). They now were able to hold additional teas and receptions and to sponsor theatre parties. The students had more opportunities to meet members of the faculty and trustees as well as their wives and friends. The Board of Managers was able to raise more funds for the purchase of books and other materials.

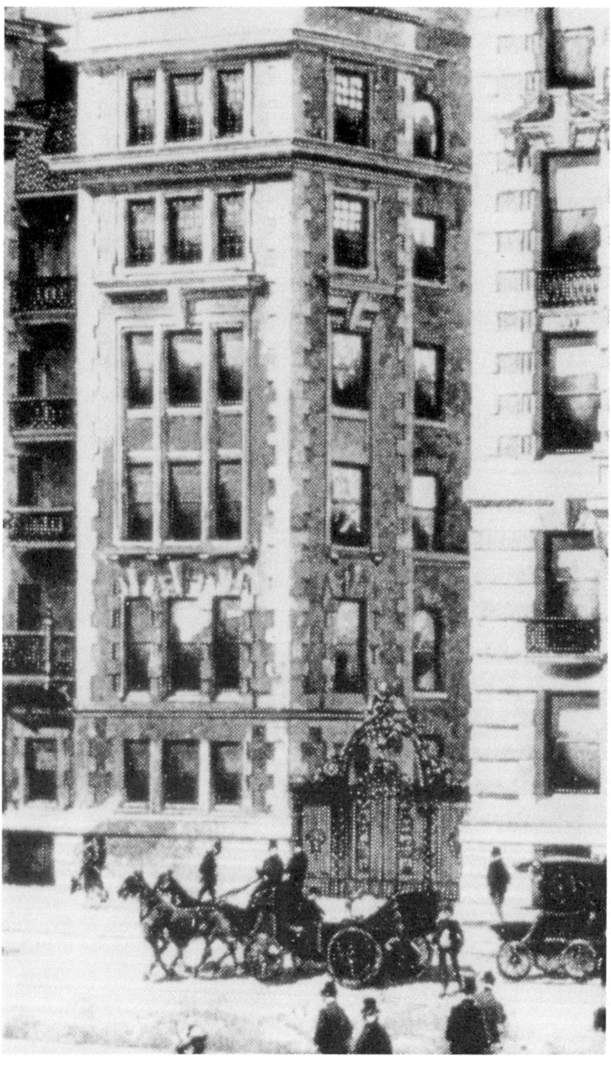

FIG. 56-1. Home of the library (1896–1898). The Hamilton and Diesinger Building was on Tenth Street between Sansom and Walnut. In this photograph, the 1907 Main Hospital is on the right, and the 1898 College Building is on the left.

During this time Thomas Seiple as a volunteer had cataloged the books in the Dewey decimal classification system. Another part-time volunteer, a Mr. Hunter, was listed as Librarian for some time up to October 1900. The women, however, were now in a position to employ a full-time librarian, and in November, 1900, W.L. Wolfinger was appointed Librarian, a post he occupied through June, 1901.

Within these few years the library boasted over 3,000 volumes. A few of these had been acquired by purchase, but a glance through the first accession book shows most had been donated. The list of donors is of interest in showing that many books had come from Dean James W. Holland and Doctors Hobart A. Hare, Henry C. Chapman, Henry W. Stellwagon, William W. Keen, George M. Gould, Nicholas Senn, and William H. Green. From the founding of the library the Philadelphia medical publishers contributed new publications; the W.B. Saunders Company and the J.B. Lippincott Company have continued this practice to the present time.

In October, 1902, Mr. Charles E. Janvrin was appointed Librarian, a position he held until June, 1907. By 1903 the Board of Managers had discontinued its responsibilities for the pool room and smoking room to devote its time and funds for the management of the Reading Rooms alone. Its efforts were apparently appreciated, for the early reports show that about 100 books were consulted every day. The students of that time applied for library cards and on the presentation of their cards could procure books from the locked cages for use in the reading room. The college catalog of 1904 noted that "not being a circulating library a deposit is required when books are taken out for overnight."[3] Longer loans were not permitted. The deposit requirement stayed in force until the early 1930s. The overnight limit continued until the late 1940s.

In May, 1906, the Board of Trustees assumed direction of the library as a college activity and hence accepted all responsibility for its maintenance and regulation. At that time the collection numbered about 4,000 volumes of textbooks, monographs, reference works, and bound journals. Over 50 of the leading medical journals of this country and Europe were being received regularly.

At the October meeting of the faculty it was voted that the librarian be paid $900 per year and that his position be put under the charge of the Dean. At the same time a Library Committee was appointed to comprise Professors Edward P. Davis, Chairman, John C. DaCosta, and George McClellan (grandson of the founder). The Board also appropriated $300 per year for the purchase of books and journals.

Charles Janvrin resigned his post as of June, 1907. It was the custom for the library to be closed for the summer. This custom continued until some time in the 1920s when it was decided to have the library closed for only one month for the librarian's vacation. It was not until the time of World War II that the library was opened the year around.

Charles L. Frankenberger, B.A.; Librarian (1907–1917)

During the summer of 1907 Charles L. Frankenberger was persuaded to leave his position as Assistant Librarian at the College of Physicians of Philadelphia (Figure 56-3). As of September 1, he was appointed Librarian at Jefferson with a salary of $900 a year. Frankenberger was born at Newport, Kentucky, on February 1, 1884, but at an early age he moved with his family to Philadelphia. He was educated at Boys High School, Pierce Business College, and Temple University. Deciding on a career as a librarian, he secured a position at the College of Physicians of Philadelphia and was trained under the direction of Charles Perry Fisher, who was probably the country's leading medical librarian of his day.

Frankenberger provided Jefferson with a decade of significant professional library service. Starting with a collection of somewhat over 4,000 volumes, he set out to increase the holdings and to improve services for the library's users. In 1909 the use of the library was extended to alumni of the college who resided in the Philadelphia area. The library report of 1909–1910 noted that "quite a number of alumni had availed themselves of the privilege."

Through purchase and donations the book stock continued to grow. At the May, 1910, meeting of the faculty it was voted that the faculty

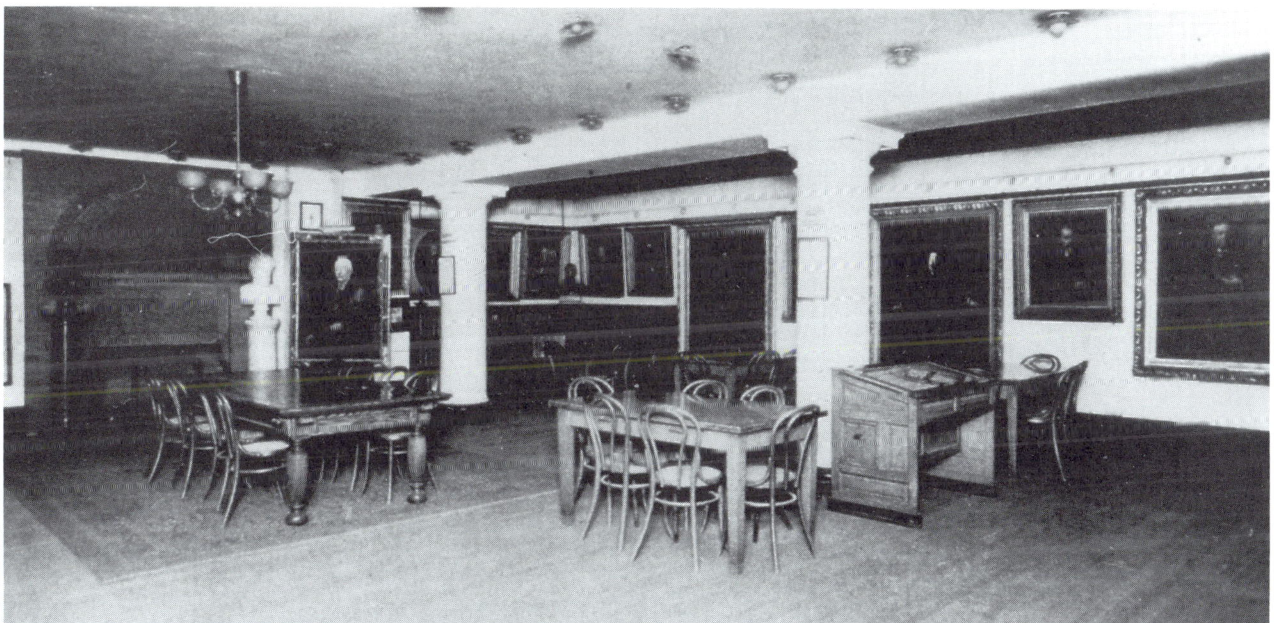

FIG. 56-2. The Reading Room in the Medical College (1898–1929).

recommend to the College Committee of the Board of Trustees, "that book cases be erected in Professor James C. Wilson's private rooms for the accommodation of books for which there is not space in the present library quarters."

Frankenberger's efforts did not go unnoticed. Abraham Flexner, who made a survey of all North American medical schools, noted in his book, *Medical Education in the United States and Canada. A report to the Carnegie Foundation for the Advancement of Teaching* (1910), "Once more it is pleasant to record exceptions: a good library, excellently administered, is to be found at Jefferson, Buffalo, and at Galveston."[4] At the November, 1911, meeting of the faculty it was "Resolved, that in view of the efficient services rendered by the present librarian, his salary be raised to $1,000.00 per year."

An announcement of the College in 1912–1914, stated:

> "The library contains over fifty-three hundred volumes of the more important medical text-books and works of reference. The reading room is supplied with sixty-five of the leading medical periodicals of this country and Europe. . . . The library is maintained without charge to the students, and is open on weekdays 9:00 A.M. to 5:30 P.M. and on Saturdays from 9:00 A.M. to 12:00 P.M. The Librarian, Mr. Charles Frankenberger, is constantly in attendance to aid workers in their investigations. The rules permit the removal of books over night."[5]

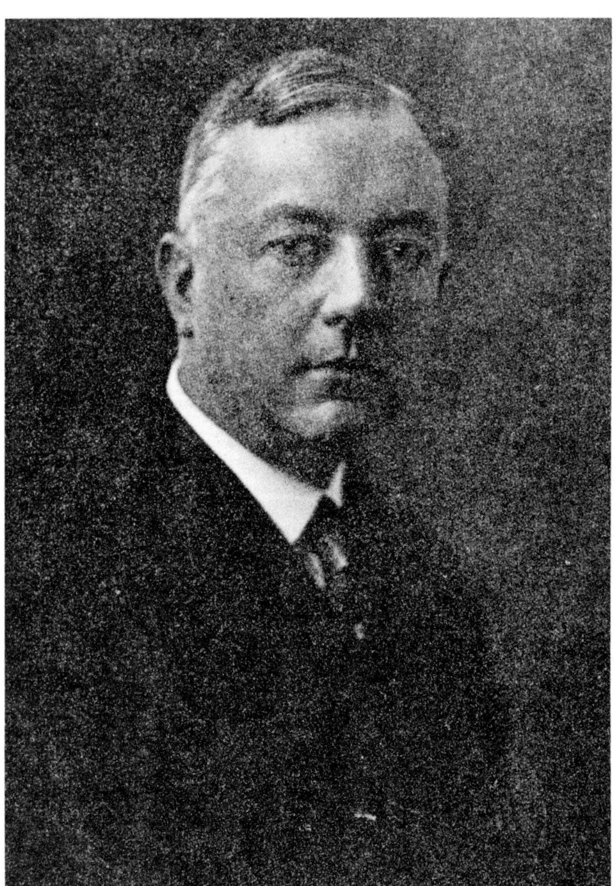

FIG. 56-3. Charles L. Frankenberger, B.A.; Librarian (1907–1917).

During 1916 Frankenberger was persuaded to assume the responsibilities as manager of the college bookstore. Before this time the various publishers of medical books had student representatives who sold the books of the individual publishers. It was not a satisfactory arrangement, and the Dean consolidated the activity in the library. This policy was continued until 1968, when the bookstore was moved to Jefferson's Alumni Hall under the University's Auxiliary Services.

Frankenberger served as Librarian until August 11, 1917, when he resigned to become the Librarian at the Medical Society of the County of Kings at Brooklyn and Consulting Librarian and Lecturer at the Long Island College of Medicine, now the State University of New York, Downstate Medical Center. He was an active member of the Medical Library Association, participating in several annual meeting programs and holding numerous committee appointments. He served as President of the association in 1934–1935. In 1943, when the Library of the Surgeon General's Office, U.S. Army, was reconstituted as the Army Medical Library, Frankenberger was appointed as a member of the Association of Honorary Consultants to the Army Medical Library. He served with this group until the time of his death. In 1946 he retired from the post of Librarian in Brooklyn because of ill health and was elected Consulting Librarian at the Library of the County of Kings Medical Society. He retained this position until his death, which occurred at his home in Brooklyn on September 16, 1951. He had married Hester Hillsley in 1915, while still at Jefferson, and she was his sole survivor.

A resolution of the Association of Honorary Consultants to the Army Medical Library referred to Charles Frankenberger as "a modest, kindly and helpful man and a true and loyal friend. He was a generous contributor to the Association, a wise counsellor, and one who held the respect of all who knew him."[6]

The Wilson Era (1917–1949)

Joseph J. Wilson was selected as the new Librarian as of September, 1917 (Figure 56-4). He was born in Philadelphia on June 21, 1879, the son of John Harrison and Sarah (Prutzman) Wilson. In 1896 he was graduated from the Central High School and later that year was employed by the Free Library of Philadelphia. The library's training courses had not yet been established, so he received his training "on the job" in the cataloging, binding, and shipping departments. For a number of years he was assigned to the Port Richmond and Widener branches of the Free Library system. With his appointment at Jefferson he continued as part-time head of the overdue book department of the Free Library until 1940.

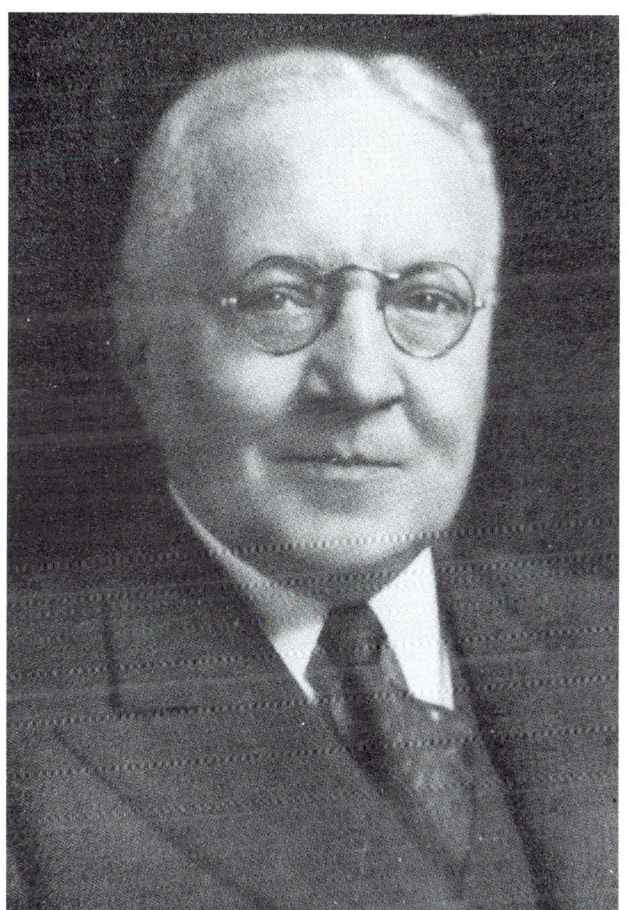

FIG. 56-4. Joseph J. Wilson; Librarian (1917-1949).

The annual salary of the librarian continued at $1,000. The salary beginning with Wilson's employment was supplemented with 50% of the income from the sale of books to students. It remained the custom to continue to close the library for the month of August, during which time Wilson regularly went to Maine to fish in his favorite lakes.

During Frankenberger's and Wilson's tenures, and even until 1960, the library maintained information about living accommodations for students in Center City Philadelphia. This was a service for students carried over from the Board of Managers and the YMCA Reading Rooms. The service was taken over with the beginning of a Student Council in the 1960s and then later by the University Housing Department. The recreation tradition continued in an unofficial way while Wilson managed several student athletic teams through the 1920s.

The library holdings in 1917 were 6,471 volumes of texts, monographs, reference works, and bound volumes of journals. The library was then receiving 61 journals. Many of these were state medical society publications that were received gratis because the college regularly placed advertisements in them. The library by modest purchases but with generous contributions from several sources continued to expand its working collection. Shortly after his appointment, Wilson arranged with Professor Albert P. Brubaker to store some of the older and less used material in the physiology department laboratory conveniently located near the Reading Room. This material, of course, remained there until the next new building was opened in 1929. Empty shelves resulting from this move were not bare for very long. Wilson witnessed the receipt of several sizable donations of the private libraries of active faculty members. Doctor Hobart Amory Hare's extensive library of therapeutics and clinical medicine literature broadened the library's holdings in these fields. Dr. Albert P. Brubaker on his retirement presented to the library a noteworthy collection on physiology, toxicology, and preventive medicine. From Professor William M. Late Coplin the college received a useful collection of books, pamphlets, and journals on pathology and general medicine. Throughout the 1920s and 1930s Doctor Pascal Brooke Bland made important donations of both current and rare historical books pertaining mostly to obstetrics and gynecology but also to the general study of medicine.

These and many other gifts of lesser amount but equal value soon caused Wilson to seek additional storage space. A room in the basement directly under the library was cleared to permit erection of shelves by the College carpenter. Again there was breathing room, but serious attention had to be given to the nagging problem of space.

Fortunately not only the library but other departments of the college were likewise cramped. Plans for a new building began to be discussed by the faculty, the administration, and the Board of Trustees. Wilson sought the assistance of his friend, Franklin Price, the Librarian of the Free Library of Philadelphia and of the consulting architect of the Board of Trustees. Together they drew up plans for a library to house a collection of 50,000 volumes. Twelve thousand volumes were to be housed in the reading room on the first floor of the new building, and 38,000 volumes in stacks in the basement directly beneath.

Samuel Parsons Scott and His Will

While the new library was under construction surprising news of a major bequest was announced. Word came to the Board of Trustees and to the Dean of the Medical School that an unknown (to Jefferson) lawyer from Hillsboro, Ohio, had died and that his will bequeathed an 8,000-volume library and the bulk of his estate to Jefferson for the establishment and maintenance of a library.

Samuel Parsons Scott (Figure 56-5) was born at Hillsboro, Highland County, Ohio, on July 8, 1846, the son of William and Elizabeth Jane (Parsons) Scott.[7] He was educated at Miami (Ohio) University, receiving the A.B. degree in 1866. At the age of 20, Mr. Scott was the valedictorian, although he was the youngest member of his class.

For one year Scott engaged in the private study of law, and in 1868 he was admitted to the Ohio bar. Then for seven years he practiced law at Leavenworth, Kansas, and at San Francisco.

During 1875 Scott retired from his law practice to return to Hillsboro. The failing health of his father and the urgent need of attention to the family business interests brought about the end of his practice. From this time on Scott's chief personal interests were in study, travel, and writing. In these endeavors he developed a major and abiding interest in Spain, and his first published work, *Through Spain,* appeared in 1886.

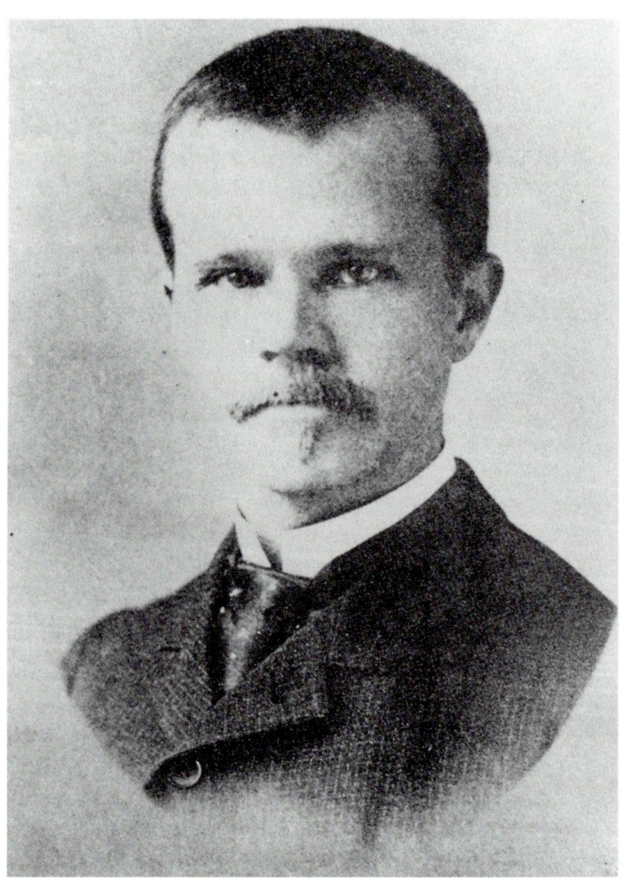

FIG. 56-5. Samuel Parsons Scott, Esq. (1846–1929), lawyer, scholar, author, and benefactor.

Though Scott had given up his law practice, he continued a strong interest in the legal profession. He was one of the founders of the Comparative Law Bureau of the American Bar Association and remained an active member of this bureau for the rest of his life. On October 10, 1895, at age 49, he married Elizabeth Woodbridge Smart of Paint Township, Ohio.

Scott's first book, *Through Spain,* laid the ground for his best-known work, *The History of the Moorish Empire in Europe,* which was published by J.B. Lippincott in 1904. This in turn led to *The Visigothic Code.* This latter book was a translation with annotations of the *Forum Judicum (Fuero Juzgo),* which was published through the Comparative Law Bureau and was the first of a series of translations by him of Spanish legal collections. Another was his translation of *Corpus Juris Civilis,* which was then the only complete translation into English. His *Las Siete Partidas,* first translated in 1912, was reprinted in a new edition shortly after his death in 1929.

Besides membership in the American Bar Association, Scott was also a member of the American Society of International Law. Among his foreign affiliations, Scott held membership in the Academie Latin des Sciences, Arts et Belles Lettres; Société Academique d'Histoire Internationale; and Société de la Renaissance Nationale, all of Paris. He was a Life Fellow of the Royal Meteorological Society of London.

Scott has been likened to the late Henry Charles Lea of Philadelphia. Both spent their retirement leisure in study and writing. It is a curious fact that both chose Spain as their chief theme, and both wrote on the same specific subject, the Moors of Spain. Scott died May 30, 1929, at age 83. His widow was his sole survivor.

In making his will, Scott bequeathed $75,000 to his widow and then wrote:

> "I do give, bequeath, and devise all the rest and residue of my estate, real and personal, of every description whatsoever, to the Board of Trustees, of Jefferson Medical College of Philadelphia, Pennsylvania, to be used for the foundation and maintenance of a library for the use of the teachers and students of said institution, and of which my entire collection of books is to form a nucleus; and the said Board of Trustees are hereby empowered to sell, to the best advantage, such of the property of my Estate as may come into their hands, which it may seem advisable to them to dispose of for that purpose. I make this bequest in grateful acknowledgement of the inestimable service rendered me by one of the Professors of said Institution, in relieving me of hay-fever, thereby prolonging my life in comparative comfort for many years."

Scott's will explained his bequest to his wife with this terse sentence: "I leave to my said wife no more than the sum above mentioned, because on account of the insults, outrages, cruelty, disgrace and humiliation which she has constantly, and without reason, during all of my entire married life, heaped upon me, she is wholly undeserving of my generosity."

The Scotts lived in a stately three-story house on the crest of a low hill at the north edge of Hillsboro, a pleasant rural county seat in south-central Ohio (Figure 56-6). The east side of the house was probably the location of Scott's library, where he also probably secluded himself, spending much of his time reading and writing. He also maintained a small office building behind the county court house, two blocks to the east of his home. This was undoubtedly a handy retreat when he required complete solitude. It is doubted that he ever spent much time in conversation or idle gossip with his fellow townspeople.

Scott's widow contested the will and after extended negotiations the legal authorities representing her and the Jefferson Board of Trustees agreed to a settlement awarding her 55% of the estate and Jefferson 45%. The estate consisted of some 20 farms and other properties in Highland County and its surrounding counties in Ohio. Most of the properties were held in the estate until Mrs. Scott's death, which occurred February 8, 1946. Jefferson's share of the estate as eventually settled was about $1,250,000. These funds have been kept intact as an endowment whose interest monies have been used for library expenses, and in the 1960s, when matching funds were needed to secure a grant for a new library building, such funds were at hand in this account.

To complete the story of the Scotts, Scott's denunciation of his wife was countered by an epitaph on the Scott family monument (Figure 56-7), which reads, "Elizabeth Woodbridge Scott, born Chillicothe, Ohio, died February 8, 1946. Loved, admired and most highly regarded by all who knew her."

The 1929 Library

Construction of the new library was completed just in time. The Scott Collection arrived in September, 1929. The books were placed on shelves in the back of the ground-floor stack-room where they remained until 1950.

The new library was opened for service on October 10, 1929 (Figure 56-8). It occupied the entire east end of the first floor of the College building. The terrazzo floor was sunken three feet below the regular floor level. The interior decorations were of Florentine design, with a color blend that was harmoniously pleasing. The room was furnished with specially designed reading tables and chairs of old English walnut. The book stacks around the entire room and the library's charging desk were of oak construction. The table lamps were of special design to conform to the proper height and angle of reflection. The posts of the lamps were monogramed with JMC as part of their design.

When the stacks were filled with multicolored books, the reading room with its colorful ceiling and overhanging beams presented an awesome and pleasant view that never failed to inspire praise from both readers and visitors.

The somewhat smaller stack area on the ground floor directly beneath the reading room contained a room for bookstore stock and for library supplies. Beyond the stockroom were four locked cases for the storage of rare books and archival materials. The remaining space contained steel storage stacks for about 38,000 volumes.

The appearance of partially filled shelves in the attractive new reading room created new interest

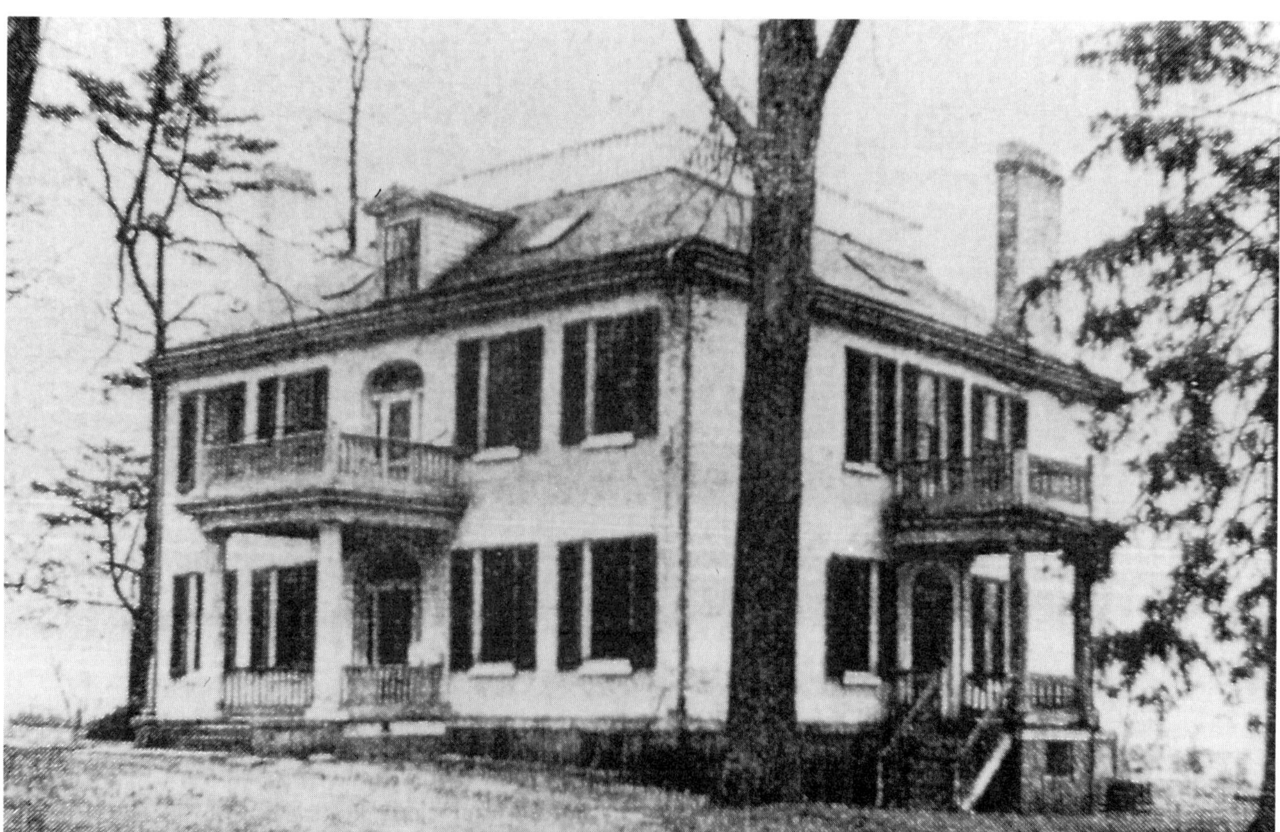

FIG. 56-6. The family home of Samuel P. Scott, Esq., Hillsboro, Ohio.

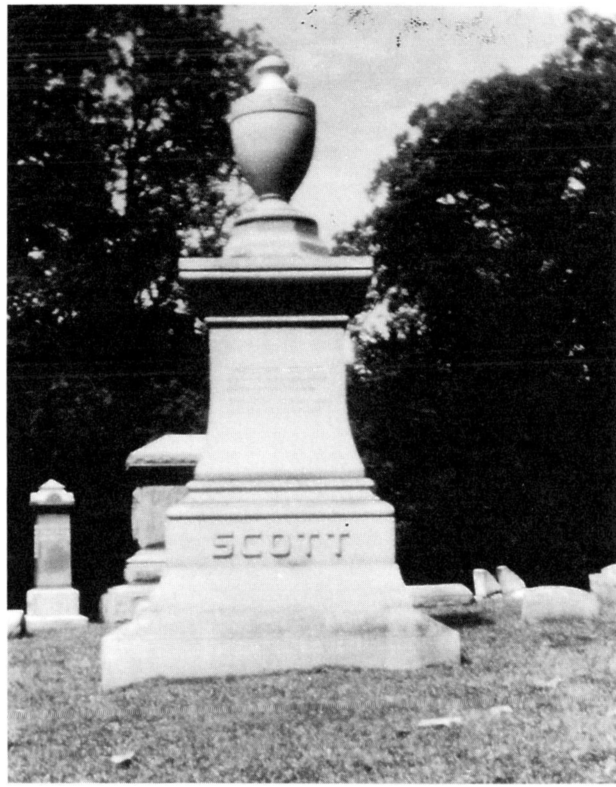

FIG. 56-7. The Scott family monument, Hillsboro (Ohio) Cemetery; site of the graves of Samuel P. Scott, Esq., and Elizabeth W. Scott.

among the faculty and graduates of the school. The shelves began to fill rapidly despite the fact that the library budget for 1930–1931 was still $300 for all expenses beyond the librarian's salary. The first budget change was an increase for the salary of an Assistant Librarian. Eight hundred dollars was appropriated for this position for the session of 1931–1932

On September 17, 1931, Robert T. Lentz, a recent graduate of Banks Business College, was employed as Assistant Librarian. The salary was set at $18 per 45-hour week. It was reasonable pay during the Great Depression, except that it would be seven long years before it would be increased. It may be of interest to note that there were no academically trained librarians at any of the Philadelphia medical schools until well into the 1940s.

With the appointment of an assistant it became possible to keep the library open over the lunch hour, so library hours were 8:45 A.M. to 5:30 P.M. Monday to Friday and from 8:45 A.M. to 1 P.M. on Saturday. Library regulations permitted faculty members to borrow books and journals for an indefinite period, to be recalled when another reader requested the same material. Students were permitted to borrow books and journals for overnight and weekend use after 3 P.M. on

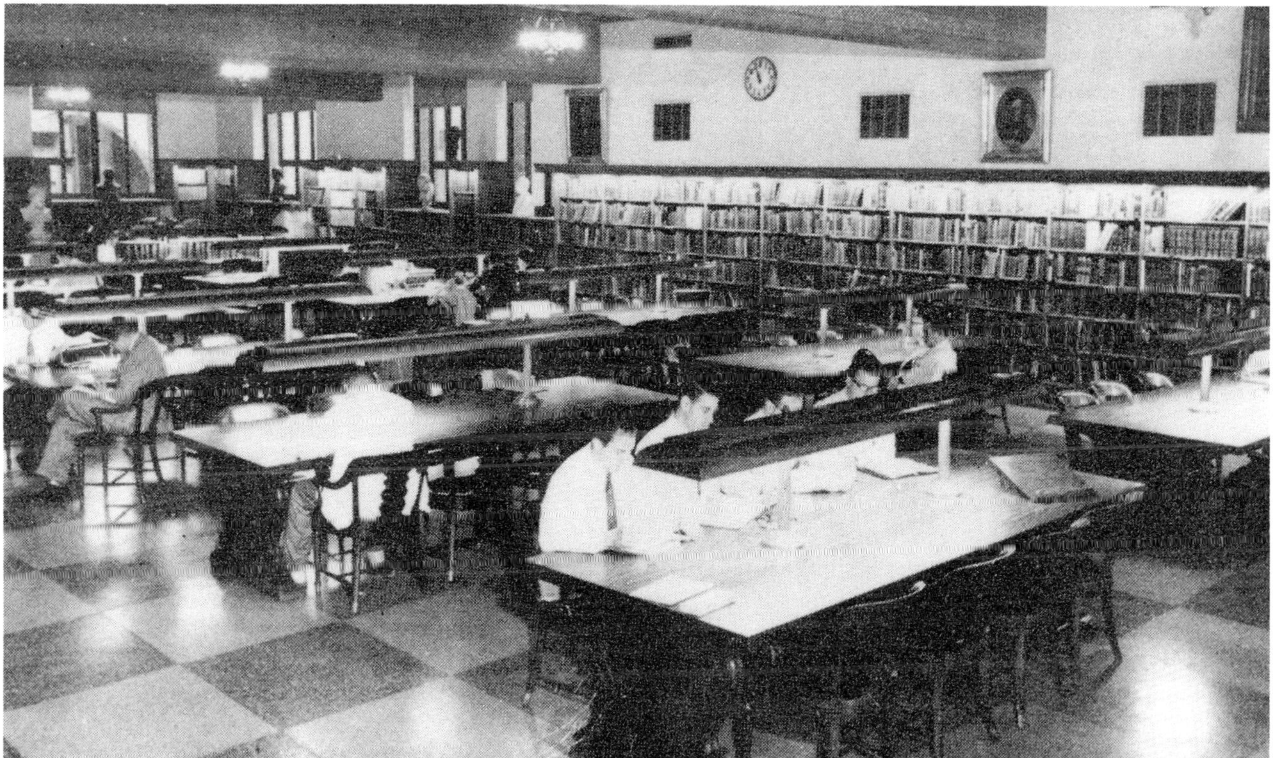
FIG. 56-8. The Reading Room in the Medical College (1929–1970).

weekdays and after noon on Saturdays. The current issue of each journal title did not circulate until the next issue was received. A deposit of $1 was required of students, and material was due back by 9 A.M. the following library day. A 10¢ fine was charged for overdue material.

The book collection was still organized by the Dewey decimal classification, book numbers being marked on labels inside the front cover. No markings were made on the spines or front covers of books. The books, of course, were more attractive on the shelves, but unfortunately it was much more difficult to keep them in order on the shelves and to find a particular book when needed.

A unique arrangement was the housing of unbound journals in about 180 small boxes with front doors located on the north end of the west wall of the reading room (Figure 56-9). It was a tidy arrangement but was somewhat of a nuisance in placing each day's receipt of journals. The major problem was that it could not be expanded, and the number of cubbyholes soon became insufficient for an expanding collection. Otherwise, throughout the 1930s there was adequate space for readers and for expansion of the library collection.

On November 16, 1931, the Board of Trustees passed a resolution designating the medical school library as the Samuel Parsons Scott Memorial Library and directed the Dean to indicate this fact by the erection of an appropriate tablet. In 1934 an oak panel with the inscription "Samuel Parsons Scott Memorial Library" was erected over the doors to the reading room.

Beginning in November, 1938, the library instituted evening hours in response to requests from students and faculty members. The library was opened on Tuesday and Thursday evenings from 7 to 10 P.M. The response by students was enough to ensure keeping the library open on this schedule during the college sessions. The next change in hours was not until 1949, when the hours became from 8:45 A.M. to 9 P.M. Monday to Friday and 8:45 A.M. to 5 P.M. on Saturday.

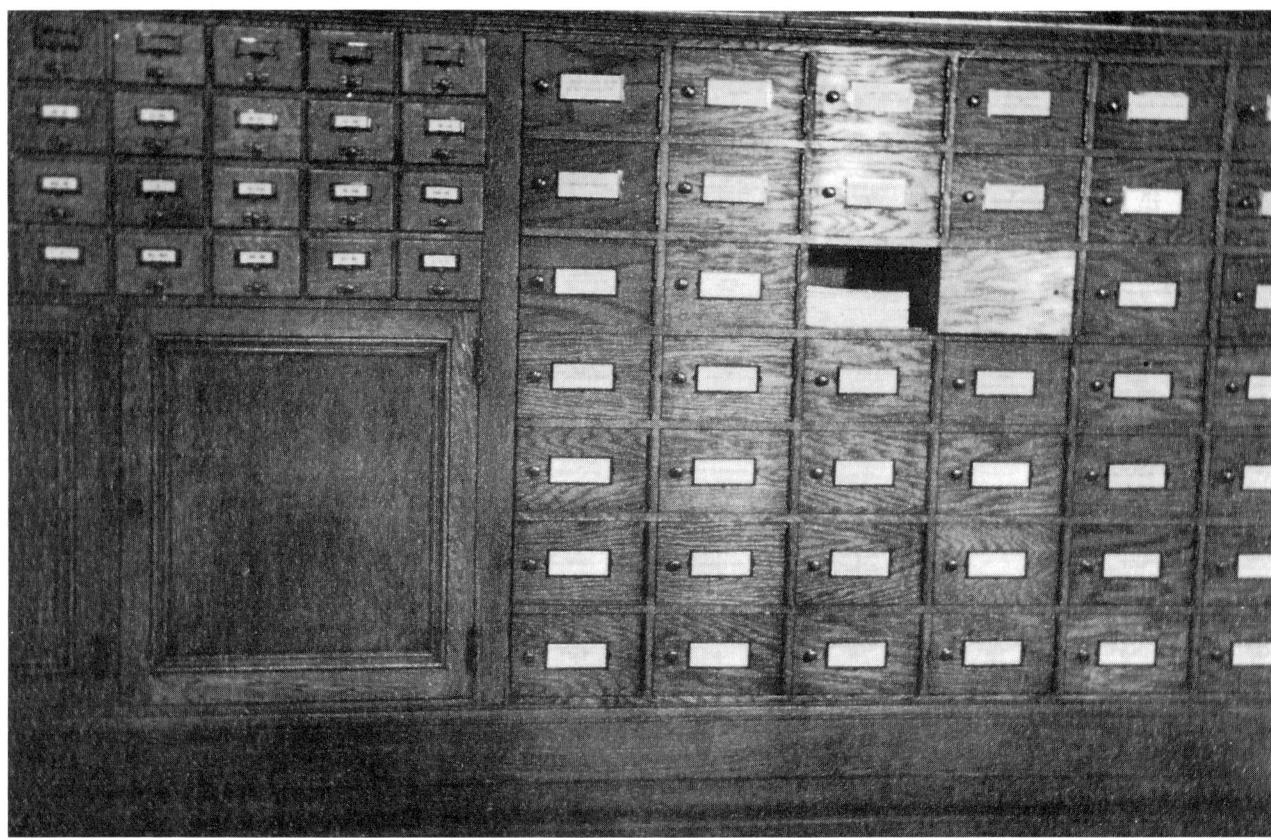

FIG. 56-9. A section of the card catalog and cubbyholes for periodicals in the 1929–1970 Reading Room.

The 1940s

A major collection of rare books came to the library following the 1940 death of Pascal Brooke Bland, Emeritus Professor of Obstetrics. Doctor Bland had been a good friend of the library. Through the 1930s he had been Chairman of the Faculty's Library Committee. His contributions of rare volumes and books of historic interest had been significant, but in January 1941 the receipt of 2,848 volumes gave the Scott Library a special collection to be envied by most of the medical schools of the country.[8]

Until the 1940s the library staff had been small and stable but this was shortly to change. In November, 1939, George McNabb was employed as a clerical assistant. He remained until 1942, when he resigned and was replaced by Walter Sczcepaniak. In January 1943, Robert Lentz was drafted for Army service. Marjorie K. Lentz, a graduate of Montclair (New Jersey) State College and a recent graduate of Emory University Library School, was employed as the Assistant Librarian. Shortly thereafter Walter Sczcepaniak was drafted, to be replaced by his sister Julia. The staff of Wilson, Marjorie Lentz, and Judy (as Julia was generally known) carried on during the remainder of the war period.

In 1942 the Library Committee decided to keep the library open throughout the summer because of the wartime accelerated curriculum. As of January 2, 1946, Robert Lentz, having survived the war in Europe, was reappointed Assistant Librarian. Majorie Lentz was designated as Reference Librarian and remained on the staff until she resigned in September, 1947.

The library budget for all purposes other than salaries was set at $300 in 1911 and was unchanged at least through the session of 1931–1932. That budget showed $300 for supplies and $1,800 for salaries. Subsequent budgets are not available, though annual budgets were presented to the Board of Trustees by the Dean; they must have been working instruments in the Dean's offices but did not appear in the minutes of the Board of Trustees or of the faculty.

During the 1930s and most of the 1940s, book and journal acquisitions followed an informal pattern. On learning of new books or journals that appeared important for the collection, or on receipt of requests from faculty members, Wilson forwarded requests to the Dean for his approval. There is no documentation of costs or that any requests were denied. From time to time requests were also presented through the Library Committee Chairman. These requests, too, were routinely approved at meetings of the faculty.

The first extant record of an increased budgeted amount for books, journals, and supplies was for the year 1947–1948, when $2,000 was approved. During 1947 George M. Ritchie was appointed Controller for the College, and he established the first Office of the Controller. Budgeting from that time on became carefully regulated. The budget for 1948–1949 was $7,060 for salaries and $2,000 for books, journals, and supplies, a total of $9,060.

After 32 years as Librarian, Joseph J. Wilson retired on June 30, 1949. He had built up the collection from about 7,000 volumes and 55 journal subscriptions to 27,351 volumes and 300 journal subscriptions. He had planned and moved into a new and attractive library. Throughout that time he had earned and retained the friendship and respect of thousands of students, faculty members, and alumni.

Joseph Wilson spent his retirement visiting his family, enjoying his flower garden, and continuing his annual Maine fishing trips. On March 21, 1957, while visiting his son Norman in Louisville, he was stricken and passed away suddenly. He was survived by his sons Joseph Herbert and Norman Miles.

Robert T. Lentz, M.S., Sc.D.; Librarian (1949–1969); First University Librarian (1969–1975)

As of July, 1949, Robert T. Lentz, longtime Assistant Librarian, was appointed as Joseph Wilson's successor (Figure 56-10).

The 1950s

Facing the 1950s it was evident that drastic steps were needed to meet the problems of vanishing shelf space. To further complicate the situation, it was obvious that the collection needed to be expanded. To begin, a program of weeding out older, antiquated, and nonused books was instituted, following standard library procedures and criteria. In addition, many of the books were shifted from the reading room to the ground-floor stack room to make space for more bound journals on the first floor. With this shift the lower-floor stacks were opened to readers for the first time.

In October, 1949, Adeline Redheffer, a graduate of the Drexel Institute School of Library Science, was employed as Assistant Librarian. An intelligent, well-trained, and experienced librarian, Redheffer made a considerable contribution in solving the immediate growing problems and in developing sound professional library procedures and library operations. Ninety-two new journal subscriptions were entered within the first year, and a program was begun to mark call numbers on the spines or front covers of all cataloged books.

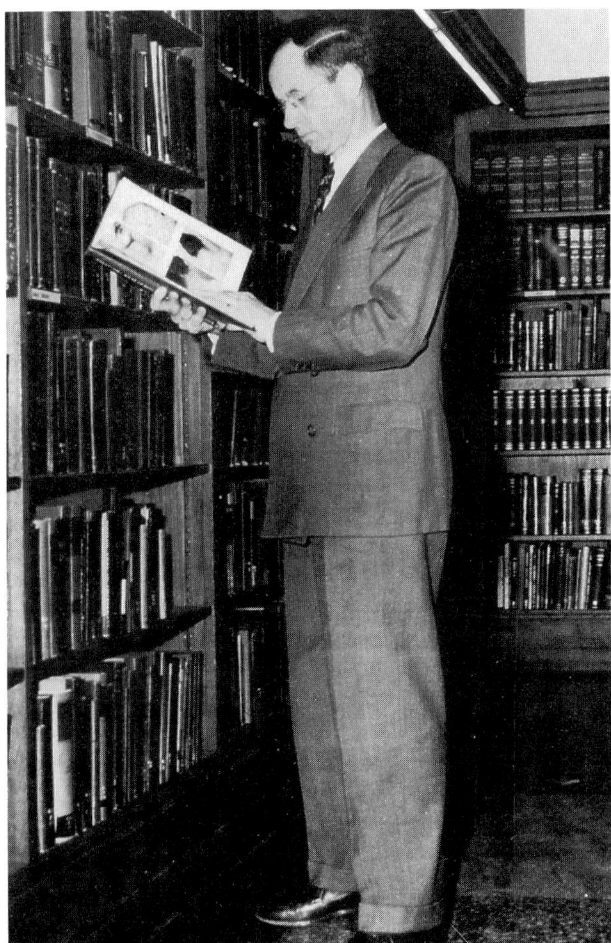

FIG. 56-10. Robert T. Lentz, B.S., M.S., Sc.D., Librarian (1949–1975).

The bookstore, which had been operated at the library's charging desk, was moved to the ground-floor stack-room, separating the commercial enterprise from the library circulation procedure.

A program of instruction to first-year medical students was instituted in January, 1951. A one-hour lecture concerning library facilities and procedures and explanations of the most generally used medical bibliographic tools was followed by two hours of demonstration and practical experience. The program was not enthusiastically welcomed by the students but increased use of the library and especially increased use of the bibliographic resources did result.

With expanded library hours begun in November, 1949, a growing collection, and increased library use, it was inevitable that the library staff of four needed to be enlarged. Over the early years of the decade of the 1950s additional assistants were employed. Alice Bruce, the first bookstore assistant, served briefly and was followed by Carmello Sarro, who continued in that capacity until the bookstore was separated from the library. Katharine Veigel was the first cataloging assistant. She was a graduate of the Drexel Institute School of Library Science who came to Jefferson from the University of Pennsylvania Library. Faye Kostenbauder Williamson, a graduate of Susquehanna University, became a member of the staff in the capacity of periodicals assistant. Janet Oswald, another Drexel graduate, was the first acquisition assistant.

Throughout this time the greatest problem was that of space. The first relief was provided when in June, 1950, the general library of Samuel Parsons Scott, numbering some 8,000 volumes, was sold to the Kress Foundation for the Bucknell University Library. This freed three complete ranges of stacks.

In the mid-1950s members of the executive faculty were invited to assist members of the library staff in making decisions as to which books should be candidates for the weeding process. Several Professors responded and were very helpful to the staff. This exercise, however, afforded only temporary relief. Plans were then drawn up to clear an area in the subbasement of the college building for the storage of older volumes of journals and of books published before 1920. After partitioning an area and erecting stacks, it was finally ready in mid-1959. Again the stress for space was relieved but not solved.

Beginning in January, 1956, the library loan regulations were relaxed to permit students to borrow books for one week and journals for three library days instead of only overnight. Faculty members had been permitted to borrow material for an indefinite time depending on their need (or perhaps their memory). The new regulation limited the loan period to one week with the privilege of three renewals as long as there were no other requests for the material. Fines were assessed to delinquent faculty members at the same rate as students, 10¢ per day for each item. These policies set by the Library Committee of the Faculty were welcomed by the students and accepted by most faculty members. As with all regulations, there are always some objectors—a few teachers refused to pay fines and were denied further borrowing privileges until they were cleared. Eventually amnesty was declared; strangely, after one episode the objectors again became cooperative library users.

At the end of June, 1958, Adeline Redheffer, Assistant Librarian, resigned to return to her first interest as a school librarian. In September, Samuel A. Davis, a graduate of the Presbyterian College, Clinton, North Carolina, and of Emory University Library School became the new Assistant Librarian with the responsibility for reference services. He had been born and educated in Brazil until his senior year of college. After receiving his library training he served in the library of the Medical College of Virginia and as Librarian at the Albany Medical College.

When in 1959 the fourth-year class of the medical school was put on a 12-month schedule, it was decided to continue the evening hours through the summer. Later, in 1967, the evening hours were extended to midnight.

During August of 1959 the Nursing School library was moved into the Scott Library. Fortunately the collection was small enough to fit into the southwest alcove of the Reading Room. The part-time nursing librarian, Robert Winship, continued to care for the collection until it was integrated into the general collection when University status was granted to Jefferson.

The 1960s

By 1961 space for periodicals, now numbering some 800, was more than critical. To relieve the situation the built-in card catalog and the cubbyholes for unbound journals were dismantled and standard oak library periodical shelving was installed in the northwest area of the Reading Room. A new freestanding card catalog, display racks for the current issues of journals, and desks for reference and interlibrary loan services were crowded into that northwest area.

The entire decade of the 1960s was involved with problems of space and plans for expansion. This was true not only for Jefferson but for all of the Philadelphia medical school libraries. The librarians of all of the local medical schools and the librarian of the College of Physicians of Philadelphia began to meet informally to discuss ways in which cooperation could help relieve the pressures of growing collections in already crowded facilities. Interlibrary loans increased considerably when a delivery service was instituted in the area. The groundwork for cooperation had been well established by this group before the Regional Medical Library Program was instituted through the National Library of Medicine.

Although regional planning was important it was urgent to begin plans for a new library at Jefferson. Early in 1963 the library staff began to develop a building program. The Librarian spoke briefly of these needs at the April, 1964, meeting of the College Committee of the Board of Trustees. As a result it was requested that a definitive program be prepared to be considered by a committee chaired by the College President. The program was completed by early fall and was presented to the President, William Bodine, and the Dean, William A. Sodeman. A committee was formed of President Bodine, Dean Sodeman, Vice President for Planning and Development George M. Norwood, Consultative Architect Roy Larson, and Librarian Lentz.

The Scott Library/Administration Building (1970)

During discussions the Administration and the Board of Trustees decided to build a dual-function structure to house the library and the medical center administration, to be built on the south side of Walnut Street opposite the main College building. The seven-level building was designed so that the library would have some space on the ground-floor level and in the basement. The second, third, and fourth floors were designed totally for library use. The fifth and sixth floors were planned for the use of the institution's administrative departments. It was decided that these upper floors be constructed to bear the weight of library stacks and materials so that when further expansion of the library became necessary, space would be available. Mr. Alfred Brandon, then the Director of the Welch Medical Library, Johns Hopkins University, was retained as library building consultant. The architectural firm of Harbeson, Hough, Livingston, and Larson was engaged because of its wide experience in planning academic libraries.

During 1965 and 1966 building plans were made final at the same time that legislation was being developed in Washington to enact the Medical Library Assistance Act of 1965, which was designed to provide funds for the support of medical library resources and to fund medical library construction. On September 12, 1966, Jefferson filed a grant application with the U.S. Public Health Service for financial support for the construction of the new Samuel Parsons Scott Memorial Library in the amount of $2,567,210 (65% of the proposed cost of construction and equipment). Jefferson's application was the first to be received by the Public Health Services, and Jefferson was selected for the first site visit. It was held on December 6, 1966, and in April, 1967 word was received that the grant had been approved and that the amount would be determined in June. Sometimes the machinery of governments grinds slowly; it was not until February, 1968 that an appropriation was announced. Since funds were not released until November, construction was not finally underway until December of that year.

The library was not completely finished when, during August and early September, 1970, the library collection was moved into its spacious and luxuriant new home. An abundance of 53,000 square feet of space contrasted to the former 9,000 square feet. At the time of moving, the collection comprised just over 68,000 volumes and the library was receiving just over 1,200 journal subscriptions. The 12-member library staff included the librarian, associate librarian, cataloger, assistant cataloger, acquisitions librarian, serials assistant, circulation assistant, interlibrary loan assistant, secretary, acquisitions clerk, xerox operator, and shelf assistant.

By the time of the opening of the session in 1970 the library was basically ready to receive the students (Figure 56-11). The grand staircase was not finished but the central core stairways and the elevators were available. Although the carpets were still being laid, the books and journals were in place. Library services were suspended for only a few days.

In the new facility several new areas and services were provided. Perhaps the most important was a reference area with desks for reference and interlibrary loan activities with special stacks for reference-type publications. Technical services had a large work space for acquisitions, periodicals, and cataloging. The circulation department now had adequate shelving for the reserve collection and a specially designed circulation desk. All of these services were located on the second floor along with the card catalog, recent books, and periodicals of the last ten years (Figure 56-12).

All earlier journals were placed on the third floor. This floor also featured a special collections room, a browsing room for recreational reading, and a conference room. The administrative offices for the library were also here with a bank of audiovisual carrels on the east wall. A cluster of five group-study rooms was located in the northwest corner. All library floors had individual study carrels around three outside walls with reading tables in areas conveniently interspersed between stack areas.

The older books of the general collection were shelved on the fourth floor. This level provided a great deal of reading and study space along with a bank of ten group-study rooms on the north wall. The library had been planned to keep the spaces open and flexible to accommodate added material and new facilities.

Since 1906, when the Board of Trustees assumed the management of the Student Reading Rooms, the library had been under the direction of the Dean of the Medical School. As of July 1, 1970, the library became a University function, the budget a part of the corporate budget, and the Librarian responsible to the President. A new library committee was established with a broad University base. Dr. Robert I. Wise, Magee Professor of Medicine, was appointed as the first chairman of the committee.

The 1970s and Beyond

The decade of the 1970s was a time for settling into the new building and for facing the new demands of the technological age. In 1966 the Librarian had published an article in the *Jefferson Medical College Alumni Bulletin* entitled "Time, Jefferson and the Information Explosion."[9] He discussed at some length the pressing problem of space for library services and also noted that the time had come to consider the technologic changes that would be required to keep the library a front-runner among medical school libraries.

Settling in meant a decided increase in the library's budget. For 1969–1970 the budget was set at $149,000. The budget for 1970–1971 was increased to $244,000. As was expected, increases were noted in all aspects of the library's operations. During 1970–1971, the collection grew by 5,751 volumes compared to 3,732 in the previous year. Eighty-three new journal titles were added to the subscription list. Four additional staff positions were filled within the year. Circulation statistics showed an increase of 5,000 and interlibrary loans shot up from 2,883 to 4,838 in one year, going on up to 6,886 in 1972–1973.

Settling in also saw the beginning of audiovisual services. A limited number of slide-tape programs

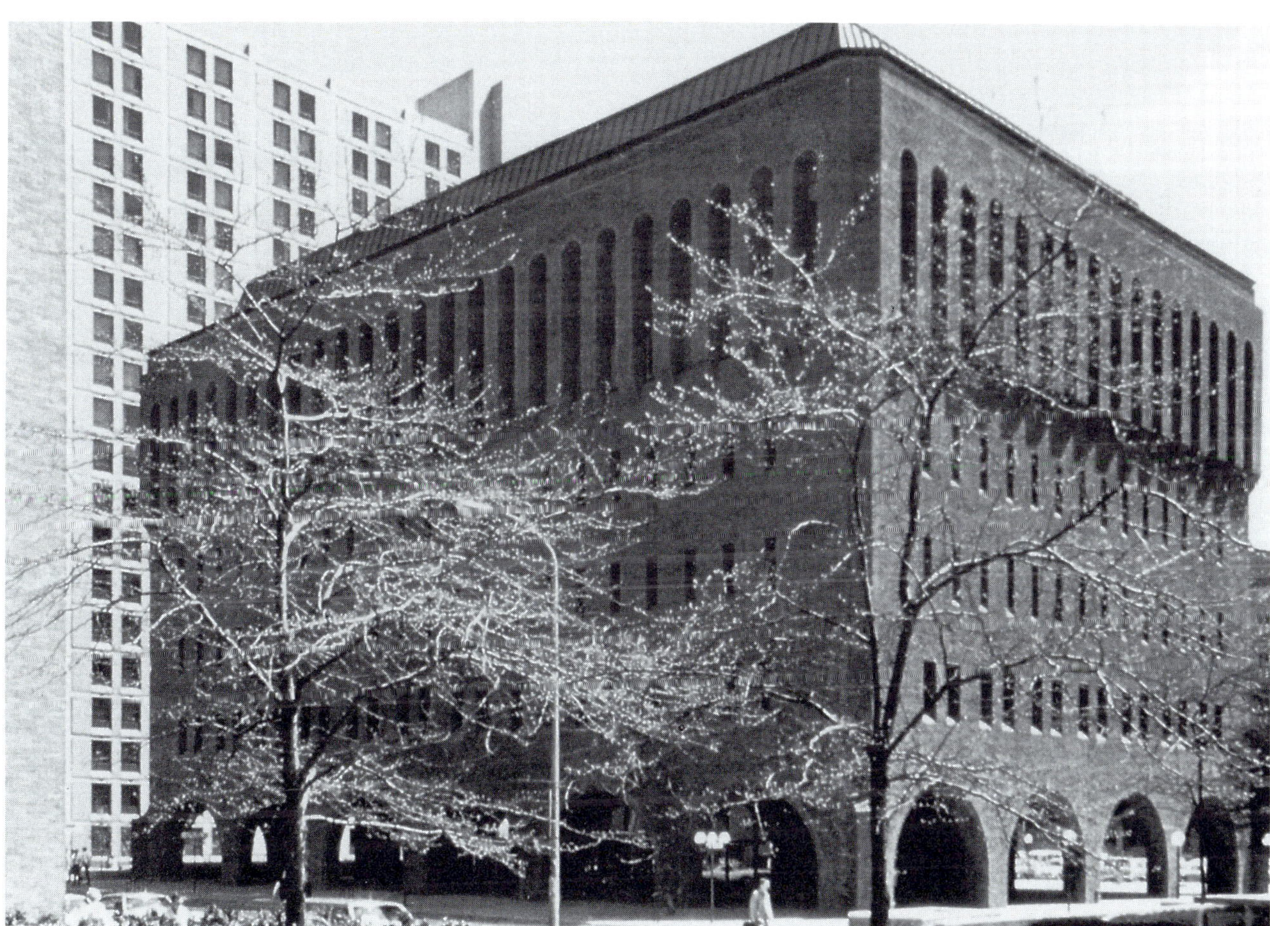

FIG. 56-11. The Scott Library (1970).

produced by or selected by members of the faculty were housed at the circulation desk to be charged out for viewing in specially designated carrels within the library. A short time later audiovisual facilities were developed in conjunction with the Department of Baccalaureate Nursing of the College of Allied Health Sciences. Viewing facilities for these programs were located in the basement of the library.

Though internal expansions were important, cooperative undertakings were not neglected. On April 29, 1971, Doctor John Killough, Associate Dean of the Medical College and members of the library staff met in the new Conference Room with the librarians of six of the hospitals affiliated with Jefferson for educational programs for its medical students. It was the first such cooperative program for any of the Philadelphia medical schools and perhaps the first countrywide as well. This session led to a series of annual meetings that continue to this time to address common problems and to seek cooperative solutions.

As the number of affiliations had grown over the years, many of the affiliated hospitals joined in consortium arrangements with neighboring academic health science and industrial libraries. These consortia developed largely because federal subsidies from the National Library of Medicine for document delivery had ceased. The current delivery service for interlibrary loans among many of these libraries is sponsored by one such consortium.

Early in 1971, Alice Mackov, a graduate of the Drexel Institute School of Library and Information Science with extensive experience in hospital laboratory and library services, was coaxed away from the staff of the Library of the College of Physicians of Philadelphia. She was appointed Reference Librarian to set up the new reference and interlibrary loan services. Having recently been trained at the National Library of Medicine, she was well acquainted with its MEDLARS (Medical Literature Analysis and Retrieval System) program and was experienced in searching the medical literature using its MEDLINE (MEDLARS' on-line data base). With a trained

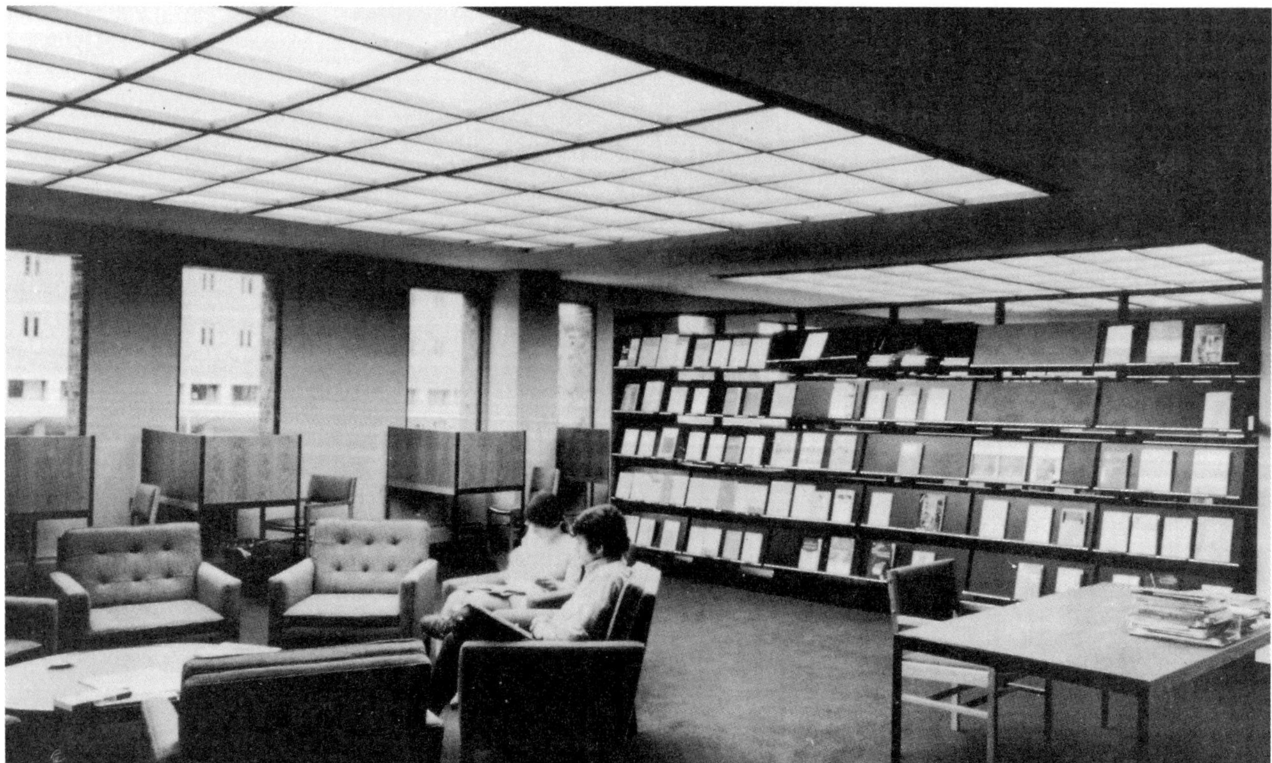

FIG. 56-12. The lounge reading area on the second floor of the Scott Memorial Library (1970).

searcher on the staff and meeting other requirements, the Scott Library became the first area medical school to acquire a MEDLINE terminal. Thus the library began its involvement with the new library automation by offering on-line access to the *Index Medicus* tapes.

A next step toward automation was taken during 1973 and 1974. The Union Library Catalogue of Philadelphia, realizing its need to automate its program, joined with other library services to form PALINET (Pennsylvania Library Network). Through PALINET Jefferson made application for an OCLC (On-Line Computer Library Center) terminal. In early 1975 the Scott Library became the first Philadelphia medical library to join this service with access to the holdings of 2,000 libraries countrywide. Included in this database are some 200 health science libraries. This service immediately became invaluable to the acquisitions, cataloging, reference, and interlibrary loan staff members. Years later, OCLC provided the machine-readable bibliographic records that became the database for the library's on-line catalog.

After 26 years as Librarian, Robert T. Lentz retired on June 30, 1975. His performance in guiding the growth and modernization of the library during these years was recognized by presentation of his portrait to the College in 1975 and the award of an honorary degree of Doctor of Science in 1980.

John A. Timour, M.A., M.L.S.; Second University Librarian (1975–1987)

The new age pushing toward automation was aided further by the appointment of John A. Timour as University Librarian and University Professor of Medical Bibliography and Library Science (Figure 56-13). Timour, a native of Connecticut, had done his undergraduate work at Miami (Ohio) University and then had earned two masters degrees, one an M.L.S. at the University of Maryland and a second, an M.A. at George Washington University. His background in medical librarianship dated back to 1966 when he was on the staff of the National Library of Medicine. Before that he had taught integrated classes for servicemen in the South. From 1969 to 1973 he directed the Regional Medical Library activities for the State of Connecticut. He came to Jefferson from the College of Physicians where he had been Director of the Mid-Eastern Regional Medical Library (1973–1975).

On coming to the Scott Library, Timour immediately became involved not only in the library but also in University and Faculty Club activities while continuing his involvement in local and national library organizations. The publication of his article in the *Jefferson Medical College Alumni Bulletin,* "Scott Library: Rearrangement Not Renovation,"[10] details much of the activity of his first few years. Perhaps his early contributions will longest be remembered for the advances he and his staff made in developing an Audiovisual Center and for instituting an automated library system.

In January, 1976, JoAnn King joined the library staff as Audiovisual Librarian. She had received her library training at Dalhousie University, Halifax, Nova Scotia. She encountered a fertile field, which she assaulted with fervor—the limited collection of software that had been housed at the circulation desk and the selected items of hardware

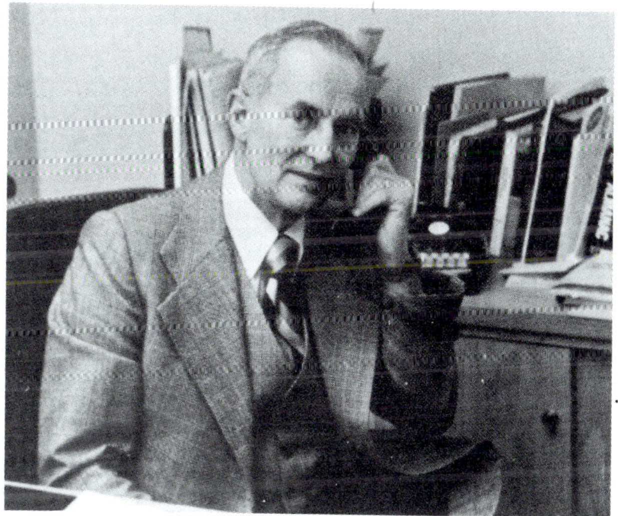

FIG. 56-13. John A. Timour, B.A., M.A., M.L.S., University Librarian, and Professor of Medical Bibliography and Library Science (1975–1987).

scattered throughout the library were gathered to form a small nucleus of an Audiovisual Center in Room 307 of the library. Standards were set for the types of media and equipment that would be best suited to a medical Audiovisual program. Additional audio and video cassettes, slide programs, and recordings in numerous medical subject fields were added and newer models of audiovisual equipment purchased. The latter included slide projectors, videocassette player/recorders, color monitors/receivers, audiocassette tape player/recorders, MacIntosh minicomputers, and an Apple II+ microcomputer. The Scott Library's Audiovisual Center became a busy and important part of the university's educational programs. The audiovisual staff compiled an extensive catalog of its holdings, its fifth edition having been published in 1986.

Late in 1980, King resigned to begin her studies for a doctorate at George Washington University in the field of manuscript and book preservation. Elaine Spyker, a graduate of Shimer College, Mt. Carroll, Illinois, and of Drexel Institute Graduate School of Library and Information Science, was employed as the new Audiovisual Librarian. Mrs. Spyker had been employed at the Chester County and Montgomery County public libraries and the Frankford Hospital Library before joining the staff at Jefferson. She remained in this position until January, 1986, when she was appointed to the new position of Systems Librarian.

Related to the development of the Audiovisual Services was a Computer Aided Instruction program that had been developed at the opening of the Scott Library by the Office of Research in Medical Education under the direction of Doctor Joseph Gonnella, later the Dean of the Medical College. Two computer terminals were installed in carrels on the fourth floor, where medical students and medical education researchers worked together to develop improved computer-assisted means for learning. The two carrels were later expanded to an adjacent room with much more sophisticated computer models and related instrumentation.

The reference department with its related interlibrary loans had begun to function well between 1971 and 1975 under the direction of Alice Mackov. The OCLC terminal added access to an important database. With the addition of a MEDLARS terminal and access to the MEDLINE tapes, a whole new age had come. During the summer of 1976 Nancy Calabretta had been employed as a cataloger, but in early 1977 she was transferred to reference services. She was a graduate of Hood College and had earned two master's degrees, one from Trenton State College in education and another from Drexel Institute in library science. At about the same time Rosalinda Ross, a graduate of St. Mary's University, San Antonio, Texas, who had received her M.A.L.S. from the University of Michigan, was added to the reference staff. In 1978 Barbara Cohen (now Barbara Laynor) joined as a reference clinical librarian for nursing. She had earned her undergraduate degree and her M.S.L.S. at the University of Pittsburgh and had served on the staff of the Medical College of Virginia and the University of Pennsylvania Medical School libraries. With four reference librarians and increased demands from the medical staff and faculty members, on-line computer searches soared. During 1975–1976, 552 searches were completed, and two years later the figure had risen to 2,848.

In January, 1980, the Scott Library established a Satellite Information Center on the third floor of the New Hospital in an effort to make access to information easier for the hospital staff. The Center, which is located on the Eleventh Street side of the Hospital, has a librarian on duty from 2 P.M. to 4 P.M. Monday through Friday. It is equipped with a computer terminal that allows the librarian to produce tailored bibliographies on a variety of subjects such as medicine, nursing, drug toxicology, psychology, hospital administration, and education. The center also has forms for ordering photocopies and for requesting interlibrary loans.

As of January, 1981, Lillian Brazin joined the reference staff. She was a graduate of Temple University and earned her library degree from the Drexel Institute. She had been Director of the Library of Daroff Division of the Einstein Medical Center and had been head of cataloging at Hershey Medical Center Library. She was named Research Resources Librarian.

By the 1980s the technical services department of the library had become well established under the supervision of Henry T. Armistead. The three sections comprised acquisitions, periodicals, and cataloging. Mr. Armistead had earned a B.A. from the University of Pennsylvania and an M.S.L.S. from Drexel's Graduate School of Library and Information Science. In the meantime he had been employed at the Northeast Regional Branch of the Free Library of Philadelphia. On completing his library degree in 1968 he joined the Scott Library staff as Acquisitions Librarian. For a time he was Head of Technical Services and is at the present time Collection Librarian.

The Periodicals Section has continued under Faye Kostenbauder Williamson since 1956. She has seen the journals file double from some 800 titles to over 1,600 in 1986.

During the 1960s and 1970s the cataloging was done by Katharine E. Veigel, in later years assisted by Esther (Mrs. Leon) Israel until 1976. Both Veigel and Israel had been trained at Drexel Institute Library School. Robert P. Lee joined the staff in 1973 as the evening circulation clerk while he completed his library school studies at Drexel Institute. On receiving his master's degree in 1974, he was promoted to cataloger. During his early years the library was involved in becoming acquainted with computerized cataloging and involved in weeding the collection, shifting material, and reclassifying most of the books. From 1980 to 1982 Joan Konrad, with a B.A. from Kutztown State College and an M.S.L.S. from Drexel University, assisted in this busy department. She left Jefferson to pursue an M.D. degree at Harvard University. In September, 1982, Elizabeth G. Mikita, B.A., Livingston College, and M.L.S., Rutgers University, became the cataloger. She had had cataloging experience at Rutgers University Library and with Baker and Taylor Company.

During this period the circulation department had continued under the direction of Muriel B. Campbell, who joined the library staff in 1959. Shortly thereafter she assumed the responsibility of managing the circulation of materials. This is the area of the library that has most contact with the library's users. She retired in 1980 after 21 years of devoted service.

At this juncture the interlibrary loan activities were transferred from Reference and joined with the circulation activities to form the Access Services Department. Margaret Devlin, with a B.A. in French and an M.L.S., both from the University of Pittsburgh, was appointed Access Services Librarian. She came to Jefferson following experience at the Temple University Library.

Automation

The first movement toward automation of library services began in 1978 with the appointment of a staff committee composed of Robert Lee, Barbara Cohen, Faye Williamson, and Muriel Campbell. Two members of the university's Management Services Department staff were added to the group, and John Timour, Director of the Library, was an ex-officio member. Two separate library functions were the first to receive the committee's attention: circulation and serials control. Within a few months it became apparent that an on-line catalog should precede an automated circulation system, or at least these two activities should be considered concurrently. The matter of serials control was prematurely resolved with the purchase of the PHILSOM II (Periodicals Held in the Library of the School of Medicine) package from the Washington University's School of Medicine Library. This punched-card system was tested for one year. It was found to be more complex and time consuming than the manual system and was discontinued.

With the assistance of the Management Services Department members, the committee investigated and tested several commercial computer systems and even attempted to develop an on-line catalog in-house. Each was determined to be too cumbersome and unwieldy for the library's purposes. Further attempts to create an on-line catalog suffered a setback when the Management Services Department members of the committee resigned from the University. No others in that department seemed available or interested, and the committee dissolved.

In 1980 a new automation committee was created and charged "to review the library's operations in order to make recommendations concerning how, where, and when automation would increase the efficiency and effectiveness of the library; to function as the library's interface with the Management Services Department (now the Department of Information Services) personnel; and to assist library staff and users to become familiar with the operation of any installed automated equipment so as to make such equipment optimally useful."[11] Robert Lee, Assistant Librarian for Technical Services, was appointed to chair the committee, which included Henry Armistead, Collection Development Librarian; Nancy Calabretta, Reference Librarian; Margaret Devlin, Access Services Librarian; and Elaine Spyker, Audiovisual Librarian.

From 1980 to 1983 the committee visited libraries with automated systems, attended workshops and seminars concerned with topics related to automation, and reviewed the available literature on the topic. By 1983 the committee had reviewed all existing turn-key integrated library systems to identify those that met the library's specifications. An initial evaluation in August, 1983, found all systems lacking at least one of the basic requirements.

By early 1984 the committee felt that significant developments had occurred in health science library automation and that other libraries had successfully replicated prototype automated systems. The Committee also noted that improvements had been made in existing turn-key systems, so they felt that some of these systems would now meet the Scott Library's requirements. At the end of June, work began on a request-for-proposal, hoping that fiscal year 1986 would be a realistic target date to establish automation.

After several months of writing, review and revision, a document was issued as a Request-for-Proposal. In December the request was released to nine vendors. Six responses were received by the February, 1985, deadline. On July 3, 1985, the committee unanimously selected Georgetown University's Library Information System (LIS) for the Scott Library's automation program. A letter of intent to negotiate for purchase was sent to Georgetown in July, 1985. The contract was finally signed in January, 1986. At that time Elaine Spyker was designated Systems Librarian for the Scott Library. During 1986, staff members were trained, equipment was ordered, delivered, and installed, and further training was begun. Bibliographic records began to be loaded, and the journal database was developed. In July, 1986, over 100,000 books and journals were bar coded by the library staff members in a ten-day period. During the same month the first MEDLINE tape was loaded and the on-line catalog was made available for staff use. By the end of 1986 the miniMEDLINE file (a subset of the MEDLINE journal citation database) was complete, training for use of the circulation and serials modules had taken place, and newly received journal issues were checked in online. Installation of all five LIS modules—acquisitions, serials, circulation, the on-line catalog, and miniMEDLINE were projected to be completed by June, 1987.

Special Collections

Mention has been made of significant donations of books and journals to the library by members of the faculty and alumni. One gift, that of Doctor Pascal Brooke Bland, was unusual in that it contained several hundred rare and historically important volumes. During Doctor Bland's later years he from time to time would select titles that he felt he could spare from his library to donate to the college library. In time, these, plus the some 2,800 volumes received after his untimely death, gave the Scott Library a very respectable rare medical book collection.

On moving into the new Scott Library Building it became possible to assemble the older and rare books in the Special Collections Room where they could more properly be cared for and displayed. At that time the library began more seriously to assemble the publications of the faculty members. This effort was aided considerably with the appointment of Samuel Davis as Special Collections Librarian in 1982. Mr. Davis had, since 1958, been Assistant and later Associate Librarian, and for a short period, from 1978 to 1982, was the Evening Librarian. With his interest and specialized training in restoration and preservation he has been able to supervise a program of proper care of the collection. He has also been able to build up the collection of books written by Jefferson faculty members. An outstanding contribution to the latter are the 34 volumes of the Peter A. Herbut, M.D., papers.

Archives

Associated with Special Collections has been the Jefferson Archives. From its early days, pieces of art, ancient and recent medical instruments, and historic artifacts, as well as historic documents, have been donated to the library. Some of this material has been displayed from time to time. Most of it, however, had collected dust in the stacks until the Jefferson Alumni Hall was occupied in 1968. Because of the library's crowded condition at that time, most of the archival material was moved to the preparation room of the Mezzanine Auditorium at Jefferson Alumni Hall.

After Robert Lentz retired as Librarian, he was asked in September, 1975, to organize the University archives on a part-time basis. The preparation room provided little more than storage space. It was a real challenge. The material was cleaned, sorted, identified when possible, packed into boxes, and labeled in preparation for a time when more space would be available. That time arrived in 1981 in the form of a room on the third floor of the Main hospital building. With double the space and with a gift of seven exhibition cases from the Atwater Kent Museum, it was much easier to sort material, and it was now possible to display some of the important holdings.

The hospital space was more temporary than expected, for in two short years, in 1983, the Archives was relocated into rooms 309 and 310 of the Scott Library. These rooms had been used for library administrative activities, which with the reference personnel's behind-the-scenes activities moved to the Mezzanine. With this move the exhibition cases were distributed about the public areas of the third floor, giving much more visibility to the Special Collection's and the Archives' treasures.

The archives work continued. A card file of matriculated students from 1825 to 1900 who were never graduated was developed to facilitate answering questions of genealogical interest. Indexes of obituaries in a newly acquired set of *Dunglison's College and Clinical Record* and the *Jeffersonian* were also prepared. Otherwise the archivist placed his emphasis on identification and filing of material for easy access. It had become evident that the collection required the services of a professionally trained archivist who would be able to use the University's historical records to help, and would know how to acquire, describe, inventory, label, and preserve the various collections.

Shortly after moving into the Scott Building, in 1983, the School of Nursing was closed and its records were deposited in the Archives. Doris Bowman, who had for some time been the Director of the School and who had overseen the closing and organization of its records, worked with the Archives of the College of Allied Health Sciences. In June of 1986 she joined the ranks of the fully retired.

During the spring of 1986 several things occurred to make it possible for the archives to take its rightful place on the University scene. First, the library conference room was assigned to the archives, giving it additional space for growth. Then, through the backing of the University Historian, Frederick B. Wagner, Jr., M.D., it was determined to employ a properly trained Archivist. During the summer and fall a search committee sought applications and interviewed qualified candidates. On December 8, 1986, Judith A. Robins, B.A. (English), University of Iowa, M.A. (History/Archives), M.A. (Library Science), University of Denver, joined the staff as Assistant Archivist. Thus began a whole new era for Jefferson's Archives.

It has been stated that "the heart of a university is its library." The miracle of Jefferson's growth and tradition is well reflected in the library's handsome architecture, its abundant collections, and its forefront management. It has supported and enhanced all aspects of medical care, education, and research for its students and faculty for nearly a century.

References

1. "History of the Jefferson Y.M.C.A.," *Jeffersonian* 5:34, May 1903.
2. "The Jefferson Students' Reading Rooms," *Jeffersonian* 1:17, April 1899.
3. Jefferson Medical College Eightieth Annual Announcement, Session of 1904–1905, p. 13.
4. Flexner, A., *Medical Education in the United States and Canada*. New York: 1910.
5. Jefferson Medical College, Announcements for the 89th Annual Session, 1913–1914, p. 82.

6. "Resolutions on Deaths of Honorary Consultants: Charles L. Frankenberger," *Bull. Med. Library Assn.* 40:100–101, 1952.
7. Lobinger, C.S., "Obituary of Samuel P. Scott," *Amer. Bar Assn. Jour.* 15:529, September 1929.
8. "Ancient Books Added to the Medical Library: New Gifts from Dr. P. Brooke Bland," *Jeff. Med. Coll. Al. Bull.* 2, No. 7, May 1940, pp. 12–18.
9. Lentz, R.T., "Time, Jefferson and the Information Explosion," *Jeff. Med. Coll. Al. Bull.* 16, No. 1, Fall 1966, p. 1922.
10. Timour, J.T., "Scott Library: Rearrangement Not Renovations," *Jeff. Med. Coll. Al. Bull.* 33, No. 3, Spring 1984.
11. Scott Memorial Library Annual Report, 1982/83, p. 49.

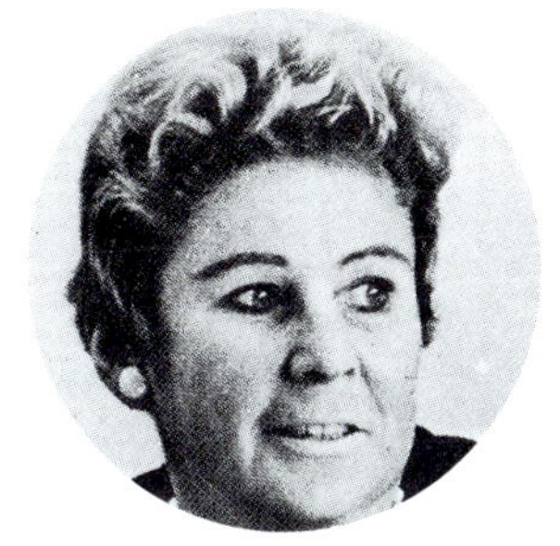

CHAPTER FIFTY-SEVEN

The Alumni Association

Nancy S. Groseclose, B.A.

"It is for the promotion of these mutual offices of kindness and courtesy that alumni associations are established . . . "

—Samuel D. Gross (1805–1884)

It was in 1870 that Doctor Samuel D. Gross (Jefferson, 1828), serving as Professor of Surgery at his alma mater, realized what power and influence could accrue to the Medical College by the creation of an Association composed of its graduates. In bringing together a distinguished group of alumni at a March 12 meeting, the first formative steps were realized. A five-member committee with Nathan Hatfield (Jefferson, 1826) as Chairman was charged with the responsibility of organization. At a subsequent meeting, just a week later, bylaws were accepted that stated: "The objects of the Association are laid down in addition to promoting the prosperity of the Jefferson Medical College to be that of awarding prizes; the publishing of meritorious theses; the endowment of scholarships for the free medical education of the sons of the alumni whose means are limited; the collection of anatomical and pathological specimens for the College Museum; the cultivation of good feelings among the alumni, and above all, the advancement of the interests of medical education and the diffusion of sound medical knowledge." Although slightly modified over the years, the bylaws still reflect the same basic philosophy. During the first few years of the Association, both the Board of Trustees and the Dean's office held reservations about the formation of this body, with unfounded fears of financial encumbrances. In 1874, however, notice of its existence was inserted into the College catalog. Since that time the administrative support has been exemplary.

The Alumni Association is governed by a President, four Vice Presidents, a Secretary, a Treasurer, and an Executive Committee. In addition, there is a Vice President for each state, except for Pennsylvania, which has three. A core of standing committees is appointed by the President to promote the ongoing programs of the organization. The Executive Committee with some variations has been in effect since the Association's founding. Although the elder Gross served as its first President for a number of years until its success was established, in succeeding years Presidents have served for just one year. Meetings of the Executive Committee are scheduled seven or eight times during the school year with an annual meeting held in February (Figure 57-1).

The history of fund raising by the Association dates as early as 1872, when a committee was appointed to secure funds for purchase of a site for Jefferson's first definitive hospital. During a time when monetary panic was sweeping the country, this effort topped $350,000. Five years later the hospital was ready for occupancy. It was one of the first in America as part of a medical school for teaching purposes. There have been similar efforts over the years, including a capital campaign initiated in 1922 to honor the Centennial of the College. At that time the founding date was regarded as 1825 but later shown to be 1824. It was in 1948, however, that the most comprehensive contribution program was conceived and implemented. Louis H. Clerf (1912), Professor of Laryngology and Broncho-Esophagology and a Past President of the Alumni Association, brought into being the Annual Giving Fund, which replaced the antiquated note system. Dr. Clerf envisioned a class agent system that would provide ongoing communication with the College through classmate/colleague direct mail solicitation. In the first year, the College realized $108,313 from this new effort. Since that time the program has grown and thrived until it has become recognized as one of the finest in the country (Figure 57-2). Several times Jefferson has been cited for its accomplishments in this connection. During the 1983 campaign the Association surpassed the $1,000,000 mark for the first time, and each succeeding year it has topped and bettered its performance. Since the program's inauguration, Jefferson has realized $14,240,551 from its Medical College Alumni.

In 1960 during the Thirteenth Roll Call, the Executive Committee approved the concept that funds would be solicited from its membership for unrestricted College use. These would provide the Dean with an active base for programs in medical education that otherwise would be unavailable to him. J. Wallace Davis (1942) has served as Chairman for the program since 1964. His efforts on behalf of the Alumni Association were recognized at the President's Club Dinner in 1978, when he was presented the University's Cornerstone Award (Figure 57-3).

Enthusiasm and ambition of the Alumni Association for Jefferson's progress were not entirely limited in 1872 to raising funds for a hospital. In that same year it commissioned the

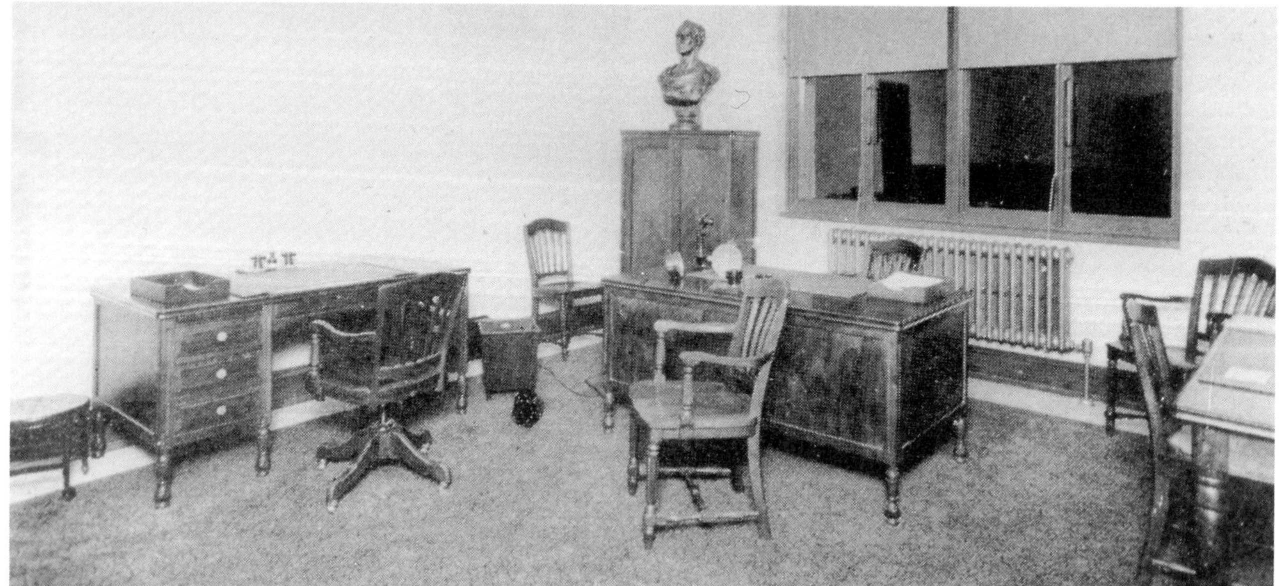

FIG. 57-1. The Alumni Office in the 1025 Walnut Street Medical College (ca. 1928). A bust of founder Samuel D. Gross can be seen in the rear.

well-known Philadelphia artist, Samuel Bell Waugh, to paint the portraits of five of its outstanding Professors: Charles Delucena Meigs, Robley Dunglison, John Barclay Biddle, Joseph Pancoast, and Samuel D. Gross. The one of Gross was presented to the Board of Trustees on the stage of the Academy of Music at the graduation exercises of March, 1875. Through the generosity of the family of Orville H. Bullitt, Jr., Ph.D., the great-great grandson of Dr. Gross and member of the Board of Trustees, the companion portrait of Mrs. Gross by the same artist was given to the University in 1987.

In 1875 Thomas Eakins, who had studied anatomy at Jefferson while an art student, admired Dr. Gross to such an extent that he painted *The Gross Clinic* on a voluntary basis without commission. This was purchased by the Alumni Association for $200 in 1878 and presented to the Board of Trustees the following year. This painting has immortalized Dr. Gross in what has come to be recognized by many as the greatest masterpiece of American art. In 1982 the Alumni Gate to Jefferson's Eakins Gallery was provided by the Alumni Association at a cost of $35,000. This specially designed wrought-iron entrance was crafted by the famous Samuel Yellin Metal Works of Philadelphia (Figure 57-4).

The Alumni Prize was established in 1894 and has been awarded each year at Commencement. The senior student who has achieved the highest cumulative average over the four-year period is so honored.

Another serious interest of the Association is the cultivation of Jefferson's current student body. A number of programs have been developed and serve as a special bond between the two memberships. The Alumni Banquet, which was first suggested at the reception at Professor Gross' home on the first anniversary of the Association,

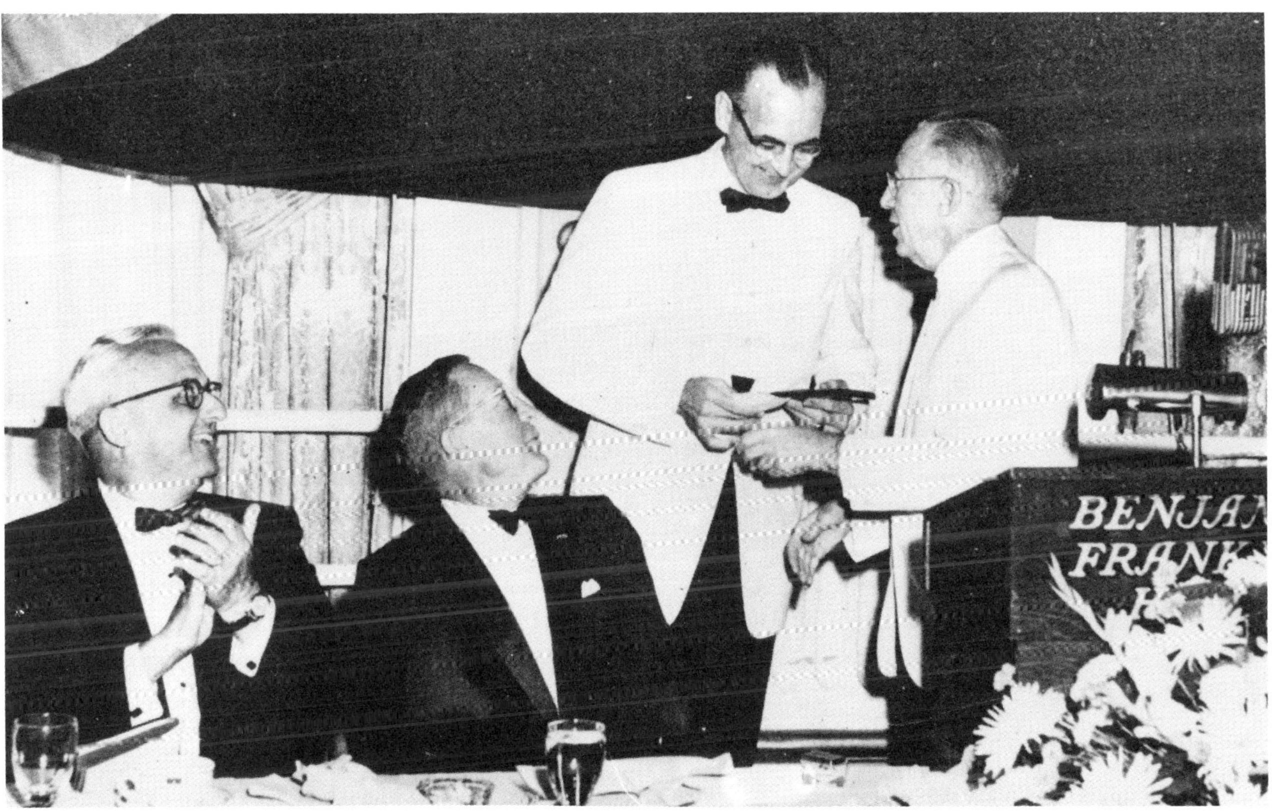

FIG. 57-2. Dr. Kenneth E. Fry, Chairman of Annual Giving, presents the plaque for First Place in total amount in the 1962 Drive to Dr. Herbert A. Luscombe, Agent for the Class of 1940. Dr. William A. Sodeman (Dean) and James M. Large (Chairman of the Board of Trustees) are shown seated left to right.

provides the membership with an opportunity to welcome the graduating class into the Association. For many years, the seniors were asked for a $5 life membership, but this was deleted from the bylaws in 1984. Originally the banquets were stag affairs. With the admittance of women in 1961, however, and with a changing social structure, this policy was changed in the early 1970s.

It was in 1964 that Benjamin Haskell (1923), then President of the Alumni Association, conceived the idea for Fathers' Day, a special program for the sophomore class. Again, as social patterns changed, the male-only program changed its format to include both parents, and the program became known as Parents' Day (1970). Faculty from the clinical and preclinical departments are invited to give morning presentations. For the luncheon that follows the students elect a speaker from the faculty and a member of their class to address the parents.

Another program to develop alumni relationship with students was initiated in 1980. Career Day was scheduled to give students an opportunity to meet with alumni/faculty in 20 specialties. It affords them a time to discuss and review on a personal and informal basis the benefits and problems in the search for postgraduate training positions.

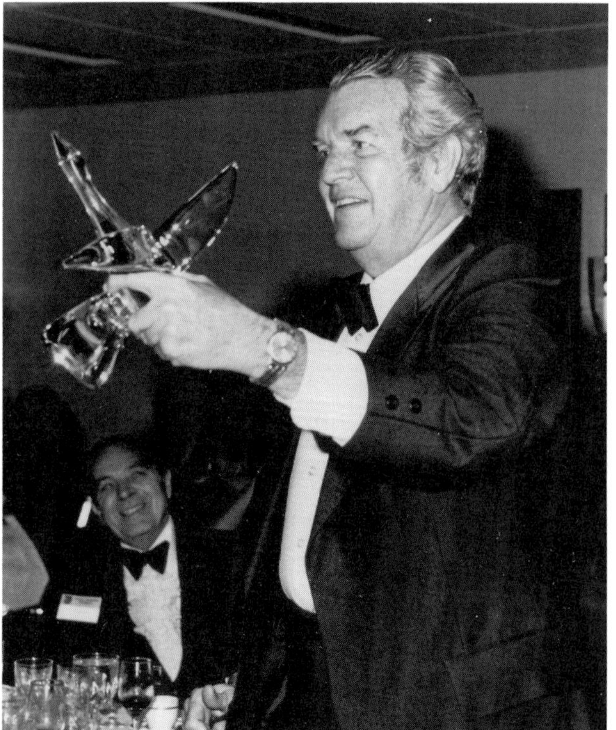

FIG. 57-3. Dr. J. Wallace Davis receives the Cornerstone Award (1978).

Wine and cheese parties are held for the freshmen and juniors to introduce them to the Association and its membership. The seniors are given certificates of membership at the time of graduation. Originally, these certificates were 24 by 19 inches but in 1961 were reduced to 11 by 14 inches. These are hand engrossed with the student's name and date of graduation and are signed by the current President and Secretary of the Association.

A housing program was inaugurated in 1980. Alumni across the country were asked to open their homes to senior students who were

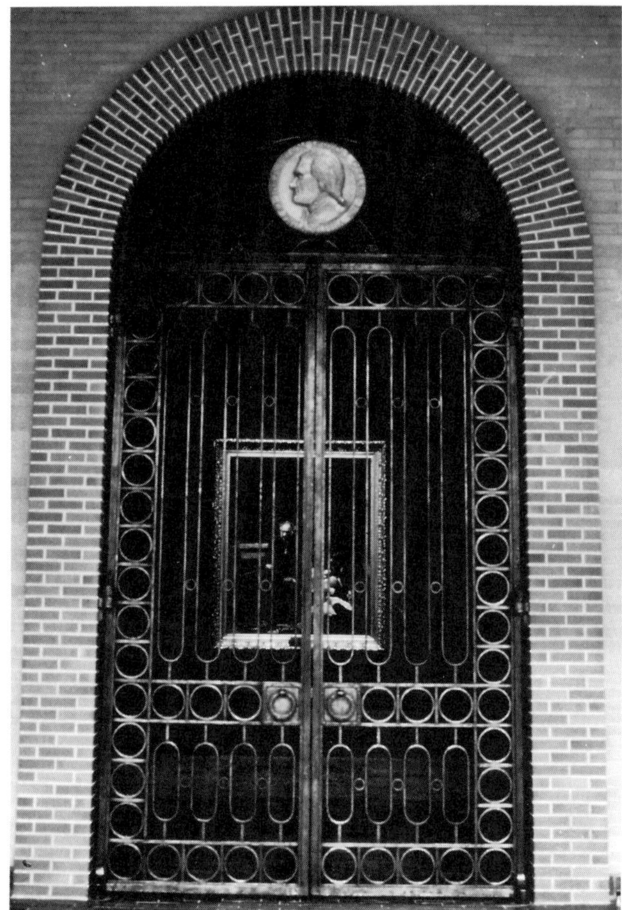

FIG. 57-4. Alumni Gate to Eakins Gallery, provided in 1982.

interviewing for postgraduate appointments. Over 1,500 alumni responded and over 100 beds are reserved annually. This program gives alumni an opportunity to meet Jefferson's recent students and allows the students to encounter Jefferson's family spirit. An endowed-bed fund was established in 1912 to offer free care to worthy alumni unable to pay for service. Due to lack of use, the Executive Committee voted in the fall of 1983 to move a percentage of this fund to complete the Gonzalo E. Aponte Professorship in Pathology, an Alumni-sponsored program.

The Alumni Association strongly endorsed the establishment of a Department of Family Medicine in 1973 with gifts of $50,000 from each annual giving campaign since that time. Dr. Paul C. Brucker was named the Alumni Professor and Chairman in May of that year. The College also has realized substantial amounts each year through a bequest program that is administered under the auspices of Jefferson's Development Office. In 1982 the Department of Obstetrics and Gynecology received $1,000,000 from the estate of P. Brooke Bland, Class of 1901 and a former Chairman of that Department. It is the largest bequest ever recorded from an alumnus.

Perhaps the most visible program of the Association is the publication of the *Alumni Bulletin,* presently issued four times each year. It is mailed to the membership, faculty, parents of current students, widows of the graduates, and friends of the Institution. The first volume was printed in December of 1922, a modest 12-page newsletter in a six by nine inches format. On the first page was a letter from William Potter, President of the Board of Trustees, to Elmer Hendricks Funk (1908), who was serving as President of the Alumni Association. It stated that the "concept of merger with any friendly rival institution of medicine (University of Pennsylvania) is not under consideration. The Administration of Jefferson Medical College is unanimous that we continue as the great independent medical school of the United States. I can conceive of no change in this fixed policy unless unhappily the alumni of Jefferson should cease to continue a vital interest in their distinguished Alma Mater."

The format for this *Bulletin,* published just twice a year in December and May, continued through the 1930s and 1940s. In January of 1949, under the first Executive Secretary, Mrs. Melrose E. Weed (Figure 57-5), the *Bulletin* was changed to an eight by eleven inches format and in 1953 a simple blue cover with the Jefferson head was added. In 1961 a photograph of commencement was used for the first time, inaugurating the use of cover design. Mrs. Joseph J. Mulone (Figure 57-6), who was serving as Executive Secretary of the Association at that time, was named Editor in 1963. She was succeeded by Miss Nancy Groseclose in 1966 (Figure 57-7).

The *Bulletin* has served as one of the finest vehicles for the dissemination of information about the College and news of the members of the alumni body. Currently the *Bulletin* schedules two to three features each issue with a general news section, class note specials, and obituaries. Special editions were published in 1950 (at which time the founding of Jefferson was still considered as 1825 instead of 1824) and 1974 commemorating

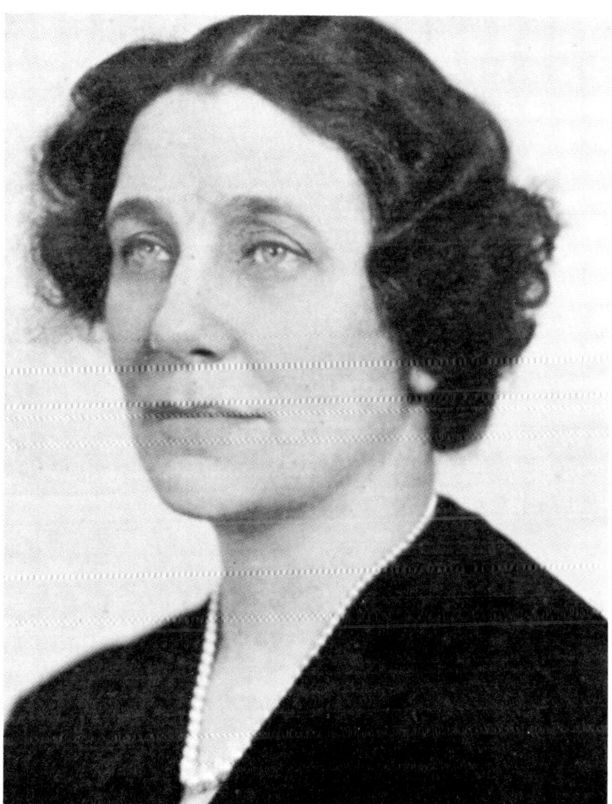

FIG. 57-5. Mrs. Melrose E. Weed, First Executive Secretary (1926–1956).

the one hundred twenty-fifth and one hundred fiftieth anniversaries of the College and again in 1970 to mark the Centennial of the Association. It was in the latter issue that a specially researched article by Associate Editor Elinor Bonner reported that nearly half of the Presidents of the United States have been attended or seen in consultation by Jefferson physicians.

In addition to Annual Giving and the *Bulletin,* the Association has maintained over the years numerous other programs to benefit its members. Each program is monitored by a standing committee and is directed by the Alumni Office. Chapter dinners have been part of the program since the early 1920s. These are geographically sponsored events organized by alumni in those areas for colleagues and classmates. Speakers from the College enhance these meetings.

During the 1930s the Executive Committee also approved allocations for renovations in the College Building, and during this period there was a $100,000 allocation for the construction of a Department of Experimental Medicine to honor J. Chalmers DaCosta (Jefferson, 1885), the first Samuel D. Gross Professor of Surgery (1910).

A graduate assembly was inaugurated in 1948. This was a midwinter Program of Continuing Medical Education sponsored and administered by the Association's Executive Committee. Before these meetings a midwinter smoker was scheduled for the membership. Presently, the annual meeting of the Association is held on the fourth Thursday in February and is open to the entire membership.

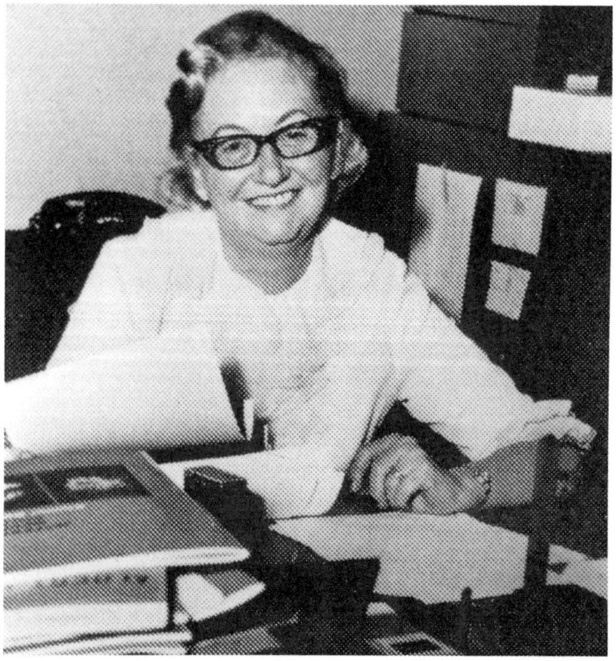

FIG. 57-6. Mrs. Joseph J. Mulone, Executive Secretary (1956–1966).

Postgraduate seminars were initiated in 1957 with a cruise out of Wilmington, North Carolina, to the Caribbean with 118 physicians aboard. Five years later, two charter planes took nearly 300 alumni, faculty, and guests to Paris. Since that time alumni have had an opportunity each year to join classmates and colleagues for trips to various parts of the world. In conjunction with these tours is a Continuing Medical Education Program involving both Jefferson and foreign faculty.

The Association has been extremely active during the times of College Anniversary Programs. It was in 1925 that the Centennial of Jefferson's founding (shown in later years to have been more correctly in 1824) was recognized by the Association with a special issue of the *Bulletin* and a banquet at the new Benjamin Franklin Hotel. Special railroad cars were chartered for New England alumni, and others from across the country attended. Merrit W. Ireland (Jefferson, 1891), who was a Surgeon General at that time, was the speaker.

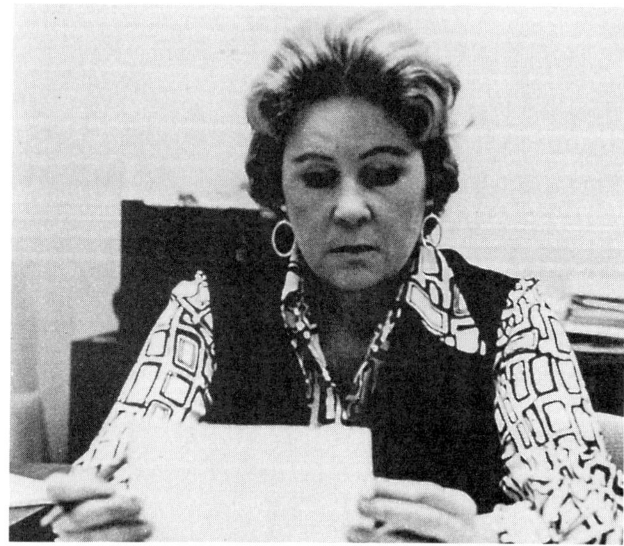

FIG. 57-7. Nancy S. Groseclose, Executive Secretary (1966–1973) and Executive Director (1973–1988).

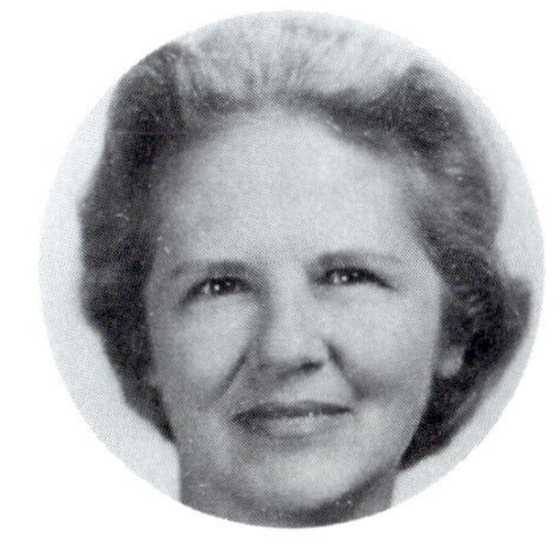

CHAPTER FIFTY-EIGHT

The Women's Board

MRS. PAUL A. BOWERS

"When society cannot afford to have what it cannot afford to be without, it is the occasion for intelligent giving."

—ALAN GREGG (1890–1957)

IN 1889 Dr. Jacob Mendes DaCosta, Chairman of Theory and Practice of Medicine, recommended to the Board of Trustees an organization of women to aid the College and Hospital. They studied the idea and on April 1, 1890, gave approval. Rules and regulations were drawn up under the aegis of the Trustees. The Maternity Department was the first to benefit when a Maternity Committee was established in 1892. In 1894 a Board of Lady Managers furnished a house at 224 South Seventh Street, on Washington Square, for maternity patients (Figure 58-1). They paid an annual rent of $1,000 plus the costs for food, domestic services, and part of the nurses' salaries. The Trustees covered expenses for fuel, light, medical needs, and some nurses' salaries. The cost of food for each patient averaged slightly more than $7 per month, and daily total costs per patient were figured at 26¢. There were no fixed time limits for the stay of a patient. Receipts came from personal contributions, board paid by some patients, Charity Ball allocation, and functions held for financial aid. There were contributions also of furniture, infant clothing, and food. The first year 74 patients were cared for by two nurses, and the following year recorded 172 births with 19 infant deaths. It must be recalled that in those days very few deliveries were performed outside the home, and most were by midwives. The purpose of the Jefferson maternity facility was not only for care but for instruction of medical students.

Until 1897 the Board of Lady Managers was under the leadership of Mrs. E.D. Gillespie, who was followed by Mrs. E.P. Davis. Mrs. E.E. Montgomery was Secretary and Mrs. Edward Weil the Treasurer. A group of 17 members met weekly in the Maternity Home. The ninth annual report requested donors to support the work as follows:

- $10 to care for a weak infant for one month
- $15 to pay a large part of the expenses of a poor woman for her confinement
- $300 to endow a bed for one year
- $1,500 to endow a bed in perpetuity

Receipts and expenses for the year averaged between $3,000 and $4,000. An appeal to the

Trustees to relieve the women of the $1,000 annual rent was approved.

In 1894 the Board of Lady Managers became involved in the Hospital, but details of their aid are lacking. In 1896 yet another group of ladies formed a committee to enhance the recreational facilities and Library of the College. They equipped a Reading Room, financed a Medical Library in the old College at Tenth and Moravian, and continued this function when the next Medical College Building was opened in 1898 at Tenth and Walnut.

Reorganization occurred in 1908 when the Board of Trustees dissolved the committees of the Board of Lady Managers and on January 9, 1909, created a new group called the Women's Auxiliary. Sub-Dean Ross V. Patterson felt at this time that the energies of the ladies would be better served in the Hospital, and the College committee was eliminated. By 1912 four major committees were active. A Hospital Committee of 30 members strove to maintain the attractiveness as well as usefulness of all areas related to care of the sick; the Maternity Committee of 24 members proposed to work for the needs of the Department; a 12-member Nurses Committee was committed to oversee the comfort and well-being of the nurses; and an Entertainment Committee, 51 strong, engaged in fund-raising and cultural events. Mrs. John Gibbon, Sr., was Treasurer of this fourth committee.

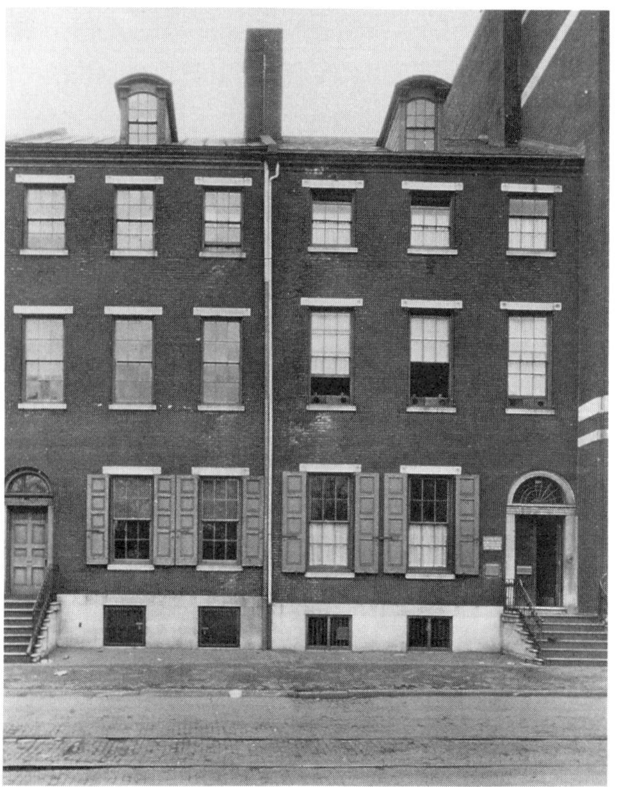

FIG. 58-1. The Maternity facility at 224 West Washington Square, established in 1894 for patient care and student instruction.

The various committees were composed of women of social standing closely related to members of the faculty or Board of Trustees. Ladies of this era who engaged in such activity were described as "social housekeepers," giving freely of time and means for their charitable services. The present-day Women's Board is the lineal successor to this Auxiliary, the records of which date from 1912. In this year the first rules of operation were printed, and a copy of the bylaws of 1925 exists.

In the surgical, medical, and "nervous" wards, 4,147 patients were treated in 1911. Of these patients 83% were free cases. Mrs. Charles M. Lea, Chairman of the Hospital Committee, noting the large census and great needs in these wards, set up a subcommittee of Public Wards. The Hospital Committee met from October through April, controlled the purchasing, and visited the hospital areas, including the wards, weekly.

In 1912 a Social Service Committee was organized through a fund provided by Ann Hinchman to aid the needy in the hospital.

By 1916 the Trustees advised that the Auxiliary could establish its own rules of organization, and in May authorized that subcommittees be abolished in favor of independent ones. In that year, the children's ward was at capacity with 100 patients—eleven had no beds and slept whereever they could be tucked in. On the international scene, that same year, Mrs. Paul Compton of the Maternity Committee lost her life when the Germans sank the *Lusitania*.

In May, 1917, the Auxiliary formed an independent committee for the preparation of surgical supplies and set up a room where 31 members could work one day a week. They were assessed $540 to buy materials for start up under the supervision of a nurse. In addition, because of the War, this committee labored to supply a Base

Hospital unit with dressings, bandages, and comfort bags and requested knitters to make 158 sweaters for the drivers of Jefferson Base Unit No. 38. Dr. John Gibbon, Sr., who was operating 16 hours a day, made an urgent request for dressings. The major sources of funding were the Charity Ball, Horse Show, and a new cooperative shop in the City.

The 1920s

Bessie (Mrs. J. Dobson) Altemus (Figure 58-2) became President of what now was called the "Women's Board" in 1921, and served in this capacity for 21 years. Records do not mention why the unofficial change in name. The annual receipts for the Board in 1922 totaled $2,282, needed for the three wards at 236–238 Pine Street. Mrs. Simon Gratz chaired the Children's Ward group, Mrs. Edward P. Davis the Maternity, Mrs. Alba B. Johnson the Social Services and Mrs. Charles Hebard the Nurses Home.

In March, 1923, the Board was notified by the Trustees through Dr. Henry K. Mohler that the establishment of Memorial Rooms was approved. They were not to be designated as such, but for a donation of $575 a brass plate would be placed on the door to read "Furnished by—."

In 1924 the Thompson Annex opened. Mrs. Simon Gratz as Chairman of the Children's Ward Committee arranged with Ellis Gimbel to provide a circus party for the children. Mrs. Brooke Anspach became Chairman of the Public Wards Committee and served until 1940. During 1924 a new Junior Committee for the Nurses' Home was formed by Mrs. Hill. Armason Harrison, a member of this committee, arranged dances and bridge parties to raise funds. Mrs. Thomas McCrae was appointed to encourage wives of new members of the College's faculty to join the Board. Mrs. Joseph Wear became Chairman of the Maternity Committee. In May, 1925, the name "Women's Board" was officially adopted.

The 1930s

Mrs. Percival Foerderer, destined to become an outstanding President in 1947, was elected to membership in 1930. Mrs. John Martin as chairman of the Maternity Committee aided the establishment of a new Antenatal Clinic, bringing an influx of 121 new patients, the largest since the founding of the Department. The outpatient maternity department moved to 2545 Wharton Street, where four senior medical students boarded and were on call to help with deliveries in patients' homes.

The Curtis Clinic opened in 1931, and in May, 1932, a new committee was formed to foster its interests. In December, 1932, an Alcove Food Facility was opened in the Thompson Annex, with proceeds to be allocated for work of the Social

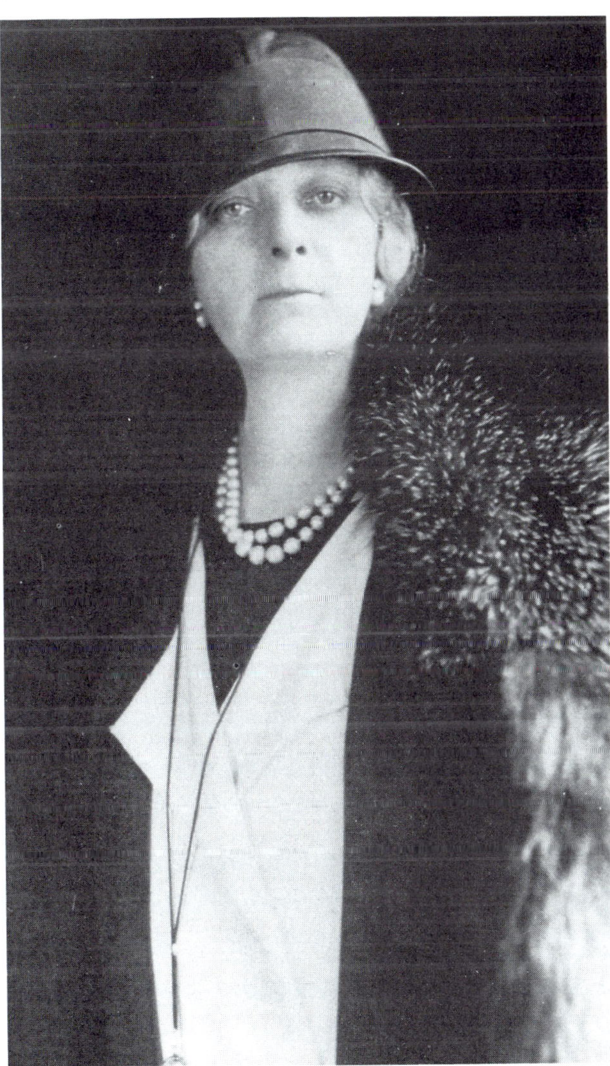

Fig. 58-2. Bessie (Mrs. J. Dobson) Altemus; President (1921–1942).

Services Committee. Staff physicians of that era will recall the camaraderie that developed in the Alcove as well as the exchange of professional information and advice.

The Philadelphia Electric Company, a longtime benefactor of the Children's Ward, provided suitable clothing for every needy child leaving the hospital. Not to be outdone, the Sewing Committee of the Women's Board on one occasion made 29 baby dresses before nightfall when an emergency rose.

In 1933, with repeal of Prohibition, the Charity Ball was an outstanding social and financial success. The Meyer Davis band played at greatly reduced cost. That year the Christmas baskets for the Pine Street Chest Hospital's needy patients and families were readied at a cost of $2.75 each. They contained a ten-pound ham, soup beans, two loaves of bread, a can of syrup, cocoa, evaporated milk, cornmeal, Mother's oats, tomatoes, onions, and macaroni.

The year 1934 (during the Great Depression) was especially poor from a financial standpoint, with only $542 received as allocation from the Cooperative Shop at 1821 Chestnut Street. Mrs. Robert Hooper on hearing this report promptly offered her home for a donation card party that raised $775.

The meetings of the Board were moved to the Roof Garden of the Thompson Annex in 1935. Upon request, a large supply of rubber gloves was purchased for the operating rooms. Operating room tables were also needed for the fourteenth floor, and the Board bought one for $79.50.

Under the Children's Ward Chairmanship of Mrs. Neff Colfelt in 1937 the Board purchased new cribs. The children of Drs. Henry K. Mohler and Elmer H. Funk saved their money to provide a party for the Children's Ward. The Public Wards Committee purchased dozens of bathrobes for the patients for $133, while the Maternity Committee bought a $400 resuscitation machine. Snellenburg's Store decorated and furnished a sitting-room for patients in a former delivery room on the fifth floor of the Tenth and Sansom Streets Hospital as a memorial to Adeline Potter Wear, who died in 1925. The home furnishings of Dean Ross V. Patterson, who died in 1938, were installed in the Nurses' Home at 1012 Spruce Street. The Emergency Aid Bazaar moved from the Penn Athletic club to the Bellevue Stratford Hotel, and the Women's Board became a participant.

The Public Wards Committee in 1938 enlarged its active membership to 35 in order to serve increased needs, especially of the surgical wards. Mrs. Percival Foerderer and E.E. Montgomery visited the "nervous" wards regularly and provided games for patients. The Maternity Committee applied to the National Youth Administration for an assistant at the Wharton Street Maternity Dispensary. The workers in this Administration received 50¢ an hour. In this year the Gray Ladies functioned as an auxiliary to the School of Nursing (Figure 58-3). They made dressings and undertook many routine tasks that released the trained nurses for the vital care of the sick.

The Maternity Committee in 1939 sponsored a luncheon at the Ritz Carlton Hotel to finance the organization of a Mother's Club to educate mothers in the care of their babies. The Blum Store gave 40 articles of clothing to "chance off," which realized $1,400. The Cooperative Shop's profit for Jefferson for the first six months was $169. The chairman of each committee of the Women's Board was made responsible to furnish workers and donations on a monthly basis. As a memorial to Dr. Harvey Righter, a Jefferson graduate of 1896 who died in 1934, the Women's Board established the custom of providing a rose to each nurse at graduation. Dr. Righter, who had been a lecturer to the nurses in bandaging, began presenting to each member of the Class of 1928 a red rose at Commencement. This eventually led to the formation of the traditional "Rose Arch" at graduation, which continued until the three-year Diploma Program was phased out in June, 1982.

The 1940s

New efforts in recruitment of members, now at 117, was instituted in 1940. There was anticipation of World War II in which Jefferson's Gray Ladies, organized by Mrs. Willard M. Rice III (Figure 58-4) and the largest such unit in the United States, was producing 200,000 dressings a year. The Pine Street Chest Hospital was provided with 24 bedside tables at a cost of $400.

Theater parties at Alden Park Manor began during the especially active year of 1941, and the first party netted $500. Jefferson participated in a Head-Dress Ball with proceeds of $1,050. Mrs. Willard Rice, Chairman of the Public Wards Committee, saw the urgent need for installation of running water in the wards. When the Trustees provided $800 for this plumbing, it released funds for the Wards group to purchase new medicine cabinets. Bessie Altemus, a political activist, was successful at Harrisburg in obtaining an allocation of $60,000 per year in State funds for the care of poor ward patients. Mrs. H. Alarik Myrin of the Curtis Clinic Committee was requested by Dr. Hayward R. Hamrick to supply 25 volunteer clerical workers. In March of the same year the hospital was making blackout preparations by a special group composed of Gray Ladies, Navy League Volunteers, and Canteen Workers. In April the Philadelphia Food Show was established with Jefferson as one of 23 hospital beneficiaries—the Women's Board sold 2,000 tickets. The Alcove Shop became self-sustaining. Plays at Alden Park Manor netted $500. The Social Service had expanded to seven subcommittees. The Junior Committee was conducting informal dances for student nurses at almost monthly intervals. The children's ward was painted at a cost of $368. Two sitting rooms in Thompson Annex were furnished in memory of Dr. P. Brooke Bland, who died in 1940. Board receipts for 1941 were $7,407, and expenditures $4,789.

No less active was 1942. Mrs. J. Howard Pew (Figure 58-5) became President and Mrs. Percival Foerderer organized the first Finance Committee. A plaque was placed in the hospital in recognition of 21 years of fruitful service by Bessie Altemus, who was also awarded the title of Honorary Chairman of the Board. Mrs. P. Brooke Bland was Chairman of the first Phantom Valentine project, which netted $1,834 and was continued for many years. She was also active in revising the bylaws,

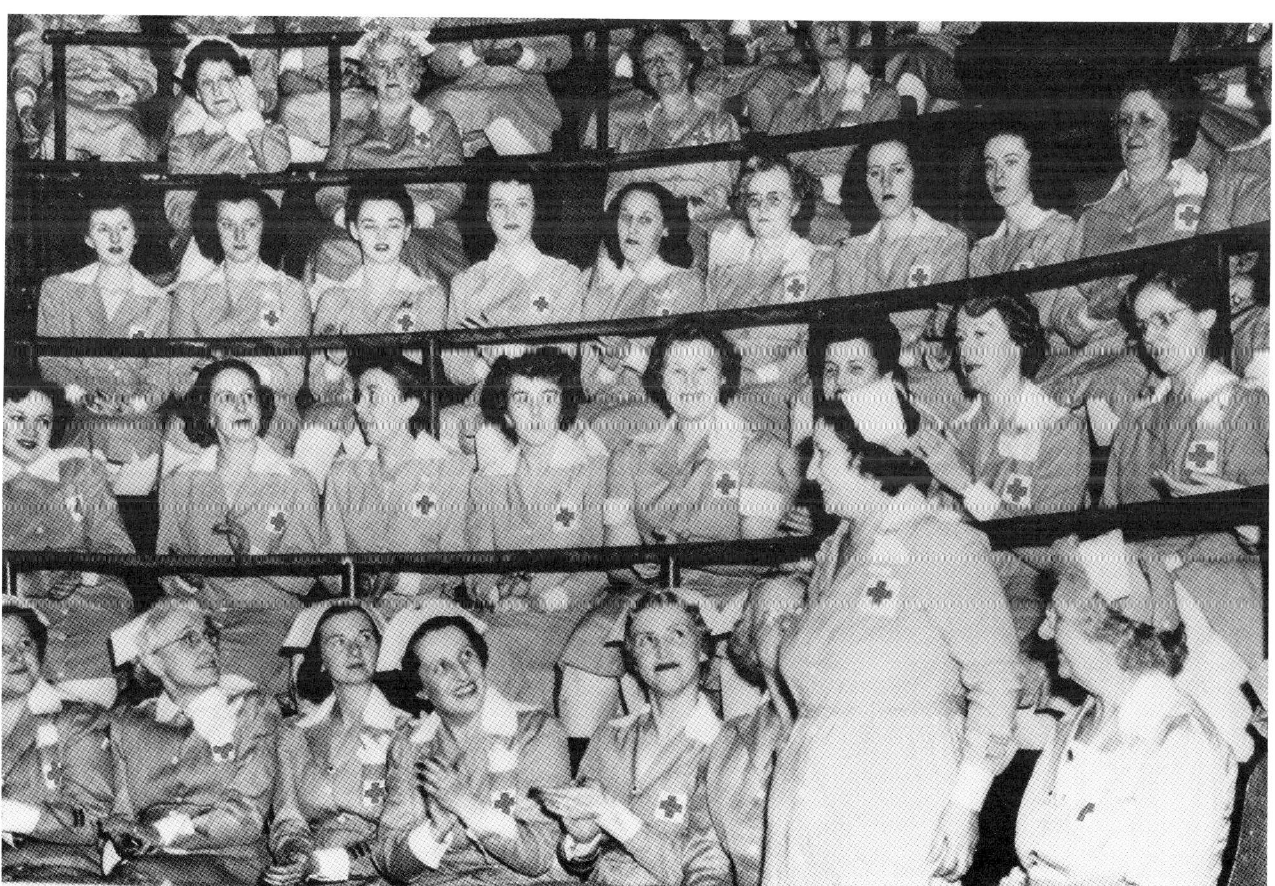

FIG. 58-3. The Gray Ladies, an auxiliary to the School of Nursing.

which now provided for active, subscribing, contributing, and honorary membership categories. Nominations from the floor were also to be recognized. Meetings increased to eight a year from the previous four. A new Executive Committee was constituted from elected officers, directors, and chairmen of the committees. There was a request from the hospital for the first time for an annual report of the Women's Board. The Maternity Committee purchased oxygen masks and gauges and provided milk for pregnant women. The Social Service volunteers made 200 sewing kits, which were requested by Dr. Baldwin Keyes for the doctors and nurses of the organizing Jefferson Base Unit No. 38. Janet Walker, the hospital dietitian, asked for funds to raise the salaries of her kitchen workers by $10 per month. Jefferson Hospital was paying $40 to $50 a month, whereas nearby stores paid $15 to $18 per week. Board volunteers gave their services in the kitchens. Mrs. Robert Liversidge replaced Mrs. Colfelt as Chairman of the Children's Ward. In April a committee toured the hospital to assess wartime preparedness in emergency situations. Windows had been painted black, and extra beds lined the halls and sitting rooms. Any shortage of nurses and household equipment was carefully noted. Mrs. Potter Wear gave the Social Service group a car for motor messages, and the Board provided gasoline and repairs. On May 15 the Jefferson Unit left for camp with 34 doctors and 34 nurses. Maternity averaged 600 patients monthly and Wharton St. Dispensary had 4,397 cases from June to September. The Curtis Clinic Committee provided shower and plumbing facilities for 17 student nurses who would reside there. The Gray Ladies gave 30,000 volunteer hours in 1942, an average of 2,500 hours a month, to maintain essential services in the hospital.

In the war effort, by early 1943 a cadet nurses corps was active in hospitals, with 26 student

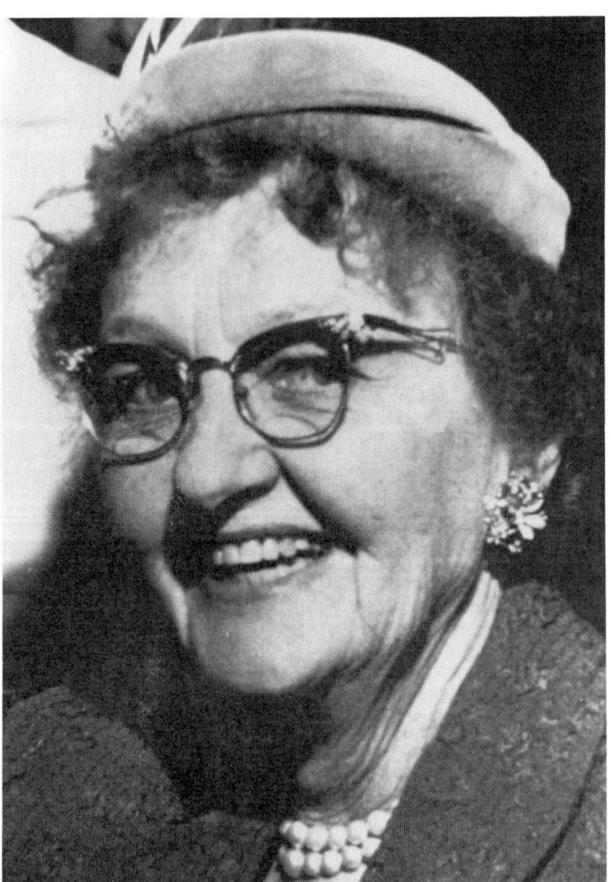

FIG. 58-4. Mrs. Willard M. Rice, III; founder of the Gray Ladies Unit at Jefferson in 1939.

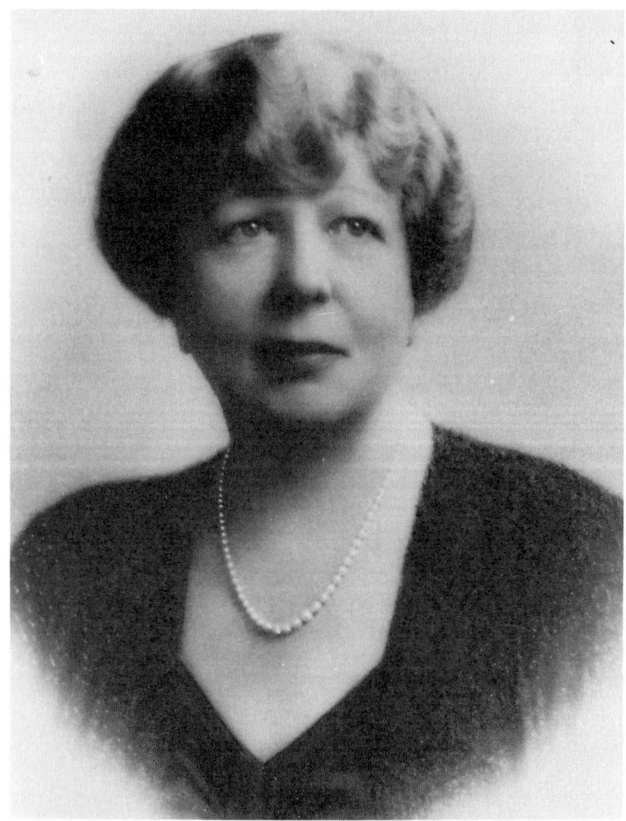

FIG. 58-5. Mrs. J. Howard Pew; President (1942–1947).

cadets at Jefferson. The tuition was paid by the government, but the cost to maintain each student was $254. The Women's Board financed one student nurse. In the fall of 1945 the cadet nurses corps was discontinued.

By February of 1944, 117 cadets resided at Tenth and Walnut Streets. A spinet piano was purchased for the wards at a cost of $231. The wards needed improvement in terms of lighting, ventilation, and floor covering. Ice water was being carried to inpatients and to clinics on litters. The House Committee supplied two volunteers daily to help sort linen, tidy the rooms, keep the drug department neat, and give sundry aid where needed. The Staff Nurses appealed to the Women's Board for support in their request for eight hours of duty instead of the existing 12, but this involvement was declined.

In 1945 the 109-member Women's Board still met in the Thompson Roof Garden. Receipts totalled $19,804 and expenditures $12,158. At year's end, six members of the Bronchoscopic Committee raised $5,000 in advertisements for the Charity Ball, the largest sum to that time. The Maternity Committee spent $2,250 for improvements in their division. The Public Wards Committee bought 100 bed lamps and 24 bedside tables. The Nurses' Home received a full tea service, and monthly teas for students began.

Mrs. Percival Foerderer (Figure 58-6) became President of the Board in 1947. She was considered a financial wizard, an innovative leader, and a superb organizer. She was responsible for first introducing a voice for the Women's Board on the Board of Trustees for establishment of the Joint Hospital Conference to further a closer working relationship. She also proposed that wives of the Trustees become members of the Executive Committee with full privileges, and that each committee should have a cochairman. The Finance Committee recommended that 5% of the total receipts in a year from any source be delegated to the Women Board's general fund, which at that time had a balance of $43.

For fund raising in 1948, a bridge party was held in McClellan Hall and a May tea and fashion show at the private residence of Mr. and Mrs. James Butt near Valley Forge. The Nurses' Home Committee established a memorial Altemus prize of $25 to be awarded annually at the graduation of the School of Nursing. The Barton Memorial Committee report of Mrs. J. Parsons Schaeffer indicated that in late 1946 the old Broad Street Hospital had been acquired and renovated, with Dr. Burgess Gordon as Medical Director. This supplanted the former 236–238 Pine Street Building for Diseases of the Chest. The Committee completely furnished the reception room with an oriental rug, love seat, chairs, lamps, mirror, and two torchéres for the lobby. Mrs. Edward L. Bauer appeared on radio station WIBG to talk about Jefferson. Receipts for 1948 totaled $15,726 and expenditures $7,720.

In 1949 the Women's Board joined a new state organization, the Pennsylvania Association of Hospital Auxiliaries under the aegis of the Pennsylvania Hospital Association. Mrs. J. Howard Pew was delegated to attend the first meeting of the Philadelphia region of this association. Mrs. Brandon Barringer was appointed Chairman for the Charity Ball, her members to consist of the Chairmen of all the

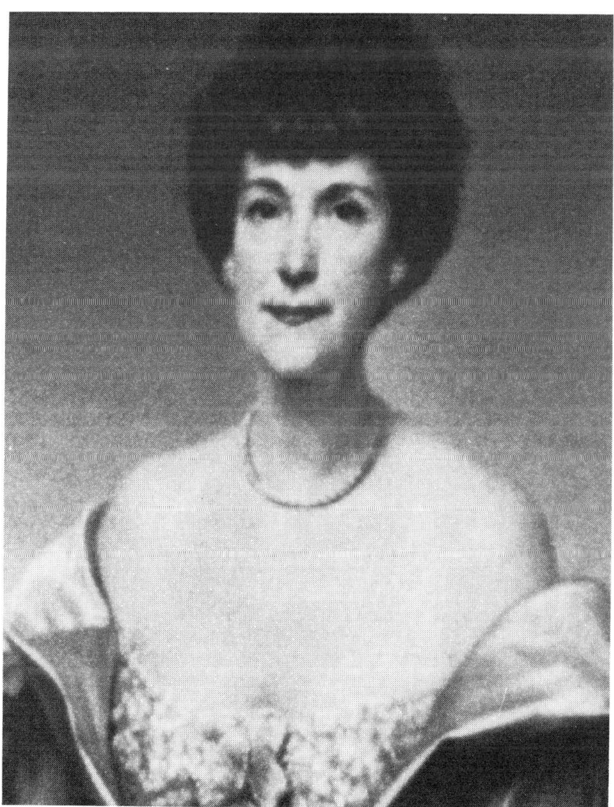

FIG. 58-6. Mrs. Percival Foerderer; President (1947–1952).

Board Committees. It was recommended also that the Board sponsor one large annual party for which all the committees would work. Receipts for the year were $15,685, and expenditures $8,391.

The 1950s

The Women's Board in 1950 had reached a membership of 261 plus seven honorary members, with Mrs. Percival Foerderer reelected as President. The Nursing School received a certificate of accreditation, which was displayed in the alcove. The Director of Nursing, Katherine Childs, requested the Board to grant scholarships in amounts of $100 to aid students through the first year of training because of economic distress in the upstate mining area from which so many promising applicants came. The Nurses' Home Committee responded with an amount of $800. The Maternity Department, under the Chairmanship of Dr. Thaddeus L. Montgomery, had 38 private and 38 ward beds. Sixteen hundred babies were delivered, of which 170 were premature. The Maternity Committee in this year started a project to photograph the newborns in addition to the footprint and the mother's thumbprint. The Public Wards Committee, grown to 27 members, was serving 250 patients on three floors. It purchased 200 bedside tables and desks for $1,196.

In January, 1951, a resolution of sympathy was sent to the family on the death of Mrs. J. Chalmers DaCosta, a founding member of the Board. On the death of Mrs. J. Dobson Altemus a plaque in her memory was installed on the ninth floor of the Thompson Annex. The Private Rooms Committee, responsible for six floors in the Thompson Annex as well as 42 scattered throughout other areas, arranged for their renovation. The Curtis Clinic Committee purchased parallel bars and a Strycher frame bed for the Physiotherapy Department at a cost of $300. Receipts for the year were $12,863, and expenditures $6,535.

Mrs. Thomas B.K. Ringe (Figure 58-7), who had been secretary of the Board for the previous ten years, became President in 1952. She was the daughter of Dr. J. Coles Brick, Professor of Proctology and a relative of the legendary Dr. J. Chalmers DaCosta. During this year the Joint Hospital Conference was operational, with the President of the Women's Board as a member.

Plans for a new hospital pavilion (Foerderer) surfaced in March, and Mrs. Joseph Eastwick was appointed Chairman of the New Building Committee. Vincent Kling, the architect, and four ladies of the Board visited hospital lobbies and furniture houses in New York for ideas in planning.

Mrs. Willard Rice, Chairman of the Public Wards Committee for 15 years, retired in 1953 as an honorary member. Ward visiting on a twice-weekly basis, instituted by her five years previously, was continued by the committee, which now numbered 35 active members. While operating the cart services in the hospital, volunteers wore the cherry red uniforms as mandated by the Association of Hospital Auxiliaries. The Junior Committee, chaired by Armason Harrison, functioned under the Nurses' Home Committee in the Cooperative Shop. It also established an endowment of $10,000 for the School of Nursing. This year marked the entry of Jefferson as a participant in the Christmas Bazaar

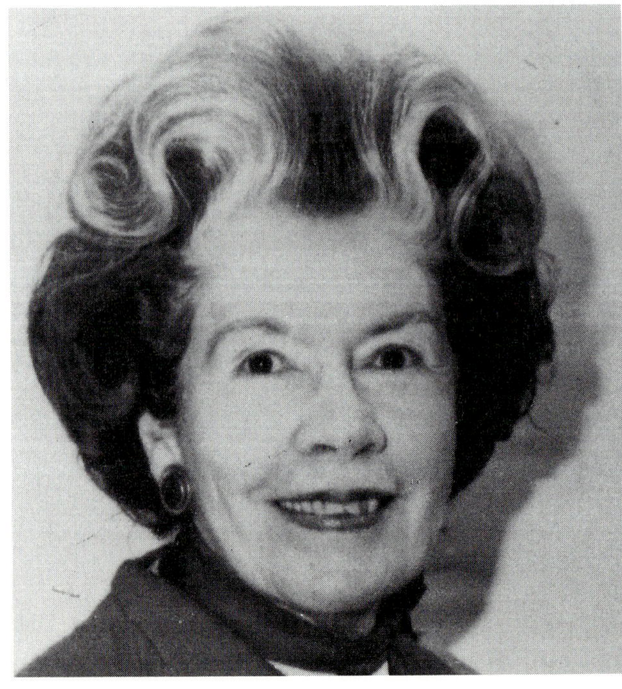

Fig. 58-7. Mrs. Thomas B.K. Ringe; President (1952–1956).

sponsored by the Emergency Aid of Pennsylvania. The Maternity Committee operated the Board's Booth and netted $1,210. From the sale of Jefferson glasses the Barton Committee gave $100 to the Nurses Alumni Fund to provide required nursing care to needy Alumni physicians. The Cooperative Shop had its best year ever, netting $38,210, with Jefferson receiving $2,302. Receipts for the year totaled $11,427, and expenditures $4,539. Mrs. Thomas James, director of the Gray Ladies for five and one half years, retired and was replaced by Virginia Metzger.

A new ruling in regard to the Charity Ball proceeds, whereby the chief beneficiary in a given year was to get one-half of the total amount (minus costs) and the remaining committees were to receive pro rata amounts, was established in 1954. Mrs. P. Brooke Bland was appointed chairman of the New Projects Committee. Annual receipts were $14,237, and expenditures $6,589. The Foerderer Pavilion, at a cost of seven and one-half million dollars, formally opened on November 8, 1954, and contained a Trustee Board Room on the fourteenth floor available to the Women's Board.

Mrs. Norman P. Russell, wife of a Trustee, was elected President in 1955. The House Committee aided in planning an ecumenical Meditation Room in the new Foerderer Pavilion. Mrs. Calvin Rankin, the new Chairman of the Public Wards Committee, reported that the wards needed remodeling at a projected cost of $500,000, but that an alternative of a new building for ward patients loomed in the future. Mrs. Ruhland Rebmann of the Social Service Committee voiced the growing need for a hospital volunteer director to coordinate the activities of the various workers, but the question of salary stymied the idea. Proceeds of $10,880 from the Charity Ball were allocated to 15 different committees. These funds were administered by Hospital Director Dr. Hayward Hamrick for the various expenditures of the committees. The Women's Board paid $100 annually to the American Hospital Association. From the Public Wards Committee there were 34 workers on the cart services, plus additional aid in other hospital services of workers from the Barton Committee, and 48 from the Social Service Committee. The Barton Committee purchased an iron lung (Figure 58-8) for $1,789, a ventilator for anesthesia for $517, and a television. Mrs. Norman Reeves became chairman of the House Committee. A new volunteer group entertained in the Children's Ward and helped to feed the children six days a week. The Curtis Clinic Committee received a grant of $10,000 from the Pew Memorial Foundation for the Emergency Room. Annual receipts were $16,949, with expenditures of $6,714.

The beginning of 1956 was saddened by the death of Mrs. James T. Haviland, a longtime devoted member of the Board. The School of Nursing Endowment Fund was given $500 as a memorial. This fund later became the Marjorie B. Haviland Fund and rapidly increased to $19,500. Three hundred copies of newly established bylaws were printed. The new Activities Committee sponsored a yearly dinner dance known as the "Salute to Spring." The first event netted $400. Miss Marian Hays was appointed Director of the Gray Ladies. The Barton Committee built and equipped a new kitchen. In connection with the construction of a new Nurses' Residence at Eleventh and Walnut Streets, the Pew, Ford, and Longwood Foundations had given $800,000. The Pew Foundation pledged an additional $200,000 if Jefferson could match this by March 1. As Building Fund chairman, Mrs. Paul Havens exceeded her $50,000 allocation by raising $76,000. In December the Meditation Room was dedicated with flowers from the Women's Board, a flag donated by the Gray Ladies, and a Bible from Mrs. Percival Foerderer. Annual receipts were $14,642, and expenditures $8,218.

In 1957 Dr. Ellsworth Browneller became the Medical Director, succeeding Dr. Hayward Hamrick, who had died the previous year. Mrs. H. Alarik Myrin (Figure 58-9), the newly elected President, obtained an Oldsmobile for $3,000, which netted a profit of $11,414 on chances. This was allocated to the new Martin Nurses' Residence. The Alcove Shop added $3,000 of accumulated funds for the same purpose. The Public Wards Committee instituted sundry improvements at a cost of $2,718. The Children's Ward Committee staged a baseball party at Connie Mack Stadium, which netted $650. The Maternity Committee gave $1,500 for air-conditioning in the nurseries. The Christmas Booth profits of $2,852 were given to the Obstetrics Department for cancer research. Annual receipts were $14,692, and expenditures $8,218.

Mrs. A. Balfour Brehman was the Board's nominee and winner of the 1958 Gimbel Award for her work with the blind. Because of the increasing importance of the Board's meetings, it was arranged for the minutes to be kept in the vaults of the Liberty Real Estate Bank and Trust Company. Agatha Rapp was appointed to the position of Volunteer Director at a salary of $3,600, one-half of which was paid by the Women's Board and the other half by the administration. Annual receipts were $17,930, and expenditures $5,590.

Mr. William Bodine became President of the College and Hospital in 1959. Dr. Ellsworth Browneller, the Medical Director, at his first meeting with the Women's Board, eulogized the members "who project the feminine genius for creating homelike atmosphere which in its way is as important as medical science in the hospital." The Public Wards Committee (Figure 58-10) initiated theater parties at Playhouse in the Park, and the first one netted $1,700. These ventures, successful for almost a decade, were eventually abandoned because of waning enthusiasm for the productions. The Maternity Committee realized $3,336 from the Christmas Booth of the Emergency Aid Bazaar and donated it for cancer research in the Department. The Board purchased a hypothermia unit for the operating room for $1,500, 33 wheelchairs for $3,000, and contributed

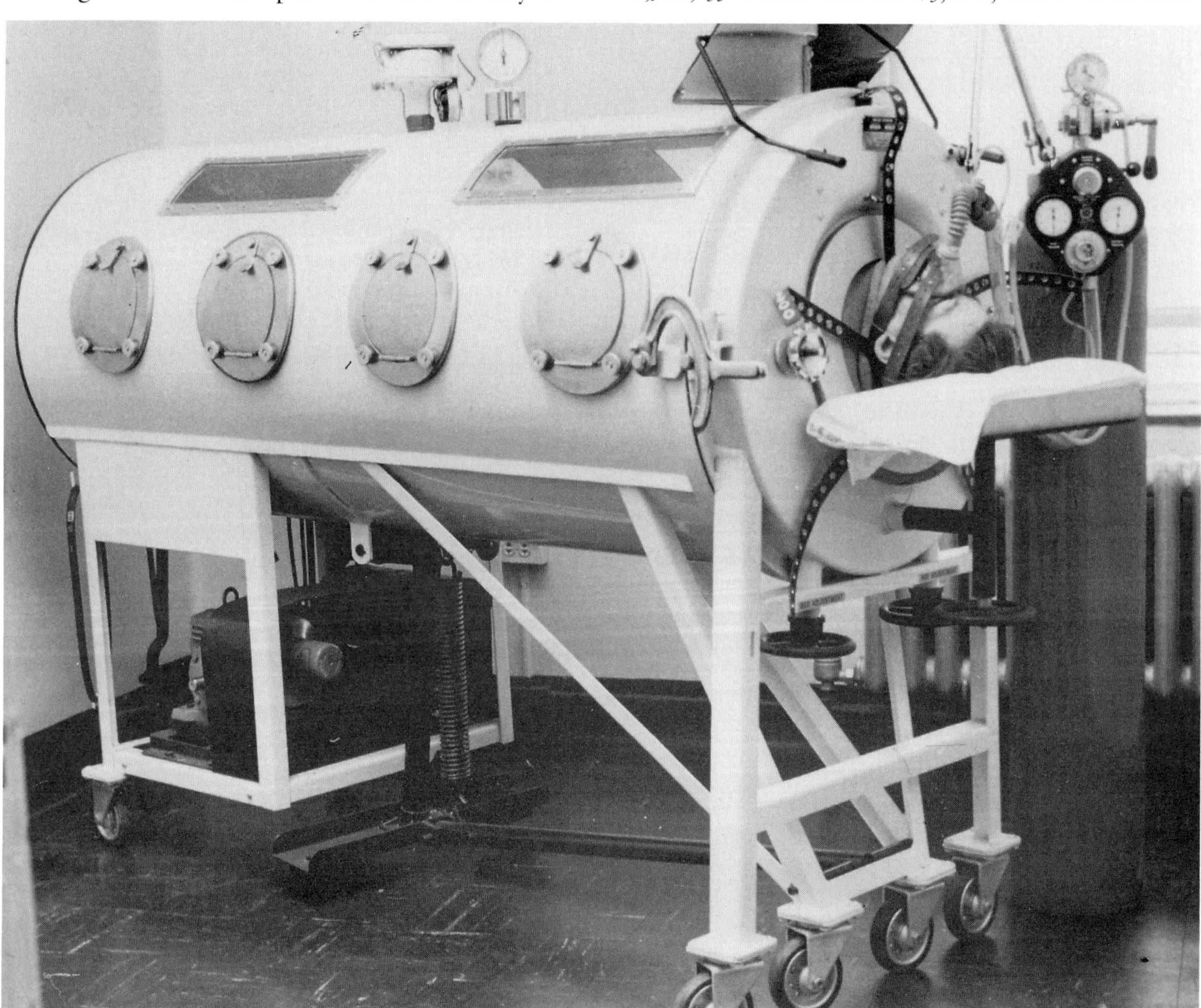

FIG. 58-8. The iron lung purchased by the Barton Committee in 1955.

She had rented a building in Ardmore for $185 a month and estimated that running expenses would average $450 a month. In its first month of operation the proceeds were $1,152. Each customer was given a bright new penny to symbolize the name of "The Pennywise Thrift Shop." A second large project, as suggested by President Bodine, was an Old Market Fair to be held in Society Hill on Head House Square. It was hoped that this unified Board event would raise $25,000 annually. At this period the administration alerted the Board concerning the growing hospital deficits, with the possible necessity of eliminating free care as well as closing the School of Nursing. A petition was sent to the Pennsylvania legislature asking full reimbursement for indigent care.

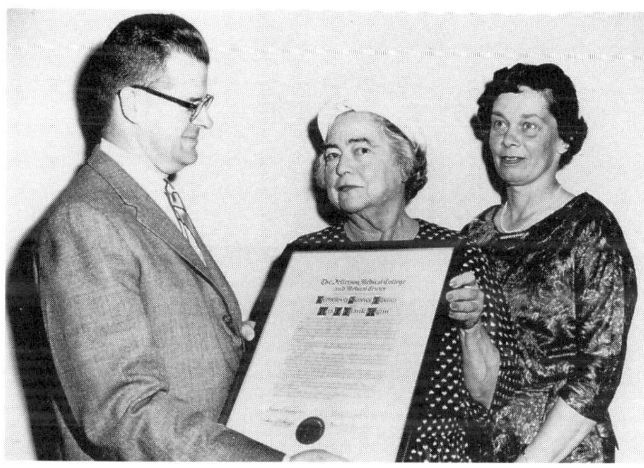

FIG. 58-12. William Bodine presents a citation to Mrs. H. Alarik Myrin and Mrs. Robert Liversidge, Incoming President.

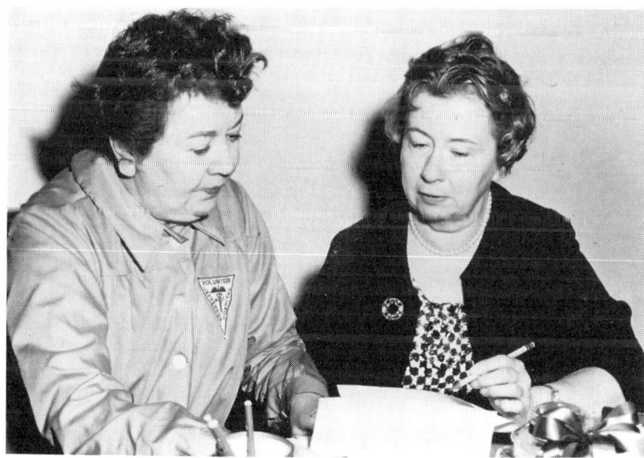

FIG. 58-13. Mrs. Calvin Rankin, Founder of the Pennywise Thrift Shop, and Thelma Reed, first Manager, 1961.

The term of Presidency was extended from two years to three, following which there would be no further eligibility for this office.

The various committees purchased labor beds, recovery stretchers, electric beds, intermittent positive pressure breathing machines, water coolers, laundry carts, stacking chairs, and rugs. A seamstress made draperies for patient rooms at $2 per pair. Twelve private rooms on the ninth, eleventh, and twelveth floors of Thompson Annex, and Star floor of the Foerderer Pavilion were redecorated. The library on the fiftheenth floor of the Foerderer Pavilion and the Library on the fifteenth floor of the Thompson Annex, where the Women's Board met, were also redecorated. The sum of $3,000 was contributed for student nurses' loans and scholarships.

Income for this year was lower because there were no more funds from the Cooperative Shop and ten committees had loaned $1,000 each to begin the intensive care unit, in which the total cost of $30,000 was born by the Board.

At the annual meeting in May, 1962, plans for the Thompson Annex expansion, at a cost of $850,000, were outlined. More significantly, a fund-raising campaign for $40 million was detailed, and Mrs. Michael Foley was appointed Chairman for the Board to raise a set quota of $225,000 for the Building Fund.

Early in the year Dr. Ellsworth Browneller resigned as Medical Director to go to Geisinger Memorial Hospital. The first President of the Faculty Wives Club, Mrs. William Sodeman, was made a member of the Executive Committee, with the agreement that succeeding presidents would be represented on the Women's Board.

The first luncheon for Pennywise Shop volunteers was held in May at the Philadelphia Country Club, where it was announced that the first year's profits from the Shop were $6,168. Need for increased space was evident, and Mrs. Myrin was to search for larger quarters. The Alcove Shop of the hospital netted $10,103.

Anesthesia equipment was 15 years old and required replacement; a new resuscitation machine for the intensive care unit, a gas machine, and a ventilator for pediatric surgery were procured. The Public Wards Committee accepted the fourteenth floor Thompson psychiatric unit as its responsibility and changed the committee name to "Martha Jefferson."

In 1963 the membership of the Board totaled 241. Mrs. Gilbert Fry (Figure 58-14) was installed as the new President. Maurice P. Coffee, Jr., became the new Medical Director of the Hospital. The Joint Hospital Conference appointed Mabel Prevost as liaison with the Women's Board for the building fund-raising campaign. The School of Nursing was accredited for six more years.

The various committees contributed their usual share of philanthropic activity, but the big event was the Board's success in the fund-raising campaign. Mrs. Robert Liversidge announced that a total of $266,831 was subscribed to the building fund by 196 members, a participation of 80%. A luncheon was held in honor of the leadership of Mrs. Michael Foley, at which President Bodine bestowed upon her the Jefferson Service Award. In surpassing its quota the Board's final total was $280,000.

The November Emergency Aid Christmas Bazaar was postponed in respect for the funeral of the assassinated President John F. Kennedy. The year 1964 began on an additional sad note with the death of Mrs. J. Howard Pew, an untiring dedicated worker for Jefferson. In January the Board gave Natalie Hubschman a citation for her work on the Charity Ball program, which netted an all-time high of $18,391 (Figure 58-15).

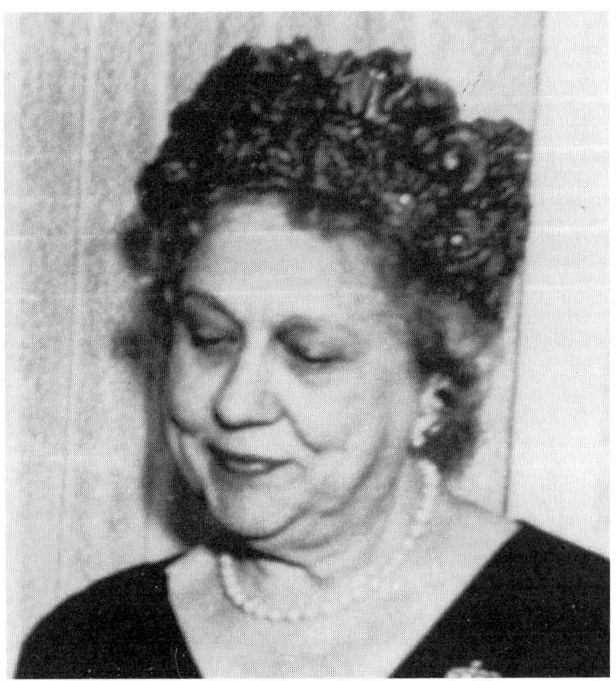

FIG. 58-14. Mrs. Gilbert Fry; President (1963–1966).

The Medical Director, Maurice Coffee, alerted the Board to the severe shortage of nurses. The salary of a nurse was $340 a month. Special efforts were made to recruit nurses from the Scranton area, where there apparently was a surplus, and Mrs. Daniel Rhoads made a visit to the Philippines where she successfully recruited for Jefferson.

President Bodine requested that the fiscal year be set to end June 30 in conformity with hospital policy.

Plans for an Old Market Fair for the following year included loans of $200 from each committee for supplies and booths. Hospital equipment was purchased, some rooms renovated, and closed-circuit television provided.

In January, 1965, the Rooms and House Committees merged, and the Children's Committee ran the Emergency Aid booth. On the ensuing March 30, Mrs. Herbert Luscombe and Mrs. Paul Bowers instituted Doctor's Day at Jefferson. Mrs. Baldwin Keyes in the previous year had asked the Board to observe this national event, established in 1958 by the U.S. Congress, by presenting carnations to the physicians. The Board purchased 300 at 12¢ each, and a committee

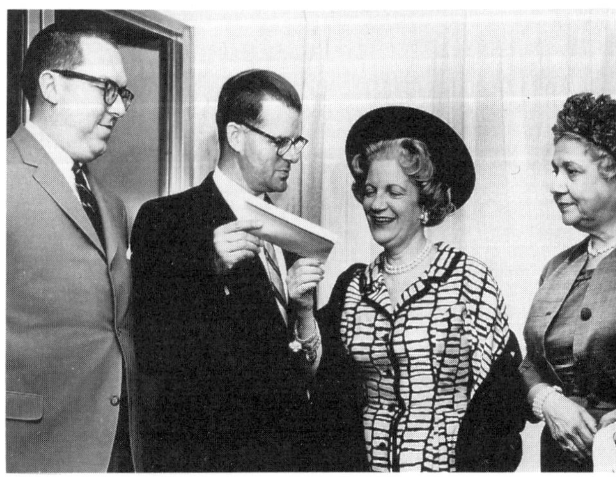

FIG. 58-15. Maurice Coffee, Hospital Director; William Bodine, President; Natalie Hubschman; and Mrs. Gilbert Fry, at the presentation to Mrs. Hubschman of a citation for a most successful Charity Ball.

distributed them at the hospital entrances. On May 1, the first Old Market Fair was held in Society Hill on a permit granted by the City. The first Chairman was Mrs. Michael Foley. Some of the workers for the booths wore colonial costumes (Figure 58-16). The event grossed $11,036, with a net profit of $7,632, and additional donations brought the final net to $10,089. These funds were allocated to upgrade the five nurseries of the Maternity Department as mandated by the City Health Department.

The Pennywise Shop profits were growing steadily and grossed $27,144 for the fiscal year ending June 30, 1965. Mrs. Myrin found a property at 57 E. Lancaster Avenue in Ardmore, to which the Shop moved when the doors closed in June. This property, at a cost of $22,000, was to be paid for from savings and a mortgage of $14,000 personally assumed by Mrs. Myrin at 4%. It was to be dissolved at $5,000 annually.

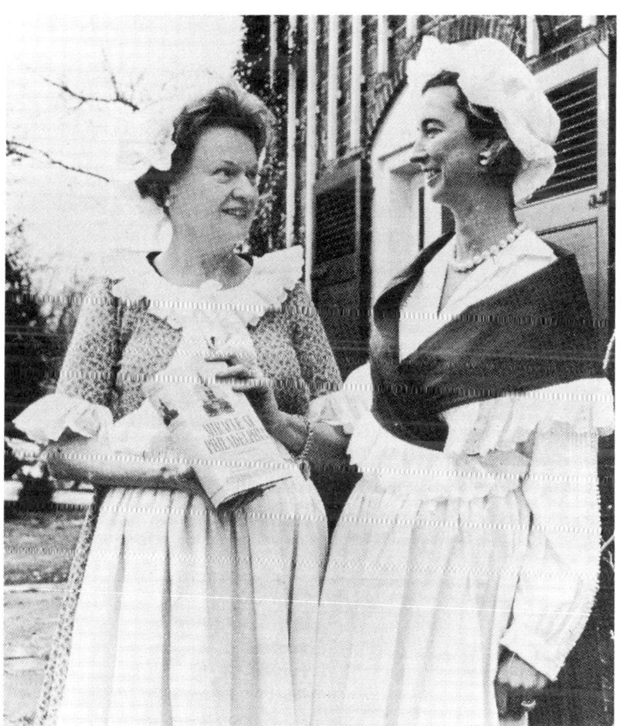

FIG. 58-16. Mrs. Michael Foley and Mrs. Samuel M.V.H. Hamilton. The Old Market Fair, 1965.

At the November meeting Mrs. Foerderer announced she had been advised by the Administration that there was no further need for the Hospital Committee and that Board members would no longer inspect hospital areas without permission. A letter expressing the Board's extreme dissatisfaction with this new policy was sent to Mr. Bodine. In compliance, however, a balance of $2,500 in the now-defunct Hospital Committee plus a gift of $5,000 from the Curtis Clinic Committee was paid to the decorator for the Foerderer Pavilion Star floor renovation.

The first significant event of 1966 was a meeting in February of Mrs. Liversidge with William Bodine and Maurice Coffee regarding inspections in the hospital with respect to maintenance, for which the Board had shown such interest and allocated so much money. A compromise was reached in that instead of the former Hospital Committee each of the various committees would send two members to visit each month. Mr. Bodine announced that he was resigning as President.

In March, three members of the Board, Lynn Dowling, Hattie Williams, and Mrs. Eloise Bowers appeared on television to advertise the approaching Old Market Fair. Twenty-five Board members were in the audience for the quiz show "Dolls and Dollars" (Figure 58-17). The affair netted $5,358, which once again was allocated to upgrading of the nurseries.

Mrs. Robert Wise became Chairman of the Pennywise Shop, and Mrs. Jane Trent was hired as Manager.

At the annual May meeting William Bodine outlined plans for the New Jefferson Hall, later to be called Jefferson Alumni Hall, to open in the summer of 1967 (Figure 58-18). James Large, Trustee, detailed the great strides made by Bodine during the seven years he was in office. He also spoke of the major goals for the upcoming eight years leading to the Sesquicentennial of the Medical College in 1974. They included construction of an Emergency Department, to cost in excess of $1 million, leading from the thruway between College and Thompson Annex into the area occupied by the amphitheater. A silver bowl as a retirement gift from the Board was presented to Mr. Bodine. Dr. Peter Herbut was to become the new President for Jefferson.

In 1967 Maurice Coffee resigned, and Dr. Francis J. Sweeney, Jr., became the Medical Director of the Hospital. This period marked the advent of Medicare and the end of ward care for patients. The fourth and sixth floors of the old Main Hospital had been condemned by state inspectors and the highest priority was given to their renovation, which would be the first in those areas for more than 60 years. Mrs. Paul Bowers and members of the Martha Jefferson Committee conducted a thorough inspection of the ward floors, to which the Administration responded by sanctioning long-overdue improvements in all areas related to patient care. Renovation costs were set at $94,000 plus more than $40,000 for decorating. The Martha Jefferson Committee pledged $10,000 to the project and Mrs. Drew Betz donated an additional $10,000. The Board voted to undertake refurbishing of the sixth floor at a cost not to exceed $40,000. A new 55-bed unit was developed for which the patient day rate was $28.

Mrs. Paul Bowers became the Jefferson representative to the Pennsylvania Association of Hospital Auxiliaries and served for 11 years in this capacity. She was also the Health Careers Program Chairman and instituted the first Health Careers Day, held in McClellan Hall for secondary public and private school students to become acquainted with the many opportunities in the health field and thus to alleviate manpower shortages. She was influential in getting Governor Raymond P. Shafer to declare November as Health Careers Month in Pennsylvania.

In the spring of 1968 the Board pledged $200,000 over a period of two years of renovate the fourth floor of the old Main Hospital. The Activities Committee auctioned a large shipment of furniture donated by Sloan's in New York, a gift arranged by Gustave Amsterdam, which netted $4,500. Mrs. Amsterdam, Chairman of the

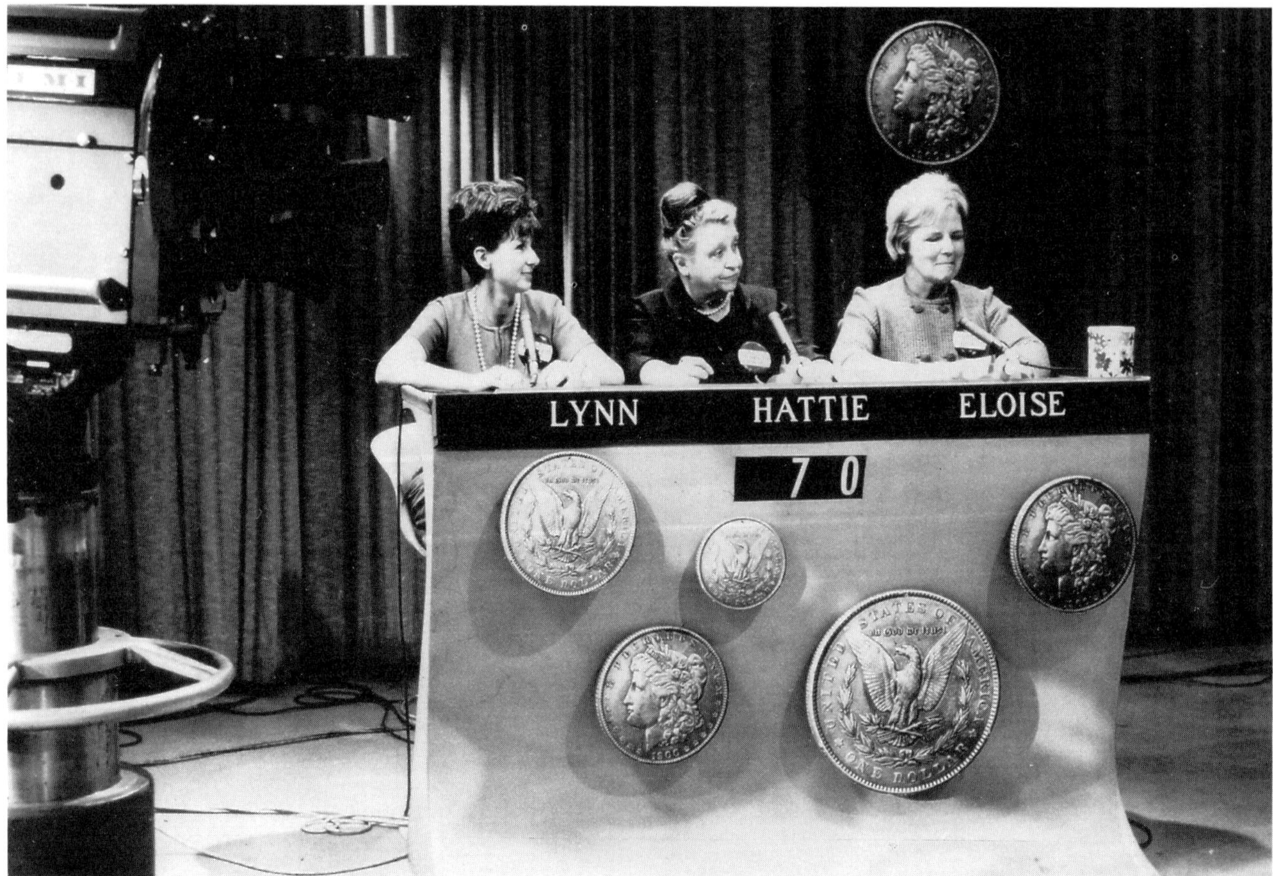

FIG. 58-17. "Dolls and Dollars," a TV Quiz Show, 1966, advertised the Old Market Fair. Left to right are Lynn Dowling, Hattie Williams and Eloise Bowers.

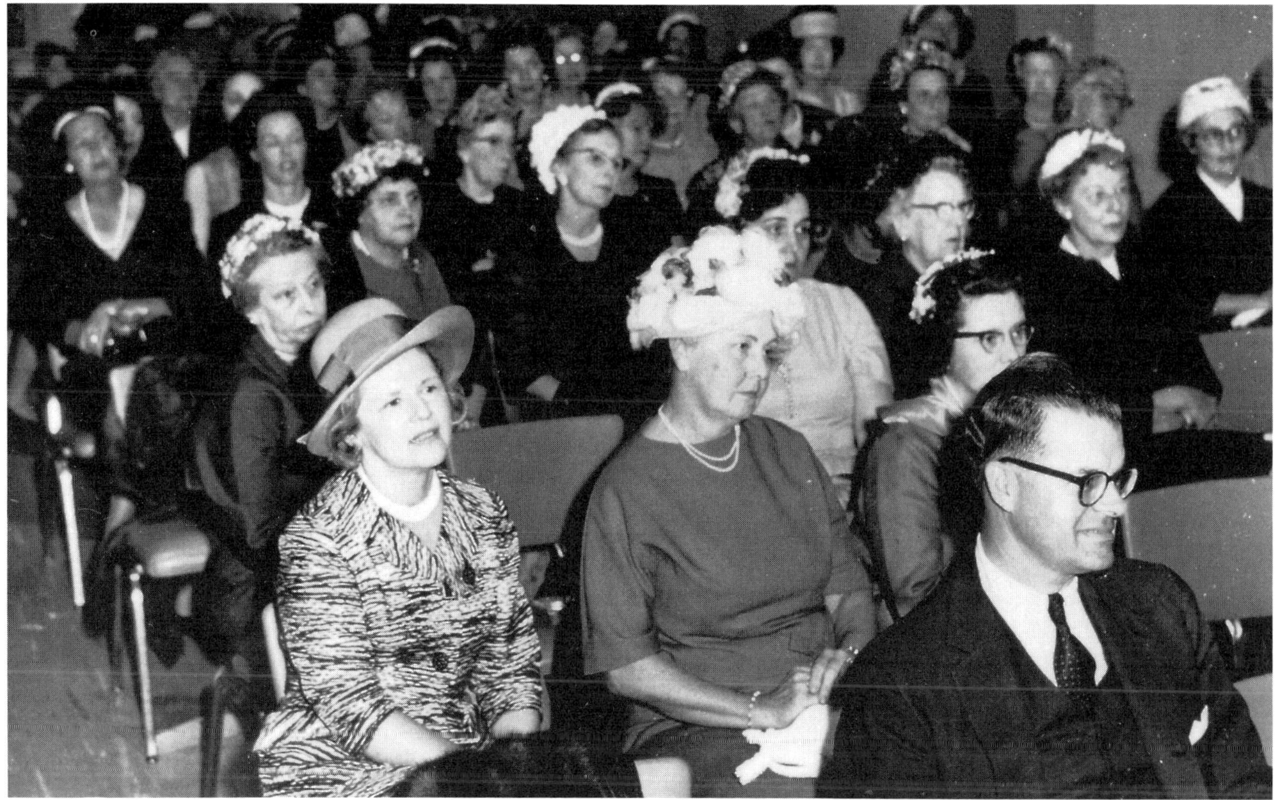

FIG. 58-18. Annual Meeting, May, 1966, in the James Martin Nurses Residence.

1968 Old Market Fair, also secured a Plymouth car to be "chanced off" (Figure 58-19). A patron's letter was started, with a mailing list of 4,000 names. The Phantom Valentine Party was eliminated, and a cocktail-fashion show at Nan Duskin, held in April as a pre-Fair event, was established. Proceeds from the Fair amounted to $36,478, with expenses of $7,892. Mrs. William Bodine was appointed Chairman for 1969. The tenth and last Playhouse in the Park event netted $1,168 for the Martha Jefferson Committee.

The Pennywise Shop grossed $36,390 with a net profit of $15,371. The Maternity Committee purchased a respiratory isolette for premature babies at $5,000, and the Bronchoscopic Committee gave an operating room table costing $3,785. New beds, furniture, and a television were also supplied.

By the end of 1968 the mortgage on the Pennywise Shop was paid in full, and the building was owned by the Board. A mortgage-burning party was held, and the ashes were saved for the cornerstone of a building that might be erected in the future (Figure 58-20). Most of the Shop's volunteers at this time were nonmembers of the Board.

In 1969 a citation was bestowed on Mrs.

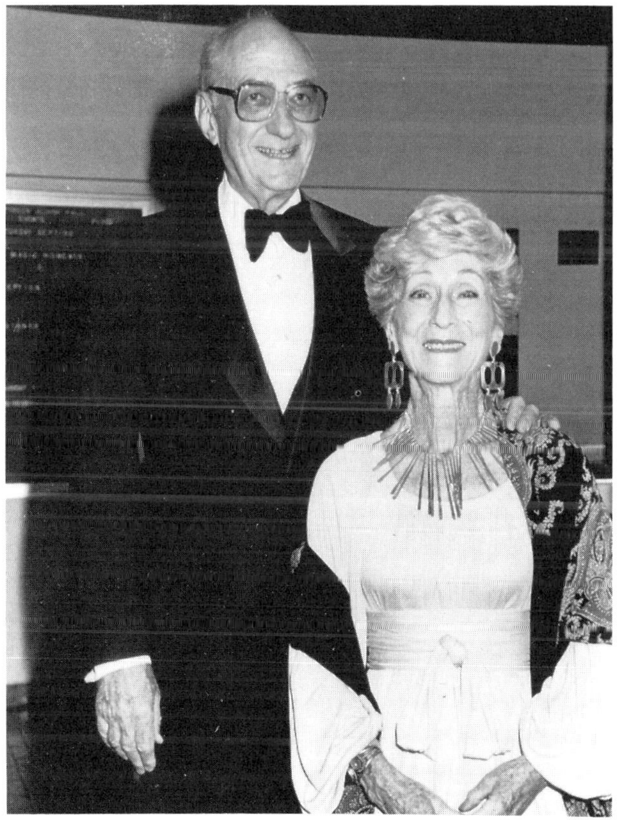

FIG. 58-19. Mr. and Mrs. Gustave Amsterdam.

Michael Foley (Figure 58-21), the outgoing President. Mrs. Samuel M.V.H. Hamilton (Figure 58-22) was installed as President. It was ruled that all past presidents would serve as an advisory council. Mrs. Horace Williams resigned after having served 15 years as Treasurer. During the summer the Pennywise Shop purchased the Pep Boys Store next door for $40,000. This wise move was justified by increasing inventory and profits. Plaques honoring the renovations by the Women's Board were installed on the fourth and sixth floors of the old Main Hospital. The Old Market Fair earned $23,175. In December, Mrs. Sherman Eger reactivated the Children's Committee. Susan B. Bland died, and her daughter donated 30 unframed paintings by her mother to the Board for use in decorating the Hospital.

The 1970s

In 1970 the Women's Board consisted of nine committees. Meetings were moved to the Thompson Annex Auditorium. Priority was given to plans for funding a heliport on top of the Foerderer Pavilion. The Martha Jefferson Committee donated $3,500 to furnish the Family Therapy Unit at the Community Health Center on Twelfth Street. A plaque to honor Lillian James, a longtime member of this Committee, was installed in this new facility.

An Eakins Exhibition and Reception in March, 1971, at the Philadelphia Museum of Art was supported by the mailing of 6,000 invitations. The Pennsylvania Association of Hospital Auxiliaries requested a member of the Jefferson Women's Board to serve as Treasurer for this organization. Mrs. Benjamin Haskell volunteered and was duly elected. Mrs. Samuel Hamilton served as Chairman of the 1971 Old Market Fair. The

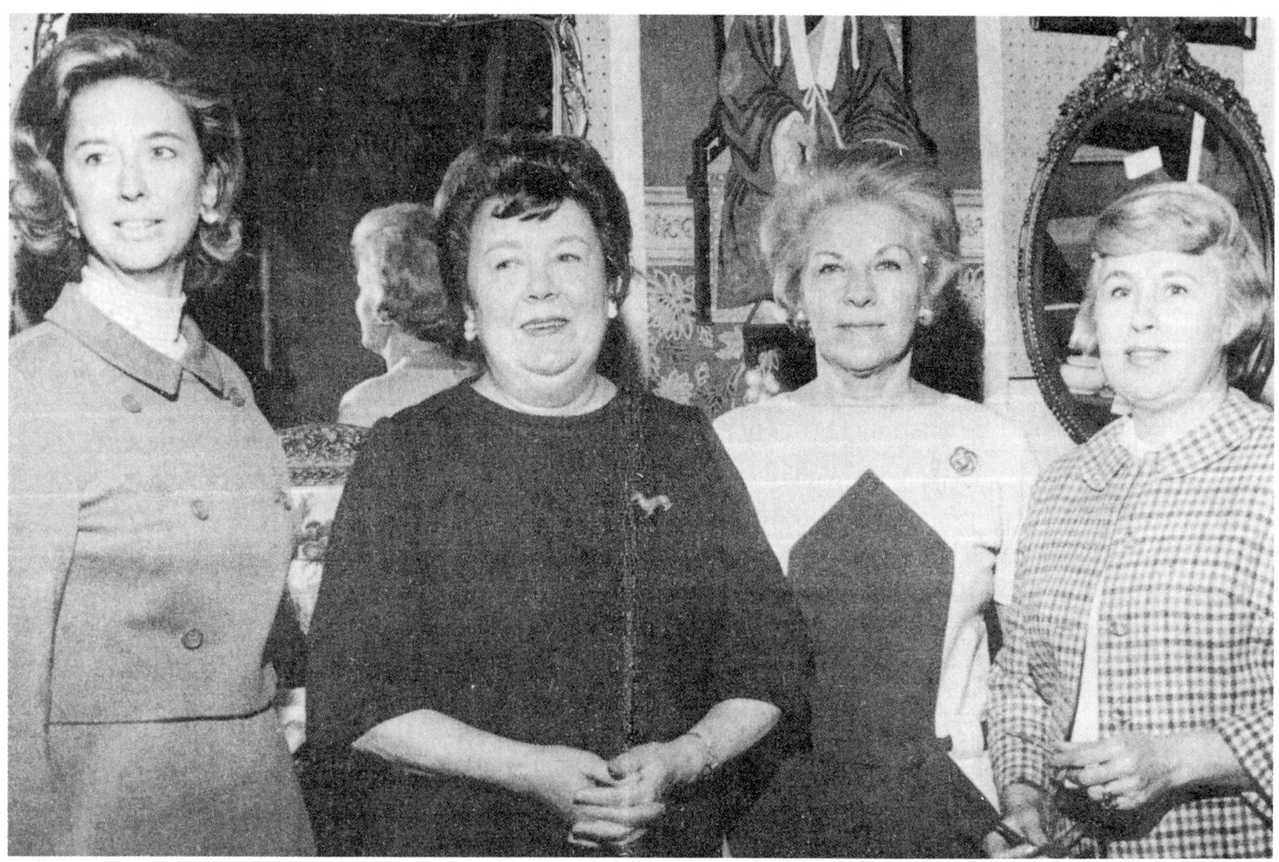

FIG. 58-20. The Mortgage-Burning Party, 1968. Left to right: Mrs. Samuel M.V.H. Hamilton, Mrs. Calvin Rankin, Mrs. Frank Fogarty, and Jane Trent.

proceeds of $10,660 were allotted to the heliport project. The Pennywise Shop (Figure 58-23) had a net profit of $35,000. The total contribution to the hospital by all the committees that year was $157,904. In September, Mabel Prevost announced to the Board that the Health Careers Program begun in 1967 would be terminated, citing an austerity policy in all hospital areas as the reason. The wards' cart service of the Martha Jefferson Committee was experiencing a shortage of volunteers. The Volunteer Department of the Hospital was called upon to take over this management.

The heliport, designed for special emergencies, was funded for $85,000 by the Women's Board and dedicated in September, 1971 (Figures 58-24 and 58-25). In November, Mrs. Calvin Rankin and Mrs. Alarik Myrin were honored at the Pennywise Shop's luncheon for the volunteers. The ten-year profit of the Shop since its inception totaled $147,000. On one occasion a Rembrandt print was sold there for $600. An unrestricted gift of $2,500 was donated to the Hospital in memory of Mrs. Myrin who had recently died.

The Salute to Spring dinner dance of the Activities Committee was held at the new Philadelphia County Medical Society building on Spring Garden Street.

In January, 1972, the Women's Board solicited the Board of Trustees for funds to buy an automobile for the Old Market Street Fair. The Charity Ball expenses were $6,000 greater this year because of the first debutante presentations, which resulted in smaller allocations to the various hospitals. A refurbished portrait of Clara Melville, former Director of Nurses, was hung in the Nurses' Residence lounge. The Curtis Clinic Committee considered disbanding after the death of Mrs. Myrin, but on advice of the

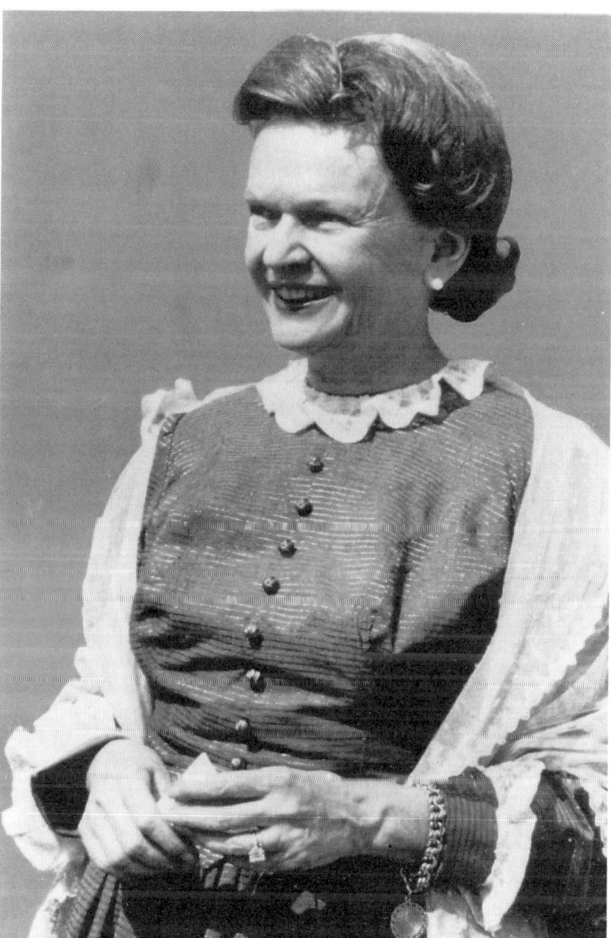

FIG. 58-21. Mrs. Michael A. Foley; President (1966–1969).

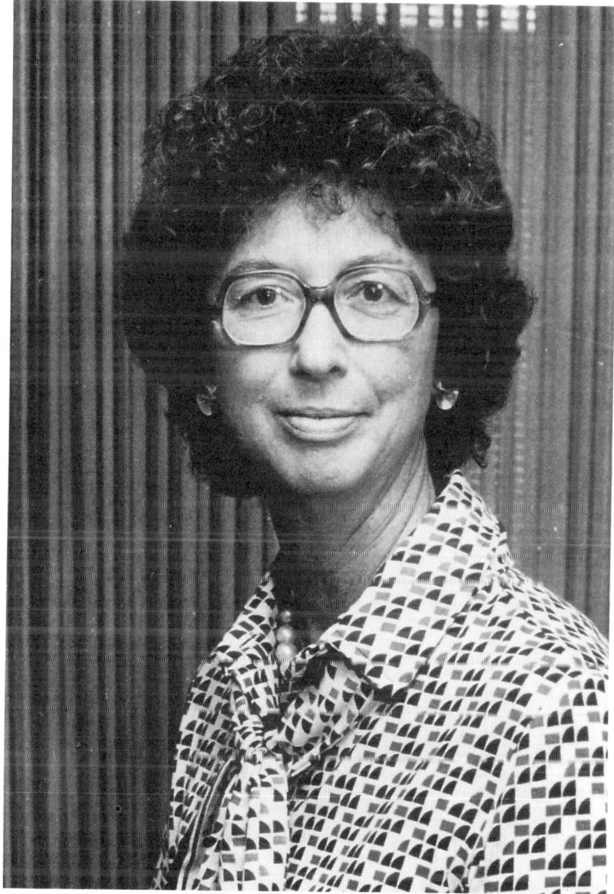

FIG. 58-22. Mrs. Samuel M.V.H. Hamilton; President (1969–1972).

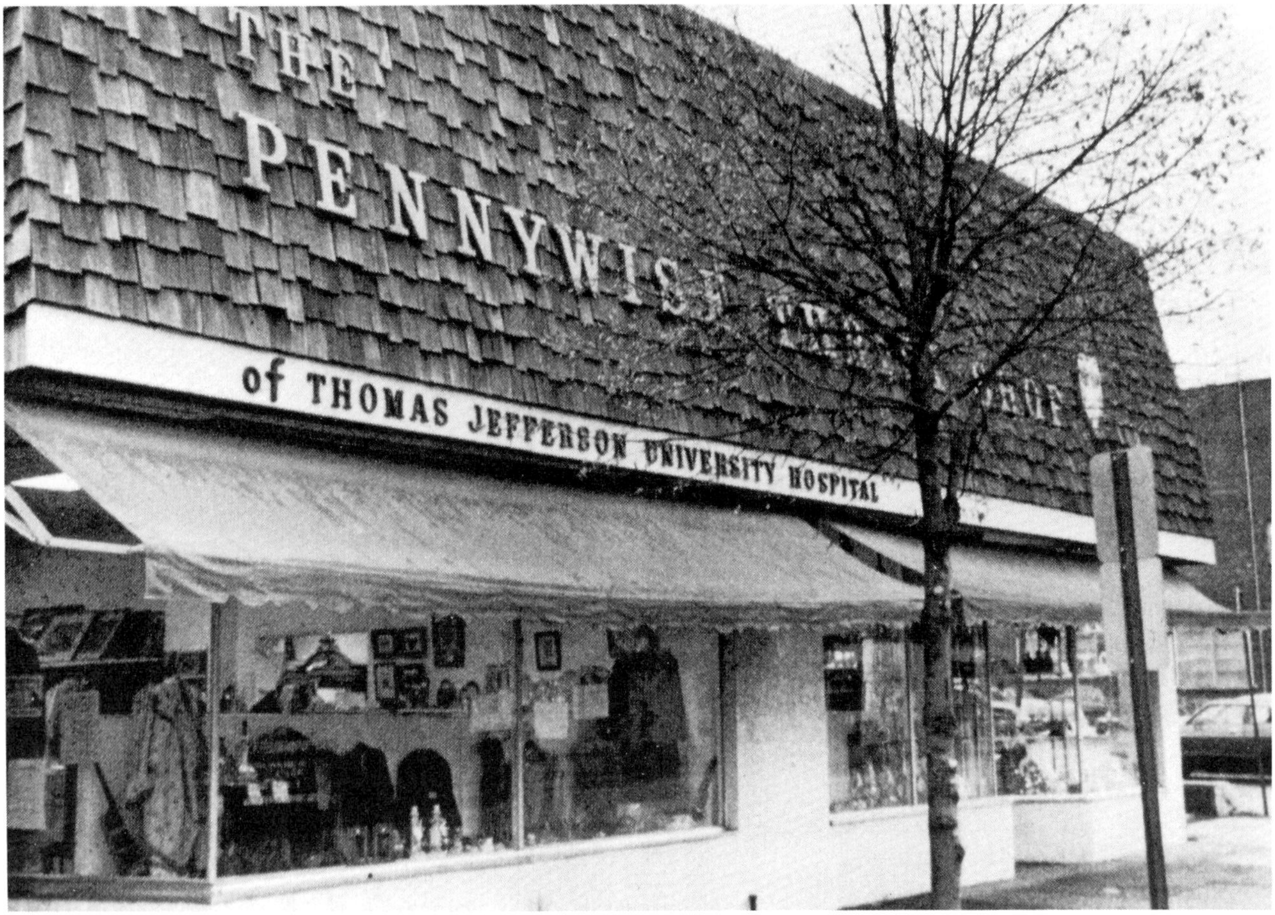

FIG. 58-23. The Pennywise Thrift Shop, Ardmore, Pennsylvania.

Administration to continue, the helm was taken by Mrs. Robert Liversidge. The Maternity Committee purchased two isolettes for $3,142 and a cardiac monitor for $2,500. It also donated $2,000 for the transport of high-risk infants to Jefferson by helicopter for patients unable to pay for this cost. An allocation of $15,000 for the kidney dialysis unit was made, and residual funds allocated for the intensive care unit of the nursery.

In May, 1972, Mrs. James P. Cavanaugh (Figure 58-26) was elected President. She reinstated the Projects Committee with Mrs. Ralph Carabasi as Chairman. By November, plans for the first Jefferson Jewel Party were underway with Mrs. James Meyers as Chairman. An exquisite brooch was donated by a New York jeweler, David Webb. In February, 1973, Mrs. Paul Bowers presented a workshop on career recruitment for the Pennsylvania Association of Hospital Auxiliaries at Presbyterian Hospital. She had previously presented a seminar for this association at the annual state conference at Penn State University. The Curtis Clinic Committee undertook the

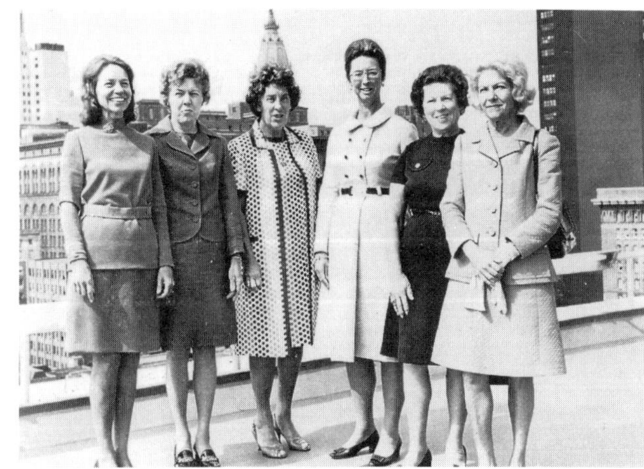

FIG. 58-24. The Jefferson Hospital Heliport Dedication, September, 1971. From left to right: Mrs. Frederick Schmidt, Mrs. John Kreemer, Mrs. Thomas Mangan, Mrs. Samuel Hamilton, Mrs. Thomas McDevitt and Mrs. Frank Fogarty.

project of furnishing the public rooms in the Edison Building at a cost of $10,000 as a memorial to Mrs. Myrin.

In May, Mrs. Samuel Vauclain became Chairman of the Pennywise Shop. In August, the shop occupied its new enlarged quarters, which included the adjacent recently purchased Pep Boys store. There was poor response to the need for more volunteers, with only 55 workers on small shifts. Theft was becoming a problem. In 1973 a Jefferson student won the scholarship initiated by Mrs. Bowers and funded through the generosity of the American Legion's Helen Fairchild Nurses Post No. 412. By then there were three male student nurses in Jefferson's freshman class.

The Women's Board was informed in October that the quota for the Sesquicentennial (1824–1974) Campaign was set at $100,000. In November, Betty Trowbridge, Charity Ball Chairman, presented a detailed accounting of the declining proceeds of this program since 1965. A serious study for further participation was recommended, but no action was taken. In December the Martha Jefferson Committee contributed $7,500 to the Ophthalmology Department for purchase of a Zeiss slit lamp for stereophotography in the care of nearly 4,000 patients yearly. At the same meeting Michael Bradley, the hospital's certified public accountant, offered free auditing of the books of the Board as well as an annual overview of the Board's financial resources. The Martha Jefferson Committee at this time established house tours in Society Hill to aid the Old Market Fair.

In January, 1974, the Pennywise Shop received an $11,000 donation that provided a new furnace and needed repairs. William Bodine explained that the goal of Sesquicentennial Campaign was a new clinical teaching facility (hospital) at a cost of $65 million. Edwin Taylor, the Medical Director, and Michael Bradley, from accounting, explained the internal revenue rulings that mandated that funds must be spent in the year raised.

The School of Nursing in October moved its offices to the Health Sciences Center and supervision of the Nurses' Residence was turned

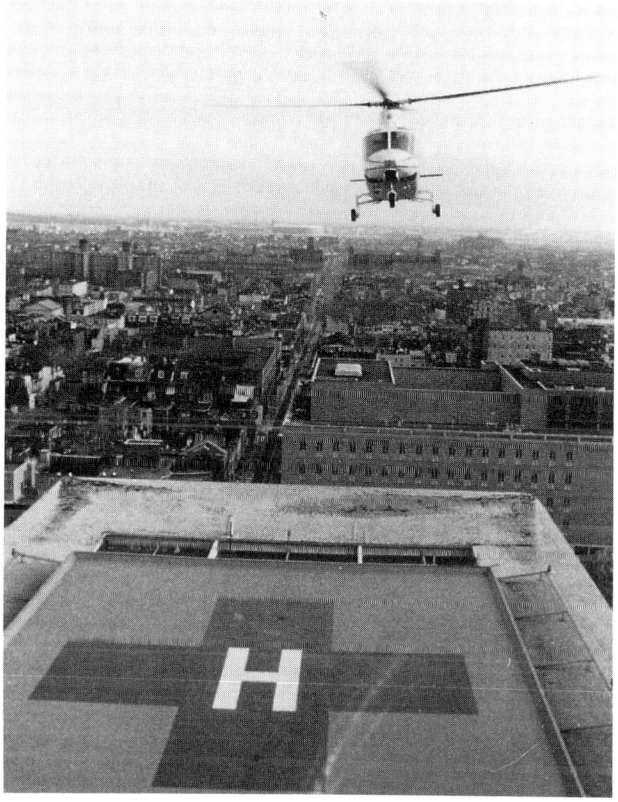

FIG. 58-25. Jefferson's heliport, dedicated September, 1971.

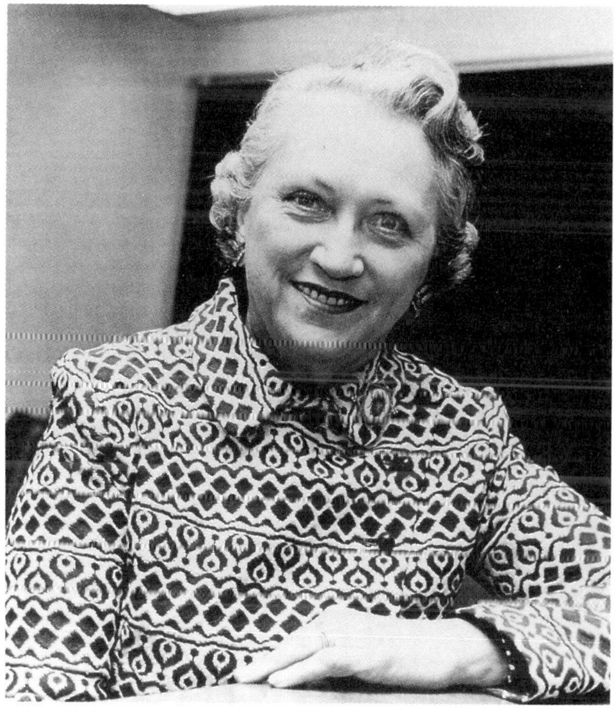

FIG. 58-26. Mrs. James P. Cavanaugh; President (1972–1975).

over to the University Housing Authority. Meetings of the Board were now held in the fourteenth floor Board Room of the Foerderer Pavilion. Revision of the bylaws was ordered.

The Martha Jefferson Committee sponsored a citywide sculpture tour with luncheon at Alden Park Manor, which was well subscribed. Each committee had the privilege of choosing its own project to support and the choices suggested by the Administration were not binding. In this year the Board allocated $75,000 for an acute respiratory care unit for the Barton Memorial Hospital. The Board contributed to Christmas decorations for the Hospital. Suggested sites for holding the second Jefferson Jewel Party were the Tonner estate and "Sugar Loaf." An unrestricted contribution of $5,000, sent by Martha Jefferson member, Mrs. Helen Lavine, was applied to the Sesquicentennial Campaign fund.

In January, 1975, the Whirly Girls, an international group of women pilots, presented the Judy Short Award to the Women's Board for establishment of the heliport at Jefferson.

The Pennywise Shop received a gift of $14,550 that was to be used for physical improvements of the building. The founder of the shop, Mrs. Calvin Rankin, died in February, and a memorial fund was established in her name.

The Sesquicentennial Campaign ended in May 1975, with $83,038 received from a 29% participation of members of the Women's Board. Medical Director Edwin Taylor reported that a new hospital with 411 beds was to be built in the next 36 to 39 months. The Board also allocated $55,000 for a new autoclave and to provide residual funds for renovation of the acute psychiatric unit. The Charity Ball was held in December at the Sheraton Hotel with proceeds of $2,188. Mrs. Samuel Vauclain, III (Figure 58-27) became the fourteenth President in May, 1975.

In January, 1976, the Martha Jefferson Committee commissioned a memorial portrait of Mrs. Calvin Rankin to be painted by Board member Mrs. Paul Poinsard. This was dedicated on May 24 and hung in the psychiatric unit. Samuel Vauclain became Treasurer of the Pennywise Shop in February, and Oliver Robbins was elected to account for consignment bookkeeping and monthly statements. A luncheon was held for the 75 volunteers on March 31 at the Merion Cricket Club, at which President Peter Herbut spoke briefly. The entire Jefferson community was shocked to learn of Dr. Herbut's sudden death later that afternoon.

The 1977 Jefferson Jewel, a diamond bracelet valued at $3,000, was purchased for $1,000. The chances netted $8,720. That year Bailey, Banks, and Biddle hosted a benefit party for the Women's Board, and Community Clothes for Charity selected Jefferson as its beneficiary. The Pennywise Shop conducted its first house sale, which netted $30,000 and reported a 40% increase in profits over the previous ten years.

At the October general meeting of the Board, Dr. Lewis Bluemle, the new University President who had assumed office in August, was introduced. He informed the Board that the State Legislature had vetoed a $750,000 appropriation to Jefferson and thus the funds provided by the Board now counted as hard dollars in terms of dependability.

For the 1977 year, $12,365 was donated for emergency room needs and $94,215 for capital needs. A plaque honoring the Board for its contributions toward renovation of the Foerderer

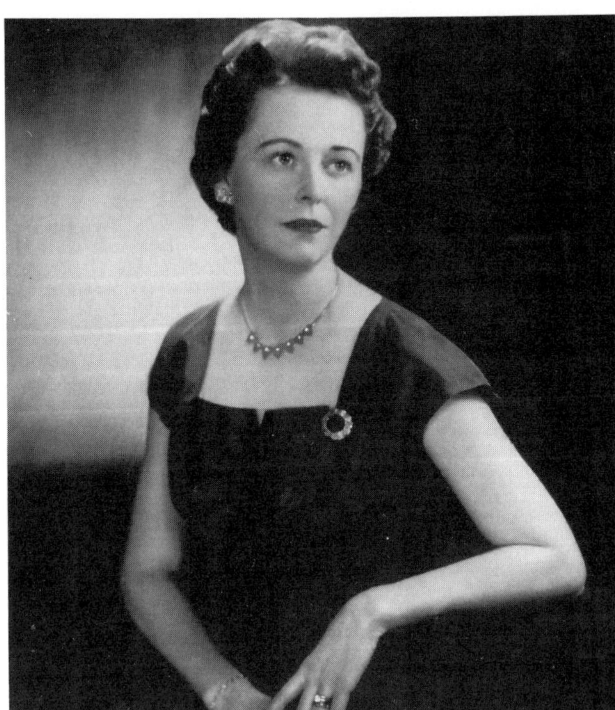

FIG. 58-27. Mrs. Samuel M. Vauclain, III; President (1975–1978).

lobby was placed in that location. The New Hospital had been dedicated on June 9 after graduation.

Mrs. John Kreemer (Figure 58-28 and 58-29) was installed as President in May, 1978. Contributions of the Board that year to the hospital totaled $144,000. The House Committee merged with the Curtis Clinic Committee. The Pennywise Shop submitted $45,000 for allocation to Board projects. The Women's Board was given office space in the New Hospital in the atrium area, Room 2020B, and furnishings were purchased for $2,045. In the fall Dr. Francis Sweeney discussed the establishment of a Health Education Committee for presenting public education on health matters to the community surrounding Jefferson together with inpatient education via the hospital's closed circuit television. The Community Clothes Charity netted $14,500 for Jefferson and the Old Market Fair grossed $13,260. The final student nurses' tea sponsored by the Board was held on December 6. The diploma program in nursing was to start phasing out in 1980.

In the spring of 1979 planning began for the Charity Ball, which would celebrate its Centennial year. The two-day Old Market Fair grossed $20,218. The Jefferson Jewel Party was held at the home of President and Mrs. Bluemle.

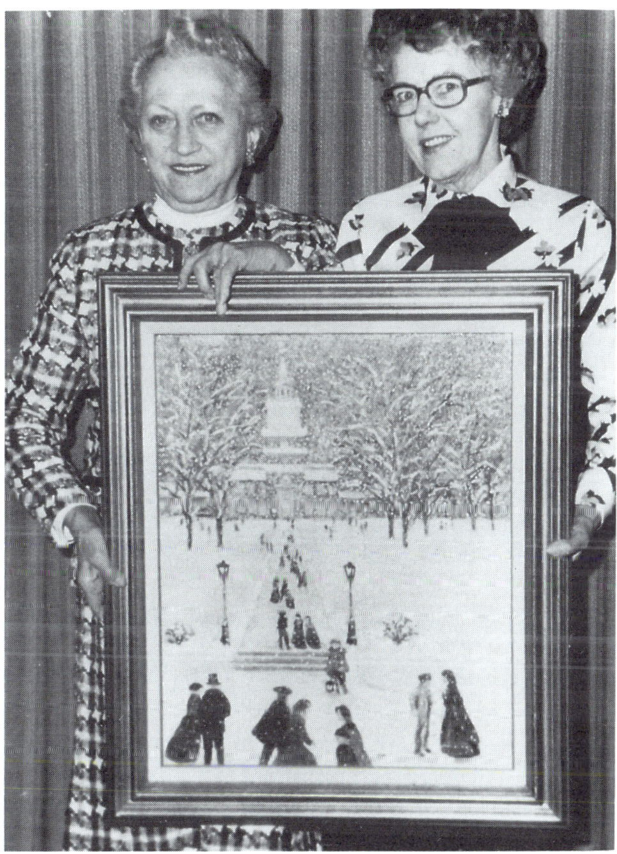

Fig. 58-28. Mrs. James P. Cavanaugh and Mrs. John I. Kreemer with a painting for the Emergency Aid Christmas Bazaar.

The 1980s

In the fall of 1980 the Women's Board received the prestigious Cornerstone Award of the University. This was bestowed at the President's Club dinner held at the Franklin Institute and subsequently placed in the Board's office.

An electric wheelchair for patients with spinal cord injury was purchased for $10,000 and other

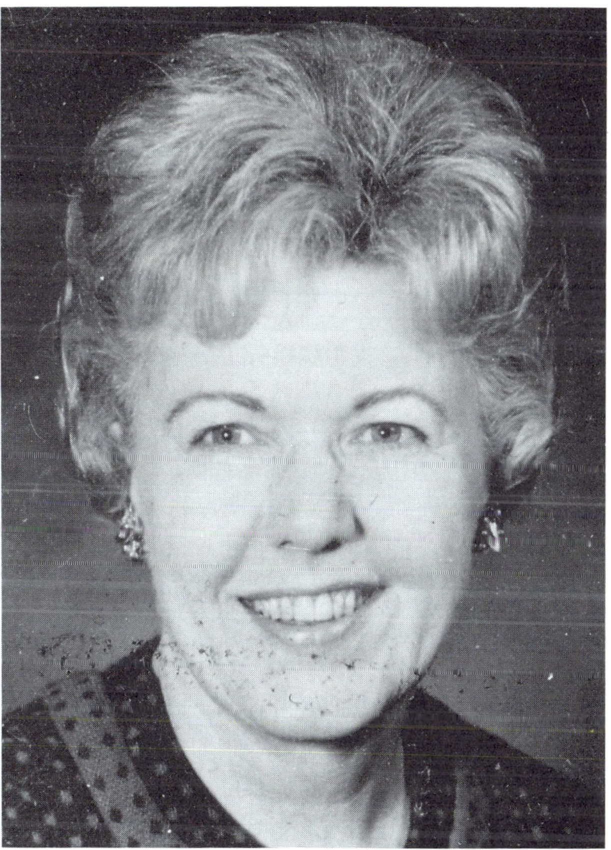

Fig. 58-29. Mrs. John I. Kreemer; President (1978–1981).

projects underwritten for a total of $84,500. Additionally, $35,000 was given to the Blood Donor Center.

The Jefferson Jewel Party was held again at the home of President and Mrs. Bluemle. The cost of chances was raised to $50 on a diamond-and-sapphire brooch valued at $4,850. The Nan Duskin Cocktail-Fashion Party was renewed (Figure 58-30). Tickets for $100 included supper at La Panetiere restaurant. In this year the School of Nursing Committee changed its name to Burt-Melville.

Mrs. Ralph A. Carabasi (Figure 58-31) was elected the sixteenth President of the Women's Board in May, 1981. Upon her resignation in August, Mrs. Paul A. Bowers (Figure 58-32) assumed the office. Meetings were then held in the Board Room of the Scott Building for the first time. The Fair proceeds of this year with its supporting events amounted to $50,000. Special emphasis was placed upon streamlining the management of the Board for efficiency as well as compliance with the financial requirements of the outside regulatory agencies and the University policies. The President initiated the Board's first *Newsletter*, and a mini-history of the Board was prepared for *Directions.*

A total of $152,300 was contributed to the Hospital for the year 1981. The projects funded by the Board were a heart-lung machine for $30,000, four dialysis machines for $18,000, a transcutaneous PO_2 monitor for $13,000, wheels program for $33,000, a blood processor for $35,000, three isolettes for $10,500, and televisions for the neurologic intensive care unit for $12,000.

In November the Board hosted a reciprocal luncheon for the Wills Eye Women's Board, at which occasion Dr. Bluemle spoke about the new Eakins Gallery. An authorization policy was established for Board members to receive

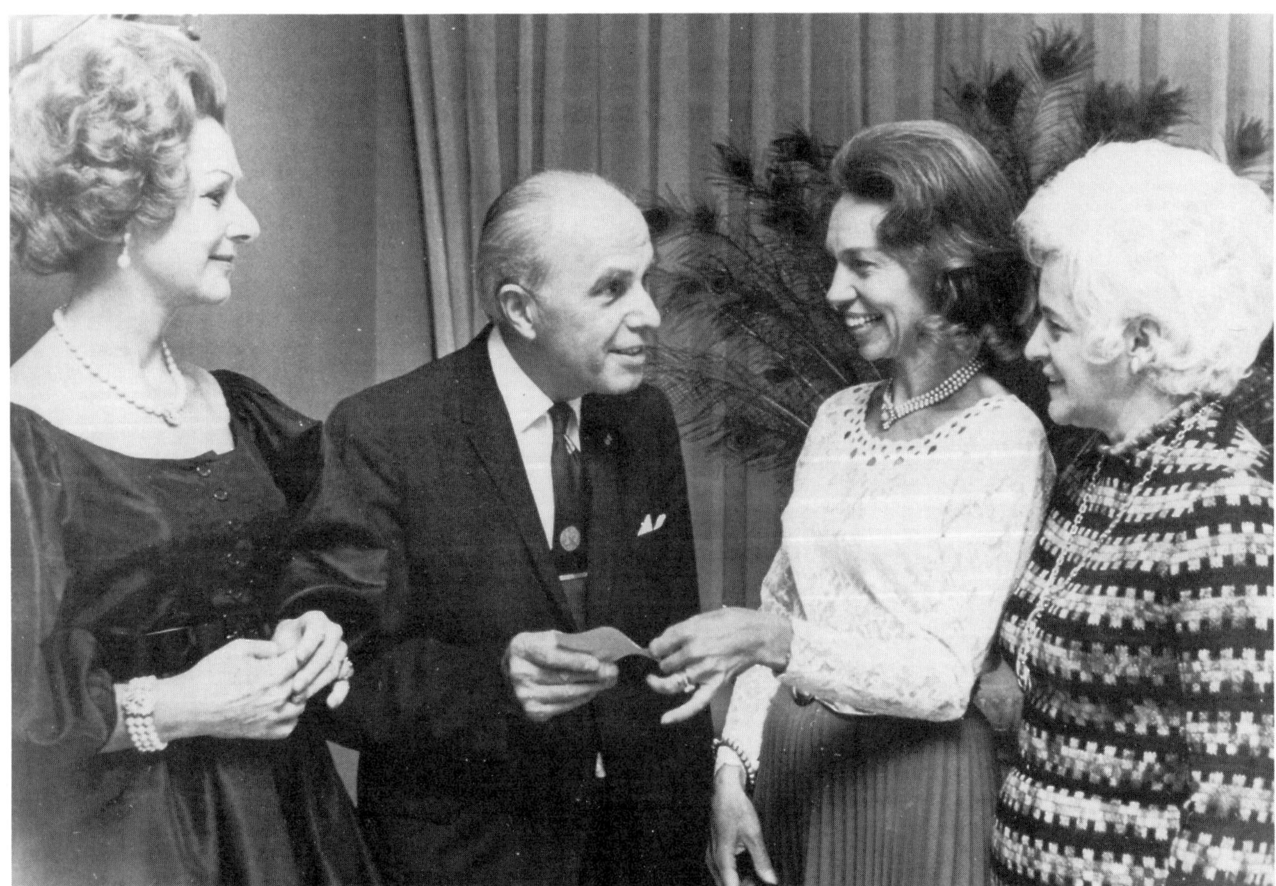

FIG. 58-30. Mrs. Ralph Carabasi, Dr. Peter Herbut, Mrs. Frederick Schmidt, and Mrs. Herbert Luscombe at Nan Duskin Cocktail-Fashion Show.

reimbursement for expenses at obligatory meetings and conventions. A volunteer coordinator was appointed to aid staffing the Pennywise Shop, which had only 12 regular volunteers since the Shop opened.

In March, 1982, the first Magic Moments dinner dance was held at the new Hershey Hotel. This event was a first venture between the Women's Board and the Board of Trustees. With 350 subscribers its grossed $56,680 and a net profit of nearly $36,000. The final nurses' graduation was held in June, and the School of Nursing closed in July.

A total of $99,300 was allocated for neonatal monitors and other accessories. For the Pennywise Shop it was a time of litigation with the township over the significant loss of parking space when the new police headquarters was built. Only 13 parking spaces were allocated for the public with a resultant loss of customers and revenue. Jefferson's legal service and the township satisfactorily resolved the problem. Roberta Pew-Bandy donated 708 shares of Sun Oil with a book value of $22,000. This money was used to purchase draperies for the renovated Foerderer Pavilion patient rooms.

In January, 1983, a special meeting was called to hear recommendations by the University's auditing department concerning financial records and reporting by the Board to conform strictly with the requirements of the Internal Revenue Service. In February the Burt-Melville Committee took over the Emergency Aid Bazaar booth. In April the Activities Committee gave notice that it was disbanding after 74 years of service. Dating back to 1909 it was the second oldest committee. A sum of $6,930 from its treasury was submitted to the Board. At this time the Maternity Committee agreed to accept the responsibilities of the inactive Children's Department. Also in April, Mrs. Norman Hayes donated $5,000 for the Rehabilitation Unit.

In May the Barton Committee ran what was to be its final Fair. After 19 years this activity was discontinued because of increasing costs and decreasing proceeds. A tomfoolery party was held at the Philadelphia College of Art, which netted $46,812, and the Pennywise Shop netted $700 from sale of clothing donated at the party. The Nan Duskin–La Panetiere Party in the fall raised

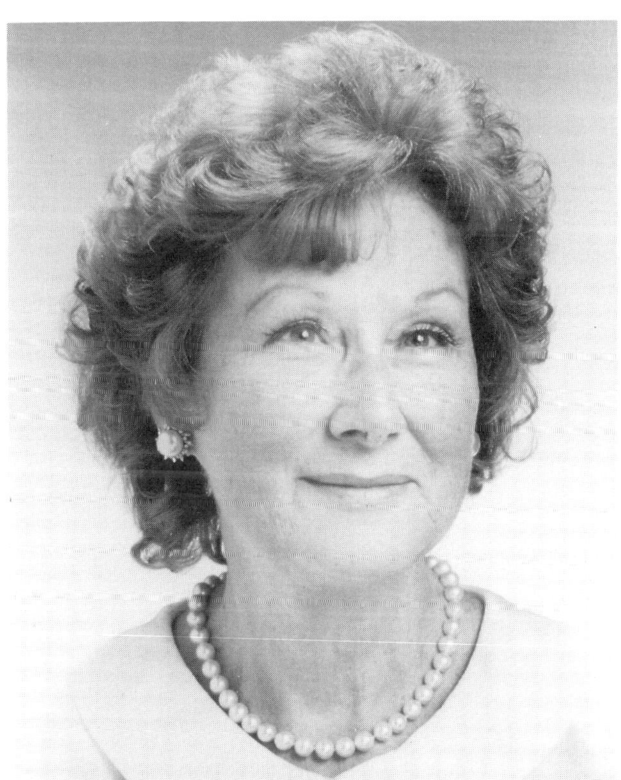

FIG. 58-31. Mrs. Ralph A. Carabasi; Jr. President (1981).

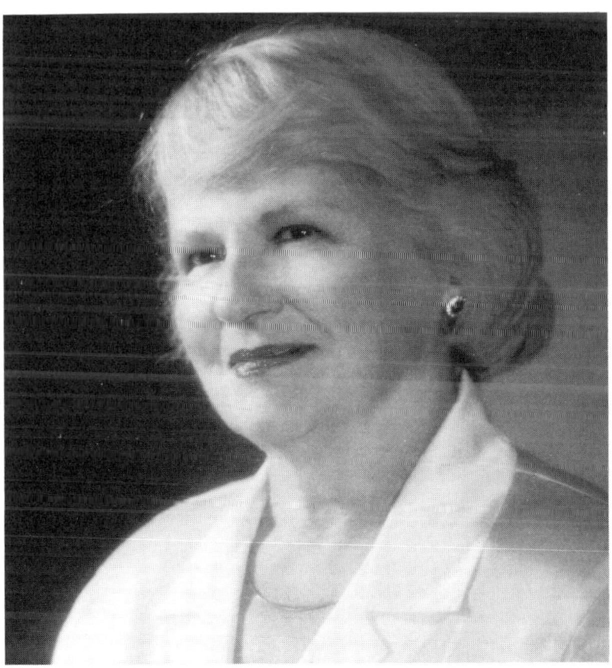

FIG. 58-32. Mrs. Paul A. Bowers; President (1981–1984).

$16,616. The Board also received a percentage of sales receipts at Nan Duskin's of $1,671.

In October the administration hosted a luncheon to celebrate the Pennywise Shop's contribution of $1 million to the hospital (Figure 58-33). The 71 volunteers in attendance witnessed the unveiling of a bronze commemorative plaque by Frederic L. Ballard, Chairman of the Board of Trustees. This plaque was to be installed in the Shop and another, listing all Presidents of the Women's Board since 1908, was to be placed in the atrium at the entrance of the Women's Board office. The Board received a gift of $35,000 from the sale of old x-ray film. The Maternity Committee netted $6,423 from its operation of the Charity Ball and reported that it had given $98,000 to the hospital during the previous six years. The projects funded during 1983 were 13 new dialysis machines at $58,000, four adult ventilators at $13,000 each, four infant respirators at $16,000, and an intensive care nursery at $26,400.

In February, 1984, the Barton Committee instituted a Phantom Fair fund-raiser that netted $4,150. In April the formal merger of the Children's Committee into the Maternity Committee was consummated. This reduced the composition of the Board to six major committees. At this time Dr. Francis Sweeney, Vice President for Health Services and Hospital Director, left for a new post at Temple University. At the annual May meeting the Presidential Report noted a record contribution of $304,000 for the year and a total of $678,958 for the previous three years. The Jefferson Jewel Party, chaired by Mrs. Samuel Vauclain, raised $97,363

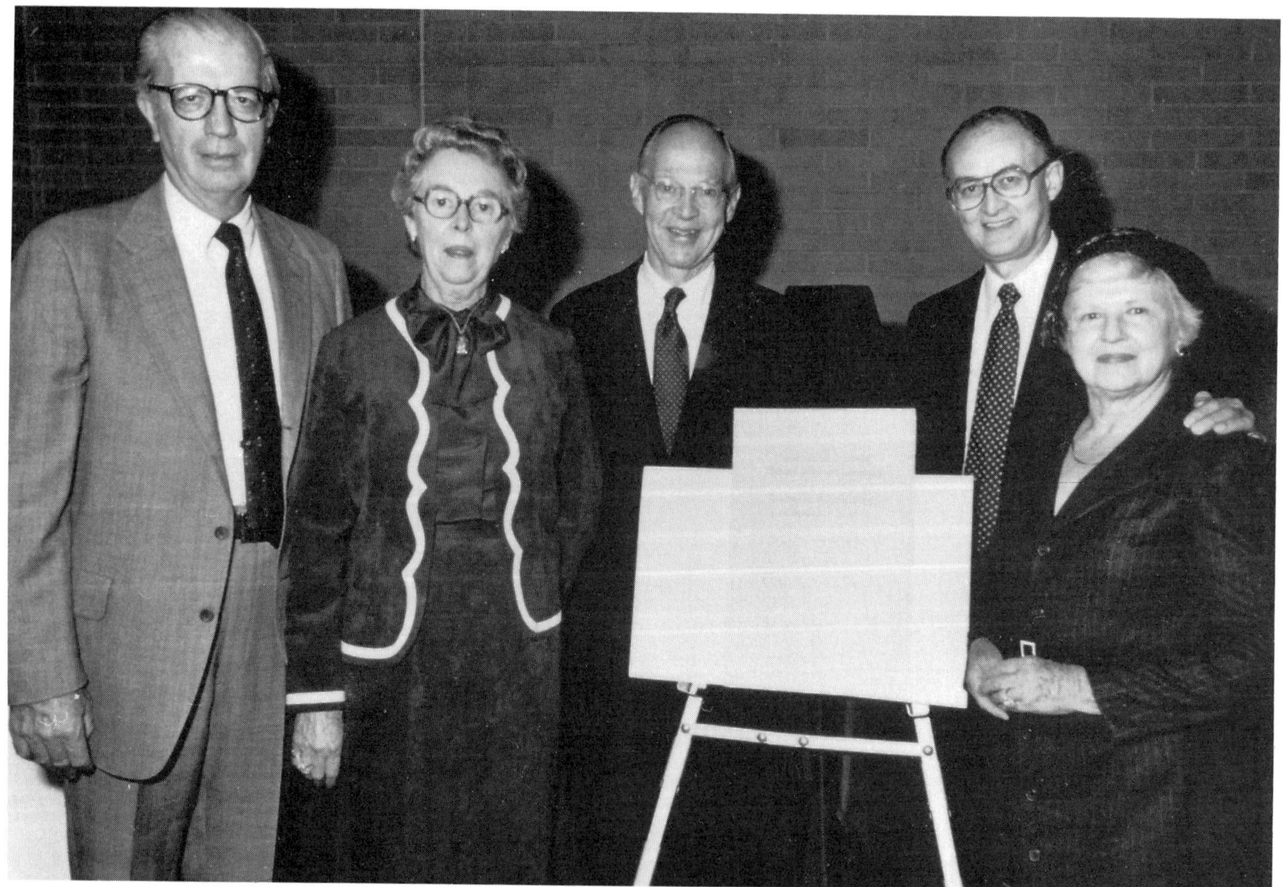

FIG. 58-33. Dr. Frank Sweeney, Mrs. Samuel Vauclain, Frederic Ballard, Esq., Dr. Lewis Bluemle, and Mrs. Paul Bowers, President, with the bronze plaque commemorating $1 million given to the Hospital by the Pennywise Shop.

for the decade of 1973–1983. The Magic Moments second dinner dance, celebrating the return of Eakins' *Gross Clinic* painting from Paris, was held in September in Jefferson Alumni Hall. The Pennywise Shop remained the major source of income with a contribution of $122,147. The Board of Trustees, in a resolution of June 4, 1984, expressed "gratitude and appreciation" to Mrs. Bowers "for her years of dedicated service and loyalty to Thomas Jefferson University" and presented to her the Jefferson Service Award.

At this meeting Mrs. Peter Theodos (Figure 58-34) was installed as the 18th President of the Women's Board. Three new projects in her term of office were a lecture series at the Philadelphia Museum of Art, a financial seminar underwritten by First Pennsylvania Bank, and "An Evening of Tennis." The Women's Board pledged the sum of $150,000 over a period of three years for the new Bodine Radiation Center at Jefferson.

The Women's Board projects for 1984–1985 were: (1) Bodine Radiation Center, $50,000; (2) Rehabilitation Unit Renovation, $121,000; and (3) Equipment for Women's and Children's Care Program, $87,000. The programs for the General Board Meetings instituted in 1982, for which physicians from various Hospital Departments and others in the University were guest speakers, continued.

The Women's Board projects for 1985–1986 were: (1) Bodine Radiation Center, $50,000; (2) medical respiratory intensive care unit monitoring center, $30,000; (3) operating microscope, $35,000; (4) 20 wheelchairs, $12,000; (5) 18 chair beds, $9,000; (6) hospital beds, $52,624; (7) ten dynamaps, $20,000; (8) E-Z movers $20,500; (9) bed-check alarm system, $12,500; (10) pediatric porch, $15,000. For this year, a total of $271,647 was contributed to the Hospital.

For 1986–1987 the Women's Board projects were: (1) Bodine Radiation Center, $50,000; (2) ten television sets for dialysis unit, $8,200; (3) intermediate cardiac care unit monitoring equipment, $8,500; (4) two dialysis machines, $7,000; (5) one operating room surgical light, $20,000; (6) one oximeter, $4,000; (7) hospitality suite for families of surgical patients, $30,000; (8) waiting room for acute dialysis unit, $1,800; (9) exercise equipment and educational materials for chronic renal disease patients, $15,000; and (10) chairs for intermediate dialysis unit, $2,800. The total amount contributed to the Hospital for the year was $165,800. Women's Board receipts for the year were $214,459.65. Departmental contributions to the Hospital totaled another $9,287.

Magic Moments IV was held in March, 1987, at the new Curtis Center (Sixth and Walnut Streets) with 214 attendees. The gross receipts totaled $36,885, and the net profit was $16,650.

In April, 1987, Michael Bradley, Executive Director of the Hospital, entertained members of the Executive Committee and past Presidents living in the area at a luncheon in the newly renovated Foerderer Board Room. A lively informative question-and-answer period followed. At the annual May meeting Annie K.V. Klotz succeeded Mrs. Theodos as President.

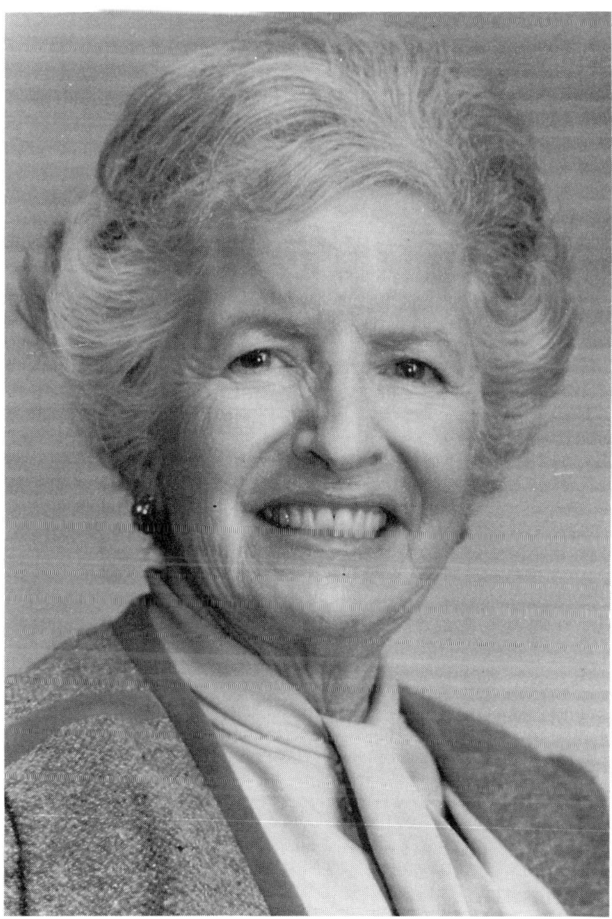

FIG. 58-34. Mrs. Peter A. Theodos; President (1984–1987).

The history of an organization is a chronicle of the sum of its achievements. The importance of nine decades must be measured in terms of events and accomplishments. The Women's Board in the rise and fall of its fortunes has maintained the vision of its small group of dedicated founders. Inspired by a fruitful heritage, the Board continues to explore how it can better serve Jefferson in times of increasing change and challenges.

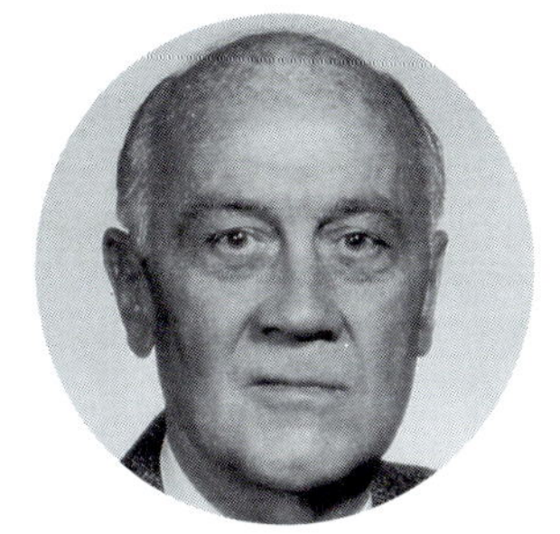

CHAPTER FIFTY-NINE

Jefferson's Military History

PAUL A. BOWERS, M.D.

"Soldiers bore operations of every kind immediately after a battle, with much more fortitude than they did at any time afterwards." —BENJAMIN RUSH (1745–1813)

WAR HAS always been a test of the strength and endurance of nations. Just as surely, however, the battlefield also tests a nation's compassion for the wounded and its capacity to care for them. For the medical profession that provides that care, the battlefield calls for a dimension of service rarely encountered in peacetime. War is a crucible by which men and women learn to practice medicine with an intensity and on a scale never repeated in the course of a professional lifetime. Hippocrates (460–370 B.C.) recognized this when he said: "He who would become a surgeon should join the army and follow it." Over the years many thousands of Jefferson graduates, students, faculty, and nurses have done that. They have committed themselves to the needs of those wounded in service of country.

Jefferson's military history is as distinguished and proud as her peacetime history. Any account of the accomplishments since Jefferson's founding would be incomplete without recognizing the dedication and skill that Jefferson people have put forth in military settings. From the time of the Civil War in the 1860s through the Vietnam conflict 100 years later, Jefferson graduates and

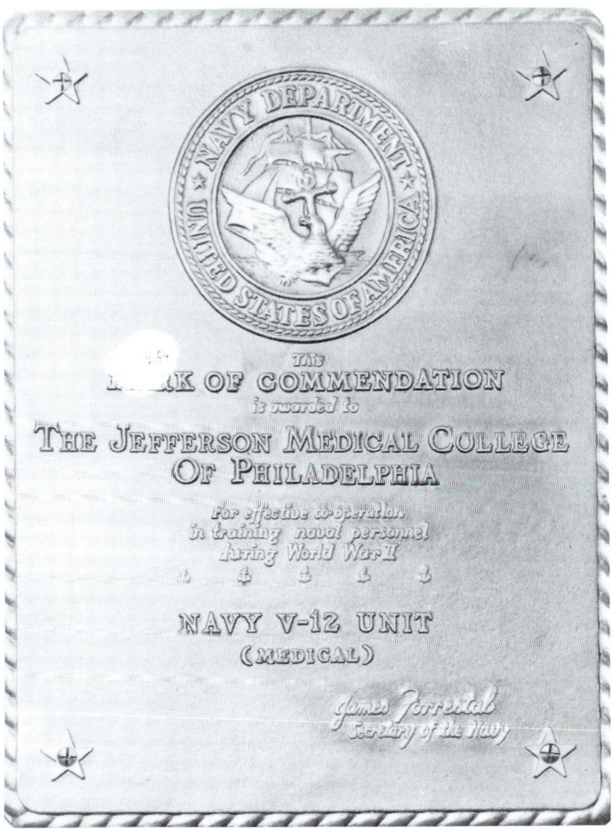

Commendation from James Forrestal, Secretary of the Navy.

staff have served in a way we have come to think of as distinctively "Jeffersonian." They have performed with a willing spirit, to the highest standards, in a cooperative effort, and with the unselfishness and pride that characterize the special place called Jefferson.

Many Jefferson physicians have experienced firsthand what General Merritt W. Ireland (Jefferson, 1891) meant when he described his experiences at an Indian post in the West. "I came to know what love of man for man is, what friendship means and what sublime faith people have in a doctor."[1] Many graduates also have seen the truth of a comment by Major General James Carr Magee (Jefferson, 1905): "A doctor at a battalion aid station cannot be a weakling; he may be the only man between this world and the next."

In this account of Jefferson's military history, some important facts and names must regretfully but pardonably be omitted. Honor is due not only to those whose deeds have won public acclaim, but also to those whose stories remain untold. Each of these Jefferson heroes evokes the deepest pride.

The First to Serve

One of Jefferson's earliest alumni, Anson Jones (Figure 59-1), earned his stripes on three fronts: in medicine, the military, and politics. Born in Great Barrington, Massachusetts, in 1798, he graduated from Jefferson in 1827 in its second class. His

BE IT KNOWN THAT THIS

CERTIFICATE OF DISTINCTION

HAS BEEN AWARDED BY THE

WAR DEPARTMENT

TO

Jefferson Medical College

FOR THE TRAINING OF SOLDIERS IN THE

ARMY SPECIALIZED TRAINING PROGRAM

DURING WORLD WAR II

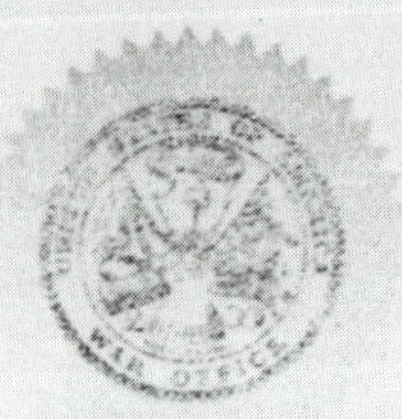

SECRETARY OF WAR

Certificate of Distinction from the War Department.

grandfather was Sir John Jones, and his grandmother was a sister of Oliver Cromwell.

When Texas declared its independence from Mexico, Jones enlisted in the Texas infantry. It was 1836, just before the Battle of San Jacinto, and Jones served as surgeon to the Second Regiment. When General Sam Houston gave the order "Fight and be damned," Jones left the hospital, joined the infantry, and entered the fray. When the battle was over, he returned to the hospital where he provided care for wounded soldiers as well as for General Houston, who had a gunshot wound in the leg.

Jones was the first Jefferson graduate to be involved in the military, and also the first to earn high political office. Capping a stormy career in public life, he became the fourth and last President of the Republic of Texas, before it was annexed to the United States.[2]

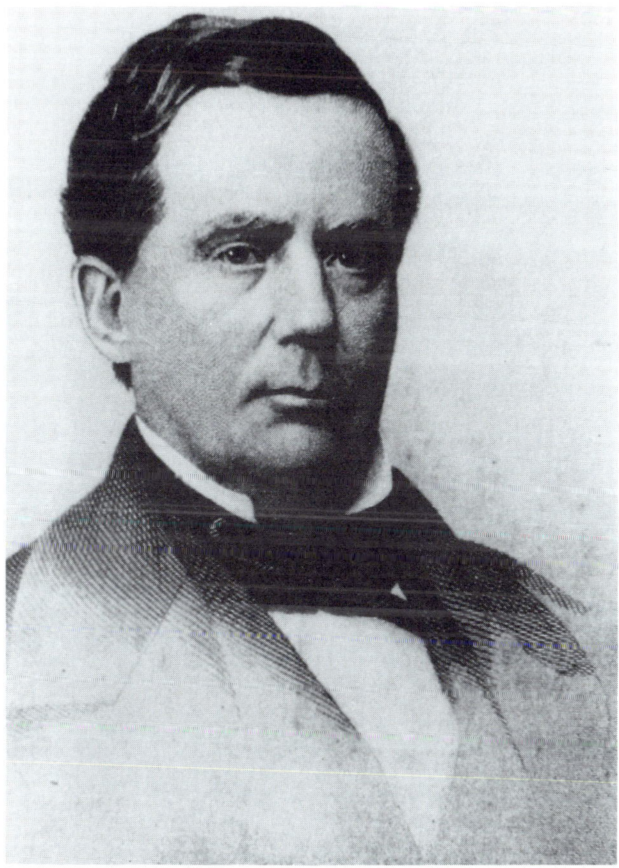

FIG. 59-1. Anson Jones (Jefferson, 1827), the last President of the Republic of Texas (1844–1846).

First Faculty Involvement

Early Jefferson records also show that William P.C. Barton (Figure 7-1) had a successful military career. Dr. Barton held Jefferson's Chair of Materia Medica from 1826 until 1829 and was also Dean from 1828 to 1829. In 1842 Barton was appointed Chief of the Bureau of Medicine and Surgery of the Navy. The post was a new one; the office of Surgeon General of the Navy had not yet been created.

Dr. Barton received his early education at Princeton, where he graduated with distinction in 1805. He studied medicine under his uncle, Dr. Benjamin Smith Barton, who was a surgeon at Pennsylvania Hospital. As early as 1809 he was recommended for appointment as a surgeon in the Navy by Drs. Benjamin Rush and Philip Syng Physick. He maintained a naval career for the rest of his life, but with long periods of shore duty he was able to conduct academic activities such as his Professorship at Jefferson. He achieved a brilliant record in the organization of the marine hospital system. In a report on the operation of these hospitals he was highly critical, particularly of the hospital at the Philadelphia Navy Yard. The report was so controversial that he was court martialed for "conduct unbecoming an officer and a gentlemen." Later, however, he was exonerated.[3]

The Civil War

The Civil War presented the nation with a crisis of unity. No less it challenged the medical profession to a test of its abilities. Disease spread widely as the battleground swept halfway across the continent. Battlefield wounds became increasingly complex, and there was an acute shortage of physicians.

Poor as it was, American medical care became the best thus far provided to the fighting man. The nation's medical schools were partly responsible for that. Jefferson was in its fourth decade by this time and had established a high level of professionalism. Its physicians contributed to the Civil War effort in ways that changed the course of military medicine. An example was Ninian Pinckney (Jefferson, 1833). Just after graduating, Pinckney enlisted in the Navy and went on eventually to become Medical Director with the rank of Commodore before retiring in 1873.

Surgeon Pinckney is known for an innovation that helped both the Army and the Navy in the Civil War. He outfitted a captured Confederate side-wheeler, the *Red Rover,* equipped it with elevators, window screens, and operating rooms, and used it as a hospital ship (Figure 59-2). Serving on it were Catholic nuns who had volunteered as nurses. This is believed to be the first Navy hospital ship that carried female nurses to care for patients.

Dr. Pinckney was also an able administrator. During his service he was responsible for the organization of medical staff rank and grade for the U.S. Navy, continually striving to improve the status of medical officers. Dr. Pinckney's prominence is indicated by the fact that in 1854 he made the Presentation Address on the occasion of Commodore Matthew Perry's presentation of the flag that had been raised on the soil of Japan after diplomatic and trade relations had been established.

Another Jefferson graduate who made a lasting mark on the military was Dr. Jonathan Letterman (Figure 59-3). Dr. Letterman's father was a Trustee of Jefferson College at Canonsburg, Pennsylvania, from which Jefferson Medical College originated. The elder Letterman wrote to the Board at Jefferson Medical College requesting that his son be accepted. He was, and the younger Letterman earned his degree in 1849. Upon graduating, Dr. Letterman entered the Army as Assistant Surgeon and became a career army man. Eventually he reached the status of Medical Director of the Army of the Potomac. He is best remembered for the system he devised to remove the wounded from the battlefield (Figure 59-4).

Before Dr. Letterman's plan, fellow soldiers transported casualties to rear hospitals in an

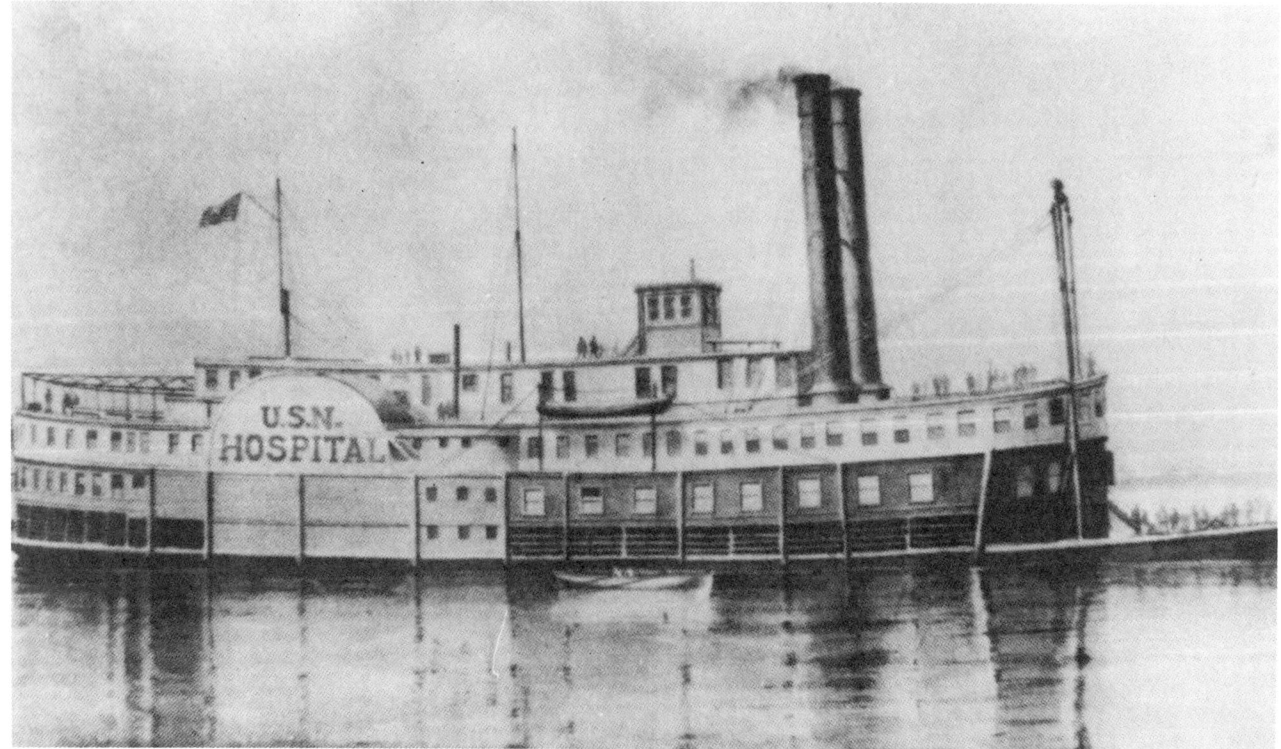

FIG. 59-2. The first Navy hospital ship, the *Red Rover,* outfitted by Dr. Ninian Pinckney (Jefferson, 1833) during the Civil War.

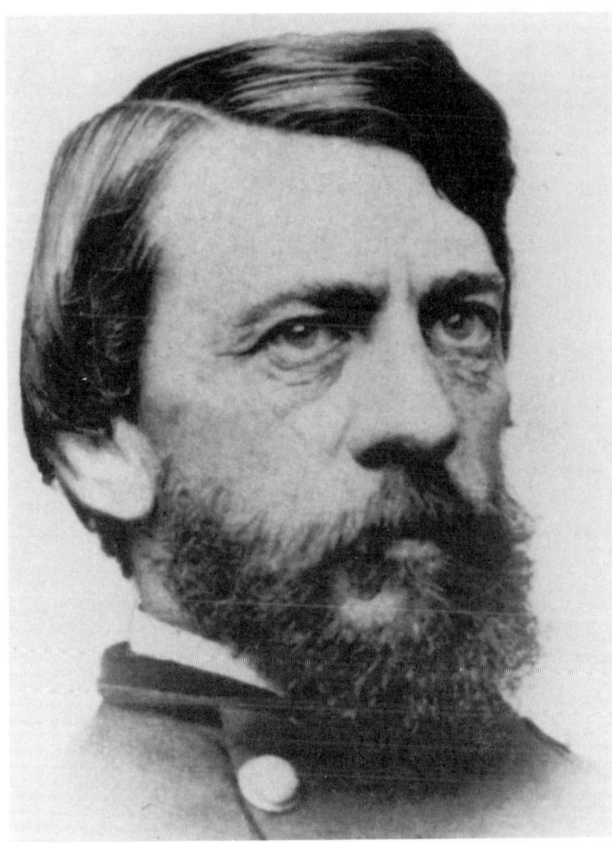

FIG. 59-3. Jonathan Letterman (Jefferson, 1849) devised a pioneer system to remove the wounded from the battlefield.

ambulance wagon. These same vehicles, however, were also used by commanders for logistical support. Medical supplies would sometimes be dumped when the vehicles were needed elsewhere. A medical organization was lacking to evacuate casualties collected by regimental units. The situation became critical in the Second Battle of Bull Run, where wounded were still on the field five days later.

At the time of Dr. Letterman's appointment as Medical Director of the Army of the Potomac, the Surgeon General remarked: "In making this assignment, I have been governed by the best interest of the service. Your energy, your determination and faithful discharge of duty in all different situations in which you have been placed during your service of 13 years, determined me to place you in the most arduous, responsible and trying position you have yet occupied. I now commit you to the health, the comfort and the lives of thousands of fellow soldiers who are fighting for the maintenance of our liberties."

Dr. Letterman proved worthy of the trust. He organized and trained an ambulance corps. The system was put into effect at Antietam in September, 1862, and it worked. Although Antietam (or Sharpsburg, in western Maryland) was the bloodiest one-day battle in the history of the American Army to that date, the field was cleared of casualties within 24 hours. Later, Dr. Letterman refined the system, organizing division hospitals, staffing them adequately, and adding

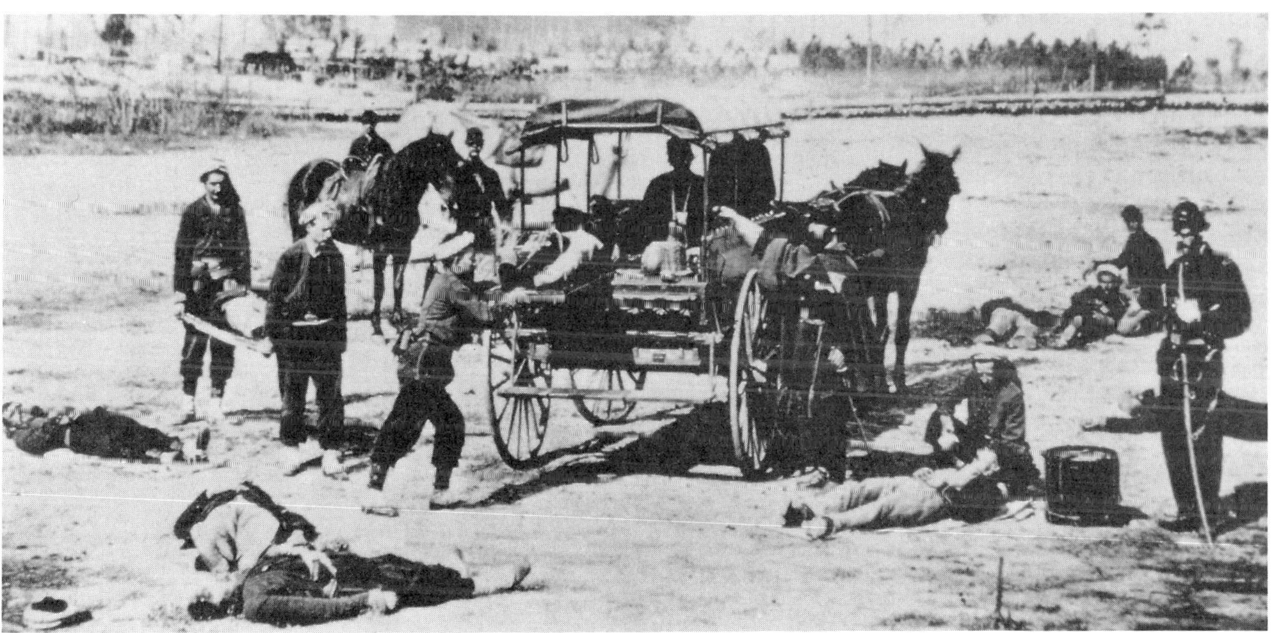

FIG. 59-4. Letterman's system in operation for removal of wounded from the battlefield.

evacuation hospitals where casualties were cared for until they were fit to travel. His 16-page plan for medical evacuation was submitted to President Lincoln. It was approved in 1864, adopted by Congress, and became law.

After the Civil War, Dr. Letterman retired to San Francisco, where he was appointed coroner for two terms and where he died at age 47. His body was later exhumed and he and his wife were reburied at Arlington National Cemetery. The stone over his grave reads: "Jonathan Letterman, who brought order and efficiency into the medical service, was an originator of modern methods of medical administration in the army." The Letterman Army Medical Center in San Francisco was named in his honor.

William W. Keen (Jefferson, 1862) became a pioneer in neurosurgery because of his findings in problems of the nervous system. He entered Jefferson in 1860, but gave up his studies temporarily to enlist in the Union Army as a Division Surgeon. At the Battle of Bull Run, Virginia, he set up an operating room at Sedley Springs Church with the aid of local women. He was then put in charge of Ekinton General Hospital near Washington, D.C. (by Dr. Letterman, who was then Medical Director of the Army of the Potomac). Later, he studied injuries of the nervous system at the Turner's Lane Hospital at Twenty-second Street and Columbia Avenue in Philadelphia. His colleagues in this clinical research endeavor were Drs. S. Weir Mitchell (Jefferson, 1850) and George R. Morehouse (Jefferson, 1850). His *Gunshot Wounds and Other Injuries of Nerves* is based on this military experience.

Although Dr. Keen wished to serve in the Spanish-American War, his services were not required because of its short duration. Amazingly, in World War I he served as a consultant medical officer at the age of 80.

At the start of the Civil War, Jefferson's enrollment included students from both the North and the South. In fact, in the 1859 class, Virginians outnumbered Pennsylvanians 46 to 28. Even before the conflict erupted, the students formed two unintegrated groups. As early as December 23, 1859, over 200 students from the South, on an offer of equal standing and free tuition, transferred to Richmond, the capital of the Confederate States. In March, 1860, fifty-six out of 140 who had matriculated graduated from the Medical College of Virginia.

This offer had apparently been arranged and organized by Dr. Hunter McGuire (Chapter 2, Figure 8). McGuire had a degree from Winchester Medical College in Virginia, Class of 1855, and practiced in Philadelphia. He conducted quiz classes for students from both Jefferson and the University of Pennsylvania. During the war, Jefferson's student body shrank from 630 to 275.[4] Jefferson and the University of Pennsylvania survived, but the Pennsylvania Medical College (McClellan's second school) dissolved by attrition.

Dr. McGuire later became Medical Director of the Army of the Shenandoah Valley and Brigadier Surgeon under Stonewall Jackson, to whom he was the personal physician. After the war, all was apparently forgiven and Dr. McGuire was awarded an honorary LL.D. degree by Jefferson Medical College in 1888. Respect for his brilliancy and honesty was never lost. In 1892 he became President of the American Medical Association.

At the end of the Civil War, many of the students from the South returned to Philadelphia to get their diplomas from Jefferson. Philadelphia had numerous military hospitals, and the facilities for obtaining training were excellent—this kept many of the graduates in the area. The Richmond School had given the Southern students adequate instruction but could not compete with Jefferson's prestige for the triumvirate of Professors Dunglison, Pancoast, and Gross.

Dr. Samuel D. Gross (Jefferson, 1828) was commissioned by the War Department to write a *Manual of Military History*. The Gross *Manual* was published in 1861 and a second edition in 1862. It was distributed to all medical personnel in the Union Army. So competent was it and so great was the need that the *Manual* was pirated by the Army of the Confederacy and reprinted for distribution to their medical personnel (Figure 59-5).[5] One Jeffersonian who could attest to the need for it was Dr. John H. Brinton (Jefferson, 1852) (Figure 59-6), who served as personal physician to Ulysses S. Grant and later founded the Army Medical Museum. His commission as Brigade Surgeon of Volunteers was signed by Abraham Lincoln, and the original is located in Jefferson's archival treasure trove (Figure 59-7). He

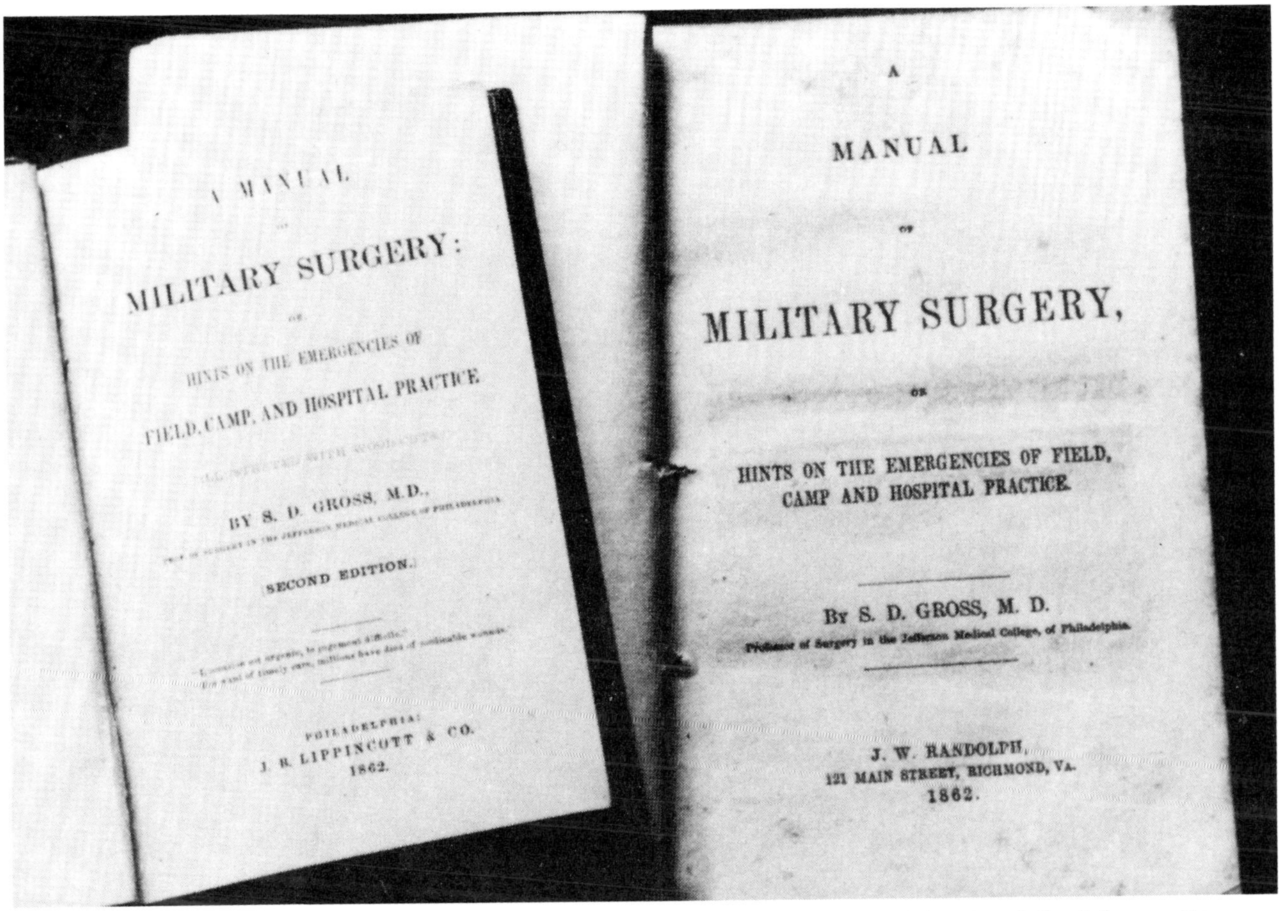

A MANUAL

OF

MILITARY SURGERY:

OR,

HINTS ON THE EMERGENCIES OF

FIELD, CAMP, AND HOSPITAL PRACTICE

BY S. D. GROSS, M.D.,

SECOND EDITION.

PHILADELPHIA:
J. B. LIPPINCOTT & CO.
1862.

A

MANUAL

OF

MILITARY SURGERY,

OR

HINTS ON THE EMERGENCIES OF FIELD,
CAMP AND HOSPITAL PRACTICE.

BY S. D. GROSS, M. D.
Professor of Surgery in the Jefferson Medical College, of Philadelphia.

J. W. RANDOLPH,
121 MAIN STREET, RICHMOND, VA.
1862.

FIG. 59-5. *The Manual of Military Surgery* by Samuel D. Gross, showing the Union and the pirated Confederate editions.

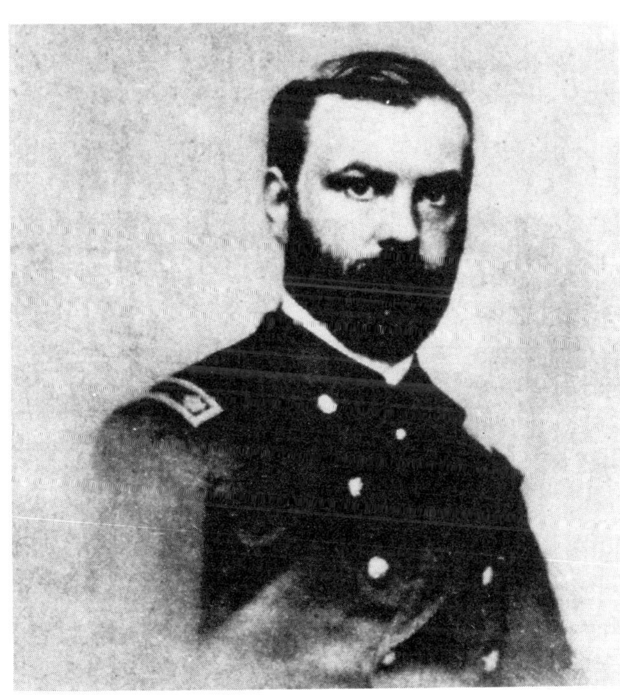

FIG. 59-6. John Hill Brinton (Jefferson, 1852), first curator of the Army Medical Museum in Washington, D.C.

encountered a Union doctor who said the first surgery he ever saw was an emergency operation he had to perform himself.[6] Brinton was a contributing author to *The Medical and Surgical History of the War of the Rebellion,* and after his death his *Personal Memoirs of the Civil War* (1914) was published. Upon the resignation of Samuel D. Gross in 1882, he served as Professor of the Practice of Surgery and Clinical Surgery at Jefferson until 1907.

A number of Jefferson graduates served with distinction in the Army of the South. Matthew W. Butler (Jefferson, 1860), father of Admiral Butler of the Medical Corps of the Navy, attended Stonewall Jackson when he was wounded at Chancellorsville, Virginia. Dr. H. Browse Trist (Jefferson, 1857), a descendent of Thomas Jefferson, served in peacetime with the U.S. Navy, and joined the Confederate Army Medical Corps when the Civil War erupted. Dr. Trist's mother (Virginia, née Randolph) was a granddaughter of Thomas Jefferson.[7]

The Era After the War

When peace came and the nation began to knit itself together, the need for the military was less immediate. Still, the country had learned to be prepared and would keep its defenses strong. In the last decades of the nineteenth century and on through the early years of the twentieth, several Jefferson graduates made notable contributions to medical military history and held the highest posts in the Army, Navy, and Public Health Services. Worthy of mention are: Commodore J. Nathan Foltz (Jefferson, 1830), who was the first Surgeon General of the Navy; Brigadier General Charles Sutherland (Jefferson, 1849), who was Surgeon General from 1890 until 1893 under President Benjamin Harrison; and Major General Merrette W. Ireland (Jefferson, 1891), who was Surgeon General of the Army from 1918 until 1931 under Presidents Wilson, Harding, Coolidge, and Hoover (Figure 59-8). Dr. Ireland was a veteran of the Philippine–Mexican expedition and went to France with the American Expeditionary Force (AEF) in 1916. He was a Chief Surgeon of the AEF in 1918 and Surgeon General that same year. General John Pershing chose Ireland as his Chief Medical Officer. He praised Ireland, calling him "abounding in vitality, mental and physical, quick and accurate in decisions and prompt in action. He understands men and knows how to work with them for the common good. He is farsighted in making plans and immeasurably able in administration. He is loyal always but courageous in promoting sound views and avoiding error." Dr. Ireland received an honorary LL.D. degree in 1919 when he addressed the graduating class at Jefferson.

A continuation of the list includes: Dr. J. Chalmers DaCosta (Jefferson, 1885), who was assigned to the ship *George Washington* as a Naval Surgeon and provided care for President Woodrow Wilson during the Peace Treaty negotiations for the League of Nations; General A.E. Bradley (Jefferson, 1887), who was the First Chief Surgeon of the AEF; and Colonel Frederick H. Mills (Jefferson, 1894), who retired at age 76 and at the time was the oldest medical officer on active duty after 45 years of service. Colonel Mills enlisted in 1898 and served in the Spanish-American War, the Philippine Insurrection, the Mexican Border War, the Boxer Rebellion, and

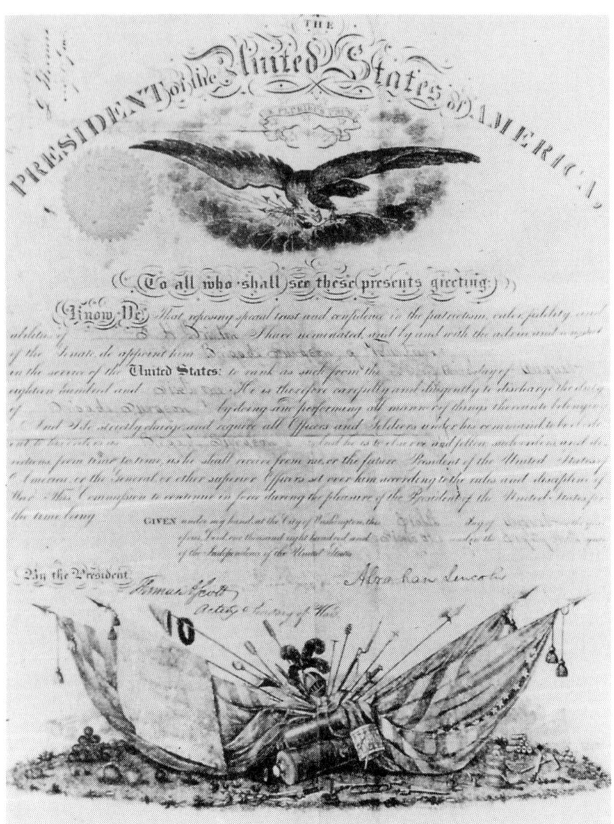
THE
PRESIDENT of the United States of AMERICA,
To all who shall see these presents greeting:
Know Ye, That reposing special trust and confidence in the patriotism, valor, fidelity and abilities of ... I have nominated, and by and with the advice and consent of the Senate do appoint him ... in the service of the United States: ...
GIVEN under my hand, at the City of Washington, ...
By the President
Abraham Lincoln

FIG. 59-7. Brinton's commission signed by Abraham Lincoln.

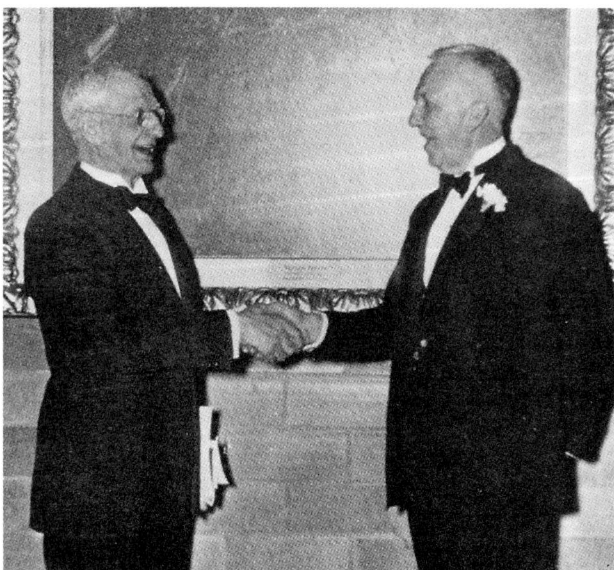

FIG. 59-8. Major General Merrette W. Ireland (Jefferson, 1867) and Board President, Robert P. Hooper, upon the occasion of the Annual William Potter Lecture in 1939.

World Wars I and II. In 1924 he became Professor of Military Service for the Reserve Officers Training Corps (ROTC) at Jefferson. In 1942 he was recalled to active duty and assigned to Jefferson. In 1945 he was selected to have his portrait presented to the College.

Additional graduates outstanding in military service were: Dr. Benjamin Lee Gordon (Jefferson, 1896), Instructor in Obstetrics from 1897 to 1901, who was a member of Keegan's Brigade in the Spanish-American War, a member of the Medical Advisory Board in World War I, and in the Volunteer Corps, and grandfather of Susan J. Gordon (Jefferson, 1966), a gastroenterologist at Jefferson; Dr. James C. Magee (Jefferson, 1905), who was Surgeon General of the Army from 1939 until 1943 under President Franklin D. Roosevelt; Major General Alexander J. Orenstein (Jefferson, 1905), who was responsible for medical service during the building of the Panama Canal and Acting Medical Director of the Medical Corps in World War II; and Colonel Thomas Leidy Rhoads (Jefferson, 1893), who had a hospital in Utica, New York, named after him. The latter was a medical officer at the White House during President Taft's administration. Colonel Rhoads saw active duty in the Spanish-American War and was Division Surgeon of the 8th Division in France during World War I. He also served as Chief Surgeon of the First Corps of the First Army.

The list concludes with unintentional omissions. Colonel Purcey M. Ashborn (Jefferson, 1893) had a hospital in McKinney, Texas, named after him. He was Inspector General of the Health Department in Panama and active in tropical medicine in the Spanish-American War. Major General William Crawford Gorgas was Surgeon General from 1913 to 1918. Although not a Jefferson graduate, he received an honorary Doctor of Science degree from Jefferson in 1909.

World War I

Military combat changed dramatically in the 50 years between the Civil War and World War I. Hand-to-hand combat was replaced by military hardware. The tank was introduced. This type of battleground constituted the first modern technological war. As warfare changed, it generated new kinds of battle injuries. Trench foot and mouth, gas poisoning, and multiple head, neck, and chest injuries from projectiles were all common. They were so new and so numerous that ways of treating them were still being developed.

It was clear that the Armed Forces Medical Corps would need assistance in coping with the anticipated massive-scale war injuries. For this reason the Red Cross organized 50 hospitals across the country to support the AEF that headed for France in 1918. The Red Cross set up and equipped base hospitals, which were to be transferred to the jurisdiction of the U.S. Army Medical Department after mobilization. The idea was to assemble a staff whose members were accustomed to working with each other, so that the unit could quickly function at an efficient level.

Jefferson asked to be one of those base hospitals. Dr. Ross V. Patterson (Jefferson, 1904) and the Honorable William Potter, Chairman of the Board of Trustees, requested an interview with Surgeon General William Gorgas concerning the establishment of a Jefferson Base Hospital. The original request was refused, but later accepted. In 1917 United States Army Base Hospital No. 38 from Jefferson was organized.[8] At that time, three other hospitals were also organized in Pennsylvania. They were: Base Hospital No. 10 from Pennsylvania Hospital; Base Hospital No. 12 from the Hospital of the University of Pennsylvania; and Base Hospital No. 34 from Episcopal Hospital. All personnel were volunteers. Major William M.L. Coplin (Figure 59-9) (Jefferson, 1886) was made Director-in-Chief of the Laboratory Division of Base Hospital No. 38, Dr. Norman J. Henry was made Chief of the Medical Division, and Major Charles F. Nassau was named Chief of the Surgical Division. The Commanding Officer was Major John S. Lambie, Medical Corps, U.S. Army, who was on active duty.

The training of the hospital personnel took place at the Second Army Regiment on North Broad Street near Susquehanna Avenue in Philadelphia. A didactic course was given by Dr. W.W. Keen, and practical instruction at several locations: Jefferson Hospital, Pennsylvania Hospital, St. Agnes Hospital, St. Joseph's Hospital, Philadelphia General Hospital, Episcopal Hospital, Frankford Hospital, Lankenau Hospital, Presbyterian Hospital, and Jewish and Samaritan Hospitals.

Jefferson Base Hospital No. 38 consisted of 35 officers, 100 registered nurses, six civilian employees, and 200 enlisted men. It had a capacity of 1,000 beds.

The hospital expected to be ordered to France. Personnel marched with their equipment to Stenton Athletic Field at Twenty-fifth street and Hunting Park Avenue. They took along tents and field kitchens. Their training lasted for nearly eight months. On June 19, 1917, a farewell dance was given at the Second Regiment Armory on Broad Street, and Base Hospital No. 38 was off to war.

Many private citizens contributed considerable sums of money for the outfitting of the unit. Adeline P. Gibson, with her husband, Henry Gibson, contributed $50,000 for the purchase of equipment. Mrs. Thomas P. Hunter contributed $5,000 to equip the operating room. Other equipment included a four-ton ice-making machine. The Women's Auxiliary of the Hospital contributed surgical dressings, bandages, and supplies. The Teachers' Association of Philadelphia gave an ambulance costing $1,500, and the Logan Improvement Association gave one costing $2,000. There was even a mascot named "Jeff," a blue-ribbon Boston terrier valued at $500.

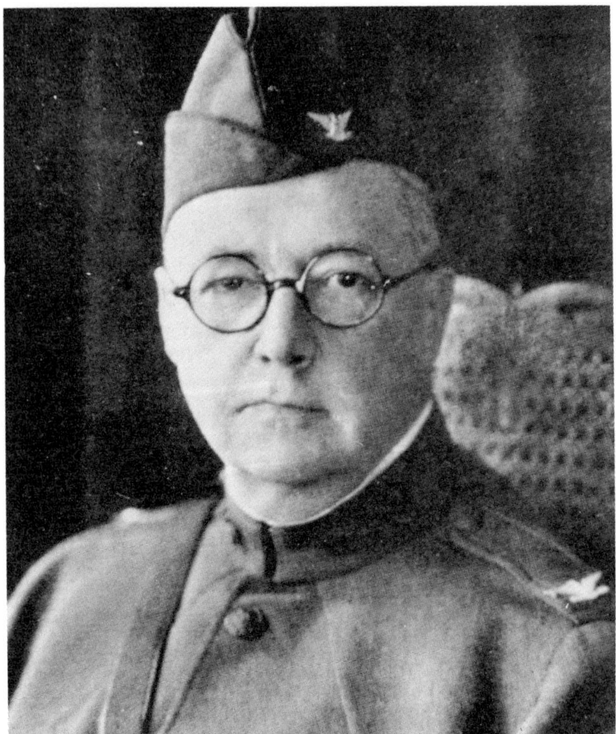

FIG. 59-9. Major William M.L. Coplin (Jefferson, 1886), Director in Chief of Laboratory Division of Base Hospital No. 38.

Prior to leaving for France on the Army transport *Saturnia* on May 19, 1918, President of the Board William Potter stated to Clara Melville, Director of Nurses, and 99 Jefferson nurses: "You will go in the holiest cause that ever angels of mercy were summoned to. You take with you the faith of the republic and your courage and your goodness." On June 21, 1918, six officers and 100 enlisted men embarked on the S.S. *Nopatin* (Figure 59-10) from New York, and another 29 officers sailed on the S.S. *President Grant*. The Base Hospital was established in Nantes, France, and served other small cities and towns in France. The hospital had 21 wards, a diet kitchen, barracks, mess hall, officers' barracks, and nurses' barracks (Figures 59-11–59-13). The nurses' mess hall and the officers' mess hall were separate. Equipment was in short supply, and much of it never arrived. Work on the building was done by officers and enlisted men who lived in an incomplete tarpaper building. By September, 1,000 patients had been admitted; in November the daily census was up to 2,412 patients. Many of the nurses were transferred to other units, and Clara Melville, Chief Nurse, had only seven nurses to assist in the operating room and to care for patients.

Nearly 9,000 patients were cared for at the Base Hospital No. 38 in Nantes, France. The primary problems encountered by the medical department were respiratory infection, effects of gassing, diphtheria, scarlet fever, mumps, and gastrointestinal problems. The surgical division had three operating room tables in each operating room, and all were busy most of the time. There were 15 wards for surgical cases and the more than 700 active cases including fractures, gunshot wounds, hemorrhage, infection, and gangrene.

The severity of the wounds and the complications were described as follows: "To die of wounds is bad enough. To die as a result of war gas is immeasurably worse. But the summation of hellish torture born of the devil's fiendish mania is wounds and gas. All fertile resources of torturing demons evolved through the

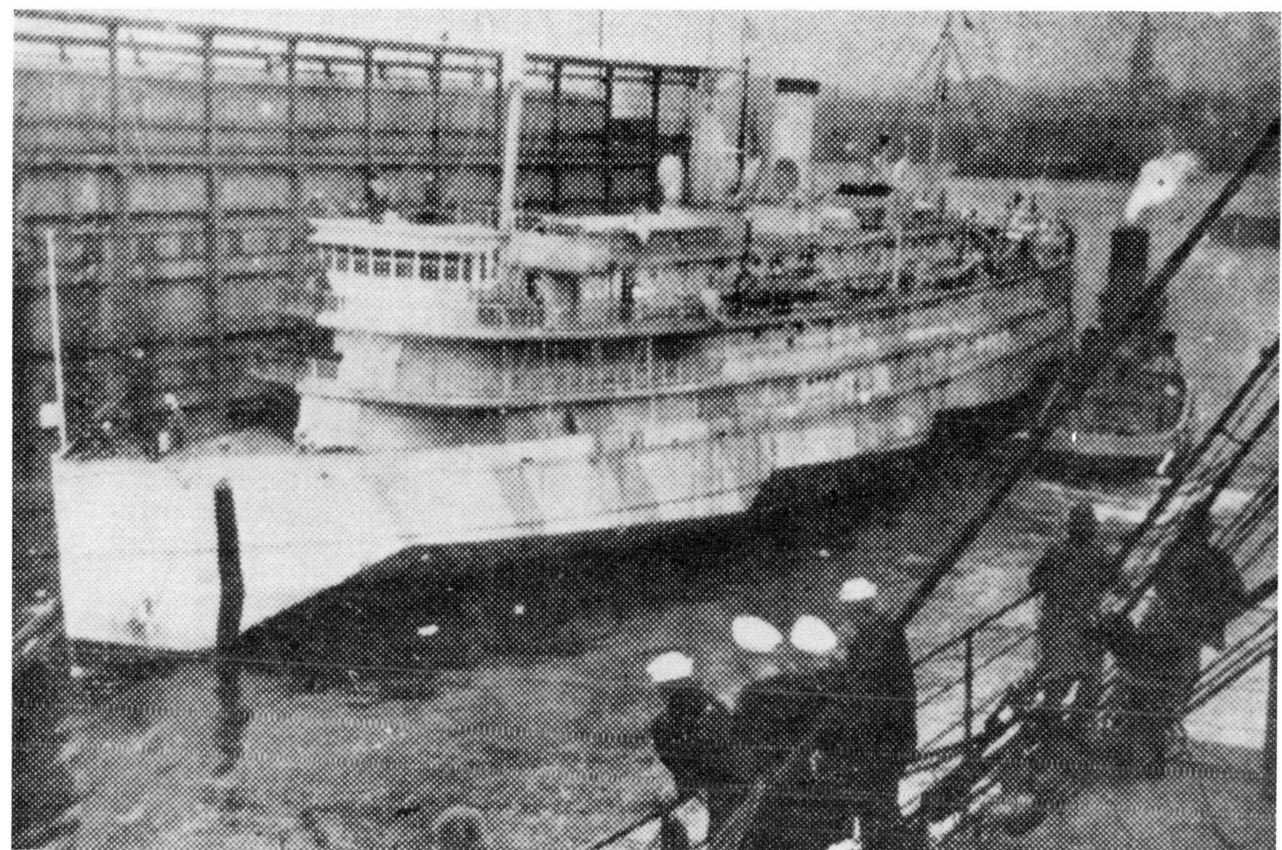

FIG. 59-10. The S.S. *Nopatin,* Jefferson troop transport to France (1918).

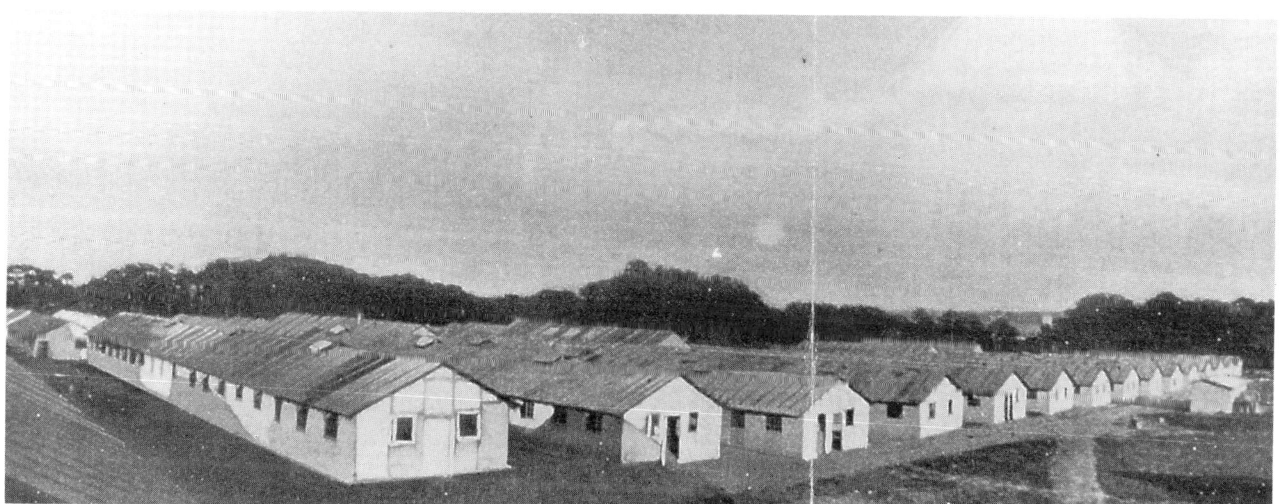

FIG. 59-11. Jefferson's Base Hospital No. 38 in World War I, established in Nantes, France.

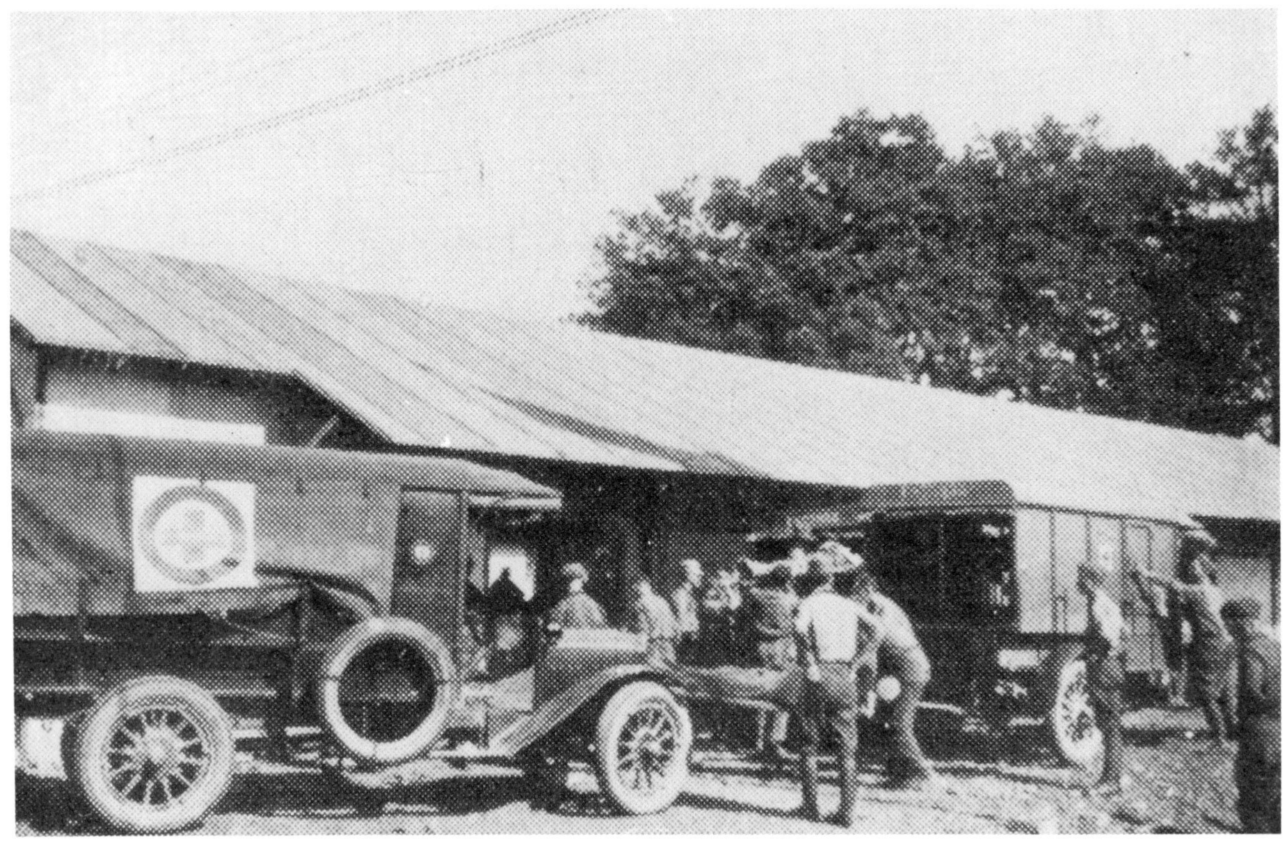

FIG. 59-12. The receiving ward of Base Hospital No. 38.

ages of unspeakable cruelty fall impotent and mild before the dragon of agonizing death."

Seven members of the Jefferson unit died in service. Adeline Pepper Gibson, who had contributed money toward the equipment of Base Hospital No. 38, accompanied the Unit to France. She died in the service of her country on June 10, 1919, from pneumonia. The memorial to her stated: "She left us one continuous period of smiling, patient helpfulness and her passing weighs upon us as one overwhelming and unforgettable service of our own great adventure. A world peopled by such souls would be sunshine and cheer without pain: a paradise."

By the war's end, 27 sons of Jefferson had given their lives. In their honor the Alumni Association presented a bronze plaque to be placed in the College building (Figure 59-14). It remains there today, just inside the main entrance. At the memorial tablet ceremony on October 7, 1920, Dr. J. Chalmers DaCosta stated: "They died to save us. Wherever man has died for man, that spot is holy ground. It is proper that names of our heroes should be commemorated. . . . It will touch our hearts to think of those brave and gallant gentlemen who made the final sacrifice to save the nation."

One of every four living Jefferson graduates served the Army in World War I. Of 5,000 living alumni, 1,286 entered the Army, and 167 the Navy (Figure 59-15). In his history of Base Hospital No. 38, Jefferson alumnus Dr. William M.L. Coplin noted: "Sixty-five percent of our graduates for the five years preceding 1918 served in the armed services. The class of 1916 had the largest number of men in service—103." Many citations and

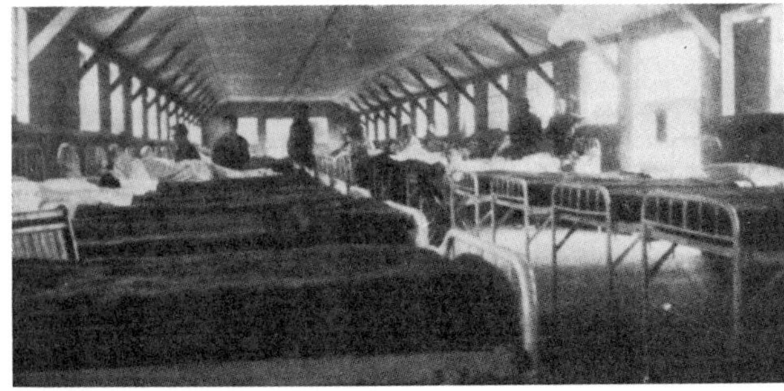

FIG. 59-13. A typical ward of Base Hospital No. 38.

decorations were awarded to Jefferson physicians. Dr. John Chalmers DaCosta noted in his address at the dedication of the memorial tablet that "Dr. Orlando H. Petty of this hospital received the well-merited, seldom given and magnificent honor of the Congressional Medal." Petty had graduated from Jefferson in 1904. When World War I started, there were only 500 medical officers in the

DEDICATED TO THE
JEFFERSON MEDICAL
WAR WHO GAVE FULL
TO THEIR COUNTRY
MIGHT
GRADUATES OF THE
COLLEGE IN THE WORLD
MEASURE OF DEVOTION
THAT CIVILIZATION
ENDURE
FREDERICK GEORGE CAROW
BOAZ BAXTER COX
REESE DAVIS
JOSEPH EDWARD DUDENHOEFER
THOMAS REED FERGUSON
FRANK HARRIS GARDNER
PERCY STEVENSON GASTON
BURGESS ALLEN GIBSON
FRANCIS FINDLAY HANBIDGE
FREDERICK ARTHUR HENDERSON
JOHN HISLOP
CARL EDWARD HOLMBERG
ROBERT LORD HULL
RICHARD LAWRENCE JETT
HARRY MILHERN LAVELLE
JUSTIN A McCARTHY
CASPER JOSEPH MIDDLEKAUFF
GUSTAV LEWIS NORSTEDT
RUSSELL CISNEY PARSON
WENDELL JAMES PHILLIPS
WILLIAM EMMET PURVIANCE
GRADY RUDISILL ROBERTS
LINDSAY COCHRANE WHITESIDE
CHESTER CAMERON WOOD
ERECTED BY THE ALUMNI ASSOCIATION
OF THE JEFFERSON MEDICAL COLLEGE
1920

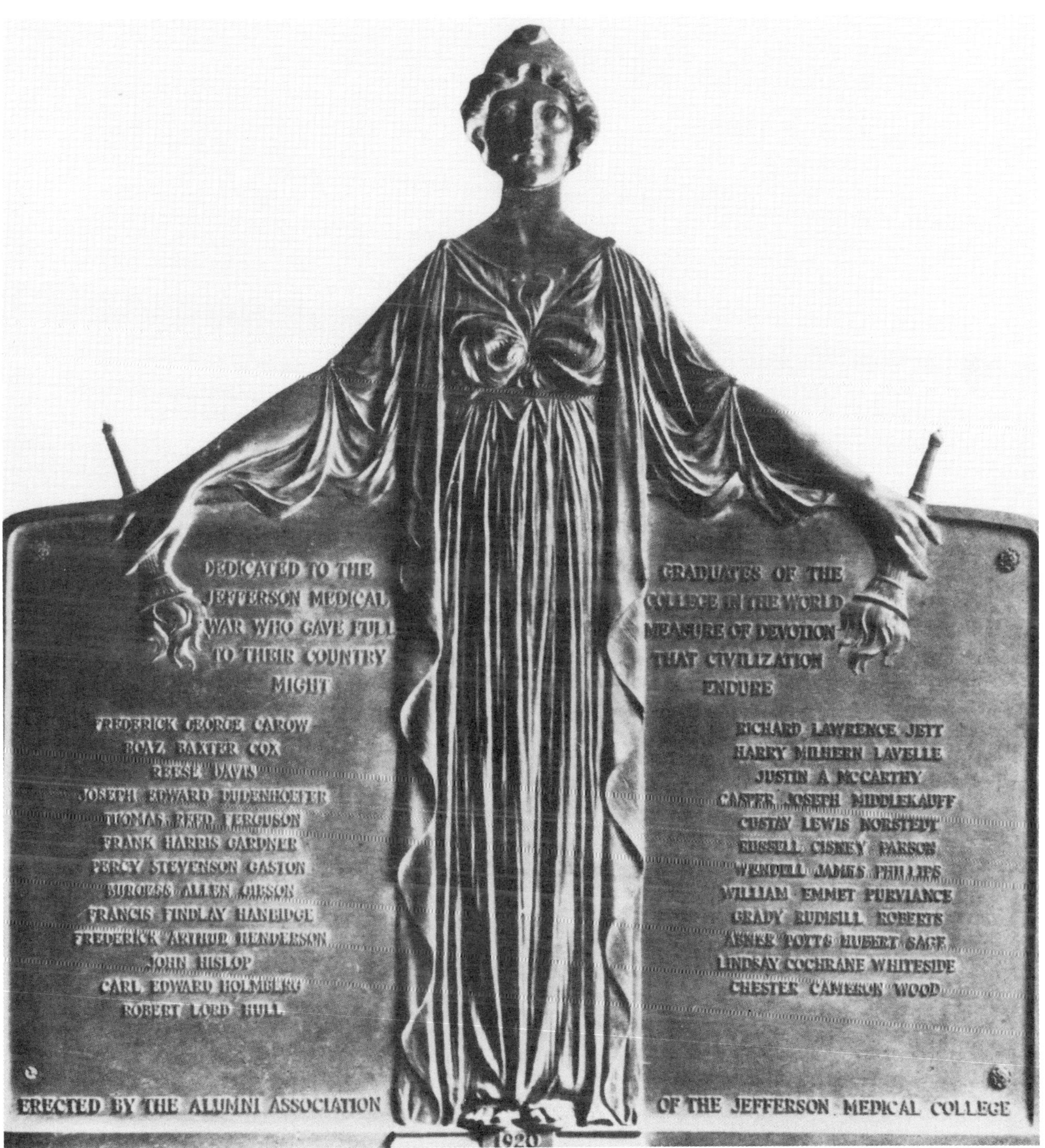

FIG. 59-14. The Alumni plaque in the College honoring the fallen in World War I.

Army. By the time of the Armistice, more than 30,000 medical officers served in the military. Five percent of those were Jefferson men.

Jefferson served the country on the home front too. Early in the war, the Army and Navy asked to send medical officers to Jefferson for graduate refresher courses. Jefferson took them in and provided dormitory room for all. In addition, there were 431 students in the Student Army Training Corps, 398 in the Army, and 33 in the Navy. In September, 1918, all Jefferson students were mobilized, and the Student Training Corps was formed for both Army and Navy units. In December, 1918, after a brief period of indoctrination into military life, the unit was demobilized as the war came to a close. The 1919 *Clinic* lists a number of Army companies and Naval units to which students were assigned.

▪ Winds of Another War

As soon after World War I as 1920, a Reserve Officers Training Corps was established at Jefferson. Students who enrolled would qualify for a commission in the medical section of the Officers' Reserve Corps of the Army on receiving the M.D. degree. Military training was not compulsory, but some 150 students enrolled. Training included six weeks of summer camp at the Carlisle Indian School barracks located at Carlisle, Pennsylvania (Figure 59-16). After less than a quarter century the nation would again depend on its medical profession to treat the wounds of another war.

World War II

The United States entered World War II on December 8, 1941, the day after the Japanese bombed Pearl Harbor. By this time systems for treating the injured had advanced considerably. The wounded were examined first at battalion aid stations just behind the lines. About a mile to the rear were collecting stations for additional emergency treatment. From there the wounded were sent to clearing stations and the gravest cases to field hospitals. These were some five miles from the combat zone. Evacuation hospitals took those who needed immediate surgery. All of these systems were mobile and moved wherever the action was. The exceptions were general hospitals,

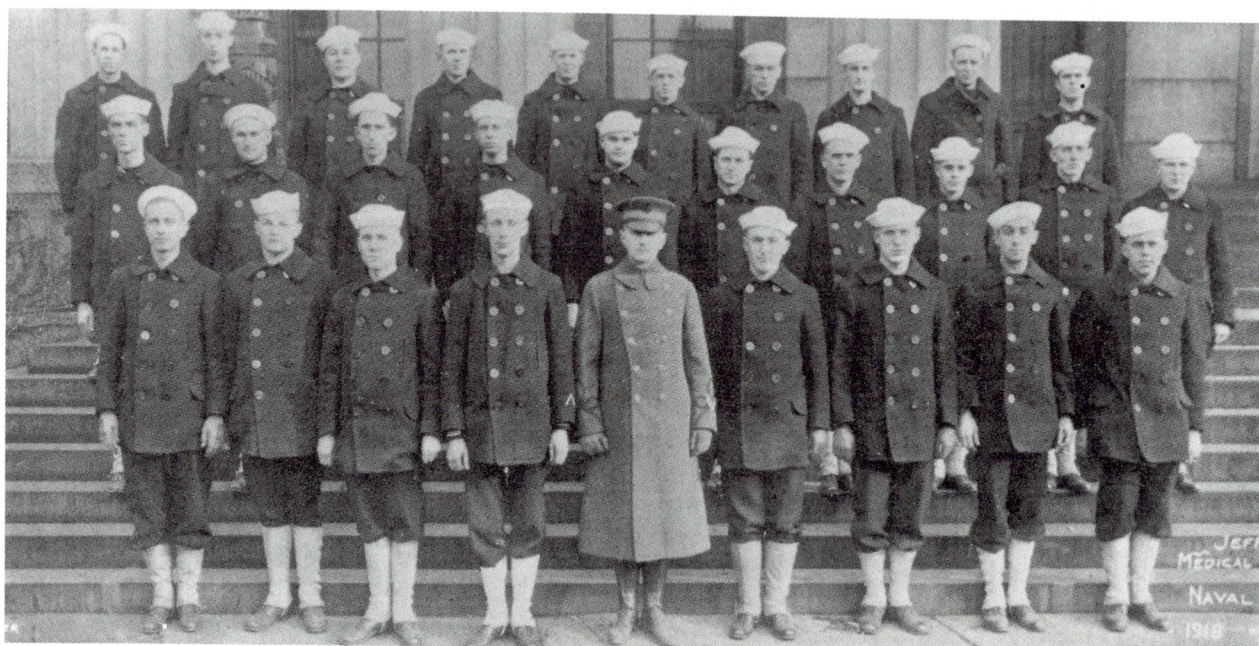

FIG. 59-15. The Jefferson Naval Unit in World War I.

which were fixed installations. One of those general hospitals was Jefferson's 38th, a reactivated version of Jefferson's World War I Base Hospital.

As in the previous war, Jefferson was ready to serve. In 1940 the Surgeon General of the Army, James Carr Magee (Jefferson, 1905) was the speaker at Jefferson's commencement. At a luncheon following the ceremony, Major General Magee asked Jefferson's Dean William H. Perkins to reorganize Jefferson Base Hospital No. 38.

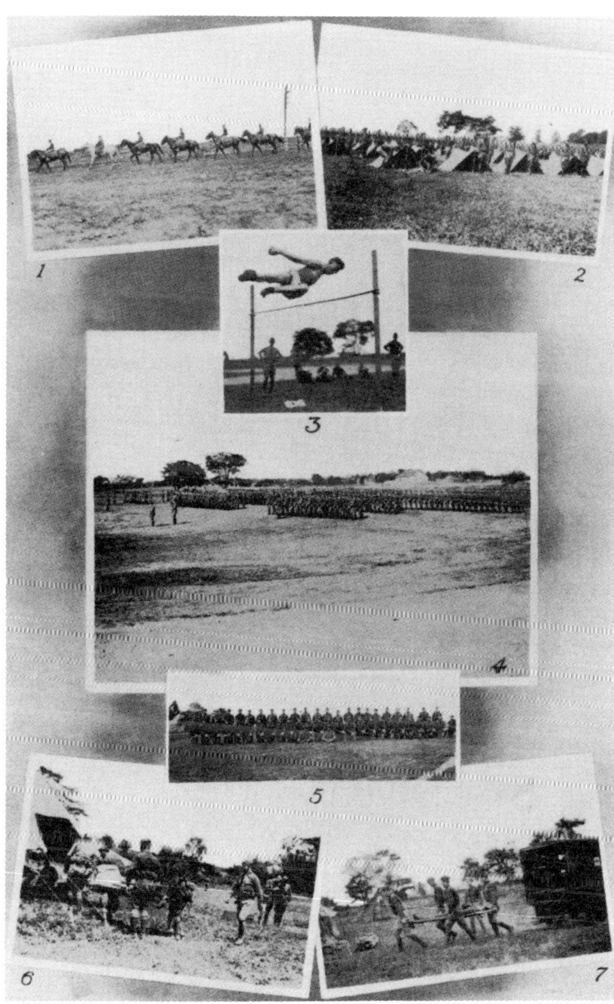

FIG. 59-16. Jefferson students in Camp Carlisle barracks (ca. 1923), (1) Equitation; (2) Tent pitching; (3) Athletics; (4) Review; (5) The Jefferson Company; (6) The Hospital station; and (7) Evacuating the wounded.

Work got underway immediately. Dr. Baldwin L. Keyes (Jefferson, 1917), a member of the Reserves since the last war, was made Commanding Officer, and Dr. Burgess L. Gordon (Jefferson, 1919) was Chief of Medical Service. Edna Scott was Director of Nurses with the rank of Major. By the time of the Pearl Harbor attack in December, 1941, Jefferson's General Hospital No. 38 was complete and ready for active duty. Dr. Keyes fulfilled his responsibility in admirable fashion, and on May 15, 1942, Jefferson's Hospital Unit left for Camp Bowie, Texas. The group rode what is described as a "ramshackle train," through hot, sticky weather in minimal accommodations.

The hospital training in Texas consisted primarily of hikes and physical activity. Colonel Forrest R. Ostrander was assigned Commanding Officer of the 38th General Hospital in August, and Dr. Keyes became Executive Officer in charge of medical affairs. In August of that year, the 38th, consisting of 56 original officers and 105 of the original nurses, left Camp Bowie by train for South Carolina

The hospital equipment was loaded aboard three ships. Two weeks later, the group was transferred to Camp Kilmer, New Jersey, and eventually to Staten Island. From there the 38th sailed over 16,000 miles, stopping at Rio de Janeiro for supplies, then moving on to Cape Town, South Africa, and up the coast of Africa through the Suez Canal to the port of Teufik, where the ship was unloaded.

The destination of the 38th was approximately 13 kilometers from Cairo, Egypt. The members called the hospital "Kilo 13" (Figures 59-17, 59-19). Dr. Keyes, in writing to Dean Perkins in 1943, stated: "Our hospital is built with locally made brick with tin roofs and ceilings of bullrushes or pressed fiber. The buildings are well scattered among the rolling sand dunes, and can only be seen all at one time by climbing on top of a large dune separating the officers' and nurses' quarters."

The hospital opened for patients on November 11, 1942, exactly 23 years from Armistice Day, the day that ended World War I. The patient load consisted of noncombatants. It had been expected that Rommel's North African Campaign would generate a number of casualties, but at the battle of Alamein in October and November of 1941, Montgomery defeated Rommel. Shortly thereafter, the African Campaign ended, and the fighting moved to Italy, beyond the hospital's operational area. The hospital, by now with Colonel Mabel Prevost as Chief Nurse, decreased in size because

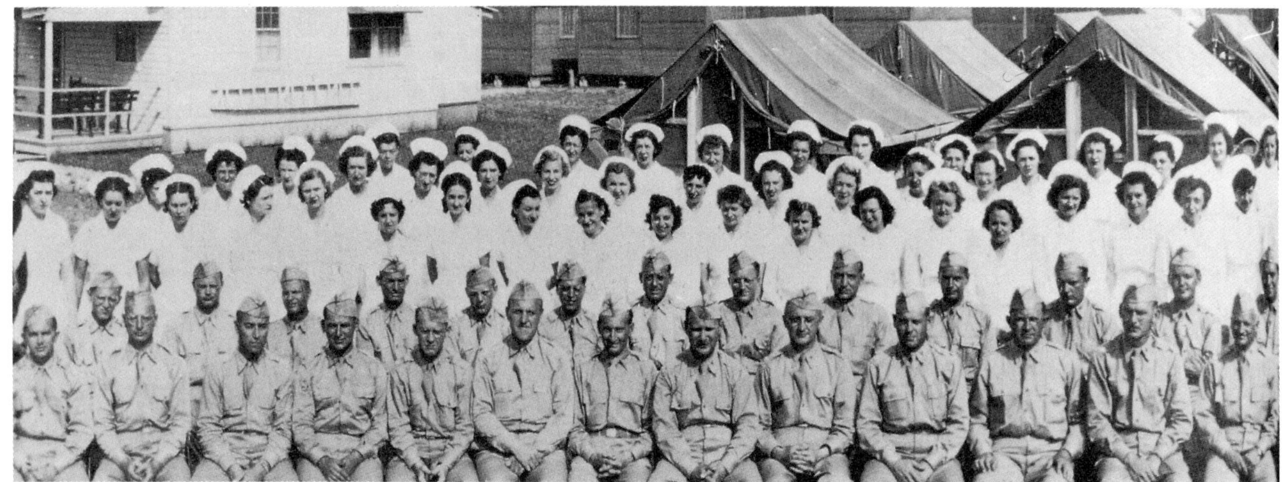

FIG. 59-17. Jefferson General Hospital No. 38 ("Kilo 13") in 1942. This is the left half of a group photograph; Dr. Baldwin L. Keyes is at the extreme lower right.

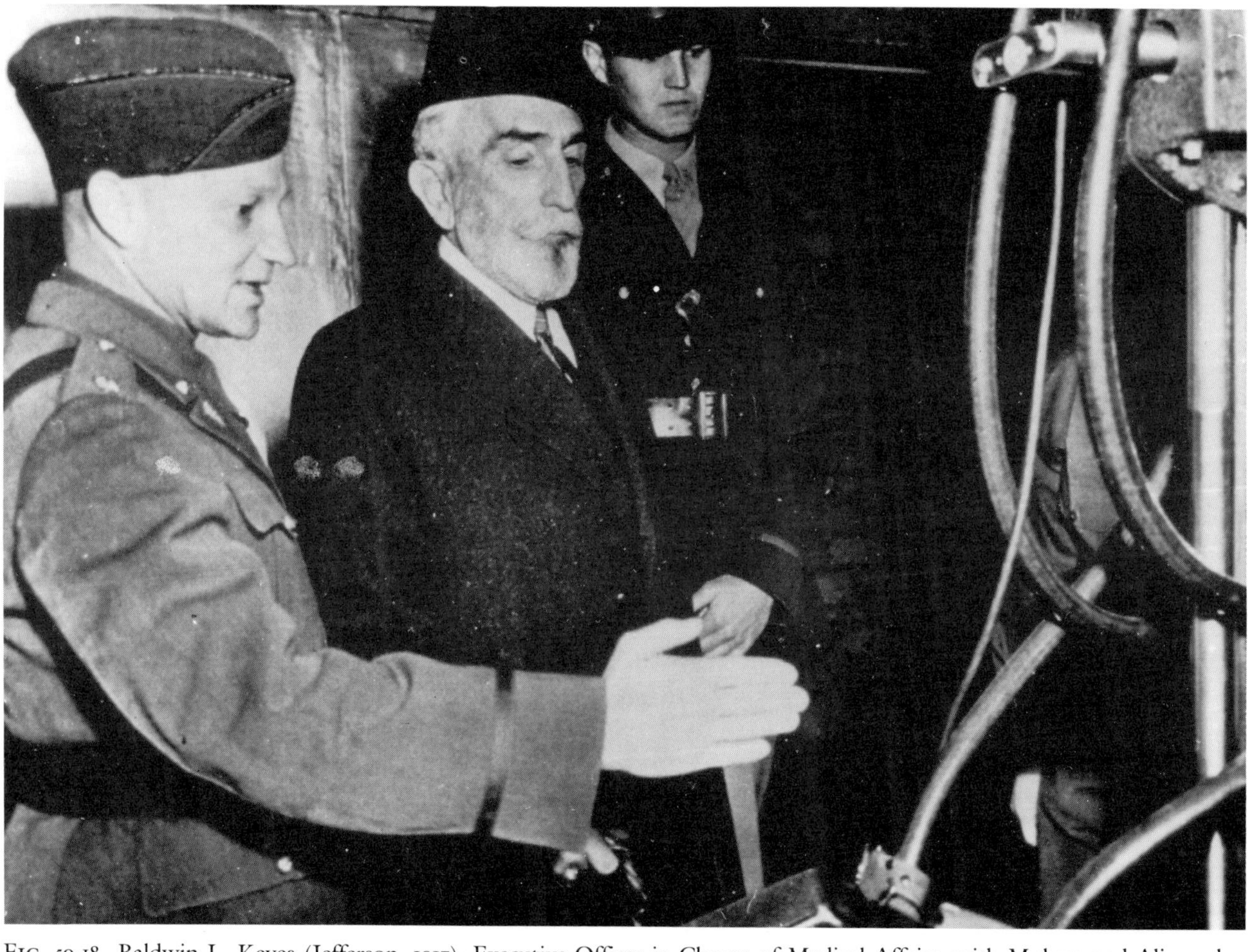

FIG. 59-18. Baldwin L. Keyes (Jefferson, 1917), Executive Officer in Charge of Medical Affairs, with Muhammed Ali, uncle of King Farouk.

it was not in a combat area. Many of the original physicians and nurses were transferred to other facilities. Dr. Keyes was transferred and promoted to Surgeon for the Delta Service Command.

One patient who passed through Jefferson General Hospital No. 38 was Associated Press Correspondent Paul K. Lee. He observed: "I have never stopped in Philadelphia in my life, but I have recently spent ten days as a patient of Jefferson Hospital of Philadelphia. The paradox is explained this way. The hospital is out on glimmering yellow-white sand somewhere between the River Nile and the Red Sea. Its official name was the 38th General Hospital, U.S. Army, but to a remarkable degree, it is still Jefferson Hospital of Philadelphia."[9] Mr. Lee's testimony simply confirms that it is the people, not the place, that gives Jefferson its special character.

The 38th General Hospital was cited for its service by Commanding General Giles of the African Middle East Theatre on May 8, 1945, with a Meritorious Service Plaque. It reads: "For superior performance of duty and the accomplishment of exceptionally difficult tasks." The Hospital was deactivated in 1949 as a Reserve General Hospital, and the designation "No. 38" was transferred to a medical school in Richmond, Virginia. Dr. Keyes' efforts to have the unit designation remain permanently associated with Jefferson were unsuccessful.

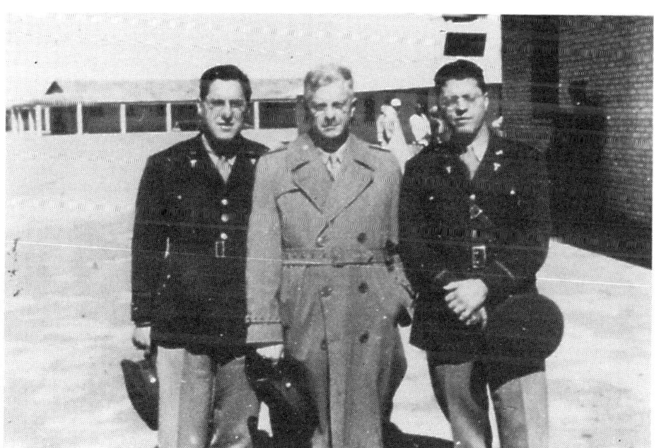

FIG. 59-19. Jacob J. Kirshner (1933), Burgess L. Gordon (1919), and Peter A. Theodos (1935) at "Kilo 13."

Jefferson contributed to the World War II effort at home as well as overseas. Early in the War, 12 beds in the hospital were set aside for the Navy by Dr. Hayward R. Hamrick (Jefferson, 1935), who was then Medical Director. Twenty corpsmen were trained in this way. Colonel Frederick H. Mills trained the students for the Army, and later Major R.H. Lackey performed this task. Registered nurses were also assigned to Jefferson for training.

In the fall of 1941, eighty-three Jefferson students from the first-year class enrolled in the Reserve Officers' Training Corps. These men spent an hour each day in military training and were commissioned as Second Lieutenants in the Student Army Training Corps. Their next year of medical school ended in April due to an accelerated program, and was followed by more stringent military training, including duty at New Cumberland, Pennsylvania. Prior to graduation these students were commissioned as First Lieutenants, Medical Corps, U.S. Army. Several later members of Jefferson's faculty, including Drs. Samuel S. Conly (Jefferson, S1944) and John J. Gartland (Jefferson, S1944), were in that unit. A Navy unit was also organized at Jefferson, but apparently military training was somewhat less rigid.

In other ways and places, Jeffersonians demonstrated competence and loyalty to country that earned them prominent military positions: Captain John H. Chambers (Jefferson, 1916), Medical Corps, U.S. Navy, was Commander of the Mobile Hospital Unit No. 2. He was present at the attack on Pearl Harbor on December 7, 1941; Captain Robert E. Duncan (Jefferson, 1919) was Commanding Officer in the Naval Hospital National Medical Center, Bethesda, Maryland; Rear Admiral Harold K. Cokely (Jefferson, 1921) was Executive Officer in a Naval Hospital in Guam, Commanding Officer of St. Alban's Hospital in New York and the U.S. Naval Hospital in Key West Florida, and Commanding Officer of the Naval Hospital in San Diego, which is the largest one in the United States; and Vice Admiral Thomas F. Cooper (Jefferson, 1924), U.S. Navy, was Inspector General and Commanding Officer of the Naval Hospital at Great Lakes, Illinois, as well as Commanding Officer of the Naval Medical Center in Bethesda.

In all, 2,122 Jefferson graduates, almost one-third of living alumni at the time, served in World War II. The great majority, 1,599, were in the U.S. Army. Another 424 were in the Navy; one in the Coast Guard; one in the British Army; and 19 in the U.S. Public Health Service. Several others were on unknown assignments.

Some alumni were killed in action or became prisoners of war: Capt. William T. Lineberry (1915), U.S. Navy (Japan); Lt. Col. Charles Leason (1918), Medical Corps, U.S. Army; Major Fred H. Beaumont (1928), (Germany); Capt. Sidney E. Seid (1933), Medical Corps (Japan); Capt. Frank Gallo (1934), Medical Corps (Japan); Capt. George A. Raider (1937), Medical Corps (Japan); Lt. J.G. Arthur Miller Barret (1938), U.S. Navy; Lt. J.G. Bey D. Landgon (1938), U.S. Navy; Dr. Richard Diamond (1943), killed or prisoner of war; Lt. Col. Clark Rodman (1943), Medical Corps, U.S. Army; Lt. J.G. Joseph A. Federowitcz (1942), U.S. Navy, killed in action.

For their heroism and devotion to their country, Jefferson graduates were awarded every decoration given to military personnel, and nearly every decoration from foreign governments. These included: Legion of Merit, Distinguished Service Medal, Commander of the Order of the British Empire, Commander of the Order of Bath, Presidential Unit Citation, Pacific Theatre Ribbon, Purple Heart, Letter of Commendation, Navy Commendation Medal, Typhus Commission Medal, European Theatre Ribbon, Bronze Arrowhead, Decoration of Aun Hai (China), American Defense Service Medal, American Theatre Medal, Victory Medal, Combat Medal Badge, European Occupation Ribbon Air Medal, Asiatic Pacific Theatre Medal, American Defense Service Medal, Philippine Liberation Ribbon, Silver Star, Brazilian War Cross, Belgian Fourrigere Liberation Ribbon, Testimonial Flag from Commanding General Chinese Army, Soldier's Medal, and Italian Medal of Valor. Many of these included Battle Stars, many with Oak Leaf Clusters, and many with palms and clasps.

In World War II, 32 Jefferson physicians were lost. Those who made this supreme sacrifice are immortalized on a plaque in the College (Figure 59-20) erected by the Alumni Association: "In Freedom's Cause. To the Eternal Memory of Those Graduates of the Jefferson Medical College Who Answered the Call of Duty and Gave Their

WORLD WAR II
IN FREEDOM'S CAUSE
TO THE ETERNAL MEMORY OF
THOSE GRADUATES OF THE
JEFFERSON MEDICAL COLLEGE
WHO ANSWERED THE CALL OF DUTY
AND GAVE THEIR LIVES WHILE SERVING
THEIR COUNTRY'S ARMED FORCES
DURING WORLD WAR II
1941 —— 1945
ABBOTT KENYON BAILEY
ARTHUR MILLER BARRETT
ALBERT JOSEPH BERTRAM
CLAYTON CALVIN EGAN CARSON
JAMES PHILIP CITTA
FOSTER LEONARD DENNIS
RICHARD CHARLES DIAMON
WILLIAM VINCENT ECKHART
JOSEPH HAROLD EISNER
JOSEPH ANTHONY FEDEROWICZ
JOHN FRANCIS GERAGHTY
SAMUEL SOLOMON GIDDING
GEORGE LEWIS GREASER
PAUL CHURCHILL JOHNSON
ABRAHAM HERMAN KOPLIN
CHARLES BYRON KORNS, JR.
ALFRED LABENSKI
ARTHUR LA ROE
CONDON CARLETON McCORNACK
LEONARD JOSEPH McGEE
THOMAS ANTHONY MARTIN, JR.
KENNETH JOSEPH MURRAY
MALCOLM LEWIS PRATT
JAMES JOSEPH QUINN
GEORGE ANDREW RADER
JOHN RICHARD SIDDALL
HARRY PAUL SINGLEY
WALTER LOW TATUM
WILLIAM JOSEPH WAGNER
HUBERT HORACE WASHBURN
GEORGE ALEXANDER WILDMANN
JOHN SCOTT WILLIAMS
ERECTED BY THE ALUMNI ASSOCIATION OF
THE JEFFERSON MEDICAL COLLEGE

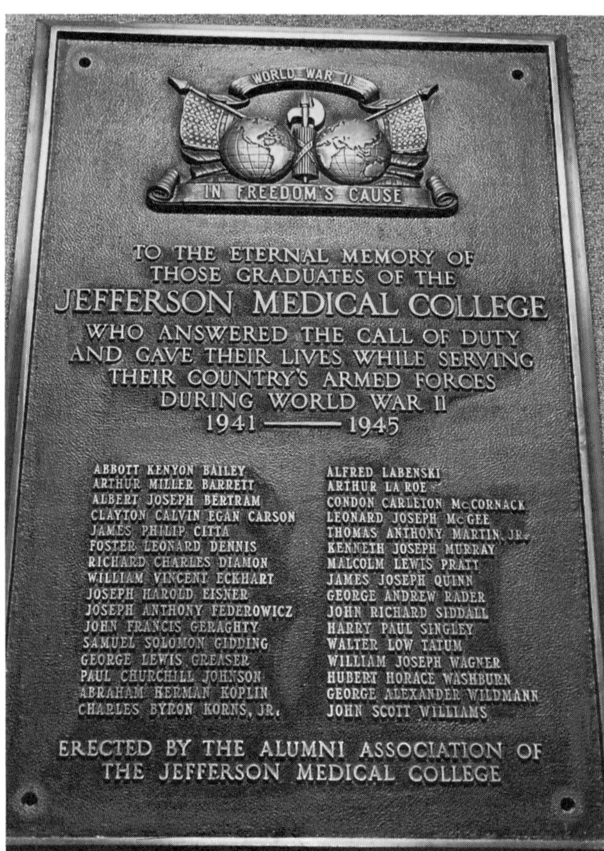

FIG. 59-20. The Alumni plaque in the College honoring the fallen in World War II.

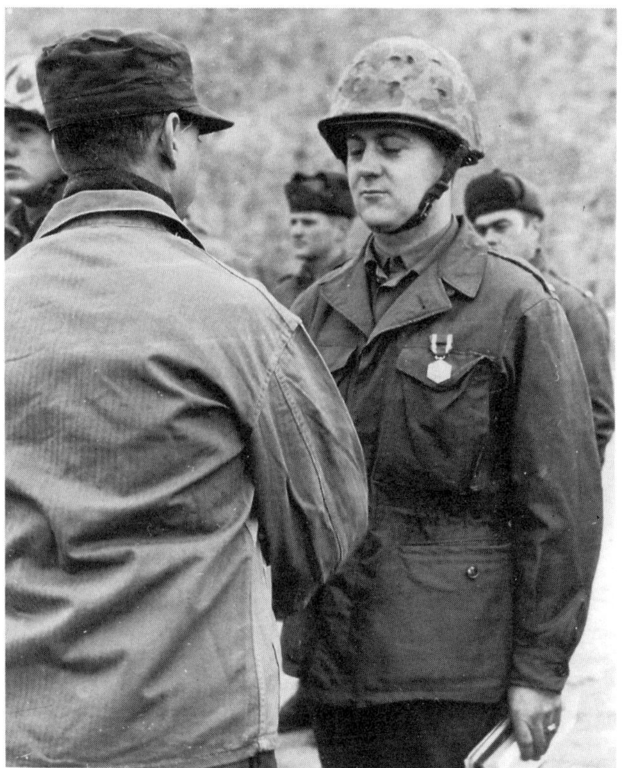

FIG. 59-21. Lt. George Farrell (1949) decorated in Korea.

Lives While Serving Their Country's Armed Forces During World War II—1941–1945."

The Korean Conflict

The mortality rate for the wounded who reached medical facilities during World War I was 8.5%. That figure was down to 4.5% by World War II. This was not only because of the increased efficiency and timing with which the injured were processed to treatment, but also because medicine by the 1940s had made significant strides.

Medical proficiency was to be put to the test again in Korea, where open hostilities broke out in 1950. Here, more than 33,000 Americans lost their lives. Certainly the number would have been greater if not for some lifesaving advances in technology. It was in Korea, for instance, that the helicopter was first used to evacuate the wounded. This timesaving factor greatly improved a soldier's chances for survival.

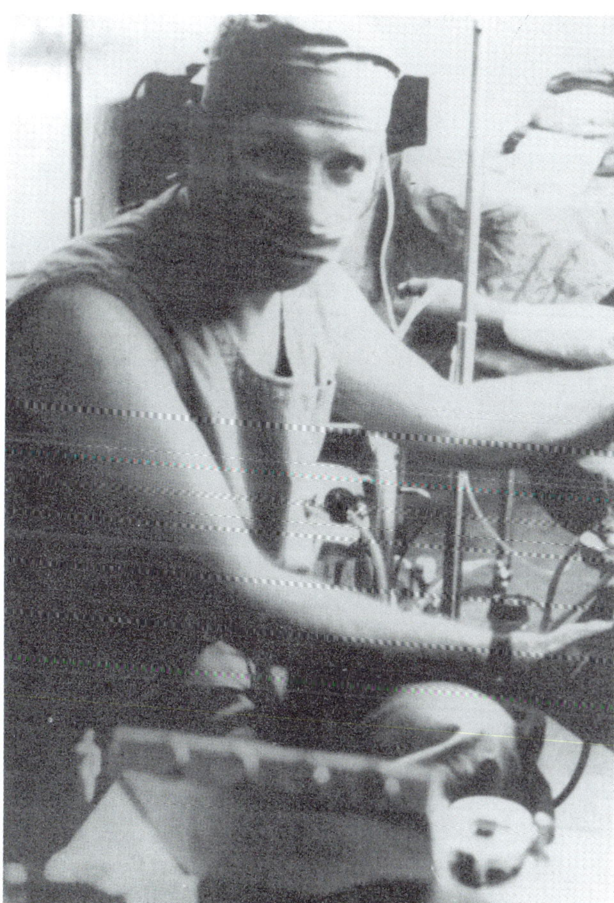

FIG. 59-22. Commander Robert A. Brown (1955), Medical Corps, U.S. Navy, administers an anesthetic at Phu Bai.

Information on the participation of Jefferson physicians in Korea is not as complete as that of earlier wars. The stories that have come to light, however, show that here too, Jefferson graduates continued the tradition of dedicated service, valor under duress, high moral character, and commitment to the country's cause. Typical is the record of Dr. Burgess A. Smith (Jefferson, 1949). Smith received the Distinguished Flying Cross for rescuing wounded men behind enemy lines in Korea.[10] On presenting the citation, the Commanding General of Medical Personnel in Korea said: "I am especially proud to present this award to you because you are one of us. It is not often that a member of the Medical Corps receives this high award." Dr. Smith was also recommended for the Silver Star. Dr. John E. Hughes (Jefferson, 1948) received a Meritorious Citation and a Secretary of War badge for general surgery in Korea. Another who unselfishly risked his life in Korea was Dr. George R. Farrell (Jefferson, 1949). Dr. Farrell received the Letter of Commendation Medal for heroism in action in Korea (Figure 59-21). He saved the lives of soldiers wounded when the First Marine Division was trapped by the Communist forces near the Changjin Reservoir.[11]

Those Jefferson men whose actions in Korea are recorded served with exceptional bravery and brilliance. Surely those Jeffersonians whose service in that conflict is not known to us also performed with the same high professional and personal standards that are fostered by the Jefferson experience.

Vietnam

By the 1960s when the United States became engaged in war in Vietnam, Jefferson had a century-long tradition of courage in combat medicine. Jefferson people had served in every war in the nation's history during that time. By now, however, it was possible to see some dramatic improvements in the survival rates of soldiers wounded in battle.

In the Civil War, the wounded often walked great distances to secure what limited medical help was available. When they reached the medical unit, amputation and palliation were often the treatment of necessity. One hundred years later, in Vietnam, it was possible to get an injured soldier to a well-equipped operating room with modern resuscitation equipment within 20 minutes of the time of injury.

Dr. Lee P. Haacker (Jefferson, 1960) has described the progress in battlefield medicine based on his firsthand experience in Vietnam.[12] As he pointed out, casualty-handling systems had greatly improved since the last war; transportation was now by helicopter and jet. Further, medicine offered better resuscitation equipment, and, most important, vast quantities of blood were accessible. Frozen blood could be stored almost indefinitely, making available larger quantities.

Even with medical and military progress, this war was no less bloody, but more men did survive. The mortality rate in Vietnam was lower than in any other major conflict. Only 2.4 percent of casualties reaching medical facilities died. Once again, Jefferson graduates helped make that possible.

Dr. Robert A. Brown (Jefferson, 1955), Commander, Medical Corps, U.S. Navy, served with the Third Marine Division during the siege of Khe Sanh in Vietnam. With enemy fire destroying the tents above ground, the medical team had to move to underground bunker space

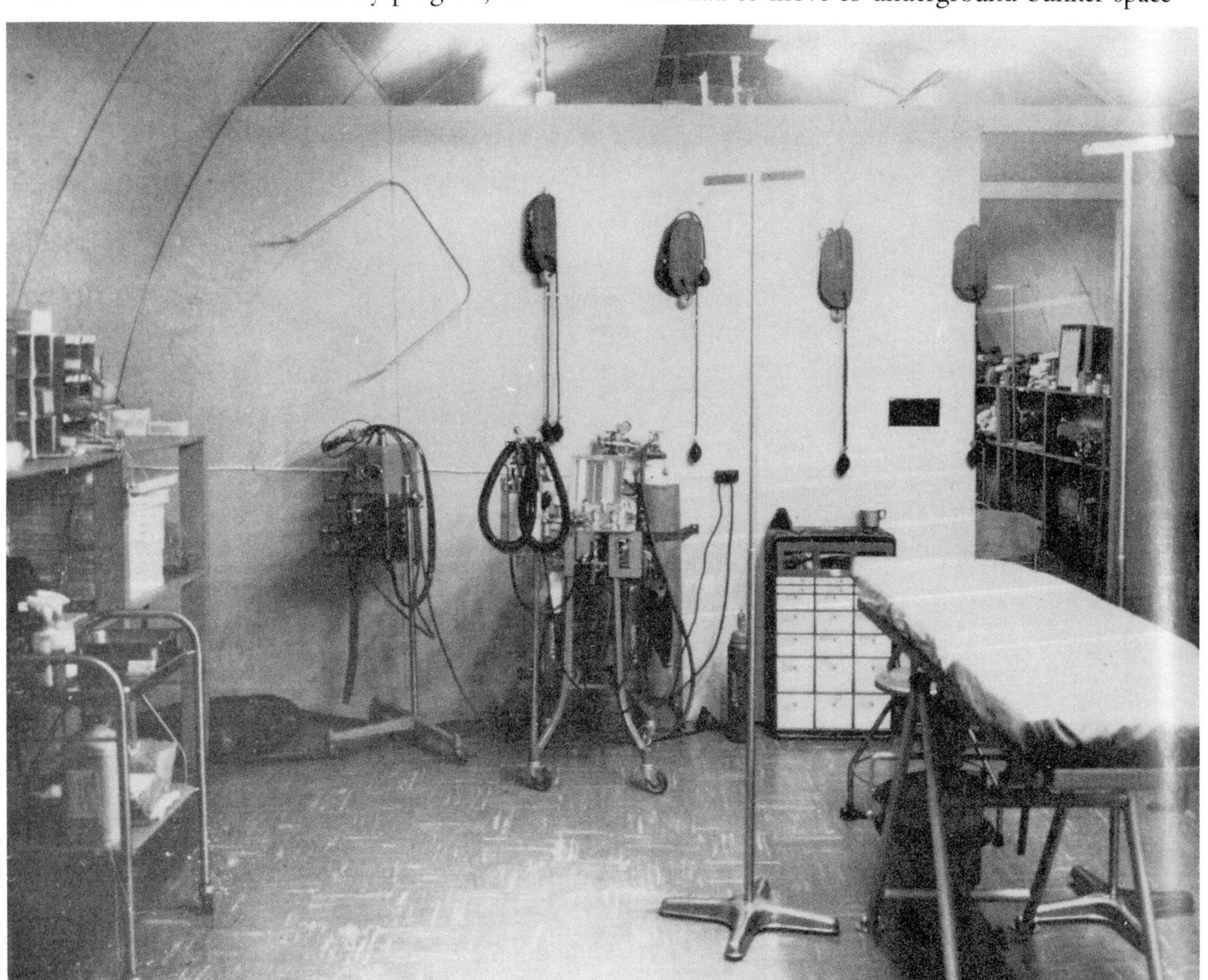

FIG. 59-23. An operating room in Vietnam.

to care for casualties when the siege began in January, 1968. During the ensuing three months the medical unit saw 2,541 patients. Most patients were wounded in action by sniper fire and shrapnel from artillery, rocket, and mortar fire (Figure 59-22). As Dr. Brown observed at the time,

> "The General Medical Officer in Vietnam adapts very rapidly to the smooth and rapid treatment of large numbers of casualties. He almost daily sees massive soft tissue trauma, with gross contamination caused by booby traps and mines and involving multiple systems of extremities, abdomen, chest and often face and neck. He learns to evaluate wounds caused by high velocity missiles and those caused by shrapnel. He automatically learns to treat the constant problem of heat exhaustion, salt depletion, malaria, dysentery, amebiasis, etc., and to consider them in his therapy in addition to the traumatic wound."[13]

Other Jefferson physicians who served in Vietnam included: Dr. Jerome Vernick (1962); Dr. Francis Madden (1967); Dr. James Holstein (1967); and Dr. Frederick J. Laucius (1967). Dr. Charles L. Deardorff, Jr. (1961) was assigned to the Seventh Surgical M.A.S.H. Hospital at CuChi for 14 months. Here he provided surgical care for casualties as well as holding weekly sick call in neighboring villages. Dr. Deardorff recalls that in traveling around to the villages, "Penicillin and soap were our main tools."[14]

The 14 doctors of the Seventh Surgical Hospital took on the casualties from Attleboro, one of the combat operations of the Vietnam War. A regiment of Vietcong had been contacted 20 miles from the hospital, and fierce fighting broke out. American casualties were high and were all flown to this hospital. The medical team treated 356 casualties in 96 hours. "Patients . . . spilled out into the field behind the hospital," Dr. Deardorff recalled. "We in the operating rooms never saw the patients we operated on before or after surgery. Other men would diagnose, resuscitate, and send the wounded into the O.R., one after the other." (Figures 59-23 and 59-24) When Attleboro was over, Dr. Deardorff was to notice in the medical personnel a deep realization: "that they had been useful, they had served their

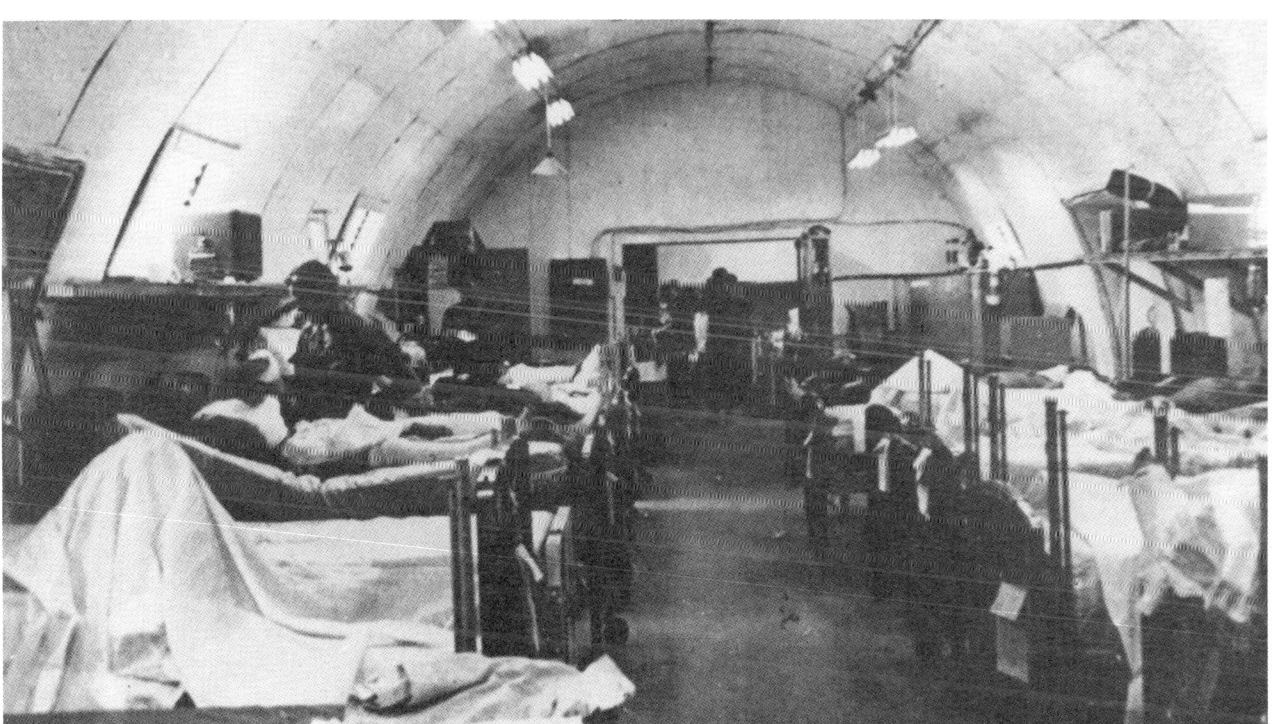

FIG. 59-24. A surgical intensive care unit and recovery room in Vietnam.

country and they were proud. . . . We have done our job."

The Class of 1970 erected a plaque in memory of their classmate, William E. Whiteman, and to those alumni who served in the Vietnam conflict (Figure 59-25).

In War and in Peace

Their names and numbers run into the thousands, those men and women of Jefferson who gave their energy, their care, and sometimes their lives when their country needed them. They gave with a spirit of generosity that was above the call of duty. They gave with a skill that makes them standard bearers for the medical profession. They gave willingly, knowing that it might require of them the highest human sacrifice.

Those educated in medicine possess a gift of healing that makes their presence indispensable when nations go to war. Perhaps none see the devastation of war as closely as those who care for its victims. An observer of World War I noted it this way: "War is the summation of all tragedies, the pinnacle of all follies, the abysmal depth of all horrors, . . . the supremacy of slaughter and starvation. It is insanity—out of which shines but one lone star, . . . the light of the Samaritan who feeds and clothes, arrests bleeding, binds wounds, bears anesthetics, sedation and opiates, nurses with tender hand, . . . takes the last faltering message to loved ones at home, and when comes the end, closes staring eyes, composes limbs, . . . covers with the flag the soldier, the fallen victim."

These were the physicians and nurses, all those who attended the battle not to destroy but to heal. It is Jefferson's privilege to have been able to serve that mission with a spirit and a distinction that represent the best of the medical profession and the best that is in us as human beings.

IN MEMORY OF
WILLIAM E. WHITEMAN, M.D. '70
KILLED OCTOBER 19, 1971
AND TO ALL ALUMNI WHO SERVED IN
THE VIET NAM CONFLICT

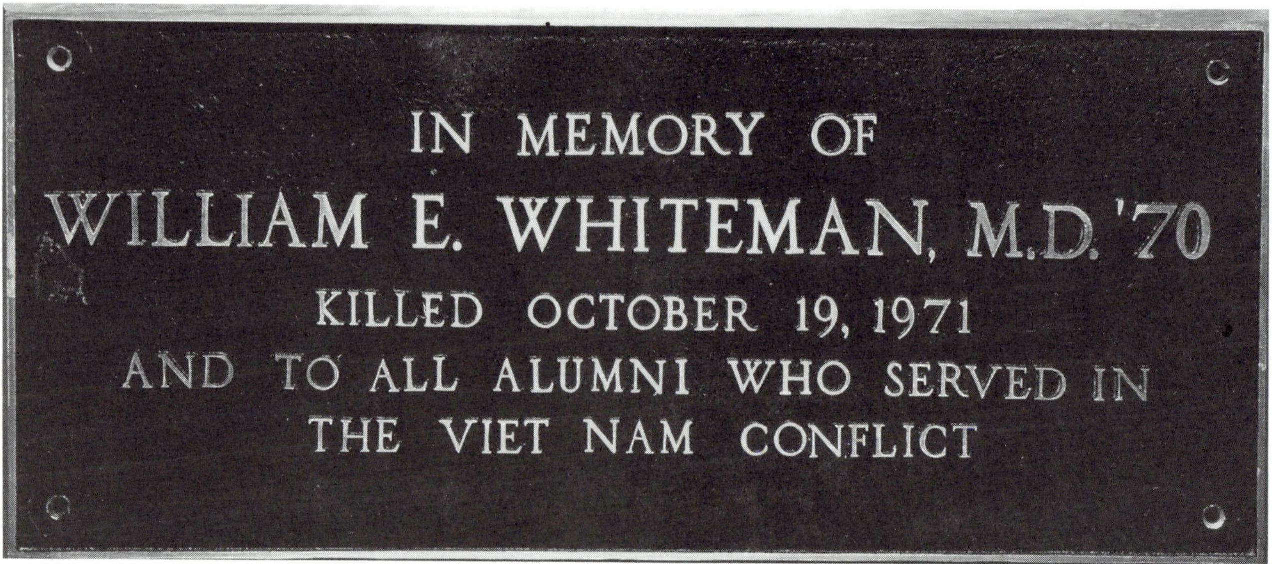

FIG. 59-25. The plaque erected by the Class of 1970.

References

1. "The William Potter Memorial Lecture," delivered at Jefferson Medical College, February 23, 1939.
2. Dalton, M., "Anson Jones, Physician-President." *The Pharos.* Winter 1986, pp. 15–20.
3. Pleadwell, F.L., "William Paul Crillon Barton, 1786–1856: Surgeon, U.S. Navy, A Pioneer in American Naval Medicine," *Military Surgeon.* March 1920, pp. 241–281.
4. Gould, G.M., *Jefferson Medical College of Philadelphia: History 1826 to 1904.* New York: Lewis Publishing Co., 1904.
5. Riordan, L., "Battlefield Medicine," *Jeff. Med. Coll. Al. Bull.,* Special Centennial Issue, 1970, pp. 10–13.
6. Ibid.
7. Ibid.
8. Coplin, W.M.L., *The American Red Cross Base Hospital No. 38.* Philadelphia: E.A. Wright Co., 1923.
9. Lee, P.K., Article in the *Philadelphia Evening Bulletin.* January 14, 1943.
10. *Jeff. Med. Coll. Al. Bull.* May 1951, p. 29.
11. *Jeff. Med. Coll. Al. Bull.* March 1951, p. 20.
12. Haacker, L.P., "Time and Its Effects on Casualties in World War II and Vietnam," *Arch. Surg.* 98:39–40, 1969.
13. Brown, R.A., "Dateline: Vietnam," *Penn. Med.* August 1968, pp. 45–53.
14. Deardorff, C.L., Jr., "A Tour of Duty," *Jeff. Med. Coll. Al. Bull.* Winter 1968, pp. 19–23.

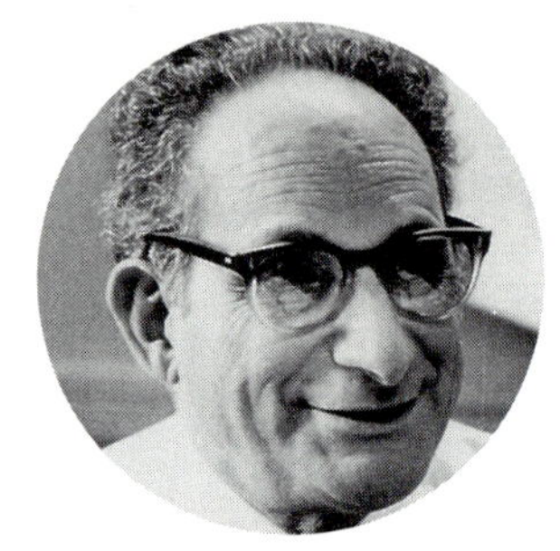

CHAPTER SIXTY

The University Art Collection

Robert J. Mandle, Ph.D.

"I trust that the Alumni Association will make it a part of their duty to adorn the College with memorials of this kind (portraiture) as a bare act of justice alike to themselves and to those who devoted their lives to the service of the school."

—Samuel D. Gross (1805–1884)

Mention of the widely known Jefferson art collection conjures up images solely of its outstanding portrait collection, one of the finest among medical schools, not only for its preeminent Eakins but also because it contains perhaps the oldest sequence of portraits of a medical college faculty. It is the largest component of the Jefferson art collection but only a part. A consideration of "Art" would include the buildings. Some, such as the Scott Library, have won awards for their architectural importance. Others are richly adorned with artistic examples such as the gargoyles on the College and Curtis Clinic buildings. Also, Jefferson's collection of sculpture, now numbering over 25 pieces, has continued to grow. Less well known are the many plaques commemorating benefactors and outstanding alumni. Many are of themselves artistic frames for the statement being presented.

The collection began with the Samuel Bell Waugh portrait of Charles D. Meigs in 1872. Frankenberger (The Librarian) in 1915 stated: "The entire collection of portraits in the possession of the College numbers twenty-four and is a valuable and most interesting one." In 1955, forty years later, there were 88 paintings, almost a threefold increase in number. These included paintings of members of the Board of Trustees, the faculty, and a few of the people who were important to the history of Jefferson, yet in neither group. The collection dated June, 1987, listed 224 paintings, a trebling in a space of only 32 years.

Paintings constitute the largest portion of Jefferson's art collection. Of the 228 paintings by 1988, a few are landscapes, but 214 are portraits. Others depict a subject that usually relates in some way to Jefferson. Most of these as well as many portraits have been given to Jefferson by friends of the University. Examples of such gifts include the painting of the front door of the Medical College building (1025 Walnut Street) by Benjamin Eisenstat and the *Osler at Old Blockley,* which, while not a gift, is on long-term loan from Wyeth Laboratories. Many of the portraits are also gifts of family or friends of faculty members, Trustees, or others thus honored.

By 1930 the collection had reached a size and importance sufficient to warrant the concern of the Board of Trustees. In essence, the Trustees were concerned about overcrowding the portraits or displaying "inferior portraits." They did not wish to have portraits accepted for hanging in the Medical College that were not "consistent with the quality of the paintings now owned and on hand." Those concerns of over one-half century ago are just as proper today. In consequence, the Dean's office, the faculty, and the Alumni Association became involved in the process of monitoring the collection and acquisitions.

Files from the 1950s indicate that a faculty committee was functioning and that it was carrying out the wishes of the Trustees with regard to the expansion, display, and maintenance of the portrait collection. The committee consisted of three or four Departmental chairmen who were concerned mainly with the "Class Portrait." The chairmen saw to it that the "Portrait Committee" of the Senior Class followed the process that would ultimately add a portrait of a distinguished "teacher" to the collection of which Jefferson is so justifiably proud. They also began to take note of conservation of a portion of the collection, especially the security of Eakins' *The Gross Clinic.*

From 1957 to July 1960 the Portrait Committee of the faculty was under the chairmanship of Dr. William Harvey Perkins. Members included Drs. Kenneth Goodner, Bernard J. Alpers, Baldwin L. Keyes, Thaddeus L. Montgomery, and Leandro M. Tocantins. Dean Sodeman was an *ex officio* member. Succeeding chairmen included Drs. Goodner, John B. Montgomery, Andrew J. Ramsay, and Peter A. Herbut. Upon his succession to the Presidency of the University, Dr. Herbut was replaced by Dr. Ramsay.

In the late 1960s the duties of the committee were assigned to the Protocol Committee of the College with Dr. Ramsay as chairman. In July, 1971, President Herbut created the "Thomas Jefferson University Committee on Art." This committee was made responsible for all aspects of art for the entire institution including the display and conservation of the portrait collection, sculptures, and plaques and approval of new acquisitions. It reported directly to the President.

In addition to Dr. Ramsay, the University Art Committee consisted of Beverly Borlandoe, the first Medical Student Representative to the Committee; Franklin C. Dalla, Director of the University Commons; Stanley Graham, Vice President for Development of the University (who shortly asked that his assistant, Oliver Robbins, be his named replacement); and Drs. John Lindquist, Robert J. Mandle, Paul J. Poinsard, Elias Schwartz, and Francis J. Sweeney, Jr. President Herbut was an *ex officio* member. Dr. Ramsay retired from the University in the fall of 1972. At that time Dr. Mandle became Chairman and remained so for nearly 16 years until July, 1986, when he too retired from the University and was replaced by Dr. Russell Schaedler.

The Portrait Collection and Other Paintings

In writing about Thomas Eakins and *The Gross Clinic* in the Summer, 1967, *Alumni Bulletin,* Elwood C. Parry, III gave an account of the beginnings of the Jefferson art collection. As he reports, after Dr. Gross had returned from a trip to Europe (1868), where he visited many famous centers for the teaching of medicine, he and Dr. Joseph Pancoast were guests of Alumni and friends at a dinner held in their honor. Dr. Gross concluded his speech to those assembled with the following remarks:

> "There is one thing that strikes an American in viewing the great literary and scientific and charitable institutions in Europe with admiration such as he cannot feel for his own. It is the respect which is everywhere shown to the memory of great and good men. Portraits, busts, and statues adorn alike the halls of learning . . . and the medical school. . . . In our city, so distinguished for its . . . institutions, there is a singular absence of everything of this kind."

The message must have been taken to heart by his audience, because two years following the founding of Alumni Association (1870) the first of five Samuel B. Waugh portraits of members of the Jefferson faculty was completed. This was a posthumous portrait of Dr. Charles D. Meigs based on a previous one by Waugh that was to be found at the College of Physicians. Thus began a tradition that continues with only slight modification today. The Meigs portrait was commissioned by "his former students" in 1872. The four others were of Drs. Joseph Pancoast (1874), Samuel D. Gross (1875), Robley Dunglison (1876), and John B. Biddle (1880). According to Elwood Parry, "there can be no doubt that Samuel B. Waugh was the official painter for the Jefferson Medical College in the 1870s."

Following Waugh, Eakins came along to take over as Jefferson's portraitist. Fortunately for Jefferson, Eakins' connections with members of its faculty had begun long before he painted the most famous of any work in the Jefferson collection: *The Gross Clinic.* Dr. Benjamin H. Rand, Professor of Chemistry, and later Dean, was Thomas Eakins' teacher and a friend of the family. For this reason and because of the admiration that Eakins felt for him as one of his teachers at Central High School, Eakins asked him to pose for a portrait, which was completed in 1874. *The Rand* portrait was entered by Eakins and selected by the committee for exhibit in the Centennial Exposition, and later Jefferson probably received the portrait from the family.

It is unfortunate that a like beneficence did not occur in the case of the Eakins' portrait of Dr. James W. Holland, *The Dean Calling the Roll.* Dr. Holland had been Dean of the Jefferson Medical College for 12 years. The family never accepted the portrait, supposedly because they disliked Eakins' realistic approach to portraiture. Eakins portrayed Dean Holland in the act of reading the names of the class while attired in his academic robe but wearing his favorite fishing shoes. This superb portrait was subsequently acquired by the Museum of Fine Arts in Boston. The Jefferson collection includes another portrait of Holland by Adolph Borie.

In 1981 Jefferson received a request from the Museum of Fine Arts (MFA) in Boston to borrow *The Gross Clinic* for an exhibit. In exchange for the loan, Jefferson was able to obtain Eakins' *The Dean Calling the Roll* for the duration of the MFA's need of the portrait of Dr. Gross, and the college placed the Holland in the space normally occupied by the perambulating *Gross Clinic.* Along with the original, Jefferson obtained a full-sized Polaroid(TM) reproduction of the original, which has been placed in the Eakins Gallery along with the other three Eakins portraits owned by the University.

The painting of Samuel David Gross by Eakins, better known as *The Gross Clinic,* has earned the respect of art historians and critics all over the world and has finally earned belated plaudits for Eakins as creator of the premier piece of American art. The University Committee on Art receives many requests each month for permission to reproduce it in textbooks or medical journals. *The Gross Clinic* has been exhibited in many cities, starting with its initial showing in Philadelphia at the time of the Centennial Exhibition in 1876. According to Carol Troyen in the catalog *A New World: Masterpieces of American Painting 1760–1910,* the painting was also exhibited in New York, 1879; St. Louis, 1904; New York and Philadelphia, 1917 (the year following the death of Eakins); Philadelphia, 1930, 1931, 1951, and 1955; Washington, D.C., 1961; Philadelphia, 1965; and New York, twice in 1970. In these shows it was usually just one of the pieces on exhibit. There have been many requests for its use in exhibits in the interim but a great reluctance over the years on the part of all of the various "committees" to allow it to travel. This was principally because of the age of the portrait, its emotional as well as its real value to Jefferson, and the attendant risks involved in allowing it to be displayed elsewhere. It was Dr. Bluemle who convinced the University Committee on Art that *The Gross Clinic* was more than a piece of important art owned by Jefferson. It was a part of Jefferson to be seen by the public and when properly exhibited would bring recognition to Jefferson. At his urging, the Committee in 1980 reluctantly agreed to allow the painting to travel to Alabama for an exhibit called "The Art of Healing: Medicine and Science in America" at the Birmingham Museum of Art. Here it was the centerpiece of the exhibit. Two years later in magnificent settings it would share the honor by being exhibited side by side with Eakins' *The Agnew Clinic* in both Philadelphia and Boston. This was as a part of an all-Eakins showing put together by the Philadelphia Museum of Art entitled "Thomas Eakins, Artist of Philadelphia." It was during this time that the reports of the art critics proclaimed *The Gross Clinic* to be the most important piece of art in America, and it was singled out for attention and high praise in the reviews of the exhibition in many newspapers and magazines.

The requests for its use in reproductions or for an exhibition escalated. With the enhancement of its position in the art world so also was there a heightened recognition of Jefferson. This reached international proportions when a request was received for its inclusion in a traveling exhibition of American art to be shown at Boston, Washington, and Paris. The exhibition was entitled, "A New World: Masterpieces of American Painting 1760–1910."

The University Committee on Art and President Bluemle in his position as an *ex officio* member had problems with this request. This was a prestigious request and not one to be turned down lightly. The exhibit was to be put together by members of the Museum of Fine Arts in Boston, the Corcoran Gallery of Art in Washington, D.C., and the Grand Palais in Paris. The pieces to be included in the exhibitions were to come from 57 public and private collections from the United States as well as the Tate Gallery in London and the Louvre. There would be eight other Eakins paintings represented in addition to works by 49 other outstanding American artists. It would be an honor to have *The Gross Clinic* included in such an exhibition, but at what risk? The work had only just returned from the tremendously successful Eakins exhibition in Philadelphia and Boston, for which it had been taken from its home in the newly constructed Eakins Gallery only one month after it initially had been installed there. If the request were to be honored, the painting would be gone from Jefferson for what would seem like an interminable ten months. The stresses placed upon the painting because of the necessity of being taken down, transported, and put up again in a different environment on four occasions might risk damage. The possibility of loss during transoceanic flight also arose. Full insurance was, however, provided which limited the dollar value that could be flown on any one plane. Was this more risky than transportation by truck on the various interstate highways to and from Boston and Washington? The decision was not an easy one, but in the end all concurred that there was an obligation to all of the viewers, American, French, and others, to include *The Gross Clinic* in this great exhibition. Inclusion would give additional recognition to Jefferson. The portrait had its own courier at each move. Mr. Roman Tybinko, himself an artist, had been associated with the Pennsylvania Academy of Fine Arts and had had similar responsibilities there. He had been engaged by Jefferson for a number of years in conserving paintings and hanging Eakins paintings. Members of Jefferson's Alumni and friends were able to view this great exhibit at each of the locations. In Washington, D.C., arrangements had been made to bring a large contingent from Philadelphia for a special viewing and refreshments. All agreed that the painting never looked better than it did in Boston and Washington.

The same unfortunately was not true for the showing in Paris. People viewing the exhibit felt that the French had shown bad taste in the manner in which the portrait was displayed. It had been hung on the back of a pillar so that it almost touched the floor and intruded into the aisles. It was placed to the rear of one's direction of progress through the exhibit and thus easily could be missed. Whoever was responsible for the choice of the location for the painting had certainly not featured it in the way it had been highlighted in the previous two exhibits. The entire exhibition was revamped from the way it had been seen in the United States, even to the changing of the cover of the catalog. The French were said to have believed that Frederick Remington's *Evening on a Candian Lake* was the work of an illustrator rather than that of a true artist, and they substituted a work by George Caleb Bingham for the cover of the French edition. Needless to say, a collective sigh of relief was heard from the University Committee on Art and President Bluemle when the portrait of Samuel Gross was safe again on the wall of the Eakins Gallery in Jefferson Alumni Hall.

The prolonged absence of *The Gross Clinic* from its usual place in the Eakins Gallery was eased somewhat by the presence of a full sized Polaroid™ reproduction in its place. During the painting's sojourn in Boston at the Eakins exhibit in 1982, Jefferson took advantage of the fact that there existed in the Museum of Fine Arts Museum in Boston a laboratory of the Polaroid Corporation. They had a unique camera capable of making full-scale color reproductions of paintings. While the exhibition was being readied, two full-sized replicas of *The Gross Clinic* were made. One of these was for use in the place of the original when it would be away from Jefferson and the other held in reserve or perhaps used for the purpose of making it available to qualified museums for teaching or display. At that same time, sets of full-scale and enlarged details of the painting were also made. These detailed prints and enlargements have enhanced the appreciation of the Eakins portrait of Dr. Gross.

Two other portraits in the collection that have interesting backgrounds are those of Thomas Jefferson and Benjamin Franklin, bearing "indecipherable inscriptions" discovered by the Historical Records Survey of Pennsylvania in December of 1939. The portraits are described in a "Fine Arts" insurance policy for the Medical College in 1951 issued by the Atlantic Mutual Insurance Company on December 8, 1951. Both the Jefferson and the Franklin are listed with the notation, under the column "Artist," "Gilbert Stuart (attributed to)."

These two portraits are said to have been given by the subjects to Jefferson College in Canonsburg, which is in western Pennsylvania. How the Jefferson Medical College got these has been detailed in an article by Doctors J. Douglas and James H. Corwin, alumni of the classes 1935 and 1956, respectively, in the "Winter 1974 Jefferson Medical College *Alumni Bulletin*." Dr. James Corwin of the Class of 1903 and Dean Ross Patterson of Jefferson in 1929 paid a visit to an "elderly Lady by the name of Roberts" who lived in Canonsburg. Dr. Corwin thought she had or knew who did have the portraits; he believed that the portraits had been kept hidden in Canonsburg after Jefferson College moved to Washington, Pennsylvania, when it merged with Washington College to create Washington and Jefferson College. The trip was highly successful, and the portraits came to Jefferson. Even though the authorship of the paintings is uncertain, their history and their association with our namesake College makes them interesting.

The Class Portraits

The highest honor that can be given to a faculty member at Jefferson is to be chosen by the senior class to have his or her portrait painted and presented to the Medical College (to the University after 1969). This is a fulfillment of the wish of Samuel D. Gross in a manner that brings honor not only to the recipient but also to the class itself. The honor is bestowed upon a member of the faculty by a vote of the graduating class. The criteria for selection have mainly been the teacher's relationship with the students and their recognition of him or her as outstanding.

The Samuel Bell Waugh portrait of Charles D. Meigs, though painted after his death, was commissioned by the students in 1872. It was given to the family, and ultimately they gave it to Jefferson. This would seem to qualify it as the first "class portrait." Three years later, the Class of 1885 commissioned Bernhard Uhle to do a portrait of William H. Pancoast, Chairman of the Department of Anatomy, who succeeded his father to this Chair. William Williams Keen was selected by the class of 1901 to have his portrait painted by artist William Merit Chase and presented to the Medical College. If one were to rank the reputation of the artists whose work is represented in the Jefferson collection, Chase would probably place second only to Thomas Eakins. Chase painted a superb life-size portrait of Dr. Keen, was an excellent teacher of art, and influenced many of the portraitists who were to paint members of the faculty in years to come.

The Classes of 1905, 1906, 1907, and 1908 asked Thomas Eakins to paint a portrait of William Smith Forbes, Chairman of Anatomy and a teacher "greatly esteemed by the students." The painting, done in 1905, was the only one to have been commissioned by four classes.

For years there were no further portraits commissioned by the students. The Class of 1924 then restored the custom by presenting the portrait of J. Chalmers DaCosta, raising funds by subscription and by the proceeds of a basketball game. The tradition continued through 1956, when the class objected to the manner of selection of the Professor for the honor and declined to participate. This caused a change in the selection process and enlarged the eligibility list to include persons below the rank of Chairman. This policy proved highly satisfactory.

For many years the portraits were paid for through the students' "laboratory fees." Ultimately the increasing cost resulted in subsidy through the office of the Dean. The selection of the artists, for a time restricted by reason of limited funding, was thus somewhat liberalized. It is appreciated that many fine artists accepted commissions at fees below their regular ones.

The mechanism for portrait presentation in recent years has included student committee input and Art Committee approval for selection of the subject and then the artist. Upon completion, the Art Committee rules upon the acceptability of the portrait before its presentation. Ceremonies usually include a biographical sketch of the subject and acceptance speeches by the Dean of the Medical College and the President or Chairman of the Board with a response by the subject being honored.

There has been a practice during the class reunions in early June to display some of the class portraits. Those portraits commissioned by the classes celebrating their twenty-fifth and fiftieth anniversaries of graduation are given places of honor for display.

This tradition is admired and copied by other colleges and is something that goes far beyond the expectations of Dr. Gross. A near-perfect record exists now of 63 years of honoring "those who devoted their lives to the service of the school." These are the portraits given not by the Alumni, as suggested by Gross, but by the students themselves.

Other Portraits And Paintings

Apart from the 62 class portraits, the remaining 201 portraits fall into one of two other categories. The first is made up of those commissioned by the Alumni Association or colleagues and friends to honor a member of the faculty or the Board of Trustees. The second category includes the many portraits and other paintings given by "Friends of Jefferson," be they former students, family of former faculty members or Trustees, or someone wishing to donate a piece of art to Jefferson.

Many examples could be given for each category. The prime piece in collection is the gift from the Alumni Association of *The Gross Clinic.* The Alumni also presented the portraits of Mr. Robert P. Hooper, a Trustee, Dr. Thomas McCrae, and Dean Ross V. Patterson. Portraits of members of the faculty given to Jefferson by colleagues and friends have in recent years constituted most of the growing number of paintings. Examples would include Dean Sodeman and the most recent addition to Jefferson's fine paintings of its faculty, the portrait of Dr. Warren Goldburgh. From members of the Alumni have come the portraits of Franklin and Jefferson and the portrait of Mrs. Burnside by her husband, the respected portraitist Cameron Burnside, contributed by Dr. Dwight Ashby, Jr. (1946).

Many families having a tie to Jefferson have generously given paintings to Jefferson. Dr. Orville H. Bullitt, Jr., a member of the Board of Trustees, recently gave a painting by Samuel Waugh of his ancestor Louisa Weissel Gross, the wife of Samuel D. Gross. Dr. Susan B. Ward (Jefferson, 1985) gave a Waugh copy of her great-great-great grandfather, Samuel D. Gross, to the University in 1988. Board President Percival Foerderer presented the portraits of his wife and himself that can be viewed in the Foederer

Pavilion. Daniel Baugh gave two portraits of himself to Jefferson for the Institute that bears his name. The paintings of Dr. John Eberle and his wife Salomé were donated by a descendant of the family and are valuable works of Jacob Eichholtz from Lancaster, who painted during the early 1800s. An alumnus, Dr. Robert Lukens, painted portraits of his former Professors including Dr. Chevalier Jackson and Dr. Randle Rosenberger and donated them to Jefferson.

Many paintings have been given by persons not directly connected with Jefferson. Molly Guion, a contemporary artist, donated two paintings. One was of Dr. Daniel Baker, Jr. (Jefferson, 1933) whom she admired—he had just been granted the Alumni Achievement Award posthumously, and she thought that it would be appropriate for Jefferson to have a copy of the portrait that she had done of him for another institution. The other was a copy of a portrait of Thomas Jefferson by Rembrandt Peale.

The sudden explosion of contemporary portraits of members of the faculty created a problem for the University Committee on Art. Proper display places were diminishing and placing portraits in storage was not desirable. To deal with this problem the University Portraits Standards Committee was formed in 1983 and specific guidelines were developed. The future care of the collection should thus be assured.

Sculpture

The Fine Arts Collection also includes 27 pieces of sculpture in addition to the gargoyles on the buildings on Walnut Street. Some of these are in fine marble, others in bronze, and some in plaster. The most recent addition has been the full-size erect statue of Thomas Jefferson by Lloyd Lilly, in bronze.

The statue that dominates the south side of Walnut Street in front of the College is *The Winged Ox,* by the Philadelphia artist Henry Mitchell. Placed on campus in the spring of 1976, it was Jefferson's fulfillment of its commitment to the Philadelphia Redevelopment Authority. Philadelphia was the first city in the United States to establish a policy that would increase the public art for the city. It mandated that developers of land made available to them by the city had to place on such property a piece of art equal to or greater in value than 1% of the cost of the building(s) to be erected. The Orlowitz and Scott Library buildings were erected on land that had been acquired in such a manner from the city. It was thus necessary for the University to obtain a piece of art that would satisfy the guidelines of the Redevelopment Authority. The senior officers of the University, in consultation with Paul Harbison, the architect of the new Scott Library, decided to hold a competition for a piece of sculpture. Henry Mitchell, the winner of the competition, chose as his subject the patron saint of both physicians and sculptors, the ox of St. Luke.

The very popular and artistically exciting statue consists of a 1,400-pound winged ox on a platform subtended by a vertical column about which is a spiral of 50 names of personages who made outstanding contributions to medicine. The list of names was compiled by George M. Norwood, then Vice President for Planning and subsequently Interim President of the University. He, with the help of the librarian, Robert Lentz, had the difficult task of paring down the list to accommodate the 50 spaces allowed by Mr. Mitchell. Among those chosen for this high honor were five alumni of Jefferson. Samuel D. Gross, Carlos Finlay, J. Marion Sims, Chevalier Jackson, and John H. Gibbon, Jr. The total weight of the statue is about 5,000 pounds, and it stands between the two buildings.

Only a few years later, the University was again responsible for a 1% Redevelopment Authority art project. The Parking Garage and the Barringer Residence for students were built on land made available to the University by the city. The University Committee on Art was asked to make recommendations to the senior officers and the Board of Trustees as to a manner in which the obligation could be met. A fountain was agreed upon and, again with the help of Paul Harbison, Jr., a competition was held. Three artists selected by the committee were asked to submit models of a fountain. The committee, unaware of the identity of the creator of each model, chose a fountain containing otters that was again the work of Henry Mitchell. The fountain was dedicated to William Bodine, Jr., Past President of the University. It was Bodine who in 1973 gave the University a fine bust of Thomas Jefferson sculpted by Rudulph Evans that now resides in the lobby of the Medical College building.

The A. Stirling Calder bronze statue of Samuel David Gross that stands on the South side of the Scott Library came to Jefferson in 1970. Previous to this it had been standing since 1897 in Smithsonian Park in Washington, D.C. Over the years it had been largely unnoticed there, and through the efforts of the Jefferson Alumni Association it was moved to the campus. It is a larger-than-life-size statue of Dr. Gross as he is seen in the Eakins portrait. He stands in the same position, addressing his students while holding in his hand the scalpel, which in this case lacks the vivid blood seen in the painting. When the statue arrived from Washington the scalpel was missing. Steve Tatti, who had been engaged by the University Committee on Art to take care of the conservation of outdoor sculptures, was able to make a very acceptable scalpel and place it in the hand of Gross.

The silver mace, symbol of authority during Commencement exercises and some other University ceremonies, is in reality a piece of sculpture. The theme of its design is the *Winged Ox* of Mitchell. A silver winged ox surmounts an ebony staff with an adornment of lapis lazuli jewels set in garlands of silver near the top and bottom. The mace was beautifully crafted by Eugene Zweigle, a remarkable silversmith, who translated Mitchell's piece into the *Jefferson Mace*. It was introduced into Jefferson's ceremonials during the commencement exercises in June, 1986.

The Slave Girl by Tadolini has been a part of the environment of the Daniel Baugh Institute of Anatomy for countless students during their introduction to human anatomy. Over the years it has been thought to be a good-luck charm for the freshmen medical students, a sort of "touchstone" for the course. This imposing marble statue is remarkable not only for the grace and form of the maiden so skillfully crafted by the artist, but also for the engineering skill manifested in the way this heavy statue is placed on its pedestal. A mechanism has been built into the top of the pedestal that allows one to rotate the statue with the effort of only a finger.

A statue of *Athena*, that stood in a niche in the lobby of the Thompson Building as long as one can remember, was moved to the anteroom of the Eakins Gallery in 1988. Investigations by Mrs. Julie Berkowitz, the University Art Researcher, suggested that this Roman work dates from somewhere between 100 B.C. and 200 A.D.

Display of the Collection

Much effort has been directed toward displaying the collection to public view rather than keeping it in storage. Risks attach to the display of any piece, whether painting or sculpture, though theft is of lesser concern than mutilation or inadvertent injury to a portrait. Damage has occurred to several paintings because of their location in areas exposed to the general public as well as to students and employees. These paintings were repaired by skilled conservators, and arrangements were made for continuing maintenance of the collection.

There is, however, great concern on the part of the Committee on Art for *The Gross Clinic*. As described elsewhere, this masterpiece escalated in value during midcentury, and in the 1960s it received the special attention it had long deserved. Through the efforts of Theodor Siegl, an outstanding conservator from the Pennsylvania Academy of Fine Arts, a complete restoration was carried out and the painting was remounted. Following this it was possible to consider the many requests for loan of the painting to major exhibitions.

The Eakins Gallery was designed by Val Lewton of the Smithsonian Institution. Its purpose was enhancement of the enjoyment of the Eakins masterpieces in addition to the provision of maximum security and preservation. The focus of attention for most people visiting the Gallery is *The Gross Clinic*. Two additions to the Gallery of three-dimensional representations of the portrait have helped visitors gain a better understanding of the scene depicted. One, a model using sculptors' figures, was made by Dr. Gary Carpenter, a member of the Committee. It helps the viewer with the perspective of the group, foreshortening the patient to aid in understanding the nature of the surgical procedure. The second model, itself a work of art, is a diorama made to a size about one-twelfth that of the painting. It is the work of Frederick W. Klotz, whose hobby is making accurate scale models of soldiers and constructing dioramas. In this one, Klotz portrays the whole scene from the perspective of one in the amphitheater at the head of the operating table. He had to imagine what the floor would look like, as well as the front of the instrument table and other details that are not seen in the two-dimensional painting. The diorama, which took about 18 months to complete, has been placed in the wall opposite the Eakins masterpiece and is itself a fine addition to the Gallery.

The Conservation of the Collection

In 1973 the Committee obtained the services of Joseph Amorotico (now deceased), who was trained by Theodor Siegl and worked with him on the restoration of *The Gross Clinic.* Mr. Amorotico examined the collection at least yearly and made recommendations for paintings needing conservation or minor cleaning and repairs, some of which could frequently be done right at Jefferson. When major restoration was required, the piece was transferred to Amorotico's conservation laboratories in the Pennsylvania Academy of the Fine Arts. This active and ongoing effort at conservation of the collection was made possible because the Jefferson art committee obtained a budget for that purpose.

Most painting conservators of the past began as practicing artists who developed a special interest in restoration. Sophisticated modern techniques have evolved in recent years that have extended their earlier efforts. Experience at Jefferson reflects the changes in emphasis from an attitude of benign neglect to one of active maintenance. In the past, records generally did not indicate how a painting was restored or by whom. Today a complete description of the painting as it was received together with photographs taken before and after the procedure as well as a description of what was done are furnished with each major conservation.

Conservation of sculpture, like that of paintings, has also evolved. Until very recently the cleaning of pieces was done by conscientious individuals in the custodial service who took the time to dust or wipe a piece, probably to its detriment. Today trained conservators of sculpture are available. A program of regular care of the outdoor pieces on the campus is under the direction of Steve Tatti, who has been trained in this highly specialized field. Care includes a form of preventive maintenance designed to prevent or minimize the deleterious effects of the environment.

The conservation of a painting or statue is an expensive undertaking. Many of the portraits have a value established for insurance purposes as little more than the value of the frame. The value to Jefferson is much more than that given by even a sympathetic insurance appraiser. For this reason, when a painting or statue is in need of conservation it gets it, often at a cost far in excess of the price or insured value of the original piece. Restoration of frames is also an art for which the application of skills is also expensive. What price can one put on a "class portrait" or on the portrait of one of Jefferson's outstanding faculty members or members of the Board of Trustees? These pieces of art are a part of the spirit of an institution and the people who make it up as well as a record of its history. As such, the Fine Arts Collection deserves the best attention that is available.

The University Committee on Art serves a very important and useful function at Jefferson. It is responsible for a unique part of Jefferson, its art collection. This includes some of the best works of American artists as well as many pieces admired for their subjects apart from their strictly artistic value. While there is a real difference in the actual dollar value of components of the collection, each and every portrait, piece of sculpture, plaque, and painting is important to Jefferson. As long as there is a living member of a class that commissioned a particular portrait or a "Friend" who contributed to the painting of a colleague, there will be a painting that has the same importance as those considered to be more monetarily valuable. The Committee's paramount concerns are the protection, display, and maintenance of the high quality of the Fine Arts Collection at Jefferson for future generations of Jeffersonians as well as for others who have an interest in the collection.

Samuel D. Gross would have been gratified to know that the Alumni Association he founded and trusted "as part of their duty to adorn the College" is underwriting a book in preparation (1988) about Jefferson's art collection. Julie Berkowitz, A.B., M.A. (History of Art), as University Art Researcher, is compiling information to author this project, estimated to require about three years.

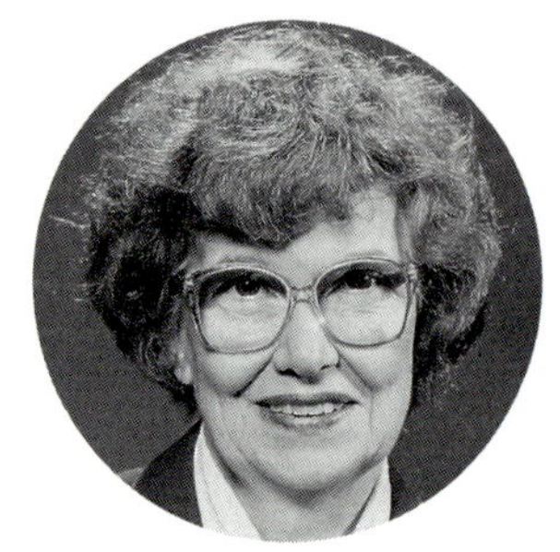

CHAPTER SIXTY-ONE

Audiovisual Services

THERESA M. POWERS, B.S.

"One picture is worth more than a thousand words."

—CHINESE PROVERB

THE USE OF teaching aids at Jefferson no doubt started with the formation of the Medical College itself in 1824, although the formal establishment of the present facility of audiovisual services did not occur until 1972. To learn of the origin and evolution of audiovisual services at medical centers in general and at Thomas Jefferson University in particular, it is interesting to look first to a period long ago when rare and valuable manuscripts were read only by the teacher and never put into the hands of the students. With the advent of printing, books and documents could be widely circulated, and teachers found it unnecessary to read to their pupils. Individual study methods were then possible, and students could be assigned various texts and related reading material. Lectures could be printed. Later, with the development of photography, the addition of still pictures to hand-drawn illustrations enhanced the written records. Motion pictures and sound next entered the field, with television only one step away. The teacher could now augment the lecture not only with chalkboard illustrations and predrawn charts, but also with professionally prepared sound recordings and visual aids. Schools early recognized their value.

Dr. Herman A. DeVry, in 1912, invented the first portable, hand-cranked, silent, motion picture projector. The first model of the projector is on exhibit at the Smithsonian Institution, and DeVry is listed, along with Thomas A. Edison, on the honor roll of the American Society of Motion Picture and Television Engineers. Dr. DeVry has been called the "Father of Visual Education." In 1925 he synchronized sound-on-disc with motion pictures and in 1933 announced 16 mm. sound-on-film projectors with sound-heads and speakers. His work in the audiovisual field had a profound influence on the use of the motion picture medium in schools and colleges as well as in industry. He founded and subsidized for years the National Conference on Visual Education, a symposium of educators, government personnel, producers, and industry representatives to study and develop more effective ways to use audiovisual media, especially sound motion pictures. This annual symposium was the creative stimulus for many highly specialized audiovisual organizations. These associations supported not only the development of better audiovisual media and equipment, but also the improvement of facilities for using them more effectively.

The terms "visual aids" and "teaching aids" were introduced into the literature prior to 1922 in reports on the comparative effectiveness of various educational methods in schools and universities of the northeastern United States. Since the early 1920s there have been countless studies of audiovisual media at leading universities throughout the United States looking toward more effective communication tools to stimulate the learning process. Summary reports were made throughout the 1930s by individual investigators. During World War II, the U.S. Government used audiovisual media extensively when the armed services faced the problem of orienting and training millions of service personnel in the shortest possible time. This led to numerous advances and technical developments.

During the nineteenth century there were two Jefferson pioneers in the field of graphic teaching and reproduction. Dr. J. Aitken Meigs (Jefferson, 1851) introduced the use of stereopticon illustrations for his teaching in the Institutes of Medicine (Physiology) during the 1870s. Dr. William Thomson (Jefferson, 1855) joined Jefferson's staff as Lecturer in Eye and Ear in 1874 after a distinguished Army career during and following the Civil War. He was one of the founders of a photographic bureau in the new Army Medical Museum and pioneered in experimental photomicrography. He devised techniques whereby prints of microscopic fields could be magnified 15 to 250 times.[1] These and other forms of graphic illustration became more widely used near the turn of the twentieth century, although primitive lantern slides became available as early as 1846.[2] As photography improved, glass lantern slides became the standard until color photography permitted the use of Kodachrome transparencies beginning in 1935. Shortly thereafter, Dr. Andrew J. Ramsay of the Department of Anatomy at Jefferson was among the first to use Kodachromes for a scientific convention presentation.

The clinical use of photography and its audiovisual successors was promoted at Jefferson by Dr. William H. Whiteley (Jefferson, 1943). Having become interested in and skilled in photography in his teens, as a medical student he quickly established a friendship with Dr. Ramsay, who taught him the elements of photomicrography. He also became friendly with Joseph Poppel in the Department of Biochemistry. Poppel did photographic work for that Department, but his services were also used extensively by other Departments for photomicrographs, for copying, and especially for lantern slides.

Another source of photographic services for the Hospital and Medical School was the Cardeza Foundation where Alan Hancock had developed skills in clinical photography. His services were soon in demand from other clinical areas. Facilities were relatively primitive, and wartime strictures limited new ventures. Dr. Whiteley, however, was called upon by colleagues with increasing frequency for clinical photography. The arrival of Dr. Rudolph Jaeger to head the Division of Neurosurgery in 1943 gave impetus to Dr. Whiteley's involvement and added to his qualifications as Dr. Jaeger's first resident in Neurosurgery.

Dr. Jaeger was already skilled in photographic art and motion picture production. In 1947 he established a photographic art studio largely furnished by Dr. Whiteley. Mary Nelson, an artist from the Johns Hopkins School of Art, joined the group and contributed sketches and illustrations for lectures. The group also prepared motion pictures and other materials for all types of teaching aids and convention exhibits.

The process remained departmentalized with Anatomy, Dermatology, Ophthalmology, Hematology, Psychiatry, and Pathology utilizing their own skills. Centralization had been planned since the 1940s but was not realized until after pioneering efforts by the Anatomy Department led the way. Dr. Andrew J. Ramsay, the new (1958) Chairman of the Department, needed a research specialist to handle the innovative audiovisual media that he envisioned as necessary for medical education. He asked Theresa M. Powers to join the Department in this role. Dr. Ramsay foresaw the need for closed circuit television, photography, projection equipment service, and medical art work. Thus, with Powers' versatility and enthusiasm, the service evolved for the Anatomy Department using a wide range of skills in producing media software. The year 1960 saw the use of television in gross anatomy, and its specialized technique of visualization through the microscope become available in the Department. It has since become widely employed.

When Jefferson Alumni Hall was opened in 1969, sophisticated techniques were built in for the Department of Anatomy. Closed circuit television linked specially designed cubicles to the entire laboratory. The television-microscopy facilities were the first in existence. Also, an x-ray apparatus with image intensification facilities was located in the embalming and cadaver storage suite. These capabilities established the base for development of a centralized service for the entire University.

In 1960 the Executive Council appointed a Supporting Facilities Committee. An immediate concern of this Committee was the development of a complete audiovisual program. An Audiovisual Subcommittee was formed that studied extensively the problems and needs and in 1970 made a complete report that established the foundation for the new Audiovisual Center. Many organizational problems remained to be solved. To aid in this purpose, Theresa Powers, Dr. Ramsay's associate in the Anatomy Department, was asked to prepare her views on the aspects of establishing a Medical Communications or Audiovisual Center and to submit a detailed proposal to the College Administration. When Dr. Ramsay retired in 1972, Dean Kellow decided to accept Powers' proposal and put the Anatomy Department capability to use for the entire Medical College. The facility was created July 1, 1972, and Powers was named its Director. Julius Robinson and Carl Goebel were designated audiovisual technicians, and Earl Spangenberg, photographic technician. The Audiovisual Office was placed under the administrative guidance of Arthur R. Owens, the Registrar, and organized in four sections:

1. The Audiovisual Section, providing projectors and recording equipment for lectures and conferences.
2. The Photographic Section, preparing slides, film strips, motion picture films, and prints.
3. The Television Section, for classrooms, laboratories, and other uses.
4. The Medical Illustration Section, assisting with graphs, charts, and diagrams.

Demands on the facilities and a rapid increase in work load resulted in two additional employees joining the staff the same year. In 1973 a close working association was established between the Supporting Facilities Committee and the Office for Audiovisual Services. In 1974 Dr. Thomas Duane presented to the Committee a proposal for a clinical learning center. Dr. Benjamin Bacharach, on March 21, 1974, submitted a report on the same proposal and, referring to the audiovisual needs, stated that an Audiovisual Center was already in operation but should be expanded to include capability for television and cinematography.

The definitive organizational plan of the Audiovisual Center evolved into the four Sections roughly in accord with the plans envisioned earlier. This included greatly expanded services and the acquisition of new equipment of markedly increased capabilities. A brief description of these sections follows:

1. The Audiovisual Equipment Service Section was made primarily responsible for the distribution of equipment for regularly scheduled Medical College activities. Dual projection equipment became routine in many classrooms. The Section serviced the new items introduced, such as battery-powered laser pointers and wireless radio-controlled units for carousel slide projectors. Maintenance and repair of equipment became a major concern of the Section. Four main access areas on the Campus provided easy distribution of the units in response to requests.
2. The Television Section acquired additional pieces of equipment, which became integrated into the existing studio system or employed for location activities. The system was frequently updated to include improvements in technology. Two videoprojectors and a film-to-videotape unit were acquired. Herbert Connor became supervisor of television production in the Audiovisual Office in 1982 following long experience in the Department of Psychiatry as a photographer. Taping of interviews and editing of material for educational and research purposes were carried out under his direction. He was joined by Ralph Woolwine with a

similar background, both having had previous experience with the Curtis Publishing Company Photographic Department before coming to Jefferson.

3. The Photographic Section under Earl Spangenberg carried on the usual photographic activities with the addition of film processing, slide duplication, and special procedures for sophisticated research purposes. Dramatic photographic results were obtained with a computer coupled with the computer image recorder, which was acquired in 1987. Spangenberg continued thorough research of modern photographic techniques and established a medical illustration unit complementing the photographic work.

4. The Medical Illustration Section expanded its services to include the use of a laser printer for the MacIntosh Computer. Many Departments including Surgery, Anatomy, Medicine, Family Medicine, the Center for Research in Medical Education and Health Care, and the College of Allied Health Sciences Department of Cytotechnology took advantage of these laser print services, thus increasing both the quantity and quality of graphic production. New computer software programs were purchased, enabling the Center to improve the understanding of computer graphic capabilities throughout the University and to encourage the use of these techniques.

Medical illustration and teaching have undergone remarkable changes. The new procedures offer students and teachers unparalleled facility for presenting and understanding the complex processes involved in medicine and its interrelated fields. The techniques of graphic representation and reproduction at Jefferson have kept pace with developments at every stage.

References

1. Zimmerman, L.E., Albert, D.M., and Blumberg, J.M., "William Thomson (1833–1907): Military Surgeon, Pioneer Photomicrographer, Clinical Ophthalmologist," *Amer. Jour. Ophthal.* 69, No. 3, 487–497, 1970.
2. Communication, Rochester, New York: Eastman Kodak, 1987.

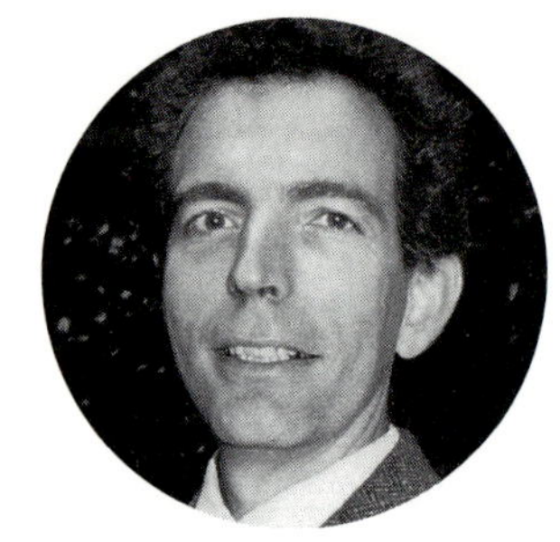

CHAPTER SIXTY-TWO

Computer Assisted Learning

F. Scott Beadenkopf, B.A., M.Ed.

"Medical education is a technical or professional discipline; it calls for the possession of certain portions of many sciences arranged and organized with a distinct practical purpose in view."

—Abraham Flexner (1886–1959)

Computers were first used in medical education at Jefferson in 1970, when Thomas Behrendt, M.D. purchased a Honeywell PDB 516 for the Department of Ophthalmology. The computer was impressive for its time, with 16 kilobytes of memory and a paper tape punch and reader for data storage. The computer was programmed to perform statistical analyses of selected student data to help in the selection of students for a tutorial review program. An authoring system was also written for the computer, and residents in the Department of Ophthalmology used the system to create instructional modules on the pharmacology of the eye and other topics.

Computer assisted learning (CAL) on a large scale was initiated at Jefferson in 1974, with the experimental use of the University of Kansas Computer Assisted Teaching System (CATS) for teaching pharmacology. In a controlled study, students using the computer-based tutorials were shown to perform as well on the National Board Examinations as did a lecture/examination control group. The experimental group required less time to finish the material and expressed enthusiasm for the method. Despite the favorable outcome of the test, the program was not continued because of the expense and the awkwardness and unreliability of the available teletype terminal and mainframe delivery system.

In 1976 two projects were undertaken: experimental use of computer-based tutorials from the Ohio State University (OSU) Health Education Network through telephone connections with their mainframe computer; and a self-assessment program created and designed at Jefferson to aid sophomore medical students in the lowest 15% of their class. The OSU hookup was discontinued in 1980, but by then a few individual faculty members had begun writing instructional programs on microcomputers for students and residents. The Self-Assessment Program continued in its mainframe version until the 1984–1985 academic year, when it was rewritten for microcomputers. The creation of the Computer Learning Laboratory that same year provided sufficient microcomputers to enable the Self-Assessment Program to be offered to the entire sophomore class.

By 1983 interest in microcomputers and CAL among both faculty and students was high. An advisory committee of faculty members was established in order to provide guidance on priorities for uses of computers for research and education in the Medical College (Figure 62-1). The committee identified a need for an individual to work directly with faculty members in the use of computers. As a result, the position of specialist in computer learning systems was created within the Center for Research in Medical Education and Health Care and filled in October 1984. Still in 1983 an experimental program of Summer Computer Fellowships was initiated. In this program seven students with a combination of interest and computer literacy were teamed with seven faculty members to develop educational computer software during the summer. Participants in the 1984 summer program were enthusiastic in their written evaluations, and the program was continued.

Although nothing can supplant the learning derived from exposure to actual patients with instruction from experienced teachers, it is reasonable to believe that computer assisted learning will have profound effects on the medical educational system in terms of effectiveness, efficiency, and cost.

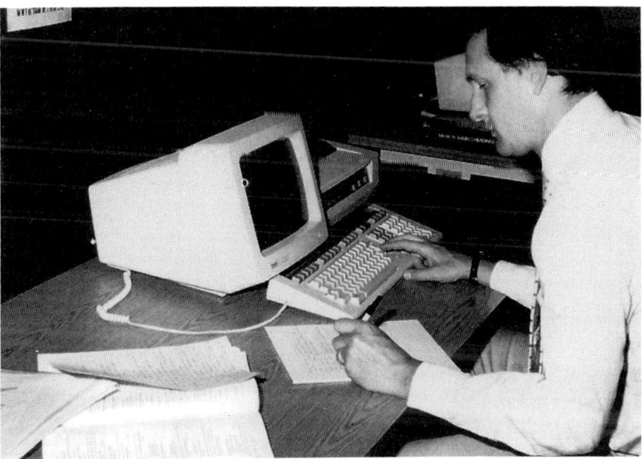

FIG. 62-1. A Resident Physician using a computer in the Scott Library to obtain research information.

CHAPTER SIXTY-THREE

Jefferson Regalia

The Black and Blue Colors

The colors, light blue and black, each of equal width, were adopted at a class meeting during the 1889–1890 session of the Jefferson graduates of 1890.[1] A revival of interest in the colors occurred when Dr. Randle Rosenberger coached the football team in 1908. James W. Holland (Dean, 1887–1916) authorized the use of the light blue and black in the cowls attached to the back of the academic gowns worn by recipients of Jefferson degrees, but the date of its inception is not recorded. Evidently Dean Holland regarded the colors as authentic, although they were never adopted officially by the Board of Trustees or the Faculty.

Mrs. Melrose E. Weed (Executive Secretary of the Alumni Association, 1926–1956) at some unrecorded point began to dress up the banquet hall for the Alumni Association's Annual Business Meetings and Commencement Dinners. Through the years it took the various forms of a football pennant, banner, or flag. The colors also were used on pins, badges, and souvenirs of Class Reunions.

The Class of 1890 acted arbitrarily, but it would be heresy to modify this entrenched color scheme.

Reference

1. Letter of Edward L. Bower, M.D. to Francis J. Sweeney, Jr., M.D., March 19, 1968. (In the archives of Thomas Jefferson University.)

The University Mace

The Thomas Jefferson University Mace was carried for the first time in the 1986 Commencement Ceremonies at the Academy of Music by Grand Marshal, Robert J. Mandle, Ph.D., Professor of Microbiology (Figure 63-1). It was designed by Howard Serlick, member of the Guild of Mastercraftsmen, Winterthur Scholar, and Chief Conservator (Gilding) of the Historical Society of Pennsylvania. Silversmith Eugene Zweigle and woodturner Michael Copeland collaborated in its crafting.

The four-foot long, 14-pound Mace is made of ebony highlighted with lapis lazulis to reflect Jefferson's black and blue colors. It features at the top a miniature of Henry Mitchell's sculpture *The Winged Ox*, symbol of St. Luke the Physician, the original of which stands on the column beside the Scott Building on Walnut Street. Mounted at the base of the staff is a profile of Thomas Jefferson. The project was coordinated by the J.E. Caldwell Company.

The Mace is carried at the head of all formal academic processions as the noble emblem of the University's heritage.

The Presidential Badge of Thomas Jefferson University

The President's Badge (Figure 63-2) was created for the Inauguration of Lewis W. Bluemle, Jr., M.D. as President of Thomas Jefferson University on September 7, 1977. It consists of four official corporate seals of Thomas Jefferson University and the predecessor corporation, The Jefferson Medical College of Philadelphia. These seals were used to mark diplomas, certificates, and other official documents and have been goldplated to form the Presidential Badge. When worn by the President they are suspended from a black and blue ribbon, the University colors, united in the form of a circle with each seal comprising a top, bottom, right, and left medallion.

The medallion on the President's right is the corporate seal of Thomas Jefferson University today and was created in 1969 when Jefferson Medical College became Thomas Jefferson University. It carries a contemporary likeness of Thomas Jefferson.

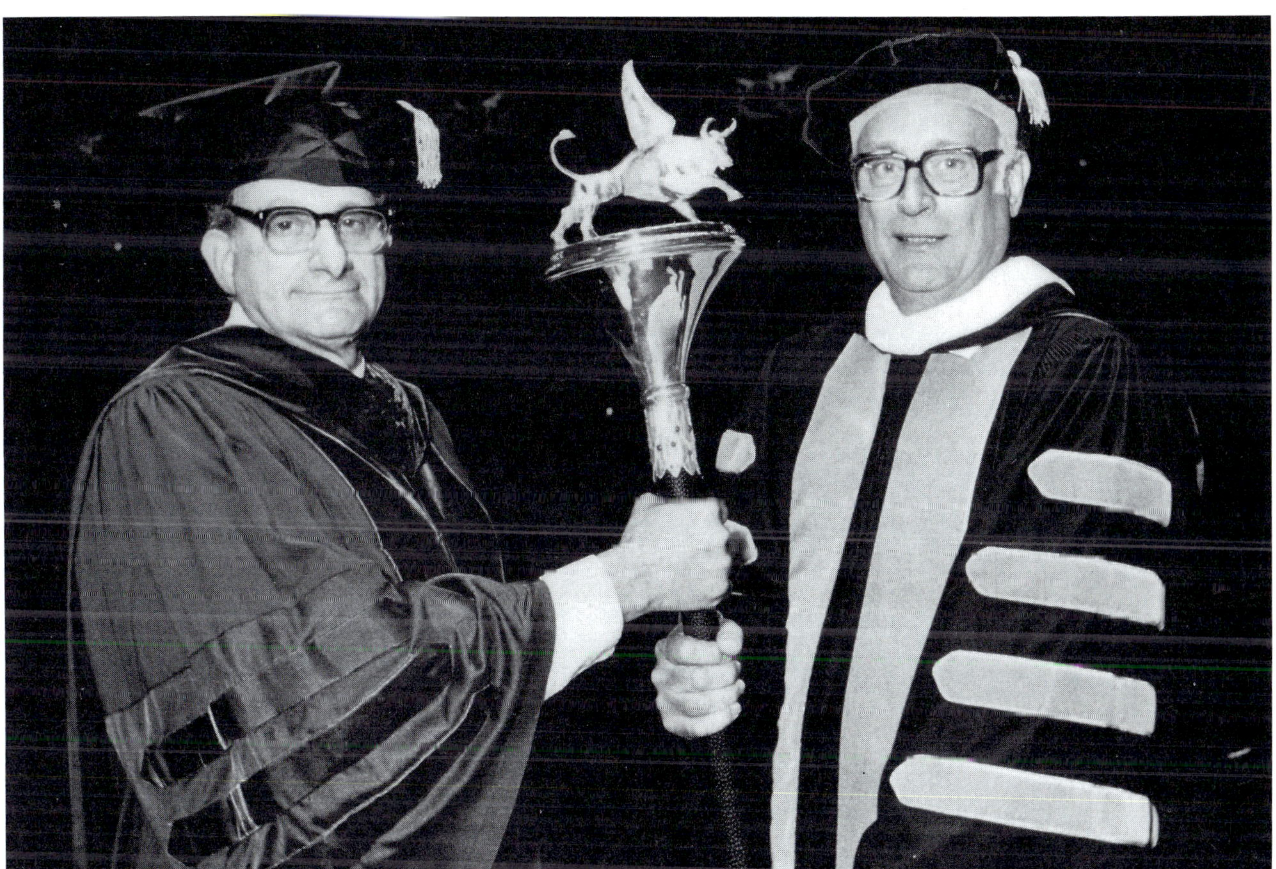

FIG. 63-1. Holding the University Mace, first carried in 1986, are Robert J. Mandle, Ph.D. (Grand Marshal) and Edward C. Driscoll (Chairman of Board of Trustees).

The other three medallions are the various seals that were used in Jefferson Medical College for many years. The oldest, at the bottom, marked every diploma that was issued by the College from 1839 to 1967. This seal carries a traditional likeness of a young Thomas Jefferson and the founding date of the College as 1826. Before 1839 the diploma of Jefferson Medical College carried the seal of the parent institution, the Jefferson College in Canonsburg, Pennsylvania. The old corporate seal on the left bears the Latin words *Sigillum Jeffersoniani Medicinae Collegii-Philadelphiae* with no date.

The seal at the top was developed in 1967 as a result of research done by the late Edward L. Bauer, Professor Emeritus of Pediatrics, who determined that the founding year of Jefferson Medical College was 1824 rather than 1826. This seal is identical to the present corporate seal except that the words "Thomas Jefferson University" are replaced by "Jefferson Medical College." It was used only for the two years of 1967 to 1969.

The Presidential Badge is on permanent display in the Scott Library and is used at all convocations of the University.

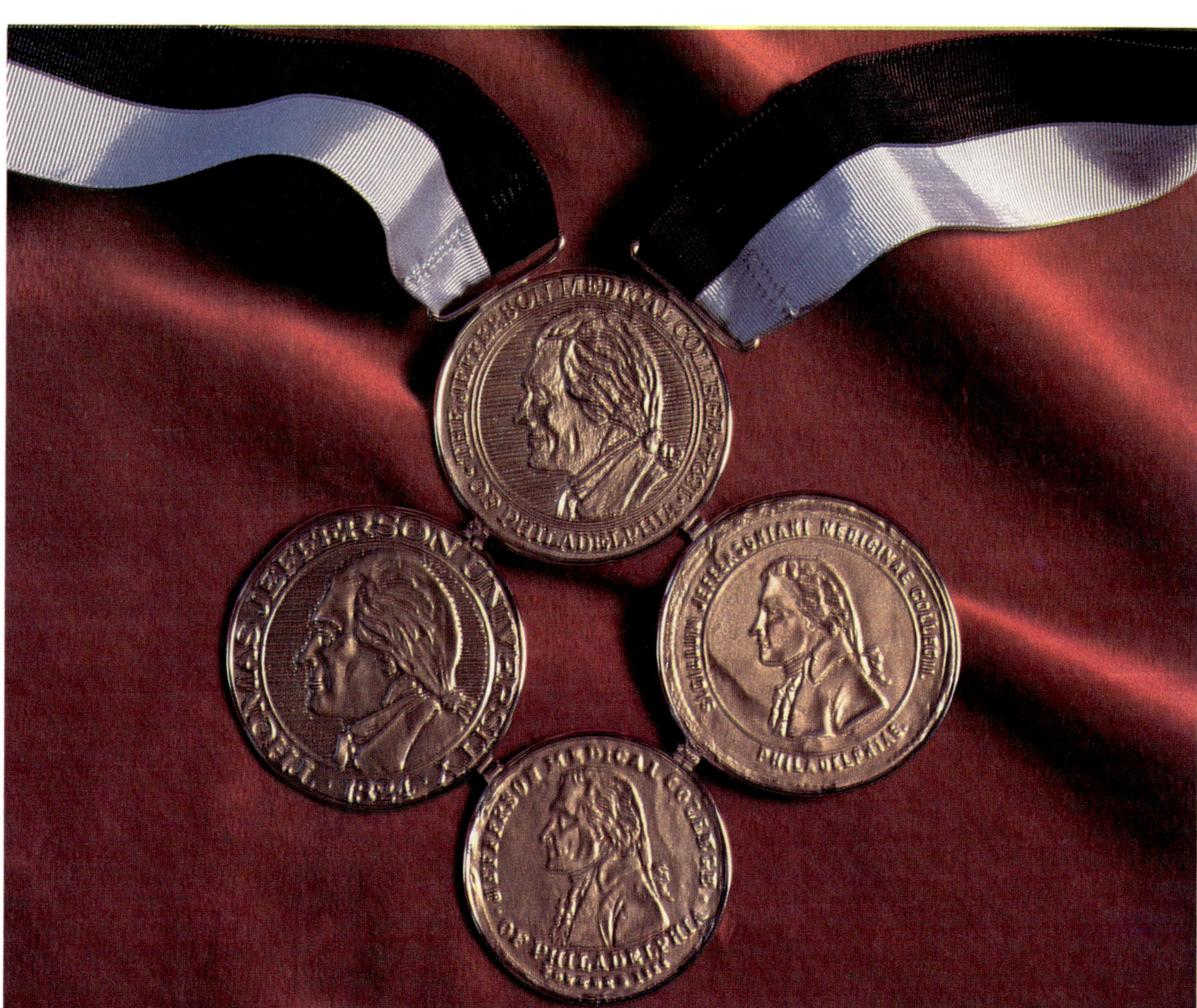

FIG. 63-2. The Presidential Badge.

Name Index

A

B

C

D

E

F

G

H

I

J

K

L

M

N

O

P

Q

R

S

T

U

V

W

Subject Index

A

B

C

D

E

F

G

H

I

J

K

L

M

N

O

P

Y

Z